TOTAL
BURN CARE

THIRD EDITION

Commissioning Editor: Geoff Greenwood
Development Editor: Sharon Nash
Project Manager: Alan Nicholson
Design Manager: Jayne Jones
Illustration Manager: Bruce Hogarth
Editorial Assistant: Kirsten Lowson
Marketing Manager(s) (UK/USA): John Canelon/Lisa Damico

TOTAL
BURN CARE

THIRD EDITION

David N. Herndon, MD, FACS

Director of Burn Services
Professor of Surgery and Pediatrics
Jesse H. Jones Distinguished Chair in Surgery
University of Texas Medical Branch
Chief of Staff and Director of Research
Shriners Burns Hospital for Children
Galveston, TX
USA

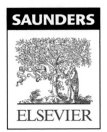

SAUNDERS

ELSEVIER

SAUNDERS
ELSEVIER

Saunders is an affiliate of Elsevier Inc.

1996 First edition
2002 Second edition
© 2007, Elsevier Inc. All rights reserved.

ISBN: 978-1-4160-3274-8

British Library Cataloguing in Publication Data
A catalogue record for this book is available from the British Library

Library of Congress Cataloging in Publication Data
A catalog record for this book is available from the Library of Congress

Notice

Medical knowledge is constantly changing. Standard safety precautions must be followed, but as new research and clinical experience broaden our knowledge, changes in treatment and drug therapy may become necessary or appropriate. Readers are advised to check the most current product information provided by the manufacturer of each drug to be administered to verify the recommended dose, the method and duration of administration, and contraindications. It is the responsibility of the practitioner, relying on experience and knowledge of the patient, to determine dosages and the best treatment for each individual patient. Neither the Publisher nor the author assume any liability for any injury and/or damage to persons or property arising from this publication.

The Publisher

Printed in China
Last digit is the print number: 9 8 7 6 5 4 3 2

Working together to grow
libraries in developing countries

www.elsevier.com | www.bookaid.org | www.sabre.org

ELSEVIER   BOOK AID International   Sabre Foundation

Contents

Contributors

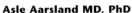

Asle Aarsland MD, PhD
Assistant Professor
Department of Anesthesiology
Co-Director, Metabolism Department
University of Texas Medical Branch
Shriners Hospital for Children
Galveston, TX
USA

Brett D. Arnoldo MD
Assistant Professor of Surgery
University of Texas
Southwestern Medical Center
Dallas, TX
USA

Juan P. Barret MD, PhD
Professor of Plastic Surgery
Head of Department
Department of Plastic Surgery and Burn
    Centre
Hospital Universitari Vall d'Hebron
Universitat Autonoma de Barcelona
Barcelona
Spain

Robert E. Barrow PhD
Professor of Surgery, Co-ordinator of
Research
University of Texas Medical Branch
Shriners Burns Hospital
Galveston, TX
USA

Orlando K. Beckum MD
Research Fellow
Department of Anesthesiology
University of Texas Medical Branch
Galveston, TX
USA

Elizabeth A. Beierle MD
Associate Professor of Surgery and Pediatrics
University of Florida
Gainesville, FL
USA

Palmer Q. Bessey MD
Professor of Surgery
Associate Director
William Randolph Hearst Burn Center
Weill Cornell Medical College
New York, NY
USA

Patricia E. Blakeney PhD
Professor
University of Texas Medical Branch
Clinical Psychologist
Shriners Hospital for Children
Galveston, TX
USA

**Michael C. Buffalo RN, MSN, CCRN,
    ACPNP**
Acute Care Pediatric Nurse Practitioner
Shriners Burns Hospital
Galveston, TX
USA

Edward Y. Chan MD
Resident Surgeon
University of Texas Medical Branch
Galveston, TX
USA

Dai H. Chung MD
Associate Professor
Department of Surgery and Pediatrics
University of Texas Medical Branch
Galveston, TX
USA

Robert H. Demling MD
Professor of Surgery
Harvard Medical School
Brigham and Women's Hospital
Boston, MA
USA

Matthias B. Donelan MD
Associate Clinical Professor of Surgery
Harvard Medical School
Chief of Plastic Surgery
Shriners Burns Hospital
Boston, MA
USA

William R. Dougherty MD, FACS
Associate Professor of Surgery
Department of Plastic Surgery
Vanderbilt University Medical Center
Nashville, TN
USA

Perenlei Enkhbaatar MD, PhD
Assistant Professor
Department of Anesthesiology
University of Texas Medical Branch
Galveston, TX
USA

E. Burke Evans MD
Professor of Surgery
Department of Orthopaedics
University of Texas Medical Branch
Galveston, TX
USA

Shawn P. Fagan MD
Assistant Professor
Shriners Hospital for Children
Boston, MA
USA

Scott Farmer MPT
Rehabilitation Services OT/PT
Shriners Hospital for Children
Galveston, TX
USA

James A. Fauerbach PhD
Chief Psychologist
Johns Hopkins Burn Center
and Associate Professor
Department of Psychiatry and Behavioral
    Sciences
and Department of Physical Medicine and
    Rehabilitation
Johns Hopkins University School of Medicine
Baltimore, MD
USA

**Dilip Gahankari MBBS, MS, MCh,
    FRCS(Edin), FRACS (Plast)**
Visiting Medical Officer
Royal Brisbane and Womens Hospital
Herston, Queensland
Australia

James J. Gallagher MD
Assistant Professor and Acute Burn Surgeon
Department of Surgery
University of Texas Medical Branch
Shriners Burns Hospitals for Children
Galveston, TX
USA

Richard L. Gamelli MD, FACS
Professor and Chairman, Department of
    Surgery
Chief, Burn Center
and Director, Burn and Shock Trauma
    Institute
Professor of Pediatrics
Department of Surgery
Loyola University Medical Center
Maywood, IL
USA

Aziz Ghahary PhD
Professor
Director, BC Professional Fire-fighters Burn
   and
Wound Healing Research Lab
Department of Surgery
University of British Columbia
Vancouver, BC
Canada

Nicole S. Gibran MD, FACS
Professor of Surgery
Department of Surgery
Division of Trauma/Burns
Harborview Medical Center
Seattle, WA
USA

Pam Gibson CPO
Hanger Inc., Prosthetics and Orthotics
Galveston, TX
USA

Cleon W. Goodwin MD
Director, Burn Services
Western States Burn Center
North Colorado Medical Center
Greeley, CO
USA

Mary D. Gordon RN, MS, CNS
Burn Clinical Nurse Specialist
Nursing Department
Shriners Hospital at Galveston
Galveston, TX
USA

Caran Graves MS, RD, CNSD
Clinical Dietitian
Nutrition Care Department
University of Utah Hospital
Salt Lake City, UT
USA

David G. Greenhalgh MD
Professor and Chief of Burns
Department of Surgery
University of California
Davis and Shriners Hospitals for Children
   Northern California
Sacramento, CA
USA

C. Edward Hartford MD
Professor of Surgery
University of Colorado Health Sciences
   Center
Director, Burn Program
Denver Children's Hospital
Denver, CO
USA

Hal H. Hawkins MD, PhD
Professor
Departments of Pathology and Pediatrics
Shriners Burns Hospital for Children
Galveston, TX
USA

John P. Heggers PhD, FAAM, BCLD
Professor Surgery (Plastic), Microbiology and
   Immunology
Shriners Hospital for Children
Galveston, TX
USA

David M. Heimbach MD, FACS
Professor of Surgery
Department
   of Surgery, Division of Trauma/Burns
Harborview Medical Center
Seattle, WA
USA

David N. Herndon MD, FACS
Director of Burn Services
Professor of Surgery and Pediatrics
Jesse H. Jones Distinguished Chair in Surgery
University of Texas Medical Branch
Chief of Staff and Director of Research
Shriners Burns Hospital for Children
Galveston, TX
USA

**Maureen Hollyoak MBBS, MMedSci,
   FRACS**
Vascular Fellow
Wilson, Queensland
Australia

Ted Huang MD, FACS
Clinical Professor of Surgery
Shriners Burns Hospital
University of Texas Medical Branch
Galveston, TX
USA

John L. Hunt MD
Professor
Department of Surgery
University of Texas Southwestern Medical
   Center
Dallas, TX
USA

Mary Jaco RN, MSN, CNAA
Nursing Director
Inpatient Services
Shriners Hospital for Children
Galveston, TX
USA

Marc G. Jeschke MD, PhD, MMS
Assistant Professor
Coordinator of Research
Shriners Hospitals for Children
University of Texas Medical Branch
Department of Surgery and Department of
Biochemistry and Molecular Biology
Galveston, TX
USA

Stephen B. Jones PhD
Professor of Physiology (Surgery)
Department of Physiology and the Burn and
   Shock Trauma Institute
Loyola University Medical Center
Maywood, IL
USA

Richard J. Kagan MD, FACS
Chief of Staff
Shriners Hospitals for Children
and Professor of Surgery
University of Cincinnati College of Medicine
And Medical Director, Skin
AlloSource, Inc.
Cincinnati, OH
USA

G. Patrick Kealy MD
Professor of Surgery
Department of Surgery
Carver College of Medicine
University of Iowa
Iowa City, IA
USA

Michael P. Kinsky MD
Assistant Professor
Department of Anesthesiology
University of Texas Medical Branch
Galveston, TX
USA

Gordon L. Klein MD, MPH
Professor of Pediatrics and Preventative
   Medicine
Department of Pediatrics
University of Texas Medical Branch
Galveston, TX
USA

George C. Kramer PhD
Director, Resuscitation Research Laboratory
and Professor
Department of Anesthesiology
University of Texas Medical Branch
Galveston, TX
USA

Jong O. Lee MD
Assistant Professor of Surgery
University of Texas Medical Branch
and Staff Surgeon
Shriners Hospitals for Children
Galveston, TX
USA

Hugo A. Linares MD
Emeritus Chief of Research Pathology
Shriners Burns Institute
Galveston, TX
USA

David B. Loran MD
General Surgery Resident
Department of Surgery
University of Texas Medical Branch
Galveston, TX
USA

Tjøstolv Lund MD, PhD
Professor of Medicine and Staff Physician
Intensive Care and Burns
Haukeland University Hospital
Bergen
Norway

James E. Lynch BS, RRT
ECMO Coordinator
University of Texas Medical Branch
Galveston, TX
USA

Robert L. McCauley MD
Professor, Departments of Surgery and
Pediatrics, University of Texas Medical
Branch
and Chief, Plastic and Reconstructive Surgery
Shriners Burns Hospital
Galveston, TX
USA

K. A. Kelly McQueen MD, MPH
Staff Anesthesiologist
and Public Health Consultant in Humanitar-
ian Aid and Disaster Management
Anesthesiologist
Valley Anesthesiology Consultants, Ltd.
Pheonix, AZ
USA

Janet Marvin RN, MN
Director of Patient Care Services
Shriners Hospitals for Children
Galveston, TX
USA

Arthur D. Mason Jr MD
Emeritus Chief
Laboratory Division
Brooke Army Medical Center
San Antonio, TX
USA

Dirk M. Maybauer MD, PhD
Department of Anesthesiology
University of Texas Medical Branch
Shriners Burns Hospital
Galveston, TX
USA

Marc O. Maybauer MD, PhD
Department of Anesthesiology
University of Texas Medical Branch
Shriners Burns Hospital
Galveston, TX
USA

Walter J. Meyer III MD
Pediatrician and Child Psychiatrist
Pediatric Endocrinologist
Gladys Kempner and RL Kempner Professor in
Child Psychiatry
University of Texas Medical Branch
and Head, Department of Psychiatric and
Psychological Services
Shriners Burns Hospital
Galveston, TX
USA

Stephen M. Milner MD
Professor of Plastic Surgery
Chief, Division of Burns
Johns Hopkins University School of Medicine
Surgical Director, Johns Hopkins Wound
Healing Center
Baltimore, MD
USA

Joseph M. Mlakar MD FACS
Private Practice,
and formerly, Director
St Joseph's Burn Center
Fort Wayne, IN
USA

Ronald P. Mlcak PhD, RRT, FAARC
Director, Respiratory Care
Shriners Hospitals for Children
and Associate Professor, Respiratory Care
University of Texas Medical Branch
Galveston, TX
USA

Dan Morgan BS
Certified Prosthetist-Orthotist
Hanger Inc., Prosthetics and Orthotics
Galveston, TX
USA

Stephen E. Morris MD, FACS
Associate Professor of Surgery
Director of Trauma
University of Utah
Salt Lake City, UT
USA

Elise M. Morvant MD
Staff Anesthesiologist
East Tennessee Children's Hospital
Knoxville, TN
USA

David W. Mozingo MD
Professor of Surgery and Anesthesiology
University of Florida Health Science Center
Gainesville, FL
USA

Thomas Muehlberger MD, PhD, FRCS
Attending Plastic Surgeon
Department of Plastic and Reconstructive
Surgery
Hannover Medical School
Hannover
Germany

Michael Muller MBBS, MMedSci, FRACS
Associate Professor in Surgery, University of
Queensland
Senior Staff General and Burns Surgeon
Royal Brisbane and Women's Hospital
Division of Surgery
Brisbane, Queensland
Australia

Erle D. Murphey DVM, PhD, Dip ACVS
Assistant Professor
Department of Anesthesiology
University of Texas Medical Branch
Galveston, TX
USA

Kuzhali Muthu PhD
Research Assistant Professor
Department of Surgery
Member, Burn and Shock Trauma Institute
Maywood, IL
USA

Andreas D. Niederbichler Dr Med
Staff Surgeon
Hannover Medical School
Department of Plastic, Hand and Reconstruc-
tive Surgery
Burn Center
Hannover
Germany

William B. Norbury MD, MRCS
Research Burn Fellow
University of Texas Medical Branch
Shriners Hospitals for Children
Galveston, TX
USA

Nora Nugent MBBCh, BAO
Specialist Registrar in Plastic Surgery
Department of Plastic Surgery
St James's Hospital
Dublin
Ireland

Sheila Ott OTR
Occupational Therapist
Department of Occupational Therapy
University of Texas Medical Branch
Galveston, TX
USA

David R. Patterson PhD
Professor of Rehabilitation Medicine
School of Medicine
University of Washington
Seattle, WA
USA

Clifford T. Pereira MD, FRCS(Eng)
Resident Physician
Department of Surgery
County of Los Angeles Harbor-UCLA Medical
Center
Torrance, CA
USA

Tam N. Pham MD
Clinical Fellow
Department of Surgery
University of Washington
Harborview Medical Center
Seattle, WA
USA

Ronald T. Plessinger MS
Medical Records Manager
AlloSource–Cincinnati
Cincinnati, OH
USA

Basil A. Pruitt Jr MD
Clinical Professor of Surgery
Department of Surgery
University of Texas Health Science Center at San Antonio
San Antonio, TX
USA

Rene Przkora MD, PhD
Anesthesiology Resident
University of Florida
Gainesville, FL
USA

Gary F. Purdue MD
Professor
Department of Surgery
University of Texas
Southwestern Medical Center
Dallas, TX
USA

Edward C. Robb AA, BS, BA, MBA
Resource Management Consultant
RMC, Inc.
Oxford, OH
USA

Rhonda Robert PhD
Associate Professor of Clinical Psychology
Division of Pediatrics
University of Texas M.D. Anderson Cancer Center
Houston, TX
USA

Laura Rosenberg PhD
Chief Clinical Psychologist
Department of Psychological and Psychiatric Services
Shriners Hospitals for Children
and Clinical Assistant Professor
Department of Psychiatry and Behavioral Sciences
University of Texas Medical Branch
Galveston, TX
USA

Marta Rosenberg PhD
Clinical Psychologist
Department of Psychological and Psychiatric Services
Shriners Hospitals for Children
and Clinical Assistant Professor
Department of Psychiatry and Behavioural Sciences
University of Texas Medical Branch
Galveston, TX
USA

Jeffrey R. Saffle MD, FACS
Professor
Burn Center
University of Utah School of Medicine
Salt Lake City, UT
USA

Arthur P. Sanford MD
Assistant Professor, Department of Surgery
University of Texas Medical Branch
Assistant Chief of Staff
Shriners Burns Hospital
Galveston, TX
USA

Paul G. Scott PhD
Professor of Biochemistry
and Adjunct Professor of Surgery
Department of Biochemistry
University of Alberta
Edmonton, AB
Canada

Michael A. Serghiou LOT
Director
Rehabilitation and Outpatient Services
Shriners Hospitals for Children
Galveston, TX
USA

Ravi Shankar PhD
Associate Professor
Department of Surgery
Loyola University Medical Center
Maywood, IL
USA

Robert L. Sheridan MD
Assistant Chief of Staff
Shriners Burns Institute
Boston, MA
USA

Edward R. Sherwood MD, PhD
Professor, James F. Arens Endowed Chair
Departments of Anesthesiology, Microbiology and Immunology
University of Texas Medical Branch
Galveston, TX
USA

Jason W. Smith MD
Resident
Loyola University Medical Center
Burn, Shock Trauma Institute
Maywood, IL
USA

Marcus Spies MD, PhD
Attending Surgeon
Assistant Chief of Staff
General Surgery, Plastic Surgery and Hand Surgery
Department of Plastic, Hand and Reconstructive Surgery
Regional Burn Center
Hannover Medical School
Hannover
Germany

Oscar E. Suman-Vejas PhD, FACSM
Assistant Professor, Department of Surgery
University of Texas Medical Branch
and Director, Children's Wellness and Exercise Center
Shriners Hospitals for Children
Galveston, TX
USA

Mark Talon MSN, CRNA
Certified Nurse Anesthetist
Department of Anesthesia
University of Texas Medical Branch
Galveston, TX
USA

Christopher R. Thomas MD, BA, FAACAP, DFAPA
Robert L. Stubblefield Professor of Child Psychiatry
Department of Psychiatry and Behavioral Sciences
University of Texas Medical Branch
Galveston, TX
USA

Tracy Toliver-Kinsky PhD
Assistant Professor
Anesthesiology
University of Texas Medical Branch
Galveston, TX
USA

Ronald G. Tompkins MD, ScD
John F. Burke Professor of Surgery
Harvard Medical School
Chief of Staff
Shriners Hospitals for Children
Boston, MA
USA

Daniel L. Traber PhD, FCCM
Charles Robert Allen Professor of Anesthesiology
Professor of Neuroscience and Cell Biology
Director, Investigative Intensive Care Unit
Department of Anesthesiology
University of Texas Medical Branch
and Shriners Hospitals for Children
Galveston, TX
USA

Edward E. Tredget MD, MSc, FRCSC
Professor
Department of Surgery
University of Alberta Hospital
Edmonton, AB
Canada

Cynthia Villarreal RPh, BSPharm
Director of Pharmacy
Department of Pharmacy
Shriners Burns Hospital
Galveston, TX
USA

Peter M. Vogt MD, PhD
Professor and Chief
Department of Plastic and Reconstructive
    Surgery
Burn Center
Hannover Medical School
Hannover
Germany

Thomas L. Wachtel MD, MMM, CPE
Clinical Professor of Surgery
General and Trauma Surgery/Burns
Shriners Hospitals for Children
Paradise Valley, AZ
USA

JianFei Wang PhD
Post-Doctoral Fellow
Department of Surgery
University of Alberta
Edmonton, AB
Canada

Glenn D. Warden MD
Emeritus Chief of Staff
Professor of Surgery
Shriners Hospital for Children
Cincinnati, OH
USA

Petra M. Warner MD
Assistant Professor
University of Cincinnati College of Medicine
and Shriners Hospital for Children
Cincinnati, OH
USA

Natalie Williams-Bouyer PhD
Assistant Professor, Department of Pathology
University of Texas Medical Branch
and Director, Clinical Laboratory Services
Shriners Hospitals for Children
Galveston, TX
USA

Steven E. Wolf MD
Betty and Bob Kelso Distinguished Professor
Department of Surgery
University of Texas Health Science Center
Director, Burn Center
US Army Institute of Surgical Research
Fort Sam Houston, TX
USA

Lee C. Woodson MD
Chief of Anesthesiology
Department of Anesthesiology
Shriners Hospitals for Children
Galveston, TX
USA

Joseph B. Zwischenberger MD
Professor Surgery, Medicine and Radiology
Le Roy Hillyer Endowed Chair in Surgery
Director, General Thoracic Surgery and
    ECMO Programs
Cardiothoracic Surgery
University of Texas Medical Branch
Galveston, TX
USA

Preface

With each subsequent edition of *Total Burn Care*, my objective has remained the same: *Total Burn Care* is designed as a text on the management of burned patients, not only for surgeons, anesthesiologists, and residents but also nurses and allied health professionals. This book has served as a sophisticated instruction manual to guide those with less experience through difficult experiences in burn care. Our hope for the future is that through multidisciplinary collaboration, scientists and clinicians will pursue solutions to the perplexing problems that burn survivors must encounter.

Contributions have been selected from a small number of institutions in order to provide a unified approach. We have allowed some repetition of concepts and techniques throughout the text so that each chapter can be self-contained in its discussion of its main topic. Themes covered elsewhere in the literature have been condensed and the bibliographies selected to assure the reader ready access to the expanded literature on current burn care.

New material is added to this book, as with every edition, reflecting the varied physiological, psychological and emotional care of acutely injured burn patients evolving through recovery, rehabilitation, and reintegration back into society and daily life activities. Almost all chapters have been totally rewritten and updated. There are many new chapters and sections in this edition, along with demonstrative color illustrations throughout the book.

The scope of burn treatment extends beyond the preservation of life and function; and the ultimate goal is the return of burn survivors, as full participants, back into their communities.

I would like to express my deep appreciation to many respected colleagues and friends for their contributions to the third edition of *Total Burn Care*. Grateful acknowledgment is given to the many authors whose time and expertise made this book possible, especially to the Shriners Hospitals for Children staff.

Sincere appreciation goes to Tiaá Bourgeois, for her excellent secretarial assistance.

I am grateful to the Elsevier publishing staff for their support and cooperation in maintaining a high standard in the development and preparation of the third edition. I wish to recognize Ms. Sharon Nash, Senior Development Editor who guided this book throughout the development process.

Finally, I would like to thank my wife, Rose, for her invaluable support.

A special thank you to Lewis Milutin, whose photographic skills produced countless of the priceless pictures presented in the book, and to Dr. Juan P. Barret, first Editor of the *Color Atlas of Burn Care*, for allowing us to reprint photos from the Atlas. The following figures were reproduced. (Plates 2.1, 3.8, 3.7, 3.9, 5.7, 5.8, 5.9, 5.10, 7.25, 7.22, 7.21, 6.26, 7.26, 7.20, 7.17, 7.30, 7.31, 7.32, 7.33, 5.38, 7.8, 7.9, 7.10, 7.11, 7.12, 7.13, 7.14, 7.15, 7.16, 7.28, 7.29, 7.27, 7.23, 7.24, 8.10, 8.2, 8.3, 8.4, 8.5, 8.6, 8.7, 7.44, 7.45, 7.35, 7.38, 7.34, 7.37, 7.42, 7.43, 7.41, 8.27, 4.41, 1.2.1.4, 6.13, 4.21, 6.14, 4.30, 4.19, 4.35, 3.8, 4.59, 8.31, 7.35, 4.57, 4.63, 8.39, 9.48, 8.39, 8.42, 6.95, 6.89, 5.39, 5.31, 9.45, 9.46, 1.1.2.2, 1.1.3.3, 1.3.3.1, 1.4.1.4, 1.4.1.5, 1.3.3.2, 1.3.4.4, 1.3.4.4, 1.4.1.6, 1.4.1.7, 3.13a, 3.13b, 3.12, 6.64, 10.12, 10.13, 9.11, 9.10, 10.44, 10.46, 10.28)

David N. Herndon
2006

Chapter 1

History of treatments of burns

Robert E. Barrow and David N. Herndon

The treatment of burns is over 3500 years old with the first direct evidence found in the cave paintings of Neanderthal man. Documentation in the Egyptian Smith papyrus of 1500 BC advocated a salve of resin and honey.[1] In 600 BC, the Chinese used tinctures and extracts from tea leaves. Nearly two hundred years later Hippocrates described the use of rendered pig fat and resin which was impregnated in bulky dressings. This was alternated with warm vinegar soaks augmented with tanning solutions made from oak bark. Celsus, in the first century AD, mentioned the use of wine and myrrh, a lotion probably used for its bacteriostatic properties. Galen, who lived from AD 130–210, used a vinegar and open wound exposure technique.[1] The Arabian physician Rhases recommended the use of cold water for the alleviation of pain associated with burns. Ambroise Paré (AD 1510–1590), who advocated a variety of ointments and poultices from medieval excremental alchemy, effectively treated burns with onions, and described a procedure for early burn wound excision. Guilhelmus Fabricius Hildanus, a German surgeon, published De Combustionibus in 1607 in which he discussed the pathophysiology of burns and made unique contributions to the treatment of contractures. In 1797, Edward Kentish published an essay describing pressure dressings as a means to relieve burn pain and blisters. Around this same period of time, Marjolin identified squamous cell carcinomas that developed in chronic open burn wounds. In the early 19th century, Dupuytren[2] reviewed the care of 50 burn patients treated with occlusive dressings and developed a classification of burn depth that remains in use today (Figure 1.1). He was perhaps the first to recognize gastric and duodenal ulceration as a complication of severe burns, a problem that was discussed in more detail by Curling of London in 1842.[3]

Dr Truman G Blocker Jr demonstrated the value of a multidisciplinary team approach to burn care and used this team approach on April 16, 1947 when two freighters loaded with ammonium nitrate fertilizer exploded at a dock in Texas City, killing 560 people and injuring more than 3000 (Figure 1.2). Dr Blocker mobilized the University of Texas Medical Branch in Galveston and soon truckloads of casualties began arriving. This 'Texas City Disaster' is still known as the deadliest industrial accident in American history. For 9 years, Drs Truman and Virginia Blocker followed more than 800 of these burn patients and published a number of papers and government reports. The Blockers became renowned for their work on burns with both receiving the Harvey Allen Distinguished Service Award from the American Burn Association. He was also recognized for his pioneering research in burns and treating children 'by cleansing, exposing the burn wounds to air, and feeding them as much as they could tolerate.' In 1962, his dedication to treating burned children convinced the Shriners of North America to build their first burn institute for children in Galveston, Texas.[4]

Most of the major advances in burn care have occurred within the last six decades. Between 1942 and 1952, shock, sepsis, and multi-organ failure caused a 50% mortality rate in children with burns covering 50% of their total body surface area.[5] Recently, burn care in children has improved survival such that a greater than 95% total body surface area burn can be survived over 50% of the time.[6] Improvements have been made in resuscitation, control of infection, support of the hypermetabolic response, nutritional support, prevention of stress ulcers, treatment of major inhalation injuries, early closure and coverage of the burn wound, effective use of anabolic agents, and the multidisciplinary team approach to burn care and rehabilitation.

Andrew M Munster became interested in measuring the quality of life after a severe burn in the 1970s, when excisional surgery and other improvements had led to a dramatic decrease in mortality (Figure 1.3). First published in 1979, his Burn Specific Health Scale became the foundation for most modern studies in burn outcome. The scale has since been improved, updated, and the scales, originally designed for adults, extended to children.

Fluid resuscitation

The foundation leading to our current fluid and electrolyte management began with the studies of Frank P Underhill who, as Professor of Pharmacology and Toxicology at Yale, studied

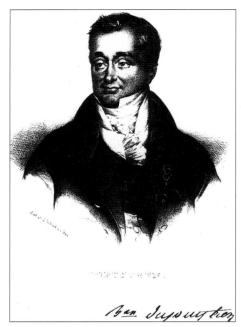

Fig. 1.1 Dupuytren.

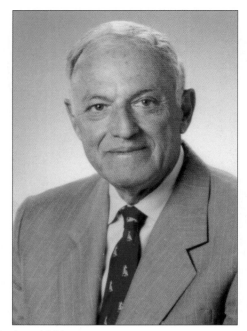

Fig. 1.3 Andrew M Munster.

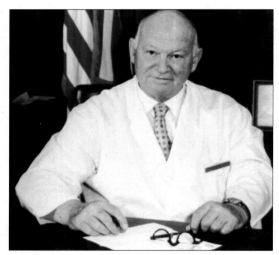

Fig. 1.2 Truman G Blocker Jr.

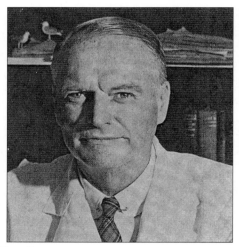

Fig. 1.4 Oliver Cope.

20 individuals burned in a 1921 fire at the Rialto Theater.[7] Underhill found that blister fluid had a composition similar to plasma and could be replicated by a salt solution containing protein. He suggested that burn patient mortality was due to loss of fluid and not, as previously thought, from toxins. In 1944, Lund and Browder estimated burn surface areas and developed diagrams by which physicians could easily draw the burned areas and derive a quantifiable percent describing the surface area burned.[8] This led to fluid replacement strategies based on surface area burned. Knaysi et al.[9] proposed a simple 'rule of nines' for evaluating the percentage of body surface area burned. In 1946, Drs Oliver Cope and Francis Moore were able to quantify the amount of fluid required for ade- quate resuscitation by analyzing young adults who were trapped inside the burning Coconut Grove Nightclub in Boston (Figure 1.4 and Figure 1.5). They postulated that the space between cells was a major recipient of plasma loss, causing swelling in both injured and uninjured tissues in proportion to the burn size.[10] Moore concluded that additional fluid, over that collected from the sheets and measured as evapora- tive water loss, was needed in the first 8 hours after burn to replace 'third space' loss. He then developed a formula for replacement of fluid based on the percent of the body surface area burned.[11] Kyle and Wallace showed the heads of children were relatively larger and the legs relatively shorter than adults and modified the fluid replacement formulas for use in

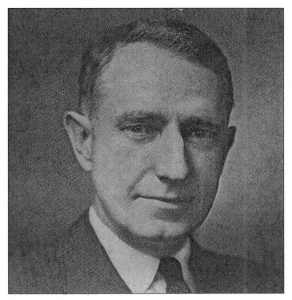

Fig. 1.5 Francis Moore.

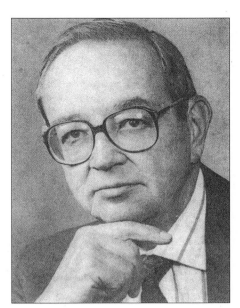

Fig. 1.6 Baxter.

TABLE 1.1			
Formula	**Crystalloid volume**	**Colloid volume**	**Free water**
Evans	mL/kg/% burn normal saline	1.0 mL/kg/% burn	2.0 liters
Brooke	1.5 ml/kg/% TBSA lactated Ringer's	0.5 mL/kg/% TBSA burn	2.0 liters
Parkland	4 mL/kg/% TBSA	None	None
Modified Brooke	2 mL/kg/% burn first 24 hours		
Hypertonic (Monafo)	250 mEq/L Na$^+$ in volume to maintain urine output @ 30 mL/hour		
Warden	Lactated Ringer's + 50 mEq NaHCO$_3$ (180 mEq Na$^+$/L for 8 hours)		
SBH-Galveston	5000 mL/m^2 burned + 1500 mL/m^2 total	None	None

children.[12] Evans and his colleagues made recommendations relating fluid requirements to body weight and surface area burned.[13] From their recommendations, normal saline (1.0 mL/kg/% burn) plus colloid (1.0 mL/kg/% burn) along with 2000 mL D5W to cover insensible water losses was infused over the first 24 hours after burn. One year later, Reiss et al presented the Brooke formula[14] which modified the Evans formula by substituting lactated Ringer's for normal saline and decreasing the amount of colloid given. Baxter and Shires developed a formula without colloid, which is now referred to as the Parkland formula (Figure 1.6).[15] This is perhaps the most widely used formula today and recommends; 4 mL of Ringer's lactate/kg/% TBSA (total body surface area) burned/24 hours after burn. All of these formulas advocate giving half of the fluid in the first 8 hours and the other half in the subsequent 16 hours after burn (Table 1.1). The greatest quantity of solute is given in the first 24 hours after burn. After that, more hypotonic solutions are given to replace evaporative water loss. Baxter and Shires discovered that after cutaneous burn, fluid is not only deposited in the interstitial space but marked intracellular edema also develops. The excess disruption of the sodium–potassium pump activity results in the inability of cells to remove excess fluid. They also showed that protein, given in the first 24 hours after injury, was not necessary and postulated that, if used, it would leak out of the vessels and cause edema to exacerbate. This was later substantiated in studies of burn patients with toxic inhalation injuries.[16]

After a severe thermal injury, fluid accumulates in the wound. Unless there is an adequate and early fluid replacement hypovolemic shock will develop. A prolonged systemic inflammatory response to severe burns can lead to multi-organ dysfunction, sepsis, and even mortality. It has been suggested that for maximum benefit, fluid resuscitation should begin as early as 2 hours after burn.[17,18] Fluid requirements in children are greater with a concomitant inhalation injury, delayed fluid resuscitation, and larger burns.

Control of infection

Another major advancement in burn care that has decreased mortality is the control of infection. Between 1966–1975, 60–80% of patients with burns over 50% of their total body surface died of bacterial sepsis. With the introduction of efficacious silver-containing topical antimicrobials, burn wound sepsis rapidly decreased. Early excision and coverage further decreased morbidity and mortality from burn wound sepsis. In 1965, Carl Moyer[19] initially used 0.5% silver nitrate soaks as a potent topical antibacterial agent for burn wounds.

Mafenide acetate (Sulfamylon), a drug used by the Germans for treatment of open wounds in World War II, was adapted for treating burns at the Institute of Surgical Research in San Antonio by microbiologist Robert Lindberg and surgeon John Moncrief.[20] This antibiotic would penetrate third-degree eschar and was extremely effective against a wide spectrum of pathogens. Simultaneously, Charles Fox[21] in New York, developed silver sulfadiazine cream (Silvadene), which was almost as efficacious as mafenide acetate cream. While mafenide penetrates the burn eschar quickly, it is a carbonic anhydrase inhibitor which can cause systemic acidosis and compensatory hyperventilation and may lead to pulmonary edema. Because of its success in controlling infection in burns combined with minimal side effects, silver sulfadiazine has become the mainstay of topical antimicrobial therapy. Nystatin in combination with silver sulfadiazine has been used to control *Candida*[22] at Shriners Burns Hospital for Children in Galveston, Texas. Mafenide acetate, however, remains useful in treating invasive wound infections.[23]

Hypermetabolic response to trauma

Major decreases in mortality have resulted from a better understanding of how to support the hypermetabolic response to severe burns. This response is characterized by an increase in the metabolic rate and peripheral catabolism. The catabolic response was described by Sneve[24] as exhaustion and emaciation and he recommended a nourishing diet and exercise. Cope et al.[25] quantified the metabolic rate in patients with moderate burns, and Francis Moore[26] advocated the maintenance of cell mass by continuous feeding to prevent catabolism after trauma and injury. Over the last 20 years the hypermetabolic response to burn has been shown to cause increased metabolism, negative nitrogen balance, glucose intolerance, and insulin resistance. In 1974, Douglas Wilmore and colleagues[27] defined catecholamines as the primary mediator of this response. He showed that catecholamines were 5 to 6-fold elevated after major burns, causing an increase in peripheral lipolysis and catabolism of peripheral protein. Hart et al.[28] further showed that the metabolic response rose with increasing burn size, reaching a plateau at a 40% TBSA burn. Bessey, in 1984, demonstrated that the stress response

required not only catecholamines but also cortisol and glucagon. Wilmore et al.[29] examined the effect of ambient temperature on the hypermetabolic response to burns and found that burn patients desired an environmental temperature of 33°C and were striving for a core temperature of 38.5°C. Thus, warming the environment from 28° to 33°C decreased the hypermetabolic response substantially, but did not abolish it. Wilmore suggested that the wound itself served as the afferent arm of the hypermetabolic response and its consuming greed for glucose and other nutrients, at the expense of the rest of the body, stimulated the stress response.[30] He felt that heat was produced by biochemical inefficiency, later defined by Robert Wolfe,[31] as futile substrate cycling. Wolfe et al. also demonstrated that burned patients were glucose-intolerant and insulin-resistant[32] with an increase in glucose transport to the periphery but a decrease in glucose uptake into the cells.[33]

Nutritional support

Shaffer and Coleman advocated high caloric feedings to burn patients as early as 1909 while Wilmore in 1971 supported supranormal feeding with a caloric intake as high as 8000 kcal/day. P William Curreri[34] retrospectively looked at a number of burned patients to quantify the amount of calories required to maintain body weight over a period of time (Figure 1.7). In a study of nine adults with 40% TBSA, he found when given a maintenance feeding at 25 kcal/kg plus an additional 40 kcal/% TBSA burned per day, their body weight could be maintained during acute hospitalization. Sutherland[35] proposed that children should receive 60 kcal/kg body weight plus 35 kcal/% TBSA burned per day. Herndon et al.[36] subsequently showed that supplemental parenteral nutrition increased both

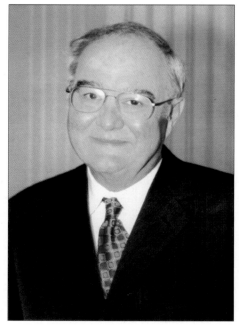

Fig. 1.7 P William Curreri.

immune deficiency and mortality, and recommended continuous enteral feeding as a standard treatment for burns.

Stress ulcers

Nearly 150 years ago, Dupuytren and Curling defined acute gastrointestinal ulcers as major problems after burn. Czaja, McAlhany, and Pruitt[37] at the Institute of Surgical Research in San Antonio studied burn patients and found gastric erosions in 86% of all burns over 40% TBSA (Figure 1.8). The incidence of gastric erosion was reduced by scheduling antacids to treat the low pH. This led to the now traditional protocol of measuring gastric pH on an hourly basis and alternating Maalox and/or Amphogel to adjust the gastric pH. This has virtually eliminated gastric ulcers as a problem in patients with a major burn. Continuous enteral feeding also helps maintain the integrity of gut mucosa, decreases bacterial translocation, and minimizes the need for antacids.

Early excision

One of the most effective therapies in decreasing mortality from major thermal injuries has been the early excision of the burn wound and its coverage.[38] Jackson and colleagues[39] pioneered excision and grafting, beginning in 1954, with burns of 3% TBSA gradually increasing up to burns covering 30% TBSA. Janzekovic,[40] working alone in Yugoslavia in the 1960s, developed the concept of removing deep second-degree burns by tangential excision with a simple uncalibrated knife (Figure 1.9). She treated 2615 patients with deep second-degree burns by tangential excision of eschars between the third and fifth day after burn and covered the excised wound with autografts which allowed patients to return to work within 2 weeks or so from the time of injury. William Monafo[41] was one of the first

Americans to advocate the use of excision and grafting techniques of larger burns (Figure 1.10). Dr John Burke,[42] while at Massachusetts General Hospital in Boston, reported an unprecedented survival after massive excision to the level of fascia in children with burns over 80% TBSA and practiced early burn excision throughout the early 1970s and 1980s using a combination of tangential excision for the smaller

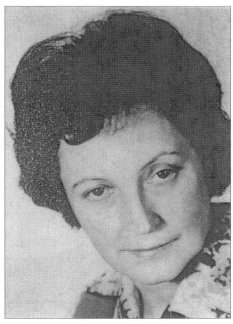

Fig. 1.9 Janzekovic.

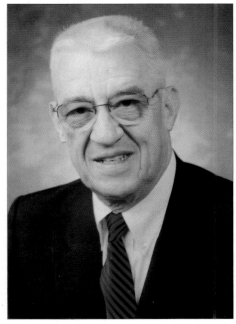

Fig. 1.8 Pruitt.

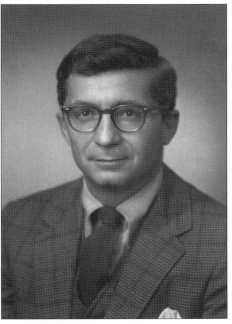

Fig. 1.10 William Monafo.

burns (Janzekovic's technique) and excision to the level of fascia for the larger burns (Figure 1.11). He showed a decrease both in length of hospital stay and mortality in massively burned patients. Lauren Engrav et al.[43] compared tangential excision versus non-operative treatment in burns of indeterminate depth. Their randomized prospective study, conducted in 1983, showed that deep second-degree burns of <20% TBSA when grafted early, allowed patients to return to work earlier, reduced hospital time, and showed less hypertrophic scarring. Herndon et al.,[44] in a randomized prospective study, showed a decrease in mortality in massively burned adults with third-degree burns when treated with early excision of the total burn wound as opposed to conservative treatment. He also reported that these massively burned children with 98% TBSA burns have a 50% survival rate.[45,46]

Skin grafting

Progress in skin grafting techniques has paralleled the developments in wound excision. A Swiss medical student, JI Reverdin, performed reproducible skin grafts[47] in 1869. The method gained widespread attention throughout Europe, but since the results were extremely variable the method quickly fell into disrepute. JS Davis[48] resurrected this technique in the United States during the 1930s and reported the use of 'small deep grafts' later known as pinch grafts. Split-thickness skin grafts were accepted during the 1930s due in part to improved and reliable instruments. The Humby knife, developed in 1936, was the first reliable dermatome, but was cumbersome. Padgett and Hood developed an adjustable dermatome which had cosmetic advantages. Padgett[49] also developed a system for categorizing skin grafts into four types based upon thickness. Tanner and colleagues,[50] in 1964, revolutionized burn wound grafting with the development of the meshed skin graft and J

Wesley Alexander[51] gave us a simple method of widely expanding autograft skin and then covering it with cadaver skin (Figure 1.12). This has since been the mainstay in the treatment of massively burned individuals. Jack Burke[52] developed an artificial skin in 1981, which is marketed today as Integra™. He first used this artificial skin on very large burns which covered over 80% of the TBSA. David Heimbach led one of the early multicenter randomized clinical trials using Integra™.[53] The development of tissue cultured grown skin by Bell et al.,[54] in combination with an artificial dermis, perhaps offers the best opportunity for better outcomes.

Inhalation injury

During the 1950s and 1960s burn wound sepsis, nutrition, kidney dysfunction, wound coverage, and shock were the main focus of burn care specialists.[55] Over the last 25 years these problems have been clinically treated with more and more success; thus, a greater interest in inhalation injury evolved. A simple classification of inhalation injury separates problems occurring in the first 24 hours after injury, which include upper airway obstruction and edema, from those which manifest after 24 hours. These include pulmonary edema and tracheobronchitis, which can progress to pneumonia, mucosal edema, and airway occlusion due to the formation of airway plugs from mucosal sloughing.[55,56] The extent of damage from the larynx to tracheobronchial tree depends upon the solubility of the toxic substance and duration of exposure. Nearly 45% of inhalation injuries are limited to the upper airways above the vocal cords while 50% have an injury to the major airways. Less than 5% have a direct parenchymal injury that results in early acute respiratory death.[55]

With the development of objective diagnostic methods the incidence of an inhalation injury in burned patients can now be

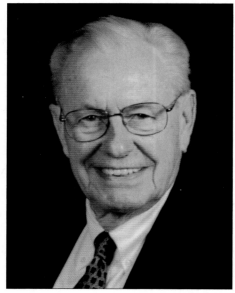

Fig. 1.11 John Burke.

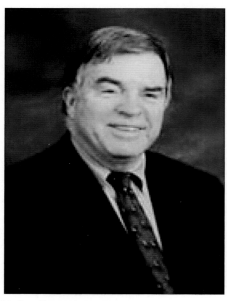

Fig. 1.12 J Wesley Alexander.

identified and its complications identified. Xenon-133, scanning was first used in 1972 in the diagnosis of inhalation injury.[57,58] When this radioisotope method is used in conjunction with a medical history the identification of inhalation injury is quite reliable. The fiberoptic bronchoscope is another diagnostic tool which under topical anesthesia can be used for early diagnosis of inhalation injury.[59] It also is capable of pulmonary lavage to remove airway plugs and particulate matter.

Shirani, Pruitt, and Mason[60] reported that smoke inhalation injury and pneumonia, in addition to age and burn size, greatly increased burn mortality. The realization that the physician should not under-resuscitate burn patients with an inhalation injury was emphasized by Navar et al.[61] and Herndon et al.[62] A major inhalation injury requires 2 mL/kg/% TBSA burn more fluid in the first 24 hours postburn to maintain adequate urine output and organ perfusion. Multicenter studies looking at patients with adult respiratory distress have advocated respiratory support at low peak pressures to reduce the incidence of barotrauma.

The high-frequency oscillating ventilator, advocated by Cioffi[63] and Cortiella et al.,[64] has added the benefit of pressure ventilation at low tidal volumes with rapid inspiratory minute volume which provides a vibration to encourage inspissated sputum to travel up the airways. The use of heparin, N-acetyl-cysteine, nitric oxide inhalation, and bronchodilator aerosols have been used with some apparent benefit at least in pediatric populations.[23,65,66]

Inhalation injury still remains one of the most prominent causes of death in thermally injured patients. In children the lethal burn area for a 10% mortality without a concomitant inhalation injury is a 73% total body surface area burn, but with an inhalation injury, the lethal burn size for a 10% mortality rate is a 50% body surface area burn.[46]

Summary

The evolution of burn treatments has been extremely exciting over the last 40 years. It is our hope that the next 10 years will witness the development of an artificial skin which combines the concepts of Burke et al.[67] with the tissue culture technology described by Bell.[54] Inhalation injury, however, remains one of the major determinants of mortality in severely burned children and adults. Further improvements in several of smoke inhalation injuries are expected through the development of arterial venous CO_2 removal and extracorporeal membrane oxygenation devices.[68] Perhaps even lung transplants will fit into the treatment regimen for end-stage pulmonary failure. Our goals continue to strive for a better understanding of the pathophysiology of contractures and hypertrophic scar formation in order to effectively treat scar formation and how to modulate it in a positive manner. Further decreases in burn mortality can be expected; however, continued advances are necessary to understand how to rehabilitate patients and return them to a productive life.

References

1. Majo G. The healing hand. Harvard: Harvard University Press; 1973.
2. Dupuytren G. Lecons orales de clinque chirorjica faites a 'l'Hotel-Dieu de Paris. Paris: Baillière; 1832: Vol. 1: pp 413–516, Vol 2: pp 1–80.
3. Curling TB. On acute ulceration of the duodenum in cases of burn. Med Chir Trans London 1842; 25:260–281.
4. Blocker TG Jr. Talk given to plastic surgery residents. Galveston, Texas, October 1, 1981, unpublished.
5. Bull JP, Fischer AJ. A study of mortality in a burns unit: a revised estimate. Ann Surg 1954; 139(95):269–274.
6. Wolf SE, Rose JK, Desai MH, et al. Mortality determinants in massive pediatric burns. Ann Surg 1997; 225(5):554–569.
7. Underhill FP. The significance of anhydremia in extensive surface burns. JAMA 1930; 95:852.
8. Lund CC, Browder NC. The estimation of areas of burns. Surg Gyn Obstet 1944; 79:352–358.
9. Knaysi GA, Crikelair GF, Cosman B. The rule of nines: it's history and accuracy. Presented to the Am Soc Plast & Reconstruct, New York City, November 6, 1967.
10. Cope O, Moore FD. The redistribution of body water. Ann Surg 1947; 126:1016.
11. Moore FD. The body-weight burn budget. Basic fluid therapy for the early burn. Surg Clin North Am 1970; 50(6):1249–1265.
12. Kyle MJ, Wallace AB. Fluid replacement in burnt children. Br J Plast Surg 1951; 194–204.
13. Evans EI, Purnell OJ, Robinett PW, et al. Fluid and electrolyte requirements in severe burns. Ann Surg 1952; 135:804.
14. Reiss E, Stirmann JA, Artz CP, et al. Fluid and electrolyte balance in burns. JAMA 1953; 152:1309.
15. Baxter CR, Shires T. Physiological response to crystalloid resuscitation of severe burns. Ann NY Acad Sci 1968; 150:874.
16. Tasaki O, Goodwin C, Saitoh D, et al. Effects of burns on inhalation injury. J Trauma 1997; 43(4):603–607.
17. Barrow RE, Jeschke MG, Herndon DN. Early fluid resuscitation improves extended outcomes in thermally injured children. Resuscitation 2000; 45:91–96.
18. Wolf SE, Rose JK, Desai MH, et al. Mortality determinants in massive pediatric burns. Ann Surg 1997; 5:554–569.
19. Moyer CA, Brentano L, Gravens DL, et al. Treatment of large human burns with 0.5 per cent silver nitrate solution. Arch Surg 1965; 90:812–867.
20. Lindberg RB, Moncreif JA, Switzer WE, et al. The successful control of burn wound sepsis. J Trauma 1965; 5(5):601–616.
21. Fox CL Jr, Ruppole B, Stanford W. The control of Pseudomonas infection in burns with silver sulfadiazine. Surg Gynecol Obstet 1969; 128:1021.
22. Heggers JP, Robson MC, Herndon DN, et al. The efficacy of nystatin combined with topical microbial agents. J Burn Care Rehabil 1989; 10(6):508–511.
23. Monafo WW, West MA. Current treatment recommendations for topical burn therapy. Drugs 1990; 40:364–373.
24. Sneve H. The treatment of burns and skin grafting. JAMA 1905; 45:1–8.
25. Cope O, Nardi GL, Quijano M, et al. Metabolic rate and thyroid function following acute thermal trauma in man. Ann Surg 1953; 137:165–174.
26. Moore FD. Burns in metabolic care of the surgical patient. Philadelphia: WB Saunders; 1959.
27. Wilmore DW, Long JM, Mason AD, et al. Catecholamines: mediators of hypermetabolic response to thermal injury. Ann Surg 1974; 180:653–669.
28. Hart DW, Wolf SE, Chinkes DL, et al. Determinants of skeletal muscle catabolism after severe burn. Ann Surg 2000; 232(4):455–465.
29. Wilmore DW, Mason AD, Johnson DW, et al. Effect of ambient temperature on heat production and heat loss in burn. J Appl Physiol 1975; 38:593–597.

30. Wilmore DW, Aulick LH, Mason AD, et al. Influence of the burn wound on local and systemic responses to injury. Ann Surg 1977; 186:444–445.

31. Wolfe RR, Durkot MJ, Wolfe MH. Effect of thermal injury on energy metabolism, substrate kinetics and hormonal concentration. Cric Shock 1982; 9:383–394.

32. Wolfe RR, Durkot MJ, Allsop JR, Burke JF. Glucose metabolism in severely burned patients. Metabolism 1979; 28(10):1031–1039.

33. Wilmore DW, Smith RJ, O'Dwyer ST. The gut: a central organ after surgical stress. Surgery 1988; 104:917–923.

34. Curreri PW, Richmond D, Marvin J, Baxter CR. Dietary requirements of patients with major burns. J Am Diet Assn 1974; 65:415–417.

35. Sutherland AB. Nitrogen requirements in the burn patient: a reappraisal. Burns 1977; 2:238–244.

36. Herndon DN, Barrow RE, Stein M, et al. Increased mortality with intravenous supplemental feeding in severely burned patients. J Burn Care Rehabil 1989; 10(4):309–313.

37. Czaja AJ, McAlhany JC, Pruitt BA. Acute gastroduodenal disease after thermal injury. An endoscopic evaluation of incidence and natural history. N Engl J Med 1974; 291(18):925–929.

38. Tompkins RG, Remensnyder JP, Burke JF, et al. Significant reductions in mortality for children with burn injuries through the use of prompt eschar excision. Ann Surg 1988; 208(5):577–585.

39. Jackson D, Topley E, Cason JS, et al. Primary excision and grafting of large burns. Ann Surg 1960; 152:167–189.

40. Janzekovic Z. A new concept in the early excision and immediate grafting of burns. J Trauma 1970; 10:1103–1108.

41. Monafo WW. Tangential excision. Clin Plast Surg 1974; 1:591–601.

42. Burke JF, Bondoc CC, Quinby WC. Primary burn excision and immediate grafting: a method of shortening illness. J Trauma 1974; 14:389–395.

43. Engrav LH, Heimbach DM, Reus JL, et al. Early excision and grafting versus non-operative treatment of burns of indeterminate depth. A randomized prospective study. J Trauma 1983; 23:1001–1004.

44. Herndon DN, Barrow RE, Rutan RL, et al. A comparison of conservative versus early excision. Ann Surg 1989; 209:547–553.

45. Herndon DN, Gore DC, Cole M, et al. Determinants of mortality on pediatric patients with greater than 70% full-thickness total body surface area thermal injury treated by early total excision and grafting. J Trauma 1987; 27:208–212.

46. Barrow RE, Spies M, Barrow LN, et al. Influence of demographics and inhalation injury on burn mortality in children. Burns 2004; 30:72–77.

47. Reverdin JL. Greffe epidermique. Bulletin de la Societe' Imperiale de Chirurgie de Paris 1869; 101:511–515.

48. Davis JS. The use of small deep skin grafts. JAMA 1914; 63:985–989.

49. Padgett FC. Indications for determination of the thickness for split skin grafts. Am J Surg 1946; 72:683–693.

50. Tanner JC, Vandeput J, Olley JF. The mesh skin graft. Plast Reconst Surg 1965; 34:287–292.

51. Alexander JW, MacMillan BG, Law E, et al. Treatment of severe burns with widely meshed skin autograft and meshed skin allograft overlay. J Trauma 1981; 21(6):433–438.

52. Burke JF, Yannas IV, Quimby WC, et al. Successful use of a physiologically acceptable artificial skin in the treatment of extensive burn injury. Ann Surg 1981; 194:413–428.

53. Heimbach D, Luterman A, Burke J, et al. Artificial dermis for major burns. A multi-center randomized clinical trial. Ann Surg 1988; 208(3):313–320.

54. Bell E, Ehrlich HP, Buttle DJ, et al. Living tissue formed in vitro and accepted as skin-equivalent tissue of full-thickness. Science 1981; 211:1052.

55. Moylan JA. Inhalation injury – a primary determinant of survival following major burns. J Burn Care Rehabil 1981; 1: 78–84.

56. Foley FD, Moncrief JA, Mason AD. Pathology of the lung in fatally burned patients. Ann Surg 1968; 167:251.

57. Moylan JA, Wilmore DW, Mouton DE, et al. Early diagnosis of inhalation injury using 133xenon lung scan. Ann Surg 1972; 176:477.

58. Agee RN, Long JM, Hunt JL, et al. Use of 133xenon in early diagnosis of inhalation injury. J Trauma 1976; 16:218.

59. Moylan JA, Adib K, Birnhaum M. Fiberoptic bronchoscopy following thermal injury. Surg Gynecol Obstet 1975; 140:541.

60. Shirani KZ, Pruitt BA, Mason AD. The influence of inhalation injury and pneumonia on burn mortality. Ann Surg 1987; 205:82.

61. Navar PD, Saffle JR, Warden GD. Effect of inhalation injury on fluid resuscitation requirements after thermal injury. Am J Surg 1985; 150(6):716–720.

62. Herndon DN, Barrow RE, Traber DL, et al. Extravascular lung water changes following smoke inhalation and massive burn injury. Surgery 1987; 102(2):324–349.

63. Fitzpatrick JC, Cioffi WG Jr. Ventilatory support following burns and smoke-inhalation injury. Resp Care Clin N Am 1997; 3(1):21–49.

64. Cortiella J, Mlcak R, Herndon DN. High frequency percussive ventilation in pediatric patients with inhalation injury. J Burn Care Rehabil 1999; 20(3):232–235.

65. Herndon DN, Traber DL, Pollard P. Pathophysiology of inhalation injury. In: Herndon DN, ed. Total burn care. London: WB Saunders; 1996:175–183.

66. Desai MH, Mlcak R, Richardson J, et al. Reduction in mortality in pediatric patients with inhalation injuries with aerosolized Heparin/N-acetylcysteine. J Burn Care Rehabil 1998; 19(3): 210–212.

67. Burke JF, Yannas IV, Quimby WC, et al. Successful use of a physiologically viable artificial skin in the treatment of extensive burn injury. Ann Surg 1981; 194:413–428.

68. Zwischenberger JB, Cardenas VJ, Tao W, et al. Intravascular membrane oxygenation and carbon dioxide removal with IVOX: can improved design and permissive hypercapnia achieve adequate respiratory support during severe respiratory failure? Artif Organs 1994; 18:833–839.

Chapter 2

Teamwork for total burn care: achievements, directions, and hopes

David N. Herndon and Patricia E. Blakeney

Chapter contents

Major burn injury evokes strong emotional responses in most lay persons and health professionals who are confronted by the spectre of pain, deformity, and potential death associated with significant burns. Severe pain and repeated episodes of sepsis followed by predictable outcomes of either death or a survival encumbered by pronounced disfigurement and disability has been the expected pattern of sequelae to serious burn injury for most of mankind's history.[1] However, these dire consequences have, over time, been ameliorated so that, while burn injury is still intensely painful and sad, the probability of resultant death has been significantly diminished. As illustrated in Table 2.1, during the decade prior to 1951, a 49% mortality rate occurred in young adults (15–43 years of age) with total body surface area (TBSA) burns of 45% or greater.[2] Forty years later, statistics from the pediatric and adult burn units in Galveston, Texas indicated that the 49% mortality rate accompanied a 70% or greater TBSA for the same age group. In 2006, those mortality figures have improved even more dramatically, so that almost all infants and children, when resuscitated adequately and quickly, can be expected to survive.[3] Although improved survival was the primary focus of burn treatment advancement for many decades, that goal has now virtually been accomplished.

Such improvement in forestalling death is a direct result of the maturation of the science of burn care. Scientifically sound analyses of patient data have led to the development of formulas for fluid resuscitation[4–7] and nutritional support.[8,9] Clinical research has demonstrated the utility of topical antimicrobials in delaying onset of sepsis, thereby contributing to decreased mortality of burn patients.[10] Prospective randomized clinical trials have determined the efficacy of early surgical therapy in improving survival for many burned patients by decreasing blood loss and by diminishing the occurrence of sepsis.[11–16] Basic science and clinical research have contributed to decreased mortality by describing pathophysiology related to inhalation injury and suggesting treatment methods which have decreased the incidence of pulmonary edema and pneumonia.[17–20] Scientific investigations of the hypermetabolic response to major burn injury have led to improved management of this life-threatening phenomenon, resulting not only in diminished loss of life but also promising improved quality of life.[21–35]

Melding scientific research with clinical care has been promoted throughout the recent history of burn care, in large part because of the aggregation of burned patients into single purpose units staffed by dedicated healthcare personnel. Dedicated burn units were first established in Great Britain in order to facilitate nursing care.[36] The first US burn center was established at the Medical College of Virginia in 1946 followed that same year by the US Army Surgical Research Unit, later renamed the US Army Institute of Surgical Research.[36] Directors of both of these centers and later the founders of the Burn Hospitals of Shriners Hospitals for Children emphasized the importance of collaboration between clinical care and basic scientific disciplines.[1] The organizational design of these centers stimulated the formation of a self-perpetuating feedback loop of clinical and basic scientific inquiry.[36] Scientists in such a system receive first-hand information about clinical problems while clinicians receive provocative ideas about patient responses to injury from experts of other disciplines. Advances in burn care attest to the value of a dedicated burn unit organized around the concept of a collegial group of basic scientists, clinical researchers, and clinical care givers, all asking questions of each other, sharing observations and information, and together seeking solutions to improve the welfare of their patients (Figure 2.1).

Findings of the group at the Army Surgical Research Institute pointed out the necessity of involving many disciplines in the treatment of patients with major burn injuries and stressed the utility of a team concept.[1] The International Society of Burn Injuries and its journal, Burns, and the American Burn Association with its publication, Journal of Burn Care and Research, have publicized to widespread audiences the notion of successful multidisciplinary work by burn teams.

Members of a burn team

As illustrated by a perusal of the contents of either of the aforementioned journals and by the contents of this volume, the burn team can include epidemiologists, molecular biolo-

TABLE 2.1 PERCENT TOTAL BODY SURFACE AREA (TBSA) BURN FOR AN EXPECTED MORTALITY OF 50% IN 1952, 1993, AND 2006			
Age (years)	1953[†] (% TBSA)	1993* (% TBSA)	2006° (% TBSA)
0–14	49	98	99
15–44	46	72	88
45–65	27	51	75
>65	10	25	33

[†]Bull, JP, Fisher, AJ. Annals of Surgery 1954;139.
*Shriners Hospital for Children and University of Texas Medical Branch, Galveston, Texas.
°Pereira CT et al. J Am Coll Surg 2006; 202(3): 536–548 and unpublished data. PP. 1138–1140 (PC65)

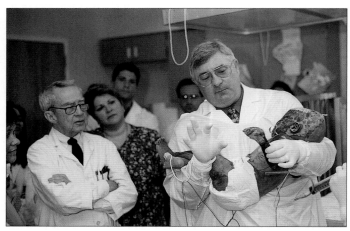

Fig. 2.1 Different experts from diverse disciplines gather together with common goals and tasks, sharing overlapping values to achieve their objectives. (Reprinted with permission from: Barret JP, Herndon DN, eds. Color atlas of burn care. London: WB Saunders; 2001.)

gists, microbiologists, physiologists, biochemists, pharmacists, pathologists, endocrinologists, nutritionists, and numerous other scientific and medical specialists. Burn injury is a complex systemic injury, and the search for improved methods of treatment leads to inquiry from many approaches. Each scientific finding stimulates new questions and potential involvement of additional specialists.

At times, the burn team can be thought of as including the environmental service workers responsible for cleaning the unit, the volunteers who may assist in a variety of ways to provide comfort for patients and families, the hospital administrator, and many others who support the day-to-day operations of a burn center and significantly impact the well-being of patients and staff. The traditional concept of the burn team, however, connotes the multidisciplinary group of direct-care providers. Burn surgeons, nurses, dietitians, and physical and occupational therapists are the skeletal core; most burn units include anesthesiologists, respiratory therapists, pharmacists, and social workers. In recent years, as mortality rates have decreased, interest has intensified in the quality of life for burn

survivors, both acutely in the hospital and for the long term. Consequently, more burn units have added psychologists, psychiatrists, and, more recently, exercise physiologists to their burn-team membership. In pediatric units, child life specialists and school teachers are significant members of the team of care takers as well.

Infrequently mentioned as members of the team, but obviously important in influencing the outcome of treatment, are the patient and the family of the patient. Persons with major burn injuries contribute actively to their own recovery, and each brings individual needs and agendas into the hospital setting which influence the ways in which treatment is provided by the professional care team.[37] The patient's family members often become active participants; obviously so in the case of children, but also in the case of adult patients. Family members become conduits of information from the professional staff to the patient; they act, at times, as spokespersons for the patient, and at other times, they become advocates for the staff in encouraging the patient to cooperate with dreaded procedures.

With so many diverse personalities and specialists potentially involved, it may appear absurd to purport to know what or who constitutes a burn team. Yet references to the 'burn team' are plentiful, and there is common agreement on some specialists whose expertise is required for excellent care of significant burn injury.

Surgeons

A burn surgeon is the key figure of the burn team. Either a general surgeon or a plastic surgeon or, perhaps, both with expertise in providing emergency and critical care, as well as the techniques of skin grafting and amputations, provides leadership and guidance for the rest of the team which may include several surgeons. The surgeon's leadership is particularly important during the early phase of patient care when moment-to-moment decisions must be made based on the surgeon's knowledge of the physiologic responses to the injury, the current scientific evidence, and the appropriate medical/surgical treatment. The surgeon must not only possess knowledge and skill in medicine but must also be able to communicate clearly, both receiving and giving information, with a diverse staff of experts in other disciplines. The surgeon cannot alone provide comprehensive care but must be wise enough to know when and how to seek counsel as well as how to give directions clearly and firmly to direct activities surrounding patient care. The senior surgeon of the team is accorded the most authority and control of any member of the team and, thus, bears the responsibility and receives the accolades for the success of the team as a whole.[37]

Nurses

The nurses of the burn team represent the largest single disciplinary segment of the burn team, providing continuous coordinated care to a patient.[36] The nursing staff is responsible for technical management of the 24-hour physical treatment of the patient. As well, they provide emotional support to the patient and patient's family and control the therapeutic milieu that allows the patient to recover. The nursing staff is often the first to identify changes in the patient's condition and initiate therapeutic interventions.[36] Because recovery from a major burn is a rather slow process, burn nurses combine the qualities of sophisticated intensive care nursing with the challenging aspects of psychiatric nursing. Nursing case management can play an important role in burn treatment, extending the coordination of care beyond the hospitalization through the lengthy period of outpatient rehabilitation.

Anesthesiologists

An anesthesiologist who is an expert in the altered physiologic parameters of the burned patient is critical to the survival of the patient, who usually undergoes multiple surgical procedures acutely. Anesthesiologists on the burn team must be familiar with the phases of burn recovery and the physiologic changes to be anticipated as the burn wounds heal.[1] Anesthesiologists play significant roles in facilitating comfort for burned patients, not only in the operating room but also in the painful ordeals of dressing changes, removal of staples, and physical exercise.

Respiratory therapists

Inhalation injury, prolonged bed rest, fluid shifts, and the threat of pneumonia concomitant with burn injury render respiratory therapists essential to the patient's welfare.[36] They evaluate pulmonary mechanics, perform therapy to facilitate breathing, and closely monitor the status of the patient's respiratory functioning.

Rehabilitation therapists

Occupational and physical therapists begin at the patient's admission to plan therapeutic interventions to maximize functional recovery. Burned patients require special positioning and splinting, early mobilization, strengthening exercises, endurance activities, and pressure garments to promote healing while controlling scar formation. These therapists must be very creative in designing and applying the appropriate appliances. Knowledge of the timing of application is necessary. In addition, rehabilitation therapists must become expert behavioral managers for their necessary treatments are usually painful to the recovering patient who will resist in a variety of ways. While the patient is angry, protesting loudly, or pleading for mercy, the rehabilitation therapist must persist with aggressive treatment in order to combat quickly forming and very strong scar contractures. The same therapist, however, typically is rewarded with adoration and gratitude from an enabled burn survivor.

Nutritionists

A nutritionist or dietitian monitors daily caloric intake and weight maintenance and recommends dietary interventions to provide optimal nutritional support to combat the hypermetabolic response of burn injury. Caloric intake as well as intake of appropriate vitamins, minerals, and trace elements must be managed to promote wound healing and facilitate recovery.

Psychosocial experts

Psychiatrists, psychologists, and social workers with expertise in human behavior and psychotherapeutic interventions provide continuous sensitivity in caring for the emotional and mental well-being of patients and their families. These professionals must be knowledgeable about the process of burn recovery as well as human behavior in order to make optimal interventions. They serve as confidants and supports for the patients, families of patients, and on occasion, for other burn team members.[38] They often assist colleagues from other disciplines in developing behavioral interventions with problematic patients which allow the colleague and the patient to achieve therapeutic success.[39] During initial hospitalization, these experts attend to managing the patient's mental status, pain tolerance, and anxiety level to provide comfort to the patient and also to facilitate physical recovery. As the patient progresses toward rehabilitation, the role of the mental health team becomes more prominent in supporting optimal psychological, social, and physical rehabilitation.

Functioning of a burn team

Gathering together a group of experts from diverse disciplines will not constitute a team.[40] In fact, the diversity of the disciplines, in addition to individual differences of gender, ethnicity, values, professional experience, and professional status render such teamwork a process fraught with opportunities for disagreements, jealousies, and confusion.[41] The process of working together to accomplish the primary goal, i.e. a burn survivor who returns to a normally functional life, is further complicated by the requirement that the patient and family of the patient collaborate with the professionals. It is not unusual for the patient to attempt to diminish his immediate discomfort by pitting one team member against another or 'splitting' the team. Much as young children will try to manipulate parents by going first to one and then to the other, patients, too, will complain about one staff member to another or assert to one staff member that another staff member allows less demanding rehabilitation exercises or some special privilege.[42] Time must be devoted to a process of trust-building among the team members. It is imperative that the team communicate — openly and frequently — or the group will lose effectiveness.

The group becomes a team when they have common goals and tasks to be accomplished and when they share, as individual members, overlapping values that will be served by accomplishing their goals.[43,44] The team becomes an efficient work group through a process of establishing mechanisms of collaboration and cooperation which facilitate focusing on explicit tasks rather than on covert distractions of personal need and interpersonal conflict.[44,45] Work groups develop best in conditions which allow each individual to feel acknowledged as valuable to the team.[46,47]

A burn team has defined and shared goals with clear tasks. For the group of burn experts to become an efficient team, skillful leadership that facilitates the development of shared values among team members and ensures the validation of the members of the team as they accomplish tasks is necessary. The burn team consists of many experts from diverse professional backgrounds; and each profession has its own culture, its own problem-solving approach, and its own language.[48] For the team to benefit fully from the expertise of the members of the team, every expert voice must be heard and acknowledged. Team members must be willing to learn from each other, eventually developing their own culture and communicating in language that all can understand. Attitudes of superiority and prejudice are most disruptive to the performance of the team.

There will be disagreement and conflict, but these can be expressed and resolved in a respectful manner. Research suggests that intelligent management of emotions is linked with successful team performance in problem solving and in conflict resolution.[49] When handled well, conflicts and disagreements can result in increased understanding and new perspectives which can, in turn, enhance working relationships[50] and lead to improved care for the patient.[51]

The acknowledged formal leader of the team is the senior surgeon who may find the arduous job of medical and social leadership difficult and perplexing. Empirical studies, with remarkable consistency, indicate that the required functions for successful leadership can be grouped into two somewhat incompatible clusters:

- to direct the group toward tasks and goal attainment; and
- to facilitate the interaction of the group members, enhancing their feelings of worth.[44,47,51–54]

Task-oriented behavior by the leader may at times clash with the needs of the group for emotional support. During those times, the team may inadvertently impede the successful performance of both the leader and the team as the group seeks alternate means of establishing feelings of self-worth. When the social/emotional needs of the group are not met, the group begins to spend more time attempting to satisfy individual needs and less time pursuing task-related activity.

Studies of group behavior demonstrate that high performance teams are characterized by synergy between task accomplishment and individual need fulfillment.[44,52] Since one formal leader cannot always attend to task and interpersonal nuances, groups allocate, informally or formally, leadership activities to multiple persons.[44,45,47,53] The literature in organizational behavior indicates that the most effective leader is one who engages the talents of others and empowers them to utilize their abilities to further the work of the group.[44,45,53] Failure to empower the informal leaders limits their abilities to contribute fully.

For the identified leader of the burn team, i.e. the senior surgeon, to achieve a successful, efficient burn team, it is important that the leader be prepared to share leadership with one or more 'informal' leaders in such a way that all leadership functions are fulfilled.[44,45,47,53,55] The prominence and the identity of any one of the informal leaders will change according to situational alteration. The successful formal leader will encourage and support the leadership roles of other members of the team, developing a climate in which the team members are more likely to cooperate and collaborate toward achievement beyond individual capacity.

For many physicians, the concept of sharing leadership and power appears at first to be threatening, for it is the physician, after all, who must ultimately write the orders and be responsible for the patient's medical needs.[56] However, sharing power does not mean giving up control.[53] The physician shares leadership by seeking information and advice from other team members and empowers them by validating the importance of their expertise in the decision-making process. The physician, however, maintains control of the patient's care and medical treatment.

Summary and hopes for the future

Centralized care provided in designated burn units has promoted a team approach to both scientific investigation and clinical care which has demonstrably improved the welfare of burn patients. Multidisciplinary efforts are imperative for the continued increase in understanding of and therapeutic responses to the emotional, psychological, and physiologic recovery and rehabilitation of the burned person. Tremendous scientific and technological advances have led to dramatically increased survivability for burn victims.

Our hopes for the future are that by following the same model of collaboration, scientists and clinicians will pursue solutions to the perplexing problems which the burn survivor must encounter. Physical discomforts such as itching still interfere with rehabilitation of the patient. New techniques for controlling hypertrophic scar and for reconstructive surgeries could do much to diminish the resultant disfigurement.[57] The combined use of anabolic agents[33,34] and supervised strength and endurance training[27,28] are currently being investigated as means of enhancing the well-being of survivors of massive burn injury. Further development of psychological expertise within burn care and increased public awareness of the competence of burn survivors may ease the survivor's transition from incapacitated patient to functional member of society. We hope that burn care in the future will continue to devote the same energy and resources which have resulted in such tremendous advances in saving lives to improving the capacity for preserving optimal quality of life for survivors.

References

1. Artz CP, Moncrief JA. The burn problem. In: Artz CP, Moncrief JA, eds. The treatment of burns. 2nd edn. Philadelphia: WB Saunders; 1969:1–21.
2. Bull JP, Fisher AJ. A study of mortality in a burns unit: a revised estimate. Ann Surg 1954; 139:269–274.
3. Pereira CT, Barrow RE, Sterns AM, et al. Age-dependent differences in survival after severe burns. J Am Coll Surg 2006; 202(3):536–548.
4. Evans EI, Purnell OJ, Robinett PW, et al. Fluid and electrolyte requirements in severe burns. Ann Surg 1952; 135:804–817.
5. Baxter CR, Marvin JA, Curreri PW. Fluid and electrolyte therapy of burn shock. Heart Lung 1973; 2:707–713.
6. Artz CR. Burns updated. J Trauma 1976; 16:2–15.
7. Carvajal HE. Fluid therapy for acutely burned child. Compr Ther 1977; 3:17–24.

8. Curreri PW, Richmond D, Marvin JA, et al. Dietary requirements of patients with major burns. J Am Diet Assoc 1974; 65:415–417.

9. Hildreth MA, Herndon DN, Desai MH, et al. Reassessing caloric requirements in pediatric burn patients. J Burn Care Rehabil 1988; 9:616–618.

10. Lindbergh RB, Pruitt BA Jr, Mason AD Jr. Topical chemotherapy and prophylaxis in thermal injury. Chemotherapy 1976; 3:351–359.

11. Janzekovic Z. A new concept in the early excision and immediate grafting of burns. J Trauma 1975; 15:42–62.

12. Burke JF, Bandoc CC, Quinby WC. Primary burn excision and immediate grafting: a method for shortening illness. J Trauma 1974; 14:389–395.

13. Engrav LH, Heimbach DM, Reus JL, et al. Early excision and grafting vs. nonoperative treatment of burns of indeterminant depth: a randomized prospective study. J Trauma 1983; 23:1001–1004.

14. Herndon DN, Barrow RE, Rutan RL, et al. A comparison of conservative versus early excision therapies in severely burned patients. Ann Surg 1989; 209:547–553.

15. Desai MH, Herndon DN, Broemeling L, et al. Early burn wound excision significantly reduces blood loss. Ann Surg 1990; 211:753–762.

16. Desai MH, Rutan RL, Herndon DN. Conservative treatment of scald burns is superior to early excision. J Burn Care Rehabil 1991; 12:482–484.

17. Shirani KZ, Pruitt BA Jr, Mason AD Jr. The influence of inhalation injury and pneumonia on burn mortality. Ann Surg 1987; 205:82–87.

18. Herndon DN, Barrow RE, Traber DL, et al. Extravascular lung water changes following smoke inhalation and massive burn injury. Surgery 1987; 102:341–349.

19. Herndon DN, Barrow RE, Linares HA, et al. Inhalation injury in burned patients: effects and treatment. Burns 1988; 14:349–356.

20. Cioffi WG Jr, Rue LW III, Graves TA, et al. Prophylactic use of high-frequency percussive ventilation in patients with inhalation injury. Ann Surg 1991; 213:575–582.

21. Wilmore DW, Long JM, Mason AD Jr, et al. Catecholamines: mediator of the hypermetabolic response to thermal injury. Ann Surg 1974; 180:653–669.

22. Herndon DN, Stein MD, Rutan TC, et al. Failure of TPN supplementation to improve liver function, immunity, and mortality in thermally injured patients. J Trauma 1987; 27:195–204.

23. Herndon DN, Barrow RE, Stein M, et al. Increased mortality with intravenous supplemental feeding in severely burned patients. J Burn Care Rehabil 1989; 10:309–313.

24. Low A, Jeschke M, Barrow R, et al. Attenuating growth delay with growth hormone in severely burned children. Seventh Vienna Shock Forum. Vienna, Austria, November 1999.

25. Low JFA, Herndon DN, Barrow RE. Effect of growth hormone on growth delay in burned children: a 3-year follow-up study. Lancet 1999; 354:1789.

26. Cucuzzo NA, Ferrando AA, Herndon DN. The effects of exercise programming vs. traditional outpatient therapy in the rehabilitation of severely burned children. J Burn Care Rehabil 2001; 22(3):214–220.

27. Celis MM, Suman OE, Huang TT, et al. Effect of a supervised exercise and physiotherapy program on surgical interventions in children with thermal injury. J Burn Care Rehabil 2003; 24(1):57–61.

28. Suman OE, Thomas SJ, Wilkins JP, et al. Effect of exogenous growth hormone and exercise on lean mass and muscle function in children with burns. J Appl Physiol 2003; 94:2273–2281.

29. Suman OE, Mlcak RP, Herndon DN. Effects of exogenous growth hormone on resting pulmonary function in children with thermal injury. J. Burn Care Rehabil 2004; 25(3):287–293.

30. Demling RH, DeSanti L. Oxandrolone induced lean mass gain during recovery from severe burns is maintained after discontinuation of the anabolic steroid. Burns 2003; 29(8):793–797.

31. Hart DW, Wolf SE, Chinkes DL, et al. Determinants of skeletal muscle catabolism after severe burn. Ann Surg 2000;232(4): 455–465.

32. Hart DW, Wolf SE, Mlcak R, et al. Persistence of muscle catabolism after severe burn. Surgery 2000; 128 (2):312–319.

33. Hart DW, Wolf SE, Ramzy PI, et al. Anabolic effects of oxandrolone following severe burn. Ann Surg 2001; 233(4):556–564.

34. Murphy KD, Thomas S, Mlcak RP, et al. Effects of long-term oxandrolone administration in severely burned children. Surgery 2004; 136(2):219–224.

35. Thomas S, Wolf SE, Murphy KD, et al. The long-term effect of oxandrolone on hepatic acute phase proteins in severely burned children. J Trauma 2004; 56(1):37–44.

36. Rutan RL. On the shoulders of giants. Galveston, TX: Shriners Burns Institute, 1994, unpublished manuscript.

37. Shakespeare PG. Who should lead the burn care team? Burns 1994; l9(6):490–494.

38. Morris J, McFadd A. The mental health team on a burn unit: a multidisciplinary approach. J Trauma 1978; 18(9):658–663.

39. Hughes TL, Medina-Walpole AM. Implementation of an interdisciplinary behavior management program. J Am Geriatr Soc 2000; 48(5):581–587.

40. Schofield RF, Amodeo M. Interdisciplinary teams in health care and human services settings: are they effective? Health and Social Work 1999; 24 (3):210

41. Fallowfield L, Jenkins V. Effective communication skills are the key to good cancer care. Eur J Cancer 1999; 35(11):1592–1597

42. Perl E. Treatment team in conflict: the wishes for and risks of consensus. Psychiatry 1997; 60(2):182.

43. Miller EJ, Rice AK. Selections from: systems of organization. In: Coleman AD, Bexton WH, eds. Group Relations Reader. Sausalito, CA: Grex; 1975:43–68.

44. Harris PR, Harris DL. High performance team management. Leadership and Organization – Development Journal 1989; 10(4):28–32.

45. Yank GR, Barber JW, Hargrove DS, et al. The mental health treatment team as a work group: team dynamics and the role of the leader. Psychiatry 1992; 55:250–264.

46. Pawlicki RE, Bertera JF, Nicholson M. Practice management: what constitutes an excellent team member. Am J Pain M 1994; 4(4):175–177.

47. Litterer JA. The analysis of organizations, 2nd edn. New York: John Wiley; 1973.

48. Hall P. Interprofessional teamwork: professional cultures as barriers. J Interprof Care 2005; 19(Suppl 1):188–196.

49. Jordan PJ, Troth AC. Managing emotions during team problem solving: emotional intelligence and conflict resolution. Human Performance 2004; 17(2):195–218.

50. Tjosvold D, Hui C, Ding DZ, et al. Conflict values and team relationships: conflict's contributions to team effectiveness and citizenship in China. J Orga Behav 2003; 24(1):69–88.

51. Van Norman G. Interdisciplinary team issues. Internet Publication, University of Washington, 1999.

52. Fleishman EA, Mumford MD, Zaccaro SJ, et al. Taxonomic efforts in the description of leader behavior: a synthesis and functional interpretation. Special issue: individual differences and leadership. Leadership Quarterly 1991; 2(4):245–287.

53. Hollander EP, Offermann LR. Power and leadership in organizations: relationships in transition. Am Psychol 1990; 45(2):179–189.

54. Krantz J. Lessons from the field: an essay on the crisis of leadership in contemporary organizations. J Appl Behav Sci 1990; 26(1):4944.

55. Glaser EM, Van Eynde DE. Human resource development, team building, and a little bit of 'Kiem Tau': Part 1. Organization Development Journal 1989:20–24.

56. Fiorelli JS. Power in work groups: team members' perspectives. Hum Relat 1988; 41(1):1–12.

57. Constable JD. The state of burn care: past, present, and future. Burns 1994; 20(4):316–324.

Chapter 3

Epidemiological, demographic, and outcome characteristics of burn injury

Basil A. Pruitt Jr, Steven E. Wolf, and Arthur D. Mason Jr

Introduction

In 2001 there were an estimated 157 078 deaths from all injuries and an estimated 29 721 821 persons with non-fatal injuries in the United States which in a total population of 286 400 669 at that time represented an age-adjusted injury death rate of 54.8/100 000 population, and an age-adjusted non-fatal injury rate of 10 378/100 000 population. Data supplied by the CDC National Vital Statistics System indicate that in 2001 there were 3 423 (1.2/100 000 population) fatal fire and burn injuries which represented 3.4% of all unintentional fatal injuries. Similarly, data supplied by the National Electronic Injury Surveillance System All Injury Program indicate that in 2001 there were 498 507 non-fatal fire and burn injuries (174/100 000 population) which represented 1.8% of all non-fatal unintentional injuries that occurred that year. There were more fatal fire and burn injuries in men (2056) than in women (1367), but the fatal fire and burn injuries in women represented a greater percentage of all fatal unintentional injuries (3.9% vs. 3.1% for men). Non-fatal fire and burn injury as a percentage of all non-fatal injuries showed essentially no gender difference, i.e. 1.8% for men and 1.9% for women.[1]

Unintentional fatal and non-fatal fire and burn injuries represent a variable percentage of all unintentional injuries as related to the population in various age groups. Fire and burn injuries represented 10.3% (1.4/100 000 population) and 3.3% (410.4/100 000 population) of all fatal and non-fatal unintentional injuries respectively in the 0 to 4-year age group, and

12.7% (0.8/100 000 population) and 1.4% (138.9/100 000 population) respectively in the 5 to 9-year age group.

The total number of non-fatal fire and burn injuries in 2001 was greatest in the 25 to 34-year age group, 91 334 (229.4/100 000 population) representing only 2.1% of all unintentional injuries, and the 35 to 44-year age group, 78 968 (174.9/100 000 population) representing only 2% of all unintentional injuries. The highest rate of non-fatal, unintentional fire and burn injury in adults, 274.6/100 000 population, was in the 20 to 24-year age group.[1]

The causes of injury in male patients with non-fatal burns were scald/thermal 198 898 (68%), chemical 45 036 (15.3%), electrical 4781 (1.6%), and radiation 39 034 (13.3%), with 6838 (2.3%) unspecified. In that same year, the causes of burns in female patients with non-fatal injuries were scald/thermal 173 205 (76.9%), chemical 25 973 (11.5%), electrical 2405 (1.1%), radiation 16 883 (7.5%), with 6744 (3%) being unspecified. As a percentage of all non-fatal burn injuries in males, scald/thermal injuries were greatest (83%) in the 0 to 14-year age group, chemical injuries were greatest (21.3%) in the 45 to 64-year age group, electric injuries were greatest (3.8%) in the 45 to 64-year age group, and radiation injuries were greatest (19.4%) in the 25 to 34-year age group. In female patients with non-fatal burns, the distribution of scald/thermal injuries appears to be bimodal, with the greatest percentage in the 0 to 14-year and the 65 and above year age groups, i.e. more than 82% in each. In female patients with non-fatal burns the highest percentage of chemical injuries, 13.6%, occurred in the 15 to 19-year age group, electrical injuries, 2.5%, in the 0 to 14-year age group, and radiation injuries, 14.5%, in the 15 to 19-year age group. Fire and burn injuries constitute 10% of all fatal, unintentional injuries in the 0 to 14-year age group, 1% in the 15 to 24-year age group, 3% in the 25 to 64-year age group, and 4% in the 65 and above age group. Fire and burn injuries can also be violence-related, but as such are relatively uncommon and for reporting purposes are grouped indistinguishably with other uncommon causes and are not cited separately.[1]

The rank of unintentional fire and burn injury as a cause of fatal and non-fatal injuries varied by both age and sex in the United States in 2001 as indicated in Table 3.1. Only in female patients is burn injury, as 10th, among the 10 leading causes of injury and then only for fatal injuries. The incidence rates of fire and burn injuries for both males and females have progressively decreased over the past two decades.[2] The incidence rate of fire and burn injuries for males has decreased from

From the US Army Institute of Surgical Research, Ft. Sam Houston, Texas and the Department of Surgery, University of Texas Health Science Center at San Antonio, San Antonio, Texas USA.

The opinions or assertions contained herein are the private views of the author and are not to be construed as official or as reflecting the views of the Department of the Army or the Department of Defense.

TABLE 3.1 RANK OF UNINTENTIONAL FIRE AND BURN INJURY IN THE TEN LEADING CAUSES OF INJURY AS RELATED TO AGE AND SEX

Age		Male	Female
<1	Fatal	6	6
	Non-fatal	4	5
1–4	Fatal	4	3
	Non-fatal	7	8
5–9	Fatal	4	3
	Non-fatal		
10–14	Fatal	10	4
	Non-fatal		
15–54	Fatal		
	Non-fatal		
55–64	Fatal	10	7
	Non-fatal		10
65–74	Fatal	7	6
	Non-fatal		10
75–84	Fatal	7	6
	Non-fatal		
≥85	Fatal	7	5
	Non-fatal		

601/100 000 population in 1985 to 276/100 000 in 2000 to 192/100 000 in 2001. The incidence rates for females decreased even more during the same time period, i.e. from 647/100 000 population in 1985 to 284/100 000 in 2000 to 158/100 000 in 2001. In a recent 1-year period, 2000–2001, the incidence rate for all burns decreased from 280/100 000 population to 175/100 000.[1,2] The magnitude of those changes reported for the one-year period, 2000 to 2001, brings the validity of the data for 2001 into question.

As would be anticipated, the upper limbs, the head and neck, and the lower limbs were the primary body parts most often affected by burns. Forty-five percent of non-fatal burns involve the arm and hand, 25% the head and neck, 16% the leg and foot, 6% the upper trunk, 3% the lower trunk, and 5% other areas. The disposition of patients with unintentional fire and burn injuries seen in emergency departments in 2001 as recorded by the National Center for Injury Prevention and Control was 'treated and released' in 480 220 (95.7%) as a reflection of the fact that the vast majority of burns are of very limited extent. In 2001, there were 17 056 (only 3.4%) of the total 501 930 patients with fire and burn injuries seen in Emergency Departments (ED) who were hospitalized or transferred to another treatment facility.[1] That estimate of burn patients admitted to hospitals is approximately one-third of that estimated below because it doesn't include patients treated in other facilities or admitted without being treated in an ED and because of lack of information on the medical chart.

In 2003 data published as the WISQARS Injury Mortality Report indicate that there were 3875 fire and burn deaths recorded in the United States which represent a crude death rate of 1.33/100 000 population in our total population of 290 810 789 in that year. Fire/burn death rates in individual states in 2003 ranged from 281 and 267 in Texas and California respectively, to a low of 4 and 1 in Hawaii and Wyoming respectively. The age-adjusted fire and burn death rates in 2003 ranged from 6.14 and 3.23 in Rhode Island and Mississippi respectively, to a low of 0.52 and 0.22/100 000 in Colorado and Wyoming respectively.[3]

The American Burn Association now maintains the National Burn Repository which contains records of 187 000 patients treated for burn injuries at 70 burn centers in the United States and Canada between January 1991 and 2005. The most recent report from this registry describes the demographics of the population of burns admitted and treated at burn centers in North America during the period 1995–2005 and includes information about associated injuries, site of injury, length of hospital stay, and mortality. The registry data indicate that 70% of the patients were men, and that 63% of the patients were Caucasian, 18% African-American, and 12.4% Hispanic. The 18% registrant rate of African-Americans exceeds by almost 50% the 12.8% African-American segment of the 2004 US population of 294 941 471. The mean age of all burn patients was 33 years with 10% of cases being under 2 years of age, and 14% of cases being 60 years of age or older. The vast majority of burns for which extent was recorded were of limited extent, i.e. 62% involved less than 10% of the total body surface, with 68% of the full-thickness burns involving less than 10% of the total body surface.[4]

The most common etiologies of burn injury were flames and scalds which together accounted for 78.5% of the reported cases. The number of scalds far exceeded the number of flame burns in the 0 to 1.9-year age group and the 2 to 4.9-year age group, but flame burns outnumbered scalds by more than a factor of 2 in all other age groups. Seventy percent of the burns in patients younger than 2 years were caused by scalding and those injuries represented 28% of all scald injuries. Contact with a hot object accounted for 8.1% of burns, chemicals for 3.2% of injuries, and electric current for 4.3% of injuries; 43.2% of the injuries occurred in the home, 8.4% at industrial sites, 16.8% on streets or highways, 4.2% during recreation and sports, 1.8% at schools, and 0.7% on farms. There were an additional 5.7% of burns for whom other rare sites of injury were specified and 19.2% for whom the site was unspecified. Circumstances of injury data indicate that 65% of the burns were sustained in non-work-related accidents, 17% in work-related accidents, 4.9% in recreation accidents, and 5% as a consequence of self-injury, abuse, or assault. Records in which transfer information was reported indicated that 61% of the patients were initially treated elsewhere and then transferred to the reporting hospital.[1]

The six surgical procedures most often performed for the registry patients were burn wound excision, skin grafts to other sites, application of wound dressing, venous catheterization, non-excision debridement, and homograft application. Other frequently performed procedures included suture of skin and subcutaneous tissue, insertion of endotracheal tube, arterial catheterization, and application of heterograft skin.[1]

Ninety-five percent of the patients entered into the registry survived and were discharged. In the 5% of cases who expired the cause of death was recorded in only 51%, and in 494 cases the cause was listed as 'treatment withheld.' The most common cause of death was multiple-organ failure, 32%, followed by burn shock, 14.6%, trauma wound, 14.2%, pulmonary failure-sepsis, 13.2%, cardiovascular failure, 12.2%, and burn wound sepsis, 4.7%. Inhalation injury was recorded in only 6.5% of burn admissions, but when present length of stay was increased as was mortality reflecting the increased risk of pneumonia and the increased need for ventilatory support.[1]

The cost of fire and burn injuries includes both medical costs and the cost of lost productivity. In 2000, total lifetime costs of the 774 376 fire and burn injuries of that year, which included 3922 fatal burns, were 7.546 billion dollars which consisted of medical costs of 1.345 billion dollars and productivity losses of 6.202 billion dollars.[2]

Epidemiology and demography

Geographic location, presumably because of regional differences in construction and heating devices as well as economic status, influences death rates from house fires. House fire death rates are higher in the Eastern part of the United States, particularly the Southeast, as compared to the West.[5] There are marked seasonal differences in house fire deaths. From 1991 to 1995, residential fire-related deaths were highest during the cold winter months (December–February) when greatest use is made of heating and lighting devices and lowest in the warm summer months (June–August).[6] Unattended and/or improperly positioned cooking and heating devices are the leading causes of residential fires.[7] House fires cause only approximately 4% of burn admissions, but the 12% fatality rate of patients hospitalized for burns sustained in house fires is higher than the 3% fatality rate for patients with burns from other causes. This difference is presumably the effect of associated inhalation injury.[8,9]

Playing with matches, cigarette lighters, and other ignition devices has been incriminated as the cause of one in ten residential fire deaths.[5] House fire death rates show little gender prominence except for an increased incidence in males age 2 to 5, a group that has the highest rate of non-fatal burns due to unsupervised play with matches.[10] In fact, among children of 9 years or less, child-play fires are the leading cause of residential fire-related death and injury. Careless smoking, which accounts for one in four residential fire deaths, is the most common cause of such fatalities.[2] Alcohol and drug intoxication, which contribute to careless smoking behavior by impairing mentation, have been reported to be a factor in 40% of residential fire deaths and appear to contribute to the high weekend frequency of house fires.[11] Arson is the second most common cause of residential fire deaths.[12] Defective or inappropriately used heating devices, which are the third most common cause, account for one in six residential fire deaths overall, and an even greater proportion in low-income areas.[12] The effect of low income on fire and burn deaths is also related to residence in older buildings, crowded living conditions, and absence of smoke detectors. Nearly 800 children, age 14 and less, died as a consequence of fire- and burn-related injury in 1996.[13] Flames and burns were considered to be responsible for one-fourth of all fire-related deaths in children. As a reflection of the effect of economic status, minority children age 0 to 19 are more than three times as likely to die in a residential fire as white children.[14] As income increases, racial differences in house fire death rates decrease.[15]

During the 5-year period, 1991 to 1995, the residential fire-related death rate in the United States decreased from 1.3 to 1.1 per 100 000 population.[6] That change and the further decrease since then has been attributed to the combined effects of improved building design, the use of safer appliances and heating devices, and the increased use of smoke and fire detectors. Data from the Centers for Disease Control Behavioral Risk Factor Surveillance System (BRFSS) indicate that the presence of smoke alarms in households in the United States is high, i.e. more than 78% of households in all 50 states. In 1995, 93.6% of all US households claimed to have at least one smoke alarm.[6] There are almost half as many fire-related deaths in homes with smoke alarms as compared to homes without those devices.[16,17]

In 1998, the Centers for Disease Control and Prevention (CDC) formed a collaboration with the US Consumer Product Safety Commission, the United States Fire Administration, and other governmental and non-governmental agencies with a stated goal of eliminating residential fire-related deaths by 2020. As a part of the larger effort, the CDC provides funds to 16 states to participate in the Smoke Alarm Installation and Fire Safety Education Program. That program, which involves installation of smoke alarms and general fire safety education, emphasizes strong partnership with local fire departments and collaboration with target communities selected on the basis of greatest risk for fire-related injury. During the program's lifetime 280 000 homes have been canvassed and over 212 000 smoke alarms have been installed in more than 160 000 high-risk homes. At 6 month follow-up, more than 90% of the alarms were functioning and program evaluation indicates the likely saving of 610 lives as a result of activation of a program alarm.[18]

The economic consequences of residential fires are also great. In 1995, property damage and other direct costs attributable to such fires were estimated to exceed four billion dollars.[19] The healthcare costs of burn injuries are also prodigious. Each year in the United States 60 000 to 80 000 people require in-hospital care for burns. The average cost of hospital care of a patient injured by flame and/or smoke inhalation ranges from $29 560.00 to $117 506.00 with much higher costs incurred by patients with extensive burns. The length of hospital stay ranges from one day to hundreds of days (mean 8.7) and for patients 80 years and above is more than twice as long as that for children under 5.[20] The estimated cost of a fire-related death, which includes the loss of future productivity ranges from $250 000.00 to 1.5 million dollars.[21–23]

Unlike fire deaths, the precise number of burn injuries which occur in the United States is unknown. Twenty-one states require that burn injuries be reported, but two require that only burns associated with assaults or arson be reported, and seven require that only larger burns (usually those involving more than 15% of the total body surface area) be reported.[24] Consequently, the total number of burns as noted above has to be estimated by extrapolation of data collected in less than one-half of the states to the entire population. Such estimates have ranged from 1.4 million to 2 million injuries due to burns and fires each year.[5,25] Because of the general improvement in living conditions in the United States, an annual incidence of approximately 1.25 million is considered to be a realistic estimate at the present time.[25] The majority of those burns are of limited extent (more than 80% of burns involve less than 20% of the total

TABLE 3.2 AMERICAN BURN ASSOCIATION MAJOR BURN INJURY CRITERIA
1. Second- and third-degree burns greater than 10% of the total body surface area in patients under 10 or over 50 years of age
2. Second- and third-degree burns greater than 20% of the total body surface area in other age groups
3. Significant burns of face, hands, feet, genitalia, or perineum and those that involve skin overlying major joints
4. Third-degree burns greater than 5% of the total body surface area in any age group
5. Inhalation injury
6. Significant electric injury including lightning injury
7. Significant chemical injury
8. Burns with significant preexisting medical disorders that could complicate management, prolong recovery, or affect mortality (e.g. diabetes mellitus, cardiopulmonary disease)
9. Burns with significant concomitant trauma (may require initial treatment in a trauma center)
10. Burn injury in patients who will require special social and emotional or long-term rehabilitative support, including cases of suspected child abuse and neglect

body surface area).[25] However, as recently as the 1980s, it was estimated that in the United States 270–300 patients per million population (67 500–75 000) per year sustained burns which, because of extent, associated injury or comorbid conditions required admission to a hospital.[27] In light of the overall decrease in the incidence of burns, it is currently estimated that only 170–230 patients per million population (50 592–68 448) will require admission to a hospital annually.[21,26]

A review of 1994 Pennsylvania statewide hospital discharge data identified 3173 cases with a fire or burn diagnosis for a rate of 263 per million population.[21] Sixty-eight percent of the patients were males and 70% of the patients were white. Hospital discharge rates showed three distinct peaks, i.e. patients of less than 5 years, patients between 25 and 39 years, and patients 65 years and older. The discharge rate for males was slightly more than twice that of females and the rate for blacks was more than twice that for whites. Scalds and hot substances were the cause of the burn in 58% of the patients. Fire and flame sources accounted for 34% of the burns (clothing ignition 15%, conflagration 12%, and controlled fire 7%). Two percent of the burns were self-inflicted and 2% were the consequence of an assault.

A smaller subset of approximately 20 000–25 000 burn patients with even more severe injuries, as defined by the American Burn Association (Table 3.2), are best cared for in a burn center.[28] Those patients consist of 42 per million population with major burns and 40 per million population having lesser burns but a complicating co-factor.[27] There are 126 self-designated burn care facilities in the United States, and 14 in Canada which are distributed in close relationship to population density and are reported to contain a total of 1811 and 125 beds respectively (Figure 3.1).[29] As described below, the geographic distribution of burn centers necessitates the use of aeromedical transfer by both rotary and fixed wing aircraft to transport patients requiring burn center care to those facilities from distant and remote areas.

In addition to economic status[30] and geographic location[30,31] the risk of being burned and the predominant cause of burn injury are related to age,[32] occupation, and participation in recreational activities.[33] Scald burns are the most frequent form of burn injury overall and cause over 100 000 patients to seek treatment in hospital emergency rooms.[34,35]

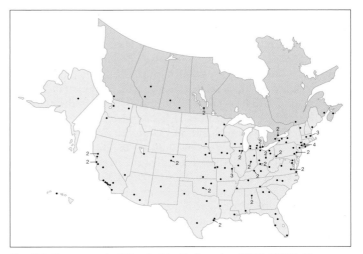

Fig. 3.1 Burn care facilities in North America 2004–2006. The numbers indicate facilities in areas where these are concentrated.

High-risk populations

Children

The number of pediatric burn patients admitted to hospitals is influenced by cultural differences, resource availability, and medical practice. Consequently, the number of pediatric burn patients admitted to a hospital for treatment varies by geographic area from a low rate of 4.4/100 000 population in America (North, Central, and South) to a high of 10.8/100 000 population in Africa. Although the incidence rate for Asia, 8.0/100 000 population, is similar to that for Europe and the Middle East, population size determines that Asia provides care for over one-half of the global pediatric burn population.[36]

It has been estimated that 83 000 children, ages 14 and under, were treated in hospital emergency rooms in the United States for burn-related injuries in 1997. Of those injuries, 59 000 were thermal burns and 24 000 scald burns.[13] An average of 16 children with scald burns die each year, and those age 4 and less account for nearly all of those deaths.[13]

Of the children age 4 and under who are hospitalized for burn-related injuries, 65% have scald burns, 20% contact burns, and the remainder flame burns. The majority of scald burns in children, especially those age 6 months to 2 years, are from hot foods and liquids, particularly coffee which may be dispensed at temperatures of up to 180°F (82.2°C), spilled in the kitchen or other places where food is prepared and served.[13] Hot tap water burns, which typically occur in the bathroom, tend to be more severe and cover a larger portion of the body surface than other scald burns. Consequently, such burns which account for nearly one-fourth of all childhood scald burns are associated with higher hospitalization and death rates than other hot liquid burns.[13] Ninety-five percent of burns among children due to the operation of microwave devices are scald burns resulting from the spillage of hot liquids or food.[13]

Among children (14 years and less) hair curlers and curling irons, room heaters, ovens and ranges, irons, gasoline, and fireworks are the most common causes of product-related burn injuries.[13] Nearly two-thirds of electric injuries in children ages 12 and under are caused by household electric cords and extension cords.[13] Contact with the current in wall outlets causes an additional 14% of such injuries.[13] Male children are at higher risk of burn-related death and injury than female children, and children ages 4 and under and children with a disability are at the greatest risk of burn-related death and injury, especially from scald and contact burns.[13] Heavy-for-age boys are more burn prone than their normal-sized counterparts. A recent retrospective study of 372 children admitted to a single burn center from January 1991 through July 1997 confirmed that males who were large for age on the basis of weight or height were over-represented in the burn population.[37] Interestingly, that same study indicated that male children at or under the fifth percentile for weight, and male and female children at or under the fifth percentile for height were also over-represented among pediatric burn patients. The authors considered the latter finding to reflect, at least in part, the effect of concomitant malnutrition or neglect.

The occurrence of tap water scalds can be prevented by adjusting the temperature settings on hot water heaters or by installing special faucet valves so that water does not leave the tap at temperatures above 120°F (48.8°C).[13,38] Thermostatic valves, which shut the hot water off if the cold water fails, are the most dependable.[39] The results of a survey in Denmark indicated that the kitchen, not the bathroom, is the most common site of burn injury (39% of burns).[40] Those burns were most commonly due to contact with hot liquids.

Home exercise treadmills represent a recently identified source of burn injury in pediatric patients. The injuries are a consequence of contact with a moving treadmill, most commonly involved the volar surface of the hand, and in two-thirds of patients required surgical intervention in the form of skin grafting.[41]

The elderly

The elderly represent an increasing segment of the population, the members of which have an increased risk of being burned and higher morbidity and mortality rates than younger patients. A recent review of medical records of patients admitted to a

burn center during a 7-year period revealed that 221 of 1557 (11%) admissions were 59 years or older.[42] Ninety-seven (44%) of that group were women, a reflection of the higher percentage of women in the elderly population. Two-thirds of the injuries were caused by flames or explosions, 20% by scalds, 6% by electricity, 2% by chemicals, and 6% by 'other causes.' Forty-one percent of the injuries occurred in the bedroom and/or living room, 28% out of doors or in the work place, 18% in the kitchen, 8% in the bathroom, and 5% in the garage or basement. Seventy-seven percent of the patients had one or more preexisting medical conditions. Sixty-four patients (29%) had smoke inhalation. In 57% of patients judgment and/or mobility were impaired. Ten percent of patients tested positive for ethanol and 29% for other drugs by toxicology screening. Survival advantage was conferred by younger age, absence of inhalation injury, absence of preexisting medical conditions, and lesser extent of burn. A review of 111 octogenarians admitted to a burn center between 1983 and 1993 revealed that scalds caused 32% of injuries, flames 30%, contact 29%, bath immersion 7%, electricity 2%, and hot oil 1%.[43] In 18% a disease such as a stroke was considered to be directly responsible for the burn injury and in an additional 50% of the patients, a preexisting disease was considered to be contributory to the injury event. The average length of stay was almost twice that of younger adults and rehabilitation of survivors was markedly prolonged.

The disabled

The disabled are a group of patients considered to be 'burn-prone.' The majority of burns in the disabled occur at home and are most often scalds. The effects of disability and preexisting disease in those patients are evident in the duration of hospital stay (27.6 days on average) and the death rate (22.2%) associated with the modest average extent of burn (10% of the total body surface area).[44] A recent report on burn injury in patients, generally elderly patients, with dementia has emphasized the need for prevention measures to reduce the incidence of burn injuries incurred when such patients are performing the activities of daily living.[45]

Military personnel

In wartime military personnel are at high risk for burn injury both combat related and accidental burn injury. The incidence of burn injury, which is related to both the type of weapons employed and the type of combat units engaged, has ranged from 2.3% to as high as 85% of casualties incurred in various periods of conflicts over the past six decades (Table 3.3). The detonation of a nuclear weapon at Hiroshima in 1945 instantaneously generated an estimated maximum of 57 700 burn patients and destroyed many treatment facilities which thereby compromised the care of those burn patients.[46] In the Vietnam conflict, as a consequence of the total air superiority achieved by the US Air Force and the lack of armored fighting vehicle activity, patients with burn injury represented only 4.6% of all patients admitted to Army medical treatment facilities or quarters from 1963 to 1975.[47] The majority (58%) of the 13 047 burn patients treated in those years were non-battle injuries, with only 5536 (42%) being battle injuries. The overall incidence of burns as the cause of injury in all United States mili-

TABLE 3.3 INCIDENCE OF BURN INJURY IN ARMED CONFLICT		
Conflict	**Casualties**	
	Percentage	**Number**
World War II Hiroshima 1945[40]	65–85	45 500–59 500
Vietnam Conflict 1965–1973[41]	4.6	13 047
Israeli Six Day War 1967[46]	4.6	
Yom Kippur War 1973[43]	10.5	
Falkland Islands War 1982 British casualties[45] Argentinian casualties[47]	14.0* 17.5	112 34 of 194
Lebanon War 1982[43]	8.6	
Panama police action 1989	2.3	6 of 259
Operation Desert Shield/Storm 1990–1991	7.9	36 of 458
*34% of all casualties from ships.		

tary forces in Vietnam during those years may well have been higher. Allen et al reported that during calendar years 1967 and 1968 a total of 1963 military burn patients from Vietnam were admitted and treated at a burn unit established in a United States Army General Hospital in Japan.[48] In consonance with the data from US Army hospitals in Vietnam, the burns in 847 (43.2%) of those patients were the result of hostile action. In the Panama police action in late 1989, the low incidence of burn injury (only 6 or 2.3% of the total 259 casualties had burns) has been attributed to the fact that the action involved only infantry and airborne infantry forces using small arms weaponry.

As exemplified by the Israeli conflicts of 1973 and 1982, and the British Army of the Rhine experience in World War II between March 1945 and the end of hostilities in Northwest Europe, the personnel in armored fighting vehicles have been at relatively high risk for burn injury.[49,50] Burns have also been common injuries in war at sea. In the Falkland Islands campaign of 1982, 34% of all casualties from the British Navy ships were burns.[51] The increased incidence of burn injuries, 10.5% and 8.6% in the Israeli conflicts of 1973 and 1982 respectively as compared to the 4.6% incidence in the 1967 Israeli conflict, is considered to reflect what has been termed 'battlefield saturation with tanks and anti-tank weaponry.'[43,49,52] The decreased incidence of burn injuries, 8.6% in the 1982 Israeli conflict as compared to the 10.5% in the 1973 Israeli conflict, has been attributed to enforced use of flame retardant garments and the effectiveness of an automatic fire extinguishing system within the Israeli tanks.[52] Those factors have also been credited with reducing the extent of the burns that did occur. In the 1973 Israeli conflict, 29% of the patients with burns had injuries that involved 40% or more of the total body surface, and only 21% had burns of less than 10% of the body surface. In the 1982 Israeli conflict those same categories of burns represented 18% and 51% respectively of all burn injuries. Modern weaponry may have eliminated the differential incidence of burn injury between armored fighting vehicle personnel and the personnel of other combat elements. One of every seven and every six casualties had burns in the British and Argentinean forces respectively in the 1982 Falkland Islands conflict in which there was little if any involvement of armored fighting vehicles.[51,53] Conversely, there were only 36 (7.8%) burn casualties in the total 458 casualties sustained by US Forces in 1990 and 1991 during Operation Desert Shield/ Desert Storm in which there was extensive involvement of armored fighting vehicles.

In the current armed conflicts, Operations Iraqi Freedom and Enduring Freedom, the US Army Burn Center has provided care for all of the patients from all branches of the armed forces who has sustained severe burns in the theaters of operation. Surgeons from the Burn Center have provided care at the Center and an Army general hospital in Landstuhl, Germany, at hospitals within the theaters of operation and during aeromedical transfers from the hospital in Europe to the Burn Center in San Antonio, Texas. During the period of March 2003 to May 2004, 109 burn casualties from those conflicts were hospitalized at the Burn Center. Twenty patients (18.3%) had burns of more than 20% of the total body surface and six patients (5.5%) had smoke inhalation injury.

During that same period of time Burn Center flight teams reactivated the Intercontinental Aeromedical Transfer System that had been organized and used effectively in the Vietnam Conflict in the first Gulf War. The teams performed 18 flights to transport 51 war-injured burn patients from the Army hospital in Landstuhl to the Burn Center in San Antonio. Those 18 missions were carried out without a death or life-threatening complication in flight.[54]

Even though the risk of burn injury in the combat population is relatively high, the distribution of burn size in other than armored fighting vehicle personnel is comparable to that in the civilian population, i.e. more than 80% of the patients have burns of less than 20% of the body surface. Even so, the number of burns that can be rapidly generated necessitates that planning for combat casualty care include augmentation of in-theater medical treatment facilities with personnel having burn-specific expertise as was done in Operation Desert Shield/Storm. Changes in both professional staffing and the patient population served at the US Army Burn Center during the period 1 January, 2001 to 1 May, 2006 are reflected in Table 3.4. Lack of on-site pediatrician support forced the Burn Center to cease function as a tertiary referral center for pediatric burn patients and reduce admission of such patients. Conversely military activity, predominantly that in Operation Iraqi Freedom, generated a marked increase in combat-related burns principally as a consequence of the ignition of improvised explosive devices.

Even in peacetime non-combat munitions incidents are common in the US Army. In a recent 7-year period there were 742 noncombat munitions incidents reported in which 894 soldiers were injured.[55] The most common types of injuries were burns which occurred in 261 or 26.7% of all the patients injured. The high incidence of burn injury in military personnel in both war and peace will generate a subset of extensively burned patients who will require tertiary burn center care to ensure optimum functional outcome and maximum survival.

TABLE 3.4 ADMISSIONS TO US ARMY INSTITUTE OF SURGICAL RESEARCH BURN CENTER JANUARY 1, 2001, TO MAY 1, 2006

Cause of burn	Age groups (years)			
	0–15	16–40	>40	Total
Hot liquids	32	89	69	190
Gasoline, diesel, and kerosene	24	228	151	403
Open flame	7	48	48	103
Structural fires	5	34	68	107
Butane, propane, natural gas explosions	6	60	47	113
Motor vehicle crashes	0	34	18	52
Smoking	0	10	27	37
Bomb, improvised explosive device, gunpowder	1	359	15	375
Contact	4	27	29	60
Electrical or electrical arc	0	60	35	95
Chemical	0	13	11	24
Welding	0	10	9	19
Intentional: Self-inflicted	0	8	11	19
Assault	0	8	3	11
Aircraft crashes	0	10	4	14
Train crashes	0	0	2	2
Sunburn	0	2	0	2
TOTAL	79	999	548	1626

Burn etiologies

Burns due to hot liquids may occur in any age group, but 77% of all hot liquid scalds have been reported to occur in children less than 3 years of age. Full-thickness injury is present in less than half of patients with hot water scalds, but present in 58% of patients with hot oil burns. Young children are most commonly injured by their pulling a container of hot water or hot cooking oil onto themselves, while older children and adults are most commonly injured by improper handling of hot oil appliances.[56–58]

Burns from scalds and contacts with hot materials cause approximately 100 deaths per year.[5] The case fatality rate of scald injury is low (presumably due to the usually modest extent and limited depth of the burn), but scalds are major causes of morbidity and associated healthcare costs, particularly in children less than 5 years of age and in the elderly. Although deaths from scalds are relatively rare in patients between the ages of 5 and 64, both rates of hospitalization for burn injury and death rates are three times higher for blacks than for Caucasians.[59]

Even though the burns of 30% of all patients requiring admission to a hospital are caused by scalding due to hot liquids,[60,61] flame is the predominant cause of burns in patients admitted to burn centers, particularly in the adult age group (Table 3.4). The misuse of fuels and flammable liquids is a common cause of burn injury. A recent retrospective review of admissions to one burn center for the multi-year period,

1978 to 1996, identified 1011 (23.3% of 4339 acute admissions) as being gasoline-related.[62] The average total extent of burn was 30% of the total body surface area with an average 14% full-thickness burn component. One hundred and forty-four of those patients expired. The unsafe use of gasoline was implicated in 87% of patients in whom the cause of the burn could be identified, and in 90 or 63% of the 144 fatalities. The use of gasoline for purposes other than as a motor fuel, and any indoor use of a volatile petroleum product should be discouraged as part of any prevention program. In one epidemiologic study in New York state, the largest number of admissions in the teenage/early adult age group (15–24 years) was related to automobiles. Ignition of fuel following a crash, steam from radiators, and contact with hot engine and exhaust parts were the most frequent causes.[61] In a review of 178 patients who had been burned in an automobile crash, it was noted that slightly more than one-third had other injuries, most commonly involving the musculoskeletal system, and that approximately 1 in 6 had inhalation injury (1 in 3 of those who died.).[63] A review of patients admitted to a referral burn center revealed that burns sustained while operating a vehicle involved an average of more than 30% of the total body surface and were associated with mechanical injuries (predominantly fractures) much more frequently than those burns incurred in the course of vehicle maintenance activities which involved an average of less than 30% of the total body surface.[64]

Contact burns from motorcycle exhaust pipes are another injury related to the use of vehicles. In Greece the incidence of burns from motorcycle exhaust pipes has been reported to be 17/100 000 person-years, or 208/100 000 motorcycle-years. The highest occurrence was in children. In adults the incidence is 60% higher in females than in males. As would be anticipated, the most frequent location of the burns was on the right leg below the knee where contact with the exhaust pipe occurs. The authors concluded that significant reduction of incidence could be achieved by wearing long pants and the use of an external exhaust pipe shield.[64,65]

Automotive-related flame burns can also be caused by fires and explosions resulting from 'carburetor-priming' with liquid gasoline; and such burns have been reported to account for 2% to 5% of burn unit admissions.[66] The burns sustained in boating accidents are also most often flash burns due to an explosion of gasoline or butane and typically affect the face and hands.[33] Bonfire and barbeque burns caused by flash ignition of a flammable liquid which is used to start or accelerate a fire affect those same areas as well as the anterior trunk.[67]

The ignition of clothing is the second leading cause of burn admissions for most ages.[61] The burn injury rate due to the ignition of clothing is influenced by poverty and is inversely related to income. The fatality rate of patients with burns due to the ignition of clothing is second only to that of patients with burns incurred in house fires.[61] Burns caused by ignition of synthetic fabrics which melt and adhere to the skin are commonly deeper than burns caused by other fabrics and typically exhibit a gravity-dependent 'runoff' pattern. More than three-quarters of deaths due to the ignition of clothing occur in patients above the age of 64.[5] Clothing ignition deaths, which were a frequent cause of death in young girls, have decreased as clothing styles have changed and are now rare among children with little overall gender difference at the present time. From 1975, when it was mandated that sleep wear sizes 0 to 6X successfully pass a standard flame test, until 1999 when that law was repealed, the percentage of clothing burns caused by sleep wear in children age 0–12 decreased from 55 to 27.[61,68] Sleep wear-related burns are being closely monitored to assess the affect of deregulation of sleep wear garments on sleep wear-related burns.

Work-related burns account for 20–25% of all serious burns. A Bureau of Labor Statistics survey in 1985 indicated that 6% of all work-related thermal burns occurred in adolescent workers (16–19 years).[69] In a 1986 study in Ohio, it was noted that the majority of hospital-treated burns in the teenage/young adult group occurred on the job.[70] A study in that same year revealed that 6 out of 10 hospitalized burn injuries in employed men in Massachusetts were work-related.[71] Restaurant-related burns, particularly those due to deep fryers, represent a major and preventable source of occupational burn morbidity, and in restaurants account for 12% of work-related injuries.[61] Almost 700 deaths annually are caused by occupation-related burns.[72,73]

A recent review of Rhode Island workers compensation claims has identified that the highest claim rate for burn injury was for workers in food service occupations. Evening and night-shift workers were at an increased risk for chemical burn injuries. The overall claim rate for burn injury was 24.3/10 000 workers and ranged from a high of 51/10 000 for workers

younger than 25 years to a low of 16.5/10 000 workers between the ages of 40 and 54.[74]

As would be anticipated, the risk of burn injury due to hot tar is greatest for roofers and paving workers. Of all accidents involving roofers and sheet metal workers, 16% are burns caused by hot bitumen, and 17% of those injuries are of sufficient severity to prevent work for a variable period of time. In the state of California, in 1979, 366 roofers and slaters sustained burn injuries.[75] The majority of hot tar burns involved the hand and upper limb.[76] Another occupation associated with an increased risk of burn injury is welding in which flash burns and explosions are the most common injury-producing events.

In the United States in 1988, there were 236 200 patients with chemical injuries of all types treated in emergency rooms. Of those patients, 35 000 or 15% were patients of all ages with chemical burns, and 6500 or 5% were children younger than 5 years with chemical burns. The limited extent of burns due to chemical content is indexed by the fact that only 800, or 2%, of the chemical burns required admission to a hospital. The effect of age (in the very young, removal of the offending agent may be delayed) on the severity of chemical injury is evident in the fact that 400 of the patients requiring admission to a hospital for the care of chemical burn injuries were children younger than 5 years.[77] The greatest risk of injury due to strong acids occurs in patients who are involved in plating processes and fertilizer manufacture. The greatest risk of injury due to strong alkalis in the work place is associated with soap manufacturing and in the home with the use of oven cleaners. The greatest risk of phenol injuries is associated with the manufacture of dyes, fertilizers, plastics, and explosives. The greatest risk of hydrofluoric acid injury is associated with etching processes, petroleum refining, and air conditioner cleaning. Anhydrous ammonia injury is most common in agricultural workers and cement injury is most common in construction workers. Injury due to petroleum distillates, which cause dilapidation, is greatest in refinery and tank farm workers, while white phosphorus and mustard gas injuries are most frequent in military personnel.[78]

Nearly 1000 deaths are caused annually by electric current. One-third of electric injuries occur in the home and one-quarter occur on farms or industrial sites.[61] The greatest incidence of electric injury caused by household current occurs in young children who insert uninsulated objects into electrical receptacles or bite or suck on electric cords in sockets.[27] Low-voltage direct current injury can be caused by contact with automobile battery terminals or by defective or inappropriately used medical equipment such as electric surgical devices,[79] external pacing devices,[80] or defibrillators.[81] Although such injuries may involve the full thickness of the skin, they are characteristically of limited extent. Caucasians, apparently because of employment patterns, are almost twice as likely to be injured by high-voltage electric current as are blacks.[73] Employees of utility companies, electricians, construction workers (particularly those working with cranes), farm workers moving irrigation pipe, oil field workers, truck drivers, and individuals installing antennae are at greatest risk of work-related high-voltage electric injury.[27] The greatest incidence of electric injury occurs during the summer as a reflection of farm irrigation activity, construction work, and work on outdoor electrical systems and equipment.[10] The current limitation and ineffectiveness of preventive measures is evident in the constancy of occurrence of high voltage injury over the past 20 years. Conversely, the use of ground-fault circuit interrupters and media-promoted awareness have reduced the incidence of low-voltage injuries.[82]

During the period 1982 to 2002, 263 patients with high-voltage injury, 143 with low-voltage injury, and 17 with lightning injury were treated at a regional burn center. The observed mortality was greatest in the patients with lightning injury, 17.6%, in contrast to 5.3% in patients of high-voltage injury, and 2.8% for patients with low-voltage injury. In the patients with high-voltage injury, 88 required fasciotomy and even so, muscle necrosis occurred in 68 with amputation necessary in 95. Pigmented urine was observed in 96 patients, and renal failure in 7. Arrhythmia was recorded in 38 patients, and cardiac arrest in 2. Neurologic deficit was recorded in 21, cataract formation in 5, and associated fractures were present in 22.[82] Another recent study reported the outcome of 195 patients with high-voltage electric injury treated at a single burn center during a 19-year period: 187 (95.9%) of the 195 patients survived and were discharged. Fasciotomy was required in the first 24 hours following injury in 56 patients, and 80 patients underwent an amputation because of extensive tissue necrosis. The presence of hemochromogens in the urine predicted the need for amputation with an overall accuracy of 73.3%.[83]

There are 30 million cloud to ground lightning strikes each year in the United States and each one represents a risk of severe injury and even death. A total of 1318 deaths were caused by lightning in the United States from 1980 through 1995.[84] Of those who died, 1125 (85%) were male and 896 (68%) were 15 to 44 years of age. The annual death rate from lightning was greatest among patients age 15 to 19 years (6 deaths per 10 million population; crude rate: 3 per 10 million) and is 7 times greater in males than females. The greatest number of deaths caused by lightning, 145 and 91, occurred in Florida and Texas respectively. However, New Mexico, Arizona, Arkansas, and Mississippi had the highest crude death rates of 10, 9, 9, and 9 per 10 000 000 population respectively. Lopez and Holle note that National Oceanic and Atmospheric Administration data identified an average of 93 deaths and 257 injuries caused by lightning occurred each year during the period 1959–1990.[85] Those authors also cited a study based on national death certificate data for 1968–1985 which reported an average of 107 lightning deaths each year and an annual death rate of 6.1 per 10 million population. Approximately 30% of persons struck by lightning die with the greatest risk of death being in those patients with cranial burns or leg burns. Ninety-two percent of lightning-associated deaths occur during the summer months (May–September) when thunderstorms are most common. Seventy-three percent of deaths occur during the afternoon and early evening when thunderstorms are most likely to occur. Fifty-two percent of patients who died from lightning injury were engaged in outdoor recreational activity such as golfing and fishing and 25% were engaged in work activities when struck. Sixty-three percent of lightning-associated deaths occur within 1 hour of injury. Virtually all lightning injuries and deaths can be prevented by taking appropriate precautions. The recent decrease in lightning-related deaths appears to be related to a decrease in the farm population, better understanding of the pathophysiology of lightning injury, and improved resuscitation techniques. Analysis of data from the Defense Medical Surveillance System by the US Army and the CDC reveals that the highest lightning-related injury rate occurred in male US military members, stationed near the East Coast or the Gulf of Mexico where lightning occurs frequently, who were subjected to outdoor exposure to thunderstorms. During 1998–2001, 350 service members were injured and one killed by 142 lightning strikes. One-half of the lightning strikes occurred during July and August and three-quarters occurred between May and September; 246 (70.1%) of the lightning injuries involved active duty personnel, with men being 3.3 times more likely to be struck than women. The overall lightning casualty rate for military personnel was 5.8/100 000 person years. Louisiana, Georgia, and Oklahoma had the highest rates of lightning injury, i.e. 39.6, 25.2, and 23.5/100 000 person-years respectively.[86]

Fireworks are another seasonal cause of burn injury. Approximately 10% of patients with fireworks injuries require in-hospital care and approximately 60% of those injuries are burns.[87] These data can be used to estimate that 1.86 to 5.82 fireworks-related burns per 100 000 persons occurred in the United States during the 4th of July holiday.[88] Extrapolation of the National Electronic Injury Surveillance System (NEISS) data indicates that 13 263 patients sustained burns in 1992 from fireworks and flares.[89] Sparklers, firecrackers, and bottle rockets caused the greatest number of burn injuries requiring hospital care.[90] Nearly 3000 children, ages 14 or less, sustained fireworks-related injuries that required treatment in hospital emergency rooms in 1996.[13] Burns accounted for approximately 60% of those injuries, and principally involved the hands, head, and eyes. As expected, 75% of such injuries occur in the month surrounding July 4.[13] Males, especially those age 10 to 14, are at the highest risk for fireworks-related injuries. Children, age 4 and under, are at highest risk for sparkler-related injuries.[13] A recent report of 7 patients with burns due to snap-cap pyrotechnic devices noted that 6 patients required hospital admission with 4 undergoing split-thickness skin grafting for closure of burns of the leg caused by explosion of multiple devices in one trouser pocket. Proposed prevention measures include reducing the explosive units per package, package warnings, and limiting the sale of the devices to children.[91] At the US Army Institute of Surgical Research Burn Center, only 4 or 0.1%, of 3628 burn patients admitted during a 15-year period had been burned by fireworks.

Burn injury can also be intentional, either self-inflicted or caused by assault. It is estimated that 4% of burns (published range 0.37–14%) are self-inflicted. A retrospective review of 5758 burn patients treated at a regional burn center during a 12-year period identified 51 patients (26 males and 25 females) with a diagnosis of self-inflicted burns.[92] In 42 patients, in whom the injury was an attempt at suicide, the burn involved from 1% to 84% of the total body surface with an average extent of 22%. Twelve, or 28%, of those patients expired. There were 9 patients in whom the injury was considered a form of self-mutilation. Those injuries typically caused by flames involved 1% to 5% of the total body surface with an average extent of 1.4%. Forty-three percent of all the injuries occurred at home, and 14 (33%) occurred while the patient was in a psychiatric institution. Seventy-three percent of the patients had a history of psychiatric disease; and these were predominantly affective disorders or schizophrenia in the suicides, and personality disorders in the self-mutilators. Fifty-five percent of the suicides had previously attempted suicide; 66% of the self-mutilators had made at least one previous attempt at self-mutilation. The authors concluded that the very fact of self-burning warranted psychiatric assessment. In a recent study the extent of such injuries was reported to be greater than that of accidental burns with the head and torso more frequently involved than in patients with accidental burns. Consequently the hospital stay was typically longer than that of patients with accidental burns.[93] Buddhist ritual burning caused by contact with smoldering incense is a traditional religious form of self-mutilation.[94] Squyres et al reported their experience in treating 17 people over a 3-year period for self-inflicted burns.[95] The average extent of burn in those patients was 29.5% of the total body surface; and 59% of them had concomitant inhalation injury. All of those patients had a psychiatric disorder which in 47% of the group, was related to substance abuse. The most frequently employed means of injury was ignition of a flammable liquid.

Assault by burning is most often caused by throwing liquid chemicals at the face of the intended victim or by the ignition of a flammable liquid with which the victim has been doused. Relatively uncommon is the infliction of burn injury by dousing the victim with hot water. Duminy and Hudson have reported their experience with 127 patients who had been intentionally injured with hot water.[96] The burns in those patients involved from 1 to 45% of the total body surface area with an average extent of 13.7%. The trunk and arms were burned in 116 of the patients, the head and neck in 84, and the legs in 27. The vast majority, 84, had only partial-thickness injuries. Fifty-one of the 94 male patients and 12 of the 33 females had been assaulted by their spouses. In cases of spouse abuse, the face or genitalia are characteristically splashed with chemicals or hot liquids while cases due to abuse or neglect in elderly, disabled, and handicapped adults resemble those in child abuse cases.[97,98] In India, a common form of spouse abuse is burning by intentional ignition of clothing. When such burns are fatal they have been called 'dowry deaths' since they have been used to establish the widower's eligibility for a new bride and dowry.

Child abuse represents a special form of burn injury most commonly inflicted by parents but also perpetrated by siblings and child care personnel. Child abuse has been associated with teenage parents, mental deficits in either the child or the abuser, illegitimacy, a single parent household, and low socio-economic status (although child abuse can occur in all economic groups). Abuse is usually inflicted upon children younger than 2 years of age who, in addition to burns, may exhibit signs of poor hygiene, psychological deprivation, and nutritional impairment.[99] The most common form (approximately one-third of cases) of child abuse thermal injury is caused by cigarettes; such injuries, because of their limited extent, frequently do not require admission to a hospital.[100] Child abuse by burning has also been inflicted by placing a small child in a microwave oven. The burn injuries produced in that manner are typically present on the body parts nearest the microwave generating element, full thickness in depth and sharply demarcated.[101] Child neglect, if not child abuse, is considered to be a factor in burns of the hand, particularly those on the dorsum of the hand, due to contact with a hot clothing iron.[102] Most often scalding causes the burns in abused children who require in-hospital care.[103] Such injuries are often associated with soft tissue trauma, fractures, and head injury. A distribution typical of child abuse immersion scald burns, i.e. feet, posterior legs, buttocks, and the hands, should heighten one's suspicion of child abuse. The presence of such burns mandates a complete evaluation of the circumstances surrounding the injury and the home situation. The importance of identifying child abuse in the case of a burn injury resides in the fact that if such abuse goes undetected and the child is returned to the abusive environment, there is a high risk of fatality due to repeated abuse. Chester et al. have recently reported that parental neglect is far more prevalent than abuse as a causative factor for burn injury in children. Children with burns that occurred as a consequence of neglect had deeper burns than children with accidental burns and were more apt to require skin grafting for wound closure. Eighty-three percent of the children with burns due to neglect had previously been referred to a child protection agency.[104]

Elder abuse can also take the form of burn injury. A congressional report published in 1991 indicated that 2 million older Americans are abused each year, and some estimates claim a 4% to 10% incidence of neglect or abuse of the elderly.[105] A recent retrospective review of 28 patients, 60 years and above, admitted to a single burn center during a calendar year, identified self-neglect in 7, neglect by others in 3, and abuse by others in 1.[106] Adult protective services were required in 2 cases. The authors of that study concluded that abuse was likely to be under-reported because of poor understanding of risk factors and a low index of suspicion on the part of the entire spectrum of healthcare personnel.

Patients may also sustain burns while in the hospital for diagnosis and treatment of other disease.[107] In addition to the electric injuries noted above, chemical burns have been produced by inadvertent application of glacial acetic acid, concentrated silver nitrate, iodine, or phenol solutions, and potassium permanganate crystals. Application of excessively hot soaks or towels or inappropriate use of heat lamps or a heating blanket are other causes of burn injury to patients.[108] Infrared heat lamps are often used in conjunction with acupuncture, but inappropriate intensity of excessive duration of exposure may cause full-thickness skin injury.[109] Much more serious are the burns and inhalation injuries caused by electrocautery or laser devices, explosion of gases (including ignition of flammable material in oxygen), or ignition of the instruments used for endotracheal and endobronchial procedures or anesthetic management.[110] Localized high-energy ultrasound may also produce coagulative necrosis as exemplified by full-thickness cutaneous injury and localized subcutaneous fat necrosis of the abdominal wall in a patient who had received focused beam high-intensity ultrasound treatment for uterine fibroids.[111] A common cause of burn injury, particularly in disoriented hospital or nursing home patients, is the ignition of bed clothes and clothing by a burning cigarette. Smoking should be banned in healthcare facilities, or at least restricted to adequately monitored situations.

A recent retrospective review of 4510 consecutive patients admitted to a burn center between January 1978 and July 1997 identified 54 patients who sustained burns while undergoing medical treatment.[112] Twenty-two patients sustained their injuries in a hospital or nursing home, most commonly (12 patients) as a consequence of a fire started by smoking activities. Fifty-eight percent of those patients expired. Another 2 patients were scalded while being bathed in nursing homes and 1 of those patients expired. Thirty-two patients were burned as a consequence of home medical therapy, including 9 vaporizer scald burns, 8 burns caused by ignition in therapeutic oxygen, and 11 caused by inappropriate application of heat. In contrast to other studies, no patients in this series sustained burns from medical lasers.

Burn patient transport and transfer

As noted above, the concordance of burn treatment facility location and population density necessitates that many patients requiring burn center care be transferred from other locations to such institutions. For transfer across short distances and in congested urban areas, ground transportation is frequently more expeditious than aeromedical transfer. Aeromedical transfer is indicated when the patient requires movement from a remote area or when such transfer will materially shorten the time during which the patient is in transit as compared to ground transportation. Helicopters are frequently employed for the aeromedical transfer of patients over distances of less than 200 miles. Vibration, poor lightning, restricted space, and noise make in-flight monitoring and therapeutic interventions difficult, a fact which emphasizes the importance of carefully evaluating the patient and modifying treatment as needed to establish hemodynamic and pulmonary stability prior to undertaking the transfer. When transfer requires movement over greater distances, fixed-wing aircraft are utilized, ideally those in which an oxygen supply is available to support mechanical ventilation. The patient compartment of such an aircraft should be well lighted, permit movement of attending personnel, and have some measure of temperature control.

In general, burned patients travel best in the immediate postburn period as soon as hemodynamic and pulmonary stability have been attained by resuscitation. This avoids the instability caused by infection, secondary hemorrhage, sepsis, or cardiac insufficiency all of which may occur later in the severely burned patient's hospital course.[113] The importance of having an experienced burn physician accompany a patient during aeromedical transfer is indicated by the findings of a study in which the management problems encountered during 124 flights to transfer 148 burn patients were reviewed.[114] More than half the patients required therapeutic interventions by the surgeon of the burn team prior to undertaking aeromedical transfer. Such interventions most commonly involved placement or adjustment of a cannula or catheter, modification of fluid therapy, or endotracheal intubation and modification of ventilatory management. In slightly more than one-third of the patients, such interventions were considered necessary to correct physiological instabilities which would have compromised patient safety during the transfer procedure. Six of the 124 patients required an escharotomy to relieve compression of the chest or a limb caused by a constricting eschar. The therapeutic alterations most commonly needed during the aeromedical transfer procedure itself were changes in fluid therapy, adjustment of a ventilator, and administration of parenteral medications exclusive of analgesics. The medical personnel effecting the burn patient transfer must bring with them all the equipment and supplies needed for pre-flight preparation and in-flight management of the patient.

Physician-to-physician case review to assess the patient's need for and ability to tolerate aeromedical transfer, prompt initiation of the aeromedical transfer mission, examination of the patient in the hospital of origin by a burn surgeon from the receiving hospital and correction of organ dysfunction prior to undertaking aeromedical transfer, and in-flight monitoring by burn experienced personnel ensure both continuity and quality of care during the transport procedure. During the 10-year period 1991–2000, US Army Institute of Surgical Research Burn Care Flight Teams using such a regimen completed 266 helicopter and fixed-wing aeromedical transfer missions to transport 310 burn patients within the continental United States without any in-flight deaths. During the same period, the Institute carried out 12 intercontinental aeromedical transfer missions in which 17 burn patients, were transported with only 1 in-flight death.

Mass casualties

Mass casualty incidents may be caused by forces of nature or by accidental or intentional explosions and conflagrations. Interest in man-made mass casualties has been heightened by recent terrorist activities and the threat of future incidents. The incidence of burn injury in a mass casualty incident varies according to the cause of the incident, the magnitude of the inciting agent, and the site of occurrence (indoors vs. outdoors). The terrorist attacks in which airplanes laden with aviation fuel crashed into the Pentagon and the World Trade Center on September 11, 2001 produced 10 patients and 39 patients respectively with burns requiring treatment at burn centers.[29,115] The terrorist attack on a nightclub in Bali in 2002 caused an explosion and fire that killed over 200 people and generated 60 burn patients who after triage and emergency care were transported by aircraft to Australia and treated at various hospitals.[116] The casualties produced in terrorist attacks often have associated blast injury and mechanical trauma in addition to burns.

Recent non-terrorist mass casualty incidents have been of greater magnitude in terms of numbers of burn casualties. In 1994 an airplane collision caused nearby military personnel to be sprayed with burning aviation fuel. Of the 130 injured soldiers, 43 required transfer to the US Army Burn Center for treatment.[117] In The Station nightclub fire in Warwick, Rhode Island in February 2003, 96 people died at the scene and 215 people were injured; 47 of the 64 burned patients evaluated at one academic medical center were admitted for definitive care.[118] Lastly, an explosion at a pharmaceutical plant in North Carolina in January 2003 killed 3 and injured more than 30 to an extent that necessitated admission to a hospital. Ten of the injured patients, all with inhalation injury and 6 with associated mechanical trauma, required admission to the regional burn center.[119] To deal effectively and efficiently with a mass casualty situation burn treatment facilities must have an operational and tested mass casualty disaster plan and be prepared to provide burn care to a highly variable number of patients injured in either natural or man-made disasters.

Outcome analysis in burn injury

The importance of extent of injury in determining burn outcome was recognized by Holmes in 1860, and discussions expressing that extent as either a measured area or as anatomical parts of the body surface appeared in the latter 19th and early 20th centuries.[120–122] Formal expression of burn size as a percentage of total body surface area, however, awaited the work of Berkow in 1924.[123] Though accorded little recognition as such, this single advance in the description of thermal injury, along with the corollary understanding that burn size is a crucial determinant of pathophysiological response, made burns the first form of trauma whose impact could be measured and easily communicated. Techniques based on this understanding produced what were in effect the first trauma indices, making assessment of the relationship between burn size and mortality, direct comparison of populations of burned patients, and rational assessment of therapy possible long before rigorous outcome analysis became feasible for any other form of injury.

The earliest comprehensive statistical technique used for such assessment was univariate probit analysis.[124,125] This approach, laborious in the days of paper files and rotary calculators, required that the population studied be arbitrarily partitioned into groups which were relatively similar in burn size and age. Such analyses yield equations describing the effect of burn size on mortality which are valid for only the particular age group studied. An early attempt to develop a multivariate evaluation was made by Schwartz, who used probit plane analysis to estimate the relative contributions of partial- and full-thickness burns to mortality. This approach also required arbitrary partitioning of the population.[126]

The advent of computers of suitable power and further development of statistical techniques have reduced the difficulty of analyzing burn mortality, removed the necessity for arbitrary partitioning, and made these techniques much more accessible.[127] Their use to assess outcome demands understanding of both the techniques themselves and the population being analyzed. The analysis of a population of 8448 patients admitted for burn care to the United States Army Institute of Surgical Research or to its predecessor, the US Army Surgical Research Unit, between January 1, 1950 and December 31, 1991 illustrates the concepts underlying such outcome analysis and depicts the trends in mortality that have been characteristic of most major burn centers in this country.

For validity, an important first step in studies of outcome is to achieve as much uniformity as possible in the population to be analyzed. These patients reached the Institute between the day of injury and postburn day 531 (mean 5.86 days, median 1 day), with burns averaging 31% (range 1–100%, median 26%) of the total body surface. Their age distribution was biphasic, with one peak at 1 year of age and another at age 20; the mean age of the entire population was 26.5 years (range 0–97 years, median 23 years). From this group, 7893

(93.4%) who had flame or scald burns were selected, excluding patients with electric or chemical injuries.

This group included patients who sustained thermal injuries in Vietnam and were first transferred to Japan and then selectively transferred to the Institute. Arriving at the Institute relatively late in their courses, these survivors of temporal cohorts in which some deaths had already occurred exhibited inordinately low mortality. Outcome is inevitably biased toward survival as the postburn time of admission lengthens. To avoid this bias, the analysis focused on the 4870 patients with flame or scald injuries who reached the Institute on or before the second postburn day, excluding later arrivals. Burn size in these patients averaged 34% (range 1–100%, median 29%), and age was again biphasic, with peaks at 1 and 21 years and a mean of 27.1 years (range 0–93 yrs, median 24 years).

One object of the analysis was to evaluate changes in burn mortality during the five decades of experience included in the study. For reliable results, some of the techniques which were used required more subjects than were available in single years; a moving 5-year interval, advancing 1 year at a time, was used to group the data. The number of patients in each of the overlapping 5-year intervals is shown in Figure 3.2. In this and subsequent plots, the data for a 5-year interval are plotted at the first year of the interval, reflecting that year and the succeeding four. The number of admissions meeting the selection criteria was small in the early years of the Institute's experience and rose in somewhat linear fashion during the second and third decades to a sustained plateau of approximately 800 (160/year).

Mean patient age is shown in Figure 3.3. Between 1950 and 1965, most of the admissions were young soldiers; mean age approximated 22.5 years and was relatively stable. During the succeeding decade, this value rose to an irregular plateau centering on 30 years of age, a change reflecting a greater number of civilian emergency admissions and increasing age in the military population.

Figure 3.4 shows the variation in mean burn size during the study interval, and Figure 3.5 shows the roughly parallel mortality. Mean burn size peaked in the two intervals spanning 1969 to 1974 and decreased steadily after that time. Mortality,

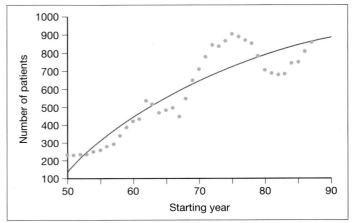

Fig. 3.2 Number of patients meeting study criteria. Values are plotted at the first year of each moving 5-year interval.

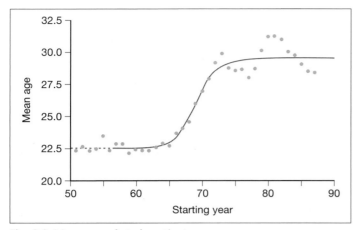

Fig. 3.3 Mean age of study patients.

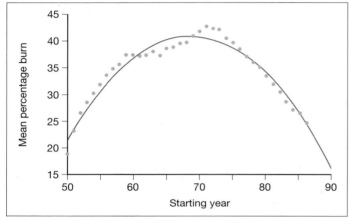

Fig. 3.4 Mean burn size in study patients.

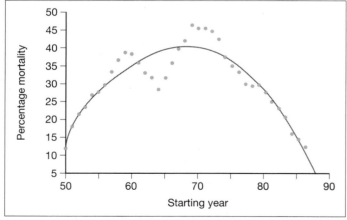

Fig. 3.5 Percent mortality in study patients in each moving 5-year interval.

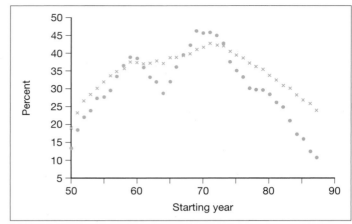

Fig. 3.6 Comparison of mean burn size (open circles) and percent mortality (solid dots).

principally due to burn wound sepsis, peaked at 46% during those years. The two data sets are shown together in Figure 3.6 and suggest a crude index of the results of burn care in this population. There were two intervals in which percent mortality exceeded mean percent burn. The first occurred in the late 1950s and early 1960s, a time when burn wound sepsis

due to *Pseudomonas aeruginosa* was uncontrolled. This was succeeded by a 6-year interval of good control of wound infection following the introduction of topical wound treatment with mafenide. In turn, this was followed by a second interval of poor control in the late 1960s and early 1970s, during which both *Pseudomonas* and a mafenide-resistant *Providencia stuartii* were major causes of sepsis; this endemic was controlled by the mid-1970s following changes in topical treatment and wound management.

Raw percent mortality, even in conjunction with burn size, is never an adequate index of the effectiveness of treatment, since the frequency of death after burn injury is also determined by prior patient condition, age, inhalation injury, and the occurrence of pneumonia and burn wound sepsis. Each of these elements, except for prior condition, can be addressed in analysis, but only burn size, age, and the presence or absence of inhalation injury are known at the time of admission. In the studied group, burn size and age were available for every patient, but data on inhalation injury were missing for patients admitted in the earlier years; we elected to use burn size and age for analysis. This choice does not exclude the impact of the complications, but does confound that impact with those of burn size and age.

For a uniform population of specific age, a plot of the relationship between burn size and percent mortality is S-shaped, or sigmoid — small burns produce relatively few deaths, but as burn size increases mortality rises steeply and then plateaus as it approaches its maximum of 100%. Figure 3.7 illustrates this dose–response relationship for 50-year-old patients admitted to the Institute between 1987 and 1991. Such curves are mathematically intractable and are usually transformed to more easily managed straight lines for analysis. Several mathematical transformations have been used to accomplish this. As previously noted, the one used in early analyses was probit transformation; in the present study, a logistic transformation, illustrated in Figure 3.8, was used. The choice between these is one of convenience as either yields essentially the same information.[128,129]

The locations of a sequence of such curves for groups of patients of increasing age move first to the right (toward larger burn size) as age increases from infancy to young adulthood,

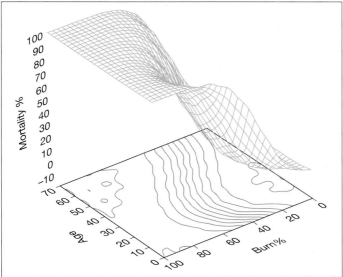

Fig. 3.14 Mortality plane for patients admitted between 1950 and 1963. Note location of contour lines in base of cube.

Logistic regression permits simple assessment of the odds ratio for mortality between the individual years and the last year of this span, with appropriate adjustment for age and burn size. Figure 3.17 depicts this ratio, which indexes the effect on mortality of everything beyond burn size and age. Peaks occurred when sepsis was uncontrolled. The lower ratios beyond 1975 reflect the additive effects of changes in treatment, environment, and infection control. No significant differences in the ratio have occurred during the 16 years between 1987 and 2002.

Though this experience conforms with that of most burn centers in the United States, it should be noted that there are still many areas of the world where the survival of patients with burns of more than 40% of the total body surface is rare. Among the patients meeting the present study criteria between 1950 and 2002, 1591 (23%) died. Had the mortality experienced since 1987 prevailed through the whole interval, only a bit more than half this number would have succumbed to their injuries. Mortality now is less than half that characterizing the first decade of the Institute's experience.

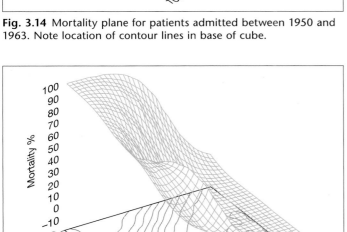

Fig. 3.15 Mortality plane for patients admitted between 1987 and 1991. Note contour locations.

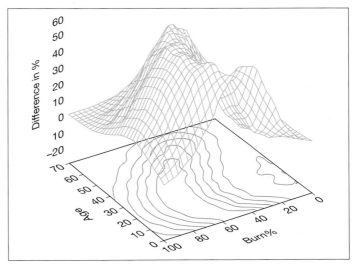

Fig. 3.16 Plane of differences in percent mortality between 1950–1963 and 1987–1991. Note location of peak.

Fig. 3.17 Odds ratio of death between individual years and 2002, adjusted for burn size and age.

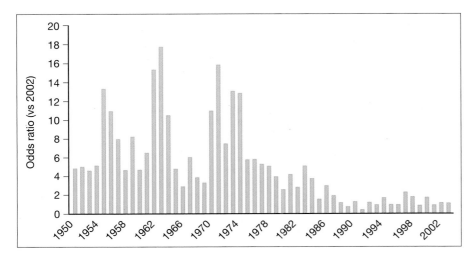

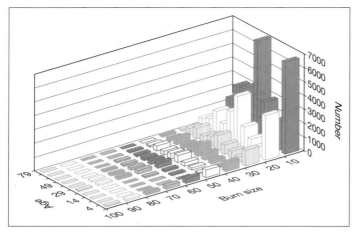

Fig. 3.18 Estimated age/burn size distribution of 70 000 annual hospital admissions.

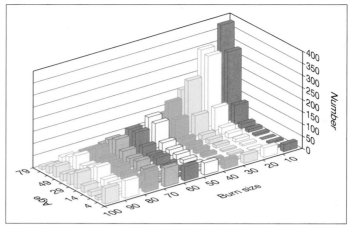

Fig. 3.19 Estimated age and burn size distribution of expected deaths among patients depicted in Figure 3.18.

As previously noted, estimates of the annual total number of burns in the United States, for which there is little reliable information, range as high as 2 000 000. A more reliable but still imperfect estimate is that between 50 000 and 70 000 acutely burned patients are admitted to hospitals in the United States each year. Figure 3.18 is based on composite data from several sources and depicts an estimate of the age and burn size distribution of these patients. Using the Institute's mortality experience between 1987 and 2002 as a basis for projecting expected mortality yields the data shown in Figure 3.19, which depicts the age and burn size distribution of the expected deaths.

According to this model, patients over 50 years of age with burns of 50% or less of the total body surface account for 19% of admissions and 50% of deaths; at the other age extreme, children under 5 account for 19% of admissions but only 12.5% of deaths.

Much has been accomplished in acute burn care during the last half century, and further improvement in outcome will probably occur as inhalation injury and pneumonia come under better control and new wound coverage techniques are developed, but such improvement will be harder won and smaller in magnitude. Preservation of function, reconstruction, and rehabilitation, areas which have received less attention in the past, appear the more likely primary targets of future burn research and may be expected to materially enhance the quality of life for burn survivors.

References

1. Vyrostek SB, Annest JL, Ryan GW. Surveillance for fatal and non-fatal injuries – United States, 2001. Office of Statistics and Programming. National Center for Injury Prevention and Control. 1600 Clifton Road N.E., MS K-59 Atlanta, GA. 30333, CDC/NCIPC/OSP; 2001.
2. Finkelstein EA, Corso PS, Miller TR, et al. The incidence and economic burden of injuries in the United States. New York, NY: Oxford University; 2006:9–169.
3. WISQARS. Injury mortality report. United States fire/burn deaths and rates per 100 000. All races, both sexes, all ages. Atlanta, GA. Centers for Disease Control and Prevention; 2003.
4. National Burn Repository. 2005 report. Data set version 2.0. Chicago: American Burn Association; 2006:35.
5. Baker SP, O'Neill B, Ginsberg NJ, et al. Fire, burns and lightning. The injury fact book, 2nd edn. New York: Oxford University; 1992:161–173.
6. Centers for Disease Control and Prevention (CDC). Deaths resulting from residential fires and the prevalence of smoke alarms — United States, 1991–1995. MMWR 1996; 47:803–806.
7. Hall JR. The US fire problem and overview report. Leading causes and other patterns and trends. Quincy, Massachusetts: National Fire Protection Association, Fire Analysis and Research Division; 1998.
8. Feck GA, Baptiste MS, Tate CL Jr. Burn injuries: epidemiology and prevention. Accid Anal Prev 1979; 11:129–136.
9. Feck GA, Baptiste MS, Tate CL Jr. An epidemiologic study of burn injuries and strategies for prevention. Atlanta, GA: Department of Health and Human Services, Public Health Services, Centers for Disease Control; 1978.
10. Baker SP, O'Neill B, Ginsberg NJ, et al. Unintentional injury. The injury fact book, 2nd edn. New York: Oxford University; 1992:39–64.
11. Runyan CW, Bangdiwala SI, Linzer MA, et al. Risk factors for fatal residential fires. N Engl J Med 1992; 327:859–863.
12. Fire in the United States, 1983 to 1990, 8th edn. Emmitsburg, MD: National Fire Data Center; October 1993.
13. Burn, injury fact sheet. 1301 Pennsylvania Avenue NW, Suite 1000, Washington DC 20004–1707: National Safe Kids Campaign. December 1998.
14. US DoH. Injury Mortality: National Summary of Injury Mortality Data. 1984–1990. Washington, DC, US: Department of Health and Human Services; June 1993.
15. Mierley MC, Baker SP. Fatal house fires in an urban population. JAMA 1983; 249:1466–1468.
16. Ahrens M. US experience with smoke detectors and other fire detectors. Quincy Massachusetts: National Fire Protection Association, Fire Analysis and Research Division; 1997.
17. Marshall S, Runyan CW, Bangdiwala SI, et al. Fatal residential fires: who dies and who survives. JAMA 1998; 279:1633–1637.
18. Ballesteros MF, Jackson ML, Martin MW. Working toward the elimination of residential fire deaths: the Centers for Disease Control and Prevention's Smoke Alarm Installation and Fire Safety Education (SAIFE) program. J Burn Care Rehabil 2005; 26:434–439.
19. Karter MJ Jr. Fire loss in the United States during 1995. Quincy Massachusetts: National Fire Protection Association, Fire Analysis and Research Division, 1996.
20. Burns causes and costs: a Burn Foundation report. Philadelphia, PA: Burn Foundation; 1989.

21. Forjuoh SN. The mechanisms, intensity of treatment, and outcomes of hospitalized burns: issues for prevention. J Burn Care Rehabil 1988; 19:456–460.

22. Rice DP, MacKenzie EJ, et al. Cost of injury in the United States: a report to Congress. University of California, San Francisco, CA, An Injury Prevention Center, The Johns Hopkins University: Institute for Health and Aging; 1989.

23. Hall JR. The Total Cost of Fire in the United States through 1991. Quincy, MA: National Fire Protection Association 1993; 1–20.

24. Hammond J. The status of statewide burn prevention legislation. J Burn Care Rehabil 1993; 14:473–475.

25. Pruitt BA Jr, Goodwin CW. Thermal injuries. In: Davis JH, Sheldon GF, eds. Surgery: a problem-solving approach, 2nd edn. St Louis: Mosby; 1995:644.

26. Brigham PA, McLoughlin E. Burn incidence and medical care use in the United States: estimate, trends, and data sources. J Burn Care Rehabil 1996; 17:95–107.

27. Pruitt BA Jr, Mason AD Jr, Goodwin CW. Epidemiology of burn injury and demography of burn care facilities. In: Gann DS, ed. Problems in general surgery. Philadelphia: JB Lippincott, 1990; 7(2):235–251.

28. Initial Assessment and Management, Chapter 1. In: Advanced Burn Life Support Course. American Burn Association. Chicago, IL 2004:22.

29. Jordan MH, Hollowed KA, Turner DG, et al. The Pentagon attack of September 11, 2001: a burn center's experience. J Burn Care Rehabil 2005; 26:109–116.

30. Henson DA, Rode H, Bloch CE. Primus stove burns in Cape Town: a costly but preventable injury. Burns 1988; 20:251–252.

31. Rioja LF, Alonso PE, Soria MD, et al. Incidence of ember burns in Andalusia (Spain). Burns 1988; 20:251–252.

32. Iregbulem LM, Nnabuko BE. Epidemiology of childhood thermal burns in Enugu, Nigeria. Burns 1993; 19:223–226.

33. Shergill G, Scerri GV, Regan PJ, et al. Burn injuries in boating accidents. Burns 1993; 19:229–231.

34. Graitcer PL, Sniezek JE. Hospitalizations due to tap water scalds 1978–1985. MMWR 1988; 37:35–38.

35. Milo Y, Robinpour M, Glicksman A, et al. Epidemiology of burns in the Tel Aviv area. Burns 1993; 19:352–357.

36. Burd A, Yuen C. A global study of hospitalized pediatric burn patients. Burns 2005; 31:432–438.

37. Barillo DJ, Burge TS, Harrington DT, et al. Body habitus as a predictor of burn risk in children: do fat boys still get burned. Burns 1998; 24:725–727.

38. Baptiste MS, Feck G. Preventing tap water burns. Am J Public Health 1980; 70:727–729.

39. Stephen FR, Murray JP. Prevention of hot tap water burns — a comparative study of three types of automatic mixing valve. Burns 1993; 19:56–62.

40. Lindblad BE, Mikkelsen SS, Larsen TK, Steinke MS. A comparative analysis of burn injuries at two burns centers in Denmark. Burns 1994; 20:173–175.

41. Han T, Han K, Kim J, et al. Pediatric hand injury induced by treadmill. Burns 2005; 31:906–909.

42. McGill V, Kowal-Vern A, Gamelli RH. Outcome for older burn patients. Arch Surg 2000; 135:320–325.

43. Cadier MA, Shakespeare PG. Burns in octogenarians. Burns 1995; 21:200–204.

44. Backstein R, Peters W, Neligan P. Burns in the disabled. Burns 1993; 19:192–197.

45. Alden NE, Rabbitts A, Yurt RW. Burn injury in patients with dementia: an impetus for prevention. J Burn Care Rehabil 2005; 26:267–271.

46. Effects on personnel. In: Glasstone S, ed. The effects of nuclear weapons. Department of the Army Pamphlet. No. 39–3. United States Atomic Energy Commission, June 1957; Ch. XI, 455–464.

47. Burns sustained in Vietnam, 1965–1973. Data tables supplied by Department of the Army. Washington, DC: The Chief of Military History and the Center of Military History 20314; 1980.

48. Allen BD, Whitson TC, Henjyoji EY. Treatment of 1963 burned patients at 106th General Hospital, Yokohama, Japan. J Trauma 1970; 10:386–392.

49. Shafir R. Burn injury and care in the recent Lebanese conflict. Presentation on behalf of The Surgeon General, Israeli Defense Forces and Staff. The Israeli Society of Plastic and Reconstructive Surgery; 1984.

50. Owen-Smith MS. Armoured fighting vehicle casualties. J Royal Army Med Corps 1977; 123:65–76.

51. Chapman CW. Burns and plastic surgery in the South Atlantic campaign 1982. J Royal Navy Med Serv 1983; 69(2):71–79.

52. Eldad A, Torem M. Burns in the Lebanon War 1982: 'the Blow and the Cure.' Military Medicine 1990; 155:130–132.

53. Carlos Sereday MD, Major, Argentine Navy Medical Corps. Personal communication, 1990.

54. Cancio LC, Horvath EE, Barillo DJ, et al. Burn support for operation Iraqi freedom and related operations, 2003–2004. J Burn Care Rehabil 2005; 26:151–161.

55. Kopchinski B. US Army noncombat munitions injuries. Military Medicine 2001; 166:135–138.

56. Hankins CL, Tang XQ, Phipps A. Hot beverage burns: an eleven-year experience of the Yorkshire Regional Burns Centre. Burns 2006; 32:87–91.

57. Hankins CL, Tang XQ, Phipps A. Hot oil burns – a study of predisposing factors, clinical course and prevention strategies. Burns 2006; 32:92–96.

58. Klein MB, Gibran NS, Emerson D, et al. Patterns of grease burn injury: development of a classification system. Burns 2005; 31:765–767.

59. Rossignol AM, Boyle CM, Locke JA, et al. Hospitalized burn injuries in Massachusetts: an assessment of incidence and product involvement. Am J Public Health 1986; 76:1341–1343.

60. Clark WR, Fromm BS. Burn mortality experienced at a regional unit. Literature review. Acta Chir Scand 1987; Suppl 357.

61. Baker SP, O'Neill B, Karpf RS. The injury fact book. Lexington, MA: Lexington Books; 1984:139–154.

62. Barillo DJ, Stetz CK, Zak AL, et al. Preventable burns associated with a misuse of gasoline. Burns 1998; 24:439–443.

63. Purdue GF, Hunt JL, Layton TR, et al. Burns in motor vehicle accidents. J Trauma 1985; 25:216–219.

64. Barillo DJ, Cioffi WG, McManus WF, et al. Vehicle-related burn injuries. Proceedings of Association for the Advancement of Automotive Medicine, 2340 Des Plaines Avenue, Suite 106, Des Plaines 1993; 11:209–218.

65. Matzavakis I, Frangakis ZE, Charalampopolulou A, et al. Burn injuries related to motorcycle exhaust pipes: a study in Greece. Burns 2005; 31:372–374.

66. Renz BM, Sherman R. Automobile carburetors- and radiator-related burns. J Burn Care Rehabil 1992; 1:414–421.

67. Regan PJ, Budny PG, Lavelle JR, et al. Bonfire and barbecue burns. Burns 1991; 17:306–308.

68. 8th Annual Flammable Fabrics Report. Washington, DC: Consumer Product Safety Commission; 1980.

69. Occupational burns among restaurant workers — Colorado and Minnesota. MMWR 1993; 42:713–716.

70. Chatterjee BF, Barancik JI, Fratianne RB, et al. Northeastern Ohio trauma study V: burn injury. J Trauma 1986; 26:844–847.

71. Rossignol AM, Locke JA, Boyle CM, et al. Epidemiology of work-related burn injuries in Massachusetts requiring hospitalization. J Trauma 1986; 26:1097–1101.

72. Personck ME. Profiles in safety and health: eating and drinking places. Monthly Labor Review 1991; 114:19–26.

73. Baker SP, O'Neill B, Ginsberg NJ, et al. Occupational injury. The injury fact book, 2nd edn. New York: Oxford University; 1992:114–133.

74. Horwitz IB, McCall BP. An analysis of occupational burn injuries in Rhode Island: workers compensation claims, 1998–2002. J Burn Care Rehabil 2005; 26:505–514.

75. Pruitt BA Jr, Edlich RF. Treatment of bitumen burns [Letter]. JAMA 1982; 247:1565.

76. Renz BM, Sherman R. Hot tar burns: 27 hospitalized cases. J Burn Care Rehabil 1994; 15:341–345.

77. Acute chemical hazards to children and adults. NEISS data highlights. Washington, DC: Directorate for Epidemiology, US Consumer Product Safety Commission; Vol. 12 January–December 1988.

78. Mozingo DW, Smith AA, McManus WF, et al. Chemical burns. J Trauma 1988; 28:642–647.

79. Leeming MN, Ray C Jr, Howland WS. Low-voltage direct current burns. JAMA 1970; 214:1681–1684.

80. Pride HB, McKinley DF. Third-degree burns from the use of an external cardiac pacing device. Crit Care Med 1990; 18:572–573.

81. Reisin L, Baruchin AM. Iatrogenic defibrillator burns. Burns 1990; 16:128.

82. Arnoldo BD, Purdue GF, Kowalske K, et al. Electrical injuries: a 20-year review. J Burn Care Rehabil 2004; 25:479–484.

83. Cancio LC, Jimenez Reyna JF, Barillo DJ, et al. One hundred ninety five cases of high-voltage electric injury. J Burn Care Rehabil 2005; 26:331–340.

84. Lightning-associated deaths – United States 1980–1995. MMWR 1998; 47:391–394.

85. Lopez RE, Holle RL. Demographics of lightning casualties. Semin Neurol 1995; 15:286–295.

86. Lightning-associated injuries and deaths among military personnel – United States, 1998–2001. MMWR 2002; 51:859–862.

87. Kale D, Harwood B. Fireworks injuries, 1981. Washington, DC: Directorate for Epidemiology, US Consumer Products Safety Commission. NEISS Data Highlights January–December 1981.

88. McFarland LV, Harris JR, Kobayashi JM, et al. Risk factors for fireworks-related injury in Washington state. JAMA 1984; 251:3251–3254.

89. Injuries associated with selected consumer products treated in hospital emergency departments calendar 1992. Washington, DC: Directorate for Epidemiology, US Consumer Products Safety Commission. NEISS Data Highlights Vol. 16, 1992.

90. Berger LR, Kalishman S, Rivara FP. Injuries from fireworks. Pediatrics 1985; 75:877–882.

91. Karamanoukian RL, Kilani M, Lozano D, et al. Pediatric burns with snap-cap fireworks. J Burn Care Rehabil 2006; 27:218–220.

92. Sonneborn CK, Vanstraelen TM. A retrospective study of self-inflicted burns. Gen Hosp Psychiatry 1992; 14:404–407.

93. Horner BM, Ahmadi H, Mulholland R, et al. Case-controlled studies of patients with self-inflicted burns. Burns 2005; 31:471–475.

94. Budny PG, Regan PJ, Riley P, et al. Ritual burns – the Buddhist tradition. Burns 1991; 17:335–337.

95. Squyres V, Law EJ, Still JM Jr. Self-inflicted burns. J Burn Care Rehabil 1993; 14:476–479.

96. Duminy FJ, Hudson DA. Assault inflicted by water. Burns 1993; 19:426–428.

97. Krob MJ, Johnson A, Jordan MH. Burned-and-battered adults. J Burn Care Rehabil 1986; 7:529–531.

98. Bowden ML, Grant ST, Vogel B, et al. The elderly, disabled and handicapped adult burned through abuse and neglect. Burns 1988; 14:447–450.

99. O'Neill JA Jr, Meacham WF, Griffin PP, et al. Patterns of injury in the battered child syndrome. J Trauma 1973; 13:332–339.

100. Showers J, Garrison KM. Burn abuse: a four-year study. J Trauma 1988; 28:1581–1583.

101. Surrell JA, Alexander RM, Kohle SD, et al. Effects of microwave radiation on living tissues. J Trauma 1987; 27:935–939.

102. Batchelor JS, Vanjari S, Budny P, et al. Domestic iron burns in children: a cause for concern? Burns 1994; 20:74–75.

103. Purdue GF, Hunt JL, Prescott PR. Child abuse by burning — an index of suspicion. J Trauma 1988; 28:221–224.

104. Chester DL, Jose RM, Adlayami E, et al. Non-accidental burns in children — are we neglecting neglect? Burns 2006; 32:222–228.

105. Elder abuse: what can be done? Select Committee on Aging, US House of Representatives, Washington, DC: Government Printing Office; 1991.

106. Bird PE, Harrington DT, Barillo DJ, et al. Elder abuse: a call to action. J Burn Care Rehabil 1998; 19:522–527.

107. Pegg SP. Can burns injuries occur in hospital? Abstract 87 in 9th Congress of International Society for Burns Injuries, Abstracts Volume. Presented at 9th Congress of the International Society for Burn Injuries, 30 June 1994, Paris, France.

108. Sadove RC, Furgasen TG. Major thermal burn as a result of intra-operative heating blanket use. J Burn Care Rehabil 1992; 13:443–445.

109. Gul A, O'Sullivan ST. Iatrogenic burns caused by infrared lamp after traditional acupuncture. Burns 2005; 31:1061–1062

110. Chang BW, Petty P, Manson PN. Patient fire safety in the operating room. Plast Reconstr Surg 1994; 93:519–521.

111. Leon-Villapalos J, Kaniorou-Larai M, Dziewulski P. Full thickness abdominal burn following magnetic resonance-guided focused ultrasound therapy. Burns 2005; 31:1054–1055.

112. Barillo DJ, Coffey EC, Shirani KZ, et al. Burns caused by medical therapy. J Burn Care Rehabil 2000; 21:269–273.

113. Pruitt BA Jr, FitzGerald BE. A military perspective. In: Bowers JZ, Purcell EF, eds. Emergency medical services: measures to improve care. Port Washington, NY: Independent Publishers Group; 1980:223–244.

114. Treat RC, Sirinek KR, Levine BE, et al. Air evacuation of thermally injured patients: principles of treatment and results. J Trauma 1980; 20:275–279.

115. Yurt RW, Bessey PQ, Bauer GJ, et al. A regional burn center's response to a disaster: September 11, 2001, and the days beyond. J Burn Care Rehabil 2005; 26:117–124.

116. Kennedy PJ, Haertsch PA, Maitz PK. The Bali burn disaster: implications and lessons learned. J Burn Care Rehabil 2005; 26:125–131.

117. Mozingo DW, Barillo DJ, Holcomb JB. The Pope Air Force Base aircraft crash and burn disaster. J Burn Care Rehabil 2005; 26:132–140.

118. Harrington DT, Biffl WL, Cioffi WG. The station nightclub fire. J Burn Care Rehabil 2005; 26:141–143.

119. Cairns BA, Stiffler A, Price F, et al. Managing a combined burn trauma disaster in the post-nine/eleven world: lessons learned from the 2003 West Pharmaceutical Plant explosion. J Burn Care Rehabil 2005; 26:144–150.

120. Holmes T, ed. A system of surgery, theoretical and practical. London: J W Parker; 1860:Vol. I, 723.

121. Suzuki S. The injuries in modern naval warfare. Boston Med Surg J CXXXVII(24): 610, December 9, 1897.

122. Weidenfeld LB. Medizinisches Vademecus 1912:206–224.

123. Berkow SG. Method of estimating extensiveness of lesions (burns and scalds) based on surface area proportions. Arch Surg 1924; 8(pt. 1):138–148.

124. Bull JP, Squire JR. A study of mortality in a burns unit: standards for the evaluation of alternative methods of treatment. Ann Surg 1949; 130(2):160–173.

125. Bull JP, Fisher AJ. A study of mortality in a burns unit: a revised estimate. Ann Surg 1954; 139(3):269–274.

126. Schwartz MS, Soroff HS, Reiss E, et al. An evaluation of the mortality and the relative severity of second- and third-degree injuries in burns. Research Report Nr 12–56. In: Research Reports. US Army Surgical Research Unit, Form Sam Houston, TX, December 1956.

127. SPSS for windows, ver.9.0. Chicago, IL: SPSS.

128. Finney DJ. Probit analysis, 3rd edn. Cambridge: Cambridge University; 1971.

129. Hosmer DW, Lemeshow S. Applied logistic regression. New York: John Wiley; 1989.

130. Moreau AR, Westfall PH, Cancio LC, et al. Development and validation of an age-risk score for mortality prediction after thermal injury. J Trauma 2005; 58(5):967–972.

Chapter 4

Prevention of burn injuries

John L. Hunt, Brett D. Arnoldo, and Gary F. Purdue

Chapter contents

Introduction

The word 'prevent' comes from the Latin word 'praevenire,' which means to anticipate. The prefix 'pre' means before and 'venire' means to come. During the last century in the United States, burn treatment had always come before burn prevention. Since burns then as now, represent such a small percent of all traumatic injuries, burn prevention has not been viewed as a high priority heath issue by a large portion of society.

Burns are still referred to as accidents by many in the medical community and society in general.[1] Believing that burns and other traumatic injuries are 'accidents' ('accident-prone' individual) implies the individual has little or no fault in the injury cause. The word 'accident' means an event that takes place without one's foresight or proceeds from an unknown cause, an unfortunate occurrence, or mishap, especially one resulting in an injury. Synonyms include misadventure, mischance, misfortune, mishap, and disaster. The word 'injury' is a more appropriate term. It is derived from the Latin word 'juris' which means not right. An injury represents damage that occurs as a result of an exposure to a physical or chemical agent at a rate greater than what the body can tolerate. Unfortunately the designation of traumatic injuries as accidents is still perpetrated in the E codes which are the supplementary classification of external causes of injury. An example is E893, Accident caused by ignition of clothing, or E898.1, Accident caused by other, burning by: candle, cigar, pipe or cigarette.

Historical perspective

The medical community in Great Britain in the first decade of the 20th century was well aware that burn injuries and deaths represented a serious public health issue.[2] Scalds and burns were noted to occur predominately in children. Unguarded fires and the flammability of flannelette, a cotton garment, were recognized as common causes of burns in children and old women. Legislation was enacted making parents liable to a fine if a child younger than 8 years was injured or died as a result of an unguarded open fire. In a review of over 3600 patients with flame burns and scalds, two-thirds occurred in and around the home, one-third were at work, 50% were children, 82% were the result of clothing fires, cottons were the common fabrics and the number of scalds about equaled that from burns, but the former were more likely to survive.[3] Approximately 50% of home accidents were judged to be preventable. Research was conducted on the design and flammability of clothing. Fabrics were treated with tin, antimony, and titanium to make them relatively flame-retardant. Statistics on common locations and causes for home 'accidents' identified the kitchen and cooking, scald burns from children pulling over containers with hot liquids, and the use of flammable liquids. Burns as a result of a seizure were recognized. Prevention efforts included education and 'propaganda' (film, radio, newspapers, exhibits, and posters), better design of housing and improving living conditions (decreasing overcrowding), safer methods of heating houses (central heating and electric fires), use of non-flammable materials in girls and women clothing, and better design of fireguards for coal fires. Better design of teapots, cups, and cooking utensils rendered them more difficult to tilt over. One author in 1946 expressed quite clearly that carelessness, neglect of normal precautions, and stupidity were human factors associated with burns.[4] It was recognized that accurate and comprehensive burn data were lacking, but necessary if long-term prevention policies were to be enacted.

Injury control

The five key areas in injury control are:
1. epidemiology,
2. prevention,
3. injury biomechanics (physical and functional responses of the victim to the energy),
4. treatment,
5. rehabilitation.[5]

The major components of epidemiology include measurement of both the frequency and distribution of the injury. This in turn is analyzed and interpreted. Next, risk factors are identified, an intervention strategy is developed and tested, and, lastly, the results analyzed.

Burn injury magnitude

The first step in any prevention program is to identify the how, who, where, and when of the injury. With this information strategic planning and implementation can be directed at reducing the risk of injury or death. In the US in 1995 the leading causes of injury deaths in their order of magnitude were motor vehicle, firearm, poisoning, fall, suffocation, drowning, and finally fire/burn.[6] In 2003 fire/burns still ranked 6th behind motor vehicle, falls, poisoning, choking, and drowning as leading causes of unintentional injury deaths.[7] Fires, flames, and smoke were the 5th leading causes of fatal injury in the home. In 1996 the number of fire deaths and injuries were 4990 and 25550 respectively. On average in the United States in 2003, a fire death occurred about every 2 hours, and someone was injured every 29 minutes.[8] Smoke inhalation accounted for the majority of fatalities in home fires. In 2001 there were 3423 and 498507 fire deaths and injuries respectively in the US.[9] This represented 3.4% and 1.8% of all fatal and non-fatal injuries reported. The rate of fatal and non-fatal fire injuries was 1.2 and 178 per 100000 populations. In 2002 there were 3363 deaths, a decrease of less than 2%. The number of fire deaths increased progressively with age and peaked at 720 over 75. The number of non-fatal injuries (almost 79000) was greatest between ages 35 to 44. Males were 1.6 times more likely to die in a fire. Populations in the lowest income levels had a greater risk of dying in a fire than people in higher income brackets. Eighty-six percent of fatalities involved a single fatality, 10% two fatalities and 4% greater than two. Seventy-four percent of fatal fires occurred in any type of structure, and 94% in residential structures or cars. The leading causes of fatal fires in residential property were incendiary/suspicious 27%, smoking 18%, and open flame 16%. The leading areas of fire origin in fatal residential structures were sleeping areas 29%, lounge 21%, and kitchen 15%. Fatal fires were more common in the winter. The time of day when most structure fires occurred was between 10 a.m. and 8 p.m.

It is well recognized that many burns treated in emergency departments are never admitted to the hospital. The National Hospital Ambulatory Medical Survey identified 516 victims of fire, flame or hot substances per 100000 emergency room visits in 2003.[10] While most of these were not life-threatening, nonetheless most were probably preventable. Unfortunately most prevention efforts are not directed at these victims. This group is worthy of future prevention efforts.

Risk factors

A number of factors must be considered when determining the fire risk to the host. Age, location, demographics, and low economic status represent important factors. The US Fire Administration expresses much of its fire data as relative risk (RR).[9] A common way to express fire deaths across different populations is to determine the RR of dying or being injured. The RR of a group (say death) is calculated by comparing its rate to the rate of the overall population. A RR of 1 is given to the general population. As a general rule of thumb, many statisticians consider a relative risk of 4 or more as important. If an RR of 4 or greater is used to identify high-risk burn populations, then based on 2001 data, prevention programs should have been directed at everyone over 85 years (RR 4.6), African-Americans (RR 6.9), and American-Indian males (RR 5.3). The RR of fire deaths in 2001 for all ages, with the exception of 0–4 years and over age 55, was less than 1. The use of RR in injury prevention may well be important when resources are limited.

In 2001 for ages 0–14 there were 599 fire deaths and 2926 fire injuries: 53.4% and 48.5% of deaths and injuries occurred in children less than 5 years. The RR of fire death for children less than 5 years was 1.2, 0.6 for ages 5 to 9, and 0.3 for 10 to 14 years.[9] The activities of children at the time of a fire injury were asleep (55%), trying to escape (26%), and unable to act, implying not understanding what was happening or how to take action (9%).

Analysis of fatal pediatric (less than 15 years) fires in Philadelphia, age of housing, income, single-parent households, and the number of children under age 15 were significant independent variables.[11] Of note the risk was greatest between 12:00 a.m. and 6:00 a.m. The common causes were playing with matches, smoking, and incendiary. The common locations were bedroom and living room. Upholstered furniture, cooking materials, bedding, mattresses, clothing, and curtains were primary materials first ignited in fatal fires. Playing with cigarette lighters, candles or near stoves with hot liquids were frequent scenarios in fatal pediatric burns. The authors stressed that identification of risk factors by analyzing population characteristics by census tract was important for burn prevention.

The 50 and older population from 2000–2050 will grow at a rate 68 times faster than the rate of growth for the total population. The number of people 65 and over is projected to rise from 13% of the total population in 2010 to nearly 20% in 2030. The elderly (over 64 years) obviously represent a high-risk group. In 2001 more than 30% of all fire deaths were in this group.[12] Their risk of dying in a fire was 2.5 times greater than the general population. The leading causes of both fire death and injuries were smoking and cooking. Additional risks included medical conditions associated with physical or mental illness – arthritis and stroke, i.e. the victim is slow or unable to escape the burn event, poor eyesight and hearing, systemic diseases such as diabetes (peripheral neuropathy with decreased or no lower extremity pain perception), Alzheimer's disease (confusion, forgetfulness), psychiatric illness (depression and suicide). Other risk factors in teenagers and adults are alcohol, and medications such as sleeping pills, tranquilizers, narcotics, and synthetic stimulant drugs such as methamphetamines.

Burn prevention involves more than just the burn community. Fire safety engineers and legislators (building code laws) and building inspectors have a vested interest in prevention. An important aspect of fire prevention is the design of fire safe buildings.[13] To do this both fire and personal characteristics associated with the greatest risks must be identified. These included the ignition factor (misuse of ignited material by children), type of material ignited (sofas, chairs, and bedding) and form of heat of ignition (electrical equipment, matches, lighters, cigarettes); personal factors were condition preventing escape, condition before injury, activity at time of injury, and location of ignition (in room of fire origin, and floor of fire origin).

Burn prevention is a worldwide problem. The United States has one of the highest fire death rates among industrialized countries. It is important to recognize worldwide prevention efforts.[14,15] The World Health Organization (WHO) reported that globally burns accounted for 238 000 deaths in 2000. Burns ranked among the 15 leading causes of death in children and young adults (5–29 years). Obviously these figures are suspect, and intuitively appear under-representations. Risk factors included cooking at floor level, open kerosene stoves, high population density, poor house construction, illiteracy, and local cultural practices (homicide by burning). Prevention programs proposed by WHO include raising or enclosing cooking areas, electrification to reduce dependency on candles and kerosene, safe stove design, improved house construction, and obviously installation of smoke detectors.

Injury prevention comes of age

The science of injury prevention took form in the middle of the last century. The energy sources involved in any injury event are classified into five physical agents: kinetic or mechanical, chemical, thermal, electrical, and radiation.[16] A common form of mechanical energy associated with a burn is a motor vehicle collision. Three risk factors associated with any injury are:
1. the vector or energy source and the way it is delivered,
2. the host or injured person, and
3. the environment, both physical and social.

A seminal article in modern injury science was published by Haddon in 1968.[17] He identified three phases of an injury event:
1. Pre-event: preventing the causative agent from reaching the susceptible host.
2. Event: includes transfer of the energy to the victim. Prevention efforts in this phase operate to reduce or completely prevent the injury.
3. Post-event: determines the outcome once the injury has occurred. This includes anything that limits ongoing damage or repairs the damage. This phase determines the ultimate outcome.

Haddon then created a matrix of nine cells which enabled the three events of the injury to be analyzed against the factors related to the host, agent or vector and environment[18] (Table 4.1). This matrix is a very useful tool for analyzing an injury-producing event and recognizing the factor(s) important in its prevention. Haddon also proposed 10 general strategies for injury control (Table 4.2). Risk factors and potential intervention strategies can be identified.

Burn intervention strategy

The emergence of the science of prevention has turned attention away from individual 'blame' and the attitude that society

TABLE 4.1 THE HADDON MATRIX FOR BURN CONTROL

	Agent or vector	Host	Environment	
			Physical	Social
Pre-event	Fire-safe cigarette	Control seizure	Non-slip tub surface	Legislation – factory preset water heater thermostats
Event	Sprinklers, smoke detectors	Flame-retardant cloths	Fire escapes	Fire drill education
Post-event	Water	First aid antibiotics	EMS	Emergency and rehabilitation services

Matrix adapted from Haddon W, Advances in the epidemiology of injuries as a basis for public policy. Public Health Reports 1980; 95:411–421.[18]

TABLE 4.2 GENERAL STRATEGIES FOR BURN CONTROL

Prevent creation of the hazard (stop producing fire crackers)

Reduce amount of hazard (decrease chemical concentration in commercial products)

Prevent release of the hazard (child-resistant butane lighters)

Modify rate or spatial distribution of the hazard (vapor-ignition resistant water heaters)

Separate release of the hazard in time or space (small spouts for hot water faucet)

Place barrier between the hazard and the host (install fence around electrical transformers, fire screen)

Modify nature of the hazard (use low conductors of heat)

Increase resistance of host to hazard (treat seizure disorder)

Begin to counter damage already done by hazard (first aid, rapid transport and resuscitation)

Stabilization, repair rehabilitation of host, example (provide acute care — burn center and rehabilitation)

General Strategies for Burn Control from Haddon W, Advances in the Epidemiology of Injuries as a Basis for Public Policy. Public Health Reports 1980; 95:411–421.[18]

has no part in the promotion of prevention to the concept that sociopolitical involvement is necessary.[19]

All burn injuries should be viewed as preventable. Public health is defined as the effort organized by society to protect, promote, and restore the people's health.[20] The public health model of injury prevention and control is divided into:

- surveillance,
- interdisciplinary education and prevention programs,
- environmental modifications,
- regulatory action, and
- support of clinical interventions.

Primary prevention is preventing the event from ever occurring. Secondary prevention includes the acute care, rehabilitation, and reducing the degree of disability or impairment as much as possible. Tertiary prevention concentrates on preventing or decreasing disability. Disability prevalence and productive activity loss are important outcome measures. There are both active and passive prevention strategies. Passive or environmental intervention is automatic; little to no cooperation or action is required by the host. This is the most effective prevention strategy. Examples include building codes requiring smoke alarms, sprinkler installation, and factory adjusted water heater temperature. Active prevention measures are voluntary, emphasize education to encourage people to change their unsafe behavior, and require repetitive educational measures to maintain individual action. Herein lays its weakness. Project Burn Prevention was a program funded by the Consumer Product Safety Commission (CPSC) in 1975.[21] It was undertaken to determine if a burn prevention program would decrease burn deaths by utilizing an educational program and media messages involving a large population base. The author concluded that there was no reduction of burn incidence or severity in their study with either the school education program or media campaign. Education to bring about and maintain personal responsibility was not sufficient. Active prevention is the least effective and most difficult strategy to maintain, especially over a long period. Examples are a home fire drill plan, and wearing goggles and gloves when handling toxic chemicals. Passive strategies are not always successful; a water heater thermostat may be raised by a homeowner and a sprinkler system or smoke alarm must be maintained. Once surveillance data have been established and collected, then prioritizing high-risk burn groups is necessary in order to identify intervention strategies.

The Four Es of Intervention comprise Engineering, Economic, Enforcement, and Education.[22]

- Engineering — focuses on the physical environment (product safety design) and the vector. Examples include fire-resistant upholstery and bedding, child-resistant multi-purpose lighters (including cigarette), and insulated electric wire.
- Economic — influences behavior, i.e. monetary incentives such as insurance rate reduction if a home has smoke alarms or sprinklers.
- Enforcement — influences behavior with laws, building codes, and regulations. Requiring fire escapes, sprinklers/smoke alarms in motels, hotels, and homes.
- Education — influences behavior through knowledge and reasoning. Examples include pamphlets, public

television programs, CPSC News Alerts. These active measures are the least effective.

In any prevention program the results must be evaluated.[23] If a prevention program does not achieve the stated goal(s) possible reasons include:

- the technique or measurement used may be inappropriate to identify the reduction caused by the prevention strategy;
- faulty program design;
- study design may have been good, but the program was carried out inappropriately.

With this background in epidemiology and prevention of injuries, important areas of challenge and opportunity in burn prevention both past, present, and future will be discussed.[24,25]

Flammable clothing

In the decade of the 1940s, publicity surrounding children sustaining burns to their legs as a result of the ignition of Gene Audry cowboy suits or 'chaps' (made of highly flammable-brushed rayon) awoke both the medical and lay community in the US to the dangers of flammable clothing.[26] This was soon reinforced when burns resulting from 'torch sweaters' worn by girls began to suddenly appear. Extensive research was conducted to determine fabric flammability.[27,28] Wool burns very slowly and doesn't ignite. It melts with a red glow, retracts from the heat source, and finally extinguishes itself. On the other hand, cotton burns like a torch and is completely destroyed in a matter of seconds. Raised cut materials were known to be very flammable. While rayon ignites easily, it does not burn as intensely as cotton. A combination of cotton and wool burns less than either by itself. Silk produces a red glow but usually goes out quite quickly. Nylon simply melts but will cling to the underlying surface. Loose-fitting clothing, particularly if the individual is in an upright position and air currents are created by moving, tends to make the burn worse. A close nap or closely woven material is more flame retardant than loose weave textiles.

In 1953 legislation regulating the manufacture and sale of wearing apparel of highly flammable clothing (the Flammability Fabrics Act) was passed in the US. As a result of the act contracts were awarded to Burn Units to collect epidemiologic data regarding flammable fabric burns, flammability testing methods were improved and standardized, and flame-retardant fabrics were developed. The initial act covered only fabrics that came in contact with the body and therefore excluded industrial fabrics. The act was amended in 1967 to include articles of wearing apparel and interior furnishings such as paper, plastic, rubber, synthetic film, and synthetic foam. In the US the chemical agent tris was the common additive used to make flame-retardant clothing. Tris was banned in 1977 by the CPSC not because of the lack of scientific proof of its effectiveness but because a 'two-year feeding study' in rodents conducted by the National Cancer Institute revealed that the agent caused cancer.[29,30] Did tris and flame-retardant sleepwear result in a decline of clothing flame burns?[31] Analysis of 6000 burns admitted to 15 burn centers in the United States between 1965 and 1969 revealed that 86% of all flame burns involved fabrics.[32] In 1977 McLoughlin et al. reported a decrease in sleepwear burns at the Shriners Burns Institute in

Boston, MA.[33] It was recognized though that accurate national statistics to support their experience were lacking. Other explanations were proposed – the change in referral patterns of patients, improved public education on the hazards of sleepwear, behavior changes not directly related to the flammability of sleepwear, changes in clothing design, and finally that burn injuries were still occurring but were less severe. Clothing burns involve three factors – flammability, the behavior of the wearer, and the heat source.[34] During this same period, make-up of clothing changed. By 1985, 87% of children's sleepwear was made of synthetics and only about 13% of sleepwear was made of cotton. In 1996 sleepwear standards for children were amended by the CPSC. The amendments permitted the sale of tight-fitting children's sleepwear and sleepwear for infants aged 9 months or under, even if the garments do not meet the flammability standards ordinarily applicable to such sleepwear. This conclusion was based on staff findings that there were virtually no injuries associated with single-point ignition incidents of tight-fitting sleepwear, or of sleepwear worn by infants under 1 year. Sleepwear for children 9 months or younger and tight-fitting garments (up to size 14 and not exceeding specified measurements for specific areas of the body) could now be sold even though they don't meet the flammability standards ordinarily applied to such sleepwear. The commission emphasized that sleepwear standards were designed to protect children from burn injuries if they came in contact with an open flame such as match or stove. Flame-resistant or snug-fit clothing does not apply for sleepwear in sizes of 9 months and under because infants wearing these sizes are 'insufficiently mobile to expose themselves to sources of fire.'[35] What about the children that don't voluntarily expose themselves to an open flame? The safest sleepwear is a snug-fitting, flame-resistant garment. In 1999 a rash of clothing burns occurred in girls, ages 2½ to 11, wearing large loose-fitting cotton T-shirts as nightdresses. The victims had been either playing with either matches or a lighter.[36]

Snug-fitting cotton and flame-resistant garments are the safest choices for children's sleepwear. Loose-fitting clothes have a large airspace between the fabric and skin. The oxygen promotes the flame. In order to meet CPSC requirements, flame-resistant implies garments don't ignite easily and must self-extinguish quickly. Snug-fitting clothes that comply with CPSC guidelines are made of fabrics that aren't flame-resistant, but don't create 'an unreasonable' risk of burn injury because they limit the airspace under the garment. The CPSC requires all snug-fitting children's sleepwear from 9 months through size 14 to have a label that reads: 'Wear Snug-Fitting, Not Flame Resistant.' A hangtag reads 'For child's safety, garment should fit snugly. This garment is not flame resistant. A loose-fitting garment is more likely to catch fire.'

The reader is encouraged to read the excellent review of sleepwear flammability and legislation in both the US and the United Kingdom by Horrocks et al.[37] The CPSC is requesting of all burn units/centers to notify the National Burn Center Reporting System (NBCRS) any burn injury in children (15 years and younger) if the clothes they were wearing ignited, melted, or smoldered. The CPSC also wants the garment sent to them. There is no specific number of cases needed to reopen hearings by the CPSC to reconsider changing sleepwear standards.

Hot water burns

Unintentional injuries are the leading cause of deaths in children. While the majority of scald burns in children aren't fatal, the exact incidence is unknown. Heretofore there has not been accurate data available. But with the institution of the American Burn Association's National Burn Repository inpatient data regarding all aspects of burn injury will be available. Unfortunately many hot liquid burns are small and don't require hospital admission. All tap water scald burns should be preventable. In 1983 the Washington state legislature required all new home water heaters be preset to 49°C [120°F].[38] The time of exposure to this temperature is sufficiently long that the victim, usually a child or elderly disabled person, is able to be removed or can climb out of the water before a severe burn can occur. An educational program was instituted to inform people to voluntarily decrease the water temperature. Follow-up in 1988 revealed there had indeed been a reduction in hot water-caused pediatric burns. Voluntary reduction of thermostat temperatures to a safe level by manufacturers has not been uniformly successful. Mandatory regulations to lower water heater temperature would be the most effective strategy, but until society is educated and convinced of its benefit, change will be slow.[39,40] Other prevention methods to reduce tap water scald burns include inserting shut-off valves in the water circuit to detect temperatures over a certain level, and the use of liquid-crystal thermometers in bathtubs to alert the caregiver of the water temperature.[41,42] Unfortunately prevention of spill burns, which represent the largest percentage of pediatric burns, is more problematic. Most spill scald burns won't be prevented by adjusting hot water thermostats. Negligence on the part of the caregiver(s) is the key issue. Preventive measures must depend on education, but how successful will behavior modification be when people forget to keep hot liquids such as coffee, soup, tea, grease or electric cords attached to pots, or deep fryers out of the reach of children? Success can be achieved through a combination of education, legislation and/or litigation regarding product safety.[43–45] Examples include ovens with a door that can be opened and climbed on by a child and an oven that is not secured to the wall. The child's weight on an open door can tip the oven forward, spilling hot liquids. Numerous active scald prevention programs have been reported. The effectiveness of active prevention has been called into question regarding effectiveness.[46] Education campaigns directed at parents and burn safety to modify behavior have been shown effective over a short period of time only. Unfortunately weaknesses of many studies include short follow up, small sample size, and no controls. Identifying why specific prevention measures are unsuccessful is as important as why some are successful. Not all scald burns involve children. Product design and installation are important. Burns occurring during bathing as a result of seizures are not uncommon.[47] Avoidable risk factors identified were shower levers were easily knocked out of position, absence of water temperature safety features, and confining shower cubicle.

Fire-safe cigarettes

A cigarette when left unattended and not even puffed can burn as long as 20–40 minutes. In 1993 30–45% of residential fire deaths were caused by the careless use of cigarettes. In 1996 smoking was the cause in 4.8 % of the 191 729 residential fires, 10.6 % of all fire injuries, 17% of the deaths, and 4.1% of the $2.6 billion lost.[6] Statistics collected from 1986–1987 revealed that positive blood alcohol levels were 7.8 times more common in fire injuries than non-injuries. Consumption of 5 or more drinks per occasion was associated with an increased risk of a fire fatality. The odds ratio of a fire injury in a house where members collectively smoked from 1 to 9 cigarettes per day was 1.5 relative to households with no smokers, from 10–19 cigarettes per day the odds ratio was 6.6 and if greater than 20 cigarettes per day the odds ratio was 3.6. Their data revealed that smoking appeared to be the more important risk factor.

Although the number of adults smoking decreased by 8.6% from 1965 to 2002, residential smoking fires still represented a major cause of fire deaths and injuries.[48] Four percent of residential fires were caused by smoking in 2002, but smoking accounted for 19% of fire fatalities and 9% of fire injuries. Tobacco material was responsible for approximately 14 450 residential fires, 520 deaths, 1330 injuries, and $371 million in residential property damage. Smoking was associated with the highest number of deaths (25 per 1000 fires), and the next highest was children playing (14 per 1000 fires).

It is no surprise that most smoking fires started in the bedroom or living/family room areas of a house. The items first ignited were upholstered furniture, trash, mattress or pillow, and bedding. The time of day of residential smoking fire deaths and injuries were 2 a.m. and 6 a.m. and 12 p.m. to noon respectively. Falling asleep, alcohol, and substance abuse were common associated factors.[49] Smoke alarm performances in residential smoking fires revealed: alarm present and operated — 39%, present and not operating — 25%, no alarm present — 36%. Alarm performance in fatal fires was — 43%, 25%, 32%.

The concept of a fire-safe cigarette was explored in the early part of the 1920s. The first federal bill mandating fire-safe cigarettes was introduced in 1974. The legislation passed the Senate but failed in the House of Representatives.[50] For the most part the concept remained dormant until 1984 when the Cigarette Safety Act created a technical study group on cigarette and little cigar fire safety.[51] This group was to determine if a fire-safe cigarette could be made and would it be commercially feasible. A number of cigarette design changes have the potential to make cigarettes less fire-prone. These include reduced tobacco density, paper porosity, cigarette circumference, and addition of citrate.[52] Two important facts emerge regarding cigarette-related burns:

1. Burn data on non-fatal cigarette fire injuries are lacking on the national level.
2. Legal liability of tobacco companies might be the most effective means of decreasing both non-fatal and fatal burns associated with cigarettes.

Unfortunately litigation against tobacco manufactures has not been very common. On January 11, 2000 Philip Morris companies announced the development of a cigarette with ultra-thin concentric paper bands that are applied to the traditional paper. The bands are referred to as 'speed bumps' and cause the cigarette to self-extinguish if it is not smoked. This is because no oxygen gets to the burning ember. This technology was first reported more than a decade ago. The production of a safe cigarette should not be voluntary, but be required by law. The state of New York implemented legislation requiring all cigarettes sold in the state after June 28, 2004 have reduced ignition propensity (RIP).[53] The US government has not yet passed fire-safe cigarette legislation. Canada passed fire-safe cigarette legislation in 2004. It was the first country to do so. Everyone is encouraged to read the article titled 'How the tobacco industry continues to keep the home fires burning' by Andrew McGuire.[54]

Carbon monoxide poisoning

Carbon monoxide (CO) inhalation is the leading cause of fatal poisoning in the industrialized world.[55] Burn injuries and fatalities are often associated with CO intoxication. Whenever a carbon-based fuel, gas, oil, wood, or charcoal is burned carbon monoxide is produced. Obviously open flames are the most common source. These include charcoal grills, gas water heaters, stoves, and lanterns. Carbon monoxide generating appliances, such as space heaters, are often used during power outages. Their use may be weather related or because home heating is shut off for financial reasons – the latter often occurring in the low-income households. If the heating source is either used improperly or ventilation is inadequate or faulty, CO levels can become toxic. The number of deaths as a result of CO poisoning is unknown because many victims may not have blood levels drawn or death may be attributed to an associated burn. In a phone survey conducted in 1003 households in the US, 97% of responders had a smoke alarm, and only 29% had a CO detector.[56] Is price a factor in the low prevalence? The cost for a single unit can be as low as $10 and $75 for a combined smoke and CO detector. A CO alarm near all sleeping areas represents an effective prevention strategy. Should any home with a smoke detector have a CO detector? Based on the success of smoke alarms, the answer is yes. But future research is needed to answer conclusively a number of questions – are they necessary, what type of CO sensor, and what level of CO gas activates the alarm, specifically the level for both a caution and dangerous or hazardous level? It is important to remember the life span of carbon monoxide detectors varies from 2 to 5 years. In addition the 'test' feature on many detectors only checks the functioning of the alarm and not the status of the detector.

Smoke detectors/alarms

Without question the use of smoke alarms has had the greatest impact in decreasing fire deaths in this country. In 1966 the percent of residential fire deaths in homes with an operating smoke alarm was 13%, 11.5% deaths occurred in homes with a non-operating alarm, and 38.5% in houses without an alarm.[6] Smoke alarm performance was not much better in one- and two-family dwellings fire fatalities — 10% had operating alarms, alarms present but not operating 10%, and no alarm 42%. Socioeconomic factors associated with lack of functioning smoke detectors include living in a non-apartment dwelling, an annual income of less than $20 000, being unmarried, and living in a non-metropolitan area, and homes with children younger than age 5. Smoke detector ownership was most often associated with not living in public housing, higher education (completing high school), maternal age (not a teenager), practice fire drills, and larger homes.[57–59]

In 1985 McLoughlin published Smoke Detector Legislation.[60] Her conclusions were smoke detector installation in new houses *appears* to be effective when mandated by a building code. Malonee et al. in 1996 collected data on a smoke detector give-away program in Oklahoma City, OK.[61] The target area for intervention had the highest rate of injuries related to residential fires in the city. The number of injuries per 100 000 population was 4.2 times higher than the rest of the city. Ten thousand-one hundred smoke alarms were distributed to 9291 homes. Over the next 4 years the annualized injury rate per 100 000 population decreased by 80% in the target area, as compared to only 8% in the rest of the city. The authors concluded that target intervention with a smoke alarm give-away program reduced residential fire injuries. Smoke alarms represent intervention before the burn event occurs. Building codes mandating installation in new homes have been proven to be a practical solution. While 'retrofit' laws would appear to be unenforceable, yet the practical solution is to require installation when a house is sold or an apartment rented. Installation in existing homes represents the ultimate goal, but this won't be accomplished by legislation. Maintenance of alarms is just as difficult.

In 2000 DiGuiseppi and Higgins questioned the benefit of injury education to promote smoke alarm usage.[62] Twenty-six published trials, 13 randomized, were reviewed. The conclusion was 'counselling and educational interventions had only a modest effect on the likelihood of owning an alarm.' Programs that gave away and installed smoke alarms appeared to decrease fire injuries, but the trials were not conclusive and the results were to be interpreted with caution. DiGuiseppi et al. conducted a randomized controlled trial to determine the effect of giving free alarms on fire rates and injuries.[63] The design was similar to the previously discussed study in Oklahoma City: 20 050 alarms, batteries, fittings, and fire safety brochures were distributed and free installation was offered. No alarms were given to the control group. Follow-up was 12–18 months after distributing alarms. The conclusion of the study was giving free smoke alarms did not reduce fire injuries. Many alarms had not been installed or maintained. Obviously a give-away program isn't the entire answer and more research is necessary. Rowland et al performed a randomized controlled trial to determine what type of fire smoke alarms were most likely to remain working and how the alarm was tolerated in households with smokers.[64] It was conducted in 2145 inner-city London households. The alarms had either ionized or optical sensors. Both sensors are very sensitive to small smoke particles; 93% of 2145 households had alarms installed; 15 months later 54% had working alarms. Reasons were a missing alarm (17%), missing battery (19%), and disconnected alarm (4%). The pattern was similar in households with smokers. Important conclusions by the authors were:

1. an alarm with an ionization sensor, lithium battery, and a pause button were most likely to remain a working alarm;
2. an alarm was less likely to work in a household with one or more smokers;
3. installing smoke alarms may not be effective use of resources.

Although evidence regarding how effective alarms are under specific circumstances is lacking, they surely represent the most effective devise yet introduced to decrease both fire injury and death.[65–67] Unfortunately even though the public knows the benefits of a smoke alarm, it is painfully clear how difficult it is to implement this preventive measure. Facts reported by the US Fire Administration's National Fire Data Center for Residential Structure Fires in 2000 revealed no smoke alarm was present in 53% of residential fires, present and operating in 32%, failed to operate in 6.7%.[9]

Fire sprinklers

Sprinklers complement smoke detectors.[68] Sprinklers are an intervention strategy that works during the event. They are the most effective method for fighting the spread of fires in their early stages Automatic fire sprinklers have been in use in the US since the later part of the 19th century. They are the most effective way of limiting the spread of fire in the early stages. As far back as 1993 the National Fire Protection Association (NFPA) estimated smoke alarms alone could reduce fire deaths by 52%; sprinklers alone could reduce fire deaths by 69% and the combination by 82%. In 1996 residential sprinklers were found in less than 2% of residential fires.[6] The NFPA estimates that occupants with a smoke alarm in the home have a 50% better change of surviving a fire than those without a smoke detector. Adding sprinklers increases the chances of surviving a fire to nearly 97%. One sprinkler is adequate to control fire in over 90% of the documented sprinkler activations in all residential fires. In 1978 San Clemente, California was the first jurisdiction in the United States to require residential sprinklers in all new structures. In 1985 in Scottsdale, Arizona required a sprinkler system in every room of all new industrial, commercial, and residential building. In 1999, 34% of public assembly properties where fires occurred in the US were equipped with sprinklers, compared with 7% of residential properties.[69] The costs for installing fire sprinkler systems in buildings 6 to 8 stories high ranges from under $1.00 to about $2.00 per square foot in most new construction and from about $1.50 to $2.50 per square foot for retrofitting sprinklers in existing buildings. At the present time, cost of a home sprinkler system in new construction is targeted at approximately $1.00 to $1.50 per square foot.[70] Table 4.3 lists components of a hotel/motel fire safety program if the structure is over 75 feet.[71] Sprinklers typically reduce both chance of dying in a fire and the average property loss by one-half to two-thirds compared to where sprinklers are not present. NFPA has no record of a fire death of more than two people in a public assembly, educational, institutional or residential building where the area was completely fitted with working sprinklers. It is estimated that 75% of high-rise and 50% of low-rise hotels have sprinkler systems. In hotels less than three stories, sprinkler requirements may not apply. As of January 2006 no new statistics were found regarding sprinkler installation. Over 200 communities in the US have residential sprinkler laws.

Evaluating the effect of burn prevention

Three important issues reappear in injury prevention literature:

1. implement what is already known, not necessarily proven,
2. passive strategies are more effective than active ones,

TABLE 4.3 COMPONENTS OF A HOTEL/MOTEL SAFETY PROGRAM (FROM HADDON[18])

Fire sprinklers
Smoke/fire detectors
Automatic alarm system
Manual alarm system (pull-boxes in stair wells and near elevators)
Fire department standpipes (a vertical pipe usually noted in stairwells that acts as a reserve in order to secure a uniform pressure in a water-supply system)
Emergency lights
Emergency exit system
Exits signs
Pressurized stairways (a fan blows air in from the exterior, thus creating a positive pressure in the stairway to keep smoke from entering into the stairway and blocking exit path. This is unnecessary if the stairway is open to the exterior of the building.)
Smoke control systems
Portable fire extinguishers
Staff fire emergency response plan
Staff training
General Strategies for Burn Control, Haddon W, Advances in the Epidemiology of Injuries as a Basis for Public Policy. Public Health Reports 1980; 95:411–421.[18]

3. new programs and their results must be subjected to more rigorous evaluation.[72,73]

Successful burn prevention includes collecting, analyzing, and then interpreting burn statistics especially mortality and even more importantly morbidity. The American Burn Association's Burn Data Repository represents a very valuable resource for everyone involved in burn prevention. Heretofore, most burn prevention has been done on a local level and without a national perspective in mind.[74] The ongoing collection of data will allow

* identification of magnitude and type of burn injury,
* monitoring the trend of specific areas of burn injuries and their prevalence,
* identification if new injury problems arise,
* development of methodologies to evaluate burn prevention or intervention efforts.

Many successful burn prevention programs have been developed on the local level using locally generated data. Behavior modification on a local level can be instituted more quickly than waiting for national societal initiatives and legislation. Unfortunately local efforts affect only a few. Prevention research should generate information which can be useful on a national level. There must be rigorous methods of evaluating research so the conclusions may be shared. Many burn prevention programs have had an insufficient number of subjects, no controls, inadequate or short follow-up periods, no control for confounders and of utmost importance, few use mortality and morbidity as outcome measures.[75] While it is difficult to conduct prospective, randomized, double-blinded studies (Class I research), nevertheless rules of good scientific research should be followed.[76] Studies with a single hypothesis should be conducted over an adequate length of time. The prevention goal should be realistic and achievable and the results must be carefully analyzed.[77] Resources must not be wasted collecting and analyzing data unless prevention initiatives are planned. The incidence of both burn injuries and deaths is decreasing throughout the United States; no single burn unit or community will have a large enough patient population to conduct meaningful prospective studies. Peck and Maley determined the population requirements necessary to conduct adequate statistical studies.[78] To undertake a study showing a decrease in injuries by 50% and 10% (alpha level of 0.05 and power of 0.08) requires a population of 9330 and 295082 subjects respectively. A 50% and 10% reduction in burn deaths would require a population of 4672000 and 148175000 subjects respectively. Wanda et al. published a review article on the effectiveness of prevention interventions in house fire injuries.[79] Various types of intervention programs were reviewed. These included school, preschool, and community education programs, fire response training programs for children, office-based counseling, home inspection programs, smoke detector give-away campaigns, and smoke detector legislation. The important conclusion was morbidity and mortality data must be used for outcome measures. There was wide variability regarding study design, data sources, and outcome measures.

Coordination of prevention strategies on a national level is necessary. Passive prevention programs are most effective, but are slow to implement. Active prevention isn't always easy, requires time, significant organizational support, and money. Unfortunately in the US it is unusual for a fire department to spend more than 5% of its budget on fire prevention.[80] Active and passive measures are not mutually exclusive and both must be utilized. All burns *should* be preventable, unfortunately the aphorism 'it is easier said than done' is true.

References

1. Doege TC. Sounding board. An injury is no accident. N Engl J Med 1978; 9:509–510.
2. Colebrook L, Colebrook V. The prevention of burns and scalds. Lancet 1949; II:181–188.
3. Colebrook L, Colebrook V, Bull JP, et al. The prevention of burning accidents. Br Med J 1956; 1:1379–1386.
4. Editorial: Death in the fire place. Lancet 1946:833–834.
5. Hennekens CH, Buring JE. Epidemiology in medicine. Boston: Little Brown; 1987:3–13, 178–194.
6. Fire in the United States 1987–1996, 17th edn. United States. Fire Administration. National Fire Data Center.
7. National Safety Council. Report on injuries in America, 2003. Data from Injury Facts®, 2004 edn. Hasca, Illinois.
8. US Fire Administration. National Fire Data Center. Topical Fire Research Series. Fire Risk December 2004.
9. US Fire Administration. National Fire Data Center. Topical Fire Research Series. Fire Risk. June 2004.
10. McCaig LF, Burt CW. National hospital ambulatory medical care survey. 2003 Emergency Department Summary 358; May 26, 2005.
11. Shai D, Lupinacci P. Fire fatalities among children: an analysis across Philadelphia's census tracts. Public Health Reports 2003; 118:115–126.
12. US Fire Administration. National Fire Data Center. Fire risk. The risk to older adults. Topical Fire Research Series. December 2004; 4(9).

13. Hasofer AM, Thomas I. Analysis of fatalities and injuries in building fire statistics. Fire Safety J 2006; 41:2–14.

14. Ahuja RB, Bhattacharya S. Burns in the developing world and burn disasters. BMJ 2004; 329:447–449.

15. Delgado J, Ramirez-Cardich ME, Gilamn RH, et al. Risk factors for burns in children: crowding, poverty, and poor maternal education. Injury Prevention 2002; 8:38–41.

16. Bonnie RJ, Fulco CE, Liverman CT. Reducing the burden of injury. Advancing prevention and treatment. Washington, DC: National Academy Press; 1999:Chapter 1.

17. Haddon W. The changing approach to the epidemiology, prevention, and amelioration of trauma: the transition to approaches etiologically rather than descriptively based. AJPH 1968; 58:1431–1438.

18. Haddon W. Advances in the epidemiology of injuries as a basis for public policy. Public Health Reports 1980; 95:411–421.

19. McKinlay JB. The promotion of health through planned socio-political change: challenges for research and policy. Soc Sci Med 1993; 36:109–117.

20. Barss P, Smith GS, Barker S, et al. Injury prevention. Epidemiology, surveillance, and policy. New York: Oxford University Press, 1998.

21. McLoughlin E, Vince CJ, Lee AM, et al. Project burn prevention: outcome and implications. Am J Public Health 1982; 72:241–247.

22. Budnick LD. Injuries. In: Cassens BJ, ed. Preventive medicine and public health. Media Pennsylvania: Harwal; 1992; 165–173.

23. McLoughlin E. Issues in evaluation of fire and burn prevention programs. J Burn Care Rehabil 1982; 3:281–284.

24. Grant EJ. Prevention of burn Injury. Problems in General Surgery. 2003; 20:16–26.

25. Liao C, Rossignol AM. Landmarks in burn prevention. Burns 2000; 26:422–434.

26. Burnett WE, Caswell HT. Severe burns from inflammable cowboy pants. JAMA 1946; 130:935–936.

27. Crikelair GF. Flame retardant clothing. J Trauma 1966; 6:422–427.

28. Crikelair GF, Agate F, Bowe A. Gasoline and flammable and non-flammable clothing studies. Pediatrics 1976; 58:585–594.

29. Blum A, Ames BN. Flame-retardant additives as possible cancer hazards. Science 1977; 95:7–23.

30. United States Consumer Product Safety Commission: CPSC bans tris-treated children's garments. News Release April 7; 1977.

31. Knudson MS, Bolieu SL, Larson DL, et al. Children's sleepwear flammability standards: have they worked? Burns 1979; 6:255–260.

32. Feller I, Tholen D, Cornell RG. Improvements in burn care, 1965 to 1979. JAMA 1980; 244:2074–2078.

33. McLoughlin E, Clarke N, Stahl K, et al. One pediatric burn unit's experience with sleepwear-related injuries. Pediatrics 1977; 60:405–409.

34. Oglesbay FB. The flammable fabrics problem. Pediatrics 1969; 44:827–895.

35. Cusick JM, Grant EJ, Kucan JO. Children's sleepwear: relaxation of the Consumer Product Safety Commission's flammability standards. J Burn Care Rehabil 1997; 18:469–476.

36. Wilson DI, Bailie FB. Night attire burns in young girls – the return of an old adversary. Burns 1999; 25:269–271.

37. Horrocks AR, Nazare S, Kandola B. The particular flammability hazards of nightwear. Fire Safety J 2004; 39:259–276.

38. Erdmann TC, Feldman KW, Rivara FP, et al. Tap water burn prevention: the effect of legislation. Pediatrics 1991; 88:572–577.

39. Clarke JA, Waller AE, Marshall SW, et al. Barriers to the reduction of domestic hot water temperatures. Safety Science 1995; 18:181–192.

40. Maley M. Scald burns associated with tap water. J Burn Care Rehabil 1989; 10:172–173.

41. Feldman KW, Schaller RT, Feldman JA, et al. Tap water scald burns in children. Pediatrics 1978; 62:1–7.

42. Katcher ML, Landry GL, Shapiro MM. Liquid-crystal thermometer use in pediatric office counseling about tap water burn prevention. Pediatrics 1980; 83:766–771.

43. Drago DA. Kitchen scalds and thermal burns in children five years and younger. Pediatrics 2005; 115:10–16.

44. Macarthur C. Evaluation of safe kid's week 2001: prevention of scald and burn injuries in young children. Injury Prevention 2003; 9:112–116.

45. Webne S, Kaplan FJ, Shaw M. Pediatric burn prevention: an evaluation of the efficacy of a strategy to reduce tap water temperature in a population at risk for scalds. Developmental Behavior Pediatr 1989; 10:187–191.

46. Corrarino JE, Walsh PJ, Nadel E. Does teaching scald burn prevention to families of young children make a difference? J Pediatr Nurs 2001; 16:256–262.

47. Unglaub F, Woodruff S, Ulrich D, Pallua N. Severe burns as a consequence of seizure while showering: risk factors and implications for prevention. Epilepsia 2005; 46:332–333.

48. MMWR – cigarette smoking-attributable morbidity — United States, 2000. Atlanta, Georgia: National Center for Chronic Disease Prevention and Health Promotion; September 2003; 52(35).

49. Ballard JE, Koepsell TD, Rivara F. Association of smoking and alcohol drinking with residential fire injuries. Am J Epid 1990; 135:26–34.

50. Barbeau EM, Kelder G, Mantuefel AV, et al. From strange bedfellows to natural allies: the shifting allegiance of fire service organizations in the push for federal fire-safe cigarette legislation. Tobacco Control 2005; 14:338–345.

51. Botkin JR. The fire-safe cigarette. JAMA 1988; 260:226–229.

52. Brigham PA, McGuire A. Progress towards a fire-safe cigarette. J Public Health Policy 1996; 16:433–439.

53. Connolly GN, Alpert HR, Rees V, et al. Effect of the New York state cigarette fire safety standard on ignition propensity, smoke constituents, and the consumer market. Tobacco Control 2005; 14:321–326.

54. McGuire A. How the tobacco industry continues to keep the home fires burning. Tobacco Control 1999; 8:67–69.

55. Varon J, Marik PE, Fromm RE, et al. Carbon monoxide poisoning: a review for clinicians. J Emerg Med 1999; 17:87–93.

56. Runyan CW, Johnson RM, Yang J, et al. Risk and protective factors for fires, burns, and carbon monoxide poisoning in US households. Am J Prev Med 2005; 28:102–108.

57. Gorman RL, Charney E, Holtzman NA, et al. A successful city-wide smoke detector give-away program. Pediatrics 1985; 75:14–18.

58. Miller RE, Reisinger KS, Blatter MM, et al. Pediatric counseling and subsequent use of smoke detectors. Am J Public Health 1982; 72:392–393.

59. Shaw KN, McCormick MC, Kustra SL, et al. Correlates of reported smoke detector usage in an inner-city population: participants in a smoke detector give-away program. Am J Public Health 1988; 78:650–653.

60. McLoughlin E, Marchone M, Hanger L, et al. Smoke detector legislation: it's effect on owner-occupied homes. Am J Public Health 1985; 75:858–862.

61. Mallonee S, Istre GR, Rosenberg M, et al. Surveillance and prevention of residential-fire injuries. N Engl J Med 1996; 335:27–31.

62. DiGuiseppi C, Higgins JP. Systematic review of controlled trials of interventions to promote smoke alarms. Arch Dis Child 2000; 82:341–348.

63. DiGuiseppi C, Roberts I, Wade A, et al. Incidence of fires and related injuries after giving out free smoke alarms: cluster randomized controlled trial. BMJ 2002; 325:995–997.

64. Rowland D, DiGuiseppi C, Roberts I, et al. Prevalence of working smoke alarms in local authority inner city housing: randomized controlled trial. BMJ 2002; 325:998–1001.

65. Haravey PA, Aitken M, Ryan GW, et al. Strategies to increase smoke alarm use in high-risk households. J Comm Health 2004; 29:375–385.

66. Stevenson MR, Lee AH. Smoke alarms and residential fire mortality in the United States: an ecologic study. Fire Safety J 2002; 38:43–52.

67. Thompson CJ, Jones AR, Davis MK, et al. Do smoke alarms still function a year after installation? A follow-up of the get-alarmed campaign. J Community Health 2004; 29:171–181.

68. Council on Scientific Affairs. Preventing death and injury from fires with automatic sprinklers and smoke detectors. JAMA 1987; 2577:1618–1620.

69. Kay RL. Letter to Editor. Let's emphasize fire sprinklers as an injury prevention technology! BMJ November 2005; 72–73.

70. Department of Home Land Security. USFA. Sprinkler systems. December 2005. Online. Available: www.USFA.FEMA/gov/safety/sprinklers.

71. The American Fire Sprinkler Association, Dallas, Texas. July 2000

72. King WJ, LeBlanc JC, Klassen TP, et al. Long term effects of a home visit to prevent childhood injury: three year follow up of a randomized trial. Inj Prev 2005; 11:106–109.

73. Peleg K, Goldman S, Sikron F. Burn prevention programs for children: do they reduce burn-related hospitalizations? Burns 2005; 31:347–350.

74. Istre GR, McCoy MA, Osborn L, et al. Deaths and injuries from house fires. N Engl J Med 2001; 344:1911–1916.

75. Tan J, Banez C, Cheung Y, et al. Effectiveness of a burn prevention campaign for older adults. J Burn Care Rehabil 2004; 25: 445–451.

76. Wards L, Tenebein M, Moffatt MEK. House fire injury prevention update. Part II. A review of the effectiveness of preventive interventions. Inj Prev 1999; 5:217–225.

77. Horan JM, Mallonee S. Injury surveillance. Epidemiol Rev 2003; 25:24–42.

78. Peck MD, Maley MP. Population requirements for statistical analysis of efficacy of burn prevention programs. J Burn Care Rehabil 1991; 12:282–284.

79. Warda L, Tenenbein M, Moffatt ME. House fire injury prevention update. Part II. A review of the effectiveness of preventive interventions. Inj Prev 1999; 5:217–225.

80. Stambaugh H, Schaenman P. International concepts of fire protection: ideas that could help US prevention. J Burn Care Rehabil 1988; 9:312–313.

Chapter 5

Burn management in disasters and humanitarian crises

Thomas L. Wachtel and K. A. Kelly McQueen

Chapter contents

Introduction

Worldwide, burns cause significant morbidity and mortality for humankind. Geography greatly impacts the resources available for disaster response and humanitarian action. These resources and actions influence the suffering and survival rate. An isolated significant burn occurring in a resource-rich country leads to a swift response and treatment, generally initiated in a matter of hours. When a similar burn occurs in a remote area or in a resource-poor country, the risk of death and disability is exponentially greater. During a burn disaster or humanitarian catastrophe, systems and resources are potentially and often overwhelmed, equalizing what would generally differentiate resource-rich and resource-poor environments. Lessons learned from disasters, humanitarian emergencies, and wars have the potential to lead to personal and systems improvement. Therefore, preparation for burn disasters and humanitarian crises based on prior disaster management and experience benefits the individual healthcare provider, the healthcare system and most of all, the burned patient, regardless of the geographic location on earth.

The concepts of disaster management and humanitarian aid are central to the discussion that follows. Most simply defined, a disaster occurs whenever need exceeds resources.[1,2] Often, outside assistance is required to restore balance to an overwhelmed system. Outside assistance takes many forms — transferring patients to another facility or another country, activating a national emergency plan or requesting assistance from international organizations. Many other definitions of disasters exist and apply specifically to burn disasters. Masellis describes a disaster as a 'serious and immediate threat to public health'.[3] He divides the management of rescue operations into thermal agent (fire) disaster and burn disaster that are linked by the common causal force — fire (Figure 5.1). A

Acknowledgment: Carey Shapiro, Librarian, Scottsdale Healthcare.

fire disaster is a serious and sudden vast ecological breakdown in the relationship between man and his environment on such a scale that the stricken community needs extraordinary efforts to cope with the disaster, and often requires outside help or international aid.[4] A burn disaster can be defined as the overall effect of massive action from a known thermal agent on living people. It is characterized by an excessive number of seriously burned patients with a high rate of disability and death[3,5] A fire causing 25 or more deaths is termed a fire catastrophe.[6]

Burn disasters are usually medical disasters for communities, states and infrequently countries, calling for medical planning, resource allocation, communication, and delegation. These disasters may become humanitarian emergencies when there is significant mechanism or when they disrupt infrastructure, government, social function, and economic resources such that the public health as well as the medical health of a community is at risk. Burn disasters can also be part of ongoing humanitarian crises, such as in Iraq where there are already stressed systems in place with very little additional capacity to deal with even a small number of burn casualties.

Public health planning for burn disasters for the most part is involved in supporting medical infrastructure and encouraging disaster planning for such emergencies. Most burn disasters will be local but when burn disasters become catastrophic (as in the event of a large explosion, use of a dirty bomb or a nuclear attack) then application of public health to the large populations becomes more important. Risk analysis reveals that these events are very unlikely but that the outcome would be disastrous. Hopefully, public health infrastructure and planning designed to prevent and react to most disasters will support the event of a large burn disaster but for many countries these systems are untested.

Burn disasters provide a true interface between medical and public health planning. While medical treatment and intervention is always part of public health planning and response, it is often a small portion of overall preparation and response for a disaster or humanitarian emergency. In natural disasters and humanitarian emergencies the public health focus includes security, provision of clean water and sanitation, prevention of disease and vaccination programs, housing, nutritional support, and medical care. In a majority of the burn disasters to date, with the exception of perhaps the 1906 San Francisco fire,[7] medical response and evacuation have been the appropriate response. But preparedness for a large-scale burn disaster remains as important in the post 9–11 world as it was during the Cold War.

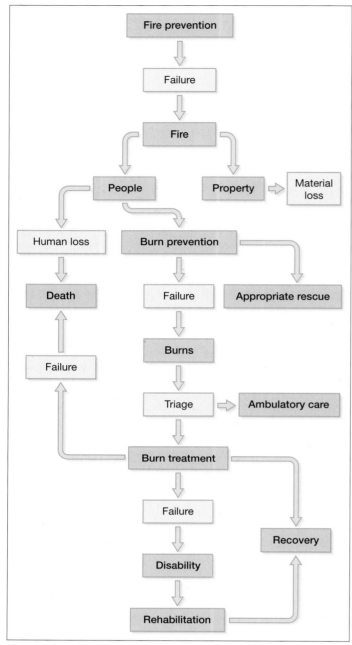

Fig. 5.1 Characteristics and consequences of a fire. Disasters increase the magnitude of the human and material losses and damages.

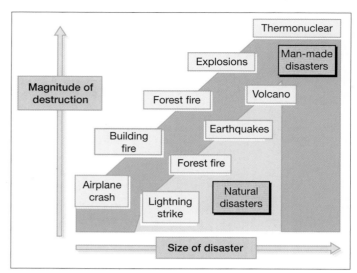

Fig. 5.2 Burn disaster sources and magnitude of destruction.

of the Geneva Conventions and Universal Declaration of Human Rights.[9] It is within this context that burn injuries commonly occur, and frequently lead to burn disasters as the health systems already in crisis are easily overwhelmed. In the current complex emergencies of Sudan, Afghanistan, and Iraq, civilians and combatants alike have been caught in the crossfire of the ongoing war, and have been targeted by insurgents with car and suicide bombs that have resulted in uncountable burns and burn deaths. Finally, terrorism and a shift in war strategies, from conventional to asymmetrical, have contributed to the burn disasters of the 21st century.[10] The events of September 11, 2001 led to many burns and while the New York City and Washington DC systems were not as overwhelmed as anticipated, the lessons learned in the aftermath of these tragedies have contributed to the overall approach of burn disaster preparedness and management for this century.[11,12]

The utilization of resources for burned patients, the most complex form of trauma, is extraordinarily high as well, when compared to other injured victims.[13] Treating two or three burn patients has the ability to stretch the capacity of even the best prepared, modern facility. Burn disasters involving 20 or more patients has the potential to overwhelm healthcare systems and require intervention from multiple well-equipped facilities and external resources.[14] Fortunately disasters involving multiple burn casualties are uncommon;[13,15] nevertheless, the potential for overwhelming burn casualties and effects on resources demand planning and preparedness.

Burn disasters and humanitarian crises are most frequently man-made as opposed to natural disasters (e.g. a volcanic eruption, lightning strike, earthquake) and, in general, are comparatively confined to a limited geographical area (Figure 5.2). The initial information needed in order to respond to a disaster revolves around a definition of the event and the geography in question. This includes information about the location as well as means of access to the location, such as points of egress from a room, a building, a field, a town or a

Burn disasters of large scale may lead to humanitarian emergencies. These are disaster situations created and/or contributed to by political, military, economic, and sometimes natural constraints but uniformly impact greater communities and result in a collapse of infrastructure, economy, and an absence or depletion of resources.[8] Since first coined as Complex Humanitarian Emergencies (CHEs) in the post-Cold War era, these crises have evolved to being simply called humanitarian emergencies and have been characterized as catastrophic public health emergencies, with high levels of violence, long-lasting and widespread, with major violations country.[16] In the modern, resource-rich world, earthquake-related flame burns and scalds are infrequent, but when they occur they are usually combined with mechanical trauma.[17] Prior to automatic gas line fail safes and protection of hazardous materials in industrialized countries with protective regulations, fire following earthquake was second only to collapse of masonry buildings as the leading cause of fatalities.[5] In under-developed areas of the world where construction is rapid, insecure and where building regulations are non-existent, fire following earthquakes still leads to a majority of casualties and fatalities. The large fire that occurred following the San Francisco earthquake of 1906 was responsible for many of the fatalities.[7] But even recently, the 1989 Loma Prieta earthquake[18] and the 1994 Northridge earthquake,[19] led to many structural fires, incidents of localized fires, and spills of volatile or explosive mixtures that resulted in fires. Explosions are common and widespread and may also cause mass burn and trauma casualties. Remote areas in resource-rich countries and most areas of resource-poor countries exponentially amplify the problems with logistics, evacuation, and treatment of burned victims and raise their morbidity and mortality.

The most recent burn disasters, in Bali and Rhode Island, revealed further lessons learned.[14,20,21] In the Bali disaster the challenges of treating expatriates, easily reachable by the resources of Australia, exposed yet another concept in evacuation and response in a country under threat of terror. Burns in Iraq, of both Americans and Iraqis, illustrate the contrast of resources and the perils of the daily threat of terrorism.[10]

Advances in science and technology have increased the risk of accidents that result in a transfer of thermal energy to people located nearby. The possible number of casualties from such accidents increases as more powerful sources of energy are harnessed.[22] Because of growth in the fields of transportation and technology, we are now confronted with a potentially rapid growth in the absolute number of burns in a mass disaster as well as heightening the possible dangers surrounding the use of thermic energy of unprecedented power such that the magnitude and consequences could be appalling.[23–26] The potential for modern-day fire catastrophes involving urban areas, high-rise buildings, large crowds collected at community events, and worldwide terrorism poses a serious challenge to fire technology and to society.[6] Such disasters normally exceed the resources of local healthcare providers and facilities,[22] especially as it relates to burns.

Every burn center needs a burn disaster plan.[27] The burn center disaster response must be integrated into the disaster planning of the hospital and its emergency department and trauma service, the prehospital system, the state emergency management system, and perhaps a national disaster plan.[15,27,28] Many hospitals, communities, states, and countries, however, will either not prepare disaster plans or will not execute the plan during an emergency. This chapter will review the epidemiology of burn disasters and humanitarian crises, elucidate public health tenets particularly as they relate to preparing a burn disaster plan for a response that will prevent or mitigate consequences, and examine the challenges of the disaster response to a real burn disaster or burn disaster exercise from two perspectives: the resource-rich or Western response and the resource-limited perspective.

Epidemiology of disasters and humanitarian crises

Epidemiology has proved most promising in disaster management.[4] Disaster epidemiology links data collection, analysis of the disaster, analysis of risk factors for adverse social and health effects, clinical investigation of the impact of diagnostic and therapeutic methods, the effectiveness of various types of the assistance, and the long-term influence of relief operations on restoration of pre-disaster conditions.[4] Disaster medicine is the study of collaborative applications of various health disciplines to the prevention, immediate response to, and rehabilitation of health problems that arise from a disaster.[4] For this kind of scientific approach and technical underpinning, special studies, surveys and applied research, social and natural science investigations, and managerial applications are necessary[4] (Table 5.1). Training people for disaster management requires courses on disaster health in addition to innate humanitarian compassion.[4] Practical application of disaster medicine is a continuous cycle of planning for disasters, exercising the plan, utilizing the practiced plan should a disaster arise, and examining the response to either an exercise or a real disaster in detail in an after-action assessment (Figure 5.3).

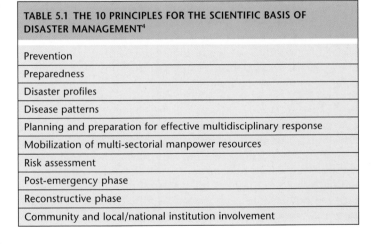

TABLE 5.1 THE 10 PRINCIPLES FOR THE SCIENTIFIC BASIS OF DISASTER MANAGEMENT[4]
Prevention
Preparedness
Disaster profiles
Disease patterns
Planning and preparation for effective multidisciplinary response
Mobilization of multi-sectorial manpower resources
Risk assessment
Post-emergency phase
Reconstructive phase
Community and local/national institution involvement

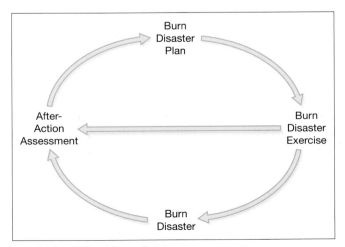

Fig. 5.3 The cycle of burn disaster management.

The incidence and distribution of burn disasters and burn injury during natural and man-made disasters was well described in the 20th century.[7,15,29–31] Despite the potential for mass disasters, conflagrations became less frequent in the United States during the last half century[6,15] while the incidence of major fires in Europe increased in recent years.[31] The 21st century brought many changes including the dawn of terrorism on a scale previously unknown, and a paradigm shift in the conduct of warfare.[10,32] Both of these realities have impacted the epidemiology of burn disasters since the year 2000. Natural events still contribute to burn disasters, and nowhere more so than in resource-poor regions of the world where the infrastructure is limited, and the fire and burn injury lessons learned and applied in the resource-rich countries have not been activated. By far, most burn disasters today are man-made and many of them intentionally applied. War and terrorism have contributed significantly to the burn disasters that have occurred since the turn of the century and will continue, it seems, for the foreseeable future. The new strategies of asymmetrical warfare alone contribute to burn disasters on a regular basis within Iraq.[10]

The large-scale burn disasters of the last century have been examined, published and the lessons learned have often led to changes in public policy, public health education campaigns, and robust disaster plans in resource-rich regions of the globe.[15] Burn injury following natural disasters has been identified, the incidence of these injuries studied, and planning for response in the initial post-disaster phase impacted.[5] The most common natural disaster contributing to burn injuries are earthquakes, which historically have led to some famous fires including the 1906 San Francisco fire.[7] These sentinel fires have led to changes in public opinion and important advances in fire prevention.[6] Changes in building codes and other regulatory interventions have resulted in a significant decrease in fires and burns following earthquakes, but in resource-poor and developing countries, construction codes and government regulations are frequently not enforced and, therefore, in these settings fires and burns may frequently contribute to morbidity and mortality. Other natural disasters may lead to downed power lines and chemical spills that may also result in burns. Early surveillance following hurricane Katrina and the floods that followed uncovered burn injuries in the early days following the event.[33]

Burn injuries during humanitarian emergencies including conflict scenarios are known to occur, but many incidents occurring in these settings often go unreported for many reasons. Medical aid in humanitarian emergencies is often provided by relief organizations, or in some cases such as Iraq, is provided to limited degree by a weakened infrastructure and a dwindling number of overworked health professionals. Recording medical events and outcomes is often a low priority in these settings.

The incidence and distribution of burn injury during natural disasters and complex humanitarian emergencies are important to this discussion. Population's increases and shifts, and global environmental changes have led to an increase in natural disasters worldwide.[34] In the 21st century the impact of humanitarian emergencies continues to provide significant challenges to the humanitarian community due almost entirely to the ongoing and unresolved crisis in Iraq,[10] with violence, trauma, and death being reported daily in the civilian and military populations.

The epidemiology of any injury is impacted by the environment where the disaster occurs. In most cases, the incidence of burn injury following a disaster tends to be higher in developing areas of the world where population density is high and prevention and preparation for such disasters is limited by resources, education and often the political will to intervene.[1] However, recent experiences in New Orleans, Louisiana, United States, revealed that even with well-developed disaster plans in place and adequate healthcare infrastructure, morbidity and mortality, including burn injury occur following natural disasters due to human and systems failures, unexecuted plans, and abandonment.[33] In addition, studies suggest that the severity of injuries among those admitted to hospitals show that either victims were able to escape rapidly and, thus, sustained relatively small burns (<30% total body surface area [TBSA]) to exposed areas of skin, or that timely escape was impossible and victims were engulfed and sustained lethal injuries (>70% TBSA).[31] One explanation is that a great number of victims are trapped in indoor fires and failed to escape. The morbidity and elevated immediate death rate in indoor disasters was mainly due to hypoxia, inhalation injuries, intoxication, and inhalation of poisonous compounds.[35,36] The effect of hydrogen cyanide and carbon monoxide has been postulated as a cause of incapacity and inability to react, and accounts for high indoor death rates.[35] No rescue people reached the severely injured in time.[35]

Burn disasters, while uncommon when compared to other natural disasters and humanitarian emergencies, are important due to the number of causalities per event, mortality rate, and economic cost of these emergencies. Burn disasters not related to natural disasters, war, and terrorism include explosions and the subsequent fires that ensue following train crashes, air crashes, underground disasters, and liquefied petroleum gas explosions.[31,35,37,38] The extreme end of the continuum of explosions and resultant burns is a nuclear event. It is such an incident, even in resource-rich parts of the world, that the magnitude of a nuclear occurrence transforms burn disasters,[23,24,26] which are approachable with adequate infrastructure, resource allocation and planning, into humanitarian crises.

Public health implications

Most burn disasters are local, impacting a small section of the population, even though the mortality rate from the event is high. When burn disasters cannot be avoided or they are intentionally deployed and become catastrophic, the tenets of public health must be employed. Public health planning for burn disasters for the most part is in supporting medical infrastructure, guiding medical resource planning, and encouraging disaster plans for such emergencies. Application of public health principles to large populations becomes important. Although risk analysis reveals that these events are very unlikely, the outcome of such an event would likely change the overall function — social, economic, and public health infrastructure for the foreseeable future.

A plan for response and mitigation must be in place (Table 5.2). Such plans vary depending on where in the world the

TABLE 5.2 DISASTER-RELATED ACTIVITIES
Pre-disaster activities
Disaster prevention
Disaster preparedness
Disaster mitigation
Emergency response
Warning
Evacuation/rescue
Emergency assistance
Post-disaster activities
Transitional period:
Repair structures and lifelines
Reclaim and clear land
Resume services
Reconstruction period:
Replace buildings
Restore service systems
Revitalize economy
Restore agriculture
From Perez E, Thompson P. Natural Hazards: causes and effects. Lesson 1 — Intro to natural disasters. Pre-Hospital Disaster Med 1994; 9(1):80–87.[39]

disaster occurs, and what resources are available. Burn disasters that occur in the United States and much of Europe are addressed systematically, and plans for surge capacity and other mass causality issues have often been addressed beforehand. In the resource-poor regions of the world, however, infrastructure is often incomplete and resources for a large-scale and rapid response are severely limited. In this case, external support and resources from international humanitarian aid disaster relief organizations are required immediately, and any delay in delivery of supplies, equipment, and personnel will adversely impact mortality rates and individual outcomes. Such scenarios must be considered, since burn disasters or other natural disasters that have the potential for many burn injuries occur more frequently in these underdeveloped areas, if only due to the vast populations that are living in these regions. For truly effective disaster management, the key is prevention and preparedness rather than a *post hoc* fire fighting type of emergency response.[4,40] This section reviews the public health aspects of prevention, preparation of a disaster plan, exercising the plan, and mitigation of the consequences of a burn catastrophe through descriptions and examples of burn disasters.

Prevention

Prevention, a most important tenet of public health, provides the best possible outcome (i.e. avoiding a burn disaster). But preventive measures were usually lacking in all disasters investigated and mistakes were observed, frequently.[35] Even in countries where long-term protection and prevention is governed by regulations, fire and building codes and education programs, systems fail and fires occur leading to burn injury. In the case of terrorism, the disaster by definition cannot be prevented due to the intentional and unpredictable nature of the strategy for promoting fear and creating instability. During the height of the Cold War when the threat of a nuclear disaster loomed as a realistic possibility, it was only the reality of world destruction and diplomacy that kept the threat in check. Prevention was only theoretical.

Ironically, the most notable immediate reward for good burn disaster planning is the template that is established for burn prevention programs. Initially, the level of prevention achieved depends on the number and effectiveness of public education and information programs that have been pursued.[41] The role of health education is to facilitate the learning of behavior patterns that will reduce risk factors and increase protection factors by means of identification of motivational elements related to behavior.[41]

Secondly, prevention must address the risk, environment, resources, and rational for fire and burn reduction technologies. Inspection of public buildings at the time of their initial construction and after any remodeling is necessary in order to ensure proper fire prevention methods. Failure to observe this axiom was crucial in the Stardust disaster[42] and Station fire.[20,21] Attention should be paid to methods of egress, as well as fire-fighting capability such as water hose reels and fire-resistant materials.[42] Posting fire escape plans within rooms of public buildings, providing adequate fire egress instructions and facilities, having fire drills in public facilities (schools, office building, hospitals,[43] operating rooms,[40] ships, airplanes,[44] racetracks,[45] etc.) are important aspects of training as well as prevention. There must be proper liaison between disaster planning departments and fire services. A fire department has to ensure that they have proper equipment to fight fires and rescue victims from all facilities and locations in their catchment area, including high-rise buildings, hospitals, schools, campsites, and recreational areas. They should be aware of buildings and locations with hazardous materials, fuel, and explosives as well as forest conditions and other fire hazards in their area. Inspections must include adherence to statutory building regulations and the laws that make these regulations effective. Fire services and local authorities must be adequately staffed, properly equipped, and appropriately trained. The payoff return for prevention is thought to be substantial, but the measurement of effectiveness and cost-effectiveness is an assessment of what could have happened and didn't because of intervention and, therefore, hard to quantify.

Preparation of the disaster plan

Preparation is the next important tenet in the overall public health infrastructure when considering burn disasters and humanitarian crises. Planning for a large-scale disaster requires preexisting public health and medical infrastructure, and the cooperation of local, state, and national agencies. In the worst-case scenario planning will need to interface civilian and military authorities, which will be the norm in disaster planning for many countries and will provide additional challenges for countries such as the United States, where the military rarely intervenes in disaster response.[28] Disaster preparedness focuses not only on structuring the response but on laying a framework for recovery as well.[39] In the case of burn disaster planning these principles all apply, and specialized burn treatment teams and facilities must take part in the plan.

The disaster plan is the best tool for preparedness. A comprehensive disaster plan is intended to provide optimal treatment of victims of a major catastrophe when there are too many patients to be treated by routine emergency services.[46] The number of people injured in a burn disaster is defined as the sum of the number admitted to hospitals with burns and the number killed outright.[31,35] For rural and wilderness areas, that number may be as few as one or two. For a modern urban burn center, in a large tertiary hospital, the ability to care for a larger number of burned victims may be enhanced. Eventually, however, even the resources of a sophisticated burns center in a multi-specialty hospital within a mature trauma system in a resource-rich environment will become exhausted, and the previous planning, preparedness, training, response, relief, rehabilitation, and reconstruction for a major burn emergency or burn disaster situation will be overwhelmed.[2] The solution will require either secondary triage of burned victims to other more distant burn and tertiary facilities (Figure 5.4) or transportation of staff, supplies, and equipment to the site of the disaster.[13] The management of mass burns remains a highly complex problem of organization.[25] The characteristics and principles of a burn disaster are shown in Table 5.3.

Fundamental planning

All disasters share common elements and therefore should be designed as a continuum to include all disaster types and scenarios.[1] However, disaster scenarios should be considered individually so that the unique elements of the scenarios can be addressed, along with the common processes.[13,25] Plans for burn disasters must be integrated into overall local, regional, national, and international disaster plans.[27] Burn disasters will require integration of medical assets and systems when they are relatively small or local, and must expand quickly to encompass all aspects of a comprehensive disaster plan when large, continuing, or catastrophic. Effective disaster planning will not only lessen property loss and social disruption caused by disaster impacts but will also reduce suffering and the distress of casualities.[47] Despite evidence available from past disasters, adequate provision for the management of burned casualties is still lacking in most disaster plans.[31] Of the 14 disasters studied by Arturson, only in the San Juanico tragedy was a disaster plan in place.[35] Disaster planning should emphasize that most burns are either minor or very extensive.[47] New developments in the organization of emergency medical service systems dictate that new approaches to disaster planning preparedness are essential in order to implement current concepts of emergency medical care delivery.[1,16,48] The important aspects of modern disaster management from the medical perspective include:

- The utilization of medical triage and treatment protocols in order to effect control and transportation of patients.

TABLE 5.3 CHARACTERISTICS AND PRINCIPLES OF A BURN DISASTER
The place the disaster occurs is not always accessible and care and assistance may not be adequate
The time interval between the accident and initiation of care must be less than 2 hours
The burns are mainly very extensive and the general condition of the victims is precarious
Triage of victims must be affected only by specialists, as only specialists are able to evaluate the immediate gravity of the burn
Inhalation of combustion gases, fumes, and hot air causes damage to the airways: and this alone can jeopardize survival
Hypovolemic shock induces a state of tissue hypoxia with irreversible damage to various organs and systems
The burn is often associated with other serious problems such as vast wounds, fractures, electrical injuries, or blast injury lesions
The overall assessment of the damage to people must be made not only on the basis of the number of dead but also on the number of people burned and suffering risk of disability
Masellis M, Ferrara MM, Gunn SWA. Fire Disaster and Burn Disaster: planning and management. Ann Burns Fire Disasters 1999; 12(2):67–82.[3]

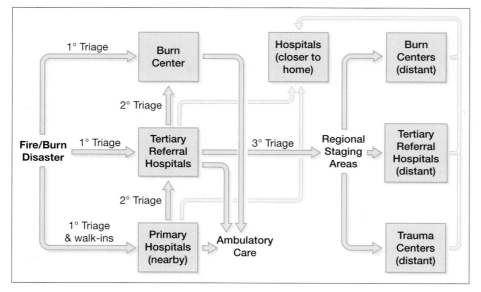

Fig. 5.4
Triage scheme for a fire/burn disaster:
1° = primary; 2° = secondary; 3° = tertiary.

- Early notification of all hospitals that could potentially receive patients.
- Transportation of patients to appropriate hospitals utilizing an existing point-of-entry plan.

This enables burn victims to be preferentially transported to facilities with burn treatment capability and available beds.[16] Three distinct phases of relief operations are necessary: immediate assistance, first aid, and organized relief. Immediate assistance is provided in the first 2–3 hours by people on the spot (trained volunteers, physicians, and nurses) and is fundamental to the prognosis of fire disaster victims. A timely, rational, safe, and effective intervention is the main guarantee *quo ad vitam* for the victims of a fire disaster.[4] A more complex body of organized relief may not be able to reach a disaster scene for at least 6 or 7 hours. When burn casualties exceed the local ability to provide adequate care, a major disaster should be declared so that all facilities can prepare for upcoming casualties.[13] Outside or even international assistance should be requested immediately. When a sovereign nation faces a disaster, international law requires that assistance be requested. It is only in the face of a humanitarian crisis that aid may be provided without national consent if the international community deems it is appropriate and necessary.

Effective disaster management can only be accomplished when a thorough disaster planning process has been conducted.[49] Such a process must include all elements and all recognized emergency response and relief agencies that could play a role in responding to a disaster.[16,48,50,51] The most important outcome of a planning exercise is that each of the agencies be educated as to the roles and responsibilities of the others so that essential links between agencies can be established.[16]

Communication

Communication during a disaster always presents unique opportunities. Sometimes sophisticated systems are available and sometimes the disaster destroys these systems and alternative and more primitive systems must be used. For planning purposes, redundancy and development of fail safe systems should be the solution. Online voice communication with a burn center, burn coordinator, burn surgeon, a trauma center, and trauma surgeon is important. Disaster plans should utilize existing reliable communication venues and have the ability to expand (i.e. bring in additional equipment and staff). Communications must be fast, practiced, and limited in scope. A point-of-entry plan ought to communicate the type of disaster: burns, burns and other trauma, trauma, spinal cord injuries, acute medical complications, poisoning, behavioral crises, neonatal patients, or pediatric victims. A consideration that impacts on incident management is the existence and utilization of a centralized reporting and notification mechanism,[16] such as the enhanced 911 centralized communication system in the United States for fire, police, and emergency medical services. The system should have the capability to contact metropolitan area ambulance services and hospitals individually or collectively through the centralized communication system. This feature allows for central collection of hospital bed availability data, relay of relevant information on the status of the disaster to hospitals, centralized coordination of the disaster response, and direction of ambulances carrying triaged patients to appropriate facilities.[16] The benefits of a comprehensive system with a centralized communications component are shown in Table 5.4.

A central data bank that stores up-to-date information on the capacity of each burn center to accept patients is imperative for disaster management. Valuable information is also provided concerning hospital capability, intensive care/burn intensive care availability, equipment availability (fluidized beds, etc.), and technical procedures. The information should be utilized on a daily basis for the distribution of burns within the geographical area under non-disaster circumstances. Such a system can then be extremely useful in the event of a disaster when the distribution of patients is urgent. The French telematic data bank for burns also includes an epidemiologic file that forms the basis for prevention campaigns. It is compatible with the International Society for Burn Injuries and the European organization.[52] The German system that is used on a daily basis responds extremely well. It was not used primarily in the Ramstein air disaster which caused criticism of their disaster management. It *was* used for secondary triage and for consultation on burned patients. The United States' system, National Disaster Management System (NDMS), was activated during Operation Desert Storm and was used by some regions for the distribution of burned patients. Operation Iraqi Freedom again stimulated tracking of daily availability of burn beds.[53] Currently the Assistant Secretary of Defense surveys burn centers electronically in the United States on a weekly basis in concert with the American Burn Association.[54] This data is available should casualty rates exceed the capacity of Department of Defense's burn center and can be used for mass casualty incidents.[53] The Italian ARGO satellite system combines a coordination center, data collection center, transportation center, and burn centers into a meshed sub-network. It is expandable and allows the organization to care for severely burned patients. The telecommunication system has high standards of reliability and survival to guarantee continuity of communications from and to a disaster area. It is divided into telephone, fax, video telecommunications networks, and a territorial data collection network. The information is continually updated and links with a national organization capable of rapid mobilization of carriers for the transport of patients. The ARGO satellite system allows immediate contact between spe-

TABLE 5.4 BENEFITS OF A COMPREHENSIVE SYSTEM WITH A CENTRALIZED COMMUNICATION COMPONENT[16]
Improved notification of the incident
Consistent initial and follow-up information
Timeliness of response
Better management of the incident
Accuracy in the collection of pertinent information concerning the incident
Analysis of the information to determine the correct level of response, triage to hospitals and specialty centers
Utilization of transport vehicles
Ultimate outcome of burn victims
From Layton TR, Elhauge ER. US Fire catastrophies of the 20th Century. J Burn Care Rehabil 1982; 3(1):21–28.[16]

cialized burn centers and the physicians treating patients in the disaster area so that support is available for staff in the field. It functions as a radio telephone in an ambulance and as an ordinary portable telephone carried by a physician.[55]

Clear, concise, honest communication with the media is important during any disaster. Embracing and embedding a public relations plan is vital.[56,57] The media can serve a very useful purpose in spreading the message for needed resources and in recording the events and responses for the after-action reports and lessons learned. Ignoring the media in the planning stages will surely disrupt the other important aspects of disaster management in the exercises and in the event of a real burn disaster.

The disaster scene

The initial task for a disaster plan is to forecast methods to identify all burned victims. A search and rescue effort involved in a disaster primarily revolves around finding, extricating, and/or transporting victims, including the injured and the dead as well as the non-injured.[47] Fire services are well positioned and structured to undertake this search and rescue role. They may need to be augmented with heavy rescue units and additional personnel. There should be significant pre-disaster planning and training for organized search and rescue, involving the fire service and a variety of local groups. Seldom does one specific community group assume complete responsibility. Timeliness is essential and stress inherent. Widespread damage to structures will result in large numbers of casualties and trapped people within an immediate disaster zone. It can be anticipated that people who are trapped will attempt to free themselves, and untrapped survivors will go to their aid. A concentrated effort to rescue trapped persons during the first few hours after a disaster will yield greater dividends in lives saved than any larger or more highly developed effort made later.[47] A larger burn disaster may require that trained rescuers operate solely in a supervisory role while large numbers of untrained workers are added to a trained nucleus in order to rapidly expand rescue capability.

Advanced planning includes availability of well-trained leadership for disaster situations.[35] Sorting or triage is performed most effectively by a clinician experienced in the care of burns, as doctors without such experience frequently overestimate the proportion of the body surface burned.[13,59] Expert triage may minimize the requirement for specialized burn beds[32] since moderate to severe burns, which are best cared for in specialized burn centers, seem to be fewer in numbers following severe fire disaster.[27,35] The French burn system, for example, incorporates this philosophy into a uniform triage system.[52]

Most disaster plans emphasize a restriction of treatment, at the site or in the emergency department/accident ward, to lifesaving measures and initial prioritization with early transfer to more sophisticated resources where reassessment can take place.[58] Delays in the dispersal of casualties may be avoided by prior planning, especially if international transfer of patients is envisioned.[31] Recent incidents involving mass burn casualties have demonstrated that the specific needs of severely burned victims demand a comprehensive plan that follows the guidelines of the Advanced Burn Life Support

(ABLS) course for initial care, assessment of burn size and depth, resuscitation, evaluation for other injuries, care of the burn wound, etc.[59]

Specific details for an incident command system that were developed for fighting forest fires in California, USA, are generally useful for organizing and implementing action for all fire and burn disasters, irregardless of size or complexity.[48] The essential figure is usually a firefighter, but other people may be involved.[60] When this system is adapted to the burns center or hospital environment it is called the Hospital Emergency Incident Command System (HEICS) and the design is compatible with the larger incident command structure.

All burn disaster response plans should include activation for explosions and industrial accidents, such as those that occur at petrochemical industries, foundries, and the like.[61] The preparation phase is characterized by mapping the industries at risk of potential flammable or toxic substances most frequently used in an area and which transit avenues are used for egress. This requires the collaboration of other experts such as engineers, chemists, physicists, toxicologists, etc., in order to coordinate all necessary data for potential fire disasters and effective disaster planning. A training phase should be carried out in close collaboration with agencies and people likely to be involved in self-protection, extinguishing of a fire, and rescue of burned victims. A didactic phase through organized meetings of volunteer personnel is required.[61] Burn centers and hospitals whose catchment area includes oil rigs or hazardous materials should plan for appropriate contingencies.[62]

A disaster plan may have to be tailored to meet the specific needs of an area or a site. In a fire disaster, the number of people involved may be so high that it is impossible to consider all victims for immediate transfer to existing specialized burn centers. Because of the limited number of beds available and because a disaster may occur some distance away,[35,63–65] the organization and establishment of a field hospital may be required. To be effective, a field hospital must have easy transport, rapid assembly, and the possibility of administering complete and effective treatment to patients. Multi-unit nomadic tents may offer the best facilities.[64,65] The reduced weights of these tents, their ease of packing, and their limited bulk represent considerable advantages, especially with regard to transportation and rapidity and simplicity of assembly. The modular composition means that their size can be adapted according to the effective needs of a disaster situation.[65] The organization and establishment of a field hospital must be based on a very precise predetermined plan that defines all the logistic and sanitary activities of a field hospital that are required to manage a disaster immediately and long term.[65] The United States Air Force Expeditionary Medical Support (EMEDS), a system of tents and equipment, from Michigan, the Carolinas and Kansas were used after hurricane Katrina to temporarily replace damaged medical facilities. The EMEDS can be transported on flatbeds with trucks or by large aircraft. Although it took some period of time to mobilize the EMEDS to the site and deploy them, the concept worked well and EMEDS could be valuable assets for a large scale fire/burn disaster.

Evacuation

Evacuation considerations depend on the number of victims and their conditions, identification of toxic substances, and other factors. Emergency transport of burned victims may be sporadic and *de novo* in a fire disaster, but more often it will involve medical rescue services such as fully equipped ambulances, helicopters, fixed wing aircraft, and water rescue craft. Most victims are transported by ground vehicles (ambulances, private vehicles, commandeered buses, trucks, etc.). For fire disasters that are up to 100 miles from medical facilities, the use of helicopter services that are fully equipped flying ambulances, often permanently based at hospitals and used exclusively for emergency purposes, are an invaluable mechanism for transport. Numerous factors have led to the creation and development worldwide of medical air rescue services and, in particular, to the widespread use of helicopter services.[66] Over 300 hospitals in the world have their own helicopter ambulances and fixed wing aircraft used exclusively for emergency transport.[66] The Italian model of helicopter rescue service is acquiring growing recognition.[66] The Italian medical evacuation is made through a single nationwide telephone number in Italy that connects qualified multilingual personnel, including physicians and other specialists, to local rescue services, hospitals, civil and military authorities, and other organizations involved in disaster relief. A sophisticated software program provides, in real time, all necessary information for rescue operations within a specific region, and if the need arises, for inter-regional coordination and transport.[66,67]

The main aim of a helicopter rescue service is to guarantee prompt arrival (maximum time 20 minutes) of a medical team specialized in resuscitation and provided with all the equipment normally available in a hospital intensive care unit. The necessary emergency therapy can be carried out on the spot or continued during transport of a patient. The transport is not necessarily to the nearest hospital, but to the hospital best equipped to receive a patient.[66,68] The communication coordination system (called emergency operations centers [EOCs] in United States' disaster systems), activated by the regional operative headquarters, coordinates transportation by ground, helicopter, or a fixed-wing aircraft for long-distance transport.

Under most circumstances, transportation must be carried out in coordination with other rescue organizations. The transport of a victim to the nearest hospital for more thorough assessment and lifesaving treatment (e.g. airway management) may occur pending possible placement in a specialized burn center. This phase is often difficult because of lack of beds for burned patients in a region, especially in the case of those requiring extensive care, and must be planned in the transportation phase of a disaster plan.[69]

Timing and coordination of transport of burned patients is critical[70] and delays may occur, especially if national or international transportation by air is envisioned, unless communication and cooperation are assured by prior agreements.[31] The personnel and material conditions, as well as the mode of transport, should be an integral part of every burn disaster plan. A burn team must consider the consequences of aeromedical transport in order to determine whether it is safe for a burned patient or what measures should be used in order to effect a safe transfer.[68,70,71] Burn casualties can best tolerate transfer on the day of the accident, so long as it does not take more than 60 minutes; and later transfers should take place by the end of the third or fourth post-burn day before sepsis can fully develop.[25] The result of an extensive traffic jam must be anticipated in a disaster plan since it may hinder the arrival of patients as well as physicians and staff who are not on duty, but who are inbound to staff or relieve current staff.[72] Long delays in transportation of patients have been the rule in most disasters.[35]

Facilities/surge capacity

Burned patients are best cared for in burn centers.[27] But the relative scarcity of specialized facilities and expertise for the treatment of extensive burns is of particular concern, such that involvement of distant burn centers may be anticipated following large disasters.[31] Even a moderate-sized disaster might fill all available burn beds and saturate the total burn capacity of a wide area. It is vital to plan for supporting hospitals in a primary inner circle and for the designated burn centers and tertiary hospitals in an outer circle to be included[20,21,35,69] (see Figure 5.4). Following very large disasters, optimal care of severely burned victims will be achieved only if distant burn centers are also involved.[73] Prior awareness of the location and capacity of specialized facilities will enhance the successful dispersal of casualties.[74]

The role played by specialized burn treatment units is significant.[25,27] Burn centers seldom plan to have low levels of occupancy that would enable them to accommodate mass burn casualties, so the emergency plan for a burn center must include emergency evacuation of existing burn, trauma, surgical, and other patients to make beds available for mass burn casualties. As a 'rule of thumb,' a burn center disaster plan should plan for expansion by one-half the number of burn beds or about 10–15 additional burn disaster patients.[27,75] The hospital must establish a control center (EOC, as part of the HEICS strategy),[20,27] discharge or move patients to alternate care, organize beds for the incoming mass casualties, and pull in extra staff, often without the knowledge of how many casualties to expect. Multiple injuries, including burns and inhalation injuries, may occur in mass casualties from explosions. A burn center should receive logistical support from the sponsoring hospital in order to provide the best treatment for a large number of burned casualties. Logistical support requires work from the hospital staff who are concerned with sterilization, pharmacy, medical and nursing care, radiological diagnosis, and intensive care.[72] Even little things, such as availability of urine dosimeters, are important!

Traditionally, hospitals have seen their role, during a burn disaster, as related to the medical management of patients admitted to them because of an incident. An expanded role has included sending teams of physicians and nurses to disaster scenes in order to aid in triage and medical management.[76,77] The role of a hospital in disaster management can be expanded further to include a strong focus on leadership within the medical component of a disaster. On-site medical management can be organized in one of two ways:

- via 'proceed-out teams' of physicians who go directly to the scene; or
- through medical direction given by radio to trained prehospital life support teams at the scene.[16]

Another responsibility that may be given to a hospital is the coordination with and medical guidance of the fire, rescue, police, and public safety components of a disaster response.[16] Few major hospitals have full comprehensive specialty services, including burn units. Sophisticated disaster plans should recognize such limitations and obtain prior consent for referral (comprehensive prearranged transfer agreements with burn centers, trauma centers, and other hospitals).[27,46] Within a hospital, the disaster plan must bring additional operating rooms online as needed for semi-urgent care of burned victims, while reserving one or two for lifesaving procedures that may be required. The goal is to match hospital resources with the needs of burned victims. In some cases, this will be driven by priorities; in others, a first-come-first-served basis will be installed. All elective admissions and all elective operative cases must be cancelled, immediately.

As an alternative to designated burn centers, patients with smaller burns may be managed in a general hospital without any particular facility for the management of burns.[78] In this case, a hospital disaster plan must be activated. The reception area and initial treatment area ought to be available for the majority of burned victims. Additional personnel should be summoned. A hospital is obliged to clear hospital beds, particularly on surgical wards and intensive care units, by transfer or discharge. If the expertise, supplies, and equipment are not adequate, secondary triage to adequate facilities and burn centers is necessary.

Personnel

Staffing is a basic requirement for the medical treatment during burn disasters. In the event of a large-scale disaster interrupting infrastructure, it must be assumed that personnel attrition will occur, and appropriate measures employed to compensate for staffing shortages. Advanced plans should be made for personnel recruitment from the community — pool staff, locums, reactivation of retired staff.

An overall disaster plan must ensure that a sufficient number of people have adequate training for initial resuscitation of burned victims. Often the medical and hospital staff who are willing to help have little experience in burn care. Training of personnel is rare, especially concerning communication links.[35] Guidance in preventive measures typically is absent, and disasters display the lack of training of personnel to cope with a tragedy.[35,79] Education concerning simple management of minor and moderate burns should be given on a broad basis to doctors and nurses outside of burn care facilities.[35] The Advanced Burn Life Support Course is an excellent tool for training such individuals.[59] Burn center staff must be available for advisory and consultation services by telephone or telex.[25] Today, some burn centers have telemedicine or televideo medicine capabilities which allows burn surgeons and knowledgeable burn personnel to view and consult on acutely burned patients. Such systems permit better decisions on which burned patients will be better served in the burn center and which can be reasonably cared for, locally. In addition, the camera and telemedicine brings remote or resource-poor environments into closer proximity with the burn center, often enabling consultation and follow-up for burned patients. Such a system was used following the Ufa train incident.[80] The burn center in Salt Lake City, Utah, United States uses televideography on a daily basis for advice and consultation as well as follow-up, saving the expense of unnecessary transfers and long-distance

travel for follow-up. A similar system is planned for Arizona, United States and will incorporate triage and distribution in times of disaster as well as a method of dissemination of basic knowledge of burn care throughout a vast area, including many rural and resource-poor environments. Expert triage is important, but healthcare professionals must be able to work effectively in primitive conditions together with other emergency helpers.[35] When admitting patients and rendering qualified specialized medical aid at a hospital, the participation of mixed physicians teams (surgeon, burn specialist, resuscitation, therapist, etc.) is advisable.

A plan must use personnel wisely and efficiently. Using a single caregiver, usually a nurse, with each patient is optimal. That person, then, stays with a burned patient through all of the initial steps of care and insures intravenous (IV) fluid administration, pain control, tetanus toxoid administration, airway maintenance, ventilation, and documentation.

Often the first thing that is asked by a burned patient is to contact relatives.[81] This task should be delegated to someone other than hands-on caregivers for the burn casualty, capable of understanding the burn injury and empathetic with relatives and friends. The handling of families, as well as mass media,[56,57] must be an integral part of every disaster plan. Major mass burn disasters, such as the Piper Alpha and Ramstein tragedies, involve the wounded and relatives from many countries.[62,81–83] Multilingual support personnel are essential under these circumstances.

Research on human behavior in critical situations has identified three different kinds of reaction: rational action, panic, and resignation. The two normal reactions when a way of escape is apparent are rational action and panic.[84] When positive action will lead to safety, resignation is a pathologic form of behavior. It is difficult to plan for the psychological reactions to a fire/burn disaster. The two main elements of this drama that have to be understood are the actual fire and the mass of people.[84] Nevertheless, experts with psychological training should be utilized for the development of psychological support for burn victims, their families and friends, rescue workers, and healthcare workers. Immediate sessions for debriefing of the rescue workers should be put in place.[1] Psychological support for healthcare workers will be necessary because of their high levels of stress and extended hours of work. The psychological support teams in the fire and burn disaster simulations can help a team rehearse the decisions that must be made in the care of large numbers of burn casualities so that the team is less likely to suffer emotional stress at the precise moment when technical skill and emotional equilibrium are most needed.[84]

Supplies/equipment

A disaster plan must be tailored to the supplies and equipment that are available. In resource-rich environments, commercial supplies and equipment may be stored and warehoused on or near the hospital or burn center. But 'just in time' management systems that move supplies and materials to the hospital as they are needed on a daily basis have decreased on-site supplies and equipment in favor of more cost-effective methods of having suppliers drop ship or furnish what is needed on a daily or very short-time delay basis. That means that as local resources are consumed more rapidly to care for the surge capacity of the burn disaster, resupply may not be able to keep up with the new local demand. Therefore, burn center and hospital disaster plans must be tailored to match the local supply system and knowledge of how to overcome the shortages in any system and speed up resupply is mandatory. Sometimes adoption of resource-poor environmental strategies may be necessary. For example, clean sheets may be torn into strips and used for bandages and various available topical antibiotics and creams may be substituted to the ideal commercial rolled gauze and topical antibiotic creams. Fiberoptic bronchoscopy may be useful in the early diagnosis of inhalation injury, but may not be available for use during a disaster.[72] An alternate plan for an individual hospital may be the need to transport some burn victims to facilities that have the capability of proper care due to the availability of appropriate equipment. That facility is usually a designated burn center. Problems in rendering aid in such extreme situations exemplify the necessity of having an organization with a separate department of catastrophe medicine.[3,35] A plan must assure that the management of individual patients will be optimal under a variety of organizational structures and supply capabilities. Compromises may be necessary in extreme circumstances, but the ideal is to develop a plan to avoid them whenever possible (i.e. patients with eyelid/facial burns are seen within 4 hours by an ophthalmic surgeon who has proper supplies; equipment or sufficient supplies and equipment are available to start physiotherapy within 48 hours).[78] Even when personnel are available, there may be a lack of specific materials. A practical kit for various procedures in the first few hours after severe burns is helpful.[85] It must incorporate the following basic features:[86]

- easy to transport to the scene of a disaster;
- easy to keep in good condition at a medical/surgical post;
- long-lasting;
- simple to use;
- robust and lightweight enough for air transport.

The contents of an emergency kit should be an integral part of a disaster preparation and be approved by burn experts on a planning committee. Preparing a kit that includes all the necessary supplies for initial care of burned patients is a significant investment of time and money to initiate and maintain. Having the kits available and stockpiled and kept up to date at a regionalized or centralized location (i.e. National Stockpile Center) would be more cost-effective and serve a wider need. Air dropping a kit was lifesaving for immediate surgical treatment and resuscitation of burned victims in remote areas without direct access to rescue teams or made up for deficiencies in medicines and medical supplies in hospitals that have admitted people with severe burns who were not immediately transferable to other hospitals.[87] Pre-positioned supplies were of significant benefit at Landstuhl Army Hospital during the Ramstein air disaster.

Education

An educational program must be based on a precise method that starts with analysis of a problem of health and safety and then encompasses epidemiological, behavioral, and educational diagnoses.[61] Health education and training programs assume particular importance in burn disaster planning. They must include the clinical, technical, and operational aspects of a disaster. Implementation of these plans must follow well-defined programs of teaching at schools, starting with primary school level, through education at civil defense courses, periodic refresher courses for physicians, nurses, volunteers, Red Cross/Crescent personnel, fire brigades, police, etc., in addition to periodic exercises with simulated fire disasters that involve the general population and local rescue forces.[67,88] Training methods may use brochures, stickers, coloring albums, posters, notices, and a variety of audiovisual means, particularly videotapes. Videotapes can recreate and simulate situations and propose actions for assistance to victims.[88] An interactive video using ordinary documentary film with educational elements can train a student in prevention as well as every element of burn care. Multimedia presentations improve a user's attention and achieve greater educational effectiveness than a usual mono-medium message; and they should be used in initial as well as refresher courses.[88]

Educational interventions to train healthcare providers for burn disasters must cover a broad range of topics; however, learning needs may vary by practice setting, work experience, and previous exposure to disaster events. Therefore, 'one size does not fit all,' and continuing education programs (the most frequently utilized method of updating knowledge skills among the healthcare professionals) may need to be tailored to meet the unique learning needs of each audience.[89]

Exercising the plan

It is important to exercise a disaster plan through coordination of simulated disasters (see Figure 5.3) involving all of the relevant public safety agencies, prehospital ambulance providers, hospital-based personnel, and proceed-out teams.[16,40] As one team reported: 'The whole operation went very smoothly. This was partly because the staff had been through several "dummy runs" of a detailed civil accident procedure and partly because they had several hours to prepare for the first casualties to arrive'.[49] Entire systems must be tested in training programs so that they are made intelligible to the public, supported by management resources, implemented properly, and promulgated to all potential first rescue workers.[88]

Where current disaster plans had been well rehearsed, effective dispersal, immediate care, and secondary transfer of severely burned patients was efficient and resulted in good outcomes.[90] When the plans are not rehearsed and expert triage is not present at the disaster site, the burden of triage falls on the nearest hospital.[20,91] There is good evidence for developing an integrated disaster response system and for exercising that response system to prepare health care, disaster relief, and humanitarian aid workers for a proper reaction to these rare events. Mass casualty training is common in countries with adequate public health and medical infrastructure and adequate resources. There is little such coordination, planning, exercises or response in many resource-poor countries.

Mitigation

When natural disasters occur in a geographic distribution and in a predictable but chaotic pattern, another public health tenet, mitigation, will lessen the impact of the events. Planning aimed at mitigating the effects on people (in terms of suffering,

TABLE 5.5 FACTORS THAT INFLUENCE THE EVOLUTION OF A DISASTER

The unpredictability of when disasters occur
The moment of a disaster (day/night, festivity, etc.)
The characteristics of a disaster (explosion, collapse of building, production of toxic gases and fumes, forest fire, etc.)
The area where a disaster occurs (city, non-urban area, accessibility, presence of material suitable for relief operations, etc.)
The type of building involved (civil dwelling, hotel, office, hospital, etc.)
The number of people injured and the type of trauma
The population's degree of preparedness to manage a disaster situation
From Masellis M, Ferrara MM, Gunn SWA. Fire Disaster and Burn Disaster: planning and management. Ann Burns Fire Disasters 1999; 12(2):67–82.[3]

disability, and risk to life) must be related to a more complete evaluation of involved damage.[3] The operational rescue plan must be developed along three lines: immediate care, medical rescue within 3 hours, and use of specific equipment and means for the rescue of burned patients. Factors that influence the evolution of a disaster are shown in Table 5.5.[3]

The disaster response

The overall disaster response combines the public health reaction providing for the basic needs of the population impacted, but not burned to dealing with the dead, as well as supplying the medical response to individual burned patients. The initial effort is to get the right patient to the right place at the right time with the right treatment, no matter how limited the resources may be. The first steps of that process are to triage patients appropriately (burned victims to burn centers in particular) and apply initial lifesaving treatment according to the resources available.

Triage

Triage, the sorting out and classification of casualties of war or other disasters, traditionally into three categories, to determine priority of need and proper place of treatment, is an important concept. Burn disasters are no exception. Triage for these events must be adjusted to accommodate the circumstances in which the burn disaster occurs. Initial triage for the Rhode Island night club fire in the United States occurring in February 2003 was set up at an inn across from the night club from which ambulances and helicopters began to ferry people.[20] The injured patients exceeded the capacity of the regional trauma center, and ultimately 15 area hospital facilities assisted in treating the 215 patients evaluated.[21] The Bali burn disaster resulted in the transfer of patients out of Indonesia and into Australia for treatment. Burns occurring from explosions in Iraq frequently overwhelm the very limited resources of the local hospitals and if Coalition military medical personnel have the capacity for assistance or transport, these patients may be treated in military hospitals or in neighboring countries.[10] If not, the severely limited resources result in minimal treatment and a poor outlook for patient survival.

The specifics of triage, therefore, depend on the location of the disaster, the accessibility of the area, the resources of the country, and the possibility of evacuation. Triage is always dependent on resources available. Therefore, it is helpful to consider triage for a burn disaster occurring in three distinct settings:

- A developed country with good medical infrastructure, communication, and disaster planning.
- A response occurring in a remote and/or severely resource-poor situation.
- A military supported response.

These three considerations illustrate that resources dictate the number and condition of patients that will be treated aggressively and those that will receive palliative care (expectant), etc.

Triage in a resource-rich environment

Triage ought to be conducted in a simple, straightforward, and experienced manner. Triage should be prognostic with a view toward singling out those among the burned who are likely to survive.[25] The two most important aspects of triage have to do with who will perform triage and where. The initial triage will most likely be at the site of a burn disaster by bystanders followed shortly thereafter by other first responders. The triage area is an important consideration. Because of the nature of some burn disasters, it is important to establish triage stations somewhat removed from an immediate scene.[16] This would be in response to hazards to the rescue and triage personnel such as bomb threats and potential explosions, interference by a crowd, or simply the fact that better facilities for triage are nearby and available. A safe triage area must be secured so that additional burn victims are not created because of lack of scene safety. The lobby of a hotel might serve as a good triage area, since it has good access and egress, appropriate space to work, and serves as a known location to all rescue workers and medical personnel.[20] Sorting should, ideally, be performed at the site by an expert in burns.[13,84,92] Expert triage may minimize the requirement for specialized burn beds.[31] Few casualties with burn wounds of 30–70% TBSA (14% of those admitted) were encountered following fire disaster.[31] Since bed availability in specialized centers is limited, it is clear that accurate triage is essential.[31] With lack of sophistication at the scene, burn victims may be taken to the nearest hospital emergency department or accident ward for triage[16] before they are transported to tertiary verified burn centers.[16,58,83,84,93–95] The rapid evacuation of casualties to nearby hospitals is a realistic aim for all but the most isolated locations, aided by the fact that most burn victims are themselves initially mobile and cooperative[50] (see Figure 5.4).

The organization of salvage work is affected by the number of casualties, the seriousness of their injuries, and the general conditions of a disaster.[25] The actual triage of patients will be influenced not only by the total number of casualties and bed availability but also by such factors as depth and locations of wounds, complications such as inhalation injury, and extremes of age.[31,52] With effective triage, the demand for care in a specialized burn center can be minimized for small minor burns. In the case of the Ramstein air disaster, the triage sites formed *de novo* where large numbers of patients were encountered, medical personnel congregated naturally, and supplies could be obtained for initial resuscitation. The patients were then carried a short distance to staging areas for helicopter pick up or for ambulance or bus loading. In the Ramstein disaster, complete triage on the scene was not possible. The triage response of emergency services at the air base was criticized,[35,82,83] mainly because most of the victims were transported by a 'load and go' system to nearby hospitals who were use to patients being treated in the prehospital setting by trained anesthesiologists.

Patients must be triaged into categories for systematic referral to appropriate facilities. The triage category is based on the severity of injury and the potential for salvage. The overall goal is to do the most good for the most people. In general, when resources are unlimited and a disaster plan incorporates additional resources, even the most severely injured burn victim will receive optimal care if the triage is accomplished in the most favorable manner. Where resources are limited, triage may require a method for selecting casualties on a true priority basis. It may mean developing an expectant category for those so severely injured that they are not likely to survive (Figure 5.5).

The problem of triage can be simplified and facilitated by a flexible adaptation of certain formulas. The gravity of burns can be expressed in terms of the extent of TBSA burned and age of the patient. In Czechoslovakia, the sum of age and extent of burn that is greater than 90 has established an empirical 50% chance of survival. By flexibly bringing this number up or down, depending on the overall situation, one can extend or narrow the number of burn casualties who ought to be transported first.[25] Immediate triage is essential in the presence of large numbers of burned patients. It has been observed that if a long period elapses before rescue teams can start triage and resuscitation, most of the severely injured die and many of the initially moderately injured develop serious complications.[35] Triage may identify five important groups for victims of burn disasters[13,59] (Table 5.6).

Field triage in a large-scale disaster, catastrophe or resource-poor environment

The Ural mountain train-gas pipeline explosion (Ufa train disaster) was a classic example of the need for field triage and secondary triage. During the initial stages following the Ufa train accident, victims were evacuated to nearby settlements where first aid was rendered, aseptic bandages placed, and fluid resuscitation started. During the second stage, victims were evacuated by medical vehicles and helicopters to Ufa and Techelyabinsk. Total evacuation took 16 hours and 45 minutes, and 806 people were admitted to hospitals and burn centers.[22] Helicopters from a nearby military training base airlifted survivors to hospitals in the regional cities of Ufa, Asha, Gorky, and Chelyabinsk. Aeroflot organized a series of special flights, evacuating 160 of the most badly burned, including 37 children, to hospitals in Moscow.[93,94] In the Ramstein air disaster, rapid initial transport to supporting hospitals was instituted, but further transport to designated hospitals and burn centers was not thought to have been carried out properly. The result was that some hospitals and burn centers were overloaded with patients while nearby hospitals and burn centers did not get any patients at all.[35,82,83] Secondary or tertiary transfers

Age/years	Burn size (% TBSA)									
	1–10%	11–20%	21–30%	31–40%	41–50%	51–60%	61–70%	71–80%	81–90%	91+%
0.1–1.99	High	High	Medium	Medium	Medium	Medium	Low	Low	Low	Expectant
2–4.99	Outpatient	High	High	High	Medium	Medium	Medium	Low	Low	Low
5–19.9	Outpatient	High	High	High	Medium	Medium	Medium	Medium	Medium	Low
20–29.9	Outpatient	High	High	Medium	Medium	Medium	Medium	Medium	Low	Low
30–39.9	Outpatient	High	High	Medium	Medium	Medium	Medium	Medium	Low	Low
40–49.9	Outpatient	High	High	Medium	Medium	Medium	Medium	Low	Low	Low
50–59.9	Outpatient	High	High	Medium	Medium	Medium	Low	Low	Expectant	Expectant
60–69.9	High	High	Medium	Medium	Medium	Low	Low	Low	Expectant	Expectant
70+	High	Medium	Medium	Low	Low	Expectant	Expectant	Expectant	Expectant	Expectant

Outpatient: survival and good outcome expected without requiring initial admission; **High** benefit/resource: survival and good outcome expected (survival ≥ 90%) with limited/short term, initial admission and resource allocation (length of stay ≥14 days, one or two surgical procedures); **Medium** benefit resource: survival and good outcome likely (survival >50%) with aggressive care and comprehensive resource allocation, including initial admission (≥14 days), resuscitation, multiple operations; **Low** benefit-resource: survival and good outcome <50% even with long-term, aggressive treatment and resource allocation; **Expectant:** survival <10% even with unlimited, aggressive treatment. CAVEAT: this is intended only for mass burn casualty disasters where responders are overwhelmed and transfer possibilities are insufficient to meet needs.

Age/TBSA Survival Grid/Table is based on national data on survival and length of stay: adopted from the *Journal of Burn Care and Research* and used with their permission and the permission of the original author, Jeffrey R. Saffle MD, Director, Intermountain Burn Center, Salt Lake City, Utah.

Fig. 5.5 Triage decision table of benefit-to-resource ratio based on patient age and total burn size. (From Gamelli RL, Purdue GF, Greenhalgh DG, et al. Disaster management and the ABA plan. J Burn Care Rehabil 2005; 26(2):183–191).[27]

TABLE 5.6 TRIAGE CRITERIA AND CARE PLANS

Triage criteria	Care plan
Minor burns/non-critical sites: <10% TBSA for children <20% TBSA for adults	Dress wounds; tetanus prophylaxis; outpatient care
Minor burns/critical sites (hands, face, perineum)	Admit, early operations, special wound care, short hospital stay
20–60% TBSA burned	Requires intravenous fluids/careful monitoring; burn unit trained personnel
Extensive burns (>60% TBSA burned); inhalation injury/associated trauma; associated medical illnesses	Mortality high; may be placed in expectant category; pain medication; psychological support
Minor burns; inhalation injury; associated injuries	Administer oxygen; measure carboxyhemoglobin; + or – intubate; ventilate; care of associated injuries

Griffiths RW. Management of multiple casualties with Burns. Br Med J 1985; 291:917–918.[13]

could have relieved the problem. The result of good secondary triage is that none of the institutions will be overly taxed in providing disaster response; this will allow uninterrupted care of all patients, including the patients who are already in a facility.

Once patients are re-triaged to a specialty burn center, a surgeon directing a major disaster plan may not be able to personally see and assign priorities to a large number of patients because the true priority cannot be assigned until the last patient has arrived. Therefore, a first-come-first-served policy may be effective, reserving some resources for severe emergency problems. The better the prehospital communications the less likely unnecessary overload or misappropriation of resources will occur. To reexamine each of the patients thoroughly by removing all dressings is distressing for the patients and time-consuming for surgeons. Surgeons, therefore, may make hurried and incomplete examinations from which some minor mistakes may result. Further, the senior surgeon directing the surgical management of a major accident should stay out of the operating theater, freeing himself of all routine commitments for the day until the last patient has left the operating theater.[46] The senior surgeon must, however, keep control of the surgical needs of the patients, interface with relatives, and arrange for transfers of patients to other hospitals if an overload occurs in the receiving hospital and also to eventually transfer patients closer to their homes when their care can be directed safely and appropriately from a hospital closer to home (see Figure 5.4).

Forty-seven patients from the Ramstein air disaster were re-triaged at the Homburg-Saar trauma center using Plan A (natural disasters, fires and explosions/departments of surgery, anesthesia, and radiology), Level II (20–50 victims, activates additional staff and an executive team of department chairs) of their hospital disaster plan. Forty-two patients arrived together on a bus less than 1 hour after the crash and activated the main secondary triage. Secondary triage took place in the triage zone of the trauma center by six emergency room shock teams. Twenty-four victims had deep dermal or full-thickness burns up to 90%. Eleven had additional trauma. Twenty-two

were classified second priority and 8 with minor injuries went home after first aid treatment in the outpatient department. Patients were prepared for transfer to nearby hospitals; but this proved to be unnecessary. Four intensive care units were reinforced with additional staff. Six burned victims were transferred by helicopter to German and American burn centers during the following 48 hours. After discussion with burn center physicians, 5 patients with severe injuries (burns in combination with other injuries) were not transferred and expired of multiple organ failure.[83] A thorough burn disaster plan addresses the contingency of disproportions between capacities and facilities as well as the ethical problems in mass burn disasters.[24,96] Secondary triage or tertiary triage may occur when burn victims can be repatriated to their domestic hospitals. Eleven of the 22 hospitalized patients at the Homburg trauma center following the Ramstein air disaster were transferred to their domestic hospitals.

Medical response

A disaster plan is especially important for burned patients; and thus, it may be helpful to illustrate the operation of such plans through examples from actual major burn disasters. Most burn disasters and burn casualties occur in more urban or at least populated areas.[35,64,72,79,83,84,97] The Ural train-gas pipeline catastrophe was an exception.[22,93,95,98–100] Thus, the arrival of the first casualty will usually occur shortly after an incident; and the flow thereafter will be proportional to the number of casualties, the distance of the incident from the receiving facilities, the ease of triage, and the transportation available. The aim of all health workers concerned with mass burns is to give each burned patient the same care they would receive if they were the only patient burned and to save and cure as many of those afflicted as possible.[25] There may be overriding conditions that may make this impossible. It is imperative when this situation occurs that a reassessment of secondary triage to other burn care facilities be entertained. The operation of a rescue plan must take into account the types, kinds, and numbers of burn victims and the type of intervention required.[3]

Putting the disaster plan into action

Triage, communication, treatment, staffing, supply, and transport are the basic problems that confront healthcare workers caring for mass burns. Immediate care is usually delivered by people on the scene of a disaster — relatives, friends, and passersby — people who may have witnessed the disaster or people who have arrived immediately at the scene. Their help is an automatic reaction derived from affection, friendship, or a spirit of human solidarity.[3] In the case of burn disasters, the first responders must know how to approach a fire, how to enter a burning building that may be full of smoke or toxic fumes, how to rescue a person whose clothes are on fire, how to treat burn wounds initially and associated trauma immediately, and how to provide medical relief.[1] One of the most troublesome confounding problems is establishing the number of casualties and the size of their burns.

Often the major management problem is a lack of information from the site of the accident.[58] The focus of patient assessment and care responsibilities shifts from hospitals to the scene of a disaster where triage, evaluations, and medical management of multiple casualties occur.[16,101] Burn disaster activities should all be coordinated centrally through one resource center utilizing a centralized communication hub with central medical emergency direction capabilities (called EOCs in the United States) (see Table 5.4).

On-scene patient management is generally organized in two distinct phases: patient triage and ambulance staging.[16] On-scene management, when organized and conducted properly, allows for controlled treatment of patients, optimal allocation of resources, and maximization of the utility of these resources for patients.[102] Guidelines for immediate care of burn victims are shown in Table 5.7.

Organized relief refers to the mobilization of all civil defense and military forces that are ready to intervene in the event of a burn disaster.[49–51] These forces arrive at the scene of an accident as rapidly as possible, but usually not within the first 3 hours. They are equipped with the necessary means and structures to enable them to perform their rescue action during the first 48–72 hours after a disaster until all the people have been evacuated.[3] These forces are trained to manage the general details of fire disasters. Special units are composed of personnel trained in the emergency care of severely burned patients and equipped with specific means and materials. These units should be in charge of preliminary triage, preparing a preliminary evacuation plan, contacting dispatching stations, selecting means of transport, organizing first aid posts, and clearing the area of the dead.[3]

All assistance to patients who have been exposed to fire and have extensive burns or inhalation injury must be specific, precise, considerate, and timely.[88] Using an established Burns Mass Disaster plan enabled improved mortality for 10 badly burned victims that were airlifted to a burns center, 1000 kilometers away in the Miri Bank explosion.[103]

Control/communications center

A region-wide disaster network should be developed, linking the communications of multiple hospitals so that each could receive all communications relevant to a disaster from the central communications center. Air and ground transportation units would be included in the link. This requires rigid communications discipline in order to ensure that only pertinent voice communication is transmitted. Priority triage of victims can be accomplished by radio contact between central communication physicians and referring physicians in local hospitals. Through this system, secondary patient triage, hospital notification, and medical control of patients coming from a disaster, as well as mobilization of ground and aeromedical transportation, can be affected. Burned patients can be secondarily transferred to burn centers with available beds, equipment, and personnel so that optimal care can be delivered to each patient.

Accounting for patients is the main function of the control/communication center after initial communications between a disaster scene and facilities have diminished. Transmittal of pertinent information regarding the condition of those patients being transferred from one facility to another tertiary care facility is important. Equally important is to accurately account for the dead. This information is crucial for handling families and friends. Appropriate communication to the media is an issue of public trust, but must follow approved public relations protocols.[56] A central data bank of patient information, including patient's pictures, may be helpful for directing relatives and friends to the correct facility. Preserving patient confidentiality versus their identity must be balanced.

Treatment

Initial care: details of the initial and continuing treatment of burned patients is the prerogative of other chapters in this textbook. A burn disaster scenario simply emphasizes the importance of the ABCs. The first order of treatment is to ensure an adequate airway and ventilation for each burned victim. This is most often a problem in patients with inhalation injury or mechanical trauma to the face, neck, or chest. Patients with respiratory problems must be identified immediately at the disaster scene and those with inhalation injuries must be noted very early in order to reduce mortality and morbidity.[78] Intubation and ventilation may be required at the scene or at any time thereafter for inadequate airway or breathing. Firemen are usually the best-trained rescue personnel and are capable of initiating care to burned victims. The kind of assistance provided by the first rescuers is of primary importance

TABLE 5.7 GUIDELINES FOR IMMEDIATE CARE OF BURN VICTIMS[88]
Self-control
Self-protection
Qualitative assessment of burns
Quantitative assessment of a patient's burns
Intravenous fluid therapy
Analgesic therapy
Bladder catheterization
Pressure-relieving incisions (escharotomy)
Reexamination of patient
Hospital (burn center) transfer
From Masellis ML. Management of mass burn casualties in disasters. Ann Medit Burns Club 1988; 1:155–159.[88]

for the prognosis of casualties. First responders must carry out the first triage of urgent cases, taking into consideration a high number of poly-traumatized patients. They must also initiate all medical and surgical procedures necessary for preliminary resuscitative therapy and initial local treatment of burns.[3]

Patients with all but minor burns should receive prompt fluid replacement in order to counteract the loss of protein-rich fluid into interstitial tissues.[13] In the Ufa train disaster, first aid was rendered to victims at the site of the accident by local inhabitants and the medical staff of hospitals located in nearby settlements. Within 12 hours, 25 teams of emergency first aid personnel from the city of Ufa and civil defense medical brigades provided additional care. Effective early management extends the time available for dispersal of casualties.[31] The two fundamental conditions for prognosis are the time interval between the accident and commencement of infusion therapy and the quality of therapy administered.[104] Effective fluid therapy during the first 24 hours provides an interval in which transfer of patients may be organized.[31] Fluid therapy should be based on the simplest, most expedient effective way of treating a problem. The extent of a burn should be assessed in terms of the percentage of the TBSA using the rule of nines[59] or the patient's hand (fingers together) as representing 1%.[13] In the enormous gas explosion in Belgium in 2004 depth of burn was determined with the assistance of laser Doppler imaging and a newly developed color-coded Lund and Browder chart adapted daily and correlated with daily digital photography. This was helpful in planning fluid resuscitation, wound care, and operative intervention.[105] The sum of the partial-thickness and full-thickness burns is used when calculating fluid requirements. The Baxter–Shires formula of 4 ml Ringer's lactate/kg body weight/ 1% TBSA second- and third-degree burn/24 hours is an effective estimate and should be started within half an hour for adults with burns greater than 20% TBSA, for children with burns greater than 10% TBSA, and patients up to the age of 4 years with burns greater than 5% TBSA. Diuresis at 0.5–0.7 mL/kg/h should be maintained.[25] The substitution of IV resuscitation by enteral therapy is possible for small burns.[25] No colloids should be administered for the first 24 hours. (Additional information on fluid resuscitation can be found in Chapter 8.)

Junior staff can set up IV infusion, administer analgesics, obtain baseline blood samples and radiographs, arrange photographic documentation, begin monitoring fluid balance, and prepare chronological documentation.[13] Adequate resuscitation was the key to a better survival rate among similar groups of patients whose medical treatment was otherwise the same in two burn units in Spain.[35,106] The Ufa train disaster provided an example of the consequences of a long delay in fluid resuscitation.[35]

Initially, burned areas should be simply covered with a clean sheet or clean transparent conforming plastic sheets of material. If a patient must remain for a period before triage, the initial facility may wish to cover a wound with dressings impregnated with silver sulfadiazine or some other effective topical agent and gauze to hold the creams/ointment in place for the transfer. The efficient work of a nursing staff in treating patients with topical antimicrobials before an exact diagnosis of depth and extent of burns is known wastes time, because the wounds will need to be uncovered in order to allow the receiving medical staff to confirm the diagnosis of size and depth of burn.[72] One must exercise judgment as to how long to leave a burn wound unprotected from topical antimicrobials so that a physician can evaluate the burn wound. Physicians may well be consumed in lifesaving measures for other burned victims for some extended period. The same could be said for the need for escharotomies. Detailed assessment of casualties will obviously take some time. Such assessment is, therefore, only practical in a clinical environment where personnel and facilities are available for management of fluid therapy and for treatment of urgent complications.[31] Early debridement of burn tissue is not necessary initially, but can be carried out within the first 5 days post burn once a patient has reached an appropriate facility. The management of burns should involve debridement and wound coverage as soon as possible.[72] However, this is a function of the tertiary receiving hospital/burn center and should only be considered as part of the eventual care of the patient, not the initial resuscitation.

Methods of treatment must be modified, and medications must be standardized and reduced to basics.[35] Initially, no prophylactic antibiotics are administered, but prophylaxis against stress ulcers should be given. Although antibiotics are not used in many burn centers for prophylaxis because of the development of resistant organisms,[107] in a situation where a large number of patients with burns arrive at a general hospital, which would be unlikely to have an endogenous supply of resistant organisms (or the capability of early detection of burn wound sepsis), it would seem advisable to use prophylaxis.[78]

Psychological considerations

An effort should be made to reduce psychological interference that might hinder the organization of rescue work and burn care. Initially, people must trust their rescue workers and be guided by them. This assists in the escape from disaster and lessens the psychological impact. The best psychological first aid is to assist and organize escape from a disaster. During and immediately after a fire/burn disaster, civic education in schools, by mass media and through other means of communication, may help lessen the psychological impact of a disaster on a community. Psychological support must be tailored to the situation of a fire/burn disaster. As in the case of the Ramstein air disaster, the audience at the air show was family-oriented with many school children witnessing the holocaust and experiencing the panic of the event. Therefore, great energy was spent in psychological debriefs in the schools where the children attended and in other public forums.

Patients admitted to a hospital should have supportive psychological counseling given early, throughout their hospital stay, and for follow-up after discharge in order to minimize the late emotional disturbances.[78] Professionally trained teams of experienced rescue workers help to control emotional problems such as panic caused by a fire disaster.[58] Most of these patients will have major emotional problems.[62,81] They are agitated, anxious, very dependent, and out of action. Their faces are not looking good. They have seen their friends go up in flames. Some survivors had heard hundreds of men screaming that they were going to die. Psychologists and social workers were drafted to offer emotional and practical help to survivors and brief families, as well as support the nurses looking after them.[81] It is only later, as the drama of the first days dies down, that nurses start to feel the strain. Talking among the healthcare givers about an incident helps.[81] Psychological support for victims, relatives, rescuers, and health workers must not be forgotten.[108] Advisors from Bradford and Kent, who had developed special services to help the bereaved in response to the Bradford fire and the Zeebrugge ferry disasters, were available to help.[81] Apart from the casualties themselves, the greatest concern was for the bereaved relatives, most of them with no body to grieve over and no ritual funeral rites to help them mourn. Many bereaved families were desperate to speak to people in the hospitals in order to find out all they could about missing relatives, now presumed dead.[81] Professionals must be available to help these people during and after a disaster. Psychological training must be given by expert psychoanalysts using group work techniques.[84]

Staffing

Initial staffing

Medical staff on duty must be able to undertake emergency care of initial victims prior to arrival of additional staff, as was the case with the Hipercor victims when traffic conditions delayed the arrival of off-duty burns and surgical staff as well as additional hospital staff to care for burned patients.[72] This can create an overwhelming task for healthcare providers. In the Ufa train disaster the average number of patients per healthcare team was 12–15.[22] Within a very short period, initial medical people (physicians, nurses, and members of voluntary organizations) must respond to victims of a burn disaster site. These medical personnel are supported by public and private organizations in the area, hospitals, casualty departments, clinics, fire brigades, and police; and they are coordinated by local authorities.[3]

When admitting patients and rendering qualified, specialized medical aid at a hospital, the participation of mixed physician teams is advisable.[22] The Disaster Medical Assistance Teams (DMATs), Burn Specialty Teams (BSTs), and United States Army Institute for Surgical Research Special Medical Augmentation Response Teams (SMART) employ this concept.[13,27,59,109] A senior surgeon should calculate the number of hours of operating room time required for proper care of all patients. A priority must be established for initial care and for any dressing changes and re-operations that are required. From that calculation, staffing requirements for the operating rooms, as well as for postoperative anesthetic care, intensive care, and ward care can be established. A senior surgeon should act as coordinator and get surgeons working as soon as patients arrive, keeping two operating theaters reserved for lifesaving operations.[46] Such calculations will drive the requirements for equipment and supplies and, with some foresight, drive the re-supply rate.

In the San Juanico tragedy, in which about 7000 people were injured, 2000 were hospitalized, 625 had severe burns, 300 died immediately, 250 died in hospitals later, and 60 000 were evacuated. Seven thousand (7000) people were involved in the rescue work during the first 48 hours. Of these, 200 were firefighters, 1000 were physicians, 1300 were paramedics, 1800 were nurses, 2000 were military personnel, and 750 were drivers and helicopter pilots.[35,79]

Volunteers will come! Assistance from volunteers may occur spontaneously from a crowd or community as it did at Ramstein and Piper Alpha or respond to a formal request as in the Ufa train disaster.

> You'll see the basic goodness in people when this sort of thing happens. Everyone rallies around. They don't think of payment. We had no problem with staffing, people just appeared. Although only a skeleton staff was on duty, the switchboard was flooded with nurses offering their services.[81]

Volunteers may need supervision and oversight to assure that they do not become overwhelmed or psychologically dysfunctional.

At Ramstein, the townspeople in Landstuhl heard the jet airplanes stop flying and many helicopters start flying and sensed a disaster. They responded to the Landstuhl Army Hospital and served as clean-up crews, traffic control, stretcher-bearers, and many other functions without being asked and often without any supervision. They just did the right things to help the effort.

Relief staffing

Relief personnel must replace or be assigned to the effort before the initial staff becomes exhausted. With so many serious cases, often the usual number of staff must be doubled. Usually there is no difficulty in finding them. Nurses often volunteer their services and the response is great.[81] A plastic surgeon who had been attending a burn conference heard news of the Piper Alpha disaster and along with six other burn specialists from all over the country came to help treat burns.[62] At Ramstein, off-duty hospital personnel augmented the initial staff and provided the relief staff needed to care for burned and mechanically traumatized victims.

Supply

Replenishing supplies used up in the care of many burned patients initially comes from warehousing facilities at or near the burn unit or hospital. Transport of additional supplies becomes crucial since the care of burned patients has high resources requirements for IV fluids, pain medications, topical antibiotics, and the like. If resupply cannot be affected, including 'just-in-time' supply systems, then there will be a decline in the care of burn victims or a need for secondary triage to a facility equipped and supplied to provide optimal care. Just-in-time supply systems may deplete usually resource-rich hospitals and burn centers, rendering them no different than a resource-poor environment.

Transportation

Coordination and mobilization of necessary transportation mechanisms (i.e. ground ambulance, aeromedical helicopter, and/or fixed-wing aeromedical transportation) and avoidance of calling in unneeded ambulances to a scene, which tends to confuse scene management, are essential.[16] The same control may be necessary for leapfrogging facilities to not overload one hospital at any given time.[111] Most patients will be transported by ground vehicles, particularly if a disaster is in an urban area. In the MGM Grand Hotel fire in Las Vegas, the ambulances lined up in appropriate staging areas controlled

TABLE 5.8 SPECIFIC PROTOCOL FOR PREPARING BURNED PATIENTS FOR MEDICAL EVACUATION

Cannulation of several venous routes of which one should be central if possible (followed by chest radiograph)
Monitoring of diuresis
Insertion of nasogastric tube
Sedation and/or analgesia
Cleansing of wounds
Tracheal intubation (if necessary)
Application of sanitary devices to prevent excessive heat loss

From Landiscina M, Bile L, Bollini C, et al. The burn patients and medically assisted helicopter transport. In: Masellis M, Gunn SWA, eds. The management of mass burn casualties and fire disasters. Dordrecht: Kluwer Academic; 1992; 251–252. With kind permission of Springer Science and Business Media.

by the on-scene fire command, while helicopters staged autonomous daring rescues. Remoteness of areas, traffic congestion, and the need for secondary triage may provide good reasons for aeromedical transfer. For a helicopter service in Italy, 2.5% of approximately 2500 flights concerned the secondary transport of burn victims while 0.5% provided direct medical assistance to burned patients at the scene of accidents.[112] Careful preparations by a hospital requesting transfers can be performed prior to air medical evacuation (Table 5.8). The size of a helicopter (or airplane) affects the optimal therapeutic access to various anatomical parts, monitoring of a patient, ventilatory assistance, and the number of patients that can be transported at one time. Larger helicopters with advanced instrumentation and excellent air speed effect the transportation during adverse meteorological conditions.[112]

Occasionally, the burn center may need to be evacuated, also. Such a plan was exercised at the Galveston Shriners' Hospital for Children during hurricane Katrina in August 2005. The patients, guardians, and staff were transferred to sister Shriners hospitals by medical jet. The repopulation of the hospital inpatients and acceptance of new acute burn referrals began approximately 40 hours after the all clear to return signal was given.[113]

After-action assessment

Disaster management must include the overall assessment of the consequences of a disaster. This assessment must be as accurate as possible whether it refers to a presumed or actual event.[3] Awareness of the scale and nature of past disasters may aid in the formulation of new plans for dealing with mass burn casualties in the future.[31] Uniform language and a framework to report and analyze disaster incidents is important and will contribute to evaluations that are more accurate.[16] The study of 10 major fire-related public transport aircraft accidents led to changes in cabin interior materials and potential filters that could provide satisfactory respiratory protection.[114] Modifications and revisions to disaster plans and disaster management can be effectively accomplished by initiating a mechanism of post-incident evaluation of disaster exercises and actual disaster responses. The central coordination of the response can be the focal point for this evaluation, which must include all of

the emergency medical services and the resources involved in a disaster response.[76]

There is no doubt that the extensive after-action reports of the MGM Grand Hotel fire followed closely by the Las Vegas Hilton fire changed fire safety and fire prevention of high-rise hotels and buildings, forever. This resulted in pressurized fire escape systems, fire control centers in hotels, hospitals, and public buildings, fire sprinkling systems, extensive smoke alarm systems, and evacuation notices in hotels, hospitals, and public buildings among other things.

All of the agencies and individuals involved in a burn disaster should be assembled routinely, immediately following incidents in order to critique the events while the facts are clear in the minds of the providers.[16] Information included in these sessions, although sometimes subjective, is usually quite candid and complete; and when combined with taped and written recordings of the incidents, it provides important lessons about the strengths and weaknesses of the management of the response.[16] Relevant lessons learned include the knowledge that all public service agencies are integrally involved in successful management of a burn disaster and must be kept informed of current burn disaster plans. A multi-agency mass disaster plan that had been formulated and rehearsed in preparation for the Pan American Games was used when a pilotless aircraft struck a hotel.[115] Such a critique depends on reliable information for successful management of the next disaster. From an in-depth review, individual facilities are able to effect changes such as directing online communications to an admitting office, preparing intensive care units and operating rooms, as well as establishing a person with authority to make decisions for the hospitals' ability to accept patients without questioning their fiscal resources. Major internal changes can be effected, based on data and corrections made, to allow a hospital to accept burn disaster victims at any hour that a disaster may occur. The practical benefit of these evaluation sessions is the fact that changes in disaster plans and operational management are made based on information learned during a disaster response critique.[16,109] Critiques often identify problems on notification of hospitals and burn centers concerning the nature and extent of injuries, as well as the number of patients they should expect. Organized relay of pertinent patient information to hospital staff or mobilization of appropriate physicians, specialists, and staff is key. Matching patients with specific injuries, such as burns, to facilities capable of treating these specific problems, such as burn centers, is the mark of a well-designed and effectively managed disaster plan. In addition, forensic information is obtained that may be useful for disaster planning as well as for industrial change.[115,116] Follow-on studies and after-action reports have helped structural and mechanical engineers understand the differences in conflagration destruction between modern integrated steel and glass and older concrete column and beam high-rise building fires.

Some important, but previously unknown, statistics have been generated from after-action reports. The total number of injured patients was more than six times higher and the number of casualties admitted to hospitals was nearly 20 times greater following outdoor disasters than indoor disasters.[35] The immediate death rate at the site was very high (74%) in indoor fires compared to outdoor disasters (35%), but the hospital death rate was lower following indoor disasters.[31,35] Sixty percent of burn victims of indoor disasters sustained burns covering less than 30% of their TBSA.[35] In a significant number of patients with very extensive burns (greater than 70% TBSA), they occurred after outdoor fires, while very few were admitted with extensive burns after indoor fires.[13] Those who failed to escape from indoor fires died rapidly from a combination of hypoxia and inhalation of poisonous compounds.[117,118] Such a mechanism was probably the initial cause of death in the Beverley Hills Supper Club fire, but the conflagration then destroyed the evidence by severely burning the dead as determined in the after-action reports. The after-action reports of the accidental release of chlorine toxic gas from a train tank car derailment showed that burn disaster planning could be exercised effectively for inhalation injuries.[119] The poor prognosis of burn victims with large burns sustained in mass disasters has been emphasized and is reflected in the high mortality following outdoor disasters.[15,31,106,120] The number of burn victims admitted with burns in the 30–70% TBSA range was consistently low, which is more important since patients with this burn size potentially obtain the greatest benefit from referral to a burn center.[27,31] In an indoor disaster of another kind, the MGM Grand Hotel fire in Las Vegas resulted in 300 hospital admissions for smoke inhalation, but no burn injuries.[121] After-action reports will allow analysis of the environmental impact of the disaster, the vulnerability of the territory, and the information, education, and participation of the population.[42] In emergencies, human behavior is a decisive factor in the creation of dangerous or harmful situations and it plays a basic role in the evolution of the effects of a disaster.[42] Retrospective studies are less helpful, but can direct future planning of burns mass disasters.[122]

The positive effect of a previous disaster on the preparedness of the people involved is substantial.[123] A disaster plan must incorporate details of disasters occurring in several scenarios. These plans may be unique to an individual area, but all should include preparations for explosions.[35,43,58,72,79,95,98,106,124] Particular procedures regarding both medical assistance and general behavior, and those that rescue workers have to perform, must include educational campaigns, refresher courses, and training sessions aimed at citizens of every social extraction starting at school age.[3] As an example, burn disaster from a forest fire would depend on the fire typology; and the variability depends on meteorological conditions.

Prior disasters and international responses to them underscore the need for a coordinated response to major burn disasters and the positive results of international cooperation.[22,125] The disasters in Armenia and Chernobyl emphasized to the Soviet Health Ministry officials the importance of having contingency plans made in advance of any accident. That experience led to the rapid triage and transport of victims from the accident site to medical centers in surrounding towns following the Ufa train disaster. The Soviet experience during the Ufa incident demonstrated that such an organization of public health services permitted the rendering of aid to the majority of victims in a rapid and appropriate time frame.[22] The Italian military have demonstrated their role in disaster relief.[50,51] Physicians and other staff members who are not familiar with burn care must have some means to assess the extent of burns and initiate therapy. Vitale et al. have prepared a clinical file and protocol for general doctors and for non-specialized hos-

pital physicians to assist burn patients.[104] Such a file should be incorporated into every disaster plan. Placing ideal or consensus disaster plans with descriptions of duties of various personnel on a government website for wide electronic distribution, either before (to help with local disaster planning) or during a disaster (to help poorly or non-trained personnel), is a necessary current procedure. Such documents should be simple and easy to understand and use. These recommendations may have national or international applications. The lessons learned provide a framework for burn disaster management, should a group be asked to provide assistance in the future.[125] All of these data are important in planning for the next burn disaster.

National response systems

There is good evidence for an integrated disaster response system and for exercising to prepare healthcare and humanitarian workers for response to rare events. Mass casuality training is common in countries with adequate public health, medical infrastructure, and resources. There is little such coordination, planning and response in many countries. Examples of national disaster plans serve as the template for other countries to develop or strengthen their national disaster response.

In 1986 the United States sent a team to Germany to study the Ramstein air disaster. This team was composed of members of the Department of Defense and the American Burn Association. The primary objective was to prepare an after-action report of lessons learned for the Department of Defense, separate, but in concert with that of the United States Air Force. The secondary, but equally important, objective was to study the German national system that had handled the Ramstein air crash so well and provide a model for the United States to incorporate a burn disaster component into the national disaster plan of the National Defense Medical System (NDMS).

The disaster plan involved dividing the United States into workable units which the American Burn Association had already begun through its regionalization program. The objective of the regionalization program was to allow burn centers in sections of the United States to work together to improve the daily care of burned patients. The initial emphasis was to provide a common language for burn centers and non-burn center emergency departments. The Advanced Burn Life Support course[59] was in its infancy, but provided the initial education required to improve the overall burn care in the United States. The onus was on individual burn centers and burn center directors to provide expertise in burn care and to promulgate burn education throughout their catchment area. Working together the burn centers and burn center directors in a given area would adopt mechanisms similar to the German national burn distribution system that would allow transport of the burned patient to the nearest available burn center. Expanding that concept was the initial development of the regional and national burn disaster plan.[69]

In the subsequent 20 years the United States and the American Burn Association have formulated a disaster management plan that, perhaps, can be used as a template for other countries' burn disaster plans and as an outline for international cooperation.[27,59] The key background facts are:

- Burn injuries are common in mass disasters and terrorist attacks.
- Burn center care is the most efficient and cost-effective care for burn injuries.
- Burn centers are not the same as trauma centers.
- Burn centers are a unique national resource.
- The American Burn Association has the capacity to be a key component in national disaster readiness for mass burn casualties.[27]

The definitions, supporting documentation, and key policy statements were published in 2005.[27,59] It defined a mass burn casualty disaster as any catastrophic event in which the number of burn victims exceeds the capacity of the local burn center to provide optimal burn care. It went on to define surge capacity as the capacity to handle up to 50% more than the normal maximum number of burn patients when there is a disaster. Primary triage is the triage that occurs at the disaster scene or at the emergency department of the first receiving hospital; however, primary triage should be handled according to local and state mass casualty disaster plans. By federal legislation, state disaster plans must incorporate burn centers into such plans. In the American Burn Association's primary triage policy, a burned patient should be triaged to a burn center within 24 hours of the incident. The disaster site incident commander should call the nearest verified burn center regarding available capability and alternate site burned center information. Furthermore, the American Burn Association's recommended triage decision diagram that is specific for burn casualty disasters is shown in the Figure 5.5.[27,59] Secondary triage is the transfer of burned patients from one burn center to another burn center when the first burn center reaches surge capacity using pre-established formal written transfer agreements. Secondary transfer is implemented within the first 48 hours of the incident by the burn center director when the burn center's surge capacity is reached.

The magnitude of the disaster will determine whether the involvement of local, state, or federal agencies is necessary. It is imperative that all elements work in concert. The disaster response in the United States is multi-tiered and ranked as follows:

- Local response disaster plan.
- State response disaster systems.
- National Disaster Medical System (NDMS):
  - Disaster Medical Assistance Teams (DMATs).
  - Burn Specialty Teams (BSTs).
- Military support to civil authorities:
  - United States Army Special Medical Augmentation Response Teams (SMARTs).

NDMS, a section of the Federal Emergency Management Agency (FEMA) in the Department of Homeland Security, manages and coordinates the federal medical response to major emergencies and federally declared disasters, including natural disasters, technological disasters, major transportation accidents, and acts of terrorism. NDMS can be activated by:

- The governor of an affected state may request a presidential declaration of disaster or emergency.
- A state health officer may request NDMS activation by the Department of Homeland Security.
- The Assistant Secretary of Defense for Health Affairs may request NDMS activation when military patient

levels exceed Department of Defense and Department of Veterans Affairs capabilities.
- At the request of the National Transportation Safety Board.[27]

NDMS has three functions:

- Medical response to the disaster site.
- Patient movement from the disaster area to unaffected areas of the nation (responsibility of the Department of Defense — global patient movement requirements center of the United States transportation command, Scott Air Force Base, Illinois).
- Definitive medical care in unaffected areas.

DMATs provide care during a disaster and are composed of physicians, nurses, technicians, and administrative support staff.[27] BSTs are specialized DMATs designed to be deployed along with a DMAT to provide burn expertise and augment existing local capabilities.[27,110] The team may assist the evaluation and resuscitation or help direct triage and transferred efforts. The BST is led by an American Burn Association member and is composed of approximately 15 burn experienced personnel, including the following:

- One surgeon (team leader).
- Six registered nurses.
- One anesthesia provider.
- One respiratory therapist.
- One administrative officer.
- Five support personnel selected based on mission requirements.[27]

Military support to civil authorities is the final tier in the nation's disaster response system. Among the many SMART team resources are the two United States Army, Institute of Surgical Research, Brooke Army Medical Center, Fort Sam Houston, Texas, burn SMART teams. The mission of the SMART teams is to provide short duration medical liaison to local, and state, federal and Department of Defense agencies responding to disasters, military–civilian cooperative actions, humanitarian assistance missions, weapons of mass destruction incidents, or chemical, biological, radiological, nuclear, or explosive incidents. These teams were particularly useful to the William Randolph Hearst Burn Center in New York following the September 11, 2001 disaster and the days beyond.[11]

Another aspect of the national burn disaster plan that was learned from the German system was a determination of bed availability. The American Burn Association's central office, working with United States Department of Health and Human Services Office of Public Health Emergency Preparedness established and maintained a real-time burn bed availability program for the nation. Initially, the American Burn Association worked with United States Army Institute of Surgical Research on a burn bed resource capability project. During times of crisis, a real-time burn bed resource capability reporting system is available. This model was further refined into a tracking system for the daily availability of burn beds for national emergencies,[53] which is currently surveilled electronically on a weekly basis by the Assistant Secretary of Defense for Health Affairs.[54]

The American Burn Association has added a number of action items on disaster preparedness to assist disaster planning at all levels.[27] And thus the United States finally has a comprehensive national disaster plan that incorporates burn disasters, is sophisticated, and serves as a model for other national disaster plans. The burn disaster subcommittee of the Committee on Organization and Delivery of Burn Care of the American Burn Association continuously updates this national burn disaster plan with recommendations. While the burn disaster plan speaks specifically to burn injuries, disasters with combined burn and trauma may require transfer to a trauma center for appropriate care. Clearly, when burn centers are overwhelmed, trauma centers serve as the next echelon of disaster relief.

Trauma systems

Burn centers should be integrated into large hospitals that are able to obtain assistance from several other specialty units from within the hospital.[72] Trauma centers must begin to fill the gap that exists between resources for emergency medical systems and a disaster response.[16] With leadership from trauma systems, meaningful planning can be accomplished among pre-hospital emergency medical systems, hospitals, and the public safety community.[16] This shift in disaster management responsibility from the public safety sector to the medical community incorporates advances made in the organization of emergency medical services.[16]

International applications

During the past two decades the response to burn disasters has improved greatly. The Ufa train disaster,[22,95] the Bali nightclub fire[14] and Operation Iraqi Freedom[10] have demonstrated that national boundaries no longer restrict burn disaster management. International cooperation during times of burn disasters, including repatriation of burn victims to their home country or to another country for optimal burn care, is a realistic expectation. Nations and non-governmental agencies look upon burn disasters as an opportunity to augment resource-poor countries and areas. Even though burn care is not optimal in all countries or even within parts of any country, the ability to move burned patients long distances, safely,[68,70,71] and transport assistance in the way of trained personnel, supplies, and equipment has changed the expectations for burn disaster management in burn disasters and humanitarian crises.[27,95]

Not all fire disasters result in mass burn casualties.[12] However, when a mass casualty event occurs involving a significant number of burned patients, an international response will be necessary to respond to the resources, materials, and manpower requirements,[22,93] and to compensate for the destruction of systems and resources and/or the inability for the system to surge further. This is likely to be the usual situation in resource-poor countries, where local infrastructure is absent or unable to respond to the needs of multiple burn victims. This was the case in Bali. Not only did Australia provide response teams to aid in the immediate aftermath but they also evacuated many of the critically ill patients to facilities in Australia for the advanced care they required.[14] The joint work of the Soviet and United States physicians during the Ufa train explosion demonstrated the efficacy of international cooperation. In planning for the care of victims of future disasters, such international cooperation should be illustrious.[125]

After needs were assessed in the Bashkir train-gas pipeline disaster, two pediatric burn teams were sent to assist in the care of burned children. These teams integrated with the host nation's medical personnel to care for the burn victims.[94,95] The United States team arrived 2 weeks after the disaster.[94] The cooperative effort allowed an increased frequency of dressings and more aggressive, rapid, and complete debridement of wounds. New techniques were introduced such as the use of a free hand skin graft knife, an air-driven dermatome, a skin graft mesher, and the use of dilute epinephrine solution for topical control of bleeding. Additional splints were made. One aspect of the burn care at Children's Hospital Nine was the role of parents providing much of the care of their children. They were present virtually all of the time on the wards. For those children whose parents were missing or children orphaned because of the disaster, others acted as surrogates. They fed the children, changed the beds and clothing, transported them around the hospitals, and received them directly from the dressing and operating rooms still partially anesthetized.[94,95] Soviet medical and paramedical staff slowly realized the large number of patients involved, the extent of their injuries, and the logistics of their care. The result was acceptance of medical help offered by burn care teams from the United States, United Kingdom, France, Israel, and Cuba, which illustrated the importance of having access to international medical support following disasters of such magnitude that local (regional and national) medical resources were exhausted.[35] Full and immediate use should be made of colleagues called out under a major disaster plan or they will disappear.

As of the United States team joined the burn surgeons at Children's Hospital Nine in caring for children from the Ufa train disaster, certain ideas and materials also necessarily came along. Project Hope provided over 7000 kg of badly needed medical supplies, drugs, and equipment, all of which arrived during the 2 weeks while the United States team was in the former Soviet Union. Such material aid permitted the Soviet surgeons to carry out usual therapy more effectively and the United States team to introduce some new ideas and techniques.[94] The Brooke Army team brought tons of much-needed supplies with them as well.[125] Authorities need to act on guidelines that provide for the stockpiling of specific mobilization materials in the most convenient location, the management of ambulance services, traffic control, the use of local and regional mass media, and the general means of transportation.[3] At Ramstein, contingency supplies specifically for a mass disaster were brought in and used for the care of burned patients.

A bonus lesson learned from after-action reporting was that burn teams working together could exchange new ideas and techniques with colleagues from other parts of the world who are not familiar with such techniques.[22,80] The effect of the combined efforts of the Soviet and United States Army medical teams who worked together at the largest hospital in the city of Ufa was that the team was able to effectively care for a large number of patients. Prior to this event, neither the hospital nor the Soviet physicians working at the hospital had had significant burn care experience.[22] Other follow-on studies directed comparative studies of the microbial spectrum of burn wounds and medicinal sensitivities of the microorganisms.[126]

References

1. Burkle FM. Mass casualty management of a large-scale bioterrorist event: an epidemiologic approach that shapes triage decisions. Emerg Med Clin N Am 2002; 20: 409–436.

2. Gunn SWA. Multilingual dictionary of disaster medicine and international relief. Dordrecht: Kluwer Academic; 1990.

3. Masellis M, Ferrara MM, Gunn SWA. Fire disaster and burn disaster: planning and management. Ann Burns Fire Disasters 1999; 12(2):67–82.

4. Gunn SWA. The scientific basis of disaster medicine. In: Masellis M, Gunn SWA, eds. The management of mass burn casualties and fire disasters: proceedings of the First International Conference on Burns and Fire Disasters. Dordrecht: Kluwer Academic; 1992: 13–18.

5. Noji E. The public health consequences of disasters. New York: Oxford University Press; 1997.

6. Layton TR, Elhauge ER. US fire catastrophes of the 20th century. J Burn Care Rehabil 1982; 3(1):21–28.

7. Hansen G. Timeline of the San Francisco earthquake: April 18–23, 1906. In: Chronology of the Great Earthquake, and the 1906–1907 graft investigations. Online. Available at: http://www.sfmuseum.net/hist/timeline.html.

8. Burkel FM. Complex humanitarian emergencies: I. Concept and participants. Pre-hospital Disaster Med. Jan–March 1995.

9. Burkel FM. Lessons learnt and future expectations of complex emergencies. Br Med J 1999; 319:14.

10. Cancio LC, Horvath EE, Barillo DJ, et al. Burn support for Operation Iraqi Freedom and related operations, 2003 to 2004. J Burn Care Rehabil 2005; 26(2):151–161.

11. Yurt RW, Bessy PQ, Bauer GJ, et al. A regional burn center's response to a disaster: September 11, 2001, and the days beyond. J Burn Care Rehabil 2005; 26(2):117–124.

12. Jordan MH, Hollowed KA, Turner DG, et al. The Pentagon attack of September 11, 2001: a burn center's experience. J Burn Care Rehabil 2005; 26(2):109–116.

13. Griffiths RW. Management of multiple casualties with burns. Br Med J 1985; 291:917–918.

14. Kennedy PJ, Haertsch PA, Maiitz PK. The Bali burn disaster: implications and lessons learned. J Burn Care Rehabil 2005; 26(2):125–131.

15. Barillo DJ. Planning for the burn disasters: what can we learn from 100 years of history? J Burn Care Res 2006; 27(2):S49.

16. Jacobs LM, Goody MM, Sinclair A. The role of a trauma center in disaster management. J Trauma 1983; 23:697–701.

17. Nakamori Y, Tanaka H, Oda J, et al. Burn injuries in the 1995 Hanshin-Awaji earthquake. Burns 1997; 23(4):319–322.

18. Benuska L, ed. Loma Prieta earthquake reconnaissance report. Earthquake Spectra 1990; 6(Suppl):1–448.

19. Hall JF. The January 17, 1994 Northridge, California. San Francisco. EQE International; 1994.

20. Harrington DT, Biffl WL, Cioffi WG. The Station nightclub fire. J Burn Care Rehabil 2005; 26(2):141–143.

21. Mahoney EJ, Harrington DT, Biffl WL, et al. Lessons learned from a nightclub fire: institutional disaster preparedness. J Trauma 2005; 58(3):487–491.

22. Kulyapin AV, Sakhautdinov VG, Temerbulatov VM, et al. Bashkiria train-gas pipeline disaster; a history of the joint USSR/USA collaboration. Burns 1990; 16(5):339–342.

23. Abend M, Bubke O, Hotop S, et al. Estimating medical resources required following a nuclear event. Comput Biol Med 1999; 29(6):407–421.

24. Kumar P, Jagetia GC. A review of triage and management of burns victims following a nuclear disaster. Burns 1994; 20(5):397–402.

25. Simko S. Reflections on the organization of mass burns treatment. Acta Chir Plast 1981; 23(3):197–200.

26. Sorensen B. Management of burns occurring as mass casualties after nuclear explosion. Burns 1979; 6:33–36.

27. Gamelli RL, Purdue GF, Greenhalgh DG, et al. Disaster management and the ABA plan. J Burn Care Rehabil 2005; 26(2):102–106.

28. Jordan MH, Mozingo DW, Gilbran NS, et al. Plenary session II: American Burn Association disaster readiness plan. J Burn Care Rehabil 2005; 26(2):183–191.

29. Coconut Grove Fire in Boston. Online. Available at: http://boston.about.com/cs/bostonnightlife/a/coconut_grove.htm

30. Cowan D, Kuenster J. To sleep with the angels : a story of a fire. Chicago: Ivan R. Dee; 1958.

31. Mackie DP, Koning HM. Fate of mass burn casualties; implications for disaster planning. Burns 1990; 16(3):203–206.

32. Barillo DJ, Cancio LC, Hutton BG, et al. Combat burn life support: a military burn-education program. J Burn Care Rehabil 2005; 26(2):162–165.

33. MMWR. Oct 14, 2005. Surveillance for injury and illness following hurricane Katrina 2005; Sept 8–25.

34. Braine T. In focus: was 2005 the year of natural disasters? Pan American Health Organization. Online. Available at: http://www.paho.org. Accessed Jan 1, 2006.

35. Arturson G. Analysis of severe fire disasters. In: Masellis M, Gunn SWA, eds. The management of mass burn casualties and fire disasters: proceedings of the First International Conference on Burns and Fire Disasters. Dordrecht: Kluwer Academic; 1992: 24–33.

36. Woolley WD, Smith PC, Fardell PJ, et al. The Stardust disco fire, Dublin 1981: studies of combustion products during simulation experiments. Fire Safety J 1984; 7:267.

37. Mozingo DW, Barillo DJ, Holcomb JB. The Pope Air Force base aircraft crash and burn disaster. J Burn Care Rehabil 2005; 26(2):132–140.

38. Cairns BA, Stiffler A, Price F, et al. Managing a combined burn trauma disaster in the post-9/11 world: lessons learned from the 2003 West Phamaceutical plant explosion. J Burn Care Rehabil 2005; 26(2):144–150.

39. Perez E, Thompson P. Natural hazards: causes and effects. Lesson 1 — Intro to natural disasters. Pre-Hospital Disaster Med 1994; 9(1):80–87.

40. Halstead MA. Fire drill in the operating room. Role playing as a learning tool. AORN J 1993; 58(4):697–706.

41. Costanzo S. Health education in disaster medicine. In: Masellis M, Gunn SWA, eds. The management of mass burn casualties and fire disasters: proceedings of the First International Conference on Burns and Fire Disasters. Dordrecht: Kluwer Academic; 1992:133–139.

42. McCollum ST. Lessons from the Dublin 1981 fire catastrophe. In: Masellis M, Gunn SWA, eds. The management of mass burn casualties and fire disasters: proceedings of the First International Conference on Burns and Fire Disasters. Dordrecht: Kluwer Academic; 1992:45–50.

43. Servais J. Fire emergency in a hospital. In: Masellis M, Gunn SWA, eds. The management of mass burn casualties and fire disasters: proceedings of the First International Conference on Burns and Fire Disasters. Dordrecht: Kluwer Academic; 1992:113–115.

44. Hill IR. An analysis of factors impeding passenger escape from aircraft fires. Avia Space Environ Med 1990; 61(3):261–265.

45. Trovato B. Fire services at a motor racing track. In: Masellis M, Gunn SWA, eds. The management of mass burn casualties and fire disasters: proceedings of the First International Conference on Burns and Fire Disasters. Dordrecht: Kluwer Academic; 1992:110–112.

46. Bliss AR. Major disaster planning. Br Med J 1984; 288:1433–1434.

47. Alley EE. Problems of search and rescue in disasters. In: Masellis M, Gunn SWA, eds. The management of mass burn casualties and fire disasters: proceedings of the First International Conference on Burns and Fire Disasters. Dordrecht: Kluwer Academic; 1992:175–176.

48. Firescope California. Fire Service Field Operations Guide, ICS 420–1. California: Incident Command System; April 1999.

49. Jenkins AL. Disaster planning. In: Jenkins AL, van de Leuv JH, eds. Emergency department organization and management 2nd edn. St Louis: Mosby; 1978:243–261.

50. Cuccinello G. The commitment of the Italian Army Medical Corps to relief of the civilian population in the event of public disasters. In: Masellis M, Gunn SWA, eds. The management of mass burn casualties and fire disasters: proceedings of the First International Conference on Burns and Fire Disasters. Dordrecht: Kluwer Academic; 1992:183–184.

51. Di Martino M. The organization of the Italian Army Medical Corps in relation to contributions to civil defense in the event of disasters. In: Masellis M, Gunn SWA, eds. The management of mass burn casualties and fire disasters: proceedings of the First International Conference on Burns and Fire Disasters. Dordrecht: Kluwer Academic; 1992:185–186.

52. Costagliola M, Laguerre J, Rouge D. Infobrul — the value of a telematic databank for burns and burns centers in the event of a disaster. In: Masellis M, Gunn SWA, eds. The management of mass burn casualties and fire disasters: proceedings of the First International Conference on Burns and Fire Disasters. Dordrecht: Kluwer Academic; 1992:190–194.

53. Barillo DJ, Jordan MJ, Joez RJ, et al. Tracking the daily availability of burn beds for national emergencies. J Burn Care Rehabil 2005; 26(2):174–182.

54. Secretary's Operations Center, Office of Emergency Operations and Security Programs, Office of Public Health and Emergency Preparedness, Department of Health and Human Services, 200 Independence Avenue, Washington, DC 20201, (202) 619–7800 [Office], (202) 619–7870 [Fax]

55. Martinelli G. The ARGO satellite system: a network for severe burns and disasters. In: Masellis M, Gunn SWA, eds. The management of mass burn casualties and fire disasters: proceedings of the First International Conference on Burns and Fire Disasters. Dordrecht: Kluwer Academic; 1992:253–259.

56. Melorio E. Mass media and serious emergencies. In: Masellis M, Gunn SWA, eds. The management of mass burn casualties and fire disasters: proceedings of the First International Conference on Burns and Fire Disasters. Dordrecht: Kluwer Academic; 1992; 301–304.

57. Mosca A, Amico M, Geraci V, et al. The role of the mass media burn prevention campaigns — psychological considerations. In: Masellis M, Gunn SWA, eds. The management of mass burn casualties and fire disasters: proceedings of the First International Conference on Burns and Fire Disasters. Dordrecht: Kluwer Academic; 1992:311–313.

58. Allister L, Hamilton GM. Cardowan coal mine explosion: experience of a mass burns event. Br Med J 1983; 287:403–405.

59. Sheridan RL, Palmieri T, Ahrenholz DH, et al. ABLS: advanced burn life support course. Chicago, IL: American Burn Association, 625 N. Michigan Avenue, Suite 2550, Chicago, IL, 60611, 2005; (312):642–9260.

60. Bovio G. Forest fires and the danger to firefighters. In: Masellis M, Gunn SWA, eds. The management of mass burn casualties and fire disasters: proceedings of the First International Conference on Burns and Fire Disasters. Dordrecht: Kluwer Academic; 1992:51–59.

61. Colombo D, Foti F, Volonte M, et al. Rescue of the burn patients and on-site medical assistance by a helicopter rescue service. In: Masellis M, Gunn SWA, eds. The management of mass burn casualties and fire disasters: proceedings of the First International Conference on Burns and Fire Disasters. Dordrecht: Kluwer Academic; 1992:249–250.

62. Rayner C. Offshore disaster on a fixed installation — the Piper Alpha disaster of 6 July 1988. In: Zellner PR, ed. Die Versorgung des Brandverletzten in Katastrophenfall. Darmstadt: Steinkopff Verlag; 1990:33–37.

63. Dioguardi D, Brienza E, Altacera M. The role of information sciences in the management of disasters. Ann Medit Burns Club 1988; 1:165–167.

64. Dioguardi D, Brienza E, Portincasa A, et al. A proposal for the strategic planning of medical services in the case of major fire disasters in the city of Bari. Ann Medit Burns Club 1989; 2(3):147–150.

65. Brienza E, Madami LM, Catalano F, et al. Organizational criteria for setting up a field hospital after a fire disaster. In: Masellis M, Gunn SWA, eds. The management of mass burn casualties and fire disasters: proceedings of the First International Conference on Burns and Fire Disasters. Dordrecht: Kluwer Academic; 1992:195–197.

66. Bianchi M, Minniti U. The use of helicopters in integrated rescue work and medical transport. In: Masellis M, Gunn SWA, eds. The management of mass burn casualties and fire disasters: proceedings of the First International Conference on Burns and Fire Disasters. Dordrecht: Kluwer Academic; 1992:246–248.

67. Meurant J. Communications in the prevention of natural and manmade disasters: the role of the national and international Red Cross and Red Crescent organizations. In: Masellis M, Gunn SWA, eds. The management of mass burn casualties and fire disasters: proceedings of the First International Conference on Burns and Fire Disasters. Dordrecht: Kluwer Academic; 1992:317–327.

68. Treat RC, Sirinek KR, Levine BA, et al. Air evacuation of thermally injured patients: principles of treatment and results. J Trauma 1980; 20(4):270–275.

69. Wachtel TL, Cowan ML, Reardon JD. Developing a regional and national burn disaster response. J Burn Care Rehabil 1989; 10(6):561–567.

70. Judkins KC. Aeromedical transfer of burned patients: a review with special reference to European civilian practice. Burns 1988; 14(3):171–179.

71. Heredero FXS. Physiopathology of burn disease during air evacuation. In: Masellis M, Gunn SWA, eds. The management of mass burn casualties and fire disasters: proceedings of the First International Conference on Burns and Fire Disasters. Dordrecht: Kluwer Academic; 1992:243–245.

72. Morrell PAG, Nasif FE, Domenech RP, et al. Burns caused by the terrorist bombing of the department store hipercor in Barcelona: Part 1. Burns 1990; 16(6):423–425.

73. Bayer M. Rampenbestrijiding verliep uitzonderlijk snel. Alert 1988; 10:2.

74. Editorial. Burn care facilities in the UK. Burns 1989; 15(3):183–186.

75. Barillo DJ. Burn disasters and mass casualty incidents. J Burn Care Rehabil 2005; 26(2):107–108.

76. Baker F. The management of mass casualty disasters. Top Emerg Med 1979; 1:149–157.

77. Orr S, Robinson W. The Hyatt disaster: two physicians' perspectives. J Emerg Nurs 1982;8: 6–11.

78. Duignan JP, McEntee GP, Scully B, et al. Report of a fire disaster — management of burns and complications. Irish Med J 1984; 77:8–10.

79. Arturson G. The tragedy of San Juanico — the most severe LPG disaster in history. Burns 1987; 13(2):87–102.

80. Remensynder JP, Astrozjnikova S, Bell L, et al. Progress in a Moscow children's burn unit: a joint Russian–American collaboration. Burns 1995; 21(5):323–335.

81. Hicks H. No stranger to disaster. Nurs Times 1988; 84(29):16–17.

82. Kossman T, Trentz O. Das Flugschau-Ungluck in Ramstein: Erfahrungbericht uber die Akutversorgung des Verletztenkontingents des Universitatsklinikums Homburg/Saar. In: Zellner PR, ed. Die Versorgung des Brandveniertzten in Katastrophenfall. Darmstadt: Steinkopff Verlag; 1990:79–83.

83. Kossmann T, Wittling I, Buhren V, et al. Transferred triage to a level 1 trauma center in a mass catastrophe of patients; many of them burns. Acta Chir Plast 1991; 33(3):145–150.

84. Amico M, Geraci V, Mosca A, et al. Psychological reactions in the disaster emergencies: hypotheses and operative guidelines. In: Masellis M, Gunn SWA, eds. The management of mass burn casualties and fire disasters: proceedings of the First International Conference on Burns and Fire Disasters. Dordrecht: Kluwer Academic; 1992:278–281.

85. Di Salvo L, Vitale R, Masellis M. Therapeutic kit and procedures for fluid resuscitation in disasters. In: Masellis M, Gunn SWA, eds. The management of mass burn casualties and fire disasters: proceedings of the First International Conference on Burns and Fire Disasters. Dordrecht: Kluwer Academic; 1992:231–238.

86. Caruso E, Crabai P, Donati L, et al. Ready-to-use emergency kit for treatment of severe burns: definition and specifications. In:

Masellis M, Gunn SWA, eds. The management of mass burn casualties and fire disasters: proceedings of the First International Conference on Burns and Fire Disasters. Dordrecht: Kluwer Academic; 1992:239–242.

87. Donati L. Campiglio GL, Garbin S, et al. Burn patients in major emergencies. The preparation of air-drop kits for emergency surgical-resuscitation use. Minerva Chir 1993; 48(9):479–483.

88. Masellis ML. Management of mass burn casualties in disasters. Ann Medit Burns Club 1988; 1:155–159.

89. Wetta-Hall R, Jost G, Cusick-Jost J. Preparing for burn disasters, a statewide continuing education training initiative in Kansas: predictors of improved self-reported competence among participants. J Burn Care Res 2006; 27(2):S50.

90. Mackie DP, Hoekstra MJ, Baruchin AM. The Amsterdam air disaster — management and fate of casualties. Harefuah 1994; 126(8):484–485.

91. Ortenwall P, Sager-Lund C, Nystrom J, et al. Disaster management lessons can be learned from the Gothenburg fire. Lakartidningen 2000; 97(13):1532–1539.

92. Barclay TL. Planning for mass burn casualties. In: Wood C, ed. Accident and emergency burns: lessons from the Bradford disaster. London: Royal Society of Medicine Services Roundtable No. 3. 1986:81–88.

93. Remensnyder JP, Ackroyd FP, Astrozjinikova S, et al. Burned children from the Bashkir train-gas pipeline disaster I. Acute management at Children's Hospital 9, Moscow. Burns 1990; 16(5):329–332.

94. Remensnyder JP, Ackroyd FP, Astrozjnikova S, et al. Burned children from the Bashkir train-gas pipeline disaster II. Follow-up experience at Children's Hospital 9, Moscow. Burns 1990; 16(5):333–336.

95. Herndon DN. A survey of the primary aid response to the Bashkir train-gas pipeline disaster. Burns 1990; 16:323–324.

96. Roding H. Ethical problems in mass burn disasters. Zentralbl Chir 1981; 106(18):1204–1209.

97. Pietersen CM, Huerta SC. Analysis of the LPG incident at San Juan Ixhuatepec, Mexico City. The Hague: TNO; 1984.

98. Benmeir P, Levine I, Shostak A, et al. The Ural train-gas pipeline catastrophe: the report of the IDF medical corps assistance. Burns 1991; 17(4):320–322.

99. Pietersen CM. De ramp met de pepleiding in de Sovjet Unie. Alert 1989; 9:3.

100. Fedorov VD, Alekseev AA. Medical care of mass burn victims: the Vishnevsky principles and organization in the Ufa disaster. In: Masellis M, Gunn SWA, eds. The management of mass burn casualties and fire disasters: proceedings of the First International Conference on Burns and Fire Disasters. Dordrecht: Kluwer Academic; 1992:222–223.

101. Mazzarella B, Scanni E, Carideo P, et al. On-site treatment of severely burned patients. In: Masellis M, Gunn SWA, eds. The management of mass burn casualties and fire disasters: proceedings of the First International Conference on Burns and Fire Disasters. Dordrecht: Kluwer Academic; 1992:224–226.

102. Cohen E. Triage 1982. J Emerg Med Ser 1982; 7:24–28.

103. Wu WT, Ngim RC. Anatomy of a burns disaster: the Miri Bank explosion. Ann Acad Med Singapore 1992; 21(5):640–648.

104. Vitale R, D'Arpa N, Conte F, et al. Clinical file and protocol for general doctors and for non-specialized hospital doctors to assist burn patients. In: Masellis M, Gunn SWA, eds. The management of mass burn casualties and fire disasters: proceedings of the First International Conference on Burns and Fire Disasters. Dordrecht: Kluwer Academic; 1992:198–221.

105. Hoeksema H, Dubrulle F, Pirayesh A, et al. Practical guidelines in burn disaster management. J Burn Care Res 2006; 27(2):S49.

106. Arturson G. The Los Alfaques disaster: a boiling-liquid, expanding-vapour explosion. Burns 1981; 7:233–251.

107. Alexander JW. Control of infection following burn injury. Arch Surg 1971; 103:435–441.

108. Anantharaman V. Burns mass disasters: aetiology, predisposing situations and initial management. Ann Acad Med Singapore 1992; 21(5):635–639.

109. Greenfield E, Winfree J. Nursing's role in the planning, preparation and response to burn disaster or mass casualty events. J Burn Care Rehabil 2005; 26(2):166–169.

110. Sheridan R, Barillo D, Herdon D, et al. Burn specialty teams. J Burn Care Rehabil 2005; 26(2):170–173.

111. Jacobs LM, Ramp JM, Breay JM. An emergency medical system approach to disaster planning. J Trauma 1979; 19(3):157–162.

112. Landiscina M, Bile L, Bollini C, et al. The burn patients and medically assisted helicopter transport. In: Masellis M, Gunn SWA, eds. The management of mass burn casualties and fire disasters: proceedings of the First International Conference on Burns and Fire Disasters. Dordrecht: Kluwer Academic; 1992: 251–252.

113. Gallagher J, Jako M, Marvin J, et al. Can burn centers evacuate safely in response to disasters? J Burn Care Res 2006; 27(2): S50.

114. Trimble EJ. The management of aircraft passenger survival in fire. Toxicology 1996; 115(1–3):41–61.

115. Clark MA, Hawley DA, McClain DL, et al. Investigation of the 1987 Indianapolis Airport Ramada Inn incident. J Forensic Sci 1994; 39(3):644–649.

116. Salomone J III, Sohn AP, Ritzlin R, et al. Correlations of injury, toxicology, and cause of death to Galaxy Flight 203 crash site. J Forensic Sci 1987; 32(5):1403–1415.

117. Davis JWL. Toxic chemical versus lung tissue — an aspect of inhalation injury revisited. The Everett Idris Evans Memorial Lecture — 1986. J Burn Care Rehabil 1986; 7(3):213–222.

118. Clark WR Jr, Nieman GF. Smoke inhalation. Burns 1988; 14(4):473–494.

119. Craft-CoffmanB, Mullins RF, Friedman B, et al. Need for preparedness and response appreciated after accidental release of toxic gas. J Burn Care Res 2006; 27(2):S51.

120. Sharpe DT, Roberts AH, Barclay TL, et al. Treatment of burns casualties after fire at Bradford City football ground. Br Med J 1985; 291:945–948.

121. Buerk CA, Batdorf JW. Cammack V, et al. The MGM Grand Hotel fire. Arch Surg 1982; 117:641–645.

122. Ngim RC. Burns mass disasters in Singapore — a three decade review with implications for future planning. Singapore Med J 1994; 35(1):47–49.

123. Sharpe DT, Foo IT. Management of burns in major disasters. Injury 1990; 21(1):41–44, discussion 55–57.

124. Brusco M. Fire in port. In: Masellis M, Gunn SWA, eds. The management of mass burn casualties and fire disasters: proceedings of the First International Conference on Burns and Fire Disasters. Dordrecht: Kluwer Academic; 1992:89–92.

125. Becker WK, Waymack JP, McManus AT, et al. Bashkirian train-gas pipeline disaster: the American military response. Burns 1990; 16(5):325–328.

126. Men'shikov DD, Zalogueva GV, Gerasimova LI, et al. The microfloral wound dynamics of the victims in the railroad disaster in Bashkiria. Zh Mikrobiol Epidemiol Immunobiol 1991; 7:32–35.

Chapter 6

Care of outpatient burns

C. Edward Hartford and G. Patrick Kealey

Introduction

Although there has been a remarkable decline in the incidence of burn injuries during the past several decades, currently in the United States each year about 700 000 individuals sustain a burn injury that requires treatment by a healthcare professional. Among these victims it is estimated that approximately 35 000 are admitted to hospitals. There are about 4500 fire- and burn-related deaths each year.[1] Therefore, thermal trauma typically results in an injury of low mortality in which the majority of care can be safely rendered in an ambulatory setting.

The outcome of burns treated in the outpatient setting is usually good. If, however, care is suboptimal, protracted morbidity or compromised function can result. The goals of therapy are to minimize pain and the risk of infection, achieve wound healing in a timely fashion, preserve physical function, minimize cosmetic deformity, and affect physical and psychosocial rehabilitation in the most expeditious manner.

Who can be managed as an outpatient?

When a patient with a burn is first evaluated, information is immediately available from which an accurate prognosis can be derived. For instance, a valuable easily remembered estimate of the probability of death from burn injury was published in 1998.[2] Using stepwise logistic regression analysis of 1665 patients, the authors identified three risk factors for death: age greater than 60 years; burns on more than 40% of the total body surface area (TBSA); and, the presence of inhalation injury. The mortality prediction for the presence of none of these risk factors is 0.3%; for the presence of one risk factor it is 3%; for two it is 33%; and, for all three it is approximately 90% (actual, 87%).

In addition to these risk factors, there are other factors — and a huge dose of common sense — which help determine the initial treatment venue. These include depth of the burn; premorbid diseases; and, co-morbid factors such as associated trauma, distribution of the burn, and injuring agent. When outpatient care is an option the patient's social situation needs to be assessed. In some instances, it may be prudent to initiate care in a hospital so that potential complicating medical problems can be sorted out or the possibility of non-accidental trauma can be excluded.

Age

Patients between 5 and 20 years of age have the most favorable survival outcome from burns. The LA_{50} (percent of total body surface area at which 50% of the patients live and 50% die) for this age cohort is 94.5% TBSA of burn.[3] Younger individuals, especially infants, have an increase in morbidity as well as mortality from burn injury. In this group, child abuse or neglect must be included in the psychosocial analysis.[4,5] The peak incidence of non-accidental burn injury is 13–24 months of age.[6] Burns that are particularly suspicious are those whose appearance suggests an injury from a cigarette, hot iron, or immersion in hot water. The latter injury is identified by a stocking/glove distribution of the burn and a sharp linear demarcation between the burned and unburned skin (Figure 6.1a,b). Scalding which has occurred in an institution or in the presence of a caregiver other than one who has a biological relationship to the victim should also heighten one's suspicion. Even with trivial injury, if the burn was sustained under suspicious circumstances or the history does not correspond with the nature or distribution of the burn, the patient should be admitted to a hospital for their protection. Cases of suspected abuse or neglect must be referred to the appropriate social services agency.

Any patient over the age of 70 years with burns is in danger of dying regardless of the extent of the burn. The LA_{50} for this age group is 29.5% TBSA of burn.[3] Therefore, admitting the older patient to a hospital to assess their response to the injury can prove invaluable before treatment is continued as an outpatient.

Extent of the burn

The larger the percent of body surface area involved by the burn, the worse the prognosis. The percent of the body surface area can be roughly estimated by using the 'rule of nines'[7] or more accurately by the technique of Lund and Browder (Table 6.1).[8] A helpful adjunct in estimating the area of burn is to use the surface area of the patient's hand. This area, which approximates 1% of the TBSA,

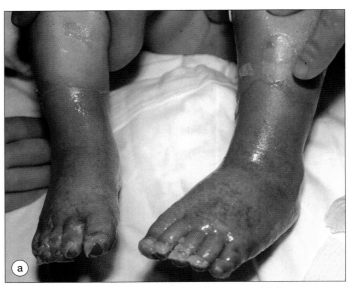
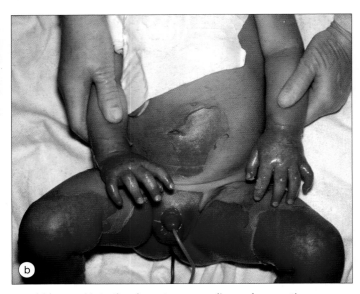

Fig. 6.1 a,b Two cases of non-accidental trauma with immersion pattern scald burns. Note the sharp transverse linear demarcation between the burned and unburned skin.

TABLE 6.1 BURN ESTIMATE — AGE VS. AREA									
Area	Birth–1 year	1–4 years	5–9 years	10–14 years	15 years	Adult	2°	3°	TBSA%
Head	19	17	13	11	9	7			
Neck	2	2	2	2	2	2			
Ant. trunk	13	13	13	13	13	13			
Post. trunk	13	13	13	13	13	13			
R. buttock	2.5	2.5	2.5	2.5	2.5	2.5			
L. buttock	2.5	2.5	2.5	2.5	2.5	2.5			
Genitalia	1	1	1	1	1	1			
R.U. arm	4	4	4	4	4	4			
L.U. arm	4	4	4	4	4	4			
R.L. arm	3	3	3	3	3	3			
L.L. arm	3	3	3	3	3	3			
R. hand	2.5	2.5	2.5	2.5	2.5	2.5			
L. hand	2.5	2.5	2.5	2.5	2.5	2.5			
R. thigh	5.5	6.5	8	8.5	9	9.5			
L. thigh	5.5	6.5	8	8.5	9	9.5			
R. leg	5	5	5.5	6	6.5	7			
L. leg	5	5	5.5	6	6.5	7			
R. foot	3.5	3.5	3.5	3.5	3.5	3.5			
L. foot	3.5	3.5	3.5	3.5	3.5	3.5			
						TOTAL			
Reproduced with permission from Surg Gynecol Obset (now J Am Coll Surg).[8]									

includes the palm together with the fingers and thumb extended and adducted.

Any burned patient who requires intravenous fluid resuscitation should be admitted to a hospital. This includes adults and older children with burns in excess of 15% of the body surface area, as well as younger children (under 5 years of age) and infants with burns in excess of 10% of the body surface area.[9] In some instances, due to premorbid dehydration caused by physical activity, an arid or semi-arid climate, alcohol, or diuretics, some patients with smaller burns may need supplemental intravenous fluids for optimal care. In the authors' practice, patients with small area burns that need intravenous fluid are often held for several hours or overnight in an observation area in the Emergency Department until their pain is controlled and fluid needs are met. Then care is continued as an outpatient.

Depth of the burn

The deeper the burn the worse is the prognosis. However, depth of small-area burns is less important in determining the need to initiate care in a hospital than the extent of the burn.

When a burn is first evaluated it is often difficult to determine its depth. The superficial injury of sunburn or its equivalent is easy to identify. Likewise, it is easy to discern a waxen, dry, inelastic, insensate, cadaveric-appearing wound as a full-thickness burn. However, it is difficult to distinguish the subtle differences between a superficial partial-thickness burn, which will heal spontaneously within 3 weeks, and a deeper partial-thickness burn which will take longer to heal. This is especially true for weeping wounds in which the blisters have ruptured. Initially, these wounds appear superficial and are perfused. However, with time, as the injured small blood vessels in the wound thrombose, the wound takes on an ischemic, cadaveric appearance of a deeper injury.[10,11] This change does not reflect invasive infection but merely the natural evolution of the wound.

Premorbid diseases

Preexisting medical conditions often have a profound influence on the clinical course and outcome of a burn injury. While any medical disorder may have an adverse effect, there are a number of conditions that occur frequently among the burned and which may play a significant role in causation or outcome. For instance, any condition or habit that alters an individual's mental state may lead to a burn injury. These include seizure disorders, senility, and psychiatric illnesses as well as the use of sedatives, controlled substances, illegal and recreational drugs, and alcohol. These usually obligate hospital admission. Medical conditions that are known to enhance morbidity of patients with burns include renal failure, congestive heart failure, cardiac dysrhythmias, hypertension, chronic obstructive pulmonary disease, diabetes mellitus, sequelae of alcoholism, morbid obesity, conditions which require the use of steroids, and other diseases which compromise the immune system.[12] The clinical status of any of these disorders must be determined and their potential influence on the outcome assessed before determining whether the patient can be safely managed as an outpatient.

Co-morbid disorders
Respiratory complications

Inhalation injury and carbon monoxide poisoning substantially magnify the burned patient's risk and may occur even with no or trivial cutaneous injury.[13,14] In addition, upper airway obstruction can be caused by the edema produced from burns of the oropharynx or the flux of fluid into the soft tissues of the upper airway resulting from deep burns of the face and/or neck. The full-blown adverse sequelae of these complications may not be immediately apparent.[15] Therefore, if the history of the accident or distribution of burns suggests any of these three complications, a period of monitored observation is warranted. Overnight observation is usually sufficient.

Associated trauma

Burns frequently occur with other forms of trauma. If the burn involves only a small area of the body, the associated trauma will dictate whether a patient needs to be admitted to a hospital.

Distribution of the burn

The location of the burn may have a profound effect on the patient's activities of daily living, and dictate the setting in which the patient receives care. For instance, the edema from a small-area superficial burn of the face may result in swelling of the eyelids, hampering the patient's vision (Figure 6.2), or burns that involve the lips or the oral cavity may inhibit efficient oral alimentation. Likewise, burns of the hands, feet, or those involving the perineum or adjacent areas may severely limit an individual's autonomy. While burns in these areas may not necessarily demand care in a hospital, there must be consideration of the assistance available to the patient when contemplating outpatient ambulatory care.

Because of fluid flux into the tissues beneath a burn, patients with circumferential burns of an extremity are in danger of ischemia of underlying and distal tissues from increased tissue pressure.[16] Except for those with very superficial burns all patients with circumferential burns of an extremity should be monitored for evidence of elevated tissue pressure. Since the clinical signs of compartment syndrome and ischemia in a burned extremity are unreliable,[17] the authors advocate measuring the tissue pressure by a direct method and uses the Stryker® Intracompartment Pressure Monitoring System. A tissue pressure above 40 mmHg is the indication for surgical decompression of the injured limb. Alternatively, a Doppler ultrasonic flow meter can be used to assess the circulatory status of the extremity.[17] A muffled first arterial sound and/

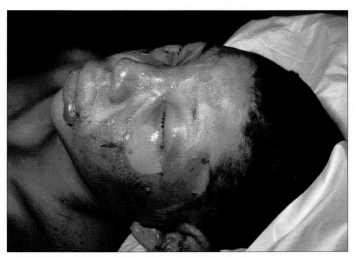

Fig. 6.2 Swelling caused by a burn that healed spontaneously without scar. For several days the edema of the eyelids prevented the patient from seeing.

or the absence of the second arterial sound is regarded as sufficient evidence of pathological elevation of the tissue pressure.

Burns across joints do not, for that reason alone, require admission to a hospital.

Injuring agent
Electricity

Patients exposed to low-voltage electricity, arbitrarily defined as less than 1000 volts (the most frequent source being household currents of 110 or 220 volts), are in great danger of dying at the accident scene from a cardiac dysrhythmia, usually ventricular fibrillation.[18] Following low-voltage electrical exposure, the most frequent residual electrocardiographic abnormality is a non-specific change in the ST-T wave segment[19] and the most troublesome dysrhythmias are among the atrial fibrillation-flutter group.[20] If the electrocardiogram is normal or becomes normal during observation, the chances of a subsequent dysrhythmia or cardiac arrest are virtually nil.

The tissue damage from low levels of electrical energy is usually small and most patients do not need to be admitted to a hospital. Occasionally, however, the damage to a child's lip, tongue, gums, and dentition from sucking on a defective energized electrical cord may preclude efficient oral alimentation. In this circumstance, hospital admission to establish satisfactory oral intake is probably wise. With an electrical burn of the lip, the injury is often deep enough to cause necrosis of the superior or inferior labial artery. The injured artery is prone to rupture between the fourth and seventh post-burn day. Therefore, the patient or caregiver must be warned of this possibility and instructed on the first aid measures for hemorrhage control.

Patients who sustain tissue damage from contact with high-voltage electricity generally require admission.

Chemicals

Although chemicals cause tissue damage by chemical reactions and not from heat, their care falls in the purview of burn care surgeons. Brushing off dry chemicals or copious lavage with water of wet chemicals are the appropriate emergency treatments.[21,22] No one knows how long lavage should be continued, but up to 1 hour has been recommended.[23] One guide is the presence of pain. The supposition is that, as long as there is pain, the chemical remains active and continues to cause damage.

In some instances, there are specific antidotes for the pain caused by a chemical. For example, with hydrofluoric acid, the injured tissues should be injected with calcium gluconate.[24] Hydrofluoric acid also serves as a good example of the many chemicals that are absorbed into the body with the potential to cause organ injury. Exposure of concentrated hydrofluoric acid to as little as 3% of the body surface area can result in a fatal dysrhythmia from hypocalcemia caused by the binding of calcium by the absorbed fluoride ion.[25] Since it is impossible to remember the systemic sequelae of all the chemicals to which an individual might be exposed, the physician should identify the chemical and seek information from the local poison control center.

After emergency local wound care, the treatment of the residual wound from a chemical is the same as the treatment for any wound.

Social circumstances

Patients whose injuries may be non-accidental need to be admitted to a hospital for their protection.

Before a patient is discharged from emergency care, the physician should ascertain that there are satisfactory resources available for supervision and care, and a way in which the patient can readily access medical care. Therefore, the distance the patient lives from care needs to be taken into consideration. For outpatients a visiting nurse can be invaluable in providing wound care and monitoring for wound complications, as well as assessing the patient's physical progress and social situation.

Treatment

Cooling the burn

The first objective in burn wound care is to dissipate the heat. As long as the temperature in the tissues is above 44°C injury continues.[26] The first step is to remove the source of heat. Both clinical and experimental evidence indicate a beneficial effect from immediate active cooling of the wound to dissipate heat.[27] Cool tap water or saline at about 8°C (46.4°F) applied in any practical manner (e.g. compress, lavage, or immersion) is as effective as any other product or method.[28–30] Colder substances, such as ice, may be detrimental.[31] The period of time that is required for active cooling is brief.[32] Typically, by the time most patients present for care, the tissues have already cooled spontaneously.

Active cooling also has several potential advantages beyond dissipation of heat. First, cooling stabilizes skin mast cells, decreasing histamine release and, thereby, decreasing edema of the wound. Secondly, in the first several hours after the injury, cooling is an effective way of controlling the pain of partial-thickness burns.[33,34] In cooling for pain control, cool, but not ice-cold,[35,36] moist compresses are applied to the painful wound. This method is applicable in the management of virtually all patients whose wounds can be safely cared for in an ambulatory setting. Because of the limited surface area of burn among most of those patients treated as outpatients, the detrimental systemic effects of active cooling, e.g. hypothermia from accelerated heat loss, should not occur. However, since water conducts heat 23 times faster than air, it makes good sense to monitor the patient's core temperature during active cooling of the wound. A limit to the surface area that is cooled is arbitrary, but a practical limit is about 10% of the TBSA.

Pain control

Burn wounds are painful. The most severe pain occurs with partial-thickness wounds devoid of epidermis. Initially it is intense and can prove to be unbearable. The pain spontaneously moderates after several hours but intensifies when wounds are manipulated during dressing changes, wound care, and physical activity. While eschar-covered burns may be insensate, when the eschar separates spontaneously or is removed, the exposed viable tissues are painful when cut into, cauterized, or manipulated.[37]

Narcotics are typically used as first-line treatment. In the emergency setting, small incremental doses of morphine can be given intravenously and titrated to effect. Subsequently, acetaminophen with codeine or oxycodone or similar analgesics, alone or in combination, are usually effective. Provided alteration of platelet function is not a concern, nonsteroidal anti-inflammatory drugs (NSAIDs) can be used. Analgesics can be supplemented with short-acting benzodiazepines, such as midazolam, to enhance sedation and provide anxiolysis. Most patients will require supplemental analgesics for wound dressing changes, physical therapy, and sleep.

Clearance of these classes of drugs is accelerated among those who regularly abuse alcohol or controlled substances.[38,39] Therefore, remarkable amounts of analgesics and sedatives may be required.

If a patient's pain cannot be controlled by oral medication, the patient may need to be admitted to a hospital. In the hospital setting, effective pain control can usually be obtained by the patient-controlled analgesia method. Even with patient-controlled analgesia, supplemental analgesia and sedation will often be required when wound dressings are changed.

Topically applied or injected local anesthetics are not recommended in the management of burns.

Local burn wound care

Loose, devitalized tissue is gently trimmed away, a practice known as épluchage. This process should not cause pain or bleeding.

Blisters

Recommendations for the management of blisters are varied and range from leaving blisters intact,[40] to removing the blistered skin immediately,[41] or delaying removal.[42]

Those who advocate removal of blistered skin cite laboratory studies that show that the blister fluid exhibits several potentially detrimental effects.[41] Immune function is depressed by impairement of polymorphonuclear leukocytes and lymphocytes. Blister fluid adversely affects neutrophil chemotaxis, opsonization, and intracellular killing. Inflammation is enhanced by the presence of metabolites of arachidonic acid in the blister fluid. A plasmin inhibitor in the blister fluid decreases vascular patency. Finally, blister fluid may provide a medium for the growth of bacteria. Based on these considerations, the case can be made that blistered skin should be removed to facilitate healing.

Conversely, these authors recommend leaving burn blisters intact. Blisters form in the stratum spinosum layer of the epidermis. An intact blister usually indicates a superficial partial-thickness wound, which will heal spontaneously within 3 weeks. If, under these circumstances, the blistered skin is removed, the wound is converted from an absolutely painless one to a painful, open wound exposed to colonization by bacteria and potential infection.[40] An infection in a burn wound covered by an intact blister rarely, if ever, occurs. Therefore, these authors prefer to leave blisters intact, and recommend that they be dressed for protection and not necessarily covered with medication.

If the blister remains intact and the wound is a superficial partial-thickness burn, spontaneous resorption of the fluid will usually begin in less than 1 week. The blistered skin will gradually wrinkle and collapse onto the healing wound surface. If the blister has ruptured, often the devitalized skin can be used as a protective dressing for the wound. Whether the blistered skin has remained intact or it has been used as a protective cover, at about the 10th day post burn, these authors inspect the underlying wound to determine its potential for healing spontaneously within the next 10 days. If it is unlikely that the wound will heal spontaneously within that time frame, surgical intervention to facilitate wound closure is undertaken.

Persistence of the blister, with no signs of spontaneous resorption of the fluid after 7–10 days, usually signifies that the underlying wound is either a deep partial-thickness or full-thickness wound.

There is often concern about large blisters in locations that limit range of motion or interfere with an efficient dressing. This concern most often occurs with a heat contact burn on the palm of the hand, a common injury among toddlers. Since contraction is a property of healing of all wounds, these authors prefer to decompress these blisters, leaving the blistered skin to protectively cover the wound. Then the palm, the thumb, and fingers can be dressed to be maintained in full extension with gentle pressure on the web spaces and the digits in moderate abduction until the danger of contraction is past. This is accomplished by several dressing methods. The hand can be immobilized in full palmar extension using an occlusive dressing consisting of triple antibiotic ointment on Adaptic® and padded with dressing sponges, including in the web spaces to maintain moderate abduction of the digits, and incorporating these dressings in a wrap of Coban®. A more secure technique is to use semi-rigid casting tape, referred to as 'Soft Cast' (3M™ Health Care, St. Paul, MN). This material consists of a polyurethane resin incorporated in a knitted fabric. Exposure to water activates the resin with a set time of 3–4 minutes. Curing is completed in about 10 more minutes. It can be removed by unwrapping or cutting it with a bandage scissors without the need to use a traditional cast saw. This is a tremendous advantage when treating young children. The technique for applying the 'Soft Cast' is shown in Figure 6.3a–h. The author keeps these casts in place for intervals of 3, 4, 7 (the most frequent interval), or 10 days, repeating the application as long as necessary to prevent contraction of the healing skin.

Cleansing the wound

For cleansing and to remove residual dirt, the wound can be gently washed with room temperature or tepid (100°F) normal saline or water with a mild, bland soap. Antiseptic solutions should not be used. The senior author's service uses Shur-Clens® Skin Wound cleanser, which is composed of poloxamer 188 (polyethylene-polypropylene glycol), a surfactant, 20%, and USP water, 80%. Shur-Clens® is a sterile cleansing solution designed for use on wounds of the skin in all areas, even around the eyes. According to the manufacturer it effectively removes contaminants from wounds without inducing tissue trauma.

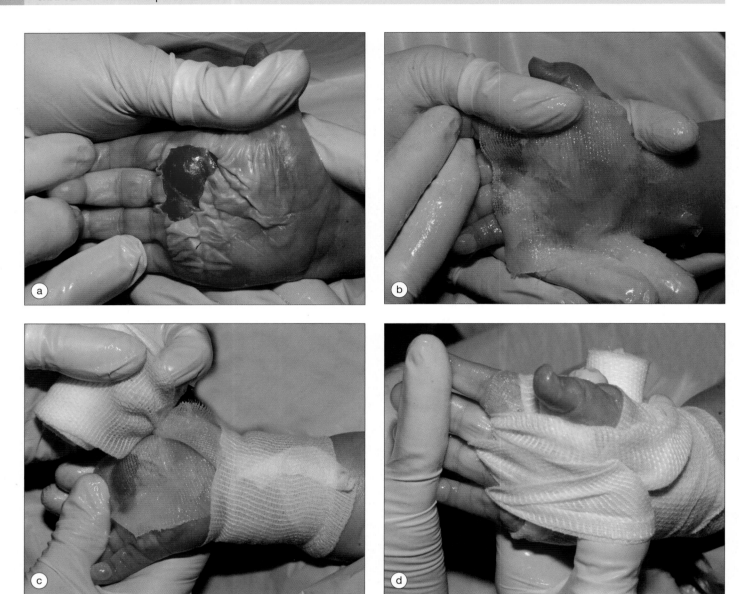

Fig. 6.3a–h 'Soft' casting technique to maintain optimal extension of the hand.
(a) Heat contact burns of the palm and tips of fingers. (b) Wound dressed with Adaptic® and triple antibiotic ointment. (c) Kling® wrap started by securing it around the wrist. (d) King® wrap threaded between fingers to prevent interdigital web formation.

In the treatment of burns from tar and asphalt, after cooling to dissipate heat, the solidified tar and asphalt can be removed by solvents that have a close structural affinity to these substances. Therefore, substances related to petrolatum (an oleaginous colloid suspension of solid microcrystalline waxes in petroleum oil) are effective. Medi-Sol™ Adhesive Remover is a citrus-based non-toxic, non-irritating Category I Medical Device solvent authorized by the FDA for use on the skin. It is an effective product for the removal of tar and asphalt.[43] It can be obtained from Orange-Sol Medical Products Division (1400 N Fiesta Blvd, Bldg. 100, Gilbert, AZ 85233–1000, phone 480–497–8822) or by using an internet search for 'Medi-Sol.' Medi-Sol™ Adhesive Remover is liberally applied and then removed by gentle wiping. Polysorbates alone or in combination with topical antibiotics[44] and topical antibiotics

in petrolatum base[45] can be used but are less effective, and repetitive applications are usually required.

Topical agents

There is a long tradition of applying substances to burn wounds in an attempt to prevent infection.[46] A large variety of antiseptics, antibiotics, and topical antibacterial (antimicrobial) agents have been advocated. Most of these agents have adverse local or systemic effects, or impede wound healing, or both. Additionally, there is no published evidence that the use of any topical agent designed to prevent or control infection will favorably influence the outcome of small burns.[47–49] In spite of this, many physicians feel obligated to apply one of these agents to the wound. All published comparative studies show no advantage of these agents over petrolatum-impregnated

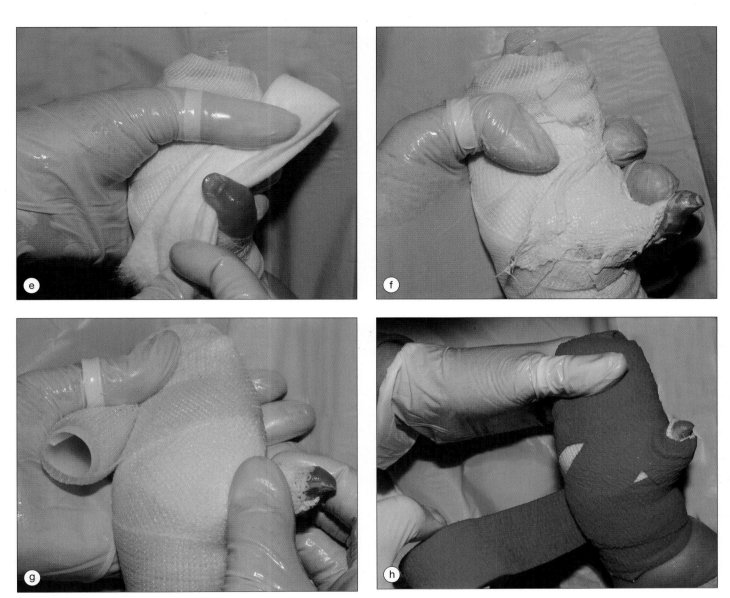

Fig. 6.3a–h—cont'd
(e) A strip of Webril™ is placed in the thumb/index finger web space preparatory to laying a strip of plaster-of-paris to maintain optimal abduction of the web space. (f) Application of the plaster-of-paris strip in the thumb/index finger web space while holding the metacarpal phalangeal joint of the thumb in optimal abduction. Because the metacarpal phalangeal joint of children is fragile, special care needs to be taken to avoid hyperextension of it. (g) Soft Cast® wrap being applied while maintaining thumb, thumb/index finger web space in optimal abduction and fingers in full extension until the Soft Cast® material sets. (h) Dressing being completed with a wrap of Coban®.

gauze.[50] However, if the treating physician believes that the use of a topical antimicrobial agent is desirable, and most do, there are several choices. Among topical antibacterial agents introduced for the treatment of burns during the past five decades, 1% silver sulfadiazine has been the most popular. However, its silver component makes it an antiseptic and, therefore, an inherent property is delay in wound healing. In comparative studies of partial-thickness burn wounds covered with dressings that do not contain antiseptics, e.g. TransCyte®,[51] Biobrane®,[52] and collagenase ointment with polymyxin B sulfate/bacitracin powder,[53] 1% silver sulfadiazine delayed spontaneous reepithelization of the wound. However, if the wound surface is covered with eschar, 1% silver sulfadiazine, among topical antiseptics recommended for burn wounds, has the fewest side effects and is probably the current best recommendation. If the patient is allergic to sulfa products, silver sulfadiazine should not be used. Because sulfonamides are known to increase the possibility of kernicterus, silver sulfadiazine is not used on pregnant women, nursing mothers, and infants less than 2 months of age. Because silver sulfadiazine impedes epithelization, it should be discontinued when healing partial-thickness wounds are devoid of necrotic tissue and evidence of reepithelization is seen.

Alternatively, there has been increasing interest in the use of combinations of antibiotics in ointment for the treatment of small-area burns. These drugs have no clinically discernible detrimental effect on wound healing. These antimicrobial combinations include triple antibiotic ointment (neomycin, 3.5 mg/g; bacitracin zinc, 400 units/g; and polymyxin B sulfate, 5000 units/g) and polysporin (polymyxin B sulfate, 10 000 units/g; and bacitracin zinc, 500 units/g). These antibiotic combinations have efficacy against the Gram-positive cocci and some of the aerobic Gram-negative bacilli that most frequently colonize small burn wounds. Occasionally, small superficial pustules caused by yeast develop on the surrounding uninjured or newly regenerated skin. Discontinuing the antimicrobial agent usually results in clearing of these lesions. The use of a topical antibiotic ointment usually decreases or eliminates the unpleasant odor often associated with the use of petrolatum-impregnated gauze alone. The senior author now uses these agents almost exclusively in the management of small-area burns when a topical antimicrobial is used.

Dressing the wound

Because there are virtually no objective studies on the subject, dogmatic recommendations for dressing small burn wounds cannot be made. Dressings serve three purposes:

1) to absorb drainage;
2) to provide protection and a measure of isolation of the wound from the environment; and
3) to decrease wound pain. In most instances these authors prefer to dress wounds and make the following suggestions.

Superficial partial-thickness burns, the equivalent of sunburn, with intact epidermis, require neither topical medication nor a dressing.

For relatively small superficial partial-thickness burns devoid of epithelium, it is generally conceded that topical antibacterial agents are not necessary.[47–49] Non-medicinal white petrolatum-impregnated fine mesh or porous mesh gauze (Adaptic®), or fine mesh absorbent gauze impregnated with 3% bismuth tribromophenate in non-medicinal petrolatum blend (Xeroform®) are satisfactory wound covers. If the burn is deeper and contains adherent necrotic tissue, a topical antimicrobial agent may be used.

For practical reasons, most burns of the face are treated without dressing. These wounds may also be treated without topical medication, allowing the wounds to dry and form a crust. Because the dry wound is often uncomfortable and heals more slowly than moist wounds, many physicians prefer to use a thin layer of bland ointment combined with a topical antibiotic, e.g. Baciquent® (bacitracin in anhydrous lanolin, mineral oil, and white petrolatum). The ointment is applied to the wound after gentle cleansing with water once or twice daily, or more frequently as needed, particularly in a dry climate. Bacitracin has activity against Gram-positive bacteria. Occasionally it causes a contact dermatitis that impedes wound healing.

Since one purpose of dressings is to absorb drainage, the thickness of the dressing is determined by the amount of drainage generated between dressing changes. In weeping superficial partial-thickness wounds, the amount of drainage is greatest soon after the injury. As the character of the wound changes and healing begins, drainage decreases. Lint-free, coarse mesh gauze, usually starting with about 20 thicknesses, is preferred by the authors.

The dressing is held in place with a gauze bandage (e.g. Kling® or Kerlix®) wrapped with sufficient tightness to hold the gauze in place but not so tightly as to impede circulation. Many use Flexinette® to secure the dressing. Stockinette, semi-impervious to liquid, can be used as an outer layer to help prevent the drainage from soaking through the dressing. As an alternative, a cohesive flexible bandage (Coflex®, Coban®, Cowrap™) can be used as an outer layer to hold a dressing securely in place and prevent drainage from seeping through. Joints are dressed to facilitate range of motion and fingers are dressed separately. However, among infants and young children, an effective way to hold the hand and fingers in extension is with a multilayer covering of one of the cohesive flexible bandages. This kind of a dressing functions as a 'soft' splint.

The frequency with which dressings are changed is arbitrary and dictated by the volume of drainage or the physical condition of the dressing. Recommendations range from twice daily, to as infrequently as once a week. Those who advocate twice-daily dressing changes do so based on the use of topical antimicrobials whose half-life is about 8 hours. Those who use petrolatum, antibiotic combinations in ointment, or bismuth-impregnated petrolatum gauze recommend less-frequent dressing changes, some extending the period to as long as 5 or 7 days.[50,54]

For inpatients, the authors prefer once-daily or every other day dressing changes to permit daily inspection and cleansing of the wound. Moreover, among inpatients after about 24–48 hours, wound dressings are often saturated or disheveled. Daily dressing changes may be used in the care of outpatients even if the patient or another layperson is responsible for the inspection, cleansing, and redressing of the wound. Cleansing of the wound can often be incorporated into general body cleansing each day. The person responsible for wound care should be instructed in the clinical manifestations of wound infections.

In the management of burns among pediatric outpatients, the senior author now has an extensive and satisfying experience with the use of triple antibiotic ointment and dressing changes done at 3-, 4- or even 7-day intervals. In many instances these dressings are changed and the progress of healing checked at clinic visits. Therefore, parents do not need to deal with the disquieting chore of changing their child's dressings and inflicting pain on them.

Biologic wound dressings

The author does not believe it is necessary or advantageous to use human cadaver allografts, xenografts, or allogenic amnion in the management of burn patients who qualify for ambulatory care. However, in certain circumstances, amniotic membranes may be plentiful and therefore useful.

Allogenic amnion

Allogenic amnion, the innermost layer of the fetal membrane, has been used as a biologic wound dressing since 1910.[55] Although fragile and technically difficult to handle, allogenic amnion is particularly effective when used as a protective dressing on partial-thickness burn wounds. It also has a good track record when used to protect and preserve a clean excised wound for subsequent autogenous skin grafting.[62] When harvested, amniotic membranes are invariably contaminated and carry a biologic risk that can never be totally eliminated. The amnion is washed, sterilized with gamma irradiation and preserved in glycerol, by lyophilization or deep freezing. The risk of biologic transmission can be diminished by systematic serologic testing of the donor for syphilis, AIDS, and hepatitis at the time of harvesting the membrane and 6 months later.[62]

Synthetic tissue-engineered wound dressings

The use of synthetic wound coverings is becoming more popular in the treatment of superficial partial-thickness burn wounds. The purported advantages are less pain, use of less pain medication, shorter wound healing time, improved compliance with scheduled outpatient visits, and lower costs.

Biobrane®

There are two prospective randomized clinical trials of small numbers of patients that show that in the treatment of superficial partial-thickness burns the use of Biobrane® results in less pain, a lower pain medication requirement, and shorter healing time when compared to those patients treated with 1% silver sulfadiazine.[56,57]

Biobrane® is a bilayer fabric composed of an inner layer of knitted nylon threads coated with porcine collagen and an outer layer of rubberized silicone, pervious to gases but not to liquids and bacteria.[58] Wounds on which Biobrane® is to be applied must be carefully selected. They must be fresh, not infected, free of eschar and debris, moist, have a sensate surface, and demonstrate capillary blanching and refill. It is applied snugly to the cleansed wound overlapping itself or fixed to unburned skin with sterile strips of adhesive tape. The key to the successful use of Biobrane® is adherence to the wound. Therefore, the burned area must be dressed or splinted, especially across a joint, to prevent shearing of the Biobrane® from the wound surface. Satisfactory adherence usually occurs in about 4 days. If, at follow-up, the Biobrane® is found to be loose, the non-adherent area can be trimmed away and new Biobrane® applied. If sterile fluid accumulates beneath the synthetic dressing, it can be aspirated. However, if the fluid is purulent, the Biobrane® must be opened to permit complete drainage. Biobrane® is left intact until the wound has reepithelized. Then it can be gently teased away. If the wound surface has even a thin veneer of residual necrotic tissue, Biobrane® will not adhere.

Hydrocolloid dressings

Hydrocolloid dressings are described as wafers, powders, or pastes composed of materials such as gelatin, pectin, and carboxymethyl-cellulose. They provide a moist environment favorable for wound healing and a barrier against exogenous bacteria. In comparison to wounds treated with 1% silver sulfadiazine, those treated with hydrocolloid occlusive dressings had more rapid wound healing, less pain, and needed fewer dressing changes.[59,60] As a result, the cost of care was lower. Hydrocolloid dressings have been effective in the treatment of small-area partial-thickness burns and are especially useful in

the terminal phase of spontaneous healing of small burns. There are a number of products made by different manufactures that are probably suitable, e.g. Cutinova® Thin (Beiersdorf-Jobst), DuoDerm® CGF Border Sterile Dressing (ConvaTec), RepliCare® Hydrocolloid Dressing (Smith & Nephew, Inc.), Restore® Wound Care Dressing (Hollister). Hydrocolloid dressings may be left in place for several days at a time.

TransCyte®

TransCyte® (Smith & Nephew, Inc.), a bioengineered skin substitute composed of human newborn fibroblasts cultured onto the nylon mesh layer of Biobrane®, is used as a dressing applied as soon as practical to eschar- and debris-free partial-thickness burn wounds. It is left in place until the wound heals. In clinical trials, TransCyte®-covered partial-thickness burn wounds healed faster than paired wounds treated with 1% silver sulfadiazine.[51,61]

Other wound dressing/covering materials

Publications are replete with technologic advances and innovations for wound dressings with the purported goal of enhancement of spontaneous wound healing or protection of the wound until it can be closed with skin grafts or with tissue-engineered delivery systems which contain cultured autogenous keratinocytes with or without fibroblasts.[62] This effort has resulted in several available products, including: Tissue Tech autograft system (Fidia Advanced Biopolymers S.r.l., Padua, Italy); Hyaff-NW (Fidia Advanced Biopolymers S.r.l.); Laserskin (Fidia Advanced Biopolymers S.r.l.); Apligraft (Organogenesis, Canton, MD); Epicell CEA (Genzyme, Cambridge, MA); Integra (Johnson and Johnson, Ratingen, Germany; Integra Life Sciences Corporation, Plainsboro NJ, USA); Alloderm (Life Cell Corporation, Woodlands, TX); Terumo (Terumo, Tokyo, Japan);[63] and, Pelnac (Kowa Company, Tokyo, Japan).[64] While the results of use of these products may be encouraging, a major limitation in their use is undoubtedly their high cost. However, among most of those treated as outpatients the area of burn wound requiring skin grafts is relatively small. Therefore, the use of these innovative products is unnecessary and standard techniques of surgical wound debridement and skin grafting suffice. Most of the clinical information about the efficacy of these products is anecdotal. However, information in medical publications can be accessed through the cost-free National Library of Medicine's online service: http://www.nlm.nih.gov/. On the search screen use the name of the product and burns as the subjects.

Elevation of the burned part

One of the most effective ways to reduce the incidence of infection in burns is to eliminate edema from the burned part. Burn injury elicits a flux of fluid into the tissues immediately subjacent to the wound. Additionally, there is a great tendency for the patient to hold the injured part immobile in a dependent position. To eliminate edema, the injured part should be exercised regularly and, when not in use, maintained slightly above the level of the heart. Merely elevating a leg off the floor to the level of the hip when in the sitting position is not sufficient. Holding the burned forearm flexed and dependent in a sling will enhance edema. Specific instructions and a demonstration of the proper position should be explicit. Patients with small burns who experience persistent edema beyond 3 days are spending too much time with the part dependent.

The most efficient position for the injured part is just slightly above the level of the heart. To elevate the burned part higher does not further enhance removal of excess tissue fluid. However, for every incremental elevation of the part there is an incremental decrease in the arterial perfusion pressure.[65]

When burns involve the lower extremity, walking and holding the leg in the dependent position often elicit severe pain. To diminish this effect, support, such as with a rubberized elastic bandage (Ace Bandage®), applied from the level of the toes to above the burn, should be used. This will also aid in reducing the accumulation of edema during walking.

Instructions and follow-up care

Before patients are released from emergency care, they are instructed in wound care, positioning, physical therapy, the clinical manifestations of infection, a convenient way to access medical care (usually by telephone), and given pain medication.

The authors often examine patients within the next several days. This allows re-inspection of the wound, assessment of the patient's compliance with instructions, and reinforcement of the principles of wound care. Often, because of pain during emergency care, the patient is distracted from fully understanding instructions. If concern remains, more frequent visits are scheduled until the physician is certain that care is being followed appropriately. After that, the patient can be seen at weekly intervals.

Definitive wound closure

A primary objective in burn care is to have all wounds healed within 1 month. Usually, this goal is easily achieved in an ambulatory setting. Burn wounds that heal spontaneously from the depth of the wound within 3 weeks have an excellent result. When this occurs, the skin functions normally with good elasticity, a nil incidence of hypertrophic scarring (scars that are red, raised, and indurated), and little, if any, alteration in pigmentation. The longer spontaneous healing takes, the worse the result. With longer healing periods, there is an increasing likelihood of developing hypertrophic scarring[66] and unsightly alterations in pigmentation. In addition, wounds that take a very long time to heal spontaneously may have unstable epithelium.

It is the surgeon's responsibility to make certain that burn wounds either heal spontaneously or are closed surgically in a timely fashion. If it is apparent that a wound will not heal spontaneously within 3 weeks, a better outcome[67,68] can usually be anticipated by surgically removing the residual necrotic tissue and any granulation tissue by tangential excision[69] and applying a skin graft. In many instances it is obvious immediately or within several days as to whether spontaneous healing will occur within 3 weeks. Among wounds in which the subtle differences between superficial and deep partial-thickness burns are not initially discernable, by 2 weeks after injury it is usually apparent whether or not the wound will heal spontaneously within the next 7–10 days. At about 10 days after injury, those wounds which are devoid of necrotic tissue and have evidence of squamous reepithelization will usually heal spontaneously within the desirable time frame. The beginning of reepithelization can be detected by seeing tiny opalescent islands of epithelium scattered throughout the wound. Inspection with a magnifying lens is helpful.

Infection and use of systemic antibiotics

There is no evidence that systemic antibiotic prophylaxis will decrease the incidence of infection in small burn wounds.[70] Antibiotics should be used only when there is evidence of infection.

The burn itself elicits inflammation. Therefore, the early manifestation of infection in the wound may be quite subtle. Mild erythema, edema, pain, and tenderness, all classic signs of infection, may be present without infection. However, when these manifestations increase over baseline, especially in the presence of lymphangitis and fever, treatment for infection should be instituted. Mainstays of treatment for infection include elevation and rest of the infected wound to control swelling and systemic antibiotic therapy. If the infection progresses the patient should be admitted to a hospital and antibiotics given intravenously.

Infections in the outpatient setting are usually caused by common skin flora. Those most frequently implicated are staphylococci. If there is evidence of infection, a culture of the surface of the wound should be obtained to identify the offending organism and narrow the spectrum of antibiotic therapy. While some burn care physicians advocate the use of burn wound biopsy quantitative culture rather than a wound surface culture,[71] the authors have not found biopsy cultures to be necessary in the treatment of outpatient burns.

Among patients with burns treated in an ambulatory setting, it is quite unusual to develop systemic sepsis. However, patients should be instructed to take their temperature twice daily, once in the morning shortly after they get up from sleep, and again late in the afternoon before they eat supper. Localized infection will be reflected in fever in the afternoon or evening. Sustained fever is suggestive of systemic sepsis. Temperatures above 38°C, especially if accompanied by symptoms of malaise and anorexia, should be reported to the physician and the patient called in for an examination.

A change in the appearance of the wound during the first several days is more likely to result from a decrease in perfusion of the wound than from wound infection. This occurs as the blood vessels injured by heat clot off. This is frequently observed with scald burns. Any further burn wound discoloration, such as the appearance of gray or black spots, especially if there are other manifestations of infection, should raise concern for invasive infection. This rarely occurs among those treated as outpatients. However, if it does occur, the patient should be admitted to a hospital, the wound biopsied for histologic and microbiological studies,[72] and treatment for infection instituted.

Burns, even minor ones, are regarded as tetanus-prone wounds.[73] Tetanus prophylaxis should be provided unless the patient has received tetanus immunization within 5 years.[74]

Pruritus

Itching is an annoying, often unrelenting manifestation of healing and healed burn wounds.

Most burn patients develop pruritus. The incidence is higher among children. The lower extremities are most frequently affected and more frequently than the upper. The face is seldom involved.[75]

Post-burn itching interferes with everything. Scratching often results in repetitive superficial wounding of both skin grafted and spontaneously healed wounds. Triggered and enhanced by environmental extremes, especially heat, physical activity, and stress, pruritus is most intense in the period immediately after wounds are healed. In most instances, it gradually diminishes and eventually stops. There are a few patients in whom it persists beyond 18 months. Patients with prolonged and chronic itching may harbor a psychogenic component.

The sensation of itch is most likely a primary sensory modality rather than, as widely held in the past, a forme fruste of pain.[76] Histamine, whose synthesis is known to be increased in healing and inflamed wounds,[77] as well as bradykinin and a series of endopeptides, have all been implicated in the genesis of itching.[78,79] Because the precise mechanism of pruritus is not known, the likelihood is that there are multiple causative factors.

Since there are no controlled trials defining the best treatment, management is by trial and error. However, antihistamines, cool compress, and lotions are the cornerstones of most attempts to relieve burn-related itching. The antihistaminic diphenhydramine hydrochloride is the most frequently prescribed first treatment.[80] This drug has an added benefit of providing mild sedation. Other antihistamines, such as cyproheptadine hydrochloride, may also be tried. Analgesics of any kind may be helpful by altering perception of itching in the central nervous system. Combinations of antihistamines and analgesics may be tried. Hydroxyzine hydrochloride, a drug used to provide relief from anxiety and emotional tension, is used by many to help ameliorate itching. Many patients find comfort in an air-conditioned environment. Cool compresses also may temporarily interrupt the itching cycle. A variety of topical agents, including aloe vera,[81] which has anti-inflammatory and antimicrobial properties, and skin moisturizing creams, such as Elta®, Vaseline Intensive Care®, Eucerin®, Nivea®, mineral oil, cocoa butter, and even lard, have been effective. Any odorless lotion free of alcohol is probably helpful. In addition, many patients prefer loose, soft clothing made from cotton.

The staff at the Shriners Burns Hospital, Galveston, Texas, uses the following protocol for the treatment of itching:

Step 1: Use moisturizing body shampoo and lotions.
Step 2: Diphenhydramine 1.25 mg/kg/dose PO q 4 h scheduled.
Step 3: Hydroxyzine 0.5 mg/kg/dose PO q 6 h and diphenyhydramine 1.25 mg/kg/dose PO q 6 h. Alter-

nate medication so that patient is receiving one itch medicine every 3 hours while awake.
Step 4: Hydroxyzine 0.5 mg/kg/dose PO q 6 h and cyproheptadine 0.1 mg/kg/dose PO q 6 h and diphenhydramine 1.25 mg/kg/dose PO q 6 h. Alternate medication so that patient is receiving one itch medicine every 2 hours while awake.

Phillips and Robson[82] advocate using penicillin in pruritus management. They observed that post-burn hypertrophic scars were much more frequently colonized with beta-hemolytic streptococcus, *Staphylococcus aureus*, and *Staph. epidermidis* compared to matched healed wounds without hypertrophic scarring. Therefore, to decrease the inflammation caused by these microorganisms, a root cause of itching, they used the following regimen: low-dose oral penicillin, 250 mg twice daily, to control the beta-hemolytic streptococcus, and aloe vera cream applied topically. As noted above, aloe vera has both anti-inflammatory and antimicrobial properties.

Traumatic blisters in reepitheliazed wounds

As the wounds reepithelialize, the delicate thin layer of epithelium is fragile and easily damaged. Itching and other mild forms of trauma may cause small blisters. Patients need to be cautioned about this potential and assured that the epithelium will gain strength and that this will not be a long-term problem. If these blisters rupture, leaving small superficial wounds, the wounds may be left exposed to form a crust. Alternatively, Adaptic® or Xeroform® and a light dressing or one of the hydrocolloid wafer products may be used.

Rehabilitative physical care

Measures to preserve strength and restore function should be incorporated into the initial treatment plan.[83] Before leaving emergency care, the patient's physical activity should be discussed and a program for range of motion exercises and muscle strengthening outlined, both verbally and in writing.

At each subsequent follow-up visit, function and strength should be assessed. If there is lack of compliance or if the patient's function begins to deteriorate, the patient should be referred for supervised physical or occupational therapy, or both. If the injury extends across a joint, or involves the hand or distal portion of the lower extremity, it is advisable to have therapists involved from the outset. When there are burns of the face that have the potential for facial dysfunction, it may be prudent to have the patient evaluated and treated by a speech pathologist.

The potential for development of contractures and hypertrophic scars among the burned treated as outpatients is the same as for those treated as inpatients.[83] The principles of prevention and treatment of these complications apply in both settings.

Outpatient treatment of moderate and major burns

Some patients classified as having moderate or even major burn injuries (Table 6.2)[84] are suitable for treatment in the

TABLE 6.2 CLASSIFICATION OF BURN SEVERITY

Minor burn

15% TBSA or less in adults

10% TBSA of less in children and the elderly

2% TBSA or less full-thickness burn in children or adults without cosmetic or functional risk to eyes, ear, face, hands, feet, or perineum

Moderate burn

15–25% TBSA in adults with less than 10% full-thickness burn

10–20% TBSA partial-thickness burn in children under 10 and adults over 40 years of age with less than 10% full-thickness burn

10% TBSA or less full-thickness burn in children or adults without cosmetic or functional risk to eyes, ears, face, hands, feet, or perineum

Major burn

25% TBSA or greater

20% TBSA or greater in children under 10 and adults over 40 years of age

10% TBSA or greater full-thickness burn

All burns involving eyes, ears, face, hands, feet, or perineum that are likely to result in cosmetic or functional impairment

All high-voltage electrical burns

All burn injury complicated by major trauma or inhalation injury

All poor-risk patients with burn injury

TBSA, total body surface area.

ambulatory setting.[85] The purported advantages include less cost, less chance of exposure to antibiotic-resistant microorganisms, and a more psychologically comfortable environment for the patient. In spite of these benefits, caution should be exercised in selecting patients with moderate and major thermal injury for early discharge from the hospital. On the other hand, as convalescence progresses, many of these patients can have the terminal phase of their acute burn care completed safely as outpatients.

The conditions that need to be met in order to consider ambulatory care for any patient include: intravenous fluid resuscitation must be completed; there must be no ongoing complication; there must be no wound or systemic manifestation of sepsis; adequate enteral nutrition must be established; and pain control must be satisfactory with medication taken by mouth. Additionally, arrangements need to be made for wound care and physical and/or occupational therapy.

Acknowledgments

Maureen L Smith RN MSN provided valuable assistance in the preparation of this manuscript.

References

1. Brigham, PA. Personal communication. December 2005 Philadelphia, Burn Foundation.
2. Ryan CM, Schoenfeld DA, Thorpe WP, et al. Objective extimates of the probability of death from burn injuries. N Engl J Med 1998; 338:362–366.
3. Saffle JR, Davis B, Williams P. Recent outcomes in the treatment of burn injury in the United States: report from the American Burn Association Patient Registry. J Burn Care Rehabil 1995; 16:219–232.
4. Rosenberg NM, Marino D. Frequency of suspected abuse/neglect in burn patients. Pediatr Emerg Care 1989; 5: 219–221.
5. Guzzetta PC, Randolph J. Burns in children: 1982. Ped Rev 1983; 4:271–278.
6. Uchiyama N, German J. Pediatric considerations. In: Achauer BM, ed. Management of the burned patient. Norwalk, CT: Appleton & Lange; 1987:203–209.
7. Evans EI, Purnell OJ, Robinett PW, et al. Fluid and electrolyte requirements in severe burns. Ann Surg 1952; 135:804–815.
8. Lund CC, Browder NC. The estimate of areas of burns. Surg Gynecol Obstet 1944; 79:352–358.
9. Herndon DN, Rutan RL, Rutan TC. Management of the pediatric patient with burns. J Burn Care Rehabil 1993; 14:3–8.
10. deCamara DL, Raine TJ, London MD, et al. Progression of thermal injury: a morphologic study. Plast Reconstr Surg 1982; 69:491–499.
11. Gatti JE, LaRossa D, Silverman DG, et al. Evaluation of the burn wound with perfusion fluorometry. J Trauma 1983; 23:202–206.
12. Krob MJ, D'Amico FJ, Ross DL. Do trauma scores accurately predict outcomes for patients with burns? J Burn Care Rehabil 1991; 12:560–563.
13. Heimbach DM, Waeckerle JF. Inhalation injuries. Ann Emerg Med 1988; 17:1316–1320.
14. Thompson PB, Herndon DN, Traber DL, et al. Effect of mortality of inhalation injury. J Trauma 1986; 26:163–165.
15. McManus WF, Pruitt BA Jr. Thermal injuries. In: Mattox KL, Moore EE, Feliciano DV, eds. Trauma. Norwalk, CT: Appleton & Lange; 1988:675–689.
16. Waymack JP, Pruitt BA Jr. Burn wound care. Adv Surg 1990; 23:261–289.
17. Moylan JA Jr, Inge WW Jr, Pruitt BA Jr. Circulatory changes following circumferential extremity burns evaluated by the ultrasonic flowmeter: an analysis of 60 thermally injured limbs. J Trauma 1971; 11:763–770.
18. Hooker DR, Kouvenhoven WB, Langworthy OR. The effect of alternating electrical currents on the heart. Am J Physiol 1933; 103:444–454.
19. Solem L, Fischer RP, Strate RG. The natural history of electrical injury. J Trauma 1977; 17:487–492.
20. Baxter CR. Present concepts in the management of major electrical injury. Surg Clin N Am 1970; 50:1401–1418.
21. Curreri PW, Asch MJ, Pruitt BA Jr. The treatment of chemical burns: specialized diagnostic, therapeutic, and prognostic considerations. J Trauma 1970; 10:634–642.
22. van Rensburg LC. An experimental study of chemical burns. S Afr Med J 1962; 36:754–759.
23. Gruber RP, Laub DR, Vistnes LM. The effect of hydrotherapy on the clinical course and pH of experimental cutaneous chemical burns. Plast Reconstr Surg 1975; 55:200–204.
24. Dibbell DG, Iverson RE, Jones W, et al. Hydrofluoric acid burns of the hand. J Bone Joint Surg 1970; 52-A:931–936.
25. Greco RJ, Hartford CE, Haith LR Jr, Patton ML. Hydrofluoric acid-induced hypocalcemia. J Trauma 1988; 28:1593–1596.

26. Moritz AR, Henriques FC Jr. Studies of thermal injury II. The relative importance of time and surface temperature in the causation of cutaneous burns. Am J Pathol 1947; 23:695–720.

27. Davies JW. Prompt cooling of burned area: a review of benefits and the effector mechanisms. Burns Incl Therm Inj 1982; 9:1–6.

28. Blomgren I, Eriksson E, Bagge U. The effect of different cooling temperatures and immersion fluids on post-burn oedema and survival of the partially scalded hairy mouse ear. Burns Incl Therm Inj 1985; 11:161–165.

29. Saranto JR, Rubayi S, Zawacki BE. Blisters, cooling, antithromboxanes, and healing in experimental zone-of-stasis burns. J Trauma 1983; 23:927–933.

30. Jandera V, Hudson DA, deWet PM, et al. Cooling the burn wound: evaluation of different modalities. Burns 2000; 26:256–270.

31. Swada Y, Urushidate D, Yotsuyangl T, et al. Is prolonged and excessive cooling of a scalded wound effective? Burns 1997; 23:55–58.

32. Demling RH, Mazess RB, Wolberg W. The effect of immediate and delayed cool immersion on burn edema formation and resorption. J Trauma 1979; 19:56–60.

33. King TC, Zimmerman JM. First-aid cooling of the fresh burn. Surg Gynecol Obstet 1965; 120:1271–1273.

34. Ofeigsson OJ. Water cooling: first-aid treatment for scalds and burns. Surgery 1965; 57:391–400.

35. Pushkar NS, Sandorminsky BP. Cold treatment of burns. Burns Incl Thermal Inj 1982; 9:101–110.

36. Purdue GF, Layton TR, Copeland CE. Cold injury complicating burn therapy. J Trauma 1985; 25:167–168.

37. Osgood PF, Szyfelbein SK. Management of burn pain in children. Pediatr Clin N Am 1989; 36: 1001–1013.

38. Goldstein JA. Mechanism of induction of hepatic drug metabolizing enzymes: recent advances. Trends Pharmacol Sci 1984; 5:290.

39. Jaffe JH. Drug addiction and drug abuse. In: Gilman AG, Rall TW, Nies AS, Taylor P, eds. Goodman and Gilman's the pharmacological basis of therapeutics, 8th edn. New York: Pergamon Press; 1990:522–573.

40. Swain AH, Azadian BS, Wakeley CJ, et al. Management of blisters in minor burns. Br Med J (Clin Res) 1987; 295:181.

41. Rockwell WB, Ehrlich HP. Should burn blister fluid be evacuated? J Burn Care Rehabil 1990; 11: 93–95.

42. Demling RH, LaLonde C. Burn trauma. In: Blaisdell FW, Trunkey DD, eds. Trauma management. New York: Thieme Medical; 1989; (IV):55–56.

43. Stratta RJ, Saffle JR, Kravitz M, et al. Management of tar and asphalt injuries. Am J Surg 1983; 146:766–769.

44. Demling RH, Buerstatte WR, Perea A. Management of hot tar burns. J Trauma 1980; 20:242.

45. Ashbell TS, Crawford HH, Adamson JE, et al. Tar and grease removal from injured parts. Plast Reconstr Surg 1967; 40:330–331.

46. Hartford CE. The bequests of Moncrief and Moyer: an appraisal of topical therapy of burns – 1981 American Burn Association presidential address. J Trauma 1981; 21:827–834.

47. Hunter GR, Chang FC. Outpatient burns: prospective study. J Trauma 1976; 16:191–195.

48. Miller SF. Outpatient management of minor burns. Am Fam Physician 1977; 16:167–172.

49. Nance FC, Lewis VL Jr, Hines JL, et al. Aggressive outpatient care of burns. J Trauma 1972; 12:144–146.

50. Heinrich JJ, Brand DA, Cuono CB. The role of topical treatment as a determinant of infection in outpatient burns. J Burn Care Rehabil 1988; 9:253–257.

51. Kumar RJ, Kimble, RM, Boots R, et al. Treatment of partial-thickness burns: a prospective randomized trial using Transcyte. ANZ J Surg 2004; 47:622–626.

52. Barret JP, Dziewulski P, Ramy PI, et al. Biobrane versus 1% silver sulfadiazine in second-degree pediatric burns. Plast Reconstr Surg 2000; 105:62–65.

53. Hansbrough JF, Achauer B, Dawson J, et al. Wound healing in partial-thickness burn wounds treated with collagenase ointment versus silver sulfadiazine cream. J. Burn Care Rehabil 1995; 16:241–247.

54. Haynes BW Jr. Outpatient burns. Clin Plastic Surg 1974; 1:645–651.

55. Rejzek A, Weyer F, Eichberger R, et al. Physical changes of amniotic membranes through glycerolization for use as an epidermal substitute. Light and electron microscopic studies. Cell Tissue Bank 2001; 2:95–102.

56. Gerding RL, Emerman CL, Effron D, et al. Outpatient management of partial-thickness burns: Biobrane® versus 1% silver sulfadiazine. Ann Emerg Med 1990; 19:121–124.

57. Barret JP, Dziewulski P, Ramy Pl, et al. Biobrane versus 1% silver sulfadiazine in second-degree pediatric burns. Plast Reconstr Surg 2000; 105:62–65.

58. Tavis MJ, Thornton JW, Bartlett RH, et al. A new composite skin prosthesis. Burns Incl Thermal Inj 1980; 7:123–130.

59. Wyatt D, McGowan DN, Najarian MP. Comparison of a hydrocolloid dressing and silver sulfadiazine cream in the outpatient management of second-degree burns. J Trauma 1990; 30:857–865.

60. Hermans MH. Hydrocolloid dressing (Duoderm) for the treatment of superficial and deep partial thickness burns. Scand J Plast Reconstr Surg Hand Surg 1987; 21:283–285.

61. Noordenbos J, Doré C, Hansborough JF. Safety and efficacy of TransCyte for the treatment of partial-thickness burns. J Burn Care Rehabil 1999; 20:275–281.

62. Bishara SA, Hayek SN, Gunn SW. New technologies for burn wound closure and healing — review of the literature. Burns 2005; 31:944–956.

63. Lee JW, Jang YC, Oh SJ. Use of artificial dermis for free radial forearm flap donor site. Ann Plast Surg 2005; 55:500–502.

64. Suzuki S, Kawai K, Ashoori F, et al. Long-term follow-up study of artificial dermis composed of outer silicone layer and inner collagen sponge. Br J Plast Surg 2000: 53:659–666.

65. Matsen FA III. Compartmental syndromes. New York: Grune & Stratton; 1980:57–58.

66. Deitch EA, Wheelahan TM, Rose MP, et al. Hypertrophic burn scars: analysis of variables. J Trauma 1983; 23:895–898.

67. Engrav LH, Heimbach DM, Reus JL, et al. Early excision and grafting vs. nonoperative treatment of burns of indeterminant depth: a randomized prospective study. J Trauma 1983; 23:1001–1004.

68. Burke JF, Bondoc CC, Quinby WC Jr, et al. Primary surgical management of the deeply burned hand. J Trauma 1976; 16:593–598.

69. Janvekovic Z. A new concept in the early and immediate grafting of burns. J Trauma 1970; 10:1103–1108.

70. Durtschi MB, Orgain C, Counts GW, et al. A prospective study of prophylactic penicillin in acutely burned hospitalized patients. J Trauma 1982; 22:11–14.

71. Loebl EC, Marvin JA, Heck EL, et al. The method of quantitative burn-wound biopsy cultures and its routine use in the care of the burned patient. Am J Clin Pathol 1974; 61:20–24.

72. Pruitt BA Jr. The diagnosis and treatment of infection in the burn patient. Burns Incl Thermal Inj 1984; 11:79–91.

73. Larkin JM, Moylan JA. Tetanus following a minor burn. J Trauma 1975; 15:546–548.

74. Committee on Trauma, American College of Surgeons. A guide to prophylaxis against tetanus in wound management, 1984 revision. Philadelphia: The American College of Surgeons; 1984.

75. Bell L, McAdams T, Morgan R, et al. Pruritus in burns: a descriptive study. J Burn Care Rehabil 1988; 9:305–308.

76. Herndon JH Jr. Itching: the pathophysiology of pruritus. Int J Dermatol 1975; 14:465–484.

77. Kahlson G, Rosengren E. New approaches to the physiology of medicine. Physiol Rev 1968; 48:155–196.

78. Keele CA, Armstrong D. Substances producing pain and itch. London: Edward Arnold; 1964:297–298.

79. Robson MC, Jellema A, Heggers JP, et al. Care of the healed burn wound: a prospective randomized study. San Antonio, TX: American Burn Association; 1980:94 (Abstract).

80. Gordon MD. Pruritus in burns. J Burn Care Rehabil 1988; 9:305–311.

81. Heimbach DM, Engrav LH, Marvin J. Minor burns: guidelines for successful outpatient management. Postgrad Med 1981; 69:22–32.

82. Phillips LG, Robson MC. Comments from Detroit Receiving Hospital, Detroit, Michigan. J Burn Care Rehabil 1988; 9:308–309.

83. Helm PA, Kevorkian G, Lushbaugh M, et al. Burn injury: rehabilitation management in 1982. Arch Phys Med Rehabil 1982; 63:6–16.

84. Guidelines for service standards and severity classification in the treatment of burn injury. Appendix B to Hospital Resources Document. ACS Bulletin 1984; 69:25–28.

85. Warden GD, Kravitz M, Schnebly A. The outpatient management of moderate and major thermal injury. J Burn Care Rehabil 1981; 2:159–161.

Chapter 7

Pre-hospital management, transportation, and emergency care

Ronald P. Mlcak and Michael C. Buffalo

Chapter contents

Introduction

Advances in trauma and burn management over the past three decades have resulted in improved survival and reduced morbidity from major burns. The cost of such care, however, is high; it requires conservation of resources such that only a limited number of burn intensive care units with the capabilities of caring for such labor-intensive patients can be found — hence, regional burn care has evolved. This regionalization has led to the need for effective pre-hospital management, transportation, and emergency care. Progress in the development of rapid, effective transport systems has resulted in marked improvement in the clinical course and survival for victims of thermal trauma.

For burn victims, there are usually two phases of transport. The first is the entry of the burn patient into the emergency medical system with treatment at the scene and transport to the initial care facility. The second phase is the assessment and stabilization of the patient at the initial care facility and transportation to the burn intensive care unit.[1] With this perspective in mind, this chapter reviews current principles of optimal pre-hospital management, transportation, and emergency care.

Pre-hospital care

Prior to any specific treatment, a patient must be removed from the source of injury and the burning process stopped. As the patient is removed from the injuring source, care must be taken so that a rescuer does not become another victim.[2] All

caregivers should be aware of the possibility that they may be injured by contact with the patient or the patient's clothing. Universal precautions, including wearing gloves, gowns, masks, and protective eye wear, should be used whenever there is likely contact with blood or body fluids. Burning clothing should be removed as soon as possible to prevent further injury.[3] All rings, watches, jewelry, and belts should be removed as they can retain heat and produce a tourniquet-like effect with digital vascular ischemia.[4] If water is readily available, it should be poured directly on the burned area. Early cooling can reduce the depth of the burn and reduce pain, but cooling measures must be used with caution, since a significant drop in body temperature may result in hypothermia with ventricular fibrillation or asystole. Ice or ice packs should never be used, since they may cause further injury to the skin or produce hypothermia.

Initial management of chemical burns involves removing saturated clothing, brushing the skin if the agent is a powder, and irrigation with copious amounts of water, taking care not to spread chemical on burns to adjacent unburned areas. Irrigation with water should continue from the scene of the accident through emergency evaluation in the hospital. Efforts to neutralize chemicals are contraindicated due to the additional generation of heat, which would further contribute to tissue damage. A rescuer must be careful not to come in contact with the chemical, i.e. gloves, eye protectors, etc., should be worn.

Removal of a victim from an electrical current is best accomplished by turning off the current and by using a non-conductor to separate the victim from the source.[5]

On-site assessment of a burned patient

Assessment of a burned patient is divided into primary and secondary surveys. In the primary survey, immediate life-threatening conditions are quickly identified and treated. The primary survey is a rapid, systematic approach to identify life-threatening conditions. The secondary survey is a more thorough head-to-toe evaluation of the patient. Initial management of a burned patient should be the same as for any other trauma patient, with attention directed at airway, breathing, circulation, and cervical spine immobilization.

Primary assessment

Exposure to heated gases and smoke from the combustion of a variety of materials results in damage to the respiratory tract. Direct heat to the upper airways results in edema formation, which may obstruct the airway. Initially, 100%-humidified oxygen should be given to all patients when no obvious signs of respiratory distress are present. Upper airway obstruction may develop rapidly following injury, and the respiratory status must be continually monitored in order to assess the need for airway control and ventilator support. Progressive hoarseness is a sign of impending airway obstruction. Endotracheal intubation should be done early before edema obliterates the anatomy of the area.[3]

The patient's chest should be exposed in order to adequately assess ventilatory exchange. Circumferential burns may restrict breathing and chest movement. Airway patency alone does not assure adequate ventilation. After an airway is established, breathing must be assessed in order to insure adequate chest expansion. Impaired ventilation and poor oxygenation may be due to smoke inhalation or carbon monoxide intoxication. Endotracheal intubation is necessary for unconscious patients, for those in acute respiratory distress, or for patients with burns of the face or neck which may result in edema which causes obstruction of the airway.[3] The nasal route is the recommended site of intubation. Assisted ventilation with 100%-humidified oxygen is required for all intubated patients.

Blood pressure is not the most accurate method of monitoring a patient with a large burn because of the pathophysiologic changes which accompany such an injury. Blood pressure may be difficult to ascertain because of edema in the extremities. A pulse rate may be somewhat more helpful in monitoring the appropriateness of fluid resuscitation.[6]

If a burn victim was in an explosion or deceleration accident, there is the possibility of a spinal cord injury. Appropriate cervical spine stabilization must be accomplished by whatever means necessary, including a cervical collar to keep the head immobilized until the condition can be evaluated.

Secondary assessment

After completing a primary assessment, a thorough head-to-toe evaluation of a patient is imperative.[7] A careful determination of trauma other than obvious burn wounds should be made. As long as no immediate life-threatening injury or hazard is present, a secondary examination can be performed before moving a patient; precautions such as cervical collars, backboards, and splints should be used.[8] Secondary assessment should examine a patient's past medical history, medications, allergies, and the mechanisms of injury.

There should never be a delay in transporting burn victims to an emergency facility due to an inability to establish intravenous (IV) access. If the local/regional emergency medical system (EMS) protocol prescribes that an IV line is started, then that protocol should be followed. The American Burn Association recommends that if a patient is less than 60 minutes from a hospital, an IV is not essential and can be deferred until a patient is at a hospital. If an IV line is established, Ringer's lactate solution should be infused at 500 mL/h in an adult and 250 mL/h in a child 5 years of age or over. In children younger than 5 years of age no IV lines are recommended.[4]

Pre-hospital care of wounds is basic and simple, because it requires only protection from the environment with an application of a clean dressing or sheet to cover the involved part. Covering wounds is the first step in diminishing pain. If it is approved for use by local/regional EMS, narcotics may be given for pain, but only intravenously in small doses and only enough to control pain. Intramuscular or subcutaneous routes should never be used, since fluid resuscitation could result in unpredictable patterns of uptake.[4] No topical antimicrobial agents should be applied in the field.[4,9] The patient should then be wrapped in a clean sheet and blanket to minimize heat loss and to control temperature during transport.

Transport to hospital emergency department

Rapid, uncontrolled transport of a burn victim is not the highest priority, except in cases where other life-threatening conditions coexist. In the majority of accidents involving major burns, ground transportation of victims to a hospital is available and appropriate. Helicopter transport is of greatest use when the distance between an accident and a hospital is 30–150 miles or when a patient's condition warrants.[10] Whatever the mode of transport, it should be of appropriate size, and have emergency equipment available as well as trained personnel, such as a nurse, physician, paramedic, or respiratory therapist.

Assessment and emergency treatment at initial care facility

The assessment of a patient with burn injuries in a hospital emergency department is essentially the same as outlined for a pre-hospital phase of care. The only real difference is the availability of more resources for diagnosis and treatment in an emergency department. As with other forms of trauma, the primary survey begins with the ABCs, and the establishment of an adequate airway is vital. Endotracheal intubation should be accomplished early if impending respiratory obstruction or ventilatory failure is anticipated, because it may be impossible after the onset of edema following the initiation of fluid therapy. Securing an endotracheal tube may be difficult because traditional methods often do not adhere to burned skin, and tubes are easily dislodged. One method of choice includes securing an endotracheal tube with woven tape, umbilical cord, under the ears as well as over the ears.[11] While doing assessments and making interventions for life-threatening problems in the primary survey, precautions should be taken to maintain cervical spine immobilization until injuries to the spine can be ruled out.

Following a primary survey, a thorough head-to-toe evaluation of a patient should be done. This includes obtaining a history as thorough as circumstances permit. The history should include the mechanism and time of the injury and a description of the surrounding environment, such as whether injuries were incurred in an enclosed space, the presence of noxious chemicals, the possibility of smoke inhalation, and any related trauma. A complete physical examination should include a careful neurological examination, as evidence of cerebral anoxic injury can be subtle. Patients with facial burns should have their corneas examined with fluorescent staining. Routine admission laboratories should include a complete blood count, serum electrolytes, glucose, blood urea nitrogen (BUN), and creatine. Pulmonary assessment should include arterial blood gases, chest X-rays, and carboxyhemoglobin.[12]

All extremities should be examined for pulses, especially with circumferential burns. Evaluation of pulses can be assisted by use of a Doppler ultrasound flowmeter. If pulses are absent, the involved limb may need urgent escharotomy for release of the constrictive, unyielding eschar (Figure 7.1). In circumferential chest burns, escharotomy may also be necessary to relieve chest wall restriction and improve ventilation. Escharotomies may be performed at the bedside under IV sedation using electrocautery. Midaxial incisions are made through the eschar but not into subcutaneous tissue of the eschar in order to assure adequate release. Limbs should be elevated above the heart level. Pulses should be monitored for 48 hours.[12]

If pulses are still present, but appear endangered, chemical escharotomy with enzymatic ointments (Accuzyme, collagenase, Elase) can be effective. Enzymatic escharotomy in hand burns may be preferred since surgical incisions risk exposure of superficial nerves, vessels, and tendons. Enzymatic escharotomy is indicated only during the first 24–48 hours postburn, and it should be used only in combination with a topical antimicrobial agent or sepsis can occur. With enzymatic escharotomy, there is usually a spike in temperature, which subsides after the enzyme is removed.

Evaluation of wounds

After the primary and secondary surveys are completed and resuscitation is underway, a more careful evaluation of burn wounds is performed. The wounds are gently cleaned, and loose skin and in large wounds blisters, greater than 2 cm, are debrided (see care of outpatient burns, Chapter 6). Blister fluid contains high levels of inflammatory mediators, which increase burn wound ischemia. The blister fluid is also a rich media for subsequent bacterial growth. Deep blisters on the palms and soles may be aspirated instead of debrided in order to improve patient comfort. After burn wound assessment is complete, the wounds are covered with a topical antimicrobial agent and appropriate burn dressings or a biological dressing is applied.

An estimate of burn size and depth assists in making a determination of severity, prognosis, and disposition of a patient. Burn size directly affects fluid resuscitation, nutritional support, and surgical interventions. The size of a burn wound is most frequently estimated by using the rule-of-nines method (Figure 7.2). A more accurate assessment can be made of a burn injury, especially in children, by using the Lund and Browder chart, which takes into account changes brought about by growth (Figure 7.3).[4,9] The American Burn Association identifies certain injuries as usually requiring a referral to a burn center. Patients with these burns should be treated in a specialized burn facility after initial assessment and treatment at an emergency department. Questions about specific patients should be resolved by consultation with a burn center physician (Box 7.1).[4,13]

Fluid resuscitation

Establishment of IV lines for fluid resuscitation is necessary for all patients with major burns including those with inhalation injury or other associated injuries. These lines are best started in the upper extremity peripherally. A minimum of two large-caliber IV catheters should be established through non-burned tissue if possible, or through burns if no unburned areas are available. Ringer's lactate solution should be infused at 2–4 mL/kg/% total body surface area (TBSA) which is burned.[1,4,9] Children must have additional fluid for maintenance.[14]

Taking into account the increased evaporative water loss in the formula for fluid resuscitation for pediatric patients, the

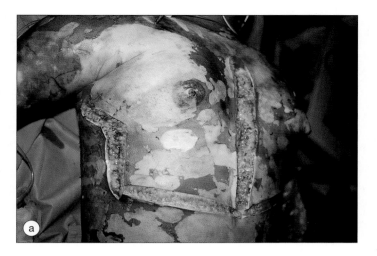

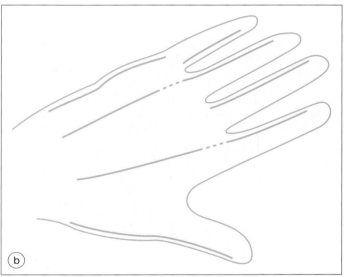

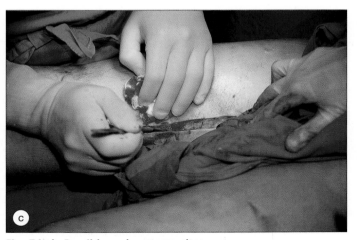

Fig. 7.1a,b Possible escharotomy sites.
(a) Chest escharotomy site.[12] (b) Escharotomy site on finger. (c) Lower limb escharotomy. (Figure 7.1a Reproduced from Herndon DN, Desai MH, Abston S, et al. Residents Manual. Galveston: Shriner's Burns Hospital, and the University of Texas Medical Branch 1992:1–17).

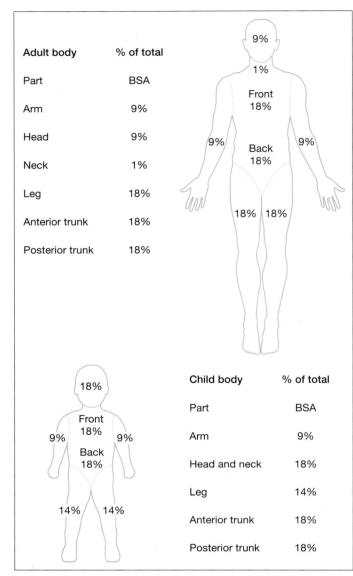

Adult body	% of total
Part	BSA
Arm	9%
Head	9%
Neck	1%
Leg	18%
Anterior trunk	18%
Posterior trunk	18%

Child body	% of total
Part	BSA
Arm	9%
Head and neck	18%
Leg	14%
Anterior trunk	18%
Posterior trunk	18%

Fig. 7.2 Estimation of burn size using the rule-of-nines. (From Advanced Burn Life Support Providers Manual. Chicago, IL. American Burn Association 2005. Reproduced with permission from American Burn Association.[4])

initial resuscitation should begin with $5000\,mL/m^2/\%$ TBSA burned/day + $2000\,mL/m^2/TBSA/day$ 5% dextrose in Ringer's lactate. This formula calls for one-half of the total amount to be given in the first 8 hours post-injury with the remainder given over the following 16 hours (Box 7.2).[14]

All resuscitation formulas are designed to serve as a guide only. The response to fluid administration and physiologic tolerance of a patient is the most important determinant. Additional fluids are commonly needed with inhalation injury, electrical burns, associated trauma, and delayed resuscitation. The appropriate resuscitation regimen administers the minimal amount of fluid necessary for maintenance of vital organ perfusion; the subsequent response of the patient over time will dictate if more or less fluid is needed so that the rate of fluid administration can be adjusted accordingly. Inadequate resuscitation can cause diminished perfusion of renal and mesenteric vascular beds. Fluid overload can produce undesired pulmonary or cerebral edema.

Urine output requirements

The single best monitor of fluid replacement is urine output. Acceptable hydration is indicated by a urine output of more than 30 mL/h in an adult (0.5 mL/kg/h) and 1 mL/kg/h in a child. Diuretics are generally not indicated during an acute resuscitation period. Patients with high-voltage electrical burns and crush injuries, with myoglobin and/or hemoglobin in the urine, have an increased risk of renal tubular obstruction. Sodium bicarbonate should be added to IV fluids in order to alkalinize the urine, and urine output should be maintained at 1–2 mL/kg/h as long as these pigments are in the urine.[1,4] The addition of an osmotic diuretic such as mannitol may also be needed to assist in clearing the urine of these pigments.

Additional assessments and treatments
Decompression of stomach

To combat the problem of gastric ileus, a nasogastric tube should be inserted in all patients with major burns in order to decompress the stomach. This is especially important for patients being transported at high altitudes.[13] Additionally, all patients should be restricted from taking anything by mouth until after the transfer has been completed. Decompression of the stomach is usually necessary because an anxious, apprehensive patient will swallow considerable amounts of air and distend the stomach. Narcotics also diminish peristalsis of the gastrointestinal tract and result in distension.

A patient must be kept warm and dry. Hypothermia is detrimental to traumatized patients and can be avoided or at least minimized by the use of sheet and blankets. Wet dressings should be avoided.

The degree of pain experienced initially by the burn victim is inversely proportional to the severity of the injury.[8] No medication for pain relief should be given intramuscularly or subcutaneously. For mild pain, acetaminophen 650 mg orally every 4–6 hours may be given. For severe pain, morphine, 1–4 mg intravenously every 2–4 hours, is the drug choice, although meperidine (Demerol) 10–40 mg by IV push every 2–4 hours may be used.[10] Recommendations for tetanus prophylaxis are based on the patient's immunization history. All patients with burns should receive 0.5 mL of tetanus toxoid. If prior immunization is absent or unclear, or if the last booster was more than 10 years ago, 250 units of tetanus immunoglobulin is also given.[4]

Transportation guidelines

The primary purpose of any transport teams is not to bring a patient to an intensive care unit but to bring that level of care to the patient as soon as possible. Therefore, the critical time involved in a transport scenario is the time it takes to get the team to the patient. The time involved in transporting a patient back to a burn center becomes secondary. Communication and teamwork are the keynotes to an effective transport system.

When transportation is required from a referring facility to a specialized burn center, a patient can be fairly well stabilized before being moved. Initially, the referring facility should be informed that all patient referrals require physician-to-

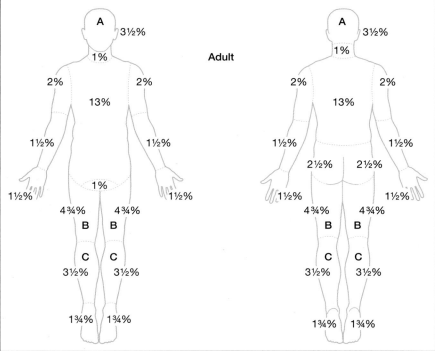

Age	0–1	1–4	5–9	10–14	15
A – ½ of head	9½%	8½%	6½%	5½%	4½%
B – ½ of one thigh	9½%	8½%	6½%	5½%	4½%
C – ½ of one leg	9½%	8½%	6½%	5½%	4½%

Fig. 7.3 Estimation of burn size using the Lund and Browder method.

BOX 7.1 Criteria for transfer of a burn patient to a burn center[4]

- Second-degree burns greater than 10% total body surface area (TBSA)
- Third-degree burns
- Burns that involve the face, hands, feet, genitalia, perineum, and major joints
- Chemical burns
- Electrical burns including lightning injuries
- Any burn with concomitant trauma in which the burn injuries pose the greatest risk to the patient
- Inhalation injury
- Patients with preexisting medical disorders that could complicate management, prolong recovery, or affect mortality
- Hospitals without qualified personnel or equipment for the care of critically burned children

Reproduced from Advanced Burn Life Supporters Manual. Chicago, IL: American Burn Association, 2005.[4]

BOX 7.2 Burn fluid resuscitation formula[14]

Fluid administration — Ringer's lactate

FIRST 24 HOURS:

- $5000\,mL/m^2$ burn + $2000\,mL$/body area m^2; administer half in 8 hours and the remaining half in 16 hours

SECOND 24 HOURS:

- $3750\,mL/m^2$ burn + $1500\,mL$/body area m^2; administer half in 8 hours and the remaining half in 16 hours
  Adjust the above rates to maintain a urine output of $1\,mL/kg/h$

Reproduced with permission from Herndon DN, Rutan R, Rutan T. The management of burned children. J Burn Care Rehabil 1993 14:3–8.[14]

---

physician discussion. Pertinent information needed will include patient demographic data; time, date, cause and extent of burn injury; weight and height; baseline vital signs; neurological status; laboratory data; respiratory status; previous medical and surgical history; and allergies.

A referring hospital is informed of specific treatment protocols regarding patient management prior to transfer. To ensure patient stability the following guidelines are offered:

- Establish two IV sites, preferably in an unburned upper extremity, and secure IV tubes with sutures.
- Insert a Foley catheter and monitor for acceptable urine output (30 mL/h adult, 1 mL/kg/h child).
- Insert a nasogastric tube and ensure that the patient remains NPO.
- Maintain body temperature between 38 and 39.0°C rectally.
- Stop all narcotics.
- For burns less than 24 hours old, only use lactated Ringer's solution. The staff physician will advise on the infusion rate, which is calculated based on the percentage of TBSA burned.

Following physician-to-physician contact and collection of all pertinent information, the physicians will make recommendations regarding an appropriate mode of transportation. The options are based on distance to a referring unit, patient complexity, and comprehensiveness of medical care required. Options include:

- Full medical intensive care unit transport with a complete team, consisting of a physician, a nurse, and a respiratory therapist from the burn facility.
- Medical intensive care transport via fixed-wing or helicopter with a team from a referring facility.
- Private plane with medical personnel to attend patient.
- Commercial airline.
- Private ground ambulance.
- Transport van with appropriate personnel.

Transport team composition

Because stabilization and care for a burned patient is so specialized, team selection is of the utmost importance. Traditionally, these patients were placed in an ambulance with an emergency medical technician and transported with few efforts made to stabilize the patient prior to transfer. As levels of care and technology have evolved, the need for specialized transport personnel has been increasingly observed. Today most transport teams are made up of one or more of the following healthcare members: a registered nurse, a respiratory therapist, and/or a staff physician or house resident. Because a large number of burned patients require some type of respiratory support due to inhalation injury or carbon monoxide intoxication, the respiratory therapist and nurse team has proven to be an effective combination. The background and training of nurses and therapists differ in many ways, so such a team provides a larger scope of knowledge and experience when both are utilized. Team members ideally should be cross-trained so that each member can function at the other's level of expertise.

Training and selection

Since the transport team will work in a high-stress environment, often with life or death consequences, these individuals must be carefully selected. The selection process should involve interviews with a nursing administrator, a director of respiratory therapy, and a medical director of a transport program.

Minimum requirements for transport team members should include:

- Transport nurse qualifications:
  - a registered nurse;
  - minimum of 6 months burn care experience;
  - current cardiopulmonary resuscitation (CPR) certification;
  - advanced cardiac life support (ACLS) or pediatric advanced life support (PALS) certification;
  - able to demonstrate clinical competency;
  - observe two transports;
  - a valid passport for international response.
- Transport respiratory therapist qualifications:
  - registered/certified respiratory therapist with 6 months burn care experience;
  - licensed by appropriate regulatory agency as a respiratory care practitioner;
  - have current CPR certification;
  - have ACLS or PALS certification;
  - able to demonstrate clinical competency;
  - observe two transports;
  - demonstrate a working knowledge of transport equipment;
  - a valid passport for international response.

Because all of the care rendered by a transport team outside a hospital is given as an extension of care from a transporting/receiving facility, specific steps must be taken to protect staff and physicians from medical liability and to provide consistent care for all patients. Strict protocols are used to guide all patient care; team members should be in constant communications with an attending physician regarding a patient's condition and the interventions to be considered. Team members must be proficient at a number of procedures, which may be needed during transport or while stabilizing a patient prior to transport. To keep up with current technology and changes, team members should be included in discussions of recent transports and current management techniques, so that they can discuss patient care issues, receive ongoing in-service education, and participate in a review of the quality of transports.

Modes of transportation

Once the need for transport of a burned patient is established, the decision must be rendered concerning what type of transportation vehicle is to be used (Table 7.1). There are two models of transport commonly used: ground (ambulance/transport vehicle), air (helicopter, fixed wing), or a combination of both. Factors to be considered when selecting a mode of transportation are the condition of the patient and the distance involved. The level of the severity of the burn mandates the speed with which the team must arrive in order the stabilize and transport a patient.[15]

Ground transport

Ground transport should be considered to cover distances of 70 miles or less; however, sometimes a patient's condition may require air transport, particularly helicopter transport, even though the distance is within the 70-mile range. The ground transport vehicle should be modified with special equipment needed for intensive care transport, and there must be enough room to comfortably seat team members and equipment.

Air transport

Air transport is used primarily when long distances or the critical nature of an injury separate a team from a patient. Air transport, however, does present its own unique set of problems. Aviation physiology is a specialty unto itself, and the gas laws play an important role in air transport and must be taken into consideration.

Dalton's law states that in a mixture of gases, the total pressure exerted by the mixture is equal to the sum of the pressures each would exert alone.[16] This is important when changing a patient's altitude because as altitude increases, barometric pressure decreases. The percentage of nitrogen, oxygen, and carbon dioxide remain the same, but the partial pressures they exert change (Table 7.2).[17]

Altitude is an important factor in the oxygenation of a transported patient and constant monitoring by a team is

TABLE 7.1 TRANSPORT CRITERIA: MODE AND TEAM COMPOSITION, BURNS ≤6 DAYS POST-BURN[15]				
Weight	% Burn	Distance (miles)	Team*	Transport mode
≤3	Any	75	C	Van, helicopter
		76–250	C	Turboprop airplane
		≥251	C	Learjet
3.1–20	≤10	75	N-RT	Van, helicopter
		76–500	N-RT	Commercial flight or turboprop airplane
		≥501	N-RT	Commercial airplane or Learjet
	≥10	75	C	Van, helicopter
		76–250	C	Turboprop airplane
		≥251	C	Learjet
20≥20	≤20	75	N	Commercial flight or turboprop airplane
		76–500	N-RT	
		≥501	N-RT	Commercial airplane or Learjet
	≥20	75	N	Van, helicopter
		76–500	C	Turboprop plane
		≥501	C	Jet

*C, Complete team (doctor, nurse, respiratory therapist); N, nurse; RT, respiratory therapist.
If any of the following criteria exist, the transport shall be changed to the fastest mode with a complete team:
- depressed mental status,
- drug depression,
- respiratory support,
- unstable cardiovascular system,
- presence of associated diseases,
- decreased urine output unresponsiveness to appropriate fluid administration,
- absent or marginal venous access,
- hypothermia unresponsive to corrective measures.

TABLE 7.2 ALTITUDE'S EFFECTS ON BLOOD GAS VALUES				
Altitude	Pressure	Tracheal P_{O_2}	Alveolar P_{O_2}	Alveolar P_{CO_2}
Sea level	760	149	103	40
5000 feet	632	122	79	38
10 000 feet	523	100	61	36
15 000 feet	429	80	46	33
20 000 feet	349	63	33	30

required under such circumstances. Boyle's law states that the volume of gas is inversely proportional to the pressure to which it is subject at a constant temperature. This gas law significantly affects patients with air leaks and free air in the abdomen, because as altitude increases, the volume of air in closed cavities also increases.[18] For this reason, all air that can be reached should be evacuated prior to an increase in altitude. Intrathoracic air and gastric air must be removed via functional chest tubes or nasogastric tubes and periodically checked during transport. Other factors that should be considered during air transport are reduced cabin pressure, turbulence, noise, and vibration, changes in barometric pressure, and acceleration/deceleration forces. Physiologic changes which affect a patient and team members include middle ear dysfunction, pressure-related problems with sinuses, air expansion in a gastrointestinal tract, and motion sickness. Utilizing transport vehicles that have pressurized cabins can reduce or eliminate most of these problems.[19]

Helicopters and fixed-wing aircraft

Helicopters and fixed-wing aircraft both have advantages and disadvantages related to patient care. Helicopters are widely used for short-distance medical air transport. Medical helicopters, because they are usually based on hospital premises, have no need to use airport facilities or ambulance services and, thereby, reduce team response time. Helicopters are able to land close to a referring hospital. Additionally, helicopters provide ease in loading and unloading patients and equipment.[15] The disadvantages of helicopter transport include its limited range, usually less than 150 miles,[20] and its non-pressurized cabin which limits the altitude at which patients can be safely carried. The low-altitude capabilities also subject the aircraft to variability in weather (i.e. fog, rain, and reduced visibility); therefore, helicopter flights experience much more interference due to the weather. Other disadvantages include noise, vibrations, reduced air speed, small working space, lower weight accommodation, and high maintenance requirements.[15]

When long distances must be traveled (greater than 150 miles) or when increased altitude is necessary, fixed-wing aircraft are considered as a viable mode of transport for patients. The advantages of using fixed-wing aircraft include: long-range capabilities, increased speed, ability to fly in most weather conditions, control of cabin pressure and temperature, larger cabin space, and more liberal weight restrictions. Disadvantages of fixed-wing aircraft include the need for an airport with adequate runway length, difficulty in loading and unloading patients and equipment, and the pressure of air turbulence and noise.

Equipment

Because medical equipment used in intensive care units has evolved tremendously in the last 10 years, there is no reason that these advances should not be extended to the equipment, which is used in a transport program. Tables 7.3 and 7.4 outline the drugs and equipment used in our successful transport system. The transport team must be able to provide ICU level care whenever needed. Most hospitals are well stocked and able to provide necessary supplies for initial patient stabilization and resuscitation; however, specialty items relating to the care of burn patients may not be present or adequate to meet the needs of burn victims. It is imperative

TABLE 7.3 MEDICAL EQUIPMENT USED IN A TRANSPORT SYSTEM

Monitor bag	Quantity	Monitor bag	Quantity
Pressure bag	1	Blood pressure tubing (NIBP)	1
EKG cable	1	Safe-cuff (NIBP — various sizes)	1 each
Pressure cable	2	Automatic blood pressure cuffs	1 each
Oxygen saturation cables	2	Temperature probe — rectal	1
Oxygen saturation probes	2	Thermometer	1
Stapler	1	Thermometer covers	1 box
Staple remover	1	Defibrillator jell tube	1
Stethoscope	1	Sphygmomanometer	1
EKG pads (adult/pedi)	9 each		
GI/GU bag	**Quantity**	**GI/GU bag**	**Quantity**
Salem sumps (10, 12, 14, 16 Fr)	1 each	Stylets adult/pedi	1
Feeding tube 8 Fr	1	Airways (sm, med, lg)	1
Surgilube	5	PEEP valves	2
Clean gloves	20	Wright respirometer	1
Umbilical tape	1 jar	Pleural drainage set	1
60 mL catheter tip syringe	2	Heimlich valves	2
Guaiac cards	10	Siemens Minimed III	1
Guaiac reagent	1 bottle	Defibrillator	1
Diastix	1 bottle	Batteries (C & D)	4 each
Benzoin swabs	5	Prepodyne swabs	4
Cal stat	1 bottle	Skin degreaser	1 bottle
Tongue blades	10	Nebulizer kit	2
Cotton swabs	10	1 inch tape roll	1
Foley's temp. (8, 10, 12, 16 Fr)	1 each	Nipple adapters	2
Sterile gloves	10	E cylinder regulator	2
pH paper	1	E cylinder wrench	2
Respiratory equipment		Suction catheters (8–14 Fr)	5 each
Resuscitation bag adult/pedi	1 each	Suction pump	1
Oxygen mask adult/pedi	1 each	Hard tip suction device	1
Venturi mask adult/pedi	1 each	Adapters (15 & 22 mm)	2 each
T-Tube adapters	2	Normal saline vials	10
CPR microshield	1	Vaponephrine solution	1 bottle
Cricothyrotomy catheter sets	1	Goggles	1
Tracheostomy tubes (00–8.0)	1 each	Clean gloves	10
Endotracheal tubes (3.0–8.0)	2 each	Humid vent adapters	2
Laryngoscope handles (1 g.sm.)	2 each	Oxygen tanks aluminum	6
Laryngoscope blades (Miller — sizes 0–4)	1 each	Oxygen tubing	2
Laryngoscope blades (MacIntosh — sizes 0–4)	2	TXP transport ventilator	1
Magill forceps adult/pedi	1	Protocol Propaq 106	1
		Defibrillator battery support system	1

TABLE 7.4 BURN TRANSPORT SUPPLY LIST

Medications	Quantity	Medications	Quantity
Epinephrine	2	Compazine	2
Atropine sulfate	2	Hep-Lock flush	5
Sodium bicarbonate	2	Heparin	1
Calcium chloride	2	Lidocaine (injectable/cardiac strip)	1
D50	2		
Lidocaine	2	Narcan	4
Bretylol	2	Albumin	2
Isoproterenol	2	Regular insulin	1
Dopamine	4	Benadryl	4
Dobutrex	2	Chloral hydrate suppository	2
Calcium gluconate	2	Chloral hydrate 500 mg/10 mL	2
Lasix	10	Tylenol 650 mg/25 mL	2
Potassium chloride	4	Tylenol suppository	2
Ranitidine	2	Lacri-Lube tube	2
Benadryl (injectable)	4	Maalox	1
Polysporin ointment	2	Phenergan	2
Elase ointment	2	Thorazine	2

Medical equipment	Quantity	Medical equipment	Quantity
IV bag 1			
D5.3NS 1000 mL	2	Needle holder	1
D10W 500 mL	1	Hemostat	1
Lactated Ringer's solution	2	0-silk suture	3
48" pressure tubing	2	Staples (10, 11, 15)	1
IV start pack	2	Solution sets (10 gtts, mL)	2
T-piece	4	Solution sets (60 gtts/mL)	2
Stopcocks	4	Minimed full set	2
Y-ports	2	Minimed half set	2
Scissors	1	Betadine (bottle)	1
IV bag 2			
D5W 250 mL	2	Syringes (1, 3, 5, 10, 35 mL)	10 each
Normal saline 250 mL	2	Needles (22 g, 20 g, 19 g, 16 g)	10 each
Pressure transducers	2	IV catheters (16 g, 18 g, 20 g, 22 g)	6 each
60 mL Luer-lock syringe	2	Medicuts (18 g, 20 g, 22 g)	1 each

Side pouch	Quantity	Side pouch	Quantity
Kerlix 6 inch	10	Burn dressing (1 g)	2
Ace wraps (6, 4 and 3 inch)	6 each	1 inch tape roll	1
Space blanket	1	2 inch tape roll	1
Urometer	1	4 × 4's (box)	2

that adequate equipment be available to handle any situation that may arise during a transport process (Figure 7.4). Extra battery packs and electrical converters on fixed-wing aircraft are recommended due to long transport times and delays caused by unforeseeable circumstances of weather or logistics.

Portable monitor

A portable ECG monitor capable of monitoring two pressure channels should accompany all patients in transport. This allows for continuous monitoring of heart rate, rhythm, and arterial blood pressure. The second pressure channel may be used for patients with a pulmonary artery catheter or those

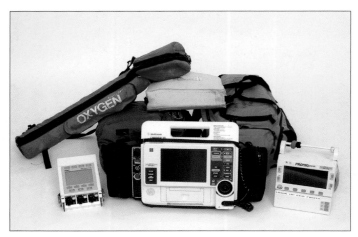

Fig. 7.4 Typical equipment used in transport of a patient.

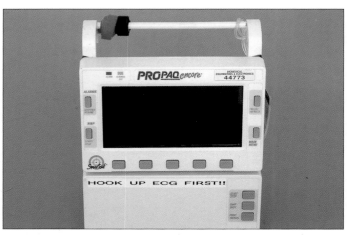

Fig. 7.5 Portable ECG monitor used in transport.

who need intracranial pressure monitoring. This monitor should be small and lightweight but able to provide a display bright enough to be seen from several feet away. The monitor should have its own rechargeable power supply which continuously charges while connected to an alternating current (AC) power supply. One suitable unit is the Protocol Systems Propaq 106 portable monitor (Figure 7.5). This monitor has two pressure channels; it provides a continuous display of ECG, heart rate, systolic, diastolic, and mean blood pressure; it can display temperature and oxygen saturation; and it is also capable of operating a non-invasive blood pressure cuff. High and low alarms for each monitored parameter can be set, silenced, or disabled by a trained operator.

Infusion pump

Continuous delivery of fluids and pharmacological agents must not be interrupted during transport. Infusion pumps can be easily attached to stretchers and are usually capable of operating for several hours on internal batteries. These devices should have alarms to warn of infusion problems and should be as small and lightweight as possible (Figure 7.6).

Ventilator

Size, weight, and oxygen consumption are the primary concerns in selecting transport ventilators. A weight under 5 pounds (2.2 kg) is desirable, and a ventilator's dimensions should make it easy to mount or to place on a bed. Orientation of controls should be along a single plane, and inadvertent movement of dials should be difficult.[21] The ventilator breathing circuit and exhalation valve should be kept simple, and incorrect assembly should be impossible. The TXP transport ventilator (Percussionaire Corporation, Sand Point, ID) is a portable pressure-limited time-cycled ventilator and is approved for in-flight use by the US Air Force (Figure 7.7). The transport ventilator weighs 1.5 pounds (0.68 kg), can be set to provide respiratory rates of between 6 and 250 breaths per minute, and provides tidal volumes of between 5 and 1500 cc. This ventilator is powered entirely by oxygen and requires no electrical power. All timing circuit gases are delivered to the patient so that operation of the ventilator does not

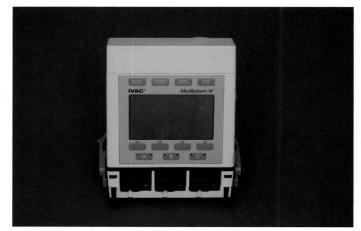

Fig. 7.6 Portable IV pump used in transport.

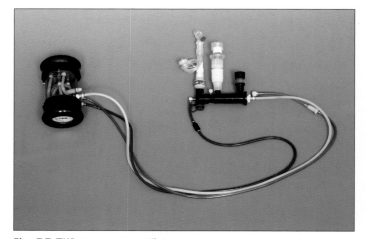

Fig. 7.7 TXP transport ventilator.

consume additional oxygen. The I:E ratios are preset at the factory from 1:1 at frequencies of 250 cycles per minute to 1:5 at a rate of 6 cycles per minute. As a result, breath stacking and undesired overinflation due to air trapping may be avoided.[22]

Stabilization

One of the primary reasons for a specialized transport team is to be able to transport a patient in as stable condition as possible. Current practice has evolved to embrace the concept that events during the first few hours following burn injury may affect the eventual outcome of the patient; this is especially true with regard to fluid management and inhalation injury. Stabilization techniques performed by the transport team have been expanded to include procedures that are usually not performed by nursing or respiratory personnel. Such techniques include interpreting radiographs and laboratory results and then conferring with fellow team members, referring physicians, and the team's own medical staff in order to arrive at a diagnosis and plan for stabilization. The transport team may perform such procedures as venous cannulation, endotracheal intubation, arterial blood gas interpretation, and management of mechanical ventilators. Team members may request new radiographs, in order to assess catheter or endotracheal tube placement or to assess the pulmonary system's condition. Team members may aid in the diagnosis of air leaks (pneumothorax) and evacuate the pleural space of the lung by needle aspiration as indicated. All of these procedures may be immediately necessary and lifesaving. Cross-training of all team members to be able to perform the others' jobs is recommended in order to safeguard patients in the event that any team member becomes incapacitated during transport. All these skills can be learned via experience in a burn intensive care unit, through formal training seminars, and via a thorough orientation program. Mature judgment, excellent clinical skills, and the ability to function under stress are characteristics needed when selecting candidates for a transport program.

Patient assessment prior to transport to a specialized burn care unit from a referring hospital

Initial assessment upon arrival of a flight team should include a list of standard procedures for determining a burned patient's current condition. First, a thorough review of the patient's history concerning the accident and past medical history must be done. This process provides the transport team with an excellent base from which to begin to formulate a plan of action. The patient will certainly have been diagnosed by a referring physician; however, a transport team often finds problems overlooked in initial evaluations. Since burn care is a specialized field, modes of treatment may very greatly outside the burn treatment community. Frequently, a referring hospital is not well versed in the treatment of burn victims and should not be expected to display the expertise found among clinicians who work with such patients everyday. Thus, the next step in stabilizing a burn patient is a physical assessment done by a transport team. These procedures should always be performed in the same order and in a structured fashion. Assessment of a burn patient begins with the ABCs of a primary survey, including airway, breathing, circulation, cervical spine immobilization, and a brief baseline neurological examination. All patients should be place on supplemental oxygen prior to transport in order to minimize the effects of altitude changes on oxygenation. Two IV lines should be started peripherally with a 16-gauge catheter or larger. Ideally, IV lines should be placed in non-burn areas but may be placed through a burn if they are the only sites available for cannulation. Intravenous lines should be sutured in place because venous access may not be available after the onset of generalized edema. The fluid of choice for initial resuscitation is lactated Ringer's solution.

In addition to initial stabilization procedures, blood should be obtained for initial laboratory studies if not already done. Initial diagnostic studies include hematocrit, electrolytes, urinalysis, chest X-ray, arterial blood gas, and carboxyhemoglobin levels. Any correction of laboratory values must be done prior to transfer and verified with repeat studies. Electrocardiographic monitoring should be instituted on any patient prior to transfer. Electrode patches may be a problem to place because the adhesive will not stick to burned skin. If alternative sites for placement cannot be found, an option for monitoring is to insert skin staples and attach the monitor leads to them with alligator clips. This provides a stable monitoring system, particularly for the agitated or restless patient who may displace needle electrodes. A Foley catheter with a urimeter should be placed to accurately monitor urine output. Acceptable hydration is indicated by a urine output of more than 30 mL/h in an adult (5 mL/kg/h) and at least 1 mL/kg/h in a child.

With the exception of escharotomies, open chest wounds, and actively bleeding wounds, management during transport consists of simply covering wounds with a topical antimicrobial agent or a biological dressing. Wet dressings are contraindicated because of the decreased thermoregulatory capacity of patients sustaining large burns and the possibility of hypothermia. To combat the problem of a gastric ileus, a nasogastric tube should be inserted in all burn patients in order to decompress the stomach. This is especially important for patients being transferred at high altitudes. Hypothermia can be avoided or minimized by the use of heated blankets and/or aluminized Mylar space blankets. The patient's rectal temperature must be kept between 37.5 and 39.0°C.

A clear, concise, chronological record of the mechanism of injury and assessment of airway, breathing, and circulation should be kept in the field and en route to the hospital. This information is vital for a referring facility to better understand and anticipate the condition of the patient. Additionally, all treatments, including invasive procedures, must be recorded, along with a patient's response to these interventions.

Summary

Burn injuries present a major challenge to a healthcare team, but an orderly, systematic approach can simplify stabilization and management. A clear understanding of the pathophysiology of burn injuries is essential for providing quality burn care in the pre-hospital setting, at the receiving healthcare facility, and at the referring hospital prior to transport. After a patient has been rescued from an injury-causing agent, assessment of the burn victim begins with a primary survey. Life-threatening injuries must be treated first, followed by a secondary survey, which documents and treats other injuries or problems. Intravenous access may be established in concert with local/regional medical control and appropriate fluid resuscitation begun. Burn wounds should be covered with clean, dry sheets; and the patient should be kept warm with blankets to prevent hypothermia. The patient should be transported to an emergency room in the most appropriate mode available.

At the local hospital, it should be determined if a burn patient needs burn center care according to the American Burn Association Guidelines. In preparing for organizing a transfer of a burn victim, consideration must be given to the continued monitoring and management of the patient during transport. In transferring burn patients, the same priorities developed for pre-hospital management remain valid. During initial assessment and treatment and throughout transport, the transport team must ensure that the patient has an adequate airway, breathing, circulation, fluid resuscitation, urine output, and pain control. Ideally, transport of burn victims will occur through an organized, protocol-driven plan that includes specialized transport mechanisms and personnel. Successful transport of burn victims, whether in the pre-hospital phase or during interhospital transfer, requires careful attention to treatment priorities, protocols, and details.

References

1. Boswick JA, ed. The art and science of burn care. Rockville, MD: Aspen Publishers; 1987.
2. Dimick AR. Triage of burn patients. In: Wachtel TL, Kahn V, Franks HA, eds. Current topics in burn care. Rockville, MD: Aspen Systems; 1983:15–18.
3. Wachtel TL. Initial care of major burns. Postgrad Med 1989; 85(1):178–196.
4. American Burn Association. Advanced burn life support providers manual. Chicago, IL: American Burn Association; 2005.
5. American Burn Association. Radiation injury. Advanced burn life support manual. Appendix 1. Chicago, IL: American Burn Association; 2005.
6. Bartholomew CW, Jacoby WD. Cutaneous manifestations of lightning injury. Arch Dermatol 1975; 26:1466–1468.
7. Committee on Trauma, American College of Surgeons. Burns. In: Advanced trauma life support course book. Chicago, IL: American College of Surgeons; 1984;155–163.
8. Rauscher LA, Ochs GM. Pre-hospital care of the seriously burned patient. In: Wachtel TL, Kahn V, Franks HA, eds. Current topics in burn care. Rockville, MD: Aspen Systems; 1983:1–9.
9. Goldfarb JW. The burn patient, Air Medical Crew national standards curriculum, Phoenix: ASHBEAMS; 1988.
10. Marvin JA, Heinback DM. Pain control during the intensive care phase of burn care. Crit Care Clin 1985; 1:147–157.
11. Mlcak RP, Helvick B. Protocol for securing endotracheal tubes in a pediatric burn unit. J Burn Care Rehabil 1987; 8:233–237.
12. Herndon DN, Desai MH, Abston S. et al. Residents manual. Galveston: Shriners Burns Hospital, and the University of Texas Medical Branch; 1992:1–17.
13. Collini FJ, Kealy GP. Burns: a review and update. Contemp Surg 1989; 34:75–77.
14. Herndon DN, Rutan R, Rutan T. The management of burned children. J Burn Care Rehabil 1993; 14:3–8.
15. Roy LR, Cunningham W. Transport. Neonatal and pediatric respiratory care. St Louis: CV Mosby; 1988:321.
16. McPhearson SP. Respiratory therapy equipment, 3rd edn. St Louis: Mosby; 1986.
17. US Navy Flight Surgeons' Manual. Government publication, 1968.
18. Jacobs B. Emergency patient care, pre-hospital ground and air procedures. New York: Macmillan; 1983.
19. McNeil EL. Airborne care of the ill and injured. New York: Springer-Verlag; 1983.
20. Federal Regulations for Pilots. Government publication, 1987.
21. Branson RD. Intrahospital transport of critically ill, mechanically ventilated patients. Respir Care 1992; 37:775–793.
22. Johanningman JA, Branson RD, Cambell RS, et al. Laboratory and clinical evaluation of the Max transport ventilator. Resp Care 1990; 35:952–959.

Chapter 8

Pathophysiology of burn shock and burn edema

George C. Kramer, Tjøstolv Lund, and Orlando K. Beckum

Chapter contents

Introduction and historical notes

Cutaneous thermal injury greater than one-third of the total body surface area (TBSA) invariably results in the severe and unique derangements of cardiovascular function called burn shock. Shock is an abnormal physiologic state in which tissue perfusion is insufficient to maintain adequate delivery of oxygen and nutrients and removal of cellular waste products. Before the 19th century, investigators demonstrated that, after a burn, fluid is lost from the blood and blood becomes thicker; and in 1897, saline infusions for severe burns were first advocated.[1,2] However, a more complete understanding of burn pathophysiology was not reached until the work of Frank Underhill.[3] He demonstrated that unresuscitated burn shock correlates with increased hematocrit values in burned patients, which are secondary to fluid and electrolyte loss after burn injury. Increased hematocrit values occurring shortly after severe burn were interpreted as a plasma volume deficit. Cope and Moore showed that the hypovolemia of burn injury resulted from fluid and protein translocation into both burned and nonburned tissues.[4]

Over the last 80 years an extensive record of both animal and clinical studies has established the importance of fluid resuscitation for burn shock. Investigations have focused on correcting the rapid and massive fluid sequestration in the burn wound and the resultant hypovolemia. The peer-reviewed literature contains a large experimental and clinical database on the circulatory and microcirculatory alterations associated with burn shock and edema generation in both the burn wound and nonburned tissues. During the last 40 years, research has focused on identifying and defining the release mechanisms and effects of the many inflammatory mediators produced after burn injury.[5]

It is now recognized that burn shock is a complex process of cardiovascular dysfunction that is not easily or fully repaired by fluid resuscitation. Severe burn injury results in significant hypovolemic shock and substantial tissue trauma, both of which cause the formation and release of many local and systemic mediators.[6–8] Burn shock results from the interplay of hypovolemia and multiple mediators of inflammation with effects on both the microcirculation as well as the function of the heart, large vessels, and lungs. Subsequently, burn shock continues as a significant pathophysiologic state, even if hypovolemia is corrected. Increases in pulmonary and systemic vascular resistance (SVR) and myocardial depression occur despite adequate preload and volume support.[8–12] Such cardiovascular dysfunctions can further exacerbate the whole body inflammatory response into a vicious cycle of accelerating organ dysfunction.[7,8,13] Hemorrhagic hypovolemia with severe mechanical trauma can provoke a similar form of shock.

This chapter examines our present understanding of the pathophysiology of the early events in burn shock, focusing on the many facets of organ and systemic effects directly resulting from hypovolemia and circulating mediators. Inflammatory shock mediators, both local and systemic, that are implicated in the pathogenesis of burn shock include histamine, serotonin, bradykinin, nitric oxide, oxygen free radicals and products of the eicosanoid acid cascade (e.g. prostaglandin, thromboxane), tumor necrosis factor, and interleukins. Additionally, certain hormones and mediators of cardiovascular function are elevated several-fold after burn injury; these include epinephrine, norepinephrine, vasopressin, angiotensin II, and neuropeptide-Y. Most certainly other mediators and unknown factors yet to be defined are also involved. Understanding the complex mechanism of the pathophysiologic actions of these mediators may lead to optimally effective therapies are designed. The hope is that an improved early treatment of burn shock, perhaps through individualized fluid resuscitation protocols and methods of mediator blockade, can be developed to ameliorate or eliminate the incidence of organ dysfunction. Effective burn resuscitation and treatment of burn shock remains a major challenge in modern medicine. Extensive efforts have been expended altering mediator release or activity, but have not met with widespread clinical utility.

Hypovolemia and rapid edema formation

Burn injury causes extravasation of plasma into the burn wound and the surrounding tissues. Burn shock is hypovolemic in nature and characterized by the hemodynamic changes similar to those that occur after hemorrhage, including decreased plasma volume, cardiac output, urine output, and an increased systemic vascular resistance with resultant reduced peripheral blood flow.[6,8,14–16] However, as opposed to a fall in hematocrit with hemorrhagic hypovolemia (due to transcapillary refill) an increase in hematocrit and hemoglobin concentration will often appear even with adequate fluid resuscitation. As in the treatment of other forms of hypovolemic shock, the primary initial therapeutic goal is to promptly restore vascular volume and to preserve tissue perfusion in order to minimize tissue ischemia. In extensive burns (>25% TBSA), fluid resuscitation is complicated not only by the severe burn wound edema but also by extravasated and sequestered fluid and protein in nonburned soft tissue. Large volumes of resuscitation solutions are required to maintain vascular volume during the first several hours after an extensive burn. Data suggests that despite fluid resuscitation normal blood volume is not restored until 24–36 hours after large burns.[17]

Edema develops when the rate by which fluid is filtered out of the microvessels exceeds the flow in the lymph vessels draining the same tissue mass. Edema formation often follows a biphasic pattern. An immediate and rapid increase in the water content of burn tissue is seen in the first hour after burn injury.[15,18] A second and more gradual increase in fluid flux of both the burned skin and nonburned soft tissue occurs during the first 12–24 hours after burn injury.[7,18] The amount of edema formation in burned skin depends on the type and extent of injury,[15,19] and whether fluid resuscitation is provided as well as the type and volume of fluid administered.[20] However, fluid resuscitation elevates blood flow and capillary pressure contributing to further fluid extravasation. Without sustained delivery of fluid into the circulation, edema fluid is somewhat self-limited as plasma volume and capillary pressure decrease. The edema development in thermal injured skin is characterized by the extreme rapid onset of tissue water content, which can double within the first hour after burn.[15,21] Leape found a 70–80% water content increase in a full-thickness burn wound 30 minutes after burn injury with 90% of this change occurring in the first 5 minutes.[16,22,23] There was little increase in burn wound water content after the first hour in the nonresuscitated animals. In resuscitated animals or animals with small wounds, adequate tissue perfusion continues to 'feed' the edema for several hours. Demling et al. used dichromatic absorptionmetry to measure edema development during the first week after an experimental partial-thickness burn injury on one hind limb in sheep.[18] Although edema was rapid, with over 50% occurring in the first hour, maximum water content did not occur until 12–24 hours after burn injury.

Normal microcirculatory fluid exchange

An understanding of the physiologic mechanisms of the rapid formation of burn edema requires an understanding of the mechanisms of microvascular fluid balance. Under normal physiologic conditions, blood pressure in capillaries causes a filtration of fluid into the interstitial space of all tissue. This fluid is then partially reabsorbed into the circulation at the venous end of capillaries and venules, while the remaining net filtration is removed from the interstitial space by lymphatic drainage.[24,25] Fluid transport across the microcirculatory wall in normal and pathological states is quantitatively described by the Landis–Starling equation:

$$J_v = K_f [(P_c - P_{if}) - \sigma(COP_p - COP_{if})]$$

This equation describes the interaction of physical forces that govern fluid transfer between vascular and extravascular compartments. J_v is the volume of fluid that crosses the microvasculature barrier. K_f is the capillary filtration coefficient, which is the product of the surface area and hydraulic conductivity of the capillary wall; P_c is the capillary hydrostatic pressure; P_{if} is the interstitial fluid hydrostatic pressure; COP_p is the colloid osmotic pressure of plasma; COP_{if} is the colloid osmotic pressure of interstitial fluid; σ is the osmotic reflection coefficient. Edema occurs when the lymphatic drainage (J_L) does not keep pace with the increased J_v (Figure 8.1).

Mechanisms of burn edema

By analyzing the factors interrelating the physiological determinants of transmicrovascular fluid flux (i.e. Landis–Starling equation), edema may theoretically be formed by: increased K_f, P_c, or COP_{if}, as well as by decreased P_{if}, σ, and COP_p. Burn edema may be unique among other types of edema, because it is only in burn edema that all of these variables change significantly in the direction required to increase fluid filtration. Each variable is discussed individually.

Capillary filtration coefficient (K_f)

Burn injury causes direct and indirect mediator-modulated changes of the permeability of blood tissue barrier of the capillaries and venules. Arturson and Mellander showed that K_f, in the scalded hind limb, immediately increases two to three times suggesting that the hydraulic conductivity (water permeability) of the capillary wall increases.[26] However, K_f is a function of both hydraulic conductivity and the capillary surface area. Thus, local vasodilation and microvascular recruitment also contribute to the increased K_f. Measuring K_f and the rate of edema formation (J_v) allowed Arturson and Mellander to determine the changes in transcapillary forces necessary to account for the increased capillary filtration. Their calculations indicated that a transcapillary pressure gradient of 100–250 mmHg was required to explain the extremely rapid edema formation that occurred in the first 10 minutes after a scald injury. They concluded that only a small fraction of the early formation of burn edema could be attributed to the changes in K_f and permeability. They further suggested that osmotically active molecules generating sufficiently large osmotic reabsorption pressures are released from burn-damaged cells. However, subsequent studies described below show that very large increases in filtration force are due to increased P_c and particularly to a large decrease in P_{if} of burn-injured skin (Table 8.1).

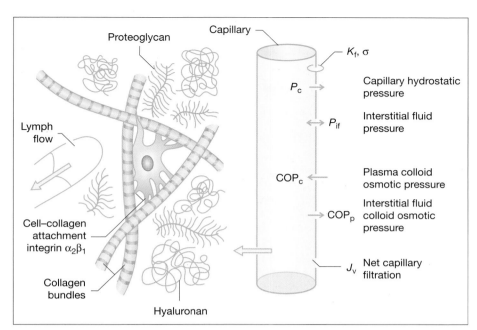

Fig. 8.1 Landis–Starling equation.

TABLE 8.1 EFFECT OF BURN INJURY ON CHANGES IN THE STARLING EQUATION VARIABLES				
Variable	Normal or baseline	Post-burn	Δ	Reference Nos
P_c	25 mmHg	50 mmHg	↑ 25 mmHg	46
COP_P	20 to 28 mmHg	15 to 18 mmHg	↓ 10 mmHg	50,51
P_i	–2 to 0 mmHg	~100 mmHg non-resuscitated non-perfused skin and –5 mmHg perfused skin	↓ 100 mmHg ↓ 3–5 mmHg	19,52 53,54
COP_{if}	10 to 15 mmHg	13–18 mmHg in burn wound ↓ and with resuscitation hypoproteinemia in nonburned skin	↑ 3 mmHg	51,53,54
σ	0.9	0.5	↓ 0.4	46,55,56
K_f	0.003 mL/min per mmHg per 100 g (leg)	↑ 2 to 3×		26,56

Notes: Enhanced microvascular blood flow typically increases capillary surface area.
Permeability typically refers to protein permeability of the microvascular exchange vessels, which is often linked to hydraulic conductivity.

Capillary pressure (P_c)

In most forms of shock, capillary pressure decreases as a result of arteriolar vasoconstriction. However, studies in which P_c was measured using vascular occlusion methods, in the scalded hind limb of dogs, showed that it doubled from ~25 mmHg to ~50 mmHg during the first 30 minutes after burn injury and slowly returned to baseline over 3 hours.[46] We are unaware of studies that have measured P_c in nonburned skin, but P_c may decrease in nonburned tissue as a result of the documented increase in peripheral resistance.

Interstitial hydrostatic pressure (P_{if})

An initial surprising, but now well-verified finding is that P_{if} in dermis becomes extremely negative after thermal injury. Using a micropipette and tissue oncometer, Lund reported that dermal P_{if} was rapidly reduced from its normal value of –1 mmHg to less than –100 mmHg in isolated skin non-perfused preparations.[19] This generation of a strongly negative interstitial fluid hydrostatic pressure constitutes a 'suction force' or imbibition pressure adding to the capillary pressure in promoting fluid filtration from the intravascular to the interstitial space. *In vivo* measurements show a temporary reduction of –20 to –30 mmHg; presumably, this number is less negative because continued tissue perfusion and fluid extravasation relieves the imbibition pressure. After resuscitation, P_{if} can be increased to a positive value of 1–2 mmHg.[47,48] On the other hand, Kinsky reported a continued negative pressure providing a partial explanation for the sustained edema for the first 4 hours post-injury (Table 8.1).[49]

Tissue volume and hydration are greatly elevated with a decrease or no change in P_{if}, implying elevated interstitial compliance, which is likely to be the main mechanism that sustains burn edema for several days. The mechanism behind this negative-pressure generation is in part related to the denaturation of collagen[47,48] and to changes in the compliance of thermally injured tissue. The release of adhesional forces (β_1-integrins) between the interstitial matrix fibers and connective tissue cells (fibroblasts) was found to cause an imbibition pressure to develop following different inflammatory reactions.[57] The cell–matrix interactions and intercellular adhesion are made up of four classes of molecules: the immunoglobulin superfamily, the cadherins, the selectins, and the integrins. Integrins are a group of cell-surface molecules which play an important role in cell–cell and cell–matrix interactions[159] and thus function as mechanoreceptors. Integrins are vital for cell migration and organization of the cytoskeleton. Antibodies towards the β_1-integrins have been shown to lower P_{if}.[160]

The magnitude of the decrease in P_{if} establishes it as the predominant mechanism responsible for both the initial rapid development of edema and the sustained edema.

Osmotic reflection coefficient (σ)

The osmotic reflection coefficient is an index of the proportion of the full osmotic pressure generated by the concentration gradient of plasma proteins across the capillary wall. A value of $\sigma = 1.0$ represents a membrane impermeable to protein; $\sigma = 0$ represents a membrane that is completely permeable to protein. In skin, the normal σ of albumin is reported to be 0.85–0.99.[25,58] Increased capillary permeability to protein causes a reduced σ, an effective reduction in the reabsorptive oncotic gradient across the capillary wall, and a resulting increase in net fluid filtration. Lymph sampled from burned skin has shown elevated protein concentrations consistent with the large and sustained increases in capillary permeability,[15,55,58] while a transient and smaller increase in capillary permeability occurs over 8–12 hours post-injury in other soft tissue not directly burned.[55] Pitt et al. estimated the σ for skin from dog hind paw using the lymph washdown technique and reported a normal σ of 0.87 for albumin and a reduction to 0.45 after scald injury.[46]

Plasma colloid osmotic pressure (COP_p)

The normal plasma protein concentration of 6–8 g/dL and its associated COP_p of 25–30 mmHg produce a significant transcapillary reabsorptive force partially outweighing the fluid filtration out of the microvasculature.[14,25] Plasma colloid osmotic pressure decreases in non-resuscitated burn injured animals as protein-rich fluid extravasates into burn wounds, while a significant volume of protein-poor transcapillary reabsorption comes from nonburned tissue such as skeletal muscle.[14,50,51,59] Plasma is further diluted and p_p is further reduced after crystalloid resuscitation. Zetterstrom and Arturson found that plasma oncotic pressure was reduced to half of the normal values in burn patients. COP_p can decrease so rapidly with resuscitation that the transcapillary colloid osmotic pressure gradient ($COP_p - COP_{if}$) will approach zero or even reverse to favor filtration and edema.[50,51] Although it is likely that some hypoproteinemia after major burn injury is inevitable, animal and clinical studies that used early colloid resuscitation maintained p_p at higher levels than crystalloid resuscitation alone.[7,59,60] The degree of hypoproteinemia and reduced COP_p were reported to correlate with the total volume of crystalloid solutions.[59] Initial therapy with colloid solution is advocated by some clinicians,[7] while the majority wait 8–24 hours post-injury, reasoning that some normalization of microvascular permeability in injured tissue must occur before colloid therapy is cost-effective.[8]

Interstitial colloid osmotic pressure (COP_{if})

The COP_{if} in skin is normally 10–15 mmHg or about one-half that of plasma in humans.[14,25] Experimental studies in animals using lymph as representative of interstitial fluid suggest that the colloid osmotic pressure in lymph from burned skin initially increases 4–8 mmHg.[55] However, more direct measurements of COP_{if} using wick sampling[14,20,51,61] or tissue sampling technique[14,25] show only modest initial increases in COP_{if} of 1–4 mmHg in the early nonresuscitated phase of burn injury. With resuscitation, COP_p falls and then COP_{if} decreases, as the protein concentration of capillary filtrate remains less than plasma despite an increased permeability. Studies show that σ decreases with burns, but never equals zero; thus, some protein sieving remains even in burn skin.[55] Compared with nonburned skin the COP_{if} remains significantly higher in the burn wound, supporting the view that sustained increases in protein permeability contributes to the persistence of burn edema.[14,25,49] However, compared with the large changes in P_c and particularly P_{if}, the increased capillary protein permeability is not the predominant mechanism for the early rapid rate of edema formation in injured skin.[47]

Nonburned tissue

Generalized edema in soft tissues that are not directly injured is another characteristic of large cutaneous burns. Brouhard et al. reported increased water content in nonburned skin even after a 10% burn, with the maximum increase occurring at 12 hours postburn.[62] Arturson reported an increased transcapillary fluid flux (lymph flow) from nonburned tissue and a transient increase in permeability, as measured by an increase in the lymph concentration of plasma protein and macromolecular dextran infused as a tracer.[15,21,58] Harms et al. extended these findings by measuring changes in lymph flow and protein transport of noninjured soft tissue for 3 days after injury.[55] They found that skin and muscle permeability (flank lymph from sheep) were elevated for up to 12 hours postburn for molecules the size of albumin and immunoglobulin G, while the microvascular permeability of the lung (lymph for caudal mediastinal node) showed no increase. Maximum increased lymph flow and tissue water content were observed to correlate with the severe hypoproteinemia occurring during the early resuscitation period of a 40% burn injury in sheep.[8,60] The sustained increase in water content and the elevated lymph flow of the nonburned tissue after the return of normal permeability is likely the result of the sustained hypoproteinemia.[50,55,58,59]

Demling and colleagues postulated that the edema could be partially attributed to alteration in the interstitial structure.[63] They suggested that interstitial protein washout increases the compliance of the interstitial space and that water transport and hydraulic conductivity across the entire blood–tissue–

lymph barrier increased with hypoproteinemia. Several clinical and animal studies have established that maintaining higher levels of total plasma protein concentration can ameliorate the overall net fluid retention and edema.[7,64] Edema in nonburned areas can also be limited by using nonprotein colloids such as dextran, if the colloid osmotic gradient is increased above normal.[8,60] However, it is not known if either the correction of hypoproteinemia or the use of either albumin or dextran can lead to improved clinical outcome. It has been reported that the use of colloids has no beneficial effect on edema in the burn wound.[49,60] Use of hypertonic saline formulations as initial fluid therapies of burn shock can dramatically reduce initial volume requirements and net fluid volume (infused minus urine out).[65,66] However, a rebound effect subsequently increasing the fluid requirements (and net fluid balance) occurred after early use of both hypertonics and colloids.[60,65] Retrospective analyses of patients correlating early albumin use versus fluid requirements show significant volume sparing during the first post-burn day, but after 48 hours the affect is not significant.[67]

Altered cellular membranes and cellular edema

In addition to a loss of capillary endothelial integrity, thermal injury also causes change in the cellular membranes. Baxter demonstrated that in burns of >30% TBSA there is a systemic decrease in cellular transmembrane potentials as measured in skeletal muscle away from the site of injury.[10] It would be expected that the directly injured cell would have a damaged cell membrane, increasing sodium and potassium fluxes, resulting in cell swelling. However, this process also appears in cells that are not directly heat-injured. Micropuncture techniques have demonstrated partial depolarization in the normal skeletal muscle membrane potential of −90 mV to levels of −70 to −80 mV; cell death occurs at −60 mV. The decrease in membrane potentials is associated with an increase in intracellular water and sodium.[68–70] Similar alterations in skeletal membrane functions and cellular edema have been reported in hemorrhagic shock[68,70] and also in the cardiac, liver, and endothelial cells.[71–73] Early investigators of this phenomenon postulated that a decrease in ATP levels or ATPase activity was the mechanism for membrane depolarization; however, other research suggests that it may result from an increased sodium conductance in membranes or an increase in sodium–hydrogen antiport activity.[69,72] Resuscitation of hemorrhage rapidly restores depolarized membrane potentials to normal, but resuscitation of burn injury only partially restores the membrane potential and intracellular sodium concentrations to normal levels, demonstrating that hypovolemia alone is not totally responsible for the cellular swelling seen in burn shock.[74] A circulating shock factor(s) is likely to be responsible for the membrane depolarization,[75–77] but, surprisingly, the molecular characterization of such a circulating factor has not been elucidated, suggesting that it has a complex structure. Data suggests it has a large molecular weight >80 KDa.[78] Membrane depolarization may be caused by different factors in different states of shock. Very little is known about the time course of the changes in membrane potential in clinical burns. More importantly, we do not know the extent to which the altered membrane potentials affect total volume requirements and organ function in burn injury or shock in general.

Mediators of burn injury

Burn injury produces a veritable cornucopia of local and circulating mediators that are produced in the blood or released by cells after thermal injury. These mediators play important and complex roles in the pathogenesis of edema and the cardiovascular abnormalities of burn injury. Many mediators alter vascular permeability directly or indirectly by increasing the microvascular hydrostatic pressure and surface area via the arteriolar vasodilation superimposed on an already altered membrane (Table 8.2). The exact mechanism(s) of mediator-induced injury are of considerable clinical importance, as this understanding would allow for the development of pharmacologic modulation of burn edema and shock by mediator inhibition.

Histamine

Histamine is most likely to be the mediator most responsible for the early phase of increased microvascular permeability seen immediately after burn. Histamine causes large endothelial gaps to transiently form as a result of the contraction of venular endothelial cells.[27] Histamine is released from mast cells in thermal-injured skin; however, the increase in histamine levels and its actions are only transient. Histamine also can cause the rise in capillary pressure (P_c) by arteriolar dilation and venular contraction. Statistically significant reductions in burn edema have been achieved with histamine blockers and mast cell stabilizers when tested in acute animal models.[27] Friedl et al. demonstrated that the pathogenesis of burn edema in the skin of rats appears to be related to the interaction of histamine with xanthine oxidase and oxygen radicals.[29] Histamine and its metabolic derivatives increased the catalytic activity of xanthine oxidase (but not xanthine dehydrogenase) in rat plasma and in rat pulmonary artery endothelial cells. In thermally injured rats, levels of plasma histamine and xanthine oxidase rose in parallel, in association with the uric acid increase. Burn edema was greatly attenuated by treating rats with the mast cell stabilizer, cromolyn, complement depletion or the H_2 receptor antagonist, cimetidine, but was unaffected by neutrophil depletion.[28,33,79] Despite encouraging results in animals, beneficial antihistamine treatment of human burn injury has not been demonstrated, although antihistamines are administered to reduce risk of gastric ulcers.

Prostaglandins

Prostaglandins are potent vasoactive autocoids synthesized from arachidonic acid. They are released from burned tissue and inflammatory cells and contribute to the inflammatory response of burn injury.[35,80] Macrophages and neutrophils are activated through the body, infiltrate the wound, and release prostaglandin as well as thromboxanes, leukotrienes, and interleukin-1. These wound mediators have both local and systemic effects. Prostaglandin E_2 (PGE_2) and leukotrienes LB_4 and LD_4 directly and indirectly increase microvascular permeability.[81] Prostacyclin (PGI_2) is produced in burn injury and

TABLE 8.2 CARDIOVASCULAR AND INFLAMMATORY MEDIATORS OF BURN SHOCK

Mediators	Central cardiovascular effects (at high concentrations)	Load tissue effects	References
Histamine	↓ Blood pressure Hypovolemia	Arteriolar dilation, and venular constriction ↑ Blood flow ↑ Permeability	27–33
Prostaglandin E$_2$ (PGE$_2$)	↓ Systemic arterial and pulmonary arterial blood pressure	Vasodilation ↑ Blood flow ↑ Permeability	27,34,35
Prostacyclin (PG1$_2$)	↓ Blood pressure	↑ Permeability	27
Leukotrienes LB$_4$ LD$_4$	Pulmonary hypertension	Vasoconstriction of pulmonary vessels	27
Thromboxane A$_2$ (TXA$_2$) Thromboxane B$_2$ (TXB$_2$)	GI ischemia Pulmonary hypertension	Vasoconstriction ↑ Permeability	34,36–38
Bradykinin	↓ Blood pressure Hypovolemia	Vasodilation, ↑ Permeability	27,32
Serotonin		↑ Permeability	31
Catecholamines Epinephrine Norepinephrine	↑ Heart rate ↑ Blood pressure ↑ Metabolism	Vasoconstriction (∝,receptors); Vasodilation (β$_2$ receptors in muscle); block ↑ permeability due to histamine and bradykinin via β receptors	27,30,39,40
Oxygen radicals: Superoxide anion (O$_2^-$) Hydrogen peroxide (H$_2$O$_2$) Hydroxyl ion (OH$^-$) Peroxynitrite (ONOO$^-$)	Cardiac dysfunction	Tissue damage ↑ Permeability	27–29,41
Platelet aggregation factor	↑ Blood pressure	Vasoconstriction	42–44
Angiotensin II	GI ischemia ↑ Blood pressure	Vasoconstriction	45
Vasopressin	GI ischemia ↑ Blood pressure	Vasoconstriction	45

is a vasodilator, but also may cause direct increases in capillary permeability. PGE$_2$ appears to be one of the more potent inflammatory prostaglandins, causing the postburn vasodilation in wounds, which, when coupled with the increased microvascular permeability, amplifies edema formation.[82,83]

Thromboxane

Thromboxane A$_2$ (TXA$_2$) and its metabolite, thromboxane B$_2$ (TXB$_2$), are produced locally in the burn wound by platelets.[27] Vasoconstrictor thromboxanes may be less important in edema formation; however, by decreasing blood flow they can contribute to a growing zone of ischemia under the burn wound and can cause the conversion of a partial-thickness wound to a deeper full-thickness wound. The serum level of TXA, and TXA$_2$/PGI$_2$ ratios are increased significantly in burn patients.[36] Heggers showed the release of TXB$_2$ at the burn wound was associated with local tissue ischemia, and that thromboxane inhibitors prevented the progressive dermal ischemia associated with thermal injury and thromboxane release.[34,84] A TXA$_2$ synthesis inhibitor, anisodamine, also demonstrated beneficial macrocirculatory effects by restoring the hemody-

namic and rheological disturbances towards normal. Demling showed that topically applied ibuprofen (which inhibits the synthesis of prostaglandins and thromboxanes) decreases both local edema and prostanoid production in burned tissue without altering systemic production.[85] On the other hand, systemic administration of ibuprofen did not modify early edema, but did attenuate the postburn vasoconstriction that impaired adequate oxygen delivery to tissue in burned sheep.[37] Although cyclooxygenase inhibitors have been used after burn injury, no convincing benefit or routine clinical use, has been reported.

Kinins

Bradykinin is a local mediator of inflammation that increases venular permeability. It is likely that bradykinin production is increased after burn injury, but its detection in blood or lymph can be difficult owing to the simultaneous increase in kininase activity and the rapid inactivation of free kinins. The generalized inflammatory response after burn injury favors the release of bradykinin.[86] Pretreatment of burn-injured animals with aprotinin, a general protease inhibitor, should have decreased the release of free kinin, but no effect on edema was noted.[87] On the other hand, pretreatment with a specific bradykinin receptor antagonist reduced edema in full-thickness burn wound in rabbits.[88]

Serotonin

Serotonin is released early after burn injury.[31] This agent is a smooth-muscle constrictor of large blood vessels. Antiserotonin agents such as ketanserin have been found to decrease peripheral vascular resistance after burn injury, but have not been reported to decrease edema.[31] On the other hand, the pretreatment effect of methysergide, a serotonin antagonist, reduces hyperemic or increased blood flow response in the burn wounds of rabbits, along with reducing the burn edema.[88] Methysergide did not prevent increases in the capillary reflection coefficient or permeability.[89] Ferrara et al. found a dose-dependent reduction of burn edema when methysergide was given preburn to dogs, but claimed that this was not attributable to blunting of the regional vasodilator response.[89] Zhang et al. reported a reduction in non-nutritive skin blood flow after methysergide administration to burned rabbits.[90]

Catecholamines

Circulating catecholamines, epinephrine and norepinephrine are released in massive amounts after burn injury.[7,91,92] On the arteriolar side of the microvessels these agents cause vasoconstriction via α_1-receptor activation, which tends to reduce capillary pressure, particularly when combined with the hypovolemia and the reduced venous pressure of burn shock.[27] Reduced capillary pressure may limit edema and induce interstitial fluid to be reabsorbed from nonburned skin, skeletal muscle, and visceral organs in nonresuscitated burn shock. Further, catecholamines, via β-agonist activity, may also partially inhibit increased capillary permeability induced by histamine and bradykinin.[27] These potentially beneficial effects of catecholamines may not be operative in directly injured tissue and may also be offset in nonburned tissue by the deleterious vasoconstrictor and ischemic effects. The hemodynamic effects of catecholamines will be discussed later in the chapter.

Oxygen radicals

Oxygen radicals play an important inflammatory role in all types of shock, including burn. These short-lived elements are highly unstable reactive metabolites of oxygen; each one has an unpaired electron, making them strong oxidizing agents.[93] Superoxide anion (O_2^-), hydrogen peroxide (H_2O_2), and the hydroxyl ion (OH^-) are produced and released by activated neutrophils after any inflammatory reaction or reperfusion of ischemic tissue. The hydroxyl ion is believed to be the most potent and damaging of the three. The formation of the hydroxyl radical requires free ferrous iron (Fe_2) and H_2O_2. Evidence that these agents are formed after burn injury is the increased lipid peroxidation found in circulating red blood cells and biopsied tissue.[28,93,94] Demling showed that large doses of deferoxamine (DFO), an iron chelator, when used for resuscitation of 40% TBSA in sheep, prevented systemic lipid peroxidation and decreased the vascular leak in nonburned tissue while also increasing oxygen utilization.[95] However, DFO may have accentuated burned tissue edema, possibly by increasing the perfusion of burned tissue.

Nitric oxide (NO), when simultaneously generated with the superoxide anion can lead to the formation of peroxynitrite ($ONOO^-$). The presence of nitrotyrosine in burn skin found in the first few hours after injury suggests that peroxynitrite may play a deleterious role in burn edema.[96] On the other hand, the blockade of NO synthase did not reduce burn edema, while treatment with the NO precursor arginine reduces burn edema.[97] NO may be important for maintaining perfusion and limiting the zone of stasis in burn skin.[98] Although the pro- and anti-inflammatory roles of NO remain controversial, it would appear that the acute beneficial effects of NO generation outweigh any deleterious effect in burn shock.

Antioxidants, namely agents that either directly bind to the oxygen radicals (scavengers) or cause their further metabolism, have been evaluated in several experimental studies.[99,100] Catalase, which removes H_2O_2 and superoxide dismutase (SOD), which removes radical O_2^-, have been reported to decrease the vascular loss of plasma after burn injury in dogs and rats.[28,99]

The plasma of thermally injured rats showed dramatic increases in levels of xanthine oxidase activity, with peak values appearing as early as 15 minutes after thermal injury. Excision of the burned skin immediately after the thermal injury significantly diminished the increase in plasma xanthine oxidase activity.[28,29] The skin permeability changes were attenuated by treating the animals with antioxidants (catalase, SOD, dimethyl sulfoxide, dimethylthiourea) or an iron chelator (DFO), thus supporting the role of oxygen radicals in the development of vascular injury as defined by increased vascular permeability.[28] Allopurinol, a xanthine oxidase inhibitor, markedly reduced both burn lymph flow and levels of circulating lipid peroxides, and further prevented all pulmonary lipid peroxidation and inflammation. This suggests that the release of oxidants from burned tissue was in part responsible for local burn edema, as well as distant inflammation and oxidant release.[94] The failure of neutrophil depletion to protect against the vascular permeability changes and the protective effects of the xanthine oxidase inhibitors (allopurinol and lodoxamide tromethamine) suggests that plasma xanthine oxidase is the more likely source of the oxygen radicals involved in the formation of burn edema. These oxygen radicals can increase vascular permeability by damaging microvascular endothelial cells.[28,29] The use of antioxidants has been extensively investigated in animals, and some clinical trials suggest benefit. Antioxidants (vitamin C and E) are routinely administered to patients at many burn centers. High doses of antioxidant ascorbic acid (vitamin C) have been found to be efficacious in reducing fluid needs in burn-injured experimental animals when administered postburn.[103–105] The use of high doses (10–20 g/day) of vitamin C was shown to be effective in one clinical trial, but ineffective in another.[101,102] High-dose vitamin C has not received wide clinical usage.

Platelet aggregation factor

Platelet aggregation (or activating) factor (PAF) can increase capillary permeability and is released after burn injury.[43,87] Ono et al. showed in scald-injured rabbits that TCV-309 (Takeda Pharmaceutical Co Ltd., Japan), a PAF antagonist, infused soon after burn injury, blocked edema formation in the wound and significantly inhibited PAF increase in the damaged tissue in a dose-dependent manner. In contrast, the superoxide dismutase content in the group treated with TCV-309 was significantly higher than that of the control group.[43] These findings suggest that the administration of large doses of a PAF antagonist immediately after injury may reduce burn wound edema and the subsequent degree of burn shock by suppressing PAF and superoxide radical formation.

Angiotensin II and vasopressin

Angiotensin II and vasopressin, also called antidiuretic hormone (ADH), are two hormones that participate in the normal regulation of extracellular fluid volume by controlling sodium balance and osmolality through renal function and thirst.[27] However, during burn shock when sympathetic tone is high and volume receptors are stimulated, both hormones can be found in supranormal levels in the blood. Both are potent vasoconstrictors of terminal arterioles with little affect on the venules. Angiotensin II may be responsible for the selective gut and mucosal ischemia, which can cause translocation of endotoxins and bacteria, the development of sepsis and even multi-organ failure.[106,107] In severely burn-injured patients angiotensin II levels were elevated two to eight times normal in the first 1–5 days after burn injury with peak levels occurring on day three.[108] Vasopressin had peak levels of 50 times normal upon admission and declined towards normal over the first 5 days after burn injury. Vasopressin, along with catecholamines, may be largely responsible for increased system vascular resistance and left heart afterload, which can occur in resuscitated burn shock. Sun et al. used vasopressin-receptor antagonist in rats with burn shock to improve hemodynamics and survival time, while vasopressin infusion exacerbated burn shock.[45]

Corticotropin-releasing factor

Corticotropin-releasing factor (CRF) has proven to be efficacious in reducing protein extravasation and edema in burned rat paw. CRF may be a powerful natural inhibitory mediator of the acute inflammatory response of the skin to thermal injury.[109]

Other approaches to pharmacological attenuation of burn edema

Many reports on edema-reducing strategies using known burn mediator-blocking agents have been previously discussed in this chapter. However, there are other hypothesized approaches to ameliorate or inhibit the fluid extravasation induced by thermal injury. Topically applied local anesthetic lidocaine/prilocaine cream has been reported to be effective in reducing albumin extravasation in small burns in experimental animals.[110] The inositol triphosphate analog α-trinositol has also been found effective in reducing postburn edema when administered after injury.[111–113] Even though α-trinositol showed promising effects in animal experiments and also seemed to reduce pain in pilot clinical projects, its routine clinical application is not established.

Hemodynamic consequences of acute burns

The cause of reduced cardiac output (CO) during the resuscitative phase of burn injury has been the subject of considerable debate. There is an immediate depression of cardiac output before any detectable reduction in plasma volume. The rapidity of this response suggests a neurogenic response to receptors in the thermally injured skin or increased circulating vasoconstrictor mediators. Soon after injury a developing hypovolemia and reduced venous return undeniably contribute to the reduced cardiac output. The subsequent persistence of reduced CO after apparently adequate fluid therapy, as evidenced by a reduction in heart rate and restoration of both arterial blood pressure and urinary output, has been attributed to circulating myocardial depressant factor(s), which possibly originates from the burn wound.[11,12] Demling et al. showed a 15% reduction in CO despite an aggressive volume replacement protocol after a 40% scald burn in sheep.[18] However, there are also sustained increases in catecholamine secretion and elevated systemic vascular resistance for up to 5 days after burn injury.[91,108] Michie et al. measured CO and SVR in anesthetized dogs resuscitated after burn injury.[114] They found that CO fell shortly after injury and then returned toward normal; however, reduced CO did not parallel the blood volume deficit. They concluded that the depression of CO resulted not only from decreased blood volume and venous return but also from an increased SVR and from the presence of a circulating myocardial depressant substance. Thus, there are multiple factors that can significantly reduce CO after burn injury. However, resuscitated patients suffering major burn injury also can have supranormal CO from 2 to 6 days postinjury. This is secondary to the establishment of a hypermetabolic state and a systemic inflammatory response syndrome (SIRS).

Myocardial dysfunction

Myocardial function can be compromised after burn injury due to right heart overload and direct depression of contractility shown in isolated heart studies.[115,116] Increases in the afterload of both the left and right heart result from SVR and PVR elevations. The left ventricle compensates and CO can be maintained with increased afterload by augmented adrenergic stimulation and increased myocardial oxygen extraction. The right ventricle has a minimal capacity to compensate for increased afterload. In severe cases, desynchronization of the right and left ventricles is deleteriously superimposed on a depressed myocardium.[117] Burn injury greater than 45% TBSA can produce intrinsic contractile defects. Several investigators reported that aggressive early and sustained fluid resuscitation failed to correct left ventricular contractile and compliance defects.[116–118] These data suggest that hypovolemia is not the sole mechanism underlying the myocardial defects observed with burn shock. Serum from patients failing to sustain a normal CO after thermal injury has exhibited a markedly negative inotropic effect on *in vitro* heart preparations, which is likely due to the previously described circulating shock factor.[119] In other patients with large burn injuries and normal cardiac indices, little or no depressant activity was detected.

Sugi et al. studied intact, chronically instrumented sheep after a 40% TBSA flame burn injury and smoke-inhalation injury, and smoke inhalation injury alone. They found that maximal contractile effects were reduced after either burn injury or inhalation injury.[120,121] Horton et al. demonstrated decreased left ventricular contractility in isolated, coronary perfused, guinea pig hearts harvested 24 hours after burn injury.[122] This dysfunction was more pronounced in hearts from aged animals and was not reversed by resuscitation with isotonic fluid. It was largely reversed by treatment with 4 mL/kg of hypertonic saline dextran (HSD), but only if administered during the initial 4–6 hours of resuscitation.[123,124] These authors also effectively ameliorated the cardiac dysfunction of thermal injury with infusions of antioxidants, arginine, and calcium channel blockers.[125–127] Cioffi and colleagues in a similar model observed persistent myocardial depression after burn when the animals received no resuscitation after burn injury.[128] As opposed to most studies, Cioffi reported that immediate and full resuscitation totally reversed abnormalities of contraction and relaxation after burn injury. Murphy et al. showed elevations of a serum marker for cardiac injury, troponin I, for patients with a TBSA >18%, despite good cardiac indices.[129] Resuscitation and cardiac function studies emphasize the importance of early and adequate fluid therapy and suggest that functional myocardial depression after burn injury may not occur in patients receiving prompt and adequate volume therapy.

The primary mechanisms by which burn shock alters myocardial cell membrane integrity and impairs mechanical function remain unclear. Oxygen-derived free radicals may play a key causative role in the cell membrane dysfunction that is characteristic of several low-flow states. Horton et al. showed that a combination therapy of the free radical scavengers SOD and catalase significantly improved burn-mediated defects in left ventricular contractility and relaxation when administered along with adequate fluid resuscitation (4 mL/kg per percent of burn). Antioxidant therapy did not alter the volume of fluid resuscitation required after burn injury.[125]

Increased systemic vascular resistance and organ ischemia

Cardiac output may remain below normal after adequate volume replacement in burn patients and experimental animals. Sympathetic stimulation and hypovolemia result in the release of catecholamines, vasopressin, angiotensin II, and neuropeptide-Y after burn injury.[45,108] These agents cause contraction of the arteriolar smooth muscle, which is systemically manifested by increased afterload and SVR. The increased SVR after burn injury is also partly the result of increased blood viscosity secondary to the hemoconcentration.

Hilton and others performed experiments in anesthetized dogs in which infusion of various peripheral vasodilators improved CO after burn injury.[114,130] They demonstrated a reduction in the peripheral vascular resistance and augmented CO after verapamil, but the myocardial force of contraction remained depressed. Pruitt et al. examined in a group of burn patients the hypothesis that increased sympathetic activity contributes to CO reduction.[131] They showed a higher CO with treatment using the vasodilator hydralazine along with the reduced SVR.

There are several organs particularly susceptible to ischemia, organ dysfunction, and organ failure when burn resuscitation is delayed or inadequate. These include the kidney and the gastrointestinal tract. Renal ischemia can result directly from hypovolemia and increased sympathetic tone,

but elevations in serum free hemoglobin and particularly myoglobin correlate with increased renal failure.[132,133] Renal failure rates have dramatically declined due to standardized regimens of fluid therapy, but when therapy is delayed or associated with hypotension acute renal failure is not uncommon.[132,133]

An occult hypoxia can result from vasoconstriction of the gastrointestinal tract, despite apparently 'adequate' resuscitation.[107,134] As a consequence of visceral ischemia and reduced mucosal pH, bacterial and endotoxin translocation can contribute to the development of sepsis.

Cerebral edema (and encephalopathies are) is not uncommon after large cutaneous burns, particularly in children, but the exact cause remains unclear. Studies in anesthetized sheep subjected to a 70% TBSA scald show that cerebral autoregulation is well maintained in the immediate postburn period, but 6 hours after resuscitation, increased cerebral vascular resistance reduced cerebral blood flow 50%.[135]

Edema in nonburned tissue
Lungs

In large burns, there is a pronounced increase in pulmonary vascular resistance (PVR) that corresponds with the increased SVR.[8,60] Pulmonary edema is not an uncommon finding and occurs more often after, than during, the fluid-resuscitation phase of burn injury. Increased capillary pressure secondary to the increased PVR occurs with both pre- and postcapillary vasoconstriction and may contribute to pulmonary edema formation. Pulmonary wedge pressure is increased more than left atrial pressure after experimental burn injury due to postcapillary venular constriction.[60,136] It is likely that some degree of left heart failure also contributes to the increased capillary pressure. However, hypoproteinemia may be the greatest contributing factor to postburn pulmonary edema.[137] There is no evidence of increased capillary permeability from analysis of lung lymph sampled in large animal models after 40% TBSA injury, although rat studies suggest that albumin sequestration increases in the lungs after a 30% cutaneous scald.[28] Clinical studies of burn-injured patients suggest that, in the absence of inhalation injury, the lungs do not develop edema[138,139] This finding is consistent with little or no change in the microvascular permeability of the lung and the fact that lung lymph rate may increase considerably to prevent interstitial fluid accumulation. Pulmonary dysfunction associated with inhalation injury is discussed in a separate chapter.

Edema and abdominal compartment syndrome

Prompt and adequate fluid resuscitation has undoubtedly improved the outcome of burn-injured patients. Despite the treatment advances of burn surgery, massive edema of burned and nonburned tissues continues to be a repercussion of large-volume fluid resuscitation. There is a physiological conflict that exists in the balance between the edema process and hypovolemia. Edema has been previously shown to occur from the massive efflux of intravascular fluid to the interstitial space due to increased capillary permeability, large differences in oncotic pressures, and other forces.

The Parkland formula for burn resuscitation, introduced by Baxter and Shires in 1968, has been the guideline to the cornerstone of early burn care.[119] Although the guidelines for burn resuscitation have changed little, fluid management has changed over the past two decades. Engrav and associates compiled data from seven burn centers.[140] The results included 50 patients with 43 ± 21% TBSA burns in which 16 had documented inhalation injuries. The authors found that 58% of patients with large burns received volumes that greatly exceeded the formula proposed by Baxter. Their patients received close to 6 mL/kg/% TBSA (2 mL/kg/% TBSA greater than the Parkland formula). Urine output also exceeded clinical targets (0.5–1 mL/kg/hour) in 64% of patients. Friedrich and associates[141] found that their patients admitted in the year 2000, compared to those in the 1970, received twice the resuscitation volume. In yet another report, the Parkland formula was exceeded in 84% of the burn-injured patients treated.[142] A meta-analysis of 23 clinical trials (1980–2003) using crystalloid burn resuscitation produced similar findings.[143] Mean fluid infused (5.0 ± 1.2 mL/kg/% TBSA) and mean urinary outputs (1.2 ± 0.4 mL/kg/hour) were both over the burn resuscitation guidelines, suggesting that well over half of all burn patients may be over-resuscitated.

This trend of providing fluid in excess of the Parkland formula has been termed 'fluid creep.'[144] Over-resuscitation and its resulting edema are not without consequences. The problems of the over-resuscitated burn patient may include eye injuries due to elevated orbital pressures,[145] pulmonary edema,[146,147] the need for prolonged mechanical ventilation, or tracheostomy,[148] graft failure or the need for fasciotomy of uninjured extremities[149] due to massive edema.

Recently, a new life-threatening complication of generalized edema has been seen with increased frequency and named abdominal compartment syndrome (ACS).[150,151] Intra-abdominal pressure exceeding 30 cmH$_2$O is an indication of intra-abdominal hypertension (IAH). ACS is defined as sustained IAH in association with a clinically tense abdomen combined with ventilation aberrations due to elevated pulmonary inspiratory pressures or oliguria despite aggressive fluid resuscitation. ACS may become fatal due to a cascade of physiological events. The syndrome typically leads to multiple organ dysfunction characterized by impaired renal and hepatic blood flow, bowel ischemia, pulmonary dysfunction, depressed cardiac output, and elevated intracranial pressures.[152,153] ACS can occur after major abdominal trauma or surgery, but this condition in the absence of abdominal injury is known as secondary ACS.[154] Severely burn-injured patients are at risk for this development due to increasingly large volumes of resuscitation fluid, decreased abdominal wall compliance due to eschar, increased capillary permeability with leakage of large plasma volumes, and massive edema formation.

Choice of fluids and generation of edema

A major factor in the increased fluid volumes delivered and the apparent associated morbidity in burn patients may be the decreased use of albumin. This has resulted from two factors. A focus on the growing costs of medical care have showed that albumin is one of the largest medical costs associated with critical care. Further, a meta-analysis of albumin use over a wide variety of indications suggested no benefit and even a trend towards increased mortality.[155,156] The meta-analysis was the subject of much controversy and its results were refuted in several more recent meta-analyses, some of a more comprehensive nature.[157,158] It remains to be seen if closer control of infusion rate using urinary outputs to establish guidelines or if early use of colloids or hypertonics or combinations of these modality can reduce edema and its complications, but it is clear that there is a renewed research focus on edema and the means to minimize it.

Summary and conclusion

Thermal injury results in massive fluid shifts from the circulating plasma into the interstitial fluid space causing hypovolemia and swelling of the burned skin. When burn injury exceeds 20–30% TBSA there is minimal edema generation in non-injured tissues and organs. The Starling forces change to favor fluid extravasation from blood to tissue. Rapid edema formation is predominating from the development of strongly negative interstitial fluid pressure (imbibition pressure) and to a lesser degree by an increase in microvascular pressure and permeability. The type of fluid resuscitation, timing, and total volume infused can influence these fluid shifts.

Secondary to the thermal insult there is release of inflammatory mediators and stress hormones. Circulating mediators deleteriously increase microvascular permeability and alter cellular membrane function by which water and sodium enter cells. Circulating mediators also favor renal conservation of water and salt, impair cardiac contractility, and cause vasoconstrictors, which further aggravates ischemia from combined hypovolemia and cardiac dysfunction. The end result of this complex chain of events is decreased intravascular volume, increased systemic vascular resistance, decreased cardiac output, end-organ ischemia, and metabolic acidosis. Early excision of the devitalized tissue appears to reduce the local and systemic effects of mediators released from burned tissue, thus reducing the progressive pathophysiologic derangements. Without early and full resuscitation therapy these derangements can result in acute renal failure, vascular ischemia, cardiovascular collapse, and death.

Edema in both the burn wound and particularly in the non-injured soft tissue is increased by resuscitation. Edema is a serious complication, which likely contributes to decreased tissue oxygen diffusion and further ischemic insult to already damaged cells with compromised blood flow increasing the risk of infection. Research should continue to focus on methods to ameliorate the severe edema and vasoconstriction that exacerbate tissue ischemia. The success of this research will require identification of key circulatory factors that alter capillary permeability, cause vasoconstriction, depolarize cellular membranes, and depress myocardial function. Hopefully, methods to prevent the release and to block the activity of specific mediators can be further developed in order to reduce the morbidity and mortality rates of burn shock.

References

1. Cockshott WP. The history of the treatment of burns. Surg Gynecol Obstet 1956; 102:116–124.
2. Haynes BW. The history of burn care. In: Boswick JAJ, ed. The art and science of burn care. Rockville, Md.: Aspen Publ; 1987: 3–9.
3. Underhill FP, Carrington GL, Kapsinov R, et al. Blood concentration changes in extensive superficial burns, and their significance for systemic treatment. Arch Intern Med 1923; 32:31–39.
4. Cope O, Moore FD. The redistribution of body water and fluid therapy of the burned patient. Ann Surg 1947; 126:1010–1045.
5. Youn YK, LaLonde C, Demling R. The role of mediators in the response to thermal injury. World J Surg 1992; 16(1):30–36.
6. Aulick LH, Wilmore DW, Mason AD, et al. Influence of the burn wound on peripheral circulation in thermally injured patients. Am J Physiol 1977; 233:H520–26.
7. Settle JAD. Fluid therapy in burns. J Roy Soc Med 1982; 1(75):7–11.
8. Demling RH. Fluid replacement in burned patients. Surg Clin North Am 1987; 67:15–30.
9. Demling RH, Will JA, Belzer FO. Effect of major thermal injury on the pulmonary microcirculation. Surgery 1978; 83(6):746–751.
10. Baxter CR. Fluid volume and electrolyte changes of the early postburn period. Clin Plast Surg 1974; 1(4):693–709.
11. Baxter CR, Cook WA, Shires GT. Serum myocardial depressant factor of burn shock. Surg Forum 1966; 17:1–3.
12. Hilton JG, Marullo DS. Effects of thermal trauma on cardiac force of contraction. Burns Incl Therm Inj 1986; 12:167–171.
13. Clark WR. Death due to thermal trauma. In: Dolecek R, Brizio-Molteni L, Molteni A, et al., eds. Endocrinology of thermal trauma. Philadelphia, PA: Lea & Febiger; 1990:6–27.
14. Lund T, Reed RK. Acute hemodynamic effects of thermal skin injury in the rat. Circ Shock 1986; 20:105–114.
15. Arturson G. Pathophysiological aspects of the burn syndrome. Acta Chir Scand 1961; 274((Suppl 1)):1–135.
16. Leape LL. Kinetics of burn edema formation in primates. Ann Surg 1972; 176:223–226.
17. Cioffi WG Jr, Vaughan GM, Heironimus JD, et al. Dissociation of blood volume and flow in regulation of salt and water balance in burn patients. Ann Surg 1991; 214(3):213–218; discussion 218–220.
18. Demling RH, Mazess RB, Witt RM, et al. The study of burn wound edema using dichromatic absorptiometry. J Trauma 1978; 18:124–128.
19. Lund T, Wiig H, Reed RK. Acute postburn edema: role of strongly negative interstitial fluid pressure. Am J Physiol 1988; 255:H1069.
20. Onarheim H, Lund T, Reed R. Thermal skin injury: II. Effects on edema formation and albumin extravasation of fluid resuscitation with lactated Ringer's, plasma, and hypertonic saline (2,400mosmol/l) in the rat. Circ Shock 1989; 27(1):25–37.
21. Arturson G, Jakobsson OR. Oedema measurements in a standard burn model. Burns 1985; 1:1–7.
22. Leape LL. Early burn wound changes. J Pediatr Surg 1968; 3:292–299.
23. Leape LL. Initial changes in burns: tissue changes in burned and unburned skin of rhesus monkeys. J Trauma 1970; 10:488–492.
24. Landis EM, Pappenheimer JR. Exchange of substances through the capillary walls. In: Hamilton WF, Dow P, eds. Handbook of physiology. Circulation. Washington, DC: Am Physiol Soc 1963:961–1034.
25. Aukland K, Reed RK. Interstitial-lymphatic mechanisms in the control of extracellular fluid volume. Physiol Rev 1993; 73(1):1–78.
26. Arturson G, Mellander S. Acute changes in capillary filtration and diffusion in experimental burn injury. Acta Physiol Scand 1964; 62:457–463.
27. Goodman-Gilman A, Rall TW, Nies AS, et al. The pharmacological basis of therapeutics. New York: Pergamon Press; 1990.
28. Till GO, Guilds LS, Mahrougui M, et al. Role of xanthine oxidase in thermal injury of skin. Am J Pathol 1989; 135(1):195–202.
29. Friedl HS, Till GO, Tentz O, et al. Roles of histamine, complement and xanthine oxidase in thermal injury of skin. Am J Pathol 1989; 135(1):203–217.
30. Dyess DL, Hunter JL, Lakey JR, et al. Attenuation of histamine-induced endothelial permeability responses after pacing-induced heart failure: role for endogenous catecholamines. Microcirculation 2000; 7(5):307–315.
31. Carvajal H, Linares H, Brouhard B. Effect of antihistamine, anti-serotonin, and ganglionic blocking agents upon increased capillary permeability following burn edema. J Trauma 1975; 15:969–975.
32. Paul W, Douglas GJ, Lawrence L, et al. Cutaneous permeability responses to bradykinin and histamine in the guinea-pig: possible differences in their mechanism of action. Br J Pharmacol 1994; 111(1):159–164.
33. Boykin Jr JV, Manson NH. Mechanisms of cimetidine protection following thermal injury. Am J Med 1987; 83(6A):76–81.
34. Heggers JP, Loy GL, Robson MC, et al. Histological demonstration of prostaglandins and thromboxanes in burned tissue. J Surg Res 1980; 28:11–15.
35. Anggard E, Jonsson CE. Efflux of prostaglandins in lymph from scalded tissue. Acta Physiol Scand 1971; 81:440–443.
36. Huang YS, Li A, Yang ZC. Roles of thromboxane and its inhibitor anisodamine in burn shock. Burns 1990; 4:249–253.
37. LaLonde C, Demling RH. Inhibition of thromboxane synthetase accentuates hemodynamic instability and burn edema in the anesthetized sheep model. Surgery 1989; 5:638–644.
38. Tokyay R, Loick HM, Traber DL, et al. Effects of thromboxane synthetase inhibition on postburn mesenteric vascular resistance and the rate of bacterial translocation in a chronic porcine model. Surg Gynecol Obstet 1992; 174(2):125–132.
39. Ding Z, Jiang M, Li S, et al. Vascular barrier-enhancing effect of an endogenous beta-adrenergic agonist. Inflammation 1995; 19(1):1–8.
40. Pollard V, Prough DS, DeMelo AE, et al. The influence of carbon dioxide and body position on near-infrared spectroscopic assessment of cerebral hemoglobin oxygen saturation. Anesth Analg 1996; 82(2):278–287.
41. Horton JW, White DJ. Role of xanthine oxidase and leukocytes in postburn cardiac dysfunction. J Am Coll Surg 1995; 181(2):129–137.
42. Wallace JL, Steel G, Whittle BJR, et al. Evidence for platelet-activating factor as a mediator of endotoxin-induced gastrointestinal damage in the rat: effects of three platelet-activating factor antagonists. Gastroenterology 1987; 93:765–773.
43. Ono I, Gunji H, Hasegawa T, et al. Effects of a platelet activating factor antagonist on edema formation following burns. Burns 1993; 3:202–207.
44. Lu Z, Wolf MB. Platelet activating factor-induced microvascular permeability increases in the cat hindlimb. Circ Shock 1993; 41(1):8–18.
45. Sun K, Gong A, Wang CH, et al. Effect of peripheral injection of arginine vasopressin and its receptor antagonist on burn shock in the rat. Neuropeptides 1990; 1:17–20.
46. Pitt RM, Parker JC, Jurkovich GJ, et al. Analysis of altered capillary pressure and permeability after thermal injury. J Surg Res 1987; 42(6):693–702.
47. Lund T, Onarheim H, Reed RK. Pathogenesis of edema formation in burn injuries. World J Surg 1992; 16:2–9.
48. Lund T, Onarheim H, Wiig H, et al. Mechanisms behind increased dermal imbibition pressure in acute burn edema. Am J Physiol 1989; 256(4 Pt 2):H940–H948.
49. Kinsky MP, Milner SM, Button B, et al. Resuscitation of severe thermal injury with hypertonic saline dextran: effects on peripheral and visceral edema in sheep. J Trauma 2000; 49(5):844–853.
50. Zetterstrom H, Arturson G. Plasma oncotic pressure and plasma protein concentration in patients following thermal injury. Acta Anaesth Scand 1980; 24:288–294.

51. Pitkanen J, Lund T, Aanderud L, et al. Transcapillary colloid osmotic pressures in injured and non-injured skin of seriously burned patients. Burns 1987; 13(3):198–203.

52. Lund T, Wiig H, Reed RK, Aukland K. A 'new' mechanism for edema generation: strongly negative interstitial fluid pressure causes rapid fluid flow into thermally injured skin. Acta Physiol Scand 1987; 129:433–435.

53. Kinsky MP, Guha SC, Button BM, et al. The role of interstitial Starling forces in the pathogenesis of burn edema. J Burn Care Rehabil 1998; 19(1 Pt 1):1–9.

54. Kinsky MP, Traber DL, Traber LD, et al. Changes in cutaneous interstitial Starling forces with large thickness scald. Proc Am Burn Assn 1994; 251.

55. Harms BA, Kramer GC, Bodai BI, et al. Microvascular fluid and protein flux in pulmonary and systemic circulations after thermal injury. Microvasc Res 1982; 23(1):77–86.

56. Dyess DL, Ardell JL, Townsley MI, et al. Effects of hypertonic saline and dextran 70 resuscitation on microvascular permeability after burn. Am J Physiol 1992; 262(6 Pt 2):H1832–H1837.

57. Reed RK, Woie K. Integrins and control of interstitial fluid pressure. News Physiol Sci 1997; 12:42–48.

58. Arturson G. Microvascular permeability to macromolecules in thermal injury. Acta Physioi Scand 1979; 463(Suppl):111–222.

59. Demling RH, Kramer GC, Harms B. Role of thermal injury-induced hypoproteinemia on edema formation in burned and non-burned tissue. Surgery 1984; 95:136–144.

60. Kramer GC, Gunther RA, Nerlich ML, et al. Effect of dextran 70 on increased microvascular fluid and protein flux after thermal injury. Circ Shock 1982; 9:529–543.

61. Lund T, Reed RK. Microvascular fluid exchange following thermal skin injury in the rat: changes in extravascular colloid osmotic pressure, albumin mass, and water content. Circ Shock 1986; 20:91–104.

62. Brouhard BH, Carvajal HF, Linares HA. Burn edema and protein leakage in the rat. I. Relationship to time of injury. Microvasc Res 1978; 15:221–228.

63. Neumann M, Demling RH. Colloid vs. crystalloid: a current perspective. Intens Crit Care Digest 1990; 9(1):3–6.

64. Kramer G, Harms B, Bodai B, et al. Mechanisms for redistribution of plasma protein following acute protein depletion. Am J Physiol 1982; 243:H803–H809.

65. Elgjo GI, Traber DL, Hawkins HK, et al. Burn resuscitation with two doses of 4 mL/kg hypertonic saline dextran provides sustained fluid sparing: a 48-hour prospective study in conscious sheep. J Trauma 2000; 49(2):251–263; discussion 263–265.

66. Elgjo GI, Poli de Figueiredo LF, Schenarts PJ, et al. Hypertonic saline dextran produces early (8–12h) fluid sparing in burn resuscitation: a 24-h prospective, double blind study in sheep. Crit Care Med 2000; 28(1):163–171.

67. Andritsos MJ, Kinsky MP, Herndon DN, et al. Albumin only transiently reduces fluid requirements following burn injury. Shock 2001; 15(1):6.

68. Shires GT, Cunningham JN Jr, Backer CR, et al. Alterations in cellular membrane dysfunction during hemorrhagic shock in primates. Ann Surg 1972; 176(3):288–295.

69. Nakayama S, Kramer GC, Carlsen RC, et al. Amiloride blocks membrane potential depolarization in rat skeletal muscle during hemorrhagic shock (abstract). Circ Shock 1984; 13:106–107.

70. Arango A, Illner H, Shires GT. Roles of ischemia in the induction of changes in cell membrane during hemorrhagic shock. J Surg Res 1976; 20(5):473–476.

71. Holliday RL, Illner HP, Shires GT. Liver cell membrane alterations during hemorrhagic shock in the rat. J Surg Res 1981; 31:506–515.

72. Mazzoni MC, Borgstrom P, Intaglietta M, et al. Lumenal narrowing and endothelial cell swelling in skeletal muscle capillaries during hemorrhagic shock. Circ Shock 1989; 29(1):27–39.

73. Garcia NM, Horton JW. L-arginine improves resting cardiac transmembrane potential after burn injury. Shock 1994; 1(5):354–358.

74. Button B, Baker RD, Vertrees RA, et al. Quantitative assessment of a circulating depolarizing factor in shock. Shock 2001; 15(3):239–244.

75. Evans JA, Darlington DN, Gann DS. A circulating factor(s) mediates cell depolarization in hemorrhagic shock. Ann Surg 1991; 213(6):549–557.

76. Trunkey DD, Illner H, Arango A, et al. Changes in cell membrane function following shock and cross-perfusion. Surg Forum 1974; 25:1–3.

77. Brown JM, Grosso MA, Moore EE. Hypertonic saline and dextran: impact on cardiac function in the isolated rat heart. J Trauma 1990; 30:646–651.

78. Evans JA, Massoglia G, Sutherland B, et al. Molecular properties of hemorrhagic shock factor (abstract). Biophys J 1993; 64:A384.

79. Tanaka H, Wada T, Simazaki S, et al. Effects of cimetidine on fluid requirement during resuscitation of third-degree burns. J Burn Care Rehabil 1991; 12(5):425–429.

80. Harms B, Bodai B, Demling R. Prostaglandin release and altered microvascular integrity after burn injury. J Surg Res 1981; 31:27–28.

81. Arturson G. Anti-inflammatory drugs and burn edema formation. In: May R, Dogo G, eds. Care of the burn wound. Basel: Karger; 1981:21–24.

82. Arturson G, Hamberg M, Jonsson CE. Prostaglandins in human burn blister fluid. Acta Physiol Scand 1973; 87:27–36.

83. LaLonde C, Knox J, Daryani R. Topical flurbiprofen decreases burn wound-induced hypermetabolism and systemic lipid peroxidation. Surgery 1991; 109:645–651.

84. Heggers JP, Robson MC, Zachary LS. Thromboxane inhibitors for the prevention of progressive dermal ischemia due to thermal injury. J Burn Care Rehabil 1985; 6:46–48.

85. Demling RH, LaLonde C. Topical ibuprofen decreases early postburn edema. Surgery 1987; 5:857–861.

86. Jacobsen S, Waaler BG. The effect of scalding on the content of kininogen and kininase in limb lymph. Br J Pharmacol 1966; 27:222.

87. Hafner JA, Fritz H. Balance antiinflammation: the combined application of a PAF inhibitor and a cyclooxygenase inhibitor blocks the inflammatory take-off after burns. Int J Tissue React 1990; 12:203.

88. Nwariaku FE, Sikes PJ, Lightfoot E, et al. Effect of a bradykinin antagonist on the local inflammatory response following thermal injury. Burns 1996; 22(4):324–327.

89. Ferrara JJ, Westervelt CL, Kukuy EL, et al. Burn edema reduction by methysergide is not due to control of regional vasodilation. J Surg Res 1996; 61(1):11–16.

90. Zhang XJ, Irtun O, Zheng Y, et al. Methysergide reduces nonnutritive blood flow in normal and scalded skin. Am J Physiol 2000; 278(3):E452–E461.

91. Wilmore DW, Long JM, Mason AD, et al. Catecholamines: mediator of the hypermetabolic response to thermal injury. Ann Surg 1974; 80:653–659.

92. Hilton JG. Effects of sodium nitroprusside on thermal trauma depressed cardiac output in the anesthesized dog. Burns Incl Therm Inj 1984; 10:318–322.

93. McCord J, Fridovieh I. The biology and pathology of oxygen radicals. Ann Intern Med 1978; 89:122–127.

94. Demling RH, LaLonde C. Early postburn lipid peroxidation: effect of ibuprofen and allopurinol. Surgery 1990; 107:85–93.

95. Demling R, Lalonde C, Knox J, et al. Fluid resuscitation with deferoxamine prevents systemic burn-induced oxidant injury. J Trauma 1991; 31(4):538–543.

96. Rawlingson A, Greenacre SA, Brain SD. Generation of peroxynitrite in localised, moderate temperature burns. Burns 2000; 26(3):223–227.

97. Lindblom L, Cassuto J, Yregard L, et al. Importance of nitric oxide in the regulation of burn oedema, proteinuria and urine output. Burns 2000; 26(1):13–17.

98. Lindblom L, Cassuto J, Yregard L, et al. Role of nitric oxide in the control of burn perfusion. Burns 2000; 26(1):19–23.

99. Slater TF, Benedetto C. Free radical reactions in relation to lipid peroxidation, inflammation and prostaglandin metabolism. In: Berti F, Veto G, eds. The prostaglandin system. New York: Plenum; 1979:109–126.

100. McCord JM. Oxygen-derived free radicals in post ischemic tissue injury. N Engl J Med 1979; 312:159–163.

101. Tanaka H, Matsuda T, Yukioka T, et al. High dose vitamin C reduces resuscitation fluid volume in severely burned patients. Proceedings of the American Burn Association 1996; 28:77.

102. Fischer SF, Bone HG, Powell WC, et al. Pyridoxalated hemoglobin polyoxyethylene conjugate does not restore hypoxic pulmonary vasoconstriction in ovine sepsis. Crit Care 1997; 25(9):1151–1159.

103. Tanaka H, Matsuda H, Shimazaki S, et al. Reduced resuscitation fluid volume for second-degree burns with delayed initiation of ascorbic acid therapy. Arch Surg 1997; 132(2):158–161.

104. Tanaka H, Lund T, Wiig H, et al. High dose vitamin C counteracts the negative interstitial fluid hydrostatic pressure and early edema generation in thermally injured rats. Burns 1999; 25(7):569–574.

105. Dubick MA, Williams CA, Elgjo GI, et al. High-dose vitamin C infusion reduces fluid requirements in the resuscitation of burn-injured sheep. Shock 2005; 24(2):139–144.

106. Fink MP. Gastrointestinal mucosal injury in experimental models of shock, trauma, and sepsis. Crit Care Med 1991; 19(5):627–641.

107. Cui X, Sheng Z, Guo Z. Mechanisms of early gastro-intestinal ischemia after burn: hemodynamic and hemorrheologic features [in Chinese]. Chin J Plast Surg Burns 1998; 14(4):262–265.

108. Crum RL, Dominic W, Hansbrough JF. Cardiovascular and neurohumoral responses following burn injury. Arch Surg 1990; 125:1065–1070.

109. Kiang JG, Wei-E T. Corticotropin-releasing factor inhibits thermal injury. J Pharmacol Exp Ther 1987; 2:517–520.

110. Jonsson A, Mattsson U, Tarnow P, et al. Topical local anaesthetics (EMLA) inhibit burn-induced plasma extravasation as measured by digital image colour analysis. Burns 1998; 24(4):313–318.

111. Lund T, Reed RK. Alpha-trinositol vitamin inhibits edema generation and albumin extravasation in thermally injured skin. J Trauma 1994; 36(6):761–765.

112. Ferrara JJ, Kukuy EL, Gilman DA, et al. Alpha-trinositol reduces edema formation at the site of scald injury. Surgery 1998; 123(1):36–45.

113. Tarnow P, Jonsson A, Mattsson U, et al. Inhibition of plasma extravasation after burns by D-myo-inositol-1,2,6-triphosphate using digital image colour analysis. Scand J Plast Reconstr Surg Hand Surg 1998;32(2):141–146.

114. Michie DD, Goldsmith RS, Mason AD Jr. Effects of hydralazine and high molecular weight dextran upon the circulatory responses to severe thermal burns. Circ Res 1963; 13:468–473.

115. Martyn JAJ, Wilson RS, Burke JF. Right ventricular function and pulmonary hemodynamics during dopamine infusion in burned patients. Chest 1986; 89:357–360.

116. Adams HR, Baxter CR, Izenberg SD. Decreased contractility and compliance of the left ventricle as complications of thermal trauma. Am Heart J 1984; 108(6):1477–1487.

117. Merriman TW Jr, Jackson R. Myocardial function following thermal injury. Circ Res 1962; 11:66–69.

118. Horton JW, White J, Baxter CR. Aging alters myocardial response during resuscitation in burn shock. Surg Forum 1987; 38:249–251.

119. Baxter CR, Shires GT. Physiological response to crystalloid resuscitation of severe burns. Ann NY Acad Sci 1968; 150:874–894.

120. Sugi K, Newald J, Traber LD. Smoke inhalation injury causes myocardial depression in sheep. Anesthesiology 1988; 69:A111.

121. Sugi K, Theissen JL, Traber LD, et al. Impact of carbon monoxide on cardiopulmonary dysfunction after smoke inhalation injury. Circ Res 1990; 66:69–75.

122. Horton JW, Baxter CR, White J. Differences in cardiac responses to resuscitation from burn shock. Surg Gynecol Obstet 1989; 168(3):201–213.

123. Horton JW, White DJ, Baxter CR. Hypertonic saline dextran resuscitation of thermal injury. Ann Surg 1990; 211(3):301–311.

124. Horton JW, Shite J, Hunt JL. Delayed hypertonic saline dextran administration after burn injury. J Trauma 1995; 38(2):281–286.

125. Horton JW, White J, Baxter CR. The role of oxygen derived free radicles in burn-induced myocardial contractile depression. J Burn Care Rehabil 1988; 9(6):589–598.

126. Horton JW, Garcia NM, White J, et al. Postburn cardiac contractile function and biochemical markers of postburn cardiac injury. J Am Coll Surg 1995; 181:289–298.

127. Horton JW, White J, Maass D, et al. Arginine in burn injury improves cardiac performance and prevents bacterial translocation. J Appl Physiol 1998; 84(2):695–702.

128. Cioffi WG, DeMeules JE, Gameili RL. The effects of burn injury and fluid resuscitation on cardiac function in vitro. J Trauma 1986; 26:638–643.

129. Murphy JT, Horton JW, Purdue GF, et al. Evaluation of troponin-I as an indicator of cardiac dysfunction following thermal injury. J Burn Care Rehabil 1997; 45(4):700–704.

130. Hilton JG. Effects of verapamil on thermal trauma depressed cardiac output in the anesthetized dog. Burns Incl Therm Inj 1984; 10:313–317.

131. Pruitt PAJ, Mason ADJ, Moncrief JA. Hemodynamic changes in the early post burn patients: the influence of fluid administration and of a vasodilator (hydralazine). J Trauma 1971; 11:36.

132. Holm C, Horbrand F, von Donnersmarck GH, et al. Acute renal failure in severely burned patients. Burns 1999; 25(2):171–178.

133. Chrysopoulo MT, Jeschke MG, Dziewulski P, et al. Acute renal dysfunction in severely burned adults. J Trauma 1999; 46(1):141–144.

134. Tokyay R, Zeigler ST, Traber DL, et al. Postburn gastrointestinal vasoconstriction increases bacterial and endotoxin translocation. J Am Physiol 1993; 74:1521–1527.

135. Shin C, Kinsky MP, Thomas JA, et al. Effect of cutaneous burn injury and resuscitation on the cerebral circulation. Burns 1998; 24:39–45.

136. Demling RH, Wong C, Jin LJ, et al. Early lung dysfunction after major burns: role of edema and vasoactive mediators. J Trauma 1985; 25(10):959–966.

137. Demling RH, Niehaus G, Perea A, et al. Effect of burn-induced hypoproteinemia on pulmonary transvascular fluid filtration rate. Surgery 1979; 85:339–343.

138. Tranbaugh RF, Lewis FR, Christensen IM, et al. Lung water changes after thermal injury: the effects of crystalloid resuscitation and sepsis. Ann Surg 1980; 192:47–49.

139. Tranbaugh RF, Elings VB, Christensen JM, et al. Effect of inhalation injury on lung water accumulation. J Trauma 1983; 23:597.

140. Engrav LH, Colescott PL, Kemalyan N, et al. A biopsy of the use of the Baxter formula to resuscitate burns or do we do it like Charlie did it? J Burn Care Rehabil 2000; 21(2):91–95.

141. Friedrich JB, Sullivan SR, Engrav LH, et al. Is supra-Baxter resuscitation in burn patients a new phenomenon? Burns 2004; 30(5):464–466.

142. Cancio LC, ChAvez S, Alvarado-Ortega M, et al. Predicting increased fluid requirements during the resuscitation of thermally injured patients. J Trauma 2004; 56(2):404–413.

143. Shah A, Kramer GC, Grady JJ, et al. Meta-analysis of fluid requirements for burn injury 1980–2002. J Burn Care Rehabil 2003; 24(2):S118.

144. Pruitt BA Jr. Protection from excessive resuscitation: 'pushing the pendulum back.' J Trauma 2000; 49(3):567–568.

145. Sullivan SR, Ahmadi AJ, Singh CN, et al. Elevated orbital pressure: another untoward effect of massive resuscitation after burn injury. J Trauma 2006; 60(1):72–76.

146. Blot S, Hoste E, Colardyn F. Acute respiratory failure that complicates the resuscitation of pediatric patients with scald injuries. J Burn Care Rehabil 2000; 21(3):289–290.

147. Zak AL, Harrington DT, Barillo DJ, et al. Acute respiratory failure that complicates the resuscitation of pediatric patients with scald injuries. J Burn Care Rehabil 1999; 20(5):391–399.

148. Coln CE, Purdue GF, Hunt JL. Tracheostomy in the young pediatric burn patient. Arch Surg 1998; 133(5):537–539; discussion 539–540.

149. Sheridan RL, Tompkins RG, McManus WF, et al. Intracompartmental sepsis in burn patients. J Trauma 1994; 36(3):301–305.

150. Ivy ME, Atweh NA, Palmer J, et al. Intra-abdominal hypertension and abdominal compartment syndrome in burn patients. J Trauma 2000; 49(3):387–391.

151. Oda J, Ueyama M, Yamashita K, et al. Hypertonic lactated saline resuscitation reduces the risk of abdominal compartment syndrome in severely burned patients. J Trauma 2006; 60(1): 64–71.

152. Bloomfield GL, Dalton JM, Sugerman HJ, et al. Treatment of increasing intracranial pressure secondary to the acute abdominal compartment syndrome in a patient with combined abdominal and head trauma. J Trauma 1995; 39(6):1168–1170.

153. Ivatury RR, Diebel L, Porter JM, et al. Intra-abdominal hypertension and the abdominal compartment syndrome. Surg Clin North Am 1997; 77(4):783–800.

154. Maxwell RA, Fabian TC, Croce MA, et al. Secondary abdominal compartment syndrome: an underappreciated manifestation of severe hemorrhagic shock. J Trauma 1999; 47(6):995–999.

155. Bunn F, Lefebvre C, Li Wan Po A, et al. Human albumin solution for resuscitation and volume expansion in critically ill patients. The Albumin Reviewers. [update in Cochrane Database Syst Rev 2002; (1):CD001208; PMID: 11869596]. Cochrane Database Syst Rev 2000(2):CD001208.

156. Wilkes MM, Navickis RJ. Patient survival after human albumin administration. A meta-analysis of randomized, controlled trials. Ann Intern Med 2001; 135(3):149–164.

157. Vincent JL, Navickis RJ, Wilkes MM. Morbidity in hospitalized patients receiving human albumin: a meta-analysis of randomized, controlled trials. Crit Care Med 2005; 33(4):915–917.

158. Bellomo R. Fluid resuscitation: colloids vs. crystalloids. Blood Purif 2002; 20(3):239–242.

159 Bosman FT: Integrins: cell adhesives and modulators of cell function. Histochem J 1993; 25:469–477.

160. Reed RK, Berg A, Gjerde EA, et al. Control of interstitial fluid pressure: role of beta1-integrins. Semin Nephrol 2001; 21: 222–230.

Chapter 9

Fluid resuscitation and early management

Glenn D. Warden

Introduction

Proper fluid management is critical to the survival of the victim of a major thermal injury. In the 1940s, hypovolemic shock or shock-induced renal failure was the leading cause of death after burn injury. Today, with our current knowledge of the massive fluid shifts and vascular changes that occur during burn shock, mortality related to burn-induced volume loss has decreased considerably. Although a vigorous approach to fluid therapy has ensued in the last 20 years and fewer deaths are occurring in the first 24–48 hours postburn, the fact remains that approximately 50% of the deaths occur within the first 10 days following burn injury from a multitude of causes, one of the most significant being inadequate fluid resuscitation therapy.[1] Knowledge of fluid management following burn shock resuscitation is also important and is often overlooked in burn education.

Burn shock resuscitation

The history of burn resuscitation began over a century ago; however, complete appreciation of the severity of fluid loss in burns was not apparent until the enlightening studies of Frank P Underhill,[2] who studied the victims of the Rialto Theater fire in 1921. His concept that burn shock was due to intravascular fluid loss was further elucidated by Cope and Moore,[3] who conducted studies on patients from the Coconut Grove disaster in 1942. They developed the concept of burn edema and introduced the body-weight burn budget formula for fluid resuscitation of burn patients. In 1952, Evans[1] developed a burn surface area–weight formula for computing fluid replacement in burns which became the first simplified formula for fluid resuscitation for burn patients. Surgeons at the Brooke Army Medical Center modified the original Evans formula and this became the standard for the next 15 years.

A number of methods for accomplishing adequate volume replacement therapy have been advocated in the more than 40 years since the introduction of the Evans' formula in 1952. This chapter will review the various methods advocated and present the rationale of each. Importantly, properly utilized, each resuscitation formula can be effective in the resuscitation of the burn patient in the immediate postburn period, provided that close attention is paid to the individual's clinical response to therapy and that fluid replacement therapy is modified according to this response. The fact that patients respond to a wide variety of resuscitative efforts is testimony to the fact that burn patients are very resilient and can be overwhelmed only under the most unfavorable circumstances.[4]

Pathophysiology of burn injury

Modern fluid resuscitation formulas originate from experimental studies in the pathophysiology of burn shock. Burn shock is both hypovolemic shock and cellular shock, and is characterized by specific hemodynamic changes including decreased cardiac output, extracellular fluid, plasma volume, and oliguria. As in the treatment of other forms of shock, the primary goal is to restore and preserve tissue perfusion in order to avoid ischemia. However, in burn shock, resuscitation is complicated by obligatory burn edema, and the voluminous transvascular fluid shifts which result from a major burn are unique to thermal trauma.

Although the exact pathophysiology of the postburn vascular changes and fluid shifts is unknown, one major component of burn shock is the increase in total body capillary permeability. Direct thermal injury results in marked changes in the microcirculation. Most of the changes occur locally at the burn site, when maximal edema formation occurs at about 8–12 hours post-injury in smaller burns and 12–24 hours post-injury in major thermal injuries. The rate of progression of tissue edema is dependent upon the adequacy of resuscitation.

Multiple mediators have been proposed to explain the changes in vascular permeability seen postburn. The mediators can produce either an increase in vascular permeability or an increase in microvascular hydrostatic pressure.[5,6] Most mediators act to increase permeability by altering membrane integrity in the venules. The early phase of burn edema formation, lasting for minutes to an hour, has been thought by some investigators to be the result of mediators, particularly histamine and bradykinin. Other mediators implicated in the changes in vascular permeability seen postburn include vasoactive amines, products of platelet activation and the complement cascade, hormones, prostaglandins, and leukotrienes. Vasoactive substances are also released which may act primarily by increasing microvascular blood flow or vascular pressures, further accentuating the burn edema.[7,8] Histamine is released in large quantities from mast cells in burned skin immediately after injury.[9] Histamine has been clearly demonstrated to increase the leakage of fluid and protein from systemic micro vessels, its major effect being on venules in which an increase in the intracellular junction space is characteristically seen.[10] However, the increase in serum histamine levels after burn is transient, peaking in the first several hours postinjury, indicating that histamine is only involved in the very early increase in permeability. The use of H_1 receptor inhibitors, e.g. diphenhydramine, has only limited success in decreasing edema. Recently, the use of an H_2 receptor antagonist has been reported to decrease burn edema in an animal model.[11]

Serotonin is released immediately postburn as a result of platelet aggregation and acts directly to increase the pulmonary vascular resistance and indirectly to amplify the vasoconstrictive effect of norepinephrine, histamine, angiotensin II, and prostaglandin.[12] The use of ketanserin, a specific serotonin antagonist, in a porcine burn shock model, improved cardiac index, decreased pulmonary pressure, and reduced arteriovenous oxygen content differences compared to a control group in the early postburn period. Serotonin antagonists should be investigated further as possible adjuvant therapeutic agents during burn shock resuscitation.[13] Prostaglandins, vasoactive products of arachidonic acid metabolism, have been reported to be released in burn tissue and to be at least in part responsible for burn edema. Although these substances do not directly alter vasopermeability, increased levels of vasodilator prostaglandins such as prostaglandin E_2 (PGE_2) and prostacyclin (PGI_2) result in arterial dilatation in burned tissue, increased blood flow and intravascular hydrostatic pressure in the injured microcirculation, and thus accentuate the edema process. Concentrations of PGI_2 and the vasconstrictor thromboxane A_2 (TXA_2) have been demonstrated in burned tissue, burn blister fluid, lymph, and wound secretion.[14,15] However, the use of prostaglandin inhibitors has produced variable results in animal studies. Arturson[16] reported a decrease in burn lymph and protein flow with the use of prostaglandin inhibitor, indomethacin. Those results have not been corroborated by other investigators and the role of thromboxane and the prostaglandins still needs to be elucidated.

The activation of the proteolytic cascades, including those of coagulation, fibrinolysis, the kinins, and the complement system, has been demonstrated to occur immediately following thermal injury. Kinins, specifically bradykinins, are known to increase vascular permeability, primarily in the venule. Rocha and co-workers[17] report increased kinin levels in burn edema fluid in the rat. The release of other mediators and the generalized inflammatory response after burns favors the activation of the kallikrein–kinin system, with the release of bradykinin into the circulation.[18] Elevation of proteolytic activity has been demonstrated in both animals and in burn patients.[19] Pretreatment with protease inhibitors significantly decreases free kinin levels but appears to have little effect on the edema process.

The end result of the changes in the microvasculature due to thermal injury is disruption of normal capillary barriers separating intravascular and interstitial compartments, and rapid equilibrium of these compartments. This results in severe depletion of plasma volume with a marked increase in extracellular fluid clinically manifested as hypovolemia.

In addition to a loss of capillary integrity, thermal injury also causes changes at the cellular level. Baxter[20] has demonstrated that in burns of >30% total body surface area (TBSA), there is a systemic decrease in cell transmembrane potential, involving nonthermally injured cells as well. This decrease in cell transmitting potential, as defined by the Nernste equation, results from an increase in intracellular sodium concentration. The cause of this is thought to be a decrease in sodium ATPase activity responsible for maintaining the intracellular–extracellular ionic gradient. Baxter further demonstrated that resuscitation only partially restores the membrane potential and intracellular sodium concentrations to normal levels, demonstrating that hypovolemia with its attendant ischemia is not totally responsible for the cellular swelling seen in burn shock. In fact, the membrane potential may not return to normal for many days postburn despite adequate resuscitation. If resuscitation is inadequate, cell membrane potential progressively decreases, resulting ultimately in cellular death. This may be the final common denominator in burn shock during the resuscitation period.

Although the etiology of burn shock is not totally understood, many authors have studied the fluid volume shifts and hemodynamic changes that accompany burn shock. Early work by Moyer,[21] and Baxter and Shires[22] established the definitive role of crystalloid solutions in burn resuscitation and delineated the fluid volume changes in the early postburn period. Moyer's original studies in 1965[21] demonstrated that burn edema sequestered enormous amounts of fluid, resulting in the hypovolemia of burn shock. In addition, he described the first crystalloid-only resuscitation formula used to treat burn shock. He noted that burn shock recovery occurred in the majority of patients studied, although hemoconcentration remained unchanged and the hematocrit was unresponsive to fluid administration despite adequate resuscitation. This became the first objective evidence that burn shock is not simply due to hypovolemia but is also influenced by extracellular sodium depletion. Baxter and Shires,[22] in 1968, using radioisotope dilution techniques, defined the fluid volume changes of the postburn period in relation to cardiac output. They first demonstrated that edema fluid in the burn wound is isotonic with respect to plasma fluid and contains protein in the same proportions as that found in blood. This confirmed Arturson's earlier findings that in major burns there is complete disruption of the normal capillary barrier, with free exchange between plasma and extravascular extracellular compartments. They measured changes in fluid compartment volumes in burned primates and dogs and demonstrated that in untreated (unresuscitated) animals, a 30–50% extracellular fluid (ECF) defect persisted at 18 hours postburn. Plasma volume decreased 23% to 27% below controls, although red cell mass changed only about 10% over the same 18-hour period. Thus, the greatest volume loss was functional intravascular extracellular fluid. Cardiac output was initially depressed very soon after injury to a level of about 25% of controls at 4 hours after a 30% TBSA burn. By 18 hours, however, the cardiac output had stabilized at around 40% of control, despite persistent defects in plasma and ECF volumes. On the basis of studies using different volumes of resuscitation fluids, they arrived at an optimal response in terms of cardiac output and restoration of ECF at the end of 24 hours in a canine model. Clinical studies using similar sodium and fluid loads immediately followed, confirming efficacy in restoring ECF to within 10% of controls within 24 hours. This became the basis for the Baxter or Parkland formula.[20] Mortality was comparable to that obtained with a colloid-containing resuscitation formula.

Baxter went on to demonstrate that during the first 24 hours postburn, plasma volume changes were independent of the type of infused fluid, whether crystalloid or colloid, but at approximately 24 hours post-injury, an infused amount of colloid would increase the plasma volume by the same amount. His findings prove that colloid-containing solutions are an unnecessary component of fluid resuscitation in the first 24 hours. He recommended their use only after capillary integrity was restored, to correct the persistent plasma volume deficit of about 20% as measured externally. While the fluid shifts were being defined by Baxter in terms of crystalloid resuscitation, Moncrief and Pruitt[4] worked to characterize the hemodynamic alterations that occur in burn shock with and without fluid resuscitation. Their efforts culminated in the Brooke formula modification which utilized 2 cc/kg/% burn during the first 24 hours. Fluid needs were initially estimated according to the modified Brooke formula, but the actual volume for resuscitation was based on clinical response. In their study, resuscitation permitted an average decrease of about 20% in both extracellular fluid and plasma volume, but no further loss accrued in the first 24 hours. In the second 24 hours postburn, plasma volume restoration occurred with the administration of colloid. Blood volume, however, was only partially restored and an ongoing loss of 9% of the red cell mass per day was found. Cardiac output, initially quite low, rose over the first 18 hours postburn, despite plasma volume and blood volume defects. These results were quite consistent with those demonstrated by Baxter in his animal studies. Peripheral vascular resistance during the initial 24 hours was initially very high but decreased as cardiac output improved, and in fact the changes were reciprocal. Once plasma volume and blood volume loss ceased, cardiac output rose to supranormal levels where it remained until healing or grafting occurred.

Moylan and associates[23] in 1973, using a canine model, defined the relationships between fluid volumes, sodium concentration, and colloid in restoring cardiac output during the first 12 hours post-injury. No significant colloid effect on cardiac output was noted in the first 12 hours post-injury. In addition, 1 mEq of sodium was found to exert an effect on cardiac output equal to 13 times that of 1 mL of salt-free volume. This experiment established the fact that any combination of sodium and volume within the broad limits of the study would effectively resuscitate a thermally injured patient.

Arturson's landmark studies in 1979[16] on vascular permeability characterized the nature of the 'leaky capillary' in the postburn period. He demonstrated in a canine model that increased capillary permeability is found both locally and in nonburned tissue at distant sites when the TBSA burn exceeded 25%. He proposed that the burn wound is characterized by rapid edema formation due to dilatation of the resistance vessels (precapillary arterioles); increased extravascular osmotic activity, due to the products of thermal injury; and increased microvascular permeability to macromolecules. The increased permeability permits molecules of up to 350 000 molecular weight to escape from the microvasculature, a size which allows essentially all elements of the vascular space except red blood cells to escape from it. Further studies by Demling and co-workers[24] have demonstrated that in 50% TBSA burns, one-half of the initial fluid resuscitation requirement may end up in nonthermally injured tissues.

Resuscitation from burn shock

Fluid resuscitation is aimed at supporting the patient throughout the initial 24-hour to 48-hour period of hypovolemia. The primary goal of therapy is to replace the fluid sequestered as a result of thermal injury. The critical concept in burn shock is that massive fluid shifts can occur even though total body water remains unchanged. What actually changes is the volume of each fluid compartment, intracellular and interstitial volumes increasing at the expense of plasma volume and blood volume. In light of all the studies on different fluid regimens, the question still remains: 'What is the best formula for resuscitation of the burn patient?'

It is quite clear that the edema process is accentuated by the resuscitation fluid. The magnitude of edema will be affected by the amount and type of fluid administered.[25] The National Institutes of Health consensus summary on fluid resuscitation in 1978 was not in agreement in regard to a specific formula; however, there was consensus in regard to two major issues — the guidelines used during the resuscitation process and the type of fluid used. In regard to the guidelines, the consensus was to give the least amount of fluid necessary to maintain adequate organ perfusion. The volume infused should be continually titrated so as to avoid both under-resuscitation and over-resuscitation.[26,27] As for the optimum type of fluid, there is no question that replacement of the extracellular salt lost into the burned tissue and into the cell is essential for successful resuscitation.[19,21]

Crystalloid resuscitation

Crystalloid, in particular lactated Ringer's solution with a sodium concentration of 130 mEq/L, is the most popular resuscitation fluid currently utilized. Proponents of the use of crystalloid solution alone for resuscitation report that other solutions, specifically colloids, are no better and are certainly more expensive than crystalloid for maintaining intravascular volume following thermal injury.[4] The most common reason given for not using colloids is that even large proteins leak from the capillary following thermal injury. However, capillaries in nonburned tissues do continue to sieve proteins, maintaining relatively normal protein permeability characteristics.

The quantity of crystalloid needed is in part dependent upon the parameters used to monitor resuscitation. If a urinary output of 0.5 cc/kg of body weight/hour is considered to indicate adequate perfusion, approximately 3 cc/kg/% burn will be needed in the first 24 hours. If 1 cc/kg of body weight/hour of urine is deemed necessary, then of course considerably more fluid will be needed and in turn more edema will result. The Parkland formula recommends 4 cc/kg/% burn in the first 24 hours, with one-half of that amount administered in the first 8 hours[9] (Table 9.1). The modified Brooke formula recommends beginning burn shock resuscitation at 2 cc/kg/% burn in the first 24 hours (Table 9.1). In major burns, severe hypo-

TABLE 9.1 FORMULAS FOR ESTIMATING ADULT BURN PATIENT RESUSCITATION FLUID NEEDS

Colloid formulas	Electrolyte	Colloid	D5W
Evans	Normal saline 1.0 cc/kg/% burn	1.0 cc/kg/% burn	2000 cc
Brooke	Lactated Ringer's 1.5 cc/kg/% burn	0.5 cc/kg	2000 cc
Slater	Lactated Ringer's 2 L/24 hours	Fresh frozen plasma 75 cc/kg/24 hours	
Crystalloid formulas			
Parkland	Lactated Ringer's	4 cc/kg/% burn	
Modified	Lactated Ringer's	2 cc/kg/% burn	
Brooke			
Hypertonic saline formulas			
Hypertonic saline solution (Monafo)	Volume to maintain urine output at 30 cc/h Fluid contains 250 mEq Na/L		
Modified hypertonic (Warden)	Lactated Ringer's + 50 mEq NaHCO$_3$ (180 mEq Na/L) for 8 hours to maintain urine output at 30–50 cc/h Lactated Ringer's to maintain urine output at 30–50 cc/h beginning 8 hours postburn		
Dextran formula (Demling)	Dextran 40 in saline — 2 cc/kg/h for 8 hours Lactated Ringer's — volume to maintain urine output at 30 cc/h Fresh frozen plasma – 0.5 cc/kg/h for 18 hours beginning 8 hours postburn		

Reproduced from Warden G.D. Burn shock resuscitation. World J Surg 1992; 16:21–23. With Kind permission of Springer Science and Business Media.[51]

proteinemia usually develops with these resuscitation regimens. The hypoproteinemia and interstitial protein depletion may result in more edema formation.

Hypertonic saline

Hypertonic salt solutions have been known for many years to be effective in treating burn shock.[28,29] Rapid infusion produces serum hyperosmolarity and hypernatremia with two potentially positive effects.[28,32] The hypertonic serum reduces the shift into the extracellular space of intravascular water. Proposed benefits include decreased tissue edema and fewer attendant complications, including escharotomies for vascular compromise or endotracheal intubation to protect the airway. Monafo[28] reported that the resuscitation of burn patients with salt solution of 240–300 mEq/L resulted in less edema because of the smaller total fluid requirements than with lactated Ringer's solution. Urine output was the indicator used during resuscitation. Demling and colleagues[30] in an animal model demonstrated that the net fluid intake was less if burned animals were resuscitated with hypertonic saline to the same cardiac output compared with lactated Ringer's. Urine output was much higher with hypertonic solution. Interestingly, soft-tissue interstitial edema in burned and nonburned tissue, as reflected by lymph flow, was increased with hypertonic saline similar to that of lactated Ringer's (LR). This can be explained by a shift of intracellular water into extracellular space as the result of the hyperosmolar solution. Extracellular edema can therefore occur at the same time as intracellular fluid defect. This may give the external appearance of less edema. Although several studies to date have reported that this intracellular water depletion does not appear to be deleterious, the issue remains controversial. Shimazaki et al.[31] resuscitated 46 patients with either LR or hypertonic saline. The sodium infusions were equivalent, but the free water load was greater with LR; 50% of the latter required endotracheal intubation. The hypertonic serum also delivers a more concentrated ultrafiltrate within the kidney. This increases urine volume and salt clearance without marked increases in the required volume of free water.

There is no consensus regarding the type of osmolarity of hypertonic resuscitation fluid. Caldwell and Bowser.[32] in 1979 reported a series of 37 patients with greater than 30% burns treated with either LR or hypertonic lactated saline (HLS), but no colloid. Total sodium balance was the same but the HLS group received 30% less free water and the reduced weight gain was maintained for 7 days. Subsequent reports from this institution reported successful HLS resuscitation in the elderly and children but no improvement in late mortality.[36,39,40]

Bartolani et al.[41] randomized 40 patients to receive LR or HLS. HLS patients received more sodium, but less total fluid than the LR group. The observed higher mortality with HLS was attributed to larger burns in this group.

The role of colloid in association with hypertonic reserve colloid for the second 24 hours, if at all, unless the patient remains poorly perfused after large infusions of crystalloid. Griswold et al.[42] reported resuscitation of 47 patients with HLS resuscitation. Of these, 29 were also given colloid as albumin or fresh frozen plasma based on burn severity, premorbid state, or poor response to HLS resuscitation. This group had larger burns, greater mean age, and higher incidence of inhalation injury, but required only 57% of the fluid volume predicted by the Parkland formula, compared to 75% of predicted volume in the HLS alone group. Both groups maintained urine volumes of 1 mL/kg/h with no significant difference in hematocrit or serum sodium levels. Jelenko et al.[43] also reported in a small series that patients given HLS and albumin required fewer escharotomies, fewer days of mechanical ventilation, and less total fluid than patients resuscitated with LR or HLS alone. Gunn et al.[33] in a series of 51 randomized patients found no difference in fluid requirements or weight gain if they were given LR or hypertonic saline, if fresh frozen plasma was administered to maintain serum albumin levels above 2 g/dL, but all patients received hypotonic enteral feedings during resuscitation.

Yoshioka et al.[34] reviewed 53 patients treated with greater than 30% burns resuscitated with LR, LR and colloid, or HLS. Fluid requirements were 4.8 mL/kg/% TBSA with LR, 3.3 mL/kg/% TBSA with LR and colloid, and 2.2 mL/kg/% TBSA with HLS. The total sodium requirements were increased 30% with LR compared to the other groups. Oxygen extraction, measured as A-VO$_2$ difference, was improved with HLS, but reduced with LR–colloid, perhaps because of protein leak across the alveoli.

Vigorous administration of hypertonic saline solutions can produce a serum sodium above 160 mEq/dL or serum osmolarity greater than 340 mOsm/dL, followed by a rapid fall in urine output.[35] Bowser-Wallace et al.[36] and Crum et al.[37] have reported 40–50% of patients treated with HLS developed hypernatremia with serum sodium greater than 160 mEq/L requiring switch to hypotonic fluids. Huang et al.[38] reported a series of deaths associated with hypernatremia and hyperosmolarity following hypertonic saline resuscitation. Serial determinations of serum sodium and serum osmolarity are required to prevent complications including sudden anuria, brain shrinkage with tearing of intracranial vessels, or excessive brain swelling following rapid correction of serum hyperosmolarity. Current recommendations are that the serum sodium levels should not be allowed to exceed 160 mEq/dL during its use. Of interest, Gunn and associates,[33] in a prospective randomized study of patients with 20% TBSA burns evaluating HSL versus LR solution, were not able to demonstrate decreased fluid requirements, improved nutritional tolerance, or decreased percent weight gain.

Children, have utilized a modified hypertonic solution in major thermal injuries >40% TBSA burn. The resuscitation fluid contains 180 mEq Na$^+$ (lactated Ringer's + 50 mEq NaHCO$_3$). The solution is utilized until the reversal of metabolic acidosis has occurred, usually by 8 hours postburn. The volume administered is begun at a rate calculated by the Parkland formula (4 cc/kg/% burn); however, volume is titrated to maintain urine output at 30–50 cc/h. After 8 hours the resuscitation is completed utilizing LR to maintain urine output at 30–50 cc/h. This hypertonic formula can be used in infants and in the elderly without the accompanying risk of hypernatremia.[44,45]

Colloid resuscitation

Plasma proteins are extremely important in the circulation since they generate the inward oncotic force that counteracts the outward capillary hydrostatic force. Without protein, plasma volume could not be maintained and massive edema would result. Protein replacement was an important component of early formulas for burn management. The Evans formula, advocated in 1952, used 1 cc/kg of body weight/% burn each for colloid and LR over the first 24 hours. The Brooke formula was clearly based on estimate rather than determined scientifically, but the formula used 0.5/kg/% burn as colloid and 1.5 cc/kg/% burn as LR. The burn budget of Moore similarly used a substantial amount of colloids.[3] Con-

siderable confusion exists concerning the role of protein in a resuscitation formula. There are three schools of thought:

1. Protein solutions should not be given in the first 24 hours because during this period they are no more effective than salt water in maintaining intravascular volume and they promote accumulation of lung water when edema fluid is being absorbed from the burn wound.[46]
2. Proteins, specifically albumin, should be given from the beginning of resuscitation along with crystalloid; it should usually be added to salt water.
3. Protein should be given between 8 and 12 hours postburn using strictly crystalloid in the first 8–12 hours because of the massive fluid shifts during this period. Demling demonstrated experimentally that restoration and maintenance of plasma protein contents were not effective until 8 hours postburn, after which adequate levels can be maintained with infusion.[47] Because nonburned tissues appear to regain normal permeability very shortly after injury and because hypoproteinemia may accentuate the edema, the action advocated by the first school appears to be least appropriate.

The choice of the type of protein solution can be confusing. Heat-fixed protein solutions, e.g. Plasmanate, are known to contain some denatured and aggregated protein, which decreases the oncotic effect. Albumin solutions would clearly be the most oncotically active solutions. Fresh frozen plasma, however, contains all the protein fractions that exert both the oncotic and the nononcotic actions. The optimal amount of protein to infuse remains undefined. Demling[47] uses between 0.5 and 1 cc/kg/% burn of fresh frozen plasma during the first 24 hours, beginning at 8–10 hours postburn.[48,49] He emphasizes that all major burns require large amounts of fluid, but notes that older patients with burns, patients with burns and concomitant inhalation injury, and patients with burns in excess of 50% TBSA not only develop less edema but also better maintain hemodynamic stability with the addition of protein.

Slater and co-workers[44] have recently utilized fresh frozen plasma during burn shock. They use lactated Ringer's, 2 liters for 24 hours, and fresh frozen plasma, 75 cc/kg/24 h (Table 9.1). Although the volume of fresh frozen plasma is calculated, the volume infused is titrated to maintain an adequate urine output. Although the authors are utilizing colloid early in the burn shock period, they emphasize that most burn patients have received LR in significant volumes during field management.

The use of albumin in burns and critically ill patients has recently been challenged by the Cochrane Central Register of Controlled Trials, which demonstrated in critical hypovolemia that there was no evidence that albumin reduces mortality when compared with cheaper alternatives such as saline.[90] Others using a meta-analysis of randomized, controlled trials found no effect of albumin on mortality and could not find a deleterious effect of albumin.[91] Most burn surgeons agree that in burn patients who have a very low serum albumin during burn shock albumin supplementation is warranted to maintain oncotic pressure.

Dextran resuscitation solutions

Dextran is a colloid consisting of glucose molecules which have been polymerized into chains to form high molecular weight polysaccharides.[49] This compound is commercially available in a number of molecular sizes. Dextran, which has an average molecular weight of 40 000 Da, is referred to as low molecular weight dextran. British dextran has a mean molecular weight of 150 000, whereas the dextran used predominantly in Sweden has a molecular weight of 70 000. Dextran is excreted at the kidneys, with 40% removed within 24 hours. The remainder is slowly metabolized. Demling and associates have utilized dextran 70 in a 6% solution to prevent edema in nonburned tissues. Dextran 70 carries some risk of allergic reaction and can interfere with blood typing. Dextran 40 actually improves the microcirculatory flow by decreasing red cell aggregation.[50] Demling and colleagues[49] demonstrated that the net requirements to maintain vascular pressure at the baseline levels with dextran 40 were about half those seen with LR alone during the first 24 hours postburn. These authors have used an infusion rate of dextran 40 and saline of 2 cc/kg/h along with sufficient LR to maintain adequate perfusion. At 8 hours an infusion of fresh frozen plasma at 0.5–1.0 cc/kg/% TBSA burn over 18 hours is instituted along with necessary additional crystalloid (Table 9.1).

In the young pediatric burn patient with major burn injury, colloid replacement is frequently required as serum protein concentration rapidly decreases during burn shock. The Shriners Hospitals for Children in Cincinnati and Galveston both routinely utilize colloid during resuscitation of children with major thermal injuries.[51,52]

Special considerations in burn shock resuscitation
Fluid resuscitation in the thermally injured pediatric patient

The burned child continues to represent a special challenge, since resuscitation therapy must be more precise than that for an adult with a similar burn. In addition, children have a limited physiological reserve. We have demonstrated that children require more fluid for burn shock resuscitation than adults with similar thermal injury; fluid requirements for children averaged 5.8 cc/kg/% burn.[53] In addition, children commonly require intravenous resuscitation for relatively small burns of 10–20% TBSA. Baxter[45] found similar resuscitation requirements in the pediatric age group. Graves and associates[54] substantiated that children received 6.3 ± 2 cc/kg/% TBSA burn. At the Shriners Burns Hospital, Cincinnati, we have utilized the Parkland formula with the addition of maintenance fluid,

to the resuscitation fluid volume, 4 mL/kg × % TBSA burn per 24 hours + 1500 cc/m² BSA per 24 hours. This is the formula used to begin burn shock resuscitation and to compare the amount of fluid needed by a particular pediatric burn patient with that needed by an unburned pediatric patient (Table 9.2). This is similar to the results reported by Graves and co-workers[54] who found that if maintenance fluids were subtracted from the resuscitation fluid requirements, the resulting resuscitation volumes would approach 4 cc/kg/% burn. At the Shriners Burns Hospital in Galveston, fluid requirements are estimated according to a formula based on total BSA and BSA burned in square meters.[52] Total fluid requirements for the first day are estimated as follows: 5000 mL/m² BSA burned per 24 hours + 2000 mL/m² BSA per 24 hours.

Recently pediatric burn surgeons have seen a problem of over-resuscitation and a 'saw-tooth resuscitation.' This appears to be due to first responders using the volume resuscitation formula as suggested by Pediatric Advanced Life Support (PALS) which recommends volume resuscitation begin with a fluid bolus of 20 mL/kg of isotonic crystalloid administered over 5 to 20 minutes — this amount is repeated if urine output is not adequate.[88] This regimen can lead to over-resuscitation. PALS actually recommends a modification of this fluid bolus resuscitation for burns utilizing 2–4 mL/kg/% of body surface area burned per 24 hours.[88] Education of first responders on the differences between these two fluid regimens is imperative.

Inhalation injury

The presence of inhalation injury increases the fluid requirements for resuscitation from burn shock after thermal injury.[55,89] We have demonstrated that patients with documented inhalation injury require 5.7 cc/kg/% burn, as compared to 3.98 cc/kg/% burn in patients without inhalation injury. These data confirm and quantitate that inhalation injury accompanying thermal trauma increases the magnitude of total body injury and requires increased volumes of fluid and sodium to achieve resuscitation from early burn shock.

Choice of fluids and rate of administration

It is clear that all the solutions reviewed are effective in restoring tissue perfusion. However, it makes no more sense to use one particular fluid for all patients than it does to use one antibiotic for all infections. Most patients with burns of <40% TBSA and patients with no pulmonary injury can be resusci-

TABLE 9.2 FORMULAS FOR ESTIMATING PEDIATRIC RESUSCITATION NEEDS			
Cincinnati Shriners Burns Hospital	4 mL × kg × % TBSA burn + 1500 cc × m² BSA	1st 8 hours	Lactated Ringer's + 50 mg NaHCO₃
		2nd 8 hours	Lactated Ringer's
		3rd 8 hours	Lactated Ringer's + 12.5 g albumin
Galveston Shriners Burns Hospital	5000 mL/m² BSA burn + 2000 mL/m² BSA	Ringer's lactate + 12.5 g albumin	

tated with isotonic crystalloid fluid. In patients with burns of >40% TBSA and in patients with pulmonary injury, hypertonic saline can be utilized in the first 8 hours postburn, following which lactated Ringer's is infused to complete burn shock resuscitation. In the pediatric and elderly burn patient population, utilizing a lower but still hypertonic concentration of sodium, i.e. 180 mEq/L, still gives the benefits of hypertonic resuscitation without the potential complications of excessive sodium retention and hypernatremia.

In patients with massive burns, young pediatric patients, and burns complicated by severe inhalation injury, a combination of fluids may be utilized to achieve the desired goal of tissue perfusion while minimizing edema. In treating such patients, we have utilized the regimen of modified hypertonic (lactated Ringer's +50 mEq NaHCO$_3$) saline fluid containing 180 mEq Na/L for the first 8 hours. After correction of the metabolic acidosis, which generally requires 8 hours, the patients are given LR only for the second 8 hours. In the last 8 hours, a 5% albumin in LR is utilized to complete resuscitation. The resuscitation solution used in Galveston for pediatric patients is an isotonic glucose-containing solution to which a moderate amount of colloid (human serum albumin) is added. The solution is prepared by mixing 50 mL of 25% human serum albumin (12.5 g) with 950 mL in an LR solution.

The monitoring of burn shock resuscitation is initiated by first responders and is generally concluded once the patient's fluid needs have decreased to a maintenance rate, based upon body size and evaporative water loss. Factors influencing monitoring needs include the extent and depth of burn, the presence of inhalation injury, associated injuries, preexisting medical illnesses, and patient age. The monitoring process can be classified based upon the intensity and frequency of observations, as well as the methods employed. While the level of monitoring must be individualized for each patient, one must weigh the risks and benefits of each modality. Young, healthy patients with minor burns may only require the occasional periodic assessment of vital signs, whereas those with more extensive burns and/or other risk factors may require more invasive techniques. A recent survey of 251 burn centers throughout the United States, Canada, United Kingdom, Australia, and New Zealand revealed that only 12% frequently used pulmonary artery catheter (PAC) monitoring during fluid resuscitation in patients with >30% TBSA burns.[56] Moreover, only 60% of the respondents who addressed treatment goals following PAC insertion indicated that they utilized predetermined physiologic parameters to direct fluid therapy.

Clinical monitoring of burn shock resuscitation has traditionally relied on clinical assessment of cardiovascular, renal, and biochemical parameters as indicators of vital organ perfusion. Heart rate, blood pressure, and electrocardiographic recordings are the primary modalities for monitoring cardiovascular status in any patient. Fluid balance during burn shock resuscitation is typically monitored by measuring hourly urine output via an indwelling urethral catheter. It has been recommended that urine output be maintained between 30 and 50 mL/h in adults,[22] and between 0.5 and 1.0 mL/kg/h in patients weighing less than 30 kg;[26] however, there have been no clinical studies identifying the optimal hourly urine output to maintain vital organ perfusion during burn shock resuscitation.

Because large volumes of fluid and electrolytes are administered both initially and throughout the course of resuscitation, it is important to obtain baseline laboratory measurements of complete blood count, electrolytes, glucose, albumin, and acid–base balance.[57] Laboratory values should be repeated as clinically indicated throughout the resuscitation period. These parameters are generally sufficient to assess the physiologic response of most burn patients during burn shock resuscitation. While clinical interpretation of the data should rely on the evaluation of trends rather than on isolated measurements, there have been no studies demonstrating which tests should be performed, how often they should be repeated, or the effect of frequent laboratory testing on the success of resuscitation.

Invasive hemodynamic monitoring permits the direct, and sometimes continuous, measurement of central venous pressure (CVP), pulmonary capillary wedge pressure (PCWP), and pulmonary vascular hemodynamics as well as the calculation of cardiac output (CO), systemic vascular resistance (SVR), oxygen delivery (DO$_2$), and oxygen consumption (VO$_2$). The decision to perform such monitoring requires consideration of risks, cost-effectiveness, and impact on clinical outcome. The Swan-Ganz catheter is most commonly utilized in patients in whom routine monitoring is felt to be ineffective, when there is a history of preexisting cardiac disease, or when there are other complicating factors.

PAC-guided therapy has been studied most extensively in trauma and critically ill surgical patients. Kirton and Civetta[58] performed a critical literature review to determine if the use of the PAC in trauma patients altered outcome. They concluded that hemodynamic data derived from the PAC appeared to be beneficial to ascertain cardiovascular performance, to direct therapy when noninvasive monitoring was felt to be inadequate, or when the endpoints of resuscitation were difficult to define. These findings were echoed at the 1997 Pulmonary Artery Catheter Consensus Conference; however; there was no unanimity that PAC-guided therapy altered mortality in trauma patients.[59]

Studies of PAC use for monitoring burn shock resuscitation are limited. Retrospective analyses of adult patients with extensive burn injuries have concluded that PCWP is a more reliable indicator of circulatory volume than CVP,[60] and that CO is more accurate in assessing the efficacy of resuscitation than hourly urine output.[61] These findings were supported by Dries and Waxman[62] who noted that urine output and vital signs monitoring did not correlate with PCWP, cardiac index (CI), SVR, DO$_2$, or VO$_2$. They concluded that PAC monitoring may be beneficial in patients at high risk for adverse outcomes due to suboptimal resuscitation. Most recently, Schiller and Bay have reported their retrospective experience in 95 patients treated over a 4-year period during which an attempt was made to maximize circulatory endpoints.[63] They concluded that early invasive monitoring facilitated more aggressive resuscitation and resulted in increased survival, and that the inability to achieve hyperdynamic endpoints predicted resuscitation failure.

PAC-guided monitoring has also been used to aid in achieving predetermined therapeutic endpoints during the resuscitation and management of trauma and critically ill patients. In a series of prospective randomized class II trials, Shoemaker et al.[64,65] demonstrated that patients resuscitated to hyperdynamic endpoints (i.e. increased CI, DO_2I, VO_2I) had decreased mortality, ICU stay, and ventilator days compared to patients who were resuscitated to normal hemodynamic values. Recent studies by Fleming[64] and Bishop[65] have not only supported these conclusions but also demonstrated a decreased incidence of organ failures.

While the data supporting hyperdynamic resuscitation are impressive, there is also strong evidence that such therapeutic goals are not associated with improved outcome. Two trials in critically ill patients[66,67] were unable to demonstrate any benefit of PAC monitoring on patient outcome. These studies were supported by prospective randomized trials[68,69] which demonstrated no statistical differences in survival, organ failure, or ICU days between the control and hyperdynamic groups.

In an evidence-based review of these and other citations, Cooper et al.[70] concluded that the existing literature had inconsistent results regarding the efficacy of goal-oriented hemodynamic therapy. This conclusion was underscored by Elliott[71] who cited a meta-analysis of seven studies in which no significant differences in mortality were noted between control and hyperdynamic resuscitation groups.

The most appropriate endpoints in burn shock resuscitation are also unresolved. As such, the goal of achieving hyperdynamic resuscitation remains controversial. While Aikawa[72] was able to resuscitate 19/21 patients (90.5%) using the PAC to reach normal hemodynamic endpoints, Bernard[73] demonstrated that the ability to sustain a supranormal CI was associated with enhanced tissue perfusion and survival. This was supported by Schiller et al.[74] who demonstrated that an inadequate or unsustained response to hyperdynamic resuscitation was associated with nonsurvival. A follow-up study by these authors[75] also demonstrated significantly reduced mortality in those patients where PAC-guided resuscitation assisted in achieving hyperdynamic endpoints. The ability to achieve adequate oxygen delivery with hyperdynamic burn shock resuscitation has also been recently evaluated by Barton et al.[76] While patients achieved significant increases in VO_2I and DO_2I, they required 63% more fluid than predicted by the Parkland formula, a mean resuscitation volume of 9.07 mL/kg/% TBSA burn, and a mean of 50.4 hours to complete resuscitation.

More than 20 human studies in critically ill patients have demonstrated that blood lactate (BL) levels are highly accurate as a guide to the efficacy of resuscitation.[71,77] Blood lactate levels directly reflect anaerobic metabolisms as a consequence of hypoperfusion, and normalizing levels have long been associated with improved survival from nonburn shock.[78] In other studies, BL has been demonstrated to distinguish survivors from nonsurvivors.[79,80] In two prospective, goal-directed studies in critically ill patients, BL proved superior to not only MAP and urine output but also to DO_2, VO_2, and CI.[81,82]

It is important to emphasize that all of the resuscitation formulas are only guidelines for burn shock resuscitation. The Parkland formula, for instance, decreases the volume administered by 50% at 8 hours postburn. The relationship between the fluid volume required and time postburn depicted by the smooth curve in Figure 9.1 represents the influence of temporal changes in microvascular permeability and edema volume on fluid needs. That curve is contrasted with the abrupt changes

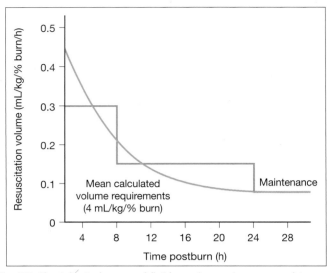

Fig. 9.1 Physiological curve of fluid requirements compared to Parkland formula, emphasizing that formulas are only guidelines for fluid therapy during burn shock. (Reproduced with permission from Warden GD. Burn shock resuscitation. World J Surg 1992; 16:21–23. With Kind permission of Springer Science and Business Media.[51]).

in fluid infusion rate as prescribed by the formula. The formulas are utilized as starting points for volume replacement and to compare the individual patient with the 'average' burn patient. Investigators from the burn center at Harborview Medical Center have demonstrated an increase in fluid administration during the recent years. This has been called 'fluid creep' by Dr. Basil Pruitt. These authors demonstrated a doubling of fluid administrated during burn shock resuscitation comparing 1975 to 2000.[92] This increase in fluid resuscitation fluid volume is associated with abdominal compartment syndrome.[93,94]

An interesting question is, 'When has burn shock resuscitation been completed successfully?' It is obvious that resuscitation is completed when there is no further accumulation of edema fluid, which generally occurs between 18 and 30 hours postburn. The resuscitation fluids are utilized until the volume of infused fluid needed to maintain adequate urine volume of 30–50 cc/h in adults and 1 cc/kg/h in children equals the maintenance fluid volume. The maintenance fluid requirements following burn shock resuscitation include the patient's normal maintenance volume plus evaporative water loss.

Failure of burn shock resuscitation

In certain patients, failure of burn shock resuscitation still occurs despite administration of massive volumes of fluid. Such patients are characterized by either extreme age and exceptionally extensive tissue trauma or by major electrical injury, major inhalation injury, delay in initiating adequate fluid resuscitation, or underlying disease that limits metabolic and cardiovascular reserve.[83] In these patients, refractory burn shock and resuscitation failure remain major causes of early mortality despite advances in emergency care and transport, resuscitation regimens, and physiologic stabilization.

We have used plasma exchange in patients with major thermal injuries who failed to respond to conventional fluid volumes during resuscitation from burn shock.[84] The indications for plasma exchange are ongoing fluid requirements exceeding twice those predicted by the Parkland formula despite conversion to hypertonic lactated saline resuscitation fluid. During a 3-year period, 22 patients underwent plasma exchange during burn shock resuscitation. A therapeutic response was documented in 21 of the 22 patients, characterized by a sharp decrease in fluid requirements from a mean of 260% above the predicted hourly volume by the resuscitation formula to within calculated requirements at a mean time of 2.3 hours following plasma exchange. Only one patient, who had a 100% TBSA burn (88% full-thickness), failed to respond to plasma exchange and expired at 18 hours postburn. Slater and Goldfarb[85] have substantiated the beneficial effect of plasma exchange in sustaining patients during the immediate postburn period when patients fail to respond appropriately to conventional fluid resuscitation. This modality offers an alternative management technique for the treatment of refractory burn shock.

Fluid replacement following burn shock resuscitation

Although the heat-injured microvessels may continue to manifest increased vascular permeability for several days, the rate of loss is considerably less than that seen in the first 24 hours. Burn edema by this time is near maximal and the interstitial space may well be saturated with sodium. Additional fluid requirements will depend on the type of fluid used during the initial resuscitation. If hypertonic salt resuscitation has been utilized during the entire burn shock period, a hyperosmolar state is produced and the addition of free water will be required to restore the extracellular space to an isoosmolar state.

If colloid has not been utilized during burn shock and the serum oncotic pressure is low due to intravascular protein depletion, protein repletion is frequently needed. The amount of protein varies with the resuscitation utilized. Requirements of 0.3–0.5 cc/kg/TBSA burn of 5% albumin during the second 24 hours are utilized with the modified Brooke formula. The Parkland formula replaces the plasma volume deficit with colloid. This deficit varies from 20 to 60% of the circulating plasma volume. We have utilized colloid replacement based on a 20% plasma volume deficit during the second 24 hours (circulating plasma volume × 20%).

In addition to colloid, the patients should receive maintenance fluids. In burn patients the maintenance fluids include an additional amount for evaporative water loss. The total daily maintenance fluid requirements in the adult patient following burn shock can be calculated by the following formula: basal (1500cc/m^2) + evaporative water loss [(25 + % burn) $\times \text{m}^2 \times 24$] = total maintenance fluid (m^2 = total body surface area in square meters). This fluid may be given via the intravenous route or with enteral feeding. The solution infused intravenously should be 50% normal saline with potassium supplements. With the loss of intracellular potassium during burn shock, the potassium requirements in adults are about 120 mEq/day. In the pediatric patient, increased fluids are required due to the differences in BSA to weight ratios compared to adults. In addition, children also require relatively larger volumes of urine for excretion of waste products. At the Cincinnati Shriners Unit, the maintenance fluid requirements are calculated by the following formula: (35 + % burn) × BSA × 24 (evaporative water loss) + 1500 mL × BSA per day (maintenance fluids). In Galveston, the recommended fluids needs are estimated as follows: 3750mL/m^2 BSA per day (burn-related losses) + 1500mL/m^2 BSA per day (maintenance fluids).

Following the initial 24–48 hours postburn period of resuscitation, urinary output is an unreliable guide to adequacy of hydration.[86] Respiratory water losses, osmotic diuresis secondary to accentuated glucose intolerance, osmotic diuresis secondary to high protein, high caloric feedings, and derangements in the ADH mechanisms all contribute to increased fluid losses despite an adequate urine output. In general, patients with major thermal injuries will require a urine output of 1500–2000 cc/24 hours in adults, and 3–4 mL/kg/h in children.

The measurement of serum sodium concentration is not only a means of diagnosing dehydration but also the best guide for planning and following successful fluid replacement. Other useful laboratory indices of the state of hydration and guides of therapy include body weight change, serum and urine nitrogen concentrations, serum and urine glucose concentrations, the intake and output record, and clinical examination.

Continuous colloid replacement may be required to maintain colloid oncotic pressure in very large burns and in the pediatric burn patient. Maintaining serum albumin levels above 2.0 g/dL is desirable.

The electrolytes calcium, magnesium, and phosphate must also be monitored. Although the replacement of these electrolytes has been studied in detail in burn patients, maintaining the values within normal limits is desirable and varies in each patient.

Summary

The volume necessary to resuscitate burn patients is dependent upon injury severity, age, physiological status, and associated injury. Consequently, the volume predicted by a resuscitation formula must commonly be modified according to the individual's response to therapy. In optimizing fluid resuscitation in severely burned patients, the amount of fluid should be just enough to maintain vital organ function without producing iatrogenic pathological changes. The composition of the resuscitation fluid, within limitations, in the first 24 hours postburn probably makes very little difference; however, it should be individualized to the particular patient. The utilization of the beneficial properties of hypertonic, crystalloid, and colloid solutions at various times postburn will minimize the amount of edema formation. The rate of administration of resuscitation fluids should maintain urine outputs of 30–50 cc in adults and 1–2 cc/kg in children. When a child weighs 30–50 kg, the urine output should be maintained at the adult level. Fluid resuscitation based on our current knowledge of the massive fluid shifts and vascular changes that occur following burn injury has markedly decreased mortality related to burn-induced volume loss. The failure rate for adequate resuscitation is <5% even for patients with burns >85% TBSA. These improved statistics, however, are derived from experience in burn centers where there is substantial knowledge of the pathophysiology of burn injury.

Inadequate volume replacement in major burns is, unfortunately, common when clinicians lack sufficient knowledge and experience in this area.

Areas of burn shock research that need further attention include:

- the definition of the postburn course of capillary permeability changes, and identification of humoral or cellular factors influencing these changes;

- the identification and evaluation of pharmacological agents that can significantly alter capillary leakage;
- elucidation of the relationships between resuscitation fluid composition and pulmonary function changes; and
- the effect of resuscitation on late organ dysfunction, such as post-resuscitation wound, renal, and pulmonary complications.[87]

References

1. Artz CP, Moncrief JA. The burn problem. In: Artz CP, Moncrief JA, eds. The treatment of burns. Philadelphia: WB Saunders, 1969:1–22.
2. Underhill FP. The significance of anhydremia in extensive surface burn. JAMA 1930; 95:852–857.
3. Moore FD. The body-weight budget. Basic fluid therapy for the early burn. Surg Clin North Am 1970; 50:1249–1265.
4. Pruitt BA Jr, Mason AD Jr, Moncrief JA. Hemodynamic changes in the early post burn patients: the influence of fluid administration and of a vasodilator (hydralazine). J Trauma 1971; 11:36–46.
5. Majno G, Palide GE. Studies on inflammation. I. The effect of histamine and serotonin on vascular permeability. J Cell Biol 1961; 11:571–578.
6. Majno G, Shea SM, Leventhal M. Endothelial contractures induced by histamine-type mediators. J Cell Biol 1969; 42:647–672.
7. Anggard E, Jonsson CE. Efflux of prostaglandins in lymph from scalded tissue. Acta Physiol Scand 1971; 81:440–447.
8. Sevitt S. Local blood flow in experimental burns. J Pathol Bact 1949; 61:427–434.
9. Leape L. Initial changes in burns: tissue changes in burned and unburned skins of Rhesus monkeys. J Trauma 1970; 10:488–492.
10. Carvajal HF, Brouhard BH, Linares HA. Effect of antihistamine-antiserotonin and ganglionic blocking agents upon increased capillary permeability following burn trauma. J Trauma 1975; 15:969–975.
11. Boykin JV Jr, Crute SL, Haynes BW Jr. Cimetidine therapy for burn shock: a quantitative assessment. J Trauma 1985; 25:864–870.
12. VanNeuten JM, Janssen PAJ, VanBeck J. Vascular effects of ketanserin (R 41 468), a novel antagonist of 5-HT$_2$ serotonergic receptors. J Pharmacol Exp Ther 1981; 218:217–280.
13. Holliman CJ, Meuleman TR, Larsen KR, et al. The effect of ketanserin, a specific serotonin antagonist, on burn shock hemodynamic parameters in a porcine burn model. J Trauma 1983; 23:867–874.
14. Heggers JP, Loy GL, Robson MC, DelBaccaro EJ. Histological demonstration of prostaglandins and thromboxanes in burned tissue. J Surg Res 1980; 28:110–117.
15. Herndon DN, Abston S, Stein MD. Increased thromboxane B$_2$ levels in the plasma of burned and septic burned patients. Surg Gynecol Obstet 1984; 159:210–213.
16. Arturson G. Microvascular permeability to macromolecules in thermal injury. Acta Physiol Scand Suppl 1979; 463:111–122.
17. Rocha E, Silva M, Antonio A. Release of bradykinin and the mechanisms of production of thermic edema (45°C) in the rat's paw. Med Exp 1960; 3:371–378.
18. Holder IA, Neely AN. Hageman factor-dependent kinin activation in burns and its theoretical relationship to postburn immunosuppression syndrome and infection. J Burn Care Rehabil 1990; 11(6):496–503.
19. Neely AN, Nathan P, Highsmith RF. Plasma proteolytic activity following burns. J Trauma 1988; 28:362–367.
20. Baxter CR. Fluid volume and electrolyte changes in the early postburn period. Clin Plast Surg 1974; 1:693–703.
21. Moyer CA, Margraf HW, Monafo WW. Burn shock and extravascular sodium deficiency: treatment with Ringer's solution with lactate. Arch Surg 1965; 90:799–811.
22. Baxter CR, Shires GT. Physiological response to crystalloid resuscitation of severe burns. Ann NY Acad Sci 1968; 150:874–894.
23. Moylan JA, Mason AB, Rogers PW, Walker HL. Postburn shock: a critical evaluation of resuscitation. J Trauma 1973; 13:354–358.
24. Demling RH, Mazess RB, Witt RM, Wolbert WH. The study of burn wound edema using dichosmatic absorptionmetry. J Trauma 1978; 18:124–128.
25. Hilton JG. Effects of fluid resuscitation on total fluid loss following thermal injury. Surg Gynecol Obstet 1981; 152:441–447.
26. Schwartz SL. Consensus summary on fluid resuscitation. J Trauma 1979; 19(11 Suppl):876–877.
27. Shires GT. Proceedings of the Second NIH Workshop on Burn Management. J Trauma 1979; 19(11 Suppl):862–863.
28. Monafo WW. The treatment of burn shock by the intravenous and oral administration of hypertonic lactated saline solution. J Trauma 1970; 10:575–586.
29. Monafo WW, Halverson JD, Schechtman K. The role of concentrated sodium solutions in the resuscitation of patients with severe burns. Surgery 1984; 95:129–135.
30. Demling RH, Gunther RA, Haines B, Kramer G. Burn edema Part II: complications, prevention, and treatment. J Burn Care Rehabil 1982; 3:199–206.
31. Shimazaki S, Yukioka T, Matsuda H. Fluid distribution and pulmonary dysfunction following burn shock. J Trauma 1991; 31:623–626.
32. Caldwell FT, Bowser BH. Critical evaluation of hypertonic and hypotonic solutions to resuscitate severely burned children: a prospective study. Ann Surg 1979; 189:546–552.
33. Gunn ML, Hansbrough JF, Davis JW, et al. Prospective randomized trial of hypertonic sodium lactate vs. lactated Ringer's solution for burn shock resuscitation. J Trauma 1989; 29:1261–1267.
34. Yoshioka T, Maemura K, Ohhashi Y, et al. Effect of intravenously administered fluid on hemodynamic change and respiratory function in extensive thermal injury. Surg Gynecol Obstet 1980; 151:503–507.
35. Shimazaki S, Yoshioka T, Tanaka N, et al. Body fluid changes during hypertonic lactated saline solution therapy for burn shock. J Trauma 1977; 17:38–43.
36. Bowser-Wallace BH, Cone JB, Caldwell FT Jr. A prospective analysis of hypertonic lactated saline vs. Ringer's lactate-colloid for the resuscitation of severely burned children. Burns Incl Therm Inj 1986; 12:402–409.
37. Crum R, Bobrow B, Shackford S, et al. The neurohumoral response to burn injury in patients resuscitated with hypertonic saline. J Trauma 1988; 28:1181–1187.
38. Huang PP, Stucky FS, Dimick AR, et al. Hypertonic sodium resuscitation is associated with renal failure and death. Ann Surg 1995; 221:543–554.
39. Bowser-Wallace BH, Cone JB, Caldwell FT Jr. Hypertonic lactated saline resuscitation of severely burned patients over 60 years of age. J Trauma 1985; 25:22–26.
40. Bowser-Wallace BH, Caldwell FT Jr. Fluid requirements of severely burned children up to 3 years old: hypertonic lactated saline vs. Ringer's lactate-colloid. Burns Incl Therm Inj 1986; 12:549–555.
41. Bartolani A, Governa M, Barisoni D. Fluid replacement in burned patients. Acta Chir Plast 1996; 38:132–136.
42. Griswold JA, Anglin BL, Love RT Jr, et al. Hypertonic saline resuscitation: efficacy in a community-based burn unit. South Med J 1991; 84:692–696.

43. Jelenko C III, Williams JB, Wheeler ML, et al. Studies in shock and resuscitation, I: use of a hypertonic, albumin-containing, fluid demand regimen (HALFD) in resuscitation. Crit Care Med 1979; 7:157–167.

44. Du G, Slater H, Goldfarb IW. Influence of different resuscitation regimens on acute weight gain in extensively burned patients. Burns 1991; 17:147–150.

45. Baxter CR. Problems and complications of burn shock resuscitation. Surg Clin North Am 1978; 58:1313–1322.

46. Goodwin CW, Dorethy J, Lam V, et al. Randomized trial of efficacy of crystalloid and colloid resuscitation on hemodynamic response and lung water following thermal injury. Ann Surg 1983; 197:520–531.

47. Demling RH. Fluid resuscitation. In: Boswick JA Jr, ed. The art and science of burn care. Rockville, MD: Aspen; 1987: 189–202.

48. Demling RH, Kramer GD, Harms B. Role of thermal injury-induced hypoproteinemia on edema formation in burned and non-burned tissue. Surgery 1984; 95:136–144.

49. Demling RH, Kramer GC, Gunther R, Nerlich M. Effect of non-protein colloid on post-burn edema formation in soft tissues and lung. Surgery 1985; 95:593–602.

50. Gelin LE, Solvell L, Zederfeldt B. The plasma volume expanding effect of low viscous dextran and Macrodex. Acta Chir Scand 1961; 122:309–323.

51. Warden GD. Burn shock resuscitation. World J Surg 1992; 16:21–23.

52. Carvajal HF. Fluid therapy for the acutely burned child. Compr Ther 1977; 3:17–24.

53. Merrell SW, Saffle JR, Sullivan JJ, et al. Fluid resuscitation in thermally injured children. Am J Surg 1986; 152:664–669.

54. Graves TA, Cioffi WG, McManus WF, et al. Fluid resuscitation of infants and children with massive thermal injury. J Trauma 1988; 28:1656–1659.

55. Navar PD, Saffle JR, Warden GD. Effect of inhalation injury on fluid resuscitation requirements after thermal injury. Am J Surg 1985; 150:716–720.

56. Mansfield MD, Kinsell J. Use of invasive cardiovascular monitoring in patients with burns greater than 30 percent body surface area: a survey of 251 centres. Burns 1996; 22:549–551.

57. Fabri PJ. Monitoring of the burn patient. Clin Plast Surg 1986; 13:21–27.

58. Kirton OC, Civetta JM. Do pulmonary artery catheters alter outcome in trauma patients? New Horizons 1997; 5:222–227.

59. Pulmonary artery catheter consensus conference: Consensus statement. Crit Care Med 1997; 25:910–25.

60. Aikawa N, Martyn JA, Burke JR. Pulmonary artery catheterization and thermodilution cardiac output determination in the management of critically burned patients. Am J Surg 1978; 135:811–817.

61. Agarwal N, Petro J, Salisbury RE. Physiologic profile monitoring in burned patients. J Trauma 1982; 23:577–583.

62. Dries DJ, Waxman K. Adequate resuscitation of burn patients may not be measured by urine output and vital signs. Crit Care Med 1991; 19:327–329.

63. Schiller WR, Bay RC. Hemodynamic and oxygen transport monitoring in management of burns. New Horizons 1996; 4:475–482.

64. Fleming AW, Bishop M, Shoemaker W, et al. Prospective trial of supranormal values as goals of resuscitation in severe trauma. Arch Surg 1992; 127:1175–1181.

65. Bishop MH, Shoemaker WC, Appel PL, et al. Prospective, randomized trial of survivor values of cardiac index, oxygen delivery, and oxygen consumption as resuscitation endpoints in severe trauma. J Trauma 1995; 38:780–787.

66. Pearson KS, Gomez MN, Moyers JR, et al. A cost/benefit analysis of randomized invasive monitoring of patients undergoing cardiac surgery. Anesth Analg 1989; 69:336–341.

67. Ontario Intensive Care Study Group. Evaluation of right heart catheterization in critically ill patients. Crit Care Med 1992; 20:928–933.

68. Yu M, Levy MM, Smith P, et al. Effect of maximizing oxygen delivery on morbidity and mortality rates in critically ill patients: a prospective, randomized, controlled study. Crit Care Med 1993; 21:830–838.

69. Gattinoni L, Brazzi L, Pelosi P, et al. A trial of goal-oriented hemo-dynamic therapy in critically ill patients. N Engl J Med 1995; 333:1025–1032.

70. Cooper AB, Goig GS, Sibbald WJ. Pulmonary artery catheters in the critically ill. An overview using the methodology of evidence-based medicine. Crit Care Clin 1996; 12:777–794.

71. Elliott DC. An evaluation of the end points of resuscitation. J Am Coll Surg 1998; 187:536–547.

72. Aikawa N, Ishbiki K, Naito C, et al. Individualized fluid resuscitation based on haemodynamic monitoring in the management of extensive burns. Burns 1982; 8:249–255.

73. Bernard F, Gueugniaud P-Y, Bertin-Maghit M, et al. Prognostic significance of early cardiac index measurements in severely burned patients. Burns 1994; 20:529–531.

74. Schiller WR, Bay RC, McLachlan JG, Sagraves SG. Survival in major burn injuries is predicted by early response to Swan-Ganz-guided resuscitation. Am J Surg 1995; 170:696–700.

75. Schiller WR, Bay RC, Garren RL, et al. Hyperdynamic resuscitation improves survival in patients with life-threatening burns. J Burn Care Rehabil 1997; 18:10–16.

76. Barton RG, Saffle JR, Morris SE, et al. Resuscitation of thermally injured patients with oxygen transport criteria as goals of therapy. J Burn Care Rehabil 1997; 18:1–9.

77. Mizock BL, Falk JL. Lactic acidosis in critical illness. Crit Care Med 1992; 20:80–93.

78. Bakker J, Coffemils M, Leon M, et al. Blood lactate levels are superior to oxygen derived variables in predicting outcome in human septic shock. Chest 1991; 99:956–962.

79. Weil MH, Afifi AA. Experimental and clinical studies on lactate and pyruvate as indicators of the severity of acute circulatory failure (shock). Circulation 1970; 41:989–1001.

80. Henning RJ, Weil MH, Weiner F. Blood lactate as a prognostic indicator of survival in patients with acute myocardial infarction. Circ Shock 1982; 9:307–315.

81. Boyd I, Grounds RM, Bennett ED. A randomized clinical trial of the effect of deliberate perioperative increase of oxygen delivery on mortality in high-risk surgical patients. JAMA 1993; 270:2699–2707.

82. Abramson D, Scalea TM, Hitchcock R, et al. Lactate clearance and survival following injury. J Trauma 1993; 35:584–588.

83. Pruitt B Jr. Fluid and electrolyte replacement in the burned patient. Surg Clin North Am 1978; 58:1291–1312.

84. Warden GD, Stratta R, Saffle JR Jr, et al. Plasma exchange therapy in patients failing to resuscitate from burn shock. J Trauma 1983; 23:945–951.

85. Schnarrs R, Cline C, Goldfarb I, et al. Plasma exchange for failure of early resuscitation in thermal injuries. J Burn Care Rehabil 1986; 7:230–233.

86. Warden GD, Wilmore D, Rogers P, et al. Hypernatremic state in hypermetabolic burn patients. Arch Surg 1973; 106:420–423.

87. Pruitt BA Jr. Fluid resuscitation of extensively burned patients. J Trauma 1981; 21(Suppl):690–692.

88. Pediatric Advanced Life Support, PALS Provider Manual. American Heart Association; 2002:146.

89. Lalonde C, Picard L, Youn YK, et al. Increased early postburn fluid requirement and oxygen demands are predictive of the degree of airways injury by smoke inhalation. J Trauma 1995 Feb; 38(2):175–84.

90. Alderson P, Bunn F, Lefevre C. Human albumin solution for resuscitation and volume expansion in critically ill patients. Cochrane Database Syst Rev 2002;(4):CD001208.

91. Wilkes MM, Navickis RJ. Patient survival after human albumin administration. A meta-analysis of randomized, controlled trials. Ann Intern Med 2001; 135(3):149–164.

92. Friedrich JB, Sullivan SR, Engrav LH, et al. Is supra-Baxter resuscitation in burn patients a new phenomenon? Burns 2004; 30(5):464–466.

93. O'Mara MS, Slater H, Goldfarb IW, et al. A prospective, randomized evaluation of intra-abdominal pressures with crystalloid and colloid resuscitation in burn patients. J Trauma 2005; 58(5): 1011–1018.

94. Oda J, Yamashita K, Inoue T, et al. Resuscitation fluid volume and abdominal compartment syndrome in patients with major burns. Burns 2006; 32(2): 151–154.

Chapter 10

Evaluation of the burn wound: management decisions

Tam N. Pham, Nicole S. Gibran, and David M. Heimbach

Introduction

Advances in the resuscitation of burn patients have greatly improved survival, so that death from burn shock has become uncommon. In the 21st century, prompt recovery and good functional outcome for the burn patient hinges, in large part, on proper management of the burn wound.

Perhaps the greatest advance in burn care to date has been the institution of early surgical excision of the burn wound with immediate or delayed wound closure strategy individualized to each patient.[1–4] For many years, burns were treated by daily washing, removal of loose dead tissue, and application of some sort of topical nostrum until wounds healed by themselves or granulation tissue appeared in the wound bed. Superficial dermal burns healed within 2 weeks and deep dermal burns healed over many weeks if infection was prevented. Full-thickness burns lost their eschar in 2–6 weeks by enzyme production from bacteria and by daily bedside débridement. Split-thickness skin grafts were applied usually 3–8 weeks after injury. A 50% graft survival was considered acceptable and repeated grafting eventually closed the wound. The prolonged and intense inflammatory response made hypertrophic scars and contractures part of normal burn treatment.

Burns that heal within 3 weeks generally do so without hypertrophic scarring or functional impairment, although long-term pigment changes may occur. Burns needing longer than 3 weeks to heal produce unsightly hypertrophic scars, and may form contractures leading to functional impairment. With few exceptions, state-of-the-art burn care now involves early excision and grafting of all burns that do not heal within 3 weeks. The challenge is to determine which burns will heal within 3 weeks.

Burn wound assessment requires an understanding of skin biology and the pathophysiological changes caused by thermal injury. The standard technique for determining burn depth in the 21st century still remains clinical assessment of the wound by an experienced burn specialist. Management decisions should take into account the mechanism of injury, as this invariably influences the healing potential of the wound, and therefore guides the timing of surgical intervention.

Pathophysiology of the burn wound

Skin biology

The skin is the largest organ in the human body and is composed of two layers: the epidermis and the dermis. The thickness of the epidermis varies among different parts of the body, from 0.05 mm on the eyelids to over 1 mm on the soles.[5] Most of the skin thickness comes from the dermis, which varies with age, gender, and body location. The skin serves as protection against fluid and electrolyte loss, infection, radiation, and provides thermal regulation. Through skin contact, the individual obtains clues to the surrounding environment via touch, perception of temperature and pain. In addition, skin appearance is a major determinant of identity and affects interpersonal interactions.

The mostly cellular epidermis is derived from ectoderm and the principal cell is the keratinocyte. These cells begin their division and differentiation at the basal layer and move progressively outward over 2–4 weeks[6] along the outer four layers of the epidermis: the stratum spinosum, the stratum granulosum, the stratum lucidum, and the stratum corneum. Keratinocytes lose their nuclei in the stratum lucidum and become flattened dead cells in the stratum corneum. Other important cells of the epidermis include melanocytes, which produce the melanin pigment essential for protection against ultraviolet radiation, and Langerhans cells, which perform phagocytosis and presentation of foreign antigens. The epidermis, because it is derived from ectoderm, is capable of regenerative healing. Thus, pure epidermal injuries heal by regeneration and without scarring. Keratinocytes proliferate from dermal appendages (hair follicles, sweat glands) and the edges of the wound to achieve reepithelialization. Depleted melanocytes after injury, however, regenerate more slowly and less predictably, which may lead to permanent pigment changes within the healed wound.[7,8]

The basement membrane zone connects the epidermis to the dermis via epidermal projections (rete ridges) that interdigitate with dermal projections (papillae). The critical structures that stabilize the epidermal–dermal junction are keratinocyte-derived collagen VII anchoring fibrils that extend into the dermis.[9,10] These anchoring fibrils may take several weeks (and sometimes months) to mature during burn wound healing. Minor shearing forces may cause shearing, blistering and sometimes epidermal loss until the interdigitations mature.

The dermis with its abundant extracellular matrix component is derived from mesoderm and is divided into the more superficial papillary dermis and the deeper reticular dermis. Collagen fibers provide the bulk of the dermal structure. Their organized orientation allows for stretching and tensile strength of the skin.[11] Elastic fibers impart the elastic recoil properties of skin. Protein turnover (by degradation, production, and remodeling) increases with mechanical stress and during healing, accounting for the high plasticity of skin. Collagen and elastin are both synthesized by fibroblasts, the principal cell of the dermis. The non-fibrous component of the dermis is called the ground substance. It is composed of glycosaminoglycans and proteoglycans such as hyaluronic acid and chondroitin sulfate, whose function is to entrap fluid to maintain the semi-fluid matrix and to regulate cellular cross-talk by binding and releasing inflammatory mediators.[12] Adnexal structures (sweat glands, sebaceous glands, and hair follicles) originate in the dermis and extend through the epidermis. Since they are lined with epidermal keratinocytes, adnexal structures provide the epithelial cells necessary for reepithelialization after a partial dermal injury. The dermal plexus of capillary vessels delivers the necessary nutrients to cellular structures in both the dermis and epidermis. After wounding, however, the endothelial cells also mediate local and systemic inflammatory responses.[13] Sensory nerves, which traverse the dermis into the epidermis, also play a significant role after injury, as they mediate pain and itching, modulate inflammation, and appear to influence the remodeling phase of wound healing.[14,15] The dermis, like other structures derived from mesoderm, heals not by regeneration but by fibrosis and scarring.

Pathophysiological changes of thermal injury

Applied heat at the cellular level causes denaturation of proteins and loss of plasma membrane integrity. Temperature and duration of contact have a synergistic effect, such that cell necrosis occurs after 1 second of exposure at 156°F (69°C), or after 1 hour at 113°F (45°C).[16] Following a burn, necrosis occurs at the center of the injury, and becomes progressively less severe at the periphery. Thus, Jackson's description in 1953 of the three zones of injury still remains our current conceptual understanding of the burn wound[17] (Figure 10.1). The zone of coagulation is at the center of the wound where no viable cells remain. Surrounding it is the zone of stasis, characterized a mix of viable and non-viable cells, capillary vasoconstriction, and ischemia. This tenuous area represents the zone 'at-risk' and may convert to necrosis with hypoperfusion, dessication, edema, and infection. With proper wound care management however, these changes may be reversed.[18] Systemic factors such as advanced age, diabetes, and other chronic illnesses also put the zone of stasis at higher risk for 'conversion.' The outer periphery of the burn wound is the zone of hyperemia, with viable cells and vasodilation mediated by local inflammatory mediators. Tissue in this zone usually recovers completely unless complicated by infection or severe hypoperfusion.

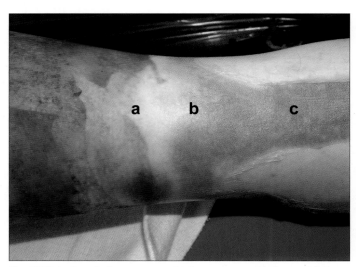

Fig. 10.1 Jackson's three zones of injury on an ankle burn: (a) the zone of coagulation, (b) the zone of stasis, and (c) the zone of hyperemia.

Since medical care, for the most part, has little impact on the outcome of the zone of coagulation, efforts have focused on the prevention of necrosis in the zone of stasis. Systemically, protection of this sensitive area is achieved with adequate fluid resuscitation, avoidance of vasoconstrictors, and prevention of infection.[19,20] Locally, optimal wound care consists of non-dessicating dressings, topical antimicrobials, and frequent monitoring of the wound.[21–23] Interest in cooling of the wound to minimize the extent of injury can be traced to antiquity,[24] but to this day, firm evidence of its efficacy is lacking. To be effective, cooling must be performed immediately after injury, and should not supersede other priorities in the evaluation of the injured patient. The optimal temperature and duration of cooling is unknown;[25–27] in fact, excessive or prolonged cooling may be harmful in that it promotes vasoconstriction and systemic hypothermia.[28,29] Current guidelines of American Burn Association recommend limiting cooling to 30 minutes in the management of minor burns.[30] Modalities to improve dermal perfusion and block injury from released inflammatory mediators have also garnered much interest. Experimental benefits have been reported for many pharmacologic agents such as heparin, steroidal and non-steroidal anti-inflammatory agents, thromboxane inhibitors, and epidermal growth factor.[31–39] Yet, all remain investigational since none has gained wide acceptance for clinical use.

Assessment of burn depth

Clinical observation

Burn injury may involve one or both layers of the skin, and may extend into the subcutaneous fat, muscle, and even bony structures.[40] Burns involving only the epidermis are erythematous and very painful but do not form blisters. Most sunburns fit this category of superficial, epidermal injury. Within 3–4 days, the dead epidermis sloughs and is replaced by regenerating keratinocytes.

Superficial dermal burns extend into the papillary dermis and characteristically form blisters. Blistering may not occur immediately following injury and burns thought to be superficial may subsequently be diagnosed as dermal burns by day.[2] Once the blister is removed from a superficial partial-thickness burn, the wound is pink, wet, and hypersensitive to touch. Wound care is often painful as uncovering the wound allows currents of air to pass over it. These wounds blanch with pressure, and the blood flow to the dermis is increased over that of normal skin due to vasodilation. With appropriate wound care, superficial dermal burns usually heal within 2–3 weeks without risk of scarring and therefore do not require operation.

Deep dermal burns extend into the reticular dermis and generally will take 3 or more weeks to heal. They also blister, but the wound surface appears mottled pink and white immediately following the injury (Figure 10.2). The patient complains of discomfort and pressure rather than pain. When pressure is applied to the burn, capillaries refill slowly or not at all. The wound is often less sensitive to pinprick than the surrounding normal skin. By the second day the wound may be white and is usually fairly dry. As a rule, partial-thickness burns that are predicted not to heal by 3 weeks should be excised and grafted.

Full-thickness burns involve the entire dermis and extend into subcutaneous tissue. Their appearance may be charred, leathery, firm, and depressed when compared to adjoining normal skin. These wounds are insensitive to light touch and pinprick. Non-charred full-thickness burns can be deceptive. Like deep dermal burns, they may be mottled in appearance. They rarely blanch on pressure, and may have a dry, white appearance. In some cases the burn may be translucent with clotted vessels visible in the depths. Some full-thickness burns, particularly immersion scalds or 'bake' injuries (caused by convective heat), may have a red appearance, and can be confused by the inexperienced observer as a superficial dermal burn. These burns, however, do not blanch with pressure. Full-thickness burns should be excised and grafted early to expedite the patient's recovery process and prevent infection and hypertrophic scarring.

The most difficult management decision involves partial-thickness burns that are intermediate in depth. In this situation, the determining factor whether these burns heal in 3 weeks may only be a matter of a few tenths of a millimeter. These burns are more aptly called 'indeterminate' burns as their healing potential becomes evident with serial assessments over several days. As evidenced by histologic studies, burn injury is a dynamic process that peaks at about 3 days.[41–43] Initial evaluation by an experienced surgeon as to whether an indeterminate dermal burn will heal in 3 weeks is only about 50–70% accurate.[44–46]

Adjuncts to clinical evaluation

An intense search for a more precise diagnosis of burn depth has been mounted ever since it became recognized that many patients would benefit from early operation. A number of techniques have been trialed based on the physiology of the skin and alterations produced by burning. These techniques take advantage of the ability to detect: dead cells or denatured collagen (biopsy, ultrasound, vital dyes);[17,47–50] the color of the wound (light reflectance);[51] physical changes, such as edema (magnetic resonance imaging);[52] and altered blood flow (fluorescein, laser Doppler imaging, and thermography).[53–55] Unfortunately, none of these techniques has been proven superior to serial clinical assessments by an experienced burn provider. Several groups, however, have recently reported clinical benefits with the use of non-contact laser Doppler imaging in indeterminate-thickness burns.[43,56] This technique provides a color perfusion map of the burn wound to add to the clinician's assessment. Since the scanner is held at a distance from the wound, this test is well tolerated and perhaps more reliable as no pressure is exerted on the wound. Furthermore, this test can be repeated over the first several days post-burn to document dynamic changes in wound bed perfusion. Although a promising tool, non-contact laser Doppler imaging has, so far, not been widely adopted into clinical practice due to variable reproducibility.

Mechanisms of thermal injury

Flash and flame burns

Flash and flame burn injuries represent approximately half of the admissions to American regional burn centers. Explosions of natural gas, propane, gasoline, and other flammable liquids cause intense heat for a very brief time. In particular, gasoline has highly flammable vapors that are 3–4 times denser than air. At room temperature, gasoline vapors can diffuse above ground and may accumulate in enclosed spaces. Victims often describe an inappropriate use of gasoline as a fire accelerant (trash burning, outdoor fire). Clothing, unless it ignites, is protective in flash burns. Hence, flash burns generally have a distribution involving all exposed skin, with the deepest areas facing the source of ignition. For the most part, flash burns reach progressive layers of the dermis in proportion to the amount and kind of fuel that explodes. While such burns will generally heal without extensive skin grafting, they may cover large areas and may be associated with thermal damage to the upper airway.

In contrast to flash injuries, flame burns are invariably deep dermal if not full-thickness because of more prolonged exposure to intense heat. Although the incidence of injuries from house fires has decreased with the advent of smoke detectors,

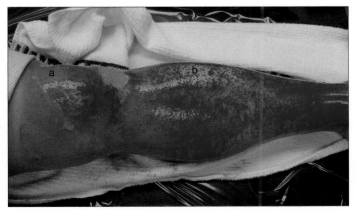

Fig. 10.2 Lower extremity burn having components of a superficial dermal burn (a) with a wet, pink, and moist appearance, as well as a deeper dermal burn (b) with mottled pink and white areas.

careless smoking, improper use of flammable liquids, automobile accidents, and clothing ignited from stoves or space heaters still exact their toll. Patients whose bedding or clothes have been on fire rarely escape without some full-thickness burns. Many victims of house fires are also prone to deeper injuries because of intoxication or confusion caused by carbon monoxide poisoning. In one study of several burn centers, 28% of flame burns occurred in patients with high blood ethanol level, and 51% of victims in fires behaved inappropriately when trying to escape.[57] Loss of consciousness may also expose the victim to convective heat inside a burning room. This type of 'bake' injury may deceptively appear shallow with intact epithelium to the inexperienced observer, but is really a full-thickness burn.

Scalds

Hot water scalds are the next most common cause of burns in the United States. Despite educational programs, the epidemiology and incidence of scalds worldwide has changed very little. The depth of scald injury depends the water temperature, the skin thickness, and the duration of contact. Water at 140°F (60°C) creates a deep dermal burn in 3 seconds but will cause the same injury in 1 second at 156°F (69°C). Freshly brewed coffee from an automatic percolator is generally about 180°F (82°C). Once in the pot, coffee temperature approximates 160°F (70°C). Boiling water often causes a deep dermal burn, unless the duration of contact is very short. Soups and sauces, which are thicker in consistency, will remain in contact longer with the skin and invariably cause deep dermal burns. In general, exposed areas tend to be burned less deeply than clothed areas. Clothing retains the heat and keeps the liquid in contact with the skin longer. As a result, scalds are often a mosaic of superficial and indeterminate dermal burns. A common example is a toddler who reaches above head level and spills hot water on himself. His face bears a superficial burn, his trunk burn is of indeterminate thickness, and his skin under his diaper has a deep dermal burn.

Immersion scalds are often deep because of the prolonged skin exposure, although the water temperature may not be as high as in spill scalds.[58,59] They occur in individuals who do not perceive the discomfort of prolonged immersion (i.e. a diabetic patient soaking his foot in hot water), or who are not able to escape from the hot water (i.e. young children, the elderly, or people with physical and cognitive disabilities). This latter group of vulnerable individuals is also susceptible to non-accidental scald burns.[60,61] Children victims of non-accidental scalds represent about 2% of all children admitted to our burn center. Circumferential extremity injuries, symmetrical burns to a child's buttocks and perineum are examples that should raise suspicion of abuse (Figure 10.3). A detailed description on the recognition and management of intentional burn injuries is available elsewhere in this text. The evaluating physician, therefore, must carefully consider whether the provided history matches the distribution and probable cause of the burn; this is best accomplished by an experienced burn surgeon who is familiar with burn distribution and etiologies.

Grease and hot oils will generally cause deep dermal or even full-thickness injuries. During cooking, grease and hot oils are

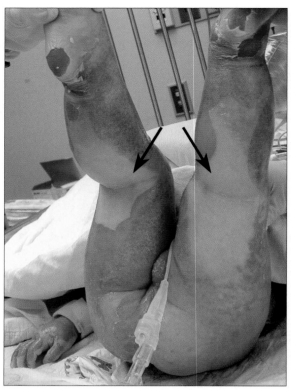

Fig. 10.3 Immersion scald burn on a child. Arrows denote sparing of bilateral popliteal fossae: the child by reflex bent his knees to avoid contact with the hot water.

heated to a level below their smoke point to avoid unpleasant odors from their decompositions. The smoke point for butter is 350°F (177°C), 400°F (204°C) for lard, and 450°F (232°C) for corn oil. Cooking oils reach their flash point at 600°F (316°C). Deep dermal burns commonly occur when a victim tries to carry the burning pan of grease outdoors and douses himself instead of putting the lid on the pan and extinguishing the fire. The extent of domestic grease injuries invariably follows a common pattern.[62] A single wrist and forearm is first affected. The panicked victim lets go of the pan and splashes himself onto his feet and sometimes thighs and trunk. The now slippery floor from spilled grease causes the victim to fall and burn his back and buttocks. Approximately 30–40% of grease burns require excision and grafting.[62,63]

Tar and asphalt are a special kind of scald. The 'mother pot' at the back of the roofing truck maintains tar at a temperature of 400–500°F (204–260°C). Burns caused by tar directly from the 'mother pot' are invariably full-thickness. By the time the tar is spread on the roof, its temperature has diminished to the point where most of the burns are deep dermal in nature. Initially evaluation consists of tar removal before injury depth can be assessed. Tar can be removed by application of petroleum-based ointment under a dressing. The dressing is changed and ointment reapplied every 2–4 hours until the tar has dissolved. Medi-Sol adhesive remover spray (Orange-Sol, Gilbert, AZ, USA) can be successfully used to remove the tar without injury to the burn wound.

Partial-thickness scald burns can be usually managed non-operatively for 10–14 days, unless they are obviously deep.

Burns should be excised and autografted as soon as it is clear that they will not heal by 3 weeks. Desai et al. confirmed the validity of this strategy in a randomized trial.[64] Children with large scald burns (approximately 25% TBSA) were either excised early (within 72 hours) or after 2 weeks post-injury. Children in the late group required excision of significantly smaller areas, while half achieved reepithelialization without surgery.

Contact burns

Contact burns result from hot metals, plastic, glass, or hot coals. Although generally small in size, contact burns are challenging in that the injury is often very deep (Figure 10.4). Burn depth can be predicted based on the temperature of the material and the duration of contact. Thus, molten materials in industrial accidents instantaneously cause a burn extending below the dermis. Likewise, an unconscious victim laying on top of a heating blanket all night will have a burn extending into fat and sometimes muscle. Industrial accidents involving presses or other hot, heavy objects may cause both contact burns and crush injuries. In these circumstances, the clinician must anticipate the possibility of extensive myonecrosis and myoglobinuria despite the relative small size of the wound. Contact burns with a hot muffler are usually full-thickness and require excision and grafting. Traffic accidents where the victim is trapped against a muffler or engine block may generate significant defects requiring flap coverage.[65]

Domestic contact burns often involve palm and finger burns in toddlers. The unsuspecting child typically puts his hands on a wood-stove, fireplace insert, iron press or oven door.[66] With aggressive wound care and hand therapy, most intermediate-depth palm burns heal in about 2–3 weeks. On the other hand, unoperated deep palm burns heal from the edges with contracture of the palm leading to permanent disability. The decision to perform excision and grafting using thick split-thickness grafts or full-thickness grafts to deep palm burns[67,68] should be tempered by the knowledge that sensory nerve endings unique to glabrous skin (Pacinian and Meissner's corpuscles) cannot be replaced by a skin graft. Therefore, an observation

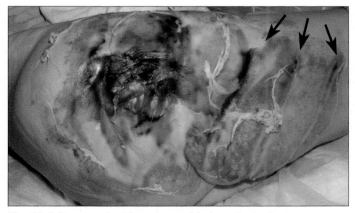

Fig. 10.4 Deep contact burn in an elderly patient who was unconscious next to a space heater. Arrows denote the imprints of the space heater grill on his lateral thigh.

period of 2–3 weeks with splinting and aggressive exercise appears prudent.

Chemical burns

Chemical burns, usually caused by strong acids or alkalis, are most often the result of industrial accidents, drain cleaners, assaults, and the improper use of harsh solvents. Chemical burns cause progressive damage until the chemicals are inactivated by reaction with the tissue or dilution by flushing with water. Although individual circumstances vary, acid burns are usually more self-limiting than alkali burns. Acid tends to 'tan' the skin, creating an impermeable barrier that limits further penetration of the acid. Alkalis, on the other hand, combine with cutaneous lipids to create soap and thereby continue 'dissolving' the skin until they are neutralized.

Initial management consists of diluting the agent with copious water, preferably at the site of the accident. To this end, many industrial workplaces are now equipped with such showers and eye wash stations. The victim ought to have the contact site irrigated for 15–20 minutes at minimum. A paper pH test applied to the patient's burn can verify that the agent has been neutralized. Attempts to neutralize alkalis with acids (and vice versa) are contraindicated because these maneuvers are dangerous and may induce an exothermic reaction leading to a thermal injury superimposed on the chemical burn. An exception to the irrigation rule is exposure to a chemical powder. In this instance, it is safer to brush the agent off. Examples of common dry chemicals include dry concrete, cement, and sodium hydroxide. A full-thickness chemical burn may appear deceptively superficial, clinically causing only a mild brownish discoloration of the skin. The skin may appear intact during the first few days post-burn, and only then begin to slough spontaneously. Unless the observer can be absolutely sure, chemical burns should be considered deep dermal or full-thickness until proven otherwise.

Burns caused by wet cement can be vexing. Workers often kneel in wet cement or spill cement inside boots or gloves and do not become symptomatic for hours.[69–71] By the time they seek medical help, the wounds are often deep and most often need grafting.

Hydrofluoric acid (HF) burns are potentially very destructive. HF is widely used in the circuit board etching, cleaning solvents, and paint removers. HF coagulates the skin at site of exposure. Fluoride ions penetrate the skin and cause deep tissue destruction by combining with cellular calcium and magnesium.[72,73] Fluoride is also a metabolic poison that inhibits key enzymes of cellular metabolism. A 10% TBSA HF burn may be life threatening due to systemic hypocalcemia;[74] this may be one instance where urgent surgical wound excision is indicated. As with cement, the worker may not become symptomatic for several hours after exposure, when severe pain develops in the involved fingers. Delayed or inadequate treatment can lead to amputation. Older recommendations of calcium-containing topical gels[75,76] and direct injection of calcium gluconate into the involved tissue have now largely been replaced by intra-arterial infusion of calcium ions into vessels perfusing the injured area.[77–80] Such treatment is almost magical, with immediate cessation of pain and minimal tissue destruction. However, once acute symptoms resolve, it has no further role in preventing tissue damage.

Electrical burns

Electrical burns are in reality thermal burns from very high-intensity heat generated as the victim's body becomes an accidental resistor. Low-voltage injuries (less than 440 volts) rarely cause significant damage beyond a small deep thermal burn at contact points. An exception to this rule is the child who chews on an active electrical connection.[81] The child's saliva completes the circuit between the positive and neutral leads. The short circuit may cause a severe burn inside the mouth and lip. Burns involving the oral commissure are at high risk for late contracture and warrant an aggressive splinting and exercise regimen.[82,83] In addition, eschar separation at the corner of the mouth by day 7–10 after injury may be associated with brisk labial artery bleeding that requires surgical control.[84] High-voltage injuries (over 1000 volts) are more apt to cause deep tissue destruction. In fact, most electrical burns are work-related (i.e. construction workers, linemen, utility and electrical workers). In this setting, extensive deep tissue destruction may take place underneath a relatively small, innocuous-appearing wound (Figure 10.5).

High resistance at skin contact points is partially protective as a dry calloused hand may provide twice the resistance of normal skin, and five times the resistance of wet skin. High resistance within the victim's body, on the other hand, causes more harm. As electricity travels through the body, electrical energy is converted to heat in direct proportion to current and electrical resistance. Deep muscle necrosis may occur adjacent to bone, which has high resistance.[85,86] A smaller body part conducting the electricity will generate more intense heat with less dissipation. Therefore, fingers, hands, forearms, feet, and lower legs are often totally destroyed, whereas the trunk usually dissipates enough current to prevent extensive damage to viscera (unless the entrance or exit wound is on the abdomen or chest).[87–89] Arc electrical burns are also common as the current takes the most direct path, rather than a longer path of seeming less resistance. These injuries occur at joints in close apposition at the time of injury. Most common are burns of the volar aspect of the wrist, the antecubital fossa when the elbow is flexed, and the axilla if the shoulder is adducted.

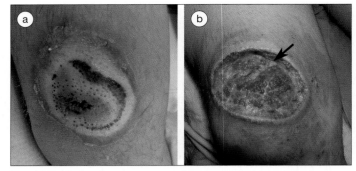

Fig. 10.5 High-voltage contact point on an electrician's knee: (a) prior to, (b) after débridement. Excision down to muscle tissue was required (arrow) to obtain a viable wound bed.

There are two reasons for early operation in the patient with electrical burns. Massive deep tissue necrosis may lead to acidosis or myoglobinuria that will not clear with standard resuscitation techniques. In this unusual circumstance, fasciotomies, major débridement, and amputation may be needed urgently. More commonly, tissue swelling raises the risk of compartment syndrome. Careful monitoring of the injured extremity is mandatory. Compartmental release is indicated with any sign of progressive peripheral neuropathy. Thus, worsening median or (less commonly) ulnar nerve deficit in the injured hand are indications for immediate median and ulnar nerve release at the wrist. The use of a technetium scan to help identify damaged and necrotic muscle has been advocated,[90] but has not achieved widespread use. This test is overly sensitive in detecting damage to deep, unexposed muscle groups that, left alone, will fibrose and not require excision.[91]

If immediate decompression or débridement is not required, definitive operations can be performed between days 3 and 5, before bacterial contamination occurs and after the tissue necrosis is delineated.[91,92] Extraordinary measures, such as vascular grafts to replace clotted arteries, and urgent free flaps may sometimes be indicated,[93,94] but the surgeon is cautioned that they may actually increase morbidity and prolong the patient's recovery. A well-fitting prosthesis might give better function than a hand or foot that is weak and has diminished sensation.

References

1. Burke JF, Bondoc CC, Quinby WC. Primary burn excision and immediate grafting: a method shortening illness. J Trauma 1974; 14(5):389–395.
2. Engrav LH, Heimbach DM, Reus JL, et al. Early excision and grafting vs. nonoperative treatment of burns of indeterminant depth: a randomized prospective study. J Trauma 1983; 23(11):1001–1004.
3. Thompson P, Herndon DN, Abston S, et al. Effect of early excision on patients with major thermal injury. J Trauma 1987; 27(2):205–207.
4. Gray DT, Pine RW, Harnar TJ, et al. Early surgical excision versus conventional therapy in patients with 20 to 40 percent burns. A comparative study. Am J Surg 1982; 144(1):76–80.
5. Southwood WF. The thickness of the skin. Plast Reconstr Surg 1955; 15(5):423–429.
6. Rudolph R, Ballantyne DL Jr. Skin grafts. In: McCarthy J, ed. Plastic surgery. Philadelphia: WB Saunders; 1990:221–274.
7. Tyack ZF, Pegg S, Ziviani J. Postburn dyspigmentation: its assessment, management, and relationship to scarring – a review of the literature. J Burn Care Rehabil 1997; 18(5):435–440.
8. de Chalain TM, Tang C, Thomson HG. Burn area color changes after superficial burns in childhood: can they be predicted? J Burn Care Rehabil 1998; 19(1 Pt 1):39–49.
9. Compton CC, Press W, Gill JM, et al. The generation of anchoring fibrils by epidermal keratinocytes: a quantitative long-term study. Epithelial Cell Biol 1995; 4(3):93–103.
10. Regauer S, Seiler GR, Barrandon Y, et al. Epithelial origin of cutaneous anchoring fibrils. J Cell Biol 1990; 111(5 Pt 1):2109–2115.
11. Yannas IV, Burke JF. Design of an artificial skin. I. Basic design principles. J Biomed Mater Res 1980; 14(1):65–81.
12. Yannas IV, Burke JF, Gordon PL, et al. Design of an artificial skin. II. Control of chemical composition. J Biomed Mater Res 1980; 14(2):107–132.

13. Gibran NS, Heimbach DM. Current status of burn wound patho-physiology. Clin Plast Surg 2000; 27(1):11–22.

14. Crowe R, Parkhouse N, McGrouther D, et al. Neuropeptide-containing nerves in painful hypertrophic human scar tissue. Br J Dermatol 1994; 130(4):444–452.

15. Dunnick CA, Gibran NS, Heimbach DM. Substance P has a role in neurogenic mediation of human burn wound healing. J Burn Care Rehabil 1996; 17(5):390–396.

16. Moritz A, Henriquez, FC. Studies of thermal injury II. Am J Pathol 1947; 23:695–720.

17. Jackson DM. The diagnosis of the depth of burning. Br J Surg 1953; 40(164):588–596.

18. Zawacki BE. Reversal of capillary stasis and prevention of necrosis in burns. Ann Surg 1974; 180(1):98–102.

19. Rico RM, Ripamonti R, Burns AL, et al. The effect of sepsis on wound healing. J Surg Res 2002; 102(2):193–197.

20. Knabl JS, Bauer W, Andel H, et al. Progression of burn wound depth by systemical application of a vasoconstrictor: an experimental study with a new rabbit model. Burns 1999; 25(8):715–721.

21. Winter GD. Formation of the scab and the rate of epithelization of superficial wounds in the skin of the young domestic pig. Nature 1962; 193:293–294.

22. Hinman CD, Maibach H. Effect of air exposure and occlusion on experimental human skin wounds. Nature 1963; 200:377–378.

23. Palmieri TL, Greenhalgh DG. Topical treatment of pediatric patients with burns: a practical guide. Am J Clin Dermatol 2002; 3(8):529–534.

24. Davies JW. Prompt cooling of burned areas: a review of benefits and the effector mechanisms. Burns Incl Therm Inj 1982; 9(1):1–6.

25. Boykin JV Jr, Eriksson E, Sholley MM, et al. Cold-water treatment of scald injury and inhibition of histamine-mediated burn edema. J Surg Res 1981; 31(2):111–123.

26. Demling RH, Mazess RB, Wolberg W. The effect of immediate and delayed cold immersion on burn edema formation and resorption. J Trauma 1979; 19(1):56–60.

27. King TC, Price PB. Surface cooling following extensive burns. JAMA 1963; 183:677–678.

28. Purdue GF, Layton TR, Copeland CE. Cold injury complicating burn therapy. J Trauma 1985; 25(2):167–168.

29. Sawada Y, Urushidate S, Yotsuyanagi T, et al. Is prolonged and excessive cooling of a scalded wound effective? Burns 1997; 23(1):55–58.

30. Practice guidelines for burn care. Outpatient management of burn patients. J Burn Care Rehabil (Suppl) 2001; 10s–13s.

31. Parsons RJ, Aldrich EM, Lehman RP. Studies on burns: effect of heparin and gravity on tissue loss from third degree burns. Surg Gyn Obstet 1950; 90:722.

32. Aldrich E. The effect of heparin on the circulating blood plasma and proteins in experimental burns. Surgery 1949; 25:686.

33. Aldrich E. Studies in burns II: observations on a vasoconstrictor substance in lymph from a burned area. Surgery 1944; 15:908–912.

34. Robson MC, Kucan JO, Paik KI, et al. Prevention of dermal ischemia after thermal injury. Arch Surg 1978; 113(5):621–625.

35. Robson MC, Del Beccaro EJ, Heggers JP. The effect of prostaglandins on the dermal microcirculation after burning, and the inhibition of the effect by specific pharmacological agents. Plast Reconstr Surg 1979; 63(6):781–787.

36. Robson MC, DelBeccaro EJ, Heggers JP, et al. Increasing dermal perfusion after burning by decreasing thromboxane production. J Trauma 1980; 20(9):722–725.

37. Ehrlich HP. Promotion of vascular patency in dermal burns with ibuprofen. Am J Med 1984; 77(1A):107–113.

38. Wang SL, Silberstein EB, Lukes S, et al. The effect of the thromboxane synthetase inhibitor Dazmegrel (UK-38,485) on wound healing, dermal ink perfusion and skin blood flow measurements in deep partial thickness burns. Burns Incl Therm Inj 1986; 12(5):312–317.

39. Brown GL, Nanney LB, Griffen J, et al. Enhancement of wound healing by topical treatment with epidermal growth factor. N Engl J Med 1989; 321(2):76–79.

40. Forage AV. The history of the classification of burns (diagnosis of depth). Br J Plast Surg 1963; 16:239–242.

41. Boykin JV, Eriksson E, Pittman RN. In vivo microcirculation of a scald burn and the progression of postburn dermal ischemia. Plast Reconstr Surg 1980; 66(2):191–198.

42. Nanney LB, Wenczak BA, Lynch JB. Progressive burn injury documented with vimentin immunostaining. J Burn Care Rehabil 1996; 17(3):191–198.

43. Riordan CL, McDonough M, Davidson JM, et al. Noncontact laser Doppler imaging in burn depth analysis of the extremities. J Burn Care Rehabil 2003; 24(4):177–186.

44. Hlava P, Moserova J, Konigova R. Validity of clinical assessment of the depth of a thermal injury. Acta Chir Plast 1983; 25(4):202–208.

45. Niazi ZB, Essex TJ, Papini R, et al. New laser Doppler scanner, a valuable adjunct in burn depth assessment. Burns 1993; 19(6):485–489.

46. Yeong EK, Mann R, Goldberg M, et al. Improved accuracy of burn wound assessment using laser Doppler. J Trauma 1996; 40(6):956–961; discussion 961–962.

47. Ho-Asjoe M, Chronnell CM, Frame JD, et al. Immunohistochemical analysis of burn depth. J Burn Care Rehabil 1999; 20(3):207–211.

48. Moserova J, Hlava P, Malinsky J. Scope for ultrasound diagnosis of the depth of thermal damage. Preliminary report. Acta Chir Plast 1982; 24(4):235–242.

49. Cantrell JH Jr. Can ultrasound assist an experienced surgeon in estimating burn depth? J Trauma 1984; 24(9 Suppl):S64–S70.

50. Kaufman T, Hurwitz DJ, Heggers JP. The india ink injection technique to assess the depth of experimental burn wounds. Burns Incl Therm Inj 1984; 10(6):405–408.

51. Heimbach DM, Afromowitz MA, Engrav LH, et al. Burn depth estimation – man or machine. J Trauma 1984; 24(5):373–378.

52. Koruda MJ, Zimbler A, Settle RG, et al. Assessing burn wound depth using in vitro nuclear magnetic resonance (NMR). J Surg Res 1986; 40(5):475–481.

53. Black KS, Hewitt CW, Miller DM, et al. Burn depth evaluation with fluorometry: is it really definitive? J Burn Care Rehabil 1986; 7(4):313–317.

54. Pape SA, Skouras CA, Byrne PO. An audit of the use of laser Doppler imaging (LDI) in the assessment of burns of intermediate depth. Burns 2001; 27(3):233–239.

55. Hackett ME. The use of thermography in the assessment of depth of burn and blood supply of flaps, with preliminary reports on its use in Dupuytren's contracture and treatment of varicose ulcers. Br J Plast Surg 1974; 27(4):311–317.

56. Jeng JC, Bridgeman A, Shivnan L, et al. Laser Doppler imaging determines need for excision and grafting in advance of clinical judgment: a prospective blinded trial. Burns 2003; 29(7):665–70.

57. Byrom RR, Word EL, Tewksbury CG, et al. Epidemiology of flame burn injuries. Burns Incl Therm Inj 1984; 11(1):1–10.

58. Ding YL, Pu SS, Pan ZL, et al. Extensive scalds following accidental immersion in hot water pools. Burns Incl Therm Inj 1987; 13(4):305–308.

59. Walker AR. Fatal tapwater scald burns in the USA, 1979–86. Burns 1990; 16(1):49–52.

60. Kumar P. Child abuse by thermal injury – a retrospective survey. Burns Incl Therm Inj 1984; 10(5):344–348.

61. Bird PE, Harrington DT, Barillo DJ, et al. Elder abuse: a call to action. J Burn Care Rehabil 1998; 19(6):522–527.

62. Klein MB, Gibran NS, Emerson D, et al. Patterns of grease burn injury: development of a classification system. Burns 2005; 31(6):765–767.

63. Murphy JT, Purdue GF, Hunt JL. Pediatric grease burn injury. Arch Surg 1995; 130(5):478–82.

64. Desai MH, Rutan RL, Herndon DN. Conservative treatment of scald burns is superior to early excision. J Burn Care Rehabil 1991; 12(5):482–484.

65. Gibran NS, Engrav LH, Heimbach DM, et al. Engine block burns: Dupuytren's fourth-, fifth- and sixth-degree burns. J Trauma 1994; 37(2):176–181.

66. Yanofsky NN, Morain WD. Upper extremity burns from woodstoves. Pediatrics 1984; 73(5):722–726.

67. Pensler JM, Steward R, Lewis SR, et al. Reconstruction of the burned palm: full-thickness versus split-thickness skin grafts – long-term follow-up. Plast Reconstr Surg 1988; 81(1):46–49.

68. Merrell SW, Saffle JR, Schnebly A, et al. Full-thickness skin grafting for contact burns of the palm in children. J Burn Care Rehabil 1986; 7(6):501–507.

69. Lewis PM, Ennis O, Kashif A, et al. Wet cement remains a poorly recognised cause of full-thickness skin burns. Injury 2004; 35(10):982–985.

70. Fisher AA. Cement burns resulting in necrotic ulcers due to kneeling on wet cement. Cutis 1979; 23(3):272–4, 370.

71. Early SH, Simpson RL. Caustic burns from contact with wet cement. JAMA 1985; 254(4):528–529.

72. Bertolini JC. Hydrofluoric acid: a review of toxicity. J Emerg Med 1992; 10(2):163–168.

73. Anderson WJ, Anderson JR. Hydrofluoric acid burns of the hand: mechanism of injury and treatment. J Hand Surg [Am] 1988; 13(1):52–57.

74. Mayer TG, Gross PL. Fatal systemic fluorosis due to hydrofluoric acid burns. Ann Emerg Med 1985; 14(2):149–153.

75. Bracken WM, Cuppage F, McLaury RL, et al. Comparative effectiveness of topical treatments for hydrofluoric acid burns. J Occup Med 1985; 27(10):733–739.

76. Chick LR, Borah G. Calcium carbonate gel therapy for hydrofluoric acid burns of the hand. Plast Reconstr Surg 1990; 86(5):935–940.

77. Siegel DC, Heard JM. Intra-arterial calcium infusion for hydrofluoric acid burns. Aviat Space Environ Med 1992; 63(3):206–211.

78. Vance MV, Curry SC, Kunkel DB, et al. Digital hydrofluoric acid burns: treatment with intraarterial calcium infusion. Ann Emerg Med 1986; 15(8):890–896.

79. Velvart J. Arterial perfusion for hydrofluoric acid burns. Hum Toxicol 1983; 2(2):233–238.

80. Pegg SP, Siu S, Gillett G. Intra-arterial infusions in the treatment of hydrofluoric acid burns. Burns Incl Therm Inj 1985; 11(6):440–443.

81. Rai J, Jeschke MG, Barrow RE, et al. Electrical injuries: a 30-year review. J Trauma 1999; 46(5):933–936.

82. Holt GR, Parel S, Richardson DS, et al. The prosthetic management of oral commissure burns. Laryngoscope 1982; 92(4):407–411.

83. al-Qattan MM, Gillett D, Thomson HG. Electrical burns to the oral commissure: does splinting obviate the need for commissuroplasty? Burns 1996; 22(7):555–556.

84. Orgel MG, Brown HC, Woolhouse FM. Electrical burns of the mouth in children; a method for assessing results. J Trauma 1975; 15(4):285–289.

85. Chilbert M, Maiman D, Sances A Jr, et al. Measure of tissue resistivity in experimental electrical burns. J Trauma 1985; 25(3):209–215.

86. Lee RC, Kolodney MS. Electrical injury mechanisms: dynamics of the thermal response. Plast Reconstr Surg 1987; 80(5):663–671.

87. Yang JY, Tsai YC, Noordhoff MS. Electrical burn with visceral injury. Burns Incl Therm Inj 1985; 11(3):207–212.

88. Branday JM, DuQuesnay DR, Yeesing MT, et al. Visceral complications of electrical burn injury. A report of two cases and review of the literature. West Indian Med J 1989; 38(2):110–113.

89. Honda T, Yamamoto Y, Mizuno M, et al. Successful treatment of a case of electrical burn with visceral injury and full-thickness loss of the abdominal wall. Burns 2000; 26(6):587–592.

90. Hunt J, Lewis S, Parkey R, Baxter C. The use of Technetium-99m stannous pyrophosphate scintigraphy to identify muscle damage in acute electric burns. J Trauma 1979; 19(6):409–413.

91. Mann R, Gibran N, Engrav L, Heimbach D. Is immediate decompression of high voltage electrical injuries to the upper extremity always necessary? J Trauma 1996; 40(4):584–587; discussion 587–589.

92. Yowler CJ, Mozingo DW, Ryan JB, et al. Factors contributing to delayed extremity amputation in burn patients. J Trauma 1998; 45(3):522–526.

93. Bartle EJ, Wang XW, Miller GJ. Early vascular grafting to prevent upper extremity necrosis after electrical burns: anastomotic false aneurysm, a severe complication. Burns Incl Therm Inj 1987; 13(4):313–317.

94. Wang XW, Bartle EJ, Roberts BB, et al. Free skin flap transfer in repairing deep electrical burns. J Burn Care Rehabil 1987; 8(2):111–114.

Chapter 11

Wound care

Palmer Q. Bessey

Chapter contents

Author's Note

I had the privilege to collaborate with Dr William W. Monafo of St. Louis on the first versions of this chapter, which were included in the first two editions of Total Burn Care. Dr Monafo was a leader in the field at the end of the 20th century. He contributed widely to the understanding and techniques of burn resuscitation and wound care. He was a founding member and the ninth president of the American Burn Association, and he led an exemplary clinical burn program for most of his career. It is to his memory and in gratitude for his support and friendship that I dedicate this version of the chapter.

> I dresst the wound . . . and God healed it.
> Ambroise Paré, 1510–1590

Introduction

The over-riding objective of acute burn care is closure of the burn wound with the patient's own epidermis. Sometimes that happens spontaneously, and sometimes it requires an operation to excise the burned tissue and ultimately cover the wound with an autologous skin graft, or autograft. When it becomes clinically apparent that the burn is a full-thickness injury or third-degree burn, common, current practice is to proceed with operation as expeditiously as possible. The subject of this chapter is the care of the burn wound in the interval between its occurrence and closure, either by spontaneous generation of new epidermis or by surgical excision.

Cutaneous wound healing

Skin biology

The skin is the largest organ of the body. It plays a major homeostatic role in maintaining body temperature and fluid balance and protecting the internal milieu from all variety of environmental dangers. It has a specialized epithelium, that is made up of epidermis, hair follicles, sebaceous glands, and sweat glands, as well as a stroma. To sustain its biologic function it constantly renews itself, and it it this renewal property that is exploited after a burn or other injury.

The outer mantle of the skin is a stratified squamous epithelium composed of keratinocytes which arise from a layer of basal cells. Cells in the basal layer of the epidermis give rise to transit amplifying cells, which function as progenitor cells for keratinocytes. They proliferate and become increasingly differentiated as they migrate outward to the skin surface elaborating proteins and lipids.[1,2] As they approach the surface, they undergo a programmed cell death,[3] and the flattened, enucleated cell skeletons (squames or corneocytes) become encased in a lipid and protein mortar to form the outer, cornified veneer. The entire process is relatively rapid. It is estimated that human epidermis — as much as $1^1/_2$–$2\,m^2$ or more of it in adults — turns over every 2 weeks.

Hair follicles are distributed throughout the epidermis and the upper or outer portions of the follicles are also covered with epidermis. The sebaceous glands are located deep to the epidermis and empty into the upper follicle and thence out onto the epidermis (Figure 11.1). Sebocytes arise from a basaloid layer of cells which are continuous with the follicular epithelium. As they differentiate and move outward they accumulate lipid and ultimately slough and are extruded onto the epidermis as sebum (holocrine secretion).[4,5] The lower portion of the hair follicle consists of an outer root sheath, an inner root sheath, and the hair shaft. The lower hair follicle has cycles of growth and quiescence. The cells in the outer root sheath are continuous with the epidermal basal cell layer. Thus, the cells in the basal layer of each or the epithelial compartments serve as lineage-restricted stem cells that give rise to other cells which then proliferate and undergo terminal differentiation resulting in epidermis, sebum, or hair.

A region of the hair follicle just below the sebaceous gland is known as the bulge (Figure 11.1). It appears to be a protected niche,[6] and the cells in it are multipotent stem cells that can give rise to the precursor cells of the epidermis, sebaceous gland, or outer root sheath.[6–11] It is currently thought that the stem cells in the bulge play little role in maintenance of the skin but serve to repopulate the various epithelial precursor cell populations following injury.[12–14]

Superficial or partial-thickness burns

The cells in the basal layer of the epidermis that give rise to the transit amplifying cells, that then proliferate and differentiate terminally into keratinocytes, qualify as epidermal

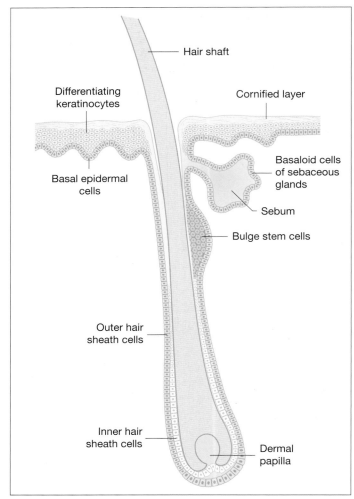

Fig. 11.1 A schematic diagram of a hair follicle. The basal cell layer of the epidermis, the basaloid cells of the sebaceous gland, and the cells of the outer hair sheath are all continuous. The cells in each compartment serve as stem cells and give rise to other cells that undergo terminal differentiation to form the cornified layer of the epidermis and sebum and also interact with the dermal papilla to form the hair shaft. Cells in the bulge region are multi-potent stem cells that can repopulate the basal cells in all compartments after injury.

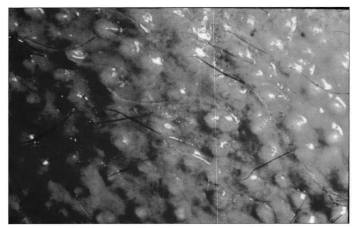

Fig. 11.2 This shows epidermal budding in a relatively deep second degree burn. Each bud of epidermis is arising from a single hair follicle. The source of the new keratinocytes is thought to be a collection of stem cells, known as 'the bulge'.

stem cells. Burns involving only the epidermis, first-degree burns, thus heal readily with the rapid emergence of new keratinocytes.

Second-degree or partial-thickness burns destroy all of the epidermis as well as a portion of the dermis and the skin appendages. If the follicular bulge region is uninjured, its cells can repopulate the epidermal basal cell layer and also give rise to new sebaceous glands and hair follicles within the new epidermis (Figure 11.2). As burn depth extends into the deeper dermis, however, the remnants of hair follicles are sparser. Deep dermal burns heal slowly, if at all, and depend to a large degree on the migration of keratinocytes from surrounding uninjured skin. This is also the mechanism whereby the interstices of meshed split-thickness skin grafts are filled in by keratinocytes that migrate from the skin bridges.

The biology of epidermal renewal is currently an area of intense research. Understanding of the basic mechanisms involved is expanding rapidly. Translation into a useful technology that will improve clinical burn care and outcomes may soon be a reality.[8,15]

Deep or full-thickness burns

Full-thickness burns involve the entire thickness of the dermis and extend into the subcutaneous fat. These do not heal spontaneously, unless they are of limited area and can reasonably be allowed to close by a combination of wound contraction and re-epithelialization by the surrounding intact epidermis. The layer of coagulated and necrotic soft tissue, eschar, varies in thickness depending on the duration and intensity of the heat exposure. Wound closure cannot occur while eschar remains *in situ*. Spontaneous eschar separation is due primarily to the action of proteases released by bacteria that proliferate beneath the eschar and do not occur in sterile full-thickness burns. For example, full-thickness burn eschar in gnotobiotic rodents may remain in place for 8 months or more.[16] Separation of eschar may be delayed by ineffective wound cleansing measures.[17,18] The thin layer of congealed necrotic debris and wound exudate that forms over deep dermal burns — referred to as a 'pseudo-eschar' — often separates spontaneously even in the absence of microorganisms as re-epithelialization proceeds beneath it.

The presence of necrotic tissue and debris and bacteria are all potent inflammatory stimuli. The burn wound soon becomes an inflammatory tissue mass containing a variety of cell types including at various times platelets, neutrophils, lymphocytes, macrophages, and fibroblasts, whose activity is regulated by a complex interplay of multiple cytokines as well as host neuro-endocrine mechanisms. The principal molecular regulators controlling the evolution of the burn wound include vascular endothelial growth factor (VEGF), platelet-derived growth factor (PDGF), and transforming growth factor-β (TGF-β). Wound cellular activities include cell recruitment and proliferation, proteolysis, bacterial killing, angiogenesis, and collagen synthesis, all of which exact a substantial metabolic price from the patient. Oxygen, energy substrate, and amino acids must be supplied to the wound to support its metabolic needs.[19]

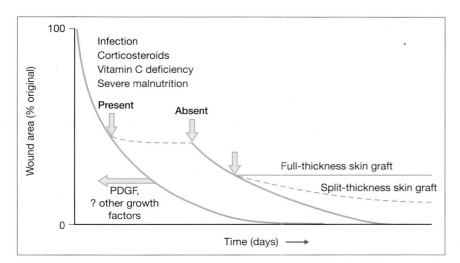

Fig. 11.3 The influence of several factors on the rate of wound contraction. Infection, severe malnutrition, and other factors impede spontaneous decrease in wound surface area. Split-thickness grafts also impede but do not prevent subsequent wound contraction. Full-thickness grafts almost abolish it.

The magnitude of these requirements is proportional to the mass of inflammatory tissue, i.e. the extent or size of the wound. The presence of a wound is a constant drain on the patient's reserves. Only with closure of the wound will these processes abate.

Deep wounds that remain open for several weeks may progressively decrease in surface area. The primary mechanism is contraction of the wound as a result of forces generated in the wound bed by differentiated fibroblasts containing contractile protein, myofibroblasts. These develop in part due to transforming growth factor-β_1 and other inflammatory mediators.[20] Another mechanism for reduction in wound surface area is ingrowth of epidermis from the wound perimeter, but this accounts for only a small portion of shrinkage of the wound, perhaps 10% or less.

Contraction may be desirable in that it reduces both the risk of infection and the metabolic drain which results from the loss of water vapor and body fluids as well as from the inflammatory processes in an open, granulating wound.[21] Wound contraction near joints, the eyelids, or the mouth is highly undesirable both functionally and cosmetically. Some factors that can alter the rate of wound contraction are schematically depicted in Figure 11.2. Successful split-thickness skin grafts slow contraction, while full-thickness ones often appear to abolish it. Split-thickness grafts have the advantage of resulting in a donor site that is akin to a superficial burn. It can heal readily by re-epithelialization in 10–14 days and does not require any surgical closure. Thick split-thickness grafts or full-thickness grafts leave deeper donor sites that do not heal readily without an additional surgical procedure. In extensive burns, it is advantageous to use thin split-thickness grafts so that the donor sites can be used for additional grafts after the initial wounds re-epithelialize in 10–14 days, Small full-thickness grafts are commonly used on the eyelids to reduce or correct severe ectropion and also for deep palmar burns in infants.[22]

Full-thickness burns are the prototypical cause of hypertrophic scar.[23] Although other mammals also heal wounds by making scar, hypertrophic scars and keloids seem to be unique to humans. Lack of a simple animal experimental model slowed progress in the understanding of the biological mecha-

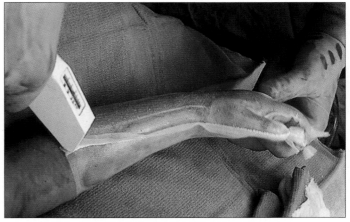

Fig. 11.4 Biobrane. The use of Biobrane has revolutionized care for second degree burns. Advantages of Biobrane include decreased pain and elimination of dressing changes.

nisms involved in the formation of hypertrophic scar, but recent studies of wound healing in fetuses have rekindled hope that it may soon be possible to control this tendency. Surgical incisions in fetuses (e.g. for prenatal correction of congenital defects) do not result in scar,[24] and that phenomenon is associated with differences in the amounts and timing of PDGF and various members of the TGF-β family.[25] In the fetal wound TGF-β_3 is elaborated in abundance, whereas TGF-β_1 is the predominant isoform in adults.

There is a tendency toward hypertrophic scar formation after any injury to the reticular dermis, but its severity is highly variable and unpredictable. Scar hypertrophy is common in deep dermal burns that are allowed to close spontaneously, at the perimeter of skin grafts, and in the interstices of meshed grafts. Unmeshed split-thickness skin grafts (sheet grafts) retard this process to some degree. Early closure of deep burns also seems to result in less hypertrophic scar than does delayed closure.

The surgical management of full-thickness wounds, the prevention and treatment of hypertrophic scar, and the physiologic support of the patient are all fully covered in other chapters in this book. The wound is central to the total care of the burn patient, and its care prior to spontaneous healing or surgical closure has at least the potential to influence other aspects of the patient's care and the later, long-term outcome of the injury.

Wound care

Burns that obviously involve the full thickness of the skin are best treated with excision and grafting as soon as feasible.[26] Most burns, however, go on to heal spontaneously and do not require operation.[27] Some are obviously superficial on presentation and re-epithelialize quickly, and others are indeterminate or of mixed depth. Some of these may ultimately require skin grafting of a portion of the wound, but that is not obvious on presentation. In that context then, the goals of burn wound care are to assure an optimal environment for epidermal renewal, if it can occur; to avoid any further injury to the skin or deeper tissues; and to avoid secondary complications, such as infection. To achieve these goals, a two-pronged approach is needed, involving both care of the wound itself and care of the patient with a wound.

Care of the patient with a wound

The wound's need for oxygen, amino acids, and energy substrate requires effective perfusion of the wound. The environment of a wound is relatively hypoxic and that serves as an early inflammatory stimulus. The cellular activity that develops in the wound, however, requires increased consumption of oxygen and nutrients. Delivery of these substances to the site of repair requires both perfusion of the wound and surrounding tissues and also diffusion from the serum through the interstitial fluid to the wound. The driving force for diffusion is determined by the gradient between the concentration of a substance in the serum and that in the wound. If the gradient is not sufficiently great, it can limit the utilization of a given substance by the cells of the wound, even if perfusion is good. This is especially important for oxygen, which is poorly soluble in aqueous solution, so that a small gradient between the pO_2 in the serum and the pO_2 in the interstitial fluid may be rate limiting. In patients with elective surgical wounds, the level of interstitial pO_2 correlated with the risk of infection and delayed wound healing,[28] and in another series, supplemental perioperative oxygen increased the interstitial pO_2, which reduced the incidence of wound infection by half.[29] Thus, a normal or somewhat elevated arterial pO_2 appears to be beneficial for wound healing.

Effective resuscitation and appropriate fluid management and measures to avoid vasoconstriction, such as maintaining a warm environment, controlling pain and anxiety, and avoidance of pressors, will help maintain perfusion. Maintenance of an arterial pO_2 near normal or slightly elevated should result in an oxygen gradient sufficient to meet the oxygen needs of the wound. In addition, provision of sufficient nutrients to meet the increased energy and protein needs of the patient and his or her wound will support wound repair and reduce the draft on the patient's metabolic reserves.

Assessing the wound

Some burns can be classified as partial- or full-thickness injuries with certainty on initial evaluation based on their appearance and on the mechanism of injury, taking into account the source of the heat and the duration of skin exposure. There are many burns, however, about which there is less certainty at the outset. These will change in appearance over the first week, so that the initial clinical assessment may be inaccurate as much as 30% of the time. Some wounds may come to seem much deeper than they did originally. The initial heat exposure coagulates a portion of the thickness of the skin and may also result in an endothelial injury of the small vessels in the tissue immediately adjacent to this.[30] The apparent increase in the burn depth may be due to an inevitable, progressive occlusion of the circulation in this 'zone of stasis' at the wound periphery where endothelial injury has occurred, to potentially preventable inadequate resuscitation and perfusion, or to compression of the dermal vessels by the edema attending injury and/or resuscitation. This highlights the importance of adequate but not excessive resuscitation. The use of subatmospheric pressure may be helpful in this regard by reducing edema and promoting perfusion.[31] Conversely, some dermal burns may appear to be quite deep early after burn and then go on to re-epithelialize well. This is often the case in burns on the palms of the hands and soles of the feet.

Clinical observation of the burn wound and its evolution remains the primary basis of wound depth assessment. Although the use of the laser Doppler may give a reasonably accurate measurement of burn depth, methodologic problems and details of standardization still need to be worked out before the potential benefits of this technique can be accurately assessed.[32]

Once a burn has been determined to be a third-degree or full-thickness injury, excision of the burn and grafting are usually carried out as soon as the patient is clinically stable. Wound care for a full-thickness wound then consists of prevention of further tissue loss or invasive infection prior to excision. All other burns as well as donor sites and wounds with fresh split-thickness grafts must in addition be maintained in such a way as to facilitate or at least not impede re-epithelialization. This includes a warm and moist environment, removal of exudate and potentially contaminated or necrotic material, and control of bacterial proliferation.

The dressing

A burn dressing has three principal functions:
- *Comfort.* Superficial burns are initially extraordinarily sensitive to air currents; and deeper burns become progressively more tender with time. Open wounds also produce a substantial amount of drainage. The dressing shields the wound surface from air currents in the environment, absorbs and contains wound secretions, and if properly constructed may also provide splinting action to maintain a desirable position of function and limit movement.
- *Metabolic.* An occlusive dressing reduces evaporative heat loss and minimizes cold stress and shivering. Because the principal cutaneous water vapor barrier resides in the epidermis, even superficial burns result in substantial water vapor loss. Intact eschar provides only a partial impediment, while excised or granulating wounds lose water vapor maximally.[11] Evaporative loss from exposed burns may be much greater than the

'normal' 150 mL/24 hours, especially if air-fluidized beds are used. This loss of water from the wound also contributes to the loss of heat by 0.58 kcal/kg water lost.[8] An occlusive dressing of reasonable thickness will impede water vapor loss appreciably, particularly if it is in turn kept covered with a dry blanket. Biological dressings such as cadaver allograft and an ever-increasing number of commercially available synthetic dressings and bioengineered materials may also minimize the water loss, but their efficacy and cost-effectiveness are controversial, especially in major burns.

- *Protective.* When skin is thermally injured the physical barrier of the epidermis to microorganisms is lost, as well as its mild antiseptic property. The result is that the environmental flora proliferate readily on the wound surface. In small burns, an effective dressing can isolate the wound so that few if any organisms are ever recoverable. As the wound area increases, however, the efficacy of a dressing's barrier function decreases.

Wound hygiene

The French word débridement ('unbridle', i.e. as in escharotomy or fasciotomy) has, in North America at least, come to signify both the formal surgical excision of devitalized tissue (including, but not limited to burns) as well as the simple piecemeal removal of bits and fragments of separating eschar, ruptured bleb fragments, foreign material, and other debris during the routine dressing change. On initial evaluation, most burn wounds will be cleansed and debrided and a dressing will be applied. After that, there are a variety of ways to manage the wounds. The method that is selected will depend in part on the type and size of the burn, but equally or more important is local experience and other factors. The field does continue to progress, but differences between techniques of wound care are usually not so marked as to counter professional opinion. Thus, the management of acute burn wounds still relies to a large degree on uncontrolled clinical observations and anecdotal personal experience.

A common approach to burn wound care consists of wound cleansing and debridement daily or twice daily and reapplication of the dressing. Additional fragments of blebs or desquamated epidermis can then be removed. The thin pseudo-eschar that forms over deep dermal burns tends to separate piecemeal as re-epithelialization occurs beneath it. Although systematic, gentle wound cleansing with removals of bits of slough, exudate, and debris would seem eminently reasonable, evidence of benefit does not exist to our knowledge. It is, however, associated with not inconsiderable pain, apprehension, and expense.

Dressing materials

The typical burn wound dressing for wounds that are cleaned and debrided frequently consists of a relatively fine mesh material that contains or is placed over an antimicrobial cream or liquid and applied directly to the wound surface. This is then wrapped in several layers of gauze in pads or rolls. Use of non-adherent materials, such as Telfa®, Exu-Dry®, Xeroform®, or Adaptic®, directly on the wound may reduce both the pain associated with removal of the dressing and the risk of pulling off migrating epidermal cells from the wound surface. The non-adherent sheet and the topical antimicrobial material together will serve as at least a partial barrier to the loss of water vapor from the wound and help provide a warm, moist environment for re-epithelialization. The dressings, however, become soaked with drainage from the wound and must be changed frequently.

Topical antimicrobial agents

General background

Burn injury not only damages the normal skin barrier but also impairs host immunological defenses. Because the eschar may be several centimeters or more distant from patent microvasculature, systemically administered antimicrobial agents may not achieve therapeutic levels by diffusion to the wound surface, where microbial numbers are usually greatest. Topically applied antimicrobials provide high concentrations of drug at the wound surface; they penetrate eschar variably, a property that should be considered in their selection. Normal skin harbors a sparse bacterial flora, consisting mainly of diphtheroids and *Staphylococcus epidermidis* and, occasionally, *S. aureus*.

Gram-negative bacteria are not usually present in normal skin. The burn wound flora changes in the post-injury interval, depending in part on the topical and/or systemic antimicrobial therapy being used and on the efficacy with which cross-contamination is prevented. After a variable initial period (days) when the wound is apparently sterile or contains only normal flora, Gram-positive organisms, mainly *S. aureus*, typically predominate. Subsequently, Gram-negative species appear. In the past, isolates of *Proteus*, *Klebsiella*, *Escherichia coli* and other enteric flora predominated, but *Pseudomonas*, *Enterobacter*, *Serratia*, and *Acinetobacter* are increasingly frequent today.[33-35] Anaerobes are infrequent, but can be encountered when large volumes of necrotic muscle are present, as in high-voltage electrical injury.

The goal of prophylactic topical therapy is initially to delay and later to minimize wound colonization.[33] With effective topical agents and the prompt excision of full-thickness eschar, the incidence of invasive burn wound infections is low. Prophylactic agents do not need to penetrate the eschar deeply, as environmental fallout is the source of contamination. They should have activity against common wound pathogens as listed above, should not retard wound healing (although some of them do so, to some extent),[36] and they should have low toxicity, which implies that systemic absorption is low. None of the topical antimicrobials, either alone or in combination, will eliminate colonization of major burn wounds. Frequent clinical observation is necessary in order to ensure that basic wound hygienic measures are being satisfactorily carried out, that the frequency of dressing changes is appropriate, and that the clinical appearance of the wounds is satisfactory.

When an established burn wound infection is present, the spectrum of activity of a proposed agent must include the organisms responsible. Concerns about toxicity, patient comfort, cost, and other factors require careful assessment. In most instances, eradication of an invasive infection will require the use of one or more topical agents, which penetrate eschar readily, as by definition microbial invasion of previously normal, unburned tissue exists. Systemic antibiotics of appropriate spectrum are also necessary; in relatively localized infections, sub-eschar antibiotic infusions are sometimes efficacious in reducing systemic septic toxicity, but excision of the eschar and infected eschar are required for cure. Invasive burn wound infections with *Staphylococcus* or *Pseudomonas* species have been frequently treated with topical mafenide acetate, which penetrates eschar readily.[34]

Specific agents

As already noted, topical therapy in most instances is prophylactic. Frequent clinical inspection is the best method of noting the clinical response. Wound surveillance bacterial culture results require clinical correlation because the distinction between colonization, which is frequent, and invasive infection, which is now uncommon, is partly a clinical one. In general, quantitative wound biopsy cultures, which exceed 100 000 organisms per gram, are consistent with, although not diagnostic of, invasive infection. The microscopic visualization of organisms invading normal tissue in a wound biopsy specimen is diagnostic, but gives no information as to the extent of the infection.[34]

0.5% Silver nitrate solution

One-half percent silver nitrate solution was introduced as an effective topical agent in the mid-1960s.[37] Together with the near-simultaneous introduction of topical mafenide, the modern era of topical burn wound therapy had begun. Shortly thereafter, silver sulfadiazine was synthesized and would become available. More recently, silver foil or mesh dressings (Acticoat® and Silverlon®) have been introduced. Silver nitrate is effective against most strains of *Staphylococcus* and *Pseudomonas*, and also has activity against many of the Gram-negative aerobes that commonly colonize burn wounds. Concentrations much above 5% are histotoxic. Most biologically important silver salts, especially the chloride and proteinate, are highly insoluble. The agent, or at least the silver moiety, does not therefore penetrate eschar significantly and silver absorption is minimal; although trace amounts have been detected in blood and tissue following protracted application, there is no significant direct toxicity.

The hypotonic solution (29.4 mmol Ag/L) leaches electrolyte, especially sodium from the wound surface. As much as 350 mmol of sodium/day/m² of body surface area treated may be lost. Continuous oral and/or intravenous (IV) electrolyte supplementation is therefore essential. Hyponatremia or hypokalemia may occur rapidly, especially in infants or children with large burns.

Another important but fortunately infrequent complication of this agent is methemoglobinemia, which occurs as a result of nitrate reduction by wound bacteria (usually Gram-negative species) with subsequent systemic absorption of the toxic nitrite. The diagnosis should be suspected if the skin or blood appears cyanotic or 'gray' but the arterial oxygen content is normal. Confirmation of the diagnosis by blood methemoglobin measurement should lead to prompt withdrawal of the agent. Additional specific treatment with reducing agents may also be required.

Silver nitrate is relatively painless on application. It is typically used to saturate gauze dressings similar to those described above. The dressings should be moistened with the silver nitrate at 2-hourly intervals to prevent silver concentrations reaching histotoxic levels. The agent stains everything it touches brown or black, including bed linens, floors, etc. Although silver nitrate is an effective prophylactic agent, it is presently not widely used routinely, principally because of its staining property. Its therapeutic effect is approximated by silver sulfadiazine, which is easier to use.

Silver sulfadiazine

Silver sulfadiazine is easily the most frequently used prophylactic agent in burn patients. It is a white, highly insoluble compound that is synthesized from silver nitrate and sodium sulfadiazine.[33,38] It is available in 1% concentration in a water-soluble cream base. The cream is relatively painless to apply and does not stain bed linens or other objects, which it contacts. Silver sulfadiazine has *in vitro* activity against a wide range of organisms including *S. aureus*, *E. coli*, *Klebsiella* species, *Pseudomonas aeruginosa*, *Proteus* species and *Candida albicans*. The drug penetrates eschar poorly. Its precise mechanism of action is unclear.

The toxicity commonly associated with sulfonamides, such as crystalluria and methemoglobinemia, is rare after silver sulfadiazine treatment. Cutaneous sensitivity reactions, typically in the form of a maculopapular rash, occur in less than 5% of patients and rarely require discontinuing the drug. Acute hemolytic anemia has been reported in a burn patient treated with silver sulfadiazine who lacked the enzyme glucose-6 phosphatase.[39]

The most frequently associated clinical finding is a transient leukopenia which occurs within several days of the initiation of therapy. This is associated with a disproportionate decrease in circulating neutrophils. The incidence is from 5 to 15% of patients treated,[40] and it has been proposed that there is a direct toxic effect of silver sulfadizine on bone marrow.[41] The leukopenia can reach alarmingly low levels — less than 1000 mm² — and because of these observations, neutropenia is listed as a toxic effect of the agent.

Despite these observations, however, no increase in the incidence of infectious complications has been identified, and the leukopenia recovers spontaneously, whether or not the agent has been discontinued.[42] An alternative hypothesis is that marked leukocyte margination in the wound occurs early after burn independent of any drug effect. Both leukocyte and platelet counts fall over the first 2–3 days following major burn and begin to recover by post-burn day 4. A recent prospective comparison between one burn center that used topical silver nitrate exclusively and another that used silver sulfadiazine invariably demonstrated equal proportions of patients with leukopenia and that in both cases the leukopenia improved spontaneously without change of topical agent.[43]

Clinical trials have suggested that silver sulfadiazine reduces wound bacterial density and delays colonization with Gram-negative bacteria, but treatment failures occur with some frequency in large burns (>40–50% body surface area). The agent is usually applied on a daily or twice-daily basis. When it is used on superficial dermal burns, a yellow-gray pseudo-eschar typically forms after several days, which can be confusing to inexperienced personnel. This film, several millimeters thick, results from interaction between the cream and the wound exudate and is harmless; it is easily lifted away, revealing a healthy, superficial wound bed beneath it.

Mafenide acetate

Mafenide was introduced as a topical burn treatment in the mid 1960s. It is available in a water-soluble cream base at 11.1% concentration, and also, more recently, as a 5% solution. It has excellent antibacterial activity against most Gram-positive species, including *Clostridium*, but limited activity against some staphylococci, particularly methicillin-resistant strains. It has a broad activity against most Gram-negative pathogens commonly isolated from burn wounds, but, importantly, has minimal antifungal activity.[44] Early enthusiasm for its prophylactic use was soon tempered because of its systemic toxicity and by the considerable pain that occurs on application. The drug is so rapidly absorbed through open wounds that local concentrations are sharply reduced, requiring usually twice-daily applications.

Mafenide is a potent carbonic anhydrase inhibitor. Thus, hyperchloremic metabolic acidosis is frequent when it is used continuously on extensive burns.[45] Moderate to severe hyperventilation as respiratory compensation for the acidosis is characteristic and the $PaCO_2$ is persistently subnormal. Minute ventilation may approach or exceed 50 L/min. Pulmonary complications are a hazard with its continuous use and toxicity increases in frequency to the wound area and treatment duration. A maculopapular rash occurs in about 5% of patients but can usually be controlled with antihistamines and may not require discontinuing the drug. Although the use of mafenide as a prophylactic agent has decreased for the reasons cited, its excellent eschar penetration makes it useful for the short-term control of invasive burn wound infections. In some centers, the drug is still used prophylactically but toxicity is minimized or avoided by alternating it with silver sulfadiazine, usually at 12-hour intervals.

Cerium nitrate–silver sulfadiazine

This agent was introduced by Fox and Monafo in the mid 1970s.[46] It is not now commercially available in the US, but a commercial preparation is available in several western European and South American countries.[47–49] It can be easily prepared by combining commercially available silver sulfadiazine with a solution of cerium nitrate. Cerium, one of the lanthanide 'rare earth' series of elements, has antimicrobial activity *in vitro* and is relatively non-toxic. Wound bacteriostasis may be more efficient with its use in major burns compared to silver sulfadiazine alone.[48] The *in vitro* antimicrobial spectrum of this agent is qualitatively similar to that of silver nitrate or silver sulfadiazine. A highly favorable effect on mortality has been reported for burn patients who have been briefly immersed in a bath of cerium nitrate shortly after admittance to the hospital.[50] Methemoglobinemia due to nitrate reduction and absorption, as with silver nitrate, is rarely observed. The cerium moiety is absorbed to a limited extent. Electrolyte disturbances are not associated with the use of cerium nitrate–silver sulfadiazine.

Wassermann et al. reported excellent results in patients with massive burns treated with cerium nitrate–silver sulfadiazine

cream.[51] That report parallels our own early experience using the cream in patients with very large, ostensible 'lethal' injuries.[52] In the era of prompt burn excision, the addition cerium to silver sulfadiazine may be helpful for patients who are clinically unstable and not candidates for prompt excision.[53,54] The cerium mixture appears to be beneficial because of its effect on eschar not because of an effect on wound infection.[55] The eschar that forms is harder and perhaps seals the wound more effectively than the eschar that forms with silver sulfadiazine alone. A randomized, prospective clinical trial in high-risk burn patients comparing the cerium nitrate–silver sulfadiazine combination to silver sulfadiazine alone is ongoing in the US.

Silver sheets/mesh

One product (Acticoat®) consists of a sheet of thin, flexible rayon/polyester to which is bonded polyethylene mesh that has been coated with a nanocrystalline film of pure silver.[56–59] When exposed to body fluids or wound exudate, silver ions are released in an even, sustained manner over at least 24 hours and possibly 48 hours. Another product (Silverlon®) utilizes silver-coated gauze mesh. The antimicrobial spectrum of these products is broad, similar to that of silver nitrate. The silver that ionizes may have an atomic structure that differs from conventional silver ions as the result of the 'sputtering' process used and may be more bactericidal as a result. Several favorable clinical trials have been conducted.[60–62] The material is relatively painless to apply and can be left in place for 48 hours, or possibly longer. To date there has been no significant toxicity or bacterial resistance reported.[63]

Other agents

Since silver sulfadiazine may retard epithelialization,[64] other agents may be preferred on wounds that seem superficial or when initially indeterminate depth wounds begin to epithelialize. Such agents include the topical antibiotic ointments of bacitracin or polymyxin B. If methicillin-resistant staphylococci are suspected, the topical antibiotic mupirocin (Bactroban®) may be useful.[65]

Enzymatic debridement

A variety of proteolytic enzymatic agents have been utilized to debride wounds, including proteases (sutilains) elaborated by *Bacillus subtilis*, collagenase, and papain-urea.[66] This approach has not gained wide acceptance in the treatment of extensive burns, because bacteremia may occur with its use in the presence of wound colonization. There is also the hypothetical disadvantage that proteolysis occurring in marginally viable tissue could increase burn depth unnecessarily. In partial-thickness burns, however, collagenase ointment mixed with polymyxin B/bacitracin powder was associated with a slight acceleration of the time to closure compared with silver sulfadiazine.[67]

Occlusive dressings

Many fresh superficial wounds such as abrasions commonly form a protective scab which separates spontaneously as the wound epithelializes. Superficial burns and donor sites can also be dressed and allowed to form a scab after initial cleansing. Fine mesh gauze or petrolatum gauze (Xeroform®) can be applied as a scaffold. Once the scab is formed, the wound is relatively impermeable and painless, but until then the pain is intense.

A number of synthetic silicone mesh products designed to adhere to the wound until re-epithelialization is complete have been developed. These are associated with much less pain than fine mesh gauze and include Biobrane®, Aquacel Ag®, and Transcyte®. These are most effective on superficial partial-thickness wounds (Figure 11.4). If the wound is deep, however, the material will not adhere and often needs to be removed at least in part to allow for effective drainage of wound exudate. Biobrane® has no inherent antimicrobial activity, but Aqaucel Ag® contains silver.[68,69] Transcyte® consists of a layer of neo-natal fibroblasts incorporated onto Biobrane®. Several centers reported quite favorable experience with it in terms of short-ened time to wound closure and apparent improvement in the quality of the resulting scar.[70] It has been recently withdrawn from the market, however, for economic reasons. It is men-tioned here, because it was used fairly widely in burn centers and might be reintroduced.

Another type of occlusive dressings includes those that adhere to uninjured skin but not to the wound. These include DuoDerm®, OpSite®, and Tegederm®. These essentially form a 'blister' in that the wound transudate collects under the mate-rial and bathes the wound. They often leak and may need to be replaced as the fluid extravasation subsides. They also must be removed if the fluid becomes colonized and purulent. They have also been associated with more rapid healing and less pain.[71]

Envoi

After a burne the scarre which remaineth is uncom-monly rough, unequal and ill-favored.
Ambroise Paré, 1510–1590

Notwithstanding the numerous advances in supportive care that have made reasonably prompt surgical burn wound closure at a time of election a realistic option, the 'rough, unequal and ill-favored' scars that Paré lamented centuries ago unfortunately still occur and remain largely as unsightly as they were then. Although prompt excision and meticulous wound care may reduce its likelihood, hypertrophic scar remains the most important unresolved problem in burn care today.

References

1. Alonso L, Fuchs E. Stem cells in the skin: waste not, want not. Genes Dev 2003; 17(10):1189–1200.
2. Fuchs E. Epidermal differentiation: the bare essentials. J Cell Biol 1990; 111(6 Pt 2):2807–2814.
3. Lippens S, Denecker G, Ovaere P, et al. Death penalty for kerati-nocytes: apoptosis versus cornification. Cell Death Differ 2005; 12 (Suppl 2):1497–1508.
4. Thody AJ, Shuster S. Control and function of sebaceous glands. Physiol Rev 1989; 69(2):383–416.
5. Zouboulis CC. Acne and sebaceous gland function. Clin Dermatol 2004; 22(5):360–366.
6. Moore KA, Lemischka IR. Stem cells and their niches. Science 2006; 311(5769):1880–1885.
7. Claudinot S, Nicolas M, Oshima H, et al. Long-term renewal of hair follicles from clonogenic multipotent stem cells. Proc Natl Acad Sci USA 2005; 102(41):14677–14682.
8. Kaur P. Interfollicular epidermal stem cells: identification, chal-lenges, potential. J Invest Dermatol 2006; 126(7):1450–1458.
9. Legue E, Nicolas JF. Hair follicle renewal: organization of stem cells in the matrix and the role of stereotyped lineages and behav-iors. Development 2005; 132(18):4143–4154.
10. Levy V, Lindon C, Harfe BD, et al. Distinct stem cell populations regenerate the follicle and interfollicular epidermis. Dev Cell 2005; 9(6):855–861.
11. Taylor G, Lehrer MS, Jensen PJ, et al. Involvement of follicular stem cells in forming not only the follicle but also the epidermis. Cell 2000; 102(4):451–461.
12. Ito M, Liu Y, Yang Z, et al. Stem cells in the hair follicle bulge contribute to wound repair but not to homeostasis of the epidermis. Nat Med 2005; 11(12):1351–1354.
13. Morasso MI, Tomic-Canic M. Epidermal stem cells: the cradle of epidermal determination, differentiation and wound healing. Biol Cell 2005; 97(3):173–183.
14. Roh C, Lyle S. Cutaneous stem cells and wound healing. Pediatr Res 2006; 59(4 Pt 2):100R–103R.
15. Barthel R, Aberdam D. Epidermal stem cells. J Eur Acad Dermatol Venereol 2005; 19(4):405–413.
16. Dugan RC, Nance FC. Enzymatic burn wound debridement in conventional and germ-free rats. Surg Forum 1977; 28:33–34.
17. Moyer CA, Brentano L, Gravens DL, et al. Treatment of large human burns with 0.5 per cent silver nitrate solution. Arch Surg 1965; 90:812–867.
18. Singer AJ, McClain SA. Persistent wound infection delays epider-mal maturation and increases scarring in thermal burns. Wound Repair Regen 2002; 10(6):372–377.
19. Hunt TK, Ellison EC, Sen CK. Oxygen: at the foundation of wound healing – introduction. World J Surg 2004; 28(3):291–293.
20. Serini G, Bochaton-Piallat ML, Ropraz P, et al. The fibronectin domain ED-A is crucial for myofibroblastic phenotype induction by transforming growth factor-beta1. J Cell Biol 1998; 142(3):873–881.
21. Cone JB, Wallace BH, Caldwell FT Jr. The effect of staged burn wound closure on the rates of heat production and heat loss of burned children and young adults. J Trauma 1988; 28(7):968–972.
22. Schwanholt C, Greenhalgh DG, Warden GD. A comparison of full-thickness versus split-thickness autografts for the coverage of deep palm burns in the very young pediatric patient. J Burn Care Rehabil 1993; 14(1):29–33.
23. Bayat A, McGrouther DA, Ferguson MW. Skin scarring. Br Med J 2003; 326(7380):88–92.
24. Bullard KM, Longaker MT, Lorenz HP. Fetal wound healing: current biology. World J Surg 2003; 27(1):54–61.
25. Ferguson MW, O'Kane S. Scar-free healing: from embryonic mech-anisms to adult therapeutic intervention. Philos Trans R Soc Lond B Biol Sci 2004; 359(1445):839–850.
26. Xiao-Wu W, Herndon DN, Spies M, et al. Effects of delayed wound excision and grafting in severely burned children. Arch Surg 2002; 137(9):1049–1054.
27. Bessey PQ. Hospitalization for burns in New York State 1995–2004. New York: Columbia University; 2006.
28. Jonsson K, Jensen JA, Goodson WH 3rd et al. Tissue oxygenation, anemia, and perfusion in relation to wound healing in surgical patients. Ann Surg 1991; 214(5):605–613.
29. Greif R, Akca O, Horn EP, et al. Supplemental perioperative oxygen to reduce the incidence of surgical-wound infection. Outcomes Research Group. N Engl J Med 2000; 342(3):161–167.
30. Tyler MP, Watts AM, Perry ME, et al. Dermal cellular inflammation in burns. An insight into the function of dermal microvascular anatomy. Burns 2001; 27(5):433–438.
31. Kamolz LP, Andel H, Haslik W, et al. Use of subatmospheric pres-sure therapy to prevent burn wound progression in human: first experiences. Burns 2004; 30(3):253–258.

32. Chatterjee JS. A critical evaluation of the clinimetrics of laser Doppler as a method of burn assessment in clinical practice. J Burn Care Res 2006; 27(2):123–130.

33. Monafo WW, West MA. Current treatment recommendations for topical burn therapy. Drugs 1990; 40(3):364–373.

34. Pruitt BA Jr, McManus AT, Kim SH, et al. Burn wound infections: current status. World J Surg 1998; 22(2):135–145.

35. Smith DJ Jr, Thomson PD. Changing flora in burn and trauma units: historical perspective – experience in the United States. J Burn Care Rehabil 1992; 13(2 Pt 2):276–280.

36. White MG, Asch MJ. Acid–base effects of topical mafenide acetate in the burned patient. N Engl J Med 1971; 284(23):1281–1286.

37. Monafo WW. The treatment of burns: principles and practice. St. Louis: Warren H Green; 1971:267.

38. Fox CL Jr. Silver sulfadiazine – a new topical therapy for *Pseudomonas* in burns. Therapy of *Pseudomonas* infection in burns. Arch Surg 1968; 96(2):184–188.

39. Eldad A, Neuman A, Weinberg A, et al. Silver sulphadiazine-induced haemolytic anaemia in a glucose-6-phosphate dehydrogenase-deficient burn patient. Burns 1991; 17(5):430–432.

40. Choban PS, Marshall WJ. Leukopenia secondary to silver sulfadiazine: frequency, characteristics and clinical consequences. Am Surg 1987; 53(9):515–517.

41. Gamelli RL, Paxton TP, O'Reilly M. Bone marrow toxicity by silver sulfadiazine. Surg Gynecol Obstet 1993; 177(2):115–120.

42. Jarrett F, Ellerbe S, Demling R. Acute leukopenia during topical burn therapy with silver sulfadiazine. Am J Surg 1978; 135(6):818–819.

43. Cartotto R, Gomez M, Leow K, et al. Silver sulfadiazine (SSD) does not cause early post burn leukopenia (EPBL): a proospective study. J Burn Care Rehabil 2005; 26(2 Suppl):S90.

44. Lindberg RB, Moncrief JA, Mason AD Jr. Control of experimental and clinical burn wounds sepsis by topical application of sulfamylon compounds. Ann N Y Acad Sci 1968; 150(3):950–960.

45. Asch MJ, White MG, Pruitt BA Jr. Acid–base changes associated with topical Sulfamylon therapy: retrospective study of 100 burn patients. Ann Surg 1970; 172(6):946–950.

46. Fox CL Jr, Monafo WW Jr, Ayvazian VH, et al. Topical chemotherapy for burns using cerium salts and silver sulfadiazine. Surg Gynecol Obstet 1977; 144(5):668–672.

47. Garner JP, Heppell PS. The use of Flammacerium in British burns units. Burns 2005; 31(3):379–382.

48. Hermans RP. Topical treatment of serious infections with special reference to the use of a mixture of silver sulphadiazine and cerium nitrate: two clinical studies. Burns Incl Therm Inj 1984; 11(1):59–62.

49. Ross DA, Phipps AJ, Clarke JA. The use of cerium nitrate–silver sulphadiazine as a topical burns dressing. Br J Plast Surg 1993; 46(7):582–584.

50. Scheidegger D, Sparkes BG, Luscher N, et al. Survival in major burn injuries treated by one bathing in cerium nitrate. Burns 1992; 18(4):296–300.

51. Wassermann D, Schlotterer M, Lebreton F, Guelfi MC. Use of topically applied silver sulphadiazine plus cerium nitrate in major burns. Burns 1989; 15(4):257–260.

52. Monafo WW, Robinson HN, Yoshioka T, et al. 'Lethal' burns. A progress report. Arch Surg 1978; 113(4):397–401.

53. Garner JP, Heppell PS. Cerium nitrate in the management of burns. Burns 2005; 31(5):539–547.

54. Vehmeyer-Heeman M, Tondu T, Van den Kerckhove E, et al. Application of cerium nitrate–silver sulphadiazine allows for postponement of excision and grafting. Burns 2006; 32(1):60–63.

55. de Gracia CG. An open study comparing topical silver sulfadiazine and topical silver sulfadiazine–cerium nitrate in the treatment of moderate and severe burns. Burns 2001; 27(1):67–74.

56. Yin HQ, Langford R, Burrell RE. Comparative evaluation of the antimicrobial activity of ACTICOAT antimicrobial barrier dressing. J Burn Care Rehabil 1999; 20(3):195–200.

57. Dunn K, Edwards-Jones V. The role of Acticoat with nanocrystalline silver in the management of burns. Burns 2004; 30 (Suppl 1): S1–S9.

58. Graham C. The role of silver in wound healing. Br J Nurs 2005; 14(19):S22, S4, S6 passim.

59. Klasen HJ. A historical review of the use of silver in the treatment of burns. II. Renewed interest for silver. Burns 2000; 26(2):131–138.

60. Fong J, Wood F, Fowler B. A silver coated dressing reduces the incidence of early burn wound cellulitis and associated costs of inpatient treatment: comparative patient care audits. Burns 2005; 31(5):562–567.

61. Tredget EE, Shankowsky HA, Groeneveld A, et al. A matched-pair, randomized study evaluating the efficacy and safety of Acticoat silver-coated dressing for the treatment of burn wounds. J Burn Care Rehabil 1998; 19(6):531–537.

62. Varas RP, O'Keeffe T, Namias N, et al. A prospective, randomized trial of Acticoat versus silver sulfadiazine in the treatment of partial-thickness burns: which method is less painful? J Burn Care Rehabil 2005; 26(4):344–347.

63. Percival SL, Bowler PG, Russell D. Bacterial resistance to silver in wound care. J Hosp Infect 2005; 60(1):1–7.

64. Muller MJ, Hollyoak MA, Moaveni Z, et al. Retardation of wound healing by silver sulfadiazine is reversed by Aloe vera and nystatin. Burns 2003; 29(8):834–836.

65. Strock LL, Lee MM, Rutan RL, et al. Topical Bactroban (mupirocin): efficacy in treating burn wounds infected with methicillin-resistant staphylococci. J Burn Care Rehabil 1990; 11(5):454–459.

66. Brett DW. A historic review of topical enzymatic debridement. New York: McMahon; 2003.

67. Hanbrough JF, Achauer B, Dawson J, et al. Wound healing in partial-thickness burn wounds treated with collagenase ointment versus silver sulfadiazine cream. J Burn Care Rehabil 1995; 16(3):241–247.

68. Jones SA, Bowler PG, Walker M, et al. Controlling wound bioburden with a novel silver-containing Hydrofiber dressing. Wound Repair Regen 2004; 12(3):288–294.

69. Caruso DM, Foster KN, Hermans MH, et al. Aquacel Ag in the management of partial-thickness burns: results of a clinical trial. J Burn Care Rehabil 2004; 25(1):89–97.

70. Kumar RJ, Kimble RM, Boots R, et al. Treatment of partial-thickness burns: a prospective, randomized trial using Transcyte. ANZ J Surg 2004; 74(8):622–626.

71. Cassidy C, St Peter SD, Lacey S, et al. Biobrane versus duoderm for the treatment of intermediate thickness burns in children: a prospective, randomized trial. Burns 2005; 31(7):890–893.

Chapter 12

Treatment of infection in burns

*James J. Gallagher, Natalie Williams-Bouyer, Cynthia Villarreal,
John P. Heggers, and David N. Herndon*

Introduction

Infection is a most undesirable partner in any operative procedure, and it is especially troublesome in burn injury. Burns become infected due to the environment at the site of the wound being ideal for the growth of the infecting organisms. The immunosuppressed status of the patient allows the microorganisms to freely multiply. A variety of factors contribute to this development of infection in the burn patient. Among these are the roles of wound management procedures, risk factors associated with infection, virulent factors of typically isolated pathogens, current problems with antibiotic resistance, as well as wound sampling.[6]

The purpose of this chapter is to describe the diagnosis and treatment of burn wound infections, as a means of providing the burn surgeon with a practical clinical guide to assist in clinical judgment. The chapter is divided into three main sections:
1. Clinical management strategies
2. The microbiology of burn wound infection
3. Pharmacology

The section on clinical management provides an overview of the clinician's thoughts on a given problem. A more in-depth discussion of the microbiology or pharmacology of a given subject can be found in their respective sections.

Clinical management strategies

The burn surgeon

It is evident that the human population is not germ-free. Health is not the absence of bacteria, but is characterized by a delicate balance between man and his microbes, to include those of the environment. Intact skin and mucous membranes are man's most significant defense. Any alterations of the integument disturb this defense, as well as the balance with the microbial flora. Infection occurs when the microbes gain access to the underlying tissue and achieve a critical number. Invasive burn wound infection rarely occurs in partial-thickness injuries; they occur with the greatest frequency in young adults (15–40 years). Invasive burn wound is defined as the presence of bacteria in unburned tissue.[1] The major objective of the burn surgeon is to prevent this microbial invasion when and wherever possible, and, when contamination occurs, to reduce microbial levels so that wound healing can continue unretarded.[2]

Pathophysiology of the burn wound

Bacteria of normal endogenous skin flora are resistant to heat injury in practically the same degrees as are the skin cells. The bacteria on the surface are heat killed, as are the tissue cells of the surface, and initial swab cultures are usually sterile. The bacteria in the hair follicles and sebaceous glands may survive (dependent on the extent of the burn injury), and the quantitative counts of biopsied specimens may show the same numbers of bacteria per gram (10^3) as found in the tissue prior to burning.[3–5]

The mean cell generation time in optimum conditions is approximately 20 minutes. Therefore, a single bacterial cell can increase in numbers within a 24-hour period to over 10 billion cells.[6] As these bacteria increase in number following the thermal injury and reach levels of greater than 10^5 bacteria per gram of tissue, they will erupt from the hair follicles and sebaceous glands and begin transmigrating over the injury colonizing the dermal–subcutaneous boundary. Perivascular growth is accompanied by thrombosis of vessels and necrosis of any remaining dermal elements, transforming partial-thickness burns to full-thickness burn injuries. Levels of bacterial growth which exceed 10^5 bacteria per gram of tissue constitute localized burn wound infection, and levels greater than 10^8–10^9 bacteria per gram of tissue may be associated with lethal burns.[3,4,7–9] As the levels of bacterial growth increase so does the incidence of invasion of viable tissue and septicemia.[7,10] Histologically, invasive infection is seen with bacteria in unburned tissue. Other signs of invasion can be the presence of hemorrhage in unburned tissue, small-vessel thrombosis and ischemic necrosis of unburned tissue, dense bacterial growth in the subeschar space and intracellular viral inclusion bodies typical of HSV-1 infections.[1]

Occasionally, unusual organisms that are related to the mechanism of injury will cause an invasive infection. By example a burn which is treated with water in an effort to minimize injury may be contaminated by waterborne organisms such as *Aeromonas* or *Flavobacterium*.[11]

Maintaining wounds at low contamination levels diminishes the frequency and duration of septic episodes caused by wound flora. This is accomplished by cleansing the wound two to three times per day by either showering or immersing the wound in cleansing solutions. Some burn facilities still immerse patients in a tub to remove the debris and exudate that has accumulated between dressing changes; however, most burn facilities no longer advocate this cleaning technique because of the potential seeding of surface bacteria to the open burn wound of other patients by an inadequately cleaned tub. We, along with other burn facilities, use the shower technique to wash down the debris from the patients. It is important to note that wound cleansing can be quite painful, cause cooling, and may be associated with hematogenous seeding causing a bacteremia. Therefore adequate monitoring and professional attention is critical with this procedure.

The natural progression of bacterial colonization as the days pass is from Gram positive to Gram negative. By the 21st day postburn 57% of burn wounds still open will be colonized with resistant Gram-negative bacteria, thus making the antibiotic choices increasingly limited.[12,13]

Infection control best practice

Additional measures can be taken to diminish the incidence of burn wound colonization. The microorganisms initially populating the burned wound represent a mixture of endogenous resident flora and airborne contaminants seeded by contact with the environment and attending personnel. Burn patients are immunosuppressed and should be protected from exposure to environmental contaminants. (For a complete discussion of immunosuppression in the burn patient see Chapter 23.) The most elaborate methods of isolation have failed to effectively minimize the incidence of infection, although they have significantly reduced the incidence of cross-contamination.[13–15] The most effective means of decreasing exposure of burned patients to exogenous bacteria is strict observation of appropriate hand washing among the healthcare providers. Face masks, waterproof gowns, and gloves should be worn whenever direct contact with body fluids and wound exudates are unavoidable, thus protecting both the patient and the healthcare provider from inadvertent contamination. All dressing materials should be maintained as patient specific. IV pumps and poles, blood pressure devices, monitoring equipment, bedside tables, and beds should be cleaned on at least a daily basis with antibacterial solutions. Terminal cleaning, following the discharge of the patient, should include the walls, ceiling, baseboards, and floors. Mattresses should be covered with vinyl or other impermeable surface that allows culturing and cleaning without soiling, and be frequently inspected for cracks in their surfaces. At our institution we use HEPA air filters with 99.99% efficiency on $0.3\,\mu m$-sized particles. They are changed regularly, and cultured if clinically indicated by infection control monitoring.

Most units now house major burned patients within individual, self-contained positive pressure isolation rooms. However, common areas exist even within these units, predominantly the bathing or showering facilities. These areas should be conscientiously cleansed between patients with an effective bactericidal agent specifically directed at the bacteria, which are common to an individual unit. Disposable liners for cleaning surfaces are encouraged or sterilizable instruments should be used for débridements.

The smaller burn early presentation

The most common burns are less than 10%. These smaller burns when presented early for treatment are typically clean. The presence of fever alone does not indicate infection as burn is associated with an elevation in the body temperature set point. The routine use of systemic antibiotics is not advocated for early small burns. The presence of cellulitis calls for topical antimicrobials as well as systemic. For an uncomplicated burn, Gram positives are covered with vancomycin added for persistent cellulitis. Broader antibiotic coverage is added, as is clinically indicated, depending on the circumstance. Figures 12.1–12.4 demonstrate a small burn with early presentation through the stages of healing without complication.

Routine prophylaxis for tetanus (*Clostridium tetani*) is tetanus toxoid (0.5 mL) if it has not been administered in the previous 3 years as part of the admission protocol to the burn center.[16,17] In addition, if their last booster was more that 10 years ago, 250 units of tetanus antitoxin is also given. Local bacteriologic control is most frequently obtained through the use of a topical application of antimicrobials such as silver sulfadiazine (SSD). In our institution Mycostatin has been added to SSD. This decreases the incidence of *Candida* in the burn wound. (Chapter 11 offers a broad list of the antimicrobial topical dressing choices.)

Alternatively, the patient may have application of a synthetic or biologic adherent dressing. At our institution Biobrane is frequently used. Prior to application, proper cleansing is done. These patients are followed closely for the first week to assure that the dressing is adherent. The routine use of

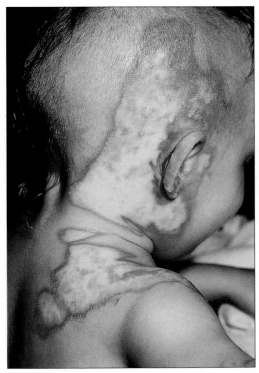

Fig. 12.1 Superficial and deep second-degree scald burns to the head, face, and shoulder. Treatment is with silver sulfadiazine.

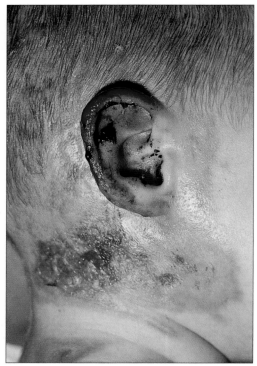

Fig. 12.2 Same patient as shown in Figure 12.1, 12 days after the injury. Note that most of the injury is healed.

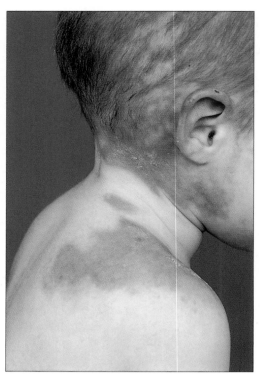

Fig. 12.4 Same patient as shown in Figure 12.1, 2 months after injury. All wounds are healed.

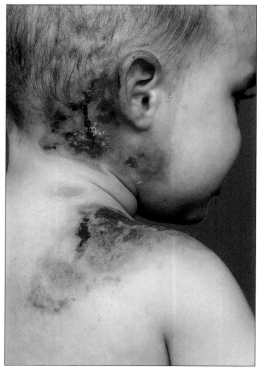

Fig. 12.3 Same patient as shown in Figure 12.1, 26 days after injury. Deep second-degree burns are still healing. Note that all superficial second-degree burns are healed and maturing.

systemic antibiotics is not advocated for wounds treated this way. During the period of observation non-adherence, the presence of cloudy exudate, surrounding cellulitis, and/or fever should make the clinician suspicious of infection. Possibly infected areas should be opened, unroofed, and cultured. The clinical management of a patient with an infected occlusive dressing must be rapid and aggressive. Late in the course of the use of Biobrane we have seen pustular lesions develop away from the burn site. Oddly this occurs after the Biobrane is adherent and the patient does not appear ill. Culture of the pus has grown methicillin-resistant *Staphylococcus aureus* (MRSA).

In general, most of these small burns will be going home. Teach the family clean technique for wound care and dressings with written instructions. Emphasize the importance of hand washing before and after caring for the patient and most importantly when performing wound care. Instruct the family to clean the bathroom, especially the bathtub and shower before and after use with strong disinfectant like bleach. Teach the signs of sepsis: fever, redness, increased pain, changes in odor or drainage, and increased swelling.[18] Our routine is to follow acutely until closed.

One area of special consideration when caring for the small burn is the small but serious complication of toxic shock syndrome (TSS). TSS is the result of a burn wound colonized with toxic shock syndrome toxin-1 producing *S. aureus*[6] (see Figure 12.5). This disease is primarily of the young child, with a burn of less than 10% that would normally be thought to heal without problem. The incidence has been reported at approximately 2.6% at a mean age of 2 years. Clinically it is characterized by a prodromal period lasting 1–2 days with pyrexia, diarrhea, vomiting, and malaise. A rash is often present; at

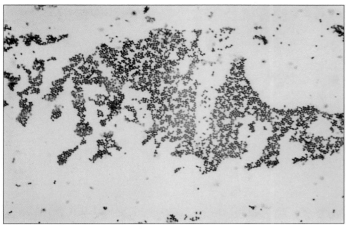

Fig. 12.5 Gram stain of *Staphylococcus aureus* (×1000).

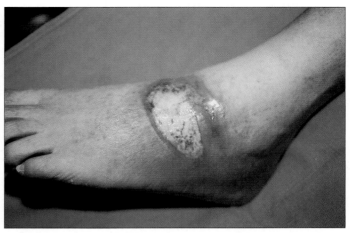

Fig. 12.7 Burn wound cellulitis caused by *Staphylococcus aureus*. Clinical findings include increased pain, local inflammatory signs, and fever. Treatment includes systemic intravenous antibiotics, excision, and autografting.

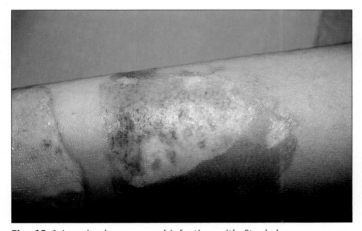

Fig. 12.6 Invasive burn wound infection with *Staphylococcus aureus*. The patient presented with extreme pain, intense inflammation to the forearm, functional impairment of forearm musculature, and high fever. Immediate excision showed purulent secretions collected in the reticular dermis and subcutaneous fat.

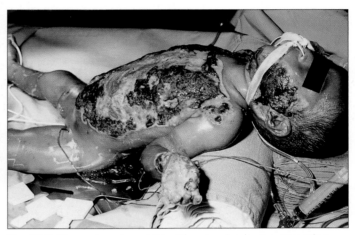

Fig. 12.8 Shown here is a child with extensive burns presenting very late. There is evidence of scar separation from the wound bed, a sign of late presentation.

this stage the burn appears clean. Shock then develops in untreated cases. This is the time of maximal illness and is usually 2–4 days after the burn injury. Once shock has developed, mortality can be as high as 50%. The main defense is knowledge and aggressive treatment.[20]

Smaller burn with a later presentation

The early burn with surrounding blanching erythema likely has an area of surrounding first-degree burn. However, the burn wound presenting late with erythema, swelling, and/or pathologic colors and odors should alert the clinician to the strong likelihood of infection. Careful clinical exam can differentiate the action needed to begin treatment. Most commonly, the wound needs only thorough cleansing and application of topical antimicrobials. With late presentation and signs of cellulitis, systemic antimicrobials are indicated (see Figures 12.6 and 12.7). The offending organism is usually *Staphylococcus*. The circumstances, appearance or history may make consideration of Gram-negative pathogens realistic and expansion

of coverage is dictated by clinical judgment. Occasionally, the severely neglected wound can progress to full thickness and even have a contained area of pus beneath a true eschar. This area needs to be opened like any other abscess. Special care should be taken with evaluation of the burn wounds in the elderly and diabetics as the inflammatory response can be blunted and the wound severely underestimated.

The larger burn

Burns over 20–30% of the body have an immunosuppressive effect which involves both the humoral and cellular lines of host defense.[6] Please see the chapter on immunosuppression in this text for a detailed discussion of the changes seen in the immune system after burn injury.

A large open wound is a favorable environment for bacterial colonization. The early management of burn must include aggressive efforts at removing the dead tissue and achieving wound closure with autograft, homograft or other biologic dressing (Figures 12.8 and 12.9). The very early burn wound,

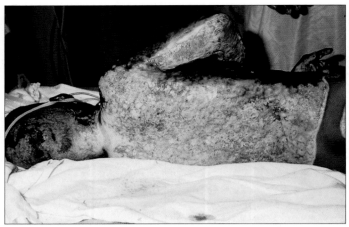

Fig. 12.9 Seventy-five percent total body surface area full-thickness burns with burn wound sepsis by *Enterococcus faecalis* and *Enterobacter cloacae*. Prompt excision and homografting, hemodynamic support, and systemic antibiotics controlled the infection.

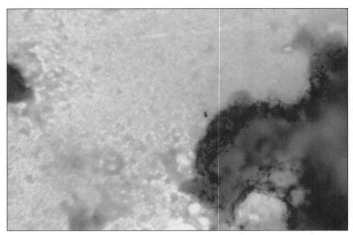

Fig. 12.10 Gram stain of biopsy revealing Gram-positive cocci. Quantitative count 6.2×10^5 organisms per gram of tissue (×1000).

less than 48 hours, normally has low colony counts. Preoperatively the patients can be held in topical antimicrobial soaking dressings until early excision of the burn wound can be undertaken. Perioperative antibiotics should be broad to cover the Gram-positive and Gram-negative organisms that are encountered in the specific care center. The antibiotics are covering bacteria from the burn wound, as well as bacteria in the gut, which both have been shown to seed the bloodstream during burn excision. Wound cultures are taken at the time of surgery for microscopic and pathologic examination to determine if colonization is present with or without invasion. The term 'colonization' indicates only the presence of viable bacteria on the surface of the wound or in the burn eschar. Although potentially dangerous, wound colonization does not imply that locally destructive or systemic infection is present. If the microorganisms successfully invade into viable tissue, they will produce a locally destructive infection and may disseminate either viable bacteria or their toxic products systemically via blood or lymphatic vessels (burn wound sepsis).

Larger burn with a late presentation

Dead tissue has no resistance to infection. It is also excellent growth media for all manner of pathogenic organisms. Control of these wounds is by surgical excision often down to fascia as the delay has ensured that the zone of stasis has converted second-degree burns to full thickness. Large burns with delayed presentation have host immunosuppression, polymicrobial colonization, and possible invasive infection. The elimination of all dead tissue including aggressive removal of dead muscle is the basis of control. The antimicrobial choice for the first operation should be broad coverage for fungus, resistant Gram-positive and Gram-negative organisms. Complete removal of dead tissue and topical antimicrobials such as silver nitrate, Sulfamylon, and topical nystatin are common choices. Here the surgeon must be aggressive as in necrotizing fasciitis, if the wound is to come under control and support grafting. Further antimicrobial management follows the culture information obtained from biopsies with persistent efforts to cover the offending organisms with adequate well-timed doses of

TABLE 12.1 BURN WOUND INFECTION: LOCAL SIGNS*
Black or dark brown focal areas of discoloration
Enhanced sloughing of burned tissue or eschar
Partial-thickness injury converted to full-thickness necrosis
Purplish discoloration or edema of skin around the margins of the wound
Presence of ecthyma gangrenosa
Pyocyanotic appearance of subeschar tissue
Subcutaneous tissue with hemorrhagic discoloration
Variable-sized abscess formation and focal subeschar inconsistency
*Reproduced with permission from Heggers JP, Robson MC. Infection control in burn patients. Clin Plast Surg 1986; 13:39–47.

cost-effective antibiotics chosen for their specific activity against the pathogen. This requires a coordinated effort of the clinician, microbiologist, and pharmacist.

Burn wound surveillance

Daily inspection of the burn wound by a burn surgeon is mandatory for decision making. Major burn wounds usually become colonized or infected within 3–5 days after admission; often infection arises from the patient's own bacterial flora and not an exogenous source. Burn wound biopsies should be taken from any area of the wound which has changed in appearance, as described in Table 12.1. In Figures 12.10 and 12.11 we see the presence of bacteria on a wound culture Gram stain. Bacterial sepsis is often heralded by changes in the color, odor or amount of exudate from the wound, while fungal invasion is clinically suggested by a rapidly emerging and spreading dark discoloration. Consequently the burn wound must be closely assessed for these manifestations. Few histologically demonstrated fungal infections are initially determined by culture; therefore treatment should be predicated on the identification of hyphae by histological examination and which may be subsequently confirmed by culture.

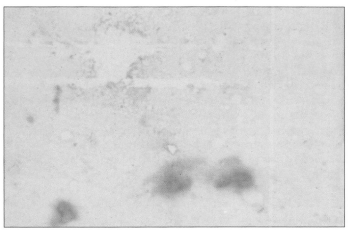

Fig. 12.11 Gram stain of biopsy revealing Gram-negative rods. Quantitative count 7.5×10^5 organisms per gram of tissue ($\times$1000).

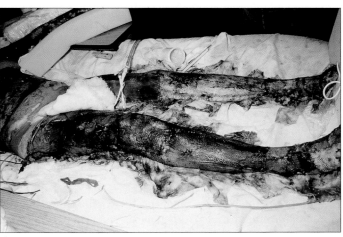

Fig. 12.14 Fungal burn wound sepsis. Systemic antifungals, topical nystatin powder, and excision of all affected areas, which usually includes fascial excision and amputations, is the treatment of choice for such deadly infections.

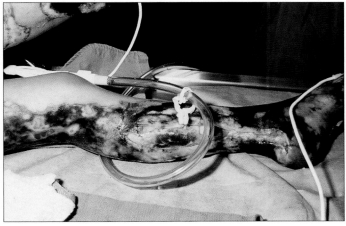

Fig. 12.12 Burn wound sepsis caused by *Aspergillus* spp. Fungal infections should be suspected in wounds presenting with dark or black discoloration and hemorrhagic areas, in patients receiving prolonged systemic broad-spectrum antibiotics and/or who come from endemic areas. This patient died of fungal sepsis, fungal pneumonia, and respiratory distress syndrome.

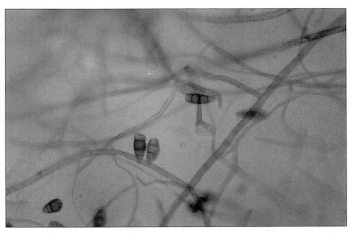

Fig. 12.15 Lactophenol blue stain of a fungus from a burn wound biopsy identified as *Curvularia* spp. ($\times$400).

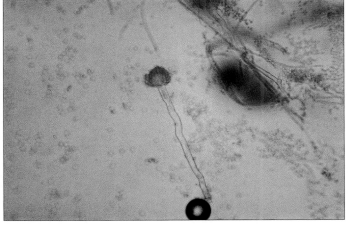

Fig. 12.13 Lactophenol blue stain of *Aspergillus* sp. isolated from a burn wound biopsy ($\times$400).

Figures 12.12–12.15 are examples of clinical and microscopic appearances of the fungal wound infection.

Many believe clinical sepsis with suspicion of the burn wound as source is a mandate for surgical control of the burn wound. Burn wound deterioration can be rapid; biopsy of changing lesions can be processed by frozen section in 1 hour or rapid prep in 24 hours. If bacteria are seen in viable tissue or in vessels, a diagnosis of burn wound sepsis is made, and wide excision of all involved areas should be completed. Surgical control can mean conversion of a tangential excision to the fascial level. The aggressive debridement of all remaining dead tissue is a minimal therapy. Dead muscle in particular can be problematic as compromised areas can be hidden from view. In the larger burn, any burden of dead tissue with loss of the skin barrier, combined with immunosuppression, makes a very aggressive surgical approach mandatory.

The major role of local burn wound infection in sepsis suggests that the diagnosis and treatment of infections should focus primarily on the burn wound. Wound colonization will progress to infection only when the surface bacterial counts exceed some critical number. Accurate quantification of the burned patient's bacterial load is therefore the foundation of infection surveillance. This is achieved through routine cultures of sputum, urine, and wound. Quantitative cultures obtained at a goal of three times weekly will provide monitoring for the progress of bacterial colonization and guidance in the event that empiric antibiotic therapy becomes necessary. If a simultaneous sample is examined by a pathologist a diagnosis of burn wound invasion in need of emergent surgical treatment can be made. Quantitative swabs, smear cultures, and/or contact plates (Rodak®) provide information regarding the potential infectious agent; quantitative wound biopsies are a better determinant of bacterial loads. Quantitative cultures showing high bacterial counts correlate with histologic evidence of burn wound infection in approximately 80% of cases.[2,3,7] If quantitative biopsies reveal greater than 10^3 organisms/g of tissue, a change in topical therapy is indicated. If bacterial counts exceed 10^5 organisms/g of tissue, localized burn wound infection should be considered and a histologic examination performed. If histologic evidence of invasion is present, systemic antibiotics should be given and the wound should be excised.[3,20,21] In addition, routine cultures of the stool are obtained to identity colonization with pathogenic organisms. These results should guide preoperative antibiotic choice and treatment of infection. The burn wound must be recognized as the site of microbial colonization which may progress to invasion with systemic dissemination if not restrained.

Wound culture, topicals, and graft take

Robson found that when colony counts were less than 10^2 per gram of wound graft, survival was greater than 90%, but when colony counts were greater than 10^5 per gram of wound, only 60% graft survival was observed.[22] We have routinely modified our topical antimicrobial therapy, alternating between silver nitrate solution and mafenide acetate when colony counts are greater than 10^5. The only exception for this rule is infection with *Streptococcus*, which may appear with just 10^3 CFU.[23] Mafenide acetate is more successful at penetration of the necrotic dermis than is silver nitrate solution. Sodium hypochlorite (NaOCl) is very effective as a cleansing agent when a foul wound is identified. Studies by Heggers and his coworkers[24] clearly defined the efficacy of NaOCl at a concentration of 0.025 % which was found to be bactericidal and non-toxic to fibroblasts and did not inhibit wound healing, provided appropriate buffers are used. However, the NaOCl is only effective over a 24-hour time frame after the buffer (0.3 N NaH_2HPO_4) is added to the NaOCl.[25] NaOCl soaks are most beneficial in reducing the bacterial numbers in a wound.

NaOCl is a broad-spectrum antiseptic and is bactericidal for *P. aeruginosa*, *S. aureus* as well as other Gram-negative and Gram-positive organisms.[24,26] It is also effective against MRSA, MRSE, and the enterococci. NaOCl can be used separately but more commonly in concert with other longer-acting antibacterials to control colonization or infection. NaOCl 0.025% also enhances wound healing and increases wound breaking strength when compared to 5% mafenide acetate (Sulfamylon).[24]

Sulfamylon is a very effective agent against bacterial wound contamination, with the added benefit of tissue penetration. It can be used both as a cream or soak. Our topical sensitivity analysis routinely indicates it as the best choice for resistant *Pseudomonas* infection. Its use in large areas is limited by its ability as a carbonic anhydrase inhibitor to cause metabolic acidosis. The aqueous soak is commonly used on the open burn wound, while the ointment is chosen for auricular chondritis. Silver nitrate aqueous solution is our most frequent choice of a soaking agent for topical bacteriologic control. Although silver nitrate does not penetrate dead tissue well, it has a reliable broad-spectrum activity. Silver nitrate solution causes a characteristic staining of normal skin because of precipitation (Figure 12.16) The double antibiotic solution of neomycin and polymyxin is also considered as an antibiotic soak and is used clinically to control wound colonization. It also lacks the tissue penetration of Sulfamylon.

Sepsis in the burn patient

Rapid and complete closure of deep burns is the best defense against the development of sepsis in the burn patient. If a comparison is made between burn patients of equal size, those who have an occurrence of sepsis during their hospitalization will have decreased lean body mass and increased mortality. We attempt to control sources of bacteria by topical antibiotics, debridement, and early closure. In addition, the idea of the gastrointestinal tract as a source of bacteria has been the motivator behind trials at selective gut decontamination. Unfortunately, this effort thus far has failed to show benefit.[28]

A major focus of rounds in the burn intensive care unit is on the identification of sepsis. There are several cardinal signs of sepsis which embody both Gram-negative as well as Gram-positive involvement (Table 12.2). Constant surveillance for these signs can provide adjunctive information concerning the etiologic agent of sepsis. A septic source can be documented as:

- burn wound biopsy with >10^5 organisms/g of tissue and/or histologic evidence of viable tissue invasion;
- positive blood culture;
- urinary tract infection with >10^5 organisms/mL of urine; or
- pulmonary infection.

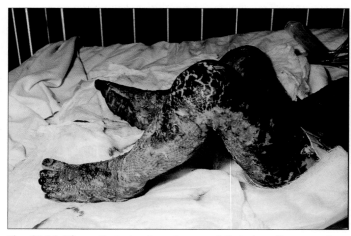

Fig. 12.16 Silver nitrate treatment as precipitated on the normal skin.

TABLE 12.2 ADDITIONAL CARDINAL SIGNS OF BURN WOUND SEPSIS*
Gram-negative sepsis
Burn wound biopsy >10⁵ organisms/g tissue and/or histologic evidence of viable tissue invasion
Rapid onset — well to ill in 8–12 hours
Increased temperature to 100–103°F (38–39°C) or may remain within normal limits (37°C)
WBC may be increased
Followed by hypothermia — 94°F (34–35°C) plus a decrease in WBC
Ileus/intolerance of tube feed
Decreased BP and urinary output
Wounds develop focal gangrene
Satellite lesions away from burn wound
Mental obtundation
Gram-positive sepsis
Burn wound biopsy >10⁵ organisms/g tissue and/or histologic evidence of viable tissue invasion
Symptoms develop gradually
Increased temperature to 105°F or higher (>40°C)
WBC 20 000–50 000
Decreased hematocrit
Wound macerated in appearance, ropy and tenacious exudate
Anorexic and irrational
Ileus/intolerance of tube feed
Decreased BP and urinary output
*Five or more signs or symptoms are definitive diagnostic parameters.

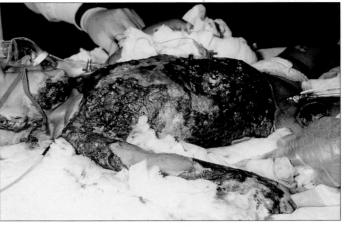

Fig. 12.17 Burn wound sepsis caused by *Pseudomonas aeruginosa.* Note the dark appearance of the burn eschar. Immediate excision after resuscitation and double antibiotic coverage against all organisms identified are mandatory.

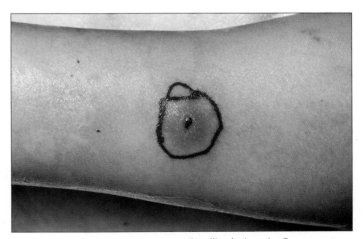

Fig. 12.18 Ecthyma gangrenosum. Satellite lesions in Gram-negative sepsis are typical and diagnostic.

In addition to the identification of a septic source, at least five or more of the following criteria should be met: tachypnea (>40 breaths/min in adults), paralytic ileus, hyper- or hypo-thermia (temperature <36.5° > 38.5°C), altered mental status, thrombocytopenia (<50 000 platelets/mm³), leukopenia or cytosis (<3.5 > 15.0 cells/mm³), acidosis or hyperglycemia. Local evidence of invasive wound infection includes black or brown patches of wound discoloration, rapid eschar separa-tion, conversion of wounds to full thickness, spreading peri-wound erythema, punctate hemorrhagic subeschar lesions, and violaceous or black lesions in unburned tissue (ecthyma gangrenosum) (Table 12.1). When a patient exhibits signs and symptoms of sepsis, immediate institution of antibiotics is obligatory while awaiting confirmatory cultures. If a patient is already on antibiotics a broadening of coverage to include highly resistant bacteria is in order if possible. Specific antibi-otic treatment should be administered if routine surveillance has identified the predominant organism. In addition to insti-tution of antibiotic treatment, there should be a rapid aggres-sive attempt at surgical source control.

Tight glycemic control is increasingly showing promise as a way of decreasing infection rates in the intensive care unit. In a recent study in pediatric burn patients this finding has been upheld and is now being recommended. This, however, remains an area of ongoing active research.[29]

Extremely virulent pathogens

Years of clinical practice in the care of burn patients following the previously outlined principles have led to rewarding out-comes. However certain pathogens have come and defied the usual measures that control other organisms. The appearance of these organisms has often returned death rates to a time before the current era of massive early excision and grafting. The following discussion is born out of the clinical manage-ment of these difficult pathogens.

Ecthyma gangrenosum is a purple-bluish black spot in previ-ously healthy tissues. Classically this is caused by invasive *Pseudomonas*. Histologically, this is characterized by throm-bosis of vessels with perivascular hemorrhage. Unfortunately, multi-drug resistant *Pseudomonas* has become a common enemy. Figures 12.17–12.25 demonstrate the clinical and histologic appearance of invasive *Pseudomonas* infection.

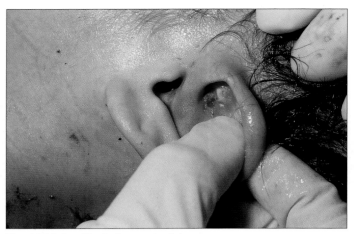

Fig. 12.19 Satellite lesion to the left ear.

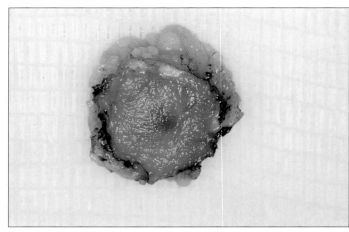

Fig. 12.20 Biopsy of ecthyma gangrenosum. The thrombolytic lesion in the center of the biopsy is characteristic of *Pseudomonas aeruginosa*.

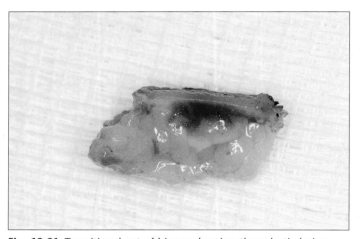

Fig. 12.21 Transitional cut of biopsy showing thrombotic lesion.

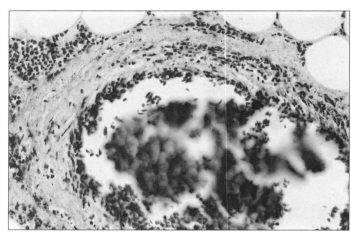

Fig. 12.22 Thrombus present in blood vessel of the biopsy with bacilli in endothelium (hematoxylin and eosin, ×400).

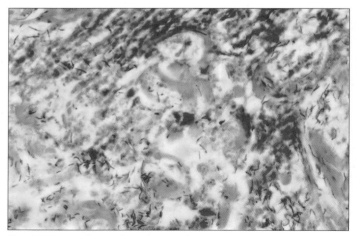

Fig. 12.23 Bacilli invading deep viable tissue. Invasion of viable tissue with histopathology confirmation is currently the only way to diagnose burn wound infection (hematoxylin and eosin, ×1000).

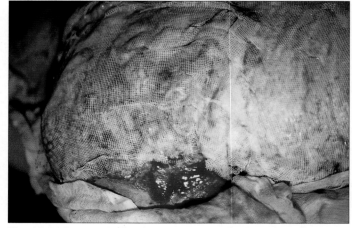

Fig. 12.24 Pyocyanic discoloration on a grafted site treated with nitrofurazone ointment.

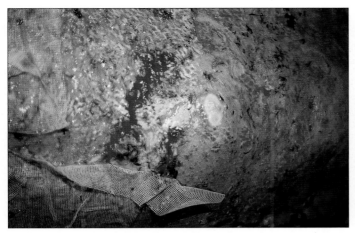

Fig. 12.25 Same patient as shown in Figure 12.24 after removal of the dressing. Cultures grew *Pseudomonas aeruginosa*. Note that all autografts have disappeared as a result of the action of the bacterial enzymes.

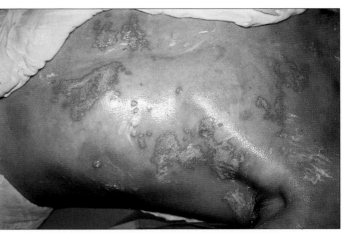

Fig. 12.26 *Candida* infection in a healing second-degree burn wound. Pain and itch is usually present in this kind of infection. Treatment with silver sulfadiazine mixed with Mycostatin has proved effective in controlling *Candida* infections in burn centers.

Invasive *Pseudomonas* in combination with vancomycin-resistant *Enterococcus* have clinically demonstrated a severe coagulopathy leading to death. The use of colistimethate has recently enabled control of multi-drug resistant *Pseudomonas*. Multi-drug resistant *Acinetobacter* has also been sensitive to colistimethate. The pharmacy section of this chapter has a complete discussion of colistimethate.

Fusarium with resistance to amphotericin has the ability to invade living tissue and create a wavefront of necrosis. This pattern is histologically recognizable by the presence of fungal hyphae extending like fingers to the border between necrotic and intact tissue, and does represent dangerous invasion of viable tissue. Very aggressive removal of all dead tissue, Voriconazole administered systemically as well as topical antifungals can be successful against this virulent organism. A similar virulent profile is possessed by *Aspergillus* spp. and *Mucor* spp. (see Figures 12.12 and 12.13).

Candida colonization will be present in 30% of burn patients with burns greater than 40% during their hospital stay. It is for this reason that nystatin was added to topical silver sulfadiazine. This change has resulted in a marked decrease in three organ involvement with *Candida* (see Figures 12.26 and 12.27). The isolation of *Candida* from three organs is usually required for the diagnosis of candidal sepsis.[29] Serum antibody titers to *Candida* have recently been advocated to assist in the early diagnosis.[31] Premortem diagnosis, confirmed with sufficient time to implement appropriate treatment, occurs in less than 40% of infected patients.[32] Because of their relatively large size, *Candida* are usually filtered out of blood at the capillary level; arterial blood cultures are recommended. Organisms are usually seen in the urine when sepsis from a distant site occurs. Candidal sepsis is considered when *C. albicans* can be isolated from any three of the following tissue sites: blood, wound, urine, bronchial washings, or by a positive retinal examination.

Candidal spores are omnipresent in the burned patient, appearing in stools, nasopharynx swabs, urine samples and cultures of intact integument. However, fewer than 20% of

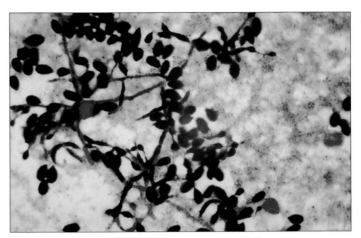

Fig. 12.27 Gram stain of *Candida albicans* (×1000).

patients with candidal wound colonization develop widespread candidiasis.[33,34] Only when the controlling bacterial populations are eradicated by systemic antibiotics or the host becomes immunosuppressed does candidal infection occur,[34] frequently following a bacterial sepsis. There is a 3–5% incidence of candidemia in the burned population[30,33,36,37] and a comparable rate of burn wound invasion.[36] Candidal infections occur most commonly in patients with large burn injuries who are hospitalized for long periods of time and have received multiple courses of antibiotics. Prophylactic treatment with oropharyngeal and topical nystatin have therefore become recommended;[30] however, fluconazole may be more effective in some cases. Mortality associated with *Candida* is usually from amphotericin-associated renal failure.

Non-bacteriologic causes of infection
Viruses

Viral infections are being more frequently clinically recognized in burned patients. Prospective and retrospective assays of sera have documented a large incidence of subclinical viral infection. Retrospectively, Linneman[38] assayed stored sera of burned children and found a four fold increase in antibodies to cytomegalovirus (CMV) in 22% of patients, 8% had increased herpes simplex titers and 5% demonstrated a rise in varicella zoster titers. The study continued in a prospective manner, with 33% of the children developing CMV infection, 25% developing herpetic infections and 17% developing adenovirus infection.

CMV infection typically occurs approximately 1 month post-burn and clinically presents as a fever of unknown origin and lymphocytosis.[39] Rarely are patients with less than 50% total body surface area burn infected. CMV infection frequently occurs concurrently with bacterial and fungal infections, but rarely alters the patient's clinical course. CMV inclusions may be identified in the cells of multiple organs, but have not been reported in the burn wound.[40] The burned patients who most commonly contract the infection are known to have received multiple blood transfusions, which represent a major source of contamination. In addition it has been shown in an animal model that cadaver skin has the ability to transmit CMV infection.

Most commonly, herpetic lesions appear in healing partial-thickness burns or split-thickness donor sites (see Figure 12.28), although other epithelial surfaces such as the oral or intestinal mucosa can be involved. In the latter case, herpetic lesions may lead to erosion and perforation. The clinical manifestations of lesions may be preceded by unexplained fever unresponsive to routine antibiotic coverage.[40] Partial-thickness burns and donor sites infected with herpes may 'convert' to full-thickness injuries requiring skin grafting for ultimate closure. Necrotizing hepatic and adrenal lesions may lead to multi-system organ failure. Mortality in patients with disseminated infection is about twice that expected for patients of similar age and burn size. Split-thickness grafts provide adequate coverage of previously infected herpetic wound.[41]

Chickenpox (varicella-zoster) infection is a frequent occurrence in school-aged children and is rapidly spread through inhalation of the virus. Varicella infections can be life-threatening in an immunocompromised host and mini-epidemics have occurred within pediatric burn units.[42] The characteristic fluid-filled lesions appear in healed or healing partial-thickness burn, as well as uninjured epithelium and mucous membranes. Due to the fragility of the newly healed or healing skin, the vesicles are much more destructive in the injured than in the uninjured skin, and may present as hemorrhagic, oozing pockmarks, which are prone to secondary infection and subsequent scarring. New, neovascularized skin grafts may be lost and further grafting procedures should be delayed until the lesions are quiescent. Herpes simplex and zoster are consistently treated with systemic acyclovir or Valtrex.

Parasites

In this age of world travel being common place, we must mention those organisms which are endemic to the patient's origin that could complicate the burn injury. Based on a study conducted by Barret et al. in 1999,[43] the authors concluded that patients being admitted from third-world countries where parasitism is endemic should be treated empirically with an antiparasite drug, preferably metronidazole or mebendazole.

Burn-associated infections

New open areas and 'ghosting' of grafts — the role of infection

New open areas in previously grafted burns, donor sites or areas that heal spontaneously can often be attributable to surface colonization (Figures 12.29 and 12.30). Typically the wounds form through blistering, which then ruptures, or through trauma from scratching. Care usually includes topical Bactroban ointment, and washing frequently with mild antibacterial soap. Swab culture is taken to identify the organism present and systemic antibiotics, if cellulitis is clinically identified. Large areas may come to re-grafting when they are clean. Folliculitis is a particular problem of the scalp and other hair-bearing areas. The same treatment algorithm applies with the addition of shaving (Figure 12.31).

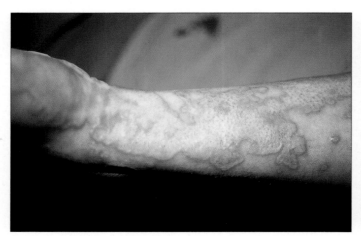

Fig. 12.28 Herpes simplex virus type I infection in a patient with 35% partial-thickness and full-thickness burns. Extreme pain and itching are typical of this infection.

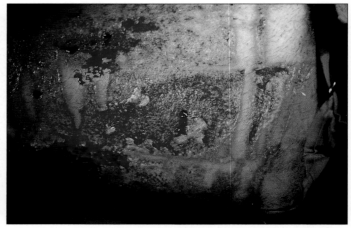

Fig. 12.29 *Staphylococcus aureus* infection in donor sites. Note the secretions and the geographic appearance of the wound, which is typical of this pathogen.

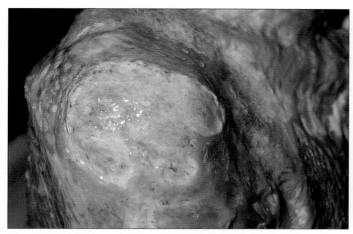

Fig. 12.30 Infection of the graft site with *Staphylococcus aureus*. Prompt topical treatment with antistaphylococcal ointment solutions stops the progression of the destruction of skin autografts.

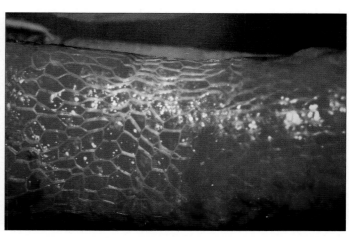

Fig. 12.32 Wound with granulating tissue grafted with 3:1 meshed autografts.

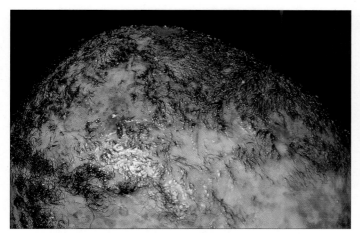

Fig. 12.31 Chronic folliculitis to the scalp, also known as the concrete scalp deformity. Hairs from hair-bearing areas are embedded in the granulation tissue of converted second-degree burns and donor sites, and microorganisms are entrapped prolonging the process. Shaving of the affected area, topical treatment, and eventually skin autografting resolve the problem.

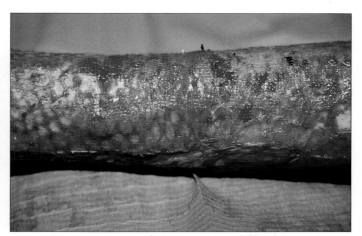

Fig. 12.33 The same wound as shown in Figure 12.32, 5 days after autografting. The mesh pattern is still visible, but the autograft is melting or vanishing. The melting graft syndrome or ghosting graft syndrome is probably related to the action of collagenases that are present in chronic wounds and wounds colonized by bacteria.

A frustrating problem for the burn surgeon is gradual loss of grafted areas that had taken through disappearance of the graft, which is commonly referred to as 'ghosting' (Figures 12.32 and 12.33). The exact etiology of this disappointing clinical phenomenon remains elusive. Enzymatic proteolysis in the presence of infection seems most likely. To combat this problem once noted, topical cultures are taken to identify the bacterial colonies present and topical soaking dressings of silver nitrate solution or equivalent are started. The series of Figures 12.34–12.37 outlines such a case. Once specific cultures are available, topical sensitivities can be obtained to more accurately treat the bacteria present. However, the causative role of bacteria in this process has not been completely established.

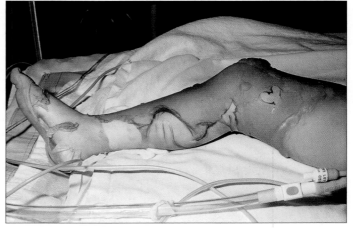

Fig. 12.34 Deep second-degree and third-degree flame burns to the lower extremities. The patient was treated with immediate excision and autografting.

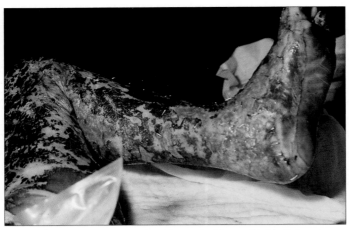

Fig. 12.35 The same wound as shown in Figure 12.34, 5 days later. Same grafts are melting due to inadequate excision of small areas. Human collagenases dissolve the remaining burn eschar and part of the autografts.

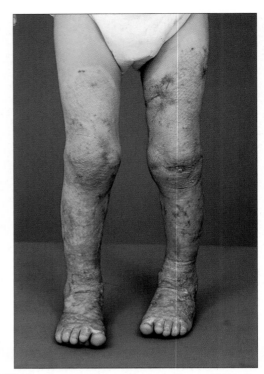

Fig. 12.37 The same patient as shown in Figure 12.34, 5 months after the injury.

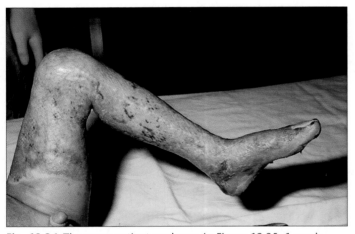

Fig. 12.36 The same patient as shown in Figure 12.35, 1 week later after treatment with silver nitrate solution. The melting or ghosting syndrome can be treated with different dressings, such as silver nitrate, normal saline, Dakin's solution, and Bactroban ointment.

Chondritis

Burns to the ear represent a clinical management challenge. Full-thickness injuries can damage the cartilage of the ear, resulting in auto-amputation of a part or the entire external auricle. Because of the auricle's comparatively low blood supply, chondritis frequently follows the progression of tissue ischemia. Chondritis is usually seen 3–5 weeks following the injury, but may be seen earlier and may occur following partial- and full-thickness injuries. The introduction of mafenide acetate has become the topical agent of choice for burned cartilagineos surfaces and since its use, the incidence of suppurative chondritis has significantly decreased (Figures 12.38 and 12.39).

Characteristically, the patient will complain of dull pain. The ear will become warm, red, tender, and edematous.

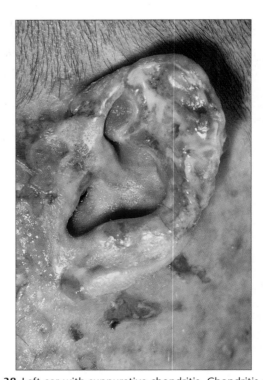

Fig. 12.38 Left ear with suppurative chondritis. Chondritis seen 3 weeks after flame burn to left ear. Note the erythema and drainage from the helical rim.

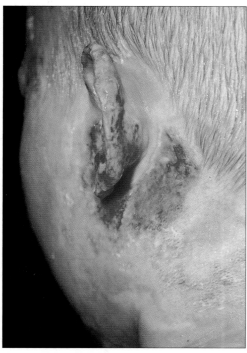

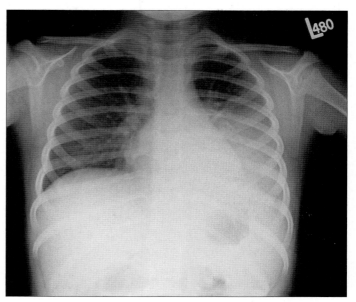

Fig. 12.40 Left lower pneumonia. Burn patient with typical radiographic picture of lobar pneumonia. The diagnosis of pneumonia in patients with inhalation injury and respiratory distress syndrome is still very difficult.

Fig. 12.39 Posterior view of the patient shown in Figure 12.38. Patients usually complain of dull pain, with warmth and tenderness to the touch. Topical mafenide acetate is the treatment of choice.

Appropriate antibiotics should be initiated immediately and if there is an identifiable site, immediate incision and drainage of the abscess should be undertaken with a culture and sensitivity obtained. Should induration and tenderness continue, a more extensive debridement is imperative. Generally the helix is bivalved at the posterior helical margin and all necrotic cartilage debrided. Difficulty may arise in distinguishing between viable and necrotic tissue and frequently normal cartilage is sacrificed in order to ensure debridement. However, infected cartilage is usually soft, while normal cartilage will feel granular on curettage. If appropriate adequate excision of the necrotic tissue is not performed, suppurative chondritis can proceed to invade the mastoid bone creating a potential for intracranial abscess formation.

Ophthalmic infections

The eyes in the burn unit are at great risk. They may have suffered an insult from the original trauma or from the time in the burn intensive care unit. The retraction of the lids from scar and the sedation that is at times necessary can interfere with the natural protective mechanism for the eye. The avascular corneal stroma is protected by one layer of epithelium. Once damaged, a perforation can mean loss of the eye. The cornerstone of treatment is prevention through treatment of abrasions with antimicrobial drops, early eyelid release, and vigilance to exposure trauma.

Pneumonia

Nosocomial pneumonia is the leading cause of death from hospital-acquired infections (Figures 12.40 and 12.41). The estimated prevalence of nosocomial pneumonia within the

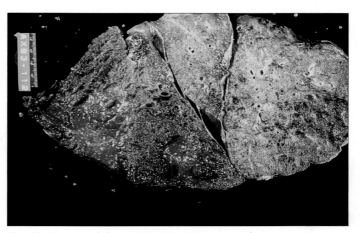

Fig. 12.41 Lower lobe pneumonia superimposed on a severe respiratory distress syndrome.

intensive care setting ranges from 10% to 65%, with fatality rates greater that 25% reported in most studies. Ventilator-associated pneumonia (VAP) specifically refers to pneumonia that develops more than 48 hours after intubation (late-onset VAP) in mechanically ventilated patients who had no clinical evidence suggesting the presence or likely development of pneumonia at the time of intubation. VAP that occurs within 48 hours of intubation is frequently the result of aspiration and usually yields a better prognosis than late-onset VAP, which is more often caused by antibiotic-resistant bacteria.

Pneumonia has two basic etiologies: direct contamination of the tracheobronchial tree via airborne or aspirated bacteria (having a better prognosis), and pneumonia spread hematogenously (Figure 12.42). Organisms cultured from pneumonia of burn patients often reflect the flora of the burn wound. In a

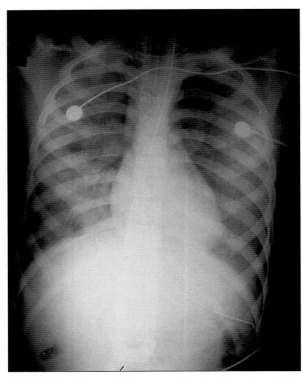

Fig. 12.42 This radiograph shows massive alveolar pneumonia. Although death by sepsis is declining in burn patients, respiratory infections are still a great concern, especially in patients with inhalation injury.

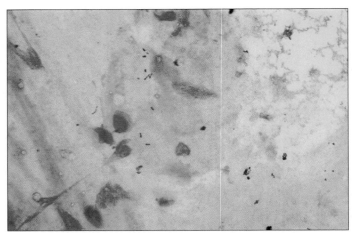

Fig. 12.43 Class III sputum with predominant Gram-positive organisms. The number of epithelial cells and neutrophils should be quantified under low power (×100) in order to maximize the diagnostic yield. Samples with more than 25 neutrophils and fewer than 10 epithelial cells contain minimal oropharyngeal contamination (Gram stain ×1000).

study by Ramzy et al., they attempted to establish the relationship of the burn wound flora to microbial pathogens in the tracheobronchial tree.[44] Management of hospital-acquired pneumonia is bolstered by surveillance quantitative wound cultures (QWC) and bronchial lavage fluid (BLF) cultures. In 30 (48%) of the 62 BLF cultures, there was a match between the organism identified in the BLF and the QWC. When strict quantitative criteria were applied, the match rate was only 9 (14%) of 62. Burn size and inhalation injury had no significant effect on match rate. Whereas the microbial pathogens were similar in the QWC and BLF, linear regression showed no value of QWC in predicting BLF culture results. The difference between qualitative and quantitative match rates suggests cross-colonization between the burn wound and tracheobronchial tree, but little to no cross-infection. The QWC and BLF cultures must be performed independently in determining antimicrobial specificity in the burned patient. This study supports the routine surveillance of the burn wound to help guide early thoughtful institution of antibiotics in a suspected pneumonia.

The diagnosis for pneumonia is often based upon clinical suspicion of infection coupled with the results of expectorated or aspirated sputum. Although these methods are readily available and often can be performed by a non-physician, the results can be misleading. If sputum expectoration is chosen, examination should include observation of the color, amount, consistency, and odor of the specimen. Mucopurulent sputum is most commonly found with bacterial pneumonia or bronchitis. Scant or watery sputum is more often noted in viral

and other atypical pneumonias. 'Rusty' sputum suggests alveolar involvement and has been most commonly associated with pneumococcal pneumonia. Dark red, mucoid sputum suggests Friedländer's pneumonia caused by encapsulated *Klebsiella pneumoniae*. Foul-smelling sputum is associated with mixed anaerobic infections most commonly seen with aspiration.[44]

Gram stain of the sputum should be ordered. In order to maximize the diagnostic yield of the sputum examination, only samples free of oropharyngeal contamination should be reviewed. As a guide, the number of neutrophils and epithelial cells should be quantitated under low power (× 100), with further examination reserved for samples containing >25 neutrophils and <10 epithelial cells. Such samples contain minimal oropharyngeal contamination. Samples with more epithelial cells and fewer neutrophils are nondiagnostic and should be disregarded. The sputum Gram stain is helpful to identify organisms other than the pneumococci. Small Gram-negative coccobacillary organisms are characteristics of *Haemophilus influenzae*. staphylococci appear as Gram-positive cocci in tetrads and grapelike clusters (Figure 12.43). Organisms of mixed morphology are characteristic of anaerobic infection. Few bacteria are seen with legionnaires' disease, mycoplasma, pneumonia and viral pneumonia.

Often the diagnosis of pulmonary infection rests with the quantitative bronchoalveolar lavage (BAL) or protected specimen brush (PSB) with a threshold of >10^4 organisms as evidence of pneumonia. The most important clinical practice is to set a unit standard and use this as a guide to treatment. In particular, to know the common pathogens in the unit as well as the surveillance wound culture of the patient and start antibiotic treatment broadly and timely. Then discontinue or narrow coverage when all the information is in.

Recently, several groups of investigators have demonstrated that mortality was greater among patients with VAP who were judged retrospectively to be receiving inadequate antibiotic therapy. These findings were based upon cultures of lower airway specimens obtained by either BAL, a PSB, or tracheal aspiration, than among patients receiving antibiotics to which the isolated bacteria were sensitive. More importantly, these studies also suggested that the increased risk or mortality persisted despite changes made to the initial antibiotic therapy after reviewing the findings from lower airway cultures.[45,46] These studies demonstrated an increased hospital mortality rate for patients who received inadequate antibiotic regimen initiated before obtaining the results of cultures, even if adjusted to cover the culture results when available. The study by Luna et al. found that subsequent changes in antibiotic therapy, based on the results of BAL fluid cultures, did not reduce the risk of hospital mortality in patients for whom inadequate antibiotic therapy was initially prescribed.[46,47]

The prevention of pneumonia can be minimized by meticulous aseptic tracheobronchial toiletry by use of effective gastric decompression to prevent emesis and aspiration during periods of ileus. Thus, it is important to limit endotracheal intubation to those patients with an absolute need for that intervention, as well as limit the duration as much as possible. Lung function should be monitored on a scheduled basis in all patients with extensive burns, particularly those with inhalation injury, with a low threshold for obtaining roentgenograms of the chest. When a pulmonary infiltrate characteristic of bronchopneumonia is identified on a chest roentgenogram, pulmonary physiotherapy and toilet should be intensified and antibiotic therapy begun with the agent showing greatest effectiveness against the predominant organism, as determined by the bacterial surveillance program if clinical infection is suspected.

Line infection

Infectious complications associated with intravenous and intra-arterial catheters represent a major problem irrespective of the constant attention to aseptic technique for insertion and appropriate maintenance.[48] The burned patient appears to be especially susceptible to this complication with catheter infection rates reported ranging from 8 to 57%.[49,50] Suppurative thrombophlebitis may be confirmed in up to 5% of patients hospitalized for burns over 20% TBSA.[51]

A prospective study documented a 50% correlation between organism cultured from the catheter tips and hubs within 48 hours of insertion and the incidence of catheter infection was inversely proportional to the distance of the insertion site from the burn wound.[52] It is interesting to note that the bacteria cultured from infected catheters could be traced to the skin in 96% of the cases. This data tend to support the hypothesis that catheter infections primarily arise from burn wound contaminants migrating down the catheter to the tip. Strict aseptic technique for insertion of intravascular catheters, the use of Teflon catheters, and rotation of the catheter site, tubing and apparatus every 72 hours have been related with a decrease in catheter infection rates.[53,54] There is currently still a debate regarding the effectiveness of antibiotic-coated catheters to reduce the number of line infections and to allow longer safe retention of a venous access point in the burn ICU. Further study is needed to elucidate the impact this technology may have on the management of intravenous access in the burn patient. It is recommended that each burn center adopt a line change protocol to standardize the management of access, and track the outcome.

Suppurative thrombophlebitis should be suspected in those patients who have persistent positive blood cultures without signs of local infection. Often suppuration can occur after the time of catheter removal so cultures at the time of removal may be an unreliable predictor of infection. Gross clinical signs of suppurative thrombophlebitis are frequently not present.[56] Careful records of previously cannulated sites can allow for sequential venotomy, examination for ultra luminal pus and histologic examination for intimal colonization. Upon confirmation of the diagnosis, immediate operative excision is essential to prevent progressive sepsis. Entire excision of a vein to the port of entry into the central circulation may be required because of the tendency of phlebitis to migrate to vein valves, leaving an apparently normal vein in between the infected foci. The subcutaneous tissue and skin should be packed open where a grossly purulent vein is removed and allowed to granulate and close by secondary intention (Figures 12.44 and 12.45).

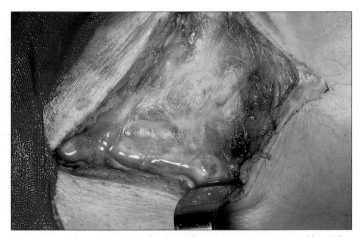

Fig. 12.44 Close-up view of infected intravenous site at ankle with suppurative thrombophlebitis. This patient with lower extremity IV access developed fever, leukocytosis, and erythema at the intravenous site.

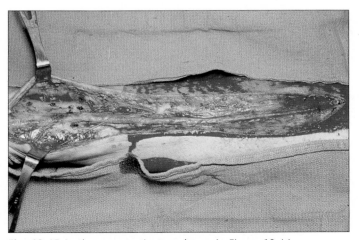

Fig. 12.45 In the same patient as shown in Figure 12.44, suppurative infection was noted along the length of vein. Proper treatment is total excision of vein from the site of infection to the point of entry into central circulation.

Urinary tract infections

Urinary tract infections are usually associated with prolonged and often unnecessary catheterization. Routine monitoring of urine from indwelling catheters should be done by needle aspirates through the rubber catheter with a 25-gauge needle on a regular basis two to three times a week. It is our practice not to use antimicrobial irrigations to prevent urinary tract infections, feeling that they are not particularly effective and may lead to infection by antibiotic-resistant organisms. When infection occurs, patients should be treated with appropriate systemic antibiotics. Candiduria is often insignificant but may reflect active infection or septicemia, especially when mycelia can be demonstrated. When present, an active infection with *Candida* species usually responds to low doses of amphotericin B, fluconazole or itraconazole.

Suppurative sinusitis

An infection of this type has become more obvious recently because of constant long-term transnasal intubation and the use of nasogastric or nasoduodenal tubes for enteral feeding. The diagnosis is usually delayed due to clinically inapparent symptoms and only after more frequent causes of fever are ruled out does it become evident. Diagnosis is confirmed based on X-rays or CT scans (Figure 12.46). Therapy with broad-spectrum antibiotics is initiated; however, surgical drainage of the involved sinuses may be necessary if the infection is unresponsive to the antibiotics. Oral intubation and nasogastric feeding may be utilized.

Subacute bacterial endocarditis

Bacteremia associated with burn wound manipulations, as well as procedures such as tooth extraction, endotracheal intubation and sigmoidoscopy, can be transient.[57,58] In healthy patients, transient bacterial showers are of little consequence. However, patients with a prior history of valvular heart disease are prone to the development of valvular vegetations. Burned patients, although usually young healthy adults prior to injury, develop a generalized immunosuppression and experience a significant number of invasive procedures which may increase the risk for endocarditis. The incidence of bacterial endocarditis appears to be increasing as we become more adept at treating major burn injuries. However, its development is usually occult and, like suppurative thrombophlebitis, frequently not noted until there are persistent positive blood cultures[51] (Figure 12.47).

Patients whose risk factor is high for the development of bacterial endocarditis are those with repetitive bacteremias, which may occur after continual instrumentation or surgical intervention. These patients should be closely monitored for the development of heart murmurs, and if found, should undergo echocardiography to determine the presence of vegetations. Blood cultures should be randomly taken for 72 hours, and then appropriate broad spectrum antibiotics initiated and continued for the next six weeks.

The abdomen

The abdomen as an infectious source in the burn patient can be a clinical challenge. Often in larger burns the abdomen is involved, which can lead to a perceived limitation in the clinical exam as compared to other similarly complex ICU patients. The defects in the overlying skin should not be allowed to interfere with a proper physical exam. Burn patients like all patients can get appendicitis, intussusception, bowel obstruction, etc. In addition, in the severe burn, peritoneal dialysis may be necessary to aid compromised renal function and potentially introduce another possible source for infection.

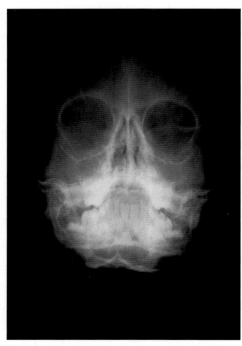

Fig. 12.46 Suppurative sinusitis after long-term intubation and tracheostomy. Note that the pneumatization of maxillary sinus has disappeared bilaterally.

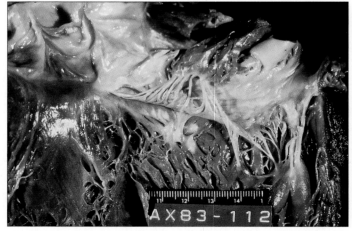

Fig. 12.47 Subacute endocarditis to the tricuspid valve. Repetitive septic showers and the microtrauma of placement of central lines and Swan-Ganz catheters put the burn patient at risk for this kind of complication.

Larger burns have episodes of hypoperfusion at times, leading to sloughing of intestinal mucosa. Heme-positive mucoid or watery stools, abdominal distension, and diminished bowel sounds often characterize this condition. Stool for reducing substances is usually positive. A patient with a very severe burn, often combined with sepsis can have critical ischemia to the gut as a result of global hypoperfusion and have progression to necrosis.

Clostridium difficile (*C.diff*) is a well-known entity in critically ill patients, especially those with a history of antibiotic use. With the ubiquitous emergence of methicillin-resistant staphylococcus, the intravenous use of vancomycin has increased to such a great degree as this may decrease our observed clinical incidence of *C.diff* diarrhea.

Necrotizing enterocolitis occurs in patients who are severely granulocytopenic from any cause. Left upper quadrant abdominal pain is usual. Irritation of the adjacent diaphragm may result in pain referred to the left shoulder. Splenic enlargement and tenderness are often present with high, spiking temperatures. Radiographic examination may reveal an elevated left hemidiaphragm, basilar pulmonary infiltrates, atelectasis, or a left pleural effusion. Shift of the colon and stomach down and to the right and extraintestinal gas, either diffusely mottled or producing an air–fluid level in the left upper quadrant, may also be seen. Ultrasonography, computed tomography, and MRI are the preferred diagnostic techniques for the evaluation of suspected splenic abscess. Initial antibiotic therapy should have a broad spectrum of activity. A combination of antibiotics that has activity against streptococci and both aerobic and anaerobic Gram-negative bacilli would be appropriate initial antimicrobial therapy.

Musculoskeletal infection

The burn patient with a large percent injury is very complex. It is possible to miss a muscular compartment syndrome. This will lead to necrosis and may become complicated by bacterial contamination and develop into a source. Diagnosis requires a high index of suspicion and liberal surgical exploration. Treatment is surgical drainage and removal of all dead tissue.

HIV and the burn patient

The world incidence of HIV infection is very common in many parts of the world. In sub-Saharan Africa, some countries have rates of 35–39% in the adult population. In the US although much less, a practice of burn care in a large city will likely have patients who are HIV infected. The HIV seems to have an additive effect on the immunosuppression of the burn as reflected in the CD4/CD8 cell counts. Graft survival is compromised greatly and infections are increased.[59]

The microbiology of burn wound infection

Selection, collection, and transport of specimens

There are several major benchmarks that must be adhered to in order to achieve reliable clinical microbiology results in its association with the thermal injury. Most important to effective microbiologic diagnosis is the appropriate selection, collection, and transport of specimens sent to the laboratory (see Table 12.3). Appropriate specimen management affects patient care in several significant ways:

- it is the key to accurate laboratory diagnosis that directly affects patient care and patient outcome;
- it influences therapeutic decisions;
- it affects hospital infection control, patient length of stay, and overall hospital costs;
- it plays a major role in laboratory costs, and influences laboratory efficiency.[60]

Before the specimen is collected for analysis, the specimen or the collection site must be selected and must represent a location of active disease. Even careful collection methods will produce a specimen of little clinical value if it is not obtained from a site where the infection is active. It must be noted that it is critical the specimen collectors know the appropriate device and collection of samples. (For specific details regarding specimen collection, it is suggested that the reader review the 8th edn. of the Manual of Clinical Microbiology, pages 55–66.[60]).

With burn wounds, it is particularly important to obtain a culture which is free from contamination from the normal flora that may be present on the surface of the injured skin. In addition, the size or amount of the specimen plays an essential role in the appropriate identification of the etiologic agent. The use of prophylactic antimicrobials, both topical and systemic, should also be noted so that appropriate inhibitors and sufficient dilutions can be prepared, or reagents added to void any effects of drug interactions. The specimen should be collected and placed in a sterile container with appropriate media for transport to the laboratory. All specimens must be promptly transported to the laboratory. To obtain optimal results, specimens should be examined immediately upon receipt in the laboratory.

TABLE 12.3 SPECIMEN SELECTION, COLLECTION, AND TRANSPORTATION GUIDELINES*

Avoid contamination from normal flora to ensure sample is representative of the infectious process
Select correct anatomic site from which to obtain the specimen
Collect adequate volumes; insufficient specimen quantities may yield false-negative results
Specimens *must* be placed in a container designed to promote survival of suspected agents and eliminate leakage and potential safety hazards
Specimens *must* be properly labeled with patient's name, identification number, source, site, date, time of collection, and initials of collector
Specimens must be promptly transported to the laboratory, preferably within 2 hours

*The information in this table is from reference 60.

Processing and presumptive examination of burn wound specimens

The first step in processing virtually all clinical material is microscopic examination. Direct examination is a rapid, cost-effective diagnostic aid. Methods for direct examination are aimed at identifying microorganisms and enumerating cells. Visible microorganisms may denote the presumptive etiologic agent, guiding the laboratory in selecting appropriate isolation media and the physician in selecting empirical antibiotic therapy. The quality of the specimen and the measure of the inflammatory response can also be evaluated. Cellular material and organisms are usually transparent and are best distinguished by the use of dyes or biological stains. The most useful and cost-effective of these stains is the Gram stain. It is the differential stain most commonly used for direct microscopic examination of specimens and bacterial colonies due to the technique having a broad staining spectrum. Since the beginning of its use in the late 19th century, the Gram stain has remained basically the same procedure and serves in dividing bacteria into two main groups: Gram-positive organisms, which retain the primary crystal violet dye and are deep blue to purple in appearance; and Gram-negative organisms, which can be decolorized, thereby losing the primary stain and subsequently taking up the counterstain safranin and appearing pink to red. The staining spectrum includes almost all bacteria, many fungi, and some parasites. The Gram reaction is used to aid in distinguishing microbial cellular characteristics, such as shape (e.g. cocci or bacilli/rod-shaped) and arrangement of the organisms. This provides clues to the preliminary identification and significance of organisms.[60]

The most reliable specimen for identification of infection in burn wounds is a tissue biopsy, which provides the best indicator of the potential pathogen in surgical sepsis. However, all specimens taken at the time of surgical intervention should be examined for the presence of potential pathogenic microorganisms. Tissue specimens should be homogenized or impression smears should be prepared, followed by microscopic examination as described above. Specimens should be inoculated to a variety of solid and liquid culture media. The liquid medium employed is generally an enriched thioglycolate medium (THIO) or brain heart infusion broth (BHIB), supplemented to facilitate the recovery of anaerobes as well as the aerobic pathogens.[60,61] Aliquots of the serial-diluted specimens are subsequently inoculated to sheep blood agar (SBA) containing phenylethyl alcohol (PEA), and MacConkey's agar (MAC). SBA is an enriched medium that contains nutrient supplements, allowing a wide variety of organisms to reproduce. The SBA with PEA is an enriched and selective medium, in that it will permit the growth of fastidious and slow-growing aerobic and anaerobic organisms from specimens containing mixed flora. MAC is a differential medium that allows for the presumptive identification of microbes based on the organism's appearance on the medium.

Each inoculated plated media should be incubated in the suspected organism's appropriate atmospheric conditions. Tissue specimens should be inoculated onto plated media, utilizing quantitative culture methods.[8,62] Quantitative cultures used in combination with histological examination provides for an indication of the predominant microorganism(s) in the burn wound, as well as the extent of the infectious process.[62]

Etiologic agents of burn wound infections

Burn wound infections are most commonly caused by bacteria, fungi, or viruses. However, bacteria cause the majority of infections in most burn care centers. Almost all burn wound infections caused by bacteria are due to aerobic microorganisms.[63] Microorganisms are transmitted from the patient's surroundings at the time of injury due to implantation or can be acquired endogenously from the patient or exogenously from hands of medical personnel, as well as fomites.[1,2] Table 12.4 describes the tissue associations of the microorganisms most often encountered in burn wound infections.

It is the design of the remaining portion of this section to describe some of the major distinguishing characteristics of the bacterial pathogens, as well as some of the fungi encountered in burn wound infection. A discussion of yeasts and viruses associated with burn injury can be found in the 'Clinical management strategies' section of this chapter.

Bacteria
Gram-positive organisms

Staphylococcus aureus is the most important cause of bacterial burn wound infections, and is well documented as a human opportunistic pathogen.[1,2,60] As a nosocomial pathogen, *S. aureus* had been a major cause of morbidity and mortality.[60] Most common infections where the etiologic agent *Staphylococcus* spp. are encountered and are considered pathognomonic are septicemia; cellulitis; impetigo; scalded skin syndrome; and postoperative wound infections. However, the most serious staphylococcal infections are puerperal sepsis; pneumonia; osteomyelitis; endocarditis; and burn wound infections. Staphylococcal pseudomembranous enterocolitis will occur most frequently as a complication of antibiotic therapy. In burn injury, the staphylococci are responsible for graft loss when the colony count of the graft bed is >10^5 CFUs per gram of tissue.[4]

Strains of *S. aureus* as well as other *Staphylococcus* species produce a wide variety of metabolites. Some are pathognomonic and also toxigenic, while those with minimal toxicity or no toxic effects at all are of some diagnostic significance. An array of byproducts such as proteinases, collegenases, and hyaluronidase digest the extracellular matrix, which serves as the structural integrity essential in wound healing.[1] Most of the human pathogens produce α- and β-lysins. Some exotoxins, which are produced by the pathogenic strains of staphylococci, include a pyrogenic toxin, a dermonecrotizing toxin, a lethal toxin, and leukocidin. These organisms can also produce an exotoxin, TSST-1 and enterotoxins A, B, and C which are risk factors for TSS in susceptible patients.[1] TSS was first described as such in 1978.[45] As previously mentioned in this chapter, the disease is characterized by sudden onset of fever, vomiting, diarrhea, shock, and a diffuse macular erythematous rash, followed by desquamation of the skin on the hand and feet as well as hyperemia of various mucous membranes. It has been our experience that although TSS is very uncommon, it can be a devastating complication of minor burns. A clinical lack of vigilance in the care of a child with TSS can lead to shock, organ failure, and death.

Another member of the *Staphylococcus* genus, *Staphylococcus epidermidis*, is a resident of human skin and mucous

TABLE 12.4 TISSUE ASSOCIATION OF MICROORGANISMS MOST COMMONLY FOUND IN BURN WOUND INFECTION*

Organism	Soft tissue skin	Upper respiratory tissue	Lower respiratory tissue	Endocardial	Gastrointestinal tissue	Urogenital tractc	Bone and joint
Staphylococcus aureus	NF, P	P, NF	P	P	P	NF, P	P
Staphylococcus epidermidis	NF, P	NF, P	P	P	P	NF, P	P
Other *Staphylococci* spp.	NF	NF, P	P	P	NF, P	NF, P	P
Streptococcus pyogenes	P, NF	P, NF	P	P	P	P	P
Other *Streptococci* spp.	NF	NF	P	P	NF	NF, P	P
Enterococcus spp.	P	P	P	P	NF, P	NF, P	P
Escherichia coli	NF, P	NF, P	P	P	NF, P	NF, P	P
Klebsiella pneumoniae	NF, P	NF, P	P	P	NF, P	NF, P	P
Enterobacter cloacae	NF, P	NF, P	P	P	NF, P	NF, P	P
Enterobacter aerogenes	NF, P	NF, P	P	P	NF, P	NF, P	P
Proteus spp.	NF, P	P	P	P	NF, P	NF, P	P
Serratia marcescens	NF, P	—	P	P	P	P	P
Other enterics	NF, P	NF, P	P	P	NF, P	P	P
Pseudomonas aeruginosa	P	NF, P	P	P	NF, P	P	P
Acinetobacter spp.	NF	NF	P	—	NF	NF	P
Candida albicans	NF	NF	P	P	NF	P,NF	P

*NF, normal flora; P, pathogens; — normally not found; however, these organisms should not be ignored when encountered.
Modified from Heggers J. Microbiology for surgeons. In: Kerstein MD, ed. Management of surgical infections. Mt Kisco, NY: Futura; 1980:27–55.

membranes and can also be associated with burn wound infection. *S. epidermidis* resembles *S. aureus* microscopically, and is tolerant of high NaCl concentrations as is *S. aureus*. However, it differs from *S. aureus* in that it is mannitol-, coagulase, and thermonuclease-negative. It is equally as pathogenic as *S. aureus*, and has been the principal etiologic agent in disease entities such as subacute bacterial endocarditis, infected surgical prosthesis, infections following bone marrow transplantation, or other states of immunosuppression such as in the thermal injury.

The streptococci are catalase-negative and produce a variety of hemolytic activity in the presence of blood. The types of hemolysis produced on SBA are frequently used as an initial means of identification for the streptococci. This hemolysis is considered a virulence factor, and quantitatively this group of organisms do not lend themselves to the standard rule of less than 10^5 for any tissue closure. The mere presence of a few β-hemolytic streptococci can cause a wound infection, failure of a primary closure, and loss of a skin graft. The major species that can be diagnosed with this particular type of hemolysis are *Streptococcus pyogenes*, β-hemolytic streptococci group

A and *S. agalactiae* β-hemolytic streptococci group B, just to mention a few. Presumptive identification of *S. pyogenes* can be made by sensitivity to bacitracin, since 90% of all *S. pyogenes* are sensitive to bacitracin.

The genus *Enterococcus* was established in 1984.[60] However, *Enterococcus faecalis* and *Enterococcus faecium* were the only two recognized species. Since that time, 12 additional species have been classified within the enterococci group.[60,65] The enterococci have become one of the most important causes of burn wound infection. This is likely due to widespread use of third-generation cephalosporins over the last decade to which enterococci are resistant. In 1986, burn wound sepsis caused by enterococci was diagnosed by recovery of at least 10^5 colony-forming units (CFUs)/g of tissue on burn wound biopsy or by recovery from blood cultures. Therefore, enterococci appear to be not only common but also virulent burn wound pathogens. The majority of the enterococci are frequently nonhemolytic, termed ?-hemolysis. However, there are some strains that produce a ?- or a-hemolysis on blood agar. All members of the enterococci group besides tolerating 6.5% NaCl and being bile esculin (BE)-positive are also pyrolidonylarylamidase (PYR)- and leucine aminopeptidase (LAP)-positive. The species are separated into three groups based on specific biochemical reactions. Group I does not hydrolyze arginine but forms acid in a manitol, sorbitol, and sorbose broth. The important species here is *Enterococcus avium*. Group II, on the other hand, hydrolyzes arginine and forms acid in mannitol and sorbitol only. The significant species in this group are *E. faecalis* and *E. faecium*. Group III, which includes *Enterococcus durans*, is negative for all tests described above.[60]

Gram-negative organisms

This family of Gram-negative rods contains a distinctive group of etiologic agents of burn wound infections. Of this group, the *Pseudomonas* species are most repeatedly encountered and are chronic or acute. Since 1960, *Pseudomonas aeruginosa* has been recognized as a major burn pathogen.[2,63,64] *Pseudomonas aeruginosa* is the second most common burn wound pathogen. *Pseudomonas* spp. have a worldwide distribution with a predilection for moist environments. Because of their ability to survive in aqueous environments, these organisms have become problematic in the hospital environment.[60] The spectrum of disease caused by this agent ranges from superficial skin infections to fulminant sepsis. *P. aeruginosa* is the leading cause of nosocomial respiratory tract infection. Patients receiving ventilatory assistance have a 20-fold higher likelihood of developing nosocomial pneumonia, with *P. aeruginosa* being the most frequently identified etiologic agent. Wound infections due to *P. aeruginosa* are particularly troublesome in burn patients. Although the incidence of such infections has declined in this patient population, the high rate of sepsis following these wound infections is responsible for significant mortality rates.[60]

Acinetobacter spp. are part of the indigenous flora of the respiratory, skin, as well as the gastrointestinal and genitourinary tracts of man and animals. They have been isolated from a diversity of clinical sources, including upper and lower respiratory tracts, urinary tract, surgical and burn wounds, and in bacteremias secondary to IV catheterization. Also occasional cases of septicemia or pneumonia have occurred in attenuated patients. Many of these patients who develop infections with this microorganism have had various manipulations including the use of respiratory therapy equipment, tracheal intubation, or bladder or central venous line catheterization. While an agent of low virulence, it has a predilection for infecting patients with dysfunctional host defense mechanisms. It develops a high degree of antimicrobial resistance. This resistance may be a direct result of previous antimicrobial therapy.

The largest and most repeatedly encountered group of microorganisms populating any burn wound environment along with the *Staphylococcus* spp. are the enterics, and they are found in the family of Enterobacteriaceae. This family contains 12 individual genera. Many of these organisms were previously categorized as non-pathogens and among these were the *Klebsiella-Enterobacter* group, *Serratia marcescens*, *Providencia* species, and *Erwinia* species.[3,6]

Eschericia coli, probably the most well-known enteric, has been responsible for a wide diversity of infectious processes. Among these are:

- frequently severe and sometimes fatal infections such as appendicitis, cystitis, pyelitis, peritonitis, septicemia, and gall bladder infections;
- surgical and burn wound sepsis, and epidemic diarrhea of children and adults; and
- 'travelers' diarrhea'.

E. coli can be identified from other members of Enterobacteriaceae by its response to the classical IMVIC (indole, methyl red, Voges-Proskauer and citrate) reaction.

The *Klebsiella-Enterobacter* group (*K-E*) are Gram-negative rods that are either motile or nonmotile. Fifty-one percent of moderately ill hospitalized patients had either *K. pneumoniae*, *Enterobacter aerogenes*, or *Enterobacter cloacae* isolated from their oropharyngeal space.[60,61,66] *K. pneumoniae* and its family are fast becoming a regular pathogen in nosocomial infections.[60,66] It is interesting that earlier isolation of the *K-E* group flora was thought to be part of the normal flora of the bronchial tree. The tribe *Klebsiella* is currently composed of the genera *Klebsiella*, *Enterobacter*, and *Serratia*.

The remaining enterics consist of three additional genera: *Proteus*, *Providencia*, and *Morganella*. The genus *Proteus* is composed of two species: *P. mirabilis* and *P. vulgaris*. Both species can be found in massive concentrations in the feces of individuals undergoing oral antibiotic therapy. This group of organisms are often accountable for surgical and burn wound infections, intra-abdominal infections, as well as bacteremias and urinary tract infections. The genus *Providencia* is composed of three species: *Providencia alcalifaciens*, *Providencia stuartii*, and *Providencia rettgeri*, which were formerly in the genus *Proteus*. *Providencia* species, like *S. marcescens*, have a broad range of pathologic involvement, from nosocomial infections to septicemias, postoperative incisional wounds, burn wounds, pneumonias, and urinary tract infections.[60,61] *P. stuartii* has been incriminated in numerous infections of patients in a burn unit, to include urinary tract infections as well.

Morganella morganii is the only species in the genus *Morganella* and was considered earlier a member of the genus *Proteus*. *M. Morganii* has been co-joined with wound infections as well as urinary tract infections.

Like the Gram-positive clinical isolates, the Gram-negative isolates from the burn wound are equally selective. While man's environment is overwhelmed with microbes, only a select smattering of Gram-negative rods predominate, which specifically includes the pseudomonads and enterics; with *P. aeruginosa* being the predominant isolate, followed by *E. coli* and the other enterics. In comparing the Gram-negative isolates for 1999 with those identified in a 1988–1989 study, we observed an increase in the number of *P. aeruginosa* isolates (53.4%) over 1988–1989 (33.6%), almost a 20% increase. Another interesting observation was the appearance of *Acinetobacter baumannii/haemolyticus*, accounting for 46.8% of the nonfermentors and, combined with *P. aeruginosa*, accounting for 53.4% of the total Gram-negative isolates. This appearance of *Acinetobacter* spp., in the ICU setting was experienced worldwide.

Anaerobes

The most repeatedly confronted organisms in this group, which may play a fearful role in surgical and burn wound infections, are *Bacteroides* spp. and *Fusobacterium* spp. They are considered normal flora of the human body, beginning at the oropharyngeal cavity and ending at the gastrointestinal (GI) and urogenital tracts. Numerically they account for the major population in the oropharyngeal region in a 5:1 ratio over the aerobes and facultative anaerobes, while in the urogenital and GI tract the ratio is more dynamic at a 1000:1.[60,61] Yet when one scrutinizes the current statistics of anaerobic infections related to locality, all but 2–5% of surgical wound infections occurring in the oropharyngeal area are caused by the anaerobic flora.[66,67] Those occurring in the GI and urogenital tract are only responsible for about 10–15% of the wound infections.[45,65] Prior surgery, malignant neoplasms, arteriosclerosis, diabetes mellitus, prior antibiotic therapy, alcoholism, improper debridement, and steroid and immunosuppressive therapy are commonly major contributors associated in these types of wound infections.[45,66] Specimens collected for anaerobic organisms should be placed in appropriate transport tubes void of atmospheric O_2 or remain in syringes with attached needles containing suspect aspirates sealed off with a rubber stopper. However, with the advent of the early excision and grafting, the incidence of anaerobic infections in the thermal injury has been significantly reduced; therefore, anaerobic cultures are uneconomical. Culturing for these anaerobes would be futile, as they require vascular tissue for survival. Their presence would only be observed if such tissue were to remain.

Anaerobic infections in burned patients are usually associated with avascular muscle found in electrical injuries, frost bite, or cutaneous flame burns with concomitant crush-type injuries.[63]

Fungi

Until the advent of topical antimicrobial agents, fungal infections were not common in burned patients. However, the incidence of mycotic invasion has doubled since the implementation of topical antimicrobial agents to control bacterial colonization.[69] The burn wound is the most commonly infected site, although local or disseminated fungal infections of the respiratory tract, urinary tract, GI tract, and vagina are increasingly common.[68,69]

Fungi are generally isolated through the inoculation of both non-selective and selective culture media. The most commonly used non-selective media includes inhibitory mold agar and Sabouraud Dextrose Brain Heart Infusion (SABHI™) agar, which permit the enhanced growth of almost all fungi, including some of the more fastidious and slowly growing fungi. The most commonly utilized selective media include those containing antimicrobial agents such as penicillin (20 U/mL) plus streptomycin (40 U/mL) or gentamicin (5 μg/mL) plus chloramphenicol (16 μg/mL) to inhibit growth of bacteria. Media containing cycloheximide (0.5 μg/mL) may also be utilized to inhibit growth of rapidly growing molds that often overgrow slower-growing dimorphic fungi; however, a medium without cycloheximide should also be used, because this agent can inhibit the growth of some medically important fungi (e.g. *Cryptococcus neoformans* and *Aspergillus fumigatus*). Additionally, Sabouraud's dextrose or potato dextrose agar is used to allow for identification of fungi through their sporulation characteristics. Yeasts are identified on the basis

of specific biochemical tests, whereas identification of molds is based on growth rate, colony structure, microscopic appearance, dimorphism at different incubation temperatures, inhibition of growth by cycloheximide, and a few biochemical tests.[66]

Candida spp. are the most common non-bacterial colonizers of the burn wound, although true fungi such as *Aspergillus*, *Penicillium*, *Rhizopus*, *Mucor*, *Rhizomucor*, *Fusarium*, and *Curvularia* are not uncommon and have a much greater invasive potential than the yeasts.[67,69]

Early diagnosis of fungal infection is difficult as clinical symptoms frequently mimic low-grade bacterial infections. Routine culture techniques may require from 7 to 14 days to identify fungal contaminants, delaying the initiation of treatment as these pathogens are frequently not recovered in culture.[67] In contrast to bacterial sepsis, venous blood cultures may not reflect the causative organism.[36] Arterial blood cultures and retinal examination for characteristic candidal lesions can be useful.

Unlike candidal infections, true fungal infections occur early in the hospital course of patients with specific predisposing characteristics. Most frequently, burned patients infected with molds are exposed to spores in the environment by either rolling on the ground or jumping into surface water at the time of injury. Other environmental foci have been cited as the source of nosocomial fungal infection, including bandaging supplies left open to air, heating, and air conditioning ducts and floor drains.[67,69] Once colonized, broad non-branching hyphae extend into subcutaneous tissue, stimulating an inflammatory response. This phenomenon is diagnostic of fungal wound infection. Vascular invasion is common and often accompanied by thrombosis and avascular necrosis, clinically observed as rapidly advancing dark discolorations of the wound margins or well-described lesions.[36] Systemic dissemination of the infection occurs with invasion of the vasculature.

Pharmacodynamics and kinetics in the burn patient

Pharmacotherapy in the control of infection in a burn patient presents many challenges for the clinician. The normal course of burn trauma effects pathophysiologic changes in the cardiovascular, renal, metabolic, hepatic, gastrointestinal, epidermal and immunological responses which changes the patient's pharmacodynamic and pharmacokinetic state.[71]

The acute or resuscitative phase

In the acute or resuscitative phase of the burn trauma which occurs within the first 48–72 hours post-burn, cardiovascular factors produce hypovolemia with decreased blood flow to organs and tissues.[71] Intravenous drug treatments during this phase will result in a slower rate of distribution and elimination through the kidneys. The burn patient will also exhibit delayed absorption of enteral, subcutaneous, and intramuscular drugs. Pharmacotherapy regimens during this acute phase will result in delayed onset of action and peak concentrations.

The hypermetabolic phase

The hypermetabolic response phase mediated by greatly increased levels of catecholamines, prostaglandins, glucagons, and cortisol occurs after the acute phase and also produces pathophysiologic changes. The burn patient will exhibit increased blood flow to organs and tissues, an increased internal core temperature and hypoproteinemia and edema formation.[71]

Intravenous drugs will have an increased onset of action due to the increased rate of distribution.[71] These drugs will also have a shorter half-life due to the enhanced glomerular filtration rate and elimination of renally excreted drugs. The antibiotic treatment of these patients requires higher doses for these drugs and perhaps a shorter dosing interval. The burn patient's antibiotic drug doses are similar to those higher doses used to treat cystic fibrosis patients. Renally excreted antibiotics such as vancomycin that are time-dependent in their ability to kill Gram-positive bacteria must be carefully monitored to ensure that they are meeting the minimum inhibitory concentration of the bacteria in the serum. Oral drugs will also exhibit an increased absorption from the GI tract and increased onset of action.[71]

The hypermetabolic phase will produce decreased levels of albumin and increased levels of acute-phase proteins.[71] Albumin binds to acidic and neutral drugs such as aminoglycosides, vancomycin, aztreonam, and cefotetan. These drugs will be tightly bound and there will be less free drug in the blood and a decreased volume of distribution. Higher drug dosages may be necessary to produce a therapeutic effect.

The hepatic response in the hypermetabolic phase will present as a decrease in phase I metabolism such as oxidation, reduction, or hydoxylation of a drug by the cytochrome P-450 system. This will affect the metabolism of many antibiotics such as the quinolones and the macrolides. The decreased activity of these hepatic drug-metabolizing enzymes as well as the decreased hepatic clearance and prolonged half-life may produce systemic toxicity. Phase II metabolism in the liver such as conjugation reactions between the drug and endogenous substrate will not be impaired.

The gastrointestinal response during the hypermetabolic phase results in increased proton secretion. It is reported that erosion of the stomach lining and duodenum occurs in 86% of adult patients within 72 hours post-injury and 40% had GI bleeding.[71] In children, the incidence of stress ulceration is twice that of adults.[71] Erosion of the stomach lining and duodenum allows the transmigration of GI bacteria from the gut into the body's bloodstream. The use of antacids, H-2 antagonists, and proton-pump inhibitors may actually permit the proliferation of bacteria that is not normally present in the gut. Transmigration of these bacteria may be found in other parts of the body such as the lungs, heart, and intestinal tract.

Diffusion resistance to water movement through burn skin is less than 1/10 that of normal skin. The burn patient will experience increased drug loss and drug absorption. This is a factor that must be weighed in the appropriate use of topical antimicrobials. Fick's law of diffusion describes the decreased resistance in burn patients:[71]

$$F = DAK/t \times (C_2 - C_1)$$

F = flux
D = diffusion coefficient
A = area
K = oil–water partition coefficient
t = thickness of the stratum corneum
C_2 = drug concentration in the vehicle
C_1 = concentration across the stratum corneum.

Other factors that affect drug absorption are the degree of hydration of the stratus corneum, the temperature, the pH of the drug, and the molecular characteristics of the drug.

Finally, the immunological response will exhibit major changes in the hypermetabolic phase. The burn patient suffers damage to the epidermis of the skin. The depression in this, the first line of defense, allows systemic microbial invasion. However, there is also depression in the second line of defense with a burn size-related depression of both cellular and humoral aspects of the immune response and phagocytic activity of fixed and bloodborne mancrophages and neutrophils. The patient suffers a release of chemical mediators, including prostaglandins, serotonin, thromboxanes, and leukotrienes which mount an inflammatory response. The patient will require a strong but specific pharmacotherapeutic regimen of antibiotics to protect the body against invasion.

Antimicrobial pharmacokinetic and pharmacodynamic parameters

The clinician should also understand key pharmacokinetic and pharmacodynamic parameters to most effectively use antibiotics in the treatment of infection. Pharmacokinetic parameters describe the action of the body on the drug. The drug is absorbed, distributed, metabolized, and eliminated by the body. Pharmacodynamic parameters describe the action of the drug on the body. They describe the relationship between drug concentration and the pharmacologic effect. They describe how an antibiotic produces its antimicrobial effects on the microbe as well as any other effects it may produce on the body. We want an antibiotic to approach the ideal pharmacokinetic parameters of 100% absorption, distribution to the site of infection, metabolism to inactive compounds, and elimination from the body. The drug should also achieve ideal pharmacodynamic parameters of a concentration in the body that is sufficient to effectively kill bacteria and maintain that effective killing concentration for a time period needed to keep the bacteria from regrowth. The pharmacodynamic parameter that describes the concentration that will effectively kill the microbe *in vitro* is the minimum inhibitory concentration or MIC while the minimum bacteriological concentration or MBC describes the concentration that will effectively kill the microbe *in vivo* and produce a clinical cure.

In order to optimize antimicrobial therapy, the clinician must also understand whether the antibiotic he has chosen produces its antimicrobial activity in a concentration dependent or independent manner, the tissue penetration of the antibiotic, whether the antibiotic is bactericidal or bacteriostatic, synergy between antibiotic agents, drug elimination dosing limitations, duration of therapy, and the use of IV versus oral therapy.

If an antimicrobial agent produces its activity in a concentration-dependent manner, it must reach the effective MBC in order to kill the microbe by producing a peak concentration that is generally about 8–10 times the MIC ($Conc_{max}$/MIC). Concentration-dependent antimicrobial agents include the aminoglycosides and metronidazole.

The relationship between an antibiotic's 24-hour area under the curve concentration divided by the MIC of a drug (AUC_{24}/MIC) describes the total exposure of the microbe to an antibiotic. This pharmacodynamic parameter best describes the efficacy of certain antibiotics such as fluoroquinolones (ciprofloxacin and levofloxacin), the ketolides and azithromycin to produce their antimicrobial effect. This parameter may be >100 for ciprofloxacin in the effective treatment of *P. aeruginosa* infections.[106]

If an antimicrobial agent produces its activity in a concentration-independent or time-dependent manner, it must maintain a concentration at least 1–2 times the MIC for the entire period between dosing intervals in order to kill the microbe and prevent its regrowth (T > MIC). Time-dependent antimicrobial agents include the β-lactam antibiotics, erythromycin, clarithromycin, the oxazolidinones, vancomycin and clindamycin.

Time-dependent antibiotics are sometimes given as continuous IV infusions to ensure that the MIC is maintained in the serum. This tactic is sometimes used in immunocompromised patients to good effect.

Tissue penetration is necessary to produce antimicrobial effect. Antibiotics that are effective against a microorganism *in vitro* but unable to reach the site of infection are of little or no benefit to the host. Antibiotic tissue penetration depends on the chemical properties of the antibiotic (e.g. lipid solubility, molecular size) and tissue (e.g. adequate blood supply, presence of inflammation). However, antibiotic tissue penetration is rarely problematic in acute infections due to increased microvascular permeability from local release of chemical inflammatory mediators. In contrast chronic infections and infections caused by intracellular pathogens often rely on the aforementioned chemical properties of an antibiotic for adequate tissue penetration. Burn wound infections are especially problematic because of the localization of infection at a poorly perfused wound site. Antibiotics cannot be expected to eradicate organisms from areas that are difficult to penetrate or have impaired blood supply, such as necrotic burn tissue, which usually require surgical excision for cure.

Antibiotics may be bacteriostatic or bactericidal. For most infections, bacteriostatic and bactericidal antibiotics inhibit/kill organisms at the same rate, and should not be a factor in antibiotic selection. Bactericidal antibiotics have an advantage in certain infections such as endocarditis, meningitis, and febrile leukopenia but there are exceptions even in these cases.

Combination therapy may be useful for drug synergy or for extending the antimicrobial spectrum from what can be obtained with a single drug. However, since drug synergy is difficult to assess and the possibility of antagonism always exists, antibiotics should be combined for synergy only if synergy is based on experience or actual testing. Synergy studies for bacterial isolates that are resistant to all or most antibiotics is especially necessary to ensure that these resistant bacterial organisms are treated appropriately.

Intravenous antibiotic therapy is preferred when a patient is first admitted to the hospital because IV therapy ensures 100% availability of the drug in the body. However, if an antibiotic is well absorbed orally then the advantages of such treatment include reduced cost, early hospital discharge, and virtual elimination of IV line infections. Drugs well suited for IV to PO switch or for treatment entirely by the oral route include doxycycline, minocycline, clindamycin, metronidazole, chloramphenicol, amoxicillin, trimethoprim/sulfamethoxazole, quinolones, and linezolid.[107]

Usual antibiotic dosing assumes normal renal and hepatic function. Patients with significant renal insufficiency and/or hepatic dysfunction may require dosage reduction in antibiotics metabolized/eliminated by these organs.

Since most antibiotics eliminated by the kidneys have a wide 'toxic-to-therapeutic ratio', dosing strategies are frequently based on formula-derived estimates of creatinine clearance (CrCl), rather than precise quantization of glomerular filtration rates. Dosage adjustments are especially important for antibiotics with narrow 'toxic-to-therapeutic' ratios (e.g. aminoglycosides), and for patients who are receiving other nephrotoxic medications or have pre-existing renal disease. For patients with renal insufficiency receiving drugs eliminated by the kidneys, the loading dose (if required) is left unchanged, and the maintenance dose and dosing interval are modified in proportion to the degree of renal insufficiency. For moderate renal insufficiency (CrCl ~ 40–60 mL/min), the maintenance dose is usually cut in half and the dosing interval is left unchanged.[107] For severe renal insufficiency (CrCl ~ 10–40 mL/min) the maintenance dose is usually cut in half and the dosing interval is doubled.[107] Dosing adjustments in renal insufficiency can be circumvented by selecting an antibiotic with a similar spectrum that is eliminated by the hepatic route.

Antibiotic dosing for patients with hepatic dysfunction is problematic since there is no hepatic counterpart to the serum creatinine to accurately assess liver function. In practice, antibiotic dosing is based on clinical assessment of the severity of liver disease, For practical purposes, dosing adjustments are usually not required for mild to moderate hepatic insufficiency. For severe hepatic insufficiency, dosing adjustments are usually made for antibiotics with hepatotoxic potential.[107] Relatively few antibiotics depend solely on hepatic inactivation/elimination, and dosing adjustment problems can be circumvented by selecting an appropriate antibiotic eliminated by the renal route.

There are no good dosing adjustment guidelines for patients with hepatorenal insufficiency. If renal insufficiency is worse than hepatic insufficiency, antibiotics eliminated by the liver are often administered at half the total daily dose. If hepatic insufficiency is worse than renal insufficiency, antibiotics eliminated by the kidneys are usually administered and dosed in proportion to renal function.

Most bacterial infections in normal hosts are treated with antibiotics for 1–2 weeks. However, the duration of therapy may have to be extended in burn patients with impaired immunity and because these patients must undergo numerous surgical procedures to excise and graft burn wounds.

Pharmacological considerations in the treatment of burn infections

The major role of an antibiotic is to help the body eliminate an agent of infection in a burn patient. The treatment of an infection is often begun based on empiric knowledge of the most common types of microbial infections seen in the burn population and the antimicrobial agents that are most efficacious in their treatment. The appropriate choice of an antibiotic to treat an infection, however, should always be based on wound cultures and sensitivities that specifically identify the infecting organism, the colony counts, and the sensitivity of that organism to specific antibiotics. Pathology studies of wound biopsies give us information on how invasive the infecting organism is in the body. A pharmacotherapeutic regimen of antibiotics should follow known parameters about specific burn wound infections in order to potentiate each antibiotic agent's mechanism of action and pharmacokinetics while decreasing its side effects and systemic toxicities.

Gram-positive bacterial infections

The three most common Gram-positive organisms responsible for burn wound infections are the streptococci, staphylococci, and enterococci.

Streptococcal infections

β-hemolytic streptococci of group A or B (*S. pyogenes or S. agalactiae*) are most commonly seen in the first 72 hours postburn. Cellulitis may develop due to streptococcal infections and usually responds to treatment with natural penicillins or first-generation cephalosporins.

The natural penicillins, which consist of penicillin G and penicillin V, and the first-generation cephalosporins are bactericidal in action. Like many other β-lactam antibiotics, the antibacterial action results from inhibition of mucopeptide synthesis in the bacterial cell wall. Resistance to these antibiotics is caused by the production of β-lactamases and/or intrinsic resistance.[72] β-lactamase enzymes inactivate these antibiotics by hydrolyzing their β-lactam ring. Intrinsic resistance can result from the presence of a permeability barrier in the outer membrane of an infecting organism or alteration in the properties of target enzymes (penicillin-binding proteins).

Should resistance or tolerance to the natural penicillins or first-generation cephalosporins develop, then culture and sensitivity data should be utilized to appropriately treat the streptococcal infection. Please see Table 12.5 to review dosing and administration parameters.

Staphylococcal infections

Staphylococcus aureus and *Staphylococcus epidermidis* are natural pathogens found on skin and therefore are the most common cause of infections in burn populations. These microbes generally produce penicillinases which break the penicillin β-lactam ring and make natural pencillins ineffective against these bacteria.

These types of infections were treated by penicillinase-resistant penicillins that were termed 'methicillin sensitive.' These antibiotics included the parenteral antibiotics, nafcillin, methicillin, and oxacillin, and the oral antibiotics, cloxacillin, dicloxacillin, nafcillin, and oxacillin. The penicillinase-resistant penicillins have a mechanism of action that is similar to other penicillins. They interfere with bacterial cell wall synthesis during active multiplication by binding to one or more of the penicillin-binding proteins. They inhibit the final transpeptidation step of peptidoglycan synthesis causing cell wall death and resultant bactericidal activity against susceptible bacteria. However, the staphylococcal bacteria resistance pattern has become such that these penicillinase-resistant penicillin are no longer very effective against these organisms. In 2005, only 31% of *S. aureus* burn wound isolates at the Shriners Burns Hospital, Galveston, Texas (SBH-G) were sensitive to oxacillin and none of the *S. epidermidis* and *S. haemolyticus* isolates were sensitive to oxacillin. The staphylococcal infections that are resistant to penicillinase-resistant penicillins are termed MRSA (methicillin-resistant *Staphylococcus aureus*) or MRSE (methicillin-resistant *Staphylococcus epidermidis*).

Vancomycin alone or in conjunction with other anti-infectives has generally been considered the treatment of choice for infections caused by methicillin-resistant staphylococci. In 2005, 100% of all staphylococcal isolates were susceptible to vancomycin at SBH-G. Vancomycin is bactericidal and appears to bind to the bacterial cell wall, causing blockage of glycopeptide polymerization. This effect, which occurs at a site different from that affected by the penicillins, produces immediate inhibition of cell wall synthesis and secondary damage to the cytoplasmic membrane.[72] However, vancomycin is a time-dependent antimicrobial which requires that the serum level of this drug must remain at all times above the minimum inhibitory concentration (MIC) in order to provide adequate bactericidal activity.

The hypermetabolic burn patient exhibits an increased glomerular filtration rate and increased excretion of the renally cleared drug, vancomycin. Because of the wide interpatient variability of vancomycin elimination in a burn patient, the dosage must be individualized in order to provide an optimal time-dependent serum concentration. The effective peak and trough levels are derived from the MIC for a particular bacterial organism. The therapeutic peak level is approximately equivalent to 5–8 times the MIC and the trough concentration is equivalent to 1–2 times the MIC. The so-called therapeutic range most often quoted for vancomycin monitoring is peak levels of 30–40 μg/mL and trough levels of 5–10 μg/mL. Because vancomycin is a concentration-independent, or time-dependent, antibiotic and because there are practical issues associated with determining a precise peak serum concentration with this multi-compartment antibiotic, most clinicians have abandoned the routine practice of determining peak serum concentrations.

The overall AUC/MIC value may be the pharmacodynamic parameter that best correlates with a successful outcome associated with the use of vancomycin, Prolonged exposure to serum levels close to the MIC are associated with the emer-

TABLE 12.5

Antibiotic (check references for neonatal dose)	Pediatric dose (do not exceed adult dose)	Adult dose	Frequency	Route	Rate of IV admin
Acyclovir PO	10 mg/kg/dose	10 mg/kg/dose	5 times a day	PO	
Acyclovir IV	10 mg/kg/dose	10 mg/kg/dose	Q8h	IVPB	60 minutes
Amikacin IV	7.5 mg/kg/dose	5 mg/kg/dose	Q8h	IVPB	30 minutes
Amoxicillin PO	8–16 mg/kg/dose	250–500 mg	Q8h	PO	
Ampicillin PO	25–50 mg/kg/dose	250–500 mg	Q6h	PO	
Ampicillin IV	25–33 mg/kg/dose	1–2 g	Q4h	IVPB	30 minutes
Amphotericin IV	0.5 mg/kg/dose	50 mg	Q24h	IVPB	4–6 hours
Augmentin (amoxicillin/clavulanate) PO	7–14 mg/kg/dose	250–500 mg	Q8–12h	PO	
Aztreonam IV	50 mg/kg/dose	2 g	Q6h	IVPB	30 minutes
Caspofungin IV (Cancidas®)	70 mg/m^2/day × 1 day then 50 mg/m^2/day	70 mg × 1 day then 50 mg	Q24h	IVPB	60 minutes
Cefazolin IV	16–33 mg/kg/dose	2 g	Q8h	IVPB	30 minutes
Cefepime IV	50 mg/kg/dose	2 g	Q8h	IVPB	30 minutes
Cefoperazone IV	50 mg/kg/dose	2 g	Q8–12h	IVPB	30 minutes
Cefotaxime IV	50 mg/kg/dose	2 g	Q6–8h	IVPB	30 minutes
Cefotetan IV	20–40 mg/kg/dose	2 g	Q12h	IVPB	30 minutes
Ceftazidime IV	50 mg/kg/dose	2 g	Q8h	IVPB	30 minutes
Ceftriaxone IV	50 mg/kg/dose	2 g	Q12h	IVPB	30 minutes
Cefuroxime PO	10 mg/kg/dose	250–500 mg	Q12h	PO	
Cefuroxime IV	25–50 mg/kg/dose	750–1500 mg	Q8h	IVPB	30 minutes
Cephalexin PO	6–25 mg/kg/dose	250–500 mg	Q6h	PO	
Chloramphenicol PO or IV	12.5–25 mg/kg/dose	250 mg	Q6h	PO or IVPB	30 minutes
Ciprofloxacin PO	10–15 mg/kg/dose	250–750 mg	Q12h	PO	
Ciprofloxacin IV	7.5–10 mg/kg/dose	200–400 mg	Q12h	IVPB	60 minutes
Clindamycin PO	5–7.5 mg/kg/dose	150–450 mg	Q6–8h	PO	
Clindamycin IV	8–10 mg/kg/dose	300–900 mg	Q6–8h	IVPB	30 minutes
Co-trimoxazole PO (Bactrim ®)	5 mg TMP/kg/dose	80–160 mg TMP	Q12h	PO	
Co-trimoxazole IV (Bactrim ®)	5 mg TMP/kg/dose	80 mg TMP	Q6–8h	IVPB	60–90 minutes
Dicloxacillin PO	6.25–12.5 mg/kg/dose	125–500 mg	Q6h	PO	
Erythromycin PO	10 mg/kg/dose	250–500 mg	Q6h	PO	
Fluconazole PO or IV	3–6 mg/kg/dose	100–200 mg	Q24h	PO or IVPB	60 minutes
Ganciclovir IV	5 mg /kg/dose	5 mg/kg/dose	Q12h	IVPB	60–120 minutes
Imipenem/cilastatin IV	<12 yrs 18.75 mg/ kg/dose ≥12 yrs 12.5 mg/kg/dose	500–1000 mg	Q6h	IVPB	30 minutes
Itraconazole PO	3–10 mg/kg/dose	200 mg	Q24h	PO	
Levofloxacin PO or IV	10 mg/kg/dose	250–500 mg	Q24h	PO or IVPB	60 minutes

TABLE 12.5—cont'd

Antibiotic (check references for neonatal dose)	Pediatric dose (do not exceed adult dose)	Adult dose	Frequency	Route	Rate of IV admin
Linezolid (Zyvox®) IV or PO	10 mg/kg/dose Q8h	600 mg Q12h	Q8–12h	PO or IV	30–120 minutes
Mebendazole PO	100 mg	100 mg	Q12h × 3 days	PO	
Metronidazole PO or IV	10–15 mg/kg/dose	250–750 mg	Q8h	PO or IVPB	60 minutes
Nafcillin IV	12.5–50 mg/kg/dose	250–1000 mg	Q4–6h	IVPB	30 minutes
Penicillin G IV	50 000–100 000 U/kg/dose	1–2 million U	Q4–6h	IVPB	30 minutes
Penicillin VK PO	8–12.5 mg/kg/dose	125–500 mg	Q6–8h	PO	
Piperacillin IV	50 mg/kg/dose	2–4 g	Q4–8h	IVPB	30 minutes
Quinupristin/dalfopristin (Synercid®) IV	7.5 mg/kg/dose	500 mg	Q8h	IVPB	60 minutes
Rifampin PO	10 mg/kg/dose	300 mg	Q12h	PO	
Timentin (ticarcillin/ clavulanate) IV	50 mg/kg/dose	3.1 g	Q4–6h	IVPB	30 minutes
Unasyn (ampicillin/ sulbactam) IV	50–100 mg/kg/dose	1.5–3 g	Q6h	IVPB	30 minutes
Vancomycin IV	10–15 mg/kg/dose	500 mg	Q6h	IVPB	60 minutes
Voriconazole IV or PO	6 mg/kg/dose × 2 doses then 4 mg/kg/dose	400 mg × 2 doses then 200 mg	Q12h	IVPB or PO	60 minutes
Zosyn (piperacillin/tazobactam) IV	50–100 mg/kg/dose	3.375 gm	Q6h	IVPB	30 minutes

gence of resistance; therefore it is important to maintain adequate serum concentrations in patients with fast or rapidly changing creatinine clearance such as burn patients. There are also certain body compartments in which penetration is poor, such as the lung and the CNS. It would, also, seem prudent to keep concentrations from being suboptimal in patients with pneumonia or meningitis, as well as in patients receiving dialysis for renal failure. The American Thoracic Society recently published guidelines for hospital-acquired, ventilator-associated, and healthcare-associated pneumonia. These guidelines recommend vancomycin trough concentrations of 15–20 μg/mL for the treatment of methicillin-resistant *Staphylococcus aureus* pneumonia.[74] These higher concentrations may be needed for sequestered infections or in situations where vancomycin penetration has been documented to be poor. Some clinicians recommend that these higher concentrations of vancomycin may be necessary in the treatment of staphylococcal infections as well. Recent testing has shown 'vancomycin MIC creep' that may necessitate higher vancomycin trough serum concentrations to eradicate these microorganisms in burn wound infections.[74]

Vancomycin is derived from *Streptomyces orientalis* bacteria and used to be termed 'Mississippi Mud' because of the brown color of the unpurified product. These protein impurities are thought to have caused the ototoxicity and nephrotoxicity that was observed with the earlier products in the 1950s. However, when newer, purer preparations were retested in the 1970s, they produced no ototoxicity and little nephrotoxicity in the animal models, unless given in combination with ami-

noglycosides.[74] In one of the largest investigations to date, Pestotnik et al. reported that the incidence of nephrotoxicity among 1750 patients was 1.4%.[74] However, in the burn patient, vancomycin is often used not only in combination with other ototoxic and nephrotoxic agents such as aminoglycosides, the loop diuretic, furosemide and the antifungal drug, amphotericin. Nephrotoxicity is manifested by transient elevations in the serum blood urea nitrogen (BUN) or serum creatinine and decreases in the glomerular filtration rate and creatinine clearance. Hyaline and granular casts and albumin may also be found in the urine.

Vancomycin is administered only by slow intravenous infusion for at least 1 hour. Although, vancomycin injection is much purer it may still cause an anaphylactoid reaction known as 'red man's syndrome' or 'red neck syndrome.' This reaction is characterized by a sudden decrease in blood pressure which can be severe and may be accompanied by flushing and/or a maculopapular or erythematous rash on the face, neck, chest, and upper extremities; the latter manifestation may also occur in the absence of hypotension. Since this is not a true 'allergic reaction,' the patient may be pretreated with acetaminophen and diphenhydramine before an extended infusion of vancomycin of at least 90–120 minutes.

The oral treatment of MRSA and MRSE may present a greater challenge to a burn clinician. Rifampin is a bactericidal antibiotic and has efficacy in the treatment of these organisms. In 2005, *S. aureus* was 64% susceptible, *S. epidermidis* was 74% and *S. haemolyticus* was 76% susceptible to rifampin at

SBH-G. Rifampin produces its action by inhibiting RNA synthesis in the bacteria, binding to the β subunit of the DNA-dependent RNA polymerase, and blocking RNA transcription.[72] However, it must be used in combination with other anti-infectives in the treatment of MRSA and MRSE due to its high resistance pattern when used alone. Other anti-infectives with a different mechanism of action against MRSA and MRSE reduce the resistance of rifampin. Oral antibiotics such as Bactrim® (sulfamethoxazole and trimethoprim) or levofloxacin are often used in conjunction with rifampin. In 2005 at SBH-G, *S. aureus* was 64% susceptible, *S. epidermidis* was 71% susceptible, and *S. haemolyticus* was only 29% susceptible to the sulfamethoxazole/trimethoprim combination antibiotic.

Sulfamethoxazole works by interfering with bacterial folic acid synthesis and growth via inhibition of dihydrofolic acid formation from para-aminobenzoic acid; trimethoprim inhibits dihydrofolic acid reduction to tetrahydrofolate, resulting in sequential inhibition of enzymes of the folic acid pathway.[72] In 2005 at SBH-G, *S. aureus* showed 47% susceptibility, *S. epidermidis* showed 49% susceptibility, and *S. haemolyticus* showed 24% susceptibility to levofloxacin. Levofloxacin produces its antibacterial action by inhibiting DNA-gyrase in susceptible organisms. This action therby inhibits relaxation of supercoiled DNA and promotes breakage of bacterial DNA strands.[72]

Linezolid is a synthetic antibacterial agent of a new class of antibiotics, the oxazolidinones, which has joined the armamentarium against MRSA and MRSE. Linezolid inhibits bacterial protein synthesis by binding to a site on the bacterial 23S ribosomal RNA of the 50S subunit and prevents the formation of a functional 70S initiation complex, which is an essential component of the bacterial translation process.[72] The results of time-kill studies have shown linezolid to be bacteriostatic against enterococci and staphylococci. For streptococci, linezolid was found to be bactericidal for the majority of the strains. *In vitro* studies, however, show that point mutations in the 23S ribosomal RNA are associated with linezolid resistance and have been reported with some strains of *Enterococcus faecium* and *Staphylococcus aureus*.[72] In 2005 at SBH-G, *S. aureus* and *S. epidermidis* both showed 96% susceptibility and *S. haemolyticus* showed 99% susceptibility to linezolid.

Adverse drug effects to linezolid include myelosuppression (e.g. anemia leukopenia, pancytopenia, and thrombocytopenia) which is generally reversible upon discontinuation of the drug and *Clostridium difficile*-associated colitis. Linezolid is also a weak, nonselective, reversible inhibitor of monoamine oxidase (MAO) and may cause increased serotonin serum levels and serotonin syndrome in patients on various serotonin re-uptake inhibitors such as fluoxetine and sertraline.

Staphylococcal infections may also be treated with quinupristin/dalfopristin (Synercid®). Quinupristin/dalfopristin is bactericidal and inhibits bacterial protein synthesis by binding to different sites on the 50S ribosomal subunit, thereby inhibiting protein synthesis in the bacterial cell.[72] In 2005 at SBH-G, *S. aureus* showed 97% susceptibility, *S. epidermidis* showed 99% susceptibility, and *S. haemolyticus* showed 100% susceptibility to this drug.

Major adverse cardiovascular effects are seen when quinupristin/dalfopristin is given concomitantly with cytochrome P-450 isoenzyme 3A4 substrates such as cyclosporine, midazolam, and nifedipine that may cause QT prolongation.[72] The concomitant administration results in increased serum concentrations of those substrates and potentially prolonged/increased therapeutic or adverse effects. *Clostridium difficile*-associated diarrhea and colitis has also been reported with this drug ranging in severity from mild to life-threatening. Adverse venous effects (e.g. thrombophlebitis) may occur; therefore, flushing infusion lines with 5% dextrose injection following completion of peripheral infusions is recommended. Do not flush with sodium chloride injection or heparin because of possible incompatibilities. Arthralgia and myalgia, severe in some cases, of unknown etiology have been reported. Some patients improved with a reduction in dosing frequency to every 12 hours.[72]

Enterococcal bacterial infections

The enterococcal microbial isolates most frequently isolated from burn wounds at the Shriners Burns Hospital are *E. faecalis* and *E. faecium*. Most enterococcal bacteria are susceptible to vancomycin. In 2005 at SBH-G, all *E. faecalis* and *E. faecium* isolates showed 100% susceptibility to vancomycin. Vancomycin-resistant enterococci, usually vancomycin-resistant *E. faecium,* or VRE, will require treatment with a combination of agents such as ampicillin and aminoglycosides. If this combination is not effective, the VRE may be treated with the quinupristin/dalfopristin (Synercid®) combination or linezolid. In 2005 at SBH-G, *E. faecalis* showed 94% susceptibility and *E. faecium* showed 96% susceptibility to quinupristin/dalfopristin. The literature also reports that the use of quinupristin/dalfopristin resulted in resistance in one study and a superinfection in another study during the treatment of VRE infection.[72] In 2005 at SBH-G, *E. faecalis* showed 94% susceptibility and *E. faecium* showed 96% susceptibility to linezolid. Linezolid, however, is a bacteriostatic agent and resistance has been reported with some strains of *E. faecium*.

Gram-negative bacterial infections

The five most common Gram-negative microbial isolates found in the burn population at the Shriners Burns Hospital, Galveston are *Pseudomonas aeruginosa, Escherichia coli, Klebsiella pneumoniae, Enterobacter cloacae,* and *Acinetobacter baumannii/haemolyticus*. The efficacy of the antibiotic arsenal varies based on the individual susceptibility of the microbial isolate. Synergy between different classes of antibiotics is often tested to determine efficacy for a multiply drug-resistant organism (MDROs). The aminoglycosides and in particular, gentamicin, were historically the antibiotics of choice in the treatment of Gram-negative infections. The synergistic activity with penicillinase-resistant penicillins and vancomycin in the treatment of staphylococcal infections further standardized its premier status before the advent of newer extended-spectrum penicillins, the fourth-generation cephalosporins, the monobactams, the carbapenems, and the quinolones. However, some Gram-negative bacteria encountered in the burn unit are now resistant to all the aforementioned antibiotic classes and must now be treated with an old drug class, the polymyxins. A discussion of each antibiotic group will elucidate the strengths and weaknesses of each group.

Aminoglycosides

Aminoglycosides are usually bactericidal in action. Although the exact mechanism has not been fully elucidated, these drugs appear to inhibit protein synthesis in susceptible bacteria by irreversibly binding to 30S ribosomal subunits. The aminoglycosides consist of amikacin, gentamicin, kanamycin, neomycin, netilmicin, paromycin, and tobramycin.

In 2005 at SBH-G, *A. baumannii/haemolyticus* showed 30% susceptibility, *E. cloacae* showed 89% susceptibility, *E. coli* showed 97% susceptibility, *K. pneumoniae* showed 92% susceptibility, and *P. aeruginosa* showed 48% susceptibility to amikacin.

Unlike some other antibiotics (e.g. β-lactams), aminoglycosides have concentration-dependent bactericidal effects against many pathogens; higher serum concentrations are associated with increased bactericidal effects. The drugs also exhibit a prolonged, concentration-dependent postantibiotic effect (PAE) against a variety of Gram-negative and Gram-positive pathogens.[72] To effectively kill Gram-negative bacteria, these antibiotics must reach a peak level that is 5–8 times the MIC of the bacterial isolate.

These antibiotics have a narrow therapeutic blood serum range that must be closely monitored to achieve efficacy. However, toxic peak serum levels may result in ototoxicity and toxic trough levels may result in nephrotoxicity especially when used in conjunction with other ototoxic and nephrotoxic medications such as amphotericin, furosemide, and vancomycin.

Current evidence suggests that once-daily dosing of aminoglycosides is as effective as, and may be less toxic than, conventional dosage regimens employing multiple daily doses of the drug. Results of several analyses of pooled data from randomized, controlled studies in adults found that once-daily administration of aminoglycosides was associated with similar or greater efficacy (e.g. bacteriologic and/or clinical cure), less nephrotoxicity, and no greater risk of ototoxicity compared with administration of multiple daily dosing of these drugs.[72] Less frequent (e.g. once-daily) dosing may minimize or prevent the occurrence of aminoglycoside-induced adaptive resistance (i.e. reversible refractoriness to the antimicrobial effects of subsequent aminoglycoside doses because of decreased uptake of the drug following the initial dose) and selection of aminoglycoside-resistant subpopulations in Gram-negative bacteria by allowing a recovery period during the dosing interval in which serum aminoglycoside concentrations are negligible.[72] However, some clinicians have suggested that use of once-daily dosing of aminoglycosides may not be advisable in patients with serious infections and impaired host defenses (e.g. *P. aeruginosa* infections in patients with neutropenia) and/or clinical conditions associated with rapid clearance or unpredictable pharmacokinetics of aminoglycosides (e.g. extensive burns, cystic fibrosis, massive ascites) since these regimens could allow prolonged intervals of undetectable aminoglycoside concentrations that could outlast the PAE. Most clinicians, therefore, recommend monitoring of aminoglycoside serum concentrations and/or peak serum concentrations/

MIC ratio in burn patients with life-threatening infections, suspected toxicity or nonresponse to treatment, decreased or varying renal function, and increased aminoglycoside clearance.

Blood specimens for peak serum concentrations should be obtained approximately 1 hour following IM administration and 30 minutes after the completion of a 30-minute IV infusion or at the completion of a 1-hour IV infusion. Blood specimens for trough drug concentrations should be obtained immediately prior to the next IM or IV dose. For gentamicin and tobramycin, a commonly defined therapeutic range of serum concentrations is represented by peak serum aminoglycoside concentrations of approximately 4–12 μg/mL, and trough concentrations of less than 2 μg/mL; peak and trough serum concentrations of 15–40 and less than 5–10 μg/mL, respectively, have been suggested for amikacin and kanamyin. The ratio of the peak serum aminoglycoside to the MIC of the pathogen also has been evaluated as an indicator of aminoglycoside bactericidal efficacy by which to adjust the aminoglycoside dosage and serum concentrations. Limited data in patients receiving multiple daily doses of aminoglycosides have suggested an association between clinical response and a peak (i.e. 1-hour post-infusion) serum concentration/MIC ratio up to 12. When MIC data are unavailable for patients receiving once-daily aminoglycoside dosing regimens, some clinicians have used a high target peak serum concentration (e.g. 20 μg/mL for gentamicin or tobramycin) to ensure optimal peak/MIC ratios.[72]

Extended-spectrum penicillins

The advent of the extended-spectrum penicillins, and their reputed synergistic effect with aminoglycosides, brought a new era of antibiotic therapy in the treatment of burn infections. The extended-spectrum penicillins which consist of carbenicilllin, mezlocillin, piperacillin and ticarcillin are a group of semi-synthetic penicillin antibiotics that, because of their chemical structure, have a wider spectra of activity than natural penicillins, penicillinase-resistant penicillins (e.g. nafcillin), and aminopenicillins (e.g. ampicillin). They are more active against Gram-negative bacteria because they are more resistant to inactivation by extended-spectrum β-lactamases (ESBLs) which are produced by Gram-negative bacteria and/or because they more readily penetrate the outer membranes of these Gram-negative organisms.

Extended-spectrum penicillins reportedly vary in their rates of bactericidal action and in the completeness of this effect. This appears to result partly from differences in drug-induced morphologic effects on susceptible bacteria and subsequent formation of bacterial variants with varying degrees of osmotic stability. For example, mezlocillin or piperacillin may be more effective in the treatment of some infections caused by Gram-negative bacteria, such as some strains of *Citrobacter*, *Enterobacter*, *Klebsiella*, *Serratia*, and *B. fragilis* that are resistant to carbenicillin and/or ticarcillin. Some clinicians suggest that α-carboxypenicillins (e.g. ticarcillin) are the preferred extended-spectrum penicillins for general use and that acyl-aminopenicllins (mezlocillin, piperacillin) should be reserved for the treatment of infections, especially, *P. aeruginosa* infections that are resistant to α-carboxypenicillins. Some clinicians further suggest that, when an extended-spectrum penicillin is indicated, mezlocillin or piperacillin may be preferred for the treatment of infections caused by Enterobacteriaceae and that piperacillin may be preferred for the treatment of infections caused by *P. aeruginosa* because this drug is more active *in vitro* on a weight basis against these organisms than other commercially available extended-spectrum penicillins.[72] Because resistant strains of some organisms, especially *P. aeruginosa*, have developed during therapy with these antibiotics, appropriate specimens should be obtained periodically during therapy with the drugs to monitor effectiveness and detect emergence of resistant organisms.

In certain severe infections (e.g. sepsis) when the causative organism is unknown or *P. aeruginosa* is suspected, some clinicians recommend that concomitant therapy with an aminoglycoside or third-generation cephalosporin be used pending results of *in vitro* susceptibility tests. Synergistic effects between extended-spectrum antibiotics and aminoglycosides or third-generation cephalosporins are generally unpredictable and should be confirmed with appropriate *in vitro* studies.

Whenever an aminoglycoside is administered in conjunction with extended-spectrum penicillins, *in vivo* mixing of the drugs in syringes or IV infusion containers should be avoided since *in vitro* studies indicate that β-lactam antibiotics, including extended-spectrum penicillins may inactivate aminoglycosides. In addition, because *in vivo* inactivation of aminoglycosides may also occur, some clinicians suggest that it may be advisable to monitor serum aminoglycoside concentrations more closely than usual in patients receiving concomitant therapy, especially when high doses of extended-spectrum penicillins are administered or when the patient has impaired renal function. In addition, because acylaminopenicillins contain less than half the sodium content of α-carboxypenicillins, piperacillin or mezlocillin may be preferred to ticarcillin in patients whose sodium intake is restricted.

The combination of ticarcillin with clavulanic acid, and piperacillin with tazobactam, two β-lactamase inhibitors, results in a synergistic bactericidal effect against many strains of β-lactamase-producing bacteria. Clavulanic acid and tazobactam have a high affinity for and irreversibly bind to certain lactamases which can inactivate the extended-spectrum penicillins, ticarcillin and piperacillin, respectively. In 2005 at SBH-G, *E. cloacae* showed 75% susceptibility, *E. coli* showed 90% susceptibility, *K. pneumoniae* showed 84% susceptibility and *P. aeruginosa* showed 69% susceptibility to piperacillin/tazobactam. During the same period at SBH-G, *A. baumannii/haemolyticus* showed 36% susceptibility, *E. cloacae* showed 62% susceptibility, *E. coli* showed 72% susceptibility, *K. pneumoniae* showed 84% susceptibility, and *P. aeruginosa* showed 39% susceptibility to ticarcillin/clavulanate.

The usage of extended-spectrum penicillin in the treatment of Gram-negative bacterial infections provide a burn population with a much less toxic antibiotic when compared to the aminoglycosides since the most frequent adverse reactions include hypersensitivity reactions, gastrointestinal effects, and local reactions.

Third- and fourth-generation cephalosporins

Cephalosporins are semisynthetic β-lactam antibiotics that are structurally and pharmacologically related to penicillins, carbacephem (e.g. loracarbef), and cephamycins (e.g. cefotetan,

cefoxitin). Cephalosporins are usually bactericidal in action. The antibacterial activity of the cephalosporins, like penicillins, carbacephems, and cephamycins, results from inhibition of mucopeptide synthesis in the bacterial cell wall. Although the exact mechanism of action of cephalosporins has not been fully elucidated, β-lactam antibiotics bind to several enzymes in the bacterial cytoplasmic membrane (e.g. carboxypeptidases, endopeptidases, transpeptidases) that are involved in cell-wall synthesis and cell division. It has been hypothesized that β-lactam antibiotics act as substrate analogs of acyl-D-alanyl-D-alanine, the usual substrate for these enzymes. This interferes with cell-wall synthesis and results in the formation of defective cell walls and osmotically unstable spheroblasts. Cell death following exposure to β-lactam antibiotics usually results in lyses, which appears to be mediated by bacterial autolysins such as peptidoglycan hydrolases.[72]

The target enzymes of β-lactam antibiotics have been classified as penicillin-binding proteins (PBPs) and appear to vary substantially among bactericidal species. The affinities of various β-lactam antibiotics for different PBPs appear to explain the differences in morphology that occur in susceptible organisms following exposure to different β-lactam antibiotics and may also explain difference in the spectrum of activity of β-lactam antibiotics that are not caused by the presence or absence of ESBLs.

Cephalosporins generally are divided into four groups ('generations') based on their spectra of activity. In this section on the treatment of Gram-negative infections, we will discuss the third- and fourth-generation cephalosporins based on their expanded spectrum against Gram-negative bacteria as compared with the first- and second-generation drugs.

The third-generation cephalosporins include cefdinir, cefditoren, cefixime, cefoperazone, cefotaxime, cefpodoxime, ceftazidime, ceftibuten, ceftizoxime, and ceftriaxone. Third-generation cephalosporins generally are active *in vitro* against Gram-negative bacteria *Citrobacter, Enterobacter, E. coli, Klebsiella, Neiserria, Proteus, Morganella, Providencia,* and *Serratia* that may be resistant to first- and second-generation cephalosporins. Cefotaxime, ceftazidime, ceftizoxime, and ceftriaxone are reported to be the drugs of choice for the treatment of infections caused by susceptible Enterobacteriaceae, including susceptible strains of *E. coli, K. pneumoniae, P. rettgeri, M. morganii, P. vulgaris,* or *P. stuartii* and are alternatives for the treatment of susceptible *Serratia.* Ceftazidime (but not cefotaxime, ceftizoxime, or ceftriaxone) is reported to be a drug of choice for the treatment of infections caused by susceptible *P. aeruginosa.* Ceftazidime is more active *in vitro* on a weight basis against *P. aeruginosa* than most other currently available cephalosporins and is active against many strains resistant to many other cephalosporins. In 2005 at SBH-G, *A. baumannii/haemolyticus* showed 30% susceptibility, *E. cloacae* showed 58% susceptibility, *E. coli* showed 78% susceptibility, *K. pneumoniae* showed 78% susceptibility, and *P. aeruginosa* showed 51% susceptibility to ceftazidime.

However, ESBLs pose a particularly acute threat because they are found in common nosocomial pathogens such as *E. coli, K. pneumoniae,* and *Enterobacter* species. Before the advent of ESBLs, most of these infections could be confidently treated with third-generation cephalosporins. These enzymes are genetically derived from several progenitor enzymes, particularly TEM and SHV β-lactamases. The use and overuse of third-generation cephalosporins have selected for ESBL-producing bacterial strains in hospitalized patients. This may have important therapeutic and epidemiological consequences. The detection of ESBLs has posed a problem for clinical microbiological laboratories; *in vitro* test results that indicate susceptibility to third-generation cephalosporins are sometimes inconsistent with clinical outcomes. New tests and new technology designed to increase the accuracy of ESBL detection have recently been introduced. These available tests are used to screen and confirm the presence of ESBL production and for distinguishing ESBLs from other β-lactamases, particularly the chromosome-mediated AmpC β-lactamases that have a phenotype similar to that of ESBLs.[75] Overall the clinical data indicate that treatment failures associated with the use of third-generation cephalosporins occur most frequently with ceftazidime. Because ESBL coding sequences are plasmid borne, they easily disseminate to other bacterial species. Effective measures to confine this highly transmissible trait promote the use of cefepime, a fourth-generation cephalosporin, β-lactam/β-lactamase inhibitors and carbapenems, while concurrently restricting the use of third-generation cephalosporins.[75]

Fourth-generation cephalosporins, which include cefepime, are active *in vitro* against some Gram-negative bacteria, including *Pseudomonas* and certain Enterobacteriaceae, that generally are resistant to third-generation cephalosprins. Cefepime has a spectrum of activity against aerobic Gram-positive and Gram-negative bacteria that is similar to that of cefotaxime, ceftriaxone, and ceftizoxime and has activity against *P. aeruginosa* that appears to approach that of ceftazidime. More importantly, cefepime is more active than third-generation cephalosporins against Enterobacteriaceae that produce inducible β-lactamases.[75] The extended spectrum of activity of cefepime is related to the fact that the drug penetrates the outer membrane of Gram-negative bacteria more rapidly and is more resistant to inactivation by chromosomally and plasmid-mediated β-lactamases than most other cephalosporins. In addition, inducible β-lactamases have a low affinity for cefepime and the drug is hydrolyzed by these enzymes at a slower rate than third-generation cephalosporins such as ceftazidime.[75] In 2005 at SBH-G, *A. baumannii/haemolyticus* showed 39% susceptibility, *E. cloacae* showed 86% susceptibility, *E. coli* showed 84% susceptibility, *K. pneumoniae* showed 80% susceptibility, and *P. aeruginosa* showed 36% susceptibility to cefepime.

Miscellaneous β-lactam antibiotics

Aztreonam is termed a synthetic monobactam antibiotic because unlike other β-lactam antibiotics which are bicyclic, it is a monocyclic β-lactam antibiotic. The antibacterial activity of aztreonam results not only from inhibition of mucopeptide synthesis in the bacterial cell wall, but in addition, aztreonam has a high affinity and preferentially binds to penicillin-binding protein 3 (PBP 3) of susceptible Gram-negative bacteria. The drug also has some affinity for PBP 1a of these bacteria, but little or no affinity for PBPs 1b, 2, 4, 5, or 6.[72] Because PBP 3 is involved in septation, aztreonam causes the formation of abnormally elongated or filamentous forms in susceptible Gram-negative bacteria. As a consequence cell division is inhibited and breakage of the cell wall occurs resulting in lyses and death.[72] Studies using *S. aureus* indicate that aztreonam does not bind to the essential PBPs of Gram-positive bacteria. Aztreonam also has poor affinity for the PBPs of anaerobic bacteria. The drug, therefore, is generally inactive against these organisms.

Aztreonam usually is bactericidal in action. Since aztreonam has a poor affinity for PBPs 1a and 1b of susceptible Gram-negative bacteria, it is not as rapidly bactericidal as some other β-lactam antibiotics (e.g. imipenem, cefotaxime, cefoxitin, ceftriaxone) against these organisms. For most susceptible Enterobacteriaceae, the minimum bactericidal concentration (MBC) of aztreonam is equal to or only 2–4 times higher than the minimum inhibitory concentration (MIC) of the drug.[72] For *P. aeruginosa*, the MBC of aztreonam is usually only two times higher than the MIC, but may be up to 125 times higher than the MIC for some strains of the organism.[72] In 2005 at SBH-G, *A. baumannii/haemolyticus* showed 21% susceptibility, *E. cloacae* showed 57% susceptibility, *E. coli* showed 80% susceptibility, *K. pneumoniae* showed 78% susceptibility, and *P. aeruginosa* showed 55% susceptibility to aztreonam.

Adverse effects reported with aztreonam are similar to those reported with other β-lactam antibiotics and the drug is generally well tolerated.

Imipenem/cilastatin sodium is a fixed combination of imipenem monohydrate (a semisynthetic carbapenem β-lactam antibiotic) and cilastatin sodium, which prevents renal metabolism of imipenem by a specific and reversible inhibitor of dehydropeptidase I which inactivates imipenem by hydrolyzing the β-lactam ring.

Imipenem usually is bactericidal in action. Imipenem has an affinity for and binds to most penicillin-binding proteins (PBPs) of susceptible organisms, including PBPs 1a, 1b, 2, 4, 5, and 6 of *Escherichia coli*; PBPs 1a, 1b, 2, 4, and 5 of *Pseudomonas aeruginosa*, and PBPs 1, 2, 3, and 4 of *Staphylococcus* aureus.[72] In susceptible Gram-negative bacteria, imipenem has the highest affinity for PBP 2 and the lowest affinity of PBP 3.[72] This results in the formation of spheroblasts or ellipsoidal cells without filament formation. Because imipenem also has a high affinity for PBPs 1a and 1b, for these organisms the spheroblasts lyse rapidly. Imipenem is able to penetrate the outer membrane of most Gram-negative bacteria and gain access to the PBPs more readily than many other currently available β-lactam antibiotics.[72]

In vitro studies also indicate that imipenem may have a post-antibiotic inhibitory effect against some susceptible organisms, although the mechanism of this PAE has not been determined to date, *in vitro* studies using *S. aureus, E. coli,* and *P. aeruginosa* indicate that following exposure to bactericidal concentrations of imipenem these organisms do not immediately resume growth after the drug is removed.[72] It is not known whether a PAE occurs *in vivo*. It has been suggested that this effect would be beneficial since imipenem may be able to prevent regrowth of susceptible organisms when drug concentrations at the site of infection fall below the MIC during a dosing interval. In 2005 at SBH-G, *A. baumannii/haemolyticus* showed 97% susceptibility, *E.*

cloacae showed 96% susceptibility, *E. coli* showed 98% susceptibility, *K. pneumoniae* showed 94% susceptibility, and *P. aeruginosa* showed 36% susceptibility to imipenem/cilastatin.

Meropenem is also a synthetic carbapenem antibiotic. Unlike imipenem, meropenem has a methyl group at position 1 of the 5-membered ring which confers stability against hydrolysis by dehydropeptidase I (DHP I) present on the brush border of proximal renal tubular cells and therefore does not require concomitant administration with a DHP I inhibitor such as cilastatin.[72]

Meropenem has a broad spectrum of activity that resembles the microbiologic activity of imipenem; however, meropenem generally is more active *in vitro* against Enterobacteriaceae and less active against Gram-positive bacteria. Meropenem appears to be susceptible to hydrolysis by metallo-β-lactamases.[72] The drug generally is inactive against methicillin-resistant staphylococci. Like imipenem, meropenem also is highly resistant to hydrolysis by a variety of β-lactamases.[72]

In vitro studies indicate that imipenem may be a potent inducer of β-lactamases and can reversibly derepress inducible, chromosomally medicated β-lactamases in *P. aeruginosa* and Enterobacteriaceae.[72]

Adverse effects with imipenem/cilastatin and meropenem are similar to those reported with other β-lactam antibiotics and the drugs are generally well tolerated although adverse nervous system effects, including seizures and myoclonus, have been reported with IV imipenem/cilastatin.

Quinolones

The quinolones class of antibiotics includes IV antibiotics ciprofloxacin, gatifloxacin, levofloxacin, moxifloxacin, ofloxacin and alatrofloxacin and oral antibiotics ciprofloxacin, gatifloxacin, levofloxacin, lomefloxacin, moxifloxacin, nalidixic acid, ofloxacin, sparfloxacin, and trofloxacin. Quinolones are usually bactericidal in action and act by inhibiting DNA topoisomerase (ATP-hydrolyzing), a type II DNA topoisomerase commonly referred to as DNA-gyrase, in susceptible organisms. DNA gyrase is necessary for bacterial DNA replication and some aspects of transcription, repair, recombination, and transposition. Inhibition of DNA-gyrase in susceptible organisms results in inhibition of ATP-dependent negative supercoiling of DNA, inhibition or ATP-independent relaxation of supercoiled DNA, and promotion of double-stranded DNA breakage.[72] Mammalian cells contain a type II topoisomerase similar to that contained in bacteria. At concentrations attained during therapy, quinolones do not appear to affect the mammalian enzyme, presumably because it functions differently than bacterial DNA-gyrase and does not cause supercoiling of DNA. Although the clinical importance has not been determined, ciprofloxacin appears to have a postantibiotic effect.[72] In 2005 at SBH-G, *A. baumannii/haemolyticus* showed 27% and 27% susceptibility, *E. cloacae* showed 92% and 89% susceptibility, *E. coli* showed 70% and 70% susceptibility, *K. pneumoniae* showed 90% and 90% susceptibility, and *P. aeruginosa* showed 36% and 36% susceptibility to levofloxacin and ciprofloxacin, respectively.

Fluoroquinolones are well absorbed orally. IV therapy with these drugs is generally reserved for patients who do not toler-

ate or are unable to take the drug orally and for other patients in whom the IV route offers a clinical advantage.

Polymyxins

The polymyxins are amphipathic molecules that interact with the lipopolysaccharide (LPS) in the bacterial outer membrane. Entry into the cell is not necessary, since polymyxin B covalently attached to agarose beads retains the ability to alter membrane permeability and inhibit bacterial respiration. Initial binding to the outer membrane takes place when the polycationic portion of polymyxin B displaces Ca^{++} and Mg^{++} bridges that normally stabilize LPS molecules in the outer leaflet of the bacterial outer membrane.[77] Binding can be antagonized by high concentrations of divalent cations. Additional complexing with LPS is facilitated by hydrophobic interaction between the lipid A portion of LPS and the fatty acid of the antibiotic. Insertion of the antibiotic into the outer membrane disrupts the membrane and releases LPS into the surrounding milieu. They also have potent antiendotoxic properties and antibacterial activity against *P. aeruginosa* and many of the Enterobacteriaceae.

According to Storm et al., the polymyxins are bacteriostatic at low concentrations and bactericidal at high concentrations. Nord and Hoeprich reported that at a concentration of $0.01\,\mu mol/mL$, polymyxin B sulfate was bactericidal to 88% of the *P. aeruginosa* strains tested.[77] Bactericidal activity against *P. aeruginosa* is not seen with colistin until its concentration reaches $0.1\,\mu mol/mL$.[77] Polymyxin B and colistin (polymyxin E) are usually given at doses of 1.5–2.5 and 5 mg/kg/day, respectively, in two divided doses. Dosing must be altered in renal failure since the kidney is the primary route of elimination. Distribution into pleural fluid, joints, and cerebrospinal fluid is poor.

Polymyxins are recommended for serious systemic infections caused by Gram-negative bacteria that are resistant to other agents and have a definite role in therapy of multi-drug-resistant Gram-negative bacterial infections. The pediatric burn hospital, Shriners Burns Hospital in Galveston, Texas reviewed the use of colistimethate sodium from 2000–2004 in 109 patients, 72 males and 37 females (median and mean age of 9 years) with a TBSA from 21% to 99% (median 60% and mean 62%). The overall survival rate was 80% in all 109 patients. Colistimethate sodium provided an important salvage option for burn patients with otherwise incompletely treated and life-threatening Gram-negative infections. In 2005 at SBH-G, *A. baumannii/haemolyticus*, *E. cloacae*, *E. coli*, and *K. pneumoniae* all showed 100% susceptibility to colistin and polymyxin B while *P. aeruginosa* showed 96% and 99% susceptibility to colistin and polymyxin B, respectively.

However, monitoring the dose-dependent nephrotoxicity and CNS toxicity associated with its systemic use is necessary to achieve a therapeutic outcome. When polymyxin B is given to animals or humans, it binds, via its free amino acid groups, to negatively charged phospholipids in tissues. Kunin and Bugg showed that binding is greatest to kidney and brain tissues, followed by liver, muscle, and lung tissues.[77] After repeated doses, the drug accumulates in tissues to concentrations four to five times higher than peak serum concentrations and persists in tissues for at least 5–7 days.[77] Removal of the drug by dialysis can be difficult due to extensive tissue binding. In our study, colistimethate sodium appears to proportionately increase the incidence of *C. difficile*-associated colitis, renal dysfunction, and neuropathies in relation to the length of its use.

Treatment of yeast and fungal infections

The five classes of systemic antifungal medications comprise the polyenes, the azoles, a nucleoside analog, an echinocandin, and an allylamine. Thus there are four potential target sites in the fungal cell for the antifungal drugs to act. The allylamine antifungal, terbinafine, which is used primarily for management of dermatophytosis and onchomycosis, and ketoconazole, which has been replaced by newer, less-toxic triazole drugs, will not be discussed.

Polyenes (amphotericin B)

Amphotericin B, an amphoteric polyene macrolide, is an antifungal antibiotic. Conventional IV amphotericin B is used for the treatment of potentially life-threatening fungal infections including aspergillosis, North American blastomycosis, systemic candidiasis, coccidioidomycosis, cryptococcosis, histoplasmosis, paracoccidioidomycosis, sporotrichosis, and zygomycosis.[72]

Amphotericin B usually is fungistatic in action at concentrations obtained clinically, but may be fungicidal in high concentrations or against very susceptible organisms. Amphotericin B exerts its antifungal activity principally by binding to sterols (e.g. ergosterol) in the fungal cell membrane. As a result of this binding, the cell membrane is no longer able to function as a selective barrier and leakage of intracellular contents occurs. Cell death occurs in part as a result of permeability changes, but other mechanisms also may contribute to the *in vivo* antifungal effects of amphotericin B against some fungi.[72] Amphotericin B is not active *in vitro* against organisms that do not contain sterols in their cell membranes (e.g. bacteria).

Binding to sterols in mammalian cells (such as certain kidney cells and erythrocytes) may account for some of the toxicities reported with conventional amphotericin B therapy. Nephrotoxicity is the major dose-limiting toxicity reported with conventional IV amphotericin B, and nephrotoxicity occurs to some degree in the majority of patients receiving the drug. Adverse renal effects include decreased renal function and renal function abnormalities such as azotemia, hypokalemia, hyposthenuria, renal tubular acidosis, and nephrocalcinosis.[72] Increased BUN and serum creatinine concentrations and decreased creatinine clearance, glomerular filtration rate, and renal plasma flow occur in most patients receiving conventional IV amphotericin.

Increased BUN and/or serum creatinine, hypokalemia, hypomagnesemia, and hypocalcemia also have been reported in patients receiving the amphotericin B cholesteryl sulfate complex, amphotericin B lipid complex, or amphotericin liposomal. While these formulations appear to be associated with a lower risk of nephrotoxicity than conventional IV amphotericin B and have been used in patients with preexisting renal impairment (in most cases resulting from prior therapy with conventional IV amphotericin B), additional experience with these drugs is necessary to more accurately determine the extent of nephrotoxicity that occurs with these formulations.[72]

Acute infusion reactions consisting of fever, shaking, chills, hypotension, anorexia, nausea, vomiting, headache, dyspnea, and tachypnea may occur 1–3 hours after initiation of IV infusions of conventional IV amphotericin B or other formulations such as amphotericin B cholesteryl sulfate, amphotericin B lipid complex, and amphotericin B liposomal. Acetaminophen, meperidine, antihistamines (e.g. diphenhydramine), or corticosteroids have been used for the treatment or prevention of these acute infusion reactions.

Azole antifungals

The azole antifungals consist of the triazole antifungal oral and intravenous drugs, fluconazole, itraconazole, and voriconazole, and the imidazole oral drug ketoconazole. These antifungal agents act by interfering with cytochrome P450 activity, decreasing ergosterol synthesis (the principal sterol in the fungal cell membrane), and inhibiting cell membrane formation.[76]

The three triazole antifungal drugs can be distinguished by differences in their spectrum of activity. Fluconazole is generally active *in vitro* against *Candida albicans*, many of the non-*albicans Candida* species, and *C. neoformans*. However it is not generally active against *Candida krusei* or *Aspergillus* species.[76] Itraconazole also has excellent anti-*Candida* activity, is more effective *in vitro* than fluconazole against the endemic fungi, *Histoplasma capsulatum*, *Sporothrix schenckii*, and *Blastomyces dermatitidis* and has fungistatic activity against *Aspergillus*.[76] Voriconazole has up to 60-fold lower MIC for *Candida* species (including resistant strains) than fluconazole, is fungicidal for *Aspergillus* and has some activity against *Fusarium* species and *Scedosporium apiospermum*.[76] None of the triazoles are active against the *Zygomycetes*.

A recently published study compared the *in vitro* activity of the three available triazoles agaist several thousand *Candida* isolates, most of which were obtained from blood or other normally sterile sites. Of note, fluconazole-resistant species were susceptible to voriconazole. Whereas only 5% of *C. krusei* were susceptible to fluconazole, 99% were susceptible to voriconazole.[76] *Candida glabrata*, which has emerged as one of the most common clinical isolates in patients with candidiasis, was susceptible to fluconazole in 60% of the cases and to voriconazole in 92%.[76] Voriconazole also had activity against fluconazole-resistant *C. albicans* isolates with the RS phenotype.[76] Thus voriconazole was a treatment option for infection with some *Candida* species that are resistant to fluconazole.

In general, the azole drugs are better tolerated than the amphotericin B formulations. Side effects of fluconazole, which are uncommon, include rash and elevations in liver function test results. In patients who receive prolonged courses of high-dose therapy, reversible alopecia and dry lips can occur. Potential side effects of itraconazole include peripheral edema, exacerbation of congestive heart failure (caused by a negative inotropic effect), hypokalemia, or rash.[76] Reported toxicities of voriconazole include elevations in liver function test results, rash, photosensitivity, and transient ocular toxicity, a unique phenomenon that has been studied extensively. The following visual disturbances have been described: blurred vision, photophobia, altered color vision, and perception of increased brightness of light. Up to one-third of patients treated with voriconazole have describes such visual disturbances, which typically occur early in the course of therapy, begin 15–30 minutes after a dose, and resolve within 30 minutes.[76] No histopathologic changes have been seen in the retinas of treated patients, and there have been no permanent sequelae of voriconazole-induced visual disturbances.[76]

Because these azole drugs are metabolized by the hepatic cytochrome P450 system, a variety of interactions can occur between these agents and other medications. The azoles inhibit the metabolism of the sulfonylureas, warfarin, digoxin, phenytoin, cyclosporine, sirolimus, tacrolimus, omeprazole, and cisapride, resulting in increased serum concentrations of these medications and the potential for drug toxicity. Conversely, serum concentrations of the triazoles are decreased by rifampin, isoniazid, phenytoin, and fosphenytoin, as well as carbamazepine.[73]

Echinocandin antifungals

Caspofungin, an echinocandin antifungal, inhibits formation of β 1, 3 glucan of the fungal cell wall. Caspofungin is effective *in vitro* against *Candida* species, including azole-resistant isolates, and *Aspergillus* species.

Caspofungin therapy is usually well tolerated. Rash or GI toxicity occurs rarely. There are relatively few drug–drug interactions with caspofungin, which is neither an inducer nor an inibitor of the cytochrome P450 system. Caspofungin does reduce the AUC and peak serum concentrations of tacrolimus by 20–25%, so tacrolimus serum concentrations should be monitored in patients taking caspofungin.[76] Cyclosporin increases the AUC of caspofungin by 35%.[76] It is suggested that caspofungin and cyclosporine not be coadministered.

Nucleoside analog antifungal (Flucytosine)

Flucytosine, the only available nucleoside analog, acts as an antifungal by disrupting pyrimidine metabolism in the fungal cell nucleus. Flucytosine is fungicidal *in vitro* against *Candida* species and *C. neoformans* but not against other commonly encountered fungi. Unfortunately, resistance emerges rapidly during flucytosine monotherapy, so use of this drug is limited to combination therapy.[76]

Flucytosine can cause bone marrow suppression and GI toxicity, although these side effects are seen less frequently with the current recommended dosage (100mg/kg/day in 4 divided doses) than with the higher dosage that was used for many years (150mg/kg/day in 4 divided doses). Flucytosine does not have any significant drug interactions.

Treatment of systemic viral infections in burn patients

Burn centers are testing for and finding more viral infections in burn patients. Linneman[38] found that in the pediatric burn population that he was studying prospectively, 33% of the children developed cytomegalovirus infections, 25% developed herpetic infections, and 17% developed adenovirus infections. In this section, we will only deal with the treatment of systemic CMV infections and mucocutaneous HSV infections.

Treatment of cytomegalovirus (CMV) infections

IV ganciclovir (Cytovene®) and oral valganciclovir (Valcyte®) are the agents that are effective in the treatment of cytomegalovirus infections. Valganciclovir is the I-valine ester of ganciclovir that allows for oral systemic absorption of this drug. Ganciclovir and valganciclovir exert their antiviral effect on human cytomegalovirus and the other human herpesviruses by interfering with DNA synthesis via competition with deoxyguanosine for incorporation into viral DNA and by being incorporated into growing viral DNA chains.[72] In addition to its activity against CMV, ganciclovir also has shown activity against herpes simplex virus types 1 and 2 (HSV-1 and HSV-2), human herpesvirus type 6 (the presumed causative agent of roseola), Epstein–Barr virus (EBV), and varicella-zoster virus (VZV).

The initial dose of ganciclovir is 10mg/kg/day divided every 12 hours for 14–21 days. The patient may be converted to the oral valganciclovir at a dose of 900mg orally twice daily to complete the recommended treatment regimen.[73]

The most common adverse effects of ganciclovir are hematologic reactions that may be severe. Neutropenia (absolute neutrophil count less than 1000/mm^3), which is potentially fatal, occurs in up to 25–50% of patients receiving ganciclovir and is the most common dose-limiting adverse effect of this drug.[72] Adverse nervous system effects have been seen in 5–17% of patients and ranged in severity from headache to seizures or coma.[72] Abnormal liver function test results (e.g. elevated aminotransferase and alkaline phosphatase concentrations) have been reported in 2–3% of patients receiving ganciclovir. Nausea and vomiting have been reported in up to 2% of patients receiving ganciclovir and diarrhea, anorexia, GI hemorrhage, and abdominal pain have been reported less frequently. Inflammation, phlebitis, and/or pain at the site of IV infusion occur commonly during ganciclovir therapy. Therefore it is recommended that veins with adequate blood flow be used to allow for rapid dilution and distribution of the drug.[72]

Treatment of herpes infections

Acyclovir sodium IV (Zovirax®) is used for the treatment of initial and recurrent mucocutaneous herpes simplex virus (HSV-1 and HSV-2) infections and the treatment of varicella-zoster infections in immunocompromised adults and children. It is also used for the treatment of HSV encephalitis and neonatal HSV infections. Acyclovir is used orally for the treatment of initial and recurrent episodes of genital herpes. It is also used for the acute treatment of herpes zoster (shingles, zoster) and varicella (chickenpox) in immunocompetent individuals.

For the treatment of mucocutaneous HSV infections in immunocompromised adults and children 12 years of age or older with normal renal function, the recommended dose is 5mg/kg/dose every 8 hours for 7–14 days; in children younger than 12 years of age, the manufacturer recommends a dosage of 10mg/kg every 8 hours for 7 days.[73]

Adverse reactions generally have been minimal following oral or IV administration of acyclovir. However, potentially serious reactions (e.g. renal failure, thrombotic thrombocytopenic/hemolytic uremic syndrome) can occur and fatalities have been reported.[72]

The use of topical antimicrobial compounds and agents

One of the most effective means to achieve a microbial balance in a colonized or infected wound is the proper use of prophylactic topical agents. Maintaining wounds at low colonization levels diminishes the frequency and duration of septic episodes caused by wound flora.[21] The introduction of topical antimicrobial agents has resulted in a significant reduction in burn mortality to date.[78,79] Recent studies have demonstrated that some agents used in the past are no longer effective in inhibiting bacterial growth *in vitro*.[80] Wounds in which the quantitative culture counts remain less than 10^2 organisms/gram tissue may remain dressed in the topical agent of choice. However, should the colony count show an increase beyond that point, a change in the topical agent is strongly recommended.

Sodium hypochlorite (NaOCl)

Currently the most effective topical antibacterial for cleansing a wound is sodium hypochlorite (NaOCl).[81] It transcends the topical antimicrobial effects and tissue toxicity of such products such as povidone-iodine, acetic acid, and hydrogen peroxide.[29] While povidone-iodine is bactericidal at 1% and 0.5% concentrations, it is toxic to fibroblasts; acetic acid at a 0.25% concentration is not bactericidal and is toxic to fibroblasts; and hydrogen peroxide at 3% and 0.3% concentrations is toxic to fibroblasts but only the 3% concentration is bactericidal.[8,81]

Studies by Heggers and his co-workers[82] reported on the efficacy of NaOCl at a concentration of 0.025%. NaOCl 0.025% solution is one-tenth the concentration of 'Half-Strength Dakins,' the formulation that is used by many hospitals as a topical antimicrobial agent. Buffered NaOCl 0.25% was formulated to mimic normal human physiologic parameters. It is an excellent cleansing agent which was found to be bactericidal, nontoxic to fibroblasts, and did not inhibit wound healing. However, the NaOCl 0.025% solution is only effective over a 24-hour time frame after the buffer ($0.3\,\mathrm{N}$ NaH_2PO_4) is added to the NaOCl.

Buffered NaOCl 0.025% solution soaks are most beneficial in reducing the bacterial numbers in a wound. NaOCl 0.025% solution is a broad-spectrum antiseptic and is bactericidal against *P. aeruginosa*, *S. aureus* microorganisms, as well as other Gram-negative and Gram-positive organisms.[82,83] It is effective against MRSA, MRSE, and the enterococci. NaOCl 0.025% solution may be used separately or in concert with other antibacterial agents to control colonization or infection. NaOCl 0.025% solution also enhances wound healing and increases wound breaking strength when compared to mafenide acetate.[82]

Silver nitrate (AgNO₃)

Silver nitrate was formerly used as a 10% solution but was found to be toxic at this concentration. It has now been reinstated as a 0.5% solution which is nontoxic, does not injure regenerating epithelium in the wound and is bacteriostatic against *S. aureus*, *E. coli*, and *P. aeruginosa* microorganisms. AgNO₃ is most effective when the wound is carefully cleansed of all emollients and other debris, and debrided of all dead tissue. Multilayered coarse-mesh dressings should be placed over the wound and saturated with the AgNO₃ solution. Like silver sulfadiazine, AgNO₃ has limited penetration since the element silver is rapidly bound to the body's natural chemical substances, such as Cl⁻.[25,78,79,84] Since it is hypotonic in nature, it can cause osmolar dilution, resulting in hyponatremia and hypochloremia. Serum electrolytes must be monitored very carefully.

AgNO₃ 0.5% solution is light-sensitive and turns black upon contact with tissues and other Cl⁻ containing compounds when it is allowed to dry out. Hyperpyrexia may also occur if AgNO₃ becomes dry and is covered with an impervious dressing.

Some institutions are combining silver nitrate with miconazole powder to produce a silver nitrate 0.5% and miconazole 2% aqueous solution that is effective in preventing fungal overgrowth in burn wounds treated with silver nitrate 0.5% solution alone.

Klebsiella species, the *Providencia* species, and other Enterobacteriaceae are not as susceptible to AgNO₃ 0.5% solution as other bacteria. The combination of AgNO₃ 0.5% solution with *E. cloacae* and other nitrate-positive organisms may cause methemoglobinemia by converting nitrate to nitrite in the body.[25,78,79,84]

Silver sulfadiazine

Silver sulfadiazine (Silvadene®, Thermazene®, Flamazine®, SSD®), a 1% water-soluble cream, is a combination of sulfadiazine and silver. The silver ion binds with the DNA of the organism, consequently releasing the sulfonamide which interferes with the intermediary metabolic pathway of the microbe.[5,85–87] It is most effective against *P. aeruginosa*, the enterics, and equally effective as any antifungal drug against *C. albicans* and *S. aureus*. However, some strains of the *Klebsiella* species have been less effectively controlled. Recently there have been reports of *P. aeruginosa* resistance to silver sulfadizene.[88] Silver sulfadiazine can be applied with equal effectiveness using either the closed or open methods. Antimicrobial effectiveness has been observed to last for up to 24 hours. More frequent changes are required if a creamy exudate forms on the wound. Some of the benefits of this topical agent are its ease of use and its ability to reduce pain. It has some tissue-penetrating ability, but is limited to the surface epidermal layer.[25,84] However, it is not associated with acid–base disturbances or pulmonary fluid overload, as is mafenide acetate.[78,79] Silver sulfadiazine can be used separately or in combination with other antibacterials and with enzymatic escharotomy compounds. It can be combined with nystatin, which enhances the antifungal capability of this agent.

By itself, silver sulfadiazine has been shown to retard wound healing; however, in conjunction with nystatin or *Aloe vera*, the wound retardant effect is reversed. The breaking strength is not affected; in fact it may be enhanced when combinations are employed (unpublished data, 1994). An adverse drug reaction may be a reversible granulocyte reduction.[25,78,79,84]

Mafenide acetate (Sulfamylon®)

Mafenide acetate is available both as an 8.5% water-soluble cream or a 5% aqueous solution. This agent has more substantial bacteriological data to support its efficacy than any other topical antimicrobial. Mafenide acetate has been shown to be effective against a broad range of microorganisms, especially against all strains of *P. aeruginosa* and *Clostridium*.[78,79,89]

After the wound has been cleansed of debris, mafenide acetate 8.5% cream is applied to the wound like 'butter' (Lindberg's butter). The treated burn surface is left exposed for maximal antimicrobial potency.[78,79,89] The cream is applied a minimum of two times a day and reapplied between applications if rubbed off the wound. Advantages of the cream are its ability to control *P. aeruginosa* wound infections, ease of application, and the absence of the need for dressings. Additionally, it has the ability to penetrate burn eschar and circumvent the colonization of the burn.

The 5% solution is used to saturate an eight-ply gauze dressing and is applied to the burn wound area. The dressing should be kept saturated with the mafenide acetate 5% solution in order to produce maximal antimicrobial effects. The dressings may be changed every 8 hours. Mafenide acetate 5% solution is proclaimed to have effective tissue-penetrating ability and appears to be especially effective after the dead tissue is removed from the granulating bed.[78,84,89,90]

However, there are several detrimental aspects to the use of mafenide acetate. Protracted use, with the low environmental pH, favors the growth of *C. albicans*. Mafenide acetate 5% solution is converted by monoamine oxidase to *p*-sulfamylvanzoic acid, a carbonic anhydrase inhibitor. Carbonic anhydrase inhibitors prevent the conversion of hydrogen ions in the body to carbonic acid, subsequently causing metabolic acidosis in the patient. If the patient has sustained an inhalation injury and developed a respiratory acidosis, the use of mafenide acetate over large areas of the body may produce a metabolic acidosis which can be fatal. This complication can also be seen when treatment with mafenide acetate occurs during septic episodes with metabolic acidosis or when applied over large areas of the body surface.[78,79,89,91] Another detrimental problem encountered with mafenide acetate is that it is painful when applied to superficial partial-thickness burns with intact free nerve endings. The open application of mafenide acetate 8.5% cream to a burn wound site for increased antimicrobial activity may be considered a disadvantage if a burn wound dressing is necessary. However, it is quite effective in burn wound areas that are not well perfused such as the ear. The 5% aqueous solution of mafenide acetate can be used in a wet dressing covered by the splint.[78,79,89,91]

Studies have reported that the use of mafenide acetate 5% solution in patients with major burns resulted in a 33% reduction of fatality.[30,92] As with silver sulfadiazine, mafenide acetate can be used individually or in conjunction with other antimicrobials. However, mafenide acetate retards wound healing and reduces the breaking strength of healed wounds.[25]

Povidone-iodine (Betadine®)

A 10% ointment of povidone-iodine was developed after the active agent demonstrated a broad spectrum of antimicrobial attributes in liquid form. Although its active antimicrobial component is iodine, there has been no documentation associated with intact skin hypersensitivity or toxic effects. It has a broad spectrum of antibacterial and antifungal activities.[25,78,79,81,93,94] Povidone-iodine ointment can be employed effectively in both the closed and open techniques. Quantitative bacteriological assessments imply that iodine is most efficacious when it is administered every 6 hours. When it is used in this manner, it is effective in controlling and/or preventing bacterial colonization.

However, there are some adverse drug effects associated with the use of this topical antimicrobial at burn wound sites. The topical application of this agent is painful. Recent studies intimate that the iodine component of this topical agent may be absorbed more extensively in burn wound sites, resulting in iodine toxicity, renal failure, and acidosis. Concomitantly, it has been shown to be cytotoxic to fibroblasts as previously described.[25,78,79,81,93,94] However, it remains a highly effective disinfectant when used on intact skin.

Gentamicin sulfate (Garamycin®)

Gentamicin sulfate is available as a 0.1% water-soluble cream and is chemically similar to other aminoglycosides, such as kanamycin and neomycin. It has a broad spectrum of antimicrobial activity. Its popular use in wounds was based on its antimicrobiocidal efficacy against *P. aeruginosa*. However, gentamicin resistance has rapidly developed due to its widespread use as a topical antimicrobial agent.[25,78,79,81,93,94]

Bacitracin/polymyxin (Polysporin®)

The topical antibiotics ointment bacitracin/polymyxin is used to 'butter' bolsters to prevent mechanical shearing of newly grafted tissue. However, this topical ointment barrier used after a grafting procedure has not been shown to be effective in controlling infection. Many surgeons rely on this topical agent for skin graft coverage because it is nontoxic and is similar to petrolatum gauze dressings, which were previously considered as a dressing for grafts. These two combined antibiotics have little or no effect on localized burn wound infections[95] (Table 12.6).

Nitrofurazone (Furacin®)

The topical antimicrobial nitrofurantoin was used in the past but had questionable value therapeutically. Recent research, however, has shown that nitrofurantoin is effective in the treatment of MRSA and other methicillin-resistant staphylococci. Nitrofurantoin has also proved to be 75% effective against Gram-negative bacterial isolates other than *P. aeruginosa* while bacitracin/polymyxin was only 21% effective[10,95] (Table 12.7).

Mupirocin (Bactroban®)

Mupirocin is one of several antibiotics derived from the fermentation of *P. fluorescens* and is also known as pseudomonic acid A. While the antimicrobial activity derived from cultures of *P. fluorescens* was first reported over a century and a half ago, this agent could not be used as an antimicrobial agent until Fuller et al.[96] executed a more complete isolation and purification of pseudomonic acid A. Further research described

TABLE 12.6 MEAN SENSITIVITY ZONES OF TOPICAL ANTIBACTERIALS AGAINST 126 BIOTYPES OF GRAM-POSITIVE ISOLATES IN THE NAWD PROCEDURE

Organism	Number tested	Zones sizes (in mm)							
		Silvadene®	Sulfamylon®	Nitrofurazone	Bactroban	Polymyxin	Silva-nystatin	Modified Dakin's	Silver nitrate
S. aureus	18	16 ± 2.72*	27 ± 4.79	32 ± 4.24	25 ± 16.32	4 ± 7.42	14 ± 5.34	3 ± 4.12	16 ± 2.94
S. auricularis	2	18	23 ± 3.53	27 ± 9.89	18 ± 10.60	0	15 ± 1.41	4 ± 5.65	18 ± 2.82
S. epidermidis	50	20 ± 3.10	27 ± 7.62	36 ± 7.26	30 ± 14.86	0	18 ± 3.87	3 ± 5.3	19 ± 2.92
S. haemolyticus	35	19 ± 0.98	31 ± 5.26	35 ± 6.10	20 ± 16.54	0	18 ± 3.46	3 ± 4.86	18 ± 1.84
S. sciuri	1	30	30	31	40	0	27	8	17
S. simulans	3	18 ± 1.52	23 ± 6.11	36 ± 5.50	23 ± 25.16	0	18 ± 1.00	0	19 ± 1.52
S. warneri	1	19	28	40	12	0	18	0	13
E. faecalis	9	17 ± 4.69	25 ± 3.67	22 ± 2.40	28 ± 6.00	0	17 ± 4.64	1 ± 3.00	12 ± 1.99
E. faecium	7	11 ± 2.73	28 ± 4.04	23 ± 3.73	29 ± 9.81	0	11 ± 5.68	0	11 ± 2.82
Total	126	100%S	97.6%	98.4%	88.9S 6.3%R 4.8%I	3% 97%R	94.4%S 2.4%I 3.2%R	12.7%S 12%I 3.26R	96.8%S 2.4%I 0.8%R

*Mean value ± standard deviation.

TABLE 12.7 MEAN SENSITIVITY ZONES OF TOPICAL ANTIBACTERIALS AGAINST 79 BIOTYPES OF GRAM-NEGATIVE ISOLATE IN THE NAWD PROCEDURE

Organism	Number tested	Zones sizes (in mm)							
		Silvadene®	Sulfamylon®	Nitrofurazone	Bactroban	Polymyxin	Silva-nystatin	Modified Dakin's	Silver nitrate
A. baumanii	8	17 ± 3.00*	23 ± 2.55	21 ± 3.02	16 ± 3.07	8 ± 0.64	17 ± 3.02	12 ± 3.02	15 ± 2.21
A. lowffii	1	16	33	30	37	8	16	12	14
C. freundii	3	16 ± 2.08	21 ± 3.46	25 ± 3.79	24 ± 7.57	3 ± 4.62	13 ± 3.79	6 ± 11.00	12 ± 3.79
E. cloacae	7	13 ± 2.7	19 ± 3.73	23 ± 0.79	26 ± 1.57	8 ± 3.78	11 ± 5.86	6 ± 4.38	10 ± 2.21
E. coli	9	14 ± 4.35	14 ± 7.30	27 ± 4.16	24 ± 4.05	2 ± 3.53	12 ± 6.51	4 ± 6.56	10 ± 6.91
P. aeruginosa	25	16 ± 5.03	29 ± 6.13	6 ± 8.15	11 ± 6.79	1 ± 2.23	14 ± 4.75	9 ± 7.55	17 ± 4.73
P. fluorescens	8	14 ± 1.67	23 ± 4.70	9 ± 7.07	12 ± 1.82	2 ± 3.7	16 ± 0.52	7 ± 5.78	16 ± 2.00
P. maltophilia	1	18	20	16	18	9	13	10	15
Other	7	11 ± 5.76	21 ± 4.05	23 ± 2.62	21 ± 6.18	4 ± 4.59	9 ± 6.41	8 ± 8.44	7 ± 7.01
Total	79	92.4%S 3.8%I 3.8%R	97.5%S 2.5%I	75%S 3.8%I 21.2%R	91.1%S 3.8%I 5.1%R	3.8%S			

*Mean value ± standard deviation.
Summary of results.

the antimicrobial activity of mupirocin as an inhibition of microbial isoleucyl t-RNA synthetase that causes inhibition of protein synthesis in the bacterial cell.[96,97]

In vitro studies have subsequently established that mupirocin has omnipotent inhibitory activity against the Gram-positive microbes, specifically *S. aureus* and *S. epidermidis*. Mupirocin's efficiency in the treatment of infection or colonization due to *S. aureus*, whether methicillin-sensitive or not,

has been shown in various clinical settings.[96–98] Rode and co-workers[99] have provided additional data regarding the efficacy of mupirocin in the treatment of established wound infections with *S. aureus* that were resistant to systemic methicillin, topical mafenide acetate, and povidone-iodine.

Recent *in vitro* and *in vivo* endeavors have shown mupirocin to be as efficacious in methicillin-resistant burn wound infections.[95] Mupirocin, while not sanctioned for Gram-negative organisms, has been shown to be 75% effective against most enteric organisms and is significantly more effective against these microorganisms than bacitracin/polymyxin[95] (Table 12.6).

Mupirocin inhibits wound healing when compared to controls by a half-life of 2 days, while the breaking strength is significantly enhanced over the control ($p < 0.05$) (unpublished data 1994).

Acticoat® A.B.

Acticoat® A.B. Dressing consists of two sheets of high-density polyethylene mesh coated with ionic silver with a rayon/polyester core. Acticoat® A.B. Dressing provides broad-spectrum antimicrobial, bactericidal coverage against VRE, MRSA, *P. aeruginosa*, *Candida* sp. and approximately 150 other organisms. It can remain intact for several days on the wound, if there is minimal exudation.[100]

Nystatin (Mycostatin®, Nilstat®)

Nystatin is an antifungal antibiotic produced by *Streptomyces noursei*. Nystatin exerts its antifungal activity by binding to sterols in the fungal cell membrane. The drug is not active against bacterial and mammalian cells because they do not contain sterols in their cell membrane. As a result of this binding, the membrane is no longer able to function as a selective barrier to prevent the loss of potassium and other cellular constituents from the fungal cell. Nystatin has fungistatic or fungicidal activity against a variety of pathogenic and non-pathogenic strains of yeasts and fungi. *In vitro*, nystatin concentrations of approximately 3 µg/mL inhibit *C. albicans* and *C. guilliermondii*. Concentrations of 6.25 µg/mL are required to inhibit *C. krusei* and *Geotrichum lactis*. In general, there is little difference between minimum inhibitory and fungicidal concentrations for a particular organism. Nystatin is not active against bacteria, protozoa, or viruses.

Nystatin is not absorbed systemically and is used orally for the treatment of intestinal candidiasis. In our burn population, nystatin 'swish and swallow' is used prophylactically to prevent the oral or perineal overgrowth of yeast and fungi in patients receiving two or three systemic antibiotics. In patients with coexisting intestinal candidiasis and vulvovaginal candidiasis, nystatin may be administered orally, in conjunction with the intravaginal application of an antifungal agent. Most evidence suggests that combined therapy does not substantially reduce the risk of recurrence of vulvovaginal candidiasis, compared with intravaginal therapy alone. However, limited evidence suggests that the reduction of intestinal candidal colonization in combination with intravaginal antifungal therapy may provide some improvement in mycologic response and reduction in recurrence rate of vulvovaginal candidiasis.

For the treatment of cutaneous or mucocutaneous candidal infections, nystatin 100 000 units/gram may be applied topically as a cream, lotion, or ointment to affected areas 2–4 times daily. The cream or lotion formulations are preferred to the ointment for use in moist, intertriginous areas. The use of occlusive dressings and ointment formulations should be avoided in the treatment of candidiasis because they favor the growth of yeast and release of its irritating endotoxin. Concomitant therapy should include attention to proper hygiene and skin care to prevent spread of infection and reinfection. In addition, the affected areas should be kept dry and exposed to air whenever possible.

Burn patients are affected by an immunocompromised system and are thus more susceptible to opportunistic infections. Depletion of the number of neutrophils, defects in neutrophil function, and T-cell defects all predispose the host to fungal infections. Aspergillosis and hyalohyphomycosis (specifically *Fusarium*) are the most common angioinvasive fungal infections in burn patients. Barret et al. examined the curative effects of direct application of nystatin powder on severely burned children affected by angioinvasive fungal infection.[101] The topical treatment of burn wounds with nystatin powder at a concentration of 6 000 000 units/gram proved to be effective in eradicating the invasive fungal infections. This new regimen of topical treatment not only is effective superficially but also eradicates invasive clusters of fungi in deep wound tissues, as documented by pathological examination. The application of the powder is easy and did not produce pain or discomfort. It did not impair wound healing and all previously autografted areas healed uneventfully.[101]

Nystatin powder may be combined with silver sulfadiazine 1% cream and mafenide acetate 5% aqueous solution to prevent the overgrowth of yeast and fungi at the wound site with continuous application of these potent topical antimicrobial agents.

Discussion

Though topical antimicrobial therapy has significantly diminished the occurrence of invasive burn wound sepsis, we must search for other methods to prevent burn wound infection. Bacterial control is imperfect at best. Burn wound biopsies, blood, and bodily fluid cultures must be coupled with early excision and grafting to prevent, diagnose, and treat the infection in a timely manner.[7,78,85,102–105]

In a recent *in vitro* study conducted at the Shriner's Childrens Hospital to assess the efficacy of eight of the aforementioned topical agents against multiresistant Gram-positive and Gram-negative isolates, silver sulfadiazine 1% cream and mafenide acetate 5% aqueous solution still remained extremely effective against both groups of organisms as determined by a modified NAWD. Among 126 Gram-positive isolates, silver sulfadiazine 1% cream was 100% effective, nitrofurazone was 98.4% effective, mafenide 5% aqueous solution was 97.6% effective, silver nitrate 0.5% aqueous solution was 96.8% effective, and silver sulfadiazine 1% cream with nystatin 100 000 units/gram in a 1:1 combination was 94.4% effective. Mupircin's susceptibility has been markedly reduced (88.9%) since Strocks et al.'s, study in 1990[82] (Table 12.6). Of the 79 Gram-negative isolates tested, which included 25 clinical isolates of *P. aeruginosa*, mafenide acetate 5% aqueous solution was 97.5% effective, silver sulfadiazine was 92.4% effective, mupirocin was 91.1% effective (an increase of 16% over the Strock et al. study).[82] The only other two topicals showing an antimicrobial effect were the silver sulfadiazine 1% cream and nystatin 100 000 units/gram in a 1:1 combination, which showed 84.8% susceptibility, and silver nitrate 0.5% aqueous solution, which showed an 83.5% susceptibility (Table 12.7).

TABLE 12.8 *IN VITRO* ANTIMICROBIAL SUSCEPTIBILITIES OF TOPICAL AGENTS AS DETERMINED BY THE NAWD TECHNIQUE

Culture	No of sample	SSD		MA		FD		MU	
		Mean	SD	Mean	SD	Mean	SD	Mean	SD
All Gram-positive	39	19.7[bcd]	3.3	25.3[a,c,d]	6.8	33.6[a,b]	6.2	30.6[a,b]	14.9
All Gram-positive	37	15.4[b]	5.8	24.2[a,c]	7.2	18.2[b]	8.5	19.7	7.7
E. coli	6	16.3[c]	3.1	17.2[c]	6.1	27.0[a,b]	4.8	23.8	4.9
P. aeruginosa	12	16.1[b]	6.4	31.4[a,c,d]	4.6	9.5[b]	8.2	13.1[b]	5.8
S. epidermidis	11	21.9[b]	3.0	24.5[a,c]	9.3	35.5[b]	2.6	30.7	14.2

*39 patients entered into the study.
38 patients survived for a 2.5% mortality rate.
Abbreviations: [a] $p < 0.05$ vs SSD (silver sulfadiazine), [b] $p < 0.05$ vs MA (matenicle acetate), [c] $p < 0.05$ vs FD (nitrofurazone), [d] $p < 0.05$ vs MU (mupirocin).

Gold et al. (unpublished data) examined the role of topical antimicrobials in decreasing morbidity and mortality in major burn injuries (>50% TBSA). Thirty-nine patients were studied who were treated with topical antimicrobials, which included silver sulfadiazine 1% cream, mafenide acetate 5% aqueous solution, nitrofurazone, and mupirocin; 38 patients survived for a mortality rate of 2.5% (Table 12.8).

References

1. Edwards-Jones V, Greenwood JE; Manchester Burns Research Group. What's new in burn microbiology? James Laing Memorial Prize Essay 2000. Burns 2003; 29:15–24.
2. Mayhall CG. The epidemiology of burn wound infections: then and now. Clin Infect Dis 2003; 7:543–550.
3. Pruitt BA Jr, McManus AT, Kim S H. Burn wound infections: current status. World J Surg 1998; 22:135–145.
4. Robson MC, Krizek TJ, Heggers JP. Biology of surgical infection. In: Ravitch MM, ed. Current problems in surgery. Chicago: Yearbook Medical; 1973:1–62.
5. Teplitz C, Davis D, Mason AD, et al. Pseudomonas burn wound sepsis. Pathogenesis of experimental pseudomonas burn wound sepsis. J Surg Res 1964; 4:200–216.
6. Robson MC. Bacterial control in the burn wound. Clin Plast Surg 1979; 6(4):515–522.
7. Artz CP, Moncrief JA. The treatment of burns. Philadelphia: WB Saunders; 1969.
8. Heggers JP, Robson MC eds. Quantitative bacteriology: its role in the armamentarium of the surgeon. 1st edn. Boca Raton, FL, CRC; 1991:139.
9. Teplitz C. The pathology of burn and fundamentals of burn wound sepsis. In: Artz CP, Moncrief JA, Pruitt BA Jr, eds. Burns: a team approach. Philadelphia: WB Saunders; 1979:45–94.
10. Burke JR, Quinby WC, Bondoc CC, et al. The contribution of a bacterial isolated environment to the prevention of infection in seriously burned patients. Ann Surg 1977; 186:377–387.
11. Perez-Cappelano R, Manelli JC, Dalayret D, et al, Evaluation of the septicaemic risk by quantitative study of the cutaneous flora in patients with burns. Burns 1976; 3:42–45.
12. Sheridan RL. Sepsis in pediatric burn patients. Pediatr Crit Care Med 2005; 6(3 Suppl):S112–S119.
13. AltoparlakU, Erol S, Akcay MN, et al. The time-related changes of antimicrobial resistance patterns and predominant bacterial profiles of burn wounds and body flora of burned patients. Burns 2004; 30:660–664.
14. Robson MC. Burn sepsis. Crit Care Clin 1988; 4(2):281–298.
15. Lowbury EJ, Babb JR, Ford PM. Protective isolation in a burn unit: the use of plastic isolators and air curtains. J Hyg 1971; 69(4):529–546.
16. Nance FC, Lewis V, Bomside GH. Absolute barrier isolation and antibiotics in the treatment of experimental burn wound sepsis. J Surg Res 1970; 10:33.
17. Sherman RT. The prevention and treatment of tetanus in the burn patient. Surg Clin North Am 1970; 50:1277–1281.
18. Larkin JM, Moylan JA. Tetanus following a minor burn. J Trauma 1975; 15:546–548.
19. Tompkins D, Rossi LA; Nursing Committee of the International Society for Burn Injuries. Care of outpatient burns. Burns 2004; 30:A7–A9.
20. White MC, Thornton K, Young AER. Early diagnosis and treatment of toxic shock syndrome in paediatric burns. Burns 2005; 31:193–197.
21. Pruitt BA, Foley FD. The use of biopsies in burn patient care. Surgery 1973; 73:887–897.
22. Parks DH, Linares HA, Thomson PD. Surgical management of burn wound sepsis. Surg Gynecol Obstet 1981; 153:374–376.
23. Robson MC, Krizek TS. Predicting skin graft survival. J Trauma 1973; 13(3):213–217.
24. Danilla S, Andrades P, Gómez ME, et al. Concordance between qualitative and quantitative cultures in burned patients analysis of 2886 cultures. Burns 2005; 31:967–971.
25. Heggers JP, Sazy JA, Stenberg BD, et al. Bactericidal and wound healing properties of sodium hypochlorite. J Burn Care Rehabil 1991; 12(5):420–424.
26. Fader RC, Maurer A, Stein MD, et al. Sodium hypochlorite decontamination of split-thickness cadaveric skin infected with bacteria and yeast with subsequent isolation and growth of basal cells to confluency in tissue culture. Antimicrob Agents Chemother 1983; 24:181–185.
27. Bruck HM, Nash G, Foley FD, et al. Opportunistic fungal infection of the burn wound with phycomycetes and Aspergillus. Arch Surg 1971; 102:476–482.
28. Barret JP, Jeschke M, Herndon DN. Selective decontamination of the digestive tract in severely burned pediatric patients. Burns 2001; 27:439–445.
29. Pham TN, Warren AJ, Pham HH, et al. Impact of tight glycemic control in severely burned children. J Trauma Inj Infect Crit Care 2005; 1148–1154.
30. Desai MH, Herndon DN, Abston S. Candida infection in massively burned patients. J Trauma 1981; 21(3):237–239.
31. Kobayashi K, Mukae N, Matsunaga Y, et al. Diagnostic value of serum antibody to Candida in an extensively burned patient. Burns 1990; 16(6):414–417.

32. Goldstein E, Hoeprich PD. Problems in the diagnosis and treatment of systemic conditions. J Infect Dis 1980; 125:190–193.

33. Kidson A, Lowbury EJL. Candida infection of burns. Burns 1980; 6:228–230.

34. Burdge JJ, Rea F, Ayers L. Noncandidal, fungal infections of the burn wound. J Burn Care Rehabil 1988; 9(6):599–601

35. Solom JS, Simmons RL. Candida infection in surgical patients. World J Surg 1980; 4:381–394.

36. Spebar MJ, Lindberg RB. Fungal infection of the burn wound. Am J Surg 1981; 21(3):237–239.

37. Prasad JK, Feller IF, Thomson PD. A ten-year review of Candida sepsis and mortality in burn patients. Surgery 1987; 101:213–216.

38. Linneman CC Jr, MacMillan BC. Viral infections in pediatric burn patients. Am J Dis 1983; 135:750–753.

39. Deepe GS Jr, MacMillan BC, Linnemann CC Jr. Unexplained fever in burned patients due to cytomegalovirus infection. JAMA 1982; 248:2299–2301.

40. Goodwin CW, McManus WF. Viral infections in burned patients. Immunol 1985; 12:3–4, 8–9.

41. Edgar P, Kravitz M, Heggers JP, et al. Herpes simplex in pediatric burn patients. Proceedings of the American Burn Association 1990; 22:56.

42. Weintraub WH, Lilly AB, Randolph JG. A chickenpox epidemic in a pediatric burn unit. Surgery 1974; 76:490–494.

43. Barrret JP, Dardano AN, Heggers JP, et al. Infestations and chronic infections in foreign pediatric patients with burns: is there a role for specific protocols? J. Burn Care Rehabil 1999; 20:482–486.

44. Ramzy PI, Herndon DN, Wolf SE, et al. Comparison of organisms found by bronchoalveolar lavage and quantitative wound culture in severely burned children. Arch Surg 1998; 133:1275–1280.

45. Mandell GL, Bennett JE, Dolin R, eds. Principles and practice of infectious diseases, 6th edn. New York: Churchill Livingstone; 2004: Vol 2.

46. Luna CM, Vukacich P, Niederman MS, et al. Impact of BAL data on the therapy and outcome of ventilator-associated pneumonia. Chest 1997; 111:676–685.

47. Kollef MH. Ventilator-associated pneumonia: the importance of initial empiric antibiotic selection. Infect Med 2000; 17(4):265–268, 278–283.

48. Hamory BH. Nosocomial sepsis related to intravascular access. Crit Care Nurs Q 1989; 11(4):58–65.

49. Samsoondar W, Freeman JB, Coultish I, et al. Colonization of intravascular catheters in the intensive care unit. Am J Surg 1985; 149:730–732.

50. Maki DG, Jarrett F, Sarafin HW. A semiquantitative culture method for identification of catheter related infection in the burn patient. J Surg Res 1977; 22:513–520.

51. Stein JM, Pruitt BA Jr. Suppurative thrombophlebitis: a lethal iatrogenic disease. N Engl J Med 1970; 282:1452–1455.

52. Franceschi D, Gerding RL, Phillips G, et al. Risk factors associated with intravascular catheter infection in burned patients; a prospective randomized study. J Trauma 1989; 29(6):811–816.

53. Smallman L, Burdon DW, Alexander-Williams J. The effect of skin preparation and care on the incidence of superficial thrombophlebitis. Br J Surg 1980; 67:861–862.

54. Sheth NK, Franson TR, Rose HD, et al. Colonization of bacteria on polyvinyl chloride and Teflon intravascular catheters in hospitalized patients. J Clin Microbiol 1983; 18:1061–1063.

55. Maki DG, Botticelli JT, LeRoy ML, et al. Prospective study of replacing administration sets for intravenous therapy at 48 to 72 hour intervals. JAMA 1987; 258:1777–1781.

56. Pruitt BA Jr, Stein JM, Foley FD, et al. Intravenous therapy in burn patients: suppurative thrombophebitis and other life threatening complications. Arch Surg 1970; 100:399–404.

57. Sasaki TM, Welch GW, Herndon DN, et al. Burn wound manipulation induced bacteremia. J Trauma 1979; 19(l):46–48.

58. Beard CH, Ribeiro CD, Jones DM. The bacteremia associated with burns surgery. Br J Surg 1975; 62:638–641.

59. Mzezewa S, Jönsson K, Sibanda E, Åberg M, Salemark L. HIV infection reduces skin graft survival in burn injuries: a prospective study. Br J Plast Surg 2003; 56:740–745.

60. Murray PR, Baron EJ, Jorgensen JH, et al., eds. Manual of clinical microbiology, 8th edn. Washington, DC: ASM; 2003.

61. Baron S. Medical microbiology, 4th edn. Galveston, Texas: University of Texas Medical Branch; 1996.

62. McManus AT, Kim SH, McManus WF, et al. Comparison of quantitative microbiology and histology in divided burn-wound biopsy specimens. Arch Surg 1987; 122:74–76.

63. Mayhall CG, ed. Hospital epidemiology and infection control, 1st edn. Baltimore, Maryland: Williams & Wilkins; 1996.

64. Sedat Y, Nursal TZ, Tarim A, et al. Bacteriological profile and antibiotic resistance: comparison of findings in a burn intensive care unit, other intensive care units, and the hospital services unit of a single center. J Burn Care Rehabil 2005; 26:488–492.

65. Koneman EW, Allen SD, Janda WM, et al, eds. Color atlas and textbook of diagnostic microbiology, 5th edn. Philadelphia, Pennsylvania: Lippincott-Raven; 1997.

66. Woods GL, Gutierrez Y, eds. Diagnostic pathology of infectious diseases, 1st edn. Malvern, Pennsylvania: Lea & Febiger; 1993.

67. Becker WK, Cioffi WG Jr, McManus AT, et al. Fungal burn wound infection. A 10-year experience. Arch Surg 1991; 126(1): 44–48.

68. Desai MH, Herndon DN, Abston S. Candida infection in massively burned patients. J Trauma 1981; 21(3):237–239.

69. Pruitt BA Jr. Phycomycotic infections. Probl Gen Surg 1984; 664–678.

70. Sheridan RL. Sepsis in pediatric burn patients. Pediatr Crit Care Med 2005; 6 (3):S112–S119.

71. Martyn, J. Clinical pharmacology and drug therapy in the burned patient. Anesthesiology 1986; 65:67–76.

72. McEvoy GK, ed. American hospital formulary service. Bethesda, MD: American Society of Health-System Pharmacists; 2003.

73. Lacy CF, Armstrong LL, Goldman MP, et al. Drug information handbook, 11th edn. Hudson, OH: Lexi; 2003.

74 Rybak MJ. The pharmacokinetic and pharmacodynamic properties of vancomycin. Clin Infect Dis 2006; 42:S35–S75.

75. Ramphal R. Developing strategies to minimize the impact of extended-spectrum β-lactamases: focus on cefepime. Clin Infect Dis 2006; 42:S151–S152.

76. McKinsey, DS. Making best use of the newer antifungal agents. Drug Benefit Trends 2004; 16:131–147.

77. Evans ME, Feola DJ, Rapp RP. Polymyxin B sulfate and colistin: old antibiotics for emerging multiresistant gram-negative bacteria. Ann Pharmacother 1999; 33:960–967.

78. Robson MC. The use of topical agents to control bacteria. In: Dimick AR, ed. The burn wound in practical approaches to burn management. Deerfield, IL: Flint Laboratories, Travenol; 1977:17–19.

79. Moncrief JA. The status of topical antibacterial therapy in the treatment of burns. Surgery 1968; 63:862.

80. Kucan IO, Smoot EC. Five percent mafenide acetate solution in the treatment of thermal injuries. J Burn Care Rehabil 1993; 14:158–163.

81. Lindberg RB, Moncrief JA, Mason AD Jr. Control of experimental and clinical burn wound sepsis by topical application of sulfamylon compounds. Am NY Acad Sci 1968; 150:950.

82. Strock LL, Lee M, Rutan RL, et al. Topical Bactroban® (mupirocin): efficacy in treating burn wounds infected with methicillin-resistant staphylococci. J Burn Care Rehabil 1990; 11(5):109–116.

83. Nash G, Foley FD, Goodwin MN Jr, et al. Fungal burn wound infection. JAMS 1971; 215:1664–1666.

84. Fuller AT, Mellows G, et al. Pseudomonic acid, an antibiotic produced by Pseudomonas fluorescens. Nature (London) 1971; 234:416–417.

85. Heggers JP: The use of antimicrobial agents. In: Krizek TJ, Robson MC, eds. Clinics in plastic surgery. Philadelphia, PA: WB Saunders; 1979: Vol. 6, 545–551.

86. Heggers, JP. Antimicrobial agents. In: Heggers JB, Robson MC, eds. Quantitative bacteriology: it's role in the armamentarium of the surgeon. Boca Raton, FL: CRC; 1991:115–125.

87. Moncrief JA. Topical antibacterial treatment of the burn wound. In: Artz CP, Moncrief JA, Pruitt BA, Jr, eds. Burns, a team approach. Philadelphia, PA: WB Saunders; 1979:250–269.

88. Buchvald J. An evaluation of topical mupirocin in moderately severe primary and secondary skin infections. J Int Med Res 1988; 16:66–70.

89. Denning DW, Haiduven-Griffiths D. Eradication of low-level resistant Staphylococcus aureus skin colonization with topical mupirocin. Infect Control Hosp Epidemiol 1988; 9(6):261–263.

90. Rode H, DeWet PM, et al. Bacterial efficacy of mupirocin in multi-antibiotic resistant Staphylococcus aureus burn wound infection. J Antimicrob Chemother 1988; 21:589–595.

91. Pruitt BA Jr, Foley F. The use of biopsies in burn patient care. Surgery 1973; 73:8878–8897.

92. Neame P, Rayner D. Mucormycosis: a report of 22 cases. Arch Pathol 1960; 70:261–268.

93. Georglade NG, Harris WA. Open and closed treatment of burns with povidone-iodine. In: Polk HC, Jr, Ebrenkranz NJ, eds. Therapeutic advances and new clinical impressions: medical and surgical antisepsis with betadine microbicides. Yonkers, NY: Purdue Frederick; 1972.

94. Krizek TJ, Davis JH, DesPrez JD, et al. Topical therapy of burns – experimental evaluation. Plast Reconstr Surg 1967; 39:248.

95. Heggers JP, Robson MC, Herndon DN, et al. The efficacy of nystatin combined with topical microbial agents in the treatment of burn wound sepsis. J Burn Care Rehabil 1989; 10:508–511.

96. Krizek TJ, Koss N, Robson MC. The current use of prophylactic antibiotics in plastic and reconstructive surgery. Plast Reconstr Surg 1975; 55:21–32.

97. Krizek TJ, Gottlieb LJ, Koss H, et al. The use of prophylactic antibacterials in plastic surgery: a 1980s update. Plast Reconstr Surg 1985; 76:953–963.

98. Richards JH. Bacteremica following irritation of foci of infection. JAMA 1932; 99:1496–1497.

99. LeFrock J, Ellis CA, Turchik JB, et al. Transient bacteremia associated with sigmoidoscopy. N Engl J Med 1973; 289:467–469.

100. Heggers JP, Villarreal C, Edgar P, et al. Ciprofloxacin, the quinolone as a therapeutic modality in pediatric burn wound infections: efficacious or contraindicated. Arch Surg 1998; 133: 1247–1250.

101. Barret JP, Ramzy PI, Heggers JP, et al. Topical nystatin powder in severe burns: a new treatment for angioinvasive fungal infection refractory to other topical and systemic agents. Burns 1999; 25(6):505–508.

102. Heggers JP, Barnes ST, Robson MC, et al. Microbial flora of orthopaedic war wounds. Milit Med 1969; 134:602.

103. Scholz D, Scharmann W, Biobet H. Leucocidic substances for Aeromonas hydrophilia. Zentralbl Bakteriol [Orig A] 1974; 228:312–316.

104. Robson MC, Duke WF, Krizek TJ. Rapid bacterial screening in the treatment of civilian wounds. J Surg Res 1973; 14:426.

105. Holder IA, Schwab M, Jackson L. Eighteen months of routine topical antimicrobial susceptibility testing of isolates from burn patients: results and conclusions. J Antimicrob Chemother 1979; 5:455–463.

Chapter 13

Operative wound management

Michael Muller, Dilip Gahankari, and David N. Herndon

Removing dead or partially devitalized tissue saves lives and improves form and function. Skin grafting of granulation tissue (the precursor of ugly scar) following eschar separation has been replaced with operative intervention within hours of injury. Skin substitutes, dermal replacements, skin culture, and bioengineering are exciting and rapidly expanding technologies that are already offering simply amazing results. This chapter deals with the pathophysiology of the burn wound, the scientific basis of wound excision, and the techniques and technologies now available to burn surgeons.

The burn wound

Dead burned tissue promotes an inflammatory response at the junction of the eschar and the underlying viable tissue. At this interface, bacterial proliferation in the eschar attracts polymorphonuclear leukocytes (neutrophils) that release large quantities of proteolytic enzymes and inflammatory mediators. Subsequent enzymatic action results in consumption or separation of the eschar leaving granulation tissue. If the burn is large, the inflammatory response at the burned site becomes generalized. This effect is described fully elsewhere. Briefly, mediators such as prostanoids, thromboxane, histamine, cytokines, and tumor necrosis factor are all produced and released from the burned site. The serum levels of these mediators become measurable and increase in proportion to the area of the burn. The hypermetabolic response with protein catabolism, increased metabolic rate, increased susceptibility to infection, marked weight loss, and poor wound healing

continue until the outpouring of mediators abates. While topical antimicrobial agents such as mafenide acetate and silver sulfadiazine have decreased the frequency and severity of systemic sepsis, these agents prolong eschar separation and therefore the hypermetabolic response.

Treatment of full-thickness burns by awaiting spontaneous eschar separation and subsequent skin grafting is a prolonged process associated with much pain and suffering, severe metabolic derangements, multiple septic episodes, and lengthy hospitalization. In the modern era, this technique should be limited to those who are so infirm that any other method cannot be contemplated.

Beneficial effects of operative wound management

Prompt wound closure has been shown repeatedly to improve survival, decrease length of hospital stay, and curb expenditure in burned patients of all ages. Children particularly have benefited from more timely and extensive surgical intervention.[1,2] There has been a remarkable increase in the burn size associated with a 50% mortality risk over recent decades such that it is now unusual for a child to succumb to burn injury of any size, even if it is associated with a smoke inhalation injury (Tables 13.1 and 13.2). Improving nutritional support and control of sepsis have also played a part in this achievement. Early surgery, however, has contributed most toward this major advance. Burke[3] reported on results of total excision of full-thickness burns in 1974. He applied homografts (cadaver skin) to seal the wound, controlled rejection by adding immunosuppressives, and cared for his patients in laminar flow chambers. Children with massive burns began surviving their injuries where they had never previously done so. Improved mortality, shorter hospital stay, and fewer metabolic complications were noted by others when early excision was retrospectively compared with late excision.[4] When 32 children, average age 7 years and mean burn size 65% total body surface area (TBSA) who underwent either total excision to fascia or serial debridement were studied: mortality, overall blood loss, and cumulative operating time were equivalent.[5] The early excision group, however, had their length of hospital stay almost halved (97 ± 8 days vs. 57 ± 5 days). Since that time, hundreds of children with burns >30% TBSA treated with early excision have exhibited a length of hospital stay less than 1 day/% TBSA burned.[6]

Mortality of adult burn patients at Massachusetts General Hospital declined from 24% in 1974 to 7% for 1979–1984 after prompt eschar excision and immediate wound closure was instituted as standard therapy in 1976.[7] Logistical regression analysis showed that this treatment significantly improved survival ($p < 0.001$). Thirty adult patients admitted to the Galveston Burn Unit with very large burns were randomized to receive either early total or staged excision. In patients with no inhalation injury, mortality was decreased with early excision. Total blood requirements were similar between groups, negating an often-used argument against excisional therapy. This study was expanded to include 85 patients, aged 17–55 years.[8] Those patients aged 17–30 years without inhalation injury showed significantly reduced mortality if treated by early excision (9%), than if treated conservatively (45%). Patients with a concomitant inhalation injury or age greater than 30 years, however, derived no survival benefit from early excision. More recently, Herndon's group have shown that delayed excision of severely burned children leads to increased hypermetabolism and all the detrimental effects that follow.[9]

Munster and colleagues[10] demonstrated a statistically significant decrease in length of hospital stay that significantly correlated with a decrease in the interval between surgical interventions over a 14-year period at his institution. Other variables such as burn size, inhalation injury, and age remained static during this time; they found that mortality rate decreased significantly while burn indices remained constant. The average annual increase of hospital charges for burn care grew at 9.6%, which was substantially lower than the hospital as a whole (10.8%). Active surgical intervention in burn care can be associated with cost containment and fewer lives lost.

Older burn patients have been shown to benefit from an early surgical approach. Deitch[11] operated upon 114 consecutive patients with an average age of 68 years, and showed a reduction of 40% in mean length of hospital stay when compared to national averages, and mortality was less than predicted. Many studies[12–16] show that early excision can be safely performed in the elderly, with clear benefit of reductions in duration of hospitalization and the number of septic episodes. Saffle[15] showed that the number of preexisting medical conditions in the elderly had no effect on survival, a salient point when planning treatment. The elderly also benefit from aggressive surgical treatment of their donor site wounds. They very commonly have loose and mobile skin. If donor sites or burns are situated on the lower abdomen, the flank, or thigh, they are amenable to excision and repair in the same manner as a reduction abdominoplasty.[17] This has the effect of reducing the area of open wound and decreasing the metabolic demand placed on their physiology.

Hypertrophic scar formation is common, with dark-skinned people and children being more prone to its development. However, the most important determinant of hypertrophic scarring is delayed wound healing. Deitch[18] has clearly shown that if wounds take more than 10 days to heal then the risk is significant and it rises to 80% if healing is delayed beyond 21 days. Surgery is therefore indicated for those whose wounds fail to heal promptly. Operative treatment is also an effective means of limiting the duration of pain that burn patients must endure. The ghastly experience of wound debridement in the tub by picking at the eschar, sometimes for many weeks, has been recounted by many as the worst part of their burn experience. Excisional therapy of the burn wound is humane, life-saving, offers improved cosmetic and functional results, is cost-effective, and more swiftly returns the patient to their normal environment.

Techniques of burn wound excision

Excising a small, deep burn

Once a burn wound is determined to be 'deep', operative intervention is indicated without further delay. 'Deep' burns are those which are clearly full-thickness or are deep dermal

---

TABLE 13.1 MORTALITY FOLLOWING BURN OVER TIME FOR DIFFERENT AGE GROUPS SHOWN AS THE BURN SIZE AT WHICH 50% LIVE OR DIE–LETHAL AREA 50 (LA50)

Age [years]	LA50 (% TBSA)		
	1942–1952	1980–1991	1992–2004
0–14	49	98	99
15–44	46	70	88
45–64	27	46	75
>65	10	19	33

TBSA = percentage of total body surface area burned.
LA50 = lethal burn area for a 50% mortality.
1992–2004: Branski LK, Barrow RE, Herndon DN, unpublished data.

TABLE 13.2 PEDIATRIC SPECIFIC MORTALITY RATES OVER TIME. NEAR-TOTAL EARLY EXCISION IS THE BASIS OF THESE EXCELLENT RESULTS. MORTALITY AND PEDIATRIC BURN PATIENTS, SHRINERS BURN INSTITUTE, GALVESTON

Years	Mortality sorted by burn size (% TBSA)							
	<20%	n	21–40%	n	41–60%	n	61–100%	n
1980–1985	<0.1%	889	1%	230	8%	105	33%	95
1986–1990	<0.1%	571	1%	224	4%	117	19%	88
1991–1995	<0.1%	522	2%	192	8%	94	20%	78
1996–2000	<0.1%	635	1%	222	3%	133	19%	114
2001–2004			2%	83	2%	121	26%	91

n = total number of patients admitted with respective burn size in given time period.

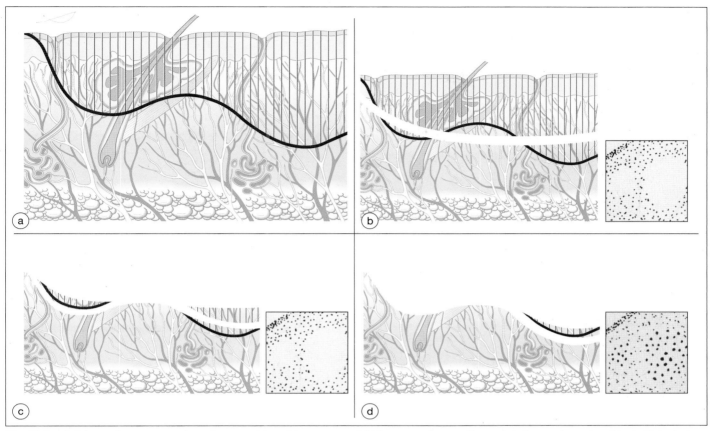

Fig. 13.1a–d Schematic representation of tangential excision; sequential slices are taken until punctate hemorrhage is evident. (Adapted from Janzekovic Z. A new concept in the early excision and immediate grafting of burns. J Trauma 1970; 10:1103–1108 with permission.)[22]

burns unlikely to heal within 14–21 days. They are typically flame and contact burns and are commonly situated on the extremities. Heimbach[19] observed that deep partial-thickness burns did not convert to full-thickness when topical antimicrobials were used to control infection. Although these wounds did eventually heal after many weeks, they showed persistent blistering, pruritus, hypertrophic scar formation, and poor functional results. These observations prompted a prospective trial of early excision and grafting versus non-operative treatment of burns of indeterminate depth of less than 20% TBSA.[20,21] Shorter hospitalization, lower cost, less time away from work, but greater use of blood products were seen in those treated operatively. Those patients treated nonoperatively required more late grafts for closure and developed more hypertrophic scarring. There was no difference in need for reconstructive procedures, range of motion, or contour irregularities.

Tangential excision

Tangential excision removes necrotic tissue while preserving as much of the underlying viable tissue as possible. Body contours are better preserved than with fascial level excision and therefore this is the usual method for small burns. The technique of tangential excision was originally described by Janzekovic,[22] who observed that deep donor sites could be overgrafted with thinner split-thickness skin harvested from another area. She then extended this concept to dermal burns by excising thin layers of burn until living tissue was reached (Figure 13.1a–d). Split skin grafts were immediately applied. This technique of tangential excision and autografting of dermal burns was a major advance. Prior to this time only full-thickness burns were excised and usually as a formal integumentectomy, taking subcutaneous fat and accompanying lymphatics down to the underlying layer of investing fascia (fascial excision) (Figure 13.2). Janzekovic analyzed the results of the use of tangential technique of excision in over 2000 patients. She found that hospital stay, pain, and reconstructive procedures were all decreased compared to fascial excision.[23]

A number of different instruments can be used to perform tangential excision. The Rosenberg knife, Goulian knife, Watson knife, and Versajet water dissector[24] are all used around the world (Figure 13.3). The Watson knife is probably the most popular instrument for tangential excision. The technique is aided by traction and counter-traction to place the area under tension. To ensure adequate depth is obtained, the excised tissue can be grasped as it appears from the top of the instrument and traction applied. Partial-thickness injuries are debrided to a white, shiny dermal surface with punctate bleeding that is fine and copious if the burn depth is superficial and less frequent from larger vessels for deep partial-thickness burns. Healthy fat has a yellow glistening appearance and it

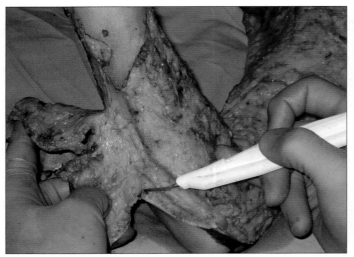

Fig. 13.2 Fascial level excision using cutting diathermy and incorporated smoke evacuator.

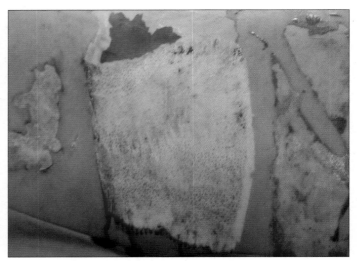

Fig. 13.4 A deep flame burn on the left thigh that is in the process of being debrided. The wound has been tumesced with 1:1000000 epinephrine in normal saline and shows minimal bleeding. The lower part of the wound demonstrates residual dead dermis with dull appearance and staining from lysed cells. The area just above demonstrates shiny yellow living fat and (mostly) surviving shiny white dermis with a few patches needing another slice.

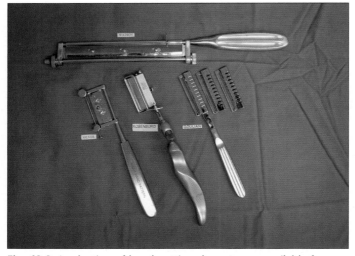

Fig. 13.3 A selection of hand-cutting dermatomes available for use for tangential excision. Most have the ability to have the aperature set to the desired depth while the Goulian has a large series of blades that are changed.

is imperative excision continues, layer by layer, until this appearance is obtained. Dullness, punctate hemorrhages, purple discoloration, or thrombosed vessels indicate nonviable tissue upon which grafts will fail and deeper excision is mandatory (Figure 13.4). When excision is performed on limbs following exsanguination with a rubber bandage and control of arterial inflow with a pneumatic tourniquet, these features are especially important. In particular, staining of the dermis with hemoglobin from lysed red cells indicates a need for deeper excision.

Controlling blood loss

Tangential excision can lead to copious blood loss unless measures are taken to limit potential hemorrhage. The simplest measure is to operate within 24 hours of injury. Vasoactive metabolites, particularly the potent vasoconstrictor thromboxane, are in abundance during this time and do much to limit blood loss.[25] This proposition is supported by a prospective trial of 318 children and adolescents with burns >30% TBSA. The average blood loss per surface area excised (mL/cm^2) was compared at various postburn periods of excision. The entire full-thickness burn, with the exception of the face and perineum, was tangentially excised with a hand knife with contiguous partial-thickness burn removed to punctate bleeding with serial passes of an electric dermatome. Patients whose blood pressure was greater or less than 40% of baseline, urine output less 0.75 mL/kg/h, or developed pulmonary edema intraoperatively, or whose hematocrit was >48 or <24% were not included in the analysis. Overall mortality was 5% for an average size burn of 60% TBSA. Notably, early excision had no adverse effect on mortality and no intraoperative deaths were recorded. Very early excision led to a halving of blood loss for both large and small burns[26,27] (Figure 13.5).

Further adjunctive measures to limit blood loss include tourniquets for the extremities, pre-debridement tumescence with weak epinephrine (adrenaline) solution, topical application of epinephrine 1:10000–1:20000 via either spray or cannula, topical application of thrombin, fibrin sealant, autologous platelet gel, calcium-enriched alginate sheets, epinephrine-soaked (~1:400000) lap-pads (sponges), and immediate bandaging with delayed grafting. Reconstituted whole blood (packed cells plus fresh frozen plasma) helps to allow extensive debridements with up to 2–3 blood volume replacement by controlling consumptive coagulopathy.[28]

All the above is predicated on normothermia being maintained.

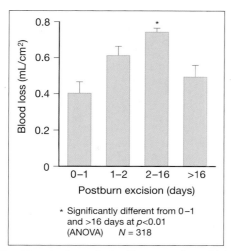

Fig. 13.5 Blood loss is almost halved by operating within 24 hours of injury. (Adapted from Desai et al. Early burn wound excision significantly reduces blood loss. Ann Surg 1990; 221:753–762. with permission.) [26]

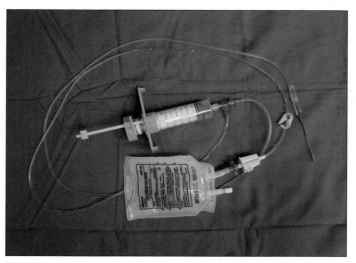

Fig. 13.6 An infuser device.

Use of a sterilizable, silicone tourniquet protected by a plastic sleeve allows for bloodless, unhurried debridement. This is a boon for the hand and fingers. The technique requires close attention to detail and some practice to recognize adequacy of debridement using the appearance of the wound bed as described above. The tourniquet can be released briefly to check adequacy of debridement and then quickly reinflated. The larger vessels are controlled by electrocautery or ligation and the wound is then flooded with a strong epinephrine solution, and covered with sheets of calcium alginate which are also soaked in a 1:100000 epinephrine solution. The tourniquet is released after 5–8 minutes. The limb should then be held elevated for about 10 minutes. Pre-excisional tumescence with epinephrine saline can be used almost everywhere except the digits. This technique is particularly useful for the trunk, scalp, and face. An infuser device speeds the process and certainly saves operator thumb strain (Figure 13.6). Pressure-bags, 'pitkin' syringes, and liposuction infusers can all be used. Delayed grafting is used in some centers to limit blood loss. If delayed grafting is undertaken, the wound bed needs to be kept moist and clean. A number of means are available: the wounds can be covered with bulky cotton dressings with tubing through the dressing to the wound surface used for continuous or intermittent irrigation with antibiotic or sulfamylon solution. Acticoat, kept moist with water via cannulae, also works. The patient returns to the operating room within 72 hours and undergoes a second procedure of harvest and application of skin grafts.

Techniques of wound closure

If the burn is small and donor sites are plentiful, skin grafts can be applied as 'sheet' or unmeshed skin. This technique requires experienced personnel to attend to the graft every few hours for a number of days to ensure that seromas and hematomas are controlled and expressed. Another less labor-intensive technique is to mesh the graft at a ratio of 1:1 or 1.5:1, but not to expand or stretch the mesh. If performed carefully, blood and seroma will drain away from the wound and a good cosmetic appearance is left. These grafts are best laid perpendicular to the long axis of limbs, particularly across joint flexural creases, which is in line with the general rule of placing potential scars perpendicular to the dominant muscle contraction in the area. This will decrease the degree of contracture if it occurs. Possible exceptions are the dorsum of the hand and forearm where some clinicians argue that longitudinally placed grafts are cosmetically superior.

If burns are huge and donor sites scarce, then areas such as the scalp, scrotum, and axillas may need to be harvested. These are meshed and widely expanded. The wound is then sealed by an overlay of unexpanded, 1.5:1 meshed, fresh or frozen partial-thickness allografts. These are applied at 90° to the autograft in a sandwich pattern as described by Alexander et al[29] (Figure 13.7a,b). The cellular immune depression associated with massive burns makes rejection phenomena to the allograft uncommon. Fresh allografts, stored at 2–4°C in nutrient media, achieve an adherence rate of 95%. Even in large burns the face, neck, and hands are sheet grafted with thick (say 15000th inch or more) split-skin if at all possible.

Advances in wound closure

When the burn has reached the fat layer, dermal replacement material such as Integra™/Terudermis are indicated. Contracture is decreased (but not eliminated) and results pleasing. Engraftment is aided by the use of negative pressure (VAC) dressings[30] (Figure 13.8a–e).

Cultured skin has a definite place in modern burn care. Munster has shown that use of cultured epithelial autografts (CEA) in the massively burned decreased mortality.[31] Herndon[32] compared the use of CEA with wide mesh autograft and allograft overlay in a group of children with enormous burns, >90% TBSA. Use of CEA was associated with a much better cosmetic result at the expense of a longer length of hospital stay and more reconstructive procedures. Successful use of CEA in the massively burned, critically ill (usually) ventilated patient is difficult. CEA is most often supplied as sheets measuring 10 cm × 15 cm. Unfortunately, it is very thin with 10–15 cell layers being the norm. This has all the strength

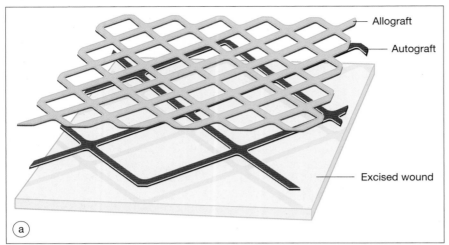

Allograft

Autograft

Excised wound

(a)

Fig. 13.7 (a) Schematic representation of 'sandwich' technique of allograft overlay. (Adapted from Alexander JW, MacMillan BG, Law E et al. Treatment of severe burns with widely meshed skin autograft and meshed skin allograft overlay. J Trauma 1981; 21(6):433–438. with permission.)[29] (b) Sandwich technique on the chest of a boy with massive deep burn having a return surgery a week after sandwich grafting. Most of the (fresh) allograft has vascularized with one piece obviously whiter than the rest. The mesh pattern of the underlying widely meshed autograft is visible.

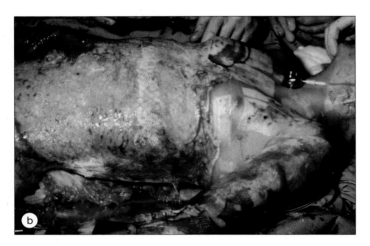

(b)

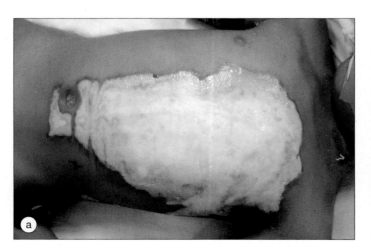

(a)

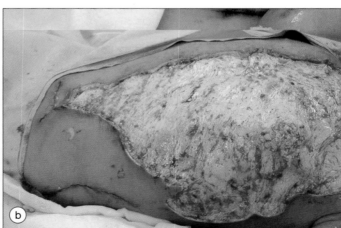

(b)

Fig. 13.8a–e Deep flame burn on a boy's chest treated with early excision and Integra with VAC.

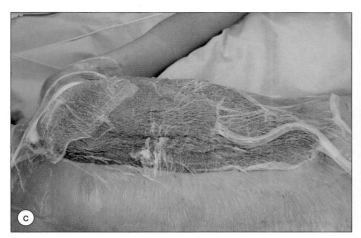

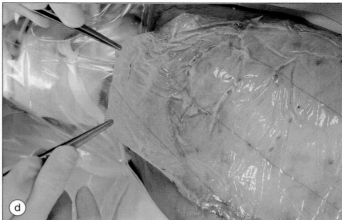

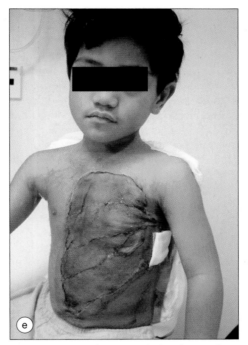

Fig. 13.8a–e – cont'd (d) The silicone layer being removed on day 12 ready for thin grafting with well-vascularized dermal template underneath. (e) The pleasing final result.

of wet tissue paper and is very prone to shearing. As CEA in this patient group is most usually applied to a wound bed devoid of dermis, anchoring of the epithelial layer is delayed and consequently shearing and blistering is common for many months. Long-term survival of CEA is therefore particularly problematic on the posterior surfaces of these massively burned patients and goes some way towards explaining the 5–50% long-term CEA engraftment rates reported in the literature. CEA does have a definite place in wound management of the massively burned and biopsies should be procured on admission and sent immediately to commence the process of culture. Areas that are less prone to shearing such as the anterior surfaces of the torso and thighs are particularly appropriate for its use. Wound excision should not be delayed whilst waiting delivery of the CEA. The wound should be temporarily closed with allograft until the CEA arrives.

Tissue engineering technology is advancing rapidly. Fetal skin constructs having been recently successfully trialled[33] and the bilaminar skin substitute of Boyce[34] is now in routine clinical use and delivering truly spectacular results. We await stem cell culture technology to deliver full cosmetic restoration for our patients.

Donor site

Selecting the best donor site region and depth is a matter of careful judgment and much controversy; even more so is the method of donor-site management. There is general agreement that, if at all possible, the face and neck should be resurfaced by grafts harvested from the 'blush' area above the line of the nipple for the best color match. Small burns in other areas allow the donor site to be hidden on the upper thigh or buttock. In children, some favor the scalp for all applications as regrowth of hair hides the area. Unfortunately, for some, this does not come with a lifelong guarantee. If a small graft is required, the mons pubis area should be considered as a potentially hidden site. The upper lateral thigh is a good compromise. The area is usually hidden from view and effective pressure garment therapy can be applied against the underlying bony structure if hypertrophic scar eventuates. The buttock donor site is easier to hide but effective pressure therapy is less assured. Good-quality grafts of consistent depth are obtained by use of a powered dermatome and certainly avoid the sawtooth pattern often seen following use of a hand knife to harvest split-skin grafts. When the burn size is huge, some unusual donor sites need to be used. The axilla and scrotum, in males, can provide useful amounts of skin graft after tumescence to produce a tight surface for harvest. The soles of the feet can also be used. It is best to shave and discard a first layer of keratin and then harvest the grafts for definitive use.

Selection of depth of split-skin grafts is influenced by a number of factors. The overall burn size may predicate a need for re-cropping and wide expansion of meshed grafts. Thinner grafts of $^{6}/_{1000}$ inch in adults should then be harvested. Massively burned patients can sometimes have such limited available donor site area that re-cropping may have to be performed repeatedly to achieve wound closure. Even if harvesting is performed at as shallow a depth as possible, there is a point at which any subsequent re-cropping is of largely nonviable skin.[35] This loss of the donor sites' regenerative capabilities has drastic implications, not only for the closure of the original burn but also for the ability to perform reconstructive procedures at some later time. Overgrafting of the donor wound with CEA sheets in patients with massive burns can allow re-cropping in a week rather than the usual 3 weeks (M Rudd, personal communication).

Donor-site management

There are as many ways of managing donor wounds as there are burn units. We present a small representative selection. The Galveston Unit favors donor sites covered by scarlet red gauze, followed by dry gauze and compression bandages if anatomically possible. Bandages are removed 6 hours later and donor sites exposed. If donor sites fail to dry or develop excess moisture, a 40 watt heat lamp is positioned 18 inches away. Heat is applied for 20 minutes each hour until dry. Smaller donor sites can be treated with occlusive or adherent dressings such as Opsite™ or Biobrane™. These dressings can be applied to larger areas with innovation and effort but they carry the risk of promoting infection if fluid accumulates beneath the occlusive layer. This can lead to conversion to full-thickness wounds. Another technique is to use alginate sheets or hydrocolloid fiber dressings. They have the advantage of promoting moist wound healing and may diminish donor-site wound pain. The trapped moisture does lend itself to Gram-negative infection, however, and this should be carefully monitored. Silver-impregnated dressings such as Acticoat™ or Acticoat Absorbent™ or Aquacel Ag™ seem to diminish bacterial overgrowth and can be used directly on the donor wound or as an intermediate layer. The slightest hint of green exudate mandates immediate removal and treatment with topical antimicrobials. Split-thickness skin graft donor sites heal primarily by epithelialization from the remaining epithelial elements. Healing is rapid with thin split-skin grafts as the residual hair follicles, sweat glands, and sebaceous glands are close together but with thicker skin grafts healing is slowed. The time to healing depends on

depth of harvest, vascularity of the donor site, wound management, and general patient factors such as age, sepsis and vasopressors. There is no regeneration of harvested dermis. This has implications particularly for patients who require harvesting of healed donor sites. There is also a greater risk of hypertrophic scarring after harvesting of deeper grafts.

Management of specific burns

Scald burns

Hot water scald burns of small or moderate size have been shown to be the exception to the general rule of early excision. Young children who had scald burns up to 20% TBSA required less area to be excised and had smaller blood transfusion requirements if operated upon in the second and third week postburn.[36] Earlier operation resulted in greater blood transfused and later operation led to much increased hospital stay. A subsequent prospective trial randomized 24 children to early or late excision if their hot water scald injury had caused burns of clinically indeterminate depth.[37] No patient experienced a significant wound infection or systemic sepsis. Only half of the delayed excision group ultimately required surgical intervention and a significantly smaller area of excision was necessary for the remainder.

In light of the foregoing evidence, children with hot water scald burns <20% TBSA can be appropriately treated with a topical antimicrobial such as silver sulfadiazine or Acticoat™ for about 2 weeks in the reasonable expectation of healing for the majority. This approach needs to be balanced by the knowledge that the longer a wound remains exposed to the environment, the greater the inflammatory response and subsequent scarring. Trauma, desiccation, and microorganisms almost certainly play a part in this process. A number of techniques are now available to cover the partial-thickness wound. When successful, they have the added advantage of eliminating a great deal of the pain associated with dressing changes. These techniques are based on adherent wound dressings in the form of skin substitutes such as Biobrane™ and Transcyte™. Glycerol or cryopreserved allograft has also been used. More superficial wounds can be covered by a polyurethane membrane such as Omiderm™. These techniques can be used on patients with burns up to about 30% TBSA. The authors favor Biobrane™ for smaller and more superficial wounds that are pink, moist, and blanch readily.[38] Biobrane™ is a nylon/silicone bilaminated composite skin substitute. At the time of the first wound dressing, all loose skin and creams are removed to leave a clean, moist surface. The skin substitute is applied under some tension (like cling wrap on a bowl) and either stapled to itself on the extremities or taped to nonburned skin. A dry, nonadherent dressing should be applied and, where possible, firmly bandaged. The material works by becoming densely adherent to the exposed dermis, thus acting as a neo-epidermis. Herndon's group report no increase in infection rates using Biobrane™ in this way.[39] If problems do occur, it follows accumulation of fluid and non-adherence which needs to be dealt with promptly or an abscess-like state can develop with pus trapped between the skin and the material. A few days of inactivity by the patient helps the development of adherence. The material needs to be applied in the first few postburn days and the normal amount of vigilance is required to watch for invasive Gram-positive infection. A toxic patient with increasing, throbbing wound pain and surrounding cellulitis are signs of this serious condition. Removal of the material, application of topical antimicrobial and appropriate systemic therapies are immediately indicated. Some centers have taken a middle ground and use Acticoat™ with great success. It has the advantage of having antimicrobial activity and only needs to be changed each 3–7 days. A series of catheters are inserted through the overlying dressing (often a retention dressing such as Hypafix/Fixomull) through which carers instill 5–10 mL of water each 4–6 hours. Another variation is to have the (adult) patient spray or immerse the material whenever they feel it becoming dried out and adhering painfully to the wound.

Slightly deeper partial-thickness scald burns up to 40% TBSA can be treated by thin tangential excision or dermabrasion and application of Transcyte™. Transcyte™ is Biobrane™ that has been placed in a culture medium of fibroblasts derived from fetal foreskin for a week. They adhere to the material and produce ground substances, collagen, and growth factors. These substances, it is said, have a modulating effect on the inflammatory response in the wound bed. It is then frozen and so has to be defrosted prior to use. Transcyte™ achieves better adherence rates than Biobrane™ and is useful in more mobile and concave areas[40] (Figure 13.9a–d).

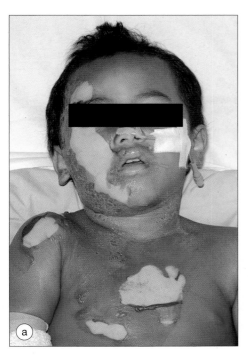

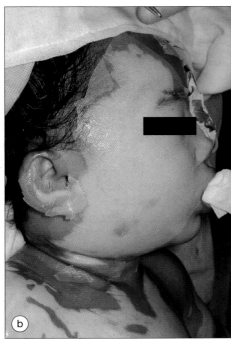

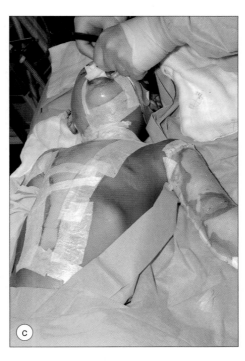

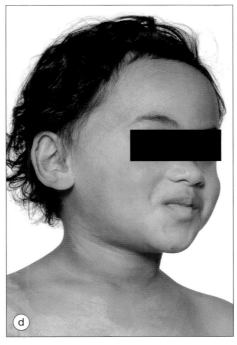

Fig. 13.9a–d Scald burn to face, chest, and arm of a young boy. The wounds were scrubbed under anesthetic within hours of injury with Transcyte™ applied to the face, neck, and chest and Biobrane™ to the arm. Tape was used extensively.

The postoperative care of either material needs to be attentive with regular examination and preemptive trimming as required. It is important that creams, gels, and ointments are not allowed in contact with the material as this prevents or loosens adherence and leads to failure. This is particularly important if the standard wound dressing is tullegras or similar. Transcyte™ and Biobrane™ can also be used as temporary wound cover for excised full-thickness wounds and in place of allograft as the overlay for widely meshed autograft. Adherence is more likely to occur and continue if the level of excision is fascia rather than subcutaneous fat — especially in very large burns.

Patients with very large scald burns, >40% TBSA, require total excision and immediate wound coverage. This may be with a combination of autograft, skin substitute, allograft, and dermal replacement (see later). Those with massive scald injury, >60% TBSA, require the same approach as the massive flame burn with selective fascial excision, widely meshed autograft and allograft overlay, dermal replacement material, and perhaps CEA.

The very large burn

Patients with deep (flame) burns between 50 and 70% TBSA pose unique challenges with many conflicting demands for available donor sites. This is even more so when the patient has suffered a concomitant smoke inhalation and is likely to require ventilation for some weeks. In general, a fascial excision is indicated unless very healthy deep dermis can be left. This may be possible in areas of thick dermis such as the back. Near total excision should be completed in the first few days after injury and certainly by the fifth day postburn. The back, buttocks, and posterior thighs are covered with autograft taken at 6/1000 in adults, thinner in children, which is meshed at an expansion ration of 4 or 6:1. This is left on the carrier, if a Zimmer™ system is used, and applied to the wound bed and then painstakingly spread. A bulb syringe is a useful tool to 'float' the spaghetti-like graft into appropriate position. 'Fresh' allograft is the best option as an overlay. The central intravenous sites — subclavian and femoral — are covered with at least a 10 cm diameter patch of narrowly meshed, 1.5:1 autograft as is the tracheostomy site.

Consideration needs to be given to the use and extent of dermal replacement such as Integra™. Dermal replacement is an expensive option, but one that leaves an excellent result — when it works. Integra™ is, to date, the material with which most units have experience. It is a bilaminar composite that has a neodermis of bovine collagen held in a matrix pattern with shark cartilage chondroitin-6-sulfate. A layer of rubberized silicone is press sealed onto this and acts as a neoepidermis. The silicone layer does not drape and bend very well and is prone to delamination by movement over joints or by external shearing forces such as rough hands. For these reasons, Integra™ lends itself to application on flat, anterior surfaces. Many centers have moved to meshing Integra™ and our experience is very positive. A cutting 1:1 (Brennan) mesher works but requires close attention or the material is mashed not meshed! The abdomen, anterior thigh, forearm, leg, and male chest are such sites (Figure 13.10a,b).

Meticulous operative technique is essential with every point of excessive electrocautery that results in tissue necrosis

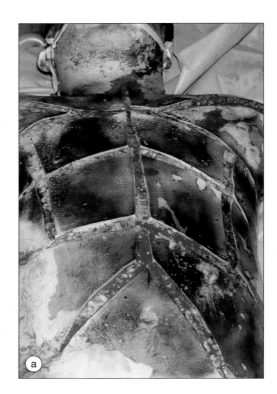

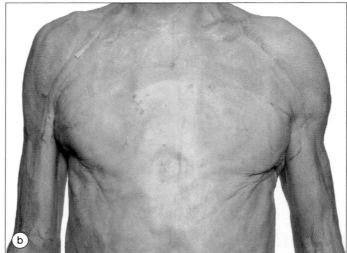

Fig.13.10 a,b High-voltage electrical flash burn treated by fascial excision and Integra™. Flat anterior surfaces are particularly amenable to use of Integra™.

leading to an area that fails. Topical epinephrine, and pinpoint accuracy with monopolar and selective use of bipolar electrocautery are the hemostatic methods of choice. Integra™ is best held in place by either a VAC or by attaching an elastic netting material (Surginet™) over it. A layer of Acticoat™ is frequently added in many centers. Further protection is then afforded with layers of netting (wedding veil, Conformant 2™, Exudry™). The neodermis is then revascularized from the underlying wound. This process takes 2–3 weeks to complete but is usually underway by 3–5 days. The neodermis often becomes a plum color due to suffusion through the matrix of red cells from minor hemorrhage. This is normal and should be left alone. Actual hematomas are recognized by lifting of the material associated with a very dark red color. The area overlying the hematoma is best excised and the edges stapled down. The Integra™ can be replaced or the area treated with Acticoat™. It must be remembered that the neodermis is inert and nonviable with no resistance to infection until neovascularization has occurred. This window of extreme vulnerability lasts about 5 days but the risk of delamination and shearing continues until the silicone neoepidermis has been replaced by epidermis.

The neodermis is 'ready' when it becomes a 'straw' color. Close inspection with magnification will reveal telangiectatic vessels dotted about. The second-stage operation involves gentle removal of the silicone layer and application of 6/1000 inch autograft which can be meshed up to an expansion of 3:1. If shortage of donor sites necessitates expansion then the harvest needs to include as little dermis as possible otherwise a mesh pattern will permanently remain. It is said that CEA can be used for epidermal cover of Integra™ neodermis.[41] It is probably best to delay this procedure to ensure adequate vascularization and enhance CEA engraftment. The author's experience with this technique in very large and massive burns with multiresistant organisms resident upon them has not been gratifying. There is benefit in performing staged, sequential replacement of the silicone layer with thin, 1:1.5 meshed autograft in sick patients with very large burns. Engraftment and graft survival seems to be more reliable in the long term and the cosmetic result enhanced; less haste but more progress. Debate continues regarding the role of Integra™ in wound coverage of patients with burns >70% TBSA. The incidence of failure due to infection rises dramatically as the burn size tops 75% TBSA. Decisions regarding its use will be influenced by the availability, or otherwise, of allograft. It cannot be stated too strongly that Integra™ cannot be left abutting unexcised wound. It all has to be removed or infection will spread relentlessly from the edge and lead to failure. Selective use of dermal replacement in areas of increased likelihood of success leaves autograft available for use on important structures such as the hand. The hands are then managed at a separate operating session on day 4 or 5 when burn edema has detumesced and the operator is fresh. While unmeshed grafts are preferable, especially for the fingers, an expansion ratio of 1.5:1 (unstretched) leaves an acceptable result and allows blood and serous exudate egress through the interstices without hindrance.

Massive burns
The operating room
The safe management of a patient undergoing a massive burn debridement requires commitment and cooperation from a large group of individuals. The procedures are long, intense, and performed under conditions that are physically and emotionally stressful. The room becomes crowded as the surgical team alone can number 6–8.

A very important perioperative issue for safe management of a patient undergoing a massive burn excision is the maintenance of body temperature. The patient is usually completely exposed and has little intact skin, especially after donor skin harvest. These areas are moist and evaporation leads to rapid heat loss. Convective heat loss also occurs at a great rate. To combat these sources of heat loss, a number of strategies can be used. The operating room should be warmed to 32°C. The latent heat of evaporation of water is 31.5°C. Above this temperature, the energy source for evaporation will come from the environment rather than the patient. This temperature, or higher, is definitely required during the process of patient preparation when the patient is being washed. Radiant heaters are also very helpful for perioperative thermoregulation. An indwelling bladder catheter temperature probe is essential to accurately monitor the patient's core temperature. Other adjunctive measures include the use of 'space blankets' — aluminum foil coverings on areas not being accessed — plastic sheeting over the head and face, and all intravenous fluids being given at 38°C through a warming coil. Repeated applications of warm blankets are also useful as are warm air blowers. Once these adjunctive measures have been put in place, the ambient temperature can often be decreased to a more comfortable (sic) 28–32°C! The operating room staff should be reminded to take fluids themselves each 30 minutes. Failure to do so leads to severe dehydration and a sickening headache.

The patient
Good vascular access is required and subclavian central and femoral arterial lines are favored. These lines need to be sutured securely to prevent dislodgment during positioning of the patient. Special attention to prevention of pressure areas is needed. The patients are often operated upon for many hours and so are at great risk of pressure necrosis. Gel pads under the heels, elbows, and occiput and an 'egg-crate' dimpled foam mattress or a Dacron-filled mattress are essential. A customized, stainless steel surgical table with a channel at the periphery, which drains fluids towards an outlet, is very useful. The ability to obtain Trendelenburg and reverse Trendelenburg positions, along with the ability to raise and lower the whole table, is essential. Scales for weighing the patient incorporated into the table are very helpful. Clipping and shaving of body hair in and around the wound and in donor sites is followed in many units with a total body wash with povidone-iodine detergent solution. The patient is then laid upon sterile drapes. This is more easily accomplished with children than with enormous adults.

The operation
During this process, loose skin and blisters are removed and cloudy burn blister fluid sent for microbiological examination. Two electrocautery dispersive devices are needed. A Megadyne mattress is a great advance. Donor skin harvest is performed early in the procedure and is often proceeded by instillation of 0.9% or 0.45% saline solution, preferably with added epinephrine, to assist in the process.

Excision commences with the patient in the prone position. Tangential or fascial excision, as appropriate, of the shoulders, back, buttocks, and upper thighs is performed. Wide-meshed autograft with allograft or Biobrane™ overlay is applied. If insufficient autograft its available, the excised wound is covered with unexpanded, 1:1.5 meshed fresh allograft. Other alternatives include skin substitutes, such as Biobrane™ or Transcyte™, or cryopreserved allograft. Dermal replacement material is prone to failure due to infection in massive burns particularly on posterior surfaces, but can be used selectively on anterior flat surfaces. Multiple layers of bulky gauze dressings are applied over the antibiotic-impregnated gauze, in the case of allografts, or Exudry™ dressings if Biobrane™ was used. Thick silk sutures are inserted in a row along the flanks and tied in a loop. Tapes are then tied to the loops and tied over the bulky gauze dressing as a bolster. Another alternative is to apply multiple layers of chlorhexidine-impregnated, Vaseline gauze (Bactigras™), held with multiple staples. The patient is then placed in the supine position. Sterilizable, silicone tourniquets are often used on the limbs to decrease blood loss. Weak epinephrine clysis, topical 1:10 000 epinephrine irrigation, topical 5–20% thrombin solution spray, epinephrine-soaked lap pads/sponges, and compression bandaging are all techniques used to limit blood loss during debridement. Electrocautery is used after a period of compression bandaging to control the residual, larger bleeding points.

Fascial level excision is required for those areas where fat has been burned and often in those with massive burns. This involves surgical removal of the full-thickness of integument, including all the subcutaneous fat, down to the layer of investing fascia. The advantages of this technique are that grafts take very well on fascia and blood loss is reduced. Episodes of sepsis lead to ischemic necrosis of subcutaneous fat subsequent to poor peripheral perfusion and microvascular stasis. This becomes problematic in patients with very large burns and leads to late graft loss and these ischemic areas become portals for invasive wound sepsis. The disadvantages of fascial excision are lymphedema and contour deformities. All lymphatics are excised, so lymphedema of dependent parts is often troublesome. The excised fat never regenerates and can give a spindly appearance to the areas excised while any increase in body fat is deposited in the remaining beds of adipose tissue. Moon faces and thick necks can result. Fascial excision is also indicated for life-threatening invasive wound sepsis particularly with fungi and yeast such as *Aspergillus* and *Candida* and also for large areas with failed graft take in a critically ill patient with massive burns.

Patients return to the operating room as soon as donor sites are healed for further autografting and replacement of nonadherent allograft or infected skin substitute. Massively burned children, when treated with recombinant human growth hormone (GH), showed donor-site wound healing accelerated by 25% even if the patients presented infected and malnourished. There is a transient hyperglycemia in a third of patients that require insulin. The GH-treated patients require less infused albumin to maintain normal serum levels and this is an indication of the net positive protein balance induced.[42] The usual hospital stay for a 30 kg patient with a 60% TBSA burn of 42 days was reduced to 32 days. This tremendous decrease in length of hospital stay realized a net saving of 15% in total costs. Salutary effects have also been documented in a group of patients treated nonoperatively. Mortality dropped from 45 to 8%.[43] Whilst it must be acknowledged that two European studies in critically ill adults of mixed etiology showed increased mortality among the GH-treated groups,

this experience has not been repeated in the massively burned, pediatric population in North America.[44] Hypertrophic scar formation has been shown to not be made worse by GH treatment.[45]

Other anabolic agents have shown promise as a means of speeding wound healing in severely injured, catabolic burn patients.[46] Oxandrolone in a dose of 20 mg/day (0.1 mg/kg in 2 divided doses) has demonstrated a positive effect on protein kinetics and wound healing in both animal models and clinical trials. Emaciated, massively burned children whose presentation was delayed by, on average, 30 days were also greatly aided by oxandrolone 0.2 mg/kg/day. Protein kinetics were normalized, further weight loss prevented, and wound healing was enhanced. Donor-site wound healing was accelerated by 20% in oxandrolone-treated severely burned adults compared to nontreated. While these pharmacological agents provide great support to the massively burned, they are only an adjunct to early, near-total excision and prompt wound coverage.

Operative management of burns in special areas

The hand

Full-thickness burns should be excised and grafted as soon as practicable after diagnosis. However, the role of early operation for partial-thickness hand burns is contentious.[47–50] If donor skin is available, and the depth of the burn indicates that wound healing will not be complete in 10–14 days, then excision and grafting is reasonable and advantageous. Thick split-thickness skin grafts have been widely used to resurface hands. However, a prospective trial by Heimbach et al. demonstrated no difference between $^{15}/_{1000}$ inch and $^{25}/_{1000}$ inch skin graft, on assessment by blinded observers (unpublished data). The thinner graft will obviously induce less donor-site morbidity and obviate the need for overgrafting. Heimbach's group have promoted the use of Integra™ and a VAC dressing for deeply burned fingers. They report fewer amputations with this technique. Indeed, some units advocate Integra™ for all deep hand burns.[51]

Deep hand burns (section author Dr Dilip Gahankari)

An alternative to Integra™ reconstruction for deep hand burns is local, pedicle, and free flap reconstruction. While microsurgical expertise is not freely available and septic burns patients not ideal candidates for microvascular anastomosis, consideration should be given to pedicle flap reconstruction for selected cases involving a devastatingly burned hand. Pedicle flaps can be performed by most surgeons and should be considered for salvage of a dominant or only remaining hand, especially when resources are meager.

Operative approach

Severe acute hand burn injury, especially from electrical injury, may cause subcutaneous tissue destruction. If, after debridement, extensor tendons or the metacarpophalangeal or interphalangeal joints are exposed and involved, skin grafts alone are inadequate for resurfacing. Small areas, usually less than 1 cm can be managed non-operatively with an emphasis on active physical rehabilitation. These small defects can be allowed to granulate and be later covered with skin grafts if necessary. As previously mentioned, Integra™ resurfacing combined with VAC suction dressings have a role and if resources are available this approach can certainly be tried in the first instance. If the areas of exposed and burnt tendon are large, we have found the technique to not always be successful. Therefore, we actively consider skin flaps during decision making for these patients.

The ideal flap for dorsal hand defects needs to be thin and supple. It needs to be well vascularized and reliable. Although a detailed account of reconstructive surgery is beyond the scope of this chapter, we would like to briefly describe some of the available options. These include, microsurgical and non-microsurgical procedures. Microsurgical reconstruction often provides well-vascularized and swift reconstruction. Although microvascular free flaps generally provide best reconstruction for hand defects, by virtue of their great versatility, they may not always be possible in severe burns for various reasons. Not uncommonly, a severely burnt upper extremity precludes the use of radial and ulnar arteries and superficial and/or deep venous systems essential for anastomosing the free flap veins. In the same context, local flap options may not be available or suitable.

In such situations, delayed pedicle flaps, like the groin flap or the abdominal flap, may be the only reliable alternatives. We frequently use these pedicle flaps with multiple delays when microvascular reconstruction options are not available. In our experience, multiple delays give an opportunity to not only make these flaps more predictable and reliable in relatively sick patients, but also to make them thin and pliable. However, the obvious disadvantage of multiple delays is inability to mobilize the hand joints adequately and expeditiously. The resultant stiff hand after the complete division of the flap requires vigorous mobilization. The key is to start early limited mobilization of the hand while it is still attached by the pedicle. The judicious use of Kirschner wires also helps to maintain the joints in functional position without being detrimental to the pedicle.

When available, a groin flap is always our first choice as it provides a much more versatile coverage and mobility of the pedicle and therefore opportunity for mobilizing the hand while still being attached by the pedicle (Figure 13.11a–e).

For both groin and abdominal flaps, preoperative planning is the key to a successful reconstruction. Bedside planning in reverse with cloth pattern (in consultation with the patient if possible), helps tremendously in getting a good functional result with minimal stages. We pay particular attention to the following aspects in pedicled flap planning.

Comfortable position of the hand at rest with pedicle attached: we always plan as long a pedicle as possible with groin flap. In most instances, the groin flap donor site can be primarily closed (up to 11 cm wide in our experience). With abdominal flap, the pedicle could be planned inferiorly, superiorly, medially or in composites of above directions depending on the resting position of the hand at the donor site and the coverage requirement (Figure 13.12a–d). It is also important to make allowance for the thickness of the flap and skin retraction. As a general rule, we add at least 0.5 cm on either side of the 'finger' extensions in case of multiple fingers

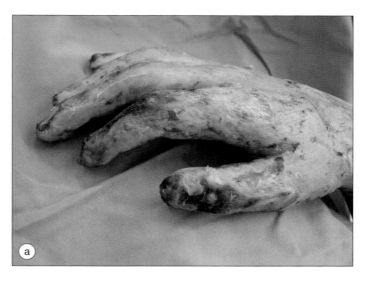

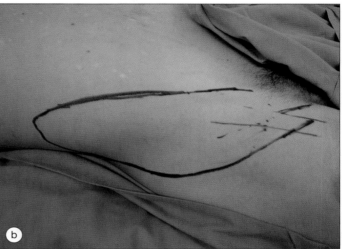

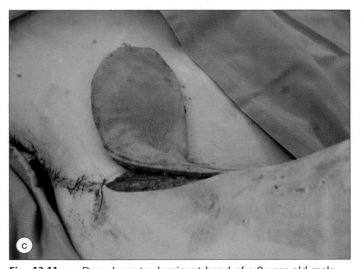

Fig. 13.11a–e Deep burn to dominant hand of a 9-year-old male with juvenile diabetes. Tendons were exposed. A 10 cm wide groin flap was used with the donor being closed primarily.

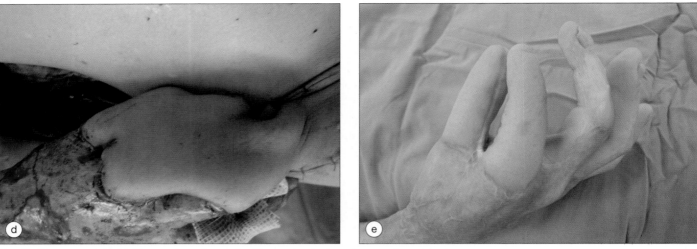

Fig. 13.11a–e – cont'd (e) The result at 6 months. He was back at work as a sale assistant.

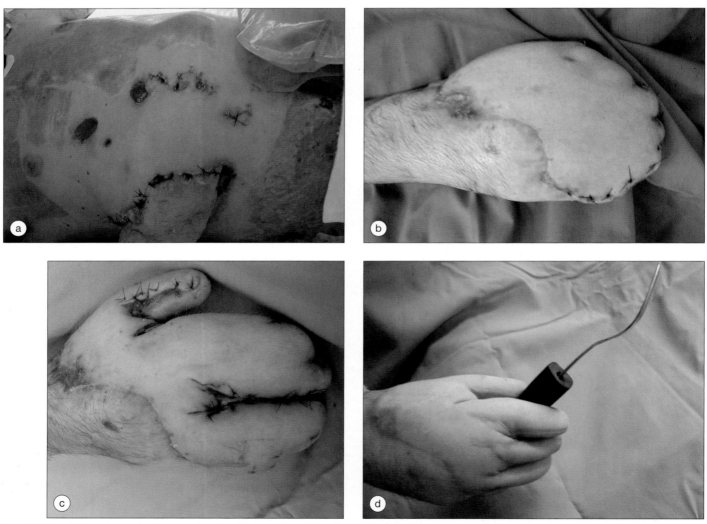

Fig. 13.12a–d Deep burns to dorsum dominant hand with all tendons and capsules exposed in a 25-year-old whose other hand was amputated and extensive deep burns (45%) elsewhere. The hand was placed in the abdomen, not far from a left-sided colostomy seen top right (a). The palmar surface partial-thickness burn was tangentially debrided and split skin grafted. Division was in three stages over a month.

coverage and at least 1 cm on either side of the dorsal or palmar margin of the defect. Both the groin flap and abdominal flaps are designed while respecting the principle of the random pattern vascularity. (Although groin flap is axial pattern flap, the useful area of groin flap used for hand coverage is the random pattern extension of the flap.) Bedside preoperative planning also permits the assessment of mobility of shoulder and elbow joints in terms of patient comfort during the period of attachment of the pedicle. This can be up to 4 weeks. We also pay specific attention to the axillary and antecubital areas if they are burnt. In such instances, we prefer to use flap coverage for axillary and antecubital areas rather than skin graft resurfacing to prevent possible contracture. These flaps are performed prior to coverage of the hand. If fingers and thumb are involved, we make an attempt to incorporate the coverage of the first web in the original planning. This prevents first web contracture and expedites the mobilization of hand after flap detachment. We exercise utmost conservatism in debridement of the tendons and the joint capsules even if they have been exposed. It is our experience that the vascularized flap coverage does normally salvage exposed extensor tendons and joints, even though they appeared clinically non-viable. Coverage of infected joints and finger tips is however a difficult problem. Joint infections and osteomyelitis in exposed joints or bones is a real risk in severely burnt patients, especially if the flap coverage is delayed for any reason. We manage this problem by addressing the specific areas by localized lavages and judicious debridement. We also attempt to preoperatively identify the risk areas and make allowance in planning of the flap so that the total period of the flap attachment is not prolonged by occurrence of the localized infection.

Finger tip coverage is a difficult area. Flap skin is usually a poor substitute for reconstruction of the nail fold or subungual skin. It is also our experience that most patients needing significant hand coverage by flap reconstruction, have poor outcome in salvage of finger tips. Hence most such hands end up in delayed amputation of finger tips. Most commonly this amputation is performed just proximal to the nail fold or at the DIP joint level. Another useful hint in finger tip flap coverage is to allow a slight extra skin coverage for the finger tips. This is keeping in line with the principle of designing these flaps on the random-pattern vascularized pedicle. The vascular status of the finger tip, especially on the dorsal aspect is often poorer in burnt hands compared to more proximal aspect of the fingers.

Abdominal and groin pedicle flaps for hand coverage: planning

For palmar coverage: whenever possible, groin flap is preferred as it allows judicious twisting of the tubed or semi-tubed pedicle. If groin flap is not available, abdominal flap is carefully planned. Both inferior pedicle as well as superior design is possible when available, but we prefer the former as it tends to have a more robust blood supply in the form of superficial inferior epigastric artery. This permits at least $1:1/2$ or $1:2$ length-to-breadth ratio and extensive thinning of the flap. For dorsal coverage, above considerations do apply; however, our preference is towards superior pedicle design of abdominal flap, if groin flap is not available. Superiorly based abdominal flap allows more deliberate mobilization of hand while still being attached by the pedicle. Uncommonly, coverage is needed on both dorsal and volar aspects and, in this situation, we prefer to use a combination of groin (superficial external pudendal artery-based) and abdominal (superficial inferior epigastric artery-based) flaps. These flaps are then raised on a common pedicle and wrapped on dorsal and volar aspects. The pedicle tubes itself well and is hence protected from kinking and twisting. If both these flaps are used jointly, donor site needs the split skin graft. For isolated fingers involvement, which quite commonly is the case for their dorsal coverage, the step-ladder pre-thinned abdominal flaps are ideal choice. Since these flaps are broad pedicle based, we divide their pedicles between 2 and 3 weeks but do not make any attempt for insetting of the flaps. This is done 1 week later when the vascularity of flaps is more stable (Figure 13.13a–d). Mobilization of the fingers and

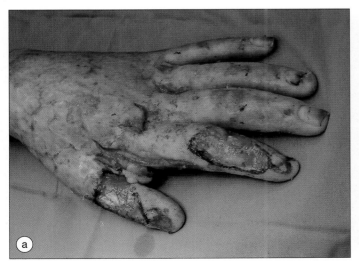

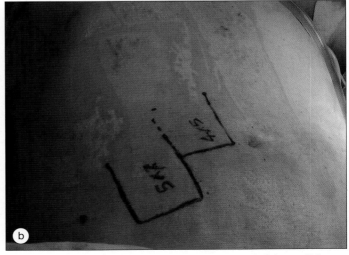

Fig. 13.13a–d Exposed tendons to the dorsum of left hand were residual defect following grafting. Thin abdominal step-ladder pedicle flaps were used to good effect.

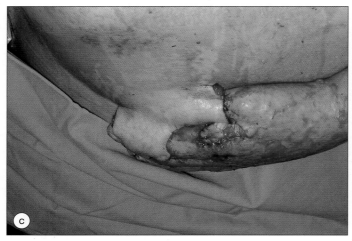

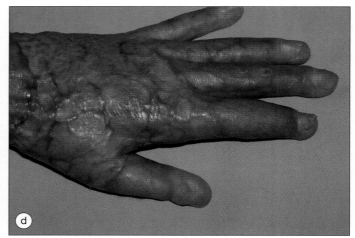

Fig. 13.13a–d – cont'd

mild compressive bandaging is, however, started immediately after the separation of the fingers.

The face

Facial burns that are obviously full-thickness and obviously require operative management are less problematic than those that are deep dermal with small patches of full-thickness injury. The face that definitely needs grafting can be scheduled for operation as soon as swelling has subsided. Some centers use face masks to exert pressure so that the grafts can be applied to a surface that more closely resembles the norm. This is a very labor-intensive exercise as the mask needs to be remolded each day to keep up with detumescence.

Selection of site and depth of donor skin harvest needs careful consideration. If at all possible, the donor skin should come from the 'blush' area above the line of the nipples for the best color match. While most favor the scalp, the potential problems of alopecia and hair growth from transplanted hair follicles are real concerns.[52] If the scalp is not available, an alternative is to harvest across the upper part of the back with subsequent overgrafting with a thin graft. Epinephrine clysis is a sensible pre-emptive measure to decrease blood loss especially if delivered in a large volume of saline.[53,54] This will make the harvesting process easier. If the skin over the upper back and shoulders is sun-damaged or freckled in fair-skinned individuals then other alternatives may need to be sought. It is best to remember also that the skin of the scalp of a bald man is usually quite thin and therefore not suitable as a donor site. If the upper back/shoulder region is selected, the donor site is best overgrafted with thin split-skin graft of, say, 6/1000 inch to prevent hypertrophic scar formation. Grafts should be taken as widely as possible so as to decrease the number of seams required.

Excising the face can be very bloody and loss of more than a total blood volume is not unknown — be prepared! Epinephrine clysis is essential to limit the exsanguinating hemorrhage. If the burn is obviously full-thickness, excision with needle-point electrocautery works well. If there is any doubt as to the depth, tangential excision with a Goulian knife is more

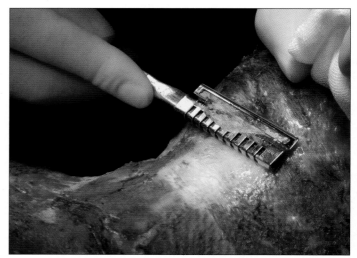

Fig. 13.14 Tangential excision being applied with a Goulian knife to the chin. Previous grafting had been largely successful. The instrument is useful for small and tricky areas.

appropriate as preservation of any viable dermal elements is essential for optimum results (Figure 13.14). Magnification with loupes aids accurate excision and graft placement. Some centers delay the reconstructive phase of the procedure to decrease graft loss from hematoma formation. Temporary wound closure with allograft is a good option if this course is chosen.[55] IMF screws can be placed into the maxilla to secure the endotracheal tube and rids the face of the tapes that inevitably rub on the grafts.

Grafts should be placed in such a fashion as to mimic the esthetic units as much as possible. Glue is useful to 'spot-weld' around the edge of the grafts and is certainly an excellent adjunct to suturing. Fibrin glue, e.g. Tisseal™, is also used routinely in some centers to increase graft adherence and limit hematoma formation.

Deep dermal facial burns were shown by Tredget[56] to be more prone to hypertrophic scarring if they took longer than

18 days to heal. This being the case, surgery can be planned for the third postburn week. At operation, the first question to be answered is what to do with unhealed/unburned areas that do not completely cover a cosmetic unit. Folklore has it that excision of a whole cosmetic unit is essential for optimum results. It is difficult to find anyone who actually uses this approach and it is one that has no appeal. The second question is what to do with the hair-bearing beard area in the adult male. If healing of this area is prolonged, folliculitis, which incites development of hypertrophic scar, is a common sequela. Excision requires removing all hair follicles as grafting a partial-thickness excision results in hair erupting through the graft, with much infection and inflammation leading to hypertrophic scarring. The answer to this conundrum remains elusive. Skin substitutes can be used for the burned face in the same fashion as described for scald burns. Transcyte™, in particular, seems to offer benefit in this situation.[57] Exposure, desiccation, trauma to fragile tissues, and presence of microorganisms are all decreased.

Eyelids

Deep burns to the eyelids should be excised and grafted early. Delay inevitably leads to cicatricial ectropion, corneal exposure, and a threat to sight.[58] Postburn cicatricial ectropion is a dangerous condition, with unconscious, ventilated patients at particular risk. Release and full-thickness grafts to the lower lid and thick, split-thickness grafts to the upper lids should be undertaken as soon as the condition is diagnosed.[59] Unconscious patients can have their corneas protected by a combination of ophthalmic lubricants and cling-film stretched over the eye socket. This creates a moisture trap and prevents exposure keratitis (unpublished data).

Genital burns

Hot water scald burns to the genitalia of both sexes, such as those in children, are best treated expectantly with spontaneous healing the usual result. Small, patchy full-thickness burns to the scrotum can be excised and closed to good effect. Most partial-thickness burns will heal spontaneously as scrotal skin is quite thick and contains multiple hair follicles. The very deep burn from flammable liquid or high-voltage electricity is often associated with full-thickness loss. Excision with electrocautery is recommended. If the tunica requires excision, temporary allografting of the testes, followed by delayed autografting, is recommended. Circumcision of full-thickness burns to the foreskin works well and is appropriate as phimosis is a common sequela. A deep burn to the glans may be best allowed to proceed to eschar separation and grafting of resultant granulation tissue as severe hemorrhage accompanies surgical debridement. Full-thickness burns to the labia majora should be excised and grafted as a delayed procedure. This will decrease the degree of contracture that would certainly develop.

Perianal burns are seen in association with extensive burns in adults and in scalded children. Early excision is required for obvious full-thickness burns. Some centers recommend diversion of the fecal stream, preferably achieved laparoscopically, to aid healing and graft take.[60] An alternative is to keep the stool liquid and maintain a rectal tube *in situ*. Another technique is to administer a bowel prep and follow surgery with an elemental diet and stool thickeners such as codeine. Bowel actions can thus be delayed for 5–7 days. If graft failure occurs, it is important to keep trying to achieve engraftment as the perianal, circular contracture that results from healing by secondary intention is difficult to fix.

The breast

The nipple-areola complex, especially in females, is another area that requires extra attention. In general, it is best left unexcised as healing can occur from the deep glandular structures that are usually preserved. Sensation is also usually preserved and this is much appreciated by patients. Absence of a nipple is very noticeable and is often the one thing remarked upon by patients of both sexes even though they have other areas of more extensive scarring. It needs to be made clear that excision of the breast mound in postpubertal, or the breast bud in prepubertal, females should be avoided if possible. Dermal replacement, such as Integra™, when applied in juxtaposition to the unexcised areola, requires close attention. Acticoat™, Lodoflex granules™, or silver nitrate 0.5% soaked gauze can be used to attempt to control infection in this situation. The relatively avascular nature of the fat and connective tissue matrix that constitutes the majority of the nonlactating breast makes careful excision of all nonviable tissue even more important than usual. Tie-over bolsters, retention and VAC dressings are useful for the isolated burn to decrease movement and increase graft take.

Conclusion

Modern burn care is based on operative wound management. The evidence is clear that prompt excision and closure is lifesaving for patients with large burns. Skin substitutes and dermal replacement have made operative wound care even more appealing and offer an attractive alternative to topical antimicrobial therapy for partial-thickness wounds. Bioengineered composite skin replacement will soon make surgical management of burn wounds the norm.

References

1. Bull JP, Fisher AJ. A study of mortality in a burns unit: a revised estimate. Ann Surg 1954; 139:269–274.
2. Muller MJ, Herndon DN. The challenge of burns. Lancet 1994; 343:216–220.
3. Burke JF, Bandoc CC, Quinby WC. Primary burn excision and immediate grafting: a method for shortening illness. J Trauma 1974; 14:389–395.
4. Pietsch JB, Netscher DT, Nagaraj HS, et al. Early excision of major burns in children: effect on morbidity and mortality. J Pediatr Surg 1985; 20(4):754–757.
5. Herndon DN, Parks DH. Comparison of serial debridement and autografting and early massive excision with cadaver skin overlay in the treatment of large burns in children. J Trauma 1986; 26(2):149–152.

6. Herndon DN, Barrow RE, Rutan RL, et al. A comparison of conservative versus early excision therapies in severely burned patients. Ann Surg 1989; 209:547–553.

7. Tompkins RG, Burke JF, Schoenfeld DA, et al. Prompt eschar excision: a treatment system contributing to reduced burn mortality. Ann Surg 1986; 204(3):272–281.

8. Thompson P, Herndon DN, Abston S, et al. Effect of early excision on patients with major thermal injury. J Trauma 1987; 27(2):205–207.

9. Xiao-Wu W, Herndon DN, Spies M, et al. Effects of delayed wound excision and grafting in severely burned children. Arch Surg 2002; 137(9):1049–1054.

10. Munster AM, Smith-Meek M, Sharkey P. The effect of early surgical intervention on mortality and cost-effectiveness in burn care, 1978–91. Burns 1994; 20(1):61–64.

11. Deitch EA, Clothier J. Burns in the elderly: an early surgical approach. J Trauma 1983; 23(10):891–894.

12. Deitch EA. A policy of early excision and grafting in elderly burn patients shortens the hospital stay and improves survival. Burns 1985; 12:109–114.

13. Hara M, Peters WJ, Douglas LG, et al. An early surgical approach to burns in the elderly. J Trauma 1990; 30(4):430–432.

14. Scott-Conner CEH, Love R, Wheeler W. Does rapid wound closure improve survival in older patients with burns. Ann Surg 1990; 56:57–60.

15. Saffle JR, Larson CM, Sullivan J, et al. The continuing challenge of burn care in the elderly. Surgery 1990; 108(3):534–543.

16. Hunt JL, Purdue CF. The elderly burn patient. Am J Surg 1992; 164:472–476.

17. Lewandowski R, Pegg SP, Fortier K, et al. Burn injuries in the elderly. Burns 1993; 19(6):513–515.

18. Ikeda J, Sugamata A, Jumbo Y, et al. A new surgical procedure for aged burn victims: applications of dermolipectomy for burn wounds and donor sites. J Burn Care Rehabil 1990; 11(1):27–31.

19. Deitch EA, Wheelahan TM, Rose MP, et al. Hypertrophic burn scars: analysis of variables. J Trauma 1983; 23(10):895–898.

20. Ong YS, Samuel M, Song C. Meta-analysis of early excision of burns. Burns 2006; 32(2):145–150.

21. Heimbach DM. Early burn excision and grafting. Surg Clin North Am 1987; 67(1):93–107.

20. Engrav LH, Heimbach DM, Reus JL, et al. Early excision and grafting vs. nonoperative treatment of burns of indeterminant depth: a randomized prospective study. J Trauma 1983; 23(11):1001–1004.

22. Janzekovic Z. A new concept in the early excision and immediate grafting of burns. J Trauma 1970; 10:1103–1108.

23. Janzekovic Z. The burn wound from the surgical point of view. J Trauma 1975; 15:42–61.

24. Klein MB, Hunter S, Heimbach DM, et al. The Versajet water dissector: a new tool for tangential excision. J Burn Care Rehabil 2005; 26(6):483–487.

25. Herndon DN, Abston S, Stein MD. Increased thromboxane B_2 levels in the plasma of burned and septic burned patients. Surg Gynecol Obstet 1984; 159:210–213.

26. Desai MH, Herndon DN, Broemeling L, et al. Early burn wound excision significantly reduces blood loss. Ann Surg 1990; 221:753–762.

27. Hart DW, Wolf SE, Beauford RB, et al. Determinants of blood loss during primary burn excision. Surgery 2001; 130(2):396–402.

28. Barret JP, Desai MH, Herndon DN. Massive transfusion of reconstituted whole blood is well tolerated in pediatric burn surgery. J Trauma 1999; 47(3):526–528

29. Alexander JW, MacMillan BG, Law E, et al. Treatment of severe burns with widely meshed skin autograft and meshed skin allograft overlay. J Trauma 1981; 21(6):433–438.

30. McEwan W, Brown TL, Mills SM, et al. Suction dressings to secure a dermal substitute. Burns 2004; 30(3):259–261.

31. Munster MA. Cultured skin for massive burns. A prospective, controlled trial. Ann Surg 1996; 224(3):372–375.

32. Barret JP, Wolf SE, Desai MH, et al. Cost-efficacy of cultured epidermal autografts in massive pediatric burns. Ann Surg 2000; 231(6):869–876.

33. Hohlfeld J, de Buys Roessingh A, Hirt-Burri N, et al. Tissue engineered fetal skin constructs for paediatric burns. Lancet 2005; 366(9488):840–842.

34. Supp DM, Boyce ST. Engineered skin substitutes: practices and potentials. Clin Dermatol 2005; 23(4):403–412.

35. Huang KF, Linares HA, Evans MJ, et al. Can donor sites be harvested indefinitely? Proc Am Burns Assoc 1992; Vol. 24.

36. Irei M, Abston S, Bonds E, et al. The optimal time for excision of scald burns in toddlers. J Burn Care Rehabil 1986; 7(6): 508–510.

37. Desai MH, Rutan RL, Herndon DN. Conservative treatment of scald burns is superior to early excision. J Burn Care Rehabil 1991; 12:482–484.

38. Barret JP, Dziewulski P, Ramzy PI, et al. Biobrane versus 1% silver sulfadiazine in second-degree pediatric burns. Plast Reconstr Surg 2000; 105:62–65.

39. Lal S, Barrow RE, Wolf SE, et al. Biobrane improves wound healing in burned children without increased risk of infection. Shock 2000; 14(3):314–318.

40. Kumar RJ, Kimble RM, Boots R, et al. Treatment of partial-thickness burns: a prospective, randomized trial using Transcyte. ANZ J Surg 2004; 74(8):622–626.

41. Boyce ST, Kagan RJ, Meyer NA, et al. Cultured skin substitutes combined with Integra artificial skin to replace skin autograft and allograft for the closure of excised full-thickness burns. J Burn Care Rehabil 1999; 20(6):453–461.

42. Gilpin DA, Barrow RE, Rutan RL, et al. Recombinant human growth hormone accelerates wound healing in children with large cutaneous burns. Ann Surg 1994; 220(1):19–24.

43. Singh KP, Prasad R, Chari PS, et al. Effect of growth hormone therapy in burn patients on conservative treatment. Burns 1998; 24(8):733–738.

44. Ramirez RJ, Wolf SE, Barrow RE, et al. Growth hormone treatment in pediatric burns: a safe therapeutic approach. Ann Surg 1998; 228(4):439–448.

45. de Oliveira GV, Sanford AP, Murphy KD, et al. Growth hormone effects on hypertrophic scar formation: a randomized controlled trial of 62 burned children. Wound Repair Regen 2004; 12(4): 404–411.

46. Demling RH, Orgill DP. The anticatabolic effects of the testosterone analog oxandrolone after severe burn injury. J Crit Care 2000; 15(1):12–17.

47. Levine BA, Sirinek KR, Peterson HD, et al. Efficacy of tangential excision and immediate autografting of deep second degree burns of the hand. J Trauma 1979; 19(9):670–673.

48. Edstrom LE, Robson MC, Macchiaverna JR, et al. Prospective randomized treatments for burned hands: non operative vs operative. Scand J Plast Reconstr Surg 1979; 13:131–135.

49. Salisbury RE, Wright P. Evaluation of early excision of dorsal burns of the hand. Plast Reconstr Surg 1982; 69(4):670–675.

50. Frist W, Ackroyd F, Burke J, et al. Long term functional results of selective treatment of hand burns. Am J Surg 1985; 149:516–521.

51. Dantzer E, Queruel P, Salinier L, et al. Dermal regeneration template for deep hand burns: clinical utility for both early grafting and reconstructive surgery. Br J Plast Surg 2003; 56(8):764–774.

52. Barret JP, Dziewulski P, Wolf SE, et al. Outcome of scalp donor sites in 450 consecutive pediatric burn patients. Plast Reconstr Surg 1999; 103(4):1139–1142.

53. Huges WB, DeClement FA, Hensell DO. Intradermal injection of epinephrine to decrease blood loss during split thickness skin grafting. J Burn Care Rehabil 1996; 171(3):243–245.

54. Sheridan RL, Szyfelbein SK. Staged high-dose epinephrine clysis is safe and effective in extensive tangential burn excisions in children. Burns 1999; 25(8):745–748.

55. Horch RE, Jeschke MG, Spilker G, et al. Treatment of second degree facial burns with allografts – preliminary results. Burns 2005; 31(5):597–602.

56. Fraulin FO, Illmayer SJ, Tredget EE. Assessment of cosmetic and functional results of conservative versus surgical management of facial burns. J Burn Care Rehabil 1996; 17(1):19–29.

57. Demling RH, DeSanti L. Management of partial thickness facial burns (comparison of topical antibiotics and bio-engineered skin substitutes). Burns 1999; 25(3):256–261.

58. Barrow RE, Jeschke MG, Herndon DN. Early release of third-degree eyelid burns prevents eye injury. Plast Reconstr Surg 2000; 105(3):860–863.

59. Astori IP, Muller MJ, Pegg SP. Cicatricial postburn ectropion and exposure keratitis. Burns 1998; 24(1):64–67.

60. Quarmby CJ, Millar AJ, Rode H. The use of diverting colostomies in paediatric peri-anal burns. Burns 1999; 25(7):645–650.

Chapter 14

Anesthesia for burned patients

*Lee C. Woodson, Edward R. Sherwood, Asle Aarsland, Mark Talon,
Michael P. Kinsky, and Elise M. Morvant*

Chapter contents

Introduction

Continuous improvement in burn care since World War II has resulted in a steady increase in the rate of survival after large burn injury.[1] These improvements have been attributed to aggressive fluid resuscitation, early excision and grafting of burn wounds, more effective antimicrobials, advances in nutritional support, and development of burn centers. Today, most patients with more than 80% total body surface area (TBSA) burned will survive if promptly treated in a modern burn unit with adequate resources. In their study of risk factors for death following burn injuries Ryan et al. identified three variables that can be used to estimate the probability of death: age greater than 60 years, burns over more than 40% of the total body surface area, and the presence of inhalation injury.[2] Mortality increased in proportion to the number of risk factors present: 0.3%, 3%, 33%, or approximately 90% mortality depending on whether zero, one, two, or three risk factors were present, respectively. The incidence of mortality is also influenced by significant coexisting disease or delays in resuscitation. O'Keefe et al. observed an approximately two-fold higher risk of death in women aged 30–59 years compared with men with similar burns and age.[3] Although it has been assumed that very young children are also at increased risk of death from burn injuries, Sheridan et al. found very low rates of mortality in children younger than 48 months who had suffered large burns.[4] Some burn patients develop refractory burn shock soon after injury and cannot be resuscitated.[9]

Major burn injury results in pathophysiological changes in virtually all organ systems. Table 14.1 lists and Figure 14.1 illustrates some of the challenges presented by the acutely burned patient during the perioperative period. In addition to the predictable challenges relating to airway management, monitoring, and vascular access, patient positioning requires close communication and teamwork. Burns involving posterior areas may require turning the patient to the prone position for optimal access (Figure 14.1). Vascular catheters and the endotracheal tube must be secured with confidence and due care given these life lines during patient turning. Several highly informative reviews of anesthetic management for burn surgery have been written during the past decade, each with its own special areas of concentration.[5–7]

Patients suffering burn injuries often require surgical treatment for years after the initial injury in order to correct functional and cosmetic sequelae. Anesthetic management for reconstructive burn surgery presents many special problems[8] but this chapter will concentrate on the care of acute burn patients. The acute phase of burn injury is defined as the period from injury until the wounds have been excised, grafted, and healed.

Modern burn care depends on coordination of a multidisciplinary team including surgeons, intensivists, nurse clinicians, nutritionists, rehabilitation therapists, pulmonary care therapists, and anesthesia providers. Rational and effective anesthetic management of acute burn patients requires an understanding of this multi-disciplinary approach so that perioperative care is compatible with the overall treatment goals for the patient. The current standard of surgical treatment calls for early excision and grafting of nonviable burn wounds, which may harbor pathogens and produce inflammatory mediators with systemic effects resulting in cardiopulmonary compromise. After an extensive burn injury, the systemic effects of inflammatory mediators on metabolism and cardiopulmonary function reduce physiological reserve and the patient's tolerance to the stress of surgery deteriorates with time. Assuming adequate resuscitation, extensive surgery is best tolerated soon after injury when the patient is most fit. However, it must be recognized that the initial resuscitation of patients with large burns results in large fluid shifts and may be associated with hemodynamic instability and respiratory insufficiency. Reynolds et al. reported that more than half of deaths after burn injuries occur due to failed resuscitation.[9] Effective anesthetic management of patients with extensive burn injuries requires an understanding of the pathophysiological changes associated with large burns and careful pre-

TABLE 14.1 PERIOPERATIVE CHALLENGES IN THE ACUTE BURN PATIENT
• Compromised airway
• Pulmonary insufficiency
• Altered mental status
• Associated injuries
• Limited vascular access
• Rapid blood loss
• Impaired tissue perfusion due to:
• Hypovolemia
• Decreased myocardial contractility
• Anemia
• Decreased colloid osmotic pressure
• Edema
• Dysrhythmia
• Impaired temperature regulation
• Altered drug response
• Renal insufficiency
• Immunosuppression
• Infection/sepsis

TABLE 14.2 MAJOR PREOPERATIVE CONCERNS IN ACUTELY BURNED PATIENTS
Age of patient
Extent of burn injuries (total body surface area)
Burn depth and distribution (superficial or full thickness)
Mechanism of injury (flame, electrical, scald, or chemical)
Airway patency
Presence or absence of inhalation injury
Elapsed time from injury
Adequacy of resuscitation
Associated injuries
Coexisting diseases
Surgical plan

TABLE 14.3 FUNCTIONS OF SKIN
1. Protection from environmental elements (e.g. radiation, mechanical irritation or trauma)
2. Immunological — antigen presentation, antibacterial products (sebum), barrier to entry of pathological organisms
3. Fluid and electrolyte homeostasis — helps maintain protein and electrolyte concentrations by limiting evaporation
4. Thermoregulation — helps control heat loss through sweating and vasomotor regulation of superficial blood flow
5. Sensory — extensive and varied sensory organs in skin provide information about environment
6. Metabolic — vitamin D synthesis and excretion of certain substances
7. Social — appearance of skin has strong influence on image and social interactions
Adapted from Williams WG, Phillips LG. Pathophysiology of the burn wound. In: Herndon DN, ed. Total burn care, 1st edn. London: WB Saunders; 1996:64.

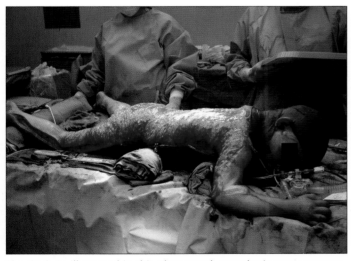

Fig. 14.1 As illustrated in this photograph anesthetic management of the acute burn patient for excision and grafting of wounds presents numerous challenges regarding monitoring, vascular access, temperature regulation, and rapid blood loss.

operative evaluation to assure that resuscitation has been optimized and an appropriate anesthetic plan has been formulated.

Preoperative evaluation

The preoperative evaluation of burn patients requires knowledge of the continuum of pathophysiological changes that occur in these patients from the initial period after injury through the time that all wounds have healed. The dramatic changes that occur in all organ systems following burn injury directly affect anesthetic management. The following discussion will describe the pathophysiological changes that occur in the acutely burned patient as they relate to the preoperative evaluation. In addition to the routine features of the preoperative evaluation, evaluation of acute burn patients requires special attention to airway management and pulmonary support, vascular access, adequacy of resuscitation, and associated injuries. The severely burned patient presents with numerous preoperative concerns (Table 14.2).

The preoperative evaluation must be performed within the context of the planned operative procedure, which will depend on the location, extent, and depth of burn wounds, time after injury, presence of infection, and existence of suitable donor sites for autografting.

Initial evaluation of burn injury

Destruction of skin by thermal injury disrupts the vital functions of the largest organ in the body. The skin provides several essential protective and homeostatic functions (Table 14.3). Treatment of patients with burn injuries must compensate for loss of these functions, until the wounds are covered and healed. As a barrier to evaporation of water, the skin helps maintain fluid and electrolyte balance. Heat loss through evaporation and impairment of vasomotor regulation in burned skin diminishes effective temperature regulation. The skin's barrier function also protects against infection by invading organisms. Wound exudate rich in protein depletes plasma proteins when large body surface areas are injured.

In addition to loss of important functions of the skin, extensive burns result in an inflammatory response with systemic effects that alter function in virtually all organ systems. Preoperative evaluation of the burn patient is guided largely by a knowledge of these pathophysiological changes.

Much of the morbidity and mortality associated with burn injuries are related to the size of the injury. The extent of the burn injury is expressed as the TBSA burned. Estimates of TBSA burned are used to guide fluid and electrolyte therapy and to estimate surgical blood loss. Percentage of the skin's surface that has been burned can be estimated by the so-called rule of nines (see Figure 14.2). Estimates are modified for pediatric patients because of age-related differences in body proportions. A knowledge of the burn depth is also critical to anticipating physiological insult, as well as planned surgical treatment. First-degree or superficial second-degree burns may heal without scarring or deformity and do not require surgical excision. Deeper second-degree and third-degree burns require surgical debridement and grafting with associated surgical blood loss.

Accurate estimates of blood loss are crucial in planning preoperative management of burn patients. With extensive wound excision or debridement, large amounts of blood can be lost rapidly. Adequate preparation in terms of monitors, vascular access, and availability of blood products is essential. Surgical blood loss depends on area to be excised (cm^2), time since injury, surgical plan (tangential vs. fascial excision), and presence of infection.[10] Blood loss from skin graft donor sites will also vary depending on whether it is an initial or repeat harvest. These variables are valuable predictors of surgical blood loss, which is a critical factor in planning anesthetic management (Table 14.4).

Airway and pulmonary function

Special attention must be paid to the airway and pulmonary function during preoperative evaluation. Burn injuries to the face and neck can distort anatomy and reduce range of mobility in ways that make direct laryngoscopy difficult or impossible. Specific alterations include impaired mouth opening, edema of the tongue, oropharynx, and larynx, as well as decreased range of motion of the neck. The tissue injury and sloughing present after severe facial burns may make mask ventilation difficult. Inhalation injury may impair pulmonary gas exchange and lead to respiratory insufficiency or failure.

The level of respiratory support must also be assessed. The level of required support may range from supplemental blow-by or mask oxygen to intubation and ventilation with high positive end-expiratory pressure (PEEP) and FIO_2. Acute lung injury can occur from inhalation of chemical irritants, systemic inflammation from burn wounds or difficulties with resuscitation, or ventilator-induced injury. Common pathologies include upper thermal airway injury with stridor,

pulmonary parenchyma damage from chemical irritants or inflammation, lower airway obstruction from mucus plugs and epithelial casts, as well as pulmonary edema due to acute lung injury or volume overload. With very high levels of PEEP or peak inspiratory pressure it must be determined if the anesthesia ventilator is adequate or if an ICU ventilator will need to be brought to the operating room. If the patient is intubated at the time of the preoperative evaluation it is essential to know what the indications for intubation were so that an appropriate plan for postoperative support can be made.

There is general recognition that smoke inhalation injury increases morbidity and mortality for burn patients.[11] The presence of an inhalation injury in combination with a cutaneous burn increases the volume of fluid required for resuscitation as much as 44%.[12] Numerous studies have also shown an increased incidence of pulmonary complications (pneumonia, respiratory failure, or ARDS) in patients with burns and inhalation injury when compared with burns alone.[13] Sequelae of inhalation injury include upper airway distortion and obstruction from direct thermal injury as well as impaired pulmonary gas exchange due to effects of irritant gases on lower airways and pulmonary parenchyma. These two components of the inhalation injury have separate time courses and pathophysiological consequences.

Foley described findings of 335 autopsies performed on patients who died from extensive burns.[14] Intraoral, palatal, and laryngeal burns were not uncommon among patients with inhalation injuries. The most common sites of laryngeal injury were the epiglottis and vocal folds where their edges were exposed. In contrast, thermal necrosis below the glottis and upper trachea was not observed in any of these patients. The lower airways are nearly always protected from direct thermal injury by the efficiency of heat exchange in the oro- and naso-pharynx unless the injury involves steam or an explosive blast. This has been demonstrated in an experimental model.[15] Inhalation injury to the lower airways and pulmonary parenchyma is due to the effect of toxic or irritant gases.

Clinical suspicion of inhalation injury is aroused by the presence of certain risk factors such as history of exposure to fire and smoke in an enclosed space or a period of unconsciousness at the accident scene, burns including the face and neck, singed facial or nasal hair, altered voice, dysphagia, oral and/or nasal soot deposits, or carbonaceous sputum. The most immediate threat from inhalation injury is upper airway obstruction due to edema. Early or prophylactic intubation is recommended when this complication threatens. However, exposure to smoke does not always lead to severe injury and in the absence of overt evidence of respiratory distress or failure it may be difficult to identify patients who will experience progressive inflammation and ultimately require intubation of the trachea. In a retrospective study, Clark et al. reported that 51% of their patients exposed to smoke inhalation did not require intubation.[16] Unnecessary intubation in the presence of an inflamed laryngeal mucosa risks further damage to the larynx and subglottic area.[17,18]

Traditional clinical predictors of airway obstruction have been found to be relatively insensitive and inadequate for identifying early severe airway inflammation and often underestimate the severity of the injury.[19,20] More objective criteria for evaluation of the risk of airway obstruction are often

BURN DIAGRAM Shriners Burns Institute – Galveston Unit

Age: _____ Sex: _____ Date of admission: _____

Type of burn: Flame ☐   Electrical ☐   Scald ☐   Chemical ☐   Inhalation injury ☐

Date of burn _____

Date completed _____

Completed by _____

Date revised _____

Revised by _____

Approved by _____

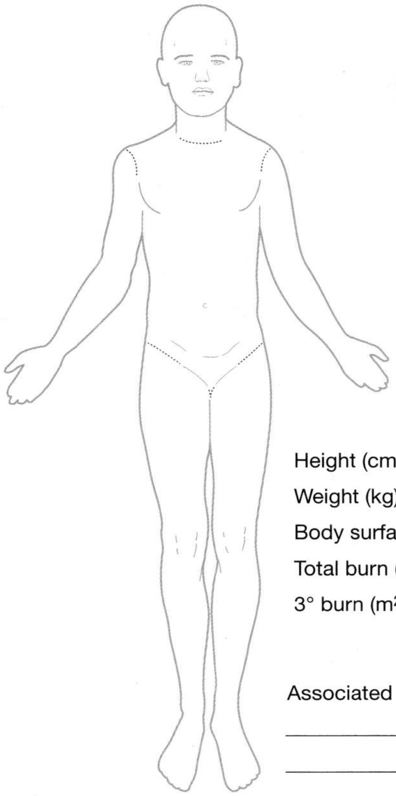

■ 3rd°

▨ 2nd°

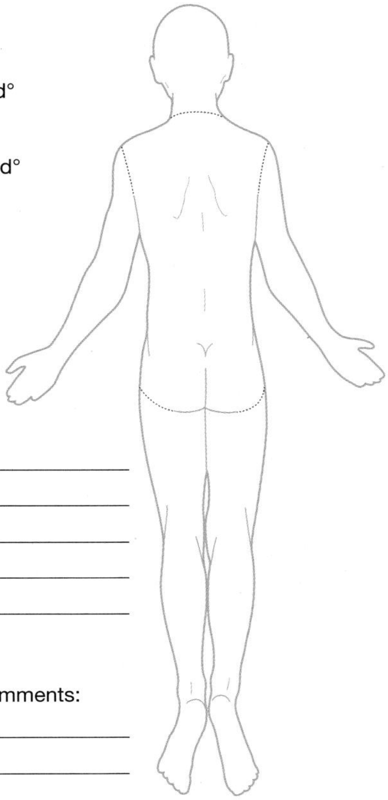

Height (cm) _____
Weight (kg) _____
Body surface (m²) _____
Total burn (m²) _____
3° burn (m²) _____

Associated injuries/comments:
_____
_____

Burn Estimate – Age vs. area

	Birth–1 year	1–4 years	5–9 1 year	10–14 years	15 years	Adult	2°	3°	TBSA%
Head	19	17	13	11	9	7			
Neck	2	2	2	2	2	2			
Anterior trunk	13	13	13	13	13	13			
Posterior trunk	13	13	13	13	13	13			
Right buttock	2.5	2.5	2.5	2.5	2.5	2.5			
Left buttock	2.5	2.5	2.5	2.5	2.5	2.5			
Genitalia	1	1	1	1	1	1			
Right upper arm	4	4	4	4	4	4			
Left upper arm	4	4	4	4	4	4			
Right lower arm	3	3	3	3	3	3			
Left lower arm	3	3	3	3	3	3			
Right hand	2.5	2.5	2.5	2.5	2.5	2.5			
Left hand	2.5	2.5	2.5	2.5	2.5	2.5			
Right thigh	5.5	6.5	8	8.5	9	9.5			
Left thigh	5.5	6.5	8	8.5	9	9.5			
Right leg	5	5	5.5	6	6.5	7			
Left leg	5	5	5.5	6	6.5	7			
Right foot	3.5	3.5	3.5	3.5	3.5	3.5			
Left foot	3.5	3.5	3.5	3.5	3.5	3.5			
						Total			

Fig. 14.2 Modified from Lund and Browder. Chart used to calculate the surface area involved by burn. It takes into account that, as one grows from infancy to adulthood, the relative surface area of the head decreases while the relative surface area of the lower extremities increases.

TABLE 14.4 CALCULATION OF EXPECTED BLOOD LOSS

Surgical procedure	Predicted blood loss
<24h since burn injury	0.45 mL/cm² burn area
1–3 days since burn injury	0.65 mL/cm² burn area
2–16 days since burn injury	0.75 mL/cm² burn area
>16 days since burn injury	0.5–0.75 mL/cm² burn area
Infected wounds	1–1.25 mL/cm² burn area

Adapted from Desai et al. Early burn wound excision significantly reduces blood loss. Ann Surg 1990; 221:753–762.[10]

needed. Hunt et al. found fiberoptic bronchoscopy to be a safe and accurate method for diagnosis of acute inhalation injury.[21] They described observations of severe supraglottic injuries associated with mucosal edema obliterating the piriform sinuses and causing massive enlargement of the epiglottis and arytenoid eminence. Haponic et al. made serial observations by nasopharyngoscopy in patients at risk for inhalation injury and found distortions of the upper airway described as compliant, edematous mucosa of the aryepiglottic folds, and arytenoid eminences that prolapsed to occlude the airway on inspiration.[22] Progressive upper airway edema in these patients was correlated with body surface area burned, resuscitative volume administered, and rate of infusion of resuscitative fluids. For patients who are at risk for inhalation injury but lack definitive indications for intubation, fiberoptic nasopharyngoscopy is effective in identifying laryngeal edema. Serial exams may help avoid unnecessary intubations and at the same time identify progressive inflammatory changes and allow intubation before severe airway obstruction and emergent conditions develop.

Lower airway and parenchymal injuries develop more slowly than upper airway obstruction. Prior to resuscitation, clinical signs and symptoms, chest X-ray, and blood gas analysis may be within normal limits despite significant injury that eventually progresses to respiratory failure requiring intubation and mechanical ventilation.[23]

Linares et al. studied the sequence of morphological changes following smoke inhalation in an experimental sheep model.[24] They observed four discrete but overlapping phases of injury described as exudative, degenerative, proliferative, and reparative. During the first 48 hours the *exudative phase* was characterized by polymorphonuclear (PMN) infiltration, interstitial edema, loss of Type I pneumocytes, and damage to the tracheobronchial epithelium in the form of focal necrosis, hemorrhage, and submucosal edema. The *degenerative phase* occurred between 12 and 72 hours and was characterized by progressive epithelial damage with shedding of necrotic tissue and formation of pseudomembranes and casts. Hyaline membranes developed over alveolar surfaces. Macrophages began to accumulate to begin absorption of necrotic debris. A *proliferative phase* was described between days 2 and 7 during which Type II pneumocytes and macrophages proliferated. After the fourth day *reparative* changes were observed with regeneration of epithelium from spared epithelium from the orifices of glands.

Demling and Chen have provided a lucid description of the pathophysiological changes following inhalation injury.[25] Decreased dynamic compliance increases the work of breathing. Increased closing volume and decreased functional residual capacity lead to atelectasis and shunt resulting in hypoxia. Airways become plugged by sloughed epithelium, casts, and mucus. Impaired ciliary action exacerbates the airway obstruction by decreasing the clearance of airway debris. These changes lead to further shunt and allow colonization and pneumonia. Treatment for inhalation injury is empiric and supportive with tracheal intubation and mechanical ventilation. The application of aggressive pulmonary toilet, high-frequency percussive ventilation, and respiratory therapy protocols designed to mobilize obstructing debris are also highly beneficial. The importance of strategies to limit ventilator-induced lung injury has been recognized.[26–30]

Carbon monoxide (CO) and cyanide are two major toxic components of smoke. The burn patient with evidence of inhalation injury should be evaluated for the presence of toxicity resulting from these compounds. CO binds hemoglobin 200 times more avidly than oxygen.[31] Therefore, CO markedly impairs the association of oxygen with hemoglobin and decreases oxygen-carrying capacity. CO also shifts the oxyhemoglobin dissociation curve to the left, thus decreasing the release of oxygen into tissues. These factors result in decreased oxygen delivery to tissues and, at critical levels, lead to anaerobic metabolism and metabolic acidosis. Signs and symptoms of CO poisoning include headache, mental status changes, dyspnea, nausea, weakness, and tachycardia. Patients suffering CO poisoning have a normal PaO_2 and oxygen saturation by routine pulse oximetry. They are not cyanotic. Carboxyhemoglobin must be detected by co-oximetry. Carboxyhemoglobin levels above 15% are toxic and those above 50% are often lethal. The major treatment approach is administration of 100% oxygen and, in severe cases, hyperbaric treatment to increase the partial pressure of oxygen in blood.[32]

Cyanide is also a component of smoke, resulting from the burning of certain plastic products.[33] Cyanide directly impairs the oxidative apparatus in mitochondria and decreases the ability of cells to utilize oxygen in metabolism. These alterations result in conversion to anaerobic metabolism and the development of metabolic acidosis. Signs and symptoms include headache, mental status changes, nausea, lethargy, and weakness. Hydrogen cyanide levels above 100 ppm are generally fatal.[34,35]

Treatment of cyanide toxicity begins with a high inspired oxygen concentration, which may increase intracellular oxygen tension enough to cause non-enzymatic oxidation of reduced cytochromes, or displace cytochrome oxidase and potentiate the effects of administered antidotes. Pharmacological intervention includes methemoglobin generators such as the nitrates (amyl nitrite inhalation 0.2 mLs, or sodium nitrite intravenous 10 mL of 3% solution for adults and 0.13–0.33 mL/kg of 3% solution for pediatrics) and dimethylaminophenol (3.25 mg/kg) to increase methemoglobin levels. Methemoglobin competes with cytochrome oxidase for cyanide. However, excessive levels of methemoglobin lead to decreased oxygen-carrying capacity and may be toxic. Direct binding agents have a high affinity for cyanide. Di-cobalt edetate (20 mL of 15% solution for adults or 0.3–0.5 mL/kg of 15% solution for pediatrics) is extremely rapid in action but has significant toxicity, whereas hydroxocobalamin (adults 5–10 g or pediatrics 70 mg/kg), the precursor of vitamin B_{12}, has been shown to be safe with few systemic side effects; it is actively metabolized by the liver and avoids renal absorption. Sulfur donors such as sodium thiosulfate (adults 25 mL of 50% solution or pediatrics 1.65 mL/kg of 25 % solution) accentuate the bodies' enzymatic conversion of cyanide to thiocyanate in the presence of the mitochondrial enzyme rhodanese, decreasing its toxicity and increasing elimination.[34,35]

Effect of burn injury on circulation

Thermal injury has profound effects on the systemic circulation, and hemodynamic management is a major component of perioperative care. It is critical for the anesthesiologist to assess the adequacy of postburn fluid resuscitation and the hemodynamic status of the patient. Important variables include blood pressure, heart rate, urine output, central venous pressure, base deficit, and blood lactate levels. In patients with pulmonary artery catheters, cardiac output, mixed venous oxygen saturation, cardiac and pulmonary filling pressures, and oxygen delivery parameters provide important information regarding the hemodynamic status of the burn patient. In addition, determination of blood hemoglobin level, fluid requirements, and the need for pressors or inotropes are important for developing an effective anesthetic plan.

After massive thermal injury, a state of burn shock develops due to intravascular hypovolemia and, in some cases, myocardial depression. This state of burn shock is characterized by decreased cardiac output, increased systemic vascular resistance, and tissue hypoperfusion.[36,37] Intravascular hypovolemia results from alterations in the microcirculation in both burned and unburned tissues, leading to the development of massive interstitial fluid accumulation. Cutaneous lymph flow increases dramatically in the immediate postburn period and remains elevated for approximately 48 hours.[38] The forces responsible for this massive fluid shift involve all components of the Starling equilibrium:[39]

$$J_v = K_f \left[(P_c - P_{if}) - \sigma(\pi_p - \pi_i) \right]$$

where: K_f is the capillary filtration coefficient, P_c is the capillary pressure, P_{if} is the interstitial hydrostatic pressure, σ is the reflection coefficient for protein, π_p is the plasma colloid osmotic pressure, and π_{if} the interstitial colloid osmotic pressure.

The specific alterations include:

- an increased microvascular permeability coefficient (k_f and s) due primarily to the release of local and systemic inflammatory mediators;
- an increase in intravascular hydrostatic pressure (P_c) due to microvascular dilatation;
- decreased interstitial hydrostatic pressure (P_{if});
- decreased intravascular oncotic pressure (π_c) due to leakage of protein from the intravascular space; and
- a relative increase in interstitial oncotic pressure due to a smaller decrease in interstitial oncotic pressure (π_i) compared to π_c.

The leakage of protein and fluid into the interstitial space often results in a washout of the interstitium and markedly increased lymph flow. The net effect of these changes is the development of massive edema during the first 24–48 hours after thermal injury with a concomitant loss of intravascular volume. The hypotension associated with burn injury is also due, in part, to myocardial depression.[40-44] The inflammatory response to thermal injury results in the release of large amounts of inflammatory mediators such as tumor necrosis factor α (TNFα), interleukin-1 (IL-1), and prostaglandins. TNFα and IL-1 are known to have myocardial suppressant effects.[45,46] These factors, and other possibly unrecognized factors, are responsible for the depression in myocardial function that often results from burn injury.

If the patient survives the initial burn shock and is adequately resuscitated, a state of hyperdynamic circulation develops that is mediated by a variety of inflammatory mediators. This state of massive inflammation has been termed the systemic inflammatory response syndrome (SIRS) and is characterized by hypotension, tachycardia, a marked decrease in systemic vascular resistance, and increased cardiac output. SIRS has a continuum of severity ranging from the presence of tachycardia, tachypnea, fever, and leukocytosis to refractory hypotension and, in its most severe form, shock and multiple organ system dysfunction. In thermally injured patients, the most common cause of SIRS is the burn itself; however, sepsis, SIRS with the presence of infection or bacteremia, is also a common occurrence.

Burn patients require large-volume fluid resuscitation in the immediate postburn period. This is due to a state of burn shock that develops in the immediate postburn period as described earlier. Several resuscitation protocols that utilize various combinations of crystalloids, colloids, and hypertonic fluids have been developed (Table 14.5). Isotonic crystalloid resuscitation is the most commonly used fluid for initial resuscitation in US burn centers. The most popular fluid resuscitation regimen, the Parkland Formula, uses isotonic crystalloid solutions and estimates the fluid requirements in the first 24 hours to be 4 mL/kg/% TBSA, although, many burn centers are administering 50% more fluid than the Parkland formula would predict.[47] Crystalloid solutions generally provide adequate volume resuscitation; however, the large volumes that are needed result in substantial tissue edema and hypoproteinemia. Therefore, interest has developed in analyzing colloid and hypertonic resuscitation regimens. Overall, colloid resuscitation within the first 24 hours of burn injury has not improved outcome compared to crystalloid resuscitation.[48,49] Furthermore, a recent meta-analysis indicated that mortality is higher in burned patients receiving albumin as part of the initial resuscitation protocol with a 2.4 relative risk of mortality compared to patients receiving crystalloid alone.[50] Because of the added cost with little established benefit, colloid solutions have not been used routinely in the United States for initial volume resuscitation in burned patients. Recently, however, in a prospective, randomized study, use of plasma for volume resuscitation has been found to limit volume infused along with intra-abdominal pressure and abdominal compartment syndrome (see below).[51] These outcome variables have not been used for comparing crystalloid and colloid resuscitation in the past. With the trend toward larger volumes for initial resuscitation it may be that the use of colloid may be beneficial for larger injuries requiring more volume.

TABLE 14.5 FORMULAS FOR ESTIMATING ADULT BURN PATIENT RESUSCITATION FLUID NEEDS

Colloid formulas	Electrolyte	Colloid	D5W
Evans	Normal saline 1.0 mL/kg/% burn	1.0 mL/kg/% burn	2000 mL/24 h
Brooke	Lactated Ringer's 1.5 mL/kg/% burn	0.5 mL/kg	2000 mL/24 h
Slater	Lactated Ringer's 2 liters/24 h	Fresh frozen plasma	75 mL/kg/24 h
Crystalloid formulas			
Parkland	Lactated Ringer's	4 mL/kg/% burn	
Modified Brooke	Lactated Ringer's	2 mL/kg/% burn	
Hypertonic saline formulas			
Hypertonic saline solution (Monafo)	Volume to maintain urine output at 30 mL/h Fluid contains 250 mEq Na/liter		
Modified hypertonic (Warden)	Lactated Ringer's +50 mEq $NaHCO_3$ (180 mEq Na/liter) for 8 hours to maintain urine output at 30–50 mL/h Lactated Ringer's to maintain urine output at 30–50 mL/h beginning 8 hours postburn		
Dextran formula (Demling)	Dextran 40 in saline — 2 mL/kg/h for 8 hours Lactated Ringer's — volume to maintain urine output at 30 mL/h Fresh frozen plasma — 0.5 mL/kg/h for 18 hours beginning 8 hours postburn		

The use of hypertonic saline, either alone or in conjunction with colloids, has also been advocated by some in the initial resuscitation of burned patients. Among the potential benefits are reduced volume requirements to attain similar levels of intravascular resuscitation and tissue perfusion compared to isotonic fluids.[52] Theoretically, the reduced volume requirements would decrease the incidence of pulmonary and peripheral edema, thus reducing the incidence of pulmonary complications and the need for escharotomy. Hypertonic saline dextran solutions have been shown to expand intravascular volume by mobilizing fluids from intracellular and interstitial fluid compartments. Although hypertonic saline dextran solutions will transiently decrease fluid requirements, there is a potential for a rebound in fluid resuscitation needs.[53,54] Therefore, most burn centers continue to employ isotonic crystalloid fluids for initial resuscitation of patients in burn shock.

Several parameters have been used to assess the adequacy of volume resuscitation in burned patients (Table 14.6). Unfortunately there is no single physiological variable that is always reliable as an endpoint to guide resuscitation in acute burn patients. The overall goal is early volume resuscitation and establishment of tissue perfusion. Traditionally, urine output (0.5–1 mL/kg/h) and normalization of blood pressure (mean arterial blood pressure of greater than 70 mmHg) have been used as endpoints. However, recent studies indicate that these parameters may be poor predictors of adequate tissue perfusion. Jeng and colleagues showed that attaining urine outputs of greater than 30 mL/h and mean blood pressures of greater than 70 mmHg correlated poorly with other global indicators of tissue perfusion such as base deficit and blood lactate levels.[55] In order to maintain perfusion of vital organs such as heart and brain, blood flow is often redistributed away from splanchnic organs. Persistent hypoperfusion of these organs ultimately results in tissue injury and may be a contributing factor to multisystem organ dysfunction. Several studies have shown that normalization of blood pressure, heart rate, and

TABLE 14.6 CRITERIA FOR ADEQUATE FLUID RESUSCITATION

- Normalization of blood pressure
- Urine output (1–2 mL/kg/h)
- Blood lactate (<2 mmol/liter)
- Base deficit (<–5)
- Gastric intramucosal pH (>7.32)
- Central venous pressure
- Cardiac index (CI) (4.5 liters/min/m²)
- Oxygen delivery index (DO_2I) (600 mL/min/m²)

urine output do not correlate with improved outcome.[56,57] Therefore, in the preoperative assessment of the burn patient, the anesthesiologist should not base the cardiovascular assessment strictly on these parameters.

Invasive cardiovascular monitors are not used routinely in burned patients to guide volume resuscitation. Most patients can be adequately resuscitated without their use. However, a small subset of patients, such as those with underlying cardiovascular disease or those who do not respond normally to volume resuscitation, may benefit from invasive monitoring. Some investigations have focused on the use of cardiac index and oxygen delivery as useful endpoints to guide volume resuscitation.[58,59] One way in which shock can be defined is oxygen debt. Therefore, maintaining an adequate cardiac index and oxygen delivery capacity such that oxygen delivery meets oxygen consumption provide useful criteria in guiding volume resuscitation. Bernard and colleagues have shown that patients surviving large burn injuries had higher cardiac indices and more effective oxygen delivery than nonsurvivors.[60] Some investigators have proposed the use of supranormal oxygen delivery as a means of assuring adequate tissue perfusion.[61,62] The preselected goals were a cardiac index of 4.5 $1/m^2$ and an oxygen delivery index of 600 mL/min/m^2. These values represent approximately 150% of normal cardiac index and oxygen delivery values. Attaining supraphysiological cardiac output and oxygen delivery has been shown to improve outcome in some studies. Schiller and colleagues demonstrated that maintaining a hyperdynamic hemodynamic state using fluids and inotropes improved survival in burn patients.[63] However, other investigations, including a meta-analysis, have shown that achieving supra-physiological levels of cardiac output and oxygen delivery did not improve mortality or decrease the incidence of organ failure in trauma and burn patients.[64–66] The use of inotropes to attain supra-physiological oxygen transport could be detrimental in some cases. One study that employed dobutamine to increase cardiac output and increase oxygen delivery demonstrated increased mortality.[67]

Estimating preload in the acutely burned patient is quite challenging. Filling pressures (central venous pressure and pulmonary artery occlusion pressure) correlate poorly with circulating blood volume especially during positive pressure ventilation.[68] A single indicator transcardiopulmonary thermo-dilution technique has been used to estimate the volume of blood in the thorax (intrathoracic blood volume or ITBV).[69] This technique has been used in burn patients during resuscitation. Holm and colleagues observed that where neither central venous pressure nor pulmonary capillary wedge pressures correlated with changes in cardiac index or oxygen delivery during fluid resuscitation of burn patients, there was a moderate correlation of these variables with ITBV.[70] This monitor was used successfully to resuscitate 24 severely burned patients. Volumes administered were significantly larger than predicted by the Parkland formula.[70] This technology is available commercially as the PiCCO system (Pulsion Medical Systems, Munich, Germany). In addition to ITBV this system also provides an estimate of extravascular lung water and continuous estimate of cardiac output and systemic vascular resistance.

Blood lactate and base deficit provide indirect metabolic global indices of tissue perfusion. Lactic acid is a byproduct of anaerobic metabolism and is an indicator of either inadequate oxygen delivery or impaired oxygen utilization. In the absence of conditions such as cyanide poisoning or sepsis that alter oxygen utilization at the cellular level, lactate production serves as a useful marker of oxygen availability. Serum lactate levels have served as a useful marker of fluid resuscitation and tissue perfusion in burn patients.[71] A recent study showed serum lactate to be the most predictive index of adequate tissue perfusion and a lactate level of less than 2 mmol/L in the first 24–72 hours after burn injury correlated with increased survival.[57] Base deficit is another indirect indicator of global tissue perfusion. The base deficit is calculated from the arterial blood gas using the Astrup and Siggard-Anderson nomograms. Although it is not directly measured, base deficit provides a readily obtained and widely available indicator of tissue acidosis and shock. Base deficit has been shown to correlate closely with blood lactate and provides a useful indicator of inadequate oxygen delivery. A retrospective study by Kaups et al. showed that base deficit was an accurate predictor of fluid requirements, burn size, and mortality rate.[73]

Lactate and base deficit serve as global markers of tissue perfusion and oxygen delivery. However, in burn patients, tissue perfusion is not uniform. Perfusion of the splanchnic beds is often sacrificed in order to maintain the perfusion of heart, brain, and kidneys. The use of gastric intramucosal pH (pH$_i$) has been advocated as a measure of splanchnic perfusion. Several studies have shown that measurement of pH$_i$ is useful in guiding resuscitation and that low pH$_i$ is a predictor of organ failure and death.[74] pH$_i$ is measured by gastric tonometry and can provide useful information regarding tissue perfusion.

Formulae for resuscitation of burns provide an approximation of fluid needs but volumes actually administered need to be individualized for each patient. Although two patients may each have 50% TBSA burns, it is not likely that their wounds will be equivalent otherwise. Several factors can increase fluid requirements (Table 14.7). Deep full-thickness burns require larger volume than partial-thickness injuries. Likewise, extensive soft tissue damage from electrical burns or crush injuries increases fluid needs. Inhalation injury can also increase fluid requirements as much as 50% as noted above.[12] These differences in wounds and fluid requirements among patients make it very difficult at times to optimize fluid administration. None of the physiological endpoints is always reliable. All available clinical information must be examined and each variable evaluated within the context of all the other variables.

It has been observed over the past several years that increased volumes of crystalloid solutions are being used for resuscitation of burn patients.[75] In many cases as much as twice the volume recommended by the Parkland formula is used. As a consequence, patients experience increased edema. During the preoperative evaluation, attention must be paid to the degree to which edema produces physiologic derangements. The edema can lead to compartment syndrome of extremities or abdomen (Figure 14.3). Blindness due to ischemic optic neuropathy has been reported as a complication of burn resuscitation.[76] Increased intra-abdominal pressure is a complication of vigorous fluid resuscitation, which may be more common than generally appreciated and may often explain difficulties with resuscitation. Greenhalgh and Warden first described the association of increased abdominal pressures and compartment syndrome with burn resuscitation.[77] Ivy and colleagues prospectively studied 10 adult patients presenting with greater than 20% TBSA burns and found that 70% of these patients had at least transient intra-abdominal hypertension.[78] Two of their patients with more than 80% TBSA burns developed

TABLE 14.7 FACTORS THAT MAY INCREASE FLUID NEEDS FOR RESUSCITATION OF PATIENTS WITH ACUTE BURN INJURIES
• Inhalation injury
• Delay in resuscitation
• Crush injury
• Electrical injury
• Large full-thickness burns
• Methamphetamine lab accidents
• Associated injuries

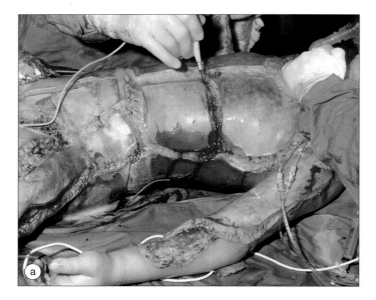

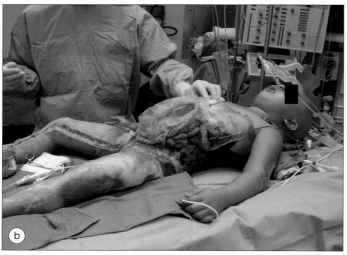

Fig. 14.3 Large volumes of crystalloid solution required for resuscitation of patients with acute burns can be associated with compartment syndrome of extremities and abdomen. (a) Escarotomies can decompress these compartments but (b) laparotomy may be required for abdominal compartment syndrome when escarotomies do not adequately decompress the abdomen.

abdominal compartment syndrome requiring surgical decompression. Several studies since then have described the common occurrence of increased intra-abdominal pressure with large-volume burn resuscitation. Increased intra-abdominal hypertension is termed abdominal compartment syndrome when it is associated with impaired respiration, circulation, and urine output. Mechanical ventilation is impaired by pressure on the diaphragm, circulation is impaired by restricted venous return due to caval compression, and urine output is impaired by compression of renal vessels. When this pattern presents the patient should be examined for elevated intra-abdominal pressure. This can be accomplished by measuring bladder pressure: 50 mL of saline is instilled into the bladder through the Foley catheter and the height of the saline column above the symphysis pubis is measured ($1.36\, cm\, H_2O = 1\, mmHg$).[79]

Conservative treatment of elevated intra-abdominal pressure includes attempts to limit the volume of intravenous fluid needed for resuscitation. The inclusion of plasma with infused fluids has been found to reduce volume required and was associated with significantly lower intra-abdominal pressures.[51] In addition adequate analgesia and sedation should be achieved. Diuresis with furosemide and muscle relaxants to reduce muscle tone have been used to reduce intra-abdominal pressure. More invasive measures include escharotomies,[80] percutaneous peritoneal dialysis catheter drainage,[81] and laparotomy.[77]

Recently several clinicians have reported a specific type of burn injury that has been associated with difficulties with resuscitation.[82–84] There has been a dramatic increase in burn injuries from explosions and fires related to methamphetamine production in illicit labs. Victims of these accidents present unique challenges for a variety of reasons. Substances used in methamphetamine production include chemicals that are corrosive and toxic (e.g. anhydrous ammonia, hydrochloric acid, red phosphorus, and ephedrine). Other ingredients are flammable (acetone, alcohol, and gasoline) and explosions can coat the victims with all these chemicals. As a result, in addition to the victim's toxic exposure, contacting incompletely decontaminated victims of these accidents has injured first responders and hospital workers.[85,86]

In addition to exposures described above, these patients are usually intoxicated with methamphetamine, as demonstrated by positive urine screen, and may have inhaled toxic fumes such as phosphine gas. Santos et al. found the incidence of inhalation injury twice as great in victims of methamphetamine-related burns as in age and burn-matched controls.[82] Among their patients requiring intubation for inhalation injury methamphetamine users also required roughly twice as many ventilator days.

Clinical studies have consistently observed increased fluid requirements for resuscitation of methamphetamine patients.[82,85] For example, Santos et al. found that resuscitation volumes were 1.8 times greater for methamphetamine users with burns than controls.[82]

Methamphetamine users with burns experienced more behavioral problems also. These patients are more often agitated and require restraints. Santos et al. reported that all their methamphetamine patients required greater than normal doses of sedatives and displayed what they referred to as 'withdrawal type syndrome.'[82] This behavior may be due to withdrawal of methamphetamine from chronic users.

Effect of burn injury on renal function

Acute renal failure (ARF) is a relatively common complication following major burn injuries. The incidence of ARF following burn injury has been reported to range from 0.5 to 30% and is most dependent on the severity of the burn and the presence of inhalation injury.[87–89] The development of ARF is a poor prognostic indicator with mortality rates as high as 100% reported by some investigators.[90] However, Jeschke and colleagues have shown a decrease in mortality in pediatric burn patients with ARF to 56% since 1984.[91] Holm and colleagues observed that ARF could be divided into early and late categories. Early ARF was defined as occurring within 5 days of burn injury.[92] The most common apparent causes were hypotension and myoglobinuria. ARF occurring after 5 days of injury was defined as late. Here, sepsis was the most common cause, with a small number of cases resulting from the administration of nephrotoxic drugs. Factors that will decrease the incidence of ARF and, if it occurs, associated mortality, include adequate fluid resuscitation, early wound excision, and prevention of infection.[93] Regardless of the cause, it is critical to assess renal function in burn patients in order to develop a comprehensive anesthetic plan. Important areas of analysis include urine output, dialysis dependence, volume status, and electrolytes; also diuretic therapy should be noted. Scheduled doses of diuretics may need to be continued during the perioperative period to maintain urine output.

Metabolic changes associated with burn injury

Increased metabolic rate is the hallmark of the metabolic alteration that takes place after thermal injury. The magnitude of the hypermetabolism is influenced by the size of the burn wound, how the burn patient is treated, and the ambient temperature of the patient.[94,95] Within the range of 30–70% TBSA burn injury the hypermetabolism tends to be proportionate to the size of the burn wound. With burns beyond this range the hypermetabolism appears to plateau and only increases in smaller increments.[96] Septic complication is an important factor that can increase the metabolic response and so does the physiologic stress of pain. It has been observed that modern day treatment of burn injuries with early excision and closed wound treatment ameliorates the hypermetabolism.[97] As mentioned earlier, burn patients increase their metabolic rate in an effort to generate heat according to a new threshold set point for the body temperature that is influenced by the size of the burn (see below: Thermoregulation in burn patients). The recognition of this fact has led to an increased awareness of the importance of the ambient temperature in modulating the hypermetabolism of the burn patient. Using indirect calorimetry in acute patients with major burn injuries that are treated according to current standards, resting energy expenditures that are 110–150% above predicted values are frequently measured.[98]

As a result of the hypermetabolic response the burned patient has an increased O_2 consumption along with an increased CO_2 production that collectively demands a higher respiratory effort. The anesthetic care of the acute burned patient has to accommodate these changes and frequently this has to be done in patients with compromised pulmonary function due to burn injury.

According to the hypermetabolism the caloric needs of the burn patient are also increased. Furthermore, numerous studies have shown that optimized nutritional care not only can ameliorate the burn-associated state of catabolism and immune suppression but also improves wound healing.[94] Oral or enteral feeding is recognized as the optimal feeding route of the burned patient. Frequently the acute burn patient has to be fed continuously over extended time periods. This is not only because of the increased caloric needs but also because of compromised gastric emptying and decreased intestinal motility that necessitates a slower feeding rate of critically ill patients. If standard guidelines for perioperative fasting are implemented recurrent operative procedures can significantly impinge on the nutritional needs of the patient and ultimately cause a caloric deficit. To accommodate the nutritional needs of the patient a continuation of duodenal nutrition perioperatively has been advocated. Studies indicate that not only is this procedure safe but it might also provide for a favorable gut oxygen balance.[99]

At the time of the withdrawal of ventilator support and extubation the metabolic state of the burn patient should be considered. The characteristic catabolic state of major burn injury spares no muscles[100] and the respiratory muscles are affected. Along with decreased muscle strength there is frequently decreased pulmonary compliance not only due to the formation of scar tissue and pulmonary interstitial changes but also due to increased intra-abdominal content. Burn-associated hepatomegaly along with gastrointestinal retention can significantly impinge on respiratory reserves.[101]

Severe insulin resistance with hyperglycemia and concurrent hyperinsulinemia is a key feature of the metabolic alterations of burn injury.[95] It is well recognized that critically ill patients with insulin resistance benefit from tight glycemic control in the ICU[102] and these findings have been expanded to the burn patient population.[103] During the intraoperative period the question is less studied. Although the benefit of tight intraoperative glycemic control has been documented in other patient populations,[104] the risk versus benefit during anesthesia has not been studied specifically in burn patients.

Thermoregulation in burn patients

Maintenance of proper body temperature is an important factor in the care of severely burned patients. The thermoregulatory system is controlled by three major components. These are the afferent system that senses changes in core body temperature and transmits this information to the brain, the central regulatory mechanisms located primarily in the hypothalamus that process afferent input and initiate responses, and the efferent limb that mediates specific biological and behavioral responses to changes in core body temperature (Figure 14.4). Temperature is sensed by $A\delta$ and C fibers present in peripheral tissues such as skin and muscle as well as core tissues such as brain, deep abdominal tissues, and thoracic viscera.[105] The vast majority of afferent input arises from the core tissues. Because the skin is in direct contact with the environment, it senses immediate changes in environmental temperature. However, the overall afferent input of the skin and other peripheral tissues is estimated to be only 5–20% of total afferent thermoregulatory input.[105] Therefore, loss of skin following a burn injury is not likely to markedly alter overall afferent input. Wallace and colleagues have shown that burn patients perceive changes in ambient temperature as effectively as normal controls.[106] This is likely due to the retained ability of burn patients to sense changes in core temperature and transmit this information to the central nervous system. Central control of temperature is a complicated system that is not well understood. The hypothalamus plays an important role in temperature regulation, but the complete mechanism of temperature control is likely to be multifaceted and is an area of intense research. Regard-

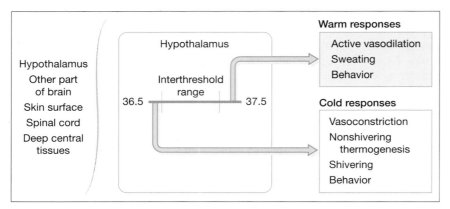

Fig. 14.4 Thermoregulatory control mechanisms. Afferent input from a variety of sites, most notably skin, central tissues, and brain, are processed in the central nervous system. Based on input, a variety of efferent thermoregulatory responses are initiated. (From: Sessler DI. Temperature monitoring. In: Miller R, ed. Anesthesia, 3rd edn. New York: Churchill Livingstone; 1990.)

less of the ultimate control mechanisms, temperature control can be divided into three main functions: threshold, gain, and maximum response intensity.

Threshold encompasses a set point at which responses to temperature change are initiated. In normal individuals the threshold range is generally near 36.5–37.5°C. In burn patients, the threshold set point is higher and the increase is proportional to the size of the burn. The work of Caldwell and colleagues predicts that the temperature set point will increase by 0.03°C/% TBSA burn.[107] This increase in temperature threshold appears to be due to the hypermetabolic state and the presence of pyrogenic inflammatory mediators such as TNF, IL-1, and IL-6 that are present after thermal injury. The elevated temperature set point can be decreased by administration of indomethacin, which suggests prostaglandins act as final common mediators of this response.[108,109]

Gain describes the intensity of response to alterations in temperature. In most cases the gain of thermoregulatory responses is very high with response intensity increasing from 10 to 90% with only a few tenths of a degree change in core temperature. This response is maintained in most burn patients, resulting in a further increase in metabolic rate.[106] Burn patients respond with a brisk increase in heat generation and metabolic rate in response to changes in core body temperature.[106] However, work by Shiozaki and colleagues has shown that burn patients who are slow to respond to postoperative hypothermia are at increased risk of mortality.[110] The decreased responsiveness may be due, in part, to tissue catabolism, poor nutrition, or sepsis. In addition, the response to relative hypothermia is characterized by increased catecholamine release, tissue catabolism, and hypermetabolism. These responses further stress burn patients, and decrease their ability to respond to their primary injury.[111]

The most important efferent responses to hypothermia are behavioral responses such as gaining shelter, covering up, and seeking a more desirable ambient temperature. In the acute postburn setting, most of these behaviors are impeded by positioning, sedation, and inability to seek a more favorable environment. Therefore, caregivers must be attentive to the patient's temperature and perception of cold so that measures can be undertaken to optimize the patient's temperature. Cutaneous vasoconstriction is another important mechanism for preserving heat and core body temperature. In unburned persons, a temperature gradient of 2–4°C exists between skin and core tissues. This gradient is maintained by cutaneous vasoconstriction. Without cutaneous vasoconstriction, heat is

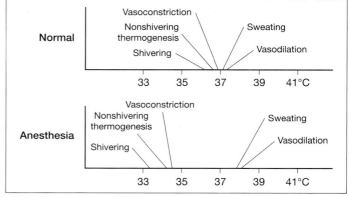

Fig. 14.5 Effects of anesthesia on thermoregulatory mechanisms. (From: Sessler DI. Temperature monitoring. In: Miller R, ed. Anesthesia, 3rd edn. New York: Churchill Livingstone; 1990.)

redistributed from the core compartment to the periphery. This heat is ultimately lost to the environment. Peripheral vasoconstriction minimizes temperature redistribution and acts to maintain core body temperature. This mechanism of heat preservation is lost with the loss of large areas of skin, particularly if cutaneous tissues are excised down to the fascial level. The loss of skin facilitates the loss of core body heat into the environment and places the burn patient at risk for core hypothermia. Another mechanism of heat loss in burn patients is evaporation. Burn patients can lose as much as 4000 mL/m² burned/day of fluids through evaporative losses.[112] Mechanisms of nonshivering heat production, and shivering remain intact in burn patients. However, shivering increases metabolic requirements and is likely deleterious.

The induction of anesthesia results in relative ablation of thermoregulatory mechanisms and puts the patient at further risk for developing hypothermia. Patients under general anesthesia exhibit a markedly decreased threshold for responding to hypothermia (Figure 14.5). This is particularly important in burn patients given their high temperature set point and the deleterious effects of further stress responses and hypermetabolism in this patient population. Most anesthetics decrease nonbehavioral responses to hypothermia such as vasoconstriction, nonshivering thermogenesis, and shivering. Of course, behavioral responses are ablated during general anesthesia. Therefore, it is the responsibility of the intraoperative caregivers to monitor and maintain patient temperature.

Actions such as maintaining higher ambient air temperature, covering extremities and head, applying warm blankets, utilizing radiant heaters and forced air warming devices, warming fluids and blood, and warming gases are usually effective in maintaining core temperature if applied aggressively. Ideally, hypothermia should be corrected prior to transport to the operating room.[113] Hypothermia revealed in the preoperative evaluation may be due to inadequate resuscitation or metabolic instability. Either situation may predispose burn patients to intolerance of anesthetic drugs or the stress of surgery.

Pharmacological considerations

General considerations

Burn injury and its treatment result in physiological changes that may profoundly alter response to drugs. These changes alter both pharmacokinetic and pharmacodynamic determinants of drug response. Altered drug response in burned patients may require deviation from usual dosages to avoid toxicity or decreased efficacy.[114] The complex nature of the pathophysiological changes, interpatient variation in the nature and extent of burn injuries, as well as the dynamic nature of these changes during healing and recovery make it difficult to formulate precise dosage guidelines for burn patients. However, an understanding of the systemic response to large burn injuries can help predict when altered drug response can be expected and how to compensate.

The two distinct phases of cardiovascular response to thermal injury can affect pharmacokinetic parameters in different ways. During the acute or resuscitation phase the rapid loss of fluid from the vascular space due to edema formation results in decreased cardiac output and tissue perfusion. Volume resuscitation during this phase dilutes plasma proteins and expands the extracellular fluid space especially, but not exclusively, around the burn injury itself. Decreased renal and hepatic blood flow during the resuscitation phase reduces drug elimination by these organs. Also, decreased cardiac output will accelerate the rate of alveolar accumulation of inhalation agents, which may result in an exaggerated hypotensive response during induction of general anesthesia.

After approximately 48 hours, the hypermetabolic and hyperdynamic circulatory phase is established with increased cardiac output, oxygen consumption, and core temperature. During this phase, increased blood flow to the kidneys and liver may increase clearance of some drugs to the point where increased doses are required.[115]

Many drugs are highly protein bound. Drug effects and elimination are often related to the unbound fraction of the drug which is available for receptor interaction, glomerular filtration, or enzymatic metabolism. The two major drug-binding proteins have disparate response to burn injury. Albumin binds mostly acidic and neutral drugs (diazepam or thiopental) and is decreased in burn patients. Basic drugs (pKa >8, propranolol, lidocaine, or imipramine) bind to α-acid glycoprotein (AAG). AAG is considered an acute phase protein and its concentration may double after burns. Since these drug-binding proteins respond in opposite ways to thermal injury it can be expected that changes in drug binding and function will depend on which of these proteins has the highest affinity for the drug in question. Martyn et al. observed decreased plasma albumin concentration and increased plasma

AAG concentration in burn patients.[116] These observations were associated with an increased unbound fraction for diazepam (bound by albumin) and a decreased unbound fraction for imipramine (bound by AAG).

Volume of distribution (V_d) can be changed by alterations of either extracellular fluid volume or protein binding. Large changes in both of these variables occur with thermal injuries. Drugs with high protein binding and/or a V_d in the range of the extracellular fluid volume may be associated with clinically significant alterations of V_d in burned patients. V_d is the most important determinant of drug response following a rapid loading dose. However, adjustments in dose to compensate for altered V_d are indicated only when V_d for the drug is small (<30 liters) because with larger V_d only a small fraction of the drug is present in the plasma.[114]

Clearance is the most important factor determining the maintenance dose of drugs and can influence the response to drugs given by infusion or repeated bolus during anesthesia. Drug clearance is influenced by four factors:
- metabolism;
- protein binding;
- renal excretion; and
- novel excretion pathways.

The characteristic hepatic extraction of a particular drug influences changes in its clearance that occur after thermal injury. Drugs vary greatly in their extraction by the liver. Hepatic clearance of drugs highly extracted by the liver depends primarily on hepatic blood flow and is insensitive to alterations in protein binding. Clearance of these drugs may increase during the hyperdynamic phase when hepatic blood flow is increased. In contrast, clearance of drugs that have a low hepatic extraction coefficient is not affected by changes in hepatic blood flow but is sensitive to alterations in plasma protein levels.[114] For these drugs it is the unbound fraction of the drug that is metabolized. As above, changes in unbound fraction depend on whether the drug is bound by albumin or AAG. Changes in protein levels produce clinically significant pharmacokinetic changes only for drugs that are highly bound (>80%).[117]

During resuscitation, renal blood flow may be reduced and renal excretion of drugs may be impaired. Later, during the hypermetabolic phase, renal blood flow is increased as a result of the elevated cardiac output. During this period excretion of certain drugs can be increased to the point that the dose may need to be increased. Loirat et al. reported increased glomerular filtration rates and reduced half-life of tobramycin in burn patients.[118] However, this was age-dependent and patients over 30 years of age did not have increased glomerular filtration or reduced half-life.

Burn patients may also experience altered drug clearance due to novel excretion pathways. Glew et al. found that 20% of a daily gentamicin dose was eliminated in the exudates lost to wound dressings.[119] In addition, rapid blood loss during surgery may speed elimination of drugs when blood loss and transfusion amount, essentially, to an exchange transfusion.

Hepatic clearance of drugs with low extraction coefficients is also sensitive to alterations of hepatic capacity (enzyme activity). There is evidence of impairment of hepatic enzyme activity in burn patients.[114] Phase I reactions (oxidation, reduction, or hydroxylation by the cytochrome P-450 system) are impaired in burn patients while phase II reactions (conjugation) seem to be relatively preserved.[115] However, these generalizations do not always produce predictable alterations in pharmacokinetic parameters. For example, contradictory observations of morphine clearance in burn patients have been reported. Morphine metabolism is by glucuronidation. This is a phase II reaction which is normally retained in thermally injured patients. Consequently, morphine clearance has been reported unchanged as predicted or decreased.[120,121] With so many variables involved, such as hepatic blood flow, V_d, plasma proteins, multiple drug exposure, and variation in burn injury, this inconsistency is not surprising. The key to effective drug therapy in burn patients is to monitor drug effects and carefully titrate the dose to the desired effect.

Muscle relaxants

In terms of anesthetic management, the most profound and clinically significant effect of burn injuries on drug response relates to muscle relaxants. Burn injuries of more than 25% total body surface area influence responses to both succinylcholine and the nondepolarizing muscle relaxants. In burned patients, sensitization to the muscle relaxant effects of succinylcholine can produce exaggerated hyperkalemic responses severe enough to induce cardiac arrest.[122-124] In contrast, burned patients are resistant to the effects of nondepolarizing muscle relaxants.[125-127] These changes are explained by up-regulation of skeletal muscle acetylcholine receptors.[128-130]

Martyn and Richtsfeld[130] have recently reviewed the mechanisms of exaggerated hyperkalemic responses to succinylcholine. There are several disease states, including burns, denervation, and immobilization, that are associated with potentially lethal hyperkalemic responses to succinylcholine. The molecular mechanism appears to be both quantitative and qualitative changes in skeletal muscle postsynaptic nicotinic acetylcholine receptors. Animal and human studies consistently demonstrate an association of increased numbers of skeletal muscle acetylcholine receptors with resistance to nondepolarizing muscle relaxants and increased sensitivity to succinylcholine. In addition, the distribution of the new receptors is altered. Nicotinic receptors are normally restricted to the neuromuscular synaptic cleft but in these disease states new receptors are distributed across the surface of the skeletal muscle membrane. The new receptors are also a distinctly different isoform (α7AChR) that has been referred to as an immature, extrajunctional, or fetal receptor. The immature receptors are more easily depolarized by succinylcholine and their ion channel stays open longer. The immature receptors are also strongly and persistently depolarized by the metabolite of acetylcholine and succinylcholine, choline. It has been suggested that the hyperkalemic response to succinylcholine after burn or denervation injury results when potassium is released from receptor-associated ion channels across the entire muscle cell membrane rather than just the junctional receptors. Depolarization persists because the channels stay open longer and the breakdown product of succinylcholine, choline, is also a strong agonist for the immature receptors.

Cardiac arrest in burned patients after succinylcholine administration was first reported in 1958.[122] It was not until 1967, however, that an exaggerated hyperkalemic effect was identified as the cause of this phenomenon.[123,124] Several clinical studies have documented exaggerated increases in potassium concentrations after succinylcholine administration in burned patients. However, considerable individual variability exists; only a few patients in these series developed dangerously high potassium levels. The size of the increase was greatest about 3–4 weeks after injury. The earliest exaggerated hyperkalemic response described occurred 9 days after injury and normal responses were observed in the remaining patients in this series for up to 14–20 days.[131] The shortest post-burn interval associated with succinylcholine-induced cardiac arrest was 21 days.[132] Controversy surrounds recommendations regarding the safe use of succinylcholine after burn injury. Various authors recommend avoidance of succinylcholine at intervals ranging from 24 hours to 21 days after burn injury.[5,133] A series of letters to the editor of Anesthesiology from experts in this area illustrates the controversy surrounding this question.[134-136] It was pointed out by Martyn[136] that at the time when the mechanism of the cardiac arrest after succinylcholine was elucidated surgical treatment of burns was delayed for approximately 2 weeks until the eschar spontaneously separated. As a result there are few clinical data regarding potassium changes during this early period. On the basis of indirect evidence from experimental data, Martyn[136] recommended avoidance of succinylcholine, starting 48 hours after injury. This seems rational and prudent. Brown and Bell[137] described supersensitivity of burned pediatric patients to the relaxant effect of succinylcholine. They observed more than 90% depression of muscle activity with 0.2 mg/kg succinylcholine without dangerous hyperkalemia. Despite these observations, Brown and Bell state that it is generally advisable not to use succinylcholine in patients with large burns. The question remains: in the presence of life-threatening laryngospasm in a burn patient, is it acceptable to give a small dose of succinylcholine (e.g. 0.1 mg/kg) and accept a theoretical risk of hyperkalemia to treat a real and immediate risk of asphyxia? There is not enough clinical evidence to answer this question conclusively and it remains a matter of clinical judgment.

When rapid sequence induction and quick onset of paralysis in burn patients is desired rocuronium is the drug of choice. A dose of 1.2 mg/kg of this drug provided good intubation conditions in 86 + 20 seconds in burned patients.[138] The problem with this choice is that muscle relaxation will persist for some time and precludes extubation after short cases and difficulty with intubation and ventilation may require emergent surgical airway access. A cyclodextrin (Org 25969) has recently been tested in man as a reversal agent with a novel mechanism of action for rocuronium.[138b] Org 25969 has been specifically designed to encapsulate rocuronium. This agent has been found to rapidly terminate neuromuscular blockade by rocuronium theoretically by sequestering it from nicotinic neuromuscular receptors. If this agent becomes approved for clinical use it may provide a way to rapidly reverse muscle relaxation with rocuronium and provide a more attractive choice for burn patients when rapid sequence induction is indicated.

Responses to nondepolarizing relaxants are also altered by burn injury. Three-to-fivefold greater doses are required to achieve adequate relaxation.[125] Resistance is apparent by 7 days after injury and peaks by approximately 40 days. Sensitivity returns to normal after approximately 70 days. Two reports described slight but measurable resistance to nondepolarizing relaxants persisting for more than a year after complete healing of the wounds. The mechanism of the altered response appears to involve pharmacodynamic rather than pharmacokinetic changes. Up-regulated immature receptors are less sensitive to nondepolarizing relaxants. Burns greater than 25% total body surface area require higher total dose and greater plasma concentrations of nondepolarizing blockers to achieve a given level of twitch depression.[126]

Proliferation of acetylcholine receptors across the muscle membrane has been used to explain both resistance to nondepolarizing muscle relaxants and the exaggerated hyperkalemic response to succinylcholine.[30] The observation of resistance of a patient to metocurine for up to 463 days after burn has been used to suggest that hyperkalemic responses to succinylcholine also could persist for more than a year.[127] However, no pathologic hyperkalemic responses to succinylcholine in burned patients have been reported more than 66 days after burns.[133]

In contrast to other nondepolarizing neuromuscular blockers, mivacurium dosage requirements in pediatric patients appear to be unchanged by burn injury. The time to onset of drug action, degree of paralysis achieved by a specific dose, and rate of infusion required to maintain a given level of relaxation were all the same in burn patients as values reported for non-burned control patients.[134,135] Plasma cholinesterase activity is reduced in burn patients.[136] In a study by Martyn, the observation of an inverse relationship between plasma cholinesterase activity and recovery time from 25 to 75% twitch tension suggests that reduction of metabolic degradation of mivacurium may compensate for other factors that induce resistance to relaxants.[134,140] This observation suggests that mivacurium can be administered to burn patients in normal doses that would avoid cardiovascular perturbations associated with required larger doses of other relaxants in burn patients.

Anesthetic management

Airway management

If injuries do not preclude conventional airway management (i.e. mask fit, jaw lift, and mouth opening), standard induction and intubation procedures are appropriate. Hu et al. reported that gastric emptying was not delayed in patients with severe burns so that a rapid sequence induction is not necessary.[141] However, attention should be given to gastric residuals during enteric feeding. Development of sepsis can slow gastric emptying which can result in retained fluids in the stomach and risk of aspiration.

When burns include face and neck, swelling and distortion may make direct laryngoscopy difficult or impossible. In addition, loss of mandibular mobility may impair airway manipulation and make mask ventilation difficult. Fiberoptic intubation while maintaining spontaneous ventilation is a safe and reliable technique under these conditions. Fiberoptic intubation can be performed in awake adults but pediatric patients are unable to cooperate and must be sedated. Since most anesthetics cause collapse of pharyngeal tissues and airway obstruction they are unsuitable for fiberoptic intubation in patients whose airway would be difficult to manage with a mask.[142] Ketamine, however, is unique among anesthetic drugs because it maintains spontaneous ventilation and airway patency (Figure 14.6).[143,144]

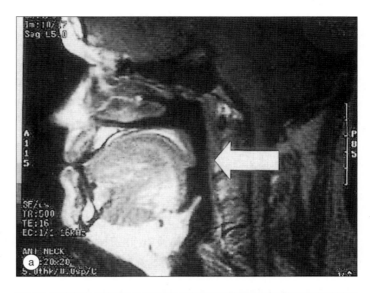
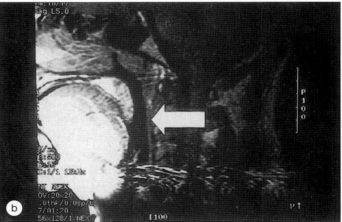
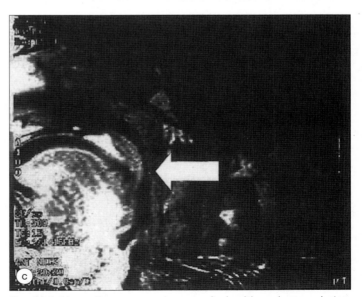

Fig. 14.6 Magnetic resonance images of a healthy volunteer during inspiration while conscious (a), or anesthetized with propofol (b) or ketamine (c). Anterior-posterior diameter of the pharynx at the level of the soft palate is marked by decreased during propofol anesthesia (b) but maintained during ketamine anesthesia (c).

Ketamine anesthesia has been found safe and effective for airway management in infants with difficult airways caused by congenital airway anomalies. Reports of successful nasotracheal intubation in infants with congenital airway malformations have been made both by manipulations guided by fiberoptic nasopharyngoscopy and the conventional technique of fiberoptic intubation with the endotracheal tube mounted on the fiberscope.[145,146] In the latter case an ultra-thin bronchoscope (2.7 mm) was required because a larger fiberscope would not fit through the appropriate-sized endotracheal tube. To facilitate intubation under ketamine anesthesia, topical anesthesia of the larynx with lidocaine prior to instrumentation of the larynx is advised. Since the ultra-thin bronchoscope lacks a working channel for administration of topical lidocaine, fiberoptic intubation with the 2.7 mm bronchoscope was preceded by nasopharyngoscopy with a 3.5 mm fiberscope for administration of topical lidocaine. At SBH Galveston we have also found this technique, utilizing two fiberscopes, effective in infants with burn injuries. Wrigley et al. evaluated the use of a 2.2 mm intubating fiberscope during halothane anesthesia in ASA 1 or 2 children aged 6 months to 7 years.[147] In this series of 40 patients a number of complications were experienced including laryngospasm and failure to achieve intubation with the fiberscope. This experience is in contrast to numerous reports of safe and effective airway management with ketamine.

Securing an endotracheal tube in a patient with facial burns presents a variety of problems and numerous techniques have been described.[148] Tape or ties crossing over burned areas will irritate the wound or dislodge grafts. A useful technique to avoid these problems involves the use of a nasal septal tie with one-eighth inch umbilical tape (Figure 14.7). The umbilical tape is placed around the nasal septum using 8 or 10 French red rubber catheters that are passed through each naris and retrieved from the pharynx by direct laryngoscopy and McGill forceps. A length of umbilical tape is tied to each of the catheters; and when the catheters are pulled back through the nose, each end of the umbilical tape is pulled out its respective naris, producing a loop around the nasal septum. Before securing with a knot, care should be taken to assure that the uvula is not captured in the loop. A knot in the nasal septal tie should be snug enough to prevent excessive movement of the endotracheal tube but loose enough to prevent ischemic necrosis of the underlying tissues.

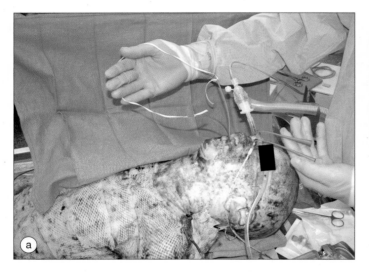

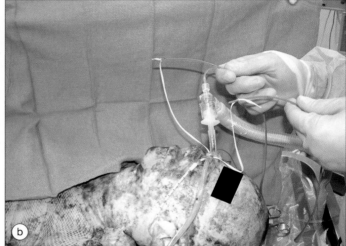

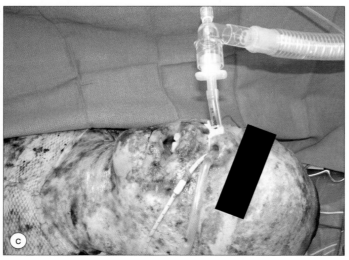

Fig. 14.7 Nasotracheal tubes can be secured with confidence by tying to umbilical tape tied in a loop around the nasal septum. (a) Red rubber catheters (8 or 10 Fr) are passed through each naris, retrieved with McGill forceps from the oropharynx, and each end of a piece of umbilical tape is tied to the catheters. (b) When the catheters are pulled out of the nares, the umbilical tape follows and, after laryngoscopy to assure the uvula has not been entrapped, a loop can be tied around the bony nasal septum. (c) Umbilical tape can be used to secure the endotracheal tube to this loop. This technique is very secure, avoids irritating facial burn wounds or grafts, and leaves the surgical field free of tape or ties.

Airway management using a laryngeal mask airway (LMA) has also been used successfully during burn surgery for children. McCall et al. reported their experience with 141 general anesthetics administered to 88 pediatric burn patients.[149] Nineteen (14.5%) of the procedures were complicated by respiratory events such as unseating, desaturation, and partial laryngospasm that required intervention. Two of these events required intraoperative intubation without sequelae, while all other events resolved with therapy. Interestingly, the presence of preoperative respiratory problems or face/neck burns did not predict intraoperative respiratory problems. These authors suggest that, in patients with upper airway mucosal injury, LMA airway management may help avoid further laryngeal injury that might occur with intubation of the trachea.

Hagberg et al. published a case report describing the successful use of an esophageal tracheal Combitube™ in a patient undergoing elective surgery for burn scars involving the mouth.[150] The patient had a Class IV oral airway by Samsoon and Young's modification of the Mallampati airway classification and limited mouth opening. A translaryngeal endotracheal tube was undesirable because tracheostomy had resulted in subglottic stenosis which could have been exacerbated by an endotracheal tube. After induction with fentanyl and propofol the Combitube™ was placed and the patient was relaxed with rocuronium and mechanically ventilated during the 60 minute procedure.

Monitors

As with any critically ill patient suffering from multiorgan system involvement, the choice of monitors in a burned patient will depend on the extent of the patient's injuries, physiological state, and planned surgery. In addition to the preoperative pathophysiology associated with thermal injuries, perioperative monitoring must be adequate to assess rapid changes in blood pressure and tissue perfusion associated with the massive blood loss that can accompany excision of burn wounds. The minimum standards of the American Society of Anesthesiologists require monitoring of circulation, ventilation, and oxygenation. Standard monitors include electrocardiography (EKG), measurement of systemic blood pressure, pulse oximetry, capnography, and inspired oxygen concentration. The ability to measure body temperature should be readily available and is highly recommended for the burn patient.

Standard EKG gel electrodes usually will not adhere to burn patients because the skin is injured or covered with antibiotic ointment. For acute burn surgery, surgical staples and alligator clips are useful. Respiratory rate can be quantitated using bioimpedance from the EKG signal or from the capnogram. Pulse oximetry in burn patients can be difficult when transmission pulse oximetry sites are either burned or within the operative field. Reflectance pulse oximetry has been suggested as an alternative in these circumstances.[151] However, an effective commercially available instrument has been slow in development.

If direct arterial pressure monitoring is not necessary, a blood pressure cuff can provide accurate measurements even if placed over bulky dressings applied to an extremity.[152] Systolic blood pressures obtained from the pressure at which the pulse oximetry signal returns during cuff deflation has also been found accurate.[153]

When blood loss is expected to be rapid and extensive, blood pressure may change more rapidly than the interval between cycles of noninvasive blood pressure measurement. In this case an arterial catheter can provide direct and continuous measurement of blood pressure. This monitor can provide much more information regarding the patient's circulatory status than just systolic and diastolic blood pressure. The arterial pressure waveform is influenced by preload, contractility, and vascular tone. Perioperative variation in the rate of rise of arterial pressure, the area under the pressure wave, position of the dicrotic notch, and beat-to-beat alterations in systolic pressure related to respiration all reflect clinically significant hemodynamic changes.[154] With experience, trends in these variables can help guide volume and vasoactive therapy. Display of the beat-to-beat arterial pressure allows measurement of systolic pressure variation (SPV). SPV is the difference between maximum and minimum systolic blood pressure during a single cycle of positive pressure mechanical ventilation. Several studies have correlated SPV with cardiac output response to volume infusion. Tavernier et al. reported that in septic patients on mechanical ventilation, SPV is a better predictor of left ventricular ejection volume response to volume loading than either pulmonary artery occlusion pressure or echocardiographic measurement of left ventricular end diastolic area.[155] Measurements are not as simple as merely 'eyeballing' the blood pressure trace because several variables influence SPV, including arrhythmias, tidal volume, and mechanical versus spontaneous ventilation. SPV provides a dynamic assessment of the interaction of preload and cardiac output.[156]

Arterial blood sampling for blood gas analysis also provides valuable information regarding pulmonary function and acid–base balance. Inadequate tissue perfusion may manifest as metabolic acidosis despite apparently adequate arterial and central venous blood pressures.

In patients with large burns a central venous catheter serves several functions. Central venous pressure can be useful for titrating blood and fluid administration. Blood samples from a central vein are not truly mixed venous but trends in central venous oxygen tension can help identify inadequate tissue perfusion. A central venous catheter sutured into place also provides very secure intravenous access and is an ideal route for administration of vasoactive infusions. A pulmonary artery catheter is usually not required for burn surgery. In some cases, however, the ability to more closely monitor ventricular function and oxygen supply/demand relationships may be helpful as when large doses of inotropes or high PEEP is required. As described above, a newer transpulmonary thermodilution catheter system is also capable of estimating thoracic and end diastolic cardiac blood volumes. These measures of preload have been reported to correlate better than filling pressures (central venous pressure or pulmonary artery occlusion pressure) with changes in cardiac index or oxygen delivery with fluid volume administration.

Urine output is the most useful perioperative monitor of renal function. Urine output of 0.5–1.0 mL/kg/h is often recommended as an endpoint for fluid management in acute burn patients. Adequate urine output is one measure of both renal and global perfusion. When intraoperative transfusion is planned, examination of the urine may be the only reliable indicator of a transfusion reaction since signs and symptoms other than hematuria are masked by general anesthesia or hemodynamic changes associated with burn surgery. Myoglobinuria may also occur after burn injury and in this case a Foley catheter is necessary to monitor response to therapy. Diuretic therapy for myoglobinuria or any other indication will negate the usefulness of urine output as an index of perfusion.

Vascular access

Securing adequate vascular access in the acutely burned patient is one of the more technically challenging procedures facing the anesthesia care team. In the pediatric age group the task can be even more difficult. Skin sites for insertion of vascular access catheters may be involved in the burn, and regional anatomy is often distorted by burn, edema, or scarring. Early in the course of an acute burn, shock leads to vasoconstriction, making cannulation of peripheral vessels nearly impossible. Later, once the patient has had several operative procedures, scarring in the area of access sites makes their placement difficult as well. Since burn patients undergo multiple debridement procedures it is necessary to attain vascular access many times in each patient. The need for frequent catheter changes between procedures to minimize catheter-related sepsis compounds the problem. The anesthesia care team is frequently involved in the maintenance of adequate vascular access during the period of acute care and therefore must be facile in their placement. When a large portion of the surface area is burned, it becomes necessary to insert catheters through burned skin. Sutures are typically necessary to secure these catheters. If the burn is deep, it may have to be debrided prior to line placement so that the catheter can be sutured to viable tissue.

For the operative excision of a large burn wound, an arterial catheter allows continuous blood pressure monitoring in the face of sudden and sometimes massive blood loss as well as during the titration of vasoactive drugs. It also allows easy access to blood samples for arterial blood gases, chemistries, and serial hematocrit determinations. For pediatric patients with large burns, arterial monitoring is essential. Achieving arterial access is often complicated by overlying burn, skin graft, or scarring. In the latter case palpation of pulses can be difficult and the use of a Doppler probe is often very helpful.

The radial artery is the most frequently used site for monitoring nonburned patients, with large numbers of patients cannulated without complications.[157] There is a relatively high rate of arterial occlusion: 8% with 20-gauge catheters and 34% with 18-gauge, but almost all completely recanalize.[158] Clearly, however, the catheter must be removed if distal hand or digit ischemia develops. In patients with severe hypotension the radial artery is not always easy to cannulate and blood pressure readings from the vessel can be inaccurate. Additionally, it is often difficult to maintain a radial arterial catheter in burn patients for more than 48 hours, particularly in pediatric patients, and, unfortunately, the hands and forearms are typically involved in a large burn wound.

Accessing the femoral artery is easier in most patients, particularly those in low perfusion states because it is a larger and more central vessel.[159,160] The groin is often spared from injury, even in a large burn, and placement of a catheter in the femoral

artery is not affected greatly by the presence of edema.[161] The duration of patency is longer than that of a radial artery catheter, and the incidence of infection in a femoral artery catheter is similar to that of any other location, about 1%.[159] The risk of mechanical complications is smaller than that of more peripheral arteries because the arterial/catheter diameter ratio is larger. Still some recommend avoiding the femoral site unless no other site is available since loss of limb, or limb length discrepancy in children, is a devastating, if rare, complication.[162]

Other sites for arterial access include the dorsalis pedis, posterior tibial, and temporal arteries, none used with great frequency, and all distal enough to give inaccurate blood pressure readings, particularly in hypotensive patients. Use of the axillary artery has the disadvantages of a relatively higher rate of infection and difficulty in maintaining correct arm positioning for proper catheter function.[163]

The incidence of complications from arterial catheters has been cited as anywhere from 0.4 to 11%, with the higher rate seen most often in pediatric patients, particularly those under 1 year of age.[164–166] Early complications include bleeding, which is usually easily controlled, and hematoma formation, which is more common if the artery is transfixed during cannulation and is avoided by an adequate period of pressure applied to the site if bleeding occurs. Damping of the arterial waveform or clotting of the catheter is more common with small catheters or small arteries; this can be lessened somewhat by continuous heparin flushing systems.[167]

The incidence of catheter-related infections with arterial catheters is generally low, quoted at anywhere from 0.4 to 2.5% until 4 days duration. The incidence of infection gradually increases to 10% by 7 days, but stays constant thereafter. This relatively low rate of infection in comparison to central venous catheters confirms the clinical impression that catheter-related infections are less commonly seen in the high-flow arterial system.[162,168]

Vascular insufficiency of the distal extremity occurs in 3–4% of patients in whom arterial catheters are placed.[163] Fortunately, most cases of ischemia resulting from vascular obstruction are evident immediately and resolve when the catheter is removed. The risk of ischemia can be minimized by selecting the smallest possible catheter that will give an accurate arterial waveform.[161] There is a marked increase in the incidence of arterial vasospasm when over 50% of the vessel lumen is occluded by the catheter.[169] This is certainly more of a problem in pediatric patients than adults. Predisposing factors to ischemia from arterial obstruction include hypotension, the use of vasoconstrictors, prolonged catheterization, age under 5 years, and insertion by cutdown.[170] Indeed, most reports of chronic sequelae have come in patients less than 1 year of age who were hypotensive at the time of catheter insertion. Other less commonly reported complications from arterial catheters include cutaneous damage, pseudoaneurysm formation, and septic arthritis of the hip.[171–173]

Central venous catheters are very useful for large-volume resuscitation in patients with burns over 30% or more of their TBSA. As with arterial catheters, burn wound, edema, and scarring all hamper the placement of central venous catheters. Normal anatomic landmarks can be totally obliterated. The problem is compounded by the need for long-term access in patients with large burns who are also at high risk for central venous catheter infections and so will require frequent line changes. Ultrasound guidance has been used successfully to guide correct placement of appropriate-size catheters into central veins but is less helpful for the subclavian approach and extensive scarring from burn wounds can degrade the ultrasound image.

Catheters placed in the subclavian vein have a lower risk of infection than those placed in the internal jugular or femoral vein, but carry a higher risk of mechanical complications during their placement.[174] The internal jugular vein is typically more difficult to access in burn patients with facial and neck burns or edema and is associated with a higher infection risk. Additionally it is a difficult position in terms of patient comfort, particularly for pediatric patients. The femoral vein is a large central vein that is usually easy to cannulate. It has several advantages, including no risk of pneumothorax, easier control of bleeding, less anatomic distortion due to edema, and the inguinal region is often spared even in a large burn. The risk of catheter-related infection is higher in the femoral vein than at other vascular access sites in some studies, and the risk of venous thrombosis is also quoted by some authors as being greater.[175-177]

Early complications with the placement of venous catheters include trauma, hematoma, bleeding, air embolus, pleural effusion, pneumothorax, or pericardial tamponade. Delayed complications include infection and thrombosis, which have been studied by many authors with often conflicting results. In one trial, 45 patients were randomized to either an upper extremity catheter group in which catheters were placed in the internal jugular or subclavian vein, or to a lower extremity catheter group in which catheters were placed in the femoral vein. No patients in the upper extremity group developed thrombosis, while six patients (25%) in the lower extremity group developed deep vein thrombosis. Additionally, another seven patients (29%) in the lower extremity group had non-diagnostic ultrasound findings.[177] In another trial involving pediatric patients, mechanical complications occurred in 9.5% of femoral venous catheters but only 1.8% of nonfemoral catheters.[178] A third study involved 162 femoral venous catheters and 233 nonfemoral venous catheters; mechanical complications were equal in the two groups, 2.5% versus 2.1%. However, three of four patients who developed thrombosis were in the femoral group, as was the one patient who developed an embolus.[176] Conversely, 1449 femoral venous catheters were maintained in 313 burn patients with no pulmonary emboli. These catheters were changed every 3 days and the authors maintain that the femoral site can successfully be used as part of a site rotation for central venous access in burn patients.[179] Another 224 pediatric burn patients with femoral venous catheters had only a 3.5% incidence of mechanical complications, including only one thrombus.[180] Finally, there has been a 20–46% incidence of femoral venous thrombosis found at autopsy in patients with femoral venous catheters left in place for a week or longer. A 67% incidence of thrombotic complications has been reported with internal jugular catheters and 61% with umbilical venous catheters when studied at autopsy.[181] It would seem safe to say that the femoral vein can be used for catheterization for short intervals with frequent line changes and diligent monitoring for thrombotic complications.[182]

When looking at the incidence of catheter-related infection from central venous catheters in burn patients, the answer is even less clear. There is an inherent difficulty when talking about the incidence of catheter-related infection in burn patients for several reasons. First, the patients with central venous catheters are the sickest patients. Secondly, the burn wound is a constant source of infection and pneumonia, and urinary tract infections are also fairly common in critically ill burn patients; in many patients catheter-related infection is a diagnosis of exclusion but burn patients always have at least one other obvious source of infection. Finally, since most catheter-related infections develop when bacteria migrate down the catheter tract from the skin, there is a higher risk of catheter infection when the insertion site is through or very near a burn wound.[183,184] To further cloud the picture, differing definitions of catheter-related infection make comparing different studies of the problem more difficult. Catheter-related infection in burn patients has been reported to have an incidence as low as 2.5% and as high as 22.4%.[183] One large study of 1183 burn patients and 1346 central venous catheters showed that the incidence of catheter-related infection was 19.5% with a mortality of 14.1%. These authors cite catheter-related infection as the second most common cause of sepsis in the burn patient after the burn wound.[185]

Many older studies recommend frequent catheter changes to decrease the incidence of infection, but several studies show no increase in infection out to as many as 7–10 days. Three large randomized trials demonstrated no difference in the incidence of catheter-related infections among groups who had lines placed at a new site every 7 days and groups who had their lines changed over a guidewire every 7 days.[175,186,187] The incidence of mechanical complications is clearly lower with guidewire exchange rather than changing to a new site. Several other trials have also indicated no advantage to routine changing of catheters before 7–10 days.[180,188,189] There are conflicting data in relation to incidence of infection and the site of the central venous catheter, although almost all studies agree that the incidence of infection is lowest if the subclavian approach is used.[175,178,189,190] Also, all studies that compared single-lumen and multilumen catheters found a lower rate of infection with single-lumen catheters.[174,189,190] Those that compared percutaneous catheter placement with placement via cutdown technique found a higher incidence of infection with cutdowns.[189-191]

Advances in vascular catheters that incorporate an antibiotic have improved the efficacy of these devices in reducing the incidence of catheter-related bloodstream infections. A recent prospective, randomized trial examined the efficacy of two types of central venous catheters that incorporate antibiotics: one catheter releases silver ions continuously and the other is impregnated with two antibiotics with different mechanisms of action, rifampin and minocycline. Both catheters were associated with low rates of catheter-related bloodstream infections.[192] Improvements in this technology would provide two significant clinical advantages. Reduced colonization of central venous catheters will reduce bloodborne infections and reduced need for changes in vascular access sites for infection control will reduce the incidence of mechanical complications of catheter insertion.

Additional measures recognized by the CDC for reducing catheter-related bloodstream infections include maximum sterile barrier technique (cap, mask, sterile gown, sterile gloves, and large sterile drape with a small opening).[193] A meta-analysis concluded that chlorhexidine gluconate is superior to providone-iodine for insertion-site disinfection.[194]

The operative debridement of a large burn wound is accompanied by rapid and sometimes considerable blood loss. Critical hypoperfusion of vital organs begins to occur when 20–30% of the blood volume is lost.[195] Irreversible shock and cellular damage can begin to occur within minutes, depending on the continuing rate of loss. The achievement of a very rapid fluid infusion rate is critical in the resuscitation of the patient undergoing operative excision of the burn wound. Clearly, adequate venous access to achieve rapid infusion rates is imperative.

The laminar nonpulsatile flow of fluid through a tube was described by Poiseuille and is expressed by the formula:

$$Q = \Delta P \pi r^4 / 8 \eta L$$

where Q is flow, ΔP is the pressure differential in the tube, r is the radius of the tube, η is viscosity of the fluid, and L is the length of the tube. From this formula, several relationships are established (Table 14.7). Flow through a tube can be increased by high-pressure gradients, tubes of large diameter and short length, and the use of low-viscosity fluids. The most significant variable is the radius of the tube, where changes result in exponential changes in flow: doubling the diameter of the tube increases flow 16 times. There have been a number of studies comparing flow rates of various catheters under different conditions. It is difficult to compare these studies directly since methods are not standardized. However, it is possible to gain from them valuable insight about the factors affecting flow. Large-diameter, short catheters maximize flow, as does a central venous location: flow is 20–40% less in a peripheral vein than in a central vein for the equivalent diameter and length catheter. Peripheral veins add resistance to flow before fluid is delivered to the central compartment.[196] Flow rates, however, are equal in hypovolemia and normovolemia for the same catheter size and length.

The high viscosity of blood diminishes flow rates considerably. Diluting one unit of packed red blood cells with 250 mL of normal saline can increase the flow of the blood by tenfold.[197] The application of a 300 mmHg pressure device to the blood unit can increase the flow rate another seven times. The diameter and length of the intravenous tubing system delivering fluid from the bag to the patient has profound effects on the rate of fluid delivery. Large-bore trauma tubing with an internal diameter of 5.0 mm allows fluid to flow three times as fast as standard blood infusion set tubing with an internal diameter of 4.4 mm, which is twice as fast as standard intravenous tubing with an internal diameter of 3.2 mm. The large-bore trauma tubing allows fluid flow rates of 1200–1400 mL/min.[198] Also, infusing blood or fluid through a 'piggyback' system into another access line can decrease flow by up to 90%

Several large studies have shown introducer catheters to be superior to all other devices for the rapid infusion of blood and intravenous (IV) fluid (Tables 14.8 and 14.9). These catheters are typically of large diameter, with thin walls and no tapering so that for any given catheter size the inner diameter is largest.[195,199,200] This finding holds especially true for pediatric patients where vessel size is limited. The flow rate of a 4-French introducer catheter is greater than a 16-gauge IV cath-

TABLE 14.8 INTRODUCER CATHETER SIZES AND FLOW RATES (FLOW RATES FOR NORMAL SALINE UNDER GRAVITY)

Catheter size	Patient size	Flow rate
4 French	5–10 kg	285 mL/min
5 French	10–15 kg	380 mL/min
6 French	15–20 kg	480 mL/min
7 French	>20 kg	585 mL/min
8.5 French	>40 kg	805 mL/min

TABLE 14.9 INTRAVENOUS CATHETER SIZES AND FLOW RATES (FLOW RATES FOR NORMAL SALINE UNDER GRAVITY)

Intravenous catheter	Flow rate
24 gauge	14 mL/min
22 gauge	24 mL/min
20 gauge	38 mL/min
18 gauge	55 mL/min
16 gauge	75 mL/min
14 gauge	93 mL/min

eter. However, the 4-French introducer, placed by the Seldinger technique, requires only a 21-gauge needle to be inserted into the vein for its placement.

When planning vascular access for perioperative anesthetic management it is important to be aware of and take into account the patient's hospital course. Choice of access site should avoid vessels previously involved in complications such as thrombosis or vascular injury. Note must be taken of when existing catheters were placed and what the local convention is with regard to timing of regular changes of access sites for infection control. The patient's hospital course must also be considered when choosing a catheter. Although introducers offer the greatest flow and may provide the anesthesiologist a sense of assurance, the patient may require continuous vascular access for months of hospitalization and may return for surgery weekly. Large vascular introducers placed weekly will not be tolerated without complications that may result in morbidity and will limit access sites for future surgery. The catheter should be large enough to transfuse appropriately for the case but catheters much larger will increase risk without benefit.

Patient transport

The safe transport of a critically ill burn patient to and from the operating room can be a formidable task. A methodical approach will help to insure patient safety and the seamless maintenance of respiratory, hemodynamic, and general support. Hemodynamic status should be optimized prior to patient transport; pharmacological support may be required. The American Society of Anesthesiologists standards mandate evaluation, treatment, monitoring, and equipment appropriate to the patient's medical condition for any transport. Depending on the patient's condition, simple observation may be appropriate. Patients requiring supplemental oxygen should be monitored by pulse oximetry. Hemodynamic monitoring is guided by the patient's hemodynamic status. Sufficient battery power must be available for uninterrupted monitor and infusion pump function during transport.

Airway supplies should be readily available, including a full oxygen cylinder, a self-inflating Ambu bag with mask, and intubation equipment. The patient's airway and ventilation as well as overall condition must be continually observed by the anesthesia care team. Drugs for resuscitation should accompany the patient on any transport. As discussed below, hypothermia is poorly tolerated by patients with an acute burn injury. It is imperative that patients be kept warm during transport in order to avoid increasing oxygen consumption and taxing limited metabolic reserve.

Selection of anesthetic agents

Many anesthetic agents have been used effectively for the induction and maintenance of anesthesia in burn patients. Intravenous agents (Table 14.10) can be used for both induction and maintenance and the specific agent used will depend primarily on the patient's hemodynamic and pulmonary status as well as the potential difficulty in securing the patient's airway. Ketamine has many advantages for use in the burn patient for induction and maintenance of anesthesia. As an induction agent, ketamine can be administered at a dose of 0.5–2.0 mg/kg. Except in patients that are catecholamine-depleted, ketamine generally preserves hemodynamic stability (Figure 14.8). In addition, ketamine preserves hypoxic and hypercapnic ventilatory responses and reduces airway resistance.[201] Compared to other IV anesthetics, airway reflexes remain more intact after ketamine administration. However, some risk of aspiration remains. Patients who do not require ventilatory support can be allowed to breathe spontaneously, which provides an additional margin of safety should inadvertent extubation occur. In fact, some clinicians have reported the use of ketamine anesthesia without instrumentation of the airway.[202,203] Patients were allowed to breath spontaneously and the airway complication rate was comparable to that of intubated patients. The use of intramuscular ketamine can be beneficial in securing the airway in pediatric burn patients or uncooperative adults who do not have vascular access. Because ketamine preserves spontaneous ventilation and induces dissociative anesthesia, it provides good conditions for securing the airway by fiberoptic bronchoscopy. Addition of other anesthetic agents, particularly potent volatile agents or opioids, should be avoided until the airway is secured because these anesthetics depress respiratory drive and relax pharyngeal muscles, thus increasing the risk of apnea, upper airway obstruction, or laryngospasm. Ketamine can also be utilized, either alone or in combination with other anesthetics, for maintenance of anesthesia either by infusion or intermittent bolus. Ketamine has potent analgesic properties and is used extensively in the operating room as well as for painful dressing changes and patient manipulations. A drying agent such as glycopyrrolate (2–5 µg/kg) is commonly given in combination with ketamine to reduce ketamine-induced secretions. In addition, benzodiazepines are often recommended in older children and adults to reduce the incidence of dysphoria sometimes associated with ketamine administration. Induction agents such as thiopental or propofol are more commonly used in patients returning for reconstructive procedures rather than in the acute phase of injury but are also sometimes chosen in patients with small burns and no evidence of airway or facial involvement when direct laryngoscopy is planned.

TABLE 14.10 DOSAGE GUIDELINES FOR THE MOST COMMONLY USED INTRAVENOUS ANESTHETIC INFUSIONS

Infusion rate			
Anesthetic	Loading dose (mg/kg)	Maintenance of anesthesia* (mg/min)	Sedation (mg/min)
Thiopental	2.0–4.0	10–20	1.0–5.0
Methohexital	1.5–3.0	5.0–8.0	0.5–2.5
Midazolam†	0.2–0.4	0.1–1.0	0.035–0.7
Etomidate	0.2–0.4	1.0–2.0	0.5–1.0
Propofol	1.5–2.0	4.0–12.0	2.0–5.0
Ketamine‡	0.5–1.0	0.7–5.4	1.0–2.0

*Adjuvant to other agents (i.e. nitrous oxide, opioids).
†Infusion rate for midazolam is highly variable. Values in the table represent more commonly used doses.
‡Ketamine is contraindicated in head-injured patients. Its inclusion in this table pertains to use in other injuries.
From Nolan JP. Intravenous agents. In: Grande CM, et al., eds. Textbook of trauma anesthesia and critical care. St Louis: Mosby Year Book; 1993.

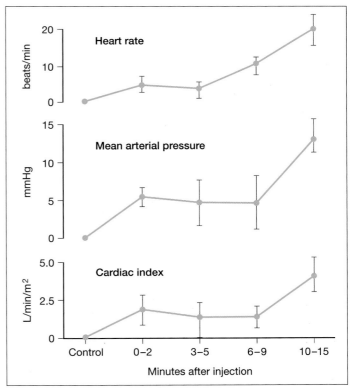

Fig. 14.8 Heart rate, mean arterial pressure, and cardiac index changes during a 15-minute period of ketamine administration to critically ill patients. (From: Nolan JP. Intravenous agents. In Grande CM, et al., eds. Textbook of trauma anesthesia and critical care. St. Louis: Mosby Yearbook; 1993.)

Volatile anesthetics may be used for both induction and maintenance of anesthesia in burn patients. In pediatric patients, mask induction with either halothane or sevoflurane is commonly used if the patient does not have injuries that may make airway manipulation difficult. In the acute setting, an anesthetic technique involving nasotracheal intubation after mask induction with halothane, nitrous oxide, and oxygen has been described.[204] The proponents particularly emphasize avoiding the potential problems associated with the ketamine-based technique. However, volatile agents produce dose-dependent cardiac depression and vasodilation (Table 14.11). In addition, hypoxic ventilatory drive is ablated by volatile anesthetics at low concentrations and a dose-dependent depression of hypercapnic drive also occurs. However, as maintenance agents, volatile anesthetics have predictable washin and washout kinetics (Figure 14.9) and provide a useful adjunct to other agents when titrated to hemodynamic and ventilatory parameters. Of the volatile agents, nitrous oxide has the least impact on cardiovascular and respiratory function and can serve as a useful component of a balanced anesthetic if the patient's oxygen requirements permit (Table 14.11).

Opioids are important agents for providing analgesia for burn patients throughout the acute phase of injury and for providing postoperative analgesia in patients undergoing reconstructive procedures. The spectrum of opioids currently available provides a wide range of potencies, durations of action, and effects on the cardiopulmonary system (Table 14.12). Burn patients experience intense pain even in the absence of movement or procedures, and opioids are the mainstay for providing analgesia in the acute phase of burn management. However, acute burn patients usually become tolerant to opioids because they receive continuous and prolonged administration of these drugs. Therefore, opioids should be titrated to effect in the acute burn patient. Most opioids have little effect on cardiovascular function but they are potent respiratory depressants. Therefore, the ventilatory status of patients receiving opioids, particularly those with challenging airways, should be monitored closely.

Regional anesthesia can be used effectively in patients with small burns or those having reconstructive procedures. In pediatric or adult patients having procedures confined to the lower extremities, lumbar epidural or caudal anesthesia can provide a useful adjunct for control of postoperative pain. In cooperative adult patients with injuries confined to lower extremities, epidural or intrathecal anesthesia may be used if no contraindications exist. For upper extremity procedures,

TABLE 14.11 CARDIOVASCULAR EFFECTS OF INHALATION AGENTS

Effect	Halothane	Enflurane	Isoflurane	Sevoflurane	Nitrous oxide
Contractibility	↓↓	↓↓	↓	↓	±
Cardiac output	↓↓	↓↓	±	±	±
Systemic vascular resistance	±	↓	↓↓	↓↓	±
Mean arterial pressure	↓↓	↓↓	↓↓	↓↓	±
Heart rate	↓	±	↑↑	↑↑	±
Sensitization to catecholamines	↑↑↑	±	±	±	±
Baroreceptor reflexes	↓↓↓	↓↓↓	↓	↓	±

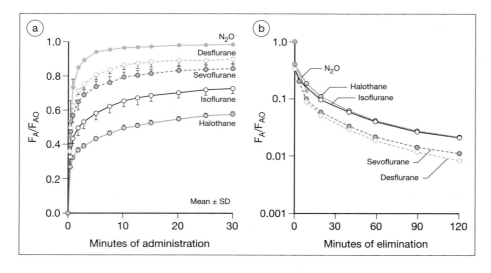

Fig. 14.9 (a) Washin curves of a variety of inhalation anesthetics. (b) Washout curve for volatile anesthetics. (Reproduced with permission from Yasuda N, et al. Comparison of kinetics of sevoflurane and isoflurane in humans. Anesth Analg 1991; 72:316–324.)

TABLE 14.12 CLINICALLY RELEVANT CHARACTERISTICS OF THE FIVE MOST COMMONLY USED OPIOIDS

	Morphine	Meperidine	Fentanyl	Sufentanil	Alfentanil
Relative potency	1.0	0.1	100–200	700–1200	30–60
LD_{50} in dogs (mg/kg)	200	700	10	4.0	59.5–87.5
Analgesic dose	70–210 µg/kg	0.7–2.1 mg/kg	1.0–2.0 µg/kg	0.25 µg/kg	4.8 µg/kg
Anesthetic dose*	0.5–3.0 mg/kg	3.0–10 mg/kg	50–100 µg/kg	5.12 µg/kg	100–300 µg/kg loading dose +25.50 µg/kg/h
MIC_{50}			15 ng/mL		270–400
MIC_{90}			25 ng/mL		
MIC_{95}			30 ng/mL		
Cardiovascular stability	±	−−	++++	++++	+++
Histamine release	++	+++	−	−	−
Respiratory depression	++	++	+++	+++	+++
Elimination half-life (h)	3.0	2.5	3.5	2.5	1.5

LD_{50} the dose that is lethal in 50% of subjects; $MIC_{50,90,95}$ minimum intra-arterial concentration that prevents response to sternotomy incision in 50%, 90%, and 95% of patients; −, no; +, yes.
*Doses used for cardiac surgery. Smaller doses combined with other drugs are sufficient for most trauma patients.
Reproduced with permission from Capan LM, et al. Principles of anesthesia for major trauma victim. In: Capan LM, Miller SM, Turndorf H, eds. Trauma: anesthesia and intensive care. Philadelphia: JP Lippincott; 1991.

brachial plexus block may be considered as the primary anesthetic or as an adjunct for postoperative pain control.

Scalp donor sites are particularly painful. Sensory nerves to the scalp are superficial and easily blocked with injections of local anesthetic and this technique has been used for awake craniotomy.[205] Scalp blocks have been used with success at our institution for donor sites in acute patients (unpublished observation) and for scalp procedures in reconstructive patients.[206]

Fluid management

Fluid management and blood transfusion for burn wound excision can be quite challenging. Fluid administration should be guided not only by intraoperative events but previous hospital course and ICU treatment goals. If early excision is performed during the first 24 hours, perioperative fluid management may involve the acute resuscitation and fluid needs will exceed replacement of shed blood. Even after this period insensible fluid requirements are increased by large open surfaces from excised wounds, hypermetabolic state, and hyperthermia. However, early in the patients' hospital course, patients are edematous from the large amounts of crystalloid solutions administered during resuscitation. At this time additional crystalloid administered during the perioperative period may be poorly tolerated and may result in complications of compartment syndrome in extremities or the abdomen. After the initial period of resuscitation, ICU therapy may include vigorous attempts to reduce edema including the use of diuretics. If the ICU staff have been administering diuretics to the patients all week in order to reduce interstitial edema it is not helpful when the patient receives several liters of fluid in the operating room. Perioperative fluid management must also take into account hypotonic clysis fluids that the surgeons may inject to facilitate donor skin harvest with the dermatome. In small children the volume of this fluid can be in excess of 50 mL/kg. State of hydration and electrolyte balance must be monitored carefully in order to maintain proper fluid balance.

Replacement of surgical blood loss during burn wound excision and grafting can be just as challenging. Unlike most general surgical procedures, during burn surgery it is impossible to accurately estimate the amount of shed blood. Shed blood is not collected in suction canisters where it can be measured. During burn surgery shed blood is concealed beneath the patient, in drapes, in sponges, or may be washed down a drain on the operating table. As discussed above regarding the initial resuscitation, there is no one physiological endpoint to titrate volume replacement. Arterial pressure may be maintained by vasoconstriction despite significant hypovolemia, central venous pressure is not a reliable index of preload, changes in urine output and hematocrit lag behind rapid reductions in blood volume, and metabolic acidosis may indicate deficient perfusion but does not identify the specific problem. All of these variables are useful, however, when evaluated together. Although, systolic blood pressure may be within the normal range, alterations in the arterial waveform and changes with the respiratory cycle may indicate hypovolemia. Even though central venous pressure correlates poorly with hemodynamic function, this variable is useful in determining if volume administration will be tolerated by the patient. If perfusion appears inadequate and central venous pressure is low or normal it is safe to give volume. If central venous pressure is elevated, volume administration may cause pulmonary edema.

The concept of transfusion trigger with regard to burn care is discussed below. It must be remembered, however, that during rapid blood loss the hematocrit may change much slower than the blood loss and often blood must be administered before the hematocrit falls below a specific trigger.

Blood transfusion

The need for blood transfusion is usually not a major concern during the immediate resuscitation phase in acutely burned patients unless other coexisting trauma exists. Nevertheless, a fall in plasma hemoglobin concentration can occur during the acute resuscitative phase due to hemodilution and blood loss from escharotomies and other invasive procedures.[207] However, major blood loss is common when patients are taken to the operating room for excision and grafting of burn wounds. Desai and colleagues reported that the amount of blood loss during burn wound excision is determined by the age of the burn, the body surface area involved, and whether infection is present (see Table 14.4).[10] In general, more blood loss was observed as the time from initial injury increased and if wounds were infected. Transfusion requirements ranging from 0.45 to 1.25 mL of packed red blood cells (PRBCs) per cm² burn area were reported. In another study, Criswell and Gamelli[212] reported an average transfusion rate of 0.89 mL PRBC/cm² burn area in a cohort of adult burn patients. A study by O'Mara and colleagues showed an average transfusion rate of 0.65 mL PRBC/cm² in a heterogeneous group of burn patients.[208]

Controversy exists regarding transfusion triggers and targets. Some authors advocate allowing hematocrit to drop to 15–20% prior to transfusion in otherwise healthy patients undergoing limited excision and transfusing at a hematocrit of 25% in patients with preexisting cardiovascular disease.[209] The same group proposed maintaining hematocrit near 25% in patients with more extensive burns, and near 30% if the patients have preexisting cardiovascular disease. A small study by Sittig and Deitch showed fewer transfused units and no increase in adverse hemodynamic or metabolic effects in patients transfused at a hemoglobin of 6–6.5 g/dL compared to patients maintained at a hemoglobin near 10 g/dL.[210] However, in general, little outcome data exist regarding the optimum transfusion trigger for blood transfusion during burn wound excision. Assessment of blood transfusion needs is best determined by evaluating the clinical status of the patient. Specifically, assessment of ongoing blood losses, preoperative hemoglobin levels, vital signs, and evidence of inadequate oxygen delivery such as hypotension, tachycardia, acidosis, and decreasing mixed venous oxygen tension provide important information regarding the oxygen balance in the patient. In addition, determinations of the patient's oxygen content needs are important in determining the transfusion trigger for an individual patient. Patients with coexisting cardiac and pulmonary disease generally require higher oxygen-carrying capacity. Oxygen requirements will be determined by the type and severity of coexisting conditions. Overall, American Society of Anesthesiologists guidelines indicate that blood transfusion is rarely required at a hemoglobin of 10 g/dL or above and is almost always indicated at a hemoglobin of less than 6 g/dL.[211] For each patient, therefore, acceptable blood loss can be determined based on preexisting diseases, preoperative hematocrit (Hct), and the patients estimated blood volume (EBV). Estimated blood volumes for different patient populations are indicated in Table 14.13.

TABLE 14.13 AVERAGE BLOOD VOLUMES	
Age	Blood volume (mL/kg)
Neonate	
Premature	95
Full-term	85
Infants	80
Adults	
Men	75
Women	65

During excision of large burn wounds, patients will often require one or more blood volumes of transfused blood to replace intraoperative blood losses. Massive blood transfusion can be associated with a variety of complications and the use of blood products is associated with significant financial costs.[212]

Several means of decreasing surgical blood loss during burn wound excision may be employed such as the use of tourniquets on limbs and compression dressings at sites of burn wound excision or skin graft harvesting.[213] Tourniquets have been shown to be an effective strategy for decreasing blood loss during burn wound excision.[208] The drawbacks of tourniquet use are that their effectiveness is limited to surgery on the extremities and tourniquets may interfere with the surgical field. Pharmacological interventions that may decrease blood loss include the use of epinephrine-soaked dressings, or topical epinephrine spray to induce local vasoconstriction. Alternatively, subcutaneous tissues may be infiltrated with epinephrine-containing fluids. The use of epinephrine may be associated with tachycardia and hypertension if significant amounts are absorbed into the systemic circulation. However, some studies have reported that the use of topical or subcutaneous epinephrine in burn patients is not associated with an increased incidence of side-effects or complications.[214] However, the effectiveness of this approach is unclear. A recent study showed that the use of topical epinephrine spray or subcutaneous epinephrine infiltration did not result in decreased blood loss during burn wound excision.[215] However, the data were quite variable and the patients also received topical thrombin. A larger study examining the effects of subcutaneous epinephrine and topical thrombin might clarify this issue. In a more recent study, Mzezewa and colleagues reported that treatment with systemic terlipressin, a vasopressin analog, decreased blood loss and transfusion requirements in a cohort of pediatric and adult burn patients[216] The authors did not report significant complications associated with this approach.

Blood components

Several blood components are available for replacement of losses incurred during burn wound excision.

Whole blood

Whole blood consists of unfractionated blood and contains all of the components of blood, including red blood cells, plasma, platelets, and white blood cells; however, whole blood stored for more than 24 hours does not contain functional white blood cells or platelets (Table 14.14). One unit of whole blood contains approximately 200 mL of red blood cells and 250 mL of plasma. Whole blood is available in some hospitals for large-volume blood transfusions (trauma, liver transplantation, burns) and treatment of hypovolemic shock. However, because of the scarcity of blood products in most communities, whole blood is not readily available. Fractionation of whole blood into its individual components is a much more efficient and cost-effective means of maximizing blood usage. When available, however, whole blood provides an excellent means of volume expansion and providing oxygen-carrying capacity in patients requiring large volume blood transfusion.

Packed red blood cells

PRBCs are the most common means of replacing RBC loss during surgical procedures. Most of the plasma and platelets are removed during processing so that PRBCs provide few plasma components, clotting factors, or platelets. A unit of PRBCs contains approximately 200 mL of red cells and 50 mL of residual plasma. A comparison of PRBC composition with whole blood is shown in Table 14.15. PRBCs provide oxygen-carrying capacity and, when reconstituted with crystalloid or plasma, volume resuscitation.

Fresh frozen plasma

In the setting of burn injury, fresh frozen plasma (FFP) is most commonly used to replace clotting factors during massive blood transfusion. FFP will replace clotting factors as well as protein S and protein C by a factor of 2–3% per unit. The initial recommended volume is 10–15 mL/kg. The use of FFP varies among different burn centers. Plasma is frozen within 6 hours of collection and each unit provides approximately 250 mL of plasma containing normal levels of all coagulation factors. A National Institutes of Health consensus conference has recommended usage guidelines for FFP (Table 14.16).

In the setting of massive blood transfusion, FFP administration is indicated if active bleeding exists and laboratory evidence of coagulation factor depletion is shown. A volume of 2–6 units is generally used depending on the severity of the coagulopathy. In some burn centers, PRBCs are reconstituted with FFP on a one-to-one basis. Although this practice has not been shown to be deleterious compared to use of PRBCs

reconstituted with crystalloid, there is no evidence that it decreases bleeding complications.[217] However, some practitioners argue that the use of FFP rather than crystalloid to reconstitute PRBCs results in less interstitial edema during the postoperative period and may enhance skin graft survival.

Platelets

Platelets are stored at room temperature to maximize viability. The incidence of bacterial contamination increases exponentially after 4 days. However, refrigerated platelets remain viable for only 24–48 hours. Platelets are obtained from either units of whole blood or by apheresis from a single donor. ABO-compatible platelets, particularly if from a single donor, should be used when possible because post-transfusion viability is improved. One unit of whole blood platelets contains approximately 5×10^{10} platelets in 50 mL of plasma. Most commonly, 6 units of platelets are combined into a single bag and transfused. A unit of single-donor platelets contains about 30×10^{10} platelets suspended in 200–400 mL of plasma. Therefore, 1 unit of single-donor platelets is equal to about 6 units of whole blood platelets. One unit of whole blood platelets will increase the platelet count by 5000–10 000/μL.

TABLE 14.15 COMPARISON OF WHOLE BLOOD AND PACKED RED BLOOD CELLS

Value	Whole blood	Packed red blood cells
Volume (mL)	517	300
Erythrocyte mass (mL)	200	200
Hematocrit (%)	40	70
Albumin (g)	12.5	4
Globulin (g)	6.25	2
Total protein (g)	48.8	36
Plasma sodium (mEq)	45	15
Plasma potassium (mEq)	15	4
Plasma acid (citric/lactic) (mEq)	80	25
Donor/recipient ratio	1 unit per patient	1 unit every 4–6 patients

TABLE 14.14 CHANGES THAT OCCUR DURING STORAGE OF WHOLE BLOOD IN CITRATE–PHOSPHATE–DEXTROSE

	Days of storage at 4°C			
	1	7	14	21
pH	7.1	7.0	7.0	6.9
PCO_2 (mmHg)	48	80	110	140
Potassium (mEq/L)	3.9	12	17	21
2,3-Diphosphoglycerate (μmol/mL)	4.8	1.2	1	1
Viable platelets (%)	10	0	0	0
Factors V and VII (%)	70	50	40	20

TABLE 14.16 INDICATIONS FOR FFP ACCORDING TO NATIONAL INSTITUTES OF HEALTH GUIDELINES

A.	Replacement of isolated factor deficiencies (as documented by laboratory evidence)
B.	Reversal of warfarin effect
C.	In antithrombin III deficiency
D.	Treatment of immunodeficiencies
E.	Treatment of thrombotic thrombocytopenia purpura
F.	Massive blood transfusion (only when factors V and VIII are 25% of normal)
G.	Requirements for indications A and F would be a prothrombin and partial thromboplastin time of 1.5 times normal

Cryoprecipitate

Cryoprecipitate is prepared by thawing FFP at 4°C and collecting the precipitate. Cryoprecipitate is rich in factors VIII and XIII, fibrinogen, and von Willebrand's factor. In the setting of massive blood transfusion, it is used primarily to treat hypofibrinogenemia. Generally, cryoprecipitate is administered when plasma fibrinogen levels fall below 100 mg/dL. One unit of cryoprecipitate will increase plasma fibrinogen levels by 5–7 mg/dL.

Complications of massive blood transfusion

Coagulopathy

Coagulopathy associated with massive blood transfusion is due to thrombocytopenia or depletion of coagulation factors. PRBCs are essentially devoid of platelets, and whole blood stored for more than 24 hours does not possess significant numbers of viable platelets. Whole blood contains essentially normal levels of coagulation factors with the exception of the volatile factors V and VIII. Because most plasma is removed from PRBCs, they provide a poor source of coagulation factors. Massive blood loss and transfusion with PRBCs or whole blood results in dilutional losses of both platelets and factors V and VIII.

Thrombocytopenia is the most common cause of nonsurgical bleeding after massive blood transfusion. In general, 15–20 units, or 2–4 blood volumes of blood or PRBCs, must be transfused before bleeding due to thrombocytopenia will develop (Figure 14.10). Observed platelet counts usually remain higher than calculated values due to release of platelets from sites of sequestration. Bleeding due to thrombocytopenia usually develops when the platelet count drops below 50–100 000

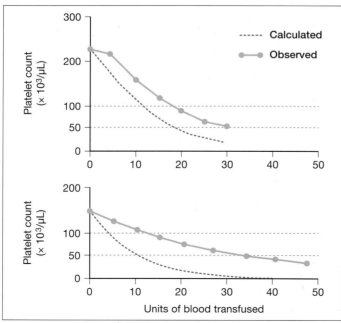

Fig. 14.10 Calculated versus observed mean platelet counts in two studies of platelet count after massive blood transfusion. (Reproduced with permission from Reed RL, et al. Prophylactic platelet administration during massive transfusion. Ann Surg 1986; 203:46.)

platelets/μL. Replacement of platelets usually requires transfusion of 6 units of whole blood platelets or 1 unit of single-donor platelets as described earlier in this chapter.

Development of coagulopathy due to depletion of coagulation factors is also possible during massive blood transfusion. Significant prolongation of the prothrombin (PT) and partial thromboplastin time (PTT) can result after transfusion of 10–12 units of PRBCs. Generally, FFP should be given to correct dilutional coagulopathy if the PT and PTT exceed 1.5 times normal levels. It is also important to know the fibrinogen level in massively transfused patients since hypofibrinogenemia can also result in prolongation of the PT and PTT. Fibrinogen may be replaced using cryoprecipitate.

Citrate toxicity

Citrate is universally used as an anticoagulant in the storage of blood because of its ability to bind calcium that is required for activation of the coagulation cascade. Citrate is metabolized by the liver and excreted by the kidneys. Patients with normal liver and kidney function are able to respond to a large citrate load much better than patients with hepatic or renal insufficiency. During massive blood transfusion, citrate can accumulate in the circulation, resulting in a fall in ionized calcium.[218] Hypocalcemia can result in hypotension, reduced cardiac function, and cardiac arrhythmias. Severe hypocalcemia can also result in clotting abnormalities. However, the level of calcium required for adequate coagulation is much lower than that necessary to maintain cardiovascular stability. Therefore, hypotension and decreased cardiac contractility occur long before coagulation abnormalities are seen. During massive blood transfusion it is generally prudent to monitor ionized calcium, especially if hemodynamic instability is present in the hypocalcemic patient.

Potassium abnormalities

During the storage of whole blood or packed red cells, potassium leaks from erythrocytes into the extracellular fluid and can accumulate at concentrations of 40–80 mEq/L. Once the RBCs are returned to the *in vivo* environment, the potassium quickly reenters RBCs. However, during rapid blood transfusion, transient hyperkalemia may result, particularly in patients with renal insufficiency. The transient hyperkalemia, particularly in the presence of hypocalcemia, can lead to cardiac dysfunction and arrhythmias. In patients with renal insufficiency, potassium load can be minimized by the use of either freshly obtained blood or washed packed RBCs. Hypokalemia can also result from massive blood transfusion due to reentry of potassium into RBCs and other cells during stress, alkalosis, or massive catecholamine release associated with large volume blood loss. Therefore, potassium levels should be monitored routinely during large-volume blood transfusions.

Acid–base abnormalities

During the storage of whole blood, an acidic environment develops due to the accumulation of lactate and citrate with a pH in the range of 6.5–6.7. Rapid transfusion of this acidic fluid can contribute to the metabolic acidosis observed during massive blood transfusion. However, metabolic acidosis in this setting is more commonly due to relative tissue hypoxia and anaerobic metabolism due to an imbalance of oxygen consumption and delivery. The anaerobic metabolism that occurs during states of hypovolemia and poor tissue perfusion results in lactic acidosis. Generally, administration of sodium bicarbonate is not indicated. The re-establishment of tissue perfusion and homeostasis is a much more important factor in re-establishing acid–base balance. In contrast, many patients receiving massive blood transfusion will develop a metabolic alkalosis during the post-transfusion phase. This is due to the conversion of citrate to sodium bicarbonate by the liver and is an additional reason to avoid sodium bicarbonate administration during massive blood transfusion except in cases of severe metabolic acidosis (base deficit >12).

Altered oxygen transport

During the storage of blood, red blood cell 2,3-diphosphoglycerate (DPG) levels decline. This results in a shift in the oxyhemoglobin dissociation curve to the left. Under these conditions, oxygen has a higher affinity for hemoglobin, and oxygen release at the tissue level is theoretically diminished. In clinical practice, this alteration in oxygen affinity has not been shown to be functionally significant.

Hypothermia

Rapid infusion of large volumes of cold (4°C) blood can result in significant hypothermia. When added to the already impaired thermoregulatory mechanisms in burn patients this can result in significant hypothermia. Potential complications of hypothermia include altered citrate metabolism, coagulopathy, and cardiac dysfunction. During large-volume blood transfusion in burn patients, fluids should be actively warmed with systems designed to effectively warm large volumes of rapidly transfused blood. In addition, the room temperature should be elevated and the patient's extremities and head covered to minimize heat loss. Body temperature should be maintained at or above 37°C in burn patients.

Pulmonary complications

Pulmonary edema is a potential complication of massive blood transfusion. This may result from volume overload and/or pulmonary capillary leak due to inflammation and microaggregates present in transfused blood. Some studies have indicated that the incidence of pulmonary edema is more related to the patient's underlying injury than to blood transfusion *per se*. However, volume status should be monitored closely during large-volume blood transfusion so that volume overload may be avoided.

Transfusion reactions

Hemolytic transfusion reactions are a relatively rare but devastating complication of blood transfusion. The incidence of transfusion reactions is approximately 1:5000 units transfused and fatal transfusion reactions occur at a rate of 1:100000 units transfused. Most severe reactions result from ABO incompatibility. The most common cause of transfusing ABO-incompatible blood is clerical error. Therefore, most hospitals have developed policies that require multiple checks of the blood prior to transfusion. A list of blood types and associated circulating antibodies is shown in Table 14.17. Massive hemolytic transfusion reactions result from destruction of transfused erythrocytes by circulating antibodies and complement. Many of the common signs and symptoms of transfusion reactions (Table 14.18), such as chills, chest pain, and nausea, cannot be detected in the patient under anesthesia. The most commonly recognized signs of transfusion reaction in the anesthetized patient are fever, hypotension, hemoglobinuria, and coagulopathy. The steps involved in the treatment of hemolytic transfusion reaction are outlined in Table 14.19. The cornerstones of treatment are to stop the transfusion, protect the kidneys with aggressive hydration and alkalinization of urine, and treat existing coagulopathy.

Delayed hemolytic transfusion reactions can occur in patients that have received prior blood transfusions and result from a secondary immune response with production of antibodies to blood antigens. This reaction can occur from 2 to 21 days after transfusion and should be suspected in patients with unexplained decreases in hematocrit during the postoperative

TABLE 14.18 FREQUENCY AND SIGNS AND SYMPTOMS FROM HEMOLYTIC TRANSFUSION REACTIONS IN 40 PATIENTS

Sign or symptom	No. of patients
Fever	19
Fever and chills	16
Chest pain	6
Hypotension	6
Nausea	2
Flushing	2
Dyspnea	2
Hemoglobinuria	1

TABLE 14.17 BLOOD GROUPS AND CROSS-MATCH

Blood group	Antigen on erythrocyte	Plasma antibodies	Incidence (%)	
			Whites	African-Americans
A	A	Anti-B	.40	27
B	B	Anti-A	11	20
AB	AB	None	4	4
O	None	Anti-A Anti-B	45	49
Rh	Rh		42	17

TABLE 14.19 STEPS FOR THE TREATMENT OF A HEMOLYTIC TRANSFUSION REACTION
1. STOP THE TRANSFUSION
2. Maintain the urine output at a minimum of 75–100 mL/h by the following methods:
a. Generously administer fluids intravenously and possibly mannitol, 12.5–50 g, given over a 5- to 15-minute period
b. If intravenously administered fluids and mannitol are ineffective, then administer furosemide, 20–40 mg IV
3. Alkalinize the urine; since bicarbonate is preferentially excreted in the urine, only 40–70 mEq/70 kg of sodium bicarbonate is usually required to raise the urine pH to 8, whereupon repeat urine pH determinations indicate the need for additional bicarbonate
4. Assay urine and plasma hemoglobin concentrations
5. Determine platelet count, partial thromboplastin time, and serum fibrinogen level
6. Return unused blood to blood bank for re-cross-match
7. Send patient blood sample to blood bank for antibody screen and direct antiglobulin test
8. Prevent hypotension to ensure adequate renal blood flow

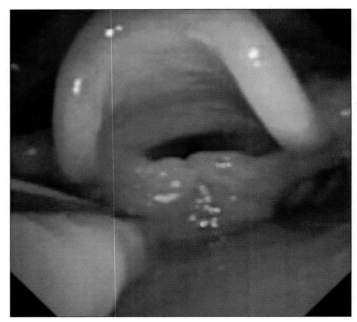

Fig. 14.11 Inflammation of the larynx caused by thermal, mechanical, or chemical irritation may result in swelling of the mucosa over the arytenoid eminences and this redundant tissue can fold into the glottic inlet and cause obstruction.

period. Renal injury is less common than in acute hemolytic reactions but adequate hydration and alkalinization of urine are usually indicated. Febrile reactions are common following blood transfusion and are generally due to contaminating leukocytes and leukocyte antigens present in transfused blood. Pure febrile reactions usually do not require termination of the transfusion but the patient should be monitored closely to assure that a more severe transfusion reaction is not developing.

Infection

Infection is a major problem in burn patients due to disruption of the cutaneous barrier and immunosuppression. Blood transfusion adds to the infection risk. Graves and colleagues showed a significant correlation between the number of blood transfusions and infectious complications in burn patients.[219] The most common source of major infection from blood products is hepatitis. Hepatitis C is the most common offender, followed by hepatitis B. The incidence of hepatitis C is approximately 3 in 10 000 units transfused. The development of rigorous screening mechanisms has markedly decreased the incidence of HIV infection to 1 in 200 000–500 000 units transfused. Cytomegalovirus (CMV) has been identified in blood products and could cause clinically significant problems in immunocompromised burn patients. However, the incidence of clinically important CMV infection is low in burn patients.

Postoperative care

Decisions regarding postoperative airway management and support of ventilation depend on several factors. Extubation is desirable as soon as it is indicated but in burn patients, for a number of reasons, it often may be even more important not to extubate when it is not indicated. If the patient came to the operating room intubated, the indication for intubation must be determined. If the initial indication has resolved, the decision to extubate depends on perioperative events. Some patients with neck and facial burns are intubated to protect the airway from obstruction by edema. The airway must be examined to be sure edematous tissues will not cause obstruction when the endotracheal tube is removed. Air leaking around a deflated endotracheal tube cuff during positive pressure ventilation is an encouraging sign that the airway may remain patent after extubation. The upper airway can also be examined by direct laryngoscopy or with an endoscope. In marginal cases the endotracheal tube can be removed while an exchanger is left in the trachea. Another technique is to extubate under direct vision with a bronchoscope with an endotracheal tube already loaded on the bronchoscope. Especially in small pediatric patients a common reason for postextubation stridor and failed extubation is edematous and redundant mucosa over the arytenoid eminences that obstruct the glottic inlet during inspiration (Figure 14.11). This condition can be exacerbated by an endotracheal tube that is too large, excessive patient motion due to inadequate sedation and analgesia, reflux of acidic gastric contents, and mechanical irritation due to compression of the posterior laryngeal structures between the endotracheal tube and gastric tubes. These irritants can also cause laryngomalacia in pediatric patients (Figure 14.12). If laryngeal obstruction persists despite attention to all these details, a short course of steroids is often effective as long as concerns regarding burn wound infection do not preclude the use of steroids (unpublished observations). Heliox has also been used successfully in this situation.[220]

After transfer of monitors and ventilatory support in the intensive care unit, a full report of the intraoperative anesthetic course is given, along with information about the patient's current condition and therapy. A chest radiograph

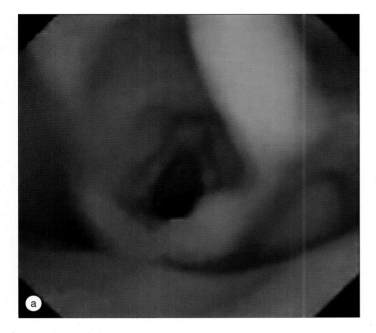

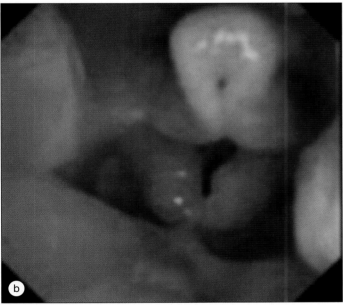

Fig. 14.12 Laryngomalacia due to local irritation and inflammation can cause dynamic inspiratory airway obstruction. (a) During exhalation the glottic opening is patent but (b) during inhalation the larynx collapses and obstructs air flow.

may be needed for vascular catheters placed in the OR or to check position of an endotracheal tube if the patient will be ventilated postoperatively. Laboratory studies including arterial blood gas, blood chemistries, renal function tests, hematocrit, platelet count, and coagulation studies are sent soon after patient arrival to the intensive care unit. These studies are particularly important if massive transfusion was required in the operating room.

One of the most important issues in the immediate postoperative period for burn patients is adequate analgesia and sedation, particularly for the intubated and mechanically ven-

tilated patient. Debridement of burned tissue and the harvesting of skin grafts are painful procedures that merit ample analgesic doses in order to insure patient comfort. It is not uncommon for burn patients to be quite tolerant to narcotic analgesics, especially after they have had several operative procedures, and in this case larger doses than normal are required.

Ongoing blood loss is unfortunately a common problem after the excision and grafting of a large burn wound, even when strict attention is placed on intraoperative hemostasis by surgical personnel. The burn wounds are necessarily excised down to bleeding tissue before skin grafts are applied. Massive intraoperative transfusion adds to the problem with dilutional thrombocytopenia and coagulopathy. Diligent postoperative care is needed to continually assess ongoing blood loss and transfuse additional blood products as they are indicated by clinical course and laboratory studies. Ongoing bleeding may manifest as hypovolemia and hypotension even in the brief period of transport from the operating room to the intensive care unit. Monitoring of central venous pressure and urine output also help in guiding postoperative blood and fluid therapy.

Adequate ventilation is essential in the postoperative period in order to minimize hypoxemia and hypercarbia. Blood gases and oxygen saturation can be used as guides to ventilator management. Patients with inhalation injury benefit not only from rational ventilator management but also from a program of inhaled bronchodilators and mucolytics combined with judicious airway suctioning. Extubated patients require supplemental oxygen for at least the first few hours postoperatively in order to maintain adequate oxygen saturation. Airway support may also be necessary initially in these patients until they are more alert and responsive.

Finally, burn patients must be recovered in a warm environment. Postoperative hypothermia can result in vasoconstriction, hypoperfusion, and metabolic acidosis. Radiant heaters, blood and fluid warmers, warm blankets, heated humidifiers for gas delivery, and high room temperature are all useful in the postoperative period to provide warmth to the recovering patient.

Summary

Anesthetic management of the burn patient presents numerous challenges. Anatomical distortions make airway management and vascular access difficult. Pathophysiological changes in cardiovascular function range from initial hypovolemia and impaired perfusion to a hyperdynamic and hypermetabolic state that develops after the resuscitative stage. These and other changes profoundly alter response to anesthetic drugs. Effective anesthetic management will depend on knowledge of the continuum of pathophysiological changes, technical skills, proper planning, and availability of proper resources. A team approach is necessary, keeping in mind that perioperative management should be compatible with ICU management and goals. This requires close communication with other members of the burn care team and is one of the most important principles of effective anesthetic management of these challenging patients.

References

1. Saffle VR. Predicting outcomes of burns. N Engl J Med 1998; 338:387–388.
2. Ryan CM, Schoenfeld DA, Thorpe WP, et al. Objective estimates of the probability of death from burn injuries. N Engl J Med 1998; 338:362–366.
3. O'Keefe GE, Hunt JL, Purdue GF. An evaluation of risk factors for mortality after burn trauma and the identification of gender-dependent differences in outcomes. J Am Coll Surg 2001; 192:153–160.
4. Sheridan RL, Remensnyder JP, Schnitzer JJ, et al. Current expectations for survival in pediatric burns. Arch Pediatr Adolesc Med 2000; 154(3):245–249.
5. MacLennan N, Heimbach DM, Cullen BF. Anesthesia for major thermal injury. Anesthesiology 1998; 89:749–770.
6. Beushausen T, Mucke K. Anesthesia and pain management in pediatric burn patients. Pediatric Surg Int 1997; 12:327–333.
7. Martyn JA, ed. Acute management of the burned patient. London: WB Saunders; 1990.
8. Woodson LC, Sherwood ER, Cortiella J, et al. Anesthesia for reconstructive burn surgery. In: McCauley RL, ed. Functional and aesthetic reconstruction of burned patients. Boca Raton, Taylor & Francis; 2005:85–103.
9. Reynolds EM, Ryan DP, Sheridan RL, et al. Left ventricular failure complicating severe pediatric burn injuries. J Pediatric Surg 1995; 30:264–269.
10. Desai MH, Herndon DN, Broemeling L, et al. Early burn wound excision significantly reduces blood loss. Ann Surg 1990; 211:753–759.
11. Thompson PB, Herndon DN, Traber DL, et al. Effect on mortality of inhalation injury. J Trauma 1986; 26:163–165.
12. Navar PD, Saffle JR, Warden GD. Effect of inhalation injury on fluid resuscitation requirements after thermal injury. Am J Surg 1985; 150:716–720.
13. Hollingsed TC, Saffle JR, Barton RG, et al. Etiology and consequences of respiratory failure in thermally injured patients. Am J Surg 1993; 166:592–597.
14. Foley FD. The burn autopsy. Am J Clin Pathol 1969; 52:1–13.
15. Moritz AR, Henriques FC, McLean R. The effects of inhaled heat on the air passages and lungs: an experimental investigation. Am J Pathol 1945; 21:311–331.
16. Clark WR, Bonaventura M, Myers W. Smoke inhalation and airway management at a regional burn unit: 1974–1983. Diagnosis and consequences of smoke inhalation. J Burn Care Rehabil 1989; 10:52–62.
17. Muehlberger T, Kunar D, Munster A, et al. Efficacy of fiberoptic laryngoscopy in the diagnosis of inhalation injuries. Arch Otolaryngol Head Neck Surg 1998; 124:1003–1007.
18. Colice GL, Munster AM, Haponik EF. Tracheal stenosis complicating cutaneous burns: an underestimated problem. Am Rev Respir Dis 1986; 134:1315–1318.
19. Clark CJ, Reid WH, Telfer ABM, et al. Respiratory injury in the burned patient; the role of flexible bronchoscopy. Anaesthesia 1983; 38:35–39.
20. Haponic EF, Lykens MG. Acute upper airway obstruction in patients with burns. Crit Care Rep 1990; 2:28–49.
21. Hunt JL, Agee RN, Pruitt BA. Fiberoptic bronchoscopy in acute inhalation injury. J Trauma 1975; 15:641–649.
22. Haponic EF, Myers DA, Munster AM, et al. Acute upper airway injury in burn patients: serial changes of flow-volume curves and nasopharyngoscopy. Am Rev Respir Dis 1987; 135:360–366.
23. Lee JM, O'Connell DJ. The plain chest radiograph after acute smoke inhalation. Clin Radiol 1988; 39:33.
24. Linares HA, Herndon DN, Traber DL. Sequence of morphologic events in experimental smoke inhalation. J Burn Care Rehabil 1989; 10:27–37.
25. Demling RH, Chen C. Pulmonary function in the burn patient. Semin Nephrol 1993; 13:371–81.
26. Sheridan RL, Kacmarek RM, McEttrick MM, et al. Permissive hypercapnia as a ventilatory strategy in burned children: effect on barotrauma, pneumonia and mortality. J Trauma 1995; 39(5):854–859.
27. Cioffi WG Jr, Rue LW III, Graves TA, et al. Prophylactic use of high-frequency percussive ventilation in patients with inhalation injury. Ann Surg 1991; 213(6):575–580; discussion 580–582.
28. Fitzpatrick JC, Cioffi WG Jr. Ventilatory support following burns and smoke-inhalation injury. Respir Care Clin N Am 1997; 3(1):21–49.
29. Reper P, Dankaert R, van Hille F, et al. The usefulness of combined high-frequency percussive ventilation during acute respiratory failure after smoke inhalation. Burns 1998; 24(1):34–38.
30. Cortiella J, Mlcak R, Herndon DN. High frequency percussive ventilation in pediatric patients with inhalation injury. J Burn Care Rehabil 1999; 20(3):232–235.
31. Ernst A, Zibrak JD. Carbon monoxide poisoning. N Engl J Med 1998; 339:1603–1608.
32. Tibbles P, Perrotta P. Treatment of carbon monoxide poisoning: a critical review of human outcome studies comparing normobaric oxygen with hyperbaric oxygen. Ann Emerg Med 1994; 24:269–276.
33. Clark CJ. Measurement of toxic combustion products in fire survivors. J Roy Soc Med 1982; 153:41–44.
34. Cummings TF. The treatment of cyanide poisoning. Occup Med 2004; 54:82–85.
35. Hardman JG, Limbird LE, Goodman Gilman A. Goodman and Gilman's the pharmacological basis or therapeutics, 10th edn. New York: Pergamon; 2001:1892–1893.
36. Deitch EA. The management of burns. N Engl J Med 1990; 323:1249–1253.
37. Horton JW, Baxter CR, White DJ. Differences in cardiac responses to resuscitation from burn shock. Surg Gynecol Obstet 1989; 168:201–213.
38. Zetterstrom H, Arturson G. Plasma oncotic pressure and plasma protein concentration in patients following thermal injury. Acta Anaesthesiol Scand 1980; 24:288–294.
39. Kinsky MP, Guha SC, Button BM, et al. The role of interstitial Starling forces in the pathogenesis of burn edema. J Burn Care Rehabil 1998; 19(1 Pt 1):1–9.
40. Baxter CR, Cook WA, Shires GT. Serum myocardial depressant factor of burn shock. Surg Forum 1966; 17:1–2.
41. Maass DL, White J, Horton JW. IL-1beta and IL-6 act synergistically with TNF-alpha to alter cardiac contractile function after burn trauma. Shock 2002; 18(4):360–366.
42. Horton JW, Tan J, White DJ, et al. Selective decontamination of the digestive tract attenuated the myocardial inflammation and dysfunction that occur with burn injury. Am J Physiol Heart Circ Physiol 2004; 287(5):H2241–H2251.
43. Horton JW. Left ventricular contractile dysfunction as a complication of thermal injury. Shock 2004; 22(6):495–507.
44. Westphal M, Noshima S, Isago T, et al. Selective thromboxane A2 synthase inhibition by OKY-046 prevents cardiopulmonary dysfunction after ovine smoke inhalation injury Anesthesiology 2005; 102(5):954–961.
45. Muller-Werdan U, Engelmann H, Werdan K. Cardiodepression by tumor necrosis factor-alpha. Eur Cytokine Netw 1998; 9:689–691.
46. Roberts AB, Vodovotz Y, Roche NS, et al. Role of nitric oxide in antagonistic effects of transforming growth factor-beta and interleukin-1 beta on the beating rate of cultured cardiac myocytes. Mol Endocrinol 1992; 6:1921–1930.
47. Cartotto RC, Innes M, Musgrave MA, et al. How well does the Parkland formula estimate actual fluid resuscitation volumes? J Burn Care Rehabil 2002; 23(4):258–265.
48. Alderson P, Schierhout G, Roberts I, et al. Colloids versus crystalloids for fluid resuscitation in critically ill patients. Cochrane Database Syst Rev 2000; 2:CD000567.
49. Nguyen TT, Gilpin DA, Meyer NA, et al. Current treatment of severely burned patients. Ann Surg 1996; 223:14–25.

50. Alderson P, Bunn F, Lefebvre C, et al. The albumin reviewers. Human albumin solution for resuscitation and volume expansion in critically ill patients. Cochrane Database Syst Rev 2000; 2: CD001208.

51. O'Mara MS, Slater H, Goldfarb IW, et al. A prospective, randomized evaluation of intra-abdominal pressures with crystalloid and colloid resuscitation in burn patients. J Trauma 2005; 58(5):1011–1018.

52. Guha SC, Kinsky MP, Button B, et al. Burn resuscitation: crystalloid versus colloid versus hypertonic saline hyperoncotic colloid in sheep. Crit Care Med 1996; 24:1849–1857.

53. Elgjo Gl, Poli de Figueiredo LF, et al. Hypertonic saline dextran produces early (8–12 hours) fluid sparing in burn resuscitation: a 24-hour prospective, double-blind study in sheep. Crit Care Med 2000; 28:163–171.

54. Suzuki K, Ogino R, Nishina M, et al. Effects of hypertonic saline and dextran cardiac functions after burns. Am J Physiol 1995; 268(2 Pt 2):H856–H864.

55. Jeng JC, Lee K, Jablonski K, et al. Serum lactate and base deficit suggest inadequate resuscitation of patients with burn injuries: application of a point-of-care laboratory instrument. J Burn Care Rehabil 1997; 18:402–405.

56. Dries DJ, Waxman K. Adequate resuscitation of burn patients may not be measured by urine output and vital signs. Crit Care Med 1991; 19:327–329.

57. Wo CC, Shoemaker WC, Appel PL, et al. Unreliability of blood pressure and heart rate to evaluate cardiac output in emergency resuscitation and critical illness. Crit Care Med 1993; 21:218–223.

58. Schiller WR, Bay RC, Garren RL, et al. Hyperdynamic resuscitation improves survival in patients with life-threatening burns. J Burn Care Rehabil 1997; 18:10–16.

59. Holm C, Melcer B, Horbrand F, et al. The relationship between oxygen delivery and oxygen consumption during fluid resuscitation of burn-related shock. J Burn Care Rehabil 2000; 21:147–154.

60. Bernard F, Gueugniaud PY, Bertin-Maghit M, et al. Prognostic significance of early cardiac index measurements in severely burned patients. Burns 1994; 20:529–531.

61. Bishop MH, Shoemaker WC, Appel PL, et al. Prospective, randomized trial of survivor values of cardiac index, oxygen delivery, and oxygen consumption as resuscitation endpoints in severe trauma. J Trauma 1995; 38:780–787.

62. Fleming A, Bishop M, Shoemaker W, et al. Prospective trial of supranormal values as goals of resuscitation in severe trauma. Arch Surg 1992; 127:1175–1179.

63. Schiller WR, Bay RC, Garren RL, et al. Hyperdynamic resuscitation improves survival in patients with life-threatening burns. J Burn Care Rehabil 1997; 18:10–16.

64. Heyland DK, Cook DJ, King D, et al. Maximizing oxygen delivery in critically ill patients: a methodologic appraisal of the evidence. Crit Care Med 1996; 24:517–524.

65. Gattinoni L, Brazzi L, Pelosi P, et al. A trial of goal-oriented hemodynamic therapy in critically ill patients. SvO2 Collaborative Group. N Engl J Med 1995; 333:1025–1032.

66. Durham RM, Neunaber K, Mazuski JE, et al. The use of oxygen consumption and delivery as endpoints for resuscitation in critically ill patients. J Trauma 1996; 41:32–39.

67. Hayes MA, Timmins AC, Yau EH, et al. Elevation of systemic oxygen delivery in the treatment of critically ill patients. N Engl J Med 1994; 330:1717–1722.

68. Hendenstierna G. What value does the recording of intrathoracic blood volume have in clinical practice? Intensive Care Med 1992; 18(3):142–147.

69. Kuntscher MV, Czermak C, Blome-Eberwein S, et al. Transcardiopulmonary thermal dye versus single thermodilution methods for assessment of intrathoracic blood volume and extravascular lung water in major burn resuscitation. J Burn Care Rehabil 2003; 24:142–147.

70. Holm C, Melcer B, Horbrand F, et al. Intrathoracic blood volume as an end point in resuscitation of the severely burned: an observational study of 24 patients. J Trauma 2000; 48(4):728–734.

71. Porter JM, Ivatury RR. In search of the optimal end points of resuscitation in trauma patients: a review. J Trauma 1998; 44:908–914.

72. Holm C, Melcer B, Horbrand F, et al. Haemodynamic and oxygen transport responses in survivors and non-survivors following thermal injury. Burns 2000; 26:25–33.

73. Kaups KL, Davis JW, Dominic WJ. Base deficit as an indicator or resuscitation needs in patients with burn injuries. J Burn Care Rehabil 1998; 19:346–348.

74. Robbins MR, Smith RS, Helmer SD. Serial pHi measurement as a predictor of mortality, organ failure, and hospital stay in surgical patients. Am Surg 1999; 65:715–719.

75. Engrav LV, Colescott PL, Kemalyan N, et al. A biopsy of the use of the Baxter formula to resuscitate burns or do we do it like Charlie did it? J Burn Care Rehabil 2000; 21(2):91–95.

76. Pirson J, Zizi M, Jacob E, et al. Acute ischemic optic neuropathy associated with and abdominal compartment syndrome in a burn patient. Burns 2004; 30:491–494.

77. Greenhalgh DG, Warden GD. The importance of intra-abdominal pressure measurements in burned children. J Trauma 1994; 36(5):685–690.

78. Ivy ME, Atweh NA, Palmer J, et al. Intra-abdominal hypertension and abdominal compartment syndrome in burn patients. J Trauma 2000; 49(3):387–391.

79. Ivatury RR, Sugerman HJ, Peitzman AB. Abdominal compartment syndrome: recognition and management. Adv Surg 2001; 35:251–269.

80. Oda J, Ueyama M, Yamashita K, et al. Effects of escharotomy as abdominal decompression on cardiopulmonary function and visceral perfusion in abdominal compartment syndrome with burn patients. J Trauma 2005; 59(2):368–373.

81. Corcos AC, Sherman HF. Percutaneous treatment of secondary abdominal compartment syndrome. J Trauma 2001; 51(6): 1062–1064.

82. Santos AP, Wilson AK, Hornung CA, et al. Methamphetamine laboratory explosions: a new and emerging burn injury. J Burn Care Rehabil 2005; 26(3):228–232.

83. Warner P, Connolly JP, Gibran NS, et al. The methamphetamine burn patient. J Burn Care Rehabil 2003; 24(5):275–278.

84. Danks RR, Wibbenmeyer LA, Faucher LD, et al. Methamphetamine-associated burn injuries: a retrospective analysis. J Burn Care Rehabil 2004; 25(5):425–429.

85. Mitka M. Meth lab fires put heat on burn centers. JAMA 2005; 294(16):2009–20010.

86. Cooper D, Souther L, Hanlon D, et al. Public health consequences among first responders to emergency events associated with illicit methamphetamine laboratories-selected states, 1996–1999. JAMA 2000; 284(21):2715–2716.

87. Davies MP, Evans J, McGonigle RJ. The dialysis debate: acute renal failure in burns patients. Burns 1994; 20:71–73.

88. Davies DM, Pusey CD, Rainford DJ, et al. Acute renal failure in burns. Scand J Plast Reconstr Surg 1979; 13:189–192.

89. Cameron JS. Disturbances of renal function in burnt patients. Proc R Soc Med 1969; 62:49–50.

90. Kim GH, Oh KH, Yoon JW, et al. Impact of burn size and initial serum albumin level on acute renal failure occurring in major burn. Am J Nephrol 2003; 23:55–60.

91. Jeschke MG, Barrow RE, Wolf SE, et al. Mortality in burned children with acute renal failure. Arch Surg 1998; 133:752–756.

92. Holm C, Horbrand F, von Donnersmarck GH, et al. Acute renal failure in severely burned patients. Burns 1999; 25:171–178.

93. Chrysopoulo MT, Jeschke MG, Dziewulski P, et al. Acute renal dysfunction in severely burned adults. J Trauma 1999; 46:141–144.

94. Herndon DN, Tompkins RG. Support of the metabolic response to burn injury. Lancet 2004; 363(9424):1895902.

95. Wolfe RR. Herman award lecture, 1996: relation of metabolic studies to clinical nutrition – the example of burn injury. Am J Clin Nutr 1996; 64(5):800–808.

96. Wilmore DW, Long JM, Mason AD Jr, et al. Catecholamines: mediator of the hypermetabolic response to thermal injury. Ann Surg 1974; 180(4):653–669.

97. Hart DW, Wolf SE, Chinkes DL, et al. Effects of early excision and aggressive enteral feeding on hypermetabolism, catabolism, and sepsis after severe burn. J Trauma 2003; 54(4):755–761, discussion 761–764.

98. Liusuwan RA, Palmieri TL, Kinoshita L, et al. Comparison of measured resting energy expenditure versus predictive equations in pediatric burn patients. J Burn Care Rehabil 2005; 26(6):464–4670.

99. Andel D, Kamolz LP, Donner A, et al. Impact of intraoperative duodenal feeding on the oxygen balance of the splanchnic region in severely burned patients. Burns 2005; 31(3):302–305.

100. Hart DW, Wolf SE, Chinkes DL, et al. Determinants of skeletal muscle catabolism after severe burn. Ann Surg 2000; 232(4):455–465.

101. Barrow RE, Hawkins HK, Aarsland A, et al. Identification of factors contributing to hepatomegaly in severely burned children. Shock 2005; 24(6):523–528.

102. Langouche L, Van den Berghe G. Glucose metabolism and insulin therapy. Crit Care Clin 2006; 22(1):119–129, vii.

103. Pham TN, Warren AJ, Phan HH, et al. Impact of tight glycemic control in severely burned children. J Trauma 2005; 59(5):1148–1154.

104. Ouattara A, Lecomte P, Le Manach Y, et al. Poor intraoperative blood glucose control is associated with a worsened hospital outcome after cardiac surgery in diabetic patients. Anesthesiology 2005; 103(4):687–694.

105. Sessler DI. Perioperative heat balance. Anesthesiology 2000; 92:578–616.

106. Wallace BH, Caldwell FT Jr, Cone JB. The interrelationships between wound management, thermal stress, energy metabolism, and temperature profiles of patients with burns. J Burn Care Rehabil 1994; 15:499–508.

107. Caldwell FT Jr, Wallace BH, Cone JB. The effect of wound management on the interaction of burn size, heat production, and rectal temperature. J Burn Care Rehabil 1994; 15:121–129.

108. Caldwell FT Jr, Graves DB, Wallace BH. Pathogenesis of fever in a rat burn model: the role of cytokines and lipopolysaccharide. J Burn Care Rehabil 1997; 18:525–530.

109. Caldwell FT Jr, Graves DB, Wallace BH. Chronic indomethacin administration blocks increased body temperature after burn injury in rats. J Burn Care Rehabil 1998; 19:501–511.

110. Shiozaki T, Kishikawa M, Hiraide A, et al. Recovery from post-operative hypothermia predicts survival in extensively burned patients. Am J Surg 1993; 165:326–330.

111. Pereira CT, Muphy KD, Herndon DN. Altering metabolism. J Burn Care Rehabil 2005; 26:194–199.

112. Zawacki BE, Spitzer KW, Mason AD, et al. Does increased evaporative loss cause hypermetabolism in burned patients? Ann Surg 1970; 171:236–240.

113. Vanni SMA, Braz JRC, Modolo NSP, et al. Preoperative combined with intraoperative skin surface warming avoids hypothermia caused by general anesthesia and surgery. J Clin Anesthesia 2003, 15:119–125.

114. Jaehde U, Sorgel F. Clinical pharmacokinetics in patients with burns. Clin Pharmacokinet 1995; 29:15–28.

115. Bonate PL. Pathophysiology and pharmacokinetics following burn injury. Clin Pharmacokinet 1990; 18:118–130.

116. Martyn JA, Abernethy DR, Greenblatt DJ. Plasma protein binding of drugs after severe burn injury. Clin Pharmacol Ther 1984; 35:535–539.

117. Blaschke TF. Protein binding and kinetics of drugs in liver disease. Clin Pharmacokinet 1977; 2:32–44.

118. Loirat P, Rohan J, Baillet A, et al. Increased glomerulo-filtration rate in patients with major burns and its effect on the pharmacokinetics of tobramycin. N Engl J Med 1978; 299:915–919.

119. Glew RH, Moellering RC Jr, Burke JF. Gentamicin dosage in children with extensive burns. J Trauma 1976; 16:819–823.

120. Perry S, Inturrisi CE. Analgesia and morphine disposition in burn patients. J Burn Care Rehabil 1983; 4:276–279.

121. Furman WR, Munster AM, Cane EJ. Morphine pharmacokinetics during anesthesia and surgery in patients with burns. J Burn Care Rehabil 1990; 11:391–394.

122. Moncrief JA. Complications of burns. Ann Surg 1958; 147:443–475.

123. Tolmie JD, Joyce TH, Mitchell GD. Succinylcholine danger in the burned patient. Anesthesiology 1967; 18:467–470.

124. Schaner PJ, Brown RL, Kirksey TD, et al. Succinylcholine-induced hyperkalemia in burned patients. Anesth Analg 1969; 48:764–770.

125. Martyn JAJ, Szyfelbein SK, Ali HA, et al. Increased d-tubocurarine requirement following major thermal injury. Anesthesiology 1980; 52:352–355.

126. Martyn JAJ, Liu LMO, Szyfelbein SK, et al. The neuromuscular effects of pancuronium in burned children. Anesthesiology 1983; 59:561–564.

127. Martyn JA, Matteo RS, Szfelbein SK, et al. Unprecedented resistance to neuromuscular blocking effects of metocurine with persistence after complete recovery in a burned patient. Anesth Analg 1982; 61:614–617.

128. Kim C, Fuke N, Martyn JA. Burn injury to rat increases nicotinic acetylcholine receptors in the diaphragm. Anesthesiology 1988; 68:401–406.

129. Martyn JA, White DA, Gronert GA, et al. Up-and-down regulation of skeletal muscle acetylcholine receptors. Effects on neuromuscular blockers. Anesthesiology 1992; 76(5):822–843.

130. Martyn JAJ, Richtsfeld M. Succinylcholine-induced hyperkalemia in acquired pathologic states. Anesthesiology 2006; 104(1):158–169.

131. Viby-Mogensen J, Hanel HK, Hansen E, et al. Serum cholinesterase activity in burned patients. II: Anaesthesia, suxamethonium and hyperkalaemia. Acta Anaesthesiol Scand 1975; 19:169–179.

132. McCaughey TJ. Hazards of anesthesia for the burned child. Can Anaesth Soc J 1962; 9:220–233.

133. Yentis SM. Suxamethonium and hyperkalemia. Anaesth Intensive Care 1990; 18:92–101.

134. Gronert GA. Letter to the editor: Succinylcholine hyperkalemia after burns. Anesthesiology 1999; 91:320.

135. MacLenna N, Heimbach DM, Cullen BF. Letter to the editor. Succinylcholine hyperkalemia after burns. Anesthesiology 1999; 91:320.

136. Martyn JA. Letter to editor in reply to: Succinylcholine hyperkalemia after burns. Anesthesiology 1999; 91:321–322.

137. Brown TCK, Bell B. Electromyographic responses to small doses of suxamethonium in children after burns. Br J Anaesth 1987; 59:1017–1021.

138. Han TY, Kim HS, Bae JY, et al. Neuromuscular pharmacodynamics of rocuronium in patients with major burns. Anesth Analg 2004; 99:386–392.

139. Viby-Mogensen J, Hanel HK, Hansen E, et al. Serum cholinesterase activity in burned patients I: biochemical findings. Acta Anaesth Scand 1975; 19:159–163.

140. Martyn JAJ, Chang Y, Goudsouzian NG, et al. Pharmacodynamics of mivacurium chloride in 13 to 18 year old adolescents with thermal injury. Br J Anaesth 2002; 89(4):580–585.

141. Hu OY, Ho ST, Wang JJ, et al. Evaluation of gastric emptying in severe, burn-injured patients. Crit Care Med 1993; 21:527–531.

142. Esch O, Lang J, Herbert ME, et al. Magnetic resonance imaging of the upper airway: Effects of propofol anesthesia and nasal continuous positive airway pressure in humans. Anesthesiology 1996; 84:275–278.

143. Lang J, Herbert M, Esch O, et al. Magnetic resonance of the upper airway: Ketamine preserves airway potency compared to propofol anesthesia in human volunteers. Anesth Analg 1997; 84:542.

144. Wilson RD, Nichols RJ, McCoy NR. Dissociative anesthesia with CI-581 in burned children. Anesth Analg 1967; 46:719–724.

145. Alfery DD, Ward CF, Harwood IR, et al. Airway management for a neonate with congenital fusion of the jaws. Anesthesia 1979; 51:340–342.

146. Kleeman PP, Jantzen JP, Bonfils P. Clinical reports: the ultra-thin bronchoscope in management of the difficult paediatric airway. Can J Anaesth 1987; 34:606–608.

147. Wrigley SR, Black AE, Sidhu VS. A fiberoptic laryngoscope for paediatric anaesthesia; a study to evaluate the use of the 2.2 mm Olympus (LF-P) intubating fiberscope. Anaesthesia 1995; 50:709–712.

148. Gordon MD, ed. Burn care protocols: anchoring endotracheal tubes on patients with facial burns. J Burn Care Rehabil 1987; 8:233–237.

149. McCall VE, Fischer CG, Schomaker E, et al. Laryngeal mask airway use in children with acute burns: intraoperative airway management. Paediatr Anaesth 1999; 9:515–520.

150. Hagberg CA, Johnson S, Pillai D. Effective use of the esophageal tracheal Combitube™ following severe burn injury. J Clin Anesth 2003; 15:463–466.

151. Sheridan RL, Prelack KM, Petras LM, et al. Intraoperative reflectance oximetry in burn patients. J Clin Monit 1995; 11(1):32–34.

152. Bainbridge LC, Simmons HM, Elliot D. The use of automatic blood pressure monitors in the burned patient. Br J Plast Surg 1990; 43(3):322–324.

153. Talke P, Nichols RJ, Traber DL. Does measurement of systolic blood pressure with a pulse oximeter correlate with conventional methods? J Clin Monit 1990; 6:5–9.

154. Murray WB, Foster PA. The peripheral pulse wave: information overlooked. J Clin Monit 1996; 12:365–377.

155. Tavernier B, Makhotine O, Lebuffe G, et al. Systolic pressure variation as a guide to fluid therapy in patients with sepsis-induced hypotension. Anesthesiology 1998; 89:1313–1321.

156. Perel A. Assessing fluid responsiveness by the systolic pressure variation in mechanically ventilated patients. Anesthesiology 1998; 89:1309–1310.

157. Slogoff S, Keats AS, Arlund C. On the safety of radial artery cannulation. Anesthesiology 1983; 59:42–47.

158. Bedford RF. Radial arterial function following percutaneous cannulation with 18- and 20-gauge catheters. Anesthesiology 1977; 47:37–39.

159. Thomas F, Burke JP, Parker J, et al. The risk of infection related to radial versus femoral sites for arterial catheterization. Crit Care Med 1983; 11:807–812.

160. Gurman GM, Kriemerman S. Cannulation of big arteries in critically ill patients. Crit Care Med 1985; 13:217–220.

161. Purdue GF, Hunt JL. Vascular access through the femoral vessels: indications and complications. J Burn Care Rehabil 1986; 7:448–450.

162. Cilley RE. Arterial access in infants and children. Semin Pediatr Surg 1992; 3:174–180.

163. Norwood SH, Cormier B, McMahon NG, et al. Prospective study of catheter-related infection during prolonged arterial catheterization. Crit Care Med 1988; 16:836–839.

164. Frezza EE, Mezghebe H. Indications and complications of arterial catheter use in surgical or medical intensive care units: analysis of 4932 patients. Am Surg 1998; 64:127–131.

165. Kocis KC, Vermilion RP, Callow LB, et al. Complications of femoral artery cannulation for perioperative monitoring in children. J Thorac Cardiovasc Surg 1996; 112:1399–1400.

166. Graves PW, Davis AL, Maggi JC, et al. Femoral artery cannulation for monitoring in critically ill children: prospective study. Crit Care Med 1990; 18:1363–1366.

167. Randolph AG, Cook DJ, Gonzales CA, et al. Benefit of heparin in peripheral venous and arterial catheters: systematic review and meta-analysis of randomized clinical trials. Br Med J 1998; 316:969–975.

168. Sheridan RL, Weber JM, Tompkins RG. Femoral arterial catheterization in pediatric burn patients. Burns 1994; 20:451–452.

169. Franken EA Jr, Girod D, Sequeira FW, et al. Femoral artery spasm in children: catheter size is the principal cause. AJR Am J Roentgenol 1982; 138:295–298.

170. Smith-Wright DL, Green TP, Lock JE, et al. Complication of vascular catheterization in critically ill children. Crit Care Med 1984; 12:1015–1017.

171. Sellden H, Nilsson K, Eksrom-Jodal B. Radial arterial catheters in children and neonates: a prospective study. Crit Care Med 1987; 15:1106–1109.

172. Miyasaka K, Edmonds JF, Conn AW. Complication of radial artery lines in the paediatric patient. Canad Anaesth Soc J 1976; 23:9–14.

173. Soderstom CA, Wasserman DH, Dunham CM, et al. Superiority of the femoral artery for monitoring. Am J Surg 1982; 144:309–312.

174. Saint S, Matthay MA. Risk reduction in the intensive care unit. Am J Med 1998; 105:515–523.

175. Hagley MT, Marin B, Gast P, et al. Infectious and mechanical complications of central venous catheters placed by percutaneous venipuncture and over guidewire. Crit Care Med 1192; 20:1426–1430.

176. Stenzel JP, Green TP, Fuhrman BP, et al. Percutaneous femoral venous catheterizations: a prospective study of complications. J Pediatr 1989; 114:411–415.

177. Trottier SJ, Veremakis C, O'Brien J, et al. Femoral deep vein thrombosis associated with central venous catheterization: results from a prospective, randomized trial. Crit Care Med 1995; 23:52–59.

178. Venkataraman ST, Thompson AE, Orr RA. Femoral vascular catheterization in critically ill infants and children. Clin Pediatr (Phila) 1997; 311:311–319.

179. Purdue GF, Hunt JL. Pulmonary emboli in burned patients. J Trauma 1988; 28:218–220.

180. Goldstein AM, Weber JM, Sheridan RL. Femoral venous access is safe in burned children: an analysis of 224 catheters. J Pediatr 1997; 130:442–446.

181. Kanter RK, Zimmerman JJ, Strauss RH et al. Central venous catheter insertion by femoral vein: safety and effectiveness for the pediatric patient. Pediatrics 1986; 77:842–847.

182. Murr MM, Rosenquist MD, Lewis RW, et al. A prospective safety study of femoral vein versus nonfermoral vein catheterization in patients with burns. J Burn Care Rehabil 1991; 12:576–578.

183. Still JM, Law E, Thiruvaiyaru D, et al. Central line-related sepsis in acute burn patients. Am Surg 1998; 64:165–170.

184. Kealey GP, Chang P, Heinle J, et al. Prospective comparison of two management strategies of central venous catheters in burns patients. J Trauma 1995; 38:344–349.

185. Lesseva M. Central venous catheter-related bacteremia in burn patients. Scand J Infect Dis 1998; 30:585–589.

186. Eyer S, Brummitt C, Crossley K, et al. Catheter-related sepsis: prospective, randomized study of three methods of long-term catheter maintenance. Crit Care Med 1990; 18:1073–1079.

187. Sheridan RL, Weber JM, Peterson HF, et al. Central venous catheter sepsis with weekly catheter change in paediatric burn patients: an analysis of 221 catheters. Burns 1995; 21:127–129.

188. Stenzel JP, Green TP, Fuhrman BP, et al. Percutaneous central venous catherization in a pediatric intensive care unit: a survival analysis of complications. Crit Care Med 1989; 17:984–988.

189. Garrison RN, Wilson MA. Intravenous and central catheter infections. Surg Clin N Am 1994; 74:557–570.

190. American Society of Anesthesiologists. Recommendations for infection control for the practice of anesthesiology. Prevention of infection during insertion and maintenance of central venous catheters. Park Ridge: ASA, 1997.

191. Ahmed Z, Mohyuddin Z. Complications associated with different insertion techniques for Hickman catheters. Postgrad Med J 1998; 868:104–107.

192. Fraenkel D, Rickard C, Thomas P, et al. A prospective, randomized trial of rifampicin-minocycline-coated and silver-platinum-carbon-impregnated central venous catheters. Crit Care Med 2006; 34(3):668–675.

193. O'Grady NP, Alexander M, Dellinger EP, et al. Guidelines for the prevention of intravascular catheter-related infections. MMWR Recomm Rep 2002; 51:1–29.

194. Chalyakunapruk N, Veenstra DL, Lipsky BA, et al. Chlorhexidine compared with providone-iodine solution for vascular catheter-site care: a meta-analysis. Ann Intern Med 2002; 136:792–801.

195. Idris AH, Melker RJ. High-flow sheaths for pediatric fluid resuscitation: a comparison of flow rates with standard pediatric catheters. Pediatr Emerg Care 1992; 8:119–122.

196. Hodge D, Delgado-Paredes C, Fleisher G. Central and peripheral catheter flow rates in 'pediatric' dogs. Ann Emerg Med 1986; 15:1151–1154.

197. de la Roche MR, Gauthier L. Rapid transfusion of packed red blood cells: effects of dilution, pressure, and catheter size. Ann Emerg Med 1993; 22:1551–1555.

198. Millikan JA, Cain TL, Hansbrough J. Rapid volume replacement for hypovolemic shock: a comparison of techniques and equipment. J Trauma 1984; 24:428–431.

199. Dutky PA, Stevens SL, Maull KI. Factors affecting fluid resuscitation with large-bore introducer catheters. J Trauma 1989; 29:856–860.

200. Beebe DS, Beck D, Belani KG. Comparison of the flow rates of central venous catheters designed for rapid transfusion in infants and small children. Paediatr Anaesth 1995; 5:35–39.

201. White PF, Way WL, Trevor AJ. Ketamine — its pharmacology and therapeutic uses. Anesthesiology 1982; 56:119–136.

202. Layon AJ, Vetter TR, Hanna PG, et al. An anesthetic technique to fabricate a pressure mask for controlling scar formation from facial burns. J Burn Care Rehabil 1991; 12:349–152.

203. Maldini B. Ketamine anesthesia in children with acute burns and scalds. Acta Anaesthesiol Scand 1996; 40:1108–1111.

204. Irving GA, Butt AD. Anaesthesia for burns in children: a review of procedures practiced at Red Cross War Memorial Children's Hospital, Cape Town. Burns 1994; 20:241–243.

205. Costello TG, Cormack JR. Anaesthesia for awake craniotomy: a modern approach. J Clin Neurosci 2004; 11(1):16–19.

206. Talon MD, Woodson LC, Sherwood E. Regional sensory nerve blocks of the scalp decrease the incidence of post-operative nausea and vomiting in reconstructive burn children: a pilot study. J Burn Care Rehabil 2006; 27(2):5149.

207. Sheridan RL, Szyfelbein SK. Trends in blood conservation in burn care. Burns 2001; 27:272–276.

208. O'Mara MS, Hayetian F, Slater H, et al. Results of a protocol of transfusion threshold and surgical technique on transfusion requirements in burn patients. Burns 2005; 31:558–561.

209. Mann R, Heimbach DM, Engrav LH, et al. Changes in transfusion practices in burn patients. J Trauma 1994; 37:220–222.

210. Sittig KM, Deitch EA. Blood transfusions: for the thermally injured or for the doctor? J Trauma 1994; 36:369–372.

211. American Society of Anesthesiologists. Practice guidelines for blood component therapy: a report by the American Society of Anesthesiologists Task Force on Blood Component Therapy. Anesthesiology 1996; 84:732–747.

212. Criswell KK, Gamelli RL. Establishing transfusion needs in burn patients. Am J Surg 2005; 189:324–326.

213. Smoot EC III. Modified use of extremity tourniquets for burn wound debridement. J Burn Care Rehabil 1996; 17:334–337.

214. Missavage AE, Bush RL, Kien ND, et al. The effect of clysed and topical epinephrine on intraoperative catecholamine levels. J Trauma 1998; 45:1074–1078.

215. Barret JP, Dziewulski P, Wolf SE, et al. Effect of topical and sub-cutaneous epinephrine in combination with topical thrombin in blood loss during immediate near-total burn wound excision in pediatric burned patients. Burns 1999; 25:509–513.

216. Mzezewa S, Jonsson K, Aberg M, et al. A prospective double blind randomized study comparing the need for blood transfusion with terlipressin or a placebo during early excision and grafting of burns. Burns 2004; 30:236–240.

217. Barret JP, Desai MH, Herndon DN. Massive transfusion of reconstituted whole blood is well tolerated in pediatric burn surgery. J Trauma 1999; 47:526–528.

218. Dzik WH, Kirkley SA. Citrate toxicity during massive blood transfusion. Transfus Med Rev 1988; 2:76–94.

219. Graves TA, Cioffi WG, Mason AD Jr et al. Relationship of transfusion and infection in a burn population. J Trauma 1989; 29:948–952.

220. Rodeberg DA, Easter AJ, Washam MA, et al. Use of a helium-oxygen mixture in the treatment of postextubation stridor in pediatric patients with burns. J Burn Care Rehabil 1995; 16(5):476–480.

Chapter 15

The skin bank

Richard J. Kagan, Edward C. Robb and Ronald T. Plessinger

History

The first skin autograft was described by Reverdin[1] in 1871 and the use of allograft skin as a clinical method for wound coverage soon followed.[2] In 1874, Thiersch published a report about a small series of patients on whom he had used partial-thickness skin grafts.[3] This led to extensive trials of harvesting extremely thin grafts, leaving some of the surface epithelium behind to aid in donor site healing. Results from the use of these small thin grafts, known as 'Thiersch grafts,' 'pinch grafts,' 'epidermis grafts,' or 'razor grafts' were generally so unsatisfactory for resurfacing large areas that they were typically limited to the treatment of small ulcerated wounds. The first successful use of allogeneic skin for burn wound coverage was reported by Girdner[4] in 1881. Five years later, Thiersch described the histologic anatomy of skin engraftment which popularized the clinical use of split-thickness skin grafts.[3]

Radical advances in the treatment of burn wounds brought about three developments in skin graft recovery techniques. First, it was noted that the dermal layer was the most important part of a skin graft in producing a new, tough, resilient surface. Secondly, it was demonstrated that after removing a partial-thickness graft, the donor-site epithelium was regenerated from deep epithelial islands within the hair follicles and sebaceous glands; therefore, thicker grafts could be harvested and transferring the upper dermis would not interfere with donor-site healing. Finally, by allowing for the recovery of thicker grafts, the design instruments for their harvesting became more feasible. These thicker grafts were termed 'split-thickness grafts,' and resulted in the coverage of large areas of the body surface. These major advances in skin graft recovery techniques permitted increased flexibility in the treatment of burn wounds so that the Thiersch, or pinch-graft, method and the use of pedicle flaps were rarely necessary for the treatment of cutaneous scar contractures. The use of split-thickness grafts permitted skin grafting to become a routine procedure.

Storage of human skin did not begin until the early 1900s, when Wentscher[5] reported his experience with the transplantation of human skin that had been refrigerated for 3–14 days; however, it wasn't until the 1930s that blood and tissue banking took their place in the clinical practice of medicine. The clinical utility of allograft skin in burn wound coverage was first described in 1938 when Bettman[6] reported his success in the treatment of children with extensive full-thickness burn injuries. Webster[7] and Matthews[8] later described the successful healing of skin autografts stored for 3 weeks at 4–7°C; however, it wasn't until 1949, following the establishment of the United States Navy tissue bank, that modern day skin banking began.

The establishment of skin banking signaled the beginning of significant research related to the processing, preservation, and storage of human tissues. Baxter[9] explored the histologic effects of freezing on human skin and discovered that the formation of ice crystals caused the destruction of skin architecture. This was followed in 1952 by the pioneering research of Billingham and Medawar[10] who demonstrated that skin could be effectively cryopreserved using glycerol. Soon afterwards, Taylor[11] was able to demonstrate that the addition of glycerol to storage solutions decreased ice crystal formation in frozen tissues. These advancements permitted Brown[12] and Jackson[13] to popularize the use of allogeneic human skin grafts as biologic dressings for extensive burns and denuded tissue. By 1966, Zaroff[14] had reported the 10-year experience using allograft skin in the treatment of thermally injured patients at the Brooke Army Medical Center. In this report, he described the mechanical and physiologic advantages of allograft skin as a biologic dressing. In 1966, Cochrane[15] reported the first successful use of frozen autologous skin grafts following controlled-rate freezing in 15% glycerol and rapid rewarming prior to implantation. This was followed by Morris'[16] report demonstrating the beneficial effects of using allogeneic skin in the treatment of infected ulcers and other contaminated wounds and Shuck et al.'s[17] report suggesting the potential use of allogeneic skin in the treatment of traumatic wounds based upon their Vietnam War experience. These increased uses of allograft skin led to further research into the beneficial effects of allograft skin on wound healing, including its association with a reduced incidence of bacterial infections[18,19] and the stimulation of wound bed neovascularization.[20]

Bondoc and Burke[21] are credited with the establishment of the first functional skin bank in 1971. Their experience with allograft skin led to a report of successful burn wound excision and allografting with temporary immunosuppression in children with extensive injuries.[22] Today, allograft skin remains an ideal temporary cover for extensive or excised cutaneous or soft tissue wounds, particularly when sufficient autograft skin is not available or when temporary wound coverage is desired.

Clinical uses of allograft skin

Coverage of extensive full-thickness wounds

The increasing use of allograft skin in specialized burn care centers has been one of the driving forces behind the growth and development of skin banks in the United States. The general indications for its use in wound management are listed in Box 15.1. Allograft skin possesses many of the ideal properties of biologic dressings and plays a major role in the surgical management of extensive wounds when autologous tissue may not be immediately available (Box 15.2). It reduces evaporative water loss and the exudation of protein-rich fluids, prevents wound desiccation, and suppresses microbial proliferation. Wound pain is lessened and is associated with better patient compliance with occupational and physical therapy. By restoring the physiologic barrier at the wound surface, the allografts reduce heat loss through the wound and mitigate the hypermetabolic response to burn injury. The frequent and unpredictable demand for allograft skin in specialized burn care centers has prompted the growth and development of local and regional skin banks throughout the world.

Fresh allograft skin represents the gold standard for all biologic dressings employed for temporary wound closure based upon a number of its distinctive properties compared to cryopreserved skin (Box 15.3). Its availability is critically important for the surgeon faced with the need to provide immediate coverage of large excised burn wounds. Allogeneic grafts are best applied unmeshed (or minimally expanded) in order to maximize their ability to temporarily close the wound. Fresh allografts become well vascularized, stimulate neovascularization in the underlying wound bed, and prepare the recipient sites for permanent coverage with autologous skin. In addition, fresh allografts tolerate modest wound contamination and adhere better to the freshly excised subcutaneous fat than do cryopreserved grafts. The allogeneic skin is usually removed once the patient's donor sites have healed sufficiently for reharvesting or once autologous cultured skin is available for permanent wound closure. Figure 15.1 depicts the quantitative use of allograft skin and, in particular, the increased use of fresh refrigerated allograft skin, in thermally-injured children treated at the Shriners Hospital for Children in Cincinnati, Ohio since 1998.

When fresh allograft is not available, cryopreserved skin is an excellent alternative for temporary wound coverage. Although frozen cryopreserved skin generally has less measurable viability than fresh skin, it is currently difficult to maintain continuous and ample stores of fresh skin beyond 14 days. It has therefore been standard skin banking practice to cryopreserve allograft skin within 7–10 days of recovery if it is not going to be utilized within the time period that viability can be maintained. Regardless of whether the allografts are fresh or cryopreserved, wide (mesh) expansion of allograft skin is rarely performed because reepithelialization of the interstices by allogeneic epidermis is uncommon. Figure 15.2 demonstrates the difference in appearance

---

BOX 15.1 Indications for allograft skin use in wound management

- Coverage of extensive wounds where autologous tissue is not available
- Coverage of widely meshed skin autografts
- Extensive partial-thickness burns
- Extensive epidermal slough.
  - Stevens–Johnson syndrome
  - Toxic epidermal necrolysis
  - Staphylococcal scalded skin syndrome
- Testing the wound bed's ability to accept autograft
- Template for the delayed application of keratinocytes

BOX 15.2 Advantages of human allograft skin use

- Reduce water, electrolyte, and protein loss
- Prevent desiccation of tissue
- Suppress bacterial proliferation
- Reduce wound pain
- Reduce energy requirements
- Promote epithelialization
- Prepare wounds for definitive closure
- Provide dermal template for epidermal grafts

BOX 15.3 Advantages of fresh allograft skin

- Rapidity and strength of adherence to the wound
- Control of microbial growth
- Rapidity of revascularization
- Reproducible clinical results

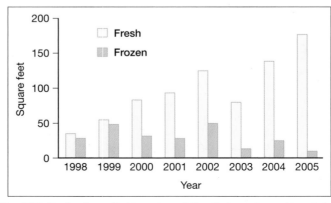

Fig. 15.1 Fresh allograft skin usage at the Shriners Burns Hospital, Cincinnati, Ohio.

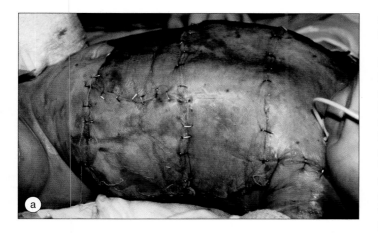

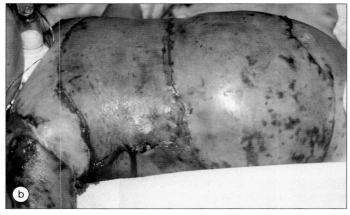

Fig. 15.2 Appearance of cryopreserved and fresh, refrigerated allograft skin on postoperative day 5. Note poor vascularization and epidermolysis in the cryopreserved skin (a) compared to the pink revascularized refrigerated allograft (b).

and vascularization of cryopreserved and fresh, refrigerated skin.

The emergence of Integra® dermal regeneration template for the treatment of excised burn wounds has been significant and in some burn centers has replaced or decreased the use of allograft skin in patients with extensive full-thickness burn injuries. Heimbach et al. reported the results of a randomized multicenter clinical trial comparing Integra® and other grafting materials.[23] When the artificial dermis was compared to allograft, there was no difference in the 'take' rates; however, 'take' was not defined in the manuscript and it is unclear whether there were equivalent rates of adherence and/or vascularization. Furthermore, it is unclear if the allografts applied were fresh or cryopreserved, although it is most likely that the allografts were frozen as the refrigeration of allograft skin was not common skin banking practice at the time of the study. A subsequent retrospective study performed at our burn center and skin bank 10 years later indicated that fresh, refrigerated allograft had a better rate of engraftment than the dermal regeneration template.[24]

Coverage of widely meshed skin autografts

Another use of allograft skin has been its application as an overlay on top of widely expanded, meshed autologous skin grafts (Figure 15.3). This technique was originally described utilizing meshed allograft[25] and provides immediate, as well as both temporary and permanent wound closure. For this reason, most burn surgeons who currently perform overlay allografting utilize nonmeshed or nonexpanded mesh allografts. This affords better protection of the underlying wound bed from desiccation and microbial contamination as this tissue is potentially exposed by the interstices of the widely meshed autograft until autologous epithelialization is complete. While this technique may play a role in the

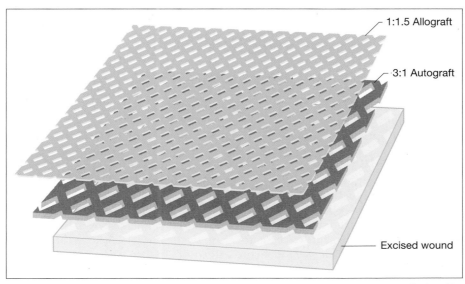

1:1.5 Allograft

3:1 Autograft

Excised wound

Fig. 15.3 Diagrammatic illustration of meshed allograft overlay technique as described by Alexander et al. The allograft is generally meshed 1.5:1 or 2:1 while the underlying autograft may be meshed 3:1 or greater. Reproduced with permission from Alexander JW, MacMillan BG, Law E, et al. Treatment of severe burns with widely meshed skin autograft and widely meshed skin allograft overlay. J Trauma 1981; 21:433–438.[25]

management of massive excised full-thickness injuries, it should be used with discretion since many surgeons have expressed concern that the overlying allograft may induce an inflammatory rejection response that can retard the rate of reepithelialization of the underlying autografts. Some have therefore advocated the use of lyophilized allograft for this purpose as it is less viable and less antigenic.[26]

Healing of partial-thickness wounds

Frozen allograft skin is an excellent wound cover when vascularization is not desired. Because it is usually less viable than fresh skin, it functions more as a biologic dressing than as a temporary skin replacement. Its adherence to the underlying wound bed results in the relief of pain and the limitation of exudative and water losses, and reduces the need for frequent dressing changes. As the partial-thickness wound reepithelializes, the allograft slowly separates without disturbing the delicate underlying epithelium. Although this application is probably not cost-effective in the management of small second-degree burns or skin graft donor sites, it is often beneficial in the treatment of extensive partial-thickness burns where its ability to prevent desiccation and promote epithelialization may reduce hospital stay and/or the need for autografting. In addition, cryopreserved allograft is an excellent biologic dressing for the management of patients with extensive cutaneous wounds resulting from drug reactions or superficial skin disorders (i.e. toxic epidermal necrolysis, Stevens–Johnson syndrome, staphylococcal scalded skin syndrome). When used for the coverage of these superficial wounds, allograft skin should be applied prior to exposing the wound to topical antibiotics since the application of these agents results in decreased allograft adherence to the wound surface.

Testing for later acceptance of autograft

Both cryopreserved and fresh allografts have been used for the care of a variety of cutaneous and soft tissue wounds. In these instances, allograft is used to provide a temporary biologic cover and to help predict the likelihood of autologous graft take later in the course of treatment. Allograft usage for this indication has been quite common in the management of deep electrical burns and purpura fulminans while the viability of the deep soft tissues is in doubt. Allograft has also been used to cover the soft tissues exposed by escharotomies and fasciotomies as well as extensive open abdominal and soft tissue wounds. Adherence or vascularization of the allograft is a reliable indication that the wound bed has sufficient blood supply to accept an autologous graft or flap.

Template for delayed application of keratinocytes

The clinical use of cultured epidermal autografts (CEA) in the care of burn patients was first described by O'Connor[27] in 1981. Since that time, there have been numerous reports supporting its use as a permanent skin replacement for patients with extensive full-thickness burn injuries. This methodology has not been without problems, however, with many authors describing variable take rates and instability of the grafts. Cuono first advocated the use of allogeneic skin with CEA, allowing the allograft skin to vascularize before removing the antigenic epidermal layer by dermabrasion.[28] Hickerson

reported his results on five burn patients demonstrating over 90% CEA take on the allogeneic dermis and supple, durable grafts up to 4 years postoperatively.[29]

The past decade has also witnessed the development of an acellular allogeneic dermal matrix (AlloDerm®) as a template for the simultaneous application of thin split-thickness autografts.[30] The potential advantage of the dermal template is reasoned to be the use of a thinner autologous skin graft resulting in more rapid donor site healing and reduced morbidity. A recently completed multicenter clinical trial demonstrated equivalence of this technique with a standard split-thickness meshed autograft; however, autograft take rates were somewhat lower than that for controls and varied from center to center.[31] In addition, the allogeneic dermal grafts measured only 36 to 116 cm^2 and were only evaluated up to 180 days post-grafting. AlloDerm® has also been used as a template for CEA; however, there have been only a few anecdotal reports related to this potential application.

Micrografting techniques

Chinese surgeons have proposed the use of micrografts using both autologous and allogeneic skin.[32] This technique involves the mincing of autologous skin into pieces less than 1 mm in diameter. These micrografts are then used to seed the dermal surface of large sheets of allogeneic skin prior to transplantation onto the excised burn wound. As the autologous epidermal cells propagate on the wound surface, the allograft skin gradually separates in a manner similar to that observed with the overlay technique. This method, while resulting in an effective skin expansion ratio approaching 1:18, has been shown to be associated with severe wound contraction that is often worse than that noted following the application of meshed skin autografts.

Potential disadvantages of allograft use

Infection

Allograft skin has been reported to cause bacterial infection.[33] It is therefore imperative that skin banks perform microbial cultures prior to releasing the tissue for transplantation. Although White has suggested that cadaver allograft containing <10^3 organisms/gram of tissue can be safely used for wound coverage,[34] current American Association of Tissue Banks (AATB) Standards[35,36] require that skin be discarded if pathogenic bacteria or fungi are present. This is particularly important given the immunocompromised status of the potential recipient and the potential for developing wound sepsis following such contamination.

There have also been reports of viral disease transmission by skin allografts. In 1987, Clarke reported what was thought to be the transmission of HIV-1 to a burn patient from an HIV-positive donor;[37] however, the results of donor testing were not known prior to skin use. Moreover, the recipient, who had a number of risk factors for HIV, had not been tested prior to receiving the allograft. To date, there have been no other reported cases of HIV or hepatitis transmission from skin allografts.

Kealey et al. recently reported the transmission of cytomegalovirus (CMV) from cadaver skin allografts.[38] Because nearly 23% of the CMV-negative patients seroconverted, they recommended the use of CMV-negative allograft skin for seronegative burn patients. Plessinger et al. reviewed 479 consecutive skin donors and found 63% of this predominantly adult donor pool to be CMV-positive.[39] They reasoned that while tissue from seronegative donors would be ideal for use in seronegative patients, such a practice would significantly limit the availability of fresh allograft skin for most thermally-injured patients. In addition, while there is good evidence to support the transmission of CMV by allograft in burn patients, there is little evidence that CMV seroconversion is clinically significant or affects outcome in thermally-injured patients.[40,41] Furthermore, Herndon and Rose[40] reiterated that the benefits of using cadaver allograft skin for the treatment of burn patients clearly outweigh the small risks associated with CMV seroconversion. At present, most burn surgeons and skin banks recommend that the decision regarding the use of allograft skin from CMV-positive donors should be made by the burn/transplanting surgeon.

Rejection

While demonstrating many characteristics of an ideal wound covering, allograft skin contains Langerhans cells which express class II antigens on their surface. These cells reside in the epidermis of the skin and are ultimately rejected as the result of an immunologic rejection response. This typically results in an acute inflammatory reaction and can lead to wound infection. Vascularized allogeneic skin grafts typically remain intact on the wound of a burn patient for 2–3 weeks although there have been reports of allograft skin survival for up to 67 days due to the inherent immunosuppression of extensive burn injury.[42] Recent improvements in immunonutrition, critical care management, and a more aggressive surgical approach to definitive wound closure, however, have made the persistence of allografts less predictable.

Efforts to prevent rejection have included methods that might reduce antigen expression by controlling the activity of the Langerhans cells in the allograft skin. Treatment of the allografts with ultraviolet light irradiation and incubation of the skin in glucocorticoids has been reported to result in a modest prolongation of allograft survival compared to non-treated skin; however, the utility of this methodology has not been substantiated. Other investigators have studied the effects of pharmacologic agents to induce immunosuppression in patients with major burn injuries. Initial clinical trials reported an improvement in both allograft and patient survival when children were treated with azathioprine and anti-thymocyte globulin;[43] however, this regimen was associated with azathioprine-induced neutropenia and the clinical outcomes have not been corroborated by others. More recently, the use of cyclosporin A has been demonstrated to prolong skin allograft survival in patients with extensive full-thickness burns.[44,45] In these studies, allograft rejection was generally observed within a few days of discontinuing treatment; however, there were instances where engraftment persisted after the completion of therapy. Further studies of these and newer immunosuppressive agents may be warranted.

The growth of skin banking

The widespread use of allograft skin in the management of patients with extensive burn, traumatic and soft tissue injuries has had a major impact on the number of skin banking facilities over the past two decades. Consequently, the majority of skin banks have been founded in close proximity to regional burn centers or within the burn center hospitals themselves. Skin banks must therefore maintain a close working relationship with regional burn centers not only to meet the specific needs of the burn surgeon but also to help generate community support for skin donation through combined educational outreach programs.

From 1969 to 1988, there was a steady growth in the number of skin banks; however, this number declined, reaching its nadir in 2002. Since that time, however, there has been a steady increase in the number of skin banking facilities to its current total of 52 AATB-accredited tissue banks that recover, process, store, and/or distribute skin for transplantation (Figure 15.4). In 1983, DeClement and May estimated that as much as 32 000 square feet of skin might be needed in burn and wound care centers.[46] This figure, however, was only a crude estimate and, over the past 6 years, there has recently been a substantial increase in the amount of skin recovered and distributed for transplantation within North America (Figure 15.5), as indicated in the AATB's

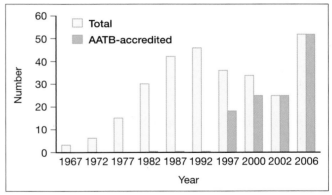

Fig. 15.4 Growth in the number of skin banks in the United States and Canada. (Data collected from AATB sources (various) with permission).

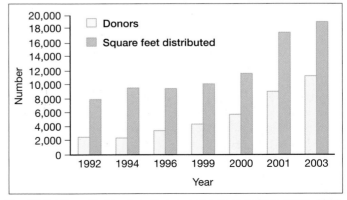

Fig. 15.5 Allograft skin donation and distribution from 1990–2003. (Data collected from AATB sources (various) with permission).

2003 Survey of accredited tissue banks. In that calendar year, skin was recovered from over 11000 donors with nearly 19000 square feet of skin distributed for human transplantation.

Role of the American Association of Tissue Banks

As skin banking facilities grew in number, it became apparent that policies and procedures required standardization. This was quite difficult initially as there was insufficient data to develop a consensus regarding standards of practice. As early as 1976, the AATB had begun to address this issue by the formation of a Skin Council. This provided a forum for the discussion of skin banking practices and was complimented by the activities of the American Burn Association's Skin Banking Special Interest Group. The Standards and Procedures Committees were created in 1977 and produced the first 'Guidelines' for tissue banking in 1979. The first Standards for Tissue Banking was published in 1984 and tissue-specific technical manuals (including skin) were developed in 1987. Since that time, the Standards have been modified and refined based upon consensus and, where available, supportive scientific research. In addition, shortly after the development and promulgation of its Standards for Tissue Banking, the AATB created an inspection and accreditation committee in 1982 and began conducting voluntary inspections in 1986. This program continues today and is important in ensuring that tissue banks adhere not only to AATB Standards but also the Food and Drug Administration (FDA) regulations governing all aspects of human tissue banking.

Technical aspects of skin banking

Donor screening

It is vitally important that complete and accurate medical information about the potential donor be obtained to ensure the safety of the tissue for transplantation. The AATB and the FDA require a comprehensive medical and social history of the donor. In this regard, the AATB developed a Donor Medical History and Behavioral Risk Assessment Questionnaire with the cooperation and assistance of other organ and tissue procurement organizations and the FDA. A thorough physical examination is also necessary to determine if the donor should be deferred for other medical reasons as well as to determine the quality of the skin and the technical feasibility of skin retrieval by evaluating the donor's size and skin condition. Box 15.4 lists disease states which are commonly associated with deferral of a potential skin donor.

While it is also necessary for the tissue bank medical director to review the results of an autopsy (if one was performed), a review of over 2200 consecutive donors recovered by our tissue bank from January 1994 through May 1998 indicated that only 11 donors (0.5%) required discard as a result of the autopsy findings.[47] Furthermore, a 10-month follow-up study of 264 donors recovered following the 1998 changes in the AATB Standards revealed that none of the donors required deferral based upon the autopsy findings alone.[47]

> **BOX 15.4 Disease states commonly associated with potential skin donor deferral**
>
> - Extensive dermatitis
> - Acute burn injuries
> - Cutaneous malignancy
> - Poor skin quality
> - Extensive tattoos
> - Collagen vascular disease
> - Toxic chemical exposure
> - Skin infections
> - Extensive skin lesions
> - Extensive skin or soft tissue trauma

A panel of serologic screening tests for transmissible viral diseases (HIV-1/2 antibody, hepatitis B surface antigen and B core antibody, and hepatitis C and HTLV-1 antibodies) is also required. Recently, skin/tissue banks have been obtaining HIV-1/2 and HCV nucleic acid tests (NAT) to add to the safety of the tissue grafts being transplanted. Ideally, the test kits should be approved for cadaveric specimens. Barnett et al. reported their 2-year experience with cadaveric skin donor discards due to positive serologic tests. In that report, they noted that 61 of 813 donors (7.5%) required tissue discard due to positive serologic tests. A positive hepatitis B core antibody test accounted for 52.3% of the serology-based discards while hepatitis B surface antigen testing accounted for 18.1%, and hepatitis C, HIV-1/2, HTLV-1, and syphilis tests accounted for 14.3%, 4.9%, 4.9%, and 5.5%, respectively.[48] This finding was substantiated by our tissue bank's 5-year review of 1235 donors, of whom 93 (7.5%) were deferred based upon positive serologic tests.[47]

Skin recovery

Once donor screening is complete and proper consents have been obtained, the recovery team must arrange the time and location for skin removal in an appropriate facility (i.e. hospital morgue or operating room, medical examiner's office, or the tissue bank). It is extremely important that the time of death and body storage conditions be accurately documented as these have a significant bearing upon skin viability and microbial contamination. Current AATB Standards require that skin retrieval begin within 24 hours of death if the donor was refrigerated within 12 hours of asystole or within 15 hours if refrigeration did not occur within the prescribed time limits.

In brief, the skin is removed under aseptic conditions. The areas from which the skin is taken are shaved of hair and cleansed with detergent solutions approved for use in operative procedures (i.e. povidone-iodine, chlorhexidine). The retrieval technician puts on a cap and mask, performs a surgical scrub, and dons a sterile gown and gloves while the circulating technician prepares tissue and transport containers. This is usually followed by a chlorhexidine prep and rinsing with 70% isopropyl alcohol, and allowing the skin surface to dry. The donor is then draped with sterile sheets and a blood sample is obtained by either a central venous or intraventricular puncture. Following this, a thin layer of sterile mineral oil (or other sterile lubricant) is applied to the surfaces from which skin is to be removed. Split-thickness skin grafts are then removed using a dermatome at a thickness of 0.012–0.018 inches. The width of the grafts generally should range from 3 to 4 inches but ideally should be determined by the preference of the transplanting surgeon(s). Skin retrieval sites are usually limited to the torso, hips, thighs, and upper calves. The amount of skin obtained may vary depending on body habitus, skin defects or lesions, and body geometry; however, an average of 4–6 square feet per donor is not unusual. After tissue is obtained from the posterior surfaces, the donor is turned to expose the anterior surface, reprepped, and draped prior to completing the retrieval process. The skin is then placed in tissue medium and maintained at 1–10°C during transport to the skin bank for processing.[49]

Skin processing
Processing environment
Skin should be processed under aseptic conditions. While current AATB Standards mandate the processing of cardiovascular tissues in a class 100 laminar flow environment, no such requirement exists for human skin banking. In fact, a study performed at our skin bank failed to demonstrate any statistically significant quantitative or qualitative difference in microbial growth whether the skin was processed and packaged in a class 100 laminar flow hood or a class 100000 clean room.[50]

Microbiologic testing
After returning to the skin bank, the procurement team should obtain cultures for aerobic and anaerobic bacteria, yeast, and fungi. Incubation of allograft skin in antibiotics remains somewhat controversial since many of these antimicrobial agents are unable to effectively kill microorganisms at 4°C and there is the potential for exposing the recipient to resistant organisms. In addition, there has been little research to determine which antibiotics are effective against most skin contaminants yet nontoxic to the cellular components of the skin. It is therefore recommended that samples should be obtained prior to exposure of the skin to antibiotics[35] using a 1 cm^2 biopsy sample for each 10% of the body surface area from which the skin has been recovered.[49,51] Testing should be conducted in accordance with the National Committee on Clinical Laboratory Standards and the skin should not be used for transplantation if it contains any of the following microorganisms:

* coagulase-positive staphylococci,
* group A, beta-hemolytic streptococci,
* enterococci,
* Gram-negative organisms,
* Clostridium sp., or
* yeast or fungi.

When fresh, non-cryopreserved allograft skin is to be released for transplantation within days of tissue recovery, the results of the microbial cultures are frequently unavailable; however, AATB Standards require that microbiology culture results not be reported before 7 days of incubation before releasing the tissues for transplantation. Since our tissue bank frequently provides allograft skin to our regional burn centers under the exceptional release provision, we reviewed the results of the

microbiologic skin cultures from 219 consecutive skin donors whose tissues were released for transplantation prior to the availability of culture results. While 14.3% of the cultures were positive for microbial growth, only 1.8% of the cultures identified organisms that required subsequent notification of the transplanting surgeon. In each of these instances, there were no adverse outcomes in any of the burn patients who received the skin transplants.[52] This issue was also addressed by Lynch et al. in their review of 939 allograft skin donors whose skin was authorized for exceptional release after only 3 days of incubation. They reported that three cases resulted in tissue recall due to positive microbiological cultures. The authors concluded that 3-day culture results do not result in significant microbiologic contamination of allograft skin.[53] Despite the results of these studies, it is strongly recommended that the tissue bank communicate all available information regarding donor and tissue suitability to the transplanting surgeon so that he/she can adequately assess the potential risks and benefits for the recipient.

Maintenance of viability
Maintenance of cell viability and structural integrity are vital for the engraftment and neovascularization of allograft skin, yet there have been no studies that have quantified the degree of viability necessary to ensure allograft 'take.' Postmortem time lapse appears to have the single greatest effect on skin viability as May demonstrated that the functional metabolic activity of the skin rapidly declined if the donor was not refrigerated within 18 hours of death.[54,55] The ideal nutrient tissue culture medium has also not yet been identified. Eagle's MEM and RPMI-1640 continue to be generally accepted; however, Cuono has demonstrated the potential benefits of University of Wisconsin (UW) solution.[56] Lastly, it remains unclear which cryoprotectants offer the greatest preservation of cell viability and structural integrity. Glycerol (10–20%) and dimethylsulfoxide (10–15%) have been reported to maintain skin viability following incubation times ranging from 30 minutes to 2 hours; however, the optimal concentrations of these cryoprotectants have not been identified nor have these agents been compared for efficacy. Factors such as age and gender do not appear to influence skin viability.

Refrigeration
'Fresh' allograft skin is the preferred biologic dressing for the temporary coverage of excised extensive full-thickness burn wounds due to its more rapid adherence and rapid vascularization. The skin is typically stored at 4°C in tissue culture medium with or without antibiotics. Refrigeration slows the metabolic rate of the viable cells and nutrient tissue culture medium supports cellular metabolic activity. The skin should be free-floating in an aseptic container with approximately 300 mL of medium per square foot of skin. Recent studies suggest that skin viability can be maintained for up to 2 weeks at 4°C if the nutrient medium is changed every 3 days.[57,58] The major shortcoming of this storage method is the limited time that viability can be maintained.

It has been common practice to cryopreserve the skin within 5–7 days of refrigeration. This has been based on the work of May et al., who demonstrated that glucose metabolism declines at a rate of 10–15% each day during refrigerated storage.[55]

Recently, we have demonstrated the benefit of a two-layer storage method utilizing 95% oxygen-enriched perfluorocarbon (O₂PFC) combined with changing the nutrient media every 3 days in an effort to prolong the viability of refrigerated skin. This method results in maintenance of skin viability for up to 41–63 days as well as maintenance of normal skin anatomy.[59] Further research in allograft skin cryopreservation techniques will be essential in order to maintain an ample supply of viable fresh tissue for clinical use.

Cryopreservation

When skin is frozen for long-term storage, it is important that the methods utilized maintain cell viability and structural integrity. If the skin is not to be used 'fresh,' it should be cryopreserved within 10 days of procurement if the nutrient media is changed every 3 days. If the media is not changed in this manner, AATB Standards dictate that the skin must be frozen within 96 hours of recovery. The skin is generally incubated in cryoprotectant solution for 30 minutes at 4°C. Skin that is to be frozen should be folded with fine mesh gauze or bridal veil covering the dermal surface prior to placement in a flat packet to ensure uniformity of the cooling process.[60] This is followed by slow-rate cooling at a rate of approximately –1°C per minute. Although computer-assisted, control-rate freezing is thought to be optimal, studies have demonstrated that cooling in a heat sink box at less than –2°C per minute is equally effective and does not compromise the metabolic activity of the skin.[61] The skin is frozen to a temperature of –70° to –100°C prior to placement in either a mechanical freezer or liquid nitrogen. Skin stored in a mechanical freezer (–70 to –100°C) can be maintained for 3–6 months, whereas storage in liquid nitrogen (–150 to –196°C) has been shown to maintain viability for up to 10 years. Although this methodology has been reported to result in 85% retention of viability, there remains a need for research to determine the optimal technology for skin preservation.[62]

Lyophilization

Skin can also be lyophilized by freeze drying or incubation in glycerol.[63] This process has been reported to decrease biologic degradation and antigenicity; however, this also results in epidermal cell destruction and the loss of barrier function. Moreover, lyophilized allograft skin has poor adherence to the excised wound bed and is far less effective than 'fresh' skin or cryopreserved skin in controlling microbial growth. Its clinical use has been further limited by its high cost of production compared to conventional allograft.

Transport

Refrigerated skin should be transported in tissue culture medium at wet ice temperatures (1–10°C) in an insulated container. Frozen allograft skin is transported on dry ice in an insulated container to prevent the skin temperature from rising to greater than –50°C. If the frozen skin is thawed at the tissue bank, it should be transported at wet ice temperatures.

Rewarming

Rewarming of frozen cryopreserved allograft skin must be performed in such a manner as to minimize cryodamage and preserve the structural integrity and viability of the skin. Early studies demonstrated that warming rates of 50–70°C/min resulted in 80–95% graft survival. Subsequent research[60] has revealed that warming should be performed in 2–4 minutes or less at a temperature of 10–37°C (127–470°C/min). Rewarming in a microwave is not recommended due to uneven heating and excessive intracellular temperatures.

The future of skin banking

Skin banking must continue to evolve as engineered skin substitutes enter the clinical arena for the temporary and permanent coverage of partial- and full-thickness wounds. A number of skin substitutes have recently received FDA approval for use in the United States and have become part of the surgeon's armamentarium. Although they are generally more costly than allograft skin, some of these products have been demonstrated to possess a number of attributes, including:

- nonantigenicity,
- ready availability,
- sterility, and
- the ability to provide a dermal equivalent as a template for the later application of ultrathin (0.006 inch) skin autografts.

Allograft skin has the potential to play a major role in permanent skin reconstruction after extensive thermal injury; however, this will require interactive research with the burn centers caring for these patients. This point is well illustrated by the studies of Rose[64] and Naoum[65] who demonstrated more rapid healing times and shorter hospital stays for children with extensive indeterminate depth scald burns when treated with early wound debridement and allografting compared to conventional topical antimicrobial therapy. Homografts acted as the best protection for damaged dermis, thus providing an environment for spontaneous epithelialization.

Skin banks must also identify ways of increasing cadaveric skin donation, ensuring recipient safety from potential disease transmission, and reducing procurement and processing costs while optimizing allograft viability. This will become increasingly difficult as it becomes necessary to perform additional and newer microbiological testing procedures to ensure recipient safety. To accomplish these goals, it may become necessary for skin banking operations to become regionalized. Such an undertaking could enhance tissue supplies and availability and result in increased clinical use by surgeons.

Allograft-based skin products

There is tremendous potential for human allograft-based skin products to be developed in the upcoming years; however, it will become increasingly important for skin banks to perform basic science and clinical research (in conjunction with burn and wound healing centers) to demonstrate the clinical indications and efficacy of allograft skin products in various clinical applications. Technological advances may include modifications to reduce immunogenicity and/or the potential for disease transmission. Newer processing techniques could sterilize the skin without injuring the viable cellular elements or the structural integrity of the tissue. In addition, with continued research, deepidermized allograft dermis could become:

- a source of growth factors and antimicrobial agents,
- a permanent full-thickness wound cover seeded with the patient's autologous keratinocytes and fibroblasts,
- a bilayer membrane system for epidermal autografting, and/or
- a readily-available permanent wound cover preseeded with non-antigenic allogeneic keratinocytes, fibroblasts, and melanocytes.

Allogeneic skin provides a source of skin cells, including keratinocytes, fibroblasts, melanocytes, and endothelial cells. These cells may be grown into large populations (greater than 1×10^{12} cells), cryopreserved in liquid nitrogen, recovered into culture, and combined with degradable biopolymers to form cultured skin substitutes.[66] Preclinical studies have shown organization of the epidermal keratinocytes to form a skin barrier,[67,68] expression of pigment by melanocytes,[69] and organization of endothelial cells into vascular analogs.[70] Clinical studies have demonstrated improved healing of chronic wounds with allogeneic skin substitutes,[71] and permanent closure of excised burns with cultured autologous grafts;[72] however, cryopreservation of multilayered grafts with keratinized epithelium remains an unachieved goal in tissue transplantation. It therefore appears likely that the principles and practices of skin banking may contribute to eventual availability of unlimited supplies of skin grown in laboratories for the treatment of a wide variety of skin-loss conditions. Collaborative research efforts will be necessary to achieve these goals in a timely and cost-effective manner as skin banks find themselves competing and/or collaborating with the tissue bioengineering industry.

References

1. Reverdin JL. Sur la greffe epidermique. CR Acad Sci 1871; 73:1280.
2. Reverdin JL. De la greffe epidermique. Arch Gen Med (Suppl) 1872; 19:276.
3. Thiersch JC. On skin grafting. Verhandl 2nd Deutsch Ges Chir 1886; 15:17–20.
4. Girdner JH. Skin grafting with grafts taken from the dead subject. Medical Record 1881; 20:119–120.
5. Wentscher J. A further contribution about the survivability of human epidermal cells. Dtsch Z Chir 1903; 70:21–44.
6. Bettman AG. Homogeneous Thiersch grafting as a life saving measure. Am J Surg 1938; 39:156–162.
7. Webster JP. Refrigerated skin grafts. Ann Surg 1944; 120:431–439.
8. Matthews DN. Storage of skin for autogenous grafts. Lancet 1945; 2:775–778.
9. Baxter H, Entin MA. Experimental and clinical studies of reduced temperatures in injury and repair in man III. Direct effect of cooling and freezing on various elements of the human skin. Plast Reconstr Surg 1948; 3:303–334.
10. Billingham RE, Medawar PB. The freezing, drying, and storage of mammalian skin. J Exp Biol 1952; 19:454–468.
11. Taylor AC. Survival of rat skin and changes in hair pigmentation following freezing. J Exp Zool 1949; 110:77–112.
12. Brown JB, Fryer MP, Tandall P, et al. Post mortem homografts as 'biological dressings' for extensive burns and denuded areas. Ann Surg 1953; 138:618–623.
13. Jackson D. A clinical study of the use of skin homografts for burns. Br J Plast Surg 1954; 7:26–43.
14. Zaroff L, Mills W, Duckett JW, et al. Multiple uses of viable cutaneous homografts in the burned patient. Surgery 1966; 59:368–372.
15. Cochrane T. The low temperature storage of skin: a preliminary report. Br J Plast Surg 1966; 21:118–125.
16. Morris PJ, Bondoc C, Burke JF. The use of frequently changed skin allografts to promote healing in the nonhealing infected ulcer. Surgery 1966; 60:13–19.
17. Shuck JM, Pruitt BA, Moncrief JA. Homograft skin for wound coverage: a study in versatility. Arch Surg 1969; 98:472–479.
18. Eade GG. The relationship between granulation tissue, bacteria, and skin grafts in burned patients. Plast Reconstr Surg 1958; 22:42–55.
19. Woods WB. Phagocytosis with particular reference to encapsulated bacteria. Bact Rev 1960; 224:41.
20. O'Donoghue MN, Zarem HA. Stimulation of neovascularization. Comparative efficacy of fresh and preserved skin grafts. Plast Reconstr Surg 1958; 48:474–477.
21. Bondoc CC, Burke JF. Clinical experience with viable frozen human skin and a frozen skin bank. Ann Surg 1971; 174:371–382.
22. Burke JF, Quinby WC, Bondoc CC, et al. Immunosuppression and temporary skin transplantation in the treatment of massive third degree burns. N Engl J Med 1975; 182:183–197.
23. Heimbach D, Luterman A, Burke J, et al. Artificial dermis for major burns. Ann Surg 1988; 208:313–320.
24. Stamper B, Plessinger RT, Rieman M, et al. A comparison of 'fresh' allograft and Integra in the management of extensive full-thickness burns. J Burn Care Rehabil 1999; 20:S196.
25. Alexander JW, MacMillan BG, Law E, et al. Treatment of severe burns with widely meshed skin autograft and widely meshed skin allograft overlay. J Trauma 1981; 21:433–438.
26. Herrmann L, Rogowitz L, Ullrich H. Basic principles of skin transplantation in burns and use of lyophilized skin transplants. Zentralbl Chir 1965; 90(26):1129–1134.
27. O'Connor NE, Mulliken JB, Banks-Schlegel S, et al. Grafting of burns with cultured epithelium prepared from autologous epidermal cells. Lancet 1981; 1:75–78.
28. Cuono C, Langdon R, McGuire J. Use of cultured autografts and dermal allografts as skin replacement after burn injury. Lancet 1986; 1:1123–1124.
29. Hickerson WL, Compton C, Fletchall S, et al. Cultured epidermal autografts and allodermis combination for permanent burn wound coverage. Burns 1994; 20:S52–S56.
30. Livesey SA, Herndon DN, Hollyoak MA, et al. Transplanted acellular allograft dermal matrix. Transplantation 1995; 60:1–9.
31. Wainwright D, Madden M, Luterman A, et al. Clinical evaluation of an acellular allograft dermal matrix in full-thickness burns. J Burn Care Rehabil 1996; 17:124–136.
32. Zhang ML, Chang ZD, Wang CY, et al. Microskin grafting in the treatment of extensive burns: a preliminary report. J Trauma 1988; 28:804–807.
33. Monafo WW, Tandon SN, Bradley RE, et al. Bacterial contamination of skin used as a biologic dressing: a potential hazard. JAMA 1976; 235:1248–1249.
34. White MJ, Whalen JD, Gould JA, et al. Procurement and transplantation of colonized cadaver skin. Am Surg 1991; 57:402–407.
35. Heck E. Operational standards and regulation for tissue banks. J Burn Care Rehabil 1997; 18:S11–S12.
36. Hornicek F. AATB standards for tissue banks, 10th edn.: AATB; April 2002:K2.220,112–113.
37. Clarke JA. HIV transmission and skin grafts. Lancet 1987; 1:983.
38. Kealey GP, Aguiar J, Lewis RW, et al. Cadaver skin allografts and transmission of human cytomegalovirus to burn patients. J Am Coll Surg 1996; 182:201–205.
39. Plessinger RT, Robb EC, Kagan RJ. Cytomegalovirus in skin donors. Proc Am Assoc Tissue Banks 1996; S6.
40. Herndon DN, Rose JK. Cadaver skin allograft and the transmission of human cytomegalovirus in burn patients: benefits clearly outweigh risks. J Am Coll Surg 1996; 182:263–264.

41. Keown PA. Cytomegalovirus infection in transplantation: a risk and management perspective. Transplantation 1996; 12: 22–23.

42. Ninnemann JL, Fisher JC, Frank HA. Prolonged survival of human skin allografts following thermal injury. Transplantation 1978; 25:69–72.

43. Burke JF, May JB, Albright N, et al. Temporary skin transplantation and immunosuppression for extensive burns. N Engl J Med 1974; 290:269–271.

44. Achauer BM, Hewitt CW, Black KS, et al. Long-term allograft survival after short-term cyclosporin treatment in a patient with massive burns. Lancet 1986; 1:14–15.

45. Sakabu SA, Hansbrough JF, Cooper ML, et al. Cyclosporin A for prolonging allograft survival in patients with massive burns. J Burn Care Rehabil 1990; 11:410–418.

46. DeClement FA, May SR. Procurement, cryopreservation and clinical application of skin. In: Glassman A, Umlas J, eds. The preservation of tissues and solid organs for transplantation. Arlington, VA: American Association of Blood Banks; 1983:29–56.

47. Plessinger RT, Robb EC, Kagan RJ. The impact of autopsy report findings on the acceptability of the potential tissue donor. Proc Am Assoc Tissue Banks 1999; 48.

48. Barnett JR, McCauley RL, Schutzler S, et al. Cadaver donor discards secondary to serology. J Burn Care Rehabil 2001; 22: 124–127.

49. Holder IA, Robb E, Kagan RJ. Antimicrobial mixtures used to store harvested skin: antimicrobial activities tested at refrigerator (4°C) temperatures. J Burn Care Rehabil 1999; 20:501–504.

50. Plessinger RT, Robb EC, Kagan RJ. Allograft skin cultures II: should allograft skin be processed in a class 10 000 or better environment? Proc Am Assoc Tissue Banks 1997; S23.

51. May SR, DeClement FA. Skin banking. Part II. Low contamination cadaveric allograft skin for temporary burn wound coverage. J Burn Care Rehabil 1981; 2:64–76.

52. Plessinger RT, Robb EC, Kagan RJ. Safe use of refrigerated allograft skin in burn patients. Proc Am Assoc Tissue Banks 2005; 29: A35.

53. Lynch JP, Williamson SA, McCauley RL. Early use of allograft skin: are three day cultures safe? J Burn Care Rehabil 2005; 26: S169.

54. May SR, DeClement FA. Skin banking. Part III. Cadaveric allograft skin viability. J Burn Care Rehabil 1981; 19:362–371.

55. May SR, DeClement FA. Development of a metabolic activity testing method for human and porcine skin. Cryobiology 1982; 19:362–371.

56. Brown W, Cuono CB. Approaches to minimizing leakage of beneficial glycosaminoglycans in processing skin for cryopreservation. Proc Am Burn Assoc 1992; 24:40.

57. Robb EC, Bechmann N, Plessinger RT, et al. A comparison of changed vs. unchanged media for viability testing of banked allograft skin. Proc Am Assoc Tissue Banks 1997; S3.

58. Robb EC, Bechmann N, Plessinger RT, et al. Storage media and temperature maintain normal anatomy of cadaveric human skin for transplantation to full-thickness skin wounds. J Burn Care Rehabil 2001; 22:393–396.

59. Koizumi T, Robb EC, Bechmann N, et al. Prolonging human skin viability using 95% oxygen-enriched perfluorocarbon (PFC). Proc Am Burn Assoc 2004; 25:S80.

60. May SR, DeClement FA. Skin banking methodology: an evaluation of package format, cooling and warming rates. Cryobiology 1980; 17:34–45.

61. Cuono CB, Langdon R, Birchall N, et al. Viability and functional performance of allograft skin preserved by slow, controlled, non-programmed freezing. Proc Am Burn Assoc 1988; 20:55.

62. Agarwal SJ, Baxter CR, Diller KR. Cryopreservation of skin: an assessment of current clinical applicability. J Burn Care Rehabil 1985; 6:69–76.

63. Mackie DP. The Euro skin bank: development and application of glycerol-preserved allografts. J Burn Care Rehabil 1997; 18: S7–S9.

64. Rose JK, Desai MH, Mlakar JM, et al. Allograft is superior to topical antimicrobial therapy in the treatment of partial-thickness scald burns in children. J Burn Care Rehabil 1997; 4:338–341.

65. Naoum JJ, Roehl KR, Wolf SE, et al. The use of homograft compared to topical antimicrobial therapy in the treatment of second-degree burns of more than 40% total body surface area. Burns 2004; 30:548–551.

66. Boyce ST, Warden GD. Principles and practices for treatment of cutaneous wounds with cultured skin substitutes. Am J Surg 2002; 183:445–456.

67. Boyce ST, Supp AP, Harriger MD, et al. Surface electrical capacitance as a noninvasive index of epidermal barrier in cultured skin substitutes in athymic mice. J Invest Dermatol 1996; 107(1):82–87.

68. Boyce ST, Supp AP, Swope VB, et al. Vitamin C regulates keratinocyte viability, epidermal barrier, and basement membrane formation in vitro, and reduces wound contraction after grafting of cultured skin substitutes. J Invest Dermatol 2002; 118:565–572.

69. Swope VB, Supp AP, Boyce ST. Regulation of cutaneous pigmentation by titration of human melanocytes in cultured skin substitutes grafted to athymic mice. Wound Rep Reg 2002; 10: 378–386.

70. Supp DM, Wilson-Landy K, Boyce ST. Human dermal microvascular endothelial cells form vascular analogs in cultured skin substitutes after grafting to athymic mice. FASEB J 2002; 16:797–804.

71. Boyce ST, Glatter R, Kitzmiller WJ. Treatment of chronic wounds with cultured cells and biopolymers: a pilot study. Wounds 1995; 7(1):24–29.

72. Boyce ST, Kagan RJ, Yakuboff KP, et al. Cultured skin substitutes reduce donor skin harvesting for closure of excised, full-thickness burns. Ann Surg 2002; 235:269–279.

Chapter 16

Alternative wound coverings

Robert L. Sheridan and Ronald G. Tompkins

Chapter contents

Introduction

The skin envelope consists of two basic layers. The epidermis, consisting of keratinocytes attached to an underlying basement membrane, provides most barrier functions. The dermal layer provides the durable and pliable characteristics of skin, which are so vital to proper function and cosmesis. When available, the replacement material of choice is the patient's own (autologous) skin as shown in an algorithm describing the decision process to treat acute burns. In smaller injuries, this can be accomplished by split-thickness sheet autograft (Figure 16.1). However in larger injuries, meshed autologous skin grafts or skin substitutes are required.

Physiologic considerations

Skin is a truly amazing organ, rarely properly appreciated until it is missing. To date, all attempts to replace it, either temporarily or permanently, have been highly imperfect. As those with serious burns survive in greater numbers, the absence of effective skin replacements is increasingly a hindrance to progress in burn care.

Structure and function of the skin

Skin, the body's largest organ, is incredibly complex. Functionally there are two layers with a highly specialized and effective bonding mechanism. Numerous appendages traverse the skin and a rich and reactive capillary network provides nutrient flow while controlling temperature. The epidermis, consisting of the strata basale, spinosum, granulosum, and corneum, provides a vapor and bacterial barrier. The dermis provides strength and elasticity. The thin epidermal layer is constantly refreshing itself from its basal layer, with new keratinocytes undergoing terminal differentiation over approximately 4 weeks to anuclear keratin-filled cells that make up

the stratum corneum, which provides much of the barrier function of the epidermis. The basal layer of the epidermis is firmly attached to the dermis by a complex bonding mechanism containing collagen types IV and VII. When this bond fails, serious morbidity results, as demonstrated by the disease processes of toxic epidermal necrolysis[1] and epidermolysis bullosa[2] (Figure 16.2).

Consequences of loss of barrier function

Loss of the epidermal barrier has serious adverse physiologic effects. Direct and evaporative fluid losses are immediately seen. If wounds are large, this quickly leads to dehydration and shock. Protein losses are also substantial, leading to loss of colloid oncotic pressure and secondary edema. Microorganisms have unimpeded access to the microcirculation with resulting systemic infection. Deep tissues become desiccated with secondary cell death and progression of wound depth. Dry wounds will not epithelialize as readily. It is clearly important for the burn surgeon to have prompt biologic closure of wounds as an important early objective.

Although it is an imperfect replacement, autologous split-thickness skin is closest to being the ideal skin substitute (Box 16.1). Because of the paucity of autologous donor skin available in patients with massive burn injuries, both the short-term and long-term problems of skin loss must be solved by alternative wound closure materials. Alternative materials can be used for either wound coverage which will be temporary or for permanent wound closure. Allogenic (cadaver) skin has been the most widely used alternative wound closure material. However, there are other choices. This is an exciting and fast-moving area which may profoundly change the care of patients with serious burns. The objective of this chapter is to review the currently available alternative skin closure materials, both temporary and permanent.

Temporary skin substitutes

Temporary skin substitutes provide transient physiologic wound closure, thereby helping to control pain, absorb wound exudate, and prevent wound desiccation. They are clinically useful in several settings in burn care:

- as a dressing on donor sites to facilitate pain control and epithelialization from skin appendages;
- as a dressing on clean superficial wounds for the same reasons;
- to provide temporary physiologic closure of deep dermal and full-thickness wounds after excision while

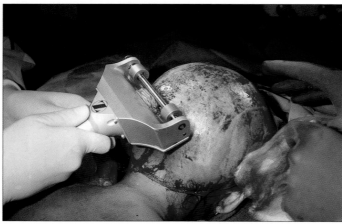

Fig. 16.1 The replacement material of choice remains the patient's own (autologous) skin.

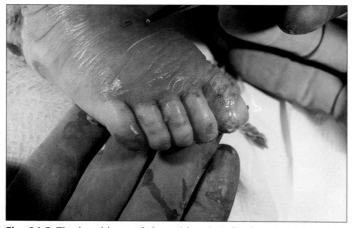

Fig. 16.2 The basal layer of the epidermis is firmly attached to the dermis by a complex bonding mechanism containing collagen types IV and VII. When this bond fails, serious morbidity results, as demonstrated here by the disease processes of dystrophic epidermolysis bullosa.

BOX 16.1 The perfect skin substitute — autologous split-thickness skin

- Prevents water loss
- Barrier to bacteria
- Inexpensive
- Long shelf life
- Can be applied in one operation
- Does not become hypertrophic
- Flexible
- Conforms to irregular wound surfaces
- Can be used 'off the shelf'
- Does not require refrigeration
- Cannot transmit viral diseases
- Does not incite inflammatory response
- Durable
- Easy to secure
- Grows with a child

---

awaiting autografting or healing of underlying widely meshed autografts; and
- as a 'test' graft in questionable wound beds.

Their principal utility is provision of temporary physiologic closure of wounds, which implies protection from mechanical trauma, vapor transmission characteristics similar to skin, and a physical barrier to bacteria. These membranes create a moist wound environment with a low bacterial density.

Human allograft

Human allograft is generally used as a split-thickness graft after being procured from organ donors. When used in a viable fresh or cryopreserved state, it vascularizes and remains the 'gold standard' of temporary wound closures.[3-5] It can be refrigerated for up to 7 days, but can be stored for extended periods when cryopreserved. It is also used in a nonviable state after preservation in glycerol or after lyophilization; however, most existing data describe results when it is used in a viable state. Viable split-thickness allograft provides durable biologic cover until it is rejected by the host, usually within 3 or 4 weeks. Prolongation of allograft survival, through the use of antirejection drugs, has been advocated,[6] but is not generally practiced for fear that antirejection drugs will increase the risk of infection.[7]

Human skin allografts are generally placed into frozen storage awaiting the return of numerous laboratory tests allowing one to safely exclude the possibility of viral disease transmission. When modern screening techniques are followed, the risk of viral disease transmission is exceedingly small. Allograft is also effectively used in combination with meshed autograft in patients with large burns, the interstices of the meshed graft being immediately closed by the overlying unexpanded allograft, possibly reducing metabolic stress and local wound inflammation (Figure 16.3).

Human amnion

Human amniotic membrane is used in many parts of the world as a temporary dressing for clean superficial wounds such as

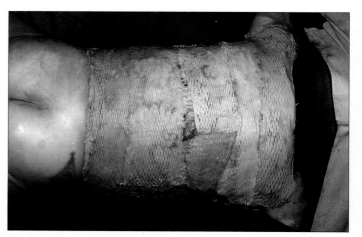

Fig. 16.3 Allograft is also effectively used in combination with meshed autograft in patients with large burns, the interstices of the meshed graft being immediately closed by the overlying unexpanded allograft, possibly reducing metabolic stress and local wound inflammation.

partial-thickness burns, donor sites, and freshly excised burns awaiting donor site availability.[8,9] Amniotic membrane is generally procured fresh and used after brief refrigerated storage.[10,11] It can also be used in a nonviable state after preservation with glycerol. It has been treated with silver to facilitate control of bacterial overgrowth.[12] Amnion does not vascularize but still can provide effective temporary wound closure.[13] The principal concern with amnion is the difficulty in screening the material for viral diseases unless preservation methods can eliminate potential viral contamination. Without the ability to screen the material in this way, the risks of disease transmission must be balanced against the clinical need and the known characteristics of the donor.

Allogenic epithelial sheets

In many centers, particularly in Europe, sheets of allogenic and autogenous epithelium are used to dress partial-thickness wounds or to cover the interstices of meshed split-thickness autografts.[14,15] These are generally applied as thin sheets placed on a gauze carrier for ease of handling. Cell suspensions in fibrin sealant have also been trailed. The concept is that the sheets will both prevent desiccation of underlying wounds and that the release of unknown growth-stimulating substances by the cells as they die will stimulate native wound healing.[16] The concept is attractive, but controlled data are not available, particularly as regards any impact on long-term outcomes.

Xenografts

Although various animal skins have been used for many years to provide temporary coverage of wounds,[17] only porcine xenograft is widely used today (Figure 16.4).[18] Porcine xeno-

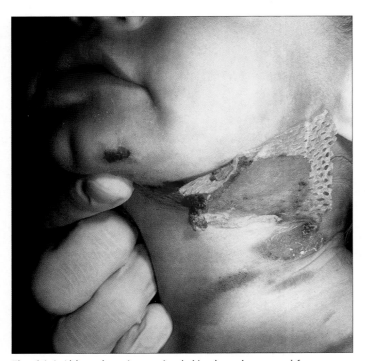

Fig. 16.4 Although various animal skins have been used for many years to provide temporary coverage of wounds, only porcine xenograft is widely used today.

graft is commonly distributed as a reconstituted product consisting of homogenized porcine dermis which is fashioned into sheets and meshed.[19] Split-thickness porcine skin is also used fresh, after brief refrigeration, after cryopreservation, or after glycerol preservation. It effectively provides temporary coverage of clean wounds such as superficial second-degree burns and donor sites[20] and has been used in patients with toxic epidermal necrolysis.[1,21] Porcine xenograft has been combined with silver to suppress wound colonization.[22,23] Porcine xenograft does not vascularize, but it will adhere to a clean superficial wound and can provide excellent pain control while the underlying wound heals.

Synthetic membranes

A number of semipermeable membrane dressings can provide a vapor and bacterial barrier and control pain while the underlying superficial wound or donor sites heal. These typically consist of a single semipermeable layer that provides a mechanical barrier to bacteria and has physiologic vapor transmission characteristics.[24,25] Biobrane™ (Dow-Hickham, Sugarland, TX) is a two-layer membrane constructed of an inner layer of nylon mesh that allows fibrovascular ingrowth and an outer layer of silastic that serves as a vapor and bacterial barrier.[26] It is widely used to provide temporary closure of superficial burns and donor sites. All synthetic membranes are occlusive and can foster infection if placed over contaminated wounds, especially in the presence of necrotic tissue.[27] Appropriate monitoring is essential to their proper use.

Hydrocolloid dressings are generally designed with a three-layer structure: a porous, gently adherent inner layer; a methyl cellulose absorbent middle layer; and a semipermeable outer layer. They foster a moist wound environment while absorbing exudate. A moist wound environment has been found to favor wound healing.[28] A variety of pastes and powders made from hydrocolloid materials are also widely available. These can be applied to superficial or deeper chronic wounds to absorb wound exudate while maintaining a moist wound environment.

Hydrofiber matts absorb wound exudate and have been used as temporary wound membranes. When combined with ionic silver (Aquacel-Ag, ConvaTec, Chester, UK), additional antimicrobial activity is seen. This membrane has been used successfully in some burn programs as an adjunct in the management of partial-thickness burns and donor sites.[29]

Combined allogenic and synthetic membranes

Epidermal growth factor, transforming growth factor-β, insulin-like growth factor (IGF), platelet-derived growth factors (PDGF), fibroblast growth factors, and other mediators play an important role in wound healing.[30] To provide some of these substances topically to wounds, investigators have placed both viable and nonviable allogenic cell types into temporary wound dressings.[31] These cells persist for no more than 14 days, but it is hoped that factors secreted by the allogeneic cells, or released upon their death and dissolution, will enhance wound healing. These membranes are generally regulated as both devices and biologics.

An allogeneic dermal–epidermal device that used a collagen lattice to culture both cell types was shown effective in an athymic mouse model[32-34] and then went into clinical trials.

Although it has not been demonstrated to have a clinical role in burn patients, the device is being explored for utility in chronic ulcers of the lower extremity.[35–39] Dow-Hickam's Biobrane™ has been used as a scaffold to support the growth of allogenic fibroblasts. This device is now marketed as Transcyte® (Smith and Nephew, La Jolla, CA) and has been successful in some burn programs as an adjunct to the management of dermal burns.[40–44] Viral transfection can be employed to modify keratinocytes so that they overexpress PDGF, human growth hormone, IGF-1, and other growth factors,[45] and it is possible that such cells might be employed as components of wound membranes over the next few years.[46] Although stimulation of wound healing by topical application of mixed growth factors in this fashion is an intriguing concept, convincing evidence of the concept's general validity is awaited.

Permanent skin substitutes

Realization of a practical permanent skin substitute will revolutionize the care of patients with burns and other difficult wounds. The perfect substitute is described in Box 16.1, but has yet to be approached by any currently available device. However, there are a number of imperfect or partial-skin substitutes available at the present time that are valuable in particular clinical settings and may be the forerunners of this hypothetical ideal.

Epidermal cells

For over 20 years it has been possible to culture vast numbers of epithelial cells from a small skin biopsy,[47,48] and this has led to the widespread clinical use of cultured epithelial grafts to cover burn wounds. Epithelial cells are procured from a full-thickness skin biopsy, the cells being separated with trypsin. The resulting epithelial cell suspension is cultured in medium containing fetal calf serum, insulin, transferrin, hydrocortisone, epidermal growth factor, and cholera toxin, overlying a layer of murine fibroblasts that have been treated with a non-lethal dose of radiation that prevents them from multiplying. Colonies of epithelial cells expand into broad sheets of undifferentiated epithelial cells. These cells are separated from the culture vessel with trypsin and taken to secondary culture using the same techniques until confluent thin sheets of undifferentiated cells are obtained. The resulting sheets are removed from the dishes after treatment with dipsase, which digests the proteins attaching the epithelial cells to the dish. The sheets of epithelial cells are attached to a petrolatum gauze carrier to ease handling.

When epithelial cultures were first used in patients with large burns it was hoped that they would provide the definitive answer to the clinical problem of the massive wound.[49–51] With more frequent use of epithelial grafts, specific liabilities have become apparent including suboptimal engraftment rates and long-term durability.[52,53] However, when faced with a very large wound and minimal donor sites, epithelial cell wound closure is a useful adjunct to split-thickness autograft, their liabilities and expense becoming more acceptable as wound size increases.

Many of the imperfections associated with epithelial cell wound closure may be attributed to the absence of a dermal element. Epithelial grafts are now commercially available. Application is generally most successful in wounds from which vascularized allograft has been removed. Despite scattered cases, application of cultured epithelial grafts onto synthetic dermal analogs has not been shown effective.

Dermal analogs

Virtually all of the characteristics of normal skin that are not related to barrier function are provided by the dermis. These characteristics include flexibility, strength, heat dissipation and conservation, lubrication, and sensation. The first dermal substitute used clinically was 'artificial skin', also called Integra™ (Integra LifeSciences Corporation, Plainsboro, NJ, USA); it has been recently approved by the US Food and Drug Administration for use in life-threatening burns. This material was developed in the early 1980s by a biomaterials research team from the Massachusetts General Hospital and Massachusetts Institute of Technology.[54] The research team, lead by surgeon John Burke from the Massachusetts General Hospital and materials scientist Ionnas Yannas from the Massachusetts Institute of Technology, had the goal of developing a wound covering that would both provide a temporary vapor and bacterial while providing a scaffold for later dermal regeneration. The material was intended to be placed on excised burn wounds and is now approved for clinical use. Its use for other indications is being explored. The inner layer of this material is a 2 mm thick combination of fibers of collagen isolated from bovine tissue and the glycosaminoglycan chondroitin-6-sulfate. This 2 mm thick inner layer has a 70–200 μm pore size that allows fibrovascular ingrowth, after which it is designed to slowly biodegrade.[55,56] To manufacture the device, glycosaminoglycan and collagen fibers are precipitated and then freeze-dried and cross-linked by glutaraldehyde. The outer layer of the membrane is 0.009-inch (0.23 mm) thick polysiloxane polymer with vapor transmission characteristics similar to normal epithelium. This membrane is intended to be placed on freshly excised full-thickness burns and the outer silicone membrane replaced with an ultra-thin epithelial autograft 2–3 weeks later (Figure 16.5).[57] Clinical reports in patients with large burns have been

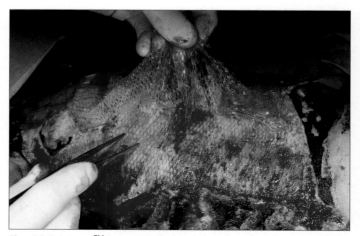

Fig. 16.5 Integra™ is intended to be placed on freshly excised full-thickness burns and the outer silicone membrane replaced with an ultra-thin epithelial autograft 2–3 weeks later.

generally favorable,[58,59] although submembrane infection must be watched for. Integra™ has also been found to be useful in selected burn reconstruction operations.[60]

Another currently available device designed as a dermal replacement is cryopreserved allogenic dermis. This material is intended to be combined with a thin epithelial autograft at the time of initial wound closure. It is marketed as AlloDerm® (LifeCell Corporation, The Woodlands, TX, USA).[61,62] Split-thickness allograft skin is obtained from cadaver donors through tissue banks after proper screening for transmissible diseases. Using hypertonic saline, the epithelial elements of the grafts are removed and the remaining dermis is treated in a detergent to inactivate any viruses and the device is freeze-dried. The process is intended to provide a nonantigenic dermal scaffold, leaving basement membrane proteins (particularly laminin and type IV and VII collagen) intact. The material is rehydrated immediately prior to placement on wounds with overlying ultra-thin epithelial autograft (Figure 16.6). Clinical experience with this material in burn surgery is limited, but early experiences have been favorable.[63,64]

Generating a dermal replacement through the prior use of human split-thickness allograft is another strategy with significant clinical support. This has been done on occasion for many years by surgeons who 'leave behind' remnants of vascularized allograft dermis when replacing allograft with thin split-thickness autografts in patients with large injuries. This has been modified for use with cultured epithelial grafts, such that the cultured epithelial cells are placed on wounds closed initially with vascularized allograft. Once allograft has vascularized, the allogeneic epithelial cells are removed by dermabrasion or tangential excision, purposefully leaving behind a vascularized but theoretically nonantigenic allogenic dermal layer.[65-67] The method has been favorably reported,[68,69] but has not been universally adopted. Perhaps the epithelial excision either leaves behind nests of antigenic epithelial cells if too superficial or removes the epidermal–dermal attachment structures if too deep.

Composite substitutes

Ideally, a skin replacement technique would provide immediate replacement of both dermal and epidermal layers. Combining epithelial cells with a dermal analog in the laboratory seems logical. A completely biologic composite skin substitute, culturing human fibroblasts in a collagen–glycosaminoglycan membrane, and then growing keratinocytes upon this, has been under development for some years.[70,71] This composite membrane has been successful in both a nude mouse model and in initial clinical series.[72,73] There is even potential to control pigment expression.[74] This exciting technology continues to be refined in laboratory and clinical investigations and may have a major impact on the field A similar project, in which autogenic epithelial cells are cultured onto allogenic dermis, shows some promise as well.[75] It remains to be seen if either technique will lead to a reliable and durable permanent skin replacement.

The future of alternative wound coverings

We are likely to see significant improvements in skin substitute technologies, both temporary and permanent, over the next few years. In temporary wound coverings, not only are improved synthetics and improved skin banking techniques probable but we may see temporary dressings containing growth factor-secreting allogenic tissues that stimulate native wound healing. Genetic modification of keratinocytes is now possible. These cells have been engineered to overexpress PDGF, human growth hormone, IGF-1, and other growth factors.[45] It is likely that they will be trialled in animal models and human wounds over the next few years.[46] If they prove efficacious, their application to healing burns and donor sites, through incorporation in temporary dressings, may become possible. It might be further possible to combine autogenous cells with modified allogenic cells such that the resulting chimeric graft benefits from transient overexpression of critical growth factors during the early stages of engraftment.

As we become increasingly successful at salvaging the lives of those with large burns, our need for a durable and reliable permanent skin substitute becomes increasingly acute. This material is needed both to truncate the acute illness through earlier wound closure and to facilitate timely and effective burn reconstruction. Just what form that substitute will take is not clear. Most likely, it would seem to be an *in vitro* combination of autologous keratinocytes and possibly fibroblasts and/or endothelial cells with a dermal analog. Whatever form the successful replacement takes, it is certain to profoundly impact the field of burn care.

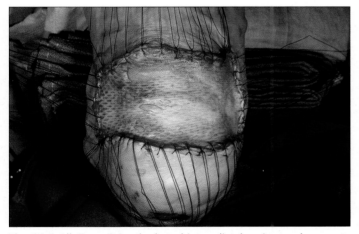

Fig. 16.6 AlloDerm® is rehydrated immediately prior to placement on wounds with overlying ultra-thin epithelial autograft.

References

1. Palmieri TL, Greenhalgh DG, Saffle JR, et al. A multicenter review of toxic epidermal necrolysis treated in U.S. burn centers at the end of the twentieth century. J Burn Care Rehabil 2002; 23(2):87–96.

2. Fine JD, Johnson LB, Cronce D, et al. Intracytoplasmic retention of type VII collagen and dominant dystrophic epidermolysis bullosa: reversal of defect following cessation of or marked improvement in disease activity. J Invest Dermatol 1993; 101:232–236.

3. Bondoc CC, Burke JF. Clinical experience with viable frozen human skin and a frozen skin bank. Ann Surg 1971; 174: 371–382.

4. Herndon DN. Perspectives in the use of allograft. J Burn Care Rehabil 1997; 18:S6.

5. Kagan RJ, Robb EC, Plessinger RT. Human skin banking. Clin Lab Med 2005; 25(3):587–605.

6. Burke JF, May JW Jr, Albright N, et al. Temporary skin transplantation and immunosuppression for extensive burns. N Engl J Med 1974; 290:269–271.

7. Bale JF Jr, Kealey GP, Ebelhack CL, et al. Cytomegalovirus infection in a cyclosporine-treated burn patient: case report. J Trauma 1992; 32:263–267.

8. Ramakrishnan KM, Jayaraman V. Management of partial-thickness burn wounds by amniotic membrane: a cost-effective treatment in developing countries. Burns 1997; 23(Suppl 1):S33–S36.

9. Subrahmanyam M. Amniotic membrane as a cover for microskin grafts. Br J Plast Surg 1995; 48:477–478.

10. Ganatra MA, Durrani KM. Method of obtaining and preparation of fresh human amniotic membrane for clinical use. J Pakistan Med Assoc 1996; 46:126–128.

11. Thomson PD, Parks DH. Monitoring, banking, and clinical use of amnion as a burn wound dressing. Ann Plast Surg 1981; 7:354–356.

12. Haberal M, Oner Z, Bayraktar U, et al. The use of silver nitrate-incorporated amniotic membrane as a temporary dressing. Burns Incl Therm Inj 1987; 13:159–163.

13. Quinby WC Jr, Hoover HC, Scheflan M, et al. Clinical trials of amniotic membranes in burn wound care. Plast Reconstr Surg 1982; 70:711–717.

14. Braye F, Oddou L, Bertin-Maghit M, et al. Widely meshed autograft associated with cultured autologous epithelium for the treatment of major burns in children: report of 12 cases. Eur J Pediatr Surg 2000; 10:35–40.

15. Horch RE, Corbei O, Formanek-Corbei B, et al. Reconstitution of basement membrane after 'sandwich-technique' skin grafting for severe burns demonstrated by immunohistochemistry. J Burn Care Rehabil 2000; 19:189–202.

16. Phillips TJ, Gilchrest BA. Cultured epidermal allografts as biological wound dressings. Prog Clin Biol Res 2000; 365:77–94.

17. Song IC, Bromberg BE, Mohn MP, et al. Heterografts as biological dressings for large skin wounds. Surgery 1966; 59:576–583.

18. Elliott RA Jr, Hoehn JG. Use of commercial porcine skin for wound dressings. Plast Reconstr Surg 1973; 52:401–405.

19. Ersek RA, Hachen HJ. Porcine xenografts in the treatment of pressure ulcers. Ann Plast Surg 1980; 5:464–470.

20. Chiu T, Burd A. 'Xenograft' dressing in the treatment of burns. Clin Dermatol 2005; 23(4):419–423.

21. Marvin JA, Heimbach DM, Engrav LH, et al. Improved treatment of the Stevens–Johnson syndrome. Arch Surg 1984; 119:601–605.

22. Ersek RA, Navarro JA. Maximizing wound healing with silver-impregnated porcine xenograft. Todays OR Nurse 1990; 12:4–9.

23. Ersek RA, Denton DR. Silver-impregnated porcine xenografts for treatment of meshed autografts. Ann Plast Surg 1984; 13:482–487.

24. Salisbury RE, Wilmore DW, Silverstein P, et al. Biological dressings for skin graft donor sites. Arch Surg 1973; 106:705–706.

25. Salisbury RE, Carnes RW, Enterline D. Biological dressings and evaporative water loss from burn wounds. Ann Plast Surg 1980; 5:270–272.

26. Demling RH. Burns. N Engl J Med 1985; 313:1389–1398.

27. Bacha EA, Sheridan RL, Donohue GA, et al. Staphylococcal toxic shock syndrome in a paediatric burn unit. Burns 1994; 20:499–502.

28. Vanstraelen P. Comparison of calcium sodium alginate (KALTO-STAT) and porcine xenograft (E-Z DERM) in the healing of split-thickness skin graft donor sites. Burns 1992; 18:145–148.

29. Caruso DM, Foster KN, Hermans MH, et al. Aquacel Ag in the management of partial-thickness burns: results of a clinical trial. J Burn Care Rehabil 2004; 25(1):89–97.

30. Greenhalgh DG. The role of growth factors in wound healing. J Trauma 1996; 41:159–167.

31. Teepe RG, Koch R, Haeseker B. Randomized trial comparing cryo-preserved cultured epidermal allografts with tulle-gras in the treatment of split-thickness skin graft donor sites. J Trauma 1993; 35:850–854.

32. Bell E, Ehrlich HP, Buttle DJ, et al. Living tissue formed in vitro and accepted as skin-equivalent tissue of full thickness. Science 1981; 211:1052–1054.

33. Nolte CJ, Oleson MA, Hansbrough JF, et al. Ultrastructural features of composite skin cultures grafted onto athymic mice. J Anat 1994; 185:325–333.

34. Hansbrough JF, Morgan J, Greenleaf G, et al. Evaluation of graftskin composite grafts on full-thickness wounds on athymic mice. J Burn Care Rehabil 1994; 15:346–353.

35. Gentzkow GD, Iwasaki SD, Hershon KS, et al. Use of dermagraft, a cultured human dermis, to treat diabetic foot ulcers. Diabetes Care 1996; 19:350–354.

36. Sacks MS, Chuong CJ, Petroll WM, et al. Collagen fiber architecture of a cultured dermal tissue. J Biomechan Engin 1997; 119:124–127.

37. Economou TP, Rosenquist MD, Lewis RW II, et al. An experimental study to determine the effects of Dermagraft on skin graft viability in the presence of bacterial wound contamination. J Burn Care Rehabil 1995; 16:27–30.

38. Falanga V, Sabolinski M. A bilayered living skin construct (APLI-GRAF) accelerates complete closure of hard-to-heal venous ulcers. Wound Repair Regen 2000; 7:201–207.

39. Wickware P. Progress from a fragile start. Nature 2000; 403:466.

40. Hansbrough JF, Morgan J, Greenleaf G, et al. Development of a temporary living skin replacement composed of human neonatal fibroblasts cultured in Biobrane, a synthetic dressing material. Surgery 1994; 115:633–644.

41. Hansbrough J. Dermagraft-TC for partial-thickness burns: a clinical evaluation. J Burn Care Rehabil 1997; 18:S25–S28.

42. Parente ST. Estimating the economic cost offsets of using Derma-graft-TC as an alternative to cadaver allograft in the treatment of graftable burns. J Burn Care Rehabil 1997; 18:S18–S24.

43. Purdue GF. Dermagraft-TC pivotal efficacy and safety study. J Burn Care Rehabil 1997; 18:S13–S14.

44. Lukish JR, Eichelberger MR, Newman KD, et al. The use of a bioactive skin substitute decreases length of stay for pediatric burn patients. J Pediatr Surg 2001; 36(8):1118–1121.

45. Morgan JR, Barrandon Y, Green H, et al. Expression of an exogenous growth hormone gene by transplantable human epidermal cells. Science 1987; 237:1476–1479.

46. Morgan JR, Yarmush ML. Bioengineered skin substitutes. Sci Med 1997; July/August:6–15.

47. Rheinwald JG, Green H. Serial cultivation of strains of human epidermal keratinocytes: the formation of keratinizing colonies from single cells. Cell 1975; 6:331–343.

48. Green H, Kehinde O, Thomas J. Growth of cultured human epidermal cells into multiple epithelia suitable for grafting. Proc Natl Acad Sci USA 1979; 76:5665–5668.

49. Green H. Cultured cells for the treatment of disease. Sci Am 1991; 265:96–102.

50. Gallico GG III, O'Connor NE, Compton CC, et al. Permanent coverage of large burn wounds with autologous cultured human epithelium. N Engl J Med 1984; 311:448–451.

51. Sheridan RL, Tompkins RG. Cultured autologous epithelium in patients with burns of ninety percent or more of the body surface. J Trauma 1995; 38:48–50.

52. Rue LW III, Cioffi WG, McManus WF, et al. Wound closure and outcome in extensively burned patients treated with cultured autologous keratinocytes. J Trauma 1993; 34:662–667.

53. Barret JP, Wolf SE, Desai MH, et al. Cost-efficacy of cultured epidermal autografts in massive pediatric burns. Ann Surg 2000; 231(6):869–876.

54. Tompkins RG, Burke JF. Progress in burn treatment and the use of artificial skin. World J Surg 1990; 14:819–824.

55. Yannas IV, Burke JF, Warpehoski M, et al. Prompt, long-term functional replacement of skin. Trans Am Soc Artif Intern Organs 1981; 27:19–23.

56. Yannas IV, Burke JF, Orgill DP, et al. Wound tissue can utilize a polymeric template to synthesize a functional extension of skin. Science 1982; 215:174–176.

57. Tompkins RG, Hilton JF, Burke JF, et al. Increased survival after massive thermal injuries in adults: preliminary report using artificial skin. Crit Care Med 1989; 17:734–740.

58. Sheridan RL, Heggerty M, Tompkins RG, et al. Artificial skin in massive burns — results at ten years. Eur J Plast Surg 1994; 17:91–93.

59. Heimbach DM, Warden GD, Luterman A, et al. Multicenter postapproval clinical trial of Integra dermal regeneration template for burn treatment. J Burn Care Rehabil 2003; 24(1):42–48.

60. Groos N, Guillot M, Zilliox R, et al. Use of an artificial dermis (Integra) for the reconstruction of extensive burn scars in children. About 22 grafts. Eur J Pediatr Surg. 2005; 15(3):187–192.

61. Wainwright DJ. Use of an acellular allograft dermal matrix (Alloderm) in the management of full-thickness burns. Burns 1995; 21:243–248.

62. Wainwright D, Madden M, Luterman A, et al. Clinical evaluation of an acellular allograft dermal matrix in full-thickness burns. J Burn Care Rehabil 1996; 17:124–136.

63. Sheridan RL, Choucair RJ. Acellular allograft dermis does not hinder initial engraftment in burn resurfacing and reconstruction. J Burn Care Rehabil 1997; 18:496–499.

64. Sheridan RL, Choucair RJ. Acellular allodermis in burn surgery: 1-year results of a pilot trial. J Burn Care Rehabil 1998; 19:528–530.

65. Langdon RC, Cuono CB, Birchall N, et al. Reconstitution of structure and cell function in human skin grafts derived from cryopreserved allogeneic dermis and autologous cultured keratinocytes. J Invest Dermatol 1988; 91:478–485.

66. Cuono CB, Langdon R, Birchall N, et al. Composite autologous-allogeneic skin replacement: development and clinical application. Plast Reconstr Surg 1987; 80:626–637.

67. Cuono C, Langdon R, McGuire J. Use of cultured epidermal autografts and dermal allografts as skin replacement after burn injury. Lancet 1986; 1:1123–1124.

68. Hickerson WL, Compton C, Fletchall S, et al. Cultured epidermal autografts and allodermis combination for permanent burn wound coverage. Burns 1994; 20 (Suppl 1):S52–S55; discussion S55–S56.

69. Compton CC, Hickerson W, Nadire K, et al. Acceleration of skin regeneration from cultured epithelial autografts by transplantation to homograft dermis. J Burn Care Rehabil 1993; 14:653–662.

70. Boyce ST, Hansbrough JF. Biologic attachment, growth, and differentiation of cultured human epidermal keratinocytes on a graftable collagen and chondroitin-6-sulfate substrate. Surgery 1988; 103:421–431.

71. Supp DM, Boyce ST. Engineered skin substitutes: practices and potentials. Clin Dermatol 2005; 23(4):403–412.

72. Cooper ML, Hansbrough JF. Use of a composite skin graft composed of cultured human keratinocytes and fibroblasts and a collagen-GAG matrix to cover full-thickness wounds on athymic mice. Surgery 1991; 109:198–207.

73. Boyce ST, Kagan RJ, Yakuboff KP, et al. Cultured skin substitutes reduce donor skin harvesting for closure of excised, full-thickness burns. Ann Surg 2002; 235(2):269–279.

74. Swope VB, Supp AP, Boyce ST. Regulation of cutaneous pigmentation by titration of human melanocytes in cultured skin substitutes grafted to athymic mice. Wound Repair Regen 2002; 10(6):378–386.

75. Sheridan RL, Morgan JR. Initial clinical experience with an autologous composite skin substitute. J Burn Care Rehabil 2000; 21:S214.

AlloDerm

Juan P. Barret

Chapter contents

AlloDerm (Life Cell Corporation, Branchburg, NJ) is an acellular dermal matrix derived from donated human skin tissue. Scientific production of this dermal-derived skin template started with research with porcine skin. The basis of the process that allowed AlloDerm production was developed in the pig model, which demonstrated that tissue rejection does not develop in an acellular allodermis.[1] Donated skin is supplied by US AATB-compliant tissue banks utilizing the standards of the American Association of Tissue Banks (AATB) and Food and Drug Administration (FDA) guidelines. It is classified as banked human tissue by the FDA since it is minimally processed and not significantly changed in structure. Human donor tissue undergoes a multistep proprietary process that removes both the epidermis and the cells that can lead to tissue rejection and graft failure, without damaging the matrix and framework of biochemical and structural components of the dermis, thus allowing the wound to regenerate and replace. Once the dermal tissue has been decellularized, the final step is preservation. The matrix is preserved with a patented freeze-drying process that prevents damaging ice crystals from forming. During this process, all cells responsible for immune response are removed, leaving a matrix ready to enable the wound to mount its own tissue regeneration process. AlloDerm allows the repair cascade to follow a more determined and guided regenerative process, restoring similar original structural, functional, and physiological conditions and minimizing scar formation. During the regeneration process, the AlloDerm matrix becomes part of the existing tissue structure by migration of stem cells in the matrix, differentiation into tissue-specific cell types, and elaboration of new matrix. Applications of AlloDerm include abdominal wall reconstruction, breast reconstruction, tissue filling, and wound coverage. The product comes in different thickness (0.17–1.8 mm and over) and sizes, some of them custom made, besides being available mesh and unmeshed. Thickness appropriate for burn wound coverage ranges from 0.18 mm to 0.34 mm.

Burn scar resurfacing with AlloDerm application

The philosophy behind the application of AlloDerm in burn scar resurfacing is the same of that with Integra dermal regeneration template; however, important differences of the technical application exist. The purpose of the technique is to remove all damage and scarred tissue, and to replace it with an even, flat, surface that will accommodate a laminar thin split-thickness skin autograft. The objective being an outcome with an exchange of hypertrophic non-pliable scar by a smooth, pliable, soft skin-like tissue. Two main points differentiate the Integra technique from the AlloDerm technique: AlloDerm resurfacing is a one-step operation (instead of the two-step Integra technique), and the nature of AlloDerm prevents it from being applicable to large wound areas. Indeed, AlloDerm is used together with a thin skin graft, which makes it appealing as a one-step operation, but the fact that all areas of AlloDerm require autograft coverage limits its use to an area of wound resurfacing that matches donor site availability. The experience with AlloDerm, although it has been on the market for many years, is still limited, with few references in acute burn surgery,[2,3] which showed good engraftment of autograft and outcomes and a decrease of length of hospital stay and donor site healing time. The applications in reconstructive surgery are most commonly retrieved as dermal or tissue filling, with few usages as reconstruction or resurfacing.[4]

Preparation of the burn wound

During the preoperative burn reconstructive visit, all areas amenable for burn scar resurfacing are outlined and discussed with the patient. An inventory of potential donor sites is developed and a decision is made on whether Integra or AlloDerm will be used. Generally speaking, indications for AlloDerm will include small areas requiring burn scar resurfacing and patients that will benefit from a one-step operation (i.e. zones of limited range of motion that require intensive and aggressive postoperative physiotherapy and occupational therapy to maintain function). A complete informed consent of the treatment proposed, which includes alternatives to the technique and the potential hazards of the product, should be obtained.

The burn scars should be completely excised to provide a clean, viable, vascularized wound bed. Hemostasis should proceed very carefully to avoid active bleeders. The area must be completely released and all joints and tendons treated with capsulotomies, ligament releases, and tenolyses when appropriate to return the area to normal anatomy. The area is kept in warm saline compresses until AlloDerm is ready for application. A thin ($^6/_{1000}$–$^8/_{1000}$ of an inch) split-thickness skin autograft is harvested from an available donor site. It should match the wound requirements, allowing for an excess to account for graft shrinkage after harvest.

Usage of AlloDerm

Prior to use, AlloDerm must be rehydrated. The rehydration procedure should begin at least half an hour ahead of intended use. Liberal amounts of warmed saline should be used in a two-step bath with light agitation. Normal rehydration is usually accomplished in 20–40 minutes depending on thickness. The first step starts by tearing and opening the outer foil bag. AlloDerm is aseptically removed from the packaging, leaving the backing on, and it is placed in the first bath of saline solution warmed at 37°C (50 mL–100 mL, depending on the total surface of AlloDerm). AlloDerm is soaked and kept submerged for a minimum of 5 minutes or until the backing separates. The backing is discarded and AlloDerm is transported to a second bath, leaving the piece submerged until it is fully rehydrated. When it is fully rehydrated, it is soft and pliable and it is ready for application to the surgical site.

AlloDerm has two distinct sides. The basement membrane is the upper side (it looks rough and dull) and the dermal surface is the lower side (it looks smooth and shiny). They can be distinguished by appearance and by the blood test. A drop of blood will infiltrate the vascular channels within the matrix after rinsing with saline, and the dermal side will look bright red, whereas the basement membrane side will look pink. The dermal side must be applied on the wound surface (placement on the wrong side will prevent engraftment), and AlloDerm is secured with absorbable sutures. Following this, the skin graft is applied on top of the basement membrane side of AlloDerm and it is secured in the usual fashion (absorbable sutures, running o not, staplers, etc.) (Figure 17.1).

Dressings and postoperative instructions

Petrolatum-based fine mesh gauze is applied on top of the graft, and is secured with bacitracin ointment. No special dressings are required. Tie-over dressings may be used, depending on location and surgeon preferences, but they are not necessary. Conversely, the vacuum assisted system may be used as well.

Grafts are inspected at day 7. Autografts will look white yellow and at this time the patient may be sent to rehabilitation services to be measured for silicone inserts, placement of interim pressure garments, and start physiotherapy and occupational therapy. Bathing and moisturizing may proceed from day 10 after surgery, when a complete stratum corneum is present. In the case of small open wounds, they are treated with gentle care and baseline or any other wound care protocol. It is seldom necessary to regraft AlloDerm; small raw areas heal spontaneously by proliferation of keratinocytes of the skin graft that seed the areas despite disintegration of the architecture of the skin graft.

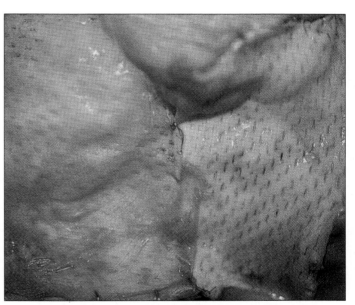

Fig. 17.1 Burn scar incision and resurfacing with AlloDerm. The dermal template integrates in the wound and behaves as true dermal tissue. The use of AlloDerm allows for the harvest of super-thin skin autografts, with rapid healing of the donor site. (Reproduced with permission from Barret JP, Herndon DN, eds. Color atlas of burn care. London: WB Saunders; 2001.)

References

1. Livesey SA, Herndon DN, Hollyoak MA, et al. Transplanted acellular allograft dermal matrix. Potential as a template for the reconstruction of viable dermis. Transplantation 1995; 60: 1–9.
2. Gore DC. Utility of acellular allograft dermis in the care of elderly burn patients. J Surg Res 2005; 125:37–41.
3. Wainwright DJ. Use of an acellular allograft dermal matrix (AlloDerm) in the management of full-thickness burns. Burns 1995; 21:243–248.
4. Barret JP, Dziewulski P, McCauley RL, et al. Dural reconstruction of a class IV calvarial burn with decellularized human dermis. Burns 1999; 25:459–462.

Chapter 18

The pathophysiology
of inhalation injury

Daniel L. Traber, David N. Herndon, Perenlei Enkhbaatar,
Marc O. Maybauer, and Dirk M. Maybauer

Introduction and epidemiology

It has been over two decades since the authors published their first manuscript on inhalation injury.[1] In the review article published the following year it was reported that inhalation injury was a main, if not *the* main, factor responsible for mortality in thermally injured patients.[2] Smoke inhalation causes 5000–10000 deaths annually in the United States and more than 23000 injuries, including approximately 5000 firefighter injuries.[3] In fact the United States has one of the highest fire death rates among industrialized countries. Inhalation injury is a serious medical problem. In the case of smoke, more than 30% of thermally injured patients admitted to burn centers in the United States have a concomitant smoke inhalation injury.[4] Similar percentages of fire victims who have sustained smoke inhalation appear in several other countries.[5–8] Despite effective management of fluid resuscitation, early surgical excision of burned tissue, and improved ventilation techniques, the mortality rate of patients who have combined burn and smoke inhalation injury is still high.[4,9–11] In patients with combined injury, the lung is a critical organ and the progressive respiratory failure associated with pulmonary edema is a pivotal determinant of mortality.[12–14] Though not as lethal, smoke inhalation alone is a serious problem. It is estimated by the World Health Organization that there are over one billion people who develop airway and pulmonary inflammation as a result of inhaling smoke from indoor cooking fires, forest fires, and burning of crops (Figure 18.1).[15,16]

The inhalation of toxic materials has been of interest for a number of years especially as the result of their use in gas warfare. In the 1940s there were two very large fires that focused interest in on the inhalation of smoke in fire victims. The first was a fire at a nightclub in Boston called 'The Cocoanut Grove' where a large number of people were trapped in a burning building and consequently sustained severe inhalation injury.[17,18] The second disaster occurred in Texas City across the bay from Galveston, Texas.[19] Here a ship exploded in a harbor and set off a chain of explosions and fires among some 50 refineries and chemical plants resulting in over 2000 hospital admissions of patients with burn injury many of whom who had simultaneously inhaled smoke as well as victims with smoke inhalation alone. In many ways the burn victims of the 9/11 disaster at the Pentagon were similar to these individuals since the burns and inhalation involved combustion of petroleum products. Among the 790 injured survivors of the terrorist attack on the Word Trade Center in NY on September 11, 2001, 49% suffered from inhalation injury. The situation was the same as the attack on the Pentagon. In both situations inhalation injury was also seen in some patients who were not burned.[20–23] Disasters like those in Boston and Galveston led to the establishment of centers for the care of burn victims and to research into the pathophysiology of burn injury.

The fire environment

Toxic smoke compounds

Smoke toxicity is an increasing concern because industrial products used today are changing from woods and natural materials towards lighter construction materials, synthetics, and petrochemical-based materials, which ignite and burn two to three times hotter and faster than conventional materials and, when heated, emit a gas or smoke that will also ignite two or three times faster and burn hotter than natural biological materials. Consequently, firefighters have less time to gain control of a fire, and victims are more likely to be incapacitated by breathing toxic gases and are more likely to sustain smoke inhalation because they have less time to escape from the burning area.[3] Inhalation injury is caused by steam or toxic inhalants such as fumes, gases, and mists. Fumes consist of small particles or droplets dispersed in air with various irritants or cytotoxic chemicals adherent to the particles. Mists consist of aerosolized irritant or cytotoxic liquids. Smoke consists of a combination of fumes, gases, mists, and hot air. Heat, toxic gases, and low oxygen levels are the most common causes of death at a fire scene. A large variety of toxic gases and chemicals can be generated, depending on the fire environment (Table 18.1).

Many of these compounds may act together to increase mortality, especially carbon monoxide and hydrogen cyanide,[24,25] where a synergism has been found to increase tissue hypoxia and acidosis[25] and may also decrease cerebral oxygen consumption and metabolism.[26,27] Hydrogen sulfide would also be predicted to synergize with carbon monoxide, since both cyanide and hydrogen sulfide are inhibitors of mitochondrial cytochrome oxidase. Victims may be incapacitated by the blinding and irritating effects of smoke, as well the decreasing oxygen concentration that occurs with combustion and results in progressive hypoxia.

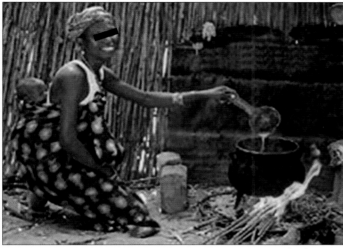
Fig. 18.1 An example of direct exposure to smoke as a result of an open fire using various materials as a fuel.

Inhalation injury can be classified into:
- upper airway injury;
- lower airways injury;
- pulmonary parenchyma injury; and
- systemic toxicity.

The extent of inhalation damage depends on fire environment: the ignition source, temperature, concentration, and solubility of the toxic gases generated. For instance, thermal and chemical compounds usually cause upper airway injury. The water-soluble materials such as acrolein and the other aldehydes damage the proximal airways and set off reactions, which are inflammatory to the bronchi and parenchyma, whereas agents with lower water solubility such as chlorine, phosgene, and nitrogen oxide, nitrogen dioxide or N_2O_3 or even N_2O_4 are more likely to cause insidious injury.[27] Toxic gases such as carbon monoxide and cyanide rarely damage the airway but affect gas exchange, producing more systemic effect. It is thus important to obtain information relative to the source of the fire and the combustion products generated when treating a fire victim (see Table 18.1). It is also important to know the duration of exposure and the extent to which the fire victim was in an enclosed area since this relates to the dose of toxic materials presented them.

TABLE 18.1 ORIGIN OF SELECTED TOXIC COMPOUNDS[24]

Gases and chemicals	Material	Source
Carbon monoxide	Polyvinyl chloride Cellulose	Upholstery, wire/pipe coating, wall, floor, furniture coverings Clothing, fabric Wood, paper, cotton
Cyanide	Wool, silk, cotton, paper, plastic, polymers Polyurethane Polyacrylonitrile Polyamide Melamine resins	Clothing, fabric, blankets, furniture Insulation, upholstery material Appliances, engineering, plastics Carpeting, clothing Household and kitchen goods
Hydrogen chloride	Polyvinyl chloride Polyester	Upholstery, wire/pipe coating, wall, floor, furniture coverings Clothing, fabric
Phosgene	Polyvinyl chloride	Upholstery, wire/pipe coating, wall, floor, furniture coverings
Ammonia	Wool, silk Polyurethane Polyamide Melamine resins	Clothing, fabric, blankets, furniture Insulation, upholstery material Carpeting, clothing Household and kitchen goods
Sulfur dioxide	Rubber	Tires
Hydrogen sulfide	Wool, silk	Clothing, fabric, blankets, furniture
Acrolein	Cellulose Polypropylene Acrylics	Wood, paper, cotton, jute Upholstery, carpeting Aircraft windows, textiles, wall coverings
Formaldehyde	Melamine resins	Household and kitchen goods
Isocyanates	Polyurethane	Insulation, upholstery material
Acrylonitriles	Polyurethane	Insulation, upholstery material

Carbon monoxide

Carbon monoxide (CO) is an odorless, colorless gas that is produced by incomplete combustion of many fuels, especially cellulolytic (cellulose products) such as wood, paper, and cotton.[28] Carbon monoxide toxicity remains one of the most frequent immediate causes of death following smoke-induced inhalation injury. The predominant toxic effect of CO is its binding to hemoglobin to form carboxyhemoglobin (COHb). The affinity of CO for hemoglobin is ~200 to 250 times higher than that of oxygen.[29] Inhalation of a 0.1% carbon monoxide mixture may result in generation of a carboxyhemoglobin level as high as 50% of the total hemoglobin. The competitive binding of CO to hemoglobin reduces delivery of oxygen to tissues, leading to severe hypoxia, especially of most vulnerable organs such as brain and heart where oxygen extraction is considerably higher than most other organs. The oxygen–hemoglobin dissociation curve loses its sigmoid shape and is shifted to the left, thus further impairing tissue oxygen availability.[24,30] In addition, the ability of CO to bind to intracellular cytochromes and to other metalloproteins contributes to CO toxicity. This competitive inhibition with cytochrome oxidase enzyme systems (most notably cytochromes a and P-450) results in an inability of cellular systems to use oxygen.[30,31] Shimazu and his colleagues have shown that extravascular binding of CO to cytochromes and other structures accounts for 10–15% of total body CO stores. This intracellular binding of CO explains the two-compartment elimination of CO from the circulation.[32] Miro and colleagues reported that CO inhibits cytochrome-c oxidase activity in lymphocytes.[33] The electron chain dysfunction by CO may cause electron leakage, leading to superoxide production and mitochondrial oxidative stress.[34]

Symptoms and diagnosis of carbon monoxide poisoning

The symptoms of CO poisoning may predominantly manifest in organ and systems with high oxygen utilization. The severity of clinical manifestations is varied depending on the concentration of CO. For instance, the central nervous system symptoms such as headache, confusion, and collapse may occur when the blood COHb level is 40–50%. Symptoms such as unconsciousness, intermittent convulsions, and respiratory failure may occur if the COHb level exceeds 60% eventually leading to death if exposure continues. The cardiovascular manifestations may result in tachycardia, increase in cardiac output, dysrhythmias, myocardial ischemia, and hypotension, depending on severity of poisoning. The correlation of clinical manifestation and severity of CO poisoning is summarized in Table 18.2.

Diagnosis should be based on direct measurement of COHb levels in arterial or venous blood by co-oximetry; it has to be taken into account that venous blood underestimates the arterial COHb content.[37] Diagnosis may be facilitated by use of on-site portable breath analyzers. The inability to differentiate oxyhemoglobin from COHb limits the use of a pulse oximeter. The use of blood gas analyzers that estimate SO_2 based on measurement of dissolved PO_2 should also be avoided. The measurements of acid–base balance, plasma lactate levels, and bicarbonate are helpful in management of CO poisoning with accompanying lactic or metabolic acidosis. It is important to note that high oxygen concentrations are usually administered

COHb%	Symptoms
0–10	None
10–20	Tightness over forehead, slight headache, dilation of cutaneous blood vessels
20–30	Headache and throbbing in the temples
30–40	Severe headache, weakness, dizziness, dimness of vision, nausea, vomiting, collapse
40–50	As above; greater possibility of collapse, syncope, increased pulse and respiratory rate
50–60	Syncope, increased pulse and respiratory rate, coma, intermittent convulsions, Cheyne–Stokes respirations
60–70	Coma, intermittent convulsions, depressed cardiac and respiratory function, possible death
70–80	Weak pulse, slow respirations, death within hours
80–90	Death in less than 1 hour
90–100	Death within minutes

TABLE 18.2 SYMPTOMS AND SIGNS AT VARIOUS CONCENTRATIONS OF CARBOXYHEMOGLOBIN[35,36]

Reproduced from Einhorn IN[35] National Institute of Environmental Health Sciences, and Schulte JH[36] Heldref publications.

to the victim in transit to hospital and some delay from cessation of exposure to measurement of CO may limit evaluation of true extent of exposure.[38] A nomogram has been developed which can relate the carboxyhemoglobin levels of a patient to the values that may have been present at the time of smoke inhalation and this can be used to estimate the true degree of inhalation injury.[39]

Treatment for CO poisoning

The half-life of carboxyhemoglobin is 250 minutes (adult male) in room air and 40–60 minutes in a person breathing 100% oxygen at 1 atmosphere.[40] Those values are 30% shorter in females.[41] Therefore all fire victims should be isolated from fire site and given 100% oxygen on route to hospital. This allows delivery of an inspired oxygen concentration of 50–60%, which is usually adequate. To adequately treat a CO poisoning it is important also to establish COHb level as early as possible. If it is necessary (loss of consciousness, cyanosis or an inability to maintain the airway), 100% oxygen should be delivered via mechanical ventilation through endotracheal tube until COHb levels drop below 10–15%. The alternative method to rapidly decrease COHb is hyperbaric oxygenation therapy (HBOT): 100% oxygen at pressure greater than 1 atmosphere in a pressure vessel. This technology has been used to treat a variety of disease states. HBOT may be necessary and beneficial for patients with smoke inhalation. If the carboxyhemoglobin level exceeds 25% or if significant clinical toxicity is present, administration of three atmospheres of pressure will reduce the carboxyhemoglobin half-life to 30 minutes. HBOT allows CO to dissociate from cytochrome a, a_3 and to increase PO_2 despite impaired hemoglobin function.[42,43] Carbon monoxide may cause xanthine dehydrase to convert to xanthine oxidase; the latter is associated with the formation of oxygen free radicals and tissue damage. Treatment with hyperbaric oxygen will convert the xanthine oxidase back to its less toxic dehydrogenase. If neurological impairment persists, this treatment may be repeated.[42,44,45] Finally, as many as 10% of survivors may demonstrate a neurological or mental deterioration delayed some months after an initial recovery. Early hyperbaric oxygen may reduce these neurological problems.[46] However, the use of HBOT in burn patients is controversial despite the benefit of this treatment for patients with smoke inhalation alone.[47] Burn patients are difficult to monitor in small chambers and are at high risk for unstable hemodynamic conditions and complications such as seizures or aspiration. A recent systematic study review has not found sufficient evidence to support or refute the effectiveness of HBOT for the management of thermal burns. Evidence from controlled trials is insufficient to provide clear guidelines for practice. Further research is needed to better define the role of HBOT in the treatment of thermal burns.[48]

Hydrogen cyanide

Hydrogen cyanide (CN), the gaseous form of cyanide, is generated by the combustion of nitrogen- and carbon-containing substances, such as wool, silk, cotton, and paper as well as synthetic substances like plastic and other polymers. Combustion of these materials may produce a rapid and lethal incapacitation of a victim at the fire source.[49] CN is a colorless gas with the odor of bitter almonds; however, it is difficult to detect at the site of a fire. The cytotoxicity of cyanide is produced by inhibition of cellular oxygenation with resultant tissue anoxia which is caused by reversible inhibition of cytochrome c oxidase.[38] CN is toxic to a number of enzyme systems. The exact chemical mechanism by which cyanide induces its toxicity includes combination with essential metal ions, formation of cyanohydrins with carbonyl compounds, and the sequestration with sulfur as a thiocyanate. However, the principal target enzyme of CN is cytochrome c oxidase, the terminal oxidase of the respiratory chain, and involves interaction with the ferric ion of cytochrome a_3. The importance of cyanide in smoke inhalation injuries is reflected by a study performed in Paris, France which shows that mean blood cyanide concentrations in both fire victims who survived (21.6 mol/L), and in those who died (116.4 mol/L) were significantly higher than those in control subjects (5.0 mol/L) and levels in fire victims who died were significantly higher than those in victims who survived.[50] A report of 144 fire victims in Dallas County, Texas, showed consistent results with the Paris study.[51] Elevated cyanide concentrations showed a direct relationship to the probability of death. Cyanide also played a greater role in mortality in the aircraft fire at Manchester International Airport, Manchester, UK in 1985. These patients were not severely burned. The majority (87%) of the 54 individuals who died had potentially lethal levels of cyanide in their blood, whereas only 21% of these fire victims had COHb levels exceeding 50%. This indicates the high possibility that, under certain conditions, cyanide can be a more important determinant of morbidity and mortality following smoke inhalation than CO, which is usually regarded as the primary toxic threat.[3] Smoke is also an often overlooked source of CN exposure in terrorist bombings. Following the World Trade Center bombing in 1993, traces of cyanide were found in the vans where the explosion originated. The Center of Disease Control and the Department of Homeland Security consider CN among the most likely agents of chemical terrorism.[52] Cyanide possesses all the attributes of an ideal terrorist weapon: it is plentiful, readily available, and easily obtainable because of its widespread use in industry and laboratories. In addition, the use of cyanide does not require any special knowledge. Cyanide is capable of causing mass incapacitation and casualties, and can cause mass confusion, panic, and social disruption.[53]

Symptoms and diagnosis of cyanide poisoning

Diagnosis at the fire scene may be difficult. Poisoning may result in central nervous, respiratory, and cardiovascular dysfunction due to inhibition of oxidative phosphorylation, depending on the concentration of cyanide inhalation (Table 18.3).

Electrocardiographic changes, such as S-T segment elevation, that mimic an acute myocardial infarction[54] may be suggestive. Laboratory findings of anion gap metabolic acidosis and lacticacidemia aid in confirming the diagnosis.[55] The lactic acidosis that is not rapidly responsive to oxygen therapy may be good indicator for cyanide poisoning.[39,50] Also, an elevated mixed venous saturation is suggestive for cyanide toxicity. Cyanide increases ventilation through carotid body and peripheral chemoreceptor stimulation. Low levels of hydrogen cyanide are routinely found in the blood of healthy individuals at levels of 0.02 μg/mL in nonsmokers and 0.04 μg/mL in smokers. Toxicity occurs at a level of 0.1 μg/mL and at 1.0 μg/mL death is likely.[56] The correlation of severity of clinical symptoms and HCN concentration is summarized in Table 18.4.

Treatment

Successful intervention for cyanide poisoning depends primarily on the concentration of exposure and the time between exposure and treatment; clearly it is critical that treatment is administered as quickly as possible after exposure. Therefore, presumptive diagnosis and empiric treatment may prove necessary. Fire victims suspected with cyanide poisoning should be removed from exposure and fully decontaminated, while

TABLE 18.3 SYMPTOMS OF CYANIDE TOXICITY	
Symptoms in low or moderate inhaled cyanide concentrations	Symptoms in moderate or high inhaled cyanide concentrations
Faintness	Prostration
Flushing	Hypotension
Anxiety	Tremors
Excitement	Cardiac arrhythmia
Perspiration	Convulsions
Vertigo	Stupor
Headache	Paralysis
Drowsiness	Coma
Tachypnea	Respiratory depression
Dyspnea	Respiratory arrest
Tachycardia	Cardiovascular collapse

TABLE 18.4 HYDROGEN CYANIDE CONCENTRATIONS IN AIR AND ASSOCIATED SYMPTOMS IN HUMANS[35,57]

HCN concentration (ppm)	Symptoms
0.2–5.0	Threshold of odor
10	(TLV-MAC)
18–36	Slight symptoms (headache) after several hours
45–54	Tolerated for $1/2$–1 hour without difficulty
100	Death in 1 hour
110–135	Fatal in $1/2$–1 hour
181	Fatal in 10 minutes
280	Immediately fatal

Einhorn IN[35] National Institute of Environmental Health Sciences, and Kimmerle G[57] University of Utah.

maintaining appropriate provider respiratory protection, restoring or maintaining airway patency, administering 100% oxygen via non-rebreathing mask or a bag valve mask. All victims should be given intravenous access and aggressive fluid resuscitation ($4 mL/kg/m^2$ body surface area when patients have burn injuries). When clinically indicated, anticonvulsants (benzodiazepines) should be given for seizures, epinephrine and antiarrhythmics to support cardiopulmonary function, and sodium bicarbonate to correct metabolic acidosis.[3] Oxygen therapy appears to have strong positive effect; however, hyperbaric oxygen therapy is not recommended for the reasons previously discussed.[54,56] Cyanide is metabolized by hepatic rhodonase, which catalyzes the donation of sulfur from the sulfane pool to cyanide to form nontoxic thiocyanate. The half-life of cyanide is ~1–3 hours in humans.[50,58] Although there is still controversy surrounding the treatment of cyanide poisoning, there are few antidotes available that can be used by first responders. Kelocyanor (dicobalt edentate) may be useful, but is dangerous in itself and requires experts to administer it.[59] A cyanide antidote appropriate for the use in smoke inhalation victims is available in Europe, but not yet in the US, where the cyanide antidote kit (Lilly-, Taylor-, or Pasadena-kit) is the only currently available antidote. The kit contains amyl nitrite, thiosulfate, and sodium nitrite. These agents may be considered in an intensive care setting, but not preclinically, since they are *methemoglobin generators*. The therapeutic goal is to convert the ferrous ion of hemoglobin to ferric ion. The resultant methemoglobin chelates cyanide to form cyanmethemoglobin. The drugs of choice in this group are sodium nitrite (IV) and amyl nitrite (inhaled). These drugs reduce oxygen-carrying capacity; therefore they should be used with caution, especially in patients with concomitant CO poisoning which induces COHb that may further compromise oxygen transport. These drugs should be also used with precautions in patients with burn shock because they are also vasodilators and can cause hypotension. In addition, there is little evidence to suggest these are effective measures, and cardiac toxicity in people with heart disease may be problematic.[60] The therapeutic goal *of sulfur donors* is to convert cyanide to thiocyanate. The drug of choice in this group is

sodium thiosulfate (IV). Toxicity is minimal other than acting as an osmotic diuretic action that in itself may be beneficial. The onset of action, however, is quite slow.[24] *Direct binding agents* are based on cobalt chemistry and chelate the cyanide ion directly. Hydroxycobalamine is the precursor of vitamin B_{12} and has very little toxicity.[24,56] Hydroxycobalamine detoxifies cyanide by binding with it to form B_{12}, and is in excess excreted in the urine.[61] However, this drug is being investigated for possible introduction in the US. Hydroxycobalamine (Cyanokit) has been available in Europe for nearly a decade. Accumulating data from an ongoing study on the prehospital use of hydroxycobalamine for cyanide poisoning suggest that it has a favorable risk benefit ratio and a reasonable safety profile. Hydroxycobalamine at a dose of 5 g appears to be effective and safe in smoke inhalation victims, as an empiric prehospital treatment.[62]

Other toxic chemicals

These may also contribute substantially to the morbidity and mortality in a burn victim. Hydrogen chloride is produced by polyvinyl chloride degradation and causes severe respiratory tract damage and pulmonary edema. Nitrogen oxides may also cause pulmonary edema and a chemical pneumonitis and may contribute to cardiovascular depression and acidosis. Aldehydes such as acrolein and acetaldehyde, which are found in wood and kerosene, may further contribute towards pulmonary edema and respiratory irritability. Toxic industrial chemicals such as, chlorine, phosgene, hydrogen sulfide, and ammonia, are of central importance. Because of their widespread availability and high toxicity, there is certain concern that these chemicals may be used as a weapon by terrorists.[63,64]

Phosgene is a colorless, non-flammable, heavier-than-air gas at room temperature with an odor of newly mown hay. Under 8°C phosgene is an odorless and fuming liquid. Phosgene's inadequate warning properties and delayed symptoms make it a potential terrorist weapon.[65,66] Phosgene is only slightly soluble in water; hence its deeper penetration in the pulmonary system. On contact with water it hydrolyzes into carbon dioxide and hydrochloric acid, resulting in direct caustic damage. It also undergoes acylation reactions with amino-, hydroxyl-, and sulfhydryl- groups of cellular macromolecules, resulting in cell damage and apoptosis.[65,67] As mentioned, phosgene has delayed effects from 20 minutes up to 48 hours depending on the intensity of exposure. Phosgene inhalation produces severe pulmonary edema. Initially victims develop upper airway irritant symptoms (eye irritation, rhinorrhea, cough) and then will develop lower respiratory symptoms such as shortness of breath, substernal burning, and chest tightness. The development of overt pulmonary edema within 4 hours of exposure portends a poor prognosis.

Chlorine is a greenish yellow gas, an oxidizing agent, and very reactive with water. It has a pungent odor. Upon contact with water, chlorine liberates hypochlorous acid, hydrochloric acid, and oxygen free radicals. It causes irritant effects throughout the respiratory tree but mostly nasal mucosa and upper airways. Cell damage is caused by its strong oxidizing capability.[68] Phosgene and chlorine were extensively used during World War I.

Ammonia is a colorless gas at room temperature with a very pungent odor. Ammonia readily dissolves in water to form ammonium hydroxide, a very caustic alkaline solution. It causes cutaneous, ocular, and pulmonary injuries. Inhaled ammonia can rapidly produce laryngeal injury and obstruction. It causes upper tracheobronchial mucosal necrosis with sloughing and severe pulmonary edema.[68] There are no specific antidotes against irritant gases (phosgene, chlorine, and ammonia) toxicity. Depending on the severity of exposure, supportive therapy such as airway management and ventilation should be provided. Early intubation is required if any significant upper airway symptoms such as stridor are present.

Pathophysiology

Injury to the oropharynx

Much of the pathophysiology that occurs with inhalation injury is related to edema formation in the oropharynx, bronchial areas, and parenchyma, and results from an increased transvascular fluid flux from these respective vascular beds. Before a discussion of the changes that occur in these structures following inhalation injury, a review of the forces responsible for the variables of the Starling–Landis equation should be given:[69,70]

$$J_v = K_f[(P_c - P_{if}) - ?\sigma(COP_p - COP_{if})]$$

This equation describes the physical forces and physiologic mechanisms that govern fluid transfer between vascular and extravascular compartments. J_v, the transvascular fluid flux, is equal to lymph flow during equilibrium states. As transvascular fluid flux increases, interstitial volume also increases (edema formation) until a new equilibrium with lymph flow occurs. K_f is the filtration coefficient, an index of the total number of pores that are filtering. The number of pores could increase if a larger area of the microcirculation were perfused or if there were more pores per given area of the microcirculation. These pores are the same size as water and electrolytes, as opposed to the larger pores associated with permeability to protein. P_c and P_{if} are the hydrostatic pressures in the microcirculation and interstitial space, respectively. The reflection coefficient, σ, is an index of microvascular permeability to protein. If σ is 1, the membrane is impermeable to protein; when σ is 0, the membrane is completely permeable to protein. COP_p and COP_{if} are the oncotic or colloid osmotic pressures in the plasma and interstitial spaces, respectively.

The major pathophysiology seen in the oropharynx following inhalation injury induces microvascular changes similar to those seen with thermal injury in other areas of the body. The heat denatures protein that, in turn, activates complement. Complement activation causes the release of histamine.[71,72] Histamine then causes the formation of xanthine oxidase, an enzyme involved in the breakdown of purines to uric acid.[73] During this conversion, reactive oxygen species are released.[74,75] Reactive oxygen species combine with NO, constitutively formed in the endothelium, to form reactive nitrogen species. The latter produce edema in the burned area by increasing the microvascular pressure and permeability to protein.[76] Eicosanoids are also released,[77,78] that, along with oxygen free radicals and IL-8, attract polymorphonuclear cells to the area.[79] These neutrophils then amplify the release of oxygen radicals, proteases, and other materials into burned areas (Figure 18.2).

The massive edema occurring in the soft tissue of the oropharynx following burns involves most of the variables in the Starling equation. There is a large increase in microvascular hydrostatic pressure,[80] a decrease in interstitial hydrostatic pressure,[81] a fall in the reflection coefficient,[80] and an increase in interstitial oncotic pressure.[81,82] The usual treatment for burn resuscitation calls for the administration of large amounts of crystalloid solutions, which has the effect of reducing the plasma oncotic pressure.[83,84] This reduction not only affects the oncotic pressure gradient in the microcirculation but also has been reported to increase the filtration coefficient.[85,86] The result of this almost complete breakdown in control of the microvascular function and the insult of fluid administration is massive edema. This is probably nowhere more apparent than in soft tissues of the face and oropharynx. The danger to the patient is extreme. The edema may obstruct the airway, not only making it laborious or impossible to breathe but also making it difficult for the physician to intubate the patient. To avoid this problem, many practitioners prophylactically intubate patients who have evidence of thermal injury to the upper airway on admission. However, intubation in itself may present problems. The tube may further damage injured areas, especially the larynx.[87] It may be time to reconsider some of these practices. Perhaps some consideration should be given to types of fluid resuscitation, which can prevent some of this soft tissue edema and reduce the volume of fluids required for resuscitation.[88,89]

Tracheobronchial area

With rare exceptions such as inhalation of steam, the injury to the airway is usually from the chemicals in smoke. The heat capacity of air is low and the upper airway circulation very

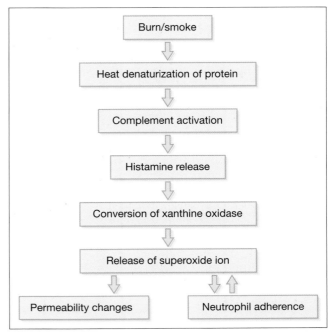

Fig. 18.2 Mechanism for edema formation in the oropharynx.

efficient in warming or cooling the airway gases so that most gasses are at body temperature as they pass the glottis.[90] Flames must almost be in direct contact with the airway to induce thermal injury.[91] The chemicals in smoke are dependent on the materials that are being burned; however, for the most part, the host response is similar. In most instances biological materials such as cotton fabric, wood, or grass contain caustic materials such as reactive oxygen and nitrogen species (ROS and RNS), organic acids, and aldehydes.[92] These chemicals interact with the airway to induce an initial response to trigger an inflammatory response.

Many of the studies that have been reported relative to the bronchial circulation following smoke inhalation injury have been performed in sheep because these animals have a single bronchial artery[93] and have a single lymphatic draining the lung that allows the measure of pulmonary transvascular fluid flux.[94] There was a 10-fold increase in bronchial blood flow within 20 minutes of smoke inhalation.[95] These same animals demonstrate a six-fold increase in pulmonary transvascular fluid flux and a fall in $PaO_2/FiO_2 = 300$, but these were delayed to 24 hours post-injury. Similar findings have been reported in patients with smoke inhalation alone or the combination of a large cutaneous thermal injury and smoke inhalation.[96]

Hyperemia (Figure 18.3a) of the airway is such a consistent finding in smoke inhalation that it is used to diagnose the injury.[97,98] Other variables that are used include injury in an enclosed space, singed nasal hair, and soot in sputum. However these latter findings may be present but the subject may still not develop the signs of low Pa and pulmonary edema characteristic of inhalation injury. Airway inflammation plays a major role in the overall response to inhalation injury.

As we have noted, there is a large sustained increase in blood flow in the airway following smoke inhalation.[99] These changes in blood flow were associated with increased bronchial microvascular permeability to protein and small particles[100] and pressure.[101] Simultaneous with the changes in the function of the bronchial microvasculature, there is a loss or shedding of the bronchial columnar epithelium.[102,103] These changes result in a profuse transudate with a protein content similar to an ultrafiltrate of the plasma.[104] There is also a copious secretion from the goblet cells.[105] Early in the response these secretions are fluid and form a foam material in the airway many have mistaken for severe pulmonary edema in patients.[106] After several hours this transudate/exudate solidifies or clots, forming obstructive materials in the airways.[107] These obstructive materials formed in the upper airway may appear (Figure 18.3b) in the lower airway and alveoli.[105] This obstructive material is problematic from several standpoints. In some rare instances of severe airway injury these materials can induce total obstruction (Figure 18.4). Table 18.5 illustrates the degree of airway obstruction in sheep subjected to burn, smoke, or combined burn and smoke inhalation injury. Occlusion of some of the bronchi or bronchioles in the setting of high production of NO (Figure 18.5) can lead to a loss of hypoxic pulmonary vasoconstriction and thus increased shunt fraction. Loss of hypoxic pulmonary vasoconstriction with inhalation injury has been reported. Furthermore, if single bronchi are occluded while the patient is on a volume-limited ventilated ventilator, there could be overstretch and barotrauma to the alveoli of the non-occluded portion of the lung.

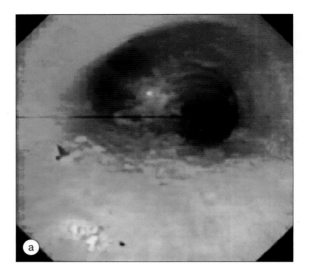

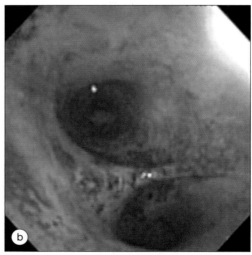

Fig. 18.3 Smoke inhalation injury in patients after burn and smoke inhalation. (a) Hyperemia of airway epithelium. (b) Formation of airway obstructive cast.

The airway is richly innervated with vasomotor and sensory nerve endings.[108] It is also known that these fibers release neuropeptides in response to caustic materials.[109] Neuropeptides release can cause activation of nitric oxide synthase, have chemokine activity, and change microvascular permeability.[110] The resultant activities lead to the formation of reactive oxygen and nitrogen species. Some of the latter are very potent oxidants that can damage DNA. Damage to DNA causes the activation of a repair enzyme poly (ADP-ribose) polymerase (PARP). This enzyme depletes the cell of high-energy phosphates and causes the activation of nuclear factor-κB (NF-κB). Activation of the nuclear factor causes the up-regulation of iNOS and IL-8, thus creating accelerated production of reactive oxygen and nitrogen species.[111] NO and 3-nitrotyrosine, an index of reactive nitrogen species, iNOS mRNA, and protein have been reported to be in the airway after smoke inhalation.[112] Poly (ADP-ribose) [PAR], the product of the constitutive enzyme PARP, was identified in the airway tissues following smoke inhalation. Inhibition of PARP prevented the formation of PAR, the up-regulation of

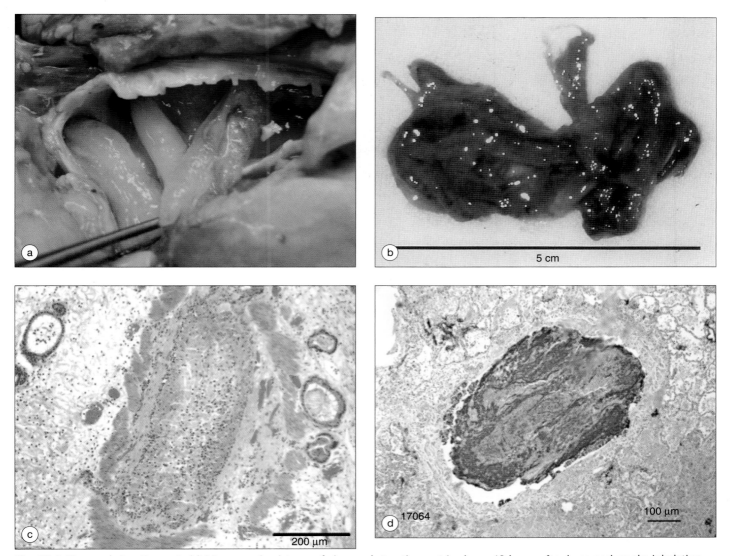

Fig. 18.4 Airway obstructive cast. (a) Macroscopic pictures of airway obstructive cast in sheep 48 hours after burn and smoke inhalation injury. (b) Macroscopic picture of airway cast taken from patient with burn and smoke inhalation injury by bronchoscope.[155] (c and d) Microscopic pictures of totally blocked by obstructive cast bronchi in sheep and bronchiole in patient after burn and smoke inhalation injury.

TABLE 18.5 MEAN LEVELS OF AIRWAY OBSTRUCTION IN UNINJURED SHEEP AND 48 HOURS AFTER BURN, SMOKE INHALATION, AND COMBINED SMOKE INHALATION AND BURN INJURY AIRWAY LEVEL

Injury	Bronchi	Bronchiole	Terminal bronchioles
Uninjured ($n = 5$)	$2.7 \pm 2.4\%$	$1.6 \pm 0.9\%$	$0.0 \pm 0.0\%$
Burn alone ($n = 6$)	$4.4 \pm 3.5\%$	$2.5 \pm 1.5\%$	$0.04 \pm 0.1\%$
Smoke alone ($n = 5$)	$18.1 \pm 10.1\%$ *†	$8.1 \pm 3.0\%$ *†	$0.3 \pm 0.4\%$*
Smoke + burn ($n = 7$)	$29.3 \pm 15.1\%$*†	$11.5 \pm 6.7\%$*†	$1.2 \pm 1.9\%$*

Data are presented as mean percent $\pm$ SD (n = number of animals in each group).
*Significantly different from uninjured animals means, Wilcoxon rank sum test, $p < 0.05$.
†Significantly different from burn injury, Wilcoxon rank sum test, $p < 0.05$.[105]

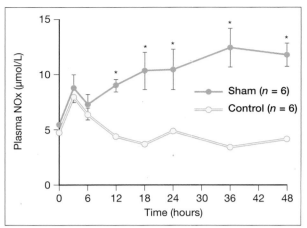

Fig. 18.5 Time changes in plasma concentration of NOx (nitrite/nitrate), a stable metabolite of nitric oxide in sheep subjected to combined burn and smoke inhalation injury. Sham, non-injured, non-treated. Control, injured (flame burn, 40% total body surface area, third degree, non-treated). $*p < 0.05$ vs. Sham.

NF-κB, and the formation of 3-nitrotyrosine.[113] It is interesting to note that in the presence of a PARP inhibitor or in mice lacking the PARP gene, airway inflammation is not seen in a typical asthma model.[114] The pathophysiology of burn and smoke inhalation-related acute lung injury is shown in Figure 18.6.

Lung parenchyma

The lung parenchyma changes, as reflected by reduced PaO_2/FiO_2 and reduced compliance, increased edema formation, are delayed. The delay is dependent on the severity of the airway injury. Lung injury is associated with an increased pulmonary transvascular fluid flux.[115] The degree of transvascular fluid is proportional to the duration of smoke exposure[92] and is independent of the levels of CO in the inhalant gas.[116] The factors responsible for fluid leak are codified in the Starling–Landis equation.[69,70] The variables of this equation relate fluid movement to pressure and permeability variations. With inhalation of smoke there is a reduction in refection coefficient (permeability to protein), an increase in filtration coefficient

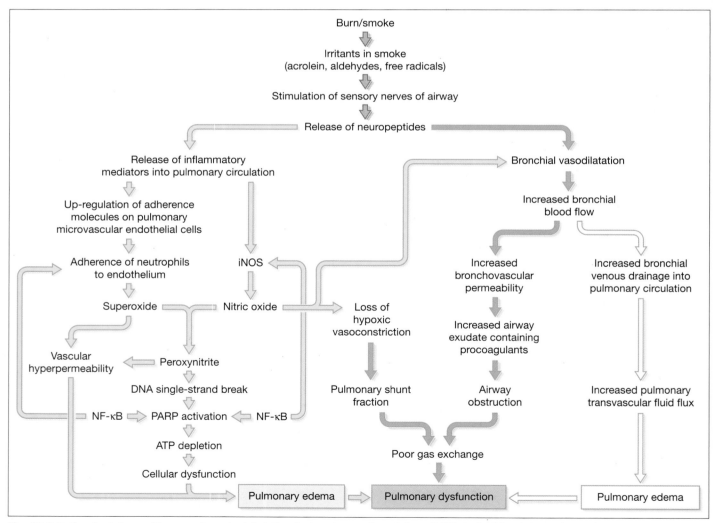

Fig. 18.6 Pathophysiology of burn and smoke inhalation-induced acute lung injury. iNOS, inducible nitric oxide synthase; PARP, poly(ADP-ribose) polymerase.

(permeability to small particles), and an increase in pulmonary microvascular pressure.[117,118]

Animals that had been exposed to smoke inhalation injury were also noted to have reduced PaO_2/FiO_2. The change in this variable showed a good relationship to the histology injury scores and the changes in transvascular fluid flux.[113] In addition, there was a loss of hypoxic pulmonary vasoconstriction in the injured animals that would help to explain the loss of oxygenation.[119] As in the airway, the injury is associated with the reduction of poly (ADP-ribose) and 3-nitrotyrosine and is markedly reduced by the administration of an iNOS or PARP inhibitors.[112,120,121]

The venous outflow of the bronchial circulation drains into the pulmonary microcirculation at the pre-capillary level.[122] Considering the fact that initial damage to the airway appeared to drive the pathophysiology of the parenchyma, led investigators to hypothesize that the bronchial blood might deliver cytotoxic materials or cells into the pulmonary microcirculation. To test this hypothesis, several investigators have tied off the bronchial artery of sheep and then exposed the animals to smoke.[100,123,124] In these studies the hypothesis was affirmed: the lung parenchymal changes were reduced.

What could be the linkage between the airway, the bronchial venous drainage, and parenchymal injury to the lung? Neutrophils activated in the bronchial circulation flow out into the bronchial venous drainage. Activated polymorphonuclear cells (PMNs), especially neutrophils, are stiff. The diameter of neutrophils that have been fixed are approximately $7\,\mu m$.[125] Since these cells have been dehydrated in alcohol as part of the fixation process, unfixed cells are much larger, on the order of $12\,\mu m$. The pulmonary capillary is small, with an average diameter of $6\,\mu m$.[125] Normally, the large neutrophil can traverse the pulmonary capillary by changing shape. However many of the neutrophils have been activated in the bronchial areas, their F-actin is activated and the cells are stiff and cannot deform. These stiff cells are carried to the pulmonary microvasculature where they are impaled by the narrow pulmonary capillaries. The activated neutrophils release reactive oxygen species and proteases that damage the parenchyma. The following evidence supports this concept of neutrophil cytotoxicity. Oxidative processes are well known following inhalation injury. There is lipid peroxidation and release of proteolytic enzymes following injury.[126–128] Administration of protease inhibitors or scavengers of reactive oxygen species will reduce the response to smoke inhalation,[127,129–131] when activated PMNs lose the L-selectin on their surface. This L-selectin shedding is prevented by the treatment with an L-selectin antibody.[132] Treatment of the cells with an antibody to L-selectin will prevent the changes in transvascular fluid flux and other aspects of parenchymal damage.[133] The final proof of this hypothesis was to deplete the animals of their neutrophils and determine how this affected the response to inhalation injury. In these studies of sheep depleted of their leukocytes, a high percentage of the response to smoke inhalation was blocked.[134]

In addition to the depletion of antioxidants discussed above, it has also been reported that burned patients are depleted of arginine.[135] When arginine levels are low, the nitric oxide synthase produces superoxide rather than nitric oxide.[136]

Administration of arginine may assist in reducing the oxidation that occurs with inhalation injury. However, the necessity of administering the arginine as arginine hydrochloride (because of solubility) limits the amount that may be given intravenously without producing acidosis.

Treatment

Some pretreatment for smoke inhalation can be accomplished. People who are chronically exposed to smoke include farmers who burn crops, individuals with fires in their huts, and firefighters. There are reports that individuals who are chronically exposed to smoke are depleted of antioxidants.[137,138] Consequently supplementation of antioxidants should be considered.[137]

In the post-inhalation period a major concern will be the airway. In the case of combined inhalation and burn injuries this is very difficult. In the burn includes the soft tissues of the face, oral pharynx, and neck, intubation is very difficult. Burn injury to these soft tissues results in an almost immediate and severe edema and swelling.[81] Intubation in such an individual requires great skill. Securing the tube is difficult. Accidental removal of the endotracheal tube is easy and may be lethal. Often, burns and/or the chemicals in smoke can damage the larynx and placement of the tube can cause damage and delay healing of such a wound. Tracheostomy is sometimes performed but can also be difficult if it has to be placed through burned skin on the neck. For information in this area, the reader is referred to two excellent chapters in a text on burn care.[139,140]

To counter obstruction, vigorous toilet should be performed. Cast material contains fibrin. Experimentally, the use of heparin has been reported to be effective in reducing airway obstruction.[141] However heparin requires the presence of antithrombin to be effective and this factor has been reported to be deficient following burn injury;[142] consequently, antithrombin has been reported to be effective in animal studies.[143] Antithrombin and may also act as anti-inflammatory agents.[144] Once obstructive materials have formed in the airway, heparin and antithrombin are ineffective in removing them. Animal studies have demonstrated that tissue plasminogen activator could be effective in removing these materials.[145] Aerosolized tissue plasminogen activator has also been reported to be effective in removing bronchial obstructive material in patients who have had Fontan procedures.[146,147] Many burn units nebulize heparin into the airway of their patients with inhalation injury.[148]

Many drugs have proven effective in reducing the injury to the lung parenchyma of in animals models of inhalation injury including cyclooxygenase inhibitors,[149] iNOS inhibitors,[120] PARP inhibitors,[113] and oxygen scavengers,[129] as well as the anticoagulant factors mentioned above. However, only the latter are in clinical use and/or clinical trial.

In many instances conventional methods of ventilation can no longer sustain the pulmonary function of burned patients. Extracorporeal membrane oxygenation has been used in these patients with some success.[150] Techniques have now been developed in animal models of inhalation injury that involve a unique form of CO_2 removal called arterial venous CO_2 removal (AVCO$_2$R). Off-the-shelf CO_2

removal devices, used in extracorporeal bypass and cardiopulmonary bypass, have been modified to be driven by the subject's own arterial pressure.[151] These were tested in animal models and shown to be very successful in reducing pathophysiology, morbidity, mortality, and days of ventilatory support of inhalation injury models.[152–154] AVCO$_2$R is now in clinical trials for the treatment of severe ARDS associated with inhalation injury.

References

1. Herndon DN, Traber DL, Niehaus GD, et al. The pathophysiology of smoke inhalation injury in a sheep model. J Trauma 1984; 24:1044–1051.
2. Herndon DN, Thompson PB, Traber DL. Pulmonary injury in burned patients. Crit Care Clin 1985; 1:79–96.
3. Alcorta R. Smoke inhalation and acute cyanide poisoning. Hydrogen cyanide poisoning proves increasingly common in smoke-inhalation victims. JEMS 2004; 29(8):suppl 6–15; quiz suppl 6–7.
4. Pruitt BA Jr, Goodwin CW, Mason AD Jr. Epidemiological, demographic and outcome characteristics of burn injury. In: Herndon DN, ed. Total burn care. London: WB Saunders; 2002: 16–32.
5. Kobayashi K, Ikeda H, Higuchi R, et al. Epidemiological and outcome characteristics of major burns in Tokyo. Burns 2005; 31(Suppl 1):S3–S11.
6. Pegg SP. Burn epidemiology in the Brisbane and Queensland area. Burns 2005; 31(Suppl 1):S27–S31.
7. Song C, Chua A. Epidemiology of burn injuries in Singapore from 1997 to 2003. Burns 2005; 31(Suppl 1):S18–S26.
8. Tung KY, Chen ML, Wang HJ, et al. A seven-year epidemiology study of 12381 admitted burn patients in Taiwan — using the Internet registration system of the Childhood Burn Foundation. Burns 2005; 31(Suppl 1):S12–S17.
9. Ware LB, Matthay MA. The acute respiratory distress syndrome. N Engl J Med 2000; 342(18):1334–1349.
10. Fodor L, Fodor A, Ramon Y, et al. Controversies in fluid resuscitation for burn management: literature review and our experience. Injury 2006; 37(5):374–379.
11. Ventilation with lower tidal volumes as compared with traditional tidal volumes for acute lung injury and the acute respiratory distress syndrome. The Acute Respiratory Distress Syndrome Network. N Engl J Med 2000; 342(18):1301–1308.
12. Shirani KZ, Pruitt BA Jr, Mason AD Jr. The influence of inhalation injury and pneumonia on burn mortality. Ann Surg 1987; 205:82–87.
13. Linares HA. A report of 115 consecutive autopsies in burned children: 1966–80. Burns 1982; 8:263–270.
14. Saffle JR, Sullivan JJ, Tuohig GM, et al. Multiple organ failure in patients with thermal injury. Crit Care Med 1993; 21(11):1673–1683.
15. Schwela DH, Goldammer JG, Morawska LH, et al. Health guidelines for vegitation fire events. Geneva: World Health Organization; 1999.
16. Schwela D. Cooking smoke: a silent killer. People Planet 1997; 6(3):24–25.
17. Saffle JR. The 1942 fire at Boston's Cocoanut Grove nightclub. Am J Surg 1993; 166(6):581–591.
18. Pittman HS, Schatzki R. Pulmonary effects of the Cocoanut Grove fire; a 5 year follow up study. N Engl J Med 1949; 241(25):1008.
19. Blocker V, Blocker TG Jr. The Texas City disaster: a survey of 3000 casualties. Am J Surg 1949; 78:756–771.
20. Jordan MH, Hollowed KA, Turner DG, et al. The Pentagon attack of September 11, 2001: a burn center's experience. J Burn Care Rehabil 2005; 26(2):109–116.
21. Yurt RW, Bessey PQ, Bauer GJ, et al. A regional burn center's response to a disaster: September 11, 2001, and the days beyond. J Burn Care Rehabil 2005; 26(2):117–124.
22. Rapid assessment of injuries among survivors of the terrorist attack on the World Trade Center, New York City, September 2001. MMWR — Morbidity & Mortality Weekly Report 2002; 51(01):1–5.
23. From the Centers for Disease Control and Prevention. Rapid assessment of injuries among survivors of the terrorist attack on the World Trade Center, New York City, September 2001. JAMA 2002; 287(7):835–838.
24. Prien T, Traber DL. Toxic smoke compounds and inhalation injury — a review. Burns 1988; 14:451–460.
25. Moore SJ, Ho IK, Hume AS. Severe hypoxia produced by concomitant intoxication with sublethal doses of carbon monoxide and cyanide. Toxicol Appl Pharmacol 1991; 109:412–420.
26. Pitt BR, Radford EP, Gurtner GH, et al. Interaction of carbon monoxide and cyanide on cerebral circulation and metabolism. Arch Environ Health 1979; 34:345–349.
27. Haponik EF. Clinical smoke inhalation injury: pulmonary effects. Occup Med 1993; 8:430–468.
28. Terrill JB, Montgomery RR, Reinhardt CF. Toxic gases from fires. Science 1978; 200(4348):1343–1347.
29. Smith RP. Toxic responses of the blood. In: Klaassen CD, Amdur MO, Doull J, eds. Casarett and Doull's toxicology, the basic science of poisons. New York: MacMillan; 1986:223–244.
30. West JB. Pulmonary pathophysiology: the essentials, 6th edn. Baltimore: Lippincott Williams & Wilkins, 2003.
31. Goldbaum LR, Orellano T, Dergal E. Mechanism of the toxic action of carbon monoxide. Ann Clin Lab Sci 1976; 6:372–376.
32. Shimazu T, Ikeuchi H, Sugimoto H, et al. Half-life of blood carboxyhemoglobin after short-term and long-term exposure to carbon monoxide. J Trauma 2000; 49(1):126–131.
33. Alonso JR, Cardellach F, Casademont J, et al. Reversible inhibition of mitochondrial complex IV activity in PBMC following acute smoking. Eur Respir J 2004; 23(2):214–218.
34. Miro O, Alonso JR, Casademont J, et al. Oxidative damage on lymphocyte membranes is increased in patients suffering from acute carbon monoxide poisoning. Toxicol Lett 1999; 110(3): 219–223.
35. Einhorn IN. Physiological and toxicological aspects of smoke produced during the combustion of polymeric materials. Environ Health Perspect 1975; 11:163–189.
36. Schulte JH. Effects of mild carbon monoxide intoxication. Arch Environ Health 1963; 7:524–530.
37. Westphal M, Morita N, Enkhbaatar P, et al. Carboxyhemoglobin formation following smoke inhalation injury in sheep is interrelated with pulmonary shunt fraction. Biochem Biophys Res Commun 2003; 311(3):754–758.
38. Charnock EL, Meehan JJ. Postburn respiratory injuries in children. Pediatr Clin North Am 1980; 27:661–676.
39. Clark CJ, Campbell D, Reid WH. Blood carboxyhaemoglobin and cyanide levels in fire survivors. Lancet 1981; 1:1332–1335.
40. Crapo RO. Smoke-inhalation injuries. JAMA 1981; 246:1694–1696.
41. Pace N, Strajman E, Walker EL. Acceleration of carbon monoxide elimination in man by high pressure oxygen. Science 1950; 111(2894):652–654.
42. Thom SR. Antagonism of carbon monoxide-mediated brain lipid peroxidation by hyperbaric oxygen. Toxicol Appl Pharmacol 1990; 105:340–344.
43. Brown SD, Piantadosi CA. Reversal of carbon monoxide-cytochrome c oxidase binding by hyperbaric oxygen in vivo. Adv Exp Med Biol 1989; 248:747–754.
44. Myers RA, Snyder SK, Linberg S, et al. Value of hyperbaric oxygen in suspected carbon monoxide poisoning. JAMA 1981; 246: 2478–2480.
45. McCord JM. Oxygen-derived radicals: a link between reperfusion injury and inflammation. Fed Proc 1987; 46:2402–2406.
46. Thom SR. Functional inhibition of leukocyte B$_2$ integrins by hyperbaric oxygen in carbon monoxide-mediated brain injury in rats. Toxicol Appl Pharmacol 1993; 123:248–256.

47. Chou KJ, Fisher JL, Silver EJ. Characteristics and outcome of children with carbon monoxide poisoning with and without smoke exposure referred for hyperbaric oxygen therapy. Pediatr Emerg Care 2000; 16(3):151–155.

48. Villanueva E, Bennett MH, Wasiak J, et al. Hyperbaric oxygen therapy for thermal burns. Cochrane Database Syst Rev 2004(3): CD004727.

49. Purser DA, Grimshaw P, Berrill KR. Intoxication by cyanide in fires: a study in monkeys using polyacrylonitrile. Arch Environ Health 1984; 39:394–400.

50. Baud FJ, Barriot P, Toffis V, et al. Elevated blood cyanide concentrations in victims of smoke inhalation. N Engl J Med 1991; 325: 1761–1766.

51. Silverman SH, Purdue GF, Hunt JL, et al. Cyanide toxicity in burned patients. J Trauma 1988; 28:171–176.

52. Biological and chemical terrorism: strategic plan for preparedness and response. Recommendations of the CDC Strategic Planning Workgroup. MMWR Recomm Rep 2000; 49(RR-4):1–14.

53. Eckstein M. Cyanide as a chemical terrorism weapon. JEMS 2004; 29(8):suppl 22–31.

54. Smith PW, Crane R, Sanders DC, et al. Effects of exposure to carbon monoxide and hydrogen cyanide. Physiological and toxological aspects of combustion products. Washington, DC: National Academy of Science; 1976:75–78.

55. Morocco AP. Cyanides. Crit Care Clin 2005; 21(4):691–705.

56. Becker CE. The role of cyanide in fires. Vet Human Toxicol 1985; 27:487–490.

57. Kimmerle G. Aspects and methodology for the evaluation of toxicological parameters during fire exposure. Polymer conference series: flammability characteristics of materials. Salt Lake City: University of Utah; 1973.

58. Kirk MA, Gerace R, Kulig KW. Cyanide and methemoglobin kinetics in smoke inhalation victims treated with the cyanide antidote kit. Ann Emerg Med 1993; 22:1413–1418.

59. Beasley DM, Glass WI. Cyanide poisoning: pathophysiology and treatment recommendations. Occup Med (Lond) 1998; 48(7): 427–431.

60. Moore SJ, Norris JC, Walsh DA, et al. Antidotal use of methemoglobin forming cyanide antagonists in concurrent carbon monoxide/cyanide intoxication. J Pharmacol Exp Ther 1987; 242:70–73.

61. Hall AH, Rumack BH. Clinical toxicology of cyanide. Ann Emerg Med 1986; 15(9):1067–1074.

62. Fortin JL, Ruttiman M, Domanski L, et al. Hydroxocobalamin: treatment for smoke inhalation-associated cyanide poisoning. Meeting the needs of fire victims. JEMS 2004; 29(8):suppl 18–21.

63. Hughart JL, Bashor MM. Industrial chemicals and terrorism: human health threat analysis, mitigation prevention. Atlanta, GA: Agency for Toxic Substances and Disease Registry, US Public Health Service.

64. Anonymous. Combating terrorism: observations on the threat of chemical and biological terrorism. Statement of Henry L. Hinton Jr, Assistant Comptroller General. In Office UGA, ed. Washington, DC: National Security and International Affairs Division; 1999.

65. Author N. Pulmonary agent. US Army Medical Research Institute of Chemical Defence Medical Management of chemical casualties handbook. Aberdeen, MA: USAMRICD; 2000:18–34.

66. Medical management for phosgene. Managing hazardous material incidents, Vol. III: agency for toxic substances and disease registry. Atlanta, GA: US Department of Health and Human Services; 2001.

67. Borak J, Diller WF. Phosgene exposure: mechanisms of injury and treatment strategies. J Occup Environ Med 2001; 43(2):110–119.

68. Burns TR, Mace ML, Greenberg SD, et al. Ultrastructure of acute ammonia toxicity in the human lung. Am J Forensic Med Pathol 1985; 6(3):204–210.

69. Starling EH. On the absorption of fluids from the connective tissue spaces. J Physiol 1896; 19:312–326.

70. Landis EM, Pappenheimer JR. Exchange of substances through the capillary walls. In: Hamilton WF, Dow P, eds. Handbook of physiology. Baltimore, MD: Williams & Wilkins; 1963:2(2):961–1034.

71. Friedl HP, Till GO, Trentz O, et al. Roles of histamine, complement and xanthine oxidase in thermal injury of skin. Am J Pathol 1989; 135:203–217.

72. Oldham KT, Guice KS, Till GO, et al. Evidence of local complement activation in cutaneous thermal injury in rats. Prog Clin Biol Res 1988; 264:421–424.

73. Schlayer HJ, Laaff H, Peters T, et al. Involvement of tumor necrosis factor in endotoxin-triggered neutrophil adherence to sinusoidal endothelial cells of mouse liver and its modulation in acute phase. J Hepatol 1988; 7:239–249.

74. Granger DN, McCord JM, Parks DA, et al. Xanthine oxidase inhibitors attenuate ischemia-induced vascular permeability changes in the cat intestine. Gastroenterology 1986; 90:80–84.

75. Granger DN. Role of xanthine oxidase and granulocytes in ischemia-reperfusion injury. Am J Physiol 1988; 255:H1269–H1275.

76. McBride AG, Brown GC. Activated human neutrophils rapidly break down nitric oxide. FEBS Lett 1997; 417:231–234.

77. DemLing RH, LaLonde C. Topical ibuprofen decreases early postburn edema. Surgery 1987; 102:857–861.

78. Herndon DN, Abston S, Stein MD. Increased thromboxane B2 levels in the plasma of burned and septic burned patients. Surg Gynecol Obstet 1984; 159:210–213.

79. Vindenes H, Ulvestad E, Bjerknes R. Increased levels of circulating interleukin-8 in patients with large burns: relation to burn size and sepsis. J Trauma 1995; 39:635–640.

80. Pitt RM, Parker JC, Jurkovich GJ, et al. Analysis of altered capillary pressure and permeability after thermal injury. J Surg Res 1987; 42:693–702.

81. Lund T. The 1999 Everett Idris Evans memorial lecture. Edema generation following thermal injury: an update. J Burn Care Rehabil 1999; 20(6):445–452.

82. Pitkanen J, Lund T, Aanderud L, et al. Transcapillary colloid osmotic pressures in injured and non-injured skin of seriously burned patients. Burns 1987; 13:198–203.

83. Zetterstrom H, Arturson G. Plasma oncotic pressure and plasma protein concentration in patients following thermal injury. Acta Anaesthesiol Scandi 1980; 24:288–294.

84. Onarheim H, Reed RK. Thermal skin injury: effect of fluid therapy on the transcapillary colloid osmotic gradient. J Surg Res 1991; 50:272–278.

85. Sheng ZY, Tung YL. Neutrophil chemiluminescence in burned patients. J Trauma 1987; 27:587–595.

86. Conhaim RL, Harms BA. A simplified two-pore filtration model explains the effects of hypoproteinemia on lung and soft tissue lymph flux in awake sheep. Microvasc Res 1992; 44: 14–26.

87. Calhoun KH, Deskin RW, Garza C, et al. Long-term airway sequelae in a pediatric burn population. Laryngoscope 1988; 98:721–725.

88. Brazeal BA, Honeycutt D, Traber LD, et al. Pentafraction for superior resuscitation of the ovine thermal burn. Crit Care Med 1995; 23:332–339.

89. DemLing RH, Kramer GC, Gunther R, et al. Effect of nonprotein colloid on postburn edema formation in soft tissues and lung. Surgery 1984; 95:593–602.

90. Baile EM, Dahlby RW, Wiggs BR, et al. Role of tracheal and bronchial circulation in respiratory heat exchange. J Appl Physiol 1985; 58:217–222.

91. Moritz AR, Henriques FC, McLean R. The effect of inhaled heat on the air passages and lungs: an experimental investigation. Am J Pathol 1945; 21:311–326.

92. Kimura R, Traber LD, Herndon DN, et al. Increasing duration of smoke exposure induces more severe lung injury in sheep. J Appl Physiol 1988; 64:1107–1113.

93. Magno MG, Fishman AP. Origin, distribution, and blood flow of bronchial circulation in anesthetized sheep. J Appl Physiol 1982; 53:272–279.

94. Staub NC, Bland RD, Brigham KL, et al. Preparation of chronic lung lymph fistulas in sheep. J Surg Res 1975; 19:315–320.

95. Abdi S, Herndon D, McGuire J, et al. Time course of alterations in lung lymph and bronchial blood flows after inhalation injury. J Burn Care Rehabil 1990; 11:510–515.

96. Herndon DN, Barrow RE, Traber DL, et al. Extravascular lung water changes following smoke inhalation and massive burn injury. Surgery 1987; 102:341–349.

97. Ramzy PI, Barret JP, Herndon DN. Thermal injury. Crit Care Clin 1999; 15(2):333–352, ix.

98. Inhalation injury: diagnosis. J Am Coll Surg 2003; 196(2): 307–312.

99. Stothert JC Jr, Ashley KD, Kramer GC, et al. Intrapulmonary distribution of bronchial blood flow after moderate smoke inhalation. J Appl Physiol 1990; 69:1734–1739.

100. Hales CA, Barkin P, Jung W, et al. Bronchial artery ligation modifies pulmonary edema after exposure to smoke with acrolein. J Appl Physiol 1989; 67:1001–1006.

101. Hinder F, Matsumoto N, Booke M, et al. Inhalation injury increases the anastomotic bronchial blood flow in the pouch model of the left ovine lung. Shock 1997; 8:131–135.

102. Linares HA, Herndon DN, Traber DL. Sequence of morphologic events in experimental smoke inhalation. J Burn Care Rehabil 1989; 10:27–37.

103. Abdi S, Evans MJ, Cox RA, et al. Inhalation injury to tracheal epithelium in an ovine model of cotton smoke exposure. Early phase (30 minutes). Am Rev Respir Dis 1990; 142:1436–1439.

104. Barrow RE, Morris SE, Basadre JO, et al. Selective permeability changes in the lungs and airways of sheep after toxic smoke inhalation. J Appl Physiol 1990; 68:2165–2170.

105. Cox RA, Burke AS, Soejima K, et al. Airway obstruction in sheep with burn and smoke inhalation injuries. Am J Respir Cell Mol Biol 2003; 29(3 Pt 1):295–302.

106. Mathru M, Venus B, Rao T, et al. Noncardiac pulmonary edema precipitated by tracheal intubation in patients with injury. Crit Care Med 1983; 11:804–806.

107. Herndon DN, Traber LD, Linares H, et al. Etiology of the pulmonary pathophysiology associated with inhalation injury. Resuscitation 1986; 14:43–59.

108. Perez Fontan JJ. On lung nerves and neurogenic injury. Ann Med 2002; 34(4):226–240.

109. Fontan JJ, Cortright DN, Krause JE, et al. Substance P and neurokinin-1 receptor expression by intrinsic airway neurons in the rat. Am J Physiol Lung Cell Mol Physiol 2000; 278(2):L344–L355.

110. Kraneveld AD, Nijkamp FP. Tachykinins and neuro-immune interactions in asthma. Int Immunopharmacol 2001; 1(9–10): 1629–1650.

111. Virag L. Poly(ADP-ribosyl)ation in asthma and other lung diseases. Pharmacol Res 2005; 52(1):83–92.

112. Soejima K, Traber LD, Schmalstieg FC, et al. Role of nitric oxide in vascular permeability after combined burns and smoke inhalation injury. Am J Respir Crit Care Med 2001; 163:745–752.

113. Shimoda K, Murakami K, Enkhbaatar P, et al. Effect of poly(ADP ribose) synthetase inhibition on burn and smoke inhalation injury in sheep. Am J Physiol Lung Cell Mol Physiol 2003; 285(1): L240–L249.

114. Boulares AH, Zoltoski AJ, Sherif ZA, et al. Gene knockout or pharmacological inhibition of poly(ADP-ribose) polymerase-1 prevents lung inflammation in a murine model of asthma. Am J Respir Cell Mol Biol 2003; 28(3):322–329.

115. Traber DL, Schlag G, Redl H, et al. Pulmonary edema and compliance changes following smoke inhalation. J Burn Care Rehabil 1985; 6:490–494.

116. Sugi K, Theissen JL, Traber LD, et al. Impact of carbon monoxide on cardiopulmonary dysfunction after smoke inhalation injury. Circ Res 1990; 66:69–75.

117. Isago T, Fujioka K, Traber LD, et al. Derived pulmonary capillary pressure changes after smoke inhalation in sheep. Crit Care Med 1991; 19:1407–1413.

118. Isago T, Noshima S, Traber LD, et al. Analysis of pulmonary microvascular permeability after smoke inhalation. J Appl Physiol 1991; 71:1403–1408.

119. Westphal M, Cox RA, Traber LD, et al. Combined burn and smoke inhalation injury impairs ovine hypoxic pulmonary vasoconstriction. Crit Care Med 2006; 34(5):1428–1436.

120. Enkhbaatar P, Murakami K, Shimoda K, et al. The inducible nitric oxide synthase inhibitor BBS-2 prevents acute lung injury in sheep after burn and smoke inhalation injury. Am J Respir Crit Care Med 2003; 167(7):1021–1026.

121. Murakami K, Enkhbaatar P, Shimoda K, et al. Inhibition of poly (ADP-ribose) polymerase attenuates acute lung injury in an ovine model of sepsis. Shock 2004; 21(2):126–133.

122. Charan NB, Turk GM, Dhand R. Gross and subgross anatomy of bronchial circulation in sheep. J Appl Physiol 1984; 57:658–664.

123. Efimova O, Volokhov AB, Iliaifar S, et al. Ligation of the bronchial artery in sheep attenuates early pulmonary changes following exposure to smoke. J Appl Physiol 2001; 88:888–893.

124. Soejima K, Schmalstieg FC, Sakurai H, et al. Pathophysiological analysis of combined burn and smoke inhalation injuries in sheep. Am J Physiol Lung Cell Mol Physiol 2001; 280:L1233–L1241.

125. Doerschuk CM, Beyers N, Coxson HO, et al. Comparison of neutrophil and capillary diameters and their relation to neutrophil sequestration in the lung. J Appl Physiol 1993; 74:3040–3045.

126. Youn YK, LaLonde C, Demling R. Oxidants and the pathophysiology of burn and smoke inhalation injury. Free Radic Biol Med 1992; 12:409–415.

127. Niehaus GD, Kimura R, Traber LD, et al. Administration of a synthetic antiprotease reduces smoke-induced lung injury. J Appl Physiol 1990; 69:694–699.

128. Traber DL, Herndon DN, Stein MD, et al. The pulmonary lesion of smoke inhalation in an ovine model. Circ Shock 1986; 18:311–323.

129. Nguyen TT, Cox CS Jr, Herndon DN, et al. Effects of manganese superoxide dismutase on lung fluid balance after smoke inhalation. J Appl Physiol 1995; 78:2161–2168.

130. Nguyen TT, Cox CS, Traber DL, et al. Free radical activity and loss of plasma antioxidants, vitamin E, and sulfhydryl groups in patients with burns: the 1993 Moyer Award. J Burn Care Rehabil 1993; 14:602–609.

131. Nguyen TT, Herndon DN, Cox CS, et al. Effect of manganous superoxide dismutase on lung fluid balance after smoke inhalation injury. Proceedings of the American Burn Association; 1993: 25,31.

132. Schenarts PJ, Schmalstieg FC, Hawkins H, et al. Effects of an L-selectin antibody on the pulmonary and systemic manifestations of severe smoke inhalation injuries in sheep. J Burn Care Rehabil 2000; 21:229–240.

133. Sakurai H, Schmalstieg FC, Traber LD, et al. Role of L-selectin in physiological manifestations after burn and smoke inhalation injury in sheep. J Appl Physiol 1999; 86(4):1151–1159.

134. Basadre JO, Sugi K, Traber DL, et al. The effect of leukocyte depletion on smoke inhalation injury in sheep. Surgery 1988; 104:208–215.

135. Yu YM, Ryan CM, Castillo L, et al. Arginine and ornithine kinetics in severely burned patients: increased rate of arginine disposal. Am J Physiol Endocrinol Metab 2001; 280:E509–E517.

136. Xia Y, Roman LJ, Masters BS, et al. Inducible nitric-oxide synthase generates superoxide from the reductase domain. J Biol Chem 1998; 273:22635–226339.

137. Bruno RS, Traber MG. Cigarette smoke alters human vitamin E requirements. J Nutr 2005; 135(4):671–674.

138. Morita N, Traber MG, Westphal M, et al. Oral supplementation of alpha-tocopherol attenuates acute lung injury following combined burn and smoke inhalation injury in sheep. Shock 2006; (In press).

139. Fitzpatrick DF, Gioffi WG. Diagnosis and treatment of inhalation injury. In: Herndon D, ed. Total burn care. New York: WB Saunders; 2002:232–242.

140. Mlcak R, Herndon D. Respiratory care. In: Herndon D, ed. Total burn care. New York: WB Saunders; 2002:242–267.

141. Brown M, Desai M, Traber LD, et al. Dimethylsulfoxide with heparin in the treatment of smoke inhalation injury. J Burn Care Rehabil 1988; 9:22–25.

142. Kowal-Vern A, McGill V, Walenga JM, et al. Antithrombin(H) concentrate infusions are safe and effective in patients with thermal injuries. J Burn Care Rehabil 2000; 21:115–127.

143. Murakami K, McGuire R, Cox RA, et al. Recombinant antithrombin attenuates pulmonary inflammation following smoke

inhalation and pneumonia in sheep. Crit Care Med 2003; 31(2): 577–583.

144. Vincent JL. Infection/inflammation and hemostasis. Curr Hematol Rep 2003; 2(5):407–410.

145. Enkhbaatar P, Murakami K, Cox R, et al. Aerosolized tissue plasminogen activator improves pulmonary function in sheep with burn and smoke inhalation. Shock 2004; 22(1):70–75.

146. Costello JM, Steinhorn D, McColley S, et al. Treatment of plastic bronchitis in a Fontan patient with tissue plasminogen activator: a case report and review of the literature. Pediatrics 2002; 109(4): e67.

147. Wakeham MK, Van Bergen AH, Torero LE, et al. Long-term treatment of plastic bronchitis with aerosolized tissue plasminogen activator in a Fontan patient. Pediatr Crit Care Med 2005; 6(1):76–78.

148. Desai MH, Mlcak R, Richardson J, et al. Reduction in mortality in pediatric patients with inhalation injury with aerosolized heparin/N-acetylcystine [correction of acetylcystine] therapy. J Burn Care Rehabil 1998; 19(3):210–212.

149. Enkhbaatar P, Murakami K, Shimoda K, et al. Inducible nitric oxide synthase dimerization inhibitor prevents cardiovascular and renal morbidity in sheep with combined burn and smoke inhalation injury. Am J Physiol Heart Circ Physiol 2003; 285(6):H2430–H2436.

150. Pierre EJ, Zwischenberger JB, Angel C, et al. Extracorporeal membrane oxygenation in the treatment of respiratory failure in pediatric patients with burns. J Burn Care Rehabil 1998; 19: 131–134.

151. Alpard SK, Zwischenberger JB, Tao W, et al. Reduced ventilator pressure and improved P/F ratio during percutaneous arteriovenous carbon dioxide removal for severe respiratory failure. Ann Surg 1999; 230:215–224.

152. Schmalstieg FC, Chow J, Savage C, et al. Interleukin-8, aquaporin-1, and inducible nitric oxide synthase in smoke and burn injured sheep treated with percutaneous carbon dioxide removal. ASAIO J 2001; 47:365–371.

153. Zwischenberger JB, Wang D, Lick SD, et al. The paracorporeal artificial lung improves 5-day outcomes from lethal smoke/burn-induced acute respiratory distress syndrome in sheep. Ann Thorac Surg 2002; 74(4):1011–1016; discussion 7–8.

154. Zwischenberger JB, Savage C, Witt SA, et al. Arterio-venous CO_2 removal (AVCO₂R) perioperative management: rapid recovery and enhanced survival. J Invest Surg 2002; 15(1):15–21.

155. Nakae H, Tanaka H, Inaba H. Failure to clear casts and secretions following inhalation injury can be dangerous: report of a case. Burns 2001; 27(2):189–191.

Chapter 19

Diagnosis and treatment of inhalation injury

Nora Nugent and David N. Herndon

Introduction

Inhalation injury remains one of the most critical injuries following thermal insult. It may occur in conjunction with cutaneous burns or in isolation. The severity of injury varies, depending on the chemical composition of the agent(s) inhaled, the duration of exposure, temperatures reached during combustion and pre-existing comorbidities.[1,2] For the most part, treatment consists of supportive respiratory and critical care measures.[3–6]

Many studies over the years have shown inhalation injury to be strongly associated with increased morbidity[6,7] and mortality in the thermally-injured patient. In one study by Shirani et al, the presence of an inhalation injury increased mortality by up to 20%, and pneumonia by up to 40%.[7] Most prediction models for mortality in burns include age extremes, burn size and presence of an inhalation injury as risk factors for increasing probability of death.[8,9] When inhalation injury and another risk factor, such as an elderly patient or an extensive burn, are both present, the influence on mortality rises.[8,10] Improvements in survival of patients with inhalation injury have been attributed to better overall burn outcomes, improved ventilatory management and improved management of pneumonias.[11]

Inhalation injuries are present in approximately one-third of major burn patients.[3,7,12,13] Early diagnosis and treatment of this injury, and the resulting complications associated with it, are required to reduce the consequent impact of this injury on morbidity and mortality rates. Clinicians involved in burn care should have a high index of suspicion for inhalation injury when assessing the burn victim, as missing or underestimating the extent of respiratory compromise can have devastating effects on the patient.

Pathophysiology of inhalation injury

Inhalation injury can occur from either the inspiration of superheated gases or steam, or the toxic, often incomplete products of combustion.[4] The respiratory tract can be injured in one or more of three zones; supraglottic, tracheobronchial and parenchymal. The supraglottic area can be injured by direct heat or chemicals. Severe edema can occur quickly, causing upper airway obstruction. Direct thermal injury to the lower airway is less common than injury due to inhalation of noxious gases, and is usually associated with steam inhalation injuries. Steam has been shown to have a heat-carrying capacity 4000 times greater than hot dry air, and also gives up heat more slowly. As a result steam-related lung injuries can be more severe.[14–16]

The toxic contents of fire smoke vary according to the source of combustion and the amount of oxygen in the environment. Carbon monoxide (CO) and several organic chemicals such as aldehydes are usually present.[3,17] Nitrogen- or halogen-containing polymers in building materials can cause release of hydrogen cyanide and inorganic acids.[17] Sulphur- and nitrogen-containing oxides are also often present.[1]

The clinical course of the patient with an inhalation injury can usually be broken into three stages. During the first phase (0–36 hours), carbon monoxide poisoning, hypoxia and thermal injury occur. Upper airway obstruction and bronchospasm can also occur here. This can result in acute pulmonary insufficiency.[1,6,18] The second phase (24–72 hours) encompasses pulmonary edema, atelectasis and tracheobronchitis.[3,4,618,19] There is damage to the airway and alveolar epithelium, with sloughing of mucosa and formation of mucous plugs and casts, which can cause obstruction and air trapping (Figure 19.1). This can result in areas of atelectasis and ventilation/perfusion (V/Q) mismatching. The normal ciliary action of the mucosa is disrupted, impairing the patient's ability to clear foreign particles from the airway. There is also an increase in capillary permeability, thus increasing lung water, causing pulmonary edema and reducing lung compliance. Surfactant can also become impaired by the noxious chemicals inhaled.[3,6,18,19] As a result of these assaults on respiratory function, gas exchange can become compromised at this time. Inflammatory mediators are released at this stage from damaged cells and inflammatory cells, such as alveolar macrophages and neutrophils. Alveolar macrophages appear to have increased production of superoxide radicals and tumor necrosis factor-α (TNFα), as well as impaired phagocytosis of bacteria.[18–20] The third phase is bronchopneumonia typically

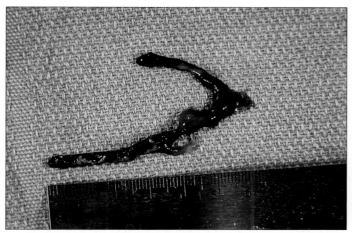

Fig. 19.1 Tracheal cast taken from the carina of a child. (From Barret JP, Herndon DN. Color atlas of burn care. Philadelphia: WB Saunders; 2001.)

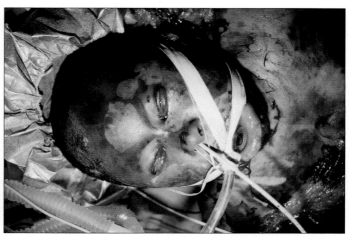

Fig. 19.2 Severe head and neck burns with marked edema. (From Barret JP, Herndon DN. Color atlas of burn care. Philadelphia: WB Saunders; 2001.)

occurring 3 to 10 days post injury, and as a result of impaired lung defenses such as the mucociliary system and alveolar macrophages, and abnormal lung function and ventilation.[5,6,18] Respiratory failure and acute respiratory distress syndrome (ARDS) can develop from the initial inhalation injury.

Diagnosis

When a burn victim is being assessed, the clinician should always be alert to the possibility of the presence of an inhalation injury. Patients with inhalation injuries may present with or without cutaneous burns. Important details in the history include if the patient was exposed to smoke in an enclosed space such as often happens in house fires or industrial accidents,[2] and also the duration of exposure to smoke. Time from injury to arrival at hospital or treatment at scene, and use of oxygen should be noted. If possible, the source of combustion should be determined, as some chemicals are more irritating than others to the airway. Carbon monoxide is usually present;[17,21] however, hydrogen cyanide and hydrochloric acid can be released from synthetic polymers used in the modern building industry such as polyvinyl chloride.[17] Zinc chloride is present in smoke bombs, and although rare, can lead to chemical pneumonitis and ARDS with a high mortality rate.[22]

During the initial assessment, the first priority is to establish if there is an immediate threat to airway patency. When a patient has hoarseness and stridor, partial airway obstruction is present, usually due to edema of the upper airway. These patients should be intubated as there is a significant risk of progression to complete airway obstruction.[3,4] Head and neck cutaneous burns may contribute to this airway problem as well as inhalation injury (Figure 19.2). This is particularly important in small children, where, due to the small diameter of the airway, even moderate edema can result in severe or complete airway obstruction. Edema can be progressive, as the body responds to injury and as resuscitation fluid is given.[4] Signs and symptoms that should evoke suspicion of an inhalation injury include dyspnea, hoarse voice, cough, anxiety or agitation, stridor, wheezing, facial burns, singed nasal hairs, production of carbonaceous sputum or presence of carbonaceous

material in the oral cavity.[4] These patients may also be disorientated or obtunded or in a coma. While the altered mental status may be as a result of CO or cyanide poisoning,[23,24] confounding factors such as intoxication with alcohol or other substances, or head trauma need to be outruled. When CO poisoning is present, cutaneous burn wounds may take on a cherry red appearance.

A carboxyhemoglobin blood level should be drawn on arrival at hospital, and the result correlated with the time from insult to treatment/use of oxygen. As CO binds to the oxygen-binding sites of hemoglobin with a greater affinity than oxygen, it reduces the oxygen-carrying capacity of blood and thus, oxygen delivery to the tissues. Systemic hypoxia develops as a result.[5,25] During this time, arterial oxygen partial pressure and oxygen saturations are often normal.[4] While an arterial blood gas should be drawn from the patient, normal oxygen values cannot be relied upon during the initial stages, and cannot be used to outrule an inhalation injury. Later as the response to injury evolves, arterial blood gas values can deteriorate, and can be used to monitor the patient's course. Blood cyanide levels may also be measured to assess exposure to hydrogen cyanide.[17,26]

Signs and symptoms indicating inhalation injury, or a history suggesting the possibility of an inhalation injury, are usually present. However, these can sometimes be unreliable, and other methods may be used to confirm the diagnosis. Chest radiography is an insensitive measure of inhalation injury. The initial radiograph is often normal,[4,27] but can be useful as baseline study. When atelectasis or pulmonary edema develop, this can show up on X-ray, as can later pneumonia and ARDS changes. Computed tomography is generally not used for the diagnosis of smoke inhalation, although atelectasis and infiltrations can show up on this scan.[28]

One of the most useful tools for the assessment of inhalation injury is the fiberoptic bronchoscope[4,29-31] (Figure 19.3). Direct visualization of the supraglottic airway as well as the tracheobronchial tree can be achieved. This allows assessment of edema of the airway mucosa and patency of the supraglottic airway, thus identifying patients at risk for airway occlusion (Figure 19.4). If deemed necessary, an endotracheal tube of

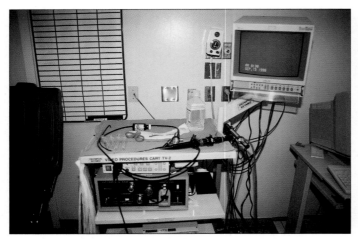

Fig. 19.3 Bronchoscope and bronchoscopy equipment. (From Barret JP, Herndon DN. Color atlas of burn care. Philadelphia: WB Saunders; 2001.)

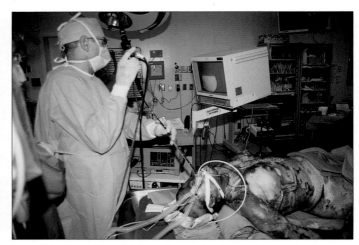

Fig. 19.5 Nasotracheal intubation under direct vision using a bronchoscope. (From Barret JP, Herndon DN. Color atlas of burn care. Philadelphia: WB Saunders; 2001.)

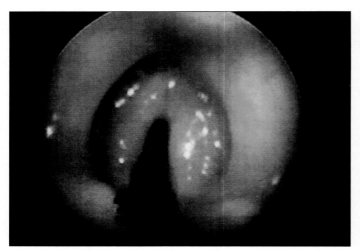

Fig. 19.4 Edematous larynx with decrease in opening but normal movement. (From Barret JP, Herndon DN. Color atlas of burn care. Philadelphia: WB Saunders; 2001.)

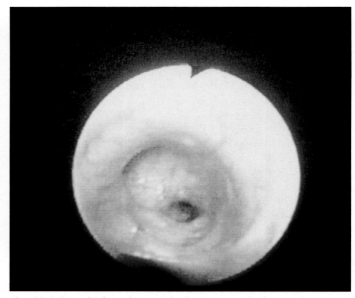

Fig. 19.6 Bronchial erythema. The lesions may be hemorrhagic and friable. (From Barret JP, Herndon DN. Color atlas of burn care. Philadelphia: WB Saunders; 2001.)

appropriate size can be placed over the bronchoscope, prior to commencement of the procedure. Then if there is a need for intubation, the tube can be slid down over the bronchoscope, and secured in place (Figure 19.5). The presence or absence of soot or carbonaceous material in the supraglottic and the tracheobronchial tree can also be seen, as can early inflammatory changes in the tracheal mucosa, such as edema, hyperemia and mucosal sloughing and breakdown (Figures 19.6–19.8). If required, biopsies can also be taken of the mucosa.[30] Bronchoscopy can be performed without sedation, as local anesthesia of the airway is adequate for most patients to tolerate the procedure. Lidocaine sprays can be used for the supraglottic area, and lidocaine can be administered to the lower airways through the appropriate channel in the bronchoscope. When photographic and video equipment are available, this becomes a useful teaching tool. In experienced hands, the complication rate of these bronchoscopies is low.[30] Complications include hemoptysis, pneumothorax, pneumonia and cardiac arrhythmias.

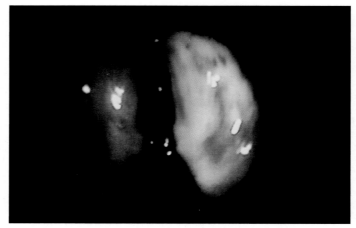

Fig. 19.7 Carbonaceous material on cords. (From Barret JP, Herndon DN. Color atlas of burn care. Philadelphia: WB Saunders; 2001.)

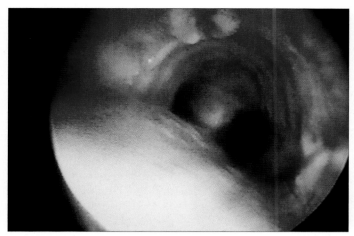

Fig. 19.8 Tracheal cast formation at the level of the carina. (From Barret JP, Herndon DN. Color atlas of burn care. Philadelphia: WB Saunders; 2001.)

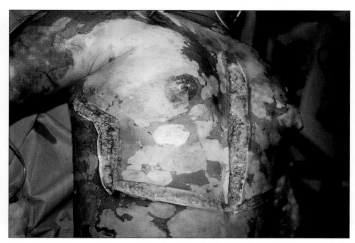

Fig. 19.9 Chest escharotomies in full-thickness burns. (From Barret JP, Herndon DN. Color atlas of burn care. Philadelphia: WB Saunders; 2001.)

Pulmonary function tests are more useful for follow-up assessments of patients with inhalation injuries than for diagnosis in the acute setting, as they are effort-dependant and it can be difficult to obtain reliable values initially. They have a useful role in evaluating patients for residual impairment in lung function following inhalation injury.[32]

Less commonly utilized, is xenon-133 ventilation-perfusion scanning. Intravenous injection of the radioisotope is performed, and then serial scintiphotograms of the chest are taken. Areas demonstrating delayed excretion of the xenon isotope by the lung indicate regions of small airway partial or total obstruction.[4,5,31,33] Patients with pre-existing respiratory disease such as chronic obstructive pulmonary disease or a pneumonia prior to thermal injury, may have unreliable results with this technique. It is useful as a confirmatory test if inhalation injury is suspected but not confirmed by other investigations.

Treatment

The management of patients with inhalation injury mostly consists of supportive treatment of the respiratory system until the patient is able to maintain adequate ventilation and gas exchange independently. For some inhaled toxins, there are additional therapeutic agents that can be used to alleviate the harm caused by their inspiration. Treatment should begin at the scene of injury. The victim must be removed from the unsafe area in a manner that does not cause further harm to them or to the rescuer. In the victim with cutaneous burns, the burning process must be halted. Next the airway needs to be assessed and if necessary secured, with protection of the cervical spine, if appropriate. Usually obstruction has not yet developed at this stage, but if the airway appears compromised, it must be protected. Oropharyngeal sweeps can clear any intraoral debris, and artificial airways such as nasopharyngeal or oropharyngeal airways can help. Sometimes, it is necessary to intubate using an endotracheal tube or in emergency situations, cricothyroidotomies. Once an adequate airway is in place, victims should receive 100% oxygen until assessed at a healthcare facility. Next, ventilation and circula-

tion need to be assessed. Appropriate intravenous access should be obtained, and fluid administration should begin at this stage.

A focused history and physical examination need to be obtained, including a neurological assessment, bearing in mind that the patient with an inhalation injury may have other, sometimes more serious and imminently life-threatening injuries. Cutaneous burns are often but not always present. The signs and symptoms of an inhalation injury need to be looked for. A blood carboxyhemoglobin level and an arterial blood gas should be obtained, along with a baseline chest radiograph. Fiberoptic bronchoscopy is useful at this stage, both to confirm the diagnosis, and to intubate the patient if this is necessary.[14,29–31] Intubation should be performed if any signs of upper airway obstruction, such as stridor, are present, if the airway appears at risk from progressive edema, or if the patient is failing to maintain adequate oxygenation. If at potential risk of airway obstruction, but no significant edema is present, the patient may be kept under close observation for a period of time, until the time of maximal risk has passed 24–36 hours post injury. If circumferential chest wall cutaneous burn eschar is present and limiting ventilation, escharotomies should be performed[4] (Figure 19.9). The incisions should adequately release both sides of the chest wall and connect transversely at the sternal notch, or costal margin. Fluid resuscitation must be commenced if significant cutaneous burns are present, to prevent hypovolemia and its associated problems. There are several resuscitation formulae that can be used to determine the fluid requirements of the patient; however, the infusion rate should be titrated to maintain an adequate urine output. Generally 0.5–1 mL urine/kg/hour is acceptable in adults, and 1–2 mL urine/kg/hour in children. Several studies have shown, that in the presence of an inhalation injury, the patient's fluid requirement is increased.[12,34,35]

Patients with inhalation injury commonly have CO and cyanide exposure. If the initial carboxyhemoglobin level is high, patients should receive 100% oxygen, until a level under 10% is reached. However, low or normal levels do not outrule inhalation injury. CO binds to iron-containing compounds such as hemoglobin and cytochromes. It has a much higher affinity for the oxygen-binding site on the hemoglobin than oxygen, and causes a leftward shift of the oxygen–hemoglobin dissociation curve, thus diminishing the amount of oxygen transported to the tissues. It also disrupts the action of cytochromes and intracellular utilization of oxygen, causing a hypoxic environment.[36] Using 100% oxygen decreases the elimination half-life ($t_{1/2}$) of CO, which is dependant on oxygen tension. On room air (FiO$_2$ 0.21), the $t_{1/2}$ is approximately 320 minutes, while on 100% normobaric oxygen, it is reduced to 80 minutes, lower in some studies.[37] When hyperbaric oxygen therapy (2–3 atmospheres) is used, this decreases to 23 minutes.[38,39] Hyperbaric oxygen therapy is usually delivered in a monoplace hyperbaric chamber. A typical regimen consists of 90 minute sessions at 2–3 atmospheres, with 10 minute airbreaks to lower the incidence of seizures due to oxygen toxicity. Patient access can be difficult in small chambers, so caution should be used in placing unstable patients under this treatment. Larger chambers expose staff to the risks of treatment.[4] Some studies have shown improvement in neurological complications of CO poisoning by using hyperbaric oxygen therapy;[40] however, a review of seven randomized trials of hyperbaric compared to normobaric oxygen therapy, published in 2005 by Juurlink et al., found mixed results for the reduction of neurological sequelae. They concluded that further research was needed to establish this effect of hyperbaric oxygen treatment.[39] For those suspected of having cyanide toxicity as a component of their inhalation injury, blood cyanide levels can be measured.[26,41,42] This assay may not be readily available in many hospitals, and by the time a result is obtained, it may not be clinically useful. The half-life of cyanide is approximately 3 hours.[43] The clinical significance of cyanide levels is controversial, with no clear correlation with mortality. Cyanide can cause hypoxia and otherwise unexplained metabolic acidosis. Therapy is also controversial, with some advocating aggressive supportive treatment, and others, the use of cyanide antidotes. The rationale behind treatment is to oxidize hemoglobin to methemoglobin, which preferentially binds cyanide to form cyanmethemoglobin. This dissociates to form free cyanide, which is metabolized by the liver mitochondria, using thiosulfate as a substrate, to thiocyanate, which is excreted in the urine.[44] Amyl nitrite or sodium nitrite and sodium thiosulfate are used to achieve this effect. However the nitrites can cause significant hypotension and cardiovascular instability, and should be used with caution in the burn patient, who is often hypovolemic. Because of this, thiosulfate is sometimes given alone, as this is safer, although its effect is much slower.[44] Chelating agents, such as hydroxycobalamin (B$_{12}$) or dicobalt edentate, have also been used as cyanide antidotes.[44,45] The use of agents to treat cyanide toxicity should be reserved for those with a confirmed or highly suspected exposure, and who are adequately resuscitated, as the therapeutic agents have significant side effects. Thiosulfate and hydroxycobalamin have fewer side effects than the other agents used. Other antidotes can be used in specific situations: for example, atropine for organophosphate exposure, or heavy metal chelators.[23]

Supplemental humidified oxygen should be used for patients suspected of having inhalation injury, the humidification helping to prevent inspissation of the airway secretions, and the head of the bed placed at a 30–45° angle. This helps reduce upper airway edema, and decreases the effect of pressure from abdominal contents on the diaphragm. Meticulous pulmonary hygiene is a vital component of the management of inhalation injury. Frequent airway suctioning, chest physiotherapy including percussive and coughing techniques, and early mobilization all help prevent build-up of secretions, which can cause airway obstruction, atelectasis and predispose to the development of pneumonias.[3,5,21] Care should be taken when suctioning to avoid hypoxia and bradycardia. Preoxygenation and suctioning for short periods of 10–15 seconds can reduce the incidence of these problems. Postural drainage can be useful, although sometimes skin graft location and fragility impede use of this technique.[46] Percussive and vibratory techniques such as high-frequency chest wall oscillation also help expectorate mucoid secretions.[46,47] It is also important to maintain good nutritional status in these patients.[6]

As a result of inhaled irritants, patients can suffer from severe bronchospasm. This can usually be managed by using inhaled beta agonists, such as albuterol or salbuterol. Sometimes intravenous bronchodilators are necessary.[4,48] Aminophylline or terbutaline can be used. Aerosolized heparin can be used as a mucolytic to help prevent inspissation of secretions and bronchial cast formation by affecting the fibrin component of the cast.[48–50] It does not appear to cause systemic anticoagulation in the doses used clinically. Aerosolized and intravenous acetylcysteine has also been used as a mucolytic and was shown to improve pulmonary antioxidant capacity in one study.[51] In a pediatric study, a combination of aerosolized heparin and acetylcysteine was used, and resulted in a significant reduction in reintubations, the incidence of atelectasis and in mortality following smoke inhalation injury.[50] When physical therapy and pharmacological agents still fail to expectorate secretions or ameliorate cast formation, fiberoptic bronchoscopy can be effective to remove secretions, and also to obtain microbiological specimens through bronchoalveolar lavage in suspected cases of pneumonia. Attempts to replace surfactant have also been studied, but are not in widespread clinical use. Antibiotics are indicated for suspected or proven pulmonary infection.[4,5] Corticosteroids are not generally used in burn patients, but may be useful in severe bronchospasm inadequately controlled by beta agonists or other bronchodilators.[4]

Mechanical ventilation is indicated when either the signs of respiratory failure are present or are imminent. These include tachypnea, use of accessory muscles of respiration, sternal retractions in children and the presence of upper airway edema. Parameters indicating inadequate ventilation or oxygenation include the following: respiratory rate >30 breaths/minute, PaO$_2$ < 65 mmHg, PaCO$_2$ > 50 mmHg and a PaO$_2$/FiO$_2$ < 200. As mentioned previously, when using a fiberoptic bronchoscope to assess the airway for inhalation injury, an endotracheal tube can be passed over the scope to secure the airway, if necessary. A nasotracheal tube may be preferable for patient comfort, oral hygiene and stability. The patient should be preoxygenated. Muscle relaxants should not be given during intubation, as if the intubation proves difficult, it may not be possible to adequately ventilate the paralyzed patient.[48]

Several different modes of ventilation can be used for the patient with an inhalation injury. The aim is to provide adequate ventilation to maintain airway and alveolar patency without causing overdistention of alveoli and barotrauma. In this patient population, airways may be narrowed by edema, and this increases airway resistance and thus, airway pressures. High airway pressures can damage already damaged airway mucosa. One technique to reduce airway pressures is to allow mild respiratory acidosis or permissive hypercapnia.[4,52] This allows lower airway pressures and smaller tidal volumes to be used when ventilating the patient, and is well tolerated when of gradual onset and the pH is kept above 7.2–7.25.[4,48] The optimal positive end-expiratory pressure (PEEP) should be determined using a pressure–volume curve. This helps maintain alveolar patency, which is important as reopening the alveoli requires higher airway pressures. The lower inflection point of the pressure–volume curve of a mechanical breath is where the slope of the lower curve begins to increase, and is the airway pressure below which the alveoli collapse. The PEEP value should be set just above this. FiO_2 should be weaned down as tolerated to reduce oxygen-related complications. The PaO_2 can be maintained between 80 and 100 mmHg, although values over 65–70 mmHg can support adequate tissue oxygenation. The ventilation rate should maximize ventilation initially, and may need to be set slightly higher than usual if lower tidal volumes or pressures are being used. Thereafter, it should be weaned to allow spontaneous ventilation.[48]

Conventional mechanical ventilation can either be volume controlled or pressure controlled. Volume-controlled ventilation delivers a consistent tidal volume and minute volume to the lungs, but this can result in variable airway pressures depending on the compliance of the lungs. Pressure-controlled ventilation limits the inflating pressure used, and thus the tidal volume varies depending on compliance and inspiratory time.[48] High-frequency percussive ventilation (HFPV) is a ventilatory mode that delivers sub-tidal breaths at a high frequency. These are superimposed on pressure-controlled ventilatory cycles. Studies of this technique have shown it to have advantages over conventional mechanical ventilation. It appears to be associated with decreased work of breathing, improved oxygenation (higher PaO_2/FiO_2 ratios) and lower peak pressures.[53–56] A pediatric study group also had a significant reduction in the incidence of pneumonia, when compared to a conventionally ventilated control group.[53] Airway pressure release ventilation (APRV) is a more recently developed pressure-controlled, time-cycled mode of ventilation, that can allow spontaneous breathing during the ventilatory cycle, without changing the preset pressure settings. It has a high-pressure and a low-pressure setting. Recruitment of alveoli and oxygenation occur at the high-pressure setting, and ventilation occurs by controlled releases to the lower pressure. The mechanical inspiratory phase can be prolonged to achieve high mean airway pressures, without high peak airway pressures. It has so far shown promising results in trauma patients and pediatric patients with mild to moderate lung disease. They achieved comparable or superior oxygenation values, while using lower peak airway pressures.[57,58] This mode may be useful in the burn population as a means to ventilate while reducing barotrauma. Extracorporeal membrane oxygenation (ECMO) is a technique, which can be used in patients with severe respiratory failure, in which the patient's blood is cir-

culated through an extracorporeal cardiopulmonary bypass circuit, that facilitates gas exchange through a semipermeable membrane. While this is taking place, low ventilatory pressures and a low FiO_2 can be used to ventilate the damaged lung. This allows the lung to heal without additional complications of mechanical ventilation such as barotrauma or oxygen toxicity. Anticoagulation is necessary during treatment. While numbers in burn patient studies are small, it may offer a salvage therapy for patients with severe respiratory disease on conventional ventilation.[59–61]

Tracheostomy may be necessary in a small number of patients. The most common indications are prolonged dependence on mechanical ventilation due to respiratory failure or pulmonary sepsis, emergent airway access, severe facial/neck burns or edema and following complications of endotracheal intubation.[62,63] In the past, high reported complication rates following tracheostomy led to controversy over its use in the burn population. However, more recent studies have shown that tracheostomy can be performed safely, without increased risk of infectious complications.[62,64] Advantages of tracheostomy include a shorter tube with reduction of dead space and airway resistance, greater ease to maintain pulmonary hygiene and a reduction in development of subglottic stenosis. Long-term endotracheal intubation is also uncomfortable for the patient. Both endotracheal intubation and tracheostomy have long-term complications associated with their use, and neither should be used unnecessarily. The decision to convert to a tracheostomy should not be taken lightly, and should take into account the characteristics of the individual patient and their injury.

Mechanical ventilation should be weaned as the patient's condition improves, and discontinued as soon as it is no longer necessary. During the weaning process, the FiO_2, PEEP and rate should be reduced as tolerated, until the patient is capable of supporting their own respiratory requirements. Parameters used as indicators for extubation include the presence of the following: an alert patient, resolution of upper airway edema with an audible air leak around the endotracheal tube with the cuff deflated, PaO_2/FiO_2 ratio greater than 200, an adequate tidal volume (6–10 mL/kg) and negative inspiratory pressure $<-20 \text{ cm H}_2\text{O}$.[4] The patient should also not be acidotic and should be hemodynamically stable. Once extubated, supplemental, humidified oxygen should be provided, and the patient should be carefully observed for any signs of respiratory compromise that might necessitate reintubation.

Complications

Complications in patients with inhalation injuries occur secondary to the original injury and due to the mechanical ventilation used to support the injured lung. Barotrauma can occur as a result of mechanical ventilation, particularly in patients that have required high peak and mean airway pressures to maintain adequate ventilation and oxygenation.[65] Sustained high airway pressures can lead to tracheal mucosal ischemia. Barotrauma can manifest itself as a pneumothorax, pneumomediastinum, pneumoperitoneum, pneumopericardium or subcutaneous emphysema.[52] Thoracostomy tubes may be required for treatment of pneumothoraces (Figure 19.10). Ventilatory strategies to reduce airway pressures, such as per-

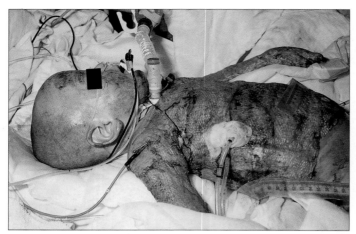

Fig. 19.10 Child with right-sided pneumothorax, treated with a chest tube. A tracheostomy is also in place. (From Barret JP, Herndon DN. Color atlas of burn care. Philadelphia: WB Saunders; 2001.)

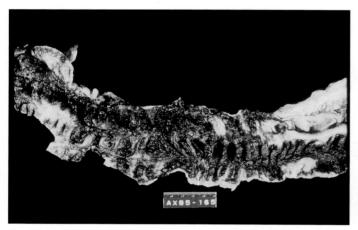

Fig. 19.11 Autopsy specimen of necrohemorrhagic tracheobronchitis. (From Barret JP, Herndon DN. Color atlas of burn care. Philadelphia: WB Saunders; 2001.)

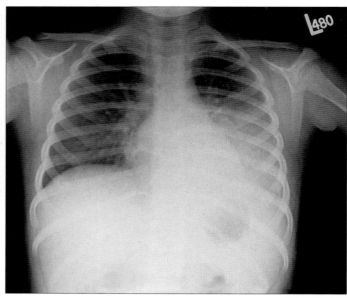

Fig. 19.12 Left lower lobe pneumonia on chest radiograph. (From Barret JP, Herndon DN. Color atlas of burn care. Philadelphia: WB Saunders; 2001.)

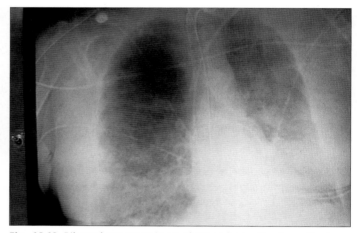

Fig. 19.13 Bilateral pneumonia on chest radiograph of a patient with inhalation injury. (Courtesy of Jaclyn Jones.) (From Barret JP, Herndon DN. Color atlas of burn care. Philadelphia: WB Saunders; 2001.)

missive hypercapnia, HFPV and APRV, aim to prevent these complications.

Infectious complications, such as tracheobronchitis or pneumonia, increase morbidity and mortality significantly (Figure 19.11). In one study, the presence of pneumonia, in thermally-injured patients with inhalation injury, substantially increased mortality up to 60%.[7] Infectious complications typically occur after the first 3–10 days post injury,[5,6] and in patients with inhalation injury, the incidence of pneumonia has varied from 38% to 60%.[52,56,66] The source of infection is generally from bacteria colonizing the oropharyngeal tract and the burn wound. Intubated patients also do not have the same capacity for self-clearing of secretions and debris from their respiratory tract as do extubated patients. The mucociliary mechanism may be damaged by the inhalation injury, alveolar macrophage function is altered, and ventilation of the lung may be impaired, due to atelectasis and small airway obstruction by secretions and casts.[5,6,18] The endotracheal tube also bypasses some of these mechanisms for self-defense, and can become colonized too. All these impairments contribute to predisposing the patient to develop pneumonia.

The diagnosis of pneumonia is based the presence of clinical signs such as fever, increased sputum or airway secretion production, laboratory values such as leukocytosis, and the presence of organisms on Gram stain and culture of sputum or bronchoalveolar lavage specimens. The chest radiograph should also show a new or altered parenchymal infiltrate[66] (Figures 19.12 and 19.13). There may also be a deterioration in the patient's oxygenation, or an increase in ventilatory requirements. Organisms colonizing the upper airway can sometimes confuse the diagnosis, as they will be commonly present and not necessarily causing pulmonary infection.[62] Treatment consists of intravenous antibiotic therapy, initially based on Gram stain from the airway specimen or previous cultures, and this is then adjusted according to the sensitivities

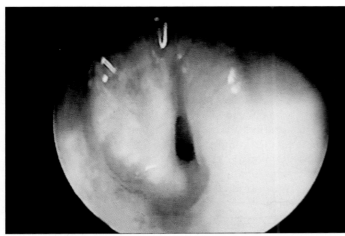

Fig. 19.14 Glottic stenosis 1-year post thermal injury. (From Barret JP, Herndon DN. Color atlas of burn care. Philadelphia: WB Saunders; 2001.)

of the organisms cultured. Ventilatory support is administered as necessary to maintain adequate ventilation and oxygenation, and meticulous pulmonary hygiene is essential. Some studies have shown a reduced incidence of pneumonia in patients receiving HFPV ventilation compared to conventional mechanical ventilation.[53,66]

Mechanical problems from endotracheal or tracheostomy tubes can also occur, and may not present acutely. As a result of injury to the upper airway epithelium, upper airway stenoses can occur. These can be supraglottic or subglottic, subglottic being more common (Figure 19.14). This is usually associated with prolonged endotracheal intubation, and theoretically should not happen with tracheostomy tubes. No treatment is necessary in mild cases; more severe cases may need dilatations or even laryngoplasties. Erosion of the tracheal cartilage can occur from cuff pressure, and lead to tracheomalacia, a weakening of the tracheal wall that can allow the airway to collapse inwards during inspiration.[62,63] Granulomatous and fibrous tissue can grow around tracheostomy sites, and this can lead to airway or tube obstruction, necessitating removal of the obstructing tissue. Tracheoesophageal fistulae and erosion into the innominate artery can occur. This can cause mediastinitis and/or exsanguinating hemorrage.[63]

Long-term pulmonary function

Post-inhalation injury, patients can have hyper-reactive airways. This has been shown to persist for at least 6 months in one study, along with inflammatory changes in the bronchial mucosa, and elevated inflammatory cytokine (TNFα, interferon (IFNγ), and interleukin-2 (IL-2)) levels in serum and broncheoalveolar lavage fluid. The majority of subjects, however, had normal pulmonary function tests.[67] Longer-term studies have, in some cases shown, development of obstructive and restrictive patterns on pulmonary function testing, indicating that normal lung function may not always be regained following recovery from inhalation injury.[32,68,69] In a pediatric burn cohort, no difference in exercise tolerance was noted between children who had sustained an inhalation injury and

those who had not; however, the children who had had an inhalation injury achieved their goal with a significantly higher respiratory rate, and had a higher incidence of abnormal lung function.[69] Conversely, an adult study did not find any evidence of altered respiratory function post-inhalation injury, or in those tested, any significant exercise intolerance.[70]

Damage to the larynx by inhaled toxins and thermal injury, and also by intubation as a treatment for inhalation injury or upper airway edema, can result in persistent hoarseness or dysphonia. Injury to the laryngeal mucosa can cause scarring that can affect the flexibility and vibratory capacity of the vocal cords, and also their ability to open and close properly. As a result, voice production may be affected, and this may not resolve without treatment. Some of the phonation problems can be helped by voice therapy, and some of the laryngeal scarring may be ameneable to surgical or laser excision.[71]

Future/investigational therapies

While the treatment of inhalation injury is currently mostly supportive, research is continuing in an effort to improve care. Attempts to improve present ventilatory and supportive strategies, as well as research into the local and systemic response to thermal and inhalation injury, are ongoing. With further understanding of the pathophysiology, it may be possible to modulate the body's response to injury, and minimize the impact of this insult to the respiratory system.

At present, the emphasis in ventilatory strategies is to adequately ventilate the lungs, while trying to reduce the airway pressures necessary to achieve this to levels that will not cause or minimize barotrauma to the patient. Methods such as HFPV and APRV appear to recruit alveoli and allow efficient gas exchange, while at the same time using lower peak airway pressures when compared to conventional mechanical ventilation.[55–58] ECMO has been used in cases of severe respiratory failure following smoke inhalation with some success in both the adult and pediatic populations.[59–61] Arteriovenous carbon dioxide removal (AVCO$_2$R), a technique utilizing an extracorporeal membrane gas exchanger to remove CO_2, while O_2 diffuses across the native alveoli by low-frequency positive pressure ventilation, has undergone animal and clinical trials, and appears to be capable of efficient CO_2 removal. This can significantly reduce ventilatory requirements, and improve arterial blood pH levels in severe respiratory failure.[72,73]

The pathophysiology of inhalation injury and the systemic response are also being explored, in conjunction with the effects of various mediators along the pathways involved. Therapies attempting to decrease airway inflammation by reducing the release of inflammatory mediators or by utilizing free radical scavengers are being investigated with varying results. Dimethylsulfoxide, a free radical scavenger, has been used alone and in conjunction with heparin. In one study, this combination, in an ovine model of smoke inhalation, improved survival and PaO$_2$/FiO$_2$ ratios. Cast formation was also reduced, and the usual increase in pulmonary lymph flow was less apparent, probably due to a reduction in free radical-induced microvascular permeability.[74] Manganese superoxide dismutase has also been evaluated for its action on free radicals. While it appears to reduce loss of protein, it does not appear to improve gas exchange or lung permeability problems.[75] Pentoxifylline[76] and lisofylline[77] (which is metabolized to pentoxifylline in the liver) have been studied for their effects on inhibition of inflammatory mediators and downregulation of leukocytes. They seem to improve ventilation-perfusion mismatching in animals and reduce ventilatory requirements. This is attributed to reduced edema formation and decreased airway damage. The use of heparin in combination with other agents such as lisofylline and dimethylsulfoxide appears to attenuate the results.

More selective inhibitors are also being evaluated, such as endotheln-1 receptor antagonists,[78] neurokinin-1 receptor antagonists (blocking the proinflammatory effect of substance P)[79] and thromboxane A_2.[80] These agents have shown potential in reducing the inflammation and pulmonary edema associated with inhalation injuries. Recombinant antithrombin[81] and tissue plasminogen activator[82] have shown beneficial effects in animals in reducing fibrin cast formation and reducing pulmonary transvascular fluid shifts and lung water. The decrease in airway obstruction as a result of less cast formation can help prevent further ventilation-perfusion mismatching and trauma to alveoli. Many other agents are also undergoing evaluation for potential benefit in treating smoke inhalation injury.

Summary

Inhalation injury is one of the leading causes of morbidity and mortality in burns. It is present in approximately one-third of burn victims, and can be present alone or in conjunction with cutaneous thermal injury. Early diagnosis and treatment are crucial to prevent complications. Diagnosis is based initially on history and physical exam. Fiberoptic bronchoscopy is a very useful diagnostic tool, and can also be utilized for an intubation aid if necessary. Treatment is mostly supportive, and must start with assessing the airway and obtaining a secure airway if needed. The patient should be removed from the source of injury and supplemental oxygen provided. Meticulous pulmonary hygiene is essential. Mechanical ventilation may need to be commenced if the patient cannot adequately support their ventilatory needs independently. Complications of inhalation injury include infectious complications such as pneumonia, and those as a result of mechanical ventilation and barotrauma.

References

1. Weiss SM, Lakshminarayan S. Acute inhalation injury. Clin Chest Med 1994; 15(1):103–116.
2. Lee-Chiong TL, Jr, Mattay RA. Burns and smoke inhalation. Curr Opin Pulm Med 1995; 1(2):96–101.
3. Herndon PB, Thompson PB, Traber DL. Pulmonary injury in burned patients. Crit Care Clin 1985; 1(1):79–96.
4. Sheridan RL. Airway management and respiratory care of the burn patient. Int Anesthesiol Clin 2000; 38(3):129–145.
5. Desai MH, Rutan RL, Herndon DN. Managing smoke inhalation injuries. Postgrad Med 1989; 86(8):69–70.
6. Demling RH. Smoke inhalation injury. New Horiz 1993; 1(3):422–434.
7. Shirani KZ, Pruitt BA Jr, Mason AD Jr. The influence of inhalation injury and pneumonia on burn mortality. Ann Surg 1987; 205(1):82–87.
8. Ryan CM, Schoenfield DA, Thorpe WP, et al. Objective estimates of the probability of death from burn injuries. N Engl J Med 1998; 338(6):362–366.
9. O'Keeffe GE, Hunt JL, Purdue GF. An evaluation of the risk factors for mortality after burn trauma and the identification of gender-dependent differences in outcomes. J Am Coll Surg 2001; 192: 153–160.
10. Leung CM, Lee ST. Morbidity and mortality in respiratory burns — a prospective study of 240 cases. Ann Acad Med Singapore 1992; 21(5):619–623.
11. Rue LW 3rd, Cioffi WG, Mason AD, et al. Improved survival of burned patients with inhalation injury. Arch Surg 1993; 128:772–778; discussion 778–780.
12. Lalonde C, Picard L, Youn YK, Demling RH. Increased early post-burn fluid requirements and oxygen demands are predictive of the degree of airways injury by smoke inhalation. J Trauma 1995; 38(2):175–184.
13. Rajpura A. The epidemiology of burns and smoke inhalation in secondary care: a population-based study covering Lancashire and South Cumbria. Burns 2002; 28:121–130.
14. Moritz A, Henritues F, McLean R. The effects of inhaled heat on the air passages and lungs: an experimental investigation. Am J Path 1944; 21:311–331.
15. Still J, Friedman B, Law E, et al. Burns due to exposure to steam. Burns 2001; 27:379–381.
16. Balakrishnan C, Tijunelis AD, Gordon DM, et al. Burns and inhalation injury caused by steam. Burns 1996; 22(4):313–315.
17. Alarie Y. Toxicity of fire smoke. Crit Rev Toxicol 2002; 32(4): 259–289.
18. Bidani A, Wang CZ, Heming TA. Early effects of smoke inhalation on alveolar macrophage function. Burns 1996; 22:101–106.
19. Enkhbaatar P, Traber DL. Pathophysiology of acute lung injury in combined burn and smoke inhalation injury. Clin Sci 2004; 107: 137–143.
20. Wright MJ, Murphy JT. Smoke inhalation enhances early alveolar leukocyte responsiveness to endotoxin. J Trauma 2005; 59:64–70.
21. Latenser BA, Iteld L. Smoke inhalation injury. Semin Respir Crit Care Med 2001; 22(1):13–22.
22. Pettila V, Takkunen O, Tukiainen P. Zinc chloride smoke inhalation: a rare cause of severe acute respiratory distress syndrome. Intensive Care Med 2000; 26:215–217.
23. Kulling P. Hospital treatment of victims exposed to combustion products. Toxicol Lett 1992; 64–65 (Spec No: 283–289).
24. Turrina S, Neri C, De Leo D. Effect of combined exposure to carbon monoxide and cyanides in selected forensic cases. J Clin Forensic Med 2004; 11(15):264–267.
25. Shirani KZ, Vaughan GM, Mason AD Jr, et al. Update on current therapeutic approaches in burns. Shock 1996; 5(1):4–16.
26. Baud FJ, Barriot P, Toffis V, et al. Elevated blood cyanide concentrations in victims of smoke inhalation. N Engl J Med 1991; 325(25):1761–1766.
27. Wittram C, Kenny JB. The admission chest radiograph after acute inhalation injury and burns. Br J Radiol 1994; 67(800): 751–754.
28. Reske A, Bak Z, Samuelsson A, et al. Computed tomography — a possible aid in the diagnosis of smoke inhalation injury? Acta Anesthesiol Scand 2005; 49:257–260.
29. Masanes MJ, Legendre C, Lioret N, et al. Fiberoptic bronchoscopy for the early diagnosis of subglottal inhalation injury: comparative value in the assessment of prognosis. J Trauma 1994; 36(1):59–67.
30. Masanes MJ, Legendre C, Lioret N, et al. Using bronchoscopy and biopsy to diagnose early inhalation injury. Macroscopic and histologic findings. Chest 1995; 107:1365–1369.
31. Pruitt BA Jr, Cioffi WG, Shimazu T, et al. Evaluation and management of patients with inhalation injury. J Trauma 1990; 30(12 Suppl):S63–S68.
32. Mlcak R, Desai MH, Robinson E, et al. Lung function following thermal injury in children — an 8-year follow up. Burns 1998; 24:213–216.
33. Moylan JA Jr, Wilmore DW, Mouton DE, et al. Early diagnosis of inhalation injury using 133 xenon lung scan. Ann Surg 1972; 176(4):477–484.

34. Inoue T, Okabayashi K, Ohtani M, et al. Effect of smoke inhalation injury on fluid requirement in burn resuscitation. Hiroshima J Med Sci 2002; 51(1):1–5.

35. Herndon DN, Barrow RE, Linares HA, et al. Inhalation injury in burned patients: effects and treatment. Burns Incl Therm Inj 1988; 14:349–356.

36. Williams J, Lewis RW II, Kealey GP. Carbon monoxide poisoning and myocardial ischemia in patients with burns. J Burn Care Rehabil 1992; 13:210–213.

37. Weaver LK, Howe S, Hopkins R, et al. Carboxyhemoglobin half-life in carbon monoxide-poisoned patients treated with 100% oxygen at atmospheric pressure. Chest 2000; 117:801–808.

38. Chou KJ, Fischer JL, Silver EJ. Characteristics and outcome of children with carbon monoxide poisoning with and without smoke exposure referred for hyperbaric oxygen therapy. Ped Emerg Care 2000; 16(3):151–155.

39. Juurlink DN, Buckley NA, Stanbrook MB, et al. Hyperbaric oxygen for carbon monoxide poisoning (review). The Cochrane Database of Systematic Reviews 2005, Issue 1. Art No.:CD002041.pub2. DOI: 10.1002/14651858.CD002041.pub2.

40. Weaver LK, Hopkins RO, Chan KJ, et al. Hyperbaric oxygen for acute carbon monoxide poisoning. N Engl J Med 2002; 347(14):1057–1067.

41. Shusterman D, Alexeef G, Hargis C, et al. Predictors of carbon monoxide and hydrogen cyanide exposure in smoke inhalation patients. J Toxicol Clin Toxicol 1996; 34(1):61–71.

42. Tung A, Lynch J, McDade WA, et al. A new biological assay for measuring cyanide in blood. Anesth Analg 1997; 85(5):1045–1051.

43. Kirk MA, Gerace R, Kulig KW. Cyanide and methemoglobin kinetics in smoke inhalation victims treated with the cyanide antidote kit. Ann Emerg Med 1993; 22(9):1413–1418.

44. Barillo DJ, Goode R, Esch V. Cyanide poisoning in victims of fire: analysis of 364 cases and review of the literature. J Burn Care Rehabil 1994; 15:46–57.

45. Houeto P, Borron SW, Sandouk P, et al. Pharmacokinetics of hydroxycobalamin in smoke inhalation victims. J Toxicol Clin Toxicol 1996; 34(4):397–404.

46. Silverberg R, Johnson J, Gorga D, et al. A survey of the prevalence and application of chest physical therapy in U.S. burn centers. J Burn Care Rehabil 1995; 16(2):154–159.

47. Koga T, Kawazu T, Iwashita K, et al. Pulmonary hyperinflation and respiratory distress following solvent aspiration in a patient with asthma: expectoration of bronchial casts and clinical improvement with high frequency chest wall oscillation. Respir Care 2004; 49(11):1335–1338.

48. McCall JE, Cahill TJ. Respiratory care of the burn patient. J Burn Care Rehabil 2005; 26(3):200–206.

49. Cox CS Jr, Zwischenberger JB, Traber DL, et al. Heparin improves oxygenation and minimizes barotrauma after severe smoke inhalation in the ovine model. Surg Gynecol Obstet 1993; 176(4):339–349.

50. Desai MH, Mlcak R, Richardson J, et al. Reduction in mortality in pediatric patients with inhalation injury with aerosolized heparin/acetylcysteine therapy. J Burn Care Rehabil 1998; 19(3):210–212.

51. Fu Z, Yang Z, Liu L, et al. The influence of N-acetyl-L-cysteine on pulmonary injury and oxygen stress after smoke inhalation injury. Zhonghua Shao Shang Za Zhi 2002; 18(3):152–154.

52. Sheridan RL, Kacmarek RM, McEttrick MM, et al. Permissive hypercapnia as a ventilatory strategy in burned children: effect on barotraumas, pneumonia, and mortality. J Trauma 1995; 39(5):854–859.

53. Cortiella J, Mlcak R, Herndon D. High frequency percussive ventilation in pediatric patients with inhalation injury. J Burn Care Rehabil 1999; 20:232–235.

54. Mlcak R, Cortiella J, Desai M, et al. Lung compliance, airway resistance, and work of breathing in children after inhalation injury. J Burn Care Rehabil 1997; 18:531–534.

55. Reper P, Van Bos R, Van Loey K, et al. High frequency percussive ventilation in burn patients: hemodynamics and gas exchange. Burns 2003; 29:603–608.

56. Reper P, Wibaux O, Van Laeke P, et al. High frequency percussive ventilation and conventional ventilation after smoke inhalation: a randomized study. Burns 2002; 28:503–508.

57. Dart BW 4th, Maxwell RA, Richart CM, et al. Preliminary experience with airway pressure release ventilation in a trauma/surgical intensive care unit. J Trauma 2005; 59:71–76.

58. Ryan Schultz T, Costarino AT, Durning SM, et al. Airway pressure release ventilation in pediatrics. Pediatr Crit Care Med 2001; 2(3):243–246.

59. Thompson JT, Molnar JA, Hines MH, et al. Successful management of adult smoke inhalation with extracorporeal membrane oxygenation. J Burn Care Rehabil 2005; 26:62–66.

60. Pierre EJ, Zwischenberger JB, Angel C, et al. Extracorporeal membrane oxygenation in the treatment of respiratory failure in pediatric patients with burns. J Burn Care Rehabil 1998; 19:131–134.

61. O'Toole G, Peek G, Jaffe W, et al. Extracorporeal membrane oxygenation in the treatment of inhalation injuries. Burns 1998; 24:562–565.

62. Barret JP, Desai MH, Herndon DN. Effects of tracheostomies on infection and airway complications in pediatric burn patients. Burns 2000; 26:190–193.

63. Hunt JL, Purdue GF, Gunning T. Is tracheostomy warranted in the burn patient? Indications and complications. J Burn Care Rehabil 1986; 7(6):492–495.

64. Coln CE, Purdue GF, Hunt JL. Tracheostomy in the young pediatric burn patient. Arch Surg 1998; 133(5):539–540.

65. Fitzpatrick JC, Cioffi WG Jr, Cheu HW, et al. Predicting ventilation failure in children with inhalation injury. J Pediatr Surg 1994; 29(8):1122–1126.

66. Rue LW III, Cioffi WG, Mason AD Jr, et al. The risk of pneumonia in thermally injured patients requiring ventilatory support. J Burn Care Rehabil 1995; 16:262–268.

67. Park GY, Park JW, Jeong DH, et al. Prolonged airway and systemic inflammatory reactions after smoke inhalation. Chest 2003; 123:475–480.

68. McElroy K, Alvarado I, Hayward PG, et al. Exercise stress testing for the pediatric patient with burns: a preliminary report. J Burn Care Rehabil 1992; 13:236–238.

69. Desai MH, Mlcak RP, Robinson E, et al. Does inhalation injury limit exercise endurance in children convalescing from thermal injury? J Burn Care Rehabil 1993; 14:16–20.

70. Bourbeau J, Lacasse Y, Rouleau MY, et al. Combined smoke inhalation and body surface burns injury does not necessarily imply long-term respiratory health consequences. Eur Respir J 1996; 9:1470–1474.

71. Casper JK, Clark WR, Kelley RT, et al. Laryngeal and phonatory status after burn/inhalation injury: a long term follow-up study. J Burn Care Rehabil 2002; 23:235–243.

72. Conrad SA, Zwischenberger JB, Grier LR, et al. Total extracorporeal arteriovenous carbon dioxide removal in acute respiratory failure: a phase I clinical study. Intensive Care Med 2001; 27:1340–1351.

73. Zhou X, Loran DB, Wang D, et al. Seventy-two hour gas exchange performance and hemodynamic properties of NOVALUNG®iLA as a gas exchanger for arteriovenous carbon dioxide removal. Perfusion 2005; 20:303–308.

74. Brown M, Desai M, Traber LD, et al. Dimethylsulfoxide with heparin in the treatment of smoke inhalation injury. J Burn Care Rehabil 1988; 9(1):22–25.

75. Maybauer MO, Kikuchi Y, Westphal M, et al. Effects of manganese superoxide dismutase nebulization on pulmonary function in an ovine model of acute lung injury. Shock 2005; 23(2):138–143.

76. Ogura H, Cioffi WG, Okerberg CV, et al. The effects of pentoxifylline on pulmonary function following smoke inhalation. J Surg Research 1992; 56:242–250.

77. Tasaki O, Mozingo DW, Dubick MA, et al. Effects of heparin and lisofylline on pulmonary function after smoke inhalation in an ovine model. Crit Care Med 2002; 30:637–643.

78. Cox RA, Enkhabaatar P, Burke AS, et al. Effects of a dual endothelin-1 receptor antagonist on airway obstruction and acute lung injury in sheep following smoke inhalation and burn injury. Clin Sci 2005; 108:265–272.

79. Wong SS, Sun NN, Lantz RC, et al. Substance P and neutral endo-peptidase in development of acute respiratory distress syndrome following fire smoke inhalation. Am J Physiol Lung Cell Mol Physiol 2004; 287:L859–866.

80. Westphal M, Noshima S, Isago T, et al. Selective thromboxane A_2 synthase inhibition by OKY-046 prevents cardiopulmonary dysfunction after ovine smoke inhalation injury. Anesthesiology 2005; 102:954–961.

81. Murakami K, McGuire R, Cox RA, et al. Recombinant antithrombin attenuates pulmonary inflammation following smoke inhalation and pneumonia in sheep. Crit Care Med 2003; 31:577–583.

82. Enthbaatar P, Murakami K, Cox R, et al. Aerosolized tissue plasminogen inhibitor improves pulmonary function in sheep with burn and smoke inhalation. Shock 2004; 22(1):70–75.

Chapter 20

Barotrauma

*Edward Y. Chan, James E. Lynch, David B. Loran and
Joseph B. Zwischenberger*

Introduction

Occasionally, the thoracic surgeon is called on to assist in the management of patients with complex pulmonary problems in the burn unit. One of the more common examples is barotrauma. To adequately manage this condition, it is important to understand the underlying mechanisms of injury. Support and specific therapies then can be administered properly. Frequently these patients are suffering from acute respiratory distress syndrome (ARDS) and are at the limits of conventional management. In this chapter we will review the etiology, incidence and management of patients with barotrauma. We will also explore adjuncts to mechanical ventilation that may act to limit injurious ventilator strategies while at the same time augmenting gas exchange. The pathophysiology of mechanical ventilation in the burn patient is complex and multifactoral, but to avoid duplication we will focus on barotrauma caused by pulmonary and non-pulmonary ARDS.

Barotrauma

In a study that included 5183 patients across 361 centers, Anzueto et al.[1] noted a 2.9% incidence of barotrauma in patients on mechanical ventilation in the intensive care unit, with highest incidence in patients with chronic interstitial lung disease (10.0%) or acute respiratory distress syndrome (ARDS) (6.5%). They also demonstrated, in a case-control analysis, an independently increased risk of mortality in patients with barotrauma (51.4 vs. 39.2%). Macklin and Macklin[2] first described the most common mechanism of injury: a small airway or alveolus ruptures and the air dissects through the bronchovascular connective tissue proximally into the mediastinum, ultimately rupturing in the pleural space.

Etiology

Although it is obvious that an air sack must rupture to produce a pneumothorax, the mechanism of that rupture is a subject of debate (Box 20.1). Most theories are based on overdistention or pressurization of the alveolus. Historically, supportive management for severe respiratory failure involved mechanical ventilation with tidal volumes of 10–15 mL/kg because Bendixen et al.[3] noted that high lung volumes minimize atelectasis and prevent deterioration in oxygenation in patients undergoing anesthesia. This strategy often requires high airway pressures (>35 cmH$_2$O) to deliver these volumes and maintain normocapnia in patients with severe lung injury. In fact, the original description of ARDS by Ashbaugh et al.[4] included high inspiratory ventilator pressures as part of the definition.

Webb and Tierney[5] first recognized ventilator-induced parenchymal lung injury as separate from the previously recognized forms of barotrauma. Rats ventilated at high airway pressures (45 cmH$_2$O) developed alveolar edema, hypoxemia, and decreased lung compliance, with death occurring within 1 hour. They proposed that interstitial edema may be caused by pulmonary interdependence and that the alveolar edema may be from depletion or inactivation of surfactant. Dreyfuss et al.[6] demonstrated increases in capillary permeability, edema and inactivation of surfactant during intermittent positive-pressure hyperventilation with high inflation pressures.

Controversy surrounds peak inspiratory pressure (PIP) as a potential cause of barotrauma. Diakun[7] reasoned that PIP requirements remain the single best predictor of barotrauma because of the higher pressures necessary to deliver an adequate minute volume when the lungs sustain a severe injury that decreases pulmonary compliance. PIP of less than 50 cmH$_2$O had initially been considered safe due to work by Peterson and Baier.[8] In comparing three groups of patients with PIP exceeding 70 cmH$_2$O, between 50 and 70 cmH$_2$O and below 50 cmH$_2$O, Peterson and Baier[8] found an incidence of barotrauma of 43%, 8% and 0%, respectively, but even this level may be too high if an underlying pulmonary pathologic condition exists that predisposes the patient to barotrauma.

More recent studies have found conflicting evidence as to what extent reducing PIP can affect mortality in patients with ARDS. Stewart et al.[9] found that in patients with ARDS, there is no mortality benefit to limiting ventilation pressures and there may be greater morbidity. In this study, 120 patients were randomly assigned to one of two groups: a limited ventilation group with PIP restricted to 30 cmH$_2$O and tidal volume no more than 8 mL/kg, or a conventional ventilation group with PIP as high as 50 cmH$_2$O and tidal volume of 10–15 mL/kg. They found no significant difference in mortality between the two groups. Additionally, patients in the limited-

BOX 20.1 Potential causes of barotraumas

High peak airway pressures
High mean airway pressures
Alveolar overdistention, increased volume
Positive end-expiratory pressure

With permission from Zwischenberger et al. Barotrauma and inhalational injuries. In: Shields T. ed. General thoracic surgery, 5th edn Philadelphia, Lippincott, Williams and Wilkins; 2000: Vol. 1; 834–839.

ventilation group required dialysis for renal failure more frequently and required more paralytic drugs. Weg et al.[10] analyzed 725 patients with sepsis-induced ARDS, 77 of whom had pneumothorax or other air leaks. In comparing the PIP, airway pressure and tidal volume of patients who had pneumothorax or other air leak to those who had no air leak, they also found no correlation between high ventilatory pressures or volumes and the development of pneumothorax. Boussarsar et al.[11] conducted a two-part study, using a randomized prospective trial of two ventilation strategies as well as a literature analysis of risk factors for barotrauma in ARDS patients. The randomized trial, which maintained plateau pressures (the pressure applied to the alveoli and small airways in positive pressure ventilation) below $35\,cmH_2O$, produced no relationship between high ventilatory pressures or volumes and barotrauma in patients with early ARDS. However, the literature analysis found a significantly higher incidence of barotrauma in patients with plateau pressure greater than $35\,cmH_2O$ and in patients with lung compliance (a static measure of lung and chest recoil) of less than $30\,mL/cmH_2O$.

Alveolar distensibility, a measure of alveolar energetics, is a precursor to barotrauma. Tsuno et al.[12] studied regional pressure-related overdistention of healthy alveoli, termed *barotrauma* or *volutrauma*, that can result in a pattern of diffuse alveolar damage that is histologically indistinguishable from other causes of ARDS. Overdistention of alveoli and distal airways, regardless of the pressure involved, has also been proposed by Hillman and Barber,[13] Hurd et al.[14] and Alpan et al.[15] as a cause of barotrauma. It occurs either through selection of a tidal volume that is too large or as a result of non-uniform lung disease. Non-uniform lung disease causes preferential ventilation of the normal alveoli, which leads to overdistention of these alveoli as they try to accommodate most of the tidal volume.

Animal studies have suggested that alveolar overdistention, whether produced by positive or negative pressure, is responsible for the initiation and/or propagation of the lung injury. Tsuno et al.[12] analyzed the histopathologic changes in lungs of baby pigs after mechanical ventilation at a PIP of $40\,cmH_2O$ for 22 ± 11 hours. Alveolar hemorrhage, alveolar neutrophil infiltration, alveolar macrophage and type II pneumocyte proliferation, interstitial congestion and thickening, interstitial lymphocyte infiltration, emphysematous change, and hyaline membrane formation were all consistent with the early stages of ARDS. Animals ventilated with conventional ventilatory parameters (tidal volume $15\,mL/kg$, PCO_2 at $44\,mmHg$) for an additional 3–6 days showed the aforementioned findings coupled with prominent organized alveolar exudates, which resemble the changes seen in the late stages of ARDS. A

control group ventilated at a PIP of $18\,cmH_2O$ showed no histopathologic changes in the lung. Dreyfuss et al.[6] likewise showed that application of high inflation pressure ventilation in rats resulted in pulmonary edema after only 20 minutes, with histologic findings similar to those seen in human ARDS.

In 2000, the landmark ARDSNet trial[16] compared traditional tidal volume (10–15 mL/kg) and maximum plateau pressure of $50\,cmH_2O$ with low tidal volume (6 mL/kg) and plateau pressure of $\leq 30\,cmH_2O$ in patients with acute lung injury and ARDS. The study was stopped after enrolling 861 of an anticipated 1000 patients because it demonstrated that the lower tidal volume group had lower mortality (31.0 vs. 38.9%, $p = 0.007$) and a greater number of ventilator-free days (mean $\pm$ SD, 12 ± 11 vs. 10 ± 11, $p = 0.007$). The lower tidal volume reduces injury related to lung overdistention and inflammatory mediator release at the expense of a greater incidence of respiratory acidosis and decreased arterial oxygenation. While the trial demonstrated decreased mortality and increased number of ventilator-free days in comparing the low tidal volume group to the high tidal volume group, they found no difference in the incidence of barotrauma between the groups. Several studies have reached findings different from that of the ARDSNet. Stewart et al.[9], as noted above, found no mortality difference when comparing 120 ARDS patients receiving limited ventilation (PIP = $30\,cmH_2O$, tidal volume of 8 mL/kg) and conventional ventilation (PIP = $50\,cmH_2O$, tidal volume of 10–15 mL/kg). Brower et al.[17] examined 52 patients with ARDS and could find no benefit to mortality, medication requirement or any other clinical outcome measure, to a lower tidal volume (5–8 mL/kg) when compared with traditional tidal volume (10–12 mL/kg). Brochard et al.[18] reached similar findings when comparing 116 patients with ARDS randomized to receive reduced tidal volume (7.1 ± 1.3 mL/kg) or traditional tidal volume (10.3 ± 1.7 mL/kg). They found no difference between the two groups in mortality, duration of mechanical ventilation or incidence of pneumothorax.

Ranieri et al.[19] studied the effects of positive end-expiratory pressure (PEEP) on alveolar recruitment in patients with respiratory distress syndrome. Observing the pressure–volume loops on zero end-expiratory pressure and PEEP, they found two populations of patients. Some patients showed evidence of alveolar recruitment as evidenced by an upward concavity of the pressure–volume curve during zero end-expiratory pressure ventilation, which increased with PEEP. Other patients demonstrated an upward convexity, noting volume displacement without alveolar recruitment. This was aggravated with PEEP. They believed that this subpopulation of patients would be susceptible to barotrauma. In the recent ARDSNet ALVEOLI trial, Brower et al.[17] randomized 549 patients with acute lung injury and ARDS to receive 6 mL/kg tidal volume and either high ($13.2 \pm 3.5\,cmH_2O$) or low ($8.3 \pm 3.2\,cmH_2O$) PEEP. They found no difference in clinical outcomes between the high and low PEEP groups. They hypothesized that while higher PEEP levels could improve oxygenation and decrease ventilator-associated lung injury, they could also cause lung injury from overdistention.

Patients at risk for barotrauma range from infants receiving physiologic continuous positive airway pressure ($5\,cmH_2O$), as reported by Alpan et al.,[15] to adults requiring controlled mechanical ventilation and high levels of PEEP, as reported by Mathru et al.[20] and Kohn and Bellamy.[21] Mathru et al.[20] and Reines[22] noted that patients who are treated with volume-cycled or controlled mechanical ventilation have a higher incidence of barotrauma when compared to patients who are treated with pressure-limited or intermittent mandatory ventilations. As pointed out by Carlon et al.[23] and Parker et al.,[24] this is due to the higher airway pressures that are generated by volume-cycled ventilators compared with pressure-limited ventilators.

Gattinoni et al.[25] observed that ARDS is a heterogeneous, not diffuse, lung injury, with areas of relatively normal lung interspersed with areas of alveolar and interstitial edema. The term 'baby lungs' has been used to describe the smaller physiologic lung volume. Exposure of relatively normal alveoli with near normal compliance characteristics to high distending pressures results in a larger delivered volume per lung unit, marked overdistention, and the possible increased risk of further lung injury. This scenario occurs regardless of which mode of ventilation generates the high inspiratory pressures.

Another potential method of pulmonary injury involves the increased production of inflammatory mediators and cytokines secondary to mechanical ventilations, dubbed 'biotrauma' by some. A study by Chiumello et al.[26] demonstrated an association between high-volume ventilation and increased levels of TNF-α and MIP-2 in the lungs and in the serum. The authors hypothesized that the increased cytokines may contribute to multiple organ dysfunction, the leading cause of death in patients with ARDS. Tremblay et al.[27] found similar results when they exposed rats to varying degrees of ventilation. They discovered increased levels of TNF-α, MIP-2, IL-1β, IL-6, IL-10 and IFN-δ associated with high-volume ventilation. These cytokines serve to initiate and propagate inflammation, stimulating the recruitment and differentiation of macrophages to the lung parenchyma and facilitating neutrophil adherence. Ranieri et al.[28] compared inflammatory cytokines in 44 patients who were randomized to either a control ventilatory strategy or a lung-protective strategy. The two strategies were significantly different (mean (SD)) in terms of tidal volume (11.1 (1.3) vs. 7.6 (1.1) mL/kg), plateau pressures (31.0 (4.5) vs. 24.6 (2.4) cmH$_2$O) and PEEP (6.5 (1.7) vs. 14.8 (2.7) cmH$_2$O). The study demonstrated significantly higher levels of TNF-α, IL-1β and IL-6 in the control ventilation group.

The role that inflammation plays in ventilator-associated lung injury is not entirely clear. Kawano et al.[29] used a saline lung lavage followed by mechanical ventilation (tidal volume of 12 mL/kg) on three groups of rabbits: a control group, a neutropenic group secondary to pretreatment with nitrogen mustard, and a nitrogen mustard group that was retransfused with granulocytes before the study was begun. The first and third groups developed a high permeability pulmonary edema with hyaline membrane formation, whereas the neutropenic group showed none of these changes. Karzai et al.[30] examined rats that were assigned to be pretreated with fucoidin (a neutrophil adhesion inhibitor), granulocyte colony-stimulating factor (G-CSF) or a placebo prior to 4 hours of low (10 mL/kg) or high (40 mL/kg) tidal volume mechanical ventilation. In the G-CSF group that received high tidal volume ventilation, 18 of 22 rats died, a significantly higher number than the 3 of 20

rats that died in the placebo high tidal volume group, while the fucoidin high tidal volume group showed no significant difference from placebo. All of the low-volume animals survived. These experimental findings suggest a prominent role for inflammatory cells and mediators in the development of lung injury and argue against an injury that is entirely mechanical.

Presentation

One of the earliest radiographic signs of barotraumas is mediastinal air. Although this finding is often a precursor of pneumothorax, not all patients with pneumomediastinum develop a pneumothorax. In addition, pneumomediastinum usually does not give a clue as to the site of origin. Once pneumomediastinum develops, vigilance is important to discover early signs of pneumothorax.

Often, the first sign of barotrauma is not seen on routine chest radiography but presents as an acute change in hemodynamics or oxygenation. Any patient with poor compliance on positive-pressure ventilation and PEEP who becomes acutely hypotensive or hypoxemic may have a pneumothorax. In patients who have severe respiratory distress syndrome, the pneumothorax may not be large. The loss of even a small amount of lung volume may be sufficient to alter the steady state. Auscultation of the chest in pneumothorax may demonstrate disparate breath sounds, which may be confirmed by chest radiography.

Management

In a patient who has acutely developed barotrauma and is hemodynamically unstable, a needle catheter thoracostomy may be diagnostic as well as lifesaving. A sterile needle placed through the second or third intercostal space lateral to the midclavicular line allows the air to escape and should stabilize the patient until a more definitive catheter or tube can be placed. A large tube, preferably 28 Fr or 32 Fr, should be placed in the fifth or sixth intercostals space at the anterior axillary line. The large tube is used to remove any high-volume leak produced. Because many of these severely ill patients also have associated effusions, the tube should be directed posteriorly.

Sometimes the surgeon is notified of a critically ill ventilated patient when the patient develops a pneumomediastinum. Because the side of origin cannot be determined in such a case, the choice is observation or bilateral tube thoracostomy. Our preference is to assemble in a room the equipment necessary for both a needle and a tube thoracostomy but to await the development of a pneumothorax and treat only that side.

Because of the underlying disease, the lungs are stiff and may not completely re-expand. However, positive-pressure ventilation is being used on these patients. Because of these two facts, negative suction on the drainage system is unnecessary. Air from the air leak escapes through the water seal. Tubes should be left in place until the compliance significantly improves and the PEEP levels are consistently below 10 cmH$_2$O.

Other management techniques

In addition to conventional ventilators, other investigators have utilized alternate ventilatory modes in attempts to improve survival. Substantial interest in high-frequency ventilation (HFV) in burn patients has existed for a number of years.[31,32] Driven by some success of high-frequency oscillatory ventilation (HFOV) in the neonatal and pediatric populations, application of various high-frequency techniques to select groups of burn patients yielded encouraging results in small case series or non-randomized trials; most reports of success have been in its use as salvage therapy for patients failing conventional ventilatory modes.[33] Recently a randomized study in adults failed to demonstrate any superiority in outcome comparing HFOV and standard therapy although a post-hoc analysis demonstrated a slight treatment benefit with HFOV in patients with higher oxygen index (OI).[34] However, Carman et al.[35] reported a decrease in the incidence of barotrauma in a randomized comparison of the Volume Diffusive Respirator® compared to conventional ventilation. More scientific study will be required prior to the recommendation of high-frequency modalities for the prevention of barotrauma can be made. HFV requires specific ventilators with trained staff. With the lack of efficacy noted, its complexity and increased costs, it cannot be recommended at this time. Airway pressure release ventilation, proportional assist ventilation and bilevel positive pressure ventilation are other alternative modes that are currently under investigation but have not been demonstrated to be superior to current LTV strategy.

For the last 15 years, our group has studied ARDS in order to develop viable alternative treatments. We have exploited mechanical ventilation to its limits, including pressure-limited ventilation (permissive hypercapnia), inverse ratio ventilation, high-frequency jet ventilation, high-frequency oscillatory ventilation, intratracheal pulmonary ventilation, and prone position ventilation. In addition, we have participated in clinical trials on partial liquid ventilation, inhaled nitric oxide and surfactant therapy. All of these therapies have shown promise toward improving arterial blood gases and limiting lung injury in the short term, but none have demonstrated significant survival benefit. Work in our animal laboratory first demonstrated a role for extracorporeal gas exchange devices in our ovine model of smoke/burn inhalation-induced ARDS.[36]

We found that avoiding high ventilation pressures ameliorated the amount of barotrauma and biotrauma induced;[37] however, this is not always possible in the acutely ill patient. Some patients would require such large reductions in ventilation to achieve a 'safe' level that the resulting hypoxia or acidosis would not be tolerated. In these patients, adjunctive measures to achieve gas exchange can be employed. Treatment modalities such as extracorporeal membrane oxygenation (ECMO) and arteriovenous carbon dioxide removal (AVCO$_2$R) allow for a more gentle ventilation strategy by providing partial or total gas exchange.

ECMO exists as an adaptation of cardiopulmonary bypass in the operating room. Early investigators reasoned if the heart and lungs could be bypassed for a few hours to facilitate repair of a congenital defect or bypass a coronary artery, this same technology could facilitate the recovery of lungs that have temporarily lost the ability to exchange gas. This theory was first tested 30 years ago by Hill et al.[38] who successfully supported an adult ARDS patient for 3 days. Although ECMO is now associated most commonly with diseases of the neonatal population, its earliest use was as a supportive therapy for

adults with severe respiratory failure. The use of ECMO in neonates has resulted in a collective experience of 23 080 patients with an 82% survival rate.[39] The experience with ECMO in children and adults with burns has been limited.

ECMO involves the placement of large catheters into the central veins or arteries of the patient, draining the blood from the body, facilitating oxygenation, removing carbon dioxide and placing it back into the circulation. In venoarterial (VA) ECMO, blood is drained from either an internal jugular vein or a femoral vein, pumped through a gas exchanger and then returned to either a carotid or femoral artery, bypassing the native lungs (Figure 20.1). This form of ECMO allows for both pulmonary and cardiac support. In venovenous (VV) ECMO, the blood is returned to a large central vein rather than an artery (Figure 20.2). Venovenous ECMO is primarily indicated in isolated pulmonary failure. Both VV and VA ECMO require patients to be fully anticoagulated with heparin.

The need for full anticoagulation would seem to exclude patients with large burns from this therapy; however, our center has had a limited experience and some degree of success in supporting this population. Recently we reported our experience with pediatric burn patients supported with ECMO at the Extracorporeal Life Support Organization annual meeting (ELSO 2005, Houston Texas). Our center has no formal inclusion criteria for ECMO; each patient is evaluated on a case-by-case basis (Box 20.2). In general, patients were placed on ECMO after maximum medical management had failed. To date, we have supported 12 pediatric patients with burns including four scald burns (3/4 survivors), seven flame burns (4/7 survivors) and a single successful case of isolated inhalational injury.

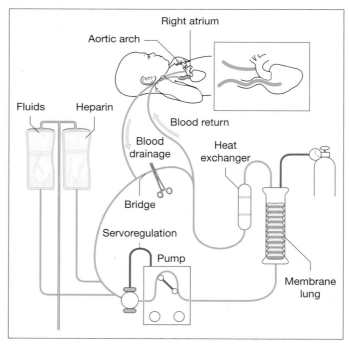

Fig. 20.1 Venoarterial extracorporeal membrane oxygenation circuit. (With permission from Alpard et al.[53] © 2004 Hodder Arnold. Reproduced with permission of Edward Arnold.)

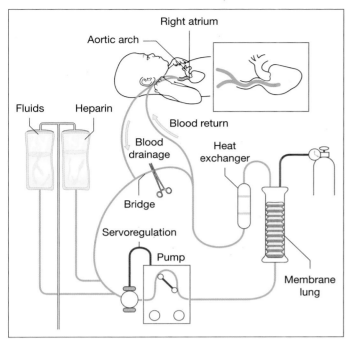

Fig. 20.2 Venovenous extracorporeal membrane oxygenation circuit. (With permission from Alpard et al.[53] © 2004 Hodder Arnold. Reproduced with permission of Edward Arnold.)

TABLE 20.1 PHYSIOLOGICAL DATA OF BURN PATIENTS SUPPORED WITH ECMO

	Survivors	Non-survivors	*p*-value
pH	7.36	7.28	ns
pCO$_2$	52	46	ns
pO$_2$	66	66	ns
PIP	48	31	ns
PEEP	14.6	8.3	ns
FiO$_2$	1.0	1.0	ns
Days of MV prior	7.4	5.8	ns

PIP = peak inspiratory pressure; PEEP = positive end-expiratory pressure; FiO$_2$ = fraction of inspired oxygen; MV = mechanical ventilation; ns = not statistically significant ($p > 0.05$).
Data presented at 2005 ELSO Conference, Houston, Texas.

BOX 20.2 ECMO burn patient selection criteria

GUIDELINES RATHER THAN CRITERIA

- Patient without PIP >50 cmH$_2$O for >24 hours
- Patient without PaO$_2$ <40 mmHg for >12 hours
- All burn wounds covered
- Has been mechanically ventilated <7 days
- Failed maximum medical management

CONTRAINDICATIONS

- CPR in progress pH <6.9 for >4 hours

*All cases evaluated on a case-by-case basis.

The most difficult aspect of utilizing ECMO to support a burn patient utilizing ECMO is deciding which patients will be successful and which will not. In a review of our experience, we found no predictive value of pre-ECMO arterial blood gases, ventilator settings, or days on mechanical ventilation (Table 20.1). As with previous studies, degree and extent of burn did not seem to affect survival ((survivors 46% (32–85), non-survivors 64% (48–60)).

Once the patient is on ECMO, the focus becomes which ones are likely to benefit from the therapy and which will not. Goretsky et al.[40] have described their experience with burns patients on ECMO and indicators that may predict a good outcome. These predictors of survival included younger age, shorter duration of ECMO support needed (<7 days) and fewer complications while on ECMO. This group also found that the extent and degree of burn had no effect on the outcome. Fur-

thermore, initial excision and allografting prior to heparinization appears beneficial. In a follow-up study, Kane et al.[41] reiterated Goretsky's findings, adding that the onset of sepsis, the requirement of blood transfusion that exceeded the patients total blood volume for 2 consecutive days, or the need for >7 days of support favored a poor outcome. Interestingly, 6 of the 8 survivors at our institution required >7 days of support and no patients required removal from ECMO for excessive bleeding. While our experience is limited to a single center, it does reiterate the need for further study in this patient population. Based on the ECMO burn experience, we will continue to offer ECMO to burned children at our institution.

The use of ECMO in burn patients has been limited for several reasons. The equipment required is expensive and requires one-on-one nursing care as well as an ECMO specialist nurse and/or a specially trained respiratory therapist. Without evidence from a randomized, controlled trial demonstrating survival benefit, some hospitals are unwilling to incur the expense associated with an ECMO program. The use of ECMO is likely to continue in specialized centers but unlikely to become a widespread treatment option for patients with burns until level I evidence-based studies show efficacy in populations other than neonates.

Occasionally, the full gas exchange support of ECMO is not needed. An adjunct to facilitate less injurious ventilator settings may be sufficient to support a patient without the need for the invasive cannulation involved with ECMO. This need can arise from the gentle ventilation techniques described by the ARDSNet trial,[16] which can result in severe respiratory acidosis. Arteriovenous carbon dioxide removal (AVCO$_2$R) is a technique that allows for CO$_2$ homeostasis without employing damaging ventilator settings. Utilizing a simple arterial-to-venous shunt with a low-resistance gas exchange device interposed, this system allows for removal of almost all metabolically produced CO$_2$ with less than a 25% shunt.[42–44]

Utilizing 'off-the-shelf' components, this form of simplified extracorporeal support provides some of the benefits of ECMO but does not require a pump, a dedicated specialist or complex equipment. A relatively small (10 Fr) cannula is placed percutaneously in the femoral artery and a slightly larger (12 Fr) cannula is placed in the femoral vein. Our early animal work

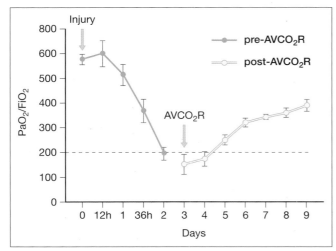

Fig. 20.3 PaO_2/FiO_2 ratio (P/F) following smoke inhalation and cutaneous flame burn injury and following placement of $AVCO_2R$. Entry criteria (P/F < 200) were met at 48 hours (194.8 ± 25.9). At the time $AVCO_2R$ was initiated P/F was 151.5 ± 40.0. After 36 hours P/F had improved to >200 and after 72 hours P/F was >300 (320.0 ± 17.8).

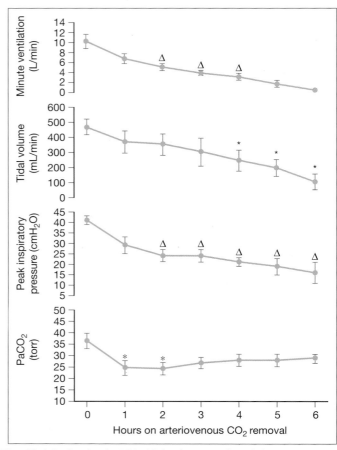

Fig. 20.4 Reduction in MV, tidal volume, and peak inspiratory pressure during arteriovenous CO_2 removal. MV reduced from 10.3 ± 1.4 L/min to 0.5 ± 0.0 L/min at 6 hours on arteriovenous CO_2 removal while maintaining normocapnia; similarly, tidal volume significantly reduced from 467 ± 53 mL/min at baseline to 102 ± 52 mL/min. With reductions in MV and tidal volume, peak inspiratory pressure significantly reduced from 40.8 ± 2.1 cmH_2O at baseline to 19.7 ± 7.5 cmH_2O at 6 hours on arteriovenous CO_2 removal (*$p < 0.05$ and ? $p < 0.01$ vs. baseline).

demonstrated that this technique was both safe and efficacious in our smoke/burn model of ARDS (Figure 20.3). Animal model studies have demonstrated that $AVCO_2R$ has allowed for increased survival time[45] and a significant decrease in ventilatory parameters (minute ventilation, tidal volume and PIP)[46] (Figures 20.4 and 20.5). Early phase I human testing showed the ability of $AVCO_2R$ to provide complete CO_2 removal during acute respiratory failure.[47] Our experience has shown that the device is safe for use in patients with severe respiratory failure, and that CO_2 removal rates of approximately 70% can be achieved.[48] As phase II clinical trials continue in this country and have struggled to meet anticipated accrual numbers, the European experience with pumpless CO_2 removal (termed pumpless extracorporeal lung assist (pECLA)) has grown significantly. Reports by Liebold et al.[49] of the first 70 patients show promise. To date over 700 patients have been supported with the pECLA system.

The gas exchanger currently used in the pECLA system has not been approved in the United States by the FDA. This hollow-fiber gas exchanger with polymethylpentane fibers allows days to weeks of support before failure and is ultra-low resistance (<10 mmHg @ 2 L/min blood flow) (Figure 20.6). Gas exchange devices used clinically in early phase I studies in the United States require change-out predictably before 72 hours of support due to 'fiber wetting,' a phenomenon attributable to the polypropylene composition of these devices. The polypropylene has hydrophilic properties which cause condensation to accumulate outside the device, thereby reducing its capacity for diffusion and gas exchange. While $AVCO_2R$ has shown success in both laboratory settings and in early trials in humans, its use is likely to remain limited. Both $AVCO_2R$ and pECLA require the patient to be anticoagulated and require the placement of a catheter in the femoral artery. This will likely limit the use of these therapies to tertiary care centers.

Prevention

Techniques to prevent barotrauma are as varied as the theories concerning its etiology. Because the major pulmonary mechanical changes in respiratory distress syndrome are decreased compliance and defect in diffusion, ventilation must be adjusted to optimize these values. Both pressure and volume determine alveolar distention and compliance. Some have theorized that peak airway pressure and PEEP are the major contributors to barotrauma. ARDSNet[16] established that tidal volumes of 6 mL/kg resulted in a lower mortality and increased number of ventilator-free days. However, Young et al.[50] surveyed three tertiary care hospitals and found that the findings from the ARDSNet trial are not being widely applied by physicians. While the tidal volumes administered by physicians after the publication of the ARDSNet trial were significantly lower compared to before publication (10.6 vs. 12.3 mL/kg of predicted body weight), they were still well above the 6 mL/kg level recommended by the study.

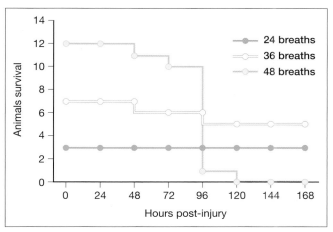

Fig. 20.5 Kaplan–Meier curve depicting the number of sheep surviving the 7-day (168 hours) study. All the sheep in the 24 breath/40% TBSA III° cutaneous flame burn group survived to 7 days: 5/7 sheep in the 36 breath/40% TBSA III cutaneous flame burn group survived to 7 days (LD_{30}). None of the sheep in the 48 breath/40% TBSA III° cutaneous flame burn group survived to 7 days. Only 1 sheep receiving 48 breaths of cotton smoke survived to day 4.

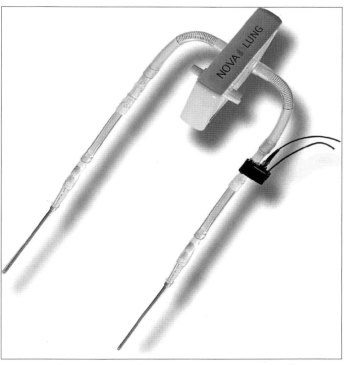

Fig. 20.6 The symmetrical lung assist device is shown with two low-resistance cannulae attached. The system's low-pressure gradient allows use without a mechanical blood pump in an arteriovenous shunt created between femoral artery and vein. (Reprinted with permission of Sage Publications Ltd from Matheis G in Perfusion 18(4) © Sage Publications Ltd 2003.)

The causes and treatments of barotrauma represent dynamic subjects. As our understanding of the pathophysiology of lung injury has progressed, so has our ability to manage and prevent these injuries. In the past, physicians had employed peak inspiratory pressures as high as 75–100 mmHg to achieve physiologically 'normal' arterial blood gas values; today, the emphasis is placed on low-volume ventilation in order to minimize alveolar overdistention at the expense of marginal arterial blood gas values. As our understanding of the molecular markers of lung injury improves, so may our ability to predict which patients are at greater risk and our knowledge of how they should best be managed.

With the body of knowledge frequently changing, it is important to bear in mind the observation by Marini and Gattinoni:[51] precise numerical guidelines for selecting PEEP, tidal volume, and ventilatory position that are applicable to any given individual patient should not be expected from the results of studies conducted in a diverse sample population. While this advice holds true, clinicians should avoid using potentially injurious ventilatory settings in an attempt to normalize blood gases. Instead more focus should be on the minimum amount of support required to provide the patient with acceptable blood gas values without inflicting further damage on their fragile lungs.

References

1. Anzueto A, Frutos-Vivar F, Esteban A, et al. Incidence, risk factors and outcome of barotrauma in mechanically ventilated patients. Intensive Care Med 2004; 30(4):612–619.
2. Macklin M, Macklin C. Malignant interstitial emphysema of the lungs and mediastinum. Medicine 1944; (23):281–352.
3. Bendixen HH, Hedley-Whyte J, Laver MB. Impaired oxygenation in surgical patients during general anesthesia with controlled ventilation. A concept of atelectasis. N Engl J Med 1963; 269:991–996.
4. Ashbaugh DG, Bigelow DB, Petty TL, et al. Acute respiratory distress in adults. Lancet 1967; 2(7511):319–323.
5. Webb HH, Tierney DF. Experimental pulmonary edema due to intermittent positive pressure ventilation with high inflation pressures. Protection by positive end-expiratory pressure. Am Rev Respir Dis 1974; 110(5):556–565.
6. Dreyfuss D, Basset G, Soler P, et al. Intermittent positive-pressure hyperventilation with high inflation pressures produces pulmonary microvascular injury in rats. Am Rev Respir Dis 1985; 132(4):880–884.
7. Diakun TA. Carbon dioxide embolism: successful resuscitation with cardiopulmonary bypass. Anesthesiology 1991; 74(6):1151–1153.
8. Peterson G, Baier H. Incidence of pulmonary barotrauma in a medical ICU. Crit Care Med 1983; 11(2):67–69.
9. Stewart TE, Meade MO, Cook DJ, et al. Evaluation of a ventilation strategy to prevent barotrauma in patients at high risk for acute respiratory distress syndrome. Pressure- and Volume-Limited Ventilation Strategy Group. N Engl J Med 1998; 338(6):355–361.
10. Weg JG, Anzueto A, Balk RA, et al. The relation of pneumothorax and other air leaks to mortality in the acute respiratory distress syndrome. N Engl J Med 1998; 338(6):341–346.
11. Boussarsar M, Thierry G, Jaber S, et al. Relationship between ventilatory settings and barotrauma in the acute respiratory distress syndrome. Intensive Care Med 2002; 28(4):406–413.
12. Tsuno K, Prato P, Kolobow T. Acute lung injury from mechanical ventilation at moderately high airway pressures. J Appl Physiol 1990; 69(3):956–961.

13. Hillman KM, Barber JD. Asynchronous independent lung ventilation (AILV). Crit Care Med 1980; 8(7):390–395.
14. Hurd TE, Novak R, Gallagher TJ. Tension pneumopericardium: a complication of mechanical ventilation. Crit Care Med 1984; 12(3):200–201.
15. Alpan G, Goder K, Glick B, et al. Pneumopericardium during continuous positive airway pressure in respiratory distress syndrome. Crit Care Med 1984; 12(12):1080–1081.
16. Ventilation with lower tidal volumes as compared with traditional tidal volumes for acute lung injury and the acute respiratory distress syndrome. The Acute Respiratory Distress Syndrome Network. N Engl J Med 2000; 342(18):1301–1308.
17. Brower RG, Shanholtz CB, Fessler HE, et al. Prospective, randomized, controlled clinical trial comparing traditional versus reduced tidal volume ventilation in acute respiratory distress syndrome patients. Crit Care Med 1999; 27(8):1492–1498.
18. Brochard L, Roudot-Thoraval F, Roupie E, et al. Tidal volume reduction for prevention of ventilator-induced lung injury in acute respiratory distress syndrome. The Multicenter Trial Group on Tidal Volume Reduction in ARDS. Am J Respir Crit Care Med 1998; 158(6):1831–1838.
19. Ranieri VM, Eissa NT, Corbeil C, et al. Effects of positive end-expiratory pressure on alveolar recruitment and gas exchange in patients with the adult respiratory distress syndrome. Am Rev Respir Dis 1991; 144(3 Pt 1):544–551.
20. Mathru M, Rao TL, Venus B. Ventilator-induced barotrauma in controlled mechanical ventilation versus intermittent mandatory ventilation. Crit Care Med 1983; 11(5):359–361.
21. Kohn S, Bellamy P. Pulmonary barotrauma in patients with adult respiratory distress syndrome (ARDS) during continuous positive pressure ventilation (CPPV). Am Rev Respir Dis 1982; 125:129A.
22. Reines HD. Manifestations of barotrauma in acute respiratory failure. Am Surg 1981; 47(10):421–425.
23. Carlon GC, Howland WS, Ray C, et al. High-frequency jet ventilation. A prospective randomized evaluation. Chest 1983; 84(5):551–559.
24. Parker JC, Hernandez LA, Peevy KJ. Mechanisms of ventilator-induced lung injury. Crit Care Med 1993; 21(1):131–143.
25. Gattinoni L, Pesenti A, Avalli L, et al. Pressure-volume curve of total respiratory system in acute respiratory failure. Computed tomographic scan study. Am Rev Respir Dis 1987; 136(3):730–736.
26. Chiumello D, Pristine G, Slutsky AS. Mechanical ventilation affects local and systemic cytokines in an animal model of acute respiratory distress syndrome. Am J Respir Crit Care Med 1999; 160(1):109–116.
27. Tremblay L, Valenza F, Ribeiro SP, et al. Injurious ventilatory strategies increase cytokines and c-fos m-RNA expression in an isolated rat lung model. J Clin Invest 1997; 99(5):944–952.
28. Ranieri VM, Suter PM, Tortorella C, et al. Effect of mechanical ventilation on inflammatory mediators in patients with acute respiratory distress syndrome: a randomized controlled trial. JAMA 1999; 282(1):54–61.
29. Kawano T, Mori S, Cybulsky M, et al. Effect of granulocyte depletion in a ventilated surfactant-depleted lung. J Appl Physiol 1987; 62(1):27–33.
30. Karzai W, Cui X, Heinicke N, et al. Neutrophil stimulation with granulocyte colony-stimulating factor worsens ventilator-induced lung injury and mortality in rats. Anesthesiology 2005; 103(5):996–1005.
31. Cioffi WG Jr, Rue LW 3rd, Graves TA, et al. Prophylactic use of high-frequency percussive ventilation in patients with inhalation injury. Ann Surg 1991; 213(6):575–580; discussion 580–572.
32. Cortiella J, Mlcak R, Herndon D. High frequency percussive ventilation in pediatric patients with inhalation injury. J Burn Care Rehabil 1999; 20(3):232–235.
33. Cartotto R, Ellis S, Smith T. Use of high-frequency oscillatory ventilation in burn patients. Crit Care Med 2005; 33(3 Suppl):S175–S181.
34. Bollen CW, van Well GT, Sherry T, et al. High frequency oscillatory ventilation compared with conventional mechanical ventilation in adult respiratory distress syndrome: a randomized controlled trial [ISRCTN24242669]. Crit Care 2005; 9(4):R430–R439.
35. Carman B, Cahill T, Warden G, et al. A prospective, randomized comparison of the Volume Diffusive Respirator vs conventional ventilation for ventilation of burned children. 2001 ABA paper. J Burn Care Rehabil 2002; 23(6):444–448.
36. Zwischenberger JB, Cox CS Jr, Minifee PK, et al. Pathophysiology of ovine smoke inhalation injury treated with extracorporeal membrane oxygenation. Chest 1993; 103(5):1582–1586.
37. Tao W, Brunston RL Jr, Bidani A, et al. Significant reduction in minute ventilation and peak inspiratory pressures with arteriovenous CO_2 removal during severe respiratory failure. Crit Care Med 1997; 25(4):689–695.
38. Hill JD, O'Brien TG, Murray JJ, et al. Prolonged extracorporeal oxygenation for acute post-traumatic respiratory failure (shock-lung syndrome). Use of the Bramson membrane lung. N Engl J Med 1972; 286(12):629–634.
39. ECMO Registry of the Extracorporeal Life Support Organization (ELSO), Ann Arbor Michigan: ECMO; (December) 2005.
40. Goretsky MJ, Greenhalgh DG, Warden GD, et al. The use of extracorporeal life support in pediatric burn patients with respiratory failure. J Pediatr Surg 1995; 30(4):620–623.
41. Kane TD, Greenhalgh DG, Warden GD, et al. Pediatric burn patients with respiratory failure: predictors of outcome with the use of extracorporeal life support. J Burn Care Rehabil 1999; 20(2):145–150.
42. Brunston RL Jr, Tao W, Bidani A, et al. Prolonged hemodynamic stability during arteriovenous carbon dioxide removal for severe respiratory failure. J Thorac Cardiovasc Surg 1997; 114(6):1107–1114.
43. Brunston RL Jr, Tao W, Bidani A, et al. Organ blood flow during arteriovenous carbon dioxide removal. ASAIO J 1997; 43(5):M821–M824.
44. Brunston RL Jr, Zwischenberger JB, Tao W, et al. Total arteriovenous CO_2 removal: simplifying extracorporeal support for respiratory failure. Ann Thorac Surg 1997; 64(6):1599–1604; discussion 1604–1595.
45. Alpard SK, Zwischenberger JB, Tao W, et al. New clinically relevant sheep model of severe respiratory failure secondary to combined smoke inhalation/cutaneous flame burn injury. Crit Care Med 2000; 28(5):1469–1476.
46. Zwischenberger JB, Alpard SK, Conrad SA, et al. Arteriovenous carbon dioxide removal: development and impact on ventilator management and survival during severe respiratory failure. Perfusion 1999; 14(4):299–310.
47. Conrad SA, Zwischenberger JB, Grier LR, et al. Total extracorporeal arteriovenous carbon dioxide removal in acute respiratory failure: a phase I clinical study. Intensive Care Med 2001; 27(8):1340–1351.
48. Zwischenberger JB, Conrad SA, Alpard SK, et al. Percutaneous extracorporeal arteriovenous CO_2 removal for severe respiratory failure. Ann Thorac Surg 1999; 68(1):181–187.
49. Liebold A, Philipp A, Kaiser M, et al. Pumpless extracorporeal lung assist using an arterio-venous shunt. Applications and limitations. Minerva Anestesiol 2002; 68(5):387–391.
50. Young MP, Manning HL, Wilson DL, et al. Ventilation of patients with acute lung injury and acute respiratory distress syndrome: has new evidence changed clinical practice? Crit Care Med 2004; 32(6):1260–1265.
51. Marini JJ, Gattinoni L. Ventilatory management of acute respiratory distress syndrome: a consensus of two. Crit Care Med 2004; 32(1):250–255.
52. Zwischenberger JB, Tao W, Alpard SK, et al. Barotrauma and inhalation injuries. In: Shields T, ed. General thoracic surgery, 5th edn. Philadelphia: Lippincott, Williams and Wilkins; 2000:Vol. 1;834–839.
53. Alpard SK, Chung DH, Zwischenberger. Extracorporeal membrane oxygenation. In: Kay PH, Munsch CM, eds. Techniques in extracorporeal circulation, 4th edn. London: Arnold; 2004:254–291.
54. Matheis G. Perfusion. London: Hodder Arnold; 2003: 18:245–251.

Chapter 21

Respiratory care

Ronald P. Mlcak and David N. Herndon

Chapter contents

Introduction

The multitude of respiratory complications caused by smoke inhalation, thermal burns, and their treatment epitomize the clinical challenges which confront respiratory care practitioners. Smoke inhalation injury and its sequelae impose demands upon the respiratory care practitioners who play a central role in its clinical management. These demands may range from intubation and resuscitation of victims in the emergency room to assistance with diagnostic bronchoscopies, to performance of pulmonary function studies, monitoring of arterial blood gases, airway maintenance, chest physiotherapy, and mechanical ventilator management.[1] Additional demands are placed upon the respiratory care practitioner in the rehabilitation phase in determining disability or limitations diagnosed by pulmonary function studies or cardiopulmonary stress testing. In some countries outside the United States, the duties of the respiratory care practitioner are augmented by a combination of physicians, nurses, and physiotherapists. It is imperative that a well-organized, protocol-driven approach to respiratory care of the burn patient be utilized so that improvements can be made, and the morbidity and mortality associated with inhalation injury can be reduced (Box 21.1). This chapter provides an overview of the common hands-on approaches to the treatment of inhalation injury, with emphasis on mucociliary clearance techniques, pharmacologic adjuncts, mechanical ventilation, infection control, and the late complications associated with inhalation injury.

Bronchial hygiene therapy

Airway clearance techniques are an essential component of respiratory management of patients with smoke inhalation. Bronchial hygiene therapy is a term used to describe several of the modalities intended to accomplish this goal. Therapeutic coughing, chest physiotherapy, early ambulation, airway suc-

tioning, therapeutic bronchoscopy, and pharmacologic agents have been effective in the removal of retained secretions.

Therapeutic coughing

Therapeutic coughing functions to promote airway clearance of excess mucus and fibrin cast in the tracheal bronchial tree. The impairment of the cough mechanism will result in retained secretions, bronchial obstruction, atelectasis, and/or pneumonia. A cough may be either a reflex or a voluntary action. The mechanisms of a cough include:
- a deep inspiration;
- the closure of the glottis;
- contraction of the muscles of the chest wall, abdomen, and pelvic floor;
- opening of the glottis; and
- a rapid expulsive exhalation phase.

During a cough, alveolar, pleural, and subglottic pressures may rise as much as $200 \, cmH_2O$. A failure of the cough mechanism may be due to an impairment of any step in the sequences described. When this occurs, it is necessary to perform techniques which are used to improve the cough.

Series of three coughs

The patient is asked to start a small breath and small cough, then a bigger breath and harder cough, and finally a really deep breath and hard cough. This technique is especially effective for postoperative patients who tend to splint from pain.[2]

Tracheal tickle

The therapist places the index and middle finger flat in the sternal notch and gently massages inward in a circular fashion over the trachea. This is most effective in obtunded patients or in patients coming out of anesthesia.[2]

Cough stimulation

Patients with artificial airways cannot cough normally since a tube is either between the vocal cords (endotracheal) or below the cords (tracheostomy). Adequate pressure cannot be built up without approximation of the cords. These patients may have a cough stimulated by inflating the cuff on the tube, giving a large, rapid inspiration by a manual resuscitation bag, holding the breath for 1–2 seconds, and rapidly allowing the bag to release and exhalation to ensue. This technique is normally performed by two persons and is made more effective by one therapist performing vibration and chest compressions from the time of the inspiratory hold, all during exhalation.[2] Cough and deep breathing exercises are encouraged every 2 hours to aid in removing retained secretions.

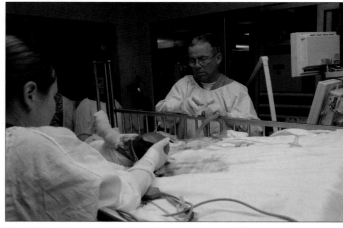

Fig. 21.1 Patient positioning for secretion mobilization.

Chest physiotherapy

Chest physiotherapy has come to mean gravity-assisted bronchial drainage with chest percussion and vibrations. Studies have shown that a combination of techniques are effective in secretion removal.[3–6]

Bronchial drainage/positioning

Bronchial drainage/positioning is a therapeutic modality that uses gravity-assisted positioning designed to improve pulmonary hygiene in patients with inhalation injury or retained secretions. There are 12 basic positions in which patients can be placed for postural drainage. Due to skin grafts, donor sites, and the use of air fluid beds, clinical judgment dictates that most of these positions are not practical. In fact, positioning in the Trendelenburg and various other positions may acutely worsen hypoxemia. Evidence has shown that a patient's arterial oxygenation may fall during positioning.[7] To accomplish the same goal it is common practice, in intensive care units, to turn patients side to side every 2 hours so as to aid in mobilizing secretions (Figure 21.1).

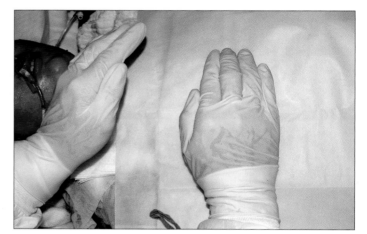

Fig. 21.2 Chest physiotherapy techniques.

Percussion

Percussion aids in the removal of secretions from the tracheal bronchial tree. Percussion is done by cupping the hand so as to allow a cushion of air to come between the percussor's hand and the patient. If this is done properly, a popping sound will be heard when the patient is percussed. There should be a towel between the patient and the percussor's hand in order to prevent irritation of the skin.[8] Percussion is applied over the surface landmarks of the bronchial segments that are being drained. The hands rhythmically and alternately strike the chest wall. Incisions, skin grafts, and bony prominences should be avoided during percussion (Figure 21.2).

Vibration/shaking

Vibration/shaking is a shaking movement used to move loosened secretions to larger airways so that they can be coughed up or removed by suctioning. Vibration involves rapid shaking of the chest wall during exhalation. The percussor vibrates the thoracic cage by placing both hands over the percussed areas

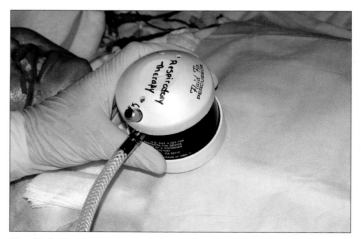

Fig. 21.3 Gentle mechanical chest vibrations.

and vibrating into the patient, isometrically contracting or tensing the muscles of their arms and shoulders. Mechanical vibrations have been reported to produce good clinical results. Gentle mechanical vibration may be indicated for patients who cannot tolerate manual percussion (Figure 21.3). Chest physiotherapy techniques should be used every 2–4 hours for patients with retained secretions. Therapy should continue until breath sounds improve.

Early ambulation

Early ambulation is another effective means of preventing respiratory complications. Patients routinely should be helped out of bed on postoperative day 5 and encouraged to ambulate and sit in a chair. With appropriate use of analgesics, even patients on continuous ventilatory support can be helped out of bed and into a chair (Figure 21.4). The rocking chair (Figure 21.5) has several beneficial effects:

* the patient can breathe with regions of the lungs which are normally hyperventilated;

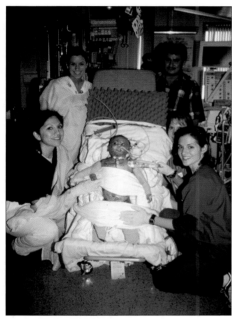

Fig. 21.4 Early ambulation.

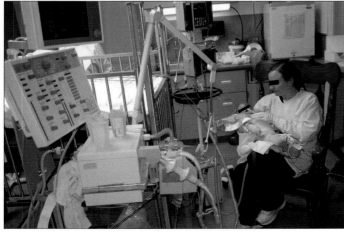

Fig. 21.5 Patient up out of bed, secretions being mobilized by rocking, and chest physiotherapy techniques.

* muscular strength and tone are preserved;
* contractions are prevented and exercise tolerance is maintained.[9]

Airway suctioning

Airway suctioning is another method of clearing an airway. Normal bronchial hygiene is usually accomplished by the mucociliary escalator process. When these methods are not effective in maintaining a clear airway, tracheobronchial suctioning is indicated.[10–13] Nasotracheal suctioning is intended to remove from the trachea accumulated secretions and other foreign material which cannot be removed by the patien's spontaneous cough or less-invasive procedures. Nasotracheal suctioning has been used to avoid intubation which was solely intended for the removal of secretions. Nasotracheal suctioning refers to the insertion of a suction catheter through the nasal passages and pharynx into the trachea in order to aspirate secretions or foreign material. The first step in this process is to hyperoxygenate the patient with 100% oxygen. The patient should be positioned in the Fowler's position and the catheter slowly advanced through the nares to a point just above the larynx. The therapist or nurse then listens for air sounds at the proximal end of the catheter. When airflow is felt to be strongest and respiratory sounds are loudest, the tip of the catheter is immediately above the epiglottis. On inspiration, the catheter is advanced into the trachea. After the vocal cords have been passed, a few deep breaths are allowed and the patient is reoxygenated. Suction is begun while the catheter is slowly withdrawn from the trachea. The patient should not be suctioned for more than 15 seconds without being reoxygenated. Suctioning is not without potential hazards.[14,15] Complications include irritation of the nasotracheal mucosa with bleeding, abrupt drops in PO_2, vagal stimulation, and bradycardia. Preoxygenating and limiting suction time have been shown to decrease or eliminate the fall in the PO_2.[12–14] Sputum cultures should be performed for microbiological identification when they are clinically indicated. Patients on mechanical ventilation should have sputum cultures performed once per week.

Therapeutic bronchoscopy

When all other techniques fail to remove secretions, the use of the fiberoptic bronchoscope has proven to be of benefit. In addition to its diagnostic functions, bronchoscopy retains important therapeutic applications. Copious secretions encountered in patients with inhalation injury may require repeated bronchoscopic procedures when more conservative methods are unsuccessful. The modern fiberoptic bronchoscope is small in diameter, flexible, and has a steerable tip that can be maneuvered into the fourth- or fifth-order bronchi for examination or specimen removal.

Pharmacologic adjuncts
Bronchodilators

Bronchodilators can be helpful in some cases. Inhalation injury to the lower airways results in a chemical tracheobronchitis which can produce wheezing and bronchospasms. This is especially true for patients with preexisting reactive airway diseases. Most drugs used in the management of bronchospasms are believed to act on the biochemical mechanism which controls bronchial muscle tone. Aerosolized sympathomimetics are effective in two ways: they result in bronchial muscle relaxation and they stimulate mucociliary clearance. The newer bronchodilators are more effective and have fewer side-effects than the older generation drugs. Some of the newer compounds used in the United States are worthy of note. First, metaproterenol is available in cartridge inhalers, as a liquid to be aerosolized, as an oral medication in tablets, or as a syrup. The recommended oral dose is 10–20 mg every 6–8 hours; as an inhaled bronchodilator, 1–2 puffs every 3–4 hours. Its duration of action as an inhaled bronchodilator is 1–5 hours.[16]

Albuterol can also be administered orally, parenterally, and by aerosol. Albuterol is available in a metered cartridge inhaler and its standard dose is 1–2 puffs three to four times daily. Aerosolized albuterol has a duration of action of approximately 4–6 hours.[17]

Racemic epinephrine is used as an aerosolized topical vasoconstrictor, bronchodilator, and secretion bond breaker. The vasoconstrictive action of racemic epinephrine is useful in reducing mucosal and submucosal edema within the walls of the pulmonary airways. A secondary bronchodilator action serves to reduce potential spasm of the smooth muscles of the terminal bronchioles. Water, employed as a diluent for racemic epinephrine, serves to lower both adhesive and cohesive forces of the retained endobronchial secretions, thus serving as a bond-breaking vehicle. Racemic epinephrine has also been used for the treatment of post-extubation stridor.[18] Its mode of action is thought to be related to the vasoconstrictive activity, with the resultant decrease in mucosal edema. Aerosolized treatments may be given every 2 hours as long as the heart rate is not increased.

Hypertonic saline offers a theoretically more effective form of mucokinetic therapy. The deposition of hypertonic droplets on the respiratory mucosa results in the osmotic attraction of fluids from the mucosal blood vessels and tissues into the airway. Thus a 'bronchorrhea' is induced, and the watery solution helps to dilute down the respiratory tract secretions and to increase their bulk, thereby augmenting expectoration. Furthermore, there is evidence that hypertonic saline has a direct effect on the mucoprotein DNA complexes, and by reducing the cohesive intramolecular forces, the salt helps reduce the viscous properties of the mucoid fluid.[19] Excessive use of hypertonic saline is not recommended because irritation can occur in the respiratory tract, absorption can occur, and burn patients who cannot tolerate the sodium load may develop edema.

Finally, aerosolized acetylcysteine is a powerful mucolytic agent in use in respiratory care. Acetylcysteine contains a thiol group; the free sulfhydryl radical of this group is a strong reducing agent which ruptures the disulfide bonds that serve to give stability to the mucoprotein network of molecules in mucus. Agents that break down these disulfide bonds produce the most effective mucolysis.[20] Acetylcysteine is an irritant to the respiratory tract. It can cause mucosal changes, and it may induce bronchospasm. For this reason, patients are evaluated for signs of bronchospasm, and a bronchodilator may be added if necessary. Acetylcysteine has proven to be effective in combination with aerosolized heparin for the treatment of inhalation injury in animal studies.[21]

Heparin/acetylcysteine combinations have been used as scavengers for the oxygen free radicals produced when alveolar macrophages are activated either directly by chemicals in smoke or by one or more of the compounds in the arachidonic cascade.[22] Animal studies have shown an increased P/F ratio, decreased peak inspiratory pressures, and a decreased amount of fibrin cast formation with heparin/acetylcystine combinations.[23] In a retrospective review, Desai et al. have shown that the use of heparin/N-acetylcysteine is effective in pediatric patients with inhalation injury.[24] Results indicate a significant decrease in the reintubation rates, incidence of atelectasis, and improved mortality for patients treated with heparin/N-acetylcysteine therapy. Therefore a standard treatment for patients with inhalation injury might include 5000–10000 units of heparin and 3 mL normal saline nebulized every 4 hours, alternating with 3–5 mL of 20% acetylcysteine for 7 days. This insures that the patient receives an aerosolized treatment every 2 hours. Baseline and daily clotting studies are recommended for the entire length of the aerosolized treatments.

A prospective randomized study on the use of nebulized heparin for the treatment of inhalation injury is necessary to validate the continued used of this mode of therapy. A multicenter study is being developed that will evaluate the effectiveness of therapy and answer some of the questions regarding the mechanism of action, safety, and affects on lung function.

Patient/family education

Burn care involves utilizing a family-centered care approach. Therefore the patient and family should be informed about the extent of the lung injury and the various treatment options available based upon evidence-based medicine or best practice.

Mechanical ventilation

Over the past 30 years, and especially over the past decade, there has been an increase in new ventilatory techniques which present alternatives for the treatment of patients with smoke inhalation. Unfortunately, although the number of options available to the clinician has appeared to increase exponentially, well-controlled clinical trials defining the specific role for each of the modes of ventilation and comparing them to other modes of ventilation have not been forthcoming. Based upon current available data, the recommendations from the American College of Chest Physicians consensus conference on mechanical ventilation generally serve as guidelines.[25] The general consensus concludes:

- The clinician should choose a ventilator mode that has been shown to be capable of supporting oxygenation and ventilation and that the clinician has experience in using.
- An acceptable oxygen saturation should be targeted.
- Based primarily on animal data, a plateau pressure of greater than 35 cmH$_2$O is cause for concern. With clinical conditions that are associated with a decreased chest wall compliance, plateau pressures greater than 35 cmH$_2$O may be acceptable.
- To accomplish the goal of limiting plateau pressures, PCO_2 values should be permitted to rise (permissive

hypercapnia) unless other contraindications exist that demand a more normal PCO_2 or pH.

- Positive end-expiratory pressure (PEEP) is useful in supporting oxygenation. An appropriate level of PEEP may be helpful in preventing lung damage. The level of PEEP required should be established by empirical trials and reevaluated on a regular basis.
- Large tidal volumes (8–10 mL/kg) with PEEP may be needed to improve oxygenation if the use of protective ventilatory strategies becomes ineffective. Peak flow rates should be adjusted as needed to satisfy patient inspiratory needs.[25] Care must be taken to avoid the consequences of utilizing high ventilator pressures if large tidal volumes are required.

A new multicenter study by the Acute Respiratory Distress Syndrome Network of the National Heart, Lung, and Blood Institute is the first large randomized study comparing high versus low tidal volumes for patients with ARDS.[47] The trial compared traditional ventilation treatment, which involved an initial tidal volume of 12 mL/kg of predicted body weight, and an airway pressure measured of 50 cmH_2O or less, to ventilation with a lower tidal volume, which involved an initial tidal volume of 6 mL/kg of predicted body weight and a plateau pressure of 30 cmH_2O or less. The volume-assist-control mode was used for the ventilation study. The trial was stopped after the enrollment of 861 patients because mortality was lower in the group treated with lower tidal volumes than in the group treated with traditional tidal volumes, and the number of days without ventilator use during the first 28 days after randomization was greater in this group.[47]

This study was the first large randomized investigation documenting a decrease in mortality with the use of lower tidal volumes for the treatment of patients with ARDS. In light of this new evidence, the tidal volumes used when initiating mechanical ventilation should be 6–8 mL/kg of predicted body weight. If the patient becomes obstructed with fibrin cast and presents with an acute increase in PCO_2 and decrease in PaO_2, the clinician should first provide aggressive pulmonary toilet, then consider changing over to volume ventilation with higher tidal volumes. If ventilation continues to worsen, tidal volumes of 8–10 mL/kg may be needed to provide adequate mechanical ventilation.

Modes of ventilation
Control mode

In the control mode of ventilation, the ventilator cycles automatically at a rate selected by the operator. The adjustment is usually made by a knob calibrated in breaths/min. The ventilator will cycle regardless of the patient need or desire for a breath, but guarantees a minimum level of minute ventilation in the apneic, sedated, or paralyzed patient. The control mode of ventilation is often utilized in patients with ARDS because of the high peak pressures needed to achieve adequate chest expansion. The major disadvantage with this mode is that the patient cannot cycle the ventilator and thus the minute ventilation must be set appropriately.

Assist-control mode

In the assist-control mode of ventilation, in which every breath is supported by the ventilator, a back-up control rate is set; however, the patient may choose any rate above the set rate. Using this mode of ventilation, the tidal volume, inspiratory flow rate, flow waveform, sensitivity, and control rate are set.[26–28] Advantages are that assist-control ventilation combines the security of controlled ventilation with the possibility of synchronizing the breathing pattern of the patient and ventilator, and it ensures ventilatory support during each breath. Disadvantages are as follows:

- Excessive patient work occurs in case of inadequate peak flow or sensitivity settings, especially if the ventilator drive of the patient is increased.[26–28]
- It is sometimes poorly tolerated in awake, nonsedated subjects and can require sedation to insure synchrony of patient and machine.
- It can cause respiratory alkalosis.
- It may worsen air trapping with patients with chronic obstructed lung disease.[24]

Synchronized intermittent mandatory ventilation

Synchronized intermittent mandatory ventilation (SIMV) combines a preset number of ventilator-delivered mandatory breaths of present tidal volume with the facility for intermittent patient-generated spontaneous breaths.[29,30]

Advantages are as follows:

- The patient is able to perform a variable amount of respiratory work and yet there is the security of a preset mandatory level of ventilation.
- SIMV allows for a variation in level of partial ventilatory support from near total ventilatory support to spontaneous breathing.
- It can be used as a weaning tool.

Disadvantages are:

- Hyperventilation with respiratory alkalosis.
- Excessive work of breathing due to the presence of a poorly responsive demand valve, suboptimal ventilatory circuits, or inappropriate flow delivery could occur.
- In each case, extra work is imposed on the patient during spontaneous breaths.

Pressure control mode

In pressure-controlled ventilation all breaths are time- or patient-triggered, pressure-limited, and time-cycled. The ventilator provides a constant pressure of air to the patient during inspiration. The length of inspiration, the pressure level, and the back-up rate are set by the operator. Tidal volume is based upon the compliance and resistance of the patient's lungs, the ventilator system, as well as on the preset pressure. Pressure control ventilation has become a frequently used mode of ventilation for the treatment of ARDS.

Pressure support ventilation

Pressure support ventilation (PSV) is a pressure-targeted, flow-cycled, mode of ventilation in which each breath must be patient-triggered. It is used both as a mode of ventilation during stable ventilatory support periods and as a weaning method.[30–34] It is primarily designed to assist spontaneous breathing and therefore the patient must have an intact respiratory drive.

Advantages are:

- It is generally regarded as a comfortable mode of ventilation for most patients.
- Pressure support reduces the work of breathing.
- It can be used to overcome the airway resistance caused by the endotracheal tube.
- Pressure support may be useful in patients who are difficult to wean.

Disadvantages are:

- The tidal volume is not controlled and is dependent on respiratory mechanics, cycling frequency, and synchrony between the patient and ventilator.
- Pressure support may be poorly tolerated in some patients with high airway resistances because of the preset high initial flow rates.

Alternate modes of ventilation

During the last decade, a new concept has emerged regarding acute lung injury. In severe cases of ARDS, only a small part of the lung parenchyma remains accessible to gas delivered by mechanical ventilation.[35,36] As a consequence, tidal volumes of 10 mL/kg or more may overexpand and injure the remaining normally aerated lung parenchyma and could worsen the prognosis of severe acute respiratory failure by extending nonspecific alveolar damage. High airway pressures may result in overdistension and local hyperventilation of more compliant parts of the diseased lung. Overdistension of lungs in animals has produced diffuse alveolar damage.[37–39] This is the reason why alternative modes of ventilation, all based on a reduction of end-inspiratory airway pressures and/or tidal volumes delivered to the patient, have been developed and are used by many clinicians caring for patients with severe forms of acute or chronic respiratory failure. Four alternative modes of ventilation — high-frequency ventilation (HFV), high-frequency percussive ventilation (HFPV), pressure control inverse ratio ventilation (PCIRV), and airway pressure release ventilation (APRV) — will be discussed.

High-frequency ventilation

High-frequency ventilation (HFV) is the administration of small tidal volumes of 1–3 mL/kg at high frequencies of 100–3000 cpm.[40] Because it is a mode of ventilation based on a marked reduction in tidal volumes and airway pressures, it has the greatest potential for reducing pulmonary barotrauma. There are a number of different types of high-frequency ventilation techniques. The two most common are high-frequency jet ventilation (HFJV) and high-frequency percussive ventilation (HFPV).

High-frequency jet ventilation is the only high-frequency mode routinely used to ventilate patients with ARDS, mainly in Europe.[25] Comparative data concerning the advantages of HFJV over conventional ventilation are limited. There is no agreement, however, that HFJV is better than conventional mechanical ventilation in ARDS.[41]

High-frequency percussive ventilation is a new technique that has shown some promise in the ventilation of patients with inhalation injury.[42–44] Clinical studies indicate that this mode of ventilation may aid in reducing pulmonary barotrauma.[42,43] In a retrospective study, Cortiella et al. have shown a decreased incidence of pneumonia, peak inspiratory pressure, and an improved *P/F* ratio in children ventilated with the use of HFPV as compared to controls.[45]

In the first prospective randomized study on HFPV, Mlcak et al. have shown a significant decrease in the peak inspiratory pressures needed to ventilate pediatric patients with inhalation injury.[46] No significant differences were found for incidence of pneumonia, *P/F* ratios, or mortality.

Based upon clinical experience, the following guidelines are given for initial set-up of the HFPV in children (Table 21.1). The pulsatile flow (PIP) rate should set at 20 cmH$_2$O. The pulse frequency (high rate) should be set between 500 and 600. The low respiratory rate should be set at about 15–20. Oscillatory PEEP levels should be initially set at about 3 cmH$_2$O, and demand PEEP set on 2 cmH$_2$O. Ventilator settings are adjusted based upon the patient's clinical condition and blood gas values. To improve oxygenation, the ventilator can be set up in a more diffusive mode (increased pulse frequency) and, to eliminate carbon dioxide, the ventilator can be set up in a more convective mode (decreased pulse frequency). With this mode of ventilation, subtidal volumes are delivered in a progressive stepwise fashion until a preset oscillatory equilibrium is reached and exhalation is passive.

Clinicians must be familiar with the technique used and its possible limitations. There must be adequate humidification of the respiratory gases or severe necrotizing tracheobronchitis can occur. Special delivery devices for providing adequate humidification during HFV are required.

Pressure control inverse ratio ventilation

Pressure control inverse ratio ventilation (PCIRV) is the use of pressure ventilation with an inspiratory/expiratory (I:E) ratio greater than 1:1. The rationale behind this is to maintain a high mean airway pressure and to hold peak alveolar pressure within a safe range. The second theoretical concept underlying PCIRV is the prolongation of inspiration to allow for recruitment of lung units with a long time constant. Deep sedation and/or paralysis is nearly always required with this mode of ventilation. At this time there is no conclusive scientific data comparing PCIRV to conventional mechanical ventilation in patients with inhalation injury.

Airway pressure release ventilation

Airway pressure release ventilation (APRV) is a pressure-regulated mode of ventilatory support that allows for time-cycled decreases in pressure to facilitate CO$_2$ elimination. This mode allows spontaneous breathing while limiting airway pressures and may therefore limit the amount of sedatives or

TABLE 21.1 HIGH-FREQUENCY PERCUSSIVE VENTILATION SET-UP GUIDELINES

Variable	Settings
Pulsatile flow rate (PIP)	20 cmH$_2$O
Pulse frequency (high rate)	500–600
Low respiratory rate	15–20
I:E ratio	1:1 or 2:1
Oscillatory PEEP	3 cmH$_2$O
Demand PEEP	2 cmH$_2$O

neuromuscular blocking agents needed. APRV is a protective ventilator strategy that uses inverse ratio ventilation at two levels of PEEP. Several limited studies have suggested that APRV may be beneficial for the treatment of burn patients who develop ARDS. Evidence-based recommendations to use this mode of ventilation await outcome studies.

Typical ventilator settings required

A large multicentered study by the NHLBI evaluated the use of volume ventilation with low versus high tidal volume on ARDS. This study documented a decreased incidence of mortality in patients with ARDS who were ventilated with small tidal volumes.[47] Based upon this study, it has become clinically accepted practice to use small tidal volumes when initially setting up mechanical ventilation (Table 21.2).

Tidal volumes

In volume-cycled ventilation, a machine-delivered tidal volume is set to be consistent with adequate gas exchange and patient comfort. The tidal volume selected for burned patients normally varies between 6 and 8 mL/kg of predicted body weight. Numerous factors, such as lung/thorax compliance, system resistance, compressible volume loss, oxygenation, ventilation, and barotrauma, are considered when volumes are selected.[46] Of critical importance is the avoidance of overdistension. This can generally be accomplished by insuring that peak airway and alveolar pressures do not exceed a maximum target. Many would agree that a peak alveolar pressure greater than 35 cmH$_2$O in adults raises concern regarding the development of barotrauma and ventilator-induced lung injury increases.[49,50] The clinician must always look at the patient to insure adequate chest expansion with the setting of the tidal volume. Expired tidal volumes should be measured for accuracy at the connection between the patient's wye and the artificial airway. This insures that the volume selected reaches the patient and is not lost in the compressible volume of the ventilator tubing.

The range of tidal volumes will vary depending on the disease process, with some diseases requiring maximum tidal volumes and others needing less. Severe interstitial diseases such as pneumonia and ARDS may require a tidal volume of 8–10 mL/kg to adequately inflate the lungs and improve gas exchange if protective ventilatory strategies become inadequate. However, the acceptable range of 6–8 mL/kg allows the clinician to make more precise adjustments in volume, as needed by the patient.

Respiratory rate

Setting of the mandatory ventilator respiratory rate is dependent on the mode of ventilation selected, the delivered tidal volume, dead space to tidal volume ratio, metabolic rate, targeted PCO$_2$ levels, and level of spontaneous ventilation. With adults, set mandatory rate normally varies between 4 and 20 breaths/min, with most clinically stable patients requiring mandatory rates in the 8–12 range.[48] In patients with inhalation injury, mandatory rates exceeding 20 per minute may be necessary, depending on the desired expired volume and targeted PCO$_2$. It is important to have targeted arterial blood gas values set to aid the clinical team in proper management (Table 21.3) Along with the PCO$_2$, pH, and patient comfort, the primary variable controlling the selection of the respiratory rate is the development of air trapping and auto PEEP.[51]

The respiratory rates of children and infants all need to be set substantially higher than those of adults. For pediatrics, the respiratory rate can be set at from 12 to 45, depending on the disease state and the level of targeted PCO$_2$ one wishes to achieve. Slower respiratory rates are useful in the patient with obstructed airways because slower rates allow more time for exhalation and emptying of hyperinflated areas.

Arterial blood gases should be checked after the patient has been on the ventilator for approximately 20 minutes and the respiratory rate adjusted accordingly.

Flow rates

The selection of peak inspiratory flow rate during volume ventilation is primarily determined by the level of spontaneous inspiratory effort. In patients triggering volume breaths, patient effort, work of breathing, and patient ventilator synchrony depend on the selection of peak inspiratory flow.[27] Peak inspiratory flows should ideally match patient peak inspiratory demands. This normally requires peak flows to be set at 40–100 L/min, depending on expired volume and the inspiratory demand.[25]

Inspiratory/expiratory (I:E) ratio

The time allowed for the inspiratory and expiratory phases of mechanical ventilation is commonly referred to as the inspiratory/expiratory (I:E) ratio. The inspiratory part of the ratio includes the time to deliver the tidal volume before the exhalation valve opens and exhalation begins. The expiratory part of the ratio includes the time necessary for the tidal volume to exit through the exhalation valve before the next inspiration begins. The inspiratory time should be long enough to

TABLE 21.2 TRADITIONAL MECHANICAL VENTILATION GUIDELINES IN CHILDREN	
Variable	Settings
Tidal volumes	6–8 mL/kg
Respiratory rate	12–45 breaths/min
Plateau pressures	<30 cmH$_2$O
I:E ratio	1:1–1:3
Flow rate	40–100 L/min
PEEP	7.5 cmH$_2$O

TABLE 21.3 ARTERIAL BLOOD GAS GOALS	
Variable	Goal
pH	7.25–7.45
PO$_2$	55–80 mmHg or SaO$_2$ of 88–95%
PCO$_2$	35–55 mmHg (permissive hypercapnia can be used as long as pH >7.25)

deliver the tidal volume at flow rates that will not result in turbulence and high peak airway pressures. The usual I:E ratio is 1:1–1:3.[52]

In severe lung disease, it is acceptable to prolong the inspiratory time to allow for better distribution of gas and enhance oxygen diffusion. When a longer inspiratory time is required, careful attention should be given to sufficient expiration to avoid stacking of breaths and impeding venous return. Prolonged inspiratory time creates a more laminar flow, which helps to keep the peak pressures lower. Fast inspiratory times are tolerated in patients with severe airway obstruction. The fast inspiratory time allows for a longer expiratory phase, which may help to decrease the amount of overinflation.

Inspired oxygen concentration

As a starting point, and until the level of hypoxemia is determined, a patient placed on a ventilator should receive an oxygen concentration of 100%. The concentration should be systematically lowered as soon as arterial blood gases dictate. In general, as a result of the concerns regarding the effects of high oxygen concentration on lung injury, the lowest acceptable oxygen level should be selected as soon as possible. In patients who are difficult to oxygenate, oxygen concentrations can be minimized by optimizing PEEP and mean airway pressures and selecting a minimally acceptable oxygen saturation.[53]

Positive end-expiratory pressure

Positive end-expiratory pressure (PEEP) is applied to recruit lung volumes, elevate mean airway pressure, and improve oxygenation.[54] The level of PEEP used varies with the disease process. PEEP levels should start at 8–10 cmH$_2$O and be increased in 2.5-cm increments. Increasing levels of PEEP, in conjunction with a prolonged inspiratory time, aids in oxygenation and allows for the safe level of oxygen to be used. The use of pressure–volume curves to determine the best PEEP level has been recommended to aid in overstretching the alveoli. This technique has certain limitations and is difficult to perform in the clinical setting. The use of PEEP trials can determine the best PEEP without causing a decrease in cardiac output.

Usually a minimum of 8 cmH$_2$O of PEEP will be indicated for use during mechanical ventilation since tracheal intubation holds the larynx constantly open, which leads to alveolar collapse and a reduction in the functional residual capacity.

Optimal PEEP is the level of end-expiratory pressure that results in the lowering of intrapulmonary shunting, significant improvement in arterial oxygenation, and only a small change in cardiac output, arteriovenous oxygen content differences, or mixed venous oxygen tension.

Extubation criteria

Standard extubation criteria include a wide variety of physiologic indices that have been proposed to guide the process of discontinuing ventilatory support. Traditional indices include:

- PaO_2/FiO_2 ratio of greater than 250.
- Maximum inspiratory pressure of greater than 60 cmH$_2$O.
- Vital capacity of at least 15–20 mL/kg.
- Tidal volume of at least 5–7 mL/kg.
- Maximum voluntary ventilation of at least twice the minute volume.[55–58]
- An audible leak around the endotracheal tube must be present.

In general, these indices evaluate a patient's ability to sustain spontaneous ventilation. They do not assess a patient's ability to protect the upper airway. For this reason, traditional indices often fail to reflect the true clinical picture of a patient with an inhalation injury. For a complete evaluation prior to extubation, bronchoscopic examination will aid in determining if the airway edema has decreased enough to attempt extubation. Prior to a scheduled extubation it is recommended that reintubation equipment be set up and that the person doing the extubation be experienced in emergency intubations.

If the patient demonstrates signs of inspiratory stridor, the use of racemic epinephrine by aerosol has been effective in reducing the mucosal edema and may prevent the patient from being reintubated.

Infection control of respiratory equipment

Infections are the leading cause of mortality in burned patients. Pneumonia has become one of the most frequent life-threatening infections and is an important determinant of survival.[57] The majority of pneumonias are nosocomial, occurring in the burned patient after 72 hours of hospitalization, and are often associated with either an inhalation injury or endotracheal intubation with exposure to respiratory care equipment, or both.[62–64] One of the most important risk factors predisposing to pneumonia in burned patients is endotracheal intubation.[65,66] The incidence of pneumonia developing is estimated to be five times higher for intubated than nonintubated patients, and tracheostomy increases this risk even higher.[67] Exposure to respiratory care equipment adds an increased risk of pneumonia above and beyond the risk associated with endotracheal intubation.[68,69] After the use of nebulization equipment in respiratory care became popular, several epidemics of nosocomial pneumonia were reported.[70] The risk of pneumonia from mechanical ventilators was significant but decreased with a better understanding of the necessity to decontaminate respiratory equipment.[71,72] Intubated patients receiving respiratory care may be at an increased risk of pneumonia because of coincidental exposure to other procedures such as suctioning and bronchoscopy. Respiratory care equipment, if not properly cared for, may provide a source of extraneous organisms that can contaminate the patient's respiratory tract.

The potential role of respiratory care equipment in providing reservoirs for organisms that are capable of infecting the lungs is well established. This problem, particularly pertaining to reservoir devices and medications, has been recognized for a number of years, and effective control strategies have been developed. Most hospitals maintain a bacteriological monitoring system, and significant contamination by this route is not likely.[73] Contamination of the compressed gases used to operate respiratory care devices is uncommon, principally because of the desiccation of gases and the inability of most bacterial species to survive such harsh treatment. Nebulization equipment delivers a fine-particle aerosol and, if contaminated, the aerosol droplets may contain bacteria. Humidification equipment provides water vapor but does not deliver a large quantity of water in particulate form. In fact, humidifiers generally remove bacteria from airstreams, because the bacteria are physically trapped in the fluid phase and are not vaporized.

Bag-mask units have been shown to allow the persistence of infectious organisms and the subsequent infection of other patients on whom the equipment has been later used.[74]

Ventilator circuits are inevitably contaminated by the patient's own respiratory tract flora during exhalation and coughing, and the fluid that collects in this tubing is thereby contaminated. However, the American Association for Respiratory Care evidence-based clinical practice guidelines suggest that ventilator circuits should not be changed routinely for infection control purposes.[75] The exact length of time that circuits can be used safely is unknown.

Handwashing

Handwashing is generally considered the single most important procedure for preventing nosocomial infections. Regardless of whatever benefits are accrued by cleaning or sterilization, they are negated if the simple process of handwashing is overlooked. The recommended handwashing procedures depend on the purpose of washing. In most situations, a vigorous brief washing with soap under a strong running water is adequate to remove transient flora. Generally, simple handwashing with soap is performed before and after contact with patients and whenever the hands are soiled.

Antimicrobial handwashing procedures are indicated before all invasive procedures, during the care of patients in strict, respiratory, or enteric isolation and before entering intensive care units. The most commonly used agents are 70% isopropyl alcohol, iodophors, and chlorhexidine. Scrub regimens such as the povidone-iodine surgical scrub are appropriate for these areas.[76]

Chemical agents for sterilization/disinfection

Disinfectants act to kill microorganisms by several methods:

- oxidating microbial cells;
- hydrolyzing;
- combining with microbial proteins to form salts;
- coagulating the proteins of microbial cells;
- denaturing enzymes; or
- modifying cell wall permeability.[77]

Aldehydes

Aldehydes contain some of the most commonly used antimicrobials in respiratory care practice. These agents achieve their antimicrobial action through the alkylation of enzymes.

The cidal action of glutaraldehyde is accomplished by disruption of the lipoproteins in the cell membrane and cytoplasm of vegetative bacterial forms. This reaction between the chemical glutaraldehyde and cell proteins is dependent on both time and contact. Items to be disinfected must be free of material that would inhibit contact, and adequate contact time is needed for the chemical reaction to be complete.

Alkaline glutaraldehyde, buffered by a 0.3% bicarbonate agent, is used as a 2% solution. Once activated with the buffering agent, it is fully potent for approximately 14 days. This solution is bactericidal, virucidal, and tuberculocidal within 10 minutes and produces sterilization when applied for 10–20 hours. Equipment disinfected or sterilized with glutaraldehyde should be thoroughly rinsed and dried prior to use, because any residue would be irritating to mucous membranes.

Glutaraldehyde solutions are commonly used for the cold disinfection or sterilization of respiratory care equipment and have a large degree of safety. These solutions can be used to disinfect bronchoscopes as well as many of the current respiratory supplies.

Alcohols

Alcohols, especially ethylene and isopropyl alcohol, are perhaps the most commonly used disinfectants. Alcohols, as a chemical family, have many desirable characteristics needed in disinfectants. They are generally bactericidal and accomplish their bactericidal activity by damaging the cell wall membrane. They also have the ability to denature proteins, particularly enzymes called dehydrogenases. For alcohol to coagulate microbial proteins, water must be present. For this reason, 70% has been considered the critical dilution for alcohol, with a rapid loss of bactericidal activity with dilutions less than 50%. Both ethyl and isopropyl alcohols are rapidly effective against vegetative bacteria and tubercle bacilli but are not sporicidal.

To be sure that the current infection control practice is effective in each institution, use of random microbiological cultures should be done whenever a problem is suspected or to test the reliability of the disinfection or sterilization techniques.

Late complications of inhalation injury

Tracheal stenosis

Tracheal complications are commonly seen and consist of tracheitis, tracheal ulcerations, and granuloma formation. The location of the stenosis is almost invariably subglottic and occurs at the site of the cuff of the endotracheal or tracheostomy tube.[78] Several problems arising after extubation represent sequelae of laryngeal or tracheal injury incurred during the period of incubation. While tracheal stenosis or tracheomalacia are usually mild and asymptomatic, in some patients they can present as severe fixed or dynamic upper airway obstructions. These conditions can require surgical correction. In the management of intubated patients, such complications should be mostly preventable by meticulous attention to the tracheostomy or endotracheal tube cuff. Inflation of the cuff should be to the minimal pressure level consistent with preventing a leak in the ventilator at end inspiration.

Obstructive/restrictive disease

Chronic airway disease is a relatively rare reported sequel of inhalation injury and its supportive treatment. Spirometry is a useful screening tool for airway obstruction. Reports in the literature for adults indicate that lung function returns to normal after inhalation injury.[79,80] However, Mlcak et al. reported pulmonary function changes following inhalation injury for up to 10 years post-injury in a group of severely burned children.[81] Fortunately, most pulmonary function abnormalities will persist for only months following lung parenchymal injury. In the great majority of cases, eventual resolution of both symptoms and physiologic abnormalities will occur. During the resolution phase, serial measurement of airflow obstruction should be obtained.[82] Desai et al. demonstrated that physiologic insults that occur as a result of thermal injury may limit exercise endurance in children.[83] Data from exercise stress testing showed evidence of a respiratory limitation to exercise. This was confirmed by a decrease in the maximal heart rate, decrease in the maximal oxygen consumption, and increased respiratory rate. In the cases of persistent severe respiratory symptoms, the severity of the impairment should be documented and the patient evaluated for a pulmonary rehabilitation program.

Conclusion

Inhalation injury and associated major burns provide a challenge for healthcare workers who provide direct hands-on care. The technical and physiologic problems which complicate the respiratory management of these patients require a practical knowledge of the possible sources of nosocomial infections. Patients with inhalation injury frequently require the use of respiratory care equipment that, if not properly cared for, can aid in the spread of infections. Important priorities for reducing the risk of infections include: an aggressive bronchial hygiene therapy program, the adherence to established infection control practices, the use of universal precautions during procedures, meticulous cleaning of respiratory care equipment, as well as routine epidemiologic surveillance of the established infection control practices within each institution.

It is imperative that a well-organized protocol-driven approach to respiratory care of the burn patient be utilized so that further improvements can be made, and the morbidity and mortality associated with inhalation injury be reduced.

References

1. Haponik E. Smoke inhalation injury: some priorities for respiratory care professionals. Resp Care 1992; 37:609.
2. Frownfelter D. Chest physical therapy and pulmonary rehabilitation, 2nd edn. Chicago: Year Book Medical; 1987.
3. Ivarez SE, Peterson M, Lansford BR. Respiratory treatments of the adult patients with spinal cord injury. Phys Ther 1981; 61:1738.
4. Chopra SK, Taplin GV, Simmons DH. Effects of hydration and physical therapy on tracheal transport velocity. Am Rev Respir Dis 1974; 115:1009–1014.
5. Marini JJ, Person DJ, Hudson LD. A prospective comparison of fiberoptic bronchoscopy and respiratory therapy. Am Rev Respir Dis 1979; 119:971–978.
6. Oldenburg FA, Dolovich MB, Montgomery JM, et al. Effects of postural drainage, exercise and cough on mucus clearance in chronic bronchitis. Am Rev Respir Dis 1979; 12:730–747.
7. Remolina C, Khan AV, Santiago TV. Positional hypoxemia in unilateral lung disease. N Engl J Med 1981; 304:522–525.
8. Soria C, Walthall W, Price H. Breathing and pulmonary hygiene techniques: pulmonary rehabilitation. Oxford: Butterworth; 1984:860.
9. Caldwell S, Sullivan K. Respiratory care – a guide to clinical practice. Philadelphia: JB Lippincott; 1977:91.
10. Albanese AJ, Toplitz AD. A hassle free guide to suctioning a tracheostomy. RN 1982; 45(4):24–30.
11. Landa JF, Kwoka M, Chapman G, et al. Effects of suctioning on mucociliary transport. Chest 1980; 77:202–207.
12. McFadden R. Decreasing respiratory compromise during infant suctioning. Am J Nurs 1981; 12:2158–2161.
13. Wanner A. Nasopharyngeal airway: a facilitated access to the trachea. Ann Intern Med 1971; 75:592–595.
14. Brandstater B, Maullem M. Atelectasis following trachea suctioning in infants. Anesthesiology 1979; 31:294–297.
15. Roper PC, Vonwiller JB, Fisk GL, et al. Lobar atelectasis after nasotracheal intubation in infants. Aust Pediat J 1982; 12:272–275.
16. Yee A, Connors G, Cress D. Pharmacology and the respiratory patient, pulmonary rehabilitation. Oxford: Butterworth; 1984:125.
17. Whitbet TL, Manion CV. Cardiac and pulmonary effects of albuterol and isoproterenol. Chest 1978; 74:251–255.
18. Zimet I. Pharmacology of drugs used in respiratory therapy. Respiratory care – a guide to clinical practice. Philadelphia: JB Lippincott; 1977:473.
19. Lieberman J, Kurnick NB. Influence of deoxyribonucleic acid content on the proteolysis of sputum and pus. Nature 1962; 196:988.
20. Hirsh SR, Zastrow JE, Kory RC. Sputum liquification agents: a comprehensive in vitro study. J Lab Clin Med 1969; 74:346.
21. Brown M, Desai MH, Mlcak R, et al. Dimethylsulfoxide with heparin in the treatment of smoke inhalation injury. J Burn Care Rehabil 1988; 9(1):22.
22. Desai MH, Mlcak R, Brown M, et al. Reduction of smoke injury with DMSO and heparin treatment. Surg Form 1985; 36:103.
23. Desai MH, Brown M, Mlcak R, et al. Nebulization treatment of smoke inhalation injury in sheep model with DMSO, heparin combinations and acetylcysteine. Crit Care Med 1986; 14:321.
24. Desai MH, Mlcak R, Nichols R, Herndon DN. Reduction in mortality in pediatric patients with inhalation injury with aerosolized heparin/N-acetylcysteine therapy. J Burn Care Rehabil 1998; 19(3):210–212.
25. Slutsky A. American College of Chest Physicians Consensus Conference: mechanical ventilation. Chest 1993; 104:1833–1859.
26. Marini JJ, Capps JS, Culver BH. The inspiratory work of breathing during assisted mechanical ventilation. Chest 1985; 87:612–618.
27. Marini JJ, Rodriquez RM, Lamb V. The inspiratory workload of patient initiated mechanical ventilation. Am Rev Respir Dis 1986; 134:902–904.
28. Ward ME, Corbeil C, Gibbons MW, et al. Optimization of respiratory muscle relaxation during mechanical ventilation. Anesthesiology 1988; 69:29–35.
29. Downs JB, Klein EF, Desautels D, et al. Intermittent mandatory ventilation: a new approach to weaning patients. Chest 1973; 64:331–335.
30. Weisman IH, Rinaldo JE, Rodgers RM, et al. Intermittent mandatory ventilation. Am Rev Respir Dis 1983; 127:641–647.
31. Hirsch C, Kacmareck RM, Stanek K. Work of breathing during CPAP and PSV imposed by the new generation mechanical ventilators. Resp Care 1991; 36:815–828.
32. Macintyre NR. Respiratory function during pressure support ventilation. Chest 1986; 89:677–683.
33. Brochard L, Harf A, Lorino H. Inspiratory pressure support prevents diaphragmatic fatique during weaning from mechanical ventilation. Am Rev Respir Dis 1989; 139:513–521.
34. Fiastro JF, Habib MP, Quan SF. Pressure support compensates for inspiratory work due to endotracheal tubes. Chest 1988; 93:499–505.
35. Brochard L, Rau F, Lorino H, et al. Inspiratory pressure support compensates for the additional work of breathing caused by the endotracheal tube. Anesthesiology 1991; 75:739–745.
36. Hickling KG. Ventilatory management of ARDS: can it affect outcome? Intensive Care Med 1990; 9:239–250.

37. Gattinoni L, Pesenti A, Avalli L, et al. Pressure–volume curve of total respiratory system in acute respiratory failure. Am Rev Respir Dis 1987; 136:730–760.

38. Dreyfuss D, Soler P, Basset G, et al. High inflation pressures, pulmonary edema, respective effects of high airway pressure, high tidal volume and PEEP. Am Rev Respir Dis 1988; 137:1159–1164.

39. Kolobow T, Moretti MP, Fumagalli R, et al. Severe impairment of lung function induced by high peak airway pressure during mechanical ventilation. Am Rev Respir Dis 1987; 135:312–315.

40. Froese AB, Bryan AC, High frequency ventilation. Am Rev Respir Dis 1987; 135:1363–1374.

41. Fusciardi J, Rouby JJ, Barakat T, et al. Hemodynamic effects of high frequency jet ventilation in patients with and without shock. Anesthesiology 1986; 65:485–491.

42. Cioffi W, Graves T, McManus W, et al. High-frequency percussive ventilation in patients with inhalation injury. J Trauma 1989; 29:350–354.

43. Cioffi W, Rue LW III, Graves T, et al. Prophylactic use of high-frequency percussive ventilation in patients with inhalation injury. Ann Surg 1991; 213:575–581.

44. Mlcak R, Cortiella J, Desai MH, Herndon DN. Lung compliance, airway resistance, and work of breathing in children after inhalation injury. J Burn Care Rehabil 1997; 18(6):531–534.

45. Cortiella J, Mlcak R, Herndon DN. High frequency percussive ventilation in pediatric patients with inhalation injury. J Burn Care Rehabil 1999; 20(3):232–235.

46. Mlcak R, Desai MH, Herndon DN. A prospective randomized study of high frequency percussive ventilation compared to conventional mechanical ventilation in pediatric patients with inhalation injury. J Burn Care Rehabil 2000; 21(1):S158.

47. The Acute Respiratory Distress Syndrome Network. Ventilation with lower tidal volumes as compared with traditional tidal volumes for acute lung injury and the acute respiratory distress syndrome. N Engl J Med 2000; 342(18):1301–1308.

48. Kacmarek RM, Vengas J. Mechanical ventilatory rates and tidal volumes. Resp Care 1987; 32:466–478.

49. Hickling KG, Henderson SJ, Jackson R. Low mortality associated with low volume, pressure limited ventilation with permissive hypercapnia in severe adult respiratory distress syndrome. Intensive Care Med 1990; 16:372–377.

50. Marini JJ. New approaches to the ventilatory management of the adult respiratory distress syndrome. J Crit Care 1992; 87:256–257.

51. Pepe PE, Marini JJ. Occult positive pressure in mechanically ventilated patients with airflow obstruction. Am Rev Respir Dis 1982; 126:166–170.

52. Kacmareck RM. Management of the patient mechanical ventilator system. In: Pierson DJ, Kacmareck RM, eds. Foundations of respiratory care. New York: Churchill Livingstone; 1992:973–997.

53. Stroller JK, Kacmareck RM. Ventilatory strategies in the management of the adult respiratory distress syndrome. Clin Chest Med 1990; 11:755–772.

54. Suter PM, Fairley HB, Isenberg MD. Optimum end-expiratory airway pressure in patients with acute respiratory failure. N Engl J Med 1975; 292:284–289.

55. Sahn SA, Lakshminarayan S. Bedside criteria for discontinuation of mechanical ventilation. Chest 1973; 63:1002–1005.

56. Tahvanainen J, Salmenpera M, Nikki P. Extubation criteria after weaning from IMV and CPAP. Crit Care Med 1983; 11:702–707.

57. Herndon DN, Lange F, Thompson P, et al. Pulmonary injury in burned patients. Surg Clin N Am 1987; 67:31.

58. Demling RH. Improved survival after major burns. J Trauma 1983; 23:179.

59. Luterman A, Dacso CC, Curreri WP. Infections in burned patients. Am J Med 1986; 81(A):45.

60. Pruitt BA Jr. The diagnosis and treatment of infection in the burned patient. Burns 1984; 11:79.

61. Pruitt BA Jr, Flemma RJ, DiVincenti FC, et al. Pulmonary complications in burned patients. J Thorac Cardiovasc Surg 1970; 59:7.

62. Foley DF, Concrief JA, Mason AD. Pathology of the lungs in fatally burned patients. Ann Surg 1968; 167:251.

63. Moylan JA, Chan C. Inhalation injury — an increased problem. Ann Surg 1978; 188:34.

64. Craven DE, Kunches LM, Kilinsky V, et al. Risk factors for pneumonia and fatalities in patients receiving controlled mechanical ventilation. Am Rev Respir Dis 1986; 133:792.

65. Garibaldi RA, Britt MR, Coleman ML, et al. Risk factors for postoperative pneumonias. Am J Med 1984; 70:677.

66. Pennington JE. Hospital acquired pneumonias. In: Wenzel RP, ed. Prevention and control of nosocomial infections. Baltimore: Williams & Wilkins; 1987:321–324.

67. Centers for Disease Control National Nosocomial Infection Study Report. Annual summary 1983. MMWR 1983; 33(259):935.

68. Schwartz SN, Dowling JN, Ben Youic C, et al. Sources of Gram-negative bacilli colonizing the trachea of intubated patients. J Infect Dis 1978; 138:227.

69. Pierce AK, Edmonson EB, McGee G, et al. An analysis of factors predisposing to Gram-negative bacillary necrotizing pneumonia. Am Rev Respir Dis 1966; 94:309.

70. Ringrose RE, McKown B, Felton FG, et al. A hospital outbreak of Serratia marcescens associated with ultrasonic equipment. Ann Intern Med 1968; 69:719–729.

71. Simmons BP, Wong ES. CDC guidelines for the prevention and control of nosocomial infections. Am J Infect Control 1983; 11:230.

72. Rhame F. The inanimate environment. In: Bennett JV, Bracham PS, eds. Hospital infections. Boston: Little Brown; 1986:223–250.

73. Cross AS, Roupe B. Role of respiratory assistance devices in endemic nosocomial pneumonia. Am J Med 1981; 70:681–685.

74. Johanson WG. Respiratory care 1982; 27:445–452.

75. Hess DR, Kallstrom TJ, Mottram CD, et al. Care of the ventilator circuit and its relation to ventilator-associated pneumonia. Respiratory Care 2003; 48(9):869–878.

76. Garner JS, Faverno MS. CDC guidelines for the prevention and control of nosocomial infections. Am J Infect Control 1986; 14:110–129.

77. Edge RS. Infection control, respiratory care practice. Chicago: Year Book Medical; 1988:574.

78. Munster AM, Wong LA. Miscellaneous pulmonary complications in respiratory injury. New York: McGraw-Hill; 1990:326.

79. Demling RH. Smoke inhalation injury. Postgrad Med 1987; 82:63.

80. Cahalane M, Demling RH. Early respiratory abnormalities from smoke inhalation. JAMA 1984; 251:771.

81. Mlcak R, Desai MH, Robinson E, et al. Inhalation injury and lung function in children – a decade later. J Burn Care Rehabil 2000; 21(1):S156.

82. Colic GL. Long term respiratory complications of inhalation injury. In: Respiratory injury, smoke inhalation and burns. New York: McGraw-Hill; 1990:342.

83. Desai MH, Mlcak R, Robinson E. Does inhalation injury limit exercise endurance in children convalescing from thermal injury. J Burn Care Rehabil 1993; 14:16–20.

The systemic inflammatory response syndrome

Edward R. Sherwood and Daniel L. Traber

Introduction

Burn patients, with or without inhalation injuries, commonly exhibit a clinical picture that is largely produced by systemic inflammation. The phrase 'systemic inflammatory response syndrome (SIRS)' has been introduced to designate the signs and symptoms of this condition. SIRS has a continuum of severity ranging from the presence of tachycardia, tachypnea, fever, and leukocytosis, to refractory hypotension and, in its most severe form, shock and multiple organ system dysfunction. In thermally injured patients, the most common cause of SIRS is the burn itself. Sepsis, defined as SIRS in the presence of infection, is also common in burn patients and is a significant cause of morbidity and mortality. Starting from a local infection at the burn wound or an infected catheter tip, the spread of microbes and their toxins can further potentiate the already activated immune system. Pathological alterations of metabolic, cardiovascular, gastrointestinal, and coagulation systems occur as a result of the hyperactive immune system. This chapter will review current understanding of SIRS and the associated immunological, cardiovascular, and pulmonary dysfunction that occurs following trauma and thermal injury.

Definition of SIRS

The phrase 'systemic inflammatory response syndrome (SIRS)' was recommended by the American College of Chest Physicians/Society for Critical Care Medicine (ACCP/SCCM) consensus conference in 1992 to describe a systemic inflammatory process, independent of its cause.[1] The proposal was based on clinical and experimental results indicating that a variety of conditions, both infectious and noninfectious (i.e. burns, ischemia-reperfusion injury, multiple trauma, pancreatitis), induce a similar host response. Two or more of the following conditions must be fulfilled for the diagnosis of SIRS to be made:

- body temperature >38°C or <36°C;
- heart rate >90 beats/min;
- respiratory rate >20/min or $PaCO_2$ <32 mmHg;
- leukocyte count >12 000/µL, <4000/µL, or >10% immature (band) forms.

All of these pathophysiologic changes must occur as an acute alteration from baseline in the absence of other known causes. This definition is very sensitive and non-specific and most of the SIRS criteria are also addressed in other scoring systems of injury-induced physiologic derangement such as the Acute Physiology and Chronic Health Evaluation (APACHE), Mortality Probability Model (MPM), and Simplified Acute Physiology Severity (SAPS) systems. Several investigators have criticized the definition of SIRS as being too sensitive and encompassing the majority of ICU patients and certainly the vast majority of patients suffering extensive thermal injury.[2,3] The initial definition of SIRS also did not address the continuum of disease severity as was defined for sepsis. Specifically, sepsis was defined by the same criteria as SIRS in patients with demonstrable infection. Criteria for the diagnosis of severe sepsis included the additional derangements of organ dysfunction, hypotension, and hypoperfusion. Evidence of hypoperfusion included, but was not limited to, the presence of lactic acidosis, oliguria, and altered mental status. Septic shock was characterized by hypotension and hypoperfusion in patients who were adequately volume resuscitated or required treatment with catecholamines or other vasoactive drugs to support cardiovascular function. Muckart and Bhagwangee,[2] in an effort to define a continuum of severity for SIRS, later proposed the categories of severe SIRS and sterile shock. These conditions were defined by the same criteria as severe sepsis and septic shock in the absence of demonstrable infection. In its most severe form, SIRS can induce organ injury and subsequent multiple organ dysfunction syndrome (MODS).

Despite the limitations in the definitions of SIRS and sepsis, most clinicians and investigators generally adopted the SIRS concept. However, it is difficult to define a specific pattern of host response. To address these issues, a second consensus conference was assembled in 2001.[4,5] The goal of the conference was to revisit the previously defined criteria for SIRS and sepsis as well as determine if revision of these criteria was indicated. The consensus was that the concepts of sepsis and

SIRS are useful but the diagnostic criteria are overly sensitive and non-specific. The participants added additional criteria that defined metabolic, biochemical and functional alterations associated with SIRS and sepsis. Among these were hyperglycemia, edema, elevated plasma C reactive protein concentration, coagulation abnormalities, thrombocytopenia, ileus and hyperbilirubinemia. This group further proposed a staging system for sepsis and SIRS that could be used to stratify patients for prediction of outcome and potential response to therapy. This staging system, termed PIRO, defined several criteria including the predisposition of patients toward poor outcome as determined by pre-morbid conditions and possible genetic factors. Other factors include the severity and type of insult, the host response to injury and the presence of organ dysfunction. The participants proposed that this model could be used to generate more specific criteria for defining the SIRS phenomenon. The validity of this approach remains to be established.

Another pitfall in the designation of SIRS is the difficulty in applying the initial criteria to children. Some of the criteria, particularly those for heart rate and respiratory rate, fall within the normal physiologic range for young children. In 2002, a consensus conference was assembled to define criteria for sepsis and SIRS in children.[6] The participants defined six age groups based on clinical and physiological characteristics (Table 22.1). SIRS was defined as the presence of at least two of the following four criteria, one of which must be abnormal temperature or leukocyte count:

- temperature >38.5°C or <36°C;
- tachycardia, defined as mean heart rate >2 SD above normal for age *or* for children <1 year, bradycardia, defined as heart rate <10% of normal for age;
- mean respiratory rate >2 SD above normal for age or requirement for mechanical ventilation;
- leukocyte count elevated or depressed for age.

The conference participants defined severe sepsis as sepsis plus one of the following: cardiovascular dysfunction, acute respiratory distress syndrome or two or more organ dysfunctions (respiratory, renal, neurologic, hematologic or hepatic). The definition of septic shock is problematic in children because children can maintain blood pressure until they become severely ill. Therefore, hypotension is not a useful criteria for diagnosing shock in children. This group proposed criteria for septic shock that included the presence of tachycardia in conjunction with signs of decreased peripheral perfusion such as decreased capillary refill, decreased peripheral pulses, decreased urine output, altered mental status and cold/mottled extremities.[6]

Several studies have been conducted with the goal of determining the prognostic value of the SIRS designation. In the acute setting, SIRS has been demonstrated in the majority of critically injured patients and the intensity of the response correlates directly with the severity of injury.[3,7] The presence of SIRS within the first 24 hours after severe injury has not served as a predictor of mortality in trauma or burn patients in some studies.[3,7] However, the presence of sterile or septic shock is an important predictor of poor outcome, particularly when associated with MODS.[2] In addition, the presence of more than two of the SIRS criteria in the setting of acute injury has correlated with increased morbidity and mortality.[8,9] A study by Rangel-Frausto et al.[9] showed that trauma patients who did not meet SIRS criteria had a mortality rate of 3% compared with 6% mortality in those with two SIRS markers. Patients with three or four SIRS criteria had mortality rates of 10 and 17%, respectively, while those with culture-negative shock had a 46% death rate. Haga et al.[10] have shown that the persistence of SIRS for more than 3 days in surgical patients is a harbinger of complications and is associated with increased morbidity. Talmor et al.[7] reported that persistence of SIRS to the second postoperative day in high-risk surgical patients correlated with an increased incidence of MODS. Additional studies have shown that persistence of SIRS criteria for more than 3 days in trauma and burn patients is associated with worse outcome.[10–13] Therefore, three important factors appear to determine the effect of SIRS on the host. The first factor is the severity of the initial inflammatory response. This response is proportional to the severity of injury. Specifically, the presence of shock or MODS within the first 24 hours after injury bears a poor prognosis. The second determinant is the persistence of SIRS beyond the first days of injury. Specifically, prolongation of SIRS beyond the second day after severe trauma or thermal injury is associated with an increased complication rate. Factors that appear to be important in decreasing the incidence of a prolonged inflammatory state include adequate fluid resuscitation within the first 24 hours of injury, aggressive excision of necrotic tissue and enteral feeding.[11–14] A further factor is the adaptive capacity of the host. Results of several studies have shown that extremes of age, either old or young, and the presence of coexisting disease will diminish the adaptive capacity of the host and predict a worse prognosis for any given severity of injury.[14,15]

The initiating event

The crucial pathophysiologic event that precipitates systemic inflammation is tissue damage. This can occur both as a result of the direct injury to tissues from mechanical or thermal trauma as well as cellular injury induced by mediators of ischemia-reperfusion injury such as oxygen free radicals. Injury results in the acute release of pro-inflammatory cytokines such as tumor necrosis factor-α (TNFα) and interleukins IL-1 and IL-6. If injury is severe, such as in extensive thermal injury, a profound release of cytokines occurs, resulting in the induction of a systemic inflammatory reaction (Figure 22.1). The ability of the host to adapt to this systemic inflammatory response is dependent on the magnitude and duration of the response as well as the adaptive capacity of the host. If the insult and host response to the insult are beyond the adaptive

TABLE 22.1 PEDIATRIC AGE GROUPS FOR SIRS CRITERIA	
Newborn	0 day to 1 week
Neonate	1 week to 1 month
Infant	1 month to 1 year
Toddler and preschool	2 to 5 years
School age	6 to 12 years
Adolescent	13 to 18 years

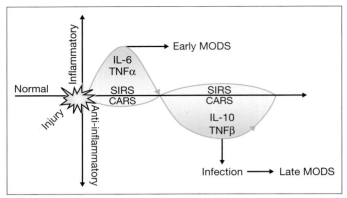

Fig. 22.1 Pathogenesis of the systemic inflammatory response syndrome (SIRS) and counter anti-inflammatory response syndrome (CARS). Tissue injury induces production of pro-inflammatory mediators such as TNFα and IL-6 resulting in SIRS. A compensatory anti-inflammatory response (CARS) may also be mounted through production of anti-inflammatory mediators such as IL-10 and TGFβ. In many cases SIRS and CARS may coexist. (From Cotran R, Kumar V, Collins T, eds. Robbins pathologic basis of disease, 6th edn. Philadelphia: WB Saunders; 1999: 75.)

capacity of the host, organ injury may ensue during the early post-injury period. Factors that have been implicated in the worsening or prolongation of SIRS include inadequate resuscitation during the acute phase following thermal injury, persistent or intermittent infection, ongoing tissue necrosis, and translocation of endotoxin across the bowel.[15,16] In many cases, SIRS may precipitate a state of immunosuppression known as the counter anti-inflammatory response syndrome (CARS). Frequently, SIRS and CARS may actually coexist (Figure 22.1). Current research indicates that the injured host responds to severe inflammation by activating anti-inflammatory pathways that are aimed at protecting the host from further inflammatory injury. Among these pathways are increased production of anti-inflammatory cytokines such as IL-10 and transforming growth factor-β (TGFβ).[17,18] However, this anti-inflammatory state may lead to immunosuppression that predisposes the host to opportunistic infections. If uncontrolled, local infections may escalate to severe systemic infections and sepsis. Sepsis can cause further inflammatory injury and serve as an additional source of organ injury in severely burned patients. The pathogenesis of injury-induced immunosuppression is discussed in detail in Chapter 23 of this text.

The two-hit hypothesis

Many investigators have described a phenomenon in which the injured host manifests an exaggerated inflammatory response if confronted with a secondary inflammatory stimulus during the post-injury period. This phenomenon has been termed the 'two-hit hypothesis.' Although the pathobiology of the two-hit hypothesis is not completely understood, monocytes and macrophages appear to play a central role in mediating the process. For example, the lymphokine α-interferon (IFN-α), produced during the initial injury, might act as the first signal and prime macrophages for a heightened inflammatory response if a second stimulus is encountered. Several changes in macrophage function, including an increase in the transcription rate of mRNA for TNFα, can be induced by exposure to IFN-α.

However, TNFα protein is not produced in large amounts in response to the first inflammatory insult. If a second stimulus, such as endotoxin, is provided in even a small dose, macrophages are triggered to become fully activated and to secrete large amounts of TNFα. Studies by Paterson et al.[19] show that macrophages have increased responsiveness to ligands for toll-like receptor 2 (TLR2) and TLR4 following burn injury. TLR2 and TLR4 are proteins that play integral roles as components of receptor complexes for various microbial products such as peptidoglycans, lipoproteins and lipopolysaccharide. Enhancement of TLR2 and TLR4 responses during the post-injury period may be one mechanism contributing to the two-hit phenomenon. T lymphocytes may also become hyper-responsive during the post-injury period. Zang et al.[20] showed an exaggerated response to bacterial superantigens at 1 day after burn injury in mice. Superantigens, such staphylococcal enterotoxins, induce polyclonal activation of T cells and cause a shock syndrome that is similar to endotoxin shock. This mechanism may also contribute to the hyper-inflammatory response seen in many patients during the post-burn period.

The exaggerated response to a secondary stimulus seen in severely injured patients appears to have functional consequences. Several studies that focused on organ injury caused by systemic inflammatory processes indicate that a phenomenon comparable to the cellular events described above can occur in severely injured patients.[21] Dehring et al. found more persistent pulmonary hypertension and an exaggerated hyperdynamic response to bacteremia in sheep when a week-old thermal injury preceded systemic bacterial challenge.[22] In a rat model of intestinal ischemia-reperfusion injury and endotoxemia, lung albumin leak and mortality rate increased only if both injuries occurred.[23] Combined administration of low doses of endotoxin and TNFα to rats caused hypotension and metabolic effects that are commonly seen after giving a highly lethal dose of either compound alone.[24] These findings are in keeping with the fact that multiple organ damage usually develops over a prolonged period of time during which several insults might occur. It also emphasizes why it is so important to prevent any subsequent ischemia or other insult that can initiate a systemic inflammatory response, particularly in patients in whom systemic inflammation is already present.

Cytokine and non-cytokine mediators of SIRS

Several proinflammatory cytokines, chemokines, and non-cytokine inflammatory mediators play a role in the pathogenesis of SIRS. Cytokines comprise a broad group of polypeptides with varied functions within the immune response (Table 22.2). The classical mediator of systemic inflammation is TNFα. TNFα is released primarily by macrophages within minutes of local or systemic injury and modulates a variety of immunologic and metabolic events.[25] At sites of local infection or inflammation, TNFα initiates an immune response that activates antimicrobial defense mechanisms and, once the infection is eradicated, tissue repair. It is a potent activator of neutrophils and mononuclear phagocytes, and also serves as a growth factor for fibroblasts and as an angiogenesis factor. However, systemic release of TNFα can precipitate a destructive cascade of events that can result in tissue injury, organ

TABLE 22.2 CYTOKINE MEDIATORS OF SYSTEMIC INFLAMMATION

Cytokine	Polypeptide size	Cell source	Cell target	Primary effects
Tumor necrosis factor-α (TNFα)	17 kDa	Monocytes, macrophages, T lymphocytes	(a) Neutrophil (b) Endothelial cell (c) Hypothalamus (d) Liver (e) Muscle, fat (f) Heart (g) Macrophages (h) T lymphocytes (i) Various tissues	Activation (inflammation) Activation (inflammation/ coagulation) Release of vasodilators (NO) Fever Acute phase response Catabolism Myocardial suppression Release of cytokines, inflammation Inflammation Apoptosis?
Interleukin-1 (IL-1)	17 kDa	Monocytes, macrophages	(a) T cells (b) Endothelial cells (c) Liver (d) Hypothalamus (e) Muscle, fat	Activation (inflammation) Activation (inflammation/coagulation) Release of vasodilators (NO) Acute phase response Fever Catabolism
Interleukin-6 (IL-6)	26 kDa	Monocytes, macrophages, T cells, endothelial cells	(a) Liver (b) B cells	Acute phase response Activation
Interleukin-8 (IL-8)	10 kDa	Monocytes, macrophages, endothelial cells	Neutrophils	Chemotaxis, activation
Interferon-γ (IFN-γ)	21–24 kDa	T cells, NK cells	Macrophages	Activation (inflammation)
Interleukin-12 (IL-12)	70 kDa	Macrophages	T cells, B cells, NK cells	Activation, differentiation
Interleukin-18 (IL-18)		Macrophages	T cells, NK cells	Activation, differentiation

dysfunction and, potentially, death. Among the systemic effects of TNFα are the induction of fever, stimulation of acute phase protein secretion by the liver, activation of the coagulation cascade, myocardial suppression, induction of systemic vasodilators with resultant hypotension, catabolism, and hypoglycemia.[25,26] Numerous studies have shown that administration of TNFα to experimental animals will mimic the systemic inflammatory response observed in sepsis and after severe injury. Another important effect of TNFα is its ability to induce apoptosis of a variety of cell types.[27] TNF-induced apoptosis may be one mechanism by which it induces tissue injury at high systemic concentrations.

TNFα is also a potent stimulus for the release of other inflammatory mediators, particularly IL-1 and IL-6. IL-1 is released primarily by mononuclear phagocytes and its physiologic effects are essentially identical to those of TNFα.[28] However, important differences between the functions of IL-1 and TNFα exist. Most notably, IL-1 does not induce tissue injury or apoptotic cell death by itself but can potentiate the injurious effects of TNFα. The IL-1 family of proteins, including IL-18, are the only group of cytokines for which known natural antagonists have been identified. The IL-1 receptor antagonists (IL-1ra) bind to the IL-1 receptor but do not induce receptor activation.[28] These proteins appear to function as competitive inhibitors of IL-1 action.

IL-6 is another protein that is commonly increased in the circulation of patients with SIRS.[28] Macrophages, endothelial cells, and fibroblasts secrete this protein. Interleukin-6 itself does not induce tissue injury but its presence in the circulation has been associated with poor outcome in trauma patients, probably because it is a marker of ongoing inflammation.[25,26] The primary effect of IL-6 is to induce secretion of acute phase proteins from the liver as well as serve as a growth and differentiation factor for B lymphocytes.

Interferon γ (IFN-γ) is a cytokine involved in the amplification of the acute inflammatory response, particularly the stimulation of cytokine secretion, phagocytosis, and respiratory burst activity by macrophages. IFN-γ is secreted primarily by T lymphocytes and natural killer (NK) cells in response to antigen presentation as well as macrophage-derived cytokines such as IL-12 and IL-18. The primary effect of IFN-γ is to amplify the inflammatory response of macrophages. In response to IFN-γ, the phagocytic and respiratory burst activity of macrophages are increased, secretion of inflammatory mediators such as TNFα and IL-1 are enhanced, and antigen presentation is potentiated by upregulation of class II major histocompatibility complex. Blockade of IFN-γ production or function has been shown to markedly decrease the deleterious inflammatory effects induced by bacterial endotoxin.[29] Therefore, IFN-γ is believed to be an important factor in the amplification of SIRS.

Chemokines are a family of proteins that function primarily as chemotactic factors for leukocytes (Table 22.3). Interleukin-8 is the most widely studied chemokine in the setting of sepsis and SIRS; it is a potent chemoattractant for neutrophils and is a major factor in recruiting neutrophils to inflammatory foci. Several studies have shown that IL-8 plays a role, particularly in the lung, in mediating tissue injury in the setting of trauma and burn injury.[30] It is likely that that other chemokines also play a role in inflammatory injury. A recent study demonstrated increased circulating levels of macrophage inflammatory protein-1α (MIP-1α) in patients with SIRS.[31]

Upregulation of most soluble mediators of inflammation is regulated at the transcriptional level. Some of the key transcription factors that control pro-inflammatory gene expression include nuclear factor-κB (NF-κB), AP-1 and STAT1 (Figure 22.2). During the last 20 years, NF-κB has emerged

TABLE 22.3 CLASSIFICATION OF CHEMOKINES

Chemokine type	Target cell	Chemokine type	Target cell
α Chemokines			
IL-8	Neutrophils	GCP-2	Neutrophils
GROα (mouse equivalent is GRO/KC)	Neutrophils	PF4	Fibroblasts
GROβ (mouse equivalent is GRO/KC)	Neutrophils	Mig	T lymphocytes
GROγ (mouse equivalent is GRO/KC)	Neutrophils	IP-10	T lymphocytes
ENA-78	Neutrophils	I-TAC	T lymphocytes
LDGF-PBP	Neutrophils, fibroblasts	SDF-1α/β	T lymphocytes
β Chemokines			
MIP-1α	Monocyte/macrophages, T lymphocytes, B cells, NK cells, basophils	DC-CK-1	T lymphocytes
MIP-1β	Same as above	MIP-3α	T lymphocytes
MDC	Monocyte, T lymphocytes	MIP-3β	T lymphocytes
TECK	Macrophages, T lymphocytes	MCP-1	T lymphocytes, monocytes
TARC	T lymphocytes	MCP-2	Same
RANTES	Monocyte/macrophages, T lymphocytes, NK cells, basophils	MCP-3	Same
HCC-1	Monocytes	MCP-4	Same
HCC-4	Monocytes, lymphocytes	Eotaxin	Eosinophils
Other chemokines			
Lymphotactin	T lymphocytes, NK cells	Fractalkine	T lymphocytes, monocytes

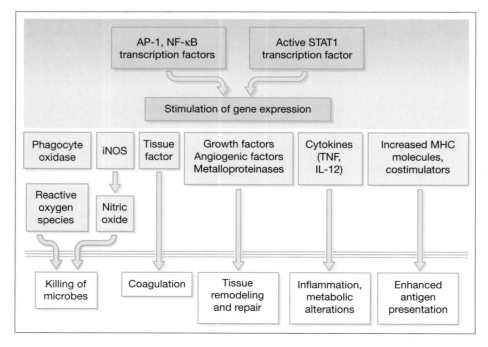

Fig. 22.2 Regulation of pro-inflammatory gene expression. Inflammatory stimuli induce activation of transcriptional pathways mediated by NF-κB, AP-1 and STAT1 that result in production of pro-inflammatory mediators. (From Cotran R, Kumar V, Collins T, eds. Robbins Pathologic basis of disease, 6th edn. Philadelphia: WB Saunders; 1999: 75.)

as a central regulator of the inflammatory process.[32] NF-κB is composed of a family of proteins including p50 (NF-κB1), p65 (RelA), C-Rel, and p52 (NF-κB2) that combine to form homo- or heterodimers and ultimately function to regulate the transcription of a variety of cytokine, chemokine, adhesion molecule, and enzyme genes involved in SIRS. Increased activation of NF-κB has been associated with poor outcome in some studies. Activation of NF-κB in peripheral blood monocytes correlates with increased mortality in septic patients, and alveolar macrophages from patients with adult respiratory distress syndrome (ARDS) exhibited greater nuclear NF-κB levels than critically ill patients without ARDS.[33,34] The AP-1 complex is activated through activation of the protein kinase JNK by stimuli that are similar to those required for NF-κB mobilization. The STAT1 pathway is induced by activation of the IFN-α receptor on phagocytes.

Several non-cytokine factors have been implicated in the pathogenesis of SIRS. Platelet activating factor (PAF) is a phospholipid autocoid released by endothelial cells that regulates the release of cytokines and amplifies the pro-inflammatory response. It appears to be an important factor in the adhesion of neutrophils to endothelial cells. The prolonged presence of PAF in the serum of patients with SIRS has correlated with poor outcome.[35] Eicosanoids are arachadonic acid metabolites that regulate many aspects of the immune response. Leukotrienes (LTC$_4$-LTE$_4$) induce contraction of endothelial cells and encourage capillary leakage.[36] Thromboxane A$_2$, a macrophage and platelet-derived factor, promotes platelet aggregation, vasoconstriction and, potentially, tissue thrombosis.[37]

The complement cascade is composed of more than 30 proteins that interact in a complex fashion to mediate inflammation and direct lysis of microbes and other cells (Figure 22.3). However, in SIRS, excessive complement activation appears to cause significant cellular injury in the host. Products of the complement cascade, most notably C3a and C5a, are potent activators of inflammation and leukocyte chemotaxis.[38] C3a

and C5a also directly activate neutrophils and promote release of reactive oxygen intermediates and proteases. Excessive release of these factors can result in significant tissue injury. The membrane attack complex (MAC) is the terminal component of the complement cascade. MAC results from the aggregation of the complement components C5–C9 on biological membranes. The accumulation of MAC on cell surfaces can result in significant tissue and cellular injury and may be a major factor in the pathogenesis of MODS.

Circulating cytokines as markers of SIRS and predictors of outcome

Numerous studies have been undertaken with the goal of using plasma cytokine levels as diagnostic and prognostic markers in patients with SIRS. This approach seems logical based on the observation that circulating cytokines have been observed in several clinical studies of trauma, sepsis, and thermal injury. Given its central role in the activation and regulation of the pro-inflammatory response, TNFα has been studied extensively as a plasma marker of SIRS. The results have been inconsistent. Martin et al.[39] showed that TNFα levels were markedly elevated in patients with septic shock and correlated with fatal outcome. However, their results also showed that trauma patients did not exhibit the same marked elevations in circulating TNFα nor did circulating TNFα concentrations correlate with increased mortality in trauma patients. In some published studies, measurement of circulating TNFα levels in burn patients has not provided a useful marker of outcome.[40,41] Overall, plasma TNFα levels have been variable and inconsistent and have not correlated with mortality or the development of MODS. However, a study by Zhang et al.[42] in 25 patients with greater than 30% total body surface area (TBSA) burns demonstrated marked increases in plasma TNFα levels in burned patients and a significant correlation between TNFα concentration and shock, MODS, and death. These findings support the results of Marano et al.,[43] who showed a significant correlation between circulating TNFα concentration and mortality in burned patients. Therefore, taken together, these results show that the value of TNFα as a marker of ongoing inflammation as well as an indicator of morbidity and mortality in the setting of burn injury remains to be established.

TNFα interacts with two known cell surface receptors designated tumor necrosis factor receptor (TNFR)-I and TNFR-II. TNFR-I, also known as TNF-R55 or p55, is expressed on a variety of cells and its activation mediates most of the activities of TNFα, including induction of apoptosis. Activation of TNFR-II (TNF-R75 or p75) results in cellular proliferation and activation. During inflammatory states, TNFR are released from cells and may serve as antagonists of TNFα. Several investigators have characterized surface-bound and soluble TNFR (sTNFR) in sepsis and trauma.[42,44,45] Hubl et al.[44] showed that surface TNFR-I were upregulated while TNFR-II were downregulated in patients with SIRS. Increased TNFR-I correlated with increased body temperature but not with survival. SIRS patients with decreased surface TNFR-II had a trend toward increased mortality. A study by Zhang et al.[42] showed a higher incidence of shock, MODS, and mortality in burn patients with increased plasma sTNFR-I and sTNFR-II levels. Presterl et al.[45] showed a correlation between sTNFR and

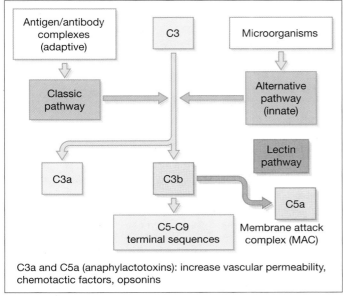

C3a and C5a (anaphylactotoxins): increase vascular permeability, chemotactic factors, opsonins

Fig. 22.3 The complement cascade. The complement cascade can be activated through three distinct mechanisms and plays an important role in innate and acquired inflammatory responses.

APACHE III scores, as well as the incidence of shock and mortality in septic patients. Overall, in the studies published to date, the presence of high levels of circulating sTNFR is a poor prognostic indicator.

Another family of proteins that has been extensively analyzed as markers of SIRS is IL-1 and IL-1 receptor antagonist (IL-1ra). In burn patients, low IL-1ra levels have correlated with mortality in two independent studies.[41,42] Plasma IL-1ra levels have been shown to correlate with body surface area burned, extent of third-degree burn, and the presence of inhalational injury.[41,46]

Of the cytokine markers studied to date, elevated levels of IL-6 appear to be one of the more consistent markers of poor outcome in burn, trauma, and septic patients. One of the primary known functions of IL-6 is induction of acute phase proteins such as C-reactive protein (CRP) by the liver. In some studies, CRP has been shown to parallel IL-6 as a marker of increased mortality.[47] Although IL-6 itself does not have any known direct injurious effects, it apparently serves as a consistent marker of ongoing inflammation. Elevated plasma IL-6 levels have correlated with increased mortality in experimental and clinical studies of thermal injury, sepsis, trauma, and hemorrhagic shock.[45,48,49] A study by Taniguchi et al.[49] showed that an increased ratio of IL-6 to the anti-inflammatory cytokine IL-10 was a predictor of poor outcome in patients with SIRS.

In trauma and burn patients it is often difficult to differentiate whether SIRS is a result of the injury itself or due to superimposed infection. Most of the clinical signs of infection, such as fever and leukocytosis, are, by definition, present in SIRS. Considerable attention has been placed on identifying indirect markers of systemic infection. The identification of circulating markers of infection that can be rapidly assessed and serve as reliable markers of the presence of infection has important implications. First, it is important clinically to identify patients with systemic infection in order to initiate antibiotic therapy in a timely fashion. Secondly, blood cultures are the gold standard for diagnosis of systemic infections. Although blood cultures provide important information regarding the presence of infection and the identity of the infecting organism, it can often take several days to obtain reliable results, and the presence of negative cultures does not assure the absence of infection. Therefore, efforts have been made to identify other markers of systemic infection. The two markers that have been most consistently elevated in patients with infection are procalcitonin and CRP. Studies have shown that increased plasma levels of procalcitonin are a sensitive marker of systemic infection.[50] Likewise, increased circulating CRP has been shown to be a sensitive marker of infection.[51,52] Both of these markers have been shown to be more reliable than clinical signs in the diagnosis of infection in high-risk surgical and trauma patients.

Overall, several markers of inflammation and infection have been identified in burn and trauma patients. Some of these markers have been shown to be consistent indicators of high-risk patients. However, cytokine and non-cytokine markers of inflammation are not used routinely in the laboratory evaluation of burned patients. With further research and demonstration of the reliability of these markers, they may become an accepted part of clinical practice. In addition, technology is evolving to measure these markers in a rapid and cost-effective manner. The combination of these factors may allow blood cytokine markers to become a component of patient management in the future.

Anti-inflammatory therapy for SIRS

Despite our increased understanding of the role of inflammatory mediators in the pathogenesis of SIRS, most anti-inflammatory drug regimens have had little success in the treatment of this problem. Neutralizing approaches to several inflammatory mediators have been studied. All of these studies have demonstrated, at best, marginal improvement in septic morbidity and mortality. One of the most widely studied approaches for the treatment of SIRS is the use of monoclonal antibodies to TNFα. Several multicenter, prospective, clinical trials have been undertaken in septic patients using several different antibodies to TNFα.[53,54] These studies did not demonstrate improved outcome in patients receiving anti-TNFα compared to placebo. One recent study evaluated the efficacy of a chimeric antibody to TNF in patients with severe sepsis.[54] Circulating levels of TNFα as well as a variety of other inflammatory mediators were assessed. Although circulating levels of TNFα were transiently decreased, anti-TNFα therapy did not result in reduction of circulating levels of other inflammatory mediators such as IL-1β, IL-1ra, sTNFR, or IL-6. In addition, evidence of systemic inflammation was not decreased and overall mortality was not improved in anti-TNFα-treated patients. Similarly, the use of sTNFR as a strategy to neutralize the systemic effects of TNFα and decrease sepsis-associated morbidity and mortality has been unsuccessful.[55,56] Other anti-inflammatory approaches that have been studied and found to be largely ineffective include the use of IL-1ra,[57,58] anti-bradykinin,[59] PAFra,[60,61] and ibuprofen.[62,63]

Because of the relative ineffectiveness of anti-inflammatory therapy aimed at neutralizing single mediators, more broad-based strategies were developed with the goal of neutralizing, removing, or inhibiting the production of several inflammatory mediators. Hemofiltration was one approach that received considerable attention. Several studies have shown that hemofiltration will increase the clearance of inflammatory mediators, particularly IL-6, from blood in patients with sepsis.[64,65] However, none of these studies has demonstrated a significant reduction in IL-6 plasma levels. A study by Kellum et al.[65] showed that continuous venovenous hemofiltration (CVVH) reduced plasma TNFα concentrations by 13%, while the use of continuous venovenous hemodialysis (CVVHD) resulted in a 32% increase in circulating TNFα levels. Overall, the use of hemofiltration has been largely ineffective in removing significant amounts of inflammatory mediators from the blood of patients with sepsis and there is currently no evidence that this approach will decrease morbidity and mortality.

The use of glucocorticoids in the treatment of sepsis has been proposed for more than 30 years. A meta-analyses[66] of studies using high-dose glucocorticoids in the treatment of sepsis was published in 1995 and later summarized by Zeni et al.[67] Overall, the use of high-dose glucocorticoids to treat sepsis and septic shock has not been beneficial. In many studies, the use of glucocorticoids in septic patients was associated with increased mortality. In burned patients, there is no evidence that administration of glucocorticoids provides effective treatment for systemic inflammation. More recent studies show that replacement dose steroids will improve survival in septic patients that have adrenal suppression.[39] Some practitioners now advocate the use of replacement dose glucocorticoids in septic patients that are refractory to conventional management.[68]

Reasons for the lack of efficacy of these anti-inflammatory strategies are likely to be multifactorial. First, the inflammatory response to injury and sepsis is mediated by a complex array of mediators that are largely interrelated. Therefore, blocking or neutralization of a single mediator is not likely to have a marked effect on the overall response. Secondly, the same mediators that are important in inducing tissue injury also play an important role in antimicrobial immunity. Blockade of these mediators may leave the host more susceptible to subsequent infection. Thirdly, many of the mediators, particularly TNFα and IL-1β, are released within minutes of injury and mobilize the inflammatory cascade shortly thereafter. Therefore, by the time that signs of SIRS or sepsis are apparent, many of the injurious effects of the inflammatory response have already been set into motion, making therapy ineffective. A recent emphasis has been placed on the identification of late mediators of inflammatory injury. This search has been prompted by the observation that SIRS and sepsis-associated death occur days after the peak effect of inflammatory cytokines. One potential late mediator that has recently been identified is high-mobility group protein-1 (HMG-1).[69] HMG-1 is released by macrophages up to 8 hours after LPS challenge and persists in the circulation for days. Administration of anti-HMG-1 in mice has been shown to improve survival. Conversely, systemic administration of HMG-1 to mice is lethal.

Whether HMG-1 plays an important role in inflammatory injury in humans remains to be determined. However, the concept of late mediators of inflammatory tissue injury may improve our understanding of the pathophysiology of SIRS.

As discussed earlier in this chapter, factors that appear to be important in limiting the extent of SIRS and, in many cases, decreasing the incidence of shock and MODS, are aggressive fluid resuscitation, excision of necrotic tissue, and adequate nutritional support.[70] There is controversy regarding the ideal fluid for volume resuscitation in trauma and burn patients. However, recent studies show that hypertonic saline has beneficial effects in modulating the SIRS-associated immunological cascade as well as restoring hemodynamic parameters and microcirculatory flow. The effect of hypertonic saline on immune function has largely centered on attenuation of post-injury immunosuppression. Recent studies have shown that resuscitation with hypertonic saline will improve macrophage and T cell function as well as increase resistance to infection in experimental models or trauma and hemorrhage.[71] Proper nutritional support is also an important factor in the treatment of severely injured patients. Enteral feeding formulas supplemented with glutamine, arginine, omega-3 fatty acids, and nucleotides have been shown to improve outcome in trauma patients.[72,73] Overall, trauma patients receiving immune-enhancing diets have been shown to have fewer infectious complications.

More recently, Metz and Tracey have described a cholinergic anti-inflammatory pathway that may be important in the regulation of inflammation and could be exploited for therapeutic benefit.[74,75] As described, local inflammation activates afferent fibers of the vagus nerve that signal the brain to elicit an anti-

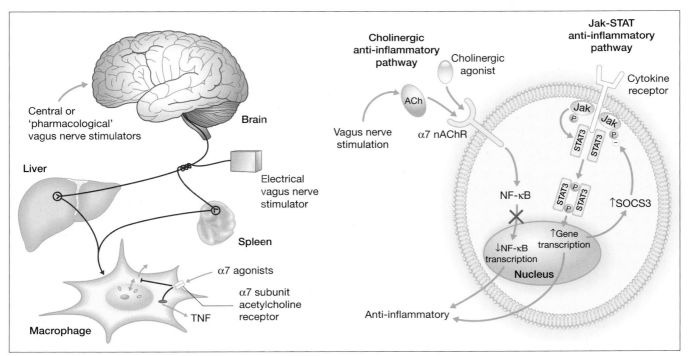

Fig. 22.4 The cholinergic anti-inflammatory pathway. Tissue inflammation sends afferent signals to the central nervous system resulting in activation of the cholinergic anti-inflammatory pathway. Release of acetylcholine by the vagus nerve induces anti-inflammatory effects by binding to nicotinic receptors on the surface of leukocytes. (Adapted from Czura CJ, Tracey KJ. Autonomic neural regulation of immunity J. Int Med 2005; 257:156–166; Metz CN and Tracey KJ. It takes nerve to dampen inflammation. Nat Immunol 2005; 6:756–757. Reprinted by permission from Macmillan Publishers Ltd.)

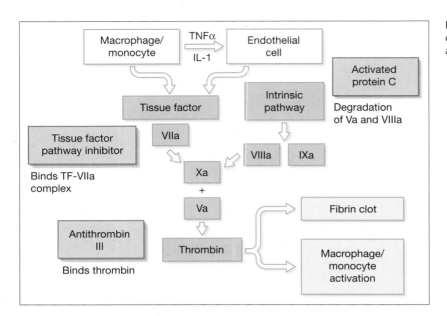

Fig. 22.5 Regulation of the coagulation cascade during inflammation. Inflammation primarily causes activation of the extrinsic coagulation pathway.

inflammatory response through efferent vagal fibers (Figure 22.4). Acetylcholine released by the vagus interacts with α7 nicotinic acetylcholine receptors (α7 nAChR) on macrophages and suppresses the production of pro-inflammatory mediators. These investigators have shown that electrical stimulation of the vagus nerve will attenuate the pro-inflammatory response induced by cecal ligation and puncture or endotoxin challenge. Acetylcholine has also been shown to inhibit the release of pro-inflammatory cytokines by cultured macrophages following endotoxin challenge.[74,75] More specific α7 nAChR agonists are under investigation for the treatment of hyperinflammatory states.

Activation of the coagulation cascade during inflammation

Inflammation and coagulation are intimately intertwined. The coagulation cascade is activated during tissue injury and during infection. It is divided into two pathways that converge and ultimately cause the activation of thrombin with subsequent cleavage of fibrinogen into fibrin (Figure 22.5). The intrinsic pathway is a series of plasma proteins that are activated by Hageman factor (factor XII), a protein synthesized in the liver that is activated by binding to collagen, basement membrane or activated platelets.[76] Activated Hageman factor triggers a cascade of proteins to become activated, resulting in the formation of thrombin. The intrinsic pathway is most commonly activated by direct tissue trauma. In contrast, the extrinsic pathway is initiated by the production of tissue factor. Recent studies indicate that the extrinsic pathway is the primary coagulation pathway activated during infection and systemic inflammation, particularly during sepsis and the SIRS.[76] Tissue factor is expressed on tissue surfaces that are not normally exposed to the vascular compartment such as subcutaneous tissues and the adventitial layer of blood vessels. In addition, endothelial cells and activated monocytes produce tissue factor during periods of inflammation in response to

TNFα, IL-1, IL-6 and CRP.[17] The presence of tissue factor causes activation of factor VII, which then forms a complex with tissue factor and ultimately causes the formation of thrombin by the activation of a series of coagulation factors (Figure 22.5). Activation of the coagulation cascade is not only important in the formation of fibrin clots but also has important effects on the pro-inflammatory response. Factor Xa, thrombin and the tissue facto—VIIa complex have been shown to elicit pro-inflammatory activity. Specifically, thrombin and the tissue factor–VIIa complex can induce production of pro-inflammatory cytokines such as TNFα by mononuclear and endothelial cells.[77] This effect appears to be mediated by the binding of these factors to protease-activated receptors on the surface of target cells. Therefore, acute inflammation causes activation of the coagulation cascade, which can then further potentiate the inflammatory response.

Activation of the clotting cascade during inflammation is limited by several factors. This is important because it prevents uncontrolled induction of procoagulant mechanisms. The most well-defined factors are antithrombin, the protein C system and the tissue factor pathway inhibitor. Antithrombin is produced in the liver and directly binds and inactivates thrombin.[78] The binding of antithrombin to thrombin is greatly potentiated by heparin and by glycosaminoglycans present on the endothelial cell surface. In rodents, interaction of antithrombin with the endothelial cell surface promotes the release of PGI$_2$, which inhibits TNFα production by monocytes through inhibition of transcription factor NF-κB activation.[79] Thus, antithrombin may have anti-inflammatory properties in addition to its function in regulating coagulation.

Protein C is a circulating protein that is activated by the thrombin–thrombomodulin complex on the surface of endothelial cells (Figure 22.6). Activation of protein C decelerates the clotting cascade by inactivating factors Va and VIIIa.[80] Activated protein C also inhibits thrombin-induced production of TNFα by monocytes by inhibiting the activation of transcription factors NF-κB and AP-1 (to be discussed).[81] There-

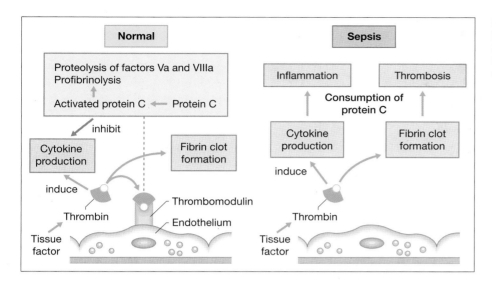

Fig. 22.6 Biology of protein C during inflammation. Activated protein C can become consumed during severe inflammation, resulting in hypercoagulability and amplification of the inflammatory response.

fore, activated protein C has both anticoagulant and anti-inflammatory properties. During sepsis, activated protein C levels can become depleted due to consumption and inflammation-induced downregulation of thrombomodulin. This results in unchecked formation of thrombin, causing accelerated coagulation and increased pro-inflammatory activity. The importance of protein C in regulating thrombin formation during sepsis is demonstrated by increased mortality in septic patients that have low activated protein C levels.[82]

A third important factor in the regulation of thrombin formation is the tissue factor pathway inhibitor (TFPI). TFPI is present on the surface of endothelial cells and bound to lipoproteins in plasma. TFPI inactivates tissue factor by forming a quaternary complex with tissue factor and factor VIIa. Factor Xa is the fourth component of the complex.[83] Inhibition of tissue factor function inhibits activation of the extrinsic clotting pathway during inflammation. Infusion of TFPI has also been shown to decrease pro-inflammatory cytokine production during endotoxin infusion in baboons, but not in humans.

The hemodynamic response

The full clinical picture of systemic inflammation after thermal injury, multiple trauma, or sepsis includes a hyperdynamic circulation. It is characterized by a low systemic vascular resistance, which requires a high cardiac output to maintain mean arterial pressure. This fall in resistance is not the result of an increase in metabolic rate. The oxygen extraction of the tissues remains the same. Blood is thus flowing to tissues that are not metabolically active. Patients who are not well resuscitated or whose heart function is compromised may not be able to increase their cardiac output to the extent needed to maintain arterial pressure during states of extensive vasodilatation and, thus, might go into shock. A reduced vascular responsiveness to vasoconstrictors finally prevents successful pharmacologic intervention and patients might die in irreversible shock. The time period from insult until the hyperdynamic response develops can vary between hours after a septic insult

or days after multiple trauma. It has been hypothesized that the development of the hyperdynamic state might be dependent on the presence of endotoxin or bacteria in the blood. An intravenous bolus injection of 4ng/kg endotoxin into healthy volunteers mimics some aspects of the hemodynamic response seen in patients.[84,85] The low systemic vascular resistance and the elevated cardiac output can also be induced in animal models by continuous infusion of low-dose endotoxin[86] or bacteria.[87] Studies in conscious sheep revealed that the hemodynamic response to continuous low-dose endotoxin can be divided into three parts.[88] The first two phases might be missed under clinical conditions most of the time due to their short duration (<3 hours).

Phase 1

Systemic vascular resistance and pulmonary vascular resistance increase markedly both upon intermittent administration of endotoxin[89] or during its continuous infusion into conscious sheep.[90] This reaction occurred within 30 minutes to 1 hour of the endotoxin administration and was attributed to the release of the potent vasoconstrictor thromboxane (TX) A_2. Lymph and plasma levels of TXB_2, the stable metabolite of the eicosanoid TXA_2, were found elevated 1 and 4 hours after challenge of sheep with 1µg/kg endotoxin.[91] Cyclooxygenase[92] and thromboxane synthetase inhibition diminished the hypertensive response.[91] Thromboxane synthetase inhibition was equally effective in preventing the marked pulmonary vasoconstriction after burn injury in pigs.[93] The high pulmonary vascular resistance during phase 1 of endotoxemia has been demonstrated to compromise myocardial function of the right heart in terms of a low ejection fraction and an increase in end-systolic diameter.[91,94] Administration of the thromboxane synthetase inhibitor OKY046 blocked these early changes in right heart function.[94]

The early systemic vasoconstriction did not occur equally throughout the vasculature. Blood flow through the superior mesenteric artery was particularly reduced.[95] Vasoconstriction of the splanchnic vessels has been associated with the release of so-called myocardial depressant factors[96] and with bacterial translocation.[95] The coincidence of markedly decreased mesenteric blood flow and bacterial translocation has also been demonstrated after burn injury[97] and multiple trauma associated with a state of circulatory shock.[98] Moreover, hypoperfusion, particularly of the ileal mucosa, was still noted during the hyperdynamic phase in a *murine* sepsis model, when blood flow to most of the splanchnic area was not decreased.[99] Bacterial translocation has been hypothesized to be one of the major factors maintaining systemic inflammation.

Phase 2

This portion of the response, between 3 and 4 hours after the endotoxin infusion has been started, is characterized more by pulmonary permeability changes (see below) than by hemodynamic alterations. In the hyperdynamic sheep model, the pulmonary artery pressure is mildly elevated and cardiac output demonstrates the lowest values throughout the experiment. The underlying mechanisms of this response are not yet clear. Many mediators of the immune system have been released by that time, including TNFα, IL-6, PAF, and peptidoleukotrienes.[100] This might indicate that these mediators are proximal elements of the mediator cascades. Although investigations into the release of many of these cytokines are few as a result of the limitations of respective assays, TNFα has been shown to be increased in both phase 1 and 2 of the response in sheep[100,101] and volunteers.[102,103] Moreover, the vasoconstrictor endothelin is elevated in the chronic sheep model of endotoxemia at that time,[104] as well as the vasodilator atrial natriuretic peptide.[105,106] Endothelin has also been correlated with reductions in cardiac output in septic humans.[107] The hemodynamic changes in phase 2 are most likely the result of the action of the mediator cocktail.

Phase 3

Continuous infusion of endotoxin into sheep and pigs resulted in a hyperdynamic circulation.[90,108,109] Beside a low systemic vascular resistance and a high cardiac output with a slightly decreased mean arterial pressure, the hyperdynamic response is further characterized by hyporesponsiveness of isolated vessels to vasoconstrictors[110] and an increased pulmonary shunt fraction in the presence of a reduced pulmonary hypoxic vasoconstriction.[90,111,112] The high cardiac output is due to an increase in heart rate in the presence of depressed myocardial contractility.[113,114]

Nitric oxide

The endothelium-derived relaxing factor, recently identified as nitric oxide (NO), has been implicated as a mediator in this reaction. NO can be synthesized from its precursor L-arginine by two different enzymes. The calcium-dependent constitutive nitric oxide synthase (NOS) is responsible for the basal release of NO, which seems to play an important role for the regulation of vascular tone under physiologic conditions (Figure 22.7). *In vitro* data suggest that this enzyme might become inactivated early after administration of endotoxin, thus accounting for some of the vasoconstrictive phenomena seen in phases 1 and 2.[115] Dependent on the species, cells producing the inducible NOS include macrophages, vascular smooth muscle cells, and vascular endothelium upon stimulation by endotoxin, TNFα, IL-1, or IFN-α.[116]

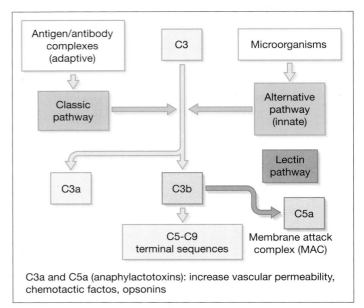

Fig. 22.7 Nitric oxide during SIRS. Activation of nitric oxide synthase isoforms, particularly eNOS and iNOS, causes vascular smooth muscle relaxation during severe inflammation.

On the other hand, it has recently been reported that the human macrophage cannot form NO under these circumstances.[117,118]

NO is a lipophilic gas which can easily enter vascular smooth muscle cells where it stimulates the soluble guanylate cyclase[119,120] to synthesize cyclic guanosine monophosphate (cGMP). High levels of cGMP stimulate cells to lower their intracellular Ca^{2+} concentration. This leads to vascular dilatation and hyporesponsiveness to vasoconstrictors. Administration of an NOS inhibitor to septic humans[121,122] and to endotoxemic sheep[90,123] increases their vascular resistance and restores their responsiveness to vasoconstrictors. It was assumed that the hemodynamic abnormalities mediated by NO formed via the inducible NOS. However, plasma concentrations of nitrite/nitrate and nitrosylated proteins were not elevated during *ovine* endotoxemia. Species specificity was also indicated by the finding that human macrophages do not produce the inducible form of NOS. However, the inducible form of the enzyme seems to be present in human hepatocytes. Elevated nitrite levels were reported in one study evaluating septic newborns.[124] There are currently no convincing data available with regard to high nitrite levels in adult humans with SIRS. Ochoa found somewhat elevated nitrite concentrations in some septic patients, but failed to demonstrate them in septic trauma patients.[125] At this point it can neither be concluded nor can it be excluded that NO mediates the hyperdynamic response during systemic inflammation.

Guanylate cyclase

The second messenger cGMP appears to play an important role in the vasodilation seen with sepsis. There have been reports of cGMP elevations in plasma of septic patients[126] and endotoxic rats.[127] cGMP was elevated in tissues removed from our animals following a continuous infusion of endotoxin.[128] The guanylate cyclase occurs in a soluble and in a particulate form.[129] The particulate form is activated by atrial natriuretic peptide (ANP).[130,131] The soluble form has a heme group that is activated by NO. This reaction is inhibited by methylene blue and hemoglobin.[132] There is a high probability that ANP is the source of the stimulation of guanylate cyclase during sepsis and endotoxemia, because the cGMP formed in some of the experiments was not inhibited by methylene blue or L-arginine analogs.

Atrial natriuretic peptide

We have reported a marked elevation in ANP after the injection of endotoxin into sheep.[105,106] We have also examined our chronic sheep models and found that the increase in plasma levels of ANP was sustained with the continuous infusion of endotoxin or bacteria. ANP has also been shown to be elevated in septic humans.[126,130] In the rat study reported above, in which the plasma levels of cGMP remained elevated despite administration of an NOS inhibitor, a marked increase in plasma levels of ANP was found.[127] ANP elevates smooth muscle cGMP[133,134] through stimulation of particulate or membrane guanylate cyclase, which is not affected by methylene blue,[129,130] and thereby produces vasodilation. ANP is released from the right atrium and might be the material responsible for the cGMP elevation that was seen in animal models of sepsis and humans with septicemia. Brigham's group has shown that cGMP levels were higher in the lung lymph than in the plasma, and higher in plasma from arterial than mixed venous blood, suggesting a thoracic origin for the second messenger.[135]

The kallikrein–kinin system

The kallikrein–kinin system, which includes several vasoactive substances, has been shown to be activated during endotoxemia in humans[136] and in sheep.[137] However, administration of a bradykinin antagonist did not change the cardiovascular or microvascular response to endotoxin in chronically instrumented sheep.[137] Therefore, activation of this mediator cascade seems rather to be an epiphenomenon of endotoxemia.

Changes in permeability

Endothelial permeability

Endotoxemia increases microvascular permeability both in the systemic[138] and in the pulmonary circulation.[139] The lung is the organ most commonly compromised during processes that lead to systemic inflammation. Edema formation due to an increase in microvascular permeability is a hallmark of the acute lung injury. The factors that determine the transvascular fluid flux are summarized in the Starling–Landis equation:[140,141]

$$J_v = K_f\,[(P_{mv} - P_i) - \alpha(\pi_{mv} - \pi_l)]$$

where: J_v is the transvascular fluid flux, K_f is the filtration coefficient (measure of the endothelial permeability to small solutes and water as well as of the permeability surface area), P_{mv} is the microvascular hydrostatic pressure, P_i is the interstitial hydrostatic pressure, α is the osmotic reflection coefficient to protein, π_{mv} is the microvascular oncotic pressure, and π_i is the interstitial oncotic pressure.

A model has been developed in sheep that allows the determination of the variables included in the Starling equation. The lymph flow draining from the efferent vessel of the caudal mediastinal lymph node has been used as a measure of the transvascular fluid flux. Using this model, changes in lymph flow and lymph protein flux were evaluated during sepsis and endotoxemia. Again, the changes in pulmonary endothelial permeability can be divided into three phases.

Phase 1

Several investigators studied lymph flow and lymph protein flux after administration of bacteria or short-time infusion of 1–2 µg/kg of endotoxin in sheep. Two phases of permeability change could be distinguished in these models.[142] During phase 1 there was a high microvascular hydrostatic pressure as defined by the Gaar equation.[143] It was associated with an increase in lung lymph flow, while the lymph protein concentration was low. It was concluded that the high microvascular hydrostatic pressure was responsible for the early increase in transvascular fluid flux. As mentioned above, TXA$_2$ had been found to be responsible for the vasoconstriction occurring during phase 1 of the response to endotoxin. Therefore, it is not surprising that administration of the thromboxane synthetase inhibitor OKY046 prevented the rise in lymph flow during phase 1.[91] This effect was also noted after blockage of the cyclooxygenase by ibuprofen.[92] Early edema formation after burns at the site of the injury might be due to a different mechanism. Recent data suggest that a marked fall in interstitial hydrostatic pressure might occur in the injured tissue, which can explain the immediate onset of edema formation after thermal injury.[144,145] These changes might be the result of an inhibition of the fibroblast β_1-integrin attachment to collagen.

Phase 2

During phase 2, lymph flow continues to be high. However, the lymph protein concentration rises considerably[142] and the pulmonary artery pressure is only mildly elevated. The oncotic pressure gradient between microvasculature and interstitial space is reduced during that period.[146] Together these data suggest that the permeability of the pulmonary endothelium to protein increases in phase 2. In fact, the reflection coefficient for total protein fell from 0.73 to 0.58, with respective changes of the reflection coefficients for albumin (0.66 to 0.5), IgG (0.76 to 0.64), and IgM (0.91 to 0.83) after 4 hours of *Escherichia coli* sepsis in sheep.[147] Confirmation of this hypothesis is still pending in models of endotoxemia, but it has been generally accepted that the changes in pulmonary transvascular fluid flux in phase 2 represent changes in microvascular permeability. The mechanisms of the increased microvascular permeability are still under discussion.

Endothelial cells play an important role in the development of vascular permeability. It has been hypothesized that endothelial cells can contract upon stimulation.[148] As a result, the intercellular gaps might increase in number and/or size, establishing the so-called capillary leak syndrome. The development of the protein-rich high-permeability edema can be ameliorated if substances are administered that raise the endothelial cell content of cyclic adenosine or guanosine monophosphate.[149,150] Endothelial cells do not merely serve as targets during systemic inflammation. They actively contribute to the ongoing inflammatory process. Their role in the inflammatory reaction has been estimated so highly that even the term 'endothelial inflammation' has been used to describe it. The endothelial cell can be stimulated by endotoxin, TNFα, or IL-1 to express E-selectin, an adhesion molecule.[151] E-selection on the surface of endothelial cells interacts with the corresponding L-selection complex on PMNs to facilitate rolling of these cells along the endothelium.[152] Moreover, endothelial cells secrete the pro-inflammatory cytokine IL-1,[153] which activates PMNs.

Conflicting data exist regarding the role of PMNs in SIRS. PMNs are usually found at the site of tissue injury, to which they migrate following a concentration gradient of chemotactic stimuli. Upon stimulation, PMNs roll along endothelial cells, and in a further step, after interaction of the PMN CD11/18 integrin with its ligand, the intercellular adhesion molecule (ICAM-1), the PMN can emigrate from the vessel into the interstitial space. Antibodies against the common CD18 β chain showed beneficial effects in an animal model of sepsis-induced lung injury.[154] On the other hand, patients who are deficient in CD18 have abundant PMNs in their alveolar spaces. In addition, the monoclonal antibody 60.3 was ineffective in completely blocking the migration of PMNs into the lung in a number of conditions.[155] We have recently reported that in chronic endotoxemia there were few PMNs in the lung but numerous macrophages.[156] Activated PMNs and macrophages secrete oxygen free radicals and proteases, which is part of their defense mechanism against bacteria. Administration of oxygen free radical scavengers and antiproteases proved to be useful in diminishing edema accumulation after endotoxin.[157,158] However, proteases and oxygen radicals are also released by macrophages, which are already present in the tissue and by monocytes that can migrate. Animals were depleted of their granulocytes by anti-PMN antiserum[159] or by treatment with nitrogen mustard.[160] This did not prevent the changes in microvascular permeability following the administration of endotoxin. Moreover, patients deficient in PMNs would still develop the adult respiratory distress syndrome associated with sepsis.[161,162] On the other hand, treatment of sheep or goats with hydroxyurea, which is another compound used to deplete granulocytes, was effective and diminished the fluid accumulation in the lung.[163] However, urea scavenges free radicals, which might explain its efficacy.[164] As the inflammatory response becomes chronic, many mediators have been released and more than one mechanism might be assumed to be responsible for the capillary leak.

Many studies were performed to evaluate the role of metabolites of the arachidonic acid for the increase in permeability. Administration of the thromboxane synthetase inhibitor OKY046 did not only reduce transvascular fluid flux in phase 1, but it was also effective in phase 2 after a bolus of endotoxin.[91] Nevertheless, this does not mean that TXA$_2$ itself had induced the increase in permeability. Indication has been reported that TXB$_2$, previously assumed to be an inactive metabolite of TXA$_2$, might cause lung damage.[165] Moreover, thromboxane synthetase blockage by OKY046 reduced the plasma-conjugated dienes, which are peroxidation products of oxygen free radicals.[91] Granulocyte chemiluminescence was elevated 4 hours after administration of 1.5 μg/kg of endotoxin

to chronically instrumented sheep, indicating the production of oxygen free radicals.[166] Oxygen free radicals can increase microvascular permeability both by activation of endothelial cell contraction[167] and by damaging the endothelial cell membrane. OKY046 has been demonstrated to reverse other forms of oxygen free radical-induced lung injury.[168,169] On the other hand, inhibition of the cyclooxygenase did not affect transvascular fluid flux during phase 2, even if TXA$_2$ is a cyclooxygenase metabolite.[92] This discrepancy is still unexplained; however, prostacyclin is elevated after endotoxin administration and this material has many actions that counter the actions of thromboxane. Administration of a cyclooxygenase inhibitor will prevent the release of this salutary eicosanoid.

Microvascular damage during systemic inflammation might also be regarded as an ischemia/reperfusion injury, particularly when it was preceded by a period of intestinal hypoperfusion. Xanthine oxidase-generated oxygen free radicals have been reported to mediate changes in microvascular and epithelial permeability.[170] Endotoxin-induced ileal and cecal permeability was associated with an increased xanthine oxidase activity and inhibition of xanthine oxidase by allopurinol has been shown to reduce intestinal mucosal damage.[171,172] Circulating xanthine oxidase after ischemia/reperfusion injury in rats was associated with pulmonary retention of PMNs and pulmonary capillary leak, which was diminished by pretreatment with allopurinol.[172] Intravenous injection of purified xanthine oxidase, however, induced pulmonary retention of PMNs without increasing microvascular permeability. Therefore, a final evaluation of the role of xanthine oxidase in ischemia/reperfusion-induced permeability changes is not yet possible.

TNFα is one of the early mediators in systemic inflammation. It has been reported to be elevated during sepsis and endotoxemia, after hemorrhagic shock or thermal injury. It is considered as one of the most important mediators in the cascade because it has the potential to stimulate or enhance most of the steps in the inflammatory response. Moreover, administration of human recombinant TNFα reproduced most of the effects of endotoxemia, including the alterations in pulmonary microvascular permeability in the chronic sheep model.[173,174] However, it has been questioned whether the *ovine* response to human TFNα was only related to the cytokine,[88] because contamination of the recombinant material with endotoxin is not uncommon.

TNFα also induces the secretion of PAF, which is a further early mediator of the systemic inflammation. PAF causes an increase in lung lymph flow and permeability to protein when it is infused into conscious sheep.[175] Administration of a PAF antagonist abolished the cardiopulmonary response that occurs during phase 1 and attenuated it during phase 2.[176] However, PAF had no direct effect on endothelial cells.[175] This suggests that it probably increased microvascular permeability through other mechanisms such as its priming effect on PMNs.[177]

Phase 3

The hyperdynamic cardiovascular response is associated with profound changes in pulmonary transvascular fluid flux in the *ovine* model of continuous endotoxemia.[109,139] The lymph protein concentration gradually decreased after phase 2 and after 24 hours of endotoxemia the reflection coefficient to protein was at baseline level, while the lymph flow was still high. Microvascular hydrostatic pressure, evaluated by Holloway's technique, was not significantly different from baseline.[178] The elevated transvascular fluid flux was attributed to a high filtration coefficient. An increase both in perfused surface area and in pore numbers might have contributed to the change in filtration. Repeated injections of endotoxin also decreased subsequent lung lymph production in response to endotoxin.[173] These changes in lung lymph flow were associated with elevations in endothelin[104,178] and atrial natriuretic peptide. However, further studies must determine if these factors affect the pulmonary microvascular changes during the late phases of sepsis and multiple organ failure.

Increased epithelial permeability

Permeability changes during systemic inflammation are not restricted to the endothelium. Loss of epithelial barrier function has been noted both in the lung and in the intestine. Administration of 2–4 ng/kg endotoxin to healthy human volunteers increased their alveolar epithelial permeability to the inhaled 492 Da molecule [^{99m}Tc] diethylenetriamine pentaacetate (DTPA) 3 hours after endotoxin had been given.[85] Human volunteers demonstrated a higher intestinal epithelial permeability to mannitol/lactulose.[179] Bacterial translocation occurred both during endotoxemia,[95] thermal injury,[93] and multiple trauma with hemorrhagic shock.[180] This might well be interpreted as a loss of intestinal barrier function. Nevertheless, one must bear in mind that epithelial permeability to molecules like lactulose/mannitol and bacterial translocation do not necessarily relate to each other. The epithelium could also be injured by ischemia/reperfusion that occurs in all of these situations.[181]

Summary

Burn injury, associated ischemia/reperfusion injury, the presence of necrotic tissue, or a septic episode might function as the initiating event of SIRS. The host response to this insult might be a localized inflammation or, if the stimulus surpasses a certain threshold, a systemic inflammatory response might occur. After a limited injury, the local tissue perfusion will increase and mediators released by macrophages and endothelial cells attract monocytes and polymorphonuclear neutrophils to the area. These cells, as well as the vascular endothelium, are stimulated to express adhesion molecules and their interaction enables the inflammatory cells to leave the vascular lumen and to enter the interstitial space. Once there, activated cells of the immune system will secrete proteolytic enzymes and oxygen radicals, phagocytize and digest bacteria and necrotic tissue, and thereby defend the organism. A side effect of this reaction is that healthy tissue will be affected by the immune attack and will be damaged. As long as the inflammatory response is localized and feedback mechanisms are effective, tissue repair will follow tissue injury as recovery ensues. When the immune system becomes extensively activated and the inflammatory mechanisms escape local control, the whole body can seriously become involved in a systemic inflammatory response. A vicious circle might evolve in which the cytotoxicity of the immune cells might contribute to early organ dysfunction. Widespread increase in microvascular permeability will lead to interstitial edema and thereby impair oxygen diffusion to the tissue. Blood flow also becomes maldistributed due to a loss of vaso-regulative function and as a result of widespread microthrombosis. Oxygenated blood does not reach the capillary bed. Moreover, oxygen utilization is impaired. The resultant hypoxic cell damage further promotes organ dysfunction. One important difference between localized and systemic inflammation is that the early dysfunction of the intestine might itself sustain the inflammatory reaction. Extensive studies have provided evidence that during a state of systemic inflammation the barrier properties of the intestine seem to fail. Similar changes might also occur in the airway barrier to bacteria. Subsequently, enteral bacteria traverse these barriers in a process called bacterial translocation. These bacteria can be cultured from the blood where they might act as potent stimuli for both the immune system and endothelial cells.

References

1. Bone RC, Balk RA, Cerra FB, et al. Definitions for sepsis and organ failure and guidelines for the use of innovative therapies in sepsis. The ACCP/SCCM Consensus Conference Committee. American College of Chest Physicians/Society of Critical Care Medicine. Chest 1992; 101:1644–1655.
2. Muckart DJ, Bhagwanjee S. American College of Chest Physicians/Society of Crit Care Med Consensus Conference definitions of the systemic inflammatory response syndrome and allied disorders in relation to critically injured patients. Crit Care Med 1997; 25(11):1789–1795.
3. Pittet D, Rangel-Frausto S, Li N, et al. Systemic inflammatory response syndrome, sepsis, severe sepsis and septic shock: incidence, morbidities and outcomes in surgical ICU patients. Intensive Care Med 1995; 21(4):302–309.
4. Levy MM, Fink MP, Marshall JC, et al. 2001 SCCM/ESICM/ACCP/ATS/SIS International Sepsis Definitions Conference. Crit Care Med 2003; 31(4):1250–1256.
5. Levy MM, Fink MP, Marshall JC, et al. 2001 SCCM/ESICM/ACCP/ATS/SIS International Sepsis Definitions Conference. Intensive Care Med 2003; 29(4):530–538.
6. Goldstein B, Giroir B, Randolph A. International pediatric sepsis consensus conference: definitions for sepsis and organ dysfunction in pediatrics. Pediatr Crit Care Med 2005; 6(1):2–8.
7. Talmor M, Hydo L, Barie PS. Relationship of systemic inflammatory response syndrome to organ dysfunction, length of stay, and mortality in critical surgical illness: effect of intensive care unit resuscitation. Arch Surg 1999; 134(1):81–87.
8. Asayama K, Aikawa N. Evaluation of systemic inflammatory response syndrome criteria as a predictor of mortality in emergency patients transported by ambulance. Keio J Med 1998; 47(1):19–27.
9. Rangel-Frausto MS, Pittet D, Costigan M, et al. The natural history of the systemic inflammatory response syndrome (SIRS). A prospective study [see comments]. JAMA 1995; 273:117–123.
10. Haga Y, Beppu T, Doi K, et al. Systemic inflammatory response syndrome and organ dysfunction following gastrointestinal surgery. Crit Care Med 1997; 25(12):1994–2000.
11. Sheridan RL, Ryan CM, Yin LM, et al. Death in the burn unit: sterile multiple organ failure. Burns 1998; 24(4):307–311.
12. Ryan CM, Schoenfeld DA, Thorpe WP, et al. Objective estimates of the probability of death from burn injuries. N Engl J Med 1998; 338(6):362–366.
13. Gando S, Nanzaki S, Kemmotsu O. Disseminated intravascular coagulation and sustained systemic inflammatory response syndrome predict organ dysfunctions after trauma: application of clinical decision analysis. Ann Surg 1999; 229(1):121–127.

14. Still JM, Law EJ, Belcher K, et al. A regional medical center's experience with burns of the elderly. J Burn Care Rehabil 1999; 20(3):218–223.

15. Wolf SE, Rose JK, Desai MH, et al. Mortality determinants in massive pediatric burns. An analysis of 103 children with > or = 80% TBSA burns (> or = 70% full-thickness). Ann Surg 1997; 225:554–565.

16. Kelly JL, O'Sullivan C, O'Riordain M, et al. Is circulating endotoxin the trigger for the systemic inflammatory response syndrome seen after injury? Ann Surg 1997; 225(5):530–541; discussion 41–43.

17. Yeh FL, Shen HD, Fang RH. Deficient transforming growth factor beta and interleukin-10 responses contribute to the septic death of burned patients. Burns 2002; 28(7):631–637.

18. Schwacha MG, Chaudry IH. The cellular basis of post-burn immunosuppression: macrophages and mediators. Int J Mol Med 2002; 10(3):239–243.

19. Paterson HM, Murphy TJ, Purcell EJ, et al. Injury primes the innate immune system for enhanced Toll-like receptor reactivity. J Immunol 2003; 171(3):1473–1483.

20. Zang Y, Dolan SM, Choileain NN, et al. Burn injury initiates a shift in superantigen-induced T cell responses and host survival. J Immunol 2004; 172(8):4883–4892.

21. Anderson BO, Harken AH. Multiple organ failure: inflammatory priming and activation sequences promote autologous tissue injury. J Trauma 1990; 30:S44–S49.

22. Dehring DJ, Lübbesmeyer HJ, Fader RC, et al. Exaggerated cardiopulmonary response after bacteremia in sheep with week-old thermal injury. Crit Care Med 1993; 21:888–893.

23. Koike K, Moore FA, Moore EE, et al. Endotoxin after gut ischemia/reperfusion causes irreversible lung injury. J Surg Res 1992; 52:656–662.

24. Ciancio MJ, Hunt J, Jones SB, et al. Comparative and interactive in vivo effects of tumor necrosis factor alpha and endotoxin. Circ Shock 1991; 33:108–120.

25. Spooner CE, Markowitz NP, Saravolatz LD. The role of tumor necrosis factor in sepsis. Clin Immunol Immunopathol 1992; 62: S11–S17.

26. Torre-Amione G, Bozkurt B, Deswal A, et al. An overview of tumor necrosis factor alpha and the failing human heart. Curr Opin Cardiol 1999; 14(3):206–210.

27. Voss M, Cotton MF. Mechanisms and clinical implications of apoptosis. Hosp Med 1998; 59(12):924–930.

28. van der Poll T, van Deventer SJ. Cytokines and anticytokines in the pathogenesis of sepsis. Infect Dis Clin North Am 1999; 13(2):413–426, ix.

29. Doherty GM, Lange JR, Langstein HN, et al. Evidence for IFN-gamma as a mediator of the lethality of endotoxin and tumor necrosis factor-alpha. J Immunol 1992; 149(5):1666–1670.

30. Laffon M, Pittet JF, Modelska K, et al. Interleukin-8 mediates injury from smoke inhalation to both the lung endothelial and the alveolar epithelial barriers in rabbits. Am J Respir Crit Care Med 1999; 160:1443–1449.

31. Stoiser B, Knapp S, Thalhammer F, et al. Time course of immunological markers in patients with the systemic inflammatory response syndrome: evaluation of sCD14, sVCAM-1, sELAM-1, MIP-1 alpha and TGF-beta 2. Eur J Clin Invest 1998; 28(8):672–678.

32. Christman JW, Lancaster LH, Blackwell TS. Nuclear factor kappa B: a pivotal role in the systemic inflammatory response syndrome and new target for therapy. Intensive Care Med 1998; 24(11):1131–1138.

33. Bohrer H, Qiu F, Zimmermann T, et al. Role of NFkappaB in the mortality of sepsis. J Clin Invest 1997; 100(5):972–985.

34. Schwartz MD, Moore EE, Moore FA, et al. Nuclear factor-kappa B is activated in alveolar macrophages from patients with acute respiratory distress syndrome. Crit Care Med 1996; 24(8):1285–1292.

35. Graham RM, Stephens CJ, Silvester W, et al. Plasma degradation of platelet-activating factor in severely ill patients with clinical sepsis. Crit Care Med 1994; 22(2):204–212.

36. Quinn D, Tager A, Joseph PM, et al. Stretch-induced mitogen-activated protein kinase activation and interleukin-8 production in type II alveolar cells. Chest 1999; 116(1 Suppl):89S–90S.

37. Heller A, Koch T, Schmeck J, et al. Lipid mediators in inflammatory disorders. Drugs 1998; 55(4):487–496.

38. Czermak BJ, Sarma V, Pierson CL, et al. Protective effects of C5a blockade in sepsis. Nat Med 1999; 5(7):788–792.

39. Annane D, Briegel J, Sprung CL. Corticosteroid insufficiency in acutely ill patients. N Engl J Med 2003; 348(21):2157–2159.

40. Cannon JG, Friedberg JS, Gelfand JA, et al. Circulating interleukin-1 beta and tumor necrosis factor-alpha concentrations after burn injury in humans. Crit Care Med 1992; 20(10):1414–1419.

41. Drost AC, Burleson DG, Cioffi WG, et al. Plasma cytokines following thermal injury and their relationship with patient mortality, burn size, and time postburn. J Trauma 1993; 35:335–339.

42. Zhang B, Huang YH, Chen Y, et al. Plasma tumor necrosis factor-alpha, its soluble receptors and interleukin-1beta levels in critically burned patients. Burns 1998; 24(7):599–603.

43. Marano MA, Fong Y, Moldawer LL, et al. Serum cachectin/tumor necrosis factor in critically ill patients with burns correlates with infection and mortality. Surg Gynecol Obstet 1990; 170:32–38.

44. Hubl W, Wolfbauer G, Streicher J, et al. Differential expression of tumor necrosis factor receptor subtypes on leukocytes in systemic inflammatory response syndrome. Crit Care Med 1999; 27(2):319–324.

45. Presterl E, Staudinger T, Pettermann M, et al. Cytokine profile and correlation to the APACHE III and MPM II scores in patients with sepsis. Am J Respir Crit Care Med 1997; 156(3 Pt 1):825–832.

46. Mandrup-Poulsen T, Wogensen LD, Jensen M, et al. Circulating interleukin-1 receptor antagonist concentrations are increased in adult patients with thermal injury. Crit Care Med 1995; 23(1):26–33.

47. Neely AN, Hoover DL, Holder IA, et al. Circulating levels of tumour necrosis factor, interleukin 6 and proteolytic activity in a murine model of burn and infection. Burns 1996; 22(7):524–530.

48. Aosasa S, Ono S, Mochizuki H, et al. Activation of monocytes and endothelial cells depends on the severity of surgical stress. World J Surg 2000; 24(1):10–16.

49. Taniguchi T, Koido Y, Aiboshi J, et al. Change in the ratio of interleukin-6 to interleukin-10 predicts a poor outcome in patients with systemic inflammatory response syndrome. Crit Care Med 1999; 27(7):1262–1264.

50. Braithwaite S. Procalcitonin: new insights on regulation and origin. Crit Care Med 2000; 28(2):586–588.

51. Miller PR, Munn DD, Meredith JW, et al. Systemic inflammatory response syndrome in the trauma intensive care unit: who is infected? J Trauma 1999; 47(6):1004–1008.

52. Clyne B, Olshaker JS. The C-reactive protein. J Emerg Med 1999; 17(6):1019–1025.

53. Abraham E, Anzueto A, Gutierrez G, et al. Double-blind randomised controlled trial of monoclonal antibody to human tumour necrosis factor in treatment of septic shock. NORASEPT II Study Group. Lancet 1998; 351(9107):929–933.

54. Clark MA, Plank LD, Connolly AB, et al. Effect of a chimeric antibody to tumor necrosis factor-alpha on cytokine and physiologic responses in patients with severe sepsis – a randomized, clinical trial. Crit Care Med 1998; 26(10):1650–1659.

55. Abraham E. Therapies for sepsis. Emerging therapies for sepsis and septic shock. West J Med 1997; 166(3):195–200.

56. Fisher CJ Jr, Agosti JM, Opal SM, et al. Treatment of septic shock with the tumor necrosis factor receptor:Fc fusion protein. The Soluble TNF Receptor Sepsis Study Group. N Engl J Med 1996; 334(26):1697–1702.

57. Fisher CJ Jr, Dhainaut JF, Opal SM, et al. Recombinant human interleukin 1 receptor antagonist in the treatment of patients with sepsis syndrome. Results from a randomized, double-blind, placebo-controlled trial. Phase III rhIL-1ra Sepsis Syndrome Study Group. JAMA 1994; 271(23):1836–1843.

58. Opal SM, Fisher CJ, Dhainaut JFA, et al. Confirmatory interleukin-1 receptor antagonist trial in severe sepsis – a phase III, randomized, double-blind, placebo-controlled, multicenter trial. Crit Care Med 1997; 25:1115–1124.

59. Fein AM, Bernard GR, Criner GJ, et al. Treatment of severe systemic inflammatory response syndrome and sepsis with a novel bradykinin antagonist, deltibant (CP-0127). Results of a random-

ized, double-blind, placebo-controlled trial. CP-0127 SIRS and Sepsis Study Group. JAMA 1997; 277(6):482–487.

60. Dhainaut JF, Tenaillon A, Hemmer M, et al. Confirmatory platelet-activating factor receptor antagonist trial in patients with severe gram-negative bacterial sepsis: a phase III, randomized, double-blind, placebo-controlled, multicenter trial. BN 52021 Sepsis Investigator Group. Crit Care Med 1998; 26(12): 1963–1971.

61. Dhainaut JF, Tenaillon A, Le Tulzo Y, et al. Platelet-activating factor receptor antagonist BN 52021 in the treatment of severe sepsis: a randomized, double-blind, placebo-controlled, multicenter clinical trial. BN 52021 Sepsis Study Group. Crit Care Med 1994; 22(11):1720–1728.

62. Bernard GR, Wheeler AP, Russell JA, et al. The effects of ibuprofen on the physiology and survival of patients with sepsis. The Ibuprofen in Sepsis Study Group. N Engl J Med 1997; 336(13): 912–918.

63. Haupt MT, Jastremski MS, Clemmer TP, et al. Effect of ibuprofen in patients with severe sepsis: a randomized, double-blind, multicenter study. The Ibuprofen Study Group. Crit Care Med 1991; 19:1339–1347.

64. Sander A, Armbruster W, Sander B, et al. Hemofiltration increases IL-6 clearance in early systemic inflammatory response syndrome but does not alter IL-6 and TNF alpha plasma concentrations. Intensive Care Med 1997; 23(8):878–884.

65. Kellum JA, Johnson JP, Kramer D, et al. Diffusive vs. convective therapy: effects on mediators of inflammation in patient with severe systemic inflammatory response syndrome. Crit Care Med 1998; 26(12):1995–2000.

66. Cronin L, Cook DJ, Carlet J, et al. Corticosteroid treatment for sepsis: a critical appraisal and meta-analysis of the literature. Crit Care Med 1995; 23(8):1430–1439.

67. Zeni F, Freeman B, Natanson C. Anti-inflammatory therapies to treat sepsis and septic shock: a reassessment. Crit Care Med 1997; 25(7):1095–1100.

68. Dellinger RP, Carlet JM, Masur H, et al. Surviving sepsis campaign guidelines for management of severe sepsis and septic shock. Crit Care Med 2004; 32(3):858–873.

69. Wang H, Bloom O, Zhang M, et al. HMG-1 as a late mediator of endotoxin lethality in mice. Science 1999; 285(5425):248–251.

70. Wolf SE, Rose JK, Desai MH, et al. Mortality determinants in massive pediatric burns. An analysis > or = 80% TBSA burns (> or = 70% full-thickness). Ann Surg 1997; 225:554–565.

71. Junger WG, Coimbra R, Liu FC, et al. Hypertonic saline resuscitation: a tool to modulate immune function in trauma patients? Shock 1997; 8(4):235–241.

72. Beale RJ, Bryg DJ, Bihari DJ. Immunonutrition in the critically ill: a systematic review of clinical outcome. Crit Care Med 1999; 27(12):2799–805.

73. Napolitano LM, Faist E, Wichmann MW, et al. Immune dysfunction in trauma. Surg Clin North Am 1999; 79(6):1385–416.

74. Metz CN, Tracey KJ. It takes nerve to dampen inflammation. Nat Immunol 2005; 6(8):756–757.

75. Pavlov VA, Tracey KJ. The cholinergic anti-inflammatory pathway. Brain Behav Immun 2005; 19(6):493–499.

76. Brunnee T, La Porta C, Reddigari SR, et al. Activation of factor XI in plasma is dependent on factor XII. Blood 1993; 81(3):580–586.

77. Pawlinski R, Pedersen B, Kehrle B, et al. Regulation of tissue factor and inflammatory mediators by Egr-1 in a mouse endotoxemia model. Blood 2003; 101(10):3940–3947.

78. Messori A, Vacca F, Vaiani M, et al. Antithrombin III in patients admitted to intensive care units: a multicenter observational study. Crit Care 2002; 6(5):447–451.

79. Okajima K. Regulation of inflammatory responses by natural anticoagulants. Immunol Rev 2001; 184:258–274.

80. Esmon CT. The protein C pathway. Chest 2003; 124(3 Suppl):26S–32S.

81. Yuksel M, Okajima K, Uchiba M, et al. Activated protein C inhibits lipopolysaccharide-induced tumor necrosis factor-alpha production by inhibiting activation of both nuclear factor-kappa B and activator protein-1 in human monocytes. Thromb Haemost 2002; 88(2):267–273.

82. Broze GJ Jr. The rediscovery and isolation of TFPI. J Thromb Haemost 2003; 1(8):1671–1675.

83. Clemenza L, Dieli F, Cicardi M, et al. Research on complement: old issues revisited and a novel sphere of influence. Trends Immunol 2003; 24(6):292–296.

84. Suffredini AF, Fromm RE, Parker MM, et al. The cardiovascular response of normal humans to the administration of endotoxin. N Engl J Med 1989; 321:280–287.

85. Suffredini AF, Shelhamer JH, Neumann RD, et al. Pulmonary and oxygen transport effects of intravenously administered endotoxin in normal humans. Am Rev Respir Dis 1992; 145:1398–1403.

86. Traber DL, Redl H, Schlag G, et al. Cardiopulmonary responses to continuous administration of endotoxin. Am J Physiol 1988; 254:H833–H839.

87. Dehring D, Lingnau W, McGuire R, et al. L-NAME transiently reverses hyperdynamic status during continuous infusion of Pseudomonas aeroginosa. Circ Shock 1993; 39:49.

88. Traber DL. Models of endotoxemia in sheep. In: Schlag G, Redl H, Traber DL, eds. Pathophysiology of shock sepsis and organ failure. New York: Springer Verlag; 1993:194–199.

89. Godsoe A, Kimura R, Herndon D, et al. Cardiopulmonary changes with intermittent endotoxin administration in sheep. Circ Shock 1988; 25:61–74.

90. Meyer J, Traber LD, Nelson S, et al. Reversal of hyperdynamic response to continuous endotoxin administration by inhibition of NO synthesis. J Appl Physiol 1992; 73:324–328.

91. Fujioka K, Sugi K, Isago T, et al. Thromboxane synthase inhibition and cardiopulmonary function during endotoxemia in sheep. J Appl Physiol 1991; 71:1376–1381.

92. Adams T Jr, Traber DL. The effects of a prostaglandin synthetase inhibitor, ibuprofen, on the cardiopulmonary response to endotoxin in sheep. Circ Shock 1982; 9:481–489.

93. Tokyay R, Loick HM, Traber DL, et al. Effects of thromboxane synthetase inhibition on postburn mesenteric vascular resistance and the rate of bacterial translocation in a chronic porcine model. Surg Gynecol Obstet 1992; 174:125–132.

94. Redl G, Abdi S, Nichols RJ, et al. The effects of a selective thromboxane synthetase inhibitor on the response of the right heart to endotoxin in sheep. Crit Care Med 1991; 19:1294–1302.

95. Navaratnam RL, Morris SE, Traber DL, et al. Endotoxin (LPS) increases mesenteric vascular resistance (MVR) and bacterial translocation (BT). J Trauma 1990; 30:1104–1113.

96. Lefer AM. Interaction between myocardial depressant factor and vasoactive mediators with ischemia and shock. Am J Physiol 1987; 252:R193–R205.

97. Morris SE, Navaratnam N, Herndon DN. A comparison of effects of thermal injury and smoke inhalation on bacterial translocation. J Trauma 1990; 30:639–643.

98. Schlag G, Redl H, Davies J, et al. Aspects of the mechanisms of bacterial translocation in a hypovolemic-traumatic shock mode in baboons. Circ Shock 1991; 34:26–27.

99. Xu D, Qi L, Guillory D, et al. Mechanisms of endotoxin-induced intestinal injury in a hyperdynamic model of sepsis. J Trauma 1993; 34:676–682.

100. Koltai M, Hosford D, Braquet PG. Platelet-activating factor in septic shock. New Horizons 1993; 1:87–95.

101. Traber DL. Endotoxin: the causative factor of mediator release during sepsis. In: Schlag G, Redl H, eds. Progress in clinical and biological research. New York: Alan R. Liss; 1987:377–392.

102. Martich GD, Danner RL, Ceska M, et al. Detection of interleukin 8 and tumor necrosis factor in normal humans after intravenous endotoxin: the effect of antiinflammatory agents. J Exp Med 1991; 173:1021–1024.

103. Michie HR, Manogue KR, Spriggs DR, et al. Detection of circulating tumor necrosis factor after endotoxin administration. N Engl J Med 1988; 318:1481–1486.

104. Morel DR, Pittet JF, Gunning K, et al. Time course of plasma and pulmonary lymph endothelin-like immunoreactivity during sustained endotoxaemia in chronically instrumented sheep. Clin Sci 1991; 81:357–365.

105. Redl G, Woodson L, Traber LD, et al. Mechanism of immunoreactive atrial natriuretic factor release in an ovine model of endotoxemia. Circ Shock 1992; 38:34–41.

106. Lübbesmeyer HJ, Woodson L, Traber LD, et al. Immunoreactive atrial natriuretic factor is increased in ovine model of endotoxemia. Am J Physiol 1988; 254:R567–R71.

107. Pittet JF, Morel DR, Hemsen A, et al. Elevated plasma endothelin-1 concentrations are associated with the severity of illness in patients with sepsis. Ann Surg 1991; 213:261–264.

108. Sloane PJ, Elsasser TH, Spath JA, et al. Plasma tumor necrosis factor-alpha during long-term endotoxemia in awake sheep. J Appl Physiol 1992; 73:1831–1837.

109. Morel DR, Lacroix JS, Hemsen A, et al. Increased plasma and pulmonary lymph levels of endothelin during endotoxin shock. Eur J Pharmacol 1989; 167:427–428.

110. Nelson S, Steward RH, Traber L, et al. Endotoxin-induced alterations in contractility of isolated blood vessels from sheep. Am J Physiol 1991; 260:H1790–H1794.

111. Theissen JL, Loick HM, Curry BB, et al. Time course of hypoxic pulmonary vasoconstriction after endotoxin infusion in unanesthetized sheep. J Appl Physiol 1991; 70:2120–2125.

112. Meyer J, Lentz CW, Stothert JC, et al. Effects of nitric oxide synthesis inhibition in hyperdynamic endotoxemia. Crit Care Med 1994; 22:306–312.

113. Sugi K, Newald J, Traber LD, et al. Cardiac dysfunction after acute endotoxin administration in conscious sheep. Am J Physiol 1991; 260:H1474–H1481.

114. Noshima S, Noda H, Herndon DN, et al. Left ventricular performance during continuous endotoxin-induced hyperdynamic endotoxemia in sheep. J Appl Physiol 1993; 74:1528–1533.

115. Myers PR, Wright TF, Tanner MA, et al. EDRF and nitric oxide production in cultured endothelial cells: direct inhibition by E. coli endotoxin. Am J Physiol 1992; 262:H710–H718.

116. Vallance P, Moncada S. Role of endogenous nitric oxide in septic shock. New Horizons 1993; 1:77–86.

117. Sakai N, Milstien S. Availability of tetrahydrobiopterin is not a factor in the inability to detect nitric oxide production by human macrophages. Biochem Biophys Res Com 1993; 193:378–383.

118. Schneemann M, Schoedon G, Hofer S, et al. Nitric oxide synthase is not a constituent of the antimicrobial armature of human mononuclear phagocytes. J Infect Dis 1993; 167:1358–1363.

119. Moncada S. Nitric oxide in the vasculature: physiology and pathophysiology. Ann NY Acad Sci 1997; 811:60–67.

120. Furchgott RF. Endothelium-derived relaxing factor: discovery, early studies, and identification as nitric oxide. Biosci Rep 1999; 19:235–251.

121. Petros A, Lamb G, Leone A, et al. Effects of a nitric oxide synthase inhibitor in humans with septic shock. Cardiovasc Res 1994; 28:34–39.

122. Geroulanos S, Schilling J, Cakmakci M, et al. Inhibition of NO synthesis in septic shock. Lancet 1992; 339:435–440.

123. Kiehl MG, Ostermann H, Meyer J, et al. Nitric oxide synthase inhibition by L-NAME in leukocytopenic patients with severe septic shock. Intensive Care Med 1997; 23(5):561–566.

124. Shi Y, Li HQ, Shen CK, et al. Plasma nitric oxide levels in newborn infants with sepsis. J Pediatr 1993; 123:435–438.

125. Ochoa JB, Udekwu AO, Billiar TR, et al. Nitrogen oxide levels in patients after trauma and during sepsis. Ann Surg 1991; 214:621–626.

126. Schneider F, Lutun P, Couchot A, et al. Plasma cyclic guanosine 3′-5′ monophosphate concentrations and low vascular resistance in human septic shock. Intensive Care Med 1993; 19:99–104.

127. Schuller F, Fleming I, Stoclet JC, et al. Effect of endotoxin on circulating cyclic GMP in the rat. Eur J Pharmacol 1992; 212:93–96.

128. Nelson SH, Dehring DJ, Ehardt JS, et al. Regional variation in content of c-GMP and associated vascular reactivity in bacteremia. Circ Shock 1993; 39:54.

129. Martin W, White DG, Henderson AH. Endothelium-derived relaxing factor and atriopeptin II elevate cyclic GMP levels in pig aortic endothelial cells. Br J Pharmacol 1988; 93:229–239.

130. Cherner JA, Singh G, Naik L. Atrial natriuretic factor activates membrane-bound guanylate cyclase of chief cells. Life Sci 1990; 47:669–677.

131. Goy MF. Activation of membrane guanylate cyclase by an invertebrate peptide hormone. J Biol Chem 1990; 265:20220–20227.

132. Boulanger C, Schini VB, Moncada S, et al. Stimulation of cyclic GMP production in cultured endothelial cells of the pig by bradykinin, adenosine diphosphate, calcium ionophore A23187 and nitric oxide. Br J Pharmacol 1990; 101:152–156.

133. Leitman DC, Agnost VL, Catalano RM, et al. Atrial natriuretic peptide, oxytocin, and vasopressin increase guanosine 3′,5′-monophosphate in LLC-PK1 kidney epithelial cells. Endocrinology 1988; 122:1478–1485.

134. Garbers DL. The guanylyl cyclase receptor family. New Biologist 1990; 2:499–504.

135. Snapper JR, Brigham KL, Heflin AC, et al. Effects of endotoxemia on cyclic nucleotides in the unanesthetized sheep. J Lab Clin Med 1983; 102:240–249.

136. DeLa Cadena RA, Suffredini AF, Page JD, et al. Activation of the kallikrein-kinin system after endotoxin administration to normal human volunteers. Blood 1993; 81:3313–3317.

137. Mann R, Woodson LC, Traber LD, et al. Role of bradykinin in ovine endotoxemia. Circ Shock 1991; 34:224–230.

138. Matsuda T, Eccleston CA, Rubinstein I, et al. Antioxidants attenuate endotoxin-induced microvascular leakage of macromolecules in vivo. Am J Physiol 1991; 70:1483–1489.

139. Nakazawa H, Noda H, Noshima S, et al. Pulmonary transvascular fluid flux and cardiovascular function in sheep with chronic sepsis. J Appl Physiol 1993; 75:2521–2528.

140. Landis EM, Pappenheimer JR. Exchange of substances through the capillary walls. In: Hamilton WF, Dow P, eds. Handbook of physiology. Baltimore, MD: Williams & Wilkins; 1963; 2(2):961–1034.

141. Starling EH. On the absorption of fluids from the connective tissue spaces. J Physiol 1896; 19:312–326.

142. Brigham KL, Bowers R, Haynes J. Increased sheep lung vascular permeability caused by Escherichia coli endotoxin. Circ Res 1979; 45:292–297.

143. Gaar KA, Taylor AE, Owens LJ, et al. Effect of capillary pressure and plasma protein on development of pulmonary edema. Am J Physiol 1967; 213:79–82.

144. Lund T, Wiig H, Reed RK, et al. A 'new' mechanism for oedema generation: strongly negative interstitial fluid pressure causes rapid fluid flow into thermally injured skin. Acta Physiol Scand 1987; 129:433–435.

145. Lund T, Wiig H, Reed RK. Acute postburn edema: role of strongly negative interstitial fluid pressure. Am J Physiol 1988; 255:H1069–H1074.

146. Traber DL, Herndon DN, Fujioka K, et al. Permeability changes during experimental endotoxemia and sepsis. In: Schlag G, Redl H, Siegel JH, et al., eds. Shock, sepsis, and organ failure: Second Wiggers Bernard conference. New York: Springer-Verlag; 1991:425–447.

147. Smith L, Andreasson S, Thoren Tolling K, et al. Sepsis in sheep reduces pulmonary microvascular sieving capacity. J Appl Physiol 1987; 62:1422–1429.

148. Oliver JA. Endothelium-derived relaxing factor contributes to the regulation of endothelial permeability. J Cell Physiol 1992; 151:506–511.

149. Farrukh IS, Gurtner GH, Michael JR. Pharmacological modification of pulmonary vascular injury: possible role of cAMP. J Appl Physiol 1987; 62:47–54.

150. Kurose I, Kubes P, Wolf R, et al. Inhibition of nitric oxide production. Mechanisms of vascular albumin leakage. Circ Res 1993; 73:164–171.

151. Leeuwenberg FM, Jeunhomme TMA, Buurman WA. Induction of an activation antigen on human endothelial cells in vitro. Eur J Immunol 1989; 19:715–720.

152. Lasky LA. Selectins: interpreters of cell-specific carbohydrate information during inflammation. Science 1992; 258:964–969.

153. Nawroth PP, Stern DM. Modulation of endothelial cell hemostatic properties by tumor necrosis factor. J Exp Med 1986; 163:740–745.

154. Walsh CJ, Carey D, Cook DJ, et al. Anti-CD18 antibody attenuates neutropenia and alveolar capillary-membrane injury during gram-negative sepsis. Surgery 1991; 110:205–212.

155. Doerschuk CM, Winn RK, Coxson HO, et al. CD18-dependent and -independent mechanisms of neutrophil emigration in the pulmonary and systemic microcirculation of rabbits. J Immunol 1990; 144:2327–2333.

156. Wang CZ, Barrow RE, Cox CS, et al. Influence of detergent aerosol on lung microvascular permeability. J Appl Physiol 1993; 74:1016–1023.

157. Traber DL. Anti-proteases in endotoxemia. Prog Clin Biol Res 1987; 236:149–157.

158. Seekamp A, LaLonde C, Zhu DG, et al. Catalase prevents prostanoid release and lung lipid peroxidation after endotoxemia in sheep. J Appl Physiol 1988; 65:1210–1216.

159. Basadre JO, Singh H, Herndon DN, et al. Effect of antibody-mediated neutropenia on the cardiopulmonary response to endotoxemia. J Surg Res 1988; 45:266–275.

160. Winn R, Maunder R, Chi E, et al. Neutrophil depletion does not prevent lung edema after endotoxin infusion in goats. J Appl Physiol 1987; 62:116–121.

161. Maunder RJ, Hackman RC, Riff E, et al. Occurrence of the adult respiratory distress syndrome in neutropenic patients. Am Rev Respir Dis 1986; 133:313–316.

162. Laufe MD, Simon RH, Flint A, et al. Adult respiratory distress syndrome in neutropenic patients. Am J Med 1986; 80:1022–1026.

163. Heflin AC Jr, Brigham KL. Prevention by granulocyte depletion of increased vascular permeability of sheep lung following endotoxemia. J Clin Invest 1981; 68:1253–1260.

164. Klausner JM, Paterson IS, Goldman G, et al. Interleukin-2-induced lung injury is mediated by oxygen free radicals. Surgery 1991; 109:169–175.

165. Goldman G, Welbourn R, Klausner JM, et al. Thromboxane mediates diapedesis after ischemia by activation of neutrophil adhesion receptors interacting with basally expressed intercellular adhesion molecule-1. Circ Res 1991; 68:1013–1019.

166. Traber DL, Schlag G, Redl H, et al. Pulmonary microvascular changes during hyperdynamic sepsis in an ovine model. Circ Shock 1987; 22:185–193.

167. Miller FN, Sims DE. Contractile elements in the regulation of macromolecular permeability. Fed Proc 1986; 45:84–88.

168. Paterson IS, Klausner JM, Goldman G, et al. Thromboxane mediates the ischemia-induced neutrophil oxidative burst. Surgery 1989; 106:224–229.

169. Turker RK, Aksulu HE, Ercan ZS, et al. Thromboxane A2 inhibitors and iloprost prevent angiotensin II-induced oedema in the isolated perfused rat lung. Arch Int Pharmacodyn Ther 1987; 287:323–329.

170. Deitch EA, Taylor M, Grisham M, et al. Endotoxin induces bacterial translocation, and increases xanthine oxidase activity. J Trauma 1989; 29:1679–1683.

171. Deitch EA, Ma L, Ma WJ, et al. Inhibition of endotoxin-induced bacterial translocation, in mice. J Clin Invest 1989; 84:36–42.

172. Terada LS, Dormish JJ, Shanley PF, et al. Circulating xanthine oxidase mediates lung neutrophil sequestration after intestinal ischemia-reperfusion. Am J Physiol 1992; 263:L394–L401.

173. Redl H, Schlag G, Lamche H. TNF- and LPS-induced changes of lung vascular permeability: studies in unanesthetised sheep. Circ Shock 1990; 31:183–192.

174. Johnson J, Meyrick B, Jesmok G, et al. Human recombinant tumor necrosis factor alpha infusion mimics endotoxemia in awake sheep. J Appl Physiol 1989; 66:1448–1454.

175. Burhop KE, Garcia JG, Selig WM, et al. Platelet-activating factor increases lung vascular permeability to protein. J Appl Physiol 1986; 61:2210–2217.

176. Sessler CN, Glauser FL, Davis D, et al. Effects of platelet-activating factor antagonist SRI 63–441 on endotoxemia in sheep. J Appl Physiol 1988; 65:2624–2631.

177. Vercellotti GM, Yin HQ, Gustavson KS, et al. Platelet activating factor primes neutrophil responses to agonists: role in promoting neutrophil-mediated endothelial damage. Blood 1988; 71:1100–1107.

178. Holloway H, Perry M, Downey J, et al. Estimation of effective pulmonary capillary pressure in intact lungs. J Appl Physiol 1983; 54(3):846–851.

179. O'Dwyer ST, Michie HR, Ziegler TR, et al. A single dose of endotoxin increases intestinal permeability in healthy humans. Arch Surg 1988; 123:1459–1464.

180. Roumen RM, Hendriks T, Wevers RA, et al. Intestinal permeability after severe trauma and hemorrhagic shock is increased without relation to septic complications. Arch Surg 1993; 128:453–457.

181. Zeigler ST, Traber DL, Herndon DN. Bacterial translocation in burns. In: Schlag G, Redl H, eds. Pathophysiology of shock, sepsis, and organ failure. New York: Springer-Verlag; 1993: 300–313.

Chapter 23

The immunological response and strategies for intervention

Erle D. Murphey, Edward R. Sherwood, and Tracy Toliver-Kinsky

Chapter contents

Introduction

Improvements in the management of burn injury have resulted in a decreased incidence of sepsis and improved survival in patients with large burn wounds. Early excision of the burn eschar coupled with wound coverage has greatly diminished the incidence of burn wound infection, and burn mortality, in the last 2 decades.[1–3] These advances in burn care have paralleled the development of broad-spectrum antibiotics, which has further decreased the incidence of life-threatening infections in burn victims. However, infections still remain a major cause of morbidity and mortality in burn patients.[4–6] Post-burn immunosuppression is thought to be a predisposing factor for the development of severe infections. Many infections in burn patients are associated with organisms considered opportunistic in nature and occur at sites other than in the burn wound, which supports the concept that immune function may be impaired in these patients. One paradigm of burn-induced immune dysfunction asserts that the initial burn injury induces an inflammatory response that is characterized by systemic release of pro-inflammatory cytokines and chemokines (Figure 23.1). This initial inflammatory response could lead to significant tissue injury and organ dysfunction. However, most burn victims survive the initial injury and enter a phase that is characterized by immune dysfunction. This state of dysfunction appears to place the burned host at increased risk of infection and further injury. Immunosuppression may be associated with the anti-inflammatory response initiated by the burned host in an effort to minimize inflammation-induced tissue injury during the acute post-burn period. Accumulation of inflammatory insults during the early post-burn period may potentiate injury-induced immunosuppression. Normalization, or enhancement, of immune function is becoming increasingly attractive because of the emergence of antibiotic-resistant microorganisms. However, few effective immunomodulatory approaches have been developed for clinical application in burn patients.

Predisposing factors

There are approximately 45 000 hospitalizations per year for burn injury in the United States (www.ameriburn.org). More than half of the hospital admissions are for burns of less than 10% total body surface area (TBSA) while 4% (~1800 admissions per year) are for burns of 60% TBSA or greater (www.ameriburn.org). Depth and size of the burn wound are well-known risk factors for burn wound infection and ultimately sepsis. The overall incidence of bacteremia in burn patients is approximately 19%[7] but rarely occurs in patients with less than 40% TBSA burns[8]. Concomitant inhalation injury is associated with an increased risk of infection, particularly pneumonia. This predisposition to infection may be due to impairment of alveolar macrophage function and the need for intubation and ventilation in many of these patients.

While studies have reported a gender effect on post-burn mortality, with females having a lower chance of survival,[9–12] there have not been any consistent data demonstrating any gender effect on the incidence of sepsis in post-burn patients. A similar study of children did not show a relationship between gender and the incidence of sepsis.[13] However, age appears to be a predisposing factor for the development of septicemia after burn injury. Not surprisingly, young children and elderly patients have the highest incidence of sepsis.[10,14]

Physical barriers are an important part of host resistance to infection. The epidermal barrier is compromised in burn patients due to the burn itself as well as the frequent insertion of intravascular catheters. Vascular access devices are significant sources of nosocomial infections in burn patients. Typical organisms associated with line sepsis include *Staphylococcus* spp. (either *S. epidermidis* or *S. aureus*) although infections with Gram-negative bacteria or yeast can also occur, especially in immunocompromised patients. Central venous catheters, relative to other catheters, are particularly prone to bacterial contamination. Approximately 25% of central venous catheters become colonized with bacteria. Lesseva et al. reported an incidence of catheter-related bacteremia of 6.6%, accounting for approximately 20% of sepsis in post-burn patients.[15] Peripheral catheters are much less likely to be associated with infection although this may be due to their shorter duration of use. Suppurative peripheral vein thrombophlebitis

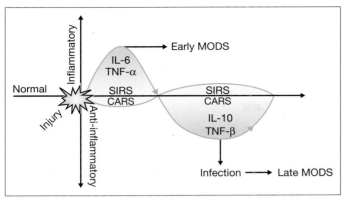

Fig. 23.1 Major injury is followed by induction of a short-lived pro-inflammatory cytokine response. During hospitalization, episodic rises in pro-inflammatory cytokines may occur in response to treatments or adverse events. However, the predominant cytokine profile in the days to weeks after a major injury is typically characterized as an immunocompromised.

was a common cause of systemic sepsis prior to the wide use of central venous catheters in critically ill patients. The risk of catheter-related infection is greatly increased if devices are inserted through infected or contaminated skin, such as burn wounds. Femoral vein catheters are more likely to become infected than subclavian or internal jugular vein catheters and catheter replacement via guidewire exchange has a higher infection rate than catheterization at a separate site.[16]

One of the most common causes of Gram-negative bacterial sepsis in hospitalized patients is urinary tract infection, especially in the presence of Foley catheters.[17] Nearly all patients with large TBSA burns require bladder catheterization. The incidence of urinary tract infection in burn patients ranges from 10% to approximately 18%.[7,18]

The incidence of respiratory infections in burn patients ranges from 20% to 40%.[7,19] Nosocomial pneumonia is frequently associated with prolonged intubation and mechanical ventilation. Gram-negative bacteria such as *Pseudomonas aeruginosa* are commonly isolated, but Gram-positive bacteria and yeast such as *Candida* spp. should also be considered.

Medications administered to burn patients may, in some instances, also be a contributing factor to post-burn immunosuppression. Prophylactic administration of systemic antibiotics has not been associated with a reduction of infections in burn patients in a number of clinical reports and, in fact, may be a predisposing factor for the development of fungal infections.[20–22] Recent experimental work suggests that administration of opiate analgesics may contribute to post-burn immunosuppression by adversely affecting T cell proliferation and altering the predominant T helper phenotype.[23] Transfusion of blood products has been reported to predispose burn victims[24] and other critically ill patients[25] to nosocomial infections. Although the exact mechanism of immunosuppression is unknown, blood transfusions have been associated with a decrease in the T-helper lymphocyte ratio, as well as adverse effects on natural killer cell activity and antigen presentation.[26,27] Finally, victims of large total body surface area burns usually require numerous operative procedures for

debridement and grafting of burn wounds. Intravenous and inhalation anesthetics have demonstrated variable and inconsistent effects on neutrophil functions including alterations in chemotaxis, endothelial adherence and transmigration, phagocytosis, and respiratory burst[28] and could contribute to post-injury immunosuppression.

Microbiology

Normal intact skin has a bacterial count of 10^5 colony-forming units (cfu)/gram without any evidence of clinical infection.[29] Loss of the epidermal barrier provides a favorable environment for bacterial growth and 10^5 microbial cfu/gram of tissue is often associated with infection[30] although some bacteria such as β-hemolytic streptococci can cause infection at significantly lower concentrations. Furthermore, polymicrobial interactions may also be a significant factor in wound infections because it has been shown that the presence of four or more bacterial species within burn wounds correlates with non-healing.[31]

Initially, wounds are colonized with commensal skin organisms. Gram-positive organisms tend to predominate in wounds during the early post-burn period. Gram-negative aerobic rods such as *Pseudomonas* spp. are typically detected later. Resident microbes of the skin that have pathogenic potential include *Staphylococcus aureus*, *Staphylococcus epidermidis*, and non-enterococcal streptococci. Bacterial flora in locations below the diaphragm are also more likely to include Gram-negative enteric organisms such as *E. coli*, as well as *Streptococcus faecalis*. Resident microbes of the oropharynx that are potentially pathogenic include *Fusobacterium*, *Haemophilus*, *Peptostreptococcus*, and *Bacteroides*, as well as *S. aureus*, *S. epidermidis* and non-enterococcal streptococcus. Fungal infections are not uncommon and can occur concurrently with bacterial infections. The most prevalent fungal organisms are *Candida* or *Aspergillus*.

Innate immune function after burn injury

After a large burn injury with extensive tissue necrosis, the immune system is activated systemically and may become ineffective or even self-destructive. Loss of some components of innate immune function after thermal injury may lead to infections in burn patients. Study of immune function in burn patients is limited by feasible tissue access and generally consists of measuring circulating soluble factors and immune cells. Not surprisingly, this provides only a limited view of the entire immune response as suggested by animal studies in which alternate tissues such as spleen and liver are available.[32] This review will highlight observational data from clinical studies and try to use results from experimental research to provide some context for these observations.

Healthy individuals resist many infectious challenges without preexisting specific (acquired) immunity because of the effectiveness of the innate immune response. Innate immunity is a protective set of rapid and primitive non-specific responses to infection including epithelial barrier defenses, cytokine elaboration, complement activation, and phagocytosis of microorganisms. These mechanisms may eradicate the infection or contain the infection during the time needed for the development of an adaptive immune response specific to the offending microbe.

Physical barriers

A mechanical barrier against invasion of microbial pathogens is provided by the epithelium of skin and mucosal tissue. This protective barrier is lost after serious burn injury, and burn wounds often have poor vascularization. The presence of necrotic tissue provides a favorable environment for microbial growth. Cellular damage may cause the release of molecules that predispose the host to bacterial infections. Syndecans are expressed by all adherent cells and their release after cellular damage may be a signal for the need of tissue repair processes including vascular permeability, angiogenesis, wound repair, and modulation of chemokine activity.[33] However, recent studies in burned mice suggest that syndecan shedding may potentiate systemic dissemination of *P. aeruginosa* from burn wound infections.[34]

Besides the loss of epidermal integrity in areas of burns, barrier function may also be compromised at other remote anatomic locations. Endothelial barrier function in the gastro-intestinal tract can be compromised after burn injury[35,36] and may be due to decreased mesenteric blood flow in the early post-burn period.[37] This may lead to systemic translocation of bacterial toxins or enteric bacteria. Increased intestinal permeability after burn injury has been associated with systemic infection in a number of studies,[37–40] and forms the basis for the therapeutic strategy of selective decontamination of the digestive tract as well as interventions aimed at improving gut barrier function such as early enteral feeding.[41] In the respiratory tract, defense mechanisms include mucus secretion and ciliary movement, which serve to trap microbes and sweep them into the upper airways and oropharynx where expulsion by coughing may occur. These defenses can be diminished after inhalation injury, or compromised by endotracheal intubation, resulting in microbial proliferation and expansion into the distal branches of the respiratory tract causing bronchitis or pneumonia.[16] Pneumonia is one of the most common infections encountered in burn patients and is associated with a higher risk of mortality.[5,19]

Epithelial cells further contribute protection by manufacturing antimicrobial peptides, including defensins, lysozymes, and cathelicidins. Defensins exert antimicrobial activity against a broad range of bacteria and fungi[42] and appear to function through disruption of the bacterial cell wall.[42,43] Although epithelial cells display some constitutive production of defensins, production is increased after microbial activation of toll-like receptors (TLRs) on the epithelial cells.[44,45] However, burn injury has been associated with a downregulation of defensin mRNA expression[46] and it is not clear that microbial stimulation would invoke an appropriate level of activation in affected areas.

Phagocytes

Beyond the physical barriers, the key cellular components of the innate immune response are the professional phagocytes, including macrophages, dendritic cells and neutrophils, that are not only important in removing microbes and debris from sites of inflammation but also are key regulators of the innate immune response (Figure 23.2). Macrophages are capable of

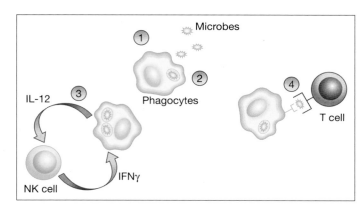

Fig. 23.2 The cellular component of innate immunity. (1) The innate immune response is initiated by recognition of microbial organisms. Toll receptors, CD14, NOD1, and NOD2 are among the specialized receptors found on immune cells to recognize molecules that are consistently found on microbes, including LPS, lipoprotein, flagellin, peptidoglycan, zymosan, and others. (2) Intracellular pathogen killing mechanisms include a variety of antimicrobial peptides, proteases, glycosidases, hydroxyl radicals, peroxynitrite, and others. (3) Intercellular communication and coordination of the cellular immune response occurs via cytokine and chemokine elaboration. (4) Macrophages and dendritic cells present microbial-derived antigen to T cells to initiate the adaptive immune response.

engulfing and killing microbes, but probably function most importantly as supervisors of the immune response to infection. They elaborate chemotactic factors for the recruitment of other cells, particularly neutrophils, to the site of infection. Macrophages also function, along with dendritic cells, to initiate the adaptive immune response by presenting antigen from the pathogen to CD4+ T cells. Neutrophils are effective at killing microbes through an arsenal of specialized antimicrobial weapons (discussed below). Because the innate immune system must react immediately in response to potential pathogens before they proliferate and disseminate, detection is dependent upon recognition of a limited number of microbial molecules that are consistently found among a vast assortment of microorganisms.

Toll-like receptors, found on mononuclear phagocytes, provide a primitive, non-specific mechanism of pathogen recognition based upon binding to conserved pathogen-associated molecular patterns rather than to specific microbial antigens.[47,48] Humans have at least 10 TLRs which recognize microbial ligands such as Gram-negative bacterial lipopolysaccharide, bacterial lipoproteins, lipotechoic acids from Gram-positive bacteria, cell-wall components of yeast and mycobacteria, unmethylated bacterial CpG DNA, and viral RNA[48,49] as well as endogenous ligands such as heat shock proteins (Table 23.1). Signaling through TLRs results in nuclear translocation of NF-κB and AP-1, which are important transcription factors that activate the promoters for a number of genes encoding inflammatory end products such as cytokines and chemokines. Interestingly, macrophages seem primed for innate immune activity after burn injury. Experimental induction of burn injury in mice causes upregulation of mRNA expression of TLR4 and increased reactivity to LPS chal-

TABLE 23.1 KNOWN HUMAN TOLL-LIKE RECEPTORS (TLRS) AND CORRESPONDING LIGANDS

TLR	Associated proteins	Described ligands
TLR1	Only signaling as a dimer with TLR2	**Exogenous**: Tri-aceylated lipopeptides (LP), phenol-soluble modulin, LP from *Mycobacterium tuberculosis*, Osp A LP from *Borrelia burgdorferi*
TLR2	CD11a/CD18, CD11b/CD18, CD14, TLR1, TLR6, dectin-1, possibly MD-2, peptidoglycan recognition proteins (PGRPs)?	**Exogenous**: LP are probably principal group activating TLR2 from wide range of species, in association with TLR1 or TLR6, inc. *M. tuberculosis*, *B. burgdorferi*, *T. pallidum*; peptidoglycans (PG) from species inc. *Staphylococcus aureus*; lipoteichoic acids, mannuronic acids, *Neisseria* porins, some rare LPS species (e.g. *P. gingivalis*), bacterial fimbriae, Yersinia virulence factors, CMV virions, measles hemagglutinin **Exogenous**: HSP60 with TLR4 **Other**: May have role in responses to oxidative stress
TLR3		**Exogenous**: Double-stranded RNA
TLR4	Lipopolysaccharide (LBP) binding protein (presents LPS to cell surface), CD14, MD-2, CD11b/CD18	**Exogenous**: LPS from a wide range of Gram-negative bacteria. Also bacterial HSP60, mannuronic acid polymers, flavolipins, teichuronic acids, *S. pneumoniae* pneumolysin, bacterial fimbriae, respiratory syncytial virus coat protein **Endogenous**: HSP60, HSP70? (LPS contamination in some preps), surfactant protein A, hyaluronan oligosaccharides, heparan sulfate fragments, fibrinogen peptides, β-defensin-2 **Drugs**: Taxol (mouse TLR4 only)
TLR5		**Exogenous**: Flagellin
TLR6	As dimer with TLR2	**Exogenous**: Di-acylated LP, ?PG, phenol-soluble modulin
TLR7		**Drugs**: Responds to imidazoquinoline antivirals. Exogenous or endogenous activators unknown
TLR8		**Drugs**: Responds to an imidazoquinoline
TLR9		**Exogenous**: Bacterial DNA as CpG motifs
TLR10		Unknown

lenge.[50,51] The importance of toll receptors in the innate immune response is illustrated by one clinical study which has suggested that post-burn patients who are at high risk for development of severe sepsis can be identified by a mutation in the TLR4 gene.[52]

Monocytes, macrophages, and neutrophils respond to bacterial invasion by migrating to the site of infection; recognizing and ingesting the microorganism; and killing and digesting the microorganism (Figure 23.3). Chemotactic gradients are provided by chemoattractants such as the complement protein C5a, endothelium-derived IL-8, and leukotrienes.[53–56] Chemoattractants and other stimuli also cause upregulation of surface phagocytic receptors.[57] Bonding between phagocyte receptors and opsonins on microbial surfaces activates cytoskeletal contractile elements resulting in invagination of the cell membrane and extension of pseudopods around the microbe. Clinical studies of neutrophils from post-burn patients demonstrate reduction in phagocytic activity.[58,59] Smoke inhalation injury may predispose to a higher incidence of bacterial pneumonia, in part, because phagocytic function of alveolar macrophages is impaired.[60,61]

Neutrophil microbicidal function

Massive neutrophil infiltration is characteristically seen in burn wounds. While this is probably an advantageous response to protect against potential pathogens, it may also be associated with some undesirable biologic effects. Oxidants and hydrolytic enzymes released from activated neutrophils can contribute to proteolysis within the wound and aid in the

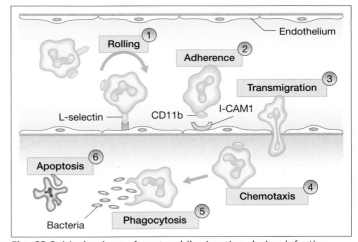

Fig. 23.3 Mechanisms of neutrophil migration during infection. Infection induces local neutrophil infiltration by causing inflammation and inducing upregulation of adherence factors on neutrophils and endothelial cells. Neutrophil surface lectins bind loosely to endothelial cell selectins to facilitate rolling of neutrophils along the blood vessel wall. Tighter neutrophil–endothelial cell bonds are formed through interaction of β integrins and intercellular adhesion molecule-1 (ICAM-1) to cause neutrophil adherence. Neutrophils then move into the interstitium by transendothelial migration, a process that is facilitated by platelet endothelial cell adhesion molecule (PECAM) and chemoattractants such as chemokines, bacterial products and leukotrienes (LTB₄). After phagocytosis and killing of microbes, neutrophils undergo apoptosis and are removed from the site of infection. (From: Seeley AJ, Pasqual JL, Christon NV. Science review: cell membrane expression (connectivity) regulates neutrophil delivery, function and clearance. Crit Care 2003; 7:291–307. Permission Biomed Central, Ltd.)

spread and dissemination of bacteria.[62,63] Abnormal neutrophil function has been associated with bacteremia in patients with burns and other major injuries.[64] Neutrophil microbicidal mechanisms are generally classified as either oxygen dependent or oxygen independent. Oxygen-independent microbicidal activity of neutrophils involves several peptides and proteins stored within the primary (azurophilic) granules, including lysozyme, bactericidal/permeability-increasing protein, β-defensins, and cathelicidin.[65] In the oxygen-dependent mechanism, NADPH oxidase within the phagosome of neutrophils (and macrophages) converts molecular oxygen into superoxide anion (O_2^-) and a series of reactions creates further oxidant products with microbicidal activity, including H_2O_2, OCl^- (hypochlorite) and NH_3Cl and RNH_2Cl (chloramines).[65] A reduction in neutrophil-mediated oxygen-dependent bacterial killing has been reported in several studies of burn patients.[58,66–68] Poor tissue perfusion and low oxygen tension in wound sites are additional factors likely to contribute to impaired oxidative killing in burn patients.

Innate lymphocytes — natural killer (NK), natural killer T (NKT), and γδ T cells

Natural killer (NK) cells are lymphoid cells that do not express clonally-expanded receptors for specific antigens.[69] NKT cells express both NK cell markers and T cell receptors (TCRs), and γδ T cells express γδ TCRs instead of the αβ TCRs found on classical T cells. All 3 innate lymphocytes are able to induce DC maturation through a combination of cell contact-dependent mechanisms and cytokine signaling. In turn, matured DCs can stimulate NK, NKT, and γδ T cells to sustain the innate immune response during the development of adaptive immunity.[70] γδ T cells, which are in found in high numbers in intestine, may play a role in recruitment of neutrophils to that site after burn injury.[71]

NK cells have been well described for their role in containing viral infections prior to the adaptive immune response, as well as assisting in the control of malignant tumors. Activated NK cells are an important source of IFNγ, which promotes the development of specific protective immune responses.[69,72] NK cells kill infected cells through the release of perforin and granzymes and through the binding of the death receptors Fas and TRAIL-R on target cells.[69,73] NK cells also interact with other cells of the immune system, including dendritic cells, by providing signals for maturation or apoptosis.[69,72] Studies of patients after burn injury have revealed a decline in NK cell activity. Most significantly, the decline in NK cell activity is most apparent more than 1 week after the occurrence of the burn injury[74,75] and corresponds with the period during which sepsis is more likely to be identified. One of these studies also noted that sera from burned patients had an inhibitory action upon NK cell activity on cells from healthy individuals.[74]

Complement

Other than toll receptors, the innate immune system has additional mechanisms for recognizing and neutralizing microbial pathogens, including the complement system, scavenger receptors, and specialized receptors on NK cells. Activation of the complement system results in production of a cascade of proteins that function to opsonize microbes and recruit phagocytes. Three distinct pathways constitute the complement

system: the classical pathway; the mannan-binding lectin pathway; and the alternative pathway (Figure 23.4). Binding of IgG or IgM to antigens on microbial surfaces activates the classical pathway. The remaining two pathways can be activated in the absence of specific antibodies. The mannan-binding lectin pathway is similar to the classical pathway but is initiated after mannan-binding lectin protein binds to mannose-containing carbohydrates on microbial surfaces.[76] The alternative pathway is dependent upon low constitutive expression of complement activity. All three of the activation pathways act on microbial surfaces to assemble a convertase that cleaves C3 to form C3b, which either binds to the surface as an opsonin, or helps activate C5 and the remainder of the complement cascade.[76–78] Opsonization facilitates the removal of microbes by macrophages and neutrophils.[77] C3a and C5a are potent chemoattractants for monocytes and neutrophils. Cleavage of C5 also leads to assembly of the membrane attack complex that causes disruption of the microbial membrane. After burn injury, neutrophil surface expression of receptors for complement are increased[79] but the complement cascade itself is diminished and may serve as a prognostic indicator. In a clinical study of severely burned patients (>60% TBSA, third-degree), serum concentrations of complement proteins were measured sequentially. All patients had decreased concentrations of C3 initially; however, serum concentrations of C3 rebounded fully in surviving patients while remaining depressed in non-survivors.[80] Diminished complement, in combination with decreased concentrations of fibronectin and serum immunoglobulins, contributed to the depression of opsonic activity in both serum and blister fluid from burn patients,[81] and likely predisposes to the development of burn wound sepsis.

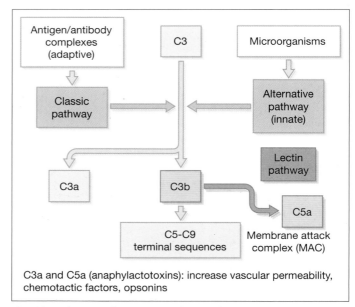

C3a and C5a (anaphylactotoxins): increase vascular permeability, chemotactic factors, opsonins

Fig. 23.4 The complement cascade (condensed). Antigen–antibody complexes or molecules on the surface of bacteria activate the complement cascade. This results in production of the anaphylacto-toxins C3a and C5a as well as the membrane attack complex. (From: Sherwood ER, Toliver-Kinsky T. Mechauisms of the inflammatory response. Best Pract Res Clin Anaesthesiol 2004; 18:385–405.

Cytokine/chemokine

Cytokines are a heterogeneous group of small polypeptide soluble mediators that are important for the regulation of antimicrobial immunity. In conjunction with hormones and neurotransmitters, cytokines regulate tissue repair and immune responses. Most cells of the immune system either release cytokines and/or respond to cytokines through specific receptors. The cytokine response evoked by microorganisms controls both innate and adaptive immune responses, including inflammation, defense against viruses, and proliferation of specific T- and B-cell clones while regulating the function and interaction of a variety of immune cells. It is interesting that cytokines do not appear to have any direct effect on microorganisms.

The description of the cytokine response after burn injury has varied widely in several clinical studies. It is likely, based upon accumulated evidence and results from well-controlled animal experiments, that burn injury by itself evokes only a modest increase in circulating cytokines. This limited cytokine response may be related to burn-induced upregulation of suppressor of cytokine signaling-3 (SOCS 3) within hours of burn injury.[82] Cytokines may be elevated within the circulation of post-burn patients, in part, because patients are subjected to a number of stresses during treatment including intubation and ventilation, surgery, transfusions, and exposure to microorganisms. In fact, there is some evidence to suggest that the cytokine response to a secondary insult may be greater after burn injury. Burn injury appears to 'prime' immune and inflammatory cells for an exaggerated response to endotoxin.[83,84] Post-burn 'hyperreactivity' in terms of cytokine production has been well described in macrophages.[85] Similar priming for an exaggerated response to LPS stimulation has been described in alveolar macrophages harvested from bronchoalveolar lavage of smoke inhalation patients or from rabbits after experimental smoke inhalation injury.[61,86] Interestingly, while surgery may potentially invoke an inflammatory response, burn wound excision has been associated with a reduction in circulating concentrations of endotoxin and cytokines[87–89] perhaps resulting from the removal of inflammatory stimuli such as necrotic tissue and bacteria.

IL-6 is one of the most consistently elevated cytokines within the circulation of post-burn patients[90,91] and in experimental animals.[92] It is unclear what function IL-6 has in the burn-induced immune response but a study in mice showed a decrease in macrophage-derived IFNγ when IL-6 was blocked in *ex vivo* experiments.[92] In another study, the pro-inflammatory response and mortality were attenuated in post-burn mice subjected to endotoxin when IL-6 was blocked.[93]

Perhaps of more importance than the burn-induced cytokine response is the secondary cytokine response to potential pathogens in the post-burn period. In this regard, burn injury may be followed by a period of attenuated expression of some cytokines that are important in the immune response to microbial organisms, and increased expression of cytokines that may hinder the immune response. For example, expression of IFNγ and a number of IFNγ-inducing cytokines including IL-2, IL-12, and IL-15 is decreased in response to a secondary immune stimulus after burn injury.[94–96] IFNγ is a cytokine with a number of beneficial effects on the immune response to microbial organisms including upregulation of class II major histocompatability complex (MHCII) proteins on many cell types. Phagocytes utilize the MHCII as a mechanism for presenting microbial antigens to CD4+ T cells at sites of inflammation.[97] Decreased monocyte expression of the MHCII is a consistent finding in septic patients. IFNγ activity also contributes to phagocytosis and microbial killing through several mechanisms. IFNγ induces IgG2a (in mice), which opsonizes bacteria, and promotes the expression of FcγR1 receptors on phagocytes.[98] IFNγ also potentiates the availability of NO, hydrogen peroxide, and superoxide in phagocytic cells[99] and promotes expression of chemotactic factors and adhesion molecules for mononuclear cell recruitment to areas of infection.[99,100] In experimental burn models, lack of IFNγ activity has been associated with diminished ability to clear bacteria.[101,102] Impaired production of IL-12 in response to endotoxin has also been described in mice after burn injury.[103] IL-12, an important product of dendritic cells and monocytes, serves to stimulate NK cell activation and production of IFNγ as well as playing a role in determining the ultimate class of T-helper lymphocyte response.

IL-10 is an anti-inflammatory cytokine that functions to attenuate the pro-inflammatory response and prevent excessive inflammation. Increased production of IL-10 may contribute to immunosuppression in the post-burn period. Immune cells from burn patients demonstrated an exaggerated IL-10 response to secondary stimulation with endotoxin or other microbial products,[104] and this finding correlated with septic episodes. Experimental studies confirm an increased IL-10 response to microbial stimuli in animals that had previously been subjected to thermal injury.[96,105] Concentrations of IL-10 have been reported to reach a peak in the plasma of patients approximately 1 week after burn injury,[106] which correlates with the time when septic episodes in post-burn patients begin to occur with increased frequency. In another clinical study, serum concentrations of IL-10 appeared to be highest in non-surviving patients with sepsis.[107]

Chemokines are a group of specialized polypeptides that play a complex role in the innate immune response by directing cell migration of immune and inflammatory cells.[53,108–110] The leukocytes and endothelial cells of most inflamed tissues can release a variety of chemokines that recruit specific sets of leukocytes to a site of infection based upon the nature of the inciting pathogen.[110,111] Chemokines also recruit leukocytes to sites of tissue injury such as the burn wound. IL-8, a neutrophil-specific chemoattractant, is one of the most widely studied chemokines. IL-8 has been reported to be significantly elevated in the circulation of post-burn patients[91] and the highest concentrations are detected in non-survivors.[106,112] Conversely, PBMC elaboration of macrophage inflammatory protein-1 alpha (MIP-1α) was diminished in post-burn patients when compared to healthy volunteers.[113] Monocyte chemoattractant protein-1 (CCL2) is upregulated in mice after thermal injury.[114]

Severe burn injury is often associated with a period of neutropenia, perhaps as a function of neutrophil activation and exit from circulation. Besides the burn wound, the lung is a preferred site for neutrophil sequestration in burn patients, even in the absence of inhalation injury. Experimentally, neutrophils can appear in lung tissue within hours of burn injury and this phenomenon can be attenuated by neutralization of complement C5a or of the chemokines keratinocyte-derived cytokine (KC) or macrophage inflammatory protein-2 (MIP-2).[115,116] MIP-2 is an IL-8 homolog in the mouse. After thermal injury, IL-8 is a major bioactive chemoattractant for neutrophils in both blister and graft donor sites of patients.[117,118] Several studies have demonstrated diminished neutrophil chemotaxis in post-burn patients which may, in part, be due to a combination of suppressive circulating soluble factors and a reduced ability to upregulate the MAC-1 (CD11b/CD18) adherence receptors on the cell surface.[119–121] A recent clinical study of burn patients demonstrated an association between the development of bacteremia and a decrease in neutrophil expression of CD11b, an adhesion molecule that functions in endothelial binding and migration from the circulation.[58]

Acquired immune function after burn injury

Whereas innate immunity provides non-specific responses that limit the growth and spread of infection, adaptive immunity provides potent, antigen-specific responses that are designed to eliminate infection and establish immunologic memory. Cytokines that are produced as a part of the innate immune response to infection can directly influence adaptive immunity. For example, production of IL-12 by antigen-presenting cells and IFNγ by natural killer cells during the innate response can influence the subsequent differentiation of CD4+ T helper cells towards a type 1 T helper (Th1) phenotype,[122,123] whereas production of IL-4, and perhaps the absence of IL-12, during innate responses can promote differentiation towards a type 2 (Th2) phenotype.[124,125] Consequently, the burn-associated alterations in innate immunity undoubtedly have an impact on subsequent adaptive immune responses both by influencing the nature of the response and also by increasing the burden that is placed on adaptive responses to eliminate infection. Indeed, there have been numerous reports of altered adaptive immune functions in burned patients. As is the case with all clinical studies, patient care precludes extensive experimental investigation, so investigators have relied on experimental models of burn injury for determining mechanisms of the immunological response to burn trauma. The current knowledge of burn-induced alterations in adaptive immune function will be reviewed, as well as information obtained from experimental models of burn injury.

Antigen presentation

Adaptive immunity is initiated upon recognition of antigen on antigen-presenting cells by antigen-specific T cell receptors. Antigenic peptides must be associated with an MHCII molecule for T cell recognition. HLA-DR is an MHCII molecule that is critical for antigen presentation in humans. A significant decrease in expression of HLA-DR has been detected in monocytes isolated from burn patients. Additionally, HLA-DR expression was further suppressed in burn patients that became septic compared to burn patients that did not develop sepsis.[126,127] In murine models of burn injury, antigen presentation is significantly impaired early after burn injury.[128] This has been associated with decreased expression of class II MHC and may be a result of diminished IFNγ,[129–131] a known inducer of class II MHC gene expression.[132]

T cell activation

The majority of observations of immune function in burn patients have come from analysis of T cells and their responses to *ex vivo* stimulation. The effects of burn injury on specific T cell subsets is not clear, and may vary depending on the time from injury, patient care, and exposure to microorganisms. One study found that the proportion of CD4+ T helper cells was significantly lower 7 days post-burn in patients that developed septicemia whereas the CD8+ cytotoxic T cell numbers were increased, and suggested that inverted CD4/CD8 ratios may be of prognostic value for septic complications.[133] However, this does not appear to be a reliable prognostic indicator since other studies have reported a decrease in CD8+ T cell numbers in burn patients.[127,134] A consistent finding among these studies was that CD4+ T helper cell numbers were decreased in burn patients, and were even further depleted in burn patients with sepsis.[135] This depletion of CD4+ T cells may be due to activation-induced apoptosis, as a significant proportion of burn patient's circulating lymphocytes were undergoing apoptosis upon analysis, and apoptosis could be further increased by mitogenic stimulation in vitro.[136] Additionally, expression of the T cell activation marker CD25 was reported to be increased both spontaneously, suggesting in vivo activation, and after mitogenic stimulation in vitro.[137] Perhaps related to these alterations are burn-associated effects on T cell phospholipid and fatty acid composition and defective transmembrane signaling.[134,138] Mouse models of burn injury have confirmed burn-induced apoptosis in T cells from various lymphoid and non-lymphoid organs, and have suggested that glucocorticoids are responsible for increased caspase-3 activity and subsequent apoptosis.[139,140] Murine burn models have also demonstrated suppressed expression of c-fos and relA, and altered activities of the AP-1 and NF-κB transcription factors that regulate genes involved in maintenance of cell survival and inflammation.[141–143]

It has been proposed that an early, 'non-specific' activation of immune cells after severe burn injury results in a subsequent impairment of their specific effector functions.[144] There appears to be at least a correlation between these early activation markers and T cell dysfunction after burn injury. T cell proliferation after mitogenic stimulation and alloreactivity in mixed leukocyte reactions have been consistently reported as being impaired in samples from burn patients.[127,137,144,145]

Significant alterations in elicited cytokine production have also been reported to occur after major burns, with a decrease in the production of Th1-associated cytokines relative to Th2 cytokines. IFNγ production by mitogen-stimulated burn patient PBMCs was significantly attenuated, whereas IL-4 production was significantly augmented.[96] Another study reported that IL-2 and IFNγ production by stimulated T cells was significantly lower in non-survivors than in survivors of severe burn injury.[146] Zedler et al.[147] found that the number of IL-4-producing CD8+ T cells was significantly higher and the number of IFNγ-producing memory T cells significantly lower in non-survivors, than in patients that survived after burn injury. Additionally, IL-10 production is reported to be higher after burn injury, and elevated plasma levels in burn patients correlated with poor prognosis.[104,126] Experimental studies in a mouse model of burn injury have demonstrated a significant increase in the activity of regulatory T cells (CD4+/CD25+)

in lymph nodes draining the burn wound. Specifically, regulatory T cells isolated from burned mice were potent suppressors of T cell proliferation and IL-2 and IFNγ production, due in part to elevated surface expression of transforming growth factor-β1 (TGF-β1). Depletion of these cells prior to burn injury ameliorated the burn-induced suppression of antigen-specific Th1-type immune responses.[148,149] While the exact significance of each of these functional impairments remains to be determined, there does appear to be a correlation between T cell dysfunction and susceptibility to infection and subsequent mortality after severe burns. In a clinical study of trauma and burn patients, those that had depressed cell proliferation of isolated T cells were at high risk for the development of multiple organ failure and mortality.[150] Teodorczyk-Injeyan et al. reported that burn patients that were unable to recover IL-2 production and T cell IL-2 receptor expression over time developed fatal sepsis.[145]

B cell-mediated immunity

Hansbrough et al. noted a defect in the ability of burn patient sera to opsonize bacteria, which subsequently affected *in vitro* phagocytosis.[151] Schluter et al. reported a decrease in expression of the B cell activation marker CD25 both before and after cytokine stimulation of burn patient samples.[137] In a clinical study, mitogen-induced immunoglobulin production was increased initially but suppressed at 3–4 weeks after burn injury. In survivors, immunoglobulin production returned to baseline, or higher, levels whereas production remained suppressed in burn patients that developed fatal septicemia.[152]

Analysis of immunoglobulin production in murine burn models has indicated that injury has a significant suppressive effect on antigen-specific antibody production. The reported effects on specific immunoglobulin subtypes vary, perhaps due

to the use of different eliciting antigens, or other experimental conditions. Production of tetanus toxoid-specific IgG, specifically IgG2a, was impaired after burn injury in mice, and could be restored by exogenous IL-12, suggesting that impaired IgG2a production after burn injury is related to impairments in Th1-associated cytokine production.[153,154] Other studies have reported that numerous B cell functions are impaired after burn injury. Specifically, antigen-specific IgM, total IgM, and total IgG production, and B cell proliferation were impaired 8 days after burn injury in mice. LPS-specific IgM could be restored to normal by cyclo-oxygenase inhibition, suggesting a role of PGE$_2$ in impaired B cell responses to antigen.[155,156] Others have reported a role of TGF-β in impairment of B cell clonal expansion, and inhibition of IgM synthesis and antigen-specific antibody production after burn injury.[148,157,158]

Hematopoiesis after burn injury

In addition to the numerous injury-associated alterations in innate and acquired immune cell functions, there are also effects of burn injury on immune cell production from bone marrow-derived progenitor cells (Figure 23.5). Analysis of burn patient peripheral blood leukocytes has revealed fluctuations in immune cell composition, with periods of neutropenia, monocytopenia, and at other times monocytosis.[159] Analysis of hematopoiesis in murine models has suggested that burn injury increases myelopoiesis in both the spleen and bone marrow, with alterations occurring at the level of the myeloid cell phenotype.[160] Burns appear to shift the hematopoietic potential of myeloid progenitor cells towards monocytopoiesis at the expense of neutrophil production.[161] These alterations may be potentiated by high norepinephrine levels seen in burned and septic patients.[162]

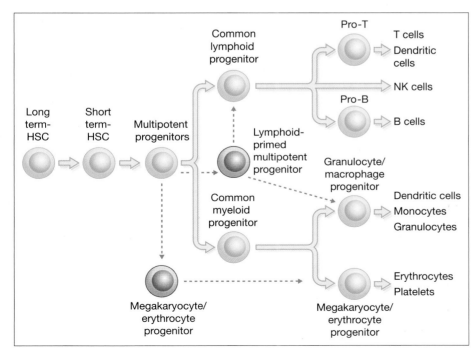

Fig. 23.5 Differentiation of hematopoietic stem cells (HSC). The conventional model of HSC differentiation (shown in bold with solid arrows) suggests that multipotent progenitor cells differentiate into strictly committed common lymphoid progenitor or common myeloid progenitor cells. The common lymphoid progenitor gives rise to T cells, dendritic cells, natural killer cells, and B cells. The common myeloid progenitor further differentiates into either a granulocyte/macrophage progenitor, which gives rise to monocytes, dendritic cells, and granulocytes, or a megakaryocyte/erythrocyte progenitor that can differentiate into erythrocytes and platelets. A recent alternative model (shown in gray with dotted lines) suggests that the megakaryocyte/erythrocyte progenitor is distinct from a 'lymphoid-primed multipotent progenitor' that further differentiates into the common lymphoid progenitor or granulocyte/macrophage progenitor.

Immunomodulation

Immunonutrition

To date, the most consistently successful intervention for enhancing immune function in burn patients is nutritional supplementation. It has been reported that early enteral feeding may decrease intestinal permeability and reduce enterogenic infection.[163] Berger et al. reported that trace element (Cu, Zn, Se) supplementation, given early, decreased the incidence of bronchopneumonia infections and decreased length of hospital stay.[164] Garrel et al. found that enteral supplementation with glutamine after burn injury significantly reduced the incidence of infections and decreased mortality.[165] Interestingly, there was no effect on PMN phagocytosis, indicating that glutamine supplementation works by some other mechanism. Arginine supplementation in burned mice was found to enhance humoral immunity (production of *P. aeruginosa*-specific antibodies) and decrease oxidative stress, but a benefit on survival was not observed in this model.[166]

Selective decontamination of digestive tract

Whether or not bacterial translocation due to changes in gut permeability is a source of infections in burned patients is controversial. In 1997 Yao et al. reported that selective decontamination of the digestive tract (SDD) in burned rats decreased bacterial translocation and endotoxemia and prevented burn-associated suppression of mitogenic responses and IL-2 production.[167] Clinically, SDD by enteral administration of antibiotics to burned children did not decrease the incidence of infections.[168] However, a recent study by De la Cal et al. reported that SDD, which included the administration of parenteral cefotaxime in addition to enteral antibiotics, significantly reduced mortality and the incidence of pneumonia in burned adults.[169]

Vaccination

A technique that may be highly effective for prevention of *P. aeruginosa* infections is vaccination with *P. aeruginosa* outer membrane proteins after burn injury. In 1970 this approach was investigated in a rat burn model,[170] and it was later demonstrated that vaccination of burned mice decreased systemic bacterial load and increased survival upon lethal infection with *P. aeruginosa*.[171] In 1983 it was reported that both active and passive vaccinations for *Pseudomonas* were effective in inducing antibodies to *Pseudomonas* and reducing mortality in both burned adults and children.[172] Since then, numerous studies have reported that vaccination of burn patients with *P. aeruginosa* outer membrane proteins is safe, significantly increases *P. aeruginosa*-specific titers, and is associated with a decrease in detection of *P. aeruginosa* by nested PCR in blood of vaccinated patients.[173–176] While this approach may be effective for decreasing *P. aeruginosa* infections, the limitation of this strategy is that it will be restricted to single bacterial species unless vaccinations against widely conserved pathogenic motifs can be developed.

Cytokine modulation

Due to the profound effects that severe burns have on pathogen-elicited cytokine production, coupled with the observed correlation between these alterations and a negative outcome in burn patients and in experimental animal models of burn injury, many attempts to modulate immune function after burns have been directed towards restoration of normal cytokine balance. One approach has been the administration of exogenous Th1 or Th1-promoting cytokines. IFNγ has been administered to burn and trauma patients in clinical studies but unfortunately has shown no benefit with respect to the incidence of infections or mortality.[177,178] Experimentally, administration of IL-12 and IL-18 has shown some benefit in animal models, but these cytokines have not been tested in the clinical scenario.[94,179,180] Adverse reactions to IL-12 in other clinical trials may preclude its introduction as an immunomodulator in burn patients.[181,182]

Another attempt at cytokine modulation has been the neutralization of cytokines believed to contribute to post-burn immunosuppression. Treatment of mice with antibodies specific for IL-10 was shown to increase resistance to infection, but only if given immediately after burn injury.[183] In a murine model of burn and sepsis, the utility of antibodies against TNF-α was found to be limited in that TNF-α neutralization was only effective during a narrow time frame after burns, and may have worsened outcome when high doses of antibodies were used.[184] Given the interactive and dynamic nature of the cytokine network, therapies targeted to modulate the levels of a single cytokine may not be sufficient to restore immunological homeostasis after severe burn injury.

Hematopoietic factors

Another approach to improving immune function in burn patients is to stimulate hematopoiesis to generate new immune cells from bone marrow-derived stem and progenitor cells. The supposition underlying this approach is that accelerated and amplified production of new effector cells may be more effective than therapies that are designed to compensate for specific burn-induced impairments in immune function. Given the propensity of burn patients to mount excessive and hazardous pro-inflammatory responses, it is imperative to consider factors that can enhance immune cell production and effector function without activation of a pronounced inflammatory response. Stimulation of macrophage and neutrophil production after burns has been investigated using granulocyte-colony stimulating factor (G-CSF), a neutrophil growth factor, and granulocyte macrophage colony-stimulating factor (GM-CSF), a growth factor for neutrophils and macrophages. Both G-CSF and GM-CSF improved immune function in animal models of burn-associated sepsis.[185,186] Treatment of burn patients with GM-CSF was shown to increase white cell counts and improve neutrophil activities, but the effect of GM-CSF on infection rate and patient outcome has not been evaluated.[187]

Another hematopoietic factor that has been examined in a mouse burn model is fms-like tyrosine kinase-3 ligand, or Flt3L, a hematopoietic cytokine and dendritic cell growth factor (Figure 23.6). Treatment of burned mice with Flt3L has been shown to stimulate the production of dendritic cells, restore pathogen-elicited Th1-associated cytokine production, and increase survival after an otherwise lethal burn wound infection. Resistance to burn wound infection could be conferred by the adoptive transfer of dendritic cells that were isolated from Flt3L-treated mice,[188] indicating that modulation of dendritic cell production and function may have future

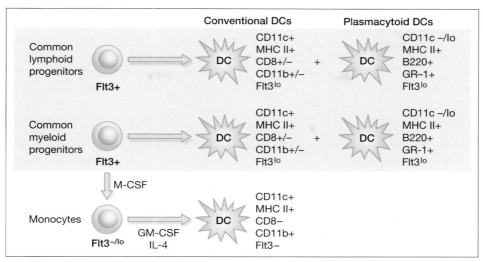

Fig. 23.6 Dendritic cell development from murine hematopoietic progenitor cells. Dendritic cells can be derived from both common lymphoid progenitor cells and common myeloid progenitor cells. The Flt3 tyrosine kinase receptor is expressed at high levels on common lymphoid and myeloid progenitors. Differentiation in response to Flt3 ligand generates both plasmacytoid (IFNα-producing cells) and 'conventional' dendritic cells (both CD8+ CD11b– and CD8– CD11b+ subtypes), all of which maintain a low level of Flt3 receptor expression. Cells that are potentially responsive to Flt3 ligand treatments are highlighted in blue. Dendritic cells can also be derived from monocytic precursors in the presence of GM-CSF and IL-4, but dendritic cells derived along this pathway do not retain Flt3 receptor expression.[208–210] M-CSF, macrophage colony-stimulating factor; GM-CSF, granulocyte–macrophage colony-stimulating factor; DC, dendritic cells.

potential for prevention of infections after major burn injury. This approach is supported by several clinical findings that suggest that decreases in dendritic cell numbers and function, due to increased apoptosis and/or decreased dendritic cell differentiation, contribute to immune dysfunction after major trauma. In one study of trauma and burn patients, decreased T cell activation in patients that eventually developed sepsis was attributed to deficient activation by dendritic cells subsequent to impaired dendritic cell differentiation from monocyte precursors.[189] Another study reported that the number of dendritic cells in spleens of patients that died from sepsis-associated complications was significantly reduced.[190] The direct relevance of these findings to burn-associated immunosuppression remains to be determined. However, in combination with the experimental studies in which dendritic cell enhancement by Flt3L was highly effective for increasing resistance to burn wound infection, these clinical observations justify further investigations of dendritic cell modulation after burn injury. It should be noted that clinical studies in healthy individuals and cancer patients have indicated that Flt3L significantly increases dendritic cell numbers in peripheral blood, with no overt toxicity.[191–193]

Other approaches

There are numerous ongoing attempts to develop prophylactic treatments to prevent infections after major burn injury. Other potential treatments have been described in clinical studies in trauma patients, since there are similarities in the immunological alterations that occur after major burns and other types of trauma. One treatment that shows promise is glucan, a β-1,3-linked glucose polymer derived from the cell wall of *Saccharomyces cerevisiae*. Glucans have been shown experimentally to decrease sepsis-induced inflammation while enhancing

microbial clearance.[194,195] Clinical studies with trauma and high-risk surgical patients have shown that glucans can decrease infectious complications and mortality in these patient populations.[196,197] Although these compounds have not yet been tested in burn patients, they have been effective in decreasing susceptibility to burn wound infection and mortality in a mouse model of burn injury.[131]

Another approach that is under investigation is the use of resuscitation fluids as immunomodulators. Junger and others have found that hypertonic saline has the ability to attenuate inflammation, decrease neutrophil-mediated lung damage, and rescue T cells from experimental trauma-associated suppression. It was reported that IL-2 production by phytohemagglutinin-stimulated human PBMCS was completely suppressed by sera from trauma patients, but that costimulation with hypertonic saline could restore IL-2 production.[198] Additionally, it was found that resuscitation of mice with hypertonic saline (compared to lactated Ringer's solution) after hemorrhagic shock decreased bacteremia and increased survival upon a subsequent cecal ligation and puncture.[199] They have proposed that leukocytes respond to hyperosmotic stress through an osmosensory system that signals a phosphorylation cascade resulting in p38 MAP kinase activation.[200,201] Clinical studies have examined resuscitation of burn patients with hypertonic saline and have reported that it is safe, provides adequate resuscitation, and may decrease severity and incidence of pulmonary dysfunction,[202–204] but the effects of hypertonic saline on inflammation and immune function have not yet been addressed in the clinical scenario.

Host defense peptides are another potential mechanism for immunomodulation after burn injury. Defense peptides are naturally occurring antimicrobial effector molecules of the innate immune system. Human β-defensins are produced in the skin by keratinocytes, and expression of one of these peptides, human beta-defensin 2, is significantly decreased in burn wounds.[205] Human cathelicidin hCAP-18/LL-37 is another class of defense peptide that is expressed in the skin. Using a rat model of burn wound infection, Jacobsen et al. showed that transient cutaneous adenoviral delivery of hCAP-18/LL-37 to infected burn wounds induced hCAP-18/LL-37 and significantly inhibited bacterial growth.[206] Future studies appear warranted to evaluate the efficacy of host defense peptides for the treatment and/or prevention of infections after burn injury.

Summary

Improvements in burn care have decreased the incidence of serious infections in burn patients. However, infectious complications remain common in severely burned patients and are one of the most common causes of mortality in patients that survive the initial burn trauma. The relatively high incidence of infections in this setting appears to be due, in part, to alterations in innate and acquired immunity. Clearly, loss of the skin barrier and the presence of invasive instrumentation contribute to the susceptibility to infection in these patients. Numerous studies suggest that alterations in cellular immunity, both innate and acquired, may also predispose burn patients to infection. Several immunomodulatory approaches have been studied in experimental models and have been shown to improve resistance to infection. This benefit may be due to reversal of immunosuppression or may simply result from augmentation of antimicrobial immune function. In either case, immunomodulatory interventions appear attractive as a means of improving host resistance to infection during the acute post-burn period, especially considering the increased prevalence of antibiotic-resistant microorganisms.

References

1. Gray DT, Pine RW, Harnar TJ, et al. Early surgical excision versus conventional therapy in patients with 20 to 40 percent burns. A comparative study. Am J Surg 1982; 144(1):76–80.
2. Pruitt BA, McManus AT, Kim SH, et al. Burn wound infections: current status. World J Surg 1998; 22(2):135–145.
3. Wolfe RA, Roi LD, Flora JD, et al. Mortality differences and speed of wound closure among specialized burn care facilities. JAMA 1983; 250(6):763–766.
4. Mason AD, McManus AT, Pruitt BA. Association of burn mortality and bacteremia — a 25-year review. Arch Surg 1986; 121(9):1027–1031.
5. Shirani KZ, Pruitt BA, Mason AD. The influence of inhalation injury and pneumonia on burn mortality. Ann Surg 1987; 205(1):82–87.
6. Peck MD, Heimbach DM. Does early excision of burn wounds change the pattern of mortality? J Burn Care Rehabil 1989; 10(1):7–10.
7. National Nosocomial Infections Surveillance (NNIS) report, data summary from October 1986–April 1997, issued May 1997. A report from the NNIS System. Am J Infect Control 1997; 25:477–487.
8. Weber JM, Sheridan RL, Pasternack MS, et al. Nosocomial infections in pediatric patients with burns. Am J Infect Control 1997; 25(3):195–201.
9. O'Keefe GE, Hunt JL, Purdue GF. An evaluation of risk factors for mortality after burn trauma and the identification of gender-dependent differences in outcomes. J Am Coll Surg 2001; 192(2):153–160.
10. Fitzwater J, Purdue GF, Hunt JL, et al. The risk factors and time course of sepsis and organ dysfunction after burn trauma. J Trauma 2003; 54(5):959–966.
11. McGwin G, George RL, Cross JM, et al. Gender differences in mortality following burn injury. Shock 2002; 18(4):311–315.
12. George RL, McGwin G, Schwacha MG, et al. The association between sex and mortality among burn patients as modified by age. J Burn Care Rehabil 2005; 26(5):416–421.
13. Barrow RE, Przkora R, Hawkins HK, et al. Mortality related to gender, age, sepsis, and ethnicity in severely burned children. Shock 2005; 23(6):485–487.
14. Bang RL, Sharma PN, Sanyal SC, et al. Burn septicaemia in Kuwait: associated demographic and clinical factors. Med Princ Pract 2004; 13(3):136–141.
15. Lesseva M. Central venous catheter-related bacteraemia in burn patients. Scand J Infect Dis 1998; 30(6):585–589.
16. Dunn DL, Rotstein OD. Diagnosis, prevention, and treatment of infection in surgical patients. In: Greenfield LJ, Mulholland MW, Oldham KT, et al, eds. Surgery: scientific principles and practice. Philadelphia: Lippincott Williams & Wilkins; 2001:178–202.
17. Bochicchio GV, Joshi M, Shih D, et al. Reclassification of urinary tract infections in critically ill trauma patients: a time-dependent analysis. Surg Infect (Larchmt) 2003; 4(4):379–385.
18. Appelgren P, Bjornhagen V, Bragderyd K, et al. A prospective study of infections in burn patients. Burns 2002; 28(1):39–46.
19. de La Cal MA, Cerda E, Garcia-Hierro P, et al. Pneumonia in patients with severe burns — a classification according to the concept of the carrier state. Chest 2001; 119(4):1160–1165.
20. Durtschi MB, Orgain C, Counts GW, et al. A prospective study of prophylactic penicillin in acutely burned hospitalized patients. J Trauma 1982; 22(1):11–14.
21. McManus AT, McManus WF, Mason AD, et al. Beta-hemolytic streptococcal burn wound infections are too infrequent to justify penicillin prophylaxis. Plast Reconstr Surg 1994; 93(3):650–651.
22. Sheridan RL, Weber JM, Pasternack MS, et al. Antibiotic prophylaxis for group A streptococcal burn wound infection is not necessary. J Trauma 2001; 51(2):352–355.
23. Alexander M, Daniel T, Chaudry IH, et al. Opiate analgesics contribute to the development of post-injury immunosuppression. J Surg Res 2005; 129(1):161–168.
24. Graves TA, Cioffi WG, Mason AD, et al. Relationship of transfusion and infection in a burn population. J Trauma 1989; 29(7):948–954.
25. Shorr AF, Jackson WL. Transfusion practice and nosocomial infection: assessing the evidence. Curr Opin Crit Care 2005; 11(5):468–472.
26. Jensen LS, Andersen AJ, Christiansen PM, et al. Postoperative infection and natural killer cell function following blood transfusion in patients undergoing elective colorectal surgery. Br J Surg 1992; 79(6):513–516.
27. Brunson ME, Alexander JW. Mechanisms of transfusion-induced immunosuppression. Transfusion 1990; 30(7):651–658.
28. Leonard SA, Redmond HP. Effects of volatile and intravenous anesthetic agents on neutrophil function. Int Anesthesiol Clin 2003; 41(1):21–29.
29. Noble WC. Ecology and host resistance in relation to skin disease. In: Freedberg I, Eisen AZ, Wolff K, eds. Dermatology in general medicine. New York: McGraw-Hill; 1999:184–191.
30. Robson MC, Heggers JP. Bacterial quantification of open wounds. Mil Med 1969; 134:19–24.
31. Trengove NJ, Stacey MC, McGechie DF, et al. Qualitative bacteriology and leg ulcer healing. J Wound Care 1996; 5(6):277–280.
32. Schwacha MG, Schneider CP, Chaudry IH. Differential expression and tissue compartmentalization of the inflammatory response following thermal injury. Cytokine 2002; 17(5):266–274.
33. Gotte M. Syndecans in inflammation. FASEB J 2003; 17(6):575–591.

34. Haynes A III, Ruda F, Oliver J, et al. Syndecan 1 shedding contributes to Pseudomonas aeruginosa sepsis. Infect Immun 2005; 73(12):7914–7921.

35. Carter EA, Tompkins RG, Schiffrin E, et al. Cutaneous thermal injury alters macromolecular permeability of rat small intestine. Surgery 1990; 107(3):335–341.

36. Horton JW. Bacterial translocation after burn injury: the contribution of ischemia and permeability changes. Shock 1994; 1(4): 286–290.

37. Herndon DN, Zeigler ST. Bacterial translocation after thermal injury. Crit Care Med 1993; 21(2):S50–S54.

38. Deitch EA. Intestinal permeability is increased in burn patients shortly after injury. Surgery 1990; 107(4):411–416.

39. Ryan CM, Yarmush ML, Burke JF, et al. Increased gut permeability early after burns correlates with the extent of burn injury. Crit Care Med 1992; 20(11):1508–1512.

40. Eaves-Pyles T, Alexander JW. Rapid and prolonged impairment of gut barrier function after thermal injury in mice. Shock 1998; 9(2):95–100.

41. La Cal MA, Cerda E, Garcia-Hierro P, et al. Survival benefit in critically ill burned patients receiving selective decontamination of the digestive tract — a randomized, placebo-controlled, double-blind trial. Ann Surg 2005; 241(3):424–430.

42. Ganz T. Defensins: antimicrobial peptides of innate immunity. Nature Rev Immunol 2003; 3(9):710–720.

43. Hoover DM, Rajashankar KR, Blumenthal R, et al. The structure of human beta-defensin-2 shows evidence of higher order oligomerization. J Biol Chem 2000; 275(42):32911–32918.

44. Vora P, Youdim A, Thomas LS, et al. beta-Defensin-2 expression is regulated by TLR signaling in intestinal epithelial cells. J Immunol 2004; 173(9):5398–5405.

45. Hertz CJ, Wu Q, Porter EM, et al. Activation of toll-like receptor 2 on human tracheobronchial epithelial cells induces the antimicrobial peptide human beta defensin-2. J Immunol 2003; 171(12):6820–6826.

46. Milner SM, Bhat S, Buja M, et al. Expression of human beta defensin 2 in thermal injury. Burns 2004; 30(7):649–654.

47. Medzhitov R, Preston-Hurlburt P, Janeway CA. A human homologue of the Drosophila Toll protein signals activation of adaptive immunity. Nature 1997; 388(6640):394–397.

48. Zarember KA, Godowski PJ. Tissue expression of human toll-like receptors and differential regulation of toll-like receptor mRNAs in leukocytes in response to microbes, their products, and cytokines. J Immunol 2002; 168(2):554–561.

49. Cohen J. The immunopathogenesis of sepsis. Nature 2002; 420(6917):885–891.

50. Maung AA, Fujimi S, Miller ML, et al. Enhanced TLR4 reactivity following injury is mediated by increased p38 activation. J Leukoc Biol 2005; 78(2):565–573.

51. Murphy TJ, Paterson HM, Kriynovich S, et al. Linking the 'two-hit' response following injury to enhanced TLR4 reactivity. J Leukoc Biol 2005; 77(1):16–23.

52. Barber RC, Aragaki CC, Rivera-Chavez FA, et al. TLR4 and TNF-alpha polymorphisms are associated with an increased risk for severe sepsis following burn injury. J Med Genet 2004; 41(11):808–813.

53. Rossi D, Zlotnik A. The biology of chemokines and their receptors. Ann Rev Immunol 2000; 18:217–243.

54. Ley K. Integration of inflammatory signals by rolling neutrophils. Immunol Rev 2002; 186:8–18.

55. Seo SM, McIntire LV, Smith CW. Effects of IL-8, Gro-alpha, and LTB4 on the adhesive kinetics of LFA-1 and Mac-1 on human neutrophils. Am J Physiol-Cell Physiol 2001; 281(5):C1568–C1578.

56. Gerard C, Gerard NP. C5A anaphylatoxin and its 7 transmembrane-segment receptor. Ann Rev Immunol 1994; 12:775–808.

57. Berger M, Oshea J, Cross AS, et al. Human neutrophils increase expression of C3Bi as well as C3B receptors upon activation. J Clin Investigat 1984; 74(5):1566–1571.

58. Babcock GF. Predictive medicine: severe trauma and burns. Cytometry B Clin Cytom 2003; 53(1):48–53.

59. Ogle CK, Ogle JD, Mao JX, et al. Effect of glutamine on phagocytosis and bacterial killing by normal and pediatric burn patient neutrophils. JPEN 1994; 18(2):128–133.

60. Herlihy JP, Vermeulen MW, Joseph PM, et al. Impaired alveolar macrophage function in smoke-inhalation injury. J Cell Physiol 1995; 163(1):1–8.

61. Bidani A, Wang CZ, Heming TA. Early effects of smoke inhalation on alveolar macrophage functions. Burns 1996; 22(2):101–106.

62. Lentsch AB, Ward PA. Regulation of inflammatory vascular damage. J Pathol 2000; 190(3):343–348.

63. Rumbaugh KP, Hamood AN, Griswold JA. Cytokine induction by the P. aeruginosa quorum sensing system during thermal injury. J Surg Res 2004; 116(1):137–144.

64. Alexander JW, Stinnett JD, Ogle CK, et al. A comparison of immunologic profiles and their influence on bacteremia in surgical patients with a high risk of infection. Surgery 1979; 86(1):94–104.

65. Tosi MF. Innate immune responses to infection. J Allergy Clin Immunol 2005; 116(2):241–249.

66. Curreri PW, Heck EL, Browne L, et al. Stimulate nitroblue tetrazolium test to assess neutrophil antibacterial function: prediction of wound sepsis in burn patients. Surgery 1973; 74:6–13.

67. Heck EL, Browne L, Curreri PW, et al. Evaluation of leukocyte function in burned individuals by in vitro oxygen consumption. J Trauma 1975; 15(6):486–489.

68. Dobke MK, Deitch EA, Harnar TJ, et al. Oxidative activity of polymorphonuclear leukocytes after thermal injury. Arch Surg 1989; 124(7):856–859.

69. Smyth MJ, Cretney E, Kelly JM, et al. Activation of NK cell cytotoxicity. Mol Immunol 2005; 42(4):501–510.

70. Munz C, Steinman RM, Fujii S. Dendritic cell maturation by innate lymphocytes: coordinated stimulation of innate and adaptive immunity. J Exp Med 2005; 202(2):203–207.

71. Toth B, Alexander M, Daniel T, et al. The role of gammadelta T cells in the regulation of neutrophil-mediated tissue damage after thermal injury. J Leukoc Biol 2004; 76(3):545–552.

72. Cerwenka A, Lanier LL. Natural killer cells, viruses and cancer. Nature Rev Immunol 2001; 1(1):41–49.

73. Sato K, Hida S, Takayanagi H, et al. Antiviral response by natural killer cells through TRAIL gene induction by IFN-alpha/beta. Eur J Immunol 2001; 31(11):3138–3146.

74. Bender BS, Winchurch RA, Thupari JN, et al. Depressed natural killer cell function in thermally injured adults: successful in vivo and in vitro immunomodulation and the role of endotoxin. Clin Exp Immunol 1988; 71(1):120–125.

75. Jira M, Polacek V, Strejcek J, et al. Natural killer cell activity following thermal injury. Scand J Plast Reconstr Surg Hand Surg 1988; 22(2):131–133.

76. Petersen SV, Thiel S, Jensenius JC. The mannan-binding lectin pathway of complement activation: biology and disease association. Mol Immunol 2001; 38(2–3):133–149.

77. Joiner KA, Brown EJ, Frank MM. Complement and bacteria — chemistry and biology in host defense. Ann Rev Immunol 1984; 2:461–491.

78. Walport MJ. Advances in immunology: complement (first of two parts). N Engl J Med 2001; 344(14):1058–1066.

79. Vindenes H, Bjerknes R. Activation of polymorphonuclear neutrophilic granulocytes following burn injury: alteration of Fcreceptor and complement-receptor expression and of opsonophagocytosis. J Trauma 1994; 36(2):161–167.

80. Kang HJ, Kim JH, Lee EH, et al. Change of complement system predicts the outcome of patients with severe thermal injury. J Burn Care Rehabil 2003; 24(3):148–153.

81. Ono Y, Kunii O, Suzuki H, et al. Opsonic activity of sera and blister fluid from severely burned patients evaluated by a chemiluminescence method. Microbiol Immunol 1994; 38(5):373–377.

82. Ogle CK, Kong F, Guo X, et al. The effect of burn injury on suppressors of cytokine signalling. Shock 2000; 14(3):392–398.

83. Pallua N, von Heimburg D. Pathogenic role of interleukin-6 in the development of sepsis. Part I: Study in a standardized contact burn murine model. Crit Care Med 2003; 31(5):1490–1494.

84. Sasaki J, Fujishima S, Iwamura H, et al. Prior burn insult induces lethal acute lung injury in endotoxemic mice: effects of cytokine inhibition. Am J Physiol Lung Cell Mol Physiol 2003; 284(2): L270–L278.

85. Schwacha MG. Macrophages and post-burn immune dysfunction. Burns 2003; 29(1):1–14.

86. Wright MJ, Murphy JT. Smoke inhalation enhances early alveolar leukocyte responsiveness to endotoxin. J Trauma 2005; 59(1):64–70.

87. Schwacha MG, Knoferl MW, Chaudry IH. Does burn wound excision after thermal injury attenuate subsequent macrophage hyperactivity and immunosuppression? Shock 2000; 14(6):623–628.

88. Barret JP, Herndon DN. Modulation of inflammatory and catabolic responses in severely burned children by early burn wound excision in the first 24 hours. Arch Surg 2003; 138(2):127–132.

89. Han TH, Lee SY, Kwon JE, et al. The limited immunomodulatory effects of escharectomy on the kinetics of endotoxin, cytokines, and adhesion molecules in major burns. Mediators Inflamm 2004; 13(4):241–246.

90. Kowal-Vern A, Webster SD, Rasmasubban S, et al. Circulating endothelial cell levels correlate with proinflammatory cytokine increase in the acute phase of thermal injury. J Burn Care Rehabil 2005; 26(5):422–429.

91. Dehne MG, Sablotzki A, Hoffmann A, et al. Alterations of acute phase reaction and cytokine production in patients following severe burn injury. Burns 2002; 28(6):535–542.

92. Durbin EA, Gregory MS, Messingham KA, et al. The role of interleukin 6 in interferon-gamma production in thermally injured mice. Cytokine 2000; 12(11):1669–1675.

93. Pallua N, Low JF, von Heimburg D. Pathogenic role of interleukin-6 in the development of sepsis. Part II: Significance of anti-interleukin-6 and anti-soluble interleukin-6 receptor-alpha antibodies in a standardized murine contact burn model. Crit Care Med 2003; 31(5):1495–1501.

94. Ami K, Kinoshita M, Yamauchi A, et al. IFN-gamma production from liver mononuclear cells of mice in burn injury as well as in postburn bacterial infection models and the therapeutic effect of IL-18. J Immunol 2002; 169(8):4437–4442.

95. Toliver-Kinsky TE, Varma TK, Lin CY, et al. Interferon-gamma production is suppressed in thermally injured mice: decreased production of regulatory cytokines and corresponding receptors. Shock 2002; 18(4):322–330.

96. O'Sullivan ST, Lederer JA, Horgan AF, et al. Major injury leads to predominance of the T helper-2 lymphocyte phenotype and diminished interleukin-12 production associated with decreased resistance to infection. Ann Surg 1995; 222(4):482–490.

97. Skoskiewicz MJ, Colvin RB, Schneeberger EE, et al. Widespread and selective induction of major histocompatibility complex-determined antigens in vivo by gamma interferon. J Exp Med 1985; 162(5):1645–1664.

98. Paludan SR. Interleukin-4 and interferon-gamma: the quintessence of a mutual antagonistic relationship. Scand J Immunol 1998; 48(5):459–468.

99. Boehm U, Klamp T, Groot M, et al. Cellular responses to interferon-gamma. Ann Rev Immunol 1997; 15:749–795.

100. Cuff CA, Schwartz J, Bergman CM, et al. Lymphotoxin alpha3 induces chemokines and adhesion molecules: insight into the role of LT alpha in inflammation and lymphoid organ development. J Immunol 1998; 161(12):6853–6860.

101. Dai WJ, Bartens W, Kohler G, et al. Impaired macrophage listericidal and cytokine activities are responsible for the rapid death of Listeria monocytogenes-infected IFN-gamma receptor-deficient mice. J Immunol 1997; 158(11):5297–5304.

102. Zantl N, Uebe A, Neumann B, et al. Essential role of gamma interferon in survival of colon ascendens stent peritonitis, a novel murine model of abdominal sepsis. Infect Immun 1998; 66(5):2300–2309.

103. Utsunomiya T, Kobayashi M, Herndon DN, et al. A mechanism of interleukin-12 unresponsiveness associated with thermal injury. J Surg Res 2001; 96(2):211–217.

104. Lyons A, Kelly JL, Rodrick ML, et al. Major injury induces increased production of interleukin-10 by cells of the immune system with a negative impact on resistance to infection. Ann Surg 1997; 226(4):450–458.

105. Mack VE, McCarter MD, Naama HA, et al. Dominance of T-helper 2-type cytokines after severe injury. Arch Surg 1996; 131(12):1303–1308.

106. Ozbalkan Z, Aslar AK, Yildiz Y, et al. Investigation of the course of proinflammatory and anti-inflammatory cytokines after burn sepsis. Int J Clin Pract 2004; 58(2):125–129.

107. Yeh FL, Lin WL, Shen HD. Changes in circulating levels of an anti-inflammatory cytokine interleukin 10 in burned patients. Burns 2000; 26(5):454–459.

108. Baggiolini M. Chemokines in pathology and medicine. J Intern Med 2001; 250(2):91–104.

109. Bacon K, Baggiolini M, Broxmeyer H, et al. Chemokine/chemokine receptor nomenclature. Cytokine 2003; 21(1):48–49.

110. Kim CH. Chemokine-chemokine receptor network in immune cell trafficking. Curr Drug Targets Immune Endocr Metabol Disord 2004; 4:343–361.

111. Glass WG, Rosenberg HF, Murphy PM. Chemokine regulation of inflammation during acute viral infection. Curr Opin Allergy Clin Immunol 2003; 3:467–473.

112. Dugan AL, Malarkey WB, Schwemberger S, et al. Serum levels of prolactin, growth hormone, and cortisol in burn patients: correlations with severity of burn, serum cytokine levels, and fatality. J Burn Care Rehabil 2004; 25(3):306–313.

113. Kobayashi M, Takahashi H, Sanford AP, et al. An increase in the susceptibility of burned patients to infectious complications due to impaired production of macrophage inflammatory protein 1 alpha. J Immunol 2002; 169(8):4460–4466.

114. Takahashi H, Tsuda Y, Kobayashi M, et al. Increased norepinephrine production associated with burn injuries results in CCL2 production and type 2 T cell generation. Burns 2004; 30(4):317–321.

115. Dries DJ, Lorenz K, Kovacs EJ. Differential neutrophil traffic in gut and lung after scald injury. J Burn Care Rehabil 2001; 22(3):203–209.

116. Piccolo MT, Wang Y, Sannomiya P, et al. Chemotactic mediator requirements in lung injury following skin burns in rats. Exp Mol Pathol 1999; 66(3):220–226.

117. Rennekampff HO, Hansbrough JF, Kiessig V, et al. Bioactive interleukin-8 is expressed in wounds and enhances wound healing. J Surg Res 2000; 93(1):41–54.

118. Garner WL, Rodriguez JL, Miller CG, et al. Acute skin injury releases neutrophil chemoattractants. Surgery 1994; 116(1):42–48.

119. Hasslen SR, Nelson RD, Ahrenholz DH, et al. Thermal injury, the inflammatory process, and wound dressing reduce human neutrophil chemotaxis to four attractants. J Burn Care Rehabil 1993; 14(3):303–309.

120. Piccolo MT, Sannomiya P. Inhibition of neutrophil chemotaxis by plasma of burned patients: effect of blood transfusion practice. Burns 1995; 21(8):569–574.

121. Rodeberg DA, Bass RC, Alexander JW, et al. Neutrophils from burn patients are unable to increase the expression of CD11b/CD18 in response to inflammatory stimuli. J Leukoc Biol 1997; 61(5):575–582.

122. Scharton TM, Scott P. Natural killer cells are a source of interferon gamma that drives differentiation of CD4+ T cell subsets and induces early resistance to Leishmania major in mice. J Exp Med 1993; 178(2):567–577.

123. Trinchieri G, Wysocka M, D'Andrea A, et al. Natural killer cell stimulatory factor (NKSF) or interleukin-12 is a key regulator of immune response and inflammation. Prog Growth Factor Res 1992; 4(4):355–368.

124. Cua DJ, Stohlman SA. In vivo effects of T helper cell type 2 cytokines on macrophage antigen-presenting cell induction of T helper subsets. J Immunol 1997; 159(12):5834–5840.

125. Manetti R, Gerosa F, Giudizi MG, et al. Interleukin 12 induces stable priming for interferon gamma (IFN-gamma) production during differentiation of human T helper (Th) cells and transient IFN-gamma production in established Th2 cell clones. J Exp Med 1994; 179(4):1273–1283.

126. Sachse C, Prigge M, Cramer G, et al. Association between reduced human leukocyte antigen (HLA)-DR expression on blood monocytes and increased plasma level of interleukin-10 in patients with severe burns. Clin Chem Lab Med 1999; 37(3):193–198.

127. Zapata-Sirvent RL, Hansbrough JF. Temporal analysis of human leucocyte surface antigen expression and neutrophil respiratory burst activity after thermal injury. Burns 1993; 19(1): 5–11.

128. Kupper TS, Green DR, Durum SK, et al. Defective antigen presentation to a cloned T helper cell by macrophages from burned mice can be restored with interleukin-1. Surgery 1985; 98(2):199–206.

129. Hershman MJ, Sonnenfeld G, Logan WA, et al. Effect of interferon-gamma treatment on the course of a burn wound infection. J Interferon Res 1988; 8(3):367–373.

130. Hultman CS, Cairns BA, Yamamoto H, et al. The 1995 Moyer Award. The effect of burn injury on allograft rejection, alloantigen processing, and cytotoxic T-lymphocyte sensitization. J Burn Care Rehabil 1995; 16(6):573–580.

131. Lyuksutova OI, Murphey ED, Toliver-Kinsky TE, et al. Glucan phosphate treatment attenuates burn-induced inflammation and improves resistance to Pseudomonas aeruginosa burn wound infection. Shock 2005; 23(3):224–232.

132. Pai RK, Convery M, Hamilton TA, et al. Inhibition of IFN-gamma-induced class II transactivator expression by a 19-kDa lipoprotein from Mycobacterium tuberculosis: a potential mechanism for immune evasion. J Immunol 2003; 171(1):175–184.

133. Rioja LF, Alonso P, de Haro J, et al. Prognostic value of the CD4/CD8 lymphocyte ratio in moderately burned patients. Burns 1993; 19(3):198–201.

134. Pratt VC, Tredget EE, Clandinin MT, et al. Alterations in lymphocyte function and relation to phospholipid composition after burn injury in humans. Crit Care Med 2002; 30(8):1753–1761.

135. Sjoberg T, Mzezewa S, Jonsson K, et al. Immune response in burn patients in relation to HIV infection and sepsis. Burns 2004; 30(7):670–674.

136. Teodorczyk-Injeyan JA, Cembrzynska-Nowak M, Lalani S, et al. Immune deficiency following thermal trauma is associated with apoptotic cell death. J Clin Immunol 1995; 15(6):318–328.

137. Schluter B, Konig W, Koller M, et al. Differential regulation of T- and B-lymphocyte activation in severely burned patients. J Trauma 1991; 31(2):239–246.

138. Faist E, Schinkel C, Zimmer S, et al. Inadequate interleukin-2 synthesis and interleukin-2 messenger expression following thermal and mechanical trauma in humans is caused by defective transmembrane signalling. J Trauma 1993; 34(6):846–853.

139. Fukuzuka K, Edwards CK, III, Clare-Salzer M, et al. Glucocorticoid and Fas ligand induced mucosal lymphocyte apoptosis after burn injury. J Trauma 2000; 49(4):710–716.

140. Fukuzuka K, Edwards CK, III, Clare-Salzler M, et al. Glucocorticoid-induced, caspase-dependent organ apoptosis early after burn injury. Am J Physiol Regul Integr Comp Physiol 2000; 278(4): R1005–R1018.

141. Horgan AF, Mendez MV, O'Riordain DS, et al. Altered gene transcription after burn injury results in depressed T-lymphocyte activation. Ann Surg 1994; 220(3):342–351.

142. O'Suilleabhain CB, Kim S, Rodrick MR, et al. Injury induces alterations in T-cell NFkappaB and AP-1 activation. Shock 2001; 15(6):432–437.

143. Phan HH, Cho K, Nelson HA, et al. Downregulation of NF-kappaB activity associated with alteration in proliferative response in the spleen after burn injury. Shock 2005; 23(1):73–79.

144. Teodorczyk-Injeyan JA, Sparkes BG, Mills GB, et al. Immunosuppression follows systemic T lymphocyte activation in the burn patient. Clin Exp Immunol 1991; 85(3):515–518.

145. Teodorczyk-Injeyan JA, Sparkes BG, Mills GB, et al. Impairment of T cell activation in burn patients: a possible mechanism of thermal injury-induced immunosuppression. Clin Exp Immunol 1986; 65(3):570–581.

146. Wolf SE, Woodside KJ, Ramirez RJ, et al. Insulin-like growth factor-I/insulin-like growth factor binding protein-3 alters lymphocyte responsiveness following severe burn. J Surg Res 2004; 117(2):255–261.

147. Zedler S, Faist E, Ostermeier B, et al. Postburn constitutional changes in T-cell reactivity occur in CD8+ rather than in CD4+ cells. J Trauma 1997; 42(5):872–880.

148. Choileain NN, Macconmara M, Zang Y, et al. Enhanced regulatory T cell activity is an element of the host response to injury. J Immunol 2006; 176(1):225–236.

149. Murphy TJ, Choileain NN, Zang Y, et al. CD4+CD25+ regulatory T cells control innate immune reactivity after injury. J Immunol 2005; 174(5):2957–2963.

150. De AK, Kodys K, Puyana JC, et al. Only a subset of trauma patients with depressed mitogen responses have true T cell dysfunctions. Clin Immunol Immunopathol 1997; 82(1):73–82.

151. Hansbrough JF, Field TO Jr, Gadd MA, et al. Immune response modulation after burn injury: T cells and antibodies. J Burn Care Rehabil 1987; 8(6):509–512.

152. Teodorczyk-Injeyan JA, Sparkes BG, Falk RE, et al. Polyclonal immunoglobulin production in burned patients – kinetics and correlations with T-cell activity. J Trauma 1986; 26(9):834–839.

153. Kelly JL, O'Suilleabhain CB, Soberg CC, et al. Severe injury triggers antigen-specific T-helper cell dysfunction. Shock 1999; 12(1):39–45.

154. Molloy RG, Nestor M, Collins KH, et al. The humoral immune response after thermal injury: an experimental model. Surgery 1994; 115(3):341–348.

155. Tabata T, Meyer AA. Immunoglobulin M synthesis after burn injury: the effects of chronic ethanol on postinjury synthesis. J Burn Care Rehabil 1995; 16(4):400–406.

156. Yamamoto H, Siltharm S, DeSerres S, et al. Effect of cyclooxygenase inhibition on in vitro B-cell function after burn injury. J Trauma 1996; 41(4):612–619.

157. Ishikawa K, Nishimura T, DeSerres S, et al. The effects of transforming growth factor-beta neutralization on postburn humoral immunity. J Trauma 2004; 57(3):529–536.

158. Nishimura T, Yamamoto H, DeSerres S, et al. Transforming growth factor-beta impairs postburn immunoglobulin production by limiting B-cell proliferation, but not cellular synthesis. J Trauma 1999; 46(5):881–885.

159. Peterson V, Hansbrough J, Buerk C, et al. Regulation of granulopoiesis following severe thermal injury. J Trauma 1983; 23(1):19–24.

160. Noel JG, Valente JF, Ogle JD, et al. Changes in bone marrow-derived myeloid cells from thermally injured rats reflect changes in the progenitor cell population. J Burn Care Rehabil 2002; 23(2):75–86.

161. Santangelo S, Gamelli RL, Shankar R. Myeloid commitment shifts toward monocytopoiesis after thermal injury and sepsis. Ann Surg 2001; 233(1):97–106.

162. Cohen MJ, Shankar R, Stevenson J, et al. Bone marrow norepinephrine mediates development of functionally different macrophages after thermal injury and sepsis. Ann Surg 2004; 240(1):132–141.

163. Peng YZ, Yuan ZQ, Xiao GX. Effects of early enteral feeding on the prevention of enterogenic infection in severely burned patients. Burns 2001; 27(2):145–149.

164. Berger MM, Spertini F, Shenkin A, et al. Trace element supplementation modulates pulmonary infection rates after major burns: a double-blind, placebo-controlled trial. Am J Clin Nutr 1998; 68(2):365–371.

165. Garrel D, Patenaude J, Nedelec B, et al. Decreased mortality and infectious morbidity in adult burn patients given enteral glutamine supplements: a prospective, controlled, randomized clinical trial. Crit Care Med 2003; 31(10):2444–2449.

166. Shang HF, Tsai HJ, Chiu WC, et al. Effects of dietary arginine supplementation on antibody production and antioxidant enzyme activity in burned mice. Burns 2003; 29(1):43–48.

167. Yao YM, Lu LR, Yu Y, et al. Influence of selective decontamination of the digestive tract on cell-mediated immune function and bacteria/endotoxin translocation in thermally injured rats. J Trauma 1997; 42(6):1073–1079.

168. Barret JP, Jeschke MG, Herndon DN. Selective decontamination of the digestive tract in severely burned pediatric patients. Burns 2001; 27(5):439–445.

169. de La Cal MA, Cerda E, Garcia-Hierro P, et al. Survival benefit in critically ill burned patients receiving selective decontamina-

tion of the digestive tract: a randomized, placebo-controlled, double-blind trial. Ann Surg 2005; 241(3):424–430.

170. Nance FC, Hines JL, Fulton RE, et al. Treatment of experimental burn wound sepsis by postburn immunization with polyvalent Pseudomonas antigen. Surgery 1970; 68(1):248–253.

171. Holder IA, Neely AN, Frank DW. PcrV immunization enhances survival of burned Pseudomonas aeruginosa-infected mice. Infect Immun 2001; 69(9):5908–5910.

172. Roe EA, Jones RJ. Active and passive immunization against Pseudomonas aeruginosa infection of burned patients. Burns Incl Therm Inj 1983; 9(6):433–439.

173. Baumann U, Mansouri E, von Specht BU. Recombinant OprF-OprI as a vaccine against Pseudomonas aeruginosa infections. Vaccine 2004; 22(7):840–847.

174. Kim DK, Kim JJ, Kim JH, et al. Comparison of two immunization schedules for a Pseudomonas aeruginosa outer membrane proteins vaccine in burn patients. Vaccine 2000; 19(9–10):1274–1283.

175. Lee NG, Jung SB, Ahn BY, et al. Immunization of burn-patients with a Pseudomonas aeruginosa outer membrane protein vaccine elicits antibodies with protective efficacy. Vaccine 2000; 18(18):1952–1961.

176. Mansouri E, Blome-Eberwein S, Gabelsberger J, et al. Clinical study to assess the immunogenicity and safety of a recombinant Pseudomonas aeruginosa OprF-OprI vaccine in burn patients. FEMS Immunol Med Microbiol 2003; 37(2–3):161–166.

177. Polk HC Jr, Cheadle WG, Livingston DH, et al. A randomized prospective clinical trial to determine the efficacy of interferon-gamma in severely injured patients. Am J Surg 1992; 163(2):191–196.

178. Wasserman D, Ioannovich JD, Hinzmann RD, et al. Interferon-gamma in the prevention of severe burn-related infections: a European phase III multicenter trial. The Severe Burns Study Group. Crit Care Med 1998; 26(3):434–439.

179. Goebel A, Kavanagh E, Lyons A, et al. Injury induces deficient interleukin-12 production, but interleukin-12 therapy after injury restores resistance to infection. Ann Surg 2000; 231(2):253–261.

180. O'Suilleabhain C, O'Sullivan ST, Kelly JL, et al. Interleukin-12 treatment restores normal resistance to bacterial challenge after burn injury. Surgery 1996; 120(2):290–296.

181. Pockros PJ, Patel K, O'Brien C, et al. A multicenter study of recombinant human interleukin 12 for the treatment of chronic hepatitis C virus infection in patients nonresponsive to previous therapy. Hepatology 2003; 37(6):1368–1374.

182. Wadler S, Levy D, Frederickson HL, et al. A phase II trial of interleukin-12 in patients with advanced cervical cancer: clinical and immunologic correlates. Eastern Cooperative Oncology Group study E1E96. Gynecol Oncol 2004; 92(3):957–964.

183. Lyons A, Goebel A, Mannick JA, et al. Protective effects of early interleukin 10 antagonism on injury-induced immune dysfunction. Arch Surg 1999; 134(12):1317–1323.

184. O'Riordain MG, O'Riordain DS, Molloy RG, et al. Dosage and timing of anti-TNF-alpha antibody treatment determine its effect of resistance to sepsis after injury. J Surg Res 1996; 64(1):95–101.

185. Gamelli RL, He LK, Liu H. Recombinant human granulocyte colony-stimulating factor treatment improves macrophage suppression of granulocyte and macrophage growth after burn and burn wound infection. J Trauma 1995; 39(6):1141–1146.

186. Molloy RG, Holzheimer R, Nestor M, et al. Granulocyte-macrophage colony-stimulating factor modulates immune function and improves survival after experimental thermal injury. Br J Surg 1995; 82(6):770–776.

187. Cioffi WG Jr, Burleson DG, Jordan BS, et al. Effects of granulocyte-macrophage colony-stimulating factor in burn patients. Arch Surg 1991; 126(1):74–79.

188. Toliver-Kinsky TE, Cui W, Murphey ED, et al. Enhancement of dendritic cell production by fms-like tyrosine kinase-3 ligand increases the resistance of mice to a burn wound infection. J Immunol 2005; 174(1):404–410.

189. De AK, Laudanski K, Miller-Graziano CL. Failure of monocytes of trauma patients to convert to immature dendritic cells is related to preferential macrophage-colony-stimulating factor-driven macrophage differentiation. J Immunol 2003; 170(12):6355–6362.

190. Hotchkiss RS, Tinsley KW, Swanson PE, et al. Depletion of dendritic cells, but not macrophages, in patients with sepsis. J Immunol 2002; 168(5):2493–2500.

191. Disis ML, Rinn K, Knutson KL, et al. Flt3 ligand as a vaccine adjuvant in association with HER-2/neu peptide-based vaccines in patients with HER-2/neu-overexpressing cancers. Blood 2002; 99(8):2845–2850.

192. Maraskovsky E, Daro E, Roux E, et al. In vivo generation of human dendritic cell subsets by Flt3 ligand. Blood 2000; 96(3):878–884.

193. Rini BI, Paintal A, Vogelzang NJ, et al. Flt-3 ligand and sequential FL/interleukin-2 in patients with metastatic renal carcinoma: clinical and biologic activity. J Immunother 2002; 25(3):269–277.

194. Browder W, Williams D, Pretus H, et al. Beneficial effect of enhanced macrophage function in the trauma patient. Ann Surg 1990; 211(5):605–612.

195. Williams DL, Li C, Ha T, Ozment-Skelton T, et al. Modulation of the phosphoinositide 3-kinase pathway alters innate resistance to polymicrobial sepsis. J Immunol 2004; 172(1):449–456.

196. Babineau TJ, Marcello P, Swails W, et al. Randomized phase I/II trial of a macrophage-specific immunomodulator (PGG-glucan) in high-risk surgical patients. Ann Surg 1994; 220(5):601–609.

197. de Felippe JJ, da Rocha e Silva Junior, Maciel FM, et al. Infection prevention in patients with severe multiple trauma with the immunomodulator beta 1–3 polyglucose (glucan). Surg Gynecol Obstet 1993; 177(4):383–388.

198. Loomis WH, Namiki S, Hoyt DB, et al. Hypertonicity rescues T cells from suppression by trauma-induced anti-inflammatory mediators. Am J Physiol Cell Physiol 2001; 281(3):C840–C848.

199. Coimbra R, Hoyt DB, Junger WG, et al. Hypertonic saline resuscitation decreases susceptibility to sepsis after hemorrhagic shock. J Trauma 1997; 42(4):602–606.

200. Junger WG, Hoyt DB, Davis RE, et al. Hypertonicity regulates the function of human neutrophils by modulating chemoattractant receptor signaling and activating mitogen-activated protein kinase p38. J Clin Invest 1998; 101(12):2768–2779.

201. Shukla A, Hashiguchi N, Chen Y, et al. Osmotic regulation of cell function and possible clinical applications. Shock 2004; 21(5):391–400.

202. Griswold JA, Anglin BL, Love RT Jr, et al. Hypertonic saline resuscitation: efficacy in a community-based burn unit. South Med J 1991; 84(6):692–696.

203. Murphy JT, Horton JW, Purdue GF, et al. Cardiovascular effect of 7.5% sodium chloride-dextran infusion after thermal injury. Arch Surg 1999; 134(10):1091–1097.

204. Shimazaki S, Yukioka T, Matuda H. Fluid distribution and pulmonary dysfunction following burn shock. J Trauma 1991; 31(5):623–626.

205. Milner SM, Ortega MR. Reduced antimicrobial peptide expression in human burn wounds. Burns 1999; 25(5):411–413.

206. Jacobsen F, Mittler D, Hirsch T, et al. Transient cutaneous adenoviral gene therapy with human host defense peptide hCAP-18/LL-37 is effective for the treatment of burn wound infections. Gene Ther 2005; 12(20):1494–1502.

Chapter 24

Hematologic, hematopoietic, and acute phase responses

Jason W. Smith, Richard L. Gamelli, and Ravi Shankar

Chapter contents

Introduction

Although our ability to care for major burns has improved over the last two decades, mortality due to septic complications still remains a major threat to the survival of severely injured patients. General physiological and cellular changes that occur immediately following a burn injury are not only important for the initial survival of the injured patients but also act as triggers for initiating the inflammatory response. Much of our understanding of the pathophysiology of burn injury has come from advances in the biology of inflammation. Well-regulated inflammation to any given insult including burn trauma is an essential part of the healing process. The inflammatory reaction allows the recruitment of leukocytes, antibodies, and other serum proteins to the site of injury which initiates the wound healing process[1,2] and serves to localize and eradicate microbial infection.[3] While controlled inflammation is an essential part of the 'healing process', uncontrolled systemic inflammatory responses, often seen during prolonged hospitalization of severely injured burn patients, represents a generalized response to trauma and can result in derangements in immune function.[4,5]

Fundamental alterations and derangements in the function and production of leukocytes and erythrocytes occur after burn injury. The primary focus of this chapter is to highlight current understanding of how severe thermal injury precipitates these hematologic and hematopoietic changes. Within this framework, we discuss recent advances in the cellular and molecular biology that have helped shed new insights into burn biology. In particular, we outline the cellular and molecu- lar mechanisms that are responsible for the dysregulated inflammatory changes that occur following severe burn injury. Lastly, we will describe how hematopoietic transcription factors can potentially play a role in the hematopoietic changes observed following severe thermal injury.

Red blood cells and erythropoiesis

Almost all hematologic parameters are significantly affected by severe burns in a characteristic biphasic manner. Following burns that are greater than 10% total body surface area (TBSA), anemia is frequently present.[6,7] The extent of anemia due to erythrocyte loss is directly proportional to the extent of the initial injury. It is estimated that patients with 15–40% full-thickness burn lose approximately 12% of their red cells within 6 hours of the injury, and as much as 18% in 24 hours.[7] Patients with severe burns continue to loose red blood cells at the rate of 1–2% per day until the burn wound is healed, primarily as a result of blood loss through multiple surgical procedures and repeated blood draws for various hematologic and biochemical tests.[6,8–10]

Several factors could explain the early onset of anemia in burn patients. First, acute red blood cell destruction occurs as a direct result of thermal injury. Secondly, extensive burns induce the formation of thrombi within the capillaries, arterioles, and venules due to the activation of complement and coagulation cascades.[11] The amount of small vessel thrombosis that results is directly proportional to the size of the burn; thus for burns of similar depth, larger burns produce a greater prothrombogenic effect. Additionally, loss of red blood cell mass can arise from burn-induced intrinsic and extrinsic alterations to the erythrocytes. Previous studies have shown that thermal energy damages the normal morphology of red blood cells not only at the site of burn wound but also within the peripheral circulation.[12,13] Systemically released oxygen free radicals and proteases from the inflammatory cells can also damage the integrity of red blood cell membrane.[13] It is hypothesized that the burn wound triggers the release of these biological mediators that compromise the integrity of red blood cell membranes to induce osmotic fragility and loss of membrane deformability. These changes in red blood cell membrane property manifest themselves as increased spherocytosis, membrane disruption, and vesiculation of erythrocytes and are apparent within a short time following severe thermal injury.[14,15] Animal studies have shown that removal of female sex hormones worsens the severity of the changes in the RBC membranes, but that the addition or subtraction of male sex hormones has no effect on membrane fragility.[16,17] If these cell membrane defects continue it may lead to red cell lysis and an increase in acute hemoglobinuria.[14,18]

Paradoxically, despite the initial and continued loss of red blood cells following burns, erythrocytosis and an increase in hematocrit are often observed in the acute phase of burn injury.[18,19] The loss of plasma volume into the extracellular space, or hemoconcentration, is the primary reason for this observed effect following thermal injury.[20,21] Nevertheless, the long-term postburn period is characterized by diminished red cell production. Under normal conditions, blood loss would stimulate the bone marrow to produce more erythrocytes. A major factor in the induction of bone marrow erythropoiesis or red blood cell production is the availability of the growth factor erythropoietin. Interestingly, despite the high circulating levels of erythropoietin, burn patients remain anemic. The defect appears to be in the ability of erythroid progenitor cells in the bone marrow to respond adequately to erythropoietin.[10,22–25] The use of exogenous erythropoietin to try and stimulate increased RBC production in these patients has not been shown to improve outcomes or change hemoglobin, hematocrit or reticulocyte counts, except in small surface area burns.[26] A possible explanation for this hyporesponsiveness is the high circulating levels of cytokines such as tumor necrosis factor-α (TNFα) and interleukin-1 (IL-1), which are often seen in severe burns. These cytokines can retard erythropoiesis by disrupting the physiologic regulation between erythropoietin and hemoglobin levels in erythroid progenitor cells.[27] Evidence from the cardiac surgery literature supports the relationship between an elevation in these cytokines and persistent anemia, which is associated with delayed RBC maturation and decreased responsiveness to erythropoietin.[28]

Burn patients may have reduced serum iron levels due to substantial loss of blood and repeated surgical procedures for purposes of skin grafting and debridement of the burn wound.[8,10,22] This reduction in serum iron levels may act as an impediment to hemoglobin synthesis and hence erythropoiesis. However, serum iron levels are unlikely to be the sole cause of burn-induced anemia, particularly among patients receiving blood transfusions during their course of burn care. Other potential explanations exist for burn-induced anemia. For example, the bone marrow's unresponsiveness to erythropoietin can stem from a yet unidentified serum factor, termed erythropoietin inhibitory factor, that inhibits erythropoietin's action on erythroid progenitor cells.[10,22,24,29] Glucocorticoids have been shown to play an important role in stress-induced erythropoiesis.[30] In burn patients and in animal models of thermal injury, high circulating levels of glucocorticoids occur simultaneously with anemia, which suggests the potential for signaling defects in erythroid differentiation in severe thermal injury. In non-burn trauma patients there is a similar failure of hematopoiesis and late, persistent anemia associated with bone marrow failure.[31] There is rodent and primate model evidence to suggest that preventing exposure to mesenteric lymph, by diverting the thoracic duct lymph flow, after severe injury, may prevent bone marrow failure and protect against injury-induced lung dysfunction.[32,33] Hence, the anemia that is observed following burns results from several factors that cause increased red blood cell destruction in the periphery and decreased production of mature red blood cells from the bone marrow.

Platelets and coagulation cascade in burns

Advances in burn and trauma care have allowed for increased success in areas of resuscitation and control of hemorrhage. It is now becoming clear that there are also elements of deranged coagulation that lead to hypercoagulability and the accumulation of thrombi in the microcirculation which contribute to the development of end-organ failure and death.[34,35] Dysregulated coagulation occurs through altered platelet maturation and function, changes in the proteins of the coagulation cascade and imbalances in the deposition and dissolution of peripheral clots.

Thermal injury causes marked reduction in circulating platelet levels during the acute phase of burn resuscitation, primarily due to the consumption of platelets during the formation of systemic microthrombi.[36,37] Although local microthrombi formation at the site of injury helps maintain the integrity of the microvasculature surrounding the burn wound, generalized systemic microthrombi formation leads to reduced end-organ perfusion and finally multiple organ failure.[35,36] In addition, dilutional effects of extensive fluid resuscitation may also contribute to a reduction in platelet counts. After the initial resuscitation, thrombocytopenia that is observed during the first week following the thermal injury is believed to be due to the diminished half-lives of platelets in circulation.[37] The thrombocytopenic phase is subsequently followed by a period of increased platelet production or bone marrow megakaryocytopoiesis during the 2–3 weeks following the initial injury that results in either a return to normal levels or to overt thrombocytosis.[38] However, in some burn patients, thrombocytopenia persists and is often considered a poor prognostic indicator.[39] Among patients with critical burn injuries who develop intravascular hemolysis an apparent thrombocytosis may be observed, which could be due to inadvertent counting of fragmented red cells and red cell microvesicles as platelets in an automated counter.[38] Therefore, in severe burns, the clinician should be aware of the possibility of spurious platelet counts in the presence of intravascular hemolysis.

In addition to the observed changes in the platelet numbers, there are significant alterations in the concentrations of coagulation proteins following thermal injury. The interplay amongst antithrombotic, prothrombotic cellular interactions, and fibrinolytic processes within the vasculature intricately control the homeostatic regulation of coagulation. Under normal physiologic conditions, the fluidity of the blood is maintained by morphological integrity of erythrocytes and the endothelial cells lining the blood vessels.[15] Normal levels of prothrombotic and antithrombotic factors, which are well regulated and remain for the most part in their quiescent state, also help maintain the homeostatic balance. In burn patients, however, both the thrombotic and fibrinolytic pathways are triggered in direct proportion to the extent of the injury.[40–42] During the early resuscitation phase of a burn injury there is a general reduction in the levels of coagulation proteins.[40] Dilutional effects of volume administration during this period and the loss of plasma proteins to the interstitium could partially explain the decrease in plasma concentrations of many coagulation proteins. This phase, however, appears to be transient in most patients as clotting factors return to normal levels 1 week post-burn.[36] Many patients suffering from major burn injuries develop a hypercoagulable state later in the postburn course, with an increase in thrombotic complications.[40] Clinical studies indicate that, in addition to elevated coagulation factors, levels of antithrombotic proteins such as antithrombin III, protein S, and protein C are decreased in burn patients.[36,40,43] These alterations prevent the normal checks on intravascular coagulation and tip the balance toward a hypercoagulable state. A significant number of studies have looked at different treatments aimed at offsetting this hypercoagulable state or replacing depleted elements of the natural anticoagulant proteins. Heparin, an extracellular matrix glycosaminoglycan, has been widely studied for anticoagulant, as well as anti-inflammatory, properties. The evidence suggests that there is a role for therapeutic doses of heparin in the care of serious burn injuries when other contraindications are not present. The benefits seem to be primarily as an anti-inflammatory agent, preventing the ongoing activation inflammation at the burn site and systemically.[43,44] Antithrombin III (ATIII) is a serine protease inhibitor that regulates hemostasis and has been shown to have anti-inflammatory properties.[45] ATIII is depleted after burn injuries as both coagulation and fibrinolysis are activated simultaneously.[46] Administration of exogenous antithrombin III to burn patients has been shown to be beneficial in reversing thrombogenicity and decreasing mortality, while animal models have suggested a role for this agent in attenuating pulmonary inflammation.[41,42,45,46]

Fibrinolytic pathways are activated in burn injuries due to the increased levels of tissue plasminogen activator protein.[40] Consumption of antithrombotic proteins by activation of fibrinolytic activities predisposes burn patients to thrombosis. Contributing to the thrombotic state in severely injured burn patients are the release of tissue phospholipids and tissue factor, activation of complement cascade, tissue ischemia, and the presence of sepsis.[36,39,40,47] As a result, patients are at increased risk for developing disseminated intravascular coagulation (DIC), which is characterized by activation of coagulation, intravascular fibrin formation and vascular thrombosis resulting in organ hypoperfusion and failure. The consumption of coagulation and anticoagulation factors leads to small vessel thrombosis and simultaneous uncontrolled bleeding.[35] It has been reported from postmortem studies that 30% of severely burned patients exhibit pathological findings of DIC with extensive microthrombi accumulation in all major organ systems. The clinical scenarios in which the autopsy evidence of DIC was present were patients with massive burns, delayed presentation, hypotension, acidosis, and/or hypothermia.[48] Retrospective clinical studies, however, report the incidence of clinically significant DIC in burns over 20% TBSA to be less than 1%.[49] Due to the high morbidity and mortality associated with episodes of DIC, a high index of suspicion needs to be maintained in this patient population when sepsis complicates the clinical course. Signs of impending DIC may include refractory shock out of proportion to apparent blood loss, bleeding from venipuncture and catheter sites and urinary and gastrointestinal bleeding. Standard laboratory values in patients with suspected DIC include prolonged prothrombin time (PT) and activated partial thromboplastin time (APTT), increased levels of fibrinogen degradation products, decreased levels of antithrombin III, and decreased platelet counts and fibrinogen levels. Vigilence must be maintained for other thromboembolic complications in this population such as deep vein thrombosis and pulmonary embolism The use of D-dimer levels has been shown to have a high negative predictive value in selecting populations for more thorough investigation.[50] The treatment modalities recommended for patients that develop DIC are primarily supportive and geared toward maintaining hemostatic parameters with replacement therapy. Future efforts in the treatment of this disease process will focus on re-establishing the balance of coagulation and fibrinolysis.[35]

Acute phase proteins

The body's reaction to injury involves the initiation of host defenses including the synthesis and release of acute phase proteins.[51] The clinical manifestations of the acute phase response include leukocytosis, fever, increased vascular permeability, increases in metabolic responses and stimulation of nonspecific host defense.[52,53] The acute phase proteins mediate these effects and therefore play a key role in protecting cells and tissues from progressive cellular injury and in restoring homeostasis (Table 24.1).[52] Acute phase proteins serve as mediators of the inflammatory process, function as transport proteins, and participate in burn wound healing.[54,55] In response to burn injury, an acute phase response also results in the activation of coagulation and complement cascades, activation of granulocytes and monocyte/macrophages, platelets, endothelial cells and fibroblasts.[36,37,56–59] The orchestration of coordinated activation is the production of proinflammatory cytokines from the burn wound and from leukocytes recruited to the wound.[51,60,61] The acute phase response stimulates the hypothalamus, which leads to pyrexia and activates the pituitary–adrenal axis to release steroid hormones.[52,62] More importantly, it induces the liver to synthesize and release acute phase proteins capable of exerting pleiotropic effects on many tissues.[52] During an acute illness or a significant injury, such as a burn injury, enhanced production of acute phase proteins serves to stimulate the healing process and is sustained by proinflammatory cytokines.[55] However, prolongation of the acute phase response and the unabated production of acute phase proteins are detrimental and can lead to a hypermetabolic state, multiple organ failure, and death.[61,63–65] The scenario is complicated by the fact that increase in acute phase proteins is sustained at the expense of constitutive hepatic proteins, propagating a vicious cycle of detrimental effects.[65–67]

Specific acute phase proteins that have been shown to be elevated in thermal injury include C-reactive protein, serum amyloid A, α_1-acid glycoprotein, α_1-antitrypsin, fibrinogen, haptoglobin, ceruloplasmin, α_1-chymotrypsin, and α_2-macroglobin.[55,68–74] Levels of constitutive proteins such as albumin, transferrin, and α_1-lipoprotein have been shown to decrease after thermal injury.[52,74–77] Generally, the greater the size of the burn, the greater is the change in acute phase proteins; however, even minor thermal burns can lead to alterations in acute phase protein.[58,78,79] The induction of acute phase proteins is driven by the proinflammatory cytokines IL-1, IL-6, and TNFα levels, with IL-6 having the most direct and significant effect.[76] IL-6 directly stimulates the production of C-reactive proteins, ceruloplasmin, haptoglobins, fibrinogen α_1-antitrypsin, and α_1-acid glycoprotein on the one hand and depresses the synthesis of hepatic constitutive proteins such as albumin, fibronectin, and

TABLE 24.1 STATUS OF ACUTE PHASE PROTEIN RESPONSE FOLLOWING THERMAL INJURY

Acute phase protein	Levels	Functions
C-reactive protein	Increased	Opsonin, complement activation, and immune modulation
Serum amyloid A	Increased	Leukocyte chemotaxis and phagocytosis
α_1-antitrypsin	Increased	Protease inhibitor of elastase and trypsin
α_1-antichymotrypsin	Increased	Inhibits chymotrypsin
α_1-acid glycoprotein	Increased	Immunomodulator, potential wound healing properties, decreases albumin clearance from circulation, transport protein, steroid binding
α_1-antiplasmin	Increased	Protease inhibitor of fibrinolysis
Ceruloplasmin	Increased	Copper transport protein, potential antioxidant properties
Haptoglobin	Increased	Hemoglobin scavenger
Fibrinogen	Increased	Mediate coagulation
C_1 inhibitor	Increased	Complement inactivation opsonization
Complement-C_3	Increased	Complement activation
α_2-macroglobulin	Decreased	Transports zinc, panproteinase inhibitor, binds growth factors and cytokines and targets them toward particular cells
α_1-lipoprotein	Decreased	Transport protein
Transferrin	Decreased	Iron transport

Reproduced from Kushner I. The phenomenon of the acute phase response. Ann N Y Acad Sci 1982; 389:39–48.[52]

transferrin on the other.[52,75] While IL-6 is the prime mediator of the acute phase response, TNFα and IL-1 play a subsidiary role through their ability to stimulate IL-6 production.[75,77] Acute phase proteins are essential in the wound healing and host defense processes, but when production becomes unregulated to the point that systemic changes in inflammatory cell function take place, the unchecked immune cell activation can have deleterious effects on the host.

Aside from its role as a regulator of acute phase protein production, IL-6 is also considered a prognostic indicator in burn patients.[79,80] Clinical studies have demonstrated that non-survivors of major burn injuries have higher levels of IL-6 than do survivors of similar burn injuries. It is hypothesized that in non-survivors acute phase protein production becomes unresponsive to IL-6 and the cytokine continues to be up-regulated because of the lack of negative feedback.[80–82] Additionally, prostaglandins, activated complement factors, cortisol, neuroendocrine, and other hormones have been implicated in the activation of acute phase proteins.[83] Future studies on the role of cytokines in the regulation and functions of acute phase proteins will add insights into their role as physiological mediators and points in the activation sequence that may allow therapeutic intervention.

Since the overproduction of proinflammatory cytokines may lead to unchecked systemic inflammation and poor outcomes, several clinical trials have been undertaken to investigate methods to attenuate the rise in these cytokines and acute phase proteins.[59,63,67,84,85] Failures of these trials clearly indicate that such anti-cytokine antibody monotherapies are not likely to be useful in modifying and controlling the prolonged acute phase response. Broader therapeutic modalities aimed at simultaneously enhancing the constitutive production of hepatic proteins (e.g. albumin, fibronectin) while inhibiting acute phase protein expression have been shown to be benefi-

cial both in animal models of thermal injury and in burn patients.[55,67–69,72,86,87] Administration of growth hormone to thermally injured rats with 40% TBSA burns decreases α1-acid glycoprotein mRNA expression and protein levels while reversing the decline in albumin production.[69] In severely burned pediatric patients, administration of recombinant human growth hormone (GH) was able to decrease the production of acute phase protein and serum TNFα and IL-1β levels without any effect on IL-6.[55] This protocol, however, did not influence the mortality rate in these studies. Since recombinant GH exerts some of its effects through its ability to stimulate insulinlike growth factor 1 (IGF-1), administration of a combination of IGF-1 and IGF-binding protein 3 (IGFBP3) was attempted as a therapeutic modality to control acute phase response in severely burned children. Similar to rGH administration, infusion of IGF-1/IGFBP3 decreased IL-1β and TNFα levels as well as type I acute phase protein production in burn patients, while increasing constitutive hepatic protein production. Interestingly, administration of cholesterol containing cationic liposomes used in gene delivery systems have been shown to attenuate the acute phase response in thermally injured rats.[88] Given the deleterious effect of unabated and prolonged acute phase response following severe burns, continued improvements in therapeutic modalities aimed at regulating this response may develop into additional tools in the care of burn and critically injured patients.

Leukocytes and burn injury

The primary effectors of host defense are the main populations of leukocytes, lymphocytes, NK cells, polymorphonuclear cells (PMN), and monocytes/macrophages. A balanced activation of these cells is important for robust host defense. Inappropriate activation of these leukocytes, especially the PMN and macrophages, can lead to tissue destruction and systemic inflammation with dire consequences to the burn patient. Over-activation of PMN and macrophages has been implicated in the development of adult respiratory distress syndrome (ARDS) and multiple organ failure.[59,89–95]

In the first 24–48 hours following burns, a leukocytosis, and more specifically a granulocytosis, is generally observed that is dependent on the size of the burn wound, with the larger burns giving rise to a greater degree of leukocytosis.[96] The initial increase in the white blood cell count (WBC) is attributable to three major factors: the acute plasma volume loss due to the burns, demargination of mature neutrophils from peripheral blood vessels, and the rapid release of bone marrow reserves. Following this initial period of leukocytosis, burn patients frequently develop leukopenia which is related to a trauma-induced failure bone marrow hematopoiesis.[31] Leukopenia is also frequently seen in burn patients whose wounds are treated with silver sulfadiazine, a common topical antimicrobial agent.[97] The severity of the leukopenia that develops from drug toxicity is directly proportional to the amount of agent that is applied to the wound and thus indirectly to the size of the burn wounds themselves. The mechanism underlying this drug-induced leukopenia is yet to be elucidated although direct bone marrow and cellular toxicity may play a role. In general, leukopenia is self-limiting and does not require discontinuation of silver sulfadiazine treatment.

Leukopenia and granulocytopenia often persist in patients when severe bacterial infection is superimposed on burn injuries, especially those with Gram-negative sepsis.[57,98,99] In the early 1970s, Newsome and Eurenius demonstrated that the initial granulocytosis was due to demargination of PMN from the blood vessels and through accelerated release of bone marrow stores in their rat model of thermal injury.[100] This granulocytosis, however, is transient and is followed by a robust bone marrow response to replenish granulocyte stores.[101–103] If the burn injury is complicated by sepsis, granulocytopenia persists.[104,105] Granulocytopenia under these conditions appears to be due to bone marrow failure.[103,104,106,107] McEuen demonstrated a significant inhibition of granulocyte colony-forming units in the bone marrow of burn septic rats.[106] In addition, serum from septic burn-injured animals retarded the granulocyte colony formation when added to bone marrow cells from normal non-septic animals.[102] In septic animals and in burn patients with sepsis, the observed granulocytopenia is not likely due to lack of available colony-stimulating factor. Granulocyte colony-stimulating factor (G-CSF) is the primary growth factor responsible for the proliferation and differentiation of bone marrow granulocyte progenitors into mature granulocytes.[108,109] In thermal injury and sepsis, the activation of macrophages, endothelial cells, and fibroblast by bacterial products and cytokines such as TNFα and IL-1 leads to increased production of G-CSF. This scenario is very similar to that seen with erythropoietin levels following thermal injury. Administration of recombinant G-CSF to burn septic animals prior to the initiation of septic insult has been shown to improve the survival rate of the burn septic mice.[110–112] However, administration of G-CSF 24 hours after the onset of septic insult had little effect on their survival.[113,114] G-CSF has been employed in cases of severely burned patients with refractory neutropenia, in particular with active HIV disease.

In addition to alterations in the kinetics of production and maturation, PMN exhibit qualitative functional changes after burn injury in animals and humans.[115–118] Some of the documented functional changes include depressed chemotaxis, phagocytosis and intracellular killing.[119–127] For example, isolated neutrophils of burn patients were shown to be defective in intracellular killing of *Pseudomonas aeruginosa* and the impairment in phagocytosis and intracellular killing are further exacerbated with sepsis.[128,129] These alterations in the production and function of PMN provide for a framework for understanding the contributing factors in the depressed immune status of severely burned patients.

Monocyte/macrophage function is also altered following severe burns, but unlike PMN where neutropenia is common, in severe burns and sepsis, monocyte counts tend to increase in both animals and humans.[24,98,130] Studies demonstrate marked monocytosis with a dramatic increase (3–5-fold) associated with sepsis.[130,131] The importance of the burn-induced monocytosis is underscored by the observation that attenuation of monocytosis as well as blunted macrophage activation results in improved survival.[132] Miller-Grazziano and Faist demonstrated that after trauma, including burns, monocyte/ macrophages could be broken down into subsets that were either hyperreactive or hyporeactive.[133,134] These cells may develop their phenotypic differences as a result of an altered monocytopoietic program within the bone marrow itself or as a result of local cytokine environments in the peripheral tissues. Ogle et al. have demonstrated that bone marrow-derived macrophages from thermal injured animals produce increased amounts of TNFα, IL-1, and PGE$_2$ compared to macrophages from non-injured animals, suggesting that thermal injury can stimulate the development of functionally different monocytes within the bone marrow.[135,136]

Patients with severe burns often suffer from suppressed cell-mediated immunity due to impairment in T cell functions.[137,138] Impairment in cell-mediated immunity has been implied by observations of delay in skin allograft rejection, suppression of the graft versus host response, and skin hypersensitivity reactions in burn patients.[139–141] The various alterations that have been reported include an overall suppression of circulating T lymphocytes, decreased mitogenesis in response to mitogens, reduced response to antigenic stimulation or activation, and redistribution of T lymphocytes within peripheral blood and tissue compartments.[138,142–144] T lymphocytes are divided into T$_{helper}$ and T$_{suppressor}$ populations based on expression of lymphokine profiles, cell surface receptors, and ability to affect functions of NK cells, T$_{cytotoxic}$ and B lymphocytes. In recent years strong evidence has emerged to support the hypothesis that burn injury-induced immune suppression is in part mediated by a shift in lymphocyte subpopulations from T$_{helper}$ to T$_{suppressor}$ subtypes.[137,139,140] Part of the initial response to a significant burn is the activation of T$_{helper}$ cells as assayed by IL-2R, HLA-2R, and transferrin receptor markers.[145,146] *In vitro* functional assays reveal that despite the initial activation of T cells, they were unable to respond to mitogenic and/or antigenic stimulation. The addition of IL-2 fails to reverse T cell anergy and fails to relieve the suppression of IL-2R.[147] In addition, thermal injury triggers the apoptotic pathway in T cells.[148,149] The exact mechanisms that initiate T lymphocyte apoptosis are still unclear. However, Fas ligand, TNFα, and

IL-2 mediated pathways have been implicated in T lymphocyte cell death.[150,151] Lastly, macrophage activation products such as PGE$_2$ and tumor transforming growth factor-β (TGFβ) can also contribute T cell suppression.

B lymphocytes also undergo functional changes with a profound reduction in immuglobin levels following thermal injury. All classes of immunoglobulins are reduced; however, IgG levels display the greatest reduction, with concentrations reaching as low as 300–400 mg/dL.[152–155] This drop in immunoglobulin is rapid and early, and is attributed to plasma leakage, increased protein turnover, and decreased IgG synthesis by the B cells. The initial deficit in immunoglobulins is slowly replenished to near-normal levels within 2 weeks.[140] Major histocompatibility complex (MHC) glycoproteins are reduced after thermal injury. Nonspecific B cell activation by burn toxins and antigen-dependent mechanisms, activation by phagocytosis of non-specific antigen, may inhibit their ability to form antigen-MHC complexes.[156] Additionally, the display of self-antigens by the B lymphocytes could contribute to antigen-dependent cell death of T lymphocytes and T cell anergy.[138,140] Previous work has shown that CD23 expression on activated B cells is abrogated in response to thermal injury.[157] IL-7 levels rise during the 1-week postburn and could account for the decreased proliferative capacity of mature B lymphocytes. Taken together, these data indicate that the functional alterations in B cells induced by thermal injury could further exacerbate the immune suppression in these high-risk patients.

Hematopoiesis and burns

Pressure is placed on the hematologic system in severely burned patients as a result of extensive tissue necrosis, fluid balance alterations, infections and repeated surgical interventions. Bone marrow hematopoiesis responds to this demand by replacing or providing additional blood cells to the circulation. A robust hematopoietic response with a balanced production of the different blood elements is required for adequate immune response, host defense and hemostasis in burn patients. In order to understand the dynamic response of the bone marrow to burn injury, a basic understanding of hematopoiesis is essential. Hematopoiesis is a dynamic orchestration of cellular events that follows a series of tightly coupled proliferation and differentiation signals. In this paradigm, the pluripotent hematopoietic stem cells (HSCs) give rise to erythrocytes, megakaryocytes, mature T cells and B cells, and cells of myeloid lineage such as neutrophils, basophils, eosinophils, and monocyte/macrophages (Figure 24.1). The process of hematopoiesis requires interactions between the pluripotent hematopoietic stem or committed progenitor cells and the stromal microenvironment.[158] The stromal environment is a source of cytokines for regulated hematopoiesis, and the proliferation and differentiation of HSCs/progenitor cells into specific terminally differentiated blood cells is dependent on the actions of both the lineage-specific early-acting and late-acting cytokines.[159] Stem cell factor and IL-3 act on bone marrow cells early in development, while erythropoietin, granulocyte-macrophage colony-stimulating factor (GM-CSF), G-CSF, macrophage colony-stimulating factor (M-CSF or CSF-1), and thrombopoietin act later in the process.[109,160]

The hematopoietic stem cell has the ability for self-renewal that insures abundant numbers of cells are present for commitment towards lineage-specific cells in response to different challenges. For example, it has been shown that during acute bacterial infection, expansion of granulocytes predominates and is attributed to increases within the stem cell compartment.[161,162] Additionally, a small percentage of the total stem cell pool that circulates in peripheral blood is activated in response to the local cytokine environment. The current consensus is that HSCs give rise to the multipotent CFU-GEMM cell, granulocyte-erythrocyte-monocyte-megakaryocyte and the lymphoid stem cell. Although the actual existence of the lymphoid stem cell has not been definitively shown, it is hypothesized that this stem cell gives rise to mature T and B cells.[163] The CFU-GEMM cell in the presence of steel factor or stem cell factor, IL-3, and GM-CSF, can develop into the myeloid-restricted bipotential cell CFU-GM, which can form either granulocytes or monocyte/macrophages depending upon the presence of G-CSF or M-CSF.[164] The terminally differentiated granulocytes in the bone marrow reserves are recruited into the circulation during periods of bacterial infection, stress, and thermal injury. Additionally, monocytes can either circulate in the peripheral blood or migrate into sites of inflammation and infection and become tissue macrophages in response to the local cytokine milieu.

Much of the knowledge of how hematopoiesis is modulated by thermal injury and sepsis has been gained through the use of animal models. Work on the cells of burn patients has demonstrated a reduction in the circulating stem cells in severely burned patients.[165] Animal models of thermal injury, however, continue to provide significant information on the status of bone marrow hematopoiesis after burns, and have allowed us to probe the overall pathophysiology of thermal injury and sepsis. For example, animal experiments have demonstrated that the initial granulocytosis observed is due to peripheral demargination and release of nondividing granulocytes from bone marrow reserves, stimulating an increase in the bone marrow CFU-G growth.[100] In the same model, burns superimposed with *P. aeruginosa* infection led to significant decreases in CFU-G colonies.[166] The serum from burn-infected animals inhibited the formation of CFU-G colonies from normal bone marrow cells.[105] These observations pointed to a primary defect in bone marrow granulocyte production, or myelopoiesis.

Although Eurenius and McEuen demonstrated that the granulocytopenia observed in their rat model of thermal injury and sepsis was due to the failure of bone marrow hematopoiesis. Gamelli et al. compared the size of burn wound, and superimposed localized *P. aeruginosa* infection, to inflammatory mediators.[104,167] Using these criteria, they demonstrated that mice exhibited peripheral leukopenia and lymphopenia on day 1 postburn and returned to normal values in 8 and 12 days.[104] Mice also exhibited diminished bone marrow and splenic cellularity following thermal injury that increased in a time-dependent manner. In addition, *in vitro* clonogenic assays showed that burn injury led to an initial depression of bone marrow and splenic cellularity. This initial decrease was followed by a consistent bone marrow and splenic hypercellularity. The bone marrow and splenic mitotic index positively correlated with the cellularity. In addition, the number of bone

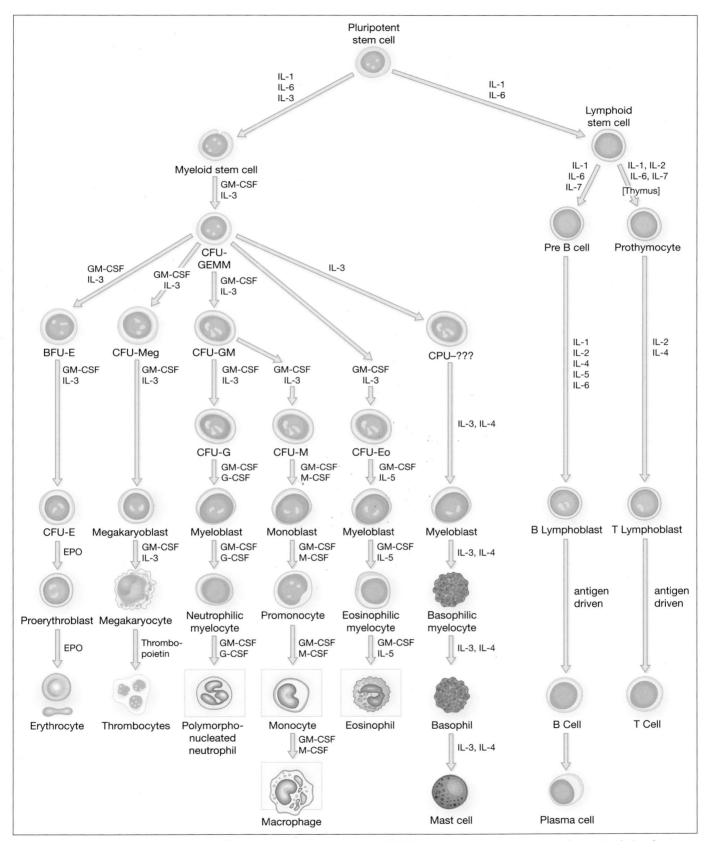

Fig. 24.1 Hematopoietic commitment paradigm: regulation by cytokines. GM-CSF, granulocyte-macrophage colony-stimulating factor; G-CSF, granulocyte colony-stimulating factor; M-CSF, monocyte colony-stimulating factor; CFU-GEEM, colony-forming unit-granulocyte, erythroid, monocyte/macrophage, megakaryocyte; BFU-E, burst forming unit-erythroid; EPO, erythropoietin; CFU-G, colony forming unit-granulocyte; CFU-M, colony forming unit-monocyte; CFU-GM, colony forming unit-granulocyte, monocyte/macrophage; CFU-Eo, colony forming unit-eosinophil; CFU-Meg, colony forming unit-megakaryocyte. (From Sandoz Pharmaceuticals Corporation.)

marrow and splenic CFU-GM cells was consistently elevated beginning days 4–12 postburn. The increased CFU-GM production within the bone marrow and splenic compartment were threefold and 100-fold, respectively.

In direct contrast to thermal injury alone, concomittent sepsis dramatically altered the bone marrow myelopoietic responses. When mice were subjected to scald injury followed by a septic challenge with *P. aeruginosa* inoculation at the burn wound site, a marked reduction (~50%) in CFU-GM growth was observed 3 days after the initial injury.[167] Interestingly, the introduction of endotoxin into normal or burned mice led to a similar decrease in CFU-GM proliferation as observed in infected burn mice. Under these conditions, the total colony-stimulating activity (CSA) was also reduced in burn-infected animals, suggesting either the levels of CSFs were low or the serum contained a potent inhibitor of colony growth.

In severe thermal injury and sepsis, however, the circulating levels of the myelopoietic growth factors such as G-CSF and M-CSF are elevated. Therefore the logical hypothesis was that the burn sera contained a potent inhibitor for clonal growth of bone marrow cells. Based on the literature evidence, PGE_2 appeared to be a logical choice for this clonal growth inhibitory substance. Prostaglandins of the E-series (PGE_1 and PGE_2) but not the prostaglandins of the F-series ($PGF_1\alpha$ and $PGF_2\alpha$) have been shown to inhibit CFC proliferation *in vitro*.[168] In addition, Pelus and his co-workers have demonstrated that administration of PGE_2 to cyclophosphamide-treated or intact mice resulted in significant suppression of myelopoiesis.[169] Pelus went on to show that inhibition of prostaglandin biosynthesis through administration of indomethacin, a cyclooxygenase inhibitor, reversed the clonal inhibitory effect of IL-1β administration.[170] Extending these observations to their murine model of thermal injury and sepsis, Gamelli et al. were able to show that administration of indomethacin could reverse burn sepsis or burn endotoxin-induced suppression in CFU-GM growth and improve survival of the septic animals.[167] While these studies directly implicated prostaglandin metabolites in burn sepsis-induced bone marrow myeloid suppression, further studies confirmed that PGE_2 is the primary mediator of this myelosuppression. Thermal injury and sepsis activate macrophages to produce PGE_2 through the induction of the enzyme cyclooxygenase-2 (COX-2).[171] Administration of a specific COX-2 inhibitor, NS-398, has been shown to both inhibit PGE_2 production of endotoxin-treated macrophages to improve the survival rate of burn septic animals compared to controls, and to restore absolute neutrophil counts and CFU-GM's proliferative capacity.[172] Similar results were also reported with the treatment of burn septic mice with a PGE_2 receptor antagonist SC-19220.[173] These results have helped establish a significant role for PGE_2 in burn-induced myelosuppression and suggest new treatment modalities for burn injury and sepsis.

Although PGE_2 has been established as a mediator of bone marrow myelosuppression in thermal injury and sepsis, until recently, no attempt has been made to explain the cellular mechanism for this myelosuppression (Figure 24.2). Using the same murine model of scald burn injury, Shoup et al. characterized the specific stages in granulopoiesis that are altered in burn sepsis.[172] The specific granulocytic cell surface marker, GR-1 was employed to document the stage of bone marrow

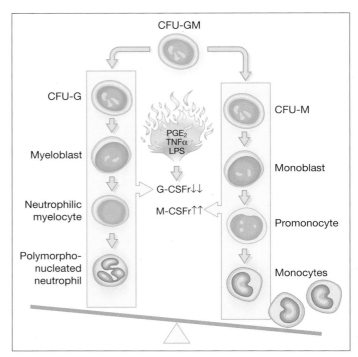

Fig. 24.2 Reprioritization of myeloid commitment following thermal injury and sepsis. PGE_2, prostagladin E_2; TNFα, tumor necrosis factor-α; LPS, lipopolysaccharide/endotoxin; CFU-GM colony forming unit-granulocyte, monocyte; CFU-M, colony forming unit-monocyte; CFU-G, colony forming unit-granulocyte; G-CSFr, G-CSF receptor; M-CSFr, M-CSF receptor (*c-fms*). (From Shoup et al. Cyclooxygenase-2 inhibitor NS-398 improves survival and restores leukocyte count in burn infection. J Trauma 1998; 45:215–220; discussion 220–221. with permission.)[172]

myeloid maturation arrest in the injured animals. The expression of GR-1, also designated as Ly-6C, progressively increases with granulocytic maturation. The lowest levels of GR-1 expression are found in myeloblasts and the highest levels in neutrophils, with promyelocytes and myelocytes expressing intermediate levels of the antigen.[174,175] The strength of GR-1 expression allowed these investigators to follow the developmental stages of granulopoiesis in sham, burn, and burn septic mice. Their results revealed that burn infection gives rise to an increased number of cells in the compartment comprising immature granulopoietic cells compared to sham or burn mice, and there was a concomitant decrease in the compartment comprising the mature granulocyte population. Using another granulocyte marker, myeloperoxidase, whose mRNA is not expressed after the promyelocyte stage in granulocyte development, they demonstrated that burn sepsis resulted in an accumulation of promyelocytes. This suggests the possibility of myeloid maturation arrest at this stage of granulopoietic development. They could further demonstrate that myelosuppression was accompanied by an attenuation of G-CSF receptor mRNA expression and G-CSF-stimulated proliferation of bone marrow cells, thereby providing a mechanistic explanation for the observed myelosuppression in thermal injury and sepsis.

Despite these data on the mechanisms regulating granulopoietic development during thermal injury and sepsis, very little information is available on the development of monocytes or monocytopoiesis in the bone marrow under the same conditions. Myelopoiesis is a development paradigm responsible for the production of granulocytes and monocytes within the bone marrow. The common myeloid committed progenitor for these lineages is the bipotential progenitor CFU-GM.[176] The CFU-GM cells under the influence of GM-CSF and M-CSF give rise to committed CFU-M progenitors and progressively differentiate into mature monocytes. The mature monocytes are released into peripheral circulation and can differentiate into tissue macrophages upon entry into tissue.[177,178] Although monocyte/macrophage activation and the resultant dysregulated cytokine milieu are considered central players in the development of systemic inflammation in severe burns and sepsis, the status of monocyte production by the bone marrow has been largely neglected. In fact, thermal injury has been shown to be associated with increased CFU-GM levels.[101,104] Patients suffering from acute peritonitis and various acute infections have also been shown to possess elevated circulating levels of CFU-GM in their blood.[71] Furthermore, increased monocytopoiesis has been documented in animal models with bacterial infections.[24,98] Recently, Santangelo et al. have specifically addressed this issue of the status of monocytopoiesis during thermal injury and sepsis.[166] These investigators took advantage of the recent development of monoclonal antibodies against monocyte developmental antigens ERMP-12 and ERMP-20.[179,180] While ERMP-12 antigen is predominantly expressed in CFU-M cells, ERMP-20 antigen is expressed primarily in monoblasts and promonocytes.[180] Through flow cytometric analysis (FACS) of ERMP-12 and ERMP-20 antigen expression, a significant increase was shown in the early monocyte progenitors expressing both ERMP-12 and ERMP-20 antigens in burn and burn septic animals compared to sham-treated animals. The burn sepsis group also showed a significant increase in the late monocyte progenitors compared to the sham and burn group. These increases in monocytopoiesis were also reflected in the peripheral blood counts. Thermal injury and sepsis stimulated absolute monocytosis and a concomitant reduction in absolute neutrophil counts in circulation. Interestingly, the creation of a localized infection without systemic involvement did not result in any changes in absolute monocyte or granulocyte counts.

This study also demonstrated that M-CSF-responsive colony growth of the total bone marrow cells, as well as ERMP-12-enriched bone marrow cells, was significantly increased in thermal injury and sepsis compared to the sham group. Similar increases were also seen with GM-CSF. Of interest, G-CSF-responsive colony growth was severely depressed in thermal injury and sepsis. More importantly, they were able to provide a mechanistic explanation for the enhanced monopoiesis in thermal injury and sepsis through the documentation of increased M-CSF receptor expression on ERMP12+/RMP-20+ enriched bone marrow cells. These studies provided a novel observation that the acute expansion of the CFU-GM compartment caused a shift in the production of the myeloid lineage toward monocytopoiesis and away from granulocytopoiesis. The observed shift led to overproduction of monocytes with concurrent underproduction of granulocytes that could be due to increased M-CSF receptor expression on monocytic lineage cells and a downregulation of G-CSF receptor expression on the cells of the granulocytic lineage. Both the increased susceptibility to infections and the maintenance of systemic

inflammatory response syndrome (SIRS) can be explained in part by the shift in myelopoiesis during severe burn injury and sepsis. Thus, these studies highlight the importance of understanding the pathophysiology of burn injury through concerted regulation of related cellular events and pave the way to new, rational therapies.

This thought process is supported by the observation that blocking PGE$_2$'s actions can reverse the preferential shift in myelopoiesis observed during the course of experimental thermal injury.[172,173] Administration of a PGE$_2$ receptor antagonist, SC-19220, that specifically blocks cellular interactions of PGE$_2$ without affecting synthesis or activation of other prostaglandins to burn septic animals restored the balance between monocytopoiesis and granulocytopoiesis toward near-normal levels. Measurement of circulating neutrophil and monocyte counts also mirrored the bone marrow myelopoietic changes. More importantly, the administration of SC-19220 improved overall survival of burn septic mice.

Aside from the hematopoietic colony-stimulating factors, other pro- and anti-inflammatory cytokines that are often elevated in burn patients can also modulate hematopoiesis. Interleukin-6, which plays a central role in the acute phase response of burn injury is also a potent stimulator of early progenitor cell proliferation without inducing differentiation.[181] Furthermore, IL-6 is a powerful mitogen for megakaryocytes and committed myeloid cells.[182–184] It also synergizes with IL-3 and GM-CSF to modulate multiple lineages within the hematopoietic hierarchy.[109,159,160] Increased IL-6 production in severely burned patients could serve to stimulate hematopoiesis so that adequate numbers of leukocytes and platelets can be produced to meet the increased demands. Similarly, TNFα can modulate myelopoiesis through its capacity to downregulate G-CSF receptor expression on granulocytic cells.[185,186] TGFβ is another cytokine that can influence hematopoiesis through its ability to suppress early hematopoietic precursor growth.[187–189] Depending on the severity of the burn injury and the presence or absence of other complicating factors such as sepsis, these and other pleiotropic cytokines in the burn milieu can significantly influence the hematopoietic commitment patterns.

In addition to thermal injury and infection, the stress response to the burn injury can also profoundly influence myelopoiesis. It has been established that the immune and hematopoietic systems are under physiologic regulation by neuroendocrine modulation. Conversely, the cytokine and hematopoietic products can alter functions of nervous system and endocrine organs. The ability of sympathetic activation to influence not only the cardiovascular and metabolic functions of the body following severe thermal injury but also its effects on the regulation of myelopoiesis are discussed elsewhere in this book.

Putative role for hematopoietic transcription factors in thermal injury

Recent advances in molecular and cellular biology have begun to describe the importance of the multitier control of pathophysiological changes that occur as a response to any injury state. The initial injury and the resultant changes in metabolic and cardiovascular responses trigger alterations in hematologic parameters, which in turn initiate the appropriate hematopoietic commitment programs. Ultimately, specific sequential and temporal gene expression patterns dictate the hematopoietic commitment. Inherent in this concept of physiological regulation is the hierarchy of genes that control proliferation, developmental fate, and functions of hematopoietic progenitor cells. These genetic processes are governed through modulations in the rate of gene transcription which are accomplished through the binding of DNA-binding proteins or transcription factors to specific regions on a gene.[190]

Transcription factors are nuclear proteins that act as control points in the conversion of a gene to a functional protein.[190] Since many key proteins are turned over rapidly to meet the changing needs of the tissues, a complex system of cell signaling architecture, with the final common pathway of gene transcription, must exist to produce bioactive proteins on demand. To exquisitely regulate the rate of protein synthesis, genes need to be quickly transcribed into RNA within the nucleus, transported to the cytoplasm, and proteins synthesized from RNA templates. Since cells respond to several signals simultaneously, and many ligand–cell interactions stimulate similar proximal signals, tight control of transcriptional initiation must exist for the proper orchestration of cellular responses.

The lineage-restricted proliferation and differentiation program in hematopoiesis is achieved through switching on and off the specific sets of genes in response to cell signals. Since thermal injury and sepsis are accompanied by hematologic and hematopoietic changes that determine the overall pathophysiological response of burn patients, it is reasonable to assume that transcriptional regulation of hematopoietic developmental genes play a significant role. Although, at present, there is little direct evidence for the role of hematopoietic transcription factors in the pathophysiology of burn injury, considerable evidence does exist to support their pivotal role in hematopoietic commitment.[191–193] Therefore a brief review of the relevant transcription factors is essential to research endeavors in burn biology. Much of our current knowledge of hematopoietic transcription factors has come from diverse fields such as hematology-oncology, immunology, mammalian virology, and signal transduction. Many concepts have been found by studying the molecular controls of leukemias, *in vitro* cell clonal assays, and various hematopoietic cell lines. The gene knockout technology has also aided in ascertaining the functional roles of characterized genes in hematopoiesis. Biological processes in cells involve changes in gene expression that manifest as altered function or cellular response. Basically, alterations in expression of a certain gene can arise from modulating its level (transcription) or changes in mRNA stability and translation (post-transcriptional mechanisms). In this section, we will review a set of transcription factors that have been shown to be essential for the normal development of many elements of hematopoietic lineage.

tal-1/SCL

The *tal-1/SCL* gene encodes a bHLH (basic helix-loop-helix) protein that was originally identified at the chromosomal breakpoint in a human acute T cell leukemia.[194,195] *tal-1/SCL* is a master gene required for devlopment of hematopoietic stem cells that eventually differentiate into lineage-specific blood cells.[196] Previous studies have revealed that the early hematopoietic stem cells (CD34+/c-kit+/Sca+ cells) express the *tal-1/SCL* gene.[196–198] T cell leukemia, which consists of a clonal cell line with the potential to differentiate into myeloid and lymphoid lineages, was shown to express tal-1/SCL protein.[195,196] In addition, mature erythrocytes, megakaryocytes, mast cells, and endothelial cells also express tal-1/SCL. These data indicate that the *tal-1/SCL* gene may play a required role in a later stage of maturation of committed progenitors. Homozygous *tal-1/SCL* gene knockout mice provided definitive evidence for its role in hematopoiesis. The homozygous *tal-1/SCL* gene deletion was lethal *in utero*.[196,199] These mice exhibited a failure in blood formation and their yolk sac contained no detectable blood elements and lacked *in vitro* clonogenic potential. These results were further confirmed by the inability of the tal-1/SCL knockout embryonic stem (ES) cells to develop into any hematopoietic lineages in culture.

GATA family

Another set of transcription factors that are essential in hematopoiesis belong to the GATA family of proteins. The GATA transcription factors are related zinc-finger DNA-binding proteins. These transcription activators bind to the canonical GATA sequence motif found in the cis-regulatory regions of many hematopoietic genes. The proteins have differential expression patterns and activate a unique set of target genes in their restricted cells. GATA-1, GATA-2, and GATA-3 proteins play pivotal roles in hematopoiesis. It was reported that GATA-2 is involved in proliferation and self-renewal of early hematopoietic stem cells. Mice engineered with a homozygous deletion of *GATA-2* gene display severe hematopoietic defects. The GATA-2 knockout mice survive to embryonic day 10–11, harbor a small number of red blood cells at that stage, undergo anemic crisis, and eventually die.[200] *In vitro* clonogenic assays revealed a drastic reduction in the number of erythroid progenitors and a substantial loss of mature erythroid and mast cell precursors. GATA-1, the other important member of this family, is expressed in erythroid, eosinophil, megakaryocyte, and mast cell progenitors.[201,202] GATA-1 appears to be critical for survival and differentiation of erythroid progenitors. Mice lacking GATA-1 protein display normal hematopoiesis, except for the erythroid lineage.[94] *In vitro* differentiation assay with the GATA-1-deficient ES cells demonstrated differentiation up to the proerythroblast stage of erythropoiesis with eventual apoptosis of the arrested cells.[94,196] Interestingly, there seems to be interrelated complex regulation among the GATA family of transcription factors. During erythroid differentiation, GATA-1 levels increase and GATA-2 expression is downregulated. Moreover, this interplay is absent in GATA-1-deficient ES cells that display high levels of GATA-2 during *in vitro* erythroid differentiation assays.[196,201,203] Aside from its role on erythroid differentiation, GATA-1 appears to have a negative regulatory role in myeloid differentiation. Increased expression of GATA-1 has been shown to negatively modulate PU.1 expression and thus suppress myeloid commitment.[193,204] Since burn injury is commonly associated with a downregulation of erythropoiesis despite increased levels of endogenous erythropoietin, studies specifically designed to correlate the strength of GATA-1 expression in progenitor cells to the status of erythropoiesis will provide novel and mechanistic information on the pathophysiology of anemia in burn injury. Lastly, mice lacking GATA-3 fail to develop normal fetal liver hematopoiesis, lack all hematopoietic lineages, except the megakaryocytic cells, and succumb to embryonic hemorrhage.[196]

PU.1

The PU.1 proto-oncogene encodes a member of the ets family of DNA-binding proteins. It was originally cloned as a sequence-specific DNA-binding protein that was found to be homologous to the *spi-1* oncogene.[205] The *spi-1* oncogene was isolated from erythroblastic leukemia cells transformed by spleen focus forming virus (SFFV). The PU.1 transcription factor contains an amino-terminal glutamine/aspartic acid-rich region (TAD) followed by PEST domain and a carboxy-terminal ets DNA-binding domain.[206] PU.1 possesses transcriptional activation potential that requires other co-activators for full potency.[207] PU.1 expression is found in monocytic, granulocytic, and B lymphoid cells.[208] Two different PU.1 knockout mice reveal the absence of monocytes, B cells, and greatly reduced neutrophil production.[209,210] Moreover, these neutrophils are unable to express some markers of fully differentiated neutrophils.[210,211] Embryonic stem cells from PU.1-deficient mice can differentiate into immature myeloid progenitors in the presence of IL-3 and G-CSF cytokines. Additionally, these PU.1 hematopoietic progenitors express low levels of mRNA for the GM-CSF, G-CSF, and M-CSF receptors.[212] The primitive hematopoietic progenitors are unable to differentiate into M-CSF and G-CSF responsive progenitors after introduction of M-CSF-R or G-CSF-R genes. Nevertheless, exogenous PU.1 expression in the PU.1-deficient hematopoietic progenitors restores myeloid differentiation. Therefore, multiple lines of evidence implicate PU.1's central role in commitment to myeloid lineage and terminal differentiation of monocytes, granulocytes, and B cells.

c-Myb

c-Myb proto-oncogene belongs to the basic helix-turn-helix (bHTH) family of DNA-binding proteins.[213] c-Myb contains an LZ motif that mediates homotypic and heterotypic protein interactions.[214] Multiple serine residues are located within the amino-terminal and carboxy-terminal regions of c-Myb that affect its DNA-binding activity and negative regulatory domain.[215–217] Studies have shown that c-myb expression is restricted to myeloid, erythroid, and immature lymphoid cells.[218–220] Collaborative data from *c-myb* knockout mice reveal the absence of all hematopoietic lineages, except within the megakaryocytic compartment. *c-myb* knockout mice exhibited normal yolk sac hematopoiesis, while liver hematopoiesis was greatly compromised and these mice die *in utero* at E14–15.[221] Detailed analysis of hematopoietic lineages revealed that functional granulocytes and monocytes were present, but they harbored 10–20-fold reduction in mature cells compared to normal mice. It is hypothesized that c-Myb functions to control quantitative effects rather than differentiation *per se* during hematopoiesis. It was also noted that c-Myb levels decrease during differentiation of hematopoietic progenitors and enforced c-Myb expression promotes proliferation and blocks hematopoietic differentiation. Hence, c-Myb plays a critical role in controlling proliferation of immature hematopoietic progenitors and its physiological downregulation is required for commitment towards lineage-specific differentiation.

C/EBPs

CCAAT/enhancer binding proteins (C/EBPs) are transcription factors that bind to core cis-regulatory sequence of CCAAT found in many regulated genes. C/EBPα was the original transcription factor described as a basic leucine zipper (bLZ) DNA-binding protein in hepatocytes and adipocytes.[222] Interestingly, C-EBP family of transcription factors, including *C-EBPα* have been shown to be elevated following thermal injury.[223] Although their expression is implicated in the acute phase response, the role of C-EBPs in the regulation of hematopoiesis during thermal injury and sepsis is yet to be delineated. Other members of this family include *C/EBPβ, C/EBPδ, C/EBPε,* and GADD153/CHOP proteins. These C/EBPs are able to homodimerize and heterodimerize with each other via the leucine zipper regions.[224] Expression studies showed that *C/EBPα* is present in monocytes, eosinophils, and neutrophils.[225,226] Moreover, human myeloid precursors and immature myeloid cell line, 32 DC13, express high levels of *C/EBPα* that decreased upon G-CSF-induced differentiation.[227,228] *C/EBPα* was shown to possess a transcriptional activation domain involved in the upregulation of mRNA from certain neutrophil genes such as G-CSF-R, lactoferrin, and collagenase. *C/EBPα* gene knockout mice are deficient in neutrophils and eosinophils, but harbor functional lymphocytes and monocytes.[229] Fetal liver cells formed M-CSF- and GM-CSF-responsive colonies, but G-CSF-induced colonies were not obtained. Hence, these studies determine that *C/EBPα* is essential for neutrophil differentiation, but not essential for monocytic differentiation. Conversely, during neutrophil differentiation of myeloid cell line, 32 DC13, *C/EBPβ* levels increase. Recently, data from the *C/EBPβ*-deficient mice revealed that hematopoiesis proceeds normally, but defects in macrophage activation and decreased B lymphocytes are observed.[230–232] Additionally, *C/EBPε* gene knockout mice exhibited abnormal neutrophilic function and deficiencies in certain key enzymes.[233] Otherwise, the mice appeared to have intact hematopoietic tissues. The preceding studies demonstrate the important regulatory function of the C/EBPs transcription factors in myelopoiesis.

c-Myc/MAD/Mxi-1

c-myc proto-oncogene is part of the bHLHLZ (basic helix-loop-helix leucine zipper) family of transcription factors.[234] c-Myc binds to canonical CANNTG DNA motifs located in many proliferative or cell cycle-regulated genes.[235] c-Myc has three transcriptional activation domains in the amino terminus and a carboxy-terminal with sequence-specific basic region and helix-loop-helix leucine zipper domains that mediate protein–protein interactions. c-Myc is required for cellular proliferation and its downregulation is essential for differentiation of many cell types.[219,234,236,237] Max is another bHLHLZ protein partner of c-Myc and this heterodimeric complex is essential for cognate DNA binding and transactivation of target genes.[238,239] Another set of genes that belong to *c-myc* family are *MAD, Mxi-1, Mxi-3,* and *Mxi-4* genes. The most important ones in hematopoiesis are *MAD* and *Mxi-1*.[240,241] MAD and

Mxi-1 proteins can heterodimerize with Max to form heterodimers that unlike Myc-Max can repress transcription at the same cognate DNA sites bound by c-Myc-Max heterodimers. Hence, within a given cell, there is a dynamic equilibrium of c-Myc-Max and MAD-Max complexes that compete for the same binding sites and the predominant complex determines whether proliferation or differentiation ensues.[239,242] During *in vitro* and *in vivo* hematopoietic differentiation, MAD/Mxi-1 levels increase, while *c-myc* expression is downregulated.[240,243,244] Recently, it was reported that *MAD* null mice have defects in myelopoiesis as demonstrated by delayed cell cycle exit during granulocytic differentiation.[245] In summary, c-Myc/MAD's roles in regulating the onset of proliferation versus differentiation are crucial for hematopoietic development.

Hox genes

The *Hox* genes encode homeobox containing transcription factors that are involved in neural development, organogenesis, and segmental development of branchial and mesoderm layers.[246] The homeodomain common to these proteins is a sequence-specific helix-turn-helix DNA-binding motif. The role of the various *Hox* genes has been examined in hematopoietic development.[247] The *Hox* genes identified in this process are *HoxA9, HoxA5, HoxA10, HoxB4,* and *HoxB7.*[247,248] In myeloid development, *HoxA9* and *HoxA10* are expressed at the highest levels in immature progenitors, and then are downregulated during differentiation.[249] *HoxA10* null mice exhibit increased levels of peripheral monocytes and neutrophils with no other apparent abnormality. Conversely, *HoxA9* knockout mice had decreased numbers of granulocytes and attenuation in G-CSF responsiveness. A recent study on *HoxA5* gene expression using antisense oligos demonstrated inhibition of neutrophil and monocytic differentiation.[250] It was hypothesized that *HoxA5* functions in early myeloid progenitors before commitment. Lastly, it was reported that *HoxB7* and *Hlx* genes might be involved in terminal differentiation or maturation of granulocytic cells.[251,252] The overall importance of the *Hox* gene family is well established in that they seem to control progression of immature myeloid precursors into mature granulocytes.

Hematologic and acute phase response: treatment strategies

Patients suffering 15% or greater body surface area burns undergo significant alterations in their circulatory status. The blood and its constituent elements must be supported, with the primary goal in the initial management phase being support of intravascular volume. A patient suffering 40% surface area burn would be subjected to a 40–50% reduction in circulating volume if not resuscitated. If the volume of resuscitation fluid is insufficient to meet the patient's needs then the patient will suffer inadequate tissue perfusion and shock, but hemo-concentration will also develop. With progressive increases in hemoglobin concentration, there is a disproportionate change in the blood's viscosity and resistance to flow through the circulatory bed. By maintaining plasma volume, perfusion will be enhanced with restoration of the rheological properties of the blood.

Patients suffering significant burns will experience some progressive decreases in their hemoglobin and hematocrit values over the first several days of hospitalization.[10,22,29,253] This is related to the reduction in red cell mass, due to the changes in red cell characteristics and erythropoietic response. Additionally, with expansion in plasma volume following successful resuscitation, there may be an element of dilution. Further reductions in hemoglobin and hematocrit concentrations are also the consequences of repeated blood sampling and blood loss related to wound manipulation. The performance of escharotomies can be associated with significant blood loss from thrombosed vessels that bleed once tissue turgor is reduced following eschar release. The characteristics of the burn wound can also contribute to ongoing hematologic loss. Patients with deep partial-thickness wounds with their associated damaged capillary bed can serve as sites for ongoing blood loss.

The optimum hematocrit for patients suffering extensive burn injuries is a matter of opinion. Many experts suggest maintaining hematocrit values of 25% or greater. In doing so, a considerable number of transfusions are likely to be required as attempts at replacement with iron and erythropoietin are typically not successful in patients with major body surface area injuries. Many patients can tolerate a hematocrit of less than 25%, and young healthy individuals whose wounds are closed will tolerate a hematocrit in the 18–22% range with a mild tachycardia and no impairment in wound healing or physiologic response. The optimum hematocrit for the individual burn patient should be adjusted to their clinical status and their co-morbid conditions. Elderly patients with significant underlying cardiac disease should be supported more aggressively with maintenance of their hemoglobin and hematocrit values above the 30%. Strategies should be invoked throughout the patient's care and surgical interventions to limit blood loss. The use of tourniquets, vasoconstrictive agents, tumescence with burn eschar excision, and fibrin sealants provide opportunities to limit operative blood loss. Additionally, the use of hemo-dilution with auto-transfusion represents another approach that can be used to limit the need for transfusions, particularly in patients who will not accept random donor transfusions.[254] Blood loss must be closely followed during the course of surgery to avoid hypotensive episodes and the development of systemic acidosis which will further compromise the patient's hemostatic capacity and exacerbate bleeding. Attention to the patient's coagulation parameters and platelet counts are important to avoid the development of coagulopathic complications due to dilutional coagulopathy. Patients receiving intensive broad-spectrum antibiotic therapy must be carefully monitored for the development of vitamin K-dependent coagulopathy. This must be corrected with the replacement of vitamin K as well as coagulation factor component therapy.

The goal of nutritional support in patients with burn injuries is to replete lean body mass and to facilitate restoration of visceral proteins. Hypo-albuminemia is a near universal response to significant burn injury. The benefit of albumin replacement therapy and how it impacts outcomes is a matter of opinion. In today's environment of cost containment, the challenge to the clinician is to provide care that is evidence based. A recent analysis by the Cochrane Injuries Group has suggested that there is no indication for the use of albumin in the management of critically ill patients.[255] Whether burn patients fall outside this recommendation remains controversial.

The response of the formed elements of the blood following burn injuries has been reviewed in great detail previously in this chapter. The impact of various interventions may also compound the pathologic response induced by the burn injury. Patients receiving heparin for the maintenance of various vascular devices may experience heparin-induced thrombocytopenia. It has been our practice for the last decade to not use heparin flushes to maintain intravascular catheters. With this approach we have had no increase in complications related to line occlusion or embolic events and no incidences of heparin-induced thrombocytopenia. Changes in leukocyte numbers occur as part of the response to injury and can be further compounded by responses to drug therapy and/or septic events. Rapid diagnosis and effective therapy for infections should be undertaken. In patients who develop profound neutropenia, current clinical experience suggests that exogenous administration of recombinant human G-CSFs is effective in supporting increases in circulating neutrophil numbers.

Following burn injury there are dilutional reductions and depletion of coagulation factors. However, after the early burn phase, the tendency for burn patients is to be hypercoagulable. A reduction in antithrombin III levels is associated with an increased propensity for microvascular thrombosis. Limited clinical trials have been performed in which there appears to be a therapeutic effect for the administration of antithrombin III in the early postburn phases.[41,42,46] The studies that have been reported suggest that there is a relative preservation of burn wound vascularity and an enhancement in the healing process. There is also some suggestion that there may be a benefit to other microvascular beds such as in the lung with preservation of pulmonary function. These studies are preliminary and provide intriguing observations that need to be confirmed in larger multicenter trials. Burn patients with intravascular devices are at risk for the development of thrombotic complications with limb ischemia as can occur with femoral arterial lines. Also, the presence of large-bore femoral venous catheters has been associated with up to a 30% incidence of deep vein thrombosis. The risk of pulmonary emboli is a recognized risk in burn patients. Preservation of circulatory volume and aggressive and early ambulation are important strategies to limit deep vein thrombotic complications and pulmonary emboli. The risk of thromboembolic complications can extend into the rehabilitation phase in patients with large burns.

Conclusion

Burn-induced changes in hematopoiesis and the induction of the acute phase response are components of the body's reaction to injury. With an extensive degree of injury, or when complications develop, the physiologic limits of this system can be exceeded. The blood and its constituent elements must provide tissue nutrition, and maintain host defenses and hemostasis. Modern day burn care allows the clinician to limit the impact of injury and provide access to various components in the form of replacement therapy. Pursuing a better understanding of the basic pathobiology of thermal injury will provide additional opportunities to intervene in the response to injury and improve patient outcome.

References

1. DiPietro LA. Wound healing: the role of the macrophage and other immune cells. Shock 1995; 4:233–240.
2. DiPietro LA, Burdick M, Low QE, et al. MIP-1alpha as a critical macrophage chemoattractant in murine wound repair. J Clin Invest 1998; 101:1693–1698.
3. Munster AM. Alterations of the host defense mechanism in burns. Surg Clin North Am 1970; 50:1217–1225.
4. Stratta RJ, Warden GD, Ninnemann JL, et al. Immunologic parameters in burned patients: effect of therapeutic interventions. J Trauma 1986; 26:7–17.
5. Winkelstein A. What are the immunological alterations induced by burn injury? J Trauma 1984; 24:S72–S83.
6. Loebl EC, Baxter CR, Curreri PW. The mechanism of erythrocyte destruction in the early post-burn period. Ann Surg 1973; 178:681–686.
7. Topley E, Jackson DM, Cason JS, et al. Assessment of red cell loss in the first two days after severe burns. Ann Surg 1962; 155:581–590.
8. Birdsell DC, Birch JR. Anemia following thermal burns: a survey of 109 children. Can J Surg 1971; 14:345–350.
9. Desai MH, Herndon DN, Broemeling L, et al. Early burn wound excision significantly reduces blood loss. Ann Surg 1990; 211:753–759; discussion 759–762.
10. Deitch EA, Sittig KM. A serial study of the erythropoietic response to thermal injury. Ann Surg 1993; 217:293–299.
11. Robb HJ. Dynamics of the microcirculation during a burn. Arch Surg 1967; 94:776–780.
12. Kimber RJ, Lander H. The effect of heat on human red cell morphology, fragility, and subsequent survival in vivo. J Lab Clin Med 1964; 64:922–933.
13. Hatherill JR, Till GO, Bruner LH, et al. Thermal injury, intravascular hemolysis, and toxic oxygen products. J Clin Invest 1986; 78:629–636.
14. Endoh Y, Kawakami M, Orringer EP, et al. Causes and time course of acute hemolysis after burn injury in the rat. J Burn Care Rehabil 1992; 13:203–209.
15. Kawakami M, Endoh Y, Orringer EP, et al. Improvements in rheologic properties of blood by fluid resuscitation after burn injury in rats. J Burn Care Rehabil 1992; 13:316–322.
16. Zaets SB, Berezina TL, Xu DZ, et al. Burn-induced red blood cell deformability and shape changes are modulated by sex hormones. Am J Surg 2003; 186:540–546.
17. Zaets SB, Berezina TL, Xu DZ, et al. Female sex hormones protect red blood cells from damage after trauma-hemorrhagic shock. Surg Infect (Larchmt) 2004; 5:51–59.
18. Dacie JV, Lewis SM. Laboratory methods used in the investigation of hemolytic anaemia II. Hereditary haemolytic anaemias. Practical haematology, 5th. edn. Edinburgh: Churchill Livingstone; 1975:202–235.
19. Wallner SF, Vautrin R. The anemia of thermal injury: mechanism of inhibition of erythropoiesis. Proc Soc Exp Biol Med 1986; 181:144–150.
20. Shoemaker WC, Vladeck BC, Bassin R, et al. Burn pathophysiology in man. I. Sequential hemodynamic alterations. J Surg Res 1973; 14:64–73.
21. Wolfe RR. Review: acute versus chronic response to burn injury. Circ Shock 1981; 8:105–115.
22. Andes WA, Rogers PW, Beason JW, et al. The erythropoietin response to the anemia of thermal injury. J Lab Clin Med 1976; 88:584–592.

23. Erslev AJ. Erythrokinetics. In: Williams WS, Beutley E, Lichtman MD, eds. Erythrokinetics. New York: McGraw-Hill; 1990:424–432.

24. Wallner S, Vautrin R, Murphy J, et al. The haematopoietic response to burning: studies in an animal model. Burns Incl Therm Inj 1984; 10:236–251.

25. MacLaren R, Gasper J, Jung R, et al. Use of exogenous erythropoietin in critically ill patients. J Clin Pharm Ther 2004; 29:195–208.

26. Still JM Jr, Belcher K, Law EJ, et al. A double-blinded prospective evaluation of recombinant human erythropoietin in acutely burned patients. J Trauma 1995; 38:233–236.

27. Jelkmann W, Wolff M, Fandrey J. Modulation of the production of erythropoietin by cytokines: in vitro studies and their clinical implications. Contrib Nephrol 1990; 87:68–77.

28. Pierce CN, Larson DF. Inflammatory cytokine inhibition of erythropoiesis in patients implanted with a mechanical circulatory assist device. Perfusion 2005; 20:83–90.

29. Wallner SF, Vautrin RM, Buerk C, et al. The anemia of thermal injury: studies of erythropoiesis in vitro. J Trauma 1982; 22:774–780.

30. Bauer A, Tronche F, Wessely O, et al. The glucocorticoid receptor is required for stress erythropoiesis. Genes Dev 1999; 13:2996–3002.

31. Livingston DH, Anjaria D, Wu J, et al. Bone marrow failure following severe injury in humans. Ann Surg 2003; 238:748–753.

32. Anjaria DJ, Rameshwar P, Deitch EA, et al. Hematopoietic failure after hemorrhagic shock is mediated partially through mesenteric lymph. Crit Care Med 2001; 29:1780–1785.

33. Deitch EA, Forsythe R, Anjaria D, et al. The role of lymph factors in lung injury, bone marrow suppression, and endothelial cell dysfunction in a primate model of trauma-hemorrhagic shock. Shock 2004; 22:221–228.

34. Dries DJ. Activation of the clotting system and complement after trauma. New Horiz 1996; 4:276–288.

35. Nimah M, Brilli RJ. Coagulation dysfunction in sepsis and multiple organ system failure. Crit Care Clin 2003; 19:441–458.

36. Bartlett RH, Fong SW, Marrujo G, et al. Coagulation and platelet changes after thermal injury in man. Burns 1981; 7:370–377.

37. Eurenius K, Mortensen RF, Meserol PM, et al. Platelet and megakaryocyte kinetics following thermal injury. J Lab Clin Med 1972; 79:247–257.

38. Lawrence C, Atac B. Hematologic changes in massive burn injury. Crit Care Med 1992; 20:1284–1288.

39. Housinger TA, Brinkerhoff C, Warden GD. The relationship between platelet count, sepsis, and survival in pediatric burn patients. Arch Surg 1993; 128:65–66; discussion 66–67.

40. Kowal-Vern A, Gamelli RL, Walenga JM, et al. The effect of burn wound size on hemostasis: a correlation of the hemostatic changes to the clinical state. J Trauma 1992; 33:50–56; discussion 56–57.

41. Kowal-Vern A, McGill V, Walenga JM, et al. Antithrombin III concentrate in the acute phase of thermal injury. Burns 2000; 26:97–101.

42. Kowal-Vern A, McGill V, Walenga JM, et al. Antithrombin(H) concentrate infusions are safe and effective in patients with thermal injuries. J Burn Care Rehabil 2000; 21:115–127.

43. Saliba MJ Jr. Heparin in the treatment of burns: a review. Burns 2001; 27:349–358.

44. Murakami K, McGuire R, Cox RA, et al. Heparin nebulization attenuates acute lung injury in sepsis following smoke inhalation in sheep. Shock 2002; 18:236–241.

45. Murakami K, McGuire R, Cox RA, et al. Recombinant antithrombin attenuates pulmonary inflammation following smoke inhalation and pneumonia in sheep. Crit Care Med 2003; 31:577–583.

46. Kowal-Vern A, Latenser BA. Antithrombin (human) concentrate infusion in pediatric patients with >50% TBSA burns. Burns 2003; 29:615–618.

47. Heideman M. The effect of thermal injury on hemodynamic, respiratory, and hematologic variables in relation to complement activation. J Trauma 1979; 19:239–247.

48. Wells S, Sissons M, Hasleton PS. Quantitation of pulmonary megakaryocytes and fibrin thrombi in patients dying from burns. Histopathology 1984; 8:517–527.

49. Barret JP, Gomez PA. Disseminated intravascular coagulation: a rare entity in burn injury. Burns 2005; 31:354–357.

50. Wahl WL, Brandt MM, Ahrns K, et al. The utility of D-dimer levels in screening for thromboembolic complications in burn patients. J Burn Care Rehabil 2002; 23:439–443.

51. Suffredini AF, Fantuzzi G, Badolato R, et al. New insights into the biology of the acute phase response. J Clin Immunol 1999; 19:203–214.

52. Kushner I. The phenomenon of the acute phase response. Ann N Y Acad Sci 1982; 389:39–48.

53. Baumann H, Gauldie J. The acute phase response. Immunol Today 1994; 15:74–80.

54. Tilg H, Dinarello CA, Mier JW. IL-6 and APPs: anti-inflammatory and immunosuppressive mediators. Immunol Today 1997; 18:428–432.

55. Jeschke MG, Barrow RE, Herndon DN. Recombinant human growth hormone treatment in pediatric burn patients and its role during the hepatic acute phase response. Crit Care Med 2000; 28:1578–1584.

56. Eurenius K, Rossi TD, McEuen DD, et al. Blood coagulation in burn injury. Proc Soc Exp Biol Med 1974; 147:878–882.

57. Emerson WA, Ieve PD, Krevans JR. Hematologic changes in septicemia. Johns Hopkins Med J 1970; 126:69–76.

58. Xia ZF, Coolbaugh MI, He F, et al. The effects of burn injury on the acute phase response. J Trauma 1992; 32:245–250; discussion 250–241.

59. Schlag G, Redl H. Mediators of injury and inflammation. World J Surg 1996; 20:406–410.

60. Dinarello CA. Interleukin-1 and the pathogenesis of the acute-phase response. N Engl J Med 1984; 311:1413–1418.

61. Guirao X, Lowry SF. Biologic control of injury and inflammation: much more than too little or too late. World J Surg 1996; 20:437–446.

62. Turchik JB, Bornstein DL. Role of the central nervous system in acute-phase responses to leukocytic pyrogen. Infect Immun 1980; 30:439–444.

63. Ertel W, Friedl HP, Trentz O. Multiple organ dysfunction syndrome (MODS) following multiple trauma: rationale and concept of therapeutic approach. Eur J Pediatr Surg 1994; 4:243–248.

64. Ching N, Grossi CE, Angers J, et al. The outcome of surgical treatment as related to the response of the serum albumin level to nutritional support. Surg Gynecol Obstet 1980; 151:199–202.

65. Brown RO, Bradley JE, Bekemeyer WB, et al. Effect of albumin supplementation during parenteral nutrition on hospital morbidity. Crit Care Med 1988; 16:1177–1182.

66. Moshage H. Cytokines and the hepatic acute phase response. J Pathol 1997; 181:257–266.

67. Jeschke MG, Herndon DN, Barrow RE. Insulin-like growth factor I in combination with insulin-like growth factor binding protein 3 affects the hepatic acute phase response and hepatic morphology in thermally injured rats. Ann Surg 2000; 231:408–416.

68. Jeschke MG, Barrow RE, Herndon DN. Insulinlike growth factor I plus insulinlike growth factor binding protein 3 attenuates the proinflammatory acute phase response in severely burned children. Ann Surg 2000; 231:246–252.

69. Jarrar D, Wolf SE, Jeschke MG, et al. Growth hormone attenuates the acute-phase response to thermal injury. Arch Surg 1997; 132:1171–1175; discussion 1175–1176.

70. Pos O, van der Stelt ME, Wolbink GJ, et al. Changes in the serum concentration and the glycosylation of human alpha 1-acid glycoprotein and alpha 1-protease inhibitor in severely burned persons: relation to interleukin-6 levels. Clin Exp Immunol 1990; 82:579–582.

71. Sevaljevic L, Glibetic M, Poznanovic G, et al. Effect of lethal scald on the mechanisms of acute-phase protein synthesis in rat liver. Circ Shock 1991; 33:98–107.

72. Jeschke MG, Herndon DN, Wolf SE, et al. Hepatocyte growth factor modulates the hepatic acute-phase response in thermally injured rats. Crit Care Med 2000; 28:504–510.

73. Sevaljevic L, Ivanovic-Matic S, Petrovic M, et al. Regulation of plasma acute-phase protein and albumin levels in the liver of scalded rats. Biochem J 1989; 258:663–668.

74. Kataranovski M, Magic Z, Pejnovic N. Early inflammatory cytokine and acute phase protein response under the stress of thermal injury in rats. Physiol Res 1999; 48:473–482.

75. Nijsten MW, Hack CE, Helle M, et al. Interleukin-6 and its relation to the humoral immune response and clinical parameters in burned patients. Surgery 1991; 109:761–767.

76. Heinrich PC, Castell JV, Andus T. Interleukin-6 and the acute phase response. Biochem J 1990; 265:621–636.

77. Fey GH, Fuller GM. Regulation of acute phase gene expression by inflammatory mediators. Mol Biol Med 1987; 4:323–338.

78. Schluter B, Konig B, Bergmann U, et al. Interleukin 6 – a potential mediator of lethal sepsis after major thermal trauma: evidence for increased IL-6 production by peripheral blood mononuclear cells. J Trauma 1991; 31:1663–1670.

79. Dickson PW, Bannister D, Schreiber G. Minor burns lead to major changes in synthesis rates of plasma proteins in the liver. J Trauma 1987; 27:283–286.

80. Biffl WL, Moore EE, Moore FA, et al. Interleukin-6 in the injured patient. Marker of injury or mediator of inflammation? Ann Surg 1996; 224:647–664.

81. Ueyama M, Maruyama I, Osame M, et al. Marked increase in plasma interleukin-6 in burn patients. J Lab Clin Med 1992; 120:693–698.

82. Guo Y, Dickerson C, Chrest FJ, et al. Increased levels of circulating interleukin 6 in burn patients. Clin Immunol Immunopathol 1990; 54:361–371.

83. Li JJ, Sanders RL, McAdam KP, et al. Impact of C-reactive protein (CRP) on surfactant function. J Trauma 1989; 29:1690–1697.

84. Livingston DH, Mosenthal AC, Deitch EA. Sepsis and multiple organ dysfunction syndrome: a clinical-mechanistic overview. New Horiz 1995; 3:257–266.

85. Pruitt JH, Copeland EM 3rd, Moldawer LL. Interleukin-1 and interleukin-1 antagonism in sepsis, systemic inflammatory response syndrome, and septic shock. Shock 1995; 3:235–251.

86. Bunn F, Lefebvre C, Li Wan Po A, et al. Human albumin solution for resuscitation and volume expansion in critically ill patients. The Albumin Reviewers. Cochrane Database Syst Rev 2000; (2): CD001208.

87. Jeschke MG, Herndon DN, Wolf SE, et al. Recombinant human growth hormone alters acute phase reactant proteins, cytokine expression, and liver morphology in burned rats. J Surg Res 1999; 83:122–129.

88. Jeschke MG, Barrow RE, Hawkins HK, et al. Biodistribution and feasibility of non-viral IGF-I gene transfers in thermally injured skin. Lab Invest 2000; 80:151–158.

89. Callery MP, Kamei T, Mangino MJ, et al. Organ interactions in sepsis. Host defense and the hepatic-pulmonary macrophage axis. Arch Surg 1991; 126:28–32.

90. Henson PM, Johnston RB Jr. Tissue injury in inflammation. Oxidants, proteinases, and cationic proteins. J Clin Invest 1987; 79:669–674.

91. Peterson VM, Rundus CH, Reinoehl PJ, et al. The myelopoietic effects of a Serratia marcescens-derived biologic response modifier in a mouse model of thermal injury. Surgery 1992; 111:447–454.

92. Goris RJ. MODS/SIRS: result of an overwhelming inflammatory response? World J Surg 1996; 20:418–421.

93. Border JR. Hypothesis: sepsis, multiple systems organ failure, and the macrophage. Arch Surg 1988; 123:285–286.

94. Weiss MJ, Keller G, Orkin SH. Novel insights into erythroid development revealed through in vitro differentiation of GATA-1 embryonic stem cells. Genes Dev 1994; 8:1184–1197.

95. Turnage RH, Nwariaku F, Murphy J, et al. Mechanisms of pulmonary microvascular dysfunction during severe burn injury. World J Surg 2002; 26:848–853.

96. Eriksson E, Straube RC, Robson MC. White blood cell consumption in the microcirculation after a major burn. J Trauma 1979; 19:94–97.

97. Gamelli RL, Paxton TP, O'Reilly M. Bone marrow toxicity by silver sulfadiazine. Surg Gynecol Obstet 1993; 177:115–120.

98. Peterson V, Hansbrough J, Buerk C, et al. Regulation of granulopoiesis following severe thermal injury. J Trauma 1983; 23:19–24.

99. Wolach B, Coates TD, Hugli TE, et al. Plasma lactoferrin reflects granulocyte activation via complement in burn patients. J Lab Clin Med 1984; 103:284–293.

100. Eurenius K, Brouse RO. Granulocyte kinetics after thermal injury. Am J Clin Pathol 1973; 60:337–342.

101. Huang WH, Wu JZ, Hu ZX, et al. Bone marrow granulopoietic response to scalds and wound infection in mice. Burns Incl Therm Inj 1988; 14:292–296.

102. Asko-Seljavaara S. Inhibition of bone marrow cell proliferation in burned mice. An in vitro study of the effect of fluid replacement and burn serum on bone marrow cell growth. Scand J Plast Reconstr Surg 1974; 8:192–197.

103. Asko-Seljavaara S. Granulocyte kinetics in burned mice. Inhibition of granulocyte studied in vivo and in vitro. Scand J Plast Reconstr Surg 1974; 8:185–191.

104. Gamelli RL, Hebert JC, Foster RS Jr. Effect of burn injury on granulocyte and macrophage production. J Trauma 1985; 25:615–619.

105. McEuen DD, Gerber GC, Blair P, et al. Granulocyte function and Pseudomonas burn wound infection. Infect Immun 1976; 14:399–402.

106. McEuen DD, Ogawa M, Eurenius K. Myelopoiesis in the infected burn. J Lab Clin Med 1977; 89:540–543.

107. Maestroni GJ. Catecholaminergic regulation of hematopoiesis in mice. Blood 1998; 92:2971; author reply 2972–2973.

108. Broxmeyer HE, Williams DE. Actions of hematopoietic colony-stimulating factors in vivo and in vitro. Pathol Immunopathol Res 1987; 6:207–220.

109. Metcalf D. The hemopoietic regulators – an embarrassment of riches. Bioessays 1992; 14:799–805.

110. Silver GM, Gamelli RL, O'Reilly M. The beneficial effect of granulocyte colony-stimulating factor (G-CSF) in combination with gentamicin on survival after Pseudomonas burn wound infection. Surgery 1989; 106:452–455; discussion 455–456.

111. Sartorelli KH, Silver GM, Gamelli RL. The effect of granulocyte colony-stimulating factor (G-CSF) upon burn-induced defective neutrophil chemotaxis. J Trauma 1991; 31:523–529; discussion 529–530.

112. Gamelli RL, He LK, Liu H. Recombinant human granulocyte colony-stimulating factor treatment improves macrophage suppression of granulocyte and macrophage growth after burn and burn wound infection. J Trauma 1995; 39:1141–1146; discussion 1146–1147.

113. Toda H, Murata A, Matsuura N, et al. Therapeutic efficacy of granulocyte colony stimulating factor against rat cecal ligation and puncture model. Stem Cells 1993; 11:228–234.

114. Smith WS, Sumnicht GE, Sharpe RW, et al. Granulocyte colony-stimulating factor versus placebo in addition to penicillin G in a randomized blinded study of gram-negative pneumonia sepsis: analysis of survival and multisystem organ failure. Blood 1995; 86:1301–1309.

115. Braquet M, Lavaud P, Dormont D, et al. Leukocytic functions in burn-injured patients. Prostaglandins 1985; 29:747–764.

116. el-Falaky MH, Abdel-Hafez A, Houtah AH. Phagocytic activity of polymorphonuclear leucocytes in burns. Burns Incl Therm Inj 1985; 11:185–191.

117. Solomkin JS. Neutrophil disorders in burn injury: complement, cytokines, and organ injury. J Trauma 1990; 30:S80–S85.

118. Grogan JB, Miller RC. Impaired function of polymorphonuclear leukocytes in patients with burns and other trauma. Surg Gynecol Obstet 1973; 137:784–788.

119. Bjerknes R, Vindenes H, Laerum OD. Altered neutrophil functions in patients with large burns. Blood Cells 1990; 16:127–141; discussion 142–123.

120. Bjerknes R, Vindenes H. Neutrophil dysfunction after thermal injury: alteration of phagolysosomal acidification in patients with large burns. Burns 1989; 15:77–81.

121. Bjornson AB, Somers SD, Knippenberg RW, et al. Circulating factors contribute to elevation of intracellular cyclic-3′,5′-adenosine monophosphate and depression of superoxide anion production in polymorphonuclear leukocytes following thermal injury. J Leukoc Biol 1992; 52:407–414.

122. Sayeed MM. Neutrophil signaling alteration: an adverse inflammatory response after burn shock. Medicina (B Aires) 1998; 58: 386–392.

123. Solomkin JS, Cotta LA, Brodt JK, et al. Neutrophil dysfunction in sepsis. III. Degranulation as a mechanism for nonspecific deactivation. J Surg Res 1984; 36:407–412.

124. Bjerknes R, Vindenes H, Pitkanen J, et al. Altered polymorphonuclear neutrophilic granulocyte functions in patients with large burns. J Trauma 1989; 29:847–855.

125. Solomkin JS, Nelson RD, Chenoweth DE, et al. Regulation of neutrophil migratory function in burn injury by complement activation products. Ann Surg 1984; 200:742–746.

126. Tchervenkov JI, Latter DA, Psychogios J, et al. Altered leukocyte delivery to specific and nonspecific inflammatory skin lesions following burn injury. J Trauma 1988; 28:582–588.

127. Duque RE, Phan SH, Hudson JL, et al. Functional defects in phagocytic cells following thermal injury. Application of flow cytometric analysis. Am J Pathol 1985; 118:116–127.

128. Mooney DP, Gamelli RL, O'Reilly M, et al. Recombinant human granulocyte colony-stimulating factor and Pseudomonas burn wound sepsis. Arch Surg 1988; 123:1353–1357.

129. Bjornson AB, Knippenberg RW, Bjornson HS. Bactericidal defect of neutrophils in a guinea pig model of thermal injury is related to elevation of intracellular cyclic-3′,5′-adenosine monophosphate. J Immunol 1989; 143:2609–2616.

130. Volenec FJ, Wood GW, Mani MM, et al. Mononuclear cell analysis of peripheral blood from burn patients. J Trauma 1979; 19:86–93.

131. Moore FD Jr, Davis CF. Monocyte activation after burns and endotoxemia. J Surg Res 1989; 46:350–354.

132. O'Riordain MG, Collins KH, Pilz M, et al. Modulation of macrophage hyperactivity improves survival in a burn-sepsis model. Arch Surg 1992; 127:152–157; discussion 157–158.

133. Miller-Graziano CL, Szabo G, Griffey K, et al. Role of elevated monocyte transforming growth factor beta (TGF beta) production in posttrauma immunosuppression. J Clin Immunol 1991; 11: 95–102.

134. Miller-Graziano CL, Szabo G, Kodys K, et al. Aberrations in posttrauma monocyte (MO) subpopulation: role in septic shock syndrome. J Trauma 1990; 30:S86–S96.

135. Ogle CK, Guo X, Wu JZ, et al. Production of cytokines and PGE$_2$ and cytotoxicity of stimulated bone marrow macrophages after thermal injury and cytotoxicity of stimulated U-937 macrophages. Inflammation 1993; 17:583–594.

136. Ogle CK, Guo X, Alexander JW, et al. The activation of bone marrow macrophages 24 hours after thermal injury. Arch Surg 1993; 128:96–100; discussion 100–101.

137. Hansbrough JF, Bender EM, Zapata-Sirvent R, et al. Altered helper and suppressor lymphocyte populations in surgical patients. A measure of postoperative immunosuppression. Am J Surg 1984; 148:303–307.

138. Sparkes BG. Immunological responses to thermal injury. Burns 1997; 23:106–113.

139. Munster AM, Eurenius K, Katz RM, et al. Cell-mediated immunity after thermal injury. Ann Surg 1973; 177:139–143.

140. Munster AM. Alteration of the immune system in burns and implications for therapy. Eur J Pediatr Surg 1994; 4:231–242.

141. Rapaport FT, Milgrom F, Kano K, et al. Immunologic sequelae of thermal injury. Ann N Y Acad Sci 1968; 150:1004–1008.

142. Munster AM. Post-traumatic immunosuppression is due to activation of suppressor T cells. Lancet 1976; 1:1329–1330.

143. Organ BC, Antonacci AC, Chiao J, et al. Changes in lymphocyte number and phenotype in seven lymphoid compartments after thermal injury. Ann Surg 1989; 210:78–89.

144. Kupper TS, Green DR. Immunoregulation after thermal injury: sequential appearance of I-J$^+$, Ly-1 T suppressor inducer cells and Ly-2 T suppressor effector cells following thermal trauma in mice. J Immunol 1984; 133:3047–3053.

145. Hansbrough JF, Zapata-Sirvent R, Hoyt D. Postburn immune suppression: an inflammatory response to the burn wound? J Trauma 1990; 30:671–674; discussion 674–675.

146. Maldonado MD, Venturoli A, Franco A, et al. Specific changes in peripheral blood lymphocyte phenotype from burn patients. Probable origin of the thermal injury-related lymphocytopenia. Burns 1991; 17:188–192.

147. Gadd MA, Hansbrough JF, Hoyt DB, et al. Defective T-cell surface antigen expression after mitogen stimulation. An index of lymphocyte dysfunction after controlled murine injury. Ann Surg 1989; 209:112–118.

148. Tenen DG, Hromas R, Licht JD, et al. Transcription factors, normal myeloid development, and leukemia. Blood 1997; 90:489–519.

149. Teodorczyk-Injeyan JA, Cembrzynska-Nowak M, Lalani S, et al. Immune deficiency following thermal trauma is associated with apoptotic cell death. J Clin Immunol 1995; 15:318–328.

150. Golstein P, Ojcius DM, Young JD. Cell death mechanisms and the immune system. Immunol Rev 1991; 121:29–65.

151. Mountz JD, Zhou T, Wu J, et al. Regulation of apoptosis in immune cells. J Clin Immunol 1995; 15:1–16.

152. Arturson G, Hogman CF, Johansson SG, et al. Changes in immunoglobulin levels in severely burned patients. Lancet 1969; 1:546–548.

153. Kohn J, Cort DF. Immunoglobulins in burned patients. Lancet 1969; 1:836–837.

154. Munster AM, Hoagland HC. Serum immunoglobulin patterns after burns. Surg Forum 1969; 20:76–77.

155. Ritzmann SE, Larson DL, McClung C, et al. Immunoglobulin levels in burned patients. Lancet 1969; 1:1152–1153.

156. Noelle RJ, Snow EC. T helper cell-dependent B cell activation. FASEB J 1991; 5:2770–2776.

157. Schluter B, Konig W, Koller M, et al. Differential regulation of T- and B-lymphocyte activation in severely burned patients. J Trauma 1991; 31:239–246.

158. Dexter TM. Introduction to the haemopoietic system. Cancer Surv 1990; 9:1–5.

159. Testa NG, Dexter TM. Cell lineages in haemopoiesis: comments on their regulation. Semin Immunol 1990; 2:167–172.

160. Metcalf D. Cellular hematopoiesis in the twentieth century. Semin Hematol 1999; 36:5–12.

161. Cheers C, Haigh AM, Kelso A, et al. Production of colony-stimulating factors (CSFs) during infection: separate determinations of macrophage-, granulocyte-, granulocyte-macrophage-, and multi-CSFs. Infect Immun 1988; 56:247–251.

162. Heyworth CM, Vallance SJ, Whetton AD, et al. The biochemistry and biology of the myeloid haemopoietic cell growth factors. J Cell Sci Suppl 1990; 13:57–74.

163. Kondo M, Weissman IL, Akashi K. Identification of clonogenic common lymphoid progenitors in mouse bone marrow. Cell 1997; 91:661–672.

164. Kozutsumi H. Special education. Oncologist 1996; 1:116–118.

165. Peterson VM, Robinson WA, Wallner SF, et al. Granulocyte stem cells are decreased in humans with fatal burns. J Trauma 1985; 25:413–418.

166. Santangelo S, Gamelli RL, Shankar R. Myeloid commitment shifts toward monocytopoiesis after thermal injury and sepsis. Ann Surg 2001; 233:97–106.

167. Gamelli RL, He LK, Liu H. Marrow granulocyte-macrophage progenitor cell response to burn injury as modified by endotoxin and indomethacin. J Trauma 1994; 37:339–346.

168. Gentile PS, Pelus LM. In vivo modulation of myelopoiesis by prostaglandin E$_2$. IV. Prostaglandin E$_2$ induction of myelopoietic inhibitory activity. J Immunol 1988; 141:2714–2720.

169. Pelus LM. Modulation of myelopoiesis by prostaglandin E$_2$: demonstration of a novel mechanism of action in vivo. Immunol Res 1989; 8:176–184.

170. Pelus LM. Blockade of prostaglandin biosynthesis in intact mice dramatically augments the expansion of committed myeloid progenitor cells (colony-forming units-granulocyte, macrophage) after acute administration of recombinant human IL-1 alpha. J Immunol 1989; 143:4171–4179.

171. Hahn EL, Tai HH, He LK, et al. Burn injury with infection alters prostaglandin E$_2$ synthesis and metabolism. J Trauma 1999; 47:1052–1057; discussion 1057–1059.

172. Shoup M, He LK, Liu H, et al. Cyclooxygenase-2 inhibitor NS-398 improves survival and restores leukocyte counts in burn infection. J Trauma 1998; 45:215–220; discussion 220–211.

173. Santangelo S, Shoup M, Gamelli RL, et al. Prostaglandin E$_2$ receptor antagonist (SC-19220) treatment restores the balance to bone marrow myelopoiesis after burn sepsis. J Trauma 2000; 48:826–830; discussion 830–821.

174. Fleming TJ, Fleming ML, Malek TR. Selective expression of Ly-6G on myeloid lineage cells in mouse bone marrow. RB6–8C5 mAb to granulocyte-differentiation antigen (Gr-1) detects members of the Ly-6 family. J Immunol 1993; 151:2399–2408.

175. Hestdal K, Ruscetti FW, Ihle JN, et al. Characterization and regulation of RB6–8C5 antigen expression on murine bone marrow cells. J Immunol 1991; 147:22–28.

176. Akashi K, Traver D, Miyamoto T, et al. A clonogenic common myeloid progenitor that gives rise to all myeloid lineages. Nature 2000; 404:193–197.

177. Van Furth R, Diesselhoff-den Dulk MC, Mattie H. Quantitative study on the production and kinetics of mononuclear phagocytes during an acute inflammatory reaction. J Exp Med 1973; 138:1314–1330.

178. Dexter TM, Coutinho LH, Spooncer E, et al. Stromal cells in haemopoiesis. Ciba Found Symp 1990; 148:76–86; discussion 86–95.

179. Leenen PJ, Melis M, Slieker WA, et al. Murine macrophage precursor characterization. II. Monoclonal antibodies against macrophage precursor antigens. Eur J Immunol 1990; 20:27–34.

180. de Bruijn MF, Slieker WA, van der Loo JC, et al. Distinct mouse bone marrow macrophage precursors identified by differential expression of ER-MP12 and ER-MP20 antigens. Eur J Immunol 1994; 24:2279–2284.

181. Ikebuchi K, Wong GG, Clark SC, et al. Interleukin 6 enhancement of interleukin 3-dependent proliferation of multipotential hemopoietic progenitors. Proc Natl Acad Sci USA 1987; 84:9035–9039.

182. Lazzari L, Henschler R, Lecchi L, et al. Interleukin-6 and interleukin-11 act synergistically with thrombopoietin and stem cell factor to modulate ex vivo expansion of human CD41+ and CD61+ megakaryocytic cells. Haematologica 2000; 85:25–30.

183. Sui X, Tsuji K, Ebihara Y, et al. Soluble interleukin-6 (IL-6) receptor with IL-6 stimulates megakaryopoiesis from human CD34(+) cells through glycoprotein (gp)130 signaling. Blood 1999; 93:2525–2532.

184. Metcalf D. Actions and interactions of G-CSF, LIF, and IL-6 on normal and leukemic murine cells. Leukemia 1989; 3:349–355.

185. Nicola NA, Vadas MA, Lopez AF. Down-modulation of receptors for granulocyte colony-stimulating factor on human neutrophils by granulocyte-activating agents. J Cell Physiol 1986; 128:501–509.

186. Walker F, Nicola NA, Metcalf D, et al. Hierarchical down-modulation of hemopoietic growth factor receptors. Cell 1985; 43:269–276.

187. Fogli M, Carlo-Stella C, Curti A, et al. Transforming growth factor beta3 inhibits chronic myelogenous leukemia hematopoiesis by inducing Fas-independent apoptosis. Exp Hematol 2000; 28:775–783.

188. Batard P, Monier MN, Fortunel N, et al. TGF-(beta)1 maintains hematopoietic immaturity by a reversible negative control of cell cycle and induces CD34 antigen up-modulation. J Cell Sci 2000; 113 (Pt 3):383–390.

189. Cashman JD, Clark-Lewis I, Eaves AC, et al. Differentiation stage-specific regulation of primitive human hematopoietic progenitor cycling by exogenous and endogenous inhibitors in an in vivo model. Blood 1999; 94:3722–3729.

190. Macfarlane WM. Demystified transcription. Mol Pathol 2000; 53:1–7.

191. Ward AC, Loeb DM, Soede-Bobok AA, et al. Regulation of granulopoiesis by transcription factors and cytokine signals. Leukemia 2000; 14:973–990.

192. Guerriero A, Langmuir PB, Spain LM, et al. PU.1 is required for myeloid-derived but not lymphoid-derived dendritic cells. Blood 2000; 95:879–885.

193. Nerlov C, Querfurth E, Kulessa H, Graf T. GATA-1 interacts with the myeloid PU.1 transcription factor and represses PU.1-dependent transcription. Blood 2000; 95:2543–2551.

194. Finger LR, Kagan J, Christopher G, et al. Involvement of the TCL5 gene on human chromosome 1 in T-cell leukemia and melanoma. Proc Natl Acad Sci USA 1989; 86:5039–5043.

195. Xia Y, Brown L, Yang CY, et al. TAL2, a helix-loop-helix gene activated by the (7; 9)(q34; q32) translocation in human T-cell leukemia. Proc Natl Acad Sci USA 1991; 88:11416–11420.

196. Shivdasani RA, Orkin SH. The transcriptional control of hematopoiesis. Blood 1996; 87:4025–4039.

197. Mouthon MA, Bernard O, Mitjavila MT, et al. Expression of tal-1 and GATA-binding proteins during human hematopoiesis. Blood 1993; 81:647–655.

198. Begley CG, Aplan PD, Denning SM, et al. The gene SCL is expressed during early hematopoiesis and encodes a differentiation-related DNA-binding motif. Proc Natl Acad Sci USA 1989; 86:10128–10132.

199. Robb L, Lyons I, Li R, et al. Absence of yolk sac hematopoiesis from mice with a targeted disruption of the scl gene. Proc Natl Acad Sci USA 1995; 92:7075–7079.

200. Tsai FY, Keller G, Kuo FC, et al. An early haematopoietic defect in mice lacking the transcription factor GATA-2. Nature 1994; 371:221–226.

201. Orkin SH. GATA-binding transcription factors in hematopoietic cells. Blood 1992; 80:575–581.

202. Visvader JE, Elefanty AG, Strasser A, et al. GATA-1 but not SCL induces megakaryocytic differentiation in an early myeloid line. EMBO J 1992; 11:4557–4564.

203. Simon MC, Pevny L, Wiles MV, et al. Rescue of erythroid development in gene targeted GATA-1- mouse embryonic stem cells. Nat Genet 1992; 1:92–98.

204. Zhang P, Behre G, Pan J, et al. Negative cross-talk between hematopoietic regulators: GATA proteins repress PU.1. Proc Natl Acad Sci USA 1999; 96:8705–8710.

205. Klemsz MJ, McKercher SR, Celada A, et al. The macrophage and B cell-specific transcription factor PU.1 is related to the ets oncogene. Cell 1990; 61:113–124.

206. Ray-Gallet D, Mao C, Tavitian A, et al. DNA binding specificities of Spi-1/PU.1 and Spi-B transcription factors and identification of a Spi-1/Spi-B binding site in the c-fes/c-fps promoter. Oncogene 1995; 11:303–313.

207. Klemsz MJ, Maki RA. Activation of transcription by PU.1 requires both acidic and glutamine domains. Mol Cell Biol 1996; 16:390–397.

208. Chen HM, Zhang P, Voso MT, et al. Neutrophils and monocytes express high levels of PU.1 (Spi-1) but not Spi-B. Blood 1995; 85:2918–2928.

209. McKercher SR, Torbett BE, Anderson KL, et al. Targeted disruption of the PU.1 gene results in multiple hematopoietic abnormalities. EMBO J 1996; 15:5647–5658.

210. Scott EW, Simon MC, Anastasi J, et al. Requirement of transcription factor PU.1 in the development of multiple hematopoietic lineages. Science 1994; 265:1573–1577.

211. Anderson KL, Smith KA, Conners K, et al. Myeloid development is selectively disrupted in PU.1 null mice. Blood 1998; 91:3702–3710.

212. DeKoter RP, Walsh JC, Singh H. PU.1 regulates both cytokine-dependent proliferation and differentiation of granulocyte/macrophage progenitors. EMBO J 1998; 17:4456–4468.

213. Biedenkapp H, Borgmeyer U, Sippel AE, et al. Viral myb oncogene encodes a sequence-specific DNA-binding activity. Nature 1988; 335:835–837.

214. Klempnauer KH, Sippel AE. The highly conserved amino-terminal region of the protein encoded by the v-myb oncogene functions as a DNA-binding domain. EMBO J 1987; 6:2719–2725.

215. Ramsay RG, Morrice N, Van Eeden P, et al. Regulation of c-Myb through protein phosphorylation and leucine zipper interactions. Oncogene 1995; 11:2113–2120.

216. Weston K, Bishop JM. Transcriptional activation by the v-myb oncogene and its cellular progenitor, c-myb. Cell 1989; 58:85–93.

217. Sakura H, Kanei-Ishii C, Nagase T, et al. Delineation of three functional domains of the transcriptional activator encoded by the c-myb protooncogene. Proc Natl Acad Sci USA 1989; 86:5758–5762.

218. Ess KC, Witte DP, Bascomb CP, et al. Diverse developing mouse lineages exhibit high-level c-Myb expression in immature cells

and loss of expression upon differentiation. Oncogene 1999; 18: 1103–1111.

219. Gonda TJ, Metcalf D. Expression of myb, myc and fos proto-oncogenes during the differentiation of a murine myeloid leukaemia. Nature 1984; 310:249–251.

220. Sheiness D, Gardinier M. Expression of a proto-oncogene (proto-myb) in hemopoietic tissues of mice. Mol Cell Biol 1984; 4:1206–1212.

221. Mucenski ML, McLain K, Kier AB, et al. A functional c-myb gene is required for normal murine fetal hepatic hematopoiesis. Cell 1991; 65:677–689.

222. Friedman AD, Landschulz WH, McKnight SL. CCAAT/enhancer binding protein activates the promoter of the serum albumin gene in cultured hepatoma cells. Genes Dev 1989; 3:1314–1322.

223. Gilpin DA, Hsieh CC, Kuninger DT, et al. Effect of thermal injury on the expression of transcription factors that regulate acute phase response genes: the response of C/EBP alpha, C/EBP beta, and C/EBP delta to thermal injury. Surgery 1996; 119:674–683.

224. Landschulz WH, Johnson PF, McKnight SL. The DNA binding domain of the rat liver nuclear protein C/EBP is bipartite. Science 1989; 243:1681–1688.

225. Scott LM, Civin CI, Rorth P, et al. A novel temporal expression pattern of three C/EBP family members in differentiating myelomonocytic cells. Blood 1992; 80:1725–1735.

226. Nerlov C, McNagny KM, Doderlein G, et al. Distinct C/EBP functions are required for eosinophil lineage commitment and maturation. Genes Dev 1998; 12:2413–2423.

227. Radomska HS, Huettner CS, Zhang P, et al. CCAAT/enhancer binding protein alpha is a regulatory switch sufficient for induction of granulocytic development from bipotential myeloid progenitors. Mol Cell Biol 1998; 18:4301–4314.

228. Wang X, Scott E, Sawyers CL, et al. C/EBPalpha bypasses granulocyte colony-stimulating factor signals to rapidly induce PU.1 gene expression, stimulate granulocytic differentiation, and limit proliferation in 32D cl3 myeloblasts. Blood 1999; 94:560–571.

229. Zhang DE, Zhang P, Wang ND, et al. Absence of granulocyte colony-stimulating factor signaling and neutrophil development in CCAAT enhancer binding protein alpha-deficient mice. Proc Natl Acad Sci USA 1997; 94:569–574.

230. Screpanti I, Romani L, Musiani P, et al. Lymphoproliferative disorder and imbalanced T-helper response in C/EBP beta-deficient mice. EMBO J 1995; 14:1932–1941.

231. Tanaka T, Akira S, Yoshida K, et al. Targeted disruption of the NF-IL6 gene discloses its essential role in bacteria killing and tumor cytotoxicity by macrophages. Cell 1995; 80:353–361.

232. Chen X, Liu W, Ambrosino C, et al. Impaired generation of bone marrow B lymphocytes in mice deficient in C/EBPbeta. Blood 1997; 90:156–164.

233. Antonson P, Stellan B, Yamanaka R, et al. A novel human CCAAT/enhancer binding protein gene, C/EBPepsilon, is expressed in cells of lymphoid and myeloid lineages and is localized on chromosome 14q11.2 close to the T-cell receptor alpha/delta locus. Genomics 1996; 35:30–38.

234. Cole MD. The myc oncogene: its role in transformation and differentiation. Annu Rev Genet 1986; 20:361–384.

235. Blackwell TK, Kretzner L, Blackwood EM, et al. Sequence-specific DNA binding by the c-Myc protein. Science 1990; 250:1149–1151.

236. Baumbach WR, Stanley ER, Cole MD. Induction of clonal monocyte/macrophage tumors in vivo by a mouse c-myc retrovirus: evidence for secondary transforming events. Curr Top Microbiol Immunol 1986; 132:23–32.

237. Delgado MD, Lerga A, Canelles M, et al. Differential regulation of Max and role of c-Myc during erythroid and myelomonocytic differentiation of K562 cells. Oncogene 1995; 10:1659–1665.

238. Blackwood EM, Eisenman RN. Max: a helix-loop-helix zipper protein that forms a sequence-specific DNA-binding complex with Myc. Science 1991; 251:1211–1217.

239. Amin C, Wagner AJ, Hay N. Sequence-specific transcriptional activation by Myc and repression by Max. Mol Cell Biol 1993; 13:383–390.

240. Ayer DE, Eisenman RN. A switch from Myc:Max to Mad:Max heterocomplexes accompanies monocyte/macrophage differentiation. Genes Dev 1993; 7:2110–2119.

241. Zervos AS, Gyuris J, Brent R. Mxi1, a protein that specifically interacts with Max to bind Myc-Max recognition sites. Cell 1993; 72:223–232.

242. Kretzner L, Blackwood EM, Eisenman RN. Transcriptional activities of the Myc and Max proteins in mammalian cells. Curr Top Microbiol Immunol 1992; 182:435–443.

243. Cultraro CM, Bino T, Segal S. Regulated expression and function of the c-Myc antagonist, Mad1, during a molecular switch from proliferation to differentiation. Curr Top Microbiol Immunol 1997; 224:149–158.

244. Larsson LG, Pettersson M, Oberg F, et al. Expression of mad, mxi1, max and c-myc during induced differentiation of hematopoietic cells: opposite regulation of mad and c-myc. Oncogene 1994; 9:1247–1252.

245. Foley KP, McArthur GA, Queva C, et al. Targeted disruption of the MYC antagonist MAD1 inhibits cell cycle exit during granulocyte differentiation. EMBO J 1998; 17:774–785.

246. McGinnis W, Garber RL, Wirz J, et al. A homologous protein-coding sequence in Drosophila homeotic genes and its conservation in other metazoans. Cell 1984; 37:403–408.

247. Lawrence HJ, Largman C. Homeobox genes in normal hematopoiesis and leukemia. Blood 1992; 80:2445–2453.

248. Helgason CD, Sauvageau G, Lawrence HJ, et al. Overexpression of HOXB4 enhances the hematopoietic potential of embryonic stem cells differentiated in vitro. Blood 1996; 87:2740–2749.

249. Lawrence HJ, Helgason CD, Sauvageau G, et al. Mice bearing a targeted interruption of the homeobox gene HOXA9 have defects in myeloid, erythroid, and lymphoid hematopoiesis. Blood 1997; 89:1922–1930.

250. Fuller JF, McAdara J, Yaron Y, et al. Characterization of HOX gene expression during myelopoiesis: role of HOX A5 in lineage commitment and maturation. Blood 1999; 93:3391–3400.

251. Lill MC, Fuller JF, Herzig R, et al. The role of the homeobox gene, HOX B7, in human myelomonocytic differentiation. Blood 1995; 85:692–697.

252. Allen JD, Adams JM. Enforced expression of Hlx homeobox gene prompts myeloid cell maturation and altered adherence properties of T cells. Blood 1993; 81:3242–3251.

253. Wallner SF, Warren GH. The haematopoietic response to burning: an autopsy study. Burns Incl Therm Inj 1985; 12:22–27.

254. McGill V, Kowal-Vern A, Gamelli RL. A conservative thermal injury treatment protocol for the appropriate Jehovah's Witness candidate. J Burn Care Rehabil 1997; 18:133–138.

255. Offringa M. Excess mortality after human albumin administration in critically ill patients. Clinical and pathophysiological evidence suggests albumin is harmful. BMJ 1998; 317:223–224.

Chapter 25

Significance of the adrenal and sympathetic response to burn injury

Stephen B. Jones, Kuzhali Muthu, Ravi Shankar, and Richard L. Gamelli

Chapter contents

Introduction

The physiological importance of the adrenal gland is most often associated with the release of epinephrine and glucocorticoids in response to cognitive stress widely recognized as the 'fight or flight' response. Such responses involving the hypothalamic–pituitary–adrenal axis begin with the hypothalamic release of corticotropin-releasing hormone (CRH) that mediates the release of adrenocorticotropic hormone (ACTH) from the pituitary that in turn stimulates cortisol synthesis and release from the adrenal cortex. Hypothalamic stimulation also initiates epinephrine and norepinephrine release from the adrenal medulla as well as the release of sympathetic neurotransmitter norepinephrine from adrenergic nerve terminals throughout the body. The action of these hormones and neurotransmitters is traditionally thought to serve in a compensatory manner facilitating heightened mental awareness along with metabolic and cardiovascular activity that supports rapid increases in muscular work.

Thermal injury, like other forms of trauma as well as infectious challenge, is a non-cognitive stimulus but also results in an elevated hormone/neurotransmitter milieu similar in magnitude to that of the cognitive 'fight or flight' responses.[1,2] However, there are important characteristics of the injury response that contrast with the fight or flight response. These include prolonged hormone/neurotransmitter elevation, the absence of increased muscle work limiting metabolic demand and the presence of massive tissue injury. Additional hormone/neurotransmitter responses may also be evoked by surgical debridement of burn wounds and skin grafting procedures. The second surge of stress hormones complicates the severe metabolic derangements and compromised immune capacity that is characteristic of the burn course during the initial 7–10 days following injury.

Regardless of the cognitive or non-cognitive nature of stress hormone stimulation, events that increase corticosteroids and catecholamines represent a stress response but may or may not involve pathology. Traumatic injury, however, clearly initiates an initial stress response with a magnitude that is proportional to the severity of injury. Under these conditions, hormone/neurotransmitter release seems to promote survival. Although such a benefit may be difficult to see in human injury, experimental animal models have provided some insights. Animals that lack stress hormones or suffer from impaired release or where hormone action is pharmacologically blocked often die of an otherwise survivable event. Similarly, overwhelming traumatic injury in man may result in stress hormone release that is detrimental to survival. Whereas this may also be difficult to document in burn patients, animal studies have demonstrated that exogenous administration of high amounts of stress hormones is detrimental.

Two historical perspectives are important to consider regarding stress and the trauma of burn injury. First is the concept described by Cuthbertson,[3] where the initial response to thermal injury is considered an 'ebb' phase characterized by reduced metabolism and tissue perfusion. Within days there is a transition to a 'flow' phase typified by increased resting energy expenditure and hypermetabolism with supportive cardiovascular function. Changes in endocrine hormone levels are important for these acute catabolic alterations. The concepts of 'stress' and release of 'stress hormones' widely used today, were clarified by the classic work of Selye.[4] His notion of stress responses include an initial 'alarm reaction' of fairly short duration with high levels of stress hormones followed by a 'resistance phase' described as a prolonged period during which there is compensation to maintain homeostasis during continued stress. Selye's final stage of 'exhaustion' is where compensation could not be maintained and death rapidly follows. The acute initial period of high-stress hormone release encompasses both Cuthbertson's ebb phase and Selye's alarm reaction and the flow phase[3] has similar features to the resistance phase.[4] These compensatory changes promote increased energy expenditure and support cardiovascular function; however, in patients with severe injury the same compensatory changes result in depletion of energy reserves, extensive muscle wasting and immune suppression; all of which are hallmarks of post-burn sequalae. This compensatory pattern is described as a hypermetabolic state with patients displaying elevated resting metabolic rates for several weeks to months following injury.[5-7] The extent of the hypermetabolic response is dependent upon the extent and depth of burn injury, septic complications and surgical interventions. Although the well-conceived concepts of ebb and flow and generalized phases of stress help to conceptualize what is happening during recovery from uncomplicated thermal injury, questions related to the magnitude of stress hormone responses and beneficial versus detrimental actions in the recovery from severe thermal injury remain unanswered.

During the last 50 years great strides have been made in the care of burn patients and with various treatment modalities attempting to exploit some of the concepts described above. Examples include:

- rapid fluid resuscitation to stabilize cardiovascular function and reduce the stimulus for continued sympathetic drive;
- nutritional support to meet metabolic demands and to support homeostasis during healing;
- elevated environmental temperatures and occlusive dressings to lessen the metabolic demands, reduce metabolic rate and cardiac output and to optimize wound healing.

Aside from the regulation of metabolic and cardiovascular function, neuro-immune interactions may be important in mediating the marked alterations in immune function that often follow severe injury. In the present chapter we have chosen to present the adrenomedullary–neurotransmitter activation and actions as separate from the adrenocortical activation and actions to clarify specific responses as we currently understand them. To this end the current chapter will review the magnitude and time course of the stress hormone/neurotransmitter responses to thermal injury as well as how the action of these substances may be integrated. How these responses may be beneficial or detrimental during the course of recovery will also be addressed. Given the cadre of pharmacologic antagonists and agonists available to the clinician, taking a mechanistic approach to understanding adrenal hormones and neurotransmitter involvement in the pathophysiology of severe thermal injury is critical to further advance the successful treatment of these patients.

Part I — Sympathetic activation and release of catecholamines following burn trauma

Although clinical observations suggested the activation of sympathetic nerves in response to thermal injury[8–10] direct evidence for such activation was not fully appreciated until the simultaneous publication of papers by both American and Swedish groups that documented these responses.[11,12] These landmark studies described marked elevations in 24-hour urinary levels of norepinephrine and epinephrine in burn patients using a bioassay system. Despite considerable variation both within individuals and between patients, the increases in urinary norepinephrine and epinephrine were proportional to the severity (size) of the injury, were highest within the first 3 days post burn and in many cases remained elevated for several weeks. Furthermore, these studies also suggested that subsequent surgical interventions and the onset of sepsis and septic shock such as hypotension or serious infections caused catecholamine secretion to increase again. Since these early reports of urinary catecholamines as measured by bioassay techniques, many studies have confirmed the initial sympathetic responses in burn patients using fluorometric, HPLC/electrochemical or radioenzymatic techniques in plasma and urine samples.[13–17] However, documenta-

tion of the striking prolongation of sympathetic activation extending from 5 to 35 weeks following thermal injury[12] has not been repeated using newer analytical techniques. With improvements in critical care medicine and the management of burn patients during the last 40 years, prolonged sympathetic activity may not occur during extended recovery. In contrast, elevations in catecholamines may still occur in transient response to surgical procedures but cardiovascular, nutritional and immune-related interventions, as part of the treatment regimen, may ameliorate the extent or impact of the hormone response (Table 25.1). Nonetheless, in the light of the strong evidence for sympathetic activation consequent to thermal injury, the compensatory or possible decompensatory consequences are important to consider.

In response to thermal injury there are acute responses in what Cuthbertson[3] described as an ebb phase and long-term responses that support a flow phase. Cardiovascular adjustments to thermal injury appear to be critical for survival following burn trauma and with initial reductions in cardiac output sympathetic responses are rapidly brought into play as reviewed by Carleton.[18] Initial sympathetic activation contributes to the dramatic increases in peripheral vascular resistance that preserves mean arterial pressure but typically limits perfusion to the kidney and splanchnic beds. Although the mechanisms for the reduction in cardiac output are not completely understood, they are in part related to the sudden loss of vascular volume as a result of fluid transudation of plasma from the wound and from non-wound vascular sites.[19,20] Movement of fluids from the vascular to interstitial spaces are compounded by the loss of plasma proteins through the incompetent capillary beds that normally act to retain ions by Donnan equilibrium.[21] Such apparent hypovolemia would initially decrease blood pressure and baroreceptor afferent nerve activity with resultant increases in efferent sympathetic nerve activity. The resultant increase in peripheral vasoconstriction and consequent increase in peripheral vascular resistance are mediated in part by nerve-stimulated release of norepinephrine but also to a significant degree by both angiotensin II (AII) and arginine vasopressin.[15,22] Since arginine vasopressin (AVP) has been shown to directly depress myocardial function in the isolated heart and this depression can be reversed pharmacologically, AVP may contribute to myocardial depression following burn injury.[23]

Myocardial depression following thermal injury can be manifest as decreased cardiac output due to decreases in vascular volume, reductions in diastolic compliance as well as decreases in myocardial contractility. Various myocardial depressant factors have also been described for many years without specific detailed identification of the actual substances. Such deficits in contractility are compounded by the increases in aortic pressure afterload that is the consequence of increased peripheral vascular resistance and, in total, contribute to the observed reductions in cardiac output. Although diastolic dysfunction has been demonstrated in patients following thermal injury, evidence for decreases in contractility are largely based on animal studies with little evidence that this occurs in patients. Consequent to decreased ventricular performance and potential intrinsic myocardial dysfunction, sympathetic drive would be important to maintain ventricular function of the non-compromised muscle upon recovery from thermal injury.

TABLE 25.1 INFLUENCE OF CATECHOLAMINES ON CARDIOVASCULAR, METABOLIC, AND IMMUNE RESPONSE TO THERMAL INJURY

Physiologic variable	Sympathetic-mediated change following burn injury
Resting metabolic rate	Increase[37] Increase[38] Increase[17] Increase (in vitro)[266]
Proteolysis	No change (urea production)[39] No change (protein oxidation)[37] Decrease[48]
Glucose production and oxidation	Decrease secondary to increase in lipid catabolism[38,267] No change[37]
Glycogenolysis	Increase (indirect evidence via cAMP)[36]
Gluconeogenesis	Increase (indirect evidence via cAMP)[36]
Lipolysis	Increase[39] Increase[37] Increase[38] Increase[41]
Cardiac output	Increase[38] Increase[39]
Peripheral vascular resistance	Unknown
Heart rate	Increase[48] Increase[39]
T-cell number and function	Unknown
B-cell number and function	Unknown
Neutrophil number and function	Unknown
Monocyte number and function	Increase (indirect — clonogenic potential)[144] Increase (indirect — clonogenic potential)[156]

Citation of studies from the current literature suggesting that sympathetic activation is involved in changing the above physiologic variables following thermal injury.

Cardiovascular disturbances might be predicted to be the dominant signal initiating a generalized sympathetic response but the persistence of such sympathetic activation after hemodynamic stabilization suggests that afferent stimulation from other sources may initiate as well as maintain this response. Hemodynamic stabilization in burn patients typically requires 1–2 days after fluid resuscitation and is followed by the flow phase of recovery characterized by low peripheral vascular resistance, elevated cardiac output, increased peripheral blood flow and increased metabolism.[24,25] The marked decrease in peripheral vascular resistance most likely drives this hyperdynamic phase by decreasing cardiac afterload, increasing cardiac preload and thus increasing cardiac output. There is abundant evidence that mediators of neural, humoral and metabolic origin are involved in driving the decrease in vascular resistance following thermal injury but which ones are dominant and details of the time sequence of release are not well defined. Specific adrenergic agonists such as epinephrine may be involved through actions on vascular β-adrenergic receptors that mediate vasodilation[26] and the specific importance of β₂-adrenergic receptors in vasodilation has recently been demonstrated using knockout mice.[27] The situation is complicated in the burn patient by the increase in nerve-stimulated release of norepinephrine which has the potential to mediate vasoconstriction. However, there is evidence that the local distribution of adrenergic receptors mediating either vasodilation or vasoconstriction will determine the effect of circulating epinephrine and nerve-stimulated norepinephrine release on peripheral vascular resistance.[28] In addition, increased tissue metabolism has been recognized for many years to produce metabolites that mediate increased blood flow by decreasing vascular resistance.[29] With markedly increased metabolism in major burns, these metabolites along with catecholamines, nitric oxide,[30] and atrial natriuretic peptide[15] may contribute to the observed decreased vascular resistance.

Typically, decreases in tissue perfusion leading to compromised organ function only occur in patients with complications related to septic events or severe metabolic acidosis. Most often in thermally injured patients there is a modest decrease in mean arterial blood pressure that is not indicative of hypoperfusion and is left untreated. Where decreases in peripheral vascular resistance become dominant with marked decreases in mean arterial pressure, pressor agents may be required to maintain adequate tissue perfusion and norepinephrine is the drug of choice providing both vasoconstrictor and inotropic effects. Clinical use of vasoconstrictor and inotropic agents are essential to counter low tissue perfusion during periods of altered hemodynamic function often seen with the onset of sepsis in burn patients.

In this regard it is interesting to note the recent work by Macarthur et al.[31] suggesting that the inactivation of catecholamines by superoxide anions contributes to the observed hypotension of septic shock. Treatment of rats with superoxide dismutase not only abrogated endotoxin-induced hypotension in anesthetized rats but also elevated circulating levels of catecholamines. These findings suggest that compensatory sympathetic activation that counteracts hypotension during conditions of sepsis may be blunted by inactivation of catecholamines by superoxides in the extracellular millieu. More recently these studies have been extended[32] to a conscious rat model with infusion of live bacteria to simulate conditions of sepsis. Furthermore, these investigators modified the activity of the superoxide dismutase mimetic agent used in their initial study by 100-fold and demonstrated its effectiveness to enhance plasma levels of catecholamines, enhance blood pressure and improve survival. In their most recent work[33] these investigators demonstrated that nitric oxide, widely recognized as a mediator of hypotension during systemic inflammation as occurs in sepsis, decreases the biological activity of norepinephrine. Furthermore, increasing NO levels in an isolated perfused mesenteric circulation was shown to decrease vascular responses to endogenously released norepinephrine (NE) without altering nerve-stimulated release. These findings may provide some insight into the clinical observations involving critically ill trauma patients where exogenous norepinephrine administration is ineffective in correcting hypotension.

Following the initial insult of thermal injury the ebb or immediate phase of recovery is characterized by decreased body temperature and decreased oxygen consumption that is accompanied with progressively elevated lactate levels and developing hyperglycemia.[34,35] The same period of recovery involves intense sympathetic stimulation suggesting the involvement of adrenergic mechanisms mediated by adenylyl cyclase and cAMP in the mobilization of liver glycogen to glucose.[36] Developing hypermetabolism that follows 1–2 days later in the flow phase can also be attributed to adrenergic influences[17,37] but does not involve increased glucose mobilization and utilization since adrenergic blockade increased glucose production and clearance under these hypermetabolic conditions.[38] The experimental studies of Wolfe and Durkot[38] suggest that adrenergic drive following thermal injury facilitates lipolysis driving increased fatty acid oxidation. These results are based on changes observed following adrenergic blockade with propranolol and further clarify that the observed increase in glucose production and clearance under such conditions reflect a shift to carbohydrate utilization in the absence of mobilized lipid. Examination of the importance of adrenergic drive on lipid metabolism following thermal injury was extended to human patients through the use of stable isotopic studies as well as adrenergic antagonists.[39–41] These results not only indicate that lipolysis following thermal injury is mediated by β_2-adrenergic receptors, but suggest increased triglyceride-fatty acid cycling with resultant heat production.

The initial description of the sustained hypermetabolic response to thermal injury[42] prompted studies to examine the role of thyroid function and catecholamines in mediating this response. Although abnormal thyroid function was not involved in the response,[42,43] Wilmore developed experimental paradigms suggesting the role of catecholamines in mediating the hypermetabolic response to thermal injury.[17] Evidence for the positive correlation of increased plasma catecholamines and whole-body oxygen consumption following thermal injury,[17] as well as the demonstration that adrenergic blockade lowers the thermal injury-induced increase in metabolic rate and cardiac output to control levels in animal models directly support this contention.[17,38] However, experimental findings using the rat suggested that the adrenal medulla is essential for high rates of heat production following thermal injury but is not responsible for the primary drive of the hypermetabolic response.[44,45] These conclusions are further supported by experiments examining hypothalamic temperature regulation that suggest an upward shift in the set or operating temperature following thermal injury. The net result of this shift is increased metabolism at room temperature. Animals with hypothalamic lesions did not increase metabolism following thermal injury and were chronically hypothermic[46] not unlike experiments where the adrenal medulla was removed prior to thermal injury.[44] These results are consistent with clinical observations in burn patients in whom reductions in heat loss were achieved with occlusive dressings; and elevated environmental temperatures have decreased metabolic rate and catecholamine secretion.[14,47]

Building on these findings that catecholamines drive postburn hypermetabolism, Herndon et al.[48] demonstrated that pediatric patients could be treated with the β-adrenergic blocker propranolol to successfully reduce metabolic rate without compromising cardiovascular function. In a more recent study by this group,[49] β-adrenergic blockade in pediatric patients for 4 weeks during recovery from severe burns decreased the elevation in resting energy expenditure and reversed the reduction in net muscle–protein balance by 82%. Such treatment also prevented the loss in fat-free whole body mass and provided for a more efficacious recovery in these children.

An important and all too frequent complication of severe thermal injury is infection that frequently leads to sepsis, septic shock, multiple organ failure and death. The development of septic complications can decrease predicted survivability by up to 50%.[50] As with thermal injury, infection results in marked sympathetic responses that are well characterized in both experimental and clinical settings. Whereas experimental paradigms of sepsis have used plasma catecholamines, nerve recordings and norepinephrine turnover to assess sympathetic activation,[51–56] human studies have primarily focused on changes in plasma catecholamines.[1] Similar to thermal injury, sympathetic responses also appear to be proportional to the degree of insult, based on experiments using incremental doses of bacterial endotoxin.[52] Furthermore, animal models of septic peritonitis suggest that initial sympathetic activation, as measured by elevated levels of plasma norepinephrine and norepinephrine turnover, persist for many hours.[51,54] Burn patients are most susceptible to infection during the second week of their hospitalization when the sympathetic response, as reflected by urinary and plasma catecholamines, has moderated but is still elevated.[13–15] Although the onset of bacterial infection and developing sepsis would be expected to cause marked increases in plasma catecholamines above that due to burn alone, longitudinal studies charting the course of plasma catecholamines following thermal injury leading to infection and progressing into septic shock are not available. While the consequences of secondary insults following the initial injury are important to consider, unfortunately no information is available comparing plasma catecholamine changes with burn and burn plus sepsis.

Sympathetic influences on immune function

Over the last 20 years experimental evidence describing the interactions between neural and immune cell systems has expanded greatly. This has important implications in our understanding of the pathobiology of thermal injury since *in vivo* sympathetic activation as well as compromised immune function both occur following thermal injury. In addition to endogenous release of catecholamines, burn patients are often treated with adrenergic pressor agents; they may be on a therapeutic regimen of β-adrenergic antagonist prior to injury or hypermetabolism may be controlled in pediatric burn patients with β-adrenergic antagonists. Thus, adrenergic modulation following thermal injury may involve therapeutic as well as endogenous mediators and may have an important impact on immune system function.

For the activation of sympathetic nerves to influence immune responses, evidence of sympathetic innervation in peripheral immune structures, namely the lymphoid organs, is important to consider. Existing anatomical evidence is based on immunohistochemical techniques to visualize tyrosine hydroxylase (the rate-limiting step in the biosynthesis of norepinephrine). These studies clearly indicate a substantial innervation of all primary (thymus and bone marrow) and secondary (spleen and lymph nodes) lymphoid organs.[57–61] Furthermore, they also show sympathetic innervation in the immune cell compartment of the spleen (the white pulp), the periarterial lymphoid sheath, marginal zone and marginal sinus areas as well as in the splenic capsule and trabeculae.[62–66] Sympathetic nerve terminals have been described in direct apposition to T cells, interdigitating dendritic cells and B cells using electron microscopic techniques.[63] The proximity of nerve terminals to immune cells may be critical in achieving the necessary local concentrations of neurotransmitters at the neural–immune junctions to modulate immune functions. In fact, that neuro–immune junction is estimated at 6 nm[65] in comparison to 20 nm in typical CNS junctions. Therefore a high enough neurotransmitter concentration could be realized across these small junctions to impact on resident immune cells.

Anatomical evidence of sympathetic innervation of the immune system is complemented by evidence for nerve-stimulated release of norepinephrine neurotransmitter in both spleen and bone marrow.[67] Whereas evidence in spleen has been recognized for many years and has been assessed in a variety of ways, norepinephrine release in bone marrow has only been recently described using norepinephrine turnover techniques based on radiotracer methods involving *in vivo* experimental paradigms.[67] In contrast, exocytosis of norepinephrine from lymph nodes has not been demonstrated. To complete the criteria for the physiologic importance of functional innervation, nerve-stimulated release of norepinephrine within lymphoid organs must increase at the appropriate time to influence the immune response and norepinephrine modulation of immune responses must be demonstrated.

β-adrenergic receptors, particularly β₂ subtypes, are known to be expressed on a number of different immune cells including activated and resting B cells, naïve CD4+ T cells, T-helper (Th1) cell clones and newly generated Th1 cells but they are not expressed in newly generated Th2 cells.[68–71] Furthermore, there is significant evidence that norepinephrine can modulate the function of CD4+ T cells, which in turn can modulate antibody production of B cells.[72] In addition, norepinephrine can directly influence B cell antibody production depending upon the time of exposure following activation.[73,74] The physiologic importance of these *in vitro* findings are supported by a series of *in vivo* experiments involving severe combined immune-deficient (*scid*) mice depleted of norepinephrine prior to reconstitution with antigen-specific Th2 and B cells. These experiments demonstrate that norepinephrine is necessary for maintaining a normal level of antibody production *in vivo*.[68] Furthermore, other recent whole animal experiments, also involving *scid* mice, provide evidence that the immune response itself stimulates the release of norepinephrine from adrenergic nerve terminals in bone marrow and spleen, that in turn can influence antibody production by B cells.[75] Although these findings fall far short of direct application to immune cell function following thermal injury they suggest the important potential of sympathetic activation in mediating immune responses.

In addition to neural influences on T and B cell function, there are direct effects on myeloid cell function particularly with respect to lipopolysaccharide (LPS)-stimulated cytokine production. The most striking examples of neural influences on macrophage function were demonstrated by the work of Spengler et al.,[76] who concluded that α-adrenergic stimulation increases tumor necrosis factor-α (TNF-α) release whereas β-adrenergic stimulation decreases such release in response to LPS. They provided further evidence to suggest that extracellular stores of catecholamines in macrophages are capable of modulating TNF-α release. Furthermore, sympathetic inhibition of TNF-α release initiated by LPS has been suggested to occur in whole animal preparations although adrenergic actions on macrophages were indirect.[32,77–82] More direct evidence of adrenergic inhibition of LPS-stimulated TNF-α production has involved whole blood.[82–87] Apart from adrenergic inhibition of LPS-stimulated TNF-α release in isolated macrophages,[88–91] similar inhibition of LPS-stimulated TNF-α production has also been demonstrated in human mast cells,[92] microglial cells,[93] astrocytes[94] and cytotoxic T lymphocytes.[95] In contrast to adrenergic stimulation of TNF-α release, experiments with isolated atria,[96,97] myenteric plexus[98] and brain tissue[99] have demonstrated that TNF-α can negatively impact on the release of norepinephrine.

Adrenergic influences on the expression and release of interleukin-6 (IL-6) has been suggested by a number of studies demonstrating increases in plasma IL-6 in response to direct or indirect stimulation.[100–102] Adrenergic enhancement of IL-6 responses to LPS has also been demonstrated *in vivo*[78,80] as well as in *ex vivo* paradigms using isolated liver.[91] In isolated cell systems, adrenergic stimulation enhances LPS-induced IL-6 response.[103,104] Catechoalmines in combination with IL-1β stimulate IL-6 release from rat C6 glioma cells and vasoactive intestinal polypeptide (VIP) has been reported to synergize with norepinephrine to induce IL-6 release in astrocytes.[105,106] In addition, adrenergic agonists have been shown to mediate IL-6 release in brown adipocytes, pituicytes, hepatocytes, astrocytes and thymic epithelial cells.[105–111]

In contrast, Nakamura et al.[94] reported that catecholamines decreased the IL-6 response to LPS and van der Poll et al.[86] demonstrated that norepinephrine inhibits the LPS-induced IL-6 response in whole blood. Other evidence for adrenergic suppression of IL-6 responses has been suggested by the work of Straub.[112–114] Using isolated splenic tissue preparation, electrically stimulated release of norepinephrine appears to inhibit IL-6 production induced by LPS or bacteria. These authors suggest that adrenergic inhibition of IL-6 is reduced under conditions simulating infection where cytokine mediation of the inflammatory response is compensatory in eradicating the bacterial load. It is apparent from these studies that catecholamines can exert a negative or a positive influence on proinflammatory cytokines, especially IL-6. However, when these different modulatory functions come into play and what role(s) they play in the pathophysiology of burn injury are unexplored.

Although the exact mechanisms of the negative modulation of proinflammatory cytokines by catecholamines are poorly understood, it may be achieved through the ability of catecholamines to induce the anti-inflammatory cytokine interleukin-10 (IL-10).[80,83,115,116] Whole animal studies involving assessment of circulating levels of IL-10,[80] as well as studies of human whole blood and mononuclear cells stimulated with LPS in the presence of adrenergic agonists,[82,83,116] support this premise. In addition, experimental neurotrauma results in increased IL-10 consequent to endogenous adrenergic stimulation in the absence of LPS or other evidence of infectious challenge.[117] The only experimental evidence suggesting an attenuation of IL-10 with adrenergic stimulation involved a macrophage cell line (RAW 264.7).[118]

Evidence that elevations of IL-10 can be blocked with inhibition of protein kinase A[116,119] is consistent with adrenergic mediation of changes in TNF and IL-6 and suggests that activation of protein kinase A is important in effecting these adrenergic modulations of cytokine release. More specifically, the recent work of Platzer et al.,[115] suggests that catecholamines in monocytic cells directly stimulate the IL-10 promoter/enhancer and provide evidence that a cAMP response element was the major target of the cAMP/protein kinase A pathway. In contrast, two recent studies from our laboratory report evidence that although adrenergic stimulation increases IL-10 release from macrophages, release of cytokines TNF-α and IL-6 are inhibited by direct adrenergic stimulation not secondary to IL-10.[120,121] These studies involved both peritoneal elicited- and bone marrow progenitor derived-macrophages under normal conditions as well as following cecal ligation and puncture injury. Macrophages from both preparations were incubated overnight with LPS both in the presence and absence of epinephrine and cytokines were determined in the conditioned media. Epinephrine attenuated TNF-α in the conditioned media but increased IL-10; however, addition of anti-IL-10 antibody did not prevent epinephrine's ability to block TNF-α reductions. Further experiments demonstrated the action of epinephrine to inhibit LPS-stimulated release of proinflammatory cytokines to be mediated by β$_2$-adrenergic receptors. The dominance of direct adrenergic inhibition of LPS-mediated proinflammatory cytokine was maintained during conditions of sepsis although such conditions elevated endogenous levels of IL-10.

Adrenergic stimulation of bacterial growth

Since the identification of mammalian hormone and neurotransmitter receptors in bacterial cells there has been considerable interest in defining a role for such signaling molecules in bacterial cells. As a consequence during the last 15 years support has emerged for the concept that release of norepinephrine within intestinal tissue promotes the growth of bacteria within the gut.[122–124] Initial experiments demonstrated the growth-promoting action of catecholamines in vitro using several different bacterial species and provided evidence that these compounds were not acting as nutritional substrates. Since growth-stimulating effects of norepinephrine were not blocked by adrenergic blocking agents, adrenergic receptors do not appear to be involved.[125,126] Further observations suggest that norepinephrine may act within an 8-hour period to induce bacterial growth, during which time stimulation of growth factors can promote bacterial growth.[127,128] Norepinephrine-stimulated bacterial growth has also been shown to produce Shiga-like enterotoxins from enterohemorrhagic strains of E.coli. Furthermore, norepinephrine promotes the expression of K99+ pilus adhesin, a virulence factor known to play a critical role in the attachment of these bacteria to the intestinal wall which initiates the infective process.[129,130] Although these studies utilize very high concentrations of norepinephrine compared to the observed plasma concentrations following thermal injury, bacteria in vivo may be exposed to high norepinephrine concentrations if such bacteria are in close proximity to the nerve terminal synapse. A related concern is the lack of information regarding the actual norepinephrine concentration within the culture media throughout the incubation period. Whereas rapidly growing bacterial cultures may generate an acid environment in which catecholamines are quite stable, initial growth conditions containing low bacterial counts and minimal nutrients may promote rapid deterioration of norepinephrine. However, high initial norepinephrine concentrations in cultures may counteract such unfavorable conditions but in turn would provide misleading dose–response information.

The extensive sympathetic innervation of the gut and associated structures has been recognized for many years with well-defined nerve terminals located primarily along blood vessels but without evidence of neruotransmitter release into the intestinal lumen. Furthermore, there is considerable evidence that once released from nerve terminals, most norepinephrine is taken back into the same terminals by uptake 1 (active) or 2 (passive) mechanisms, metabolized into a non-active form or diffuses through tissues to reach blood vessels to become part of the circulation.[131] Thus, even though intestinal bacterial growth has the potential to be enhanced by the neurotransmitter norepinephrine, transport of the norepinephrine into the intestinal lumen would seem problematic. However, since massive catecholamine release is such a consistent component of burn patients, especially those with superimposed sepsis, the hypothesis that bacterial growth can be enhanced by norepinephrine is very appealing.

Important *in vivo* findings strengthen this concept by demonstrating that cecal bacterial growth increases dramatically following massive *in vivo* release of norepinephrine and that passage of bacteria through the gut enhance their growth response to norepinephrine. In the first case[124] mice were treated with 6-hydroxydopamine, a neurotoxin that displaces norepinephrine from adrenergic nerve terminals causing a transient but massive sympathetic reaction. At 24 hours post treatment cecal bacterial growth was elevated 3–4 degrees of magnitude compared to vehicle-treated controls but bacterial growth returned to control levels by 14 days. In the second study[129] an attenuated strain of *Salmonella typhimurium* was administered to rhesus monkeys whereupon isolated fecal bacterial cultures from these animals displayed increased *in vitro* growth response to norepinephrine. To elucidate whether this hypothesis has a role in the pathophysiology of thermal injury with sepsis, future studies must build on experimental paradigms of thermal injury to demonstrate that endogenous norepinephrine enhances bacterial growth leading to sepsis.

Evidence for norepinephrine regulation of myelopoiesis in experimental thermal injury with sepsis

Patients with severe burn trauma often display significant impairment in cell-mediated immunity involving defective neutrophil chemotaxis, phagocytosis and superoxide production.[132–135] Patients with sepsis and systemic inflammatory response may also present with monocytosis and neutropenia.[136,137] While neutropenia and defective neutrophil functions may compromise host defense, monocytosis has the potential to fuel excessive cytokine production through increased availability of circulating and tissue monocyte/macrophages. For the past 15 years our laboratory has been investigating bone marrow following thermal injury with sepsis to understand mechanisms that govern leukocyte production and how they might contribute to the observed defects in leukocyte functions. The potential for sympathetic activation to modulate myelopoiesis following thermal injury and sepsis is supported by previous studies where adrenergic stimulation has been shown to participate in the regulation and control of hematopoiesis.[138,139] Maestroni[139] has not only provided evidence for the presence of adrenergic receptors on bone marrow immune cells but also that adrenergic agonists stimulate lymphopoiesis while attenuating myelopoiesis under normal non-injury conditions. These findings are further strengthened by animal experiments where adrenergic agents have been shown to modulate both lympho- and myelopoiesis.[140–143] Another important factor supporting the possible adrenergic regulation of myelopoiesis following thermal injury is that sympathetic activation can occur directly within the bone marrow compartment with nerve-stimulated release of norepinephrine in close proximity to developing immune cells. We have documented a significant increase in murine bone marrow norepinephrine release in response to either cold exposure or bacteria through the use of traditional pulse-chase experiments.[67] Furthermore, we have extended these measurements to our

murine model of thermal injury with sepsis and demonstrate increased bone marrow norepinephrine release in response to thermal injury with sepsis.[144]

These findings suggest that sympathetic activation has the capacity to drive events within the bone marrow and adrenergic-mediated expansion of leukocyte production could conceivably contribute to heightened inflammatory responses with immune challenge following thermal injury with sepsis. Experimental evidence suggesting that adrenergic stimulation inhibits myelopoiesis under normal conditions[139] but is shifted following injury to enhanced monocyte development[144] is a most interesting phenomenon. Whether adrenergic stimulation within the bone marrow functions in a compensatory or a decompensatory way toward the host following thermal injury is also interesting to consider. Is adrenergic stimulation involved in the immunosupression of patients with severe burns through functional alterations in circulating and tissue leukocytes?[145–151] These and other important questions are likely to involve events that occur within the bone marrow as it serves as a major source of new leukocytes both in the circulation and in tissues following thermal injury with sepsis.

Alterations in bone marrow hematopoietic progenitor cells have been the focus of our work and have involved our murine model of thermal injury (15% TBSA) using *Pseudomonas aeruginosa* applied directly to the wound site to establish sepsis. Following the demonstration of a shift in bone marrow myeloid commitment toward monocytopoiesis and away from granulocytopoiesis in thermal injury and sepsis,[152,153] we began to focus on the potential significance of the increased nerve-stimulated release of norepinephrine within the bone marrow under these same experimental conditions. We tested the premise that neural stimulation was modulating myeloid lineage function by manipulating the peripheral stores of norepinephrine prior to injury. Peripheral norepinephrine levels were reduced by using 6-hydroxydopamine (6-OHDA) and then animals were subjected to thermal injury with sepsis. Following thermal injury and sepsis, femoral bone marrow cells from mice with reduced norepinephrine content demonstrated a significant decrease in monocytopoietic potential compared to mice with intact bone marrow norepinephrine stores.[144] In addition, reduction of peripheral norepinephrine content prior to the injury protocol resulted in a significant survival benefit compared to animals with intact norepinephrine content.

The influence of norepinephrine on bone marrow monocyte progenitor differentiation following thermal injury with sepsis was assessed by cell surface expression patterns of ER-MP12 and ER-MP20. While ER-MP12 is a surface antigen expressed in early monocyte progenitors and represents predominantly CFU-M, progressively more ER-MP20 antigen is expressed from the CFU-M stage onwards but disappears after the monocytic stage.[154] By following the distribution pattern of the expression of these two antigens on bone marrow cells the phenotypic separation and identification of bone marrow monocyte precursors have been demonstrated.[155] Results of ER-MP12 and ER-MP20 expression patterns in animals with intact norepinephrine stores suggests that there is a significant decrease in immature monocyte progenitors following thermal injury with sepsis compared to sham. Furthermore, there is a significant population of cells in the intermediate stage of development under normal conditions and this population increases significantly following thermal injury with sepsis. In contrast, norepinephrine-depleted animals present an entirely different distribution pattern of monocyte progenitors using these markers. The norepinephrine-depleted sham group has very few cells in the immature and intermediate compartments with most cells staining for the mature monocyte progenitor cells. Thermal injury in norepinephrine-depleted animals resulted in further increases in mature monocyte progenitors. Taken together these results suggest that monocyte maturation pathways may be greatly influenced by the presence of norepinephrine and that stimulation of such pathways may be involved in the pathobiology of thermal injury with sepsis.

The potential site of adrenergic action within the hierarchy of bone marrow macrophage progenitor cells has been addressed in more recent work.[156] Whereas initial work examined the monocytopoietic potential of total bone marrow cells, Cohen et al. examined very early progenitors not committed to the myeloid lineage that express the CD117 marker.[156] In addition they also examined cells expressing ER-MP12 antigen which are early myeloid committed progenitors that differentiate either into neutrophils or monocytes. The monocytopoietic potential of both progenitor types were enhanced above control values following thermal injury and thermal injury with sepsis; however, this enhancement was greatly reduced by depletion of norepinephrine prior to the injury protocol. These findings suggest that myeloid bone marrow progenitors as well as early progenitors that are not committed to the myeloid lineage can be stimulated by endogenous norepinephrine release following thermal injury and sepsis to enhance proliferation.

Another important aspect of Cohen et al.,[156] is the demonstration that progenitor-derived macrophages express enhanced cytokine release following thermal injury and sepsis. Both CD117- and ER-MP12-enriched progenitors were taken from mice 72 hours after burn injury protocol and they were then differentiated into macrophages *in vitro* during a 7-day incubation with GM- and M-CSF. These progenitor-derived macrophages were then stimulated with bacterial endotoxin (LPS) and both TNF-α and IL-6 determined in the conditioned media. Expression of both TNF-α and IL-6 were significantly reduced in progenitor-derived macrophages from animals with depleted norepinephrine prior to the injury protocol. These results suggest that endogenous norepinephrine released during conditions of burn and sepsis impact the phenotype of differentiated macrophages and enhanced amounts of proinflammatory cytokines released could contribute to systemic inflammation. Collectively, the work of Cohen et al.[156] suggest that adrenergic stimulation during experimental thermal injury and sepsis contributes to enhanced numbers of macrophages as well as the expression of pro-inflammatory cytokines in bone marrow progenitor-derived macrophages.

In order for norepinephrine to act on bone marrow progenitor cells such cells should express functional adrenergic receptors. In fact specific β-adrenergic receptors on bone marrow hematopoietic progenitor cells enriched for ER-MP20 antigen have been characterized using conventional pharmacologic binding techniques, and values of total receptors (B_{MAX}) and affinity (K_D) were determined. Furthermore, the effect of thermal injury and sepsis on these receptors was determined at 72 hours following thermal injury and sepsis.[157] Thermal injury and sepsis resulted in significant reductions in cell surface β-adrenergic receptors (B_{MAX}) but binding affinity was increased (decreased K_D values). This paradoxical change was resolved by agonist stimulation of intracellular cAMP, which showed that agonist coupling was increased in burn sepsis. Increased cAMP production under conditions of decreased receptor number but increased affinity suggests the dominant effect of changes in affinity in the bone marrow monocyte progenitor cells. Although these findings do not provide evidence that β-adrenergic–cAMP coupling alters the phenotype of these progenitors *in vivo*, additional *in vitro* experiments demonstrate that adrenergic stimulation during differentiation of ER-MP20 progenitors significantly alters the phenotype of mature macrophages. These changes in phenotype expression with adrenergic stimulation could be reversed with the selective β2-adrenergic blocker.[157]

Although the murine animal model reflects important clinical features of thermal injury with infection, there may be important limitations. Whereas the murine animal model involves immediate infection following thermal injury, burn patients typically develop septic complications in the second week of their hospitalization. This does not, however, change the interpretation of these experimental findings that increased sympathetic activation in the bone marrow may result in both increased myelopoietic potential and altered cellular phenotype following thermal injury with sepsis. This frame of reference suggests that immune responses following injury should be considered in the context of potential action of sympathetic neurotransmitters on cellular events that occur during cellular differentiation in the bone marrow compartment.

Part II — Adrenal cortical steroids following burn trauma

Release of glucocorticoids

Whereas the acute ebb phase of recovery from thermal injury is mainly dependent upon re-establishment of cardiovascular function following circulatory disruption, the flow phase is considered to be dependent upon an adequate metabolic response. These responses are mediated in part by adrenal cortical steroids, of which cortisol is the dominant glucocorticoid hormone (Table 25.2). Elevation of glucocorticoids occurs in response to most forms of trauma,[158] including burn injury, with rapid increases in blood and urine levels.[8,159] During the first 2 weeks following burn injury, the extent of elevation of total plasma cortisol concentration is proportional to the severity of the injury. Early studies observed that glucocorticoid levels were excessively high in severely burned patients and remained high in non-surviving patients.[160] In burn patients where recovery is likely, plasma glucocorticoid levels are moderately elevated or are in the upper normal range and can persist for up to 36 days[161,162] and return to normal as healing progresses.[159] In contrast, patients with severe injury (90% TBSA) have markedly lower levels of glucocorticoid concentration, suggesting that they are unable to mount an adequate response.[162]

TABLE 25.2 INFLUENCE OF GLUCOCORTICOIDS ON METABOLIC AND IMMUNE RESPONSE TO THERMAL INJURY

Physiologic variable	Glucocorticoid-mediated change following burn injury
Resting energy expenditure	Increased[5–7]
Oxygen consumption	Increased[268,269]
Primary fuel	Lipids, glucose[216]
Proteolysis	Increased in skeletal muscle[190,191,193,194,270]
Acute phase protein synthesis	Increased[170,271,272]
Nitrogen excretion	Increased[269]
Glycogenolysis	Increased via effect on glucagons[186,188]
Gluconeogenesis	Increased[182,183,271]
Lipolysis	Increased[217]
Ketone body formation	Normal[219]
Triglyceride level	Increased[219,271]
Thymic changes	Involution[238]
T-cell population	Decreased[237,273]
T-cell proliferation	Inhibited[239,240,272]
B-cell population	Not conclusive from current data
Neutrophil population	Increased[242,273,274]
Chemotaxis	Suppressed[242]
Demargination	Increased[242,245]
Bactericidal activity	Suppressed[246]
Monocyte population	Increased transiently with corticosteroids but decreased in burn patients[137,274,275]
Chemotaxis	Suppressed[243]
Bactericidal activity	Suppressed[243,276]
Bone formation	Decreased[225]

Citation of studies from the current literature suggesting that glucocorticoid release is involved in changing the above physiologic variables following thermal injury.

Glucocorticoids circulate in the body bound to cortisol binding protein (CBG) or transcortin, as an inactive complex. Only 1–10% of total plasma cortisol circulates unbound and it is this free fraction that is responsible for the biological activity of glucocorticoids. Burn injury results in a shift in the equilibrium between unbound cortisol and total cortisol towards an elevation in the unbound fraction.[162] Serum CBG as well as CBG binding capacity are low in burn injury, severe infection and septic shock.[162–164] In burn patients, CBG levels have been shown to decrease markedly with lowest values occurring 48 hours after injury.[165] Even a minor burn such as 3% TBSA results in the reduction of serum CBG levels by 30%,[166] which return to normal levels 1–2 weeks later. The net effect of the decrease in CBG levels following thermal injury may not only result in increased free levels of cortisol but also in the amount of excreted cortisol, which is reflected in high urinary corticosteroid levels in burn patients. Additional explanations for the increased levels of corticosteroids in burn patients may be due to the direct inhibitory effect of corticosteroids on the biosynthesis of CBG.[167–169] Furthermore, the proinflammatory cytokine IL-6 which is known to be elevated following massive burns has also been implicated in reducing CBG synthesis. Human hepatoma-derived cells (HepG2) respond to IL-6 by decreasing CBG protein and mRNA.[170]

The hypothalmic–pituitary–adrenal axis displays a biphasic pattern during the course of critical illness. In the initial phase, excessive cortisol levels are associated with elevated levels of ACTH. In the second phase, which occurs 3–5 days after the initial injury, ACTH levels decline while cortisol remains elevated.[2,171] There is some evidence to suggest that cortisol elevation with decreased ACTH may be driven by endothelin or atrial natriuretic peptide/hormone (ANP/H). Vermes et al.[171] demonstrated that both plasma endothelin and ANP levels were significantly elevated for 8 days following hospitalization in severely ill patients with sepsis or trauma. In addition, infusion of ANP in humans has been shown to block CRH-stimulated secretion of ACTH and cortisol[172] while endothelin-1 and endothelin-3 enhance secretion of steroid hormones from the adrenal cortex.[173] Furthermore, endothelin-3 has been reported to elevate ACTH and corticosterone levels in rats[174] while endothelin-1 results in elevated ACTH in humans.[175] Based on this information, Vermes et al.[171] suggest that endothelin may be responsible for stimulating steroid secretion while ANP's action on the hypothalmic–pituitary axis may suppress ACTH secretion, thus explaining the paradoxical increase in cortisol with concomitant low ACTH levels in severely stressed patients.

Release of C_{19} steroids

Dehydroepiandrosterone sulfate (DHEAS), a weak androgen, is the major secretory product of the human adrenal cortex. Despite the increase in cortisol secretion by the adrenals in burn patients, there is a distinct decrease in serum DHEAS levels.[176] This is due to a reduction in the synthesis and secretion rather than an effect of enhanced metabolism or excretion.[177] While serum DHEAS levels decrease gradually, testosterone and androstenedione levels decrease abruptly. In some burn patients, subnormal testosterone levels persist for 3–18 months following the burn injury whereas cortisol levels return to normal earlier.[177] The decrease in testosterone secretion may be due to a direct effect of excessive cortisol levels on the testis.[178,179]

It appears that synthesis of C_{19} steroids by the adrenals and testes is compromised as a result of enhanced production of the C_{21} steroids such as cortisol. Aldosterone levels are also subnormal despite elevated plasma renin activity. This suggests a shift of pregnenolone metabolism away from mineralocorticoid and adrenal androgen pathways towards the glucocorticoid pathway.[176] The low level of DHEAS may also contribute to the suppressed state of the immune system in burn patients and will be discussed later.

Influence on metabolic pathways

High energy expenditure and hyperglycemia are hallmarks of thermal injury. The heavy demand for energy is due to the increase in essential functions such as the synthesis of proteins required for wound healing, the synthesis of acute phase proteins and inflammatory mediators. In addition, severe burns exert a burden on the metabolism to generate heat which in part compensates for the loss through the wound site. Part of the elevation in resting energy expenditure in burn patients is due to the increase in substrate cycling. This occurs when enzymes catalyzing opposing reactions of the same pathway are active simultaneously: for example, the conversion of glucose to glucose-6-phosphate and back to glucose. The demand for energy is increased in order to resynthesize ATP used in this and similar reactions. In burn patients the rate of glucose production and glycolysis as well as lipolysis and reesterification of triglycerides are elevated.[40] This cycling of substrates generates heat due to the hydrolysis of high-energy phosphate bonds in ATP, thus contributing to thermogenesis as well as increased energy requirement in burn patients. Keeping burn patients thermally comfortable lowers the metabolic rate and thus the demand for energy can also be lowered.[180] Increased glucocorticoid levels during severe burns can orchestrate multiple metabolic pathways to meet this energy demand. In order to understand how glucocorticoids may influence major metabolic pathways following thermal injury to facilitate the hypermetabolic state, in this section we will review the effects of glucocorticoids on glucose, protein and fatty acid metabolism as they pertain to thermal injury.

Glucocorticoids and glucose metabolism

Glucocorticoids can contribute to hyperglycemia, which persists for several days, by enhancing endogenous production of glucose in the liver.[6,181–183] In burn injury, elevated glucose levels are predominantly sustained through gluconeogenesis and impaired glucose utilization. Increased levels of plasma lactate produced by peripheral tissues following thermal injury, as documented by Wolfe et al.,[184] is an essential substrate for gluconeogenesis by the liver. Recent evidence further confirms that thermal injury causes metabolic adaptations to enhance gluconeogenesis. Burn injury causes intrinsic alterations in the liver, which increases the flow of pyruvate to oxaloacetate at the expense of non-tricarboxylic acid cycle sources.[185] Mobilization of glucose stored as glycogen and skeletal muscle amino acids as substrates for gluconeogenesis requires glucagon secretion,[186,187] which is stimulated by glucocorticoids.[186–188] In addition to gluconeogenesis, insulin resistance can also play a role in sustaining high circulating levels of glucose in burn patients. For example, glucose utilization is impaired in burn patients who do not respond to insulin infusion.[6]

Glucocorticoids and protein metabolism

In severe burn injury, protein catabolism is a part of the hypermetabolic state resulting in negative nitrogen balance. Cuthbertson's landmark studies[189] were the first to suggest the important concept that nitrogen loss is a whole-body response rather than a local burn-wound response. The increase in proteolysis seen in burn injury is, at least partly, mediated by glucocorticoids. In humans,[190] and in animal models,[191] administration of glucocorticoids enhances muscle proteolysis. Further, burn injury-induced muscle proteolysis can be inhibited by a glucocorticoid receptor antagonist.[192] Amino acids mobilized from peripheral tissues are transported to the liver,

where unlike in other tissues, cortisol stimulates protein synthesis. The increased hepatic protein synthesis in response to cortisol can drive the new synthesis of gluconeogenic enzymes and acute phase proteins in response to injury.

Specific mechanisms involved in burn-mediated alterations in protein metabolism following thermal injury are not known. However, some information could be gleaned from studies on other states of excessive catabolism. In conditions such as metabolic acidosis, adrenalectomy halts muscle proteolysis and does not increase expression of components of the ubiquitin-proteasome pathway.[193,194] These effects can be reversed by dexamethasone administration. Further support for this premise is provided by in vitro studies, which show that dexamethasone-induced increases in proteolytic degradation in myocytes can be abolished by the glucocorticoid receptor inhibitor RU486.[195] Ding et al.[196] suggest that partial inhibition of the ubiquitin-proteasome pathway may be beneficial in enhanced catabolic states. Taken together these data suggest that interaction of glucocorticoids and the ATP requiring ubiquitin-proteosome system may play an important role in burn-induced proteolysis.[196–201]

Another important aspect of protein catabolism following thermal injury is the generation of gluconeogenic amino acids. In fact, following thermal injury plasma levels of alanine are increased.[202] Nitrogen produced as a result of transaminating alanine to the gluconeogenic intermediate pyruvate is converted into glutamine and then to urea for excretion by the liver. Glutamine is one of the major participants in the translocation of amino acids from peripheral tissues to the liver for nitrogen excretion. Expression of the enzyme responsible for synthesis of this amino acid, glutamine synthase, is increased to compensate for the glutamine depletion in peripheral tissues. Following burn injury, glutamine synthase mRNA is increased first in the lung and later in muscle.[203] This is further supported by the observation that adrenalectomy partially decreases burn injury-induced glutamine synthase mRNA.[201] This is a tissue-specific response as no such effect is seen in the kidney or liver. There is evidence to suggest that glucocorticoids may augment glutamine synthesis. In lung and muscle tissues glucocorticoid administration increases glutamine production.[204] Mobilization of protein from peripheral tissues is also indicated by the increase in phenylalanine in the blood of burn patients.[202] Phenylalanine is the only amino acid that is not degraded by peripheral tissue and hence accumulates in the circulation when uptake by the liver is compromised.

The hypermetabolic and catabolic states seen in thermal injury remain long after the burn wound is completely healed.[5–7,205,206] In a recent study by Hart et al.,[205] stable isotopic methodology and gas chromatography-mass spectrometry analysis were used to measure muscle kinetics in burned children. Reduction in protein catabolism and enhancement of lean body mass were only seen 9–12 months after the initial injury.[205] This suggests that treatment to alter growth deficiency must be prolonged long after early wound healing is complete.

Other more indirect effects of glucocorticoids on glucose levels in thermal injury include modulation of insulin-like growth factor-1 (IGF-1), an important mediator of growth hormone (GH) action.[207,208] Marked depression of all components of the IGF-1 complex are seen in burn injury.[209–213] Elevated glucocorticoid levels in burn patients may contribute to the suppression of the acid labile subunit (ALS) of the IGF-1 complex. Treatment of rats with dexamethasone results in low levels of serum ALS as well as liver ALS mRNA.[214,215]

In addition to the use of amino acids released from peripheral tissue to increase endogenous glucose production, body fat is the major source of energy in traumatic situations.[216] Free fatty acids are released from adipose tissue to be used as an alternate source of fuel during times of crisis, as is the case in thermal injury. Cortisol stimulates lipolysis[217] enabling the release of free fatty acids. In burned children and adults increased lipolysis is reflected in the elevated plasma levels of palmitic and oleic aicd.[41,218,219]

Influence on bone metabolism

Aside from combating the increased demand for energy, glucocorticoids also affect bone development, which has profound effects in children. Abnormal bone metabolism in burn injury has been demonstrated in animals and humans.[220,221] In children, the reduction in bone mineral density persists for at least 5 years after severe burn injury (>40% TBSA) and results in permanent retardation of linear growth.[222,223] The reasons for loss of bone mineral density include increased production of endogenous glucocorticoids, the inflammatory response, immobilization, aluminium loading and production of cytokines such as IL-1 and IL-6 that facilitate bone resorption.[224]

Glucocorticoids have potent effects on bone formation and resorption resulting in loss of bone mass. Weinstein et al.[225] investigated the long-term (equivalent to 3–4 human years) effects of glucocorticoids on bone metabolism in an animal model and reported a reduction in osteoclastogenesis causing reduced bone turnover and a reduction in osteoblastogenesis resulting in reduced bone formation. Enhanced osteoclast and osteoblast apoptosis was observed in mice subjected to long-term glucocorticoid administration as well as in patients with glucocorticoid-induced osteoporosis.[225] This depletion in the bone cell population limits the number of cells that can synthesize matrix proteins. In addition, glucocorticoids directly downregulate expression of type I collagen and upregulate expression of collagenase-3 in chondrocytes.[226] On the other hand, IGF-1 enhances expression of type I collagen and suppresses the expression of collagenase-3.[227] Thus the massive increase in glucocorticoids and the corresponding decrease in IGF-1 in burn injury has the ability to profoundly alter bone and cartilage formation.

The mechanisms by which glucocorticoids mediate bone resorption are not clear. One possible mechanism is that glucocorticoids increase osteoclast apoptosis.[228] Glucocorticoids may also mediate bone resorption by its dual capacity to initially inhibit osteoclast synthesis but later stimulate osteoclast synthesis coupled with an increase in bone resorption.[229] Yet another mechanism by which cortisol may influence bone resorption is by suppression of IGF-1 or GH-induced chondrocyte proliferation.[230] The antiproliferative effect of glucocorticoids may be mediated through downregulation of the GH receptor and binding affinity as well as suppression of the local production of IGF-1 by these cells. These effects illustrate probable mechanisms by which glucocorticoids may impair the growth stimulatory effects of GH.

Influence on immune suppression

Severely burned patients are susceptible to opportunistic infections and sepsis is a major cause of death associated with burn injury. Immune suppression occurs soon after burn injury, perhaps to prevent over-responsiveness. This, however, leaves the patient extremely vulnerable to bacterial infection through a number of routes. Patients can be infected through the wound site and by translocation of gut bacteria.[231] Surgery and other life-supporting procedures such as nutritional supplementation and ventilation are also fertile sources of infection. The glucocorticoid response to thermal injury appears to play an important role in immune dysfunction with impairment of both specific and non-specific defences. Corticosteroids reduce lymphocyte, eosinophil and basophil numbers, alter lymphocyte subpopulations, depress immunoglobulin production by B cells and suppress neutrophil and monocyte/macrophage activity.

Acute thymic involution[232,233] and a reduction of the total T-cell population occurs soon after burn injury.[232–235] During initial thymic involution in an animal model there is marked depression of $CD4^+CD8^+$ lymphocytes. $CD4^-CD8^-$ cell numbers are also reduced with recovery in the ensuing thymic regeneration phase during the next 2 weeks. Thymic involution is a common response to various types of stress and trauma.[236] In humans, the depression of T lymphocytes is reflected by reduction of both $CD4^+$ as well as $CD8^+$ cell numbers.[234] In an animal model[232] $CD4^+CD8^-$ cells are reported to be more sensitive to the effects of thermal injury than $CD4^-CD8^+$ cells. $CD4^+CD8^-$ cell numbers remain constantly depressed during a 2-week period following burn injury, whereas $CD4^-CD8^+$ cell numbers are variable and can even be increased in comparison to control animals not subjected to thermal injury.

Thymic changes following exogenous administration of glucocorticoids are similar to that seen in burn injury[237,238] in that exogenous hypercortisolism in non-injury states or that following burn injury is associated with decreasing $CD4^+CD8^+$ and elevating $CD4^+CD8^-$ thymocytes.[233] The reduction of $CD4^+CD8^+$ cell numbers during the first 24 hours after thermal injury is due to glucocorticoid-mediated apoptosis since burn injury-induced thymocyte apoptosis is suppressed by adrenalectomy or administration of a glucocorticoid receptor antagonist (RU486).[233] Other factors contributing to lymphocyte dysfunction and immunosuppression resulting from elevated corticosteroid levels may include the ability to directly inhibit T-cell proliferation, IL-2 production[239,240] as well as the ability to alter lymphocyte membrane fluidity.[241]

Apart from these effects on lymphocytes, glucocorticoids also enhance susceptibility to infections by altering monocyte and neutrophil functions at several stages. Movement of circulating inflammatory cells to the site of infection is suppressed by the ability of glucocorticoids to reduce the cellular response to chemotactic stimuli,[242–244] diminish neutrophil adherence[245] and induce a shift from marginal to circulating cells.[242] Glucocorticoids also suppress bactericidal activity of monocytes[243] and neutrophils,[246] perhaps through impairment of lysosomal function.[247]

Although severe burns are associated with alterations in B-cell production and function, there is considerable inconsistency in the status of literature concerning B-cell biology.[248–253]

For example, in rats subjected to 30% burn injury, splenic lymphocytes respond poorly to LPS and immunoglobulin synthesis is reduced in comparison to control animals.[254] Others have found an increase in circulating B cells early after burn injury.[250,255] Interestingly, administration of methylprednisolone to normal volunteers for 2–4 weeks also reduces serum immunoglobulin levels.[256] Changes in the B-cell population parallel changes in urine 17-hydroxysterol levels and increase in stress hormones in the early stages of burn injury may result in the release of B cells from lymphoid organs.

Aside from glucocorticoids, adrenal androgens such as DHEAS, also have profound influence on the immune responses. In fact, a role for DHEAS as a potent modulator of the immune response is now well established.[257–260] DHEAS which has immunosuppresive properties on Th1 helper cells, are low during severe illness.[176] In vitro treatment of human T cells with DHEAS increases IL-2 production (which is required for clonal expansion) and IL-2 mRNA synthesis.[260] It is interesting to note that this effect was seen only in $CD4^+CD8^-$ and not in $CD4^-CD8^+$ cells. DHEAS-treated cells were also able to mediate a more potent cytotoxic effect than cells without DHEAS treatment.

Yet another factor that profoundly influences the immune status and adrenal steroid secretion in burn patients is the neurotransmitter dopamine. Dopamine is often used in the treatment of critically ill patients because of its vasopressor, renal vasodilating, and cardiac inotropic properties. However several studies indicate that dopamine treatment may undermine an already depressed immune system. This effect appears to act via the suppression of prolactin release from the anterior pituitary. Dopamine suppresses serum prolactin and DHEAS levels but not cortisol concentration.[261,262] In vitro, prolactin has a synergistic effect on ACTH-induced DHEAS secretion by human adrenal cells.[263] Thus it is possible that the dopamine-induced suppression of prolactin is responsible for lowering DHEAS levels and therefore suppression of the T-cell proliferative response. The in vitro proliferative response of T cells from patients on dopamine therapy is diminished[261] and cells treated with DHEAS mediate a more potent T cell cytotoxic effect.[260] Dopamine levels are elevated under conditions of severe physical stress and chronic illness.[264,265] This may be partly responsible for the anergic state of the immune system during severe stress.

The present review affirms that catecholamines and adrenal steroid hormones are integral parts of the physiologic response to thermal injury that are thought to support recovery through compensatory cardiovascular, metabolic and immunologic changes. Although adrenergic mechanisms are important for their ability to influence intracellular signaling pathways, their role as modulators of gene expression is still being explored. On the other hand, while much is known about the modulation of gene expression by glucocorticoids, very little is known about their modulation of gene expression consequent to severe thermal injury or other forms of trauma. Future studies hold great promise of providing important new information in these areas as to how these bioactive compounds may influence responses to thermal injury and how such information can be lead to the development of new treatment modalities.

References

1. Benedict CR, Grahame-Smith DG. Plasma noradrenaline and adrenaline concentrations and dopamine-beta-hydroxylase activity in patients with shock due to septicaemia, trauma and haemorrhage. Q J Med 1978; 47:1–20.
2. Murton SA, Tan ST, Prickett TC, et al. Hormone responses to stress in patients with major burns. Br J Plast Surg 1998; 51:388–392.
3. Cuthbertson D. Post-shock metabolic response. Lancet 1942; 1:433–436.
4. Selye H. A syndrome produced by diverse nocuous agents. Nature 1936; 138:32–33.
5. Cunningham JJ, Hegarty MT, Meara PA, et al. Measured and predicted calorie requirements of adults during recovery from severe burn trauma. Am J Clin Nutr 1989; 49:404–408.
6. Khorram-Sefat R, Behrendt W, Heiden A, et al. Long-term measurements of energy expenditure in severe burn injury. World J Surg 1999; 23:115–122.
7. Soroff HS, Pearson E, Artz C. An estimation of nitrogen requirements for equilibrium in burned patients. Surg Gynecol Obstet 1961; 2:159.
8. Evans EI, Butterfield WJH. The stress response in the severely burned. Ann Surg 1951; 134:588–613.
9. Moore FD. Adaptation of supportive treatment to needs of the surgical patient. JAMA. 1949; 141:646–653.
10. Taylor FHL, Levenson SM, Adams MA. Abnormal carbohydrate metabolism in human thermal burns. N Engl J Med 1944; 231:437.
11. Birke G, Duner H, Liljedahl SO, et al. Histamine, catecholamines and adrenocortical steroids in burns. Acta Chir Scand 1958; 114:87–98.
12. Goodall M, Stone C, Haynes BW. Urinary output of adrenaline and noradrenaline in severe thermal burns. Ann Surg 1957; 145:479–487.
13. Becker RA, Vaughan GM, Goodwin CW Jr, et al. Plasma norepinephrine, epinephrine, and thyroid hormone interactions in severely burned patients. Arch Surg 1980; 115:439–443.
14. Birke G, Carlson LA, von Euler US, et al. Studies on burns. XII. Lipid metabolism, catecholamine excretion, basal metabolic rate, and water loss during treatment of burns with warm dry air. Acta Chir Scand 1972; 138:321–333.
15. Crum RL, Dominic W, Hansbrough JF, et al. Cardiovascular and neurohumoral responses following burn injury. Arch Surg 1990; 125:1065–1069.
16. Wilmore DW, Aulick LH. Metabolic changes in burned patients. Surg Clin North Am 1978; 58:1173–1187.
17. Wilmore DW, Long JM, Mason AD Jr, et al. Catecholamines: mediator of the hypermetabolic response to thermal injury. Ann Surg 1974; 180:653–669.
18. Carleton SC. Cardiac problems associated with burns. Cardiol Clin 1995; 13:257–262.
19. Michie D, Goldsmith R, Mason A. Hemodynamics of the immediate post-burn period. J Trauma 1963; 3:111–119.
20. Pruitt BA Jr. Current treatment of thermal injury. South Med J 1971; 64:657–662.
21. Ganrot K, Jacobsson S, Rothman U. Transcapillary passage of plasma proteins in experimental burns. Acta Physiol Scand 1974; 91:497–501.
22. Carvajal HF, Reinhart JA, Traber DL. Renal and cardiovascular functional response to thermal injury in dogs subjected to sympathetic blockade. Circ Shock 1976; 3:287–298.
23. Boyle WA, Segel LD. Direct cardiac effects of vasopressin and their reversal by a vascular antagonist. Am J Physiol 1986; 251:H734–H741.
24. Asch MJ, Feldman RJ, Walker HL, et al. Systemic and pulmonary hemodynamic changes accompanying thermal injury. Ann Surg 1973; 178:218–221.

25. Szabo K. Cardiac support in burned patients with heart disease. Acta Chir Plast 1989; 31:22–34.

26. Bevan J, Pegram B, Prehn J, et al. β-adrenergic receptor-mediated vasodilatation. In: Vanhoutte P, Leusen I, eds. Mechanisms in vasodilatation. New York: S Karger; 1977:258–265.

27. Chruscinski AJ, Rohrer DK, Schauble E, et al. Targeted disruption of the beta2 adrenergic receptor gene. J Biol Chem 1999; 274:16694–16700.

28. Jacob G, Costa F, Shannon J, et al. Dissociation between neural and vascular responses to sympathetic stimulation: contribution of local adrenergic receptor function. Hypertension 2000; 35:76–81.

29. Sheperd J. Circulation to skeletal muscle. In: Geiger S, Sheperd J, Abboud F, eds. Handbook of physiology section 2: the cardiovascular system: peripheral circulation and organ blood flow. Maryland: American Physiological Society; 1983:vol 3, 319–370.

30. Kilbourn RG, Traber DL, Szabo C. Nitric oxide and shock. Dis Mon 1997; 43:277–348.

31. Macarthur H, Westfall TC, Riley DP, et al. Inactivation of catecholamines by superoxide gives new insights on the pathogenesis of septic shock. Proc Natl Acad Sci USA 2000; 97:9753–9758.

32. Macarthur H, Couri DM, Wilken GH, et al. Modulation of serum cytokine levels by a novel superoxide dismutase mimetic, M40401, in an Escherichia coli model of septic shock: correlation with preserved circulating catecholamines. Crit Care Med 2003; 31:237–245.

33. Kolo LL, Westfall TC, Macarthur H. Nitric oxide decreases the biological activity of norepinephrine resulting in altered vascular tone in the rat mesenteric arterial bed. Am J Physiol Heart Circ Physiol 2004; 286:H296–H303.

34. Wolfe RR, Miller HI. Cardiovascular and metabolic responses during burn shock in the guinea pig. Am J Physiol 1976; 231:892–897.

35. Wolfe RR, Miller HI, Elahi D, et al. Effect of burn injury on glucose turnover in guinea pigs. Surg Gynecol Obstet 1977; 144:359–364.

36. Arturson G. Metabolic changes and nutrition in children with severe burns. Prog Pediatr Surg 1981; 14:81–109.

37. Breitenstein E, Chiolero RL, Jequier E, et al. Effects of beta-blockade on energy metabolism following burns. Burns 1990; 16:259–264.

38. Wolfe RR, Durkot MJ. Evaluation of the role of the sympathetic nervous system in the response of substrate kinetics and oxidation to burn injury. Circ Shock 1982; 9:395–406.

39. Herndon DN, Nguyen TT, Wolfe RR, et al. Lipolysis in burned patients is stimulated by the beta 2-receptor for catecholamines. Arch Surg 1994; 129:1301–1304; discussion 1304–1305.

40. Wolfe RR, Herndon DN, Jahoor F, et al. Effect of severe burn injury on substrate cycling by glucose and fatty acids. N Engl J Med 1987; 317:403–408.

41. Wolfe RR, Herndon DN, Peters EJ, et al. Regulation of lipolysis in severely burned children. Ann Surg 1987; 206:214–221.

42. Cope O, Nardi G, Ouijano M, et al. Metabolic rate and thyroid function following acute thermal trauma in man. Ann Surg 1953; 137:165–174.

43. Caldwell FT Jr, Ostermann H, Sower N, et al. Metabolic response to thermal trauma of normal and thyroprivic rats at three environmental temperatures. Ann Surg 1959; 150:976–988.

44. Caldwell FT Jr. Energy metabolism following thermal burns. Arch Surg 1976; 111:181–185.

45. Chance WT, Nelson JL, Foley-Nelson T, et al. The relationship of burn-induced hypermetabolism to central and peripheral catecholamines. J Trauma 1989; 29:306–312.

46. Caldwell FT Jr, Graves DB, Wallace BH, et al. Alteration in temperature regulation induced by burn injury in the rat. J Burn Care Rehabil 1989; 10:486–493.

47. Neely WA, Petro AB, Holloman GH Jr, et al. Researches on the cause of burn hypermetabolism. Ann Surg 1974; 179:291–294.

48. Herndon DN, Barrow RE, Rutan TC, et al. Effect of propranolol administration on hemodynamic and metabolic responses of burned pediatric patients. Ann Surg 1988; 208:484–492.

49. Herndon DN, Hart DW, Wolf SE, et al. Reversal of catabolism by beta-blockade after severe burns. N Engl J Med 2001; 345:1223–1229.

50. Shirani KZ, Pruitt BA Jr, Mason AD Jr. The influence of inhalation injury and pneumonia on burn mortality. Ann Surg 1987; 205:82–87.

51. Jones SB, Kovarik MF, Romano FD. Cardiac and splenic norepinephrine turnover during septic peritonitis. Am J Physiol 1986; 250:R892–R897.

52. Jones SB, Romano FD. Dose- and time-dependent changes in plasma catecholamines in response to endotoxin in conscious rats. Circ Shock 1989; 28:59–68.

53. Jones SB, Westfall MV, Sayeed MM. Plasma catecholamines during E. coli bacteremia in conscious rats. Am J Physiol 1988; 254:R470–R477.

54. Kovarik MF, Jones SB, Romano FD. Plasma catecholamines following cecal ligation and puncture in the rat. Circ Shock 1987; 22:281–290.

55. Zhou ZZ, Jones SB. Involvement of central vs. peripheral mechanisms in mediating sympathoadrenal activation in endotoxic rats. Am J Physiol 1993; 265:R683–R688.

56. Zhou ZZ, Wurster RD, Jones SB. Arterial baroreflexes are not essential in mediating sympathoadrenal activation in conscious endotoxic rats. J Auton Nerv Syst 1992; 39:1–12.

57. Calvo W. The innervation of the bone marrow in laboratory animals. J Anatomy 1968; 123:315–328.

58. Felten SY, Felten DL, Bellinger DL, et al. Noradrenergic sympathetic innervation of lymphoid organs. Prog Allergy 1988; 43:14–36.

59. Reilly FD, McCuskey PA, Miller ML, et al. Innervation of the periarteriolar lymphatic sheath of the spleen. Tissue Cell 1979; 11:121–126.

60. Van Oosterhout AJ, Nijkamp FP. Anterior hypothalamic lesions prevent the endotoxin-induced reduction of beta-adrenoceptor number in guinea pig lung. Brain Res 1984; 302:277–280.

61. Williams JM, Felten DL. Sympathetic innervation of murine thymus and spleen: a comparative histofluorescence study. Anat Rec 1981; 199:531–542.

62. Ackerman KD, Felten SY, Bellinger DL, et al. Noradrenergic sympathetic innervation of the spleen: III. Development of innervation in the rat spleen. J Neurosci Res 1987; 18:49–54.

63. Felten DL, Ackerman KD, Wiegand SJ, et al. Noradrenergic sympathetic innervation of the spleen: I. Nerve fibers associate with lymphocytes and macrophages in specific compartments of the splenic white pulp. J Neurosci Res 1987; 18:28–36.

64. Felten DL, Felten SY, Carlson SL, et al. Noradrenergic and peptidergic innervation of lymphoid tissue. J Immunol 1985; 135:755s–765s.

65. Felten SY, Olschowka J. Noradrenergic sympathetic innervation of the spleen: II. Tyrosine hydroxylase (TH)-positive nerve terminals form synapticlike contacts on lymphocytes in the splenic white pulp. J Neurosci Res 1987; 18:37–48.

66. Livnat S, Felten SY, Carlson SL, et al. Involvement of peripheral and central catecholamine systems in neural-immune interactions. J Neuroimmunol 1985; 10:5–30.

67. Tang Y, Shankar R, Gamelli R, et al. Dynamic norepinephrine alterations in bone marrow: evidence of functional innervation. J Neuroimmunol 1999; 96:182–189.

68. Kohm AP, Sanders VM. Suppression of antigen-specific Th2 cell-dependent IgM and IgG1 production following norepinephrine depletion in vivo. J Immunol 1999; 162:5299–5308.

69. Ramer-Quinn DS, Baker RA, Sanders VM. Activated T helper 1 and T helper 2 cells differentially express the beta-2-adrenergic receptor: a mechanism for selective modulation of T helper 1 cell cytokine production. J Immunol 1997; 159:4857–4867.

70. Sanders VM. The role of adrenoceptor-mediated signals in the modulation of lymphocyte function. Adv Neuroimmunol 1995; 5:283–298.

71. Sanders VM, Baker RA, Ramer-Quinn DS, et al. Differential expression of the beta2-adrenergic receptor by Th1 and Th2 clones: implications for cytokine production and B cell help. J Immunol 1997; 158:4200–4210.

72. Swanson MA, Lee WT, Sanders VM. IFN-gamma production by Th1 cells generated from naive CD4+ T cells exposed to norepinephrine. J Immunol 2001; 166:232–240.

73. Kasprowicz DJ, Kohm AP, Berton MT, et al. Stimulation of the B cell receptor, CD86 (B7–2), and the beta 2-adrenergic receptor intrinsically modulates the level of IgG1 and IgE produced per B cell. J Immunol 2000; 165:680–690.

74. Melmon KL, Bourne HR, Weinstein Y, et al. Hemolytic plaque formation by leukocytes in vitro. Control by vasoactive hormones. J Clin Invest 1974; 53:13–21.

75. Kohm AP, Tang Y, Sanders VM, et al. Activation of antigen-specific CD4+ Th2 cells and B cells in vivo increases norepinephrine release in the spleen and bone marrow. J Immunol 2000; 165:725–733.

76. Spengler RN, Chensue SW, Giacherio DA, et al. Endogenous norepinephrine regulates tumor necrosis factor-alpha production from macrophages in vitro. J Immunol 1994; 152:3024–3031.

77. Beno DW, Kimura RE. Nonstressed rat model of acute endotoxemia that unmasks the endotoxin-induced TNF-alpha response. Am J Physiol 1999; 276:H671–H678.

78. Hasko G, Elenkov IJ, Kvetan V, et al. Differential effect of selective block of alpha 2-adrenoreceptors on plasma levels of tumour necrosis factor-alpha, interleukin-6 and corticosterone induced by bacterial lipopolysaccharide in mice. J Endocrinol 1995; 144:457–462.

79. Monastra G, Secchi EF. Beta-adrenergic receptors mediate in vivo the adrenaline inhibition of lipopolysaccharide-induced tumor necrosis factor release. Immunol Lett 1993; 38:127–130.

80. Szabo C, Hasko G, Zingarelli B, et al. Isoproterenol regulates tumour necrosis factor, interleukin-10, interleukin-6 and nitric oxide production and protects against the development of vascular hyporeactivity in endotoxaemia. Immunology 1997; 90:95–100.

81. Szelenyi J, Kiss JP, Vizi ES. Differential involvement of sympathetic nervous system and immune system in the modulation of TNF-alpha production by alpha2- and beta-adrenoceptors in mice. J Neuroimmunol 2000; 103:34–40.

82. van der Poll T, Coyle SM, Barbosa K, et al. Epinephrine inhibits tumor necrosis factor-alpha and potentiates interleukin 10 production during human endotoxemia. J Clin Invest 1996; 97:713–719.

83. Bergmann M, Gornikiewicz A, Sautner T, et al. Attenuation of catecholamine-induced immunosuppression in whole blood from patients with sepsis. Shock 1999; 12:421–427.

84. Guirao X, Kumar A, Katz J, et al. Catecholamines increase monocyte TNF receptors and inhibit TNF through beta 2-adrenoreceptor activation. Am J Physiol 1997; 273:E1203–E1208.

85. Severn A, Rapson NT, Hunter CA, et al. Regulation of tumor necrosis factor production by adrenaline and beta-adrenergic agonists. J Immunol 1992; 148:3441–3445.

86. van der Poll T, Jansen J, Endert E, et al. Noradrenaline inhibits lipopolysaccharide-induced tumor necrosis factor and interleukin 6 production in human whole blood. Infect Immun 1994; 62:2046–2050.

87. Yoshimura T, Kurita C, Nagao T, et al. Inhibition of tumor necrosis factor-alpha and interleukin-1-beta production by beta-adrenoceptor agonists from lipopolysaccharide-stimulated human peripheral blood mononuclear cells. Pharmacology 1997; 54:144–152.

88. Chou RC, Stinson MW, Noble BK, et al. Beta-adrenergic receptor regulation of macrophage-derived tumor necrosis factor-alpha production from rats with experimental arthritis. J Neuroimmunol 1996; 67:7–16.

89. Hu XX, Goldmuntz EA, Brosnan CF. The effect of norepinephrine on endotoxin-mediated macrophage activation. J Neuroimmunol 1991; 31:35–42.

90. Ignatowski TA, Spengler RN. Regulation of macrophage-derived tumor necrosis factor production by modification of adrenergic receptor sensitivity. J Neuroimmunol 1995; 61:61–70.

91. Liao J, Keiser JA, Scales WE, et al. Role of epinephrine in TNF and IL-6 production from isolated perfused rat liver. Am J Physiol 1995; 268:R896–R901.

92. Bissonnette EY, Befus AD. Anti-inflammatory effect of beta 2-agonists: inhibition of TNF-alpha release from human mast cells. J Allergy Clin Immunol 1997; 100:825–831.

93. Hetier E, Ayala J, Bousseau A, et al. Modulation of interleukin-1 and tumor necrosis factor expression by beta-adrenergic agonists in mouse ameboid microglial cells. Exp Brain Res 1991; 86:407–413.

94. Nakamura A, Johns EJ, Imaizumi A, et al. Regulation of tumour necrosis factor and interleukin-6 gene transcription by beta2-adrenoceptor in the rat astrocytes. J Neuroimmunol 1998; 88:144–153.

95. Kalinichenko VV, Mokyr MB, Graf LH Jr, et al. Norepinephrine-mediated inhibition of antitumor cytotoxic T lymphocyte generation involves a beta-adrenergic receptor mechanism and decreased TNF-alpha gene expression. J Immunol 1999; 163:2492–2499.

96. Abadie C, Foucart S, Page P, et al. Interleukin-1 beta and tumor necrosis factor-alpha inhibit the release of [3H]-noradrenaline from isolated human atrial appendages. Naunyn Schmiedebergs Arch Pharmacol 1997; 355:384–389.

97. Foucart S, Abadie C. Interleukin-1 beta and tumor necrosis factor-alpha inhibit the release of [3H]-noradrenaline from mice isolated atria. Naunyn Schmiedebergs Arch Pharmacol 1996; 354:1–6.

98. Hurst SM, Collins SM. Mechanism underlying tumor necrosis factor-alpha suppression of norepinephrine release from rat myenteric plexus. Am J Physiol 1994; 266:G1123–G1129.

99. Ignatowski TA, Noble BK, Wright JR, et al. Neuronal-associated tumor necrosis factor (TNF alpha): its role in noradrenergic functioning and modification of its expression following antidepressant drug administration. J Neuroimmunol 1997; 79:84–90.

100. DeRijk RH, Boelen A, Tilders FJ, et al. Induction of plasma interleukin-6 by circulating adrenaline in the rat. Psychoneuroendocrinology 1994; 19:155–163.

101. Takaki A, Huang QH, Somogyvari-Vigh A, et al. Immobilization stress may increase plasma interleukin-6 via central and peripheral catecholamines. Neuroimmunomodulation 1994; 1:335–342.

102. van Gool J, van Vugt H, Helle M, et al. The relation among stress, adrenalin, interleukin 6 and acute phase proteins in the rat. Clin Immunol Immunopathol 1990; 57:200–210.

103. Gornikiewicz A, Sautner T, Brostjan C, et al. Catecholamines upregulate lipopolysaccharide-induced IL-6 production in human microvascular endothelial cells. FASEB J 2000; 14:1093–1100.

104. von Patay B, Loppnow H, Feindt J, et al. Catecholamines and lipopolysaccharide synergistically induce the release of interleukin-6 from thymic epithelial cells. J Neuroimmunol 1998; 86:182–189.

105. Maimone D, Cioni C, Rosa S, et al. Norepinephrine and vasoactive intestinal peptide induce IL-6 secretion by astrocytes: synergism with IL-1 beta and TNF alpha. J Neuroimmunol 1993; 47:73–81.

106. Zumwalt JW, Thunstrom BJ, Spangelo BL. Interleukin-1beta and catecholamines synergistically stimulate interleukin-6 release from rat C6 glioma cells in vitro: a potential role for lysophosphatidylcholine. Endocrinology 1999; 140:888–896.

107. Burysek L, Houstek J. beta-Adrenergic stimulation of interleukin-1alpha and interleukin-6 expression in mouse brown adipocytes. FEBS Lett 1997; 411:83–86.

108. Christensen JD, Hansen EW, Frederiksen C, et al. Adrenaline influences the release of interleukin-6 from murine pituicytes: role of beta2-adrenoceptors. Eur J Pharmacol 1999; 378:143–148.

109. Jung BD, Kimura K, Kitamura H, et al. Norepinephrine stimulates interleukin-6 mRNA expression in primary cultured rat hepatocytes. J Biochem (Tokyo) 2000; 127:205–209.

110. Norris JG, Benveniste EN. Interleukin-6 production by astrocytes: induction by the neurotransmitter norepinephrine. J Neuroimmunol 1993; 45:137–145.

111. von Patay B, Kurz B, Mentlein R. Effect of transmitters and cotransmitters of the sympathetic nervous system on interleukin-6 synthesis in thymic epithelial cells. Neuroimmunomodulation 1999; 6:45–50.

112. Straub RH, Herrmann M, Berkmiller G, et al. Neuronal regulation of interleukin 6 secretion in murine spleen: adrenergic and opioidergic control. J Neurochem 1997; 68:1633–1639.

113. Straub RH, Herrmann M, Frauenholz T, et al. Neuroimmune control of interleukin-6 secretion in the murine spleen. Differential beta-adrenergic effects of electrically released endogenous norepinephrine under various endotoxin conditions. J Neuroimmunol 1996; 71:37–43.

114. Straub RH, Linde HJ, Mannel DN, Scholmerich J, Falk W. A bacteria-induced switch of sympathetic effector mechanisms augments local inhibition of TNF-alpha and IL-6 secretion in the spleen. FASEB J 2000; 14:1380–1388.

115. Platzer C, Docke W, Volk H, et al. Catecholamines trigger IL-10 release in acute systemic stress reaction by direct stimulation of its promoter/enhancer activity in monocytic cells. J Neuroimmunol 2000; 105:31–38.

116. Siegmund B, Eigler A, Hartmann G, et al. Adrenaline enhances LPS-induced IL-10 synthesis: evidence for protein kinase A-mediated pathway. Int J Immunopharmacol 1998; 20:57–69.

117. Woiciechowsky C, Asadullah K, Nestler D, et al. Sympathetic activation triggers systemic interleukin-10 release in immunodepression induced by brain injury. Nat Med 1998; 4:808–813.

118. Hasko G, Nemeth ZH, Szabo C, et al. Isoproterenol inhibits Il-10, TNF-alpha, and nitric oxide production in RAW 264.7 macrophages. Brain Res Bull 1998; 45:183–187.

119. Suberville S, Bellocq A, Fouqueray B, et al. Regulation of interleukin-10 production by beta-adrenergic agonists. Eur J Immunol 1996; 26:2601–2605.

120. Deng J, Muthu K, Gamelli R, et al. Adrenergic modulation of splenic macrophage cytokine release in polymicrobial sepsis. Am J Physiol Cell Physiol 2004; 287:C730–736.

121. Muthu K, Deng J, Gamelli R, et al. Adrenergic modulation of cytokine release in bone marrow progenitor-derived macrophage following polymicrobial sepsis. J Neuroimmunol 2005; 158:50–57.

122. Lyte M. The role of catecholamines in gram-negative sepsis. Med Hypotheses 1992; 37:255–258.

123. Lyte M. The role of microbial endocrinology in infectious disease. J Endocrinol 1993; 137:343–345.

124. Lyte M, Bailey MT. Neuroendocrine-bacterial interactions in a neurotoxin-induced model of trauma. J Surg Res 1997; 70:195–201.

125. Lyte M, Ernst S. Alpha and beta adrenergic receptor involvement in catecholamine-induced growth of gram-negative bacteria. Biochem Biophys Res Commun 1993; 190:447–452.

126. Lyte M, Ernst S, Driemeyer J, et al. Strain-specific enhancement of splenic T cell mitogenesis and macrophage phagocytosis following peripheral axotomy. J Neuroimmunol 1991; 31:1–8.

127. Freestone PP, Haigh RD, Williams PH, et al. Stimulation of bacterial growth by heat-stable, norepinephrine-induced autoinducers. FEMS Microbiol Lett 1999; 172:53–60.

128. Lyte M, Frank CD, Green BT. Production of an autoinducer of growth by norepinephrine cultured Escherichia coli O157:H7. FEMS Microbiol Lett 1996; 139:155–159.

129. Lyte M, Arulanandam BP, Frank CD. Production of Shiga-like toxins by Escherichia coli O157:H7 can be influenced by the neuroendocrine hormone norepinephrine. J Lab Clin Med 1996; 128:392–398.

130. Lyte M, Erickson AK, Arulanandam BP, et al. Norepinephrine-induced expression of the K99 pilus adhesin of enterotoxigenic Escherichia coli. Biochem Biophys Res Commun 1997; 232:682–686.

131. Iverson L. Neuronal and extraneuronal catecholamine uptake mechanisms. In: Usdin E, Snyder S, eds. Frontiers in catecholamine research. London: Pergamon; 1973:403–408.

132. Duque RE, Phan SH, Hudson JL, et al. Functional defects in phagocytic cells following thermal injury. Application of flow cytometric analysis. Am J Pathol 1985; 118:116–127.

133. Sartorelli KH, Silver GM, Gamelli RL. The effect of granulocyte colony-stimulating factor (G-CSF) upon burn-induced defective neutrophil chemotaxis. J Trauma 1991; 31:523–529; discussion 529–530.

134. Solomkin JS. Neutrophil disorders in burn injury: complement, cytokines, and organ injury. J Trauma 1990; 30:S80–S85.

135. Warden GD, Mason AD Jr, Pruitt BA Jr. Evaluation of leukocyte chemotaxis in vitro in thermally injured patients. J Clin Invest 1974; 54:1001–1004.

136. Peterson V, Hansbrough J, Buerk C, et al. Regulation of granulopoiesis following severe thermal injury. J Trauma 1983; 23:19–24.

137. Volenec FJ, Wood GW, Mani MM, et al. Mononuclear cell analysis of peripheral blood from burn patients. J Trauma 1979; 19:86–93.

138. Maestroni GJ. Adrenergic regulation of haematopoiesis. Pharmacol Res 1995; 32:249–253.

139. Maestroni GJ, Conti A. Modulation of hematopoiesis via alpha 1-adrenergic receptors on bone marrow cells. Exp Hematol 1994; 22:313–320.

140. Dresch C, Minc J, Mary JY. In vivo protection of normal mouse hematopoiesis by a beta 2 blocking agent during S-phase chemotherapy. Cancer Res 1984; 44:493–497.

141. Dresch C, Minc J, Poirier O, et al. Effect of beta adrenergic agonists and beta blocking agents on hemopoiesis in human bone marrow. Biomedicine 1981; 34:93–98.

142. Maestroni GJ, Conti A, Pedrinis E. Effect of adrenergic agents on hematopoiesis after syngeneic bone marrow transplantation in mice. Blood 1992; 80:1178–1182.

143. Togni M, Maestroni GJ. Hematopoietic rescue in mice via α1-adrenoceptors on bone marrow B cell precursors. Int J Oncol 1996:313–318.

144. Tang Y, Shankar R, Gamboa M, et al. Norepinephrine modulates myelopoiesis after experimental thermal injury with sepsis. Ann Surg 2001; 233:266–275.

145. Ayala A, Chaudry IH. Immune dysfunction in murine polymicrobial sepsis: mediators, macrophages, lymphocytes and apoptosis. Shock 1996; 6:S27–S38.

146. Faist E. The mechanisms of host defense dysfunction following shock and trauma. Curr Top Microbiol Immunol 1996; 216:259–274.

147. Faist E, Schinkel C, Zimmer S, et al. Inadequate interleukin-2 synthesis and interleukin-2 messenger expression following thermal and mechanical trauma in humans is caused by defective transmembrane signalling. J Trauma 1993; 34:846–853; discussion 853–844.

148. Miller CL, Baker CC. Changes in lymphocyte activity after thermal injury. The role of suppressor cells. J Clin Invest 1979; 63:202–210.

149. Miller-Graziano CL, Fink M, Wu JY, et al. Mechanisms of altered monocyte prostaglandin E_2 production in severely injured patients. Arch Surg 1988; 123:293–299.

150. Miller-Graziano CL, Szabo G, Kodys K, et al. Aberrations in post-trauma monocyte (MO) subpopulation: role in septic shock syndrome. J Trauma 1990; 30:S86–S96.

151. Miller-Graziano CL, Zhu D, Kodys K. Differential induction of human monocyte transforming growth factor beta 1 production and its regulation by interleukin 4. J Clin Immunol 1994; 14:61–72.

152. Santangelo S, Gamelli RL, Shankar R. Myeloid commitment shifts toward monocytopoiesis after thermal injury and sepsis. Ann Surg 2001; 233:97–106.

153. Shoup M, Weisenberger JM, Wang JL, et al. Mechanisms of neutropenia involving myeloid maturation arrest in burn sepsis. Ann Surg 1998; 228:112–122.

154. Leenen PJ, Melis M, Slieker WA, Van Ewijk W. Murine macrophage precursor characterization. II. Monoclonal antibodies against macrophage precursor antigens. Eur J Immunol 1990; 20:27–34.

155. de Bruijn MF, Slieker WA, van der Loo JC, et al. Distinct mouse bone marrow macrophage precursors identified by differential expression of ER-MP12 and ER-MP20 antigens. Eur J Immunol 1994; 24:2279–2284.

156. Cohen MJ, Shankar R, Stevenson J, et al. Bone marrow norepinephrine mediates development of functionally different macrophages after thermal injury and sepsis. Ann Surg 2004; 240:132–141.

157. Muthu K, Deng J, Romano F, et al. Thermal injury and sepsis modulates beta-adrenergic receptors and cAMP responses in monocyte-committed bone marrow cells. J Neuroimmunol 2005; 165:129–138.

158. Moore FD. Hormones and stress. New York: Academic Press; 1957.

159. Hume DM, Nelson DH, Miller DW. Blood and urinary 17-hydroxycorticosteroids in patients with severe burns. Ann Surg 1956; 143:316–329.

160. Moore FD. Metabolic care of the surgical patient. Philadelphia: WB Saunders; 1959.

161. Bane JW, McCaa RE, McCaa CS, et al. The pattern of aldosterone and cortisone blood levels in thermal burn patients. J Trauma 1974; 14:605–611.

162. Wise L, Margraf HW, Ballinger WF. Adrenal cortical function in severe burns. Arch Surg 1972; 105:213–220.

163. Mortensen RF, Johnson AA, Eurenius K. Serum corticosteroid binding following thermal injury. Proc Soc Exp Biol Med 1972; 139:877–882.

164. Pugeat M, Bonneton A, Perrot D, et al. Decreased immunoreactivity and binding activity of corticosteroid-binding globulin in serum in septic shock. Clin Chem 1989; 35:1675–1679.

165. Garrel DR. Corticosteroid-binding globulin during inflammation and burn injury: nutritional modulation and clinical implications. Horm Res 1996; 45:245–251.

166. Garrel DR, Zhang L, Zhao XF, et al. Effect of burn injury on corticosteroid-binding globulin levels in plasma and wound fluid. Wound Rep Reg 1993; 1:10–14.

167. Feldman D, Mondon CE, Horner JA, et al. Glucocorticoid and estrogen regulation of corticosteroid-binding globulin production by rat liver. Am J Physiol 1979; 237:E493–E499.

168. Frairia R, Agrimonti F, Fortunati N, et al. Influence of naturally occurring and synthetic glucocorticoids on corticosteroid-binding globulin-steroid interaction in human peripheral plasma. Ann N Y Acad Sci 1988; 538:287–303.

169. Smith CL, Hammond GL. Hormonal regulation of corticosteroid-binding globulin biosynthesis in the male rat. Endocrinology 1992; 130:2245–2251.

170. Emptoz-Bonneton A, Crave JC, LeJeune H, et al. Corticosteroid-binding globulin synthesis regulation by cytokines and glucocorticoids in human hepatoblastoma-derived (HepG2) cells. J Clin Endocrinol Metab 1997; 82:3758–3762.

171. Vermes I, Beishuizen A, Hampsink RM, et al. Dissociation of plasma adrenocorticotropin and cortisol levels in critically ill patients: possible role of endothelin and atrial natriuretic hormone. J Clin Endocrinol Metab 1995; 80:1238–1242.

172. Kellner M, Wiedemann K, Holsboer F. Atrial natriuretic factor inhibits the CRH-stimulated secretion of ACTH and cortisol in man. Life Sci 1992; 50:1835–1842.

173. Hinson JP, Vinson GP, Kapas S, et al. The role of endothelin in the control of adrenocortical function: stimulation of endothelin release by ACTH and the effects of endothelin-1 and endothelin-3 on steroidogenesis in rat and human adrenocortical cells. J Endocrinol 1991; 128:275–280.

174. Hirai M, Miyabo S, Ooya E, et al. Endothelin-3 stimulates the hypothalamic–pituitary–adrenal axis. Life Sci 1991; 48:2359–2363.

175. Vierhapper H, Hollenstein U, Roden M, et al. Effect of endothelin-1 in man – impact on basal and stimulated concentrations of luteinizing hormone, follicle-stimulating hormone, thyrotropin, growth hormone, corticotropin, and prolactin. Metabolism 1993; 42:902–906.

176. Parker CR Jr, Baxter CR. Divergence in adrenal steroid secretory pattern after thermal injury in adult patients. J Trauma 1985; 25:508–510.

177. Lephart ED, Baxter CR, Parker CR Jr. Effect of burn trauma on adrenal and testicular steroid hormone production. J Clin Endocrinol Metab 1987; 64:842–848.

178. Doerr P, Pirke KM. Cortisol-induced suppression of plasma testosterone in normal adult males. J Clin Endocrinol Metab 1976; 43:622–629.

179. Welsh TH Jr, Bambino TH, Hsueh AJ. Mechanism of glucocorticoid-induced suppression of testicular androgen biosynthesis in vitro. Biol Reprod 1982; 27:1138–1146.

180. Wallace BH, Caldwell FT Jr, Cone JB. The interrelationships between wound management, thermal stress, energy metabolism, and temperature profiles of patients with burns. J Burn Care Rehabil 1994; 15:499–508.

181. Allison SP, Hinton P, Chamberlain MJ. Intravenous glucose-tolerance, insulin, and free-fatty-acid levels in burned patients. Lancet 1968; 2:1113–1116.

182. Plager JE, Matsui N. An in vitro demonstration of the anti-insulin action of cortisol on glucose metabolism. Endocrinology 1966; 78:1154–1158.

183. Wolfe RR, Durkot MJ, Allsop JR, et al. Glucose metabolism in severely burned patients. Metabolism 1979; 28:1031–1039.

184. Wolfe RR, Miller HI, Spitzer JJ. Glucose and lactate kinetics in burn shock. Am J Physiol 1977; 232:E415–E418.

185. Yarmush DM, MacDonald AD, Foy BD, et al. Cutaneous burn injury alters relative tricarboxylic acid cycle fluxes in rat liver. J Burn Care Rehabil 1999; 20:292–302.

186. Shuck JM, Eaton P, Shuck LW, et al. Dynamics of insulin and glucagon secretions in severely burned patients. J Trauma 1977; 17:706–713.

187. Vaughan GM, Becker RA, Unger RH, et al. Nonthyroidal control of metabolism after burn injury: possible role of glucagon. Metabolism 1985; 34:637–641.

188. Marco J, Calle C, Roman D, et al. Hyperglucagonism induced by glucocorticoid treatment in man. N Engl J Med 1973; 288:128–131.

189. Cuthbertson DP. Observations on disturbance of metabolism produced by injury to the limbs. QJM 1932; 25:233–246.

190. Darmaun D, Matthews DE, Bier DM. Physiological hypercortisolemia increases proteolysis, glutamine, and alanine production. Am J Physiol 1988; 255:E366–E373.

191. Kayali AG, Young VR, Goodman MN. Sensitivity of myofibrillar proteins to glucocorticoid-induced muscle proteolysis. Am J Physiol 1987; 252:E621–E626.

192. Fang CH, James HJ, Ogle C, et al. Influence of burn injury on protein metabolism in different types of skeletal muscle and the role of glucocorticoids. J Am Coll Surg 1995; 180:33–42.

193. May RC, Kelly RA, Mitch WE. Metabolic acidosis stimulates protein degradation in rat muscle by a glucocorticoid-dependent mechanism. J Clin Invest 1986; 77:614–621.

194. Price SR, England BK, Bailey JL, et al. Acidosis and glucocorticoids concomitantly increase ubiquitin and proteasome subunit mRNAs in rat muscle. Am J Physiol 1994; 267:C955–C960.

195. Isozaki U, Mitch WE, England BK, et al. Protein degradation and increased mRNAs encoding proteins of the ubiquitin-proteasome proteolytic pathway in BC3H1 myocytes require an interaction between glucocorticoids and acidification. Proc Natl Acad Sci USA 1996; 93:1967–1971.

196. Ding X, Price SR, Bailey JL, et al. Cellular mechanisms controlling protein degradation in catabolic states. Miner Electrolyte Metab 1997; 23:194–197.

197. Bailey JL, Wang X, England BK, et al. The acidosis of chronic renal failure activates muscle proteolysis in rats by augmenting transcription of genes encoding proteins of the ATP-dependent ubiquitin-proteasome pathway. J Clin Invest 1996; 97:1447–1453.

198. Medina R, Wing SS, Goldberg AL. Increase in levels of polyubiquitin and proteasome mRNA in skeletal muscle during starvation and denervation atrophy. Biochem J 1995; 307:631–637.

199. Mitch WE, Medina R, Grieber S, et al. Metabolic acidosis stimulates muscle protein degradation by activating the adenosine triphosphate-dependent pathway involving ubiquitin and proteasomes. J Clin Invest 1994; 93:2127–2133.

200. Price SR, Bailey JL, Wang X, et al. Muscle wasting in insulinopenic rats results from activation of the ATP-dependent, ubiquitin-proteasome proteolytic pathway by a mechanism including gene transcription. J Clin Invest 1996; 98:1703–1708.

201. Wing SS, Goldberg AL. Glucocorticoids activate the ATP-ubiquitin-dependent proteolytic system in skeletal muscle during fasting. Am J Physiol 1993; 264:E668–E676.

202. Aulick LH, Wilmore DW. Increased peripheral amino acid release following burn injury. Surgery 1979; 85:560–565.

203. Abcouwer SF, Lohmann R, Bode BP, et al. Induction of glutamine synthetase expression after major burn injury is tissue specific and temporally variable. J Trauma 1997; 42:421–427; discussion 427–428.

204. Abcouwer SF, Bode BP, Souba WW. Glucocorticoids regulate rat glutamine synthetase expression in a tissue-specific manner. J Surg Res 1995; 59:59–65.

205. Hart DW, Wolf SE, Mlcak R, et al. Persistence of muscle catabolism after severe burn. Surgery 2000; 128:312–319.

206. Milner EA, Cioffi WG, Mason AD, et al. A longitudinal study of resting energy expenditure in thermally injured patients. J Trauma 1994; 37:167–170.

207. Casanueva FF. Physiology of growth hormone secretion and action. Endocrinol Metab Clin North Am 1992; 21:483–517.

208. Rosen CJ, Pollak M. Circulating IGF-1: new perspectives for a new century. Trends Endocrinol Metab 1999; 10:136–141.

209. Abribat T, Brazeau P, Davignon I, et al. Insulin-like growth factor-I blood levels in severely burned patients: effects of time post injury, age of patient and severity of burn. Clin Endocrinol (Oxf) 1993; 39:583–589.

210. Bereket A, Wilson TA, Blethen SL, et al. Regulation of the acid-labile subunit of the insulin-like growth factor ternary complex in patients with insulin-dependent diabetes mellitus and severe burns. Clin Endocrinol (Oxf) 1996; 44:525–532.

211. Davies SC, Wass JA, Ross RJ, et al. The induction of a specific protease for insulin-like growth factor binding protein-3 in the circulation during severe illness. J Endocrinol 1991; 130:469–473.

212. Ghahary A, Fu S, Shen YJ, et al. Differential effects of thermal injury on circulating insulin-like growth factor binding proteins in burn patients. Mol Cell Biochem 1994; 135:171–180.

213. Moller S, Jensen M, Svensson P, et al. Insulin-like growth factor 1 (IGF-1) in burn patients. Burns 1991; 17:279–281.

214. Dai J, Baxter RC. Regulation in vivo of the acid-labile subunit of the rat serum insulin-like growth factor-binding protein complex. Endocrinology 1994; 135:2335–2341.

215. Dai J, Scott CD, Baxter RC. Regulation of the acid-labile subunit of the insulin-like growth factor complex in cultured rat hepatocytes. Endocrinology 1994; 135:1066–1072.

216. Al Shamma GA, Goll CC, Baird TB, et al. Changes in body composition after thermal injury in the rat. Br J Nutr 1979; 42:267–275.

217. Fain SN, Scow RO, Chernick SS. Effects of glucocorticoids on metabolism of adipose tissue in vitro. J Biol Chem 1963; 238:54–58.

218. Galster AD, Bier DM, Cryer PE, et al. Plasma palmitate turnover in subjects with thermal injury. J Trauma 1984; 24:938–945.

219. Harris RL, Frenkel RA, Cottam GL, et al. Lipid mobilization and metabolism after thermal trauma. J Trauma 1982; 22:194–198.

220. Klein GL, Herndon DN, Rutan TC, et al. Bone disease in burn patients. J Bone Miner Res 1993; 8:337–345.

221. Schaffler MB, Li XJ, Jee WS, et al. Skeletal tissue responses to thermal injury: an experimental study. Bone 1988; 9:397–406.

222. Klein GL, Herndon DN, Langman CB, et al. Long-term reduction in bone mass after severe burn injury in children. J Pediatr 1995; 126:252–256.

223. Rutan RL, Herndon DN. Growth delay in postburn pediatric patients. Arch Surg 1990; 125:392–395.

224. Klein GL, Wolf SE, Goodman WG, et al. The management of acute bone loss in severe catabolism due to burn injury. Horm Res 1997; 48:83–87.

225. Weinstein RS, Jilka RL, Parfitt AM, et al. Inhibition of osteoblastogenesis and promotion of apoptosis of osteoblasts and osteocytes by glucocorticoids. Potential mechanisms of their deleterious effects on bone. J Clin Invest 1998; 102:274–282.

226. Canalis E. Clinical review 83: Mechanisms of glucocorticoid action in bone: implications to glucocorticoid-induced osteoporosis. J Clin Endocrinol Metab 1996; 81:3441–3447.

227. Canalis E, Rydziel S, Delany AM, et al. Insulin-like growth factors inhibit interstitial collagenase synthesis in bone cell cultures. Endocrinology 1995; 136:1348–1354.

228. Dempster DW, Moonga BS, Stein LS, et al. Glucocorticoids inhibit bone resorption by isolated rat osteoclasts by enhancing apoptosis. J Endocrinol 1997; 154:397–406.

229. Manelli I, Giustina I. Glucocorticoid-induced osteoporosis. Trends Endocrinol Metab 2000; 11:79–85.

230. Jux C, Leiber K, Hugel U, et al. Dexamethasone impairs growth hormone (GH)-stimulated growth by suppression of local insulin-like growth factor (IGF)-I production and expression of GH- and IGF-I-receptor in cultured rat chondrocytes. Endocrinology 1998; 139:3296–3305.

231. Herndon DN, Zeigler ST. Bacterial translocation after thermal injury. Crit Care Med 1993; 21:S50–S54.

232. Colic M, Mitrovic S, Dujic A. Thymic response to thermal injury in mice: I. Alterations of thymocyte subsets studied by flow cytometry and immunohistochemistry. Burns 1989; 15:155–161.

233. Nakanishi T, Nishi Y, Sato EF, et al. Thermal injury induces thymocyte apoptosis in the rat. J Trauma 1998; 44:143–148.

234. Maldonado MD, Venturoli A, Franco A, et al. Specific changes in peripheral blood lymphocyte phenotype from burn patients. Probable origin of the thermal injury-related lymphocytopenia. Burns 1991; 17:188–192.

235. Organ BC, Antonacci AC, Chiao J, et al. Changes in lymphocyte number and phenotype in seven lymphoid compartments after thermal injury. Ann Surg 1989; 210:78–89.

236. Selye H. Thymus and adrenals in the response of organism to injuries and intoxications. Br J Exp Pathol 1936; 17.

237. Blomgren H, Andersson B. Characteristics of the immunocompetent cells in the mouse thymus: cell population changes during cortisone-induced atrophy and subsequent regeneration. Cell Immunol 1970; 1:545–560.

238. Cowan WK, Sorenson DG. Electron microscopic observations of acute thymic involution produced by hydrocortisone. Lab Invest 1964; 13:353–370.

239. Gillis S, Crabtree GR, Smith KA. Glucocorticoid-induced inhibition of T cell growth factor production. I. The effect on mitogen-induced lymphocyte proliferation. J Immunol 1979; 123:1624–1631.

240. Taniguchi T. Regulation of cytokine gene expression. Annu Rev Immunol 1988; 6:439–464.

241. Tolentino MV, Sarasua MM, Hill OA, et al. Peripheral lymphocyte membrane fluidity after thermal injury. J Burn Care Rehabil 1991; 12:498–504.

242. Dale DC, Fauci AS, Wolff SM. Alternate-day prednisone. Leukocyte kinetics and susceptibility to infections. N Engl J Med 1974; 291:1154–1158.

243. Rinehart JJ, Balcerzak SP, Sagone AL, et al. Effects of corticosteroids on human monocyte function. J Clin Invest 1974; 54:1337–1343.

244. Ward PA. The chemosuppression of chemotaxis. J Exp Med 1966; 124:209–226.

245. MacGregor RR, Spagnuolo PJ, Lentnek AL. Inhibition of granulocyte adherence by ethanol, prednisone, and aspirin, measured with an assay system. N Engl J Med 1974; 291:642–646.

246. Mandell GL, Rubin W, Hook EW. The effect of an NADH oxidase inhibitor (hydrocortisone) on polymorphonuclear leukocyte bactericidal activity. J Clin Invest 1970; 49:1381–1388.

247. Hibbs JB Jr. Heterocytolysis by macrophages activated by bacillus Calmette-Guerin: lysosome exocytosis into tumor cells. Science 1974; 184:468–471.

248. Arturson G, Hogman CF, Johansson SG, et al. Changes in immunoglobulin levels in severely burned patients. Lancet 1969; 1:546–548.

249. Bjornson AB, Altemeier WA, Bjornson HS. Changes in humoral components of host defense following burn trauma. Ann Surg 1977; 186:88–96.

250. Kagan RJ, Bratescu A, Jonasson O, et al. The relationship between the percentage of circulating B cells, corticosteroid levels, and other immunologic parameters in thermally injured patients. J Trauma 1989; 29:208–213.

251. Kawakami M, Meyer AA, deSerres S, et al. Effects of acute ethanol ingestion and burn injury on serum immunoglobulin. J Burn Care Rehabil 1990; 11:395–399.

252. Kohn J, Cort DF. Immunoglobulins in burned patients. Lancet 1969; 1:836–837.

253. Munster AM, Hoagland HC, Pruitt BA Jr. The effect of thermal injury on serum immunoglobulins. Ann Surg 1970; 172:965–969.

254. Kawakami M, deSerres S, Meyer AA. Immunoglobulin synthesis by cultured lymphocytes from spleen and mesenteric lymph nodes after thermal injury. J Burn Care Rehabil 1991; 12:474–481.

255. Sakai H, Daniels JC, Beathard GA, et al. Mixed lymphocyte culture reaction in patients with acute thermal burns. J Trauma 1974; 14:53–57.

256. Butler WT, Rossen RD. Effects of corticosteroids on immunity in man. I. Decreased serum IgG concentration caused by 3 or 5 days of high doses of methylprednisolone. J Clin Invest 1973; 52:2629–2640.

257. Araneo BA, Shelby J, Li GZ, et al. Administration of dehydroepiandrosterone to burned mice preserves normal immunologic competence. Arch Surg 1993; 128:318–325.

258. Blauer KL, Poth M, Rogers WM, et al. Dehydroepiandrosterone antagonizes the suppressive effects of dexamethasone on lymphocyte proliferation. Endocrinology 1991; 129:3174–3179.

259. Daynes RA, Meikle AW, Araneo BA. Locally active steroid hormones may facilitate compartmentalization of immunity by regulating the types of lymphokines produced by helper T cells. Res Immunol 1991; 142:40–45.

260. Suzuki T, Suzuki N, Daynes RA, et al. Dehydroepiandrosterone enhances IL2 production and cytotoxic effector function of human T cells. Clin Immunol Immunopathol 1991; 61:202–211.

261. Devins SS, Miller A, Herndon BL, et al. Effects of dopamine on T-lymphocyte proliferative responses and serum prolactin concentrations in critically ill patients. Crit Care Med 1992; 20:1644–1649.

262. Van den Berghe G, de Zegher F, Wouters P, et al. Dehydroepiandrosterone sulphate in critical illness: effect of dopamine. Clin Endocrinol (Oxf) 1995; 43:457–463.

263. Higuchi K, Nawata H, Maki T, et al. Prolactin has a direct effect on adrenal androgen secretion. J Clin Endocrinol Metab 1984; 59:714–718.

264. Van Loon GR, Schwartz L, Sole MJ. Plasma dopamine responses to standing and exercise in man. Life Sci 1979; 24: 2273–2277.

265. Viquerat CE, Daly P, Swedberg K, et al. Endogenous catecholamine levels in chronic heart failure. Relation to the severity of hemodynamic abnormalities. Am J Med 1985; 78:455–460.

266. Wang XM, Yang L, Chen KM. Catecholamines: important factors in the increase of oxidative phosphorylation coupling in rat-liver mitochondria during the early phase of burn injury. Burns 1993; 19:110–112.

267. Durkot MJ, Wolfe RR. Effects of adrenergic blockade on glucose kinetics in septic and burned guinea pigs. Am J Physiol 1981; 241: R222–R227.

268. Wilmore DW, Aulick LH, Mason AD, et al. Influence of the burn wound on local and systemic responses to injury. Ann Surg 1977; 186:444–458.

269. Bessey PQ, Watters JM, Aoki TT, et al. Combined hormonal infusion simulates the metabolic response to injury. Ann Surg 1984; 200:264–281.

270. Batstone GF, Levick PL, Spurr E, et al. Changes in acute phase reactants and disturbances in metabolism after burn injury. Burns Incl Therm Inj 1983; 9:234–239.

271. Batstone GF, Alberti KGMM, Hinks L, et al. Metabolic studies in subects following thermal injury. Burns 1976; 2:207–225.

272. Sevaljevic L, Petrovic M, Bogojevic D, et al. Acute-phase response to scalding: changes in serum properties and acute- phase protein concentrations. Circ Shock 1989; 28:293–307.

273. Calvano SE, Albert JD, Legaspi A, et al. Comparison of numerical and phenotypic leukocyte changes during constant hydrocortisone infusion in normal humans with those in thermally injured patients. Surg Gynecol Obstet 1987; 164:509–520.

274. Webel ML, Ritts RE Jr, Taswell HF, et al. Cellular immunity after intravenous administration of methylprednisolone. J Lab Clin Med 1974; 83:383–392.

275. Wallner S, Vautrin R, Murphy J, et al. The haematopoietic response to burning: studies in an animal model. Burns Incl Therm Inj 1984; 10:236–251.

276. Rinehart JJ, Sagone AL, Balcerzak SP, et al. Effects of corticosteroid therapy on human monocyte function. N Engl J Med 1975; 292:236–241.

Chapter 26

The hepatic response to a thermal injury

Marc G. Jeschke

Liver damage and morphological changes

After a thermal injury a variable degree of liver injury is present, and it is usually related to the severity of the thermal injury. Fatty changes, a very common finding, are per se reversible and their significance depends on the cause and severity of accumulation (Figure 26.1a–e).[5] However, autopsies of burned children have shown that fatty liver infiltration was associated with increased bacterial translocation, liver failure and endotoxemia and thus delineating the crucial role of the liver during the postburn response (unpublished observations).

In a recent study in 102 children, 41 females and 61 males with a total body burn size of $58 \pm 2\%$, third-degree burn was $45 \pm 2\%$, we found that liver size and weight significantly increased during the first week postburn ($+85 \pm 5\%$), peeked at 2 weeks post burn ($+126 \pm 19\%$), and was at discharge increased by $+89 \pm 10\%$, $p < 0.05$. At 6, 9 and 12 months liver weight was increased by 40–50% compared to predicted liver weight. In addition liver protein synthesis was impaired over a 6-month period with a shift from constitutive hepatic proteins to acute phase proteins.[6] Liver enzymes were significantly elevated over the first 3 weeks postburn, normalizing over time. However, in a larger clinical trial we found that the hepatic acute phase response is not limited to a short period of time. In contrast, we found that the synthesis of constitutive hepatic proteins was decreased over a period of 8 weeks, while acute phase proteins were increased during the same time period, indicating the perseverance of the hepatic acute phase response.

Immediately after burn the damage of the liver may be associated with an increased hepatic edema formation. We have shown that the liver weight and liver/body-weight significantly increased 2–7 days after burn when compared to controls. As hepatic protein concentration was significantly decreased in burned rats we suggest that the liver weight gain is due to increased edema formation rather than increases in the number of hepatocytes or protein levels. An increase in edema formation may lead to cell damage, with the release of the hepatic enzymes (Table 26.1).[7]

Liver function tests and diagnostic tools

The so-called liver function tests evaluate liver activity by assessing the degree of functional impairment. They do not provide a pathological diagnosis and the extreme functional reserve of the organ occasionally produces normal results in the face of significant lesions. Many of these tests do not measure a specific function of the liver, and other organ systems may be implicated. False-positive results for each of the tests are found in about 10% of hospital controls. False-negative tests also occur in about 10% of most tests.[1–5] Diagnostic tools are:

- Ultrasonography: diagnosis of morphological changes and blood flow (duplex).
- Computed tomography (CT scan): morphological lesions (with the use of vascular enhancement).
- Magnetic resonance imaging (MRI): vascular lesions or intrahepatic focal lesions.
- Scintigrams: dynamic measures.
- Angiography: vascular patterns for the diagnosis of morphological changes.
- Needle biopsy of the liver: pathological diagnosis.

Enzymes

The three enzymes that achieve abnormal serum levels in hepatic disease and have been studied widely are alkaline phosphatase, serum glutamic oxalacetic transaminase (SGOT), and serum glutamic pyruvic transaminase (SGPT). SGOT is present in the liver, myocardium, skeletal muscles, kidney and pancreas. Cellular damage in any of the above-mentioned tissues results in elevation of the serum level. In reference to the liver, the most marked increases accompany acute cellular damage regardless of cause, and extremely high levels are noted in patients with hepatitis. SGOT is only moderately increased in cirrhosis and biliary obstruction. SGPT is more particularly applicable to the evaluation of liver disease, since the hepatic content greatly exceeds myocardial concentration. Elevations accompany acute hepatocellular damage. Lactic acid dehydrogenase (LDH) levels may also be elevated. Serum alkaline phosphatase is found in many tissues, including the liver, bile ducts, intestines, bones, kidneys, placenta, and white blood cells, provides an elevation of the patency of the bile channels at all levels, intrahepatic and extrahepatic. Elevation is demonstrated in 94% of patients with obstruction of the

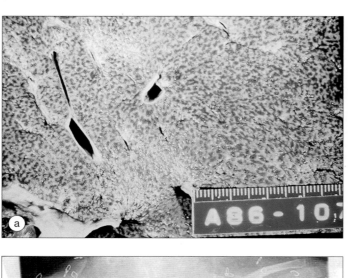

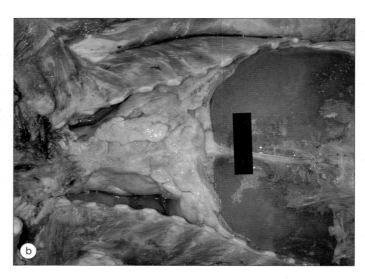

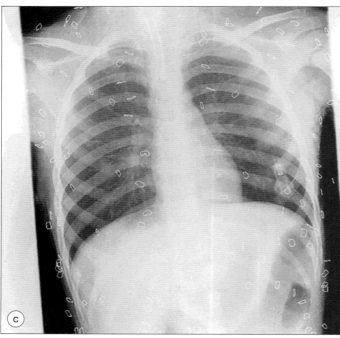

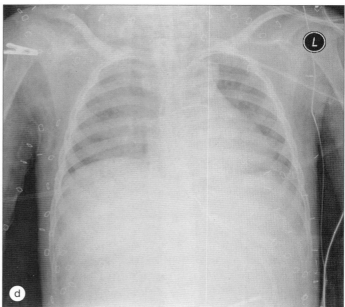

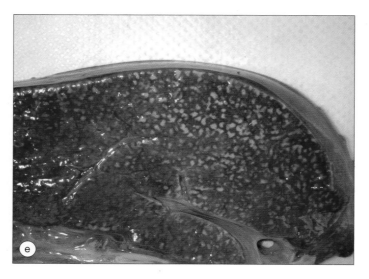

Fig. 26.1 (a) Histological section of a fatty liver after thermal injury at autopsy. The liver appears to be yellow and enriched with fat. (b) Massive enlargement of the liver in burn patient with greater than 90% TBSA. Liver was 2.68 × expected at autopsy. (c) Admission chest radiograph shows normal lung expansion. (d) Chest radiograph 2 days prior to death shows loss of thoracic domain. (e) At autopsy, liver is enlarged with central lobular necrosis.

TABLE 26.1 LIVER WEIGHT, LIVER WEIGHT/100 g BODY WEIGHT, AND LIVER PROTEIN CONTENT FOR CONTROL AND BURNED RATS

	Control days postburn				Burn days postburn			
	1 (n = 5)	2 (n = 5)	5 (n = 5)	7 (n = 5)	1 (n = 14)	2 (n = 14)	5 (n = 14)	7 (n = 14)
Liver weight (g)	13.0 ± 0.9	12.4 ± 0.8	13.2 ± 0.3	13.1 ± 0.4	13.1 ± 0.5	15.3 ± 0.7*	13.6 ± 0.4	13.6 ± 0.5
Liver weight/body weight (%)	3.4 ± 0.1	3.4 ± 0.3	3.8 ± 0.2	3.9 ± 0.2	3.5 ± 0.1	4.1 ± 0.1*	3.6 ± 0.1	3.7 ± 0.1
Liver protein content (mg/mL)	0.98 ± 0.01	0.97 ± 0.01	1.04 ± 0.02	1.0 ± 0.01	0.88 ± 0.02*	0.90 ± 0.02*	0.92 ± 0.01*	0.88 ± 0.01*

Data presented as means ± SEM. *Significant difference vs. control at corresponding day, $p < 0.05$.

extrahepatic biliary tract due to neoplasm and 76% of those in whom the obstruction is caused by calculi. Intrahepatic biliary obstruction and cholestasis also cause a rise in the enzyme level. In the presence of space-occupying lesions such as metastases, primary hepatic carcinoma, and abscesses, the alkaline phosphatase level (ALP) is also increased. The overall correlation between metastatic carcinoma of the liver and an elevated enzyme level is as high as 92%. Sixty percent of patients with primary hepatic carcinoma also demonstrate a significant increase. ALP is also elevated in several non-hepatic disease states, such as bone tumor, pregnancy, and growth.

Liver damage has been associated with increased hepatocyte cell death.[7] In general cell death occurs by two distinctly different mechanisms — programmed cell death (apoptosis) or necrosis.[8] Apoptosis is characterized by cell shrinkage, DNA fragmentation, membrane blebbing, and phagocytosis of the apoptotic cell fragments by neighboring cells or extrusion into the lumen of the bowel without inflammation. This is in contrast to necrosis, which involves cellular swelling, random DNA fragmentation, lysosomal activation, membrane breakdown and extrusion of cellular contents into the interstitium. Membrane breakdown and cellular content release induce inflammation with the migration of inflammatory cells and release of pro-inflammatory cytokines and free radicals, which leads to further tissue breakdown. Pathological studies found that about 10–15% of thermally injured patients have liver necrosis at autopsy.[9,10] The necrosis is generally focal or zonal, central or paracentral, sometimes microfocal, and related to burn shock and sepsis. The morphological differences between apoptosis and necrosis are used to differentiate the two processes.

A cutaneous thermal injury induces liver cell apoptosis.[7] This increase in hepatic programmed cell death is compensated by an increase in hepatic cell proliferation, suggesting that the liver attempts to maintain homeostasis (Figure 26.2). Despite the attempt to compensate increased apoptosis by increased hepatocyte proliferation the liver cannot regain hepatic mass and protein concentration (we found a significant decrease in hepatic protein concentration in burned rats). It has been shown that a cutaneous burn induces small bowel epithelial cell apoptosis.[11] In the same study the authors showed that small bowel epithelial cell proliferation was not increased, leading to a loss of mucosal cells and hence mucosal mass.[11] Similar findings were demonstrated in the heart.[12] Burn

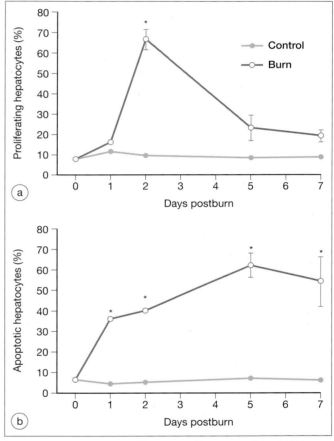

Fig. 26.2 (a) Percent of proliferating cells measured by PCNA. *Significant difference between burn vs. control, $p < 0.05$. Data presented as means ± SEM. (Burned animals $n = 7$ and controls $n = 2$ per time point). (b) Apoptotic cells measured by TUNEL assay 1, 2, 5 and 7 days after burn expressed as positive apoptotic hepatocytes per 1000 hepatocytes. Burned rats had significantly higher rates of hepatocyte apoptosis when compared to controls. Data presented as means ± SEM. (Burned animals $n = 7$ and controls $n = 2$ per time point.) *Significant difference between burn and control, $p < 0.05$.

induced cardiocyte apoptosis; however, cardiocyte proliferation remained unchanged, causing cardiac impairment and dysfunction.[12]

The mechanisms whereby a cutaneous burn induces programmed cell death in hepatocytes are not defined. Studies suggested that in general hypoperfusion and ischemia-reperfusion are associated to promote apoptosis.[13-15] After a thermal injury it has been shown that the blood flow to the bowel decreases by nearly 60% of baseline and stays decreased for approximately 4 hours.[16] It can be surmised that the hepatic blood flow also decreases, thus causing programmed cell death. In addition pro-inflammatory cytokines such as IL-1 and TNF-α have been described to be an apoptotic signal.[17,18] We have shown in our burn model that after a thermal injury serum and hepatic concentration of pro-inflammatory cytokines such as IL-1α/β, IL-6 and TNF-α are increased.[19] We therefore suggest that two possible mechanisms are involved in increased hepatocyte apoptosis: decreased splanchnic blood flow and elevation of pro-inflammatory cytokines, initiating intracellular signaling mechanisms. Signals that may be involved encompass many signals that play an important role during the acute phase response (see below).

Therapeutic possibilities could be the administration of anabolic growth factors, such as GH, IGF-I or HGF, which all have been shown to be anti-apoptotic.[19-22] In exerting an anti-apoptotic effect these growth factors could improve hepatic morphology, function, and thus homeostasis after a thermal injury.

Biliary formation

Bile secretion is an active process, relatively independent of total liver blood flow, except in conditions of shock. Bile is formed at two sites:

- the canalicular membrane of the hepatocyte, and
- the bile ductules or ducts.

Total unstimulated bile flow in a 70 kg man has been estimated as 0.41–0.43 mL/min. Eighty percent of the total daily production of bile (approximately 1500 mL) is secreted by hepatocytes and 20% is secreted by the bile duct epithelial cells. The principal organic compounds in bile are the conjugated bile acids, cholesterol, phospholipid and protein. As bile passes through the biliary ductules or ducts it is modified by secretion or absorption of epithelial cells. The highest cells in the biliary ductules have functions and architecture in common with both hepatocytes and ductular cells, and are called cholangiocytes. The best characterized hormone to stimulate bile secretion is secretin. The bile is then being secreted into the gallbladder, whose only function is to concentrate and store bile during fasting. Approximately 90% of the water in gallbladder bile is absorbed in 4 hours. Cholecystokinin appears to be the principal physiological stimulator of gallbladder concentration. Cholinergic stimulation causes contraction of the gallbladder and relaxation of the sphincter of Oddi, which means that bile is secreted into the intestine. Most of the bile salt is being absorbed into the enterohepatic circulation. The liver extracts the bile acids and transports them back to the canalicular membrane where they are resecreted back into the biliary system. Total bile pool size in humans is 2–5 grams and undergoes this circulation 2–3 times per meal and 6–10 times a day, depending on the dietary habit. In addition, 0.2–0.6 grams are lost in the stool per day, and this quantity is replaced by newly synthesized bile acids.[3]

Bilirubin is a breakdown product of heme and is almost completely excreted in the bile. With hepatocellular disease or extrahepatic biliary obstruction, free bilirubin may accumulate in blood and tissues. Approximately 75% of bilirubin is derived from senescent red blood cells. Bilirubin circulates bound to albumin, which protects tissue from its toxicity. It is rapidly removed from the plasma by the liver through a carrier transport system. In the hepatocyte, bilirubin is conjugated with glucuronide and secreted in bile. Conjugated bilirubin may form a covalent bond with albumin, so called delta bilirubin. In the intestine, bilirubin is reduced by bacteria to mesobilirubin and stercobilirubin, collectively termed urobilinogen. These are both excreted in the stool. A part of urobilinogen is oxidized to urobilin, which is a brown pigment and gives stool its normal color.

In trauma and sepsis intrahepatic cholestasis occurs frequently and appears to be an important pathophysiological factor without demonstrable extrahepatic obstruction. This phenomenon has been described in association with a number of processes, such as hypoxia, drug toxicity, or total parenteral nutrition.[23] The mechanisms of intrahepatic cholestasis seem to be associated with an impairment of basolateral and canicular hepatocyte transport of bile acids and organic anions.[24] This is most likely due to decreased transporter protein and RNA expression, thus leading to increased bile. Intrahepatic cholestasis, which is one of the prime manifestations of hepatocellular injury, was present in 26% in one clinical study.[10] All of these were concurrent with sepsis. The cellular damage observed in sepsis is most likely the result of decreased hepatic blood flow than direct cellular damage.[25]

Energy, carbohydrate, insulin, and lipid metabolism

(See Chapter Metabolic responses to burn injury.)

Most of the body's metabolic needs are regulated in some ways by the liver. The liver expends approximately 20% of the body's energy and consumes 20–25% of the total utilized oxygen, which is due to the remarkable hepatic architecture and the blood supply. The hepatocellular organelles in plasma membranes permit specific functions and, at the same time, interrelate with an extracellular matrix, which facilitates metabolic exchange between blood and hepatocytes.[2] The liver does not only conduct a large number of functions but also manufactures many substances, which serve other organs or tissues. The liver collects such substrates to meet the fuel requirements of other tissues in response to multiple metabolic signals. It is the only organ producing acetoacetate for use by muscle, brain, and kidney, but not itself. The energy-related functions of the liver are regulated by hormones, other agonists and substrates coming to and from the liver.

The liver has a central role in energy metabolism: it supports as a glucose source energy requirements of the central nervous system and red blood cells. During the fed state, results of intestinal carbohydrates digestion, glucose (80%), galactose and fructose (20%), are delivered to the liver. The latter two are rapidly converted into glucose. Glucose absorbed by the hepatocyte is converted directly into glycogen for storage up to a maximum 65 grams of glycogen per kilogram of liver mass. Excess glucose is converted to fat. Glycogen is also produced by muscle, but this is not available for use by any other tissues. During the fasting state, this glycogen is the primary source of glucose. However, after 48 hours of fasting, liver glycogen is exhausted, and proteins mobilized primarily from muscle, mainly alanine, are converted by the liver to glucose.

Lactate, by anaerobic metabolism, is metabolized only in the liver. Ordinarily it is converted to pyruvate and subsequently back into glucose. This shuttling of glucose and lactate between liver and peripheral tissue is carried out in the Cori cycle. The brain does not participate in the cycle and a continuous source of glucose for the brain must come at the expense of muscle proteins.

In liver disease the metabolism of glucose is often deranged. Frequently, in patients with cirrhosis the portal-systemic shunting causes decreased exposure of portal blood to the hepatocytes, producing an abnormal result of the oral glucose tolerance test (OGTT). Hypoglycemia is rare in chronic liver disease since the synthetic capacity of hepatocytes is preserved until late in the disorder. In fulminate hepatic failure, however, there is extensive loss of hepatocyte mass and function, and hypoglycemia supervenes as gluconeogenesis fails.

Glycogenesis, glycogen storage, glycogenolysis, and the conversion of galactose into glucose all represent hepatic functions. Hypoglycemia is a rare accompaniment of extensive hepatic disease, but the amelioration of diabetes in patients with hemochromatosis is considered an indication of neoplastic change. The more common effect of hepatic disease is the deficiency of glycogenesis of resulting hyperglycemia. An hepatic enzyme system is responsible for the conversion of galactose into glucose, and abnormal galactose tolerance tests are seen in hepatitis and active cirrhosis. In rare instances a familial deficiency in this enzyme system accounts for spontaneous galactosemia accompanied by an obstructive type of jaundice that appears after the first week of life and subsides when lactose is removed from the diet.

There are three sources of free fatty acids available to the liver: fat absorbed from the gut, fat liberated from adipocytes in response to lipolysis, and fatty acids synthesized from carbohydrates and amino acids. These fatty acids are etherified with glycerol to form triglyceride. The export of triglycerides is dependent on the synthesis of very low density lipoproteins. In cases of excess supply of fatty acid, there is lipid accumulation in the liver because there is an imbalance of triglyceride relative to very low density lipoproteins. This is seen in obesity, corticosteroid use, pregnancy, diabetes and total parenteral nutrition. Simple protein malnutrition or protein-calories imbalance may also result in fatty change of liver, based on decreased export of triglycerides, because of limited supply of precursors for hepatic synthesis of lipoproteins.

Synthesis of both the phospholipid and cholesterol takes place in the liver, and the latter serves as a standard for the determination of lipid metabolism. The liver is the major organ involved in the synthesis, esterification, and excretion of cholesterol. In the presence of parenchymal damage, both the total cholesterol and the percentage of esterified fraction decreases. The biliary obstruction results in the rise in cholesterol, and the most pronounced elevations are noted in the primary biliary cirrhosis and the cholangiolitis accompanying toxic reactions to the phenothiazine derivatives.[3,4]

Vitamin metabolism

The liver has many important roles of uptake, storage, and mobilization of vitamins. Most important are the fat-soluble vitamins A, E, D, and K. The absorption of these is dependent on bile salts. The vitamins appear in the thoracic duct 2–6 hours after oral administration. Vitamin A is exclusively stored in the liver, and excess ingestion of vitamin A may be associated with significant liver injury. A role for storage of vitamin A in the Ito cells has been suggested. The initial step in vitamin D activation occurs in the liver where vitamin D_3 is converted 25-hydroxycholecalciferol.

Of particular surgical significance was the discovery of vitamin K. This vitamin is essential for the gamma-carboxylation of the vitamin K-dependent coagulation factors II, VII, IX and X. These factors are inactive without gamma-carboxylation.[3,4] Vitamins play an important role in wound healing, energy, metabolism, inflammation and antioxidants. Postburn hypermetabolism causes a vitamin deficiency requiring substitution.[26]

- There are decreased vitamin A levels in burn patients. This is maybe due to a reduction of retinol binding protein (RBP, see proteins section), which is a vitamin A transporter. Vitamin A has been shown to enhance wound healing; thus its substitution is important for dermal wound repair.
- Vitamin E encompasses antioxidant properties and in animal experiments its administration has been shown to reduce lung injury. After a thermal injury its concentration is decreased; thus its substitution is suggested.
- Vitamin D, with its crucial function in the ossear cascade, is also decreased after burn injury; however, its substitution has not been proven.
- Thiamin and riboflavin are vitamins that affect energy and protein metabolism and wound healing. Both factors are decreased after trauma. Thiamin serves as a co-factor in the Krebs cycle and for the oxidation of glucose; thus its need is related to the energy intake. Thiamin is further necessary for the lysyl oxidase function to form collagen. Riboflavin is involved as a co-enzyme in oxidation–reduction reactions. Riboflavin is decreased after burn and an increased need for burn victims has been shown.[26]
- Folic acid is depleted after a burn and can lead to impaired synthesis of DNA and RNA. Inadequate supplies of vitamin B_{12} and the indispensable amino acid methionine, impair folate utilization. Thus, a deficiency of either of these nutrients can produce signs of folate deficiency.
- Vitamin B complex with B_6 and B_{12} serve as co-enzymes in the energy and protein metabolic process. Vitamin B_6 is involved in amino acid metabolism, vitamin B_{12} in the catabolism of odd-chain long fatty acids. Both should be substituted in the form of a multi-vitamin complex, as both are decreased in the postburn hypermetabolic response.
- Vitamin C plays an important role during the postburn hypermetabolic response. During that period oxygen free radicals, such as superoxide, peroxide and hydroxyl, may cause increased postburn vascular permeability. Vitamin C administration, a free radical scavenger, has thus been suggested to be beneficial in terms of reducing microvascular permeability and thus required fluid volume. In recent studies vitamin C has been described to enhance wound healing in skin, bones and other tissues.

Table 26.2 gives a therapeutic guideline for vitamin substitution according to our institute.[27]

Coagulation and clotting factors

The liver produces multiple coagulation factors, which can be altered or are defective in the state of liver disease. In the state of jaundice vitamin K resorption is decreased, resulting in a decreased synthesis of prothrombin, or when the liver is severely damaged, in the state of hepatocellular dysfunction prothrombin is not synthesized at all. The diagnosis of pathological prothrombin synthesis is made by the prothrombin time. Decreases in factors V, VII, IX and fibrinogen also have been noted in hepatic disease.[4] Homeostasis of clotting is complex and has been recently investigated in thermally injured patients.[27] Thrombotic and fibrinolytic mechanisms are activated after burn and the extent of activation increases with the severity of the thermal injury. Most homeostatic markers fall during the early shock phase of burns due to dilutional effects, loss and degradation of plasma proteins. Clotting factors return to normal levels after the aggressive resuscitation period. Later in the postburn course, thrombogenicity has been suggested as being increased due to a decrease in antithrombin III, protein C, and protein S levels, while fibrinolysis activation occurs via increases in tissue plasminogen activation factor, thus leading to an increased risk of thrombosis. The hypercoagulable state places many thermally injured patients at risk for disseminated intravascular coagulation (DIC). DIC has been described postmortem in 30% of the examined cases. At our institute, heparin is administered as a prophylaxis for deep venous thrombosis and thus for the onset of DIC (Fraxiparine 0.5 mL s.c.). If needed, fresh frozen plasma is therapeutically administered to improve coagulation.

Hepatic acute phase response

Proteins

The acute phase response is a cascade of events initiated to prevent tissue damage and to activate repair processes; the release of pro-inflammatory cytokines by phagocytic cells, fibroblasts, and endothelial cells leads to the systemic phase of the acute phase response. The systemic reaction affects:

- the hypothalamus — which leads to fever,
- the pituitary–adrenal axis — which leads to the release of steroid hormones,
- the liver — which causes the synthesis and secretion of acute phase proteins,
- the bone marrow — which promulgates further hematopoietic responses, and
- the immune system — which allows the activation of the reticuloendothelial system and the stimulation of lymphocytes.

However, a crucial step in this cascade of reactions involves the interaction between the site of injury and the liver, which is the principal organ responsible for producing acute phase proteins and modulating the systemic inflammatory response.

After major trauma, such as a severe burn, hepatic protein synthesis shifts from hepatic constitutive proteins, such as albumin, pre-albumin, transferrin, and retinol-binding protein, to acute phase proteins.[1–5,7] Acute phase proteins are divided into type I acute phase proteins, such as haptoglobin and α_1-acid glycoprotein, mediated by IL-1-like cytokines (IL-1α/β, TNF-α/β) and type II acute phase proteins, such as α_2-macroglobulin and fibrinogen, which are mediated by IL-6-like cytokines (IL-6, IL-11).[7] The up-regulation of acute phase proteins represents a redirection of the liver in order to fulfill immune functions, coagulation and wound healing processes (Figures 26.3 and 26.4).[2,3,8,9]

In contrast to acute phase proteins, constitutive hepatic proteins are down-regulated.[28–32] After a thermal injury, albumin and transferrin decrease by 50–70% below normal levels.[29–32] Studies have shown that two mechanisms are responsible for the decrease of constitutive hepatic proteins:

- the liver re-prioritizes its protein synthesis from constitutive hepatic proteins to acute phase proteins. This could be shown in many studies in which the mRNA synthesis for constitutive hepatic proteins is decreased.
- the other mechanism for decreased constitutive hepatic protein concentration is the capillary leakage and the

Vitamins and minerals	0–2 years	2–12 years	> 12 years
Multivitamin	Poly Vi Sol 1 mL	Poly Vi Sol 1 mL	Vi Deylin 5 mL or Theragran
Ascorbic acid	250 mg QD	250 mg QD	500 mg QD
Folic acid	1 mg QMWF	1 mg QMWF	1 mg QMWF
Vitamin A	2500 U	5000 U	10 000 U
Vitamin E	5 mg	5 mg	10 mg
Zinc sulfate	55 mg	110 mg	220 mg
Elemental iron	<30 kg dose = 2 mg/kg/dose PO TID >30 kg dose = 65 mg PO TID or FeSO$_4$ 325 mg PO TID		

TABLE 26.2 MEDICATION GUIDELINE FOR VITAMIN AND MINERAL SUPPLEMENTATION[26]

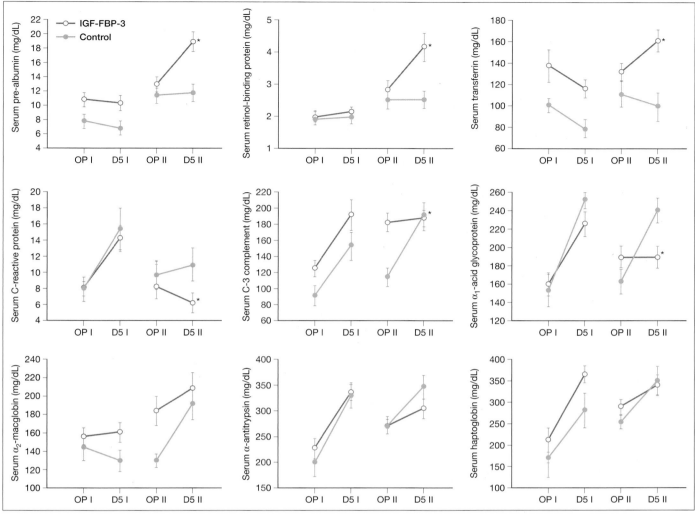

Fig. 26.3 Serum constitutive hepatic proteins (upper line), type I acute phase proteins (middle line), and type II acute phase proteins after thermal injury. The figures depict a clinical study in which the complex IGF-I/BP-3 was determined. All pediatric patients received after saline (control) from OP I to D 5 I. After this first control period patients received either IGF-I/BP-3 or saline OP II to D 5 II. Upper line: all constitutive hepatic proteins were decreased after burn (period I and II). IGF-I/BP-3 increased constitutive hepatic proteins during the second study period, as saline did not. Normal levels: pre-albumin: 25–45 mg/dL, retinol-binding protein: 3–6 m/dL, transferrin: 203–430 mg/dL. Middle line: all type I acute phase proteins are increased after thermal injury during the control and the study period. IGF-I/BP-3 decreased type I acute phase proteins when compared to controls. Normal levels: C-reactive protein: <5 mg/dL, C-3 complement: 50–90 mg/dL, α_1-acid glycoprotein: 55–140 mg/dL. Lower line: type II acute phase proteins are also increased after burn and stay elevated. IGF-I/BP-3 had no effect on type II acute phase proteins when compared with controls. Normal levels: α_2-macroglobulin: 100–150 mg/dL, α-antitrypsin: 150–250 mg/dL, haptoglobin: 50–300 mg/dL. Values are presented as means ± SEM. *Significant between IGF-I/BP-3 vs. controls, $p < 0.05$.

loss of these proteins into the massive extravascular space and burn wound.

Albumin and transferrin, however, have important physiological functions as they serve as transporter proteins and contribute to osmotic pressure and plasma pH.[29,30] Their down-regulation after trauma has been described as potentially harmful and the synthesis of these proteins has been used as a predictor of mortality, nutritional status, and severity of stress and as an indicator of improved recovery.[30,33–35] As albumin could be drastically decreased after burn injury we administered human albumin to maintain albumin levels at 2.5 mg/dL at our institute. Other studies discussed albumin substitution controversially and suggested not to substitute albumin.

The therapeutic guideline at our institute is: serum albumin is measured daily at 4:30 a.m. If serum albumin concentrations are less than 2.0 g/dL, albumin is supplemented based upon age and body weight to maintain colloid osmotic pressure at 2.0 g/dL. Children <2 years of age and <20 kg body weight receive 6.25 g/day exogenous albumin over 6 hours, children 2–9 years old weighing >20 kg but <40 kg receive 12.5 g/day over 6 hours, and children 10–18 years old weighing >40 kg receive 25 g/day. Total albumin infused, albumin infused per day and grams of albumin infused per meter square burn are recorded.

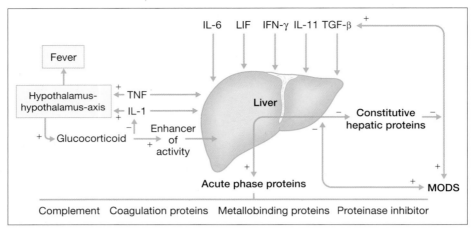

Fig. 26.4 Signal cascade of the hepatic acute phase response. Type I acute phase proteins, such as haptoglobin and α_1-acid glycoprotein, are mediated by IL-1-like cytokines (IL-1α/β, TNF-α/β) and type II acute phase proteins, such as α_2-macroglobulin and fibrinogen, are mediated by IL-6-like cytokines (IL-6, IL-11). In several studies the biphasic time course of pro-inflammatory cytokines has been demonstrated. Immediately after burn IL-1, IL-6, IL-8 and TNF-α increase 2- to 10-fold above normal levels, decrease slightly after approximately 12 hours, increase again, and then start to decrease. Cytokines bind to their receptors, activate intracellular signals by tyrosine phosphorylation, for the type I acute phase response c-jun/c-fos, hepatic nuclear factor-kappa B (NF-κB) or the CCAAT/enhancer-binding-proteins (C/EBPs). The intracellular signal cascade for type II has been shown to be a tyrosine phosphorylation and activation of intracellular tyrosine kinases (JAKs), latent cytoplasmic transcription factors, STAT1, STAT3, and STAT5 (signal transducer and activator of transcription), or mitogen-activated protein (MAP). These signals activate transcription, translation and expression of acute phase proteins. Particularly, IL-6 has been speculated to be the main mediating cytokine. IL-6 activates glycoprotein 130 (gp 130) and the JAK kinases (JAK-1) leading to activation of STAT 1 and 3 translocating to the nucleus. Intranuclear, the genes for acute phase proteins are turned on.

Mediators of the acute phase response

Mediators of the acute phase response are cytokines. Type I acute phase proteins, such as haptoglobin and α_1-acid glycoprotein, are mediated by IL-1-like cytokines (IL-1α/β, TNF-α/β) and type II acute phase proteins, such as α_2-macroglobulin and fibrinogen, are mediated by IL-6-like cytokines (IL-6, IL-11).[28] In several studies the biphasic time course of pro-inflammatory cytokines has been demonstrated. Immediately after burn IL-1, IL-6, IL-8 and TNFα increase 2- to 10-fold above normal levels, decrease slightly after approximately 12 hours, increase again, and then start to decrease. Animal and human studies demonstrated that cytokines can either approach normal levels within 2 days after trauma or can be elevated up to 2 weeks after thermal injury. Cytokine elevation has been shown to be dependent upon the extent of the burn and concomitant injuries.

The signal cascade of cytokines is the following: the cytokines bind to their receptors, activate intracellular signals by tyrosine phosphorylation, for the type I acute phase response c-jun/c-fos, hepatic nuclear factor-kappa B (NF-κB) or the CCAAT/enhancer-binding-proteins (C/EBPs).[35–47] The intracellular signal cascade for type II has been shown to be a tyrosine phosphorylation and activation of intracellular tyrosine kinases (JAKs), latent cytoplasmic transcription factors, STAT1, STAT3, and STAT5 (signal transducer and activator of transcription), or mitogen-activated protein (MAP).[28,36–48] These signals activate transcription, translation and expression of acute phase proteins. Particularly, IL-6 has been speculated to be the main mediating cytokine. IL-6 activates glycoprotein 130 (gp 130) and the JAK-kinases (JAK-1), leading to activation of STAT 1 and 3 translocating to the nucleus. Intranuclear, the genes for acute phase proteins are turned on (Figure 26.4).

The aim of the acute phase response is to protect the body from further damage, and the aim will be achieved when all elements of the acute phase response coalesce in a balanced fashion. However a prolonged increase in pro-inflammatory cytokines and acute phase proteins has been shown to be associated with a hypercatabolic state, increased risk of sepsis, multi-organ failure, morbidity and mortality.[33–35] Therefore, an important therapeutic approach to improve trauma mortality may be the modulation of the acute phase response by decreasing acute phase proteins and pro-inflammatory cytokines and increasing constitutive hepatic proteins.[33–36] The use of antibodies against pro-inflammatory cytokines such as tumor necrosis factor (TNF), interleukin-1β (IL-1β), or their receptors showed promising results *in vitro* and in animal models by increasing survival rates in the state of septicemia.[49–51] However, when these approaches entered clinical trials it became evident that these promising animal data couldn't be found in humans. A possible explanation that the anti-inflammatory agents used failed to control the exaggerated synthesis of pro-inflammatory cytokines may be because they focused on only one pathway or mediator in the inflammatory cascade, leading to a compensation through other pathways.[53–55] Another cause of the failure may have been that the anti-inflammatory cascade did not undergo intensive studies. It has not been until recently that investigations speculated about the importance of a balance between pro- and anti-inflammatory agents.[54,55] Two studies demonstrated that non-survivors with pancreatitis had decreased interleukin-6 (IL-6) to interleukin-10 (IL-10) ratios when compared with survivors.[54,55] The relevance of cytokine ratios in the pathogenesis and the prediction of trauma, sepsis and shock still need to be defined; however, individual effects have been investigated. A prolonged and increased inflammatory response contributes to multi organ failure and mortality.[33–35] The overexpression of pro-inflammatory cytokines, such as IL-1, IL-6 and TNF, inhibit the growth hormone–insulin-like growth factor-I (IGF-I) axis and increase the hypermetabolic response with resulting increases in morbidity and mortality.[56–58]

In contrast to pro-inflammatory cytokines, anti-inflammatory cytokines appear to have protective characteristics. Interleukin-2 (IL-2) and interferon-γ (IFN-γ) are signals in the TH-1 response and play a critical role in initiating and maintaining cellular immune responses, in the defense against intracellular pathogens.[59] Interleukin-4 (IL-4) and interleukin-10 (IL-10) are TH-2 cytokines, characterized by production of B-cell activating cytokines.[59] TH-2 responses enhance the production of antibodies, which are crucial for the humoral immune response, e.g. in preventing disseminated infections. Administration of IL-10 can protect against lethal doses of endotoxin in mice and decreases the release of endotoxin-induced IL-6 and IL-1.[34,60,61] Thus, IL-10 administration may ameliorate the endotoxemic shock and may improve survival. The effect of anti-inflammatory cytokines in burns still need to be defined.

Currently research focuses on new mediators and their modulation. Wang and Tracey showed that hypermobility-shift group protein-1 (HMG-1) is a late mediator responsible for lethality in the state of septicemia.[62] They suggest that blocking HMG-1 maybe a new approach to improve survival. Another group showed that macrophage inhibitory factor (MIF) plays a crucial role in the pro-inflammatory cascade and its attenuation may also improve survival after massive trauma.[63] Despite the research focusing on attenuating the pro-inflammatory acute phase response the optimal treatment for severely injured trauma patients needs to be defined. Our group has been studying the effect of growth factors, such as growth hormone (GH), hepatocyte growth factor (HGF), insulin-like growth factor-I (IGF-I), and insulin-like growth factor-I in combination with its principal binding protein-3 (IGF-I/BP-3), on the hepatic acute phase response and cytokine expression as a physiological approach to attenuate the pro-inflammatory cascade.[19–22]

Growth factors

Over the last years our group has investigated the effect of growth factors, such as growth hormone, hepatocyte growth factor, insulin-like growth factor-I, and insulin-like growth factor-I in combination with its principal binding protein-3 on the hepatic acute phase response. Our hypothesis was that physiological anabolic agents would improve constitutive hepatical protein synthesis and thus equilibrate the pro- to anti-inflammatory hepatic response. We have shown that the growth factors tested all had different effects on hepatic cytokine and protein synthesis.[19–22]

Recombinant human growth hormone (rhGH)

The effect of rhGH on the hepatic acute phase response has been tested in animal models and pediatric burn patients.[19,20,64] Data showed in burned children that GH modulated the acute phase response by decreasing both serum TNF-α and IL-1β. Decreases in serum TNF-α and IL-1β were associated with decreased type I acute phase proteins serum amyloid A (SAA) and C-reactive protein (CRP). rhGH did not affect IL-6 con-

centration and neither its dependent acute phase proteins haptoglobin, α₁-antitrypsin, or α₂-macroglobulin. The mechanisms by which rhGH modulates the acute phase response are not entirely defined; however, it has been demonstrated that rhGH binds to its cell surface receptor (GHR) and leads to tyrosine phosphorylation of CCAAT/enhancer-binding-proteins (C/EBPs), the AP-1 family of transcription factors, intracellular tyrosine kinases (JAKs), octamer-binding-proteins and STATs (signal transducer and activator of transcription).[42,44,48,63–69] These signal transcription factors translocate to the nucleus where they can interact with specific DNA sequences to modulate the gene expression of c-fos/c-jun and nuclear factor-kappa B (NF-κB), which regulate the expression of constitutive hepatic and acute phase proteins.[70,71] Interestingly, cytokines regulate constitutive hepatic and acute phase protein expression through a similar cascade.[28] IL-1-like cytokines bind to their receptors, leading to an activation/phosphorylation, which results in activation of cellular signals AP-1, NF-κB and C/EBPβ.[28] The stimulation of these signals leads to an activation of the transcription and translation of type I acute phase protein genes. Given the fact, that rhGH decreases IL-1-like cytokines, it is unknown whether rhGH decreases type I acute phase proteins through a direct down-regulation of AP-1, NF-κB or C/EBPβ, or through modulation of the IL-1-like cytokine expression which decrease these cellular signals and consecutively type I acute phase proteins.[44,70,71]

rhGH administration increased endogenous albumin levels, reducing the amount of required exogenous substitution to maintain normal serum albumin levels. Similar to acute phase proteins, the mechanisms by which rhGH increases endogenous albumin concentrations are unknown; however, rhGH might exert this effect through activation of C/EBPα.[44,73] C/EBPα is a trans-activator of liver specific genes such as albumin and its mRNA concentration decreases during trauma and stress and can be considered as a negative regulated acute phase gene.[42–44,73–75] Recently, C/EBPα mRNA levels, which are decreased after trauma, were shown to increase with rhGH.[44] Thus, a stimulation of the α isoform may consecutively lead to a stimulation of constitutive hepatic proteins, such as albumin and retinol-binding protein.[44]

Despite the advantages seen with rhGH administration Takala et al. reported increased mortalities in septic adult patients.[76] We have not found any evidence that rhGH increases mortality in pediatric burned patients; however, based on Takala et al.'s data, rhGH should not be given in septic patients or patients with multi organ failure (MOF). Another side effect of rhGH that has been recently delineated is an increase in hepatic triglyceride concentration and development of a fatty liver.[19,77] rhGH administration over 10 days increased hepatic triglyceride concentration by nearly 50% in burned rats[19] The mechanisms have been discussed in clinical studies, where the authors speculated that rhGH increased peripheral lipolysis and, due to a lack of transporter proteins (LDL, HDL), triglycerides accumulate in the liver.[77] We demonstrated in pediatric burn patients that rhGH increased free fatty acid concentration when compared to placebo, indicating that rhGH stimulates peripheral lipolysis and, subsequently, free fatty acid concentration.[64]

In summary, rhGH modulates the acute phase response by affecting pro-inflammatory IL-1-like cytokine expression followed by decreased type I acute phase proteins and increasing constitutive hepatic proteins. No effect on IL-6-like cytokines and type II acute phase proteins could be demonstrated. Given the fact that the acute phase response is a contributor to mortality after trauma, rhGH administration appears not to cause an increase in mortality in severely burned children as described by Takala et al. in trauma and septic patients as rhGH does not cause an increased and prolonged acute phase response.[76]

Hepatocyte growth factor

Hepatocyte growth factor (HGF) has been shown to accelerate hepatic regeneration and improve hepatic function in rats after trauma.[78] HGF and its receptor *c-met* (HGFR) are known to modulate the acute phase response in primary hepatocyte cultures.[79] HGF stimulates in vitro synthesis of constitutive hepatic proteins and decreases the synthesis of acute phase proteins.[79,80] Within 30–60 minutes of injury plasma HGF is elevated, presumably sending a strong mitogenic signal to the hepatocytes, which are already primed by interleukin-6 (IL-6), tumor necrosis factor-α (TNF-α), or insulin.[81] The cause of the increase in plasma HGF is currently unknown; however, it has been postulated to be due either to increased production of HGF in extrahepatic organs, such as lung, spleen, kidney, or gut, or to a decrease in hepatic HGF excretion.[81,82] The rapid increase in HGF stimulates hepatocyte mitogenesis, motogenesis, and DNA synthesis.[81] HGF administered to normal rats only stimulates a small number of hepatocytes to enter the DNA synthesis cycle, indicating that hepatocytes in normal livers are not ready to respond to mitogenic signals without the priming events that switch them into a responsive mode.[81]

We have shown that HGF administration stimulates constitutive hepatic proteins after burn injury in vivo.[21] In fact, serum transferrin reached normal levels 7 days after injury with HGF treatment, whereas in saline-treated animals serum transferrin remained low. Serum albumin levels decreased; however, beginning at day 2 after burn, HGF attenuated this drop in serum albumin. The exact mechanisms by which HGF stimulates constitutive hepatic proteins are unknown; however HGF is capable of stimulating the synthesis of C/EBPα, which regulates constitutive hepatic proteins.[68]

In contrast to recent in vitro studies, where the authors demonstrated that HGF decreased acute phase proteins, we showed in vivo that HGF increased serum α2-macroglobulin (type II acute phase protein), with no effect on α1-acid glycoprotein and haptoglobin (type I acute phase proteins).[79,80] Type II acute phase proteins are mediated through IL-6-like cytokines, including cytokines such as IL-6 and IL-11.[28] IL-6 secreted by Kupffer cells in the liver is capable of regulating the synthesis of transcription factors that have response elements in the 5′-flanking region of the HGF gene that may be potentially utilized in inducing HGF gene expression at the transcriptional level.[81,83–85] Therefore, IL-6 appears likely to substantially and quickly up-regulate HGF mRNA and HGF mRNA receptor expression.[83] However, the interaction between HGF and IL-6 in vitro has been shown to be complex and controversial.[79,84,87] In our study, we demonstrated that administration of rhHGF stimulated serum IL-6, along with an increase in its dependent type II acute phase protein, serum α2-macroglobulin and TNF-α.[21] TNF-α is another important mediator during the acute phase response, which has been shown to modulate type I acute phase proteins and to stimulate IL-6, HGF and HGF-receptor gene expression.[78,81,83,86,87] TNF-α is a pro-inflammatory cytokine, associated with increased catabolic activity and mortality.[88] However, a recent study suggested that increased TNF-α concentrations after liver injury play an important role in the early signaling pathways of liver regeneration.[81] In support of this hypothesis, we found that serum and hepatic gene expression for TNF-α was significantly elevated with HGF. This finding suggests that HGF stimulates IL-6, TNF-α and type II acute phase proteins. Increased TNF-α could not be shown to contribute to any detectable adverse side effects; however, one may speculate that body weight loss may be due to elevated TNF-α.

HGF exerted beneficial effects after thermal injury by increasing liver weight, liver weight per 100 g body weight and higher total hepatic protein content compared to rats receiving saline.[21] HGF, furthermore, demonstrated no increase in liver triglyceride content, a phenomenon associated with thermal injury.[20,77] These findings are most likely due to the strong mitogenic effect of HGF on hepatocytes.

HGF has been shown to have some beneficial effects and be a potential therapeutic agent; however, more studies need to be done before this growth factor can be applied in patients.

Insulin-like growth factor-I in combination with its principal binding protein-3

Insulin-like growth factor-I is a 7.7-kDa single chain polypeptide of 70 amino acids with sequence homology to proinsulin.[89] In the system 95–99% of IGF-I is bound and transported with one of its six binding proteins IGFBP 1–6.[90] The majority of IGF-I is bound to IGFBP-3. Administration of the IGF-I/BP-3 complex as a therapeutic agent provides several advantages over the administration of IGF-I alone, because when IGF-I is already bound to IGFBP-3, it rapidly transforms into a ternary complex which confers decreased serum clearance and it allows the delivery of significantly larger amounts of IGF-I without inducing hypoglycemia and electrolyte imbalances. In general, IGF-I has been shown to improve cell recovery, wound healing, peripheral muscle protein synthesis, and gut and immune function after thermal injury.[91–93] Recent evidence suggests that IGF-I is instrumental in the early phases of liver regeneration after trauma and modulates the hepatic acute phase response in burned rats.[22]

As administration of IGF-I in therapeutic dosages causes adverse side effects a new complex has been recently developed, in which IGF-I is bound to its principal binding protein-3 (IGFBP-3) in a 1:1 molar ratio. This complex has been shown to be safe and efficacious.[22] Thus, we investigated the effect of IGF-I/BP-3 in thermally injured pediatric patients.[94] IGF-I in combination with IGF-I/BP-3 decreased pro-inflammatory cytokines IL-1β and TNF-α, with subsequent decreases in type I acute phase proteins, C-reactive protein, complement C-3 and α1-acid glycoprotein.[94] As we did not observe an increase in IL-6 or type II acute phase proteins we suggest that IGF-I effectively decreased IL-1β and TNF-α without compensatory elevation of IL-6 and type II acute phase proteins. Decreased acute phase protein and pro-inflammatory cytokines concentration was associated with increased synthesis of constitutive hepatic proteins, such as pre-albumin, retinol-binding protein, and transferrin.[94]

IGF-I appears to have anti-apoptotic, pro-mitogenic effects on multiple cell lines, such as hepatocytes, small bowel epithelial cells, and hematopoietic progenitor cells.[95–97] Therefore, IGF-I seems to affect extra- and intracellular signaling pathways. Recent studies demonstrated that IGF-I decreases the C/EBPβ subtype, which increases after trauma and regulates cytokine and protein synthesis.[74] In contrast IGF-I increases the C/EBPα subtype, which decreases after trauma and regulates constitutive hepatic protein synthesis.[47] IGF-I has been furthermore shown to affect nuclear factor-κB (NF-κB). NF-κB controls the transcriptional regulation of many pro-inflammatory cytokines and acute phase proteins which contain NF-κB response elements in their promoter region.[28,38,40] NF-κB has also been shown as one of the most potent anti-apoptotic transcription factors in several organs. We have recently demonstrated that IGF-I increases hepatic NF-κB concentration and decreases hepatocyte apoptosis after trauma.[97] IGF-I further affects nitric oxide, JAK/STAT, Gp 130 and many more transcription and translation factors.[46,47] We therefore suggest that IGF-I plays a major role after trauma by maintaining organ homeostasis and function. In thermally injured children rhIGF-I in combination with its principal binding protein modulates the hepatic acute phase response by decreasing pro-inflammatory cytokines IL-1β and TNF-α, followed by a decrease in type I acute phase proteins. IGF-I/BP-3 had no effect on IL-6 and type II acute phase proteins (Figure 26.3). Decreases in acute phase protein and pro-inflammatory cytokine synthesis were associated with increases in constitutive hepatic protein synthesis. Attenuating the hepatic acute phase response with IGF-I/BP-3 modulated the hypermetabolic response, which may prevent MOF and improve clinical outcome after a thermal injury without any detectable adverse side effects. Data shown would make IGF-I/BP-3 an ideal therapeutic agent; however, recently our group found that IGF-I/BP-3 increased the risk for peripheral neuropathies, thus limiting the use of this agent (unpublished observations).

Insulin

In our first study we determined the effect of insulin therapy on inflammation, hepatic function, structure and hepatic mRNA and protein cytokine expression during the hypermetabolic cascade post burn.[98] Rats received a thermal injury and were randomly divided into the insulin or control group. Our outcome measures encompassed the effect of insulin on cytokines, hepatic proteins, hepatic pro- and anti-inflammatory cytokines mRNA and proteins, hepatocyte proliferation including Bcl-2 and hepatocyte apoptosis with caspases-3 and caspases-9. We found that insulin significantly improved hepatic protein synthesis by increasing albumin and decreasing C-reactive protein and fat, while insulin decreased the hepatic inflammatory response signal cascade by decreasing hepatic pro-inflammatory cytokines mRNA and proteins IL-1β and TNF at pre-translational levels (Figure 26.5). Insulin increased hepatic cytokine mRNA and protein expression of IL-2 and IL-10 at a pre-translational level when compared with controls. In addition, insulin affected hepatic signal transcription factors and attenuated on a molecular level inflammation (Figure 26.6). Insulin increased hepatocyte proliferation along

with Bcl-2 concentration, while decreasing hepatocyte apoptosis along with decreased caspases-3 and -9 concentration, thus improving liver morphology (Figure 26.7). From this animal study we concluded that insulin attenuates the inflammatory response by decreasing the pro-inflammatory and increasing the anti-inflammatory cascade, thus restoring hepatic homeostasis. The subsequent study examined whether the observed effects of insulin are limited to a thermal injury or whether insulin exerts positive effects during other pathophysiological states. We chose the model of endotoxemia (LPS administration).[99] Endotoxemic rats were divided to receive either saline or insulin. Hepatic morphology and function was determined by measuring the effect of insulin on liver proteins, enzymes, hepatocyte apoptosis and proliferation including caspases-3 and -9 and Bcl-2. Intrahepatic ATP, glucose and lactate concentrations were determined by bioluminescence. To determine possible molecular and biochemical mechanisms the effect of insulin on hepatic cytokine mRNA and gene profile analysis was performed. Insulin significantly improved hepatic protein while it attenuated hepatic damage as shown by decreased AST and ALT. Improved liver morphology was probably due to decreased hepatocyte apoptosis along with decreased caspase-3 concentration and increased hepatocyte proliferation along with Bcl-2 concentration. Insulin decreased the hepatic inflammatory response signal cascade by decreasing hepatic IL-1β, IL-6 and MIF. Bioluminescence showed that insulin improved hepatic glucose metabolism and glycolysis. Gene chip analysis revealed a strong anti-inflammatory effect of insulin on inflammatory mediators. These data provide insight that insulin improves hepatic integrity, glucose metabolism and function by increasing cell survival and attenuating the hepatic inflammatory response in endotoxemic rats. In order to confirm our animal data we went on and conducted a human study.[100] Thirteen thermally injured children received insulin to maintain blood glucose at a range from 120 to 180 mg/dL; fifteen children received no insulin with blood glucose levels also at range from 120 to 180 mg/dL and served as controls. Our outcome measures encompassed the effect of insulin on pro-inflammatory mediators, the hepatic acute phase response, fat and the IGF-I system. Insulin administration decreased pro-inflammatory cytokines and proteins, while increasing constitutive hepatic proteins. Burned children receiving insulin required significantly less albumin substitution to maintain normal levels compared to control. Insulin decreased free fatty acids and serum triglycerides when compared to controls. Serum IGF-I and IGFBP-3 significantly increased with insulin administration. In conclusion, several studies have shown that insulin attenuates the inflammatory response by decreasing the pro-inflammatory and increasing the anti-inflammatory cascade, thus restoring systemic homeostasis, which has been shown critical for organ function and survival in critically ill patients. Insulin appears to be a safe and efficacious drug to affect hepatic dysfunction. Even more so, as tight euglycemic control has been shown to be advantageous over low-dose insulin treatment. Studies in this area are warranted.[101]

Propranolol

A new therapeutic option to attenuate hepatic swelling and dysfunction appears to be a non-selective β1/β2 blocker. Beta

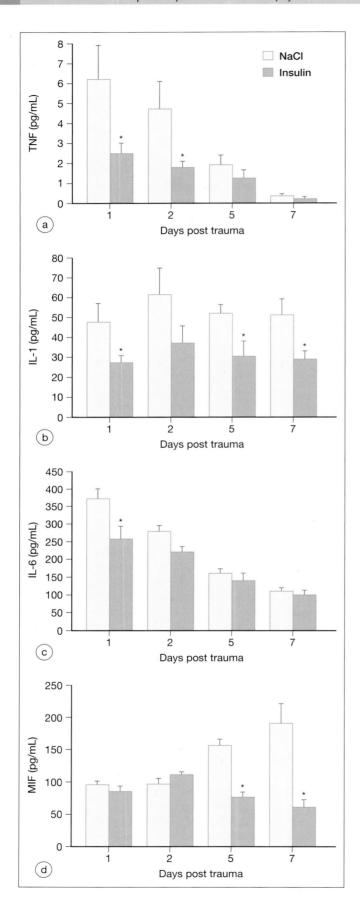

Fig. 26.5 Serum pro-inflammatory cytokines after a 30% TBSA thermal injury. (a) Serum TNF. Insulin prevented an increase of serum TNF on days 1 and 2 when compared with controls. Normal serum TNF: 0–2 pg/mL. (b) Serum IL-1 remained elevated during the study period. Insulin decreased serum IL-1 concentration on days 1, 2 and 7 after trauma when compared with animals receiving saline. Normal IL-1: 0–20 pg/mL. (c) Insulin significantly decreased serum IL-6 concentrations 1 day after burn compared to controls, which were almost 300 times elevated above normal levels. Normal IL-6: 0–10 pg/dL. (d) Macrophage inhibitory factor (MIF) was found to be increased immediately after burn, but further increased over the study period by almost 100% in the control group. Insulin significantly decreased serum MIF 5 and 7 days after trauma. Normal MIF: 0–20 pg/mL. *Significant difference between insulin and control, $p < 0.05$. Data presented as means ± SEM.

blockade results in a decrease in urinary nitrogen loss, decreased peripheral lipolysis and whole body urea production,[102] decreased resting energy expenditure, and improved skeletal muscle protein kinetics.[103] Furthermore, propranolol preserved fat-free mass when compared to controls.[103]

Another study from our group showed that propranolol decreased hepatic fat storage by limiting fatty acid delivery in severely burned pediatric patients.[104] In addition, we showed that propranolol decreased peripheral lipolysis and improved insulin responsiveness.[105] Recently we further showed that propranolol has a profound effect on fat infiltration of the liver. The effect of propranolol on attenuating, and even reversing, hepatomegaly is shown in Figure 26.8. In control patients 39 of 45 livers increased in size during acute hospitalization, whereas only 4 of 35 livers with propranolol therapy increased in size ($p = 0.0001$ between groups). We propose that propranolol reduces hepatomegaly by inhibiting lipolysis and reducing liver blood flow, in turn delivery of fatty acids to the liver. The effect of propranolol on the hepatic acute phase response, systemic inflammatory reaction and immune system is being examined in current clinical studies at our institute. In summary, for a long time hepatic dysfunction was tolerated without any treatment option. In the field of burns, it appears that there will be new treatment options available to successfully attenuate the hypermetabolic hepatic acute phase response.

Enzymes

Liver enzymes, such as aspartate aminotransferase (AST) and alanine aminotransferase (ALT), are the most sensitive indicators of hepatocyte injury. Both AST and ALT are normally present in low concentrations. However, with cellular injury or changes in cell membrane permeability, these enzymes leak into circulation. Of the two, the ALT is the more sensitive and specific test for hepatocyte injury as AST can be also elevated in the state of cardiac arrest or muscle injury. Serum glutamate dehydrogenase (GLDH) is also a marker and is elevated in the state of severe hepatic damage. Serum alkaline phosphatase (ALKP) provides an elevation of the patency of the bile channels at all levels, intrahepatic and extrahepatic. Elevation is demonstrated in patients with obstruction of the extrahepatic biliary tract or caliculi. In general, serum levels are elevated in hepatobiliary disease.[106]

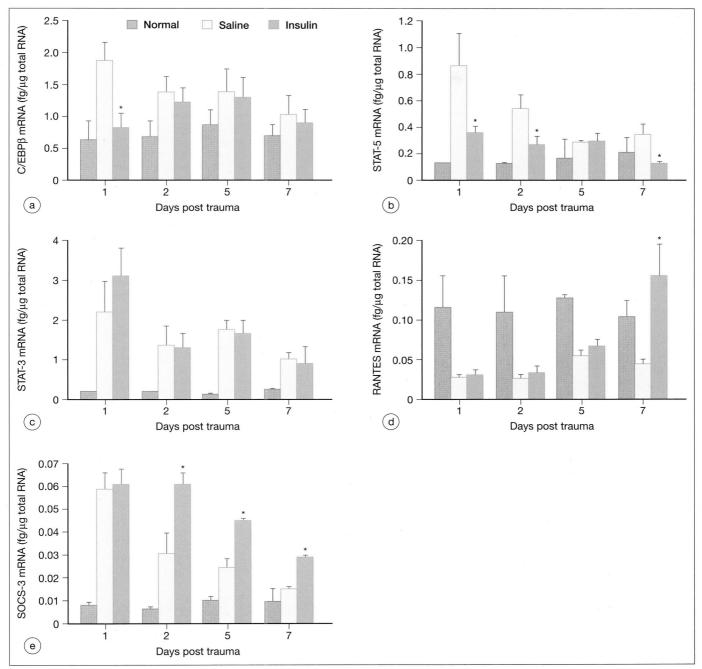

Fig. 26.6 Hepatic mRNA expression of signal transcription factors quantified by light cycler analysis. (a) C/EBPβ mRNA expression increased after burn and remained elevated during the study period. Insulin decreased hepatic C/EBPβ mRNA expression on the first day after thermal injury. (b) Hepatic STAT-5 mRNA expression increased after the burn trauma. Insulin significantly decreased STAT-5 mRNA expression on days 1, 2 and 7 when compared to controls. (c) Hepatic mRNA expression of STAT-3 increased after trauma, but differences between controls and insulin could be shown. (d) Hepatic RANTES mRNA expression was decreased with the thermal trauma. Insulin increased RANTES mRNA, which approached normal levels 7 days post trauma compared to rats receiving saline. (e) SOCS-3 mRNA was found to be increased with burn injury. Insulin further increased hepatic mRNA expression of SOCS-3 2, 5 and 7 days after burn. *Significant difference between insulin and control, $p < 0.05$. Data presented as means ± SEM.

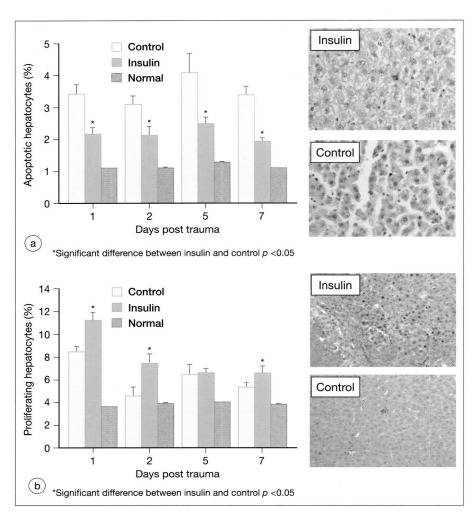

(a)

*Significant difference between insulin and control p <0.05

(b)

*Significant difference between insulin and control p <0.05

Fig. 26.7 Hepatic morphology determined by measuring hepatocyte proliferation, apoptosis and resulting hepatocyte net balance. (a) Thermal injury caused a significant increase in hepatocyte apoptosis by the biological factor 4 compared to normal. Insulin decreased apoptosis on all study days by 50% compared to controls, $p < 0.05$. Beside the figure, two representative histological sections stained for apoptosis. While in control sections many apoptotic hepatocytes could be identified, only few where found positive in the insulin sections. (b) Hepatocyte proliferation increased in the control and the insulin immediately after burn and remained elevated throughout the entire study period. Insulin had a mitotic effect on hepatocytes and significantly increased proliferation compared to controls on days 1, 2, and 7 after thermal trauma. Beside the figure, two representative histological sections stained with Ki67 for proliferation. While in control sections few proliferating hepatocytes could be identified, many hepatocytes were found positive in the insulin sections.

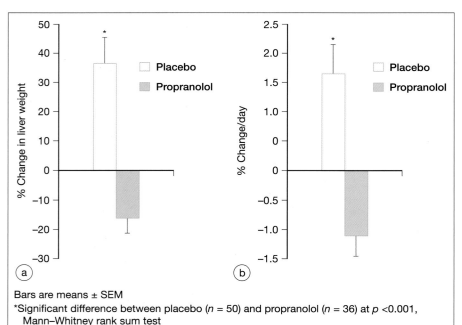

(a)

(b)

Bars are means ± SEM

*Significant difference between placebo (*n* = 50) and propranolol (*n* = 36) at *p* <0.001, Mann–Whitney rank sum test

Fig. 26.8 (a) Percent change in liver weights. *Significant difference between placebo (*n* = 50) and propranolol therapy (*n* = 36) at $p < 0.001$. Confidence intervals for differences are 30.242, 75.358. Mean ± SEM days after burn until the first measurement was 12.8 ± 1.3 days (range, 2–28 days). (b), Percent change per day in liver weights. *Significant difference between placebo (*n* = 49) and propranolol therapy (*n* = 36) at $p < 0.0001$. Confidence intervals for differences are 1.927, 4.063. (Reproduced with permission Barrow RE, Wolfe RR, Dasu MR, et al. The use of beta-adrenergic blockade in preventing trauma-induced hepatomegaly. Ann Surg 2006; 243(1):115–120.[104])

TABLE 26.3 LOCALIZATION OF HEPATIC ENZYMES AND THEIR FUNCTION IN HEPATIC DAMAGE DIAGNOSIS[97]

Localization			
Enzyme	Cytoplasma	Mitochondrial	Liver specific
AST	+	+	No: heart, muscle
ALT	+	–	Yes
GLDH	–	+	Yes
ALKP	Combination of several isoenzymes	No: bone, growth, pregnancy, etc.	

Reproduced from Jeschke MG, Herndon DN, Vita R, et al. IGF-1/BP-3 administration preserved hepatic hemeostasis after thermal injury which is associated with increases in NO and hepatic NF-κB. Shock 2001; 16:373–379.[97]

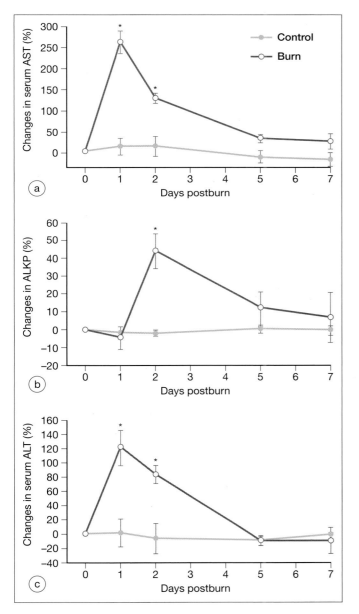

Fig. 26.9 Serum AST (a), ALKP (b) and ALT (c) levels were determined in controls and thermally injured rats. Serum AST and ALT increased during the first day after burn, whereas ALKP increased 2 days after burn when compared with controls. Data presented as means ± SEM. * Significant difference between burn and controls, $p < 0.05$.

As mentioned earlier liver damage occurs after a thermal injury. The elevation of hepatic enzymes correlates with the severity and extend of the hepatic injury. Small hepatic injury leads to a predominantly elevation of the cytoplasmatic enzymes ALT and only little elevation of AST. The so-called de Ritis ratio GOT/GPT <1. In a state of severe hepatic damage, mitochondrial bound enzymes are strongly elevated and the de Ritis ratio GOT/GPT >1 (Table 26.3).[106]

Thermal injury causes liver damage by edema formation, hypoperfusion, pro-inflammatory cytokines or other cell death signals with the release of the hepatic enzymes. Others and we have shown that serum AST, ALT and ALKP are elevated between 50 to 200% when compared with normal levels (Figure 26.9). We observed that serum AST and ALT peaked during the first day postburn and ALKP during the second day postburn. During hepatic regeneration all enzymes returned to baseline between 10–14 days postburn. If liver damage persists, enzymes stay elevated. There is no need for therapeutic intervention to decrease elevated enzymes. Enzymes can only be used as markers and the effect of therapeutics can be studied.

Summary

The liver plays a crucial role in the aftermath of a thermal injury. The synthesis of constitutive hepatic proteins, acute phase proteins, cytokines and other mediators makes it a determining factor for survival. A new approach for improving hepatic function may be the use of anabolic, anti-inflammatory agents; however, there is no effective treatment for hepatic dysfunction.

References

1. Moll KJ. Anatomie. Leber. München: Jungjohann Verlag; 366–375.
2. Winkeltau G, Kraas E. Leber. In: Schumpelick V, Bleese NM, Mommsen U, eds. Chirurgie. Stuttgart: Enke Verlag; 658–675.
3. Schwartz SI. Liver. In: Schwartz SI, Shires GT, Spencer FC, et al. (eds). Principles of surgery. New York: McGraw-Hill Companies, Inc.: 1395–1436.
4. Küttler T. Biochemie. München: Jungjohann Verlag; 240–265.
5. Linares HA. Autopsy findings in burned children. In: Carvajal HF, Parks DH, eds. Burns in children. Chicago: Year Book Medical; 1988.
6. Jeschke MG, Mlcak RP, Herndon DN. Morphologic changes of the liver after a severe thermal injury. Surgery 2006 (in review).
7. Jeschke MG, Low JFA, Spies M, et al. Cell proliferation, apoptosis, NF-κB expression, enzyme, protein, and weight changes in livers of burned rats. Am J Physiol 2001; 280:1514–1521.
8. Steller H. Mechanisms and genes of cellular suicide. Science 1995; 267:1445–1449.
9. Teplitz C. The pathology of burns and the fundamental of burn wound sepsis. In: Artz CL, Moncrief JA, Pruitt BA, eds. Burns: a team approach. Philadelphia: WB Saunders; 1979:45.
10. Linares HA. Sepsis, disseminated intravascular coagulation and multi organ failure: catastrophic events in severe burns. In: Schlag G, Redl H, Siegl JH, et al., eds. Shock, sepsis, and organ failure. Berlin: Springer Verlag; 1991:370–398.
11. Wolf SE, Ikeda H, Matin S, DebRoy MA, et al. Cutaneous burn increases apoptosis in the gut epithelium of mice. J Am Coll Surg 1999; 188:10–16.
12. Lightfoot E Jr, Horton JW, Maass DW, et al. Major burn trauma in rats promotes cardiac and gastrointestinal apoptosis. Shock 1999; 11:29–34.
13. Baron P, Traber DL, Traber LD, et al. Gut failure and translocation following burn and sepsis. J Surg Res 1994; 57:197–204.
14. Ikeda H, Suzuki Y, Suzuki M, et al. Apoptosis is a major mode of cell death caused by ischemia and ischemia/reperfusion injury to the rat intestinal epithelium. Gut 1998; 42:530–537.
15. Noda T, Iwakiri R, Fujimoto R, et al. Programmed cell death induced by ischemia-reperfusion in rat intestinal mucosa. Am J Physiol 1998; 274:G270–G276.
16. Ramzy PI, Irtun O, Wolf SE, et al. Gut epithelial apoptosis after severe burn: effects of gut hypoperfusion. J Am Coll Surg 2000; 190(3):281–287.
17. Beg AA, Finco TS, Nantermet PV, et al. Tumor necrosis factor and interleukin-1 lead to phosphorylation and loss of I kappa B alpha: a mechanism for NF-kappa B activation. Mol Cell Biol 1993; 13:3301–3310.
18. Bellas RE, FitzGerald MJ, Fausto N, et al. Inhibition of NF-kappa B activity induces apoptosis in murine hepatocytes. Am J Pathol 1997; 151:891–896.
19. Jeschke MG, Herndon DN, Wolf SE, et al. Recombinant human growth hormone alters acute phase reactant proteins, cytokine expression and liver morphology in burned rats. J Surg Res 1999; 83:122–129.
20. Jeschke MG, Wolf SE, DebRoy MA, et al. The combination of growth hormone with hepatocyte growth factor alters the acute phase response. Shock 1999; 12:181–187.
21. Jeschke MG, Herndon DN, Wolf SE, et al. Hepatocyte growth factor (HGF) modulates the hepatic acute phase response in thermally injured rats. Crit Care Med 2000; 28:504–510.
22. Jeschke MG, Herndon DN, Barrow RE. Insulin-like growth factor-I plus insulin-like growth factor binding protein-3 affects the hepatic acute phase response and hepatic morphology in thermally injured rats. Ann Surg 2000; 231:408–416.
23. Cano N, Gerolami A. Intrahepatic cholestasis during total parenteral nutrition. Lancet 1983; 1:985.
24. Bolder U, Ton-nu HT, Schteingart CD, et al. Hepatocyte transport of bile acids and organic anions in endotoxemic rats: impaired uptake and secretion. Gastroenterology 1997; 112:214–225.
25. Hurd T, Lysz T, Dikdan G, et al. Hepatic cellular dysfunction in sepsis: an ischemic phenomenon? Curr Surg 1988; 45:114–119.
26. Manning AJ, Meyer N, Klein GL. Vitamin and trace element homeostasis following burn injury. In: Herndon DN. Total burn care. Philadelphia: WB Saunders; 2001:251–255.
27. Wolf SE, Sanford A. Daily work. In: Wolf SE, Herndon DN. Handbook of burn care. Austin: Landes Bioscience; 1999:122.
28. Moshage H. Cytokines and the hepatic acute phase response. J Pathol 1997; 181:257–266.
29. Fey G, Gauldie J. The acute phase response of the liver in inflammation. In: Popper H, Schaffner F, eds. Progress in liver disease. Philadelphia: WB Saunders; 1990:89–116.
30. Rothschild MA, Oratz M, Schreiber SS. Serum albumin. Hepatology 1988; 8:385–401.
31. Hiyama DT, Von Allmen D, Rosenblum L, et al. Synthesis of albumin and acute-phase proteins in perfused liver after burn injury in rats. J Burn Care Rehabil 1991; 12:1–6.
32. Gilpin DA, Hsieh CC, Kunninger DT, et al. Regulation of the acute phase response genes alpha$_1$-acid glycoprotein and alpha$_1$-antitrypsin correlates with sensitivity to thermal injury. Surgery 1996; 119(6):664–673.
33. Livingston DH, Mosenthal AC, Deitch EA. Sepsis and multiple organ dysfunction syndrome: a clinical-mechanistic overview. New Horizons 1995; 3:276–287.
34. Selzman CH, Shames BD, Miller SA, et al. Therapeutic implications of interleukin-10 in surgical disease. Shock 1998; 10:309–318.
35. De Maio A, de Mooney ML, Matesic LE, et al. Genetic component in the inflammatory response induced by bacterial lipopolysaccharide. Shock 1998; 10:319–323.
36. Yin MJ, Yamamoto Y, Gaynor RB. The anti-inflammatory agents aspirin and salicylate inhibit the activity of I (kappa) B kinase-beta. Nature 1998; 6706:77–80.
37. Shakhov AN, Collart MA, Vassalli P, et al. Kappa B-type enhances are involved in lipopolysaccharide-mediated transcriptional activation of the tumor necrosis factor alpha gene in primary macrophages. J Exp Med 1990; 171:35–47.
38. Siebenlist U, Franzoso G, Brown K. Structure, regulation and function of NF-κB. Ann Rev Cell Biol 1994; 10:405–455.
39. Yao J, Mackman N, Edgington TS, et al. Lipopolysaccharide induction of tumor necrosis factor alpha promoter in human monocyte cells: regulation by Erg-1, c-jun, and NF-κB transcription factors. J Biol Chem 1997; 272:17795–17801.
40. Dinarello CA. Biologic basis for interleukin-1 in disease. Blood 1996; 87:2095–2147.
41. Kishimoto T, Taga T, Akira S. Cytokine signal transduction. Cell 1994; 76:325–328.
42. Gilpin DA, Hsieh CC, Kuninger DT, et al. Effect of thermal injury on the expression of transcription factors that regulate acute phase response genes: the response of C/EBPα, C/EBPβ, and C/EBPδ to thermal injury. Surgery 1996; 119:674–683.
43. Alam T, An MR, Papaconstantinou J. Differential expression of three C/EBP isoforms in multiple tissues during the acute phase response. J Biol Chem 1992; 267:5021–5024.
44. Jarrar D, Herndon DN, Wolf SE, et al. Growth hormone treat-ment after burn affects expression of C/EBPs, regulators of the acute phase response J Burn Care Rehabil 1998; 19: S163.
45. Umayahara Y, Ji C, Centrella M, et al. CCAAT/enhancer-binding protein delta activates insulin-like growth factor-I gene transcription in osteoblasts. Identification of a novel cyclic AMP signaling pathway in bone. J Biol Chem 1997; 272:31793–31800.
46. Nolten LA, Steenbergh PH, Sussenbach JS. Hepatocyte nuclear factor 1 alpha activates promoter 1 of the human insulin-like growth factor I gene via two distinct binding sites. Mol Endocrinol 1995; 9:1488–1499.
47. Nolten LA, van Schaik FM, Steenbergh PH, et al. Expression of the insulin-like growth I gene is stimulated by the liver-enriched transcription factors C/EBP alpha and LAP. Mol Endocrinol 1994; 8:1636–1645.

48. Thomas MJ, Gronowski AM, Berry SA, et al. Growth hormone rapidly activates rat serine protease inhibitor 2.1 gene transcription and induces a DNA-binding activity distinct from those of STAT1, -3, and -4. Mol Cell Biol 1995; 15:12–18.

49. Tracey KJ, Fong Y, Hesse DG, et al. Anti-cachectin/TNF monoclonal antibodies prevent septic shock during lethal bacteraemia. Nature 1987; 330:662–664.

50. Beutler B, Milsark IW, Cerami AC. Passive immunization against cachectin/tumor necrosis factor protects mice from lethal effect of endotoxin. Science 1985; 229:869–871.

51. Alexander HR, Doherty GM, Buresh CM. A recombinant human receptor antagonist to interleukin 1 improves survival after lethal endotoxemia in mice. J Exp Med 1991; 173:1029–1032.

52. Pruitt JH, Copeland EM, Moldawer LL. Interleukin-1 and interleukin-1 antagonism in sepsis systemic inflammatory response syndrome and septic shock. Shock 1995; 3:235–251.

53. Williams G, Giroir B. Regulation of cytokine gene expression: tumor-necrosis factor, interleukin-1, and the emerging biology of cytokine receptors. New Horizons 1995; 2:276–287.

54. Taniguchi T, Koido Y, Aiboshi J, et al. Change in the ratio of interleukin-6 to interleukin-10 predicts a poor outcome in patients with systemic inflammatory response syndrome. Crit Care Med 1999; 27:1262–1264.

55. Simovic MO, Bonham MJ, Abu-Zidan FM, et al. Anti-inflammatory cytokine response and clinical outcome in acute pancreatitis. Crit Care Med 1999; 27:2662–2665.

56. Thissen JP, Verniers J. Inhibition by interleukin-1β and tumor necrosis factor-α of the insulin-like growth factor I messenger ribonucleic acid response to growth hormone in rat hepatocyte primary culture. Endocrinology 1997; 138:1078–1084.

57. Lang CH, Fan J, Cooney R, et al. IL-1 receptor antagonist attenuates sepsis-induced alterations in the IGF system and protein synthesis. Am J Physiol 1996; 270:E430–E437.

58. Delhanty PJ. Interleukin-1 beta suppresses growth hormone-induced acid-labile subunit mRNA levels and secretion in primary hepatocytes. Biochem Biophys Res Com 1998; 243:269–272.

59. Salgame P, Abrams JS, Clayberger C, et al. Differing lymphokine profiles of functional subsets of human CD4 and CD8 T cell clones. Science 1991; 254:279–282.

60. de Waal Malefyt R, Abrams J, Bennett B. Interleukin 10 (IL-10) inhibits cytokine synthesis by human monocytes: an autoregulation role of IL-10 produced by monocytes. J Exp Med 1991; 174:1209–1220.

61. Kusske AM, Rongione AJ, Reber HA. Cytokines and acute pancreatitis. Gastroenterology 1996; 110:639–642.

62. Wang T, Tracey KJ. HMG-1 a late mediator of endotoxin lethality. Science 1999; 285:248–250.

63. Calandra T, Echtenacher B, Le Roy D, et al. Protection from septic shock by neutralization of macrophage migration inhibitory factor. Nature Med 2000; 2:164–170.

64. Jeschke MG, Barrow RE, Herndon DN. Recombinant human growth hormone (rhGH) treatment in pediatric burn patients and its role during the acute phase response. Crit Care Med 2000; 28:1578–1584.

65. Postel-Vinay MC, Finidori J. Growth hormone receptor: structure and signal transduction. Eur J Endocrinol 1995; 133:654–659.

66. Waxman DJ, Zhao S, Choi HK. Interaction of a novel sex-dependent, growth hormone-regulated liver nuclear factor with CYP2C12 promoter. J Biol Chem 1996; 271:29978–29987.

67. Kelly PA, Diane J, Postel-Vinay MC. The prolactin/growth hormone receptor family. Endocr Rev 1991; 12:235–251.

68. Seth A, Gonzalez FA, Gupta S. Signal transduction within the nucleus by mitogen-activated protein kinase. J Biol Chem 1992; 267:24796–24804.

69. Han Y, Leaman DW, Watling D. Participation of JAK and STAT proteins in growth hormone-induced signaling. J Biol Chem 1996; 271:5947–52.

70. Haeffner A, Thieblemont N, Deas O. Inhibitory effect of growth hormone on TNF-α secretion and nuclear factor-kappa B translocation in lipopolysaccharide-stimulated human monocytes. J Immunol 1997; 158: 1310–1314.

71. Sumantran VN, Tsai ML, Schwartz J. Growth hormone induces c-fos and c-jun expression in cells with varying requirements for differentiation. Endocrinology 1992; 130:2016–2024.

72. Clarkson RW, Chen CM, Harrison S. Early responses of trans-activating factors to growth hormone in preadipocytes: differential regulation of CCAAT enhancer-binding protein-beta (C/EBP beta) and C/EBP delta. Mol Endocrinol 1995; 9:108–120.

73. Schwander JC, Hauri C, Zapf J. Synthesis and secretion of insulin-like growth factor and its binding protein by the perfused rat liver: dependence on growth hormone status. Endocrinology 1983; 113:297–305.

74. Alam T, An MR, Mifflin RC. Trans-activation of the α_1-acid glycoprotein gene acute phase response element by multiple isoforms of C/EBP and glucocorticoid receptor. J Biol Chem 1993; 268: 15681–15688.

75. Xia ZF, Coolbaugh MI, Kuninger DT, et al: Regulation of the acute phase response genes alpha$_1$-acid glycoprotein and alpha$_1$-antitrypsin correlates with sensitivity to thermal injury. Surgery 1996; 119:664–673.

76. Takala J, Ruokonen E, Webster N, et al. Increased mortality associated with growth hormone treatment in critically ill adults. N Engl J Med 1999; 341:785–792.

77. Aarsland A, Chinkes D, Wolfe RR. Beta-blockade lowers peripheral lipolysis in burn patients receiving growth hormone. Rate of hepatic very low density lipoprotein triglyceride secretions remains unchanged. Ann Surg 1996; 223:777–789.

78. Ishii T, Sato M, Sudo K. Hepatocyte growth factor stimulates liver regeneration and elevates blood protein level in normal and partially hepatectomized rats. J Biochem 1995; 117:1105–1112.

79. Guillén MI, Gomez-Lechon MJ, Nakamura T. The hepatocyte growth factor regulates the synthesis of acute-phase proteins in human hepatocytes: divergent effect on interleukin-6 stimulated genes. Hepatology 1996; 23:345–1352.

80. Pierzchalski P, Nakamura T, Takehara T. Modulation of acute phase protein synthesis in cultured rat hepatocytes by human recombinant hepatocyte growth factor. Growth Factors 1992; 7:161–165.

81. Michalopoulos GK, DeFrances MC. Liver regeneration. Science 1997; 276:60–66.

82. Michalopoulos GK, Appasamy R. Metabolism of HGF-SF and its role in liver regeneration. EXS 1993; 65:275–283.

83. Zarnegar R. Regulation of HGF and HGFR gene expression. In: Goldberg ID, Rosen EM, eds. Epithelial-mesenchymal interactions in cancer. Basel: Birkhauser Verlag; 1995.

84. Ohira H, Miyata M, Kuroda M. Interleukin-6 induces proliferation of rat hepatocytes in vivo. J Hepatol 1996; 25:941–947.

85. Chen-Kiang S, Hsu W, Natkunman Y. Nuclear signaling by interleukin-6. Curr Opin Immunol 1993; 5:124–128.

86. Castell JV, Gomez-Lechon MJ, David M. Interleukin 6 is the major regulator of acute phase protein synthesis in adult human hepatocytes. FEBS Lett 1989; 242:237–239.

87. Rai RM, Zhang JX, Clemens M. Gadolinium chloride alters the acinar distribution of phagocytosis and balance between pro- and anti-inflammatory cytokines. Shock 1996; 6:243–247.

88. Frost RA, Lang CH, Gelato MC. Transient exposure of human myeloblasts to tumor necrosis factor-α inhibits serum and insulin-like growth factor-I stimulated protein synthesis. Endocrinology 1997; 138:4153–4159.

89. Humbel RE. Insulin-like growth factor-I and factor-II. Eur J Biochem 1990; 190:445–462.

90. Baxter RC. Circulating levels and molecular distribution of the acid-labile (alpha) subunit of the high molecular weight insulin-like growth factor-binding protein complex. J Clin Endocrinol Metab 1990; 70:1347–1353.

91. Huang KF, Chung DH, Herndon DN. Insulin-like growth factor-I (IGF-I) reduces gut atrophy and bacterial translocation after severe burn injury. Arch Surg 1993; 128:47–54.

92. Strock LL, Singh H. Abdullah A. The effect of insulin-like growth factor-1 on postburn hypermetabolism. Surgery 1990; 108: 161–164.

93. Steenfos HH. Growth factors and wound healing. Scand J Plast Reconstr Hand Surg 1994; 28:95–105.

94. Jeschke MG, Barrow RE, Herndon DN. IGF-I/IGFBP-3 attenuates the pro-inflammatory acute phase response in severely burned children. Ann Surg 2000; 231(2):246–252.

95. Pugazhenti S, Miller E, Sable C, et al. Insulin-like growth factor-I induces bcl-2 promoter through the transcription factor cAMP response element-binding protein. J Biol Chem 1999; 274:27529–27535.

96. Delaney CL, Cheng HL, Feldman EL. Insulin-like growth factor-I prevents caspase-mediated apoptosis in Schwann cells. J Neurobiol 1999; 41:540–548.

97. Jeschke MG, Herndon DN, Vita R, et al. IGF-I/BP-3 administration preserves hepatic homeostasis after thermal injury which is associated with increases in NO and hepatic NF-κB. Shock 2001; 16:373–379.

98. Klein D, Schubert T, Horch RE, et al. Insulin treatment improves hepatic morphology and function after severe trauma. Ann Surg 2004; 240:340–349.

99. Jeschke MG, Klein D, Rensing H, et al. Insulin prevents liver damage and preserves liver function during endotoxemia. J Hepatol 2005; 42(6):870–879.

100. Jeschke MG, Klein D, Herndon DN. Insulin treatment improves the systemic inflammatory reaction and hepatic acute-phase-response to severe thermal injury. Ann Surg 2004; 239(4):553–560.

101. Van den Berghe G P, Wouters F, Weekers C, et al. Intensive insulin therapy in critically ill patients. N Engl J Med 2001; 345:1359–1367.

102. Herndon DN, Nguyen TT, Wolfe RR, et al. Lipolysis in burned patients is stimulated by the beta 2-receptor for catecholamines. Arch Surg 1994; 129:1301–1304; discussion 1304–1305.

103. Herndon DN, Hart DW, Wolf SE, et al. Reversal of catabolism by beta-blockade after severe burns. N Engl J Med 2001; 345:1223–1229.

104. Barrow RE, Wolfe RR, Dasu MR, et al. The use of beta-adrenergic blockade in preventing trauma-induced hepatomegaly. Ann Surg 2006; 243(1):115–120.

105. Morio B, Irtun O, Herndon DN, et al. Propranolol decreases splanchnic triacylglycerol storage in burn patients receiving a high-carbohydrate diet. Ann Surg 2002; 236:218–225.

106. Herold G. Lebererkrankungen. In: Herold G, ed. Innere medizin 2000. Köln: Herold Verlag; 2000:411–460.

Chapter 27

Effects of burn injury on bone and mineral metabolism

Gordon L. Klein, Rene Przkora, and David N. Herndon

Importance of bone metabolism and function after burn

Burn injury exceeding 40% total body surface area (TBSA) is very disruptive to bone and calcium metabolism. Long-term consequences include an increased risk of fracture postburn resulting from long-term loss of bone calcium and a chronic, progressive vitamin D deficiency with inability of the skin to synthesize normal quantities of vitamin D from sunlight exposure. More immediately postburn, calcium homeostasis is disrupted and patients become magnesium depleted. These are in part consequences of burn-induced hypoparathyroidism and development of end-organ resistance to parathyroid hormone. This chapter will deal in detail with normal homeostasis of calcium, phosphorus, and magnesium, how the burn injury disrupts them and how these disruptions can be managed. It will then go on to discuss the known effects of burn injury on bone structure and bone biology, deal with the consequences of the damage to bone and the management of this problem as it has been worked out to date.

Metabolic functions of calcium, phosphorus, and magnesium

The effects of burn injury on homeostasis of three critical minerals (calcium, phosphorus, and magnesium) have not been studied in great detail. These three minerals play key roles in metabolism and also are stored in bone, a tissue that is significantly affected by burn injury. All three of these minerals play important roles in intracellular and extracellular metabolism.

Calcium

Calcium (Ca) plays a major role in neuromuscular impulse propagation and membrane depolarization and, consequently, in muscle contractility. Ca may also serve as a second messenger, mediating the secretory release of peptides such as amylase, insulin, and aldosterone via intracellular pathways utilizing calmodulin, an intracellular calcium receptor protein, or protein kinase C. From the standpoint of extracellular metabolism, Ca serves as a co-factor in blood coagulation, specifically in the conversion of prothrombin to thrombin and the activation of several factors in the coagulation cascade. Ca also contributes to plasma membrane stability by binding to phospholipids.[1-3]

Phosphorus

Phosphorus (P) plays a major role in intracellular energy metabolism. P, in the form of phosphate esters, is a constituent of purine nucleotides, an important source of intracellular energy. Phosphorylation of various metabolic intermediate products is also the means of intracellular energy transfer. In the form of phospholipids, P is also a major structural component of cell membranes.[1]

Magnesium

Magnesium (Mg), primarily stored in mitochondria, is a vital co-factor for the function of enzymes involved in the transfer of phosphate groups; and thus, it is important for all reactions which require adenosine triphosphate (ATP) and in reactions involving replication, transcription, and translation of nucleic acids.[1] Extracellular Mg is important in plasma membrane excitability.

Homeostasis of calcium, phosphorus, and magnesium

Calcium

Absorption of Ca is generally well regulated by the body. With high Ca intake, absorption can be as low as 20%, while with low Ca intake, absorption can reach 70%.[4] The mechanism for this regulation is shown in Figure 27.1. With high Ca intake, there is a transient hypercalcemia followed by a suppression

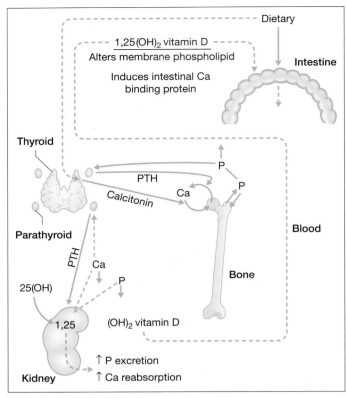

Fig. 27.1 Vitamin D and calcium metabolism.

of parathyroid hormone (PTH) secretion, and consequently a suppression of PTH-stimulated renal conversion of 25-hydroxyvitamin D, the chief circulating form of the vitamin, to calcitriol, or 1,25-dihydroxyvitamin D. With low Ca intake, the reverse occurs. There is a transient reduction in serum Ca concentration, followed by a rapid, within 5 minutes, rise in PTH secretion. PTH will under normal circumstances stimulate bone resorption and increase renal tubular Ca reabsorption in order to raise serum Ca concentration. Furthermore, it stimulates the renal enzyme 25-hydroxyvitamin D-1-α hydroxylase to convert 25-hydroxyvitamin D to calcitriol. Calcitriol then binds to intestinal epithelial cells and increases transcellular Ca absorption by altering cell membrane phospholipid and by facilitating the intracellular passage of the absorbed Ca by stimulating the cellular synthesis of *calcium binding proteins*. Thus, the efficiency of Ca absorption is improved.

Ca, given intravenously, bypasses the intestinal control mechanism and suppresses PTH production by the parathyroids as well as production of calcitriol by the kidney. The bone stores 99% of the body's Ca.[1]

Phosphorus

In contrast to Ca, the intestine plays no significant regulatory role in P absorption. Approximately 80% of dietary phosphate is absorbed and the bone stores approximately 90% of the body's phosphate.

Homeostatic control appears to rest primarily within the kidney.[5,6] The regulatory mechanisms are most likely PTH-independent.[5,6] Thus, the renal excretory rate of phosphate

will primarily regulate the serum P concentration and maintain it within a normal range. Fibroblast growth factor (FGF)-23 evolves to be one key regulator of phosphate and vitamin D metabolism in humans.[7] Studies demonstrated that mutations in the FGF-23 gene cause autosomal dominant hypophosphatemic rickets (ADHR), a phosphate wasting disorder. The exact molecular pathway of FGF-23 mediated actions is currently under intense investigations.[7]

Magnesium

Approximately 60% of the body's Mg is stored in the skeleton,[9] although not at sites where matrix is calcified. Mg absorption, like P, varies directly with dietary intake, with about 40% of an average daily load being absorbed.[10] The relationship between Ca and Mg absorption is described as inverse, but the mechanism of this is unclear. Renal excretion is the main route of Mg elimination and it may vary with serum Mg concentration.[11] Thus, hypermagnesemia and hypercalcemia inhibit renal tubular reabsorption of Mg while hypomagnesemia and PTH increase Mg reabsorption.[11]

Effect of burn injury on calcium, phosphorus, and magnesium homeostasis

The effects of burn injury on mineral homeostasis have not been studied in great detail. Data from the studies at the University of Texas Medical Branch and the Shriners Burns Hospital in Galveston most completely describe some of the developments in this area.

A study of children burned >30% total body surface area demonstrated that serial measurements of blood ionized Ca were a mean of 5% below the lower limits of normal.[11] These levels were associated with serum levels of PTH that were too low for the ionized Ca concentration in the blood indicative that these patients were hypoparathyroid following acute burn injury. Furthermore, administration of a standard amount of PTH failed to produce the expected increases in urinary cyclic AMP and phosphate excretion,[12] providing evidence for PTH resistance in these patients. Mg depletion, encountered in all of the patients studied,[12,13] is known to impair secretion of PTH in response to hypocalcemia and to result in resistance to PTH infusion. A recent study at our hospital indicates that aggressive parenteral Mg supplementation will replete approximately 50% of the burn victims admitted to our institution. However, Mg repletion failed to improve the hypoparathyroidism.[13] Therefore, the cause of the postburn hypoparathyroidism remains unknown. Recent data obtained from animal studies show that there is an up-regulation of the parathyroid gland Ca-sensing receptor, which is associated in humans with decreased circulating Ca level necessary to suppress PTH secretion.[14] This phenomenon is known as a *reduced set point* for Ca suppression of PTH secretion. The underlying mechanisms are shown in Figure 27.2.

In data collected from 11 adult patients in the burn unit between December 1989 and January 1992[15] low serum concentrations of ionized Ca, P, and Mg were far more common than high serum levels of these minerals and is consistent with the abnormalities observed in their calcium homeostasis. Six patients had low serum concentrations of ionized Ca, three of them manifesting the hypocalcemia during the first 48 hours

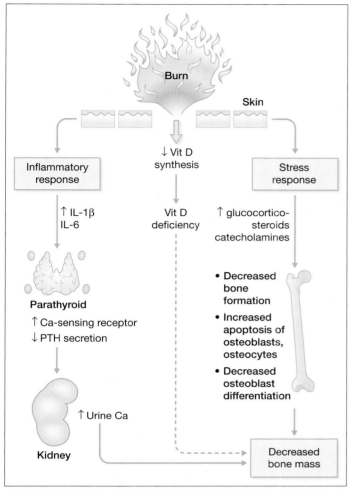

Fig. 27.2 Mechanisms of bone loss after severe burn.

postburn. Four of these patients were hypophosphatemic; this was most prevalent on day 7 postburn. Five of the patients were hypomagnesemic, with this finding most likely to be present on day 3 postburn. In contrast, only one patient demonstrated hypercalcemia and one hyperphosphatemia. No one was hypermagnesemic. In each case, the elevated serum level of either ionized Ca or P was transient. The studies in adults are not as yet as detailed as the studies in children have been in this regard.

Hypocalcemia cannot be diagnosed from determinations of total serum Ca concentration, due to the variability of serum albumin concentrations postburn. Determination of serum ionized Ca concentration should be encouraged, if available, for a more accurate diagnosis. Several possible mechanisms for hypocalcemia have been proposed. One is a shift of Ca from the extracellular to the intracellular compartment, as has been suggested by the accumulation of Ca in the erythrocyte of the burn patient,[16] a manifestation of what is termed the 'sick cell' syndrome. Alternative hypotheses include increased urinary calcium excretion, which has been documented to occur in burned children,[17] but is consistent with the documented hypoparathyroidism.[12] Losses of Ca in tissue exudate could also theoretically contribute to hypocalcemia. While it

has been argued that the amount of Ca in wound exudate is probably insufficient to entirely account for postburn hypocalcemia,[18] there are not enough studies that actually measure Ca content of the burn wound exudate.

While fecal Ca losses can be high in burn patients[18] and the large amount of endogenous corticosteroids produced by burn injury may impair intestinal Ca absorption,[19] there is no evidence to suggest that hypocalcemia is caused by corticosteroid-induced impairment of intestinal reabsorption of Ca secreted into the intestinal lumen. Other proposed mechanisms include reduced bone turnover.[15,20] The possibility of the reduced set point for calcium suppression of PTH secretion as a contributor to postburn hypocalcemia, while preliminary,[14] is an attractive hypothesis.

Studies investigating the metabolism of 25-hydroxyvitamin D and 1,25-dihydroxyvitamin D in 24 children with massive burns demonstrated a low serum concentration of 25-hydroxyvitamin D at 14 months and up to 7 years after trauma, correlating with low bone mineral density (BMD) z-scores. In contrast, concentrations of 1,25-dihydroxyvitamin D were normal 2 years after burn but showed a decrease to lower levels at 7 years after burn. This process suggests that these patients are becoming progressively vitamin D deficient.[21]

Possible explanations for postburn hypophosphatemia include intracellular accumulation of phosphate, inadequate phosphate intake, excessive urinary phosphate excretion, not likely in view of the documented hypoparathyroidism, or phosphate loss into the extravascular fluid. In a review of the subject, Dolecek[18] found increased urinary phosphate excretion only during the third and fourth weeks postburn in adults, while hypophosphatemia was documented to occur earlier. Thus, it is possible that the increased urinary phosphate excretion, seen later postburn, is more a function of increased tissue breakdown and filtered load than of inappropriate or excessive urinary phosphate losses. There is little documentation of inadequate phosphate intake following burns. Burn victims at our institution have been documented to take in a minimum of 1.6 g phosphate per day in enteral feedings alone.[15] Loss of significant phosphate in the extravascular fluid, excessive secretion of phosphate into the intestine with failure to reabsorb, and intracellular accumulation are all theoretically possible explanations for hypophosphatemia, but remain unproven. Similarly, the cause of sustained hypomagnesemia occurring postburn is unknown, although excessive urinary and fecal losses have been reported in adults[18] and excessive losses in the burn wound have also been described.[22]

One potential explanation for acute hypomagnesemia is resuscitation with Ringer's lactate, which does not contain Mg.[14]

Rationale for therapy

Because of their importance in the maintenance of bodily metabolic processes, low serum levels of ionized Ca, P, and Mg should be treated (Figure 27.3). Hypocalcemia, especially in the immediate postburn period during the resuscitation effort, can potentiate abnormalities of cardiac muscle produced by hyperkalemia[23] and cause unresponsiveness to repletion in shock.[23] If a patient is not hypocalcemic, there is insufficient evidence of benefit following provision of

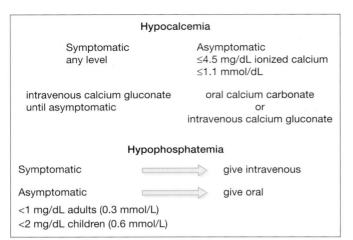

Fig. 27.3 Treatment algorithm for hypocalcemia and hypophosphatemia.

parenteral Ca during resuscitation[24–26] unless the patient has hyperkalemia, hypomagnesemia, or Ca channel blocker toxicity.[27] Similarly, while caution should be exercised during massive transfusion with citrate-containing blood, Ca therapy may not be necessary if the patient is normocalcemic and if hepatic and renal function are only minimally impaired. The liver will clear citrate, which may transiently chelate Ca, at a rate of 1 unit of blood transfused every 5 minutes.[28] Only when clinical and electrocardiographic evidence suggests hypocalcemia should treatment be initiated. Ca infusions, when given, should be administered slowly, since rapid replacement of Ca has resulted in cardiac arrhythmias.[23,28]

Hypophosphatemia may result in tissue hypoxemia due to increased hemoglobin affinity for oxygen and decreased tissue ATP, metabolic encephalopathy, hemolysis, shortened platelet survival time, myalgias, weakness, and possible impairment of myocardial contractility.[29] Hypomagnesemia, or Mg depletion with normal serum Mg, can blunt the effect of parathyroid hormone secreted in response to hypocalcemia on target organs and can impair the secretion of parathyroid hormone itself.[30] Mg deficiency can also cause generalized convulsions, muscle tremors, and weakness.[30]

Treatment options to maintain mineral homeostasis

Acute symptomatic hypocalcemia should be treated with intravenous Ca. In adults, 90–180 mg of elemental Ca over 5–10 minutes is given so as to reverse twitching. In infants or children, Ca chloride in a 20 mg/kg dose or Ca gluconate in a 200–500 mg/kg/dose in four divided doses is suggested.[30,31] Caution should attend the use of parenteral chloride since it may cause phlebitis and/or acidosis. While hypocalcemia is asymptomatic and patients can tolerate enteral feedings, milk and/or infant formula, can provide as much as 3 g/day of bioavailable Ca.[15] If, as we and others have found, hypocalcemia can occur despite enteral provision of such a large quantity of Ca, intermittent parenteral administration of Ca salts will be necessary. While the amounts given to each patient must be determined individually, as an example of what may be needed,

six of our recent patients with burns exceeding 40% TBSA received 0.9 to 15 grams of 10% calcium gluconate per day over the first 5 weeks following burn injury. Treatment was given an average of twice daily on approximately 75% of the days during those 5 weeks.

Symptomatic hypophosphatemia requires parenteral treatment with a starting dose of 2 mg/kg infused over 6 hours and treatment continued until serum P concentrations exceed 1.0 mg/dL (0.3 mmol/L).[29] Infants and children with symptomatic hypophosphatemia should receive 5–10 mg/kg infused over 6 hours followed by 15–45 mg/kg given by infusion over 24 hours or until the serum P concentration rises above 2.0 mg/dL (0.6 mmol/L).[32]

Our adult patients who tolerated enteral feedings and consumed an average of 1.6 g/day of phosphate should have consumed enough to treat asymptomatic hypophosphatemia.[15] Hypophosphatemia has not been reported to be prolonged in burn patients; however, in such cases where this may occur, parenteral supplementation would be necessary.

Patients who have signs or symptoms of Mg deficiency with serum Mg concentration below 1.5 mEq/L (1.8 mg/dL or 0.8 mmol/L) usually require parenteral therapy.[30–33] A treatment plan is displayed in Figure 27.3.

Bone

The main Ca storage depot in the body is bone. Both linear growth and bone remodeling are adversely affected by burn injury. Linear growth at the epiphysis of the long bones usually occurs by means of proliferation of cartilage cells with production of extracellular matrix; these chondrocytes and matrix undergo a series of biochemical changes which lead to the appearance of ossification centers, which appear as single expanding foci. As these ossifications expand, cartilaginous tissue is replaced by bone in a vascular supply system, which provides for the delivery of nutrients, hormones, and growth factors.

It has been reported by Rutan and Herndon[34] that linear growth velocity is retarded in children with severe burns. The mechanism for this effect of burn injury is unknown, but it has been established that the rate of growth does return to normal.[34] The effects of burn injury on bone remodeling are profound and long-lasting. In a study of 12 adult patients with burns of greater than 50% total body surface area, there was a marked reduction in bone formation.[15] In children the findings are more dramatic. Iliac crest bone biopsies from 18 children burned over 40% of their total body surface area revealed even more markedly depressed bone formation[20] and a cross-sectional study of children undergoing biopsy a mean of 5 years after suffering a similar-sized burn injury revealed that fully 50% of them had persistent decreased bone formation.[35] To put these findings in perspective, it is necessary to discuss the normal process of bone remodeling.

Bone remodeling is a continuous process of breakdown of calcified bone matrix by osteoclasts and formation of new bone matrix by osteoblasts and the mineralization of that matrix by calcium and phosphate forming a mature crystal lattice of calcium phosphate hydroxyapatite. One remodeling cycle takes about 4 months in an adult. Bone resorption and formation are normally biochemically and, perhaps mechanically, linked. All the details of this linkage are not known, but, as an example, parathyroid hormone receptors have been identified on osteoblasts but have so far not been identified on osteoclasts.[36] Thus, parathyroid hormone can increase the number of osteoblasts on bone surfaces in both humans[37] and animals.[38] Therefore, osteoblasts, which are bone-forming cells, must serve as an intermediary in the process of parathyroid hormone-mediated bone resorption. One way in which osteoblasts could act in this direction is to produce a ligand of the receptor activator of nuclear factor-κB (NF-κB), (RANK ligand or RANKL), to stimulate osteoclastogenesis in the bone marrow.[39]

The reduced bone formation following burn injury was first identified on bone biopsies in adults between 9 weeks and 9 months postburn.[15] By administering tetracycline to the patients in two doses separated by 2 weeks, we found that the newly-mineralized bone surface taking up tetracycline was markedly reduced in burned patients compared to age- and sex-matched controls[15] In contrast, the distance between the two tetracycline fluorescent labels in the bone was not significantly reduced. The distance between the tetracycline bands represents the *mineral apposition rate*, and is an index of osteoblast function. The mineral apposition rate when multiplied by the percentage of bone surface taking up tetracycline is the *bone formation rate*,[40] and is an index of osteoblast number as well as function. Thus, in the adult burn patients, bone formation is reduced possibly due to a reduced number of osteoblasts rather than to reduced osteoblast function. Also consistent with these findings is the reduced amount of osteoid or unmineralized bone matrix, a product of osteoblasts (Figures 27.4 and 27.5). There appears to be a dissociation of bone formation and bone resorption. In children, there is no separation between tetracycline labels,[20] indicating that osteoblast function as well as osteoblast number may be impaired. Furthermore, in the children biochemical markers of both bone formation and bone resorption are reduced,[20] suggesting lower

bone turnover that is seen with chronic elevation of glucocorticoid production,[41] which has been identified in these patients. Bone biopsies in adults are consistent with these findings.

The consequences of the reduced bone formation include chronically diminished bone mineral density of the lumbar spine.[17,20] This results in an increased fracture risk[17] and possible reduction in *peak bone* mass.[17] A reduction in peak bone mass would put a burned child at risk to develop adult-onset osteoporosis (Figure 27.6). Cross-sectional studies of bone mineral density of the lumbar spine were performed using dual-energy X-ray absorptiometry (DEXA) in 68 children:[17] 16 were burned between 15 and 36% of total body surface area, 22 were burned over 40% of total body surface area and studied within 8 weeks of their burn, and 30, also with burns over 40% of total body surface area, were studied a mean of 5 years following burn injury. The bone density z-scores (standard deviation scores) were less than −1 in 60% of the severely burned patients and less than −2 in 27% of the same group with no difference between those studied within 8 weeks and

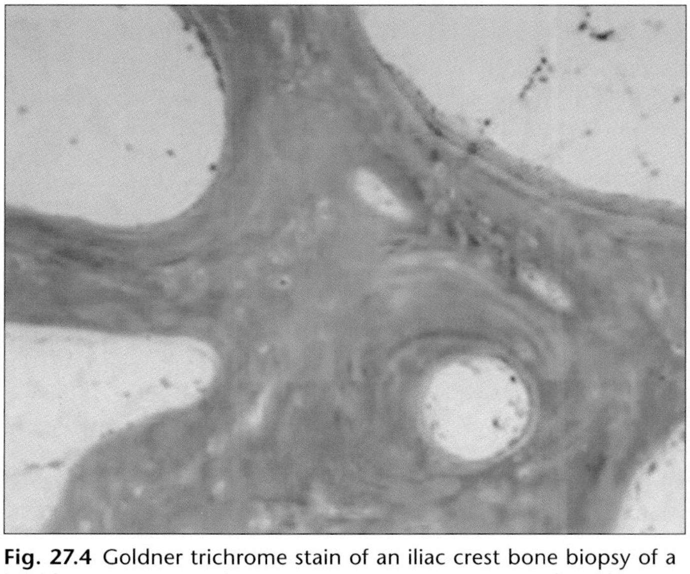

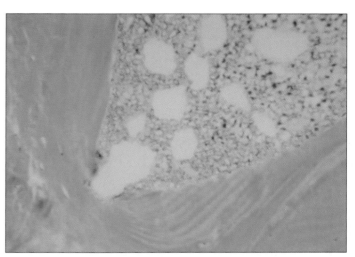

Fig. 27.5 Goldner trichrome stain of an iliac crest bone biopsy of a burned patient. The blue-green area represents mineralized bone. Compared to the previous figure, note that osteoblasts are absent on the osteoid surface.

Fig. 27.4 Goldner trichrome stain of an iliac crest bone biopsy of a healthy person. The blue-green area represents mineralized bone. The red area represents unmineralized osteoid. Spindle-shaped cells on the osteoid surface are osteoblasts.

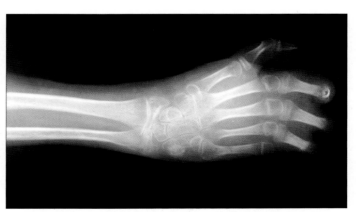

Fig. 27.6 X-ray as an example of burn-induced osteoporosis 1 year after trauma.

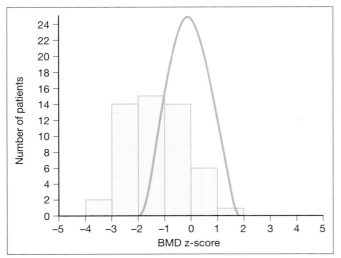

Fig. 27.7 Distribution of lumbar spine bone mineral density (BMD) z-scores of severely burned children compared to a standard distribution curve. Note that the distribution after burn is shifted to the negative side.

those studied a mean of 5 years following burn injury (Figure 27.7). Z-scores were not as low for those receiving moderate burns. These data suggest that the bone density in the severely burned children compared to age-related normal children is decreased[17] and that there is no significant improvement of bone density over time. Longitudinal studies are currently in progress in order to better define the issues causing the prolonged reduction in bone density.

There are several potential contributing factors to this pathology, including the production of pro-inflammatory cytokines, especially interleukins-1β and -6[20] immobilization, which induces bone resorption and decreases formation.[42] However, while bone resorption maybe transiently stimulated by cytokines and elevated glucocorticoids, which stimulate RANKL production by the osteoblasts, the extent of apoptosis of osteoblasts and the lack of differentiation in the bone marrow, eventually eliminate the production of RANKL and lead to chronic low turn-over disease.[41] Another possible contributing factor is aluminum loading, which can cause reduced bone formation in uremic patients[43] and in those receiving total parenteral nutrition.[44–50]

Treatment options for bone catabolism after severe burn

Studies have been conducted to address bone mass wasting after a massive thermal injury. Attempts to use high-dose recombinant human growth hormone (rhGH), 0.2 mg/kg/day subcutaneously during the course of hospitalization for the acute burn injury led to a rise in circulating levels of insulin-like growth factor 1 (IGF-1). However, serum levels of osteocalcin, a vitamin D- and vitamin K-dependent peptide produced by osteoblasts and which serves as an index of bone formation remained low following a 6-week period of treatment. The failure of rhGH to improve bone formation despite producing a rise in circulating IGF-1 may be attributable to GH-independent high circulating levels of IGF-binding protein-4 (IGFBP-

4), a binding protein that can block access of IGF-1 to local tissue receptors. Similarly, circulating levels of IGFBP-5, a binding protein that can help bind IGF-1 to hydroxyapatite matrix of bone, is initially low following a burn, rising to normal by time of hospital discharge.[51]

In contrast, the use of rhGH at a dose of 0.05 mg/kg/day subcutaneously from hospital discharge to 12 months in children after burn resulted in a significant improvement in linear height as well as bone mineral content when compared to placebo treatment. These beneficial observations continued in the second year after burn while the drug was discontinued. No adverse side effects such as rebound phenomena on growth and bone formation once rhGH was stopped were noted. This treatment with rhGH over an extended period during the rehabilitation phase after burn caused a significant increase in serum concentrations of anabolic acting hormones such as growth hormone, IGF-1, and IGFBP-3, while IGFBP-4 remains elevated, suggesting that this protein was not the cause of failure to increase osteocalcin induction as previously thought.[52] In contrast, serum concentrations of cortisol were significantly decreased in patients who received rhGH. The capacity of anabolic agents to reverse posttraumatic bone catabolism is supported by a study performed in children with a TBSA ≥40% receiving oxandrolone, an anabolic steroid, from discharge to 12 months after burn.[53,54] In this study oxandrolone was given at a dose of 0.1 mg/kg/bid daily and treated patients showed significant improvements in growth percentiles as well as in bone mineral content when compared to patients treated with placebo.[54] In each case, the increase in bone mineral content was preceded 6 months by a rise in lean body mass, reflective of muscle mass. It is possible that the effects of anabolic agents on bone are indirectly resulting from increased skeletal loading following an increase in skeletal muscle mass.[52,54] In addition to anabolic agents, therapies used successfully in the treatment of menopause-associated osteoporosis are also shown to be beneficial in burn-induced bone catabolism. In a randomized, double-blind, placebo-controlled clinical trial, severely burned children with a TBSA ≥40% received pamidronate at a dose of 1.5 mg/kg intravenously within 10 days of the burn and again 1 week later. At hospital discharge, lumbar spine bone mineral content was significantly improved in patients who received the bisphosphonate pamidronate. While this significant difference continued, total bone mineral content was additionally significantly improved at 6 months after burn. Bone histomorphometry and urine concentrations of Ca and free deoxypyridinoline were not affected by pamidronate. The treatment did not reveal any negative side effects such as hypocalcemia.[55]

In comparison to the past, we now have therapies available to attenuate bone loss after severe burn. Independent from the time phase after burn, these treatment options can be used during the acute hospitalization such as pamidronate or during the rehabilitation in the months after burn such as rhGH and oxandrolone. Future directions include the investigation of additional agents such as vitamin D supplementation on the acquisition of bone mass as it has been shown that serum levels of 25-hydroxyvitamin D correlate with bone density[21] and that the skin of burned patients is not able to convert 7-dehydrocholesterol to adequate circulating levels of active vitamin D, suggesting an absolute need to supplement this vitamin.[56]

References

1. Broadus AE. Mineral balance and homeostasis. In: Favus MJ, ed. Primer on the metabolic bone diseases and disorders of mineral metabolism, 4th edn. Philadelphia: Lippincott Williams and Wilkins; 1999:74–79.
2. Joff GA, Rosenberg RB. Physiology of hemostasis, the fluid phase. In: Nathan DG, Oski FA, eds. Hematology of infancy and childhood. Philadelphia: WB Saunders; 1993:1534–1560.
3. Rasmussen H. The calcium messenger system. N Engl J Med 1986; 314:1094–1101.
4. Neer RM. Calcium and inorganic phosphate homeostasis. In: DeGroot LJ, ed. Endocrinology. Philadelphia: WB Saunders; 1989:927–953.
5. Klein GL, Coburn JW. Parenteral nutrition: effect on bone and mineral homeostasis. Annu Rev Nutr 1991; 11:93–119.
6. Portale AA, Halloran BP, Murphy MM, et al. Oral intake of phosphorus can determine the serum concentration of 1,25-dihydroxyvitamin D by determining production rate in humans. J Clin Invest 1986; 77:7–12.
7. Shimda T, Yamazaki Y, Takahashi M, et al. Vitamin D receptor-independent FGF23 actions in regulating phosphate and vitamin D metabolism. Am J Physiol Renal Physiol 2005; 289: F1088–F1095.
8. Yu X, Ibrahimi O, Goetz R, et al. Analysis of the biochemical mechanisms for the endocrine actions of fibroblast growth factor–23. Endocrinology 2005; 146(11):4647–4656.
9. Silverberg SJ. The distribution and balance of calcium, magnesium and phosphorus. In: Favus MJ, ed. Primer on the metabolic bone diseases and disorders of mineral metabolism, 1st edn. Kelseyville, CA: American Society for Bone and Mineral Research; 1990: 32–36.
10. Lemann J Jr, Favus MJ. The intestinal absorption of calcium, magnesium, and phosphate. In: Favus MJ, ed. Primer on the metabolic bone diseases and disorders of mineral metabolism, 4th edn. Philadelphia: Lippincott Williams and Wilkins; 1999:63–66.
11. Bushinsky DA. Calcium, magnesium, and phosphorus: renal handling and urinary excretion. In: Favus MJ, ed. Primer on the metabolic bone diseases and disorders of mineral metabolism, 4th edn. Philadelphia: Lippincott Williams and Wilkins; 1999:67–73.
12. Klein GL, Nicolai M, Langman CB, et al. Dysregulation of calcium homeostasis after severe burn injury in children: possible role of magnesium depletion. J Pediatr 1997; 131:246–251.
13. Klein GL, Langman CB, Herndon DN. Persistent hypoparathyroidism following magnesium repletion of burn-injured children. Pediatr Nephrol 2000; 14:301–304.
14. Murphey ED, Chattopadhyay N, Bai M, et al. Up-regulation of the parathyroid calcium-sensing receptor after burn injury in sheep: A potential contributory factor to postburn hypocalcemia. Crit Care Med 2000; 28(12):3885–3890.
15. Klein GL, Herndon DN, Rutan TC, et al. Bone disease in burn patients. J Bone Miner Res 1993; 8: 337–345
16. Baar S. The effect of thermal injury on the loss of calcium from calcium loaded cells: its relationship to red cell function and patient survival. Clin Chem Acta 1982; 126:25–39.
17. Klein GL, Herndon D N, Langman CB, et al. Long-term reduction in bone mass following severe burn injury in children. J Pediatr 1995; 126:252–256.
18. Dolecek R. Calcium-active hormones and postburn low-calcium syndrome. In: Dolecek R, Brizio-Moltens L, Moltens A, et al., eds. Endocrinology of thermal trauma: pathophysiologic mechanisms and clinical interpretation. Philadelphia: Lea and Febiger; 1990: 216–237.
19. Hahn TJ, Halstead LR, Teitelbaum SI, et al. Altered mineral metabolism in glucocorticoid induced osteopenia. Effect of 25-hydroxyvitamin D administration. J Clin Invest 1979; 64:655–665.
20. Klein GL, Herndon DN, Goodman WG, et al. Histomorphometric and biochemical characterization of bone following acute severe burns in children. Bone 1995; 17:455–460.
21. Klein GL, Langman CB, Herndon DN. Vitamin D depletion following burn injury in children: a possible factor in postburn osteopenia. J Trauma 2002; 52(2):346–350.
22. Berger MM, Rothen C, Cavadini C, et al. Exudative mineral losses after serious burns: a clue to the alterations of magnesium and phosphate metabolism. Am J Clin Nutr 1997; 65:1473–1481.
23. British Committee for Standardization in Haematology Blood Transfusion Task Force. Guidelines for transfusion for massive blood loss. Clin Lab Haematol 1988; 10:265–273.
24. Stueven H, Thompson BM, Aprahamian C, et al. Use of calcium in pre-hospital cardiac arrest. Ann Emerg Med 1983; 12:136–139.
25. Stueven HA, Thompson BM, Aprahamian C, et al. Calcium chloride, reassessment of use in asystole. Ann Emerg Med 1984; 13: 820–822.
26. Harrison EE, Amey BD. Use of calcium in electromechanical dissociation. Ann Emerg Med 1984; 13:844–845.
27. Harinan RJ, Mangiardi LM, McAllister RG, et al. Reversal of cardiovascular effects of verapamil by calcium and sodium. Differences between electrophysiologic and hemodynamic response. Circulation 1979; 59:797–804.
28. Dzik WH, Kirkley SA. Citrate toxicity during massive blood transfusion. Transfusion Med Rev 1988; 2:76–94.
29. Hruska KA, Lederer E. Hyperphosphatemia and hypophosphatemia In: Favus MJ, ed. Primer on the metabolic bone diseases and disorders of mineral metabolism, 4th edn. Philadelphia: Lippincott Williams and Wilkins; 1999:245–253.
30. Rude RK. Magnesium depletion and hypermagnesemia. In: Favus MJ, ed. Primer on the metabolic bone disease and disorders of mineral metabolism, 4th edn. Philadelphia: Lippincott Williams and Wilkins; 1999:241–244.
31. Shane E. Hypocalcemia: pathogenesis, differential diagnosis, and management. In: Favus MJ, ed. Primer on the metabolic bone diseases and disorders of mineral metabolism, 4th edn. Philadelphia: Lippincott Williams and Wilkins; 1999:223–225.
32. Carpenter TO. Neonatal hypocalcemia. In: Favus MJ, ed. Primer on the metabolic bone diseases and disorders of mineral metabolism, 4th edn. Philadelphia: Lippincott Williams and Wilkins; 1999:235–237.
33. Greene MG. In: The Harriet Lane handbook. St Louis, MO: Mosby-Yearbook; 1991:150–244.
34. Rutan RL, Herndon DN. Growth delay in postburn pediatric patients. Arch Surg 1990; 125:392–395.
35. Klein GL, Wolf SE, Goodman WG, et al. The management of acute bone loss in severe catabolism due to burn injury. Hormone Res 1997; 48(Suppl 5):83–87.
36. Simmons DJ, Seitz PK, Kidder LS, et al. Partial characterization of marrow stromal cells. Calcif Tissue Int 1991; 48:326–334.
37. Parisien M, Charhon SA, Arlot M, et al. Evidence for a toxic effect of aluminum on osteoblasts: a histomorphometric study in hemodialysis patients with aplastic bone disease. J Bone Miner Res 1988; 3:259–267.
38. Rodriguez M, Felsenfeld AJ, Llach F. Aluminum administration in the rat separately affects the osteoblast and bone mineralization. J Bone Miner Res 1990; 5:59–67.
39. Hofbauer LC, Gori F, Riggs BL, et al. Stimulation of osteoprotegerin ligand and inhibition of osteoprotegerin production by glucocorticoids in human osteoblastic lineage cells: potential paracrine mechanisms for glucocorticoid-induced osteoporosis. Endocrinology 1999; 140:4382–4389.
40. Parfitt AM, Drezner MK, Glorieux FH, et al. Bone histomorphometry: standardization of nomenclature symbols and units. Report of the ASBMR Histomorphometry Nomenclature Committee. J Bone Miner Res 1987; 2:595–610.
41. Klein GL, Bi LX, Sherrard DJ, et al. Evidence supporting a role of glucocorticoids in short-term bone loss in burned children. Osteoporos Int 2004; 15:468–474.
42. Ishimi Y, Miyausa C, Jin CH, et al. IL-6 is produced by osteoblasts and induces bone resorption. J Immunol 1990; 145: 3297–3303.
43. Ott SM, Maloney NA, Coburn JW, et al. The prevalence of bone aluminum deposition in renal osteodystrophy and its relation to the response to calcitriol therapy. N Engl J Med 1982; 307: 709–713.

44. Ott SM, Maloney NA, Klein GL, et al. Aluminum is associated with low bone formation in patients receiving chronic parenteral nutrition. Ann Intern Med 1983; 98:910–914.

45. Milliner DS, Shinaberger JH, Shuman P, et al. Inadvertent aluminum administration during plasma exchange due to aluminum contamination of albumin replacement solutions. N Engl J Med 1985; 312:165–167.

46. Sedman AB, Klein GL, Merritt RJ, et al. Evidence of aluminum loading in infants receiving intravenous therapy. N Engl J Med 1985; 312:1337–1343.

47. Koo WWK, Kaplan LA, Horn J, et al. Aluminum in parenteral nutrition solutions – sources and possible alternatives. J Parenter Enter Nutr 1986; 10:591–595.

48. Klein GL, Herndon DN, Rutan TC, et al. Risk of aluminum loading in burn patients and ways to reduce it. J Burn Care Rehabil 1994; 15:354–358.

49. Arnaud SB, Sherrard DJ, Maloney NA, et al. Effects of one-week head-down tilt bed rest on bone formation with calcium endocrine system. Aviat Space Environ Med 1992; 63:14–20.

50. Leukens S, Arnaud SB, Taylor AK, et al. Immobilization causes an acute and sustained increase in markers of bone resorption. Clin Res 1990; 38:123A.

51. Klein GL, Wolf SE, Langman CB, et al. Effect of therapy with recombinant human growth hormone on insulin-like growth factor system components and serum levels of biochemical markers of bone formation in children following severe burn injury. J Clin Endocrinol Metab 1998; 83:21–24.

52. Hart DW, Wolf SE, Klein GL, et al. Attenuation of post-traumatic muscle catabolism and osteopenia by long-term growth hormone therapy. Ann Surg 2001; 233(6):827–834.

53. Murphy KD, Thomas S, Mlcak RP, et al. Effects of long-term oxandrolone administration in severely burned children. Surgery 2004; 136(2):219–224.

54. Przkora R, Jeschke MG, Barrow RE, et al. Metabolic and hormonal changes of severely burned children receiving long-term oxandrolone treatment. Ann Surg 2005; 242(3):384–389.

55. Klein GL, Wimalawansa SJ, Kulkarni G, et al. The efficacy of acute administration of pamidronate on the conservation of bone mass following severe burn injury in children: a double-blind, randomized, controlled study. Osteoporos Int 2005; 16(6):631–635.

56. Klein GL, Chen TC, Holick MF, et al. Synthesis of vitamin D in skin after burns. Lancet 2004; 363(9405):291–292.

Chapter 28

Vitamin and trace element homeostasis following severe burn injury

Gordon L. Klein, Rene Przkora, and David N. Herndon

Importance of vitamins and trace elements

Trace elements and vitamins are a key part in nearly every cell mechanism of the human body. However, there remains very little understood about the effects of burn injury on trace element and vitamin metabolism and post-burn requirements. The limited research that has been done has concentrated on homeostasis of trace elements and vitamins after burn injury, wound healing in relation to trace elements, vitamins, and the antioxidant properties of various of the trace elements and vitamins. We will examine each of these aspects in the context of available data.

Homeostasis of trace elements and vitamins and role in burns

There are limited data regarding trace element loss following burn injury. The major trace elements studied are zinc and copper, although a limited amount of work has also been done on selenium status post-burn.

Several groups have reported low serum concentrations of zinc and copper, as well as albumin and ceruloplasmin, their respective associated binding proteins.[1-6] Urine and skin are considered major routes of loss of these elements.[3,5,7] Thus, Cunningham et al.[5] and Boosalis et al.[8] found that patients with moderate to severe burns had excessive urinary zinc excretion associated with reduced plasma zinc levels, especially the plasma subfraction bound to albumin.[5] Zinc supplementation by means of total parenteral nutrition resulted in hyperzincuria, although not as pronounced as if zinc supplementation were given orally.[5,8] In contrast, increased urinary copper excretion was not found despite parenteral delivery of supplemental copper, although both plasma copper and ceruloplasmin were reduced. Only a few studies documented an increase in urinary copper excretion.[1,9] Voruganti et al.[9] found elevated urinary copper and zinc excretion in severely burned children at admission as well as at hospital discharge. The

pediatric burn patients in this study received up to three times the suggested oral intake of zinc and copper compared to the dietary reference intakes. Thus it would appear as if while there is a consensus that plasma copper and zinc concentrations fall post-burn, the observation of urinary losses of micronutrients such as zinc and copper vary and the functional impact remains unexplained.

With regard to cutaneous losses of zinc, Berger et al.[7] found that the losses through wound exudate greatly exceeded excretory losses over the first week post-burn. Guo et al.[1] also detected elevated quantities of zinc in wound exudate. These observations have been confirmed additionally in children. Wound zinc and copper concentrations exceeded plasma concentrations in six children with a mean total body surface area (TBSA) of 54%.[9] The other explanation offered for the uniformly reported fall in plasma zinc levels post-burn is the redistribution of zinc within the body. In a study in which rats given ^{65}Zn received a 20% TBSA burn, van Rij et al.[10] reported that there was a rapid uptake of ^{65}Zn by spleen, kidney, wound, and, particularly, liver, while there was a decrease in ^{65}Zn in brain, muscle, and, particularly, bone. Zinc-binding protein was demonstrated in the liver cytosol, suggesting that there is a flow of zinc to the liver at the expense of plasma, bone and, even wound, after burn injury. Agay et al.[11] reported a redistribution of zinc and copper to the liver without significant changes in the muscle and brain. This study analyzed additionally related antioxidant enzymes such as the superoxide dismutase and found a decrease of activity mainly in the plasma after burn. It was also found by Cunningham et al.[5] that zinc supplementation exacerbates the urinary zinc excretion, suggesting that the body cannot take up the supplemental zinc and perhaps suggesting that rather than zinc depletion, zinc redistribution is largely responsible for the low plasma levels. Consistent with this, zinc is also involved in the inflammatory response and could be redistributed to sites of barrier disruption such as skin to be lost subsequently in the wound exudate.

With regard to copper, it is clear that reduced plasma copper concentrations are associated with reduced circulating levels of ceruloplasmin.[2,6] Even though ceruloplasmin is an acute phase reactant stimulated by pro-inflammatory cytokines such as interleukin-1,[12] which is known to be elevated in the post-burn inflammatory state,[13,14] there is also evidence that ceruloplasmin, in addition to copper, can be lost in the burn wound exudate as Cunningham et al.[2] reported a strong relationship between the size of the open wound and the amount of circulating ceruloplasmin. Gosling et al.[4] reported that copper concentration in severe burns varied inversely with burn surface area, in contrast to circulating zinc levels, which showed no such correlation. Furthermore, ceruloplasmin, like albumin, may be extravasated from the intravascular compartment and carry the copper with it.

Loss of zinc and copper following burn injury are of potential significance due to the important roles of each as antioxidants, especially as components of the enzyme superoxide dismutase, and the additional roles of zinc in wound healing, collagen cross-linking, which may affect skeletal calcification[13] and immune function.[15] Clearly, further studies will be required to elucidate the mechanism of hypocupremia and hypozincemia. Despite the supplementation of zinc and copper in patients after burn, the plasma concentrations remain low, probably requiring a higher intake. In a preliminary study, Voruganti et al.[9] supplemented pediatric patients with 40% TBSA burn with 22.5 mg zinc per day according to the reference intake given by Pochon,[16] who recommended 10–30 mg of zinc sulfate per day in children with >20% burn surface area. However, this quantity failed to raise plasma zinc levels. Based on this observation, we would recommend at least an intake of 30 mg zinc sulfate per day in these children. Additionally, in the study reported by Voruganti et al.,[9] the copper intake was 2–3 times higher than the dietary reference intake, which is 3 mg per day for 4–8 years old children and 5 mg per day for 9–13 years old children, without attaining normal plasma concentrations. In parallel with the zinc intake, the intake of copper should be further increased. Appropriate criteria have yet to be determined on which to base adequacy of copper and zinc supplementation.

Another trace element which acts as an antioxidant is selenium. In 1984, Hunt et al.[17] reported that plasma and erythrocyte selenium concentrations were reduced following burn injury, as was urinary selenium excretion. Boosalis et al.[18] confirmed these findings in 1986 and suggested that urinary selenium loss was not the chief explanation for the post-burn selenium deficiency. They postulated that there may be an antagonistic relationship between selenium and the silver that is administered to the burn wounds. A possible redistribution between different organ compartments after burn may be another explanation for the observed changes in selenium levels as reported by Agay et al. in burned rats.[11]

A trace element that is reported to be elevated following burn injury is aluminum. Klein et al.[19] reported elevated serum aluminum concentration in adults suffering severe burn injury (>40% TBSA), even finding some aluminum deposition in the bones of burn patients as few as 8 days post-burn.[20] While aluminum is toxic to bone and is a known inhibitor of bone formation,[20] it is clearly not the only contributor to post-burn osteopenia and increased fracture risk. Nonetheless, the sources of aluminum contamination in burn treatment have been published[21] and attempts to minimize aluminum loading in these patients may hasten their skeletal recovery from burn injury.

Studies of the homeostasis of vitamins following burn injury are sparse. Rettmer et al.[22] performed functional testing for thiamin, riboflavin, and pyridoxine in burn patients and found them all to be normal. However, many adult burn victims are alcoholic and will require the standard thiamine supplementation of 50 mg/day. In a study of serum vitamin K levels in severely burned pediatric patients, Jenkins et al.[23] reported that 91% of the 48 children studied demonstrated circulating vitamin K levels below expected norms. These low levels were correlated with days of antibiotic therapy, percentage body surface area excised, and administration of blood products. However, there was no relationship between serum vitamin K concentration and prothrombin time. Therefore, it is not certain if the low circulating levels of vitamin K are clinically significant. It should be pointed out, however, that osteocalcin, a protein produced by osteoblasts, is a vitamin K-dependent gamma carboxylated protein that is used as a standard index of new bone formation. Osteocalcin is documented to be low in burned children during the same time period covered by the study of Jenkins et al.,[23] i.e. the first 4 weeks post-burn. Thus, the possibility remains open that low circulating vitamin K levels may contribute to low osteocalcin in the serum, although bone formation has been documented to be low by other studies as well (see Chapter 27).

Serum levels of other vitamins have also been measured within 2–3 weeks post-burn. These were vitamin A (retinol), vitamin E (alpha tocopherol), and vitamin C (ascorbic acid). Nguyen et al.[24] reported low serum vitamin E levels during the first 14 days post-burn as part of a study examining peroxidation products following thermal injury. Similar findings were noted by Rock et al.[25] not only for vitamin E but also for vitamins A and C. However, serum levels of all these vitamins improved with enteral supplementation.

Circulating levels of vitamin D have been low but so has vitamin D-binding protein.[20,26] Serum calcitriol (1,25(OH)$_2$-vitamin D) levels have been slightly low, but calcitriol, the metabolically active form of vitamin D, is bound to albumin in serum. Therefore, in light of the post-burn hypoproteinemia it is difficult to assess the short-term significance of the marginally low levels of circulating vitamin D. However, preliminary data suggest that burn patients do develop vitamin D deficiency after they are discharged from the hospital due to the recommendation that they minimize their exposure to sunlight.[27] However, it is now reported that skin from burn scars and adjacent areas cannot synthesize normal amounts of vitamin D following exposure to ultraviolet light.[27] Thus, vitamin D supplementation is mandatory although the amount required is still under study. A more detailed description of the metabolism of vitamin D is given in Chapter 27.

Effect of therapy on wound healing, fluid requirements, and the immune response

Despite the well-known role that zinc plays in wound healing, relatively little is known of the effects of zinc depletion post-burn on healing of the burn wound. A recent *in vivo* study in rats by Li et al.[28] indicated that dietary zinc supplementation by itself may not be sufficient to improve wound healing. However, zinc applied directly to the experimental wound may accelerate healing. This subject is very difficult to evaluate, however, because of the evolving nature of wound management, including artificial skin, antibiotic therapy, and surgical intervention. There has also been a report suggesting that nicotinamide may increase capillary density and rapidity of wound healing in rats.[29]

With regard to other potentially beneficial effects of supplementation with trace elements of vitamins, there are conflicting studies regarding whether administration of ascorbic acid alters the volume of fluid required for initial burn resuscitation.[30–32] In a study from Japan by Tanaka et al.,[30] infusion of ascorbic acid during the initial 24 hours post-burn in adults burned over 30% TBSA lessened the amount of fluid required to maintain heart rate and blood pressure and cut by 50% the amount of body weight gain. This is consistent with an earlier report by Nelson et al.,[31] who found that guinea pigs given large quantities of dietary ascorbic acid following burn injury had improved weight gain and reduced metabolic rates compared to controls. In contrast, a study involving infusion of ascorbic acid into dogs given graded scald burns of the paw failed to reduce paw weight gain.[32] However, this study was limited to a local burn injury involving the paw and did not take into account other systemic factors that might affect body fluid accumulation after a more extensive burn. In addition, a report by Chen et al.[33] showed that pre-treatment of rats and mice with 1,25-dihydroxyvitamin D (calcitriol) lessens fat pad edema and pulmonary vascular permeability. However, this has limited practical value in that data are not available for human post-burn treatment with calcitriol.

Contradictory reports have also been published with regard to the effects of vitamin E on the immune response. Kuroiwa et al.[34] failed to demonstrate a difference in lymphocyte response to phytohemagglutinin or in ear thickness response to 2,4-dinitrofluorobenzene in guinea pigs following a 30% burn and vitamin E supplements ranging from 0 to 100 mg/kg/day, although those receiving vitamin E supplements were less anemic than those that did not. In contrast, Haberal et al.[35] showed in patients with a >20% partial- or full-thickness burn injury, vitamin E supplementation for 3 days resulted in an increased number of circulating T cells compared to normal and in contrast to burn patients who did not receive vitamin E. In agreement with Kuroiwa et al.,[33] Berger et al.,[36] studying severely burned adults, reported that supplementation of these patients 30 days post-burn with zinc, copper, and selenium for 8 days failed to alter lymphocyte proliferation to mitogens but the number of pulmonary infections in the supplemented group decreased, resulting in a shorter hospital stay when data were normalized for burn size.

In summary, there is much to learn regarding the homeostasis of trace elements and vitamins in response to burn injury and how changes in the status of these micronutrients affect wound healing, fluid resuscitation requirements, the immune response, and skeletal recovery. This area remains wide open to advances in research that could potentially hasten recovery and improve the quality of life for victims of severe burn injury.

References

1. Guo Z, Li L, Zhao L. [Changes in contents of Zn, Cu, Fe, Ca, Mg in serum, urine and blister fluid after burn surgery]. Chung Hua Zhonghua Zheng Xing Shao Shang Wai Ke Za Zhi 2000; 13:195–198. [in Chinese]
2. Cunningham JJ, Lydon MK, Emerson R, et al. Low ceruloplasmin levels during recovery from major burn injury: influence of open wound size and copper supplementation. Nutrition 2000; 12:83–88.
3. Selmanpakoglu AN, Cetin C, Sayal A, et al. Trace element (Al, Se, Zn, Cu) levels in serum, urine and tissues of burn patients. Burns 1994; 20:99–103.
4. Gosling P, Rothe HM, Sheehan TM, et al. Serum copper and zinc concentrations in patients with burns in relation to burn surface area. J Burn Care Rehabil 1995; 16:481–486.
5. Cunningham JJ, Lydon MK, Briggs SE, et al. Zinc and copper status of severely burned children during TPN. J Am Coll Nutr 1991; 10:57–62.
6. Shewmake KB, Talbert GE, Bowser-Wallace BH, et al. Alterations in plasma copper, zinc, and ceruloplasmin levels in patients with thermal trauma. J Burn Care Rehabil 1988; 9:13–17.
7. Berger MM, Cavadini C, Bart A, et al. Cutaneous copper and zinc losses in burns. Burns 1992; 18:373–380.
8. Boosalis MG, Solem LD, Cerra FB, et al. Increased urinary zinc excretion after thermal injury. J Lab Clin Med 1991; 118(6):538–545.
9. Voruganti VS, Klein GL, Lu HX, et al. Impaired zinc and copper status in children with burn injuries: need to reassess nutritional requirements. Burns 2005; 31:711–716.
10. Van Rij AM, Hall MT, Bray JT, et al. Zinc as an integral component of the metabolic response to trauma. Surg Gynecol Obstet 1981; 153:677–682.
11. Agay D, Anderson RA, Sandre C, et al. Alterations of antioxidant trace elements (Zn, Se, Cu) and related metallo-enzymes in plasma and tissues following burn injury in rats. Burns 2005; 31:366–371.
12. Daffada AA, Young SP. Coordinated regulation of ceruloplasmin and metallothionein mRNA by interleukin-1 and copper in HepG2 cells. FEBS Lett 1999; 457:214–218.
13. Klein GL, Herndon DN, Goodman WG, et al. Histomorphometric and biochemical characterization of bone following acute severe burns in children. Bone 1995; 17:455–460.
14. Kupper TJ, Deitch EA, Baker CC, et al. The human burn wound as a primary source of interleukin-1 activity. Surgery 1986; 100:409–415.
15. Keen CL, Gershwin ME. Zinc deficiency and immune function. Annu Rev Nutr 1990; 10:415–431.
16. Pochon JP. Zinc- and copper-replacement therapy – a must in burns and scalds in children? Prog Pediatr Surg 1981; 14:151–72.
17. Hunt DR, Lane HW, Beesinger D, et al. Selenium depletion in burn patients. J Parenter Enteral Nutr 1984; 8:695–699.
18. Boosalis MG, Solem LD, Ahrenholz DH, et al. Serum and urinary selenium levels in thermal injury. Burns Incl Therm Inj 1986; 12:236–240.
19. Klein GL, Herndon DN, Rutan TC, et al. Elevated serum aluminum levels in severely burned patients receiving large quantities of albumin. J Burn Care Rehabil 1990; 11:526–530.
20. Klein GL, Herndon DN, Rutan TC, et al. Bone disease in burn patients. J Bone Miner Res 1993; 8:337–345.
21. Klein GL, Herndon DN, Rutan TC, et al. Risk of aluminum accumulation in burn patients and ways to reduce it. J Burn Care Rehabil 1994; 15:354–358.
22. Rettmer RL, Williamson JC, Labbe RF, et al. Laboratory monitoring of nutritional status in burn patients. Clin Chem 1992; 38:334–337.
23. Jenkins ME, Gottschlich MM, Kopcha R, et al. A prospective analysis of serum vitamin K in severely burned pediatric patients. J Burn Care Rehabil 1998; 19:75–81.
24. Nguyen TT, Cox CS, Traber DL, et al. Free radical activity and loss of plasma antioxidants, vitamin E, and sulfhydryl groups in patients with burns: the 1993 Moyer Award. J Burn Care Rehabil 1993; 14:602–609.
25. Rock CL, Dechert RE, Khilnani R, et al. Carotenoids and antioxidant vitamins in patients after burn injury. J Burn Care Rehabil 1997; 18:269–278.

26. Klein GL, Langman CB, Herndon DN. Vitamin D depletion following burn injury in children: a possible factor in post-burn osteopenia. J Trauma 2002; 52(2):346–350.

27. Klein GL, Chen TC, Holick MF, et al. Synthesis of vitamin D in skin after burns. Lancet 2004; 363(9405):291–292.

28. Li L, Guo Z, Zhao L. [Effects of supplement Zn on levels of Zn in serum, growth hormone and hydroxyproline]. Zhonghua Zheng Xing Shao Shang Wai Ke Za Zhi 1998; 14:425–428. [in Chinese]

29. Smith YR, Klitzman B, Ellis MN, et al. The effect of nicotinamide on microvascular density and thermal injury in rats. J Surg Res 1989; 47:465–469.

30. Tanaka H, Matsuda T, Miyagantani Y, et al. Reduction of resuscitation fluid volumes in severely burned patients using ascorbic acid administration: a randomized, prospective study. Arch Surg 2000; 135:326–331.

31. Nelson JL, Alexander JW, Jacobs PA, et al. Metabolic and immune effects of enteral ascorbic acid after burn trauma. Burns 1992; 18:92–97.

32. Aliabadi-Wahle S, Gilman DA, Dabrowski GP, et al. Postburn vitamin C infusions do not alter early postburn edema formation. J Burn Care Rehabil 1999; 20:7–14.

33. Chen SF, Ruan YJ. 1 alpha, 25-dihydroxyvitamin D_3 decreases scalding-and-platelet-activating factor-induced high vascular permeability and tissue oedema. Pharmacol Toxicol 1995; 76: 365–367.

34. Kuroiwa K, Nelson JL, Boyce ST, et al. Metabolic and immune effect of vitamin E supplementation after burn. J Parenter Enteral Nutr 1991; 15:22–26.

35. Haberal M, Hamaloglu E, Bora S, et al. The effects of vitamin E on immune regulation after thermal injury. Burns Incl Therm Inj 1988; 14:388–393.

36. Berger MM, Cavadini C, Chiolero R, et al. Influence of large intakes of trace elements on recovery after major burns. Nutrition 1994; 10:327–334.

Chapter 29

Hypophosphatemia

David W. Mozingo and Arthur D. Mason Jr.

Certain humoral and metabolic responses to thermal and mechanical trauma that maintain homeostasis and prevent cellular dysfunction also produce alterations in electrolyte balance. An example is renal retention of sodium during the resuscitative phase of burn injury, which alters sodium balance in the course of preserving intravascular volume. Despite the markedly increased cardiac output and renal plasma flow that occur in the subsequent flow phase, a decrease in blood volume persists and results in sustained elevation of plasma renin activity, secretion of antidiuretic hormone, and sodium retention.[1] Conversely, the severe hypophosphatemia that often follows major injury occurs concomitantly with a 50–100% increase in resting energy expenditure, leading to a possible deficiency in the high-energy phosphate compounds essential for cellular metabolism. Thermal injury induces a precipitous decrease in serum phosphate concentration that reaches its nadir between the second and fifth postburn days. This phenomenon has been recognized for quite some time[2] and was recently confirmed by the authors in a large series of burn patients.[3] Despite aggressive phosphorus supplementation, normal levels of serum phosphorus are rarely reached prior to the tenth postburn day (Figure 29.1). Of 550 patients studied, 175 had serum phosphorus concentrations below 2.0 mg/dL, and of these 49 were below 1.0 mg/dL, with the lower limit of normal serum phosphorus being 3.0 mg/dL. Such hypophosphatemia is not exclusive to thermal injury, having been described following multiple trauma,[4] head injury,[5] and elective surgery.[6] The exact mechanism by which thermal injury or severe stress induces hypophosphatemia is unknown. Several events associated with burn injury, however, affect phosphorus metabolism, and these may combine to produce hypophosphatemia.

Etiology of postburn hypophosphatemia

Many of the pathophysiological changes and therapeutic interventions that occur during the first postburn week influence serum phosphorus concentration (Box 29.1). Hypophosphatemia does not necessarily imply phosphorus depletion; in the case of burn injury, most patients are healthy prior to injury and presumably have normal phosphorus stores. Nor do simple calculations of phosphate balance explain the dramatic decrease in serum levels; simultaneous reduction of urinary phosphate excretion is observed, suggesting an extrarenal mechanism. The fractional excretion of phosphate, however, increases during the early period of diuresis following burn injury (postburn days 2–4), potentially contributing to the decline in serum levels. The pathophysiological events and therapeutic interventions discussed below are associated with hypophosphatemia in other disease states and in certain experimental animal models, but the extent of their contributions to the postburn decrease in serum phosphorus has not been critically evaluated and is, at present, undefined.

Stress response

In the early postburn period, the classic 'fight or flight' response occurs, with elevation of plasma catecholamines, glucose, glucagon, and cortisol. Exogenous epinephrine administration has been associated with the development of hypophosphatemia, and the profound catecholamine release accompanying thermal injury may contribute to the early decrease in serum phosphorus. The mechanism by which this occurs is uncertain but may be a consequence of the accompanying hyperglycemia, resulting in a redistribution of phosphorus from the extracellular to the intracellular compartment (see section on Metabolic support). In acute clinical states of glucagon excess, tubular reabsorption of phosphate is impaired in both the proximal and distal nephron, leading one to expect renal phosphate wastage.[7] Since urinary excretion of phosphate is usually decreased in the early post-injury period, the importance of hyperglucagonemia remains uncertain. Administration of pharmacological doses of glucocorticoids enhances phosphorus excretion and impairs phosphate absorption by the gut and reabsorption by the kidney. Whether or not the adrenocortical response significantly contributes to the hypophosphatemia after burn injury is not known.

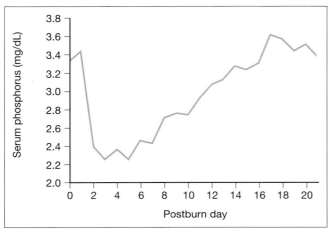

Fig. 29.1 Serum phosphorus levels abruptly decline with a nadir between postburn days 2 and 5. The data were obtained from 550 consecutive burn patients admitted to the US Army Institute of Surgical Research.

Box 29.1 Possible causes of postburn hypophosphatemia

FLUID RESUSCITATION
• volume loading
• lactate administration

CARBOHYDRATE ADMINISTRATION
• enteral alimentation
• parenteral hyperalimentation
• 5% dextrose

ELEVATED CATECHOLAMINES

PHOSPHATE-BINDING ANTACIDS/SUCRALFATE

ACID–BASE DISTURBANCE

ELECTROLYTE IMBALANCE
• hypokalemia
• hypomagnesemia
• hypocalcemia

CARBONIC ANHYDRASE INHIBITION (MAFENIDE ACETATE)

Resuscitation and topical therapy

Administration of large doses of sodium lactate for initial burn resuscitation may decrease the serum phosphorus concentration by several mechanisms.[8] Lactate is converted to glucose in the liver, a process requiring high-energy phosphate availability. Additionally, though it does not usually occur clinically, metabolic alkalosis induced by lactate infusion may result in depression of serum phosphorus concentration. Alkalosis is associated with an increase in glycolysis that promotes transfer of phosphorus to the intracellular space. During resuscitation, alkalemia is uncommon and patients are more likely to manifest a mild metabolic acidosis, which is compensated by hyperventilation, resulting in a normal or mildly alkaline blood pH. Acidosis markedly inhibits renal phosphate reabsorption, resulting in phosphaturia. The contribution of this mechanism to postburn hypophosphatemia is probably minor; early renal phosphate wastage is not observed, perhaps being obscured by diminished glomerular filtration early in burn injury. In addition, the *p*-carboxy metabolite of mafenide acetate strongly inhibits carbonic anhydrase. Such inhibition diminishes proximal tubular reabsorption of phosphate and probably occurs following topical burn wound treatment with mafenide, but the magnitude of the effect is unknown.

Expansion of the extracellular fluid volume is also associated with inhibition of proximal tubular phosphate reabsorption. A tight coupling exists between sodium and phosphate transport across the renal epithelial cell. In patients with burns, mobilization and excretion of the large edema volume usually begins by the second postburn day and continues throughout the next week to 10 days. In contrast to the relative paucity of phosphate excretion during the first 24 hours after injury, when glomerular filtration is markedly reduced, a modest loss of phosphate may occur with diuresis of the edema fluid. In fact, the diuretic phase is associated with an increase in the fractional excretion of phosphate despite a concomitant reduction in the serum phosphate concentration.[9] Phosphorus excretion during the natriuretic phase of early burn injury is consistent with the tight coupling observed in other diuretic states.

Ulcer prophylaxis

Effective prophylaxis against Curling's ulcers with H_2-antagonists and antacid buffering has been a mainstay of burn care for the past two decades. Significant degrees of hypophosphatemia and phosphate depletion occur during continuous or chronic administration of phosphate-binding agents containing magnesium, calcium, and aluminum. These agents bind not only dietary phosphate but also phosphate secreted into the intestinal lumen, often resulting in a net negative phosphate balance. The severity of such hypophosphatemia clearly depends on the dose of phosphate-binding agents, dietary phosphorus intake, and pre-existing phosphate balance. To reduce alimentary scavenging of dietary and secreted phosphate, buffering with antacids containing aluminum phosphate salts (Al_2PO_4), which do not bind any additional phosphate, may be utilized. Sucralfate, which is also effective in preventing upper gastrointestinal stress ulceration following thermal injury, is not a buffering agent, but as a complex salt of aluminum hydroxide, is capable of binding phosphate. Its administration has also been associated with the development of hypophosphatemia in critically ill patients.[10]

Hyperventilation

Respiratory alkalosis is often present during the first week postburn and may be enhanced by anxiety or pain, and even by the inhibition of carbonic anhydrase induced by mafenide acetate burn cream. As fluid resuscitation progresses, respiratory rate and tidal volume progressively increase, resulting in minute ventilation that may be twice normal. Mild hyperventilation induces only a slight decline of serum phosphorus levels; prolonged, intense hyperventilation, however, may result in serum phosphorus values less than 1.0 mg/dL.[11] During respiratory alkalosis, phosphorus virtually disappears from the urine, eliminating renal losses as the causative mechanism. Respiratory alkalosis induces a rapid movement of carbon dioxide from the intracellular to the extracellular space. Intracellular pH increases, activating glycolysis and increasing the formation of intracellular phosphorylated carbohydrate compounds. The readily diffusible inorganic phosphate pool supplies the required phosphorus, and serum phosphorus concentrations consequently fall abruptly. The extent to which this mechanism contributes to postburn hypophosphatemia is uncertain.

Metabolic support

Administration of carbohydrates may play a major role in the development of postburn hypophosphatemia. Infusion of glucose solutions or oral intake of carbohydrates produces mild hypophosphatemia in healthy individuals. This decrease in serum phosphate is associated with an increase of inorganic phosphate, ATP, and glucose 6-phosphate in muscle cells. The mechanism by which such carbohydrate administration induces hypophosphatemia is somewhat speculative. Experience with phosphate-deficient total parenteral nutrition and subsequent development of hypophosphatemia has provided some insight into the etiology.[12,13] As carbohydrates are absorbed, insulin secretion increases, shifting phosphorus from the extracellular to the intracellular space. If phosphate reserve is low, ATP is poorly regenerated since hypophosphatemia inhibits glucose 3-phosphate dehydrogenase. Inorganic phosphates in the intracellular pool become further diminished because of incorporation, initially as newly synthesized ATP, but eventually as triose phosphates when the ATP is consumed in the hexokinase reaction. Glucose utilization by red blood cells requires ATP at the hexokinase and phosphofructokinase steps, but regeneration of ATP does not occur during phosphate deficiency or acute hypophosphatemia due to a block at the glucose 3-phosphate dehydrogenase step. In states of phosphate depletion, the scant phosphate that enters the red blood cell is incorporated into 1,3-diphosphoglycerate, but most is diverted to 2,3-diphosphoglycerate, also preventing complete glycolysis to regain the ATP consumed.

In thermally injured patients, infusion of dextrose-containing solutions usually begins 24 hours postburn, and enteral nutrition, in which most of the calories are supplied as carbohydrates, is initiated within several days of injury. These interventions are temporally correlated with the rapid descent of serum phosphorus concentrations. In other clinical states, severe hypophosphatemia following the initiation of enteral or parenteral nutrition is most commonly associated with the feeding of patients with advanced protein-calorie malnutrition. When total body phosphorus is depleted by starvation, serum phosphorus levels usually remain normal, but carbohydrate administration produces a rapid marked decline in serum phosphorus concentration. If untreated, this may result in multisystem organ dysfunction, respiratory and cardiac failure, or death. Thermally injured patients are usually well nourished prior to burn injury and the clinical scenario of refeeding hypophosphatemia may not apply to them. Similar findings, however, have been described recently in previously well-nourished surgical intensive care unit patients in whom the initiation of isotonic enteral feedings resulted in a decrease of serum phosphorus from normal levels to approximately 1 mg/dL, a level that is considered to be dangerously low and to require prompt supplementation.[14,15] In addition, the authors have reported that hypophosphatemia in thermally injured patients is exacerbated by the initiation of enteral feeding and occurs regardless of the postburn day when feeding is initiated.[3] This further reduction of serum phosphorus during the first postburn week, when levels are already low, may be particularly hazardous and speaks for aggressive phosphorus supplementation prior to and during the initiation of enteral alimentation.

Burn wound physiology

In patients recovering from thermal injury, the burn wound itself may act as a significant phosphorus sink. Despite the overall catabolism accompanying major injury and loss of lean body mass, healing burn wounds and skin grafts are anabolic and require phosphorus for normal repair. In addition, the continued loss of fluid and protein through the burn wound surface is a potential source of unquantified phosphorus loss and may contribute to hypophosphatemia.[16] In a comparison between burn patients and traumatically injured patients, it was shown that urinary phosphorus clearance, fractional excretion of phosphorus and renal threshold phosphate concentrations were not different between the two groups; however, persistent hypophosphatemia persisted in the thermally injured patients. This may further implicate the wound as a source of early phosphorus loss.[17]

Acute phase response and sepsis

Burn injury is characterized by an abrupt increase in acute phase proteins as patients enter the hypermetabolic phase of burn injury. These same responses are similar to those observed in the sepsis syndrome. Recently, the development of hypophosphatemia has been characterized in patients with the acute phase response syndrome.[17] Similar findings have been documented in patients with sepsis and infection, and correlation to increase in levels of cytokines such as tumor necrosis factor alpha and interleukin-6 has been made.[18] Similar findings were observed in patients with a variety of infectious diseases, and correlation of high levels of C-reactive protein and white blood cell count was made with the magnitude of hypophosphatemia.[19] Though these reports did not include burn injured patients, one may infer that activation of the inflammatory cascades such as occurs in major thermal injury may contribute to the development of hypophosphatemia.

Other electrolytes

Disorders of electrolyte balance may contribute to the development of hypophosphatemia. Experimental magnesium deficiency in animals may lead to phosphaturia and phosphorus deficiency, but intentional magnesium deficiency in man results in no change or a slight rise in serum phosphate.[20,21] In chronic alcoholics, however, hypomagnesemia and hypophosphatemia are coexistent. Hypokalemia, which is also exacerbated by magnesium deficiency, may result in phosphate wasting and hypophosphatemia. The mechanism is uncertain, but may be related to coexistent metabolic alkalosis, diuretic use, or the underlying illness. Changes in calcium and phosphate homeostasis, and in the regulating hormones calcitonin and parathyroid hormone, have been described after thermal injury.[22] Coincident with the early depression of serum phosphorus, the fraction of ionized calcium was shown to decrease and remain low, but within the normal range, for the 14 postburn days studied. Urinary calcium output was low, about 4.5 mmol/day, and urinary phosphate output was as high as 30 mmol/day, despite a low serum phosphorus. Serum calcitonin levels were significantly elevated for up to 2 weeks post-injury, whereas parathyroid hormone remained within the normal range. The magnitude of the contribution of the classic regulating hormones of calcium and phosphorus homeostasis to the observed decrease in serum phosphorus after severe injury is not known with certainty. Catecholamines and glucagon are known to induce an increase in calcitonin secretion, and the administration of pharmacological doses of calcitonin results in phosphaturia. A direct effect of calcitonin on phosphate transport in the nephron has been demonstrated. In those burn patients, it was notable that ionized calcium decreased slightly though still within the normal range, despite very high levels of calcitonin and normal parathyroid hormone concentrations. A slight, though statistically significant, increase in parathyroid hormone was observed around the fourth postburn day and may be related, albeit indirectly through calcium regulation, to the observed postburn decrease in serum phosphorus concentration.

Summary

Clearly, multiple factors influence the serum phosphorus level following burn injury. Fluid resuscitation and subsequent mobilization of interstitial edema fluids, catecholamine excess, respiratory alkalosis, the use of phosphate-binding antacids or sucralfate, hypokalemia, hypomagnesemia, and the initiation of enteral nutrition have all been associated with hypophosphatemia in other illnesses and experimental models. All or most of these factors may be encountered in the early treatment of burn patients and the contribution and relative importance of individual factors to the depression of serum phosphorus is difficult to analyze. Most likely, carbohydrate administration, respiratory alkalosis, and diuresis of edema fluid are the more important etiologic factors contributing to hypophosphatemia in the early postburn course.

Consequences of hypophosphatemia

The clinical manifestations of hypophosphatemia (Box 29.2) are mainly those of organ system hypofunction. These responses have been defined through clinical observation and laboratory studies in circumstances in which hypophosphatemia occurred as a relatively isolated event. Phosphorus supplementation has been reported to reverse these abnormalities, suggesting a cause and effect relationship. Hypofunction of organ systems associated with phosphorus depletion has been attributed to a lack of available inorganic phosphate for synthesis of high-energy phosphorus compounds; breakdown of stored ATP occurs, and the inorganic phosphate is diverted to

---

Box 29.2 Clinical manifestations of hypophosphatemia

CNS
- lethargy, malaise, neuropathy, seizures, coma

CARDIOVASCULAR
- impaired cardiovascular contractility
- decreased response to pressor agents
- hypotension
- acute cardiac decompensation

PULMONARY
- tachypnea
- decreased vital capacity
- respiratory failure

GASTROINTESTINAL
- anorexia, dysphagia

RENAL
- glycosuria, calciuria, magnesuria, renal tubular acidosis

MUSCULOSKELETAL
- weakness, myalgia, arthralgia, rhabdomyolysis

---

other intracellular pathways. Organ system dysfunction after thermal injury is characterized by early hypofunction and later hyperfunction of most organ systems. Whether hypophosphatemia contributes significantly to the early postburn depression of function that occurs in multiple organs is not known. Clearly, some of the clinical manifestations shown in Box 29.2 are commonly observed in thermally injured patients, while others are not usually associated with such injury. Most patients reported to have had complications of hypophosphatemia have also had a coexistent and severe illness. It is important to remember that prior cellular injury has been prerequisite in most instances in which hypophosphatemia has been implicated as a cause of organ system dysfunction. The following discussions of organ system abnormalities should be interpreted in light of the specific circumstances under which the observations were made.

Cardiac dysfunction

Although the early depression of cardiac function following burn injury has been attributed to an initial decrease in circulating blood volume, the search for intrinsic myocardial depression after burn injury and for mediators of such depression continues. In experimental studies and in clinical material, a correlation between hypophosphatemia and cardiac decompensation has been reported. Cardiac output, measured by bolus thermodilution, was impaired in seven critically ill hypophosphatemic patients and improved significantly with phosphorus supplementation.[4] In one experimental study, myocardial contractility was impaired by phosphorus deficiency and reversed by phosphorus repletion, suggesting that phosphorus deficiency may be a cause of heart failure in certain clinical conditions.[23] Hypophosphatemic cardiac depression has been described as occurring in 28.8% of surgical intensive care patients.[24] Despite these reports, there appears to be little evidence that hypophosphatemic cardiomyopathy is a frequently encountered clinical entity; most patients in whom this mechanism is invoked have already had a number of other causes for myocardial dysfunction.[25]

Neuromuscular dysfunction

Varying degrees of areflexic paralysis, paresthesias, sensory loss, weakness, and respiratory insufficiency have been reported to be associated with acute hypophosphatemia, usually induced with feeding malnourished patients.[12] A reduction in available ATP to support respiratory muscle contraction has been suggested as a mechanism for acute respiratory failure, and diaphragmatic contractility has been reported to improve with phosphorus repletion in mechanically ventilated hypophosphatemic patients.[26] Profound generalized muscle weakness associated with isolated phosphorus depletion has been observed in both clinical and laboratory studies.[27,28] In a study of hypophosphatemia and muscle phosphate metabolism in patients with burns or mechanical trauma, no direct correlation was demonstrated between the serum phosphorus concentration and the high-energy phosphate content of muscle cells; all these patients, however, were receiving phosphorus supplementation during the study.[29] If acute hypophosphatemia is superimposed on pre-existing cellular injury, potentially reversible muscle cell dysfunction may extend to irreversible necrosis.[30] Several authors have reported severe rhabdomyolysis associated with severe hypophosphatemia following burns and major trauma.[31,32] This spectacular clinical event is rare but may occur to a lesser, subclinical, extent in critically ill patients.[30,33] Hypophosphatemia as the underlying etiology may often be dismissed since muscle cell destruction results in release of phosphate and elevation of serum phosphorus. In the absence of significant hemochromogenuria, the diagnosis may not even be suspected. Further investigation is required to determine whether this 'asymptomatic' rhabdomyolysis is, in fact, an important clinical entity, or merely an obligate manifestation of critical illness.

Hematologic dysfunction

When untreated, severe hypophosphatemia may lead to red blood cell dysfunction by alterations in cell shape, survival, and physiological function. Lack of high-energy phosphate results in a decrease in erythrocyte 2,3-diphosphoglycerate and subsequent leftward shift of the dissociation curve, with a consequent risk of tissue hypoxia.[7] Clinical hypophosphatemia, with or without previous phosphate depletion, results in reduced production of 2,3-diphosphoglycerate, erythrocyte ATP, and other phosphorylated intermediates of red blood cell glycolysis. In a variety of experimental and clinical situations, including burn injury and mechanical trauma, red blood cell 2,3-diphosphoglycerate has been shown to be reduced in the presence of hypophosphatemia.[34,35] In thermally injured patients it has been demonstrated that postburn disturbance of red cell phosphate metabolism may be prevented by administration of phosphorus in the early postburn course.[35] Hypophosphatemia has also been associated with decreased red cell survival and decreased red cell deformability, with impaired capillary transit and the potential for further deficiency of tissue oxygenation.

White blood cell dysfunction also has been observed as a result of hypophosphatemia induced by the initiation of phosphate-free parenteral nutrition and was associated with depressed chemotactic, phagocytic, and bactericidal activity of granulocytes.[35] A reduction in granulocyte ATP content was also documented and amelioration of these white blood cell abnormalities was coincident with phosphorus repletion. Any correlation between these observations and an increased risk of infection remains speculative for hypophosphatemic patients in general and burn patients in particular.

Summary

Though it is clear that organ system dysfunction may be a manifestation of severe untreated hypophosphatemia, the relationship between these specific abnormalities and those observed in either the hypodynamic or the hyperdynamic phases of burn injury remains unclear. Clinical experience dictates that even when severe hypophosphatemia is avoided, the scenario of early organ system hypofunction and later hyperfunction persists. This is not to say that the marked hypophosphatemia observed following burn injury is part and parcel of the disease process, without bearing on the postburn physiological response, but that thus far, the pathophysiological milieu following thermal injury has not permitted definition of the contribution of hypophosphatemia to the overall postburn response. Until cause and effect relationships are defined through ongoing research, aggressive phosphorus repletion should be approached cautiously following thermal injury. Such therapy does, however, clearly ameliorate red blood cell 2,3-diphosphoglycerate depletion, which, in and of itself, supports treatment.

Prevention and treatment of hypophosphatemia

An unequivocal recommendation to treat hypophosphatemia in thermally injured patients should be supported by evidence that the treatment is of benefit. Such evidence is somewhat lacking in thermally injured patients, but in many analogous instances of hypophosphatemia from other causes, a direct benefit has been ascribed to repletion.

Serum phosphorus levels should be measured daily during the early phase of burn care and intravenous phosphate repletion initiated when levels drop below 2.0 mg/dL (Figure 29.2). Most of the severe adverse effects of hypophosphatemia occur with concentrations below 1.0 mg/dL, and this replacement strategy should prevent the development of clinically significant hypophosphatemia. Correction of severe hypophosphatemia with serum phosphorus levels less than 1.0 mg/dL requires intravenous replacement, usually with solutions of sodium or potassium phosphate containing 0.16 mmol/kg body weight (5 mg/kg body weight) of elemental phosphorus over 6 hours. The dose may be halved for patients with serum phosphorus levels between 1.0 and 2.0 mg/dL.[36] Following completion of the infusion, a repeat serum phosphorus determination should be obtained, and further treatment based on the post-infusion plasma concentration. A potential hazard associated with intravenous administration of phosphate salts is hyperphosphatemia, which may induce metastatic deposition of calcium phosphate salts and hypocalcemia. Additionally, when

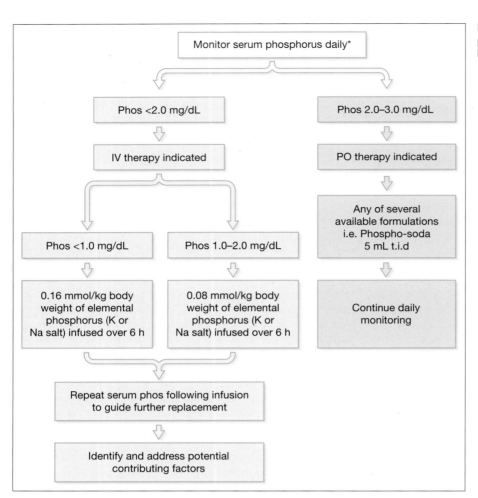

Fig. 29.2 The use of this algorithm permits prompt detection and timely correction of hypophosphatemia following burn injury.

potassium phosphate salts are used, care must be taken to avoid excessive or too rapid administration of potassium. Phosphorus replacement should be carefully monitored and proceed with great caution in patients with impaired renal function or evidence of soft tissue injury or necrosis.

Prevention of hypophosphatemia may be facilitated by beginning oral phosphorus replacement prior to interventions such as the initiation of either enteral or parenteral carbohydrate administration, gastric acid neutralization with phosphate-binding antacids or sucralfate, and the administration of diuretics. The nadir of serum phosphorus concentration typically occurs between 3 and 5 days postburn, during the period of edema mobilization, and the need to initiate phosphorus supplementation should be anticipated in this interval. Additionally, to temper the gastrointestinal losses due to administration of phosphate-binding antacids, substitution of, or alternation with, antacids containing aluminum phosphate should be considered.

For mild asymptomatic hypophosphatemia or for prophylaxis when worsening of hypophosphatemia is expected, oral supplementation with any of several available formulations is recommended. Such oral regimens have been shown to be cost-effective.[37] Five milliliters of Phospho-soda, containing 4.2 mmol/mL of elemental phosphorus, is commonly administered three times daily. Correction of other electrolyte abnor-

malities, most notably hypomagnesemia, hypocalcemia, and hypokalemia, as well as maintenance of acid–base normality, may prevent further renal phosphate losses and maintain the extracellular phosphate pool. After the 10th postburn day, the phosphorus delivered in standard liquid enteral formulas and hospital diets is usually sufficient to maintain serum phosphorus levels above 3.0 mg/dL.

Summary

Thermal injury induces a precipitous decrease in serum phosphate concentration that reaches its nadir between the second and fifth postburn days. This phenomenon has been recognized for some time, but interest in the problem has been limited. The organ system dysfunctions induced by hypophosphatemia are in many ways similar to certain of the pathophysiological changes observed following burn injury. The contribution of hypophosphatemia to these manifestations remains undefined. Wound fluid losses, increased circulating catecholamines, intracellular phosphate redistribution, and increased fractional excretion of urinary phosphate, as well as iatrogenic induction of hypophosphatemia through various therapeutic interventions, have been implicated as contributing to postburn hypophosphatemia. There may be other pathways regarding phosphorus regulation that have not been explored in this patient population. Phosphatonins have been shown to be important mediators of phosphorus homeostasis and could be important mediators in this phenomenon seen in burn patients.[40] Frequent serum phosphate measurement and prompt phosphorus replacement when hypophosphatemia is recognized should minimize any sequelae of this potentially deleterious electrolyte deficiency.

References

1. Cioffi WG, Vaughan GM, Heironimus JD, et al. Dissociation of blood volume and flow in regulation of salt and water balance in burn patients. Ann Surg 1991; 214(3):213–218.
2. Nordstrom H, Lennquist S, Lindell B, et al. Hypophosphataemia in severe burns. Acta Chir Scand 1977; 143:395–399.
3. Mozingo DW, Cioffi WG, Mason AD Jr, et al. Initiation of continuous enteral feeding induces hypophosphatemia in thermally injured patients. Proceedings of the 35th World Congress of Surgery/International Society of Surgery/International Surgical Week, 22–27 August 1993.
4. O'Connor LR, Weeler WS, Bethune JE. Effects of hypophosphatemia on myocardial performance in man. N Engl J Med 1977; 297:901.
5. Polderman KH, Bloemers FW, Peerdeman SM, et al. Hypomagnesemia and hypophosphatemia at admission in patients with severe head injury. Crit Care Med 2000; 28(6):2022–2025.
6. England PC, Duari M, Tweedle DET, et al. Postoperative hypophosphatemia. Br J Surg 1979; 66:340.
7. Lau K. Phosphate disorders. In: Kokko JP, Tannen RL, eds. Fluids and eletrolytes. Philadelphia, PA: WB Saunders; 1986:398–471.
8. Knochel JP. The pathophysiology and clinical characteristics of severe hypophosphatemia. Arch Intern Med 1977; 137:203–220.
9. Lennquist S, Lindell B, Nordstrom H, et al. Hypophosphatemia in severe burns. A prospective study. Acta Chir Scand 1979; 145:1–6.
10. Miller SJ, Simpson J. Medication–nutrient interactions: hypophosphatemia associated with sucralfate in the intensive care unit. Nutr Clin Pract 1991; 6:199–201.
11. Mostellar ME, Tuttle EP Jr. The effects of alkylosis on plasma concentration and urinary excretion of inorganic phosphate in man. J Clin Invest 1964; 43:138–149.
12. Solomon SM, Kirby DF. The refeeding syndrome: a review. J Parenter Enter Nutr 1990; 14(1):90–97.
13. Sheldon GF, Grzyb S. Phosphate depletion and repletion: relation to parenteral nutrition and oxygen transport. Ann Surg 1975; 182(6):683–689.
14. Hayek ME, Eisenberg PG. Severe hypophosphatemia following the institution of enteral feedings. Arch Surg 1989; 124:1325–1328.
15. Marik PE, Bedigian MK. Refeeding hypophosphatemia in critically ill patients in an intensive care unit. A prospective study. Arch Surg 1996; 131(10):1043–1047.
16. Berger MM, Rothen C, Cavadini C, et al. Exudative mineral losses after serious burns: a clue to the alteration of magnesium and phosphate metabolism. Am J Clin Nutr 1997; 65(5):1473–1481.
17. Dickerson RN, Gervasio JM, Sherman JJ, et al. A comparison of renal phosphorus regulation in thermally injured and multiple trauma patients receiving specialized nutrition support. J Parenter Enteral Nutr 2001; 25(3):152–159.
18. da Cunah DF, dos Santos VM, Monterio JP, et al. Hypophosphatemia in acute-phase response syndrome patients. Preliminary data. Miner Electrolyte Metab 1998; 24(5):337–340.
19. Barak V, Schwartz A, Kalickman I, et al. Prevalence of hypophosphatemia in sepsis and infection: the role of cytokines. Am J Med 1998; 104(1):40–47.
20. Haglin L, Burman LA, Nilsson M. High prevalence of hypophosphatemia amongst patients with infectious diseases. A retrospective study. J Intern Med 1999; 246(1):45–52.
21. Whang R, Welt LG. Observations in experimental magnesium depletion. J Clin Invest 1963; 42:305–313.
22. Shils ME. Experimental human magnesium depletion. Medicine 1969; 48:61–82.
23. Loven L, Nordstrom H, Lennquist S. Changes in calcium and phosphate and their regulating hormones in patients with severe burn injuries. Scand J Plast Reconstr Surg 1984; 18:49–53.
24. Fuller TJ, Nichols WW, Brenner BJ, et al. Reversible depression in myocardial performance in dogs with experimental phosphorus deficiency. J Clin Invest 1978; 62:1194–2000.
25. Zazzo JF, Troche G, Ruel P, et al. High incidence of hypophosphatemia in surgical intensive care patients: efficacy of phosphorus therapy on myocardial function. Intensive Care Med 1995; 21(10):826–831.
26. Knochel JP. The clinical status of hypophosphatemia. N Engl J Med 1985; 313(7):447–449.
27. Aubier M, Murciano D, Lecocguic Y, et al. Effect of hypophosphatemia on diaphragmatic contractility in patients with acute respiratory failure. N Engl J Med 1985; 313:420–424.
28. Lotz M, Nay R, Bartter FC. Osteomalacia and debility resulting from phosphorus depletion. Trans Assoc Am Physicians 1964; 77:281–295.
29. Lotz M, Zisman E, Bartter FC. Evidence for a phosphorus depletion syndrome in man. N Engl J Med 1968; 278:409.
30. Loven L, Lennquist S, Liljedahl SO. Hypophosphataemia and muscle phosphate metabolism in severely injured patients. Acta Chir Scand 1983; 149:743–749.
31. Knochel JP, Barcenas C, Cotton JR, et al. Hypophosphatemia and rhabdomyolysis. J Clin Invest 1978; 62:1240–1246.
32. Guechot J, Cynober L, Lioret N, et al. Rhabdomyolysis and acute renal failure in a patient with thermal injury. Intensive Care Med 1986; 12:159–160.
33. Pfeifer PM. Acute rhabdomyolysis following surgery for burns. Anaesthesia 1986; 41:614–669.
34. Singhal PC, Kumar A, Desroches L, et al. Prevalence and predictors of rhabdomyolysis in patients with hypophosphatemia. Am J Med 1992; 92:458–464.
35. Loven L, Anderson E, Larsson J, et al. Muscular high-energy phosphates and red-cell 2.3-DPG in post-traumatic hypophosphataemia. Acta Chir Scand 1983; 149:735–741.
36. Loven L, Larsson L, Nordstrom H, et al. Serum phosphate and 2,3-diphosphoglycerate in severely burned patients after phosphate supplementation. J Trauma 1986; 26(4):348–352.
37. Perreault MM, Ostrop NJ, Tierney MG. Efficacy and safety of intravenous phosphate replacement in critically ill patients. Ann Pharmacother 1997; 31(6):683–688.
38. Mathews JJ, Aleem RF, Gamelli RL. Cost reduction strategies in burn nutrition services: adjustment dietary treatment of patients with hyponatremia and hypophosphatemia. J Burn Care Rehabil 1999; 20(1 Pt 1):80–84.
39. Craddock PR, Yawata Y, VanSanten L, et al. Acquired phagocyte dysfunction. A complication of the hypophosphatemia of parenteral hyperalimentation. N Engl J Med 1974; 290(25):1403–1407.
40. Berndt TJ, Schiavi S, Kumar R. 'Phosphatonins' and the regulation of phosphorus homeostasis. Am J Physiol Renal Physiol 2005; 289:F1170–F1182.

30 Nutritional support of the burned patient

Jeffrey R. Saffle and Caran Graves

Chapter contents

Introduction

The metabolic consequences of major burn injury are profound and constitute an ongoing challenge to successful burn treatment. Metabolic rates of burn patients can exceed twice normal and cause tremendous wasting of lean body mass within a few weeks of injury. Failure to satisfy these energy and protein requirements results in impaired wound healing, organ dysfunction, susceptibility to infection, and ultimately death. Provision of aggressive nutritional support is an essential component of burn care, which can reduce mortality and complications, optimize wound healing, and minimize the devastating effects of hypermetabolism and catabolism.

Nutritional therapy is more successful when it is provided within a comprehensive protocol.[1–3] Every burn center should develop a multidisciplinary protocol that standardizes the initial and ongoing assessment, initiation, and monitoring of nutritional support for patients with all sizes of burn injury.

This chapter provides practical guidelines for addressing the nutritional needs of burn patients. In attempting to interpret recent research, two difficulties are apparent. First, research dealing specifically with burn patients is far from complete. More data are available from trauma and other ICU populations, and it is often necessary to extrapolate some information from one group to another, which may not always be accurate. While burns have long been considered a paradigm for acute stress, burn injury has some special features which require unique nutritional solutions. We will attempt to discuss these issues as they arise.

Second, results of original research are not always consistent; studies of similar therapies may reach contradictory conclusions, especially in different populations. Such findings often underscore our imperfect understanding of the complexities of nutritional physiology. We will summarize new concepts in this field but also try to distinguish them from 'tried and true' therapies which are widely accepted. The reader is referred to excellent reviews summarizing the evidence for current clinical recommendations.[1,4] Nutritional support, like many areas in burn care, is a moving target. The reader will need to interpret this chapter, and future readings, in this light.

The hypermetabolism of burn injury

Over 70 years ago, Cuthbertson documented that traumatic injury produced increased energy utilization and accelerated losses of body nitrogen.[5] In the 1970s, burn patients were found to exhibit the most severe hypermetabolism of any group, with energy expenditure from 60 to 100% above normal following a major burn, and concomitant catabolism of protein stores.[6,7] These studies also demonstrated the so-called ebb and flow response to injury (see Figure 30.1), in which an initial (12–24 hour) reduction in metabolic rate is followed by a crescendo–decrescendo curve of sustained hypermetabolism that can persist for weeks.

Attempts to nourish burn patients with oral diets often failed due to altered mental status, gastrointestinal dysfunction, and inhalation injury. Even patients who could eat were rarely able to tolerate the amount of nutrition necessary for adequate support. As a consequence, patients with major burns predictably incurred weight loses of 20% or greater within the first few weeks of injury,[8,9] with associated immune compromise and delayed wound healing. This inanition often proved fatal as patients succumbed to respiratory failure, pneumonia, and systemic infection[9] (Figure 30.2).

Mediators of hypermetabolism

The hypermetabolism following burn injury is a consequence of several predominant hormonal changes.[10,11] As described by Long et al.[6] and Wilmore et al.,[7] burn trauma stimulates major increases in the catabolic hormones epinephrine, cortisol and glucagon, resulting in greatly accelerated gluconeogenesis, glycogenolysis, and muscle proteolysis.[12] Catabolic hormones counteract the effect of insulin; as a result, blood sugar levels rise, and protein synthesis and lipogenesis are inhibited. Growth hormone is similarly antagonized and less effective.

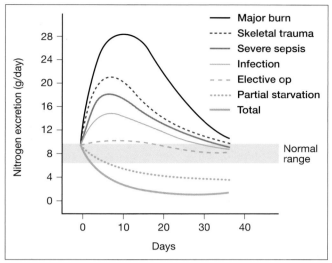

Fig. 30.1 This is a classic illustration of nitrogen excretion following injury compared to starvation and other conditions. Burn injury evokes the most pronounced catabolism of any clinical condition, with nitrogen excretion exceeding 25 g/day (150 g of protein, almost a half-pound of lean body mass!). Notice also the dynamic, 'crescendo–decrescendo' nature of this process: nitrogen excretion (and metabolic rate) rises from near-normal levels just after injury to reach a maximum at 7–14 days postburn, thereafter declining slowly throughout recovery. This illustrates the impossibility of using static formulas to estimate nutritional requirements accurately at every point throughout the course of burn treatment. (Reproduced with permission from Long et al. Metabolic response to injury and illness: estimation of energy and protein needs from indirect calorimetry and nitrogen balance. JPEN 1979; 3:452–456.[6])

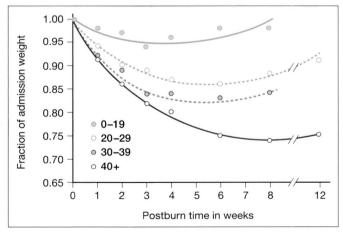

Fig. 30.2 Weight loss following burn injury as documented in the era before routine nutritional support. Dramatic losses of lean body mass occur within a week or two of injury, and progress continuously in the absence of effective nutritional support. By 4–6 weeks postburn, patients with major burns have lost 15% of lean body mass or more — a fatal degree of inanition. (Reproduced with permission from Wilmore et al. Ann Surg 1974: 180:653–658.[7])

In this environment, skeletal muscle is the major obligatory fuel for hypermetabolism. In contrast to starvation (in which metabolic rate falls, and lipolysis and ketosis provide energy and protect muscle reserves), burn injury reduces the body's ability to utilize fat as an energy source. Lipids have limited protein-sparing effect. Instead, a diet composed largely of carbohydrates is required to reduce protein catabolism, and even glucose is limited in its ability to prevent protein wasting.[13]

Although these hormonal changes provide a major challenge to the provision of adequate nutrition, they also provide mechanisms by which hypermetabolism can be reduced to facilitate metabolic support. In recent years, investigators have attempted to ameliorate burn-induced hypermetabolism by several methods, including blocking catecholamines with propranolol, administering counter-regulatory agents such as insulin and insulin-like growth factor-1 (IGF-1), or use of anabolic hormones such as growth hormone, testosterone, or synthetic anabolic agents such as oxandrolone.[14,15] This rapidly-evolving area of research is discussed in detail in other chapters of this book. Although some of these methods show promise for clinical use, it must be remembered that the hormonal milieu which accompanies burn injury is complex and incompletely understood. Additional research will be needed to confirm the efficacy and safety of these techniques.

Modern burn care and metabolic requirements

Modern methods of burn treatment do not appear to have altered the *nature* of burn-induced hypermetabolism but have significantly reduced its *magnitude*. Maneuvers as simple as maintaining high ambient temperature and relative humidity can reduce caloric requirements by up to 20%.[7] Antibiotics and routine early burn wound excision have reduced infection and modulated hypermetabolism. Although excisional surgery has not been shown to directly reduce energy expenditure,[16] covering burn wounds with autograft, allograft, or synthetic substitutes certainly shortens the duration of hypermetabolism. Other therapies, including mechanical ventilation and chemical sedation/paralysis, also reduce energy requirements.[17]

As a result, numerous recent reports using indirect calorimetry document metabolic rates which, though still increased, are now more likely to approximate 120–150% of normal, rather than the 160–200% previously reported.[18,19] Nonetheless, both temporal and patient-specific variations in energy expenditure make it difficult to predict requirements for individual patients.

Assessment of nutritional needs

Initial assessment

Patients suffering from systemic diseases such as cancer and AIDS often present with serious pre-existing nutritional depletion which must be addressed before the underlying disease can be treated. A variety of nutritional assessment techniques have been used in population-based surveys, including careful clinical evaluation, serum proteins, anthropometric measurements, tests of immune function, etc.

Pre-existing malnutrition can also exist in burn patients and can compromise wound healing and survival.[20] However, extensive initial nutritional assessments may not be necessary in burned patients for several reasons. Burn injury induces major abnormalities in nutritional indices which confound assessment of pre-burn status: swelling and eschar preclude accurate anthropometric measurements, serum proteins are altered quickly, and immune function is similarly disturbed. A careful nutritional history, calculation of body mass index (BMI), and functional status may be the most meaningful assessments to perform.[21] Moreover, satisfying *ongoing* requirements is far more important — and probably more difficult to determine — than compensating for *pre-existing* deficiencies. Attempting to 'catch up' by providing excess calories and/or protein is ineffective and likely to increase such complications as hyperglycemia, CO_2 retention, and azotemia (see 'overfeeding,' below). Therefore, the primary goal of nutritional support in burn patients is to satisfy *ongoing*, burn-specific requirements. Pre-existing deficiencies can be addressed after the acute phase resolves.

Formulas for estimating caloric requirements

Any protocol for nourishing burn patients must begin with estimation of their nutritional needs. An array of regimens for this purpose have been developed.[22] One of these, the Curreri formula,[23] has been widely (and successfully) used, though its accuracy is open to question. To create the formula, Curreri's group examined only nine patients and calculated backwards to estimate the calories which would have been needed to make up for patients' lost weight. As will be discussed, this is a dubious assumption at best.

Several popular formulas for adult nutrition are reviewed in Table 30.1.[23–28] As can be seen, they use different variables to predict different caloric requirements for specific patients, and reach very different estimate of energy needs. Because modern burn treatment has blunted the magnitude of hypermetabolism, older formulas like Curreri's significantly overestimate energy requirements.[18] Moreover, static formulas inevitably fail to account for the major differences in energy expenditure invariably documented between patients, within individuals, and over time. Dickerson et al. reviewed 46 published methods for predicting energy expenditure in burn patients.[29] They found that *none* of the methods reviewed correlated precisely (= 15% error) with measured energy expenditure in a group of 24 patients. Because postburn energy expenditure fluctuates (see Figure 30.1), formulas are likely to result in overfeeding early and late in the postburn course and may underfeed patients during periods of peak energy utilization.

TABLE 30.1 COMMONLY USED FORMULAS FOR ESTIMATING CALORIC REQUIREMENTS IN ADULT BURN PATIENTS

Formula name	Formula[a]	Daily caloric estimate (kcal), 25-year-old male (80 kg; BSA = 2.0 m² with 60% TBSA burn)	Comment
Harris–Benedict[2,25]	**Basal energy expenditure:** **Men:** 66.5 + (13.8)W + (5)H − (6.76)A **Women:** 655 + (9.6)W + (1.85)H − (4.68)A **Adjust for stress by multiplying BEE by a factor of 1.2–2.0**	Basal rate = 1915 If factor is 1.2 = 2299 If factor is 1.2 = 2299 If factor is 2.0 = 3830	The Harris–Benedict formula is an accepted standard for estimating *basal* energy expenditure (BEE). For burn patients, multiplying BEE by an arbitrary factor introduces significant inaccuracy. A factor of 1.2–1.5 should be sufficient for all but the largest burn injuries
Curreri formula[23]	**Age 16–59:** (25)W + (40)TBSA **Age ≥ 60:** (20)W + (65)TBSA	4400	This widely used formula probably overestimates modern energy requirements significantly. A modification for elderly patients is included
Davies and Lilijedahl[24]	(20)W + (70) TBSA	5800	This formula will grossly overestimate energy requirements for patients with very large injuries
RDI[28]	37(W)	2960	'One size fits all' is convenient, but inaccurate for most patients, particularly the elderly and obese
Ireton-Jones[26]	**Ventilated patient:** 1784 − 11(A) + 5(W) + 244(S) + 239 (T) + 804 (B) **Non-ventilated patient:** 629 − 11(A) + 25(W) − 609(O) =	2957 2384	This complex formula permits calculation of energy requirements for trauma and burn patients, and includes a factor for obesity
Toronto[27]	−4343 + (10.5 × TBSA) + (0.23 × CI) + (0.84 × HBE) + (114 × T) − (4.5 × PBD)	2782	Another complicated formula which requires ongoing collection of patient data

[a]For all formulas, W = weight in kilograms; H = height in centimeters; A = age in years; S = sex (male = 1, female = 0); T = trauma (present = 1, absent = 0); B = burn (present = 1, absent = 0); O = obesity (present = 1, absent = 0); TBSA = burn size (percent total body surface area); CI = calorie intake the previous day; HBE = Harris–Benedict estimates; T = temperature (°C).

Pediatric formulas

Numerous formulas have also been created to address the energy requirements of burned children; several commonly used formulas are presented in Table 30.2.[30-34] As needs change with age, pediatric formulas differ by age. Even with this accommodation, however, predictive equations yield very different caloric requirements for the same patients. These formulas share the same inherent limitations of adult formulas.

Indirect calorimetry

In recent decades, improved technology for performance of indirect calorimetry (IC) has permitted routine measurement of energy expenditure at the bedside. IC devices measure the volume of expired gas, along with inhaled and exhaled concentrations of oxygen and carbon dioxide, permitting calculation of oxygen consumption (VO_2) and carbon dioxide production (VCO_2), and thus metabolic rate.[35] Measurements made through tight-fitting face masks, hoods, or by connection to mechanical ventilators have proven reliable and reproducible over a wide range of metabolic rates and FiO_2.

IC can also detect significant under- or overfeeding through calculation of the respiratory quotient (RQ) – the ratio of carbon dioxide produced to oxygen consumed (VCO_2/VO_2).[36]

The body's metabolism of specific substrates affects this ratio, providing information about metabolic supply and demand. For example, in unstressed starvation, utilization of fat as a major energy source produces an RQ of 0.7 or less;[37] in normal metabolism of mixed substrates, RQ = 0.75–0.90; the synthesis of fat from carbohydrate, which typifies overfeeding, results in an RQ of 1.0 or greater. In this way, overfeeding can contribute to difficulty weaning from ventilatory support.[38]

IC is used widely to measure caloric requirements for burn patients and to detect significant under- or overfeeding.[39,40] Resting energy expenditure (REE) is usually measured in the early morning with patients at bed rest. Fluctuations in energy utilization associated with activity must be factored into nutritional support, and are usually estimated by increasing measured metabolic rate by 10–20%.[41]

Delivering estimated needs: How close is 'close enough'?

Recent studies in ICU patients found that less than 80% of prescribed calories were actually delivered.[42,43] Enteral nutrition was less successful than TPN, because of more frequent interruptions for diarrhea, tube dislodgement, surgery, etc. In

TABLE 30.2 COMMONLY USED FORMULAS FOR ESTIMATING CALORIC REQUIREMENTS IN PEDIATRIC BURN PATIENTS

			Daily caloric estimate (kcal) for patients with 40% TBSA burn			
Formula name	Age (years)	Formula[a]	1 month old 10 kg BSA = 0.5 m²	3 year old 12 kg BSA = 0.6 m²	10 year old 30 kg BSA = 1.1 m²	14 year old 60 kg BSA = 1.6 m²
BEE (WHO)[b]	Females 0–3	(61.0 kg) − 51	559			
	3–10	(22.5 kg) + 499		769		
	10–18	(12.2 kg) + 746			1112	1478
	Males 0–3	(60.9 kg) − 54	555			
	3–10	(22.7 kg) + 495		767		
	10–18	(17.5 kg) + 651			1176	1701
Recommended dietary intake (RDI)[3,28]	0–6 months	108 × (W)				
	months to 1 year	98 × (W)	980			
	1–3	102 × (W)		1224		
	4–10	90 × (W)			2700	
	11–14 (male)	55 × (W)				3300
	(female)	47 × (W)				2820
Curreri junior[30]	< 1	(RDA + 15 kcal/TBSA)	1580			
	1–3	(RDA + 25 kcal /TBSA)		2224		
	4–15	(RDA + 40 kcal /TBSA)			4300	4900
Galveston infant[32]	0–1	2100 kcal/m² + 1000 kcal/m² burn	1250			
Galveston revised[31]	1–11	1800 kcal/m² + 1300 kcal /m²burn		1392	2552	
Galveston adolescent[33]	≥12	1500 kcal/m² + 1500 kcal/m²burn			3360	

[a]For all formulas, W = weight in kilograms; H = height in centimeters; A = age in years; BSA = body surface area; TBSA = burn size (percent total body surface area).
[b]WHO pediatric nutrition handbook, 5th edn. Ronald E. Kleinman, ed. American Academy of Pediatrics; 243.

both types of nutrition, hyperglycemia sometimes required reducing nutrition, while dextrose-containing IV fluids added unplanned, 'empty' calories. These studies illustrate the ubiquitous practical difficulties of actually giving patients the nutrition that is prescribed for them — difficulties which can compromise the success of nutritional support.

This experience raises an important question: How close is 'close enough' in feeding critically ill patients? Despite the limitations inherent in static formulas, the superiority of IC-based nutrition has not been proven clinically.[1,44] Many patients have been successfully nourished using the Curreri and other formulas, and abundant experience demonstrates that either formulas or indirect calorimetry can be used to nourish burn patients successfully, particularly if this is done within a multidisciplinary regimen of support. Many units use a goal of delivering nutrition within 10% of measured (or calculated) needs as a quality assurance indicator, despite the lack of evidence for such a policy.

Specific nutrient requirements

Carbohydrates

The major energy source for burn patients should be carbohydrates. Glucose is the preferred fuel for healing wounds, and accessory metabolic pathways to provide glucose, including the alanine and Cori cycles, are active in burn patients.

The major complication of carbohydrate feeding under stress is glucose intolerance. Aggressive control of hyperglycemia is emerging as a critically important aspect of optimal patient care. Even patients with relatively normal tolerance may have caloric requirements that exceed the body's ability to assimilate glucose, which is estimated at approximately 7 g/kg/day (2240 kcal for an 80-kg man).[45] Patients often require significant amounts of supplemental insulin with aggressive (or 'tight') glucose control now recommended (see below). However, refractory hyperglycemia can still occur and require reduction or even discontinuation of nutrition until blood sugar can be controlled. Providing a limited amount of dietary fat reduces requirements for carbohydrates and can improve glucose tolerance significantly.

Table 30.3, discussed below, lists the composition of a number of commonly available enteral nutrition products which should help in understanding the quantities of nutrients required for support.

Requirements and uses of fat

A certain (small) quantity of fat is an essential nutrient. Essential fatty acid deficiency is a well-documented complication of patients given long-term TPN;[10] modern TPN contains significant amounts of lipid for this reason. In addition, providing a substantial proportion of fat calories reduces the required glucose load and associated VCO_2. However, the hormonal environment of burn-injured patients suppresses lipolysis and limits the extent to which lipids can be utilized for energy. For this reason, most authorities recommend that fat constitutes no more than about 30% of non-protein calories, or about 1 g/kg/day of intravenous lipids in TPN.[10]

It may be desirable to give even less fat. In an animal model, adverse effects on immune function occurred when diets contained more than 15% lipids.[46] Some clinical research supports this finding,[47] leading some authorities to recommend low-fat diets for use in burn patients. Commercially available nutritional supplements are listed in Table 30.3; popular 'stress formulas' contain 25–40% of calories as fat, while some 'specialty' formulas — for renal failure, respiratory failure, or diabetes — contain even more fat, which limits their usefulness in burn patients. Patients given TPN may be better off if fat is withheld entirely for short periods of time (as little as once weekly),[1,48] though this may result in aggravated glucose intolerance.

The composition of administered fat may be even more important than the quantity. Most common lipid sources contain mostly omega-6 fatty acids (ω-6 FFAs) such as linoleic acid which are metabolized through synthesis of arachidonic acid, a precursor of pro-inflammatory cytokines such as prostaglandin E_2. Lipids such as fish oil containing a high proportion of omega-3 fatty acids (ω-3 FFAs) are metabolized without elaborating pro-inflammatory compounds. Diets high in ω-3 FFAs have been associated with improved immune response, possible improved outcomes,[49] and may reduce problems with hyperglycemia.[50] Most experience with ω-3 FFAs has been obtained with 'immune-enhancing diets,' of which they are a major component (see below). Both the optimal composition and dose of fat in nutritional support remain topics of substantial controversy.

Protein

The hormonal environment of burn injury greatly increases proteolysis. Provision of carbohydrate and fat calories is only partially successful in reducing protein catabolism; some loss of lean body mass is obligatory following injury.[51] Increased protein must be supplied to satisfy ongoing demands, and provide amino acids for wound healing, enzymes, immunocompetence, and other functions. When calories are limited, protein will be used as an energy source rather than to replenish lost protein stores. The converse, however, is not true: providing calories in excess of need will not lead to increased protein retention or synthesis — it will just lead to overfeeding with its associated risks. Protein intake above required needs (as in extremely high protein/low carbohydrate diets) also results in protein's use as a fuel source through gluconeogenic pathways.

Protein catabolism in burn patients can exceed 150 grams/day, or almost a half-pound of skeletal muscle. Although feeding supranormal amounts of protein may not reduce breakdown of endogenous protein stores,[52] it facilitates protein synthesis, and reduces negative nitrogen balance. In burned children, a diet including increased protein (23% of total calories) was associated with improved immune function, less bacteremia, and increased survival.[53] As burn size increases, progressively more protein is required for positive nitrogen balance.[54,55]

Current recommendations call for 1.5–2.0 grams of protein per kilogram body weight per day for adult burn patients, and up to 3.0 g/kg/day in children.[39,56] With provision of sufficient non-protein calories, this should result in a calorie:nitrogen ratio of 100:1 or less, typical of the 'stress' formulas listed below. Measurement of nitrogen balance and visceral protein markers may be helpful in assessing the adequacy of nutritional support (see below).

TABLE 30.3 COMPOSITION OF COMMERCIALLY AVAILABLE ADULT AND PEDIATRIC ENTERAL NUTRITION PRODUCTS (PER 1000 KCAL OF FEEDINGS)

I. Adult formulas[a]

Brand name (manufacturer)	mL/ 1000 kcal	%RD	Carbs g	%kcal	Protein g	%kcal	Cal:N2	Fat g	%kcal	ω6ω3	Comments
'Immune-enhancing' and healing adult formulas											
Crucial™ (Nestle)	667	100	90	36	63	25	67:1	45	39	2:1	Elemental, hypertonic, concentrated enhanced with arginine
Impact™ (Novartis)	1000	67	130	53	56	22	71:1	28	25	1.4:1	Widely used 'immune-enhancing' formula; supplemented with arginine; high in ω-3 FFAs
Replete™ (Nestle)	1000	100	113	45	63	25	75:1	34	30	3:1	Inexpensive, high-protein formula
TraumaCal™ (Mead-Johnson)	667	33	95	38	55	22	91:1	45	40	6.3:1	High-protein, concentrated. Relatively high proportion of ω-6 FFAs. Deficient in some vitamins
Standard adult formulas											
Isocal-HN™ (Mead-Johnson)	943	80	117	46	42	17	125:1	43	37	N/a	Isotonic 'all purpose' feeding, without fiber
Jevity™ (Ross)	943	67	146	54	42	17	125:1	33	29	4.2:1	Isotonic, with fiber
'Specialty' adult formulas											
Nepro™ (Ross)	500	52	111	43	35	14	154:1	48	43	N/a	Widely used 'renal failure' formula; low in potassium, phosphorus, protein. Can be supplemented with protein for burn patients
Glucerna™ (Ross)	1000	70	96	34	42	17	125:1	54	49	10.8:1	Low-carbohydrate formula for diabetics; relies on high-fat content, which is of limited efficacy in burn patients
Pulmocare™ (Ross)	667	70	71	28	42	17	125:1	62	55	4:1	Customized formula for pulmonary failure relies on high fat content to avoid excessive VCO$_2$; limited efficacy in burn patients
Peptamen™ (Nestle)	1000	67	127	51	40	16	131:1	39	33	7:1	Semi-elemental, isotonic

TABLE 30.3—cont'd

II. Pediatric formulas[a]

Brand name (Manufacturer)	mL	% RDI per 1000 mL	Carbs		Protein		Fat		Comments
			g	%kcal	g	%kcal	g	%kcal	
Pediasure™ (Ross)	1000	67–100	110	44	30	12	50	44	
Kidercal™ (Mead-Johnson)	943	106	127	52	28	11	42	37	
Pediatric Vivonex™ (Novartis)	1250	108–120	163	63	30	12	30	25	Free amino acids, semi-elemental
Compleat Pedatric™ (Novartis)	900	111	130	50	38	15	39	35	

[a]Abbreviations: mL = milliliters of formula to contain 1000 kcal; % RDI per 1000 mL = percent of recommended dietary intake of micronutrients contained in 1000 mL of formula. Includes micronutrients not listed; g = grams; %kcal percentage of total calories; Cal:N2 = calorie-to-nitrogen ratio; ω6ω3 = ratio of ω-6 to ω-3 fatty acids. Information from manufacturers' websites as of December 2005.

Glutamine

Several amino acids have enhanced roles in energy delivery following injury. Alanine and glutamine (GLU) are important transport amino acids, created in large quantities from skeletal muscle to supply energy to the liver and to healing wounds.[51] GLU also serves as a primary fuel for both enterocytes and lymphocytes and is thus important in maintaining small bowel integrity, preserving gut-associated immune function, and limiting intestinal permeability following acute injury.[57,58] While the clinical significance of bacterial translocation in humans remains unresolved, glutamine may reduce passage of intact bacteria, and probably prevents translocation of endotoxin and secondary elaboration of inflammatory mediators by gut mucosa.[58,59] In addition, glutamine is a precursor of glutathione, an important antioxidant, and also improves elaboration of heat shock proteins, which provide cellular protection following stress and trauma.[60]

GLU is quickly depleted from both serum and muscle following burn injury, which may limit visceral protein synthesis, leading to the suggestion that GLU be considered a 'conditionally essential' amino acid in burns.[51,61] Importantly, GLU is almost totally absent from parenteral nutrition owing to its instability in solution; this may explain some of the inferiority of TPN, including a higher rate of systemic infections, compared to enteral nutrition.

In a number of clinical trials, GLU supplementation produced some improved outcomes in patients with cancer, AIDS, surgery, trauma, or burns.[58,62] However, the benefits of GLU supplementation were not consistently seen in comparisons between postoperative and ICU patients, provision of 'low-dose' (<0.20 g/kg/day) vs. 'high dose' (>0.20 g/kg/day) GLU, or parenteral vs. enteral administration.[60] The best data supporting GLU supplementation comes from burn patients, in whom provision of 25 g GLU/kg/day or more, given parenterally[63] or enterally,[64,65] was associated with reduced infections, improved visceral protein levels, and reduced mortality and length of hospitalization. This effect of GLU may be relatively specific to burn injuries.

At this time, supplementation of enteral nutrition with GLU for burn patients is not routinely practiced, although this has been suggested.[1] Provision of the large amounts of GLU given in these trials (0.25–0.50 g/kg/day) could interfere with delivery of other amino acids, so it might be preferable to give GLU *in addition* to the usual quantity of protein (1.5–2.0 g/kg/day in adults) required in burn patients.[58] Obviously, many questions persist regarding the clinical utility of GLU supplementation in burn care. Further clinical trials of this amino acid will be needed to clarify this issue.

Arginine and 'immunonutrition'

Arginine (ARG) is also important in postburn metabolism. ARG stimulates T-lymphocytes, enhances natural killer cell function, and stimulates synthesis of nitric oxide (NO), which is important in resistance to infection.[66,67] ARG supplementation of enteral diets has been associated with improved immune responsiveness and wound healing.[68]

Even the earliest efforts to nourish burn patients sought to define an 'ideal' nutritional mixture. Early diets were simply supplemented with eggs or milk.[22] Modern efforts have focused on combining components that appear to improve immune function and wound healing. In a study in burned children, a formula enhanced with ω-3 FFAs, histidine, ARG, RNA, and vitamins was associated with reduced infectious morbidity and improved survival.[69] This experience quickly led to commercial production of similar multi-ingredient 'immune-enhancing diets' (IEDs).

Subsequent studies have evaluated IEDs in a variety of clinical settings; some have demonstrated improvements in immunity and wound healing, and/or clinical parameters, including infection rates, incidence of multiple organ failure, or hospital stay.[70,71] However, others have not been uniformly favorable. It appears that these diets may have very different consequences in different patient groups, with improved outcomes following trauma or elective surgery,[72,73] but deleterious or no effects in patients with sepsis or pneumonia.[1,70,74] Much of the blame for these inconsistent results has been attributed to ARG, the exact dosing of which may influence its effects greatly, as too much could stimulate excessive NO production and exaggerated inflammation.[75]

Little information has been obtained on the use of IEDs in burn patients. One randomized trial comparing a highly publicized IED (Impact™) with another high-protein 'stress' solution found no differences in major outcome variables.[76] Though both solutions contained significant amounts of ω-3 FFAs, they differed in contents of vitamin A, ARG, and RNA; both feedings also contained significantly more fat than the modular tube feeding of Gottschlich et al.[69]

This experience illustrates that our understanding of complex nutritional physiology is still limited and may have been hindered by the rush to create commercially viable 'cocktails' for clinical use before understanding the real actions (and interactions) of their components, their optimal doses, and in what settings they might even be harmful to patients. At present, use of IEDs, particularly ARG, is not recommended.[1] This issue must await clarification from future well-designed and large-scale clinical trials.

Branched-chain amino acids

The branched-chain amino acids (BCAAs) leucine, isoleucine, and valine, have been postulated to spare endogenous muscle catabolism by stimulating protein synthesis and serving as energy substrates. In clinical trials in trauma and ICU patients, BCAA-enriched nutrition has been associated with improved nitrogen balance but has had no effect on survival.[77] In both animal and clinical studies in burn injury, BCAA-enriched feedings have not produced improvements in outcome, protein synthesis, or immune function,[78] and are therefore not recommended for use.

Micronutrients: vitamins and trace elements

In addition to major nutrients, metabolism of many so-called 'micronutrients' — vitamins and trace elements which are important in wound healing and immunity — is also affected by burn injury.[79] These compounds have not been evaluated extensively in clinical studies, though depressed serum levels of some compounds have been documented following burns. Limited data suggest that supplementation of some substances (vitamin A, vitamin C) may be beneficial. Table 30.4 contains a list of the most important micronutrients, their recommended daily allowances (RDAs), and the contents of several commonly used enteral formulas.

A complete listing of micronutrients and their functions is beyond the scope of this chapter; excellent reviews are available.[79,80] A few of the most important compounds are now discussed:

- Vitamin A is important in wound healing and epithelial growth. Vitamin A also functions as an antioxidant, and in preventing free radical damage. Decreased levels of vitamin A have been demonstrated following burn injury,[81] and supplementation has been recommended for burn patients.[82] However, toxicity of vitamin A can also occur.

- Vitamin C or ascorbic acid is essential for synthesis and cross-linking of collagen and thus for wound healing. It also functions as a circulating antioxidant. Some data support vitamin C supplementation in burn patients, and toxicity does not appear to be a clinical problem.[80] Supplementation of up to 1000 mg per day (over 20 times RDA) in burn patients has been recommended.[82]
- Vitamin D: considerable recent research has demonstrated that bone resorption and osteopenia is a significant problem following burn injury.[83] Disorders of vitamin D metabolism, as well as immobilization, may contribute to this problem, which is discussed in another chapter in this book.
- Iron is essential in oxygen-carrying proteins and also acts as a cofactor for a number of important enzymes. Burn patients are prone to iron deficiency, partially due to blood loss, but it should also be remembered that blood transfusions deliver a significant amount of iron.
- Zinc is required for the function of many metalloenzymes. Several aspects of wound healing appear to be affected by the availability of zinc, including DNA/RNA replication and lymphocyte function. Zinc deficiency has been documented during the first several days after burn injury.[84] Supplementation of up to 220 mg/day (15 times RDA) has been recommended.[82]
- Selenium is important in the function of lymphocytes, and hence, in cell-mediated immunity. Selenium is lost through the skin following burn injury; selenium deficiency in burn patients has been documented.[85]

A recent survey found that many burn centers provide some supplementation of trace elements, though both indications and specific doses vary among units.[86] Current reviews recommend supplementing at least the micronutrients listed above, and perhaps others.[11] However, remember that many commercially available tube feedings contain substantial quantities of these micronutrients (Table 30.4), which can approximate the recommendations for supplementation listed by Mayes et al.[82] The addition of a daily multivitamin tablet, or liquid multivitamins to tube feedings or TPN, will provide far more than RDA for most of these micronutrients at minimal cost and risk. It is unclear whether additional supplementation is of benefit of burn patients. Remember also that blood transfusions provide substantial amounts of iron, chromium, and some other micronutrients.

Formulas for enteral nutrition

Successful nutrition has been provided to burn patients with very simple concoctions of milk, eggs, and other nutrients.[22] However, commercially prepared enteral formulas offer several advantages. They are carefully composed to contain appropriate quantities of all necessary nutrients. Canned enteral diets can be infused through narrow feeding tubes with minimal clogging. Most are reasonably inexpensive, though some specialized formulas can be quite costly. Table 30.3 lists the nutrient composition of a number of popular enteral formulas.

A bewildering array of additional products are available, including fiber-containing diets, elemental diets, supplements,

TABLE 30.4 MICRONUTRIENT REQUIREMENTS AND COMPOSITION OF COMMERCIALLY AVAILABLE PRODUCTS[a,b]

Recommended daily intake by age:[3,28]

Age group	Vit A (µg)	Vit C (mg)	Vit E (mg α-TE)	Vit D (IU)	Vit K (µg)	Folate (µg)	Iron (mg)	Calcium (mg)	Phosphorus (mg)	Zinc (mg)	Selenium (µg)
<1	506	50	4	200	2.5	80	11	270	275	3	15
1–3	300	15	6	200	30	150	7	500	460	3	20
4–8	400	25	7	200	50	200	10	800	500	5	30
Adult	900	75	15	400	90–100	400	8–18	1000–1200	700	8–11	55

Recommended supplementation for burn patients[b] (per 1000 kcal; in addition to a daily multivitamin)

Age group	Vit A (µg)	Vit C (mg α-TE)	Vit E (mg	Vit D (IU)	Vit K (µg)	Folate (µg)	Iron (mg)	Calcium (mg)	Phosphorus (mg)	Zinc (mg)	Selenium (µg)
<3	1500			500					110		
>3	1000								220		

Contents of pediatric nutritional formulas (per 1000 kcal)

Formula	Vit A (µg)	Vit C (mg)	Vit E (mg α-TE)	Vit D (IU)	Vit K (µg)	Folate (µg)	Iron (mg)	Calcium (mg)	Phosphorus (mg)	Zinc (mg)	Selenium (µg)
Compleat pediatric™	3300	96	21	330	38	350	13	1440	1000	12	52
Pediasure™	1600	100	23	510	60	300	14	970	840	6	32
Pediatric Vivonex™	3125	125	38	625	50	250	12.5	1213	1000	15	38

Contents of adult nutritional formulas (per 1000 kcal)

Formula	Vit A (µg)	Vit C (mg)	Vit E (mg α-TE)	Vit D (IU)	Vit K (µg)	Folate (µg)	Iron (mg)	Calcium (mg)	Phosphorus (mg)	Zinc (mg)	Selenium (µg)
Crucial™	4000	667	67	267	50	360	12	667	667	24	67
Impact™	6700	80	60	270	67	400	12	800	800	15	100
Replete™	5000	340	60	272	50	540	18	1000	1000	24	100
Trauma-Cal™	1667	99	25	133	85	133	6	500	500	10	N/A
Osmolite-HN™	3575	217	33	288	58	429	13.2	717	717	17	51
Cernevit-12™ (liquid vitamin supplement for enteral nutrition)	3500	125	11.2	200	0	414	–	–	–	–	–

[a]Abbreviations and conversions: Vit = Vitamin; IU = International units; mg = milligrams; µg = micrograms. To convert from, the following factors were used: Vit D: 1 µg = 40 IU; Vit A: 0.3 (IU) = 1 µgRE (retinol equivalent); Vit E: 1 IU = 1 mg α-TE (alpha-tocopherol). Data extrapolated from Enteral product reference guide. 2001 by Nestle Clinical Nutrition, Deerfield, IL.
[b]From Mayes et al.[82]

and specialized diets for patients with renal failure, hepatic failure, glucose intolerance, etc. Many of these products do not meet the nutrient needs for burn patients and often limit protein while providing excess amounts of fat and carbohydrate. As an example, Table 30.5 shows the effects of changing either the volume of enteral nutrition and intravenous fluids (a major source of calories for some patients) delivered, or switching to one of the 'diabetic' formulas available. Clearly, the choice of formula can greatly influence both the success of nutrition, and the type and magnitude of complications encountered. This illustrates the need to have the burn center dietician involved in evaluating and selecting the products used to feed each patient.

TABLE 30.5 EFFECT OF DIFFERING VOLUME AND TYPE OF ENTERAL NUTRITION ON PROTEIN AND CARBOHYDRATE INTAKE

Example 1[a]
Maintenance feeding and IV

	Feedings	IV dextrose	Total
mL/h	100	200	300
kcal/d	2400	680	3080
Protein g/d	150	0	150
Carbs g/d	271	240	511
Fat g/d	82	0	82

Example 2
Decrease feeding, increase IV

	Feedings	IV dextrose	Total
mL/h	50	250	300
kcal/d	1200	1020	2220
Protein g/d	75	0	75
Carbs g/d	136	300	436
Fat g/d	41	0	41

Example 3[b]
Changing formula to Glucerna™

	Feedings	IV dextrose	Total
mL/h	100	200	300
kcal/d	2400	680	3080
Protein g/d	100	0	100
Carbs g/d	229	240	469
Fat g/d	131	0	131

[a]Typical 'maintenance' regimen for a patient with major burns, consisting of 100 mL/h of a high-protein 'stress' formula (Replete™), plus dextrose-containing crystalloid solutions to deliver a total fluid volume of 300 mL/h. Note that in Example 2, decreasing enteral nutrition, which is sometimes done to reduce glucose intolerance, results in relatively little decrease in total carbohydrate calories.

[b]Result of changing enteral products, using a formula designed for patients with glucose intolerance. These formulas are typically high-fat diets, resulting in fewer carbohydrate calories, but more fat and less protein, which is far from ideal for a stressed burns patient. The total amount of carbohydrates 'saved' by this adjustment is about 42 grams, or about three servings of starch per day.

Formulas for TPN

Solutions for TPN must be composed of elemental components that do not require digestion. Dextrose is the main calorie source, and the high concentrations require delivery through central venous catheters. Protein is supplied as prepared amino acid solutions. As mentioned previously, glutamine is not a component of TPN. In recent years, lipid emulsions have been perfected for intravenous use, and lipids can constitute a significant proportion of the calories in TPN.

The exact composition of TPN must be ordered by the physician. This permits exact tailoring of the solution to individual patient needs. Box 30.1 is an example of a protocol for ordering and administering TPN used at the University of Utah using a 'standard' TPN solution (70% dextrose, 15% amino acids, and 20% lipid emusion). Electrolytes, vitamins, and minerals can be custom-ordered, or standard 'packages' can be used. Medications such as insulin and H_2 blockers can be added as well.

Methods of nutritional support

Route of nutrition: parenteral vs. enteral

It is ironic that the development of TPN in the 1960s and 1970s actually preceded many enteral nutritional techniques. At the peak of TPN's popularity, it was estimated that over 500 000 patients were treated yearly, at a cost of over 3 billion dollars.[87] This included burn patients, for whom TPN was widely advocated.[22,88]

Use of TPN has now been largely replaced by enteral nutrition (EN) for both theoretical and practical reasons. Enteral nutrition directly nourishes the bowel mucosa; some nutrients (e.g. glutamine) may be particularly important in this regard. Also, the presence of even small amounts of nutrients within the bowel lumen stimulates the function of intestinal cells, maintains the architecture of intestinal microvilli and normal mucosal function, and may help preserve normal blood supply to the intestine.[89] Together, these effects may reduce bacterial translocation and sepsis and preserve gut-associated immune function.[90-92] In contrast, TPN appears to be associated with increased secretion of tumor necrosis factor and other proinflammatory mediators.[93] Lipids added to TPN may enhance inflammatory response as well, particularly in pulmonary dysfunction.[48]

In clinical trials, early and aggressive enteral nutrition has been associated with decreased infectious complications in trauma and ICU patients.[94,95] In burn patients, TPN supplementation of enteral nutrition has been associated with substantially increased mortality.[96,97] This is in contrast to a recent meta-analysis which showed no increased mortality associated with TPN in ICU patients.[98] The difference in these findings may be due to metabolic characteristics which are unique to burn patients, or may simply reflect more selective use of TPN in burn units, where it is limited to the sickest patients and therefore serves as a surrogate for severity of illness. As reviewed in Chapter 26, fatty infiltration of the liver is enhanced following burn injury; hepatomegaly and cholestasis can become massive, particularly in association with systemic infections.[99] This appears to be true regardless of the route of nutrition used but may be particularly severe in association with use of TPN.

In addition to maintaining gut integrity, EN provides 'first-pass' delivery of nutrients to the liver, which reduces hyperglycemia and hyperosmolarity. TPN requires central venous access, with the inherent risks of pneumo/hemothorax, bacteremia, endocarditis, air embolism, etc. Last, but by no means unimportant, TPN solutions are a great deal more costly than enteral formulas, require more expensive delivery systems, and more frequent monitoring of glucose and other blood chemistries. For all these reasons, *enteral nutrition should be considered the route of choice for the nutritional support of all burn patients with functioning (or even partially functioning) gastrointestinal tracts*.[1,100] TPN supplementation of EN is also not recommended, unless intolerance of maintenance EN is prolonged.

Early enteral feeding

A 1984 study in burned guinea pigs demonstrated that immediate EN improved maintenance of small bowel mass and

Box 30.1 A protocol for administration of TPN in burn patients

(Adapted from the 'Adult Parenteral Nutrition Orders', University of Utah)

STEP ONE: CALCULATED REQUIRED ENERGY AND PROTEIN NEEDS:

Example: 25-year-old man, 80 kg in weight. Body surface area = 2.2 m^2.
- Indirect calorimetry indicates energy expenditure of 2400 kcal/24 hours. To account for fluctuations in energy expenditure, increase measured value by 20% (480 kcal); total = 2880 nonprotein kcal/day.
- Estimate protein requirements at 2.0 g/kg/day = 160 g protein

STEP TWO: ORDER TPN SOLUTION

- Carbohydrates: carbohydrates are supplied as 70% dextrose (D70), which contains 2.4 kcal/mL. To give 75% of nonprotein calories as dextrose, calculate:

$$[(2880 \text{ total kcal}) \times (0.75 \text{ calories as dextrose})] / 2.4 \text{ kcal/mL} = 900 \text{ mL D70}$$

- Fat: The remainder of nonprotein calories will be given as lipid emulsion. This is commonly available as 10% (1.0 kcal/mL) or 20% (2.0 kcal/mL) solution. To give 25% of nonprotein calories as lipid, calculate:

$$[(2880 \text{ total kcal}) \times (0.25 \text{ calories as lipid})] / 2.0 \text{ kcal/mL} = 360 \text{ mL } 20\% \text{ lipid emulsion}$$

- Protein: protein is supplied as crystalline amino acid solutions at a concentration of 10% (0.1 g/mL), or 15% (0.15 g/mL). To give 160 g of protein, calculate:

$$(160 \text{ g protein}) / 0.15 \text{ g/mL} = 1067 \text{ mL of } 15\% \text{ amino acid solution}$$

- Total volume = 900 mL D70 + 360 mL lipids + 1067 mL amino acids = 2327 mL.
- Add electrolytes: these can be ordered as customized additions in any quantity, but a standard electrolyte 'package' contains (per liter of TPN):
  Sodium chloride: 35 mEq
  Potassium phosphate: 15 mM (22 mEq potassium)
  Magnesium sulfate: 8 mEq
  Calcium gluconate: 5 mEq
- Add vitamins: a standard vitamin 'package' contains approximately 100% of recommended dietary allowances of vitamins A, C, D, E, and B$_{12}$, pyridoxine, thiamine, riboflavin, niacin, pantothenic acid, folate, and biotin.
- Add trace elements: a standard 'package' contains:
  Zinc: 2.5 mg
  Copper: 1.0 mg
  Manganese: 0.25 mg
  Chromium: 10 μg
- Add additional water, and calculate infusion rate. If patients require additional fluid, water can be added to the TPN solution as desired. If no additional water is required, then the goal rate for infusion is 2327 mL / 24 hours = 97 mL/h.

STEP THREE: PROTOCOL FOR ADMINISTRATION

- Begin infusion at 20 mL/h via central vein.
- Increase rate every 4–6 hours by 10–20 mL/h until rate of 120 mL/h is achieved.

STEP FOUR: BEGIN MONITORING ON NUTRITIONAL SUPPORT

Blood glucose:
- As infusion is initiated, measure blood glucose every 4 hours.
- If glucose is ≥120 mg/dL, begin administration of exogenous insulin by 'sliding scale', or continuous drip. Consider oral hypoglycemic agents.
- After goal rate is achieved, measure blood glucose every 6 hours.

Daily:
- Serum electrolytes, blood urea nitrogen, creatinine.

Twice weekly:
- Hepatic enzymes (lactate dehydrogenase, alkaline phosphatase, total bilirubin, transaminases)
- 24-hour urine for nitrogen balance
- Serum transferrin or prealbumin
- Serum phosphorus, magnesium, and calcium

reduced hypermetabolism to levels approximating normal.[101] Other studies in animals and humans have not confirmed significant amelioration of hypermetabolism with early EN.[102,103] However, it appears clear that enteral feedings can be started safely within hours of injury in patients of all ages and that doing so reduces the accumulated 'calorie deficit,' improves nitrogen balance and overall nutrition.[104–106] Duodenal or jejunal feedings can be continued even during surgical procedures without increased risk of aspiration, which facilitates achievement of caloric goals, and may also reduce infectious complications.[107] For all these reasons, tube feedings should be started as soon as practically possibly following injury, and certainly within 48 hours. To enhance success, begin feedings at a rate of 20–40 mL/h (as little as 5 mL/hour in infants) and try to reach the therapeutic goal rate within 24 hours; the schedule is similar to that used for TPN in Table 30.5.

Gastric vs. intestinal feeding

Both gastric and intestinal feedings are widely used for delivery of EN; both have advantages and disadvantages. Gastric feeding can be instituted through large-diameter tubes placed blindly, which simplifies early feeding and minimizes clogging. Blenderized diets and intermittent bolus feedings can also be given into the stomach, reducing expense and the inconvenience of infusion pumps. A major disadvantage is the tendency of the stomach to develop ileus, both immediately postburn and in conjunction with sepsis or stress.

Intestinal feeding requires placement of a tube beyond the pylorus. While this can be done blindly, small enteric tubes have been placed inadvertently into the lung, with catastrophic consequences.[108] Many facilities prefer fluoroscopic or endoscopic tube placement, which is safer but inconvenient. Naso-enteric tubes are small and comfortable, but clog rather easily and often dislodge and migrate into the stomach. It is controversial whether aspiration is more common with gastric vs. intestinal feedings.[109,110] Any regimen of EN, however, requires careful ongoing monitoring for intolerance and pulmonary complications.

Many clinicians employ 'pro-motility' agents such as metoclopramide, erythromycin, or cisapride in conjunction with enteral nutrition. These agents, particularly erythromycin, may help enteral tubes pass spontaneously into the small intestine and can also ameliorate gastric ileus and feeding intolerance.[111]

Developing a program of nutritional support

Nutritional support can be provided most effectively by developing a comprehensive protocol that involves all members of the burn team and defines their roles and responsibilities. As stated previously, it has been repeatedly shown in ICU populations that adherence to such protocols increases both the success of nutrition and overall patient outcomes.

The level of support required by various patients differs greatly. For each patient, the goal is to provide adequate nutrition using the simplest and most physiological method. All patients need frequent reassessment to assure that they are achieving nutritional goals, to detect complications, and to determine if support can be simplified or if escalation is required. A simple algorithm for determining the level of nutritional support is displayed in Figure 30.3. Applying such an algorithm proactively may prevent problems from developing.

Patients with relatively small injuries (20–25% TBSA) and who are not intubated will generally be able to eat, though it

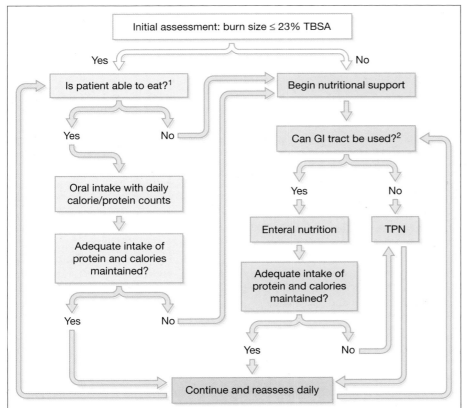

Fig. 30.3 An algorithm for determining the route of nutritional support for burn patients (see text).
[1] On admission, patients may require 3–4 days to tolerate adequate oral intake. Patients who require longer should be considered for nutritional support.
[2] Patients should be given some enteral nutrition even if they still require TPN for the balance of nutritional support.

may take several days for initial ileus and nausea to resolve. Patients with large partial-thickness burns may have more difficulty due to effects of pain and pain medications. In this circumstance, a few days of inadequate nutrition can be permitted if it appears the patient will soon be able to eat. Patients who are failing to progress with oral intake, who require major surgery, or who develop complications will benefit from the early institution of more formal nutritional support. Early initiation of enteral feeds may actually prevent development of ileus. Patients given TPN should be reassessed frequently for evidence of GI function; patients who cannot tolerate all their nutrition enterally should be given low-rate 'trophic' feeds if at all possible. These help preserve small bowel integrity and function, and facilitate gradually increasing enteral nutrition (and decreasing TPN) as the bowel recovers. Similarly, some oral intake should be permitted when possible in patients given enteral nutrition. Oral intake — even sips of liquid — is of great psychological benefit to patients and encourages them to wean from tube feedings quickly as recovery progresses.

Several patient populations merit special consideration in providing adequate nutritional support:

- Infants/children: children, like adults, demonstrate increased calorie and protein requirements following burn injury. However, adult enteral products provide high renal solute loads, large protein intakes, and vitamin and mineral levels incompatible with current recommendations for children. Most infants require relatively high fluid volumes and should not receive concentrated formulas; infant formulas are more dilute and generally provide 20 or 24 kcal/oz (0.66–0.8 kcal/mL). Some popular pediatric enteral formulas are compared in Table 30.3. Oral intake in small children is often difficult due to pain, anxiety, and an inability to comprehend the need for adequate intake. Many prefer drinking to eating and offering high-calorie, nutritionally complete fluids is helpful. However, early initiation of enteral nutritional support can meet nutrient needs and reduce the stress associated with pushing oral intake.
- The elderly: elderly patients are more likely to have pre-existing nutritional conditions and malnutrition than other adult burn patients.[20] Diabetes and its complications – heart disease, poor dentition, etc. – all affect nutritional status and provision of adequate nutrition. Resting metabolic rates decrease with age and may not rise dramatically postburn. Reliance on standard formulas to calculate energy and protein needs will likely result in overfeeding, glucose intolerance, and azotemia. Similarly, many high-protein 'stress' products provide excessive intakes of calories and protein for the elderly; using a standard product may be more appropriate in this setting. Examples of such products are included in Table 30.3. The clinician also needs to evaluate the need for restrictions (e.g. potassium, fat) in these patients.
- Pre-existing conditions: the increasing prevalence of diabetes, metabolic syndrome, and obesity in Americans affects burn patients as well. Metabolic syndrome (also called syndrome X) is a complex metabolic disorder which includes diabetes, lipid abnormalities, and hypertension, all associated with insulin resistance, and is often associated with central obesity ('apple-shaped' body habitus). The prevalence of syndrome X makes hyperglycemia more common in burn patients, and renders glucose control more difficult.
- Obese patients are often falsely presumed to be well-nourished. In fact, they often have poor muscle mass and visceral protein stores, and they continue to need calories for nutrition as metabolic changes limit the body's ability to utilize stored body fat. Underfeeding will lead to loss of muscle as in other patients. Several formulas exist to estimate calorie needs in obese individuals though the clinical relevance has not been established; indirect calorimetry and nitrogen balance studies can provide more timely information about calorie and protein needs.

Monitoring and complications

Monitoring of nutritional support

Comprehensive nutritional support in burn patients must include ongoing monitoring of its adequacy and success. As mentioned previously, the physiological changes which accompany burn injury render many monitors of nutrition difficult or impossible to interpret. In addition, most of these markers do not correlate highly with outcomes. *Careful assessment of clinical status*, including vital signs, respiratory status, functional improvement, and wound healing, remains the most important aspect of nutritional monitoring. The tests described below are most useful in identifying and monitoring trends (as opposed to point estimates) in nutritional status.

Body weight

Change in body weight is the best predictor of overall nutritional status for the general population, and significant weight loss — particularly rapid and unplanned — is a powerful predictor of mortality.[112] However, weight is often misleading in burn patients. Initial fluid resuscitation routinely adds 20–30 kilograms to patients' weights and much greater increases are common. Theoretically, this fluid will dissipate with diuresis, but the time course for this is unpredictable, particularly if resuscitation volume is high.[113] Fluid increases may mask ongoing loss of lean body mass so that patients can suffer significant inanition and still weigh more than at the time of admission. In addition, fluid shifts associated with infections, ventilator support, hypoproteinemia, and elevations in aldosterone and antidiuretic hormone lead to wide fluctuations in weight that have little to do with nutritional status. Even weeks after injury, patients have increased total body water and have almost always lost more lean body mass than is apparent from weight alone.[114] Along with increases in fluid, patients may have increased fat mass without changes in weight. In ICU patients, aggressive TPN did not prevent loss of over 12% of protein mass despite weight gain as fat.[115] In burned adults, increasing caloric intake to almost twice measured energy expenditure did not reduce ongoing muscle breakdown; increased caloric intake resulted only in accumulation of body fat.[116] In following weights, try to recognize long-term trends more than daily variations, and continue monitoring during the often long rehabilitation phase.

Nitrogen balance

Providing sufficient protein intake is a major goal of nutritional support. Because patients differ widely in their protein requirements, some ongoing monitor of this parameter is desirable. In addition to serum protein measurements (described below), a widely-used test is the assessment of nitrogen balance. Measurements should be obtained at least weekly and require accurate collections of urine for determination of urea nitrogen along with concomitant recording of nitrogen intake. Twenty-four-hour collections are often used, though shorter times can also provide accurate data.[117] Nitrogen balance (N_2 bal) can then be calculated by formulas such as the following:[118]

$$N_2 \text{ bal} = N_2I - (1.25 \times (UUN + 4))$$

where N_2I = 24-hour nitrogen intake.

Most formulas contain two constants, which can introduce significant error to calculations. Urinary urea nitrogen (UUN) is increased by 4 g/dL (2 g/dL is used for children less than 4 years old, and 3 g/dL for children 4–10 years) to approximate total urinary nitrogen (TUN). However, TUN may exceed this value in burn patients,[119] leading to underestimation of nitrogen losses. The formula provided also multiplies estimated TUN by 1.25, to account for significant loss of protein-rich exudates from burn wounds. Many formulas which estimate nitrogen balance do not account for it. Actual burn wound losses can exceed these estimates, again leading to overly-optimistic estimation of the adequacy of protein intake. Thus these formulas provide only an approximation of actual nitrogen balance.

Attainment of positive or even neutral nitrogen may not always be possible, especially in the absence of exercise. Inactivity causes muscle wasting and increased nitrogen excretion even in healthy people.[120] In the early postburn period, patients are often bedridden and sedated, and may even be chemically paralyzed; increasing levels of protein intake only result in increased nitrogen excretion. This emphasizes the importance of a comprehensive, team-based plan of care in which nutritional and physical therapy are equally important in maintaining muscle mass.

Serum proteins

The acute response to burn injury shifts metabolic pathways away from maintenance of visceral proteins often cited as 'nutritional markers.'[121] Albumin, an important indicator of *chronic* nutritional status, is of much less value in assessing *acute* changes. In burn patients, serum albumin levels are both immediately and chronically depressed; even successful nutrition will not produce rising albumin levels for long periods. Administration of supplemental albumin, to improve colloid oncotic pressure and control edema, has not improved clinical or nutritional outcomes.[122,123]

Some other proteins have been advocated as more useful markers of nutrition. Prealbumin (or transthyretin) has a short half-life, making it theoretically more responsive to nutritional changes.[121] However, prealbumin levels also fall quickly post-injury, and rebound slowly. Levels may correlate with susceptibility to infection, but may not reflect ongoing nutritional status.[39,124] Serum transferrin, retinol-binding protein, and others have also been used, but their clinical usefulness appears equally limited.[53,121,125] Measurement of these proteins may be expensive or not routinely available. Protein markers, if used at all, should be interpreted in the context of patients' clinical condition and, like body weight, evaluated serially to indicate trends.

Other parameters

Abnormalities of immune function and susceptibility to infection are major consequences of malnutrition. In the past, markers of immune competence have been advocated for use in nutritional assessment, including total lymphocyte count[82] and measurement of delayed-type hypersensitivity (DTH) to antigens injected into the dermis.[126,127] These markers have not proved very useful, particularly in burn patients. Acute thermal injury is itself profoundly immunosuppressive; anergy can also be produced by infection, old age, or other complicating factors and does not itself constitute evidence of inadequate nutrition.

A number of other parameters should be followed routinely in all patients receiving nutritional support. Burn injury produces accelerated evaporative water losses, so hydration should be monitored closely. Electrolyte abnormalities, and levels of phosphorus, magnesium, and calcium should also be assessed regularly. Liver function abnormalities can result from overfeeding but can also indicate other serious conditions which complicate burn treatment including hepatitis and acalculous cholecystitis. The large protein loads required by burn patients result in increased urinary excretion of nitrogenous wastes and predispose to elevations of blood urea nitrogen. Table 30.5 illustrates a protocol for administration of TPN to a burn patient, including the recommended monitoring of nutritional status.

Some new, technically-advanced methods are now available for nutritional monitoring as well. Bioimpedance analysis (BIA) measures the body's resistance to the passage of electrical currents; from this information total body water, and the body's fat-free cell mass can be calculated.[128,129] Dual X-ray absorptiometry (DEXA) scanning measures precise absorption of radiation by various tissues; it has been used to measure bone density as well as fat-free mass in clinical studies.[130] Both of these techniques are currently useful primarily in research but may be utilized more widely in clinical care in the future.

As this information suggests, no single laboratory test is universally applicable or reliable for nutritional monitoring of burn patients. A survey of nutrition practices in 46 burn centers[131] indicated that the most commonly-used parameters were body weight (100% of centers), serum albumin (93%), nitrogen balance (70%), transferrin (41%), and prealbumin (26%). In establishing a nutrition protocol, it remains essential to follow clinical course and wound healing, and it is probably reasonable to monitor at least body weight and possibly one or two indices of protein status, such as nitrogen balance, transferrin, or prealbumin. Other tests probably don't add much additional information, and can be reserved for research studies.

Overfeeding

While almost any disorder of fluids, electrolytes or homeostasis can occur with nutritional support, one of the most frequent complications of modern nutrition is overfeeding. As noted previously, it can be difficult both to estimate the nutrition needed by burn patients and to deliver these nutrients successfully. Nutrition is often inadequate in the early postburn period, a time when ileus and nausea interfere with enteral nutrition, and hyperglycemia complicates both EN and TPN. Aggressive efforts to feed patients in the early postburn period can lead to unintended overfeeding as metabolic rate declines and regimens become more successful. Significant overfeeding, especially for long periods, can produce three major complications.

Increased production of CO₂

As noted above, overfeeding carbohydrates results in fat synthesis, increased VCO_2, and elevation in repiratory quotient (RQ). Patients with ongoing respiratory compromise may demonstrate difficulty weaning from ventilatory support. This problem can be particularly severe with use of TPN.[132] Regular monitoring of RQ with indirect calorimetry will detect this problem. Nutritional support can be tapered to match measured values, or glucose administration reduced by giving a more calories as fat, or both. If it is possible to switch patients on TPN to enteral nutrition: this may be helpful, though overfeeding of enteral nutrition can occur as well.

Fatty liver

Excess carbohydrate or fat administration leads to deposition of fat in the liver parenchyma.[133] Some degree of hepatic enzyme elevation is common in burn patients, and this may also be more pronounced with TPN. Enzymes should be monitored regularly, and feeding evaluated carefully if enzymes become elevated above 2–3 times normal. Pronounced elevations can suggest other disorders (hepatitis, acalculous cholecystitis, etc.), and may be unavoidably associated with sepsis.[99]

Azotemia

The large amounts of protein required by burn patients can lead to elevation of blood urea nitrogen (BUN), particularly if dehydration occurs.[134] Acute renal failure is one of the most dreaded complications of sepsis, with a persistently high mortality rate. Monitor fluid intake, urine output, and blood chemistries frequently in burn patients who require nutritional support. An increase in BUN in excess of 30% above baseline may indicate relative dehydration or overfeeding of protein, particularly if nitrogen balance is positive; reduce the amount of protein being given. Even in established renal failure, patients continue to require large amounts of protein. Protein restriction should be avoided, even if doing so commits the patient to hemodialysis.[1]

Hyperglycemia

Hyperglycemia is extremely common following critical illness. Approximately 10–20% of patients admitted to ICUs have pre-existing diabetes. Far more important, however, is that up to 90% of all ICU patients develop elevated blood glucose values during their hospital stay.[135] In burn patients, insulin's effects are overwhelmed by catabolic hormones, causing relative insulin resistance and hyperglycemia which can be both profound and sustained — the 'diabetes of injury.' Prolonged elevations in blood sugar are clearly associated with immune deficiency and increased susceptibility to infection; this may also be true for acute hyperglycemia.[135] And, since infection exaggerates glucose intolerance, infection and hyperglycemia often potentiate each other.

Recent evidence has emphasized the value of maintaining glucose levels as close to normal as possible. In a landmark study, surgical ICU patients randomized to a regimen of 'intensive' glucose control (maintaining glucose levels at 80–110 mg/dL), compared to more traditional control (180–200 mg/dL) had substantial reductions in multiple organ failure, infection, renal failure, polyneuropathy, length of stay, and mortality.[136] This experience has been confirmed repeatedly.[137,138] In addition to lowering blood sugar, insulin exerts a number of beneficial effects of its own, including reducing circulating levels of C-reactive protein and other pro-inflammatory compounds,[139,140] which may explain some of the benefits shown in these studies.

Thus, meticulous control of blood sugar is emerging as a cost-effective way to improve outcomes in critical care. It is reasonable to assume that similar benefits can be expected in burn care, though there are as yet no large studies in burn patients. Many units are now adopting comprehensive protocols for intensive monitoring and treatment of blood sugar values; an example from our burn center is given in Figure 30.4. Because hyperglycemia is often resistant to therapy, effective glucose control may require substantial insulin doses, glucose monitoring, and nursing time, even in patients not receiving nutritional support. Hyperglycemia is both more common and more severe with TPN as opposed to enteral nutrition, and this alone constitutes a powerful argument for avoiding parenteral nutrition. Reassessing patients' calorie needs (with changes in clinical status and/or over time) and reducing the quantity of infused calories if appropriate is probably the first step in managing hyperglycemia. A number of other adjuncts can contribute to effective blood sugar maintenance as well, including controlling infections, increasing patient activity, and restricting oral intake of sweets. Oral hypoglycemic agents and anabolic agents may ultimately prove to have major benefit in this effort.[141] Adherence to strict policies for blood sugar monitoring and control is likely to emerge as a major focus of quality assurance in burn care in the years to come.

Complications of enteral nutrition

Enteral feeding complications fall into two categories: metabolic and mechanical. Major metabolic complications of nutritional support are reviewed in Table 30.6. Mechanical complications include misplaced feeding tubes, gastric distension, nausea, and aspiration. All tube placements should be verified prior to use, and clinicians must monitor gastrointestinal function frequently. Surgically-placed gastrostomy or jejunostomy tubes eliminate problems with tube migration, but are associated with (generally low) risks of dislodgement, leakage, and bowel perforation. Some units add blue dye to tube feeds in an effort to detect aspiration more efficiently. Unfortunately, blue dye has a low specificity and sensitivity

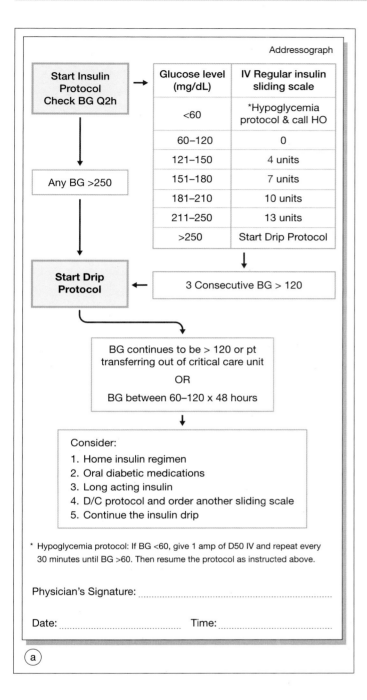

Insulin drip protocol

Step 1: initiate insulin infusion
- Standard insulin drip: Regular insulin 100 units/100 mL of NS
- Give IV bolus as indicated and initiate insulin drip based on the following table:

Initiation of insulin drip protocol only

Blood glucose	Regular insulin bolus	Regular insulin dose
121–140	0 units	1 unit/h
141–169	6 units	1 unit/h
170–249	8 units	2 units/h
250–299	10 units	3 units/h
300–399	10 units	4 units/h
400–500	10 units	5 units/h
>500	10 units	6 units/h

Important note:
All patients receiving IV insulin drip therapy must have a continuous source of glucose (continuous tube feeds OR TPN unless ordered by MD)

Step 2: monitoring
- Check BG *Q1h* timed such that BG are checked 1 hour after drip initiation or rate change.
- If 3 consecutive BG within 80–120 with no change in therapy, reduce checks to *Q2h*.
- Then, if 3 consecutive BG within 80–120 with no change in therapy and insulin rate is ≤2 units/h, reduce checks to *Q4h*.

Step 3: ongoing infusion
- Make adjustments based on the following table:

Blood glucose	Infusion rate adjustment
<60	Hold drip. Give 1/2 amp D50. Recheck Q30min, repeat 1/2 amp D50 until BG >60
60–79	Hold drip. Check BG in 1 hour. *if BG >80, restart at 1/2 rate prior to holding drip*
80–120	No change
121–140	↑ rate by 0.2 unit/h
141–170	↑ rate by 1 unit/h
171–250	Give 8 units regular insulin bolus and ↑ rate by 1 unit/h
>250	Give 10 units regular insulin bolus and ↑ rate by 1 unit/h

Note: If blood glucose <60 on glucometer send sample to the lab for measurement per policy

Step 4: important nursing information
- If BG decreases by ≥100 mg/dL from previous level, ↓ rate by 1/2 and recheck in 1 hour.
- If BG ≤150 mg/dL and subsequent level decreases by ≥30 mg/dL, ↓ rate by 1/2.
- If patient's enteral or parenteral nutrition is discontinued, hold insulin drip and check BG Q2h and restart sliding scale on previous page.

Step 5: discontinuation
- After insulin drip is discontinued, check BG *Q2h*.
- Begin appropriate insulin sliding scale and/or oral diabetic agents (i.e. home regimen).

An adequate physician order is 'Insulin per Protocol'. Reference protocol copies will be available on the units.

Fig. 30.4 Hyperglycemia Management Guidelines, Burn Intensive Care Unit, University of Utah.

TABLE 30.6 METABOLIC COMPLICATIONS OF NUTRITIONAL SUPPORT (PARTICULARLY TPN)

Complication	Description/cause	Frequency	Severity	Diagnosis/treatment
Hyperglycemia	Occurs to some degree in almost all patients on nutritional support; more common and more severe with TPN. Any nutritional support regimen should be started slowly, and monitored regularly	Common	Moderate to very severe	Blood glucose *must* be monitored regularly in all patients. Insulin added to TPN solution can be helpful; patients may also require a rigorous protocol using supplemental insulin and oral hypoglycemic agents. Sustained hyperglycemia may require slowing/holding TPN until controlled
Hyperosmolarity	Occurs almost exclusively with TPN: prolonged hyperglycemia can cause dehydration, mental status changes; coma	Rare	Can be life-threatening	A complication of untreated hyperglycemia. Close attention to glucose control should prevent this. Treat by stopping TPN, hydrating, controlling glucose
Hyperkalemia	Excessive administration of potassium; often occurs when a 'standard' electrolyte solution is added to TPN without considering patient-specific issues (i.e. renal failure)	Uncommon	Can be life-threatening	Routinely monitor potassium, especially during initiation of TPN. Occurs in association with hyperglycemia, renal dysfunction, sepsis. Severe hyperkalemia (≥ 6.0 mEq/L) causes T-wave elevation, can be fatal. This is a medical emergency, and mandates discontinuation of TPN, or change to a low-potassium enteral formula
Hypokalemia	Low serum potassium. Can occur if electrolytes are not added during TPN ordering. The institution of TPN causes uptake of potassium and sudden hypokalemia. This occurs along with hypophosphatemia and hypomagesemia — the 'refeeding' syndrome	Uncommon	Moderate to serious	Routinely monitor potassium, especially during initiation of TPN. Institution of aggressive glucose control can cause this. Can cause weakness arrhythmias. Treat by potassium supplementation. Magnesium deficiency can contribute to hypokalemia as well
Hyponatremia/fluid overload	Occurs usually when dilute solutions are used for TPN. Can result in pulmonary failure, ascites, edema. Use of 'peripheral' TPN requires large fluid loads, particularly in children, and should be avoided. Additional fluids given with antibiotics and resuscitation can compound this problem	Moderately common	Moderate to serious	Monitor intake/output, serum sodium. Nutritional support in renal failure should be continued, but may require more frequent dialysis. Severe hyponatremia from any cause must be corrected gradually (≤ 0.5 mEq/L/hour) to avoid severe neurologic complications
Hypernatremia/dehydration	Can occur when insufficient free water is given. Burn patients may have significant requirements over and above the fluids required for TPN	Moderately common	Moderate to serious	Monitor intake/output, serum sodium. Additional free water can be added to TPN or given separately. Persistent hyperglycemia causes obligatory diuresis and dehydration
Hypermagnesemia	Presents with lethargy, weakness, prolongation of P-R and Q-T, AV-block	Rare	Moderate to serious	Usually occurs in the setting of renal failure
Hypomagnesemia	Presents with perioral tingling, weakness, tetany, arrhythmias. Magnesium is consumed during protein synthesis, and institution of nutrition, particularly TPN, can precipitate hypomagnesemia — the 'refeeding syndrome'. Diuretics also cause this	Moderately common	Moderate to serious	Monitor magnesium routinely, especially during institution of nutritional support. May require substantial supplementation

TABLE 30.6—cont'd

Complication	Description/cause	Frequency	Severity	Diagnosis/treatment
Hyperphosphatemia	Usually occurs in the setting of renal failure	Uncommon	Moderate	Renal dysfunction may require removal of all phosphate from TPN and use of phosphate binders, or change to a low-phosphate enteral formula
Hypophosphatemia	Presents with weakness, particularly of jaw muscles, lethargy, obtundation. Often occurs early postburn even without nutrition, but phosphorus is consumed into protein with TPN — part of the 'refeeding syndrome'	Common	Moderate	Monitor phosphorus levels routinely, especially during institution of nutrition. Patients may require frequent monitoring and supplementation
Trace element deficiency	Copper deficiency can cause anemia and neutropenia; zinc deficiency causes skin lesions, hair loss, impaired immunity. Deficiencies of selenium, cobalt, manganese, and others have been described	Rare	Moderate to serious	Trace element deficiencies usually occur only with prolonged TPN. Standard trace element 'packages' contain more than enough for maintenance. Blood transfusions also contain significant amounts of copper, chromium, and some others
Vitamin deficiency	A variety of vitamin deficiencies have been described, almost exclusively in patients on long-term TPN	Rare	Moderate to serious	Fat-soluble vitamins (A, D, E, K) and water-soluble 'B' vitamins should all be included in standardized vitamin 'packages' for TPN supplementation. Individual vitamins can be given as well
Essential fatty acid deficiency	Presents with malabsorption/diarrhea, dry skin, anemia, thrombocytopenia. Hyperinsulinemia prevents fatty acid mobilization, so deficiency can develop in as little as 10 days of TPN	Uncommon	Moderate to severe	Use of medium-chain triglycerides (MCTs) do not prevent this, but modern lipid solutions contain long-chain triglycerides as well. Lipid emulsion should be given at least once weekly
Fatty liver dysfunction	Presents with hepatomegaly, right upper quadrant pain, and elevation of hepatic enzymes. May occur to a mild extent in many patients, but becomes worse with prolonged overfeeding and TPN; can lead to cirrhosis	Common	Mild to severe	Avoid overfeeding, particularly fats. Monitor liver enzymes routinely. More common and more severe in septic patients

for detecting aspiration. Reports of blue dye-associated mortality have led the FDA and others to recommend eliminating blue dye for this purpose.[142]

Bowel necrosis and perforation

Several reports have documented bowel necrosis and perforation as a rare complication of enteral nutrition in the critically ill, including burn patients.[143,144] It is likely that continued administration of tube feedings in the face of decreased bowel motility causes distension, interfering with intestinal blood supply. Bacterial overgrowth of stagnant tube feedings, and administration of narcotics and antidiarrheal agents also contribute to this complication.[89] Fever, leukocytosis, tachycardia, and abdominal distension may precede frank peritonitis. Abdominal CT scanning can confirm perforation, which mandates laparotomy, and usually intestinal resection. Mortality rates approximate 50%.[144]

Diarrhea

Tube feedings are frequently blamed for diarrhea, which can range from a minor problem, to a major source of patient discomfort, morbidity, fluid and electrolyte imbalance, and other complications. Often the cause is multifactorial.[145] The high glucose loads of hypertonic tube feedings may contribute to diarrhea, though diluting feedings has generally not proved helpful in treatment. Enteral medications including antacids, phosphates, antibiotics, and others contribute to diarrhea as well. Infectious causes include cytomegalovirus infection[146] and pseudomembranous colitis caused by *Clostridium difficile*.[147] A prospective study found an association between the concentration of fat in tube feedings and the incidence of diarrhea;[148] diarrhea was reduced in a group of children fed a low-fat 'immune-enhancing diet.'[69] Because the gut's tolerance of tube feedings is limited, diarrhea is increased with overfeeding, and can be controlled by reducing infusion rate.

A variety of compounds have been suggested for treatment of diarrhea, including opiates (Imodium™, Lomotil™, Paregoric, etc.), bulk agents (Metamucil™), and others. Some clinicians advocate use of fiber-containing tube feedings to reduce this complication. Fiber is a normal component of nutrition, and its presence may help prevent bacterial overgrowth and stasis.[149] However, these compounds have also been blamed for intestinal stasis and bowel necrosis.[150] In addition, fiber-containing feedings sometimes clog small-diameter tubes. In our experience, attempts to control diarrhea with medications are frequently either ineffective or lead to constipation and distension. Infectious diarrheas may be worsened by slowing intestinal transit. Most diarrhea is self-limited and does not require pharmacological therapy. Try altering the tube formula, stopping enteral medications, reducing the infusion rate, or simply waiting a day or two. It may be necessary to hold feedings temporarily to permit refractory diarrhea to resolve, then restart them gradually. Diarrhea unresponsive to simple measures should prompt evaluation for an infectious source inside or outside the bowel.[151]

Complications of parenteral nutrition

Technical complications of TPN are those associated with line placement and maintenance. These complications can be life-threatening, and demand close attention to protocols for line care. Complications occurring at the time of line placement include pneumothorax, hemothorax, pericardial tamponade, hydrothorax, and catheter misplacement. These complications can also occur later if lines erode through venous structures.

Indwelling central venous lines can cause hemorrhage or air embolism if disconnected inadvertently. In addition, central lines can develop serious infections, including catheter sepsis, septic thrombophlebitis, and even endocarditis; not surprisingly, these infectious complications are more common when catheters are placed through cutaneous burn wounds.[152] Central lines used for TPN are particularly prone to infectious problems, and risk is increased if lines are left in place for long periods, and if they are used for multiple purposes (blood draws, hemodynamic monitoring, antibiotics, maintenance fluids, etc.). Consider changing central venous catheters — especially TPN lines — in any patients with persistent, unexplained fevers, or other evidence of infection.

Metabolic complications of TPN can be both severe and difficult to treat. Because TPN often represents the only fluid and electrolyte therapy given to patients, the body's ability to compensate for deficiencies/excesses is severely limited, which can allow almost any disorder of electrolyte or vitamin deficiency or excess to develop. In addition, a number of common complications of any nutritional regimen can be either more frequent or more severe when associated with TPN use as opposed to enteral nutrition. Such complications are outlined in Table 30.6.[153]

Conclusion

Although nutritional support following a major burn continues to evolve, several aspects are clear. Enteral nutrition and high protein intake are important, though there is no 'one-size-fits-all' solution — needs vary with each individual, and change throughout the course of care. A thorough protocol involving all team members that includes ongoing and systematic assessment can tailor support to changing needs, and provide optimal care to every patient.

References

1. Heyland DK, Dhaliwal R, Drover JW, et al. Canadian clinical practice guidelines for nutrition support in mechanically ventilated, critically ill adult patients. JPEN 2003; 27(5):355–373.
2. Heyland DK, Dhaliwal R, Day A, et al. Validation of the Canadian clinical practice guidelines for nutrition support in mechanically ventilated, critically ill adult patients: results of a prospective observational study. Crit Care Med 2004; 32(11):2260–2266.
3. Barr J, Hecht M, Flavin KE, et al. Outcomes in critically ill patients before and after the implementation of an evidence-based nutritional management protocol. Chest 2004; 125(4):1446–1457.
4. Guidelines for the use of parenteral and enteral nutrition in adult and pediatric patients. JPEN J Parenter Enteral Nutr 2002; 26(1 Suppl):1SA–138SA.
5. Cuthbertson D. The disturbance of metabolism produced by bony and nonbony injury with notes of certain abnormal conditions of bone. Biochem J 1930; 24:1244–1263.
6. Long C, Schaffel N, Geiger C, et al. Metabolic response to injury and illness: estimation of energy and protein needs from indirect calorimetry and nitrogen balance. JPEN 1979; 3:452–456.
7. Wilmore D, Long J, Mason A, et al. Catecholamines: mediators of the hypermetabolic response to thermal injury. Ann Surg 1974; 180:653–658.
8. Newsome T, Mason A, Pruitt B. Weight loss following thermal injury. Ann Surg 1973; 178:215–217.
9. Wilmore DW. Nutrition and metabolism following thermal injury. Clin Plast Surg 1974; 1(4):603–619.
10. Demling R, Seigne P. Metabolic management of patients with severe burns. World J Surg 2000; 24:673–680.
11. Kudsk K, Brown R. Nutritional support. In: Mattox K, Feliciano D, Moore E, eds. Trauma. New York: McGraw-Hill; 2000: 1369–1405.
12. Bessey P, Jiang Z, Johnson D, et al. Posttraumatic skeletal muscle proteolysis: the role of the hormonal environment. World J Surg 1989; 13:465–470.
13. Long C, Kinney J, Geiger C. Nonsuppressibility of gluconeogenesis by glucose in septic patients. Metabolism 1976; 25:193.
14. Demling R, Signe P. Metabolic management of patients with severe burns. World J Surg 2000; 24:673–680.
15. Hart DW, Wolf SE, Chinkes DL, et al. Determinants of skeletal muscle catabolism after severe burn. Ann Surg 2000; 232(4):455–465.
16. Rutan T, Herndon D, VanOsten T, et al. Metabolic rate alterations in early excision and grafting versus conservative treatment. J Trauma 1986; 26:140–146.
17. Barton R, Craft W, Saffle J. Chemical paralysis reduces energy expenditure in mechanically ventilated trauma patients. J Burn Care Rehabil 1997; 18:461–468.
18. Saffle J, Medina E, Raymond J, et al. Use of indirect calorimetry in the nutritional management of burn patients. J Trauma 1985; 25:32–39.

19. Hildreth M, Herndon D, Desai M, et al. Current treatment reduced calories required to maintain weight in pediatric patients with burns. J Burn Care Rehabil 1990; 11:405–409.

20. Demling RH. The incidence and impact of pre-existing protein energy malnutrition on outcome in the elderly burn patient population. J Burn Care Rehabil 2005; 26(1):94–100.

21. Baker JP, Detsky AS, Wesson DE, et al. Nutritional assessment: a comparison of clinical judgment and objective measurements. N Engl J Med 1982; 306(16):969–972.

22. Ireton-Jones C, Gottschlich M. The evolution of nutrition support in burns. J Burn Care Rehabil 1993; 14:272–280.

23. Curreri P, Richmond D, Marvin J, et al. Dietary requirements of patients with major burns. J Am Diet Assoc 1974; 65:415–417.

24. Davies J, Lilijedahl S. Metabolic consequences of an extensive burn. In: Polk H, ed. Contemporary burn management. Boston: Little, Brown; 1971:415–417.

25. Harris J, Benedict F. A biometric study of basal metabolism in man. Washington, DC: Carnegie Institute of Washington; 1919.

26. Ireton-Jones C, Jones JD. Improved equations for predicting energy expenditure in patients: the Ireton-Jones Equations. Nutr Clin Pract 2002; 17(1):29–31.

27. Allard JP, Pichard C, Hoshino E, et al. Validation of a new formula for calculating the energy requirements of burn patients. JPEN 1990; 14(2):115–118.

28. Dietary Reference Intakes, Food and Nutrition Board, Institute of Medicine. In: National Academy Press; 1997, 1998, 2002.

29. Dickerson RN, Gervasio JM, Riley ML, et al. Accuracy of predictive methods to estimate resting energy expenditure of thermally-injured patients. JPEN 2002; 26(1):17–29.

30. Day T, Dean P, Adams M, et al. Nutritional requirements of the burned child: The Curreri Junior formula. Proceedings of the American Burn Association 1986; 18:86.

31. Hildreth M, Herndon D, Desai M, et al. Current treatment reduces calories required to maintain weight in pediatric patients with burns. J Burn Care Rehabil 1990; 11:405–409.

32. Hildreth M, Herndon D, Desai M, et al. Caloric requirements of patients with burns under one year of age. J Burn Care Rehabil 1993; 14:108–112.

33. Hildreth M, Herndon D, Desai M, et al. Caloric needs of adolescent patients with burns. J Burn Care Rehabil 1989; 10:523–526.

34. Food and Nutrition Board: National Research Council Recommended Dietary Allowances. Washington, DC: National Academy of Science; 1980.

35. Bursztein S, Glaser P, Trichet B, et al. Utilization of protein, carbohydrate, and fat in fasting and postabsorptive subjects. Am J Clin Nutr 1980; 33:998–1001.

36. Ireton-Jones CS, Turner WW Jr. The use of respiratory quotient to determine the efficacy of nutrition support regimens. J Am Diet Assoc 1987; 87:1880–1883.

37. Shaw-Delanty S, Elwyn D, Askanazi J, et al. Resting energy expenditure in injured, septic, and malnourished adult patients on intravenous diets. Clin Nutr 1990; 9:305–312.

38. Hester D, Lawson K. Suggested guidelines for use by dietitians in the interpretation of indirect calorimetry data. J Am Diet Assoc 1989; 89:100–101.

39. Peck M. Practice guidelines for burn care: nutritional support. J Burn Care Rehabil 2001; 22:59S–66S.

40. Gottschlich M, Alexander J, Bower R. Enteral nutrition in patients with burns or trauma. In: Rombeau J, Caldwell M, eds. Enteral and tube feeding. Philadelphia: WB Saunders; 1984:306–324.

41. Swinamer D, Phang P, Jones R, et al. Twenty-four hour energy expenditure in critically ill patients. Crit Care Med 1987; 15:637–641.

42. De Jonghe B, Appere-De-Vechi C, Fournier M, et al. A prospective survey of nutritional support practices in intensive care unit patients: what is prescribed? What is delivered? Crit Care Med 2001; 29(1):8–12.

43. Adam S, Batson S. A study of problems associated with the delivery of enteral feed in critically ill patients in five ICUs in the UK. Intensive Care Med 1997; 23(3):261–266.

44. Saffle JR, Larson CM, Sullivan J. A randomized trial of indirect calorimetry-based feedings in thermal injury. J Trauma 1990; 30(7):776–82; discussion 82–83.

45. Wolfe R, Allsop J, Burke J. Responses to intravenous glucose infusion. Metabolism 1979; 28:210–217.

46. Mochizuki H, Trocki O, Dominioni L, et al. Optimal lipid content for enteral diets following thermal injury. JPEN 1984; 8:638–646.

47. Garrel D, Razi M, Lariviere R. Improved clinical status and length of care with low-fat nutrition support in burn patients. JPEN 1995; 19:482–491.

48. Battistella FD, Widergren JT, Anderson JT, et al. A prospective, randomized trial of intravenous fat emulsion administration in trauma victims requiring total parenteral nutrition. J Trauma 1997; 43(1):52–58; discussion 58–60.

49. Alexander J, Saito H, Trocki O, et al. The importance of lipid type in the diet after burn injury. Ann Surg 1986; 204:1–8.

50. Huschak G, Zur Nieden K, Hoell T, et al. Olive oil based nutrition in multiple trauma patients: a pilot study. Intensive Care Med 2005; 31(9):1202–1208.

51. Soeters PB, van de Poll MC, van Gemert WG, et al. Amino acid adequacy in pathophysiological states. J Nutr 2004; 134(6 Suppl):1575S–1582S.

52. Wolfe R, Goodenough R, Burke J, et al. Response of proteins and urea kinetics in burn patients to different levels of protein intake. Ann Surg 1983; 197:163–171.

53. Alexander J, MacMillan B, Stinnet J, et al. Beneficial effects of aggressive protein feeding in severely burned children. Ann Surg 1980; 192:505–517.

54. Matsuda T, Kagan R, Hanumadass M, et al. The importance of burn wound size in determining the optimal calorie:nitrogen ratio. Surgery 1983; 94:562–568.

55. Prelack K, Cunningham J, Sheridan R, et al. Energy and protein provisions for thermally injured children revisited: an outcome-based approach for determining requirements. J Burn Care Rehabil 1997; 18:117–181.

56. Waymack J, Herndon D. Nutritional support of the burned patient. World J Surg 1992; 16:80–86.

57. Souba W. Glutamine: a key substrate for the splanchnic bed. Ann Rev Nutr 1991; 11:285–289.

58. De-Souza DA, Greene LJ. Intestinal permeability and systemic infections in critically ill patients: effect of glutamine. Crit Care Med 2005; 33(5):1125–1135.

59. Wischmeyer PE. Can glutamine turn off the motor that drives systemic inflammation? Crit Care Med 2005; 33(5):1175–1178.

60. Novak F, Heyland DK, Avenell A, et al. Glutamine supplementation in serious illness: a systematic review of the evidence. Crit Care Med 2002; 30(9):2022–2029.

61. Gore D, Jahoor F. Glutamine kinetics in burn patients. Arch Surg 1994; 129:1318–1323.

62. Houdijk AP, Rijnsburger ER, Jansen J, et al. Randomized trial of glutamine-enriched enteral nutrition on infectious morbidity in patients with multiple trauma. Lancet 1998; 352:772–776.

63. Wischmeyer PE, Lynch J, Liedel J, et al. Glutamine administration reduces Gram-negative bacteremia in severely burned patients: a prospective, randomized, double-blind trial versus isonitrogenous control. Crit Care Med 2001; 29(11):2075–2080.

64. Zhou YP, Jiang ZM, Sun YH, et al. The effect of supplemental enteral glutamine on plasma levels, gut function, and outcome in severe burns: a randomized, double-blind, controlled clinical trial. JPEN 2003; 27(4):241–245.

65. Garrel D. The effect of supplemental enteral glutamine on plasma levels, gut function, and outcome in severe burns. JPEN 2004; 28(2):123; author reply 123.

66. Hishikawa K, Nakaki T, Tsuda M, et al. Effect of systemic L-arginine administration on hemodynamics and nitric oxide release in man. Japan Heart J 1992; 33:41–48.

67. Kirk S, Barbul A. Role of arginine in trauma, sepsis, and immunity. JPEN 1990; 14:226S–229S.

68. Barbul A, Larzarrow S, Efron O. Arginine enhances wound healing and lymphocyte immune response in humans. Surgery 1990; 108:331–335.

69. Gottschlich MM, Jenkins M, Warden GD, et al. Differential effects of three enteral dietary regimens on selected outcome variables in burn patients. JPEN J Parenter Enteral Nutr 1990; 14(3):225–236.

70. Heys SD, Walker LG, Smith I, et al. Enteral nutritional supplementation with key nutrients in patients with critical illness and cancer: a meta-analysis of randomized controlled clinical trials. Ann Surg 1999; 229(4):467–477.

71. Bower RH, Cerra FB, Bershadsky B, et al. Early enteral administration of a formula (Impact) supplemented with arginine, nucleotides, and fish oil in intensive care unit patients: results of a multicenter, prospective, randomized, clinical trial. Crit Care Med 1995; 23(3):436–449.

72. Moore FA, Moore EE, Kudsk KA, et al. Clinical benefits of an immune-enhancing diet for early postinjury enteral feeding. J Trauma 1994; 37(4):607–615.

73. Daly JM, Lieberman MD, Goldfine J, et al. Enteral nutrition with supplemental arginine, RNA, and omega-3 fatty acids in patients after operation: immunologic, metabolic, and clinical outcome. Surgery 1992; 112(1):56–67.

74. Heyland DK, Samis A. Does immunonutrition in patients with sepsis do more harm than good? Intensive Care Med 2003; 29(5):669–671.

75. Luiking YC, Poeze M, Ramsay G, et al. The role of arginine in infection and sepsis. JPEN J Parenter Enteral Nutr 2005; 29(1 Suppl):S70–S74.

76. Saffle J, Wiebke G, Jennings K, et al. Randomized trial of immune-enhancing enteral nutrition in burn patients. J Trauma 1997; 42:793–802.

77. Cerra F, Mazuski J, Chute E, et al. Branched-chain metabolic support: a prospective, randomized, double-blind trial in surgical stress. Ann Surg 1984; 199:286–291.

78. Yu Y, Wagner D, Walesreswi J, et al. A kinetic study of leucine metabolism in severely burned patients. Comparison between conventional and branched-chain amino acid enriched nutritional therapy. Ann Surg 1987; 207:421–490.

79. Gamliel Z, DeBiasse M, Demling R. Essential microminerals and their response to burn injury. J Burn Care Rehabil 1996; 17:264–272.

80. Gottschlich M, Warden G. Vitamin supplementation in the patient with burns. J Burn Care Rehabil 1990; 11:275–279.

81. Rock C, Dechert R, Khilnani R, et al. Carotenoids and antioxidant vitamins in patients after burn injury. J Burn Care Rehabil 1997; 18:269–278.

82. Mayes T, Gottschlich M, Warden G. Clinical nutrition protocols for continuous quality improvement in the outcomes of patients with burns. J Burn Care Rehabil 1997; 18:365–368.

83. Gottschlich MM, Mayes T, Khoury J, et al. Hypovitaminosis D in acutely injured pediatric burn patients. J Am Diet Assoc 2004; 104(6):931–941, quiz 1031.

84. Selmanpakoglu A, Sayal A, Isimer A. Trace element (Al, Se, Zn, Cu) levels in serum, urine, and tissues of burn patients. Burns 1994; 20:99–103.

85. Hunt D, Lane H, Beesinger D, et al. Selenium depletion in burn patients. JPEN 1984; 8:695–699.

86. Shippee R, Wilson S, King N. Trace mineral supplementation of burn patients: a national survey. J Am Diet Assoc 1987; 87:300–303.

87. Steinberg E, Anderson G. Implications of Medicare's prospective payment system for specialized nutrition services: the 'Hopkins' report. Nutr Clin Pract 1986; 1:12–28.

88. Popp M, Law E, MacMillan B. Parenteral nutrition in the burned child: a study of twenty-six patients. Ann Surg 1974; 179:219–225.

89. Andel H, Rab M, Andel D, et al. Impact of duodenal feeding on the oxygen balance of the splanchnic region during different phases of severe burn injury. Burns 2002; 28:60–64.

90. Alverdy J, Aoys E, Moss G. Total parenteral nutrition promotes bacterial translocation from the gut. Surgery 1988; 104:185–190.

91. Saito H, Trocki O, Alexander J, et al. The effect of route of nutrient administration on the nutritional state, catabolic hormone secretion and gut mucosal integrity after burn injury. JPEN 1987; 11:1–7.

92. Magnotti L, Deitch E. Burns, bacterial translocation, gut barrier function, and failure. J Burn Care Rehabil 2005; 26:383–391.

93. Fong Y, Marano M, Barber E, et al. Total parenteral nutrition and bowel rest modify the metabolic response to endotoxin in humans. Ann Surg 1989; 210:449–454.

94. Kudsk K, Croce M, Fabian T, et al. Enteral vs. parenteral feeding: effects on septic morbidity following blunt and penetrating abdominal trauma. Ann Surg 1992; 215:503–508.

95. Moore F, Feliciano, D, Andrassy, R, et al. TEN vs TPN following major abdominal trauma – reduced septic morbidity. J Trauma 1989; 29:916–922.

96. Herndon D, Stein M, Rutan T, et al. Failure of TPN supplementation to improve liver function, immunity, and mortality in thermally injured patients. J Trauma 1987; 27:195–204.

97. Herndon DN, Barrow RE, Stein M, et al. Increased mortality with intravenous supplemental feeding in severely burned patients. J Burn Care Rehabil 1989; 10(4):309–313.

98. Heyland DK, MacDonald S, Keefe L, Drover JW. Total parenteral nutrition in the critically ill patient: a meta-analysis. JAMA 1998; 280(23):2013–2019.

99. Barret JP, Jeschke MG, Herndon DN. Fatty infiltration of the liver in severely burned pediatric patients: autopsy findings and clinical implications. J Trauma 2001; 51(4):736–739.

100. Andel H, Kamolz LP, Horauf K, et al. Nutrition and anabolic agents in burned patients. Burns 2003; 29(6):592–595.

101. Mochizuki H, Trocki O, Dominioni L, et al. Mechanism of prevention of postburn hypermetabolism and catabolism by early enteral feeding. Ann Surg 1984; 200:297–310.

102. Chiarelli A, Enzi G, Casadei A, et al. Very early nutrition supplementation in burned patients. Am J Clin Nutr 1990; 213:177–183.

103. Peck MD, Kessler M, Cairns BA, et al. Early enteral nutrition does not decrease hypermetabolism associated with burn injury. J Trauma 2004; 57(6):1143–1149.

104. Gottschlich M, Jenkins M, Mayes T, et al. The 2002 Clinical Research Award: an evaluation of the safety of early vs. delayed enteral support and effects on clinical nutritional, and endocrine outcomes after severe burns. J Burn Care Rehabil 2002; 23:401–415.

105. Trocki O, Michelini JA, Robbins ST, et al. Evaluation of early enteral feeding in children less than 3 years old with smaller burns (8–25 per cent TBSA). Burns 1995; 21(1):17–23.

106. Moore E, Jones T. Benefits of immediate jejunostomy feeding after major abdominal trauma– a prospective, randomized study. J Trauma 1988; 26:874–881.

107. Jenkins M, Gottschlich M, Mayes T, et al. Enteral feeding during operative procedures. J Burn Care Rehabil 1994; 15:199–205.

108. Dobranowski J, Fitzgerald JM, Baxter F, et al. Incorrect positioning of nasogastric feeding tubes and the development of pneumothorax. Can Assoc Radiol J 1992; 43(1):35–39.

109. Kearns PJ, Chin D, Mueller L, et al. The incidence of ventilator-associated pneumonia and success in nutrient delivery with gastric versus small intestinal feeding: a randomized clinical trial. Crit Care Med 2000; 28(6):1742–1746.

110. Mentec H, Dupont H, Bocchetti M, et al. Upper digestive intolerance during enteral nutrition in critically ill patients: frequency, risk factors, and complications. Crit Care Med 2001; 29(10):1955–1961.

111. Booth CM, Heyland DK, Paterson WG. Gastrointestinal promotility drugs in the critical care setting: a systematic review of the evidence. Crit Care Med 2002; 30(7):1429–1435.

112. Shopbell J, Hopkins B, Shronts E. Nutrition screening and assessment. In: Gottschlich M, ed. The science and practice of nutrition support: a case-based core curriculum. Silver Springs, MD: Society of Parenteral and Enteral Nutrition; 2001.

113. Gump F, Kinney J. Energy balance and weight loss in burned patients. Arch Surg 1971; 103:442–448.

114. Zdolsek HJ, Lindahl OA, Angquist KA, et al. Non-invasive assessment of intercompartmental fluid shifts in burn victims. Burns 1998; 24(3):233–240.

115. Streat SJ, Beddoe AH, Hill GL. Aggressive nutritional support does not prevent protein loss despite fat gain in septic intensive care patients. J Trauma 1987; 27(3):262–266.

116. Hart DW, Wolf SE, Herndon DN, et al. Energy expenditure and caloric balance after burn: increased feeding leads to fat rather than lean mass accretion. Ann Surg 2002; 235(1):152–161.

117. Graves C, Saffle J, Morris S. Comparison of urine urea nitrogen collection times in critically ill patients. Nutr Clin Pract 2005; 20(2):271–275.

118. Rodriguez D. Inaccuracy of nitrogen balance determinations in thermal injury with calculated total urinary nitrogen. J Burn Care Rehabil 1992; 13:254–260.

119. Konstantinides F, Radmer W, Becker W, et al. Inaccuracy of nitrogen balance determinations in thermal injury with calculated total urinary nitrogen. J Burn Care Rehabil 1992; 13:254–260.

120. LeBlanc A, Gogia P, Schneider V, et al. Calf muscle area and strength changes after five weeks of horizontal bed rest. Am J Sports Med 1988; 16(6):624–629.

121. Rettmer R, Williamson J, Labbe R, et al. Laboratory monitoring of nutrition status in burn patients. Clin Chem 1992; 38:334–337.

122. Sheridan RL, Prelack K, Cunningham JJ. Physiologic hypoalbuminemia is well tolerated by severely burned children. J Trauma 1997; 43(3):448–452.

123. Greenhalgh DG, Housinger TA, Kagan RJ, et al. Maintenance of serum albumin levels in pediatric burn patients: a prospective, randomized trial. J Trauma 1995; 39(1):67–73.

124. Cynober L, Prugnaud O, Lioret H, et al. Serum transthyretin levels in patients with burn injury. Surgery 1991; 109:640–644.

125. Manelli J, Abdetii C, Botti G, et al. A reference standard for plasma proteins is required for nutritional assessment of adult burn patients. Burns 1998; 24:337–345.

126. Meakins J, Pietsch J, Bubekik O. Delayed hypersensitivity: indicator of acquired failure of host defenses in sepsis and trauma. Ann Surg 1977; 186:241–250.

127. Pietsch J, Meakins J. Delayed hypersensitivity response: application in clinical surgery. Surgery 1988; 82:349–355.

128. Kyle UG, Bosaeus I, De Lorenzo AD, et al. Bioelectrical impedance analysis – part I: review of principles and methods. Clin Nutr 2004; 23(5):1226–1243.

129. Kyle UG, Bosaeus I, De Lorenzo AD, et al. Bioelectrical impedance analysis – part II: utilization in clinical practice. Clin Nutr 2004; 23(6):1430–1453.

130. Bachrach LK. Dual energy X-ray absorptiometry (DEXA) measurements of bone density and body composition: promise and pitfalls. J Pediatr Endocrinol Metab 2000; 13(Suppl 2):983–988.

131. Williamson J. Actual burn nutrition care practices: a national survey (Part II). J Burn Care Rehabil 1989; 10:185–194.

132. Askanazi J, Rosenbaum S, Hyman A, et al. Respiratory changes induced by the large glucose loads of total parenteral nutrition. JAMA 1980; 243:1444–1447.

133. Lowry S, Brennan M. Abnormal liver function during parenteral nutrition: relation to infusion excess. J Surg Res 1979; 26:300–307.

134. Iapichino G, Radrizzani D. Parenteral nutrition. In: Webb A, Shapiro M, Singer M, et al., eds. Oxford textbook of critical care. New York: Oxford University Press; 1999:398–401.

135. Turina M, Fry DE, Polk HC Jr. Acute hyperglycemia and the innate immune system: clinical, cellular, and molecular aspects. Crit Care Med 2005; 33(7):1624–1633.

136. van den Berghe G, Wouters P, Weekers F, et al. Intensive insulin therapy in the critically ill patients. N Engl J Med 2001; 345(19):1359–1367.

137. Lewis KS, Kane-Gill SL, Bobek MB, et al. Intensive insulin therapy for critically ill patients. Ann Pharmacother 2004; 38(7–8):1243–1251.

138. Khoury W, Klausner JM, Ben-Abraham R, et al. Glucose control by insulin for critically ill surgical patients. J Trauma 2004; 57(5):1132–1138.

139. Wu X, Thomas SJ, Herndon DN, Sanford AP, et al. Insulin decreases hepatic acute phase protein levels in severely burned children. Surgery 2004; 135(2):196–202.

140. Solano T, Totaro R. Insulin therapy in critically ill patients. Curr Opin Clin Nutr Metab Care 2004; 7(2):199–205.

141. Gore DC, Wolf SE, Sanford A, et al. Influence of metformin on glucose intolerance and muscle catabolism following severe burn injury. Ann Surg 2005; 241(2):334–342.

142. FDA Public Health Advisory, Sept 29, 2003. Reports of blue discoloration and death in patients receiving enteral feedings tinted with the dye, FD&C blue No. 1. Online. Available at: www.cfsan.fda.gov/dms/col-ltr2.html.

143. Kowal-Vern A, McGill V, Gamelli R. Ischemic necrotic bowel disease in thermal injury. Arch Surg 1997; 132:440–443.

144. Marvin R, McKinley B, McQuiggan M, et al. Nonocclusive bowel necrosis occurring in critically-ill trauma patients receiving enteral nutrition manifests no reliable clinical signs for early detection. Am J Surg 2000; 179:7–12.

145. Eisenberg P. Causes of diarrhea in tube-fed patients: a comprehensive approach to diagnosis and management. Nutr Clin Pract 1993; 8:119–123.

146. Kealey G, Aguillar J, Lewis R, et al. Cadaver skin allografts and transmission of human cytomegalovirus to burn patients. J Am Coll Surg 1996; 182:201–205.

147. Grube BJ, Heimbach DM, Marvin JA. Clostridium difficile diarrhea in critically ill burned patients. Arch Surg 1987; 122(6):655–661.

148. Gottschlich M, Warden G, Michel M, et al. Diarrhea in tube-fed burn patients: incidence, etiology, nutritional impact, and prevention. JPEN 1988; 12:338–345.

149. Frankenfeld D, Beyer P. Dietary fiber and bowel function in tube-fed patients. J Am Diet Assoc 1991; 91:590–596.

150. Scaife CL, Saffle JR, Morris SE. Intestinal obstruction secondary to enteral feedings in burn trauma patients. J Trauma 1999; 47(5):859–863.

151. Wolf SE, Jeschke MG, Rose JK, et al. Enteral feeding intolerance: an indicator of sepsis-associated mortality in burned children. Arch Surg 1997; 132(12):1310–1313; discussion 1313–1314.

152. Gottschlich M, Warden G. Parenteral nutrition in the burned patient. In: Fischer J, ed. Total parenteral nutrition. Boston: Little, Brown; 1991.

153. Grant J, Ross L. Parenteral nutrition. In: Charnow B, ed. Essentials of critical care pharmacology. Baltimore, MD: Williams and Wilkins; 1994:535–560.

Chapter 31

Modulation of the hypermetabolic response after burn injury

William B. Norbury and David N. Herndon

Chapter contents

Introduction

Severe thermal injury leads to a change in patient metabolism that may be seen for more than 12 months after the initial event. The ensuing period of hypermetabolism and catabolism following a burn leads to impaired immune function, decreased wound healing, erosion of lean body mass, and hinders rehabilitative efforts delaying reintegration into normal society. Strategies for attenuating this maladaptive response may be divided into pharmacological and non-pharmacological. Non-pharmacological approaches include prompt, early excision and closure of wounds, pertinacious surveillance for and treatment of sepsis, early commencement of high-protein, high-carbohydrate enteral feeding, elevation of the immediate environmental temperature to 31.5°C (±0.7°C); and early institution of an aerobic resistive exercise program. Several pharmacotherapeutic options are also available to further reduce erosion of lean body mass; these include anabolic agents such as recombinant human growth hormone (rhGH), insulin, and oxandrolone and also beta blockade using propranolol. This chapter will discuss the metabolic changes seen following a major burn and how different treatment options effect outcome (Figure 31.1).

Metabolic alterations following burn injury

The hypermetabolic response

Severe burns lead to a hypermetabolic response far in excess of that seen in any other disease state.[1] Patients admitted with multiple traumatic wounds have an increase in metabolic rate that rises further when placed on a ventilator to between 30 and 75% that of normal.[2,3] However, those admitted with burns involving more than 40% of the total body surface area (TBSA) have increases in metabolic rate of between 80 and 200% of normal, leaving the patient with a nitrogen deficit of up to 30g/day.[4] Initially, over the first 3 days, there is a reduction in metabolic rate — called the 'ebb' phase; this is followed by an increase in metabolic rate that lasts for more than 9 months after the burn injury.[5] The hypermetabolic or 'flow' phase is characterized by a hyperdynamic circulation,[6] increased core temperature,[7] increased oxygen and glucose consumption,[8,9] carbon dioxide production,[9] glycogenolysis,[10] lipolysis,[11] proteolysis,[12,13] and futile substrate cycling.[14,15] The intensity of the response is dependent on the percentage TBSA burned, body weight at admission, and time from injury to excision of eschar.[16] Moreover, the magnitude of the ensuing catabolic process is dependent on the severity of the hypermetabolism and development of sepsis during hospital stay.[16] The resting metabolic rate of patients with large burns increases in a curvilinear fashion from close to normal predicted levels for TBSA < 10% to twice that of normal predicted levels at 40% TBSA and above. In those patients with burns greater than 40% TBSA the resting metabolic rate at thermal neutrality (33°C) reaches 180% of predicted basal rate during their acute admission, this reduces to 150% once the wounds are fully healed, 140% at 6 months after injury, 120% at 9 months postburn, and 110% after 12 months (Figure 31.2).[5]

This rise in metabolic rate and resulting loss of total body protein results in decreased immune defenses, decreased wound healing, and exhaustion, which hinders rehabilitation.[5]

Mediators of hypermetabolism

The cause of the hypermetabolic response is unclear; however, endotoxin, platelet-activating factor, tumor necrosis factor, interleukins 1 and 6, arachadonic acid metabolites using the cyclooxygenase and lipooxygenase pathways, neutrophil-adherence complexes, reactive oxygen species, nitric oxide and the coagulation and complement cascades have all been implicated in regulating this response.[17] More recently the cortisol releasing factor (CRF) type-2 receptor ligand had been

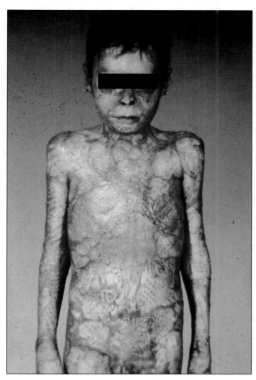

Fig. 31.1 Major burn injury.

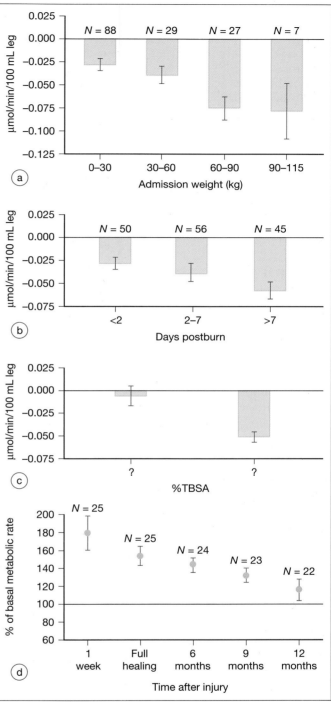

Fig. 31.2 (a) Association between admission weight and negative protein balance. Data presented as mean ± SEM.[16] (b) Association between time to primary wound excision and negative protein net balance. Data presented as mean ± SEM.[16] (c) Influence of burn size >0.40% total body surface area on catabolism. Data presented as mean ± SEM. *$P = 0.0001$ by Student's t test.[16] (d) Resting energy expenditure. Indirect calorimetry was used to measure energy expenditure in a resting state at admission, full healing, and 6, 9, and 12 months after burn. At all time points, the energy expenditure was higher than the basal metabolic rate predicted for age-, sex-, weight-, and height-matched individuals by the Harris–Benedict equation. Error bars represent 95% confidence intervals. (Figures (a–c) reproduced with permission from Hart et al.[16] Ann Surg 2000; 232(4):455–465. Figure (d) reproduced with permission from Hart et al.[5] Surgery 2000; 128(2):312–319.)

proposed as integral to maintenance of the hypermetabolism associated with burns.[18]

The change in regulation of skeletal muscle during the stress response following major trauma is due to the activation of pathways of protein breakdown. Recent studies have shown one of the chief protagonists to be the ubiquitin-proteasome pathway.[19] Ubiquitin is a common 8 kDa peptide found throughout all eukaryotic cells (hence the name). During skeletal muscle degradation it is activated in a stepwise process to covalently attach to other proteins, reducing their ability to disassociate from proteosomes and subsequently leading to degradation of the protein it has attached to. Ubiquitin has seven lysine residues, the use of which confers different functions. Chains of ubiquitin peptides linked via lysine 48 lead to degradation of the target protein by the proteasome.[20] However, those linked by lysine 63 appear to confer signaling functions in the nuclear factor-kappaB (NF-κB) pathway,[21,22] and act as mediators in DNA repair[23] and the stress response.[24] The role of ubiquitin peptides linked by other lysine residues is still unclear. The ubiquitin pathway is stimulated by TNF and the rise in glucocorticoids seen following severe thermal injury.[25] The other main reason for the net loss of skeletal muscle is due to an imbalance in the rate of amino acid production secondary to protein breakdown and the ability of the cell to retain and reuse these amino acids.[26] A study comparing the protein turnover in patients suffering from massive burns with that in normal individuals found an increase in both muscle protein degradation and muscle protein synthesis in the burns group. However there was an 83% increase in muscle protein degradation compared with a 50% increase in muscle protein synthesis. In the same study they found that the absolute values of inward transport of phenylalanine, leucine, and lysine were not significantly different in the two groups. However, the ability of transport systems to take up amino acids from the bloodstream, as assessed by dividing inward transport by amino acid delivery to leg muscle, were 50–63% lower in the patients. In contrast, outward phenylalanine and lysine transport were 40% and 67% greater in the patients than in the controls, respectively.[27] These results suggest that the increased protein synthesis seen is secondary to the rise in amino acid concentration; however, this synthetic rate is unable to keep up with the acceleration in protein breakdown. The increased net efflux of amino acids from the cell is facilitated by accelerated outward transmembrane transport and impaired influx due to the hyperdynamic circulation caused by the rise in catecholamine release.[27]

Hormonal changes seen following trauma

Cortisol levels increase in response to stress in patients, this increase is accompanied by an increase in cortisol binding in skeletal muscle. In a recent study we identified a rise in cortisol following a major burn injury (>40% TBSA); this rise was greater in male patients, but both male and female patients returned to near-normal cortisol levels at around 3 months following injury. The significance of adrenal and sympathetic response to burn injury is described in more detail in the previous chapter, including the hyperdynamic circulation, peripheral lipolysis and increases in fatty infiltration of the liver. These responses can be attenuated by the use of β-adrenergic receptor antagonists such as propranolol.

Alterations in metabolism of carbohydrate, protein and fat

The increase in energy expenditure is mirrored by substrate oxidation resulting from increases in ATP consumption. Increases in catecholamine, glucagon and glucocorticoid production lead to enhanced glycogenolysis and protein breakdown in both the liver and skeletal muscle. This in turn leads to increases in triglyceride, urea and glucose production (gluconeogenesis) which consequently leads to hyperglycemia. The process of substrate cycling leads to increased thermogenesis[14] which raises core and skin temperature to 2°C above that of normal, unburned patients. Raised catecholamine levels also increase peripheral lipolysis and subsequent triglyceride-fatty acid cycling, leading to fatty infiltration of the liver such that the liver weight increases by 120%. This has been associated with an increased incidence of sepsis; however, no causative effect has been found (Figure 31.3, Table 31.1).[28]

A large proportion of the glucose produced by the liver is directed towards the burn wound, where it is consumed by anaerobic metabolism of inflammatory cells, fibroblasts, and endothelial cells; this in turn produces lactate, which is recycled back to the liver and into gluconeogenic pathways. The catabolism of protein in skeletal muscle produces three-carbon amino acids such as alanine that are also recycled to the liver to contribute to gluconeogenic pathways. The release of catecholamines increases glucagon secretion, which in turn promotes gluconeogenesis. The relative insulin resistance seen

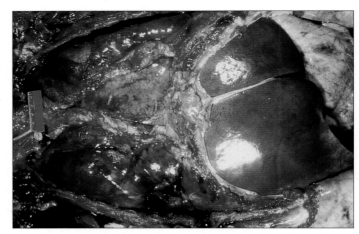

Fig. 31.3 Significant enlargement of the liver and fatty deposition therein are common findings in severe and fatal burns. (Reprinted with permission from Barret JP, Herndon DN, eds. Color atlas of burn care. London: WB Saunders; 2001:133, Plate 8.38.)

TABLE 31.1 LIVER WEIGHT PER BODY WEIGHT FOR NORMAL VS. BURNED PATIENTS (2 MONTHS TO 15 YEARS OF AGE)

	Full-thickness burn (%)	Liver wt/BW (g/kg)	Weight increase (%)
Normal (n = 14)	0	34.3 ± 1.1	
Burn (n = 14)	76 ± 5	75.6 ± 6.0*	120

Burn size and liver weight ratios are means ± SE.
BW = body weight.
*Significant difference at p < 0.001.

following a major burn combined with increased hepatic gluconeogenesis leads to hyperglycemia;[10] patients in this situation have been shown to have an increased rate of muscle protein breakdown.[29] A study measuring whole body protein flux in normal individuals showed a three-fold increase in the rate of protein catabolism with no accompanying alteration in protein synthesis during a period of hyperglycemia.[30] Endogenous anabolic hormone levels change with both IGF-I and IGFBP-3 significantly lower immediately after burn, and neither reaching normal levels after 40 days postburn. Serum insulin levels are significantly increased during the same time period with female patients producing up to 3 times normal levels; however, in the presence of insulin resistance, hyperglycemia remains a problem. Endogenous growth hormone levels also fall 4–5-fold initially and remain below half the normal level during the first 40 days. The result of these levels combined with relative insulin resistance in the burns patient leads to a marked reduction in protein synthetic ability which can only be reversed by restoration of more normal levels from an exogenous source.

Nutritional support

Patients with burns greater than 40% TBSA can lose up to 25% of their body weight in the first 3 weeks following injury if sustained on an oral diet alone. Numerous formulae have been developed to calculate the requirements of each patient; the caloric requirement is based on size of burn, the total surface area of the patient, the presence or not of sepsis and body weight: 25 kcal/kg/day plus 40 kcal/%TBSA/day would provide enough calories to maintain body weight in an adult patient; for children the requirement is 1800 kcal/day plus 2200 kcal/m^2 burn/day. Ideally this calorific intake should be all via enteral feeding, with parenteral feeding held in reserve for those with prolonged ileus or intolerance of enteral feeding.

Methods
Parenteral vs. enteral

The route of delivery of nutrition is just as important as the composition. Early enteral nutrition is associated with reduced postoperative septic morbidity rates compared with those administered by parenteral nutrition alone.[31] An increase in mortality, impairment of liver function and reduced immune response has been shown when using both enteral and parenteral feeding combined to reach caloric intake when compared with enteral feeding alone.[32,33] The use of total parenteral nutrition (TPN) in burns patients increases mortality threefold and decreases the amount of enteral calories that are tolerated.[32,33] Therefore it may only be used in the presence of mitigating circumstances where enteral feeding is not feasible such as Ogilvie's syndrome, bowel obstruction, ischemic enterocolitis or a protracted ileus. An attenuation of the catecholamine response and maintenance of gut mucosal integrity with consequent reduction in bacterial translocation has been shown with immediate enteral nutrition but not with parenteral nutrition. The associated risk of vomiting, reported as 2.8% in one study, was not linked to any increase in aspiration pneumonia.

Gastric vs. intestinal feeding

The ileus associated with severe thermal injury is not as common as previously thought; that which derives from mesenteric hypoperfusion prior to adequate resuscitation is reversed once the patient is suitably volume replete. Postburn ileus does not affect the small bowel as profoundly as the stomach. Therefore feeding using a nasoduodenal tube passed through the pylorus, or a nasojejunal tube advanced past the ligament of Treitz, can be initiated as soon as possible and preferably within the first 6 hours following injury (Figure 31.4).[34,35] This approach also allows continuous feeding during operations and physical therapy sessions. The initiation of immediate enteral feeding allowed the delivery of calculated caloric requirements by the third day postburn.[36] Other studies have shown a reduction in hypermetabolism when enteral feeding is commenced immediately after burn injury; this reduction in metabolic rate was associated with prevention of elevations in glucagon, cortisol, and catecholamines.[37]

Specific requirements

All patients with a significant burn require increased caloric intake and are placed on a high-protein, high-carbohydrate diet. Those with burns in excess of 30% TBSA should be

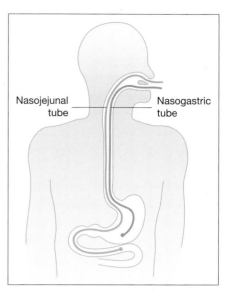

Fig. 31.4 Diagram showing position of nasogastric and nasojejunal tubes.

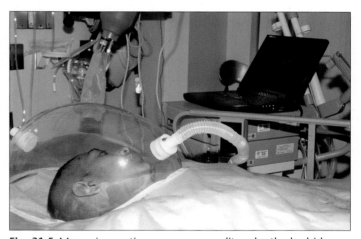

Fig. 31.5 Measuring resting energy expenditure by the bedside.

placed on tube feeds to allow for constant feeding in the initial period. In order to calculate the calorific requirements of each patient, resting energy expenditure (REE) is measured directly at the bedside by indirect calorimetry using portable calorimeters. The mode of testing should be via ventilator, mouthpiece, mask, or canopy[38] (as shown below) and carried out by trained personnel as per the AARC Clinical Practice Guidelines.[39] Oxygen consumption and carbon dioxide production are measured and used to calculate the energy expenditure (Figure 31.5).[9]

In pediatric patients with burns in excess of 40% TBSA receiving 1.4 times the measured resting energy expenditure (MREE in kcal/m^2/day) the body weight is maintained. Optimum nutritional support in a convalescent burns patient should be 1.2 times the MREE.[40] Any increase in calorific delivery above 1.4 times the MREE results in additional weight gain though solely due to fat deposition (Figure 31.6).[41]

In the absence of access to indirect calorimetry there are other formulas to estimate the caloric needs of a burns patient; unfortunately, these normally overestimate the needs considerably. A recent comparison of three such formulas with MREE found that the World Health Organization × 2 multiplier (WHO × 2) was the closest to MREE × 1.3 (Table 31.2).[42]

Two of the above equations are then multiplied by a factor to take into account the increased energy requirements due to the burn: WHO × 2 and Harris–Benedict × 2. The Mayes formulas take the burn into account at the original calculation.

- The Galveston formula for estimating caloric requirements in pediatric patients is derived from retrospective analyses of dietary intake, which was associated with maintenance of body weight averaged over hospital admission (Table 31.3).
- The Curreri formula used in Galveston for the calculation of energy requirement in adult patients has been reached following linear regression analysis of weight change vs. predicted dietary intakes in adults at 25 kcal/kg/day + 40 kcal/%TBSA/day[43] (Table 31.4).

Carbohydrates

In pediatric burns patients with burns in excess of 40% TBSA a high carbohydrate diet (3% fat, 82% carbohydrate, and 15%

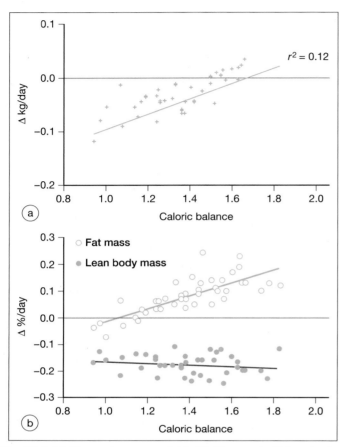

Fig. 31.6 (a) Change in gross weight. (b) Changes in % lean body mass and % fat mass. (Reproduced with permission from Hart et al. Ann Surg 2002; 235(1):152–161.[41])

TABLE 31.3 GALVESTON FORMULA FOR CALCULATION OF CALORIFIC REQUIREMENTS FOLLOWING BURN INJURY

Age range	Equation
0–1	$(2100 \text{ kcal/m}^2\text{TBSA/day}) + (1000 \text{ kcal/m}^2\text{TBSA/day})$
1–11	$(1800 \text{ kcal/m}^2\text{TBSA/day}) + (1300 \text{ kcal/m}^2\text{TBSA/day})$
12–18	$(1500 \text{ kcal/m}^2\text{TBSA/day}) + (1500 \text{ kcal/m}^2\text{TBSA/day})$

TABLE 31.4 THE CURRERI FORMULA FOR CALCULATION OF CALORIFIC REQUIREMENTS FOLLOWING BURN INJURY IN ADULTS[43]

Age range	Equation
16–60	25 kcal/kg/day + 40 kcal/%TBSA/day
60	25 kcal/kg/day + 65 kcal/%TBSA/day

Reprinted from Curreri et al. J Am Diet Assoc 1974; 65(4):415–417.[43] with permission from The American Dietetic Association.

TABLE 31.2 COMMONLY USED EQUATIONS FOR CALCULATING ENERGY REQUIREMENTS IN THE ABSENCE OF INDIRECT CALORIMETRY

Equation	Age and gender	Formula
Harris–Benedict	Male Female	$66.5 + (13.75 \times W) + (5.003 \times H) - (6.775 \times A)$ $655.1 + (9.563 \times W) + (1.850 \times H) - (4.676 \times A)$
WHO	Male <3 Male 3–10 Female <3 Female 3–10	$(60.9*W) - 54$ $(22.7*W) - 495$ $(61*W) - 51$ $(22.5*W) - 499$
Mayes 1	<3 (M & F)	$108 + 68W + 3.9*\%TBSA$
Mayes 2	<3 (M & F)	$179 + 66W + 3.2*\%3rdTBSA$
Mayes 3	5–10 (M & F)	$818 + 37.4W + 9.3*TBSA$
Mayes 4	5–10 (M & F)	$950 + 38.5W + 5.9*TBSA$

W = weight in kg.
H = height in cm.
A = age in years.
Adapted from Liusuwan et al. J Burn Care Rehabil 1990; 11(5):400–404[42] with permission.

protein) stimulates protein synthesis secondary to increases in endogenous insulin production and improves lean body mass accretion, relative to isocaloric-isoprotein but high-fat enteral diet.[44] We have reduced the delivery of high-fat diets in our patients due to those findings. We also aim to reduce substrate for lipolysis and the subsequent generation of fatty deposition in the liver, a serious problem in burns patients.

Protein

Sufficient protein intake is vital to maintain lean body mass as the rate oxidation of most amino acids in burned patients can reach as high as 50% higher than rates seen in healthy individuals in a fasting state. Therefore raising protein intake by more than 50% from 1 g/kg/day to between 1.5 and 2 g/kg/day will ensure adequate supply in adults; the same cannot be said for children, however, who may increase urea production without any beneficial anabolic effect. One study in burns patients showed that a balance between protein synthesis and catabolism could be achieved with a protein intake of 1.4 g protein/kg/day.[45] Additional delivery of protein above 1.5 g/kg/day has been shown to only increase urinary excretion of urea.[46]

Particular attention must however be paid to supplementation of amino acids in the diet of those patients with severe burns. Leucine, important in signaling the initiation of protein synthesis,[47] is oxidized at an increased rate in critically ill patients.[45] Acute administration of leucine initiates cellular protein synthesis by its activation of the mammalian target of rapamycin (mTOR) cell-signaling pathway; however, a recent study in rats has shown that chronic administration of leucine, via drinking water over 12 days, led to an increase in protein synthesis in adipose tissue, skeletal muscle, and liver without notable adaptive changes in signaling proteins or metabolic enzymes.[48] Myocardial dysfunction, a common problem associated with severe burns, has been shown to be reversed at least in part by oral administration of leucine in the early postburn period. Enteral glutamine supplementation in adult burn patients has been shown to result in reduced positive blood cultures by a factor of three, prevent bacteremia with *Pseudomonas aeruginosa*, and may decrease mortality rate. However, it had no effect on level of consciousness and did not appear to influence phagocytosis by circulating polymorphonuclear cells.[49]

New areas of development in nutrition for burns
Fat

A novel enteral feed containing an altered lipid profile and enhanced antioxidants moderated the severity of the initial inflammatory response in the lungs of patients developing acute respiratory distress syndrome (ARDS), a common problem among burns patients with smoke inhalation injury. The beneficial effects of the eicosapentaenoic acid, gamma-linolenic acid diet on pulmonary neutrophil recruitment, gas exchange, requirement for mechanical ventilation, length of intensive care unit stay, and the reduction of new organ failures suggest that this enteral nutrition formula would be a useful adjuvant therapy in the clinical management of patients with or at risk of developing ARDS.[50] However, a follow-up study showed that although enteral nutrition with the experi-

mental diet for at least 4–7 days did not reduce oxidative stress as measured, it did restore plasma levels of beta-carotene and alpha-tocopherol to normal or higher levels and appeared to protect ARDS patients from further lipid peroxidation.[51]

Micronutrients/vitamins

Burns patients have been shown to suffer significant trace element deficiencies involving predominantly copper, iron, selenium, and zinc.[52] Early trace element supplementation has been shown to be beneficial is a study involving patients with burns greater than 40% TBSA. It was associated with a significant decrease in number of bronchopneumonia infections and shorter length of hospital stay.

Altered copper levels seem to be of particular importance in the burn patient. Through its interaction with enzymes such as lysyl oxidase, copper is essential in collagen synthesis and therefore wound healing. It also takes part in antioxidant defense via its action on superoxide dismutase.[53] Ceruloplasmin, an acute phase protein induced by IL-1 and IL-6, is normally in short supply during times of copper deficiency and both normally increase in concentration in response to stress. However, following a severe burn of >30% TBSA, copper is lost in large quantities through the burn wound, resulting in a 20–40% reduction from normal levels within the first week postburn.[54] The copper deficit may remain for many weeks and is inversely proportional to burn size.[55] Copper deficiency is further associated with the use of silver sulfadiazine, a commonly applied topical agent in burns, is antagonistic to the actions of copper, and further reduces serum concentrations.[56] Zinc, long known as essential to wound healing, particularly for ulcers, is an indispensable supplement in burns nutrition, although the quantities needed have yet to be clarified. Carbonic anhydrase, DNA and RNA polymerases and proteases all rely on zinc to play a central role in their efforts to improve wound healing and tissue regeneration.[57] Supplements containing copper and zinc have been shown in an animal model that, given following early wound excision, reduced lipid peroxidation and subsequently the quantities of lipid peroxide delivered to distant tissues.[58]

A study looking at the presence of trace elements in burn wounds found increased levels of manganese, a trace element involved in mucopolysaccharide and glycoprotein synthesis, as well as in the mitochondrial antioxidant defense (Mn SOD), indicating that its antioxidant function might be important during wound healing.[59]

Environmental support

A proportion of the energy generated during the hypermetabolic response is to offset heat losses secondary to evaporation through the burn eschar; this loss of body water can be up to 4000 mL/m^2 TBSA/day. The body tries to raise the core and skin temperature by 2°C secondary to a hypothalamic reset mechanism similar to that seen in cold acclimatization. Therefore the hypermetabolic response may be reduced by warming the ambient temperature to thermal neutrality (33°C) at which point the heat for evaporation is derived from the environment, taking the burden away from the patient. Raising the immediate environmental temperature can reduce the

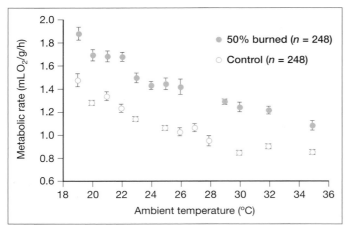

Fig. 31.7 Effect of ambient temperature on metabolic rate. (Reproduced with permission: Herndon DN. Mediators of metabolism. J Trauma 1981; 21:701–705.)

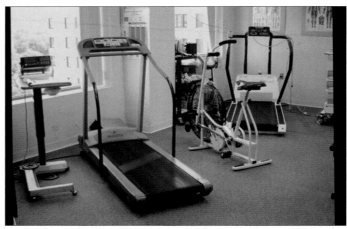

Fig. 31.9 Some of the exercise equipment used for the supervised exercise training program.

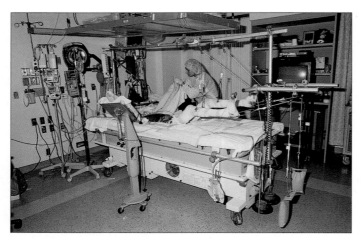

Fig. 31.8 Heating panel shown suspended from the ceiling in an intensive care room. (Reprinted with permission from Barret JP, Herndon DN, eds. Color atlas of burn care. London: WB Saunders; 2001:150, Plate 9.48)

magnitude of the hypermetabolic response from 2.0 to 1.4 times the resting energy expenditure in burns >40% TBSA[60] (Figures 31.7 and 31.8).

Exercise

Initial excision and grafting, followed by prompt treatment of infection and sepsis together with early enteral feeding, are all integral parts of immediate interventions for a patient with severe burns. However, once past the initial acute phase, patients enter into a long period of rehabilitation that normally includes reconstructive operations to increase movement and allow the patient a more normal life. The early institution of a balanced physical therapy program is essential in reducing contractures and restoring metabolic variables. Progressive resistance exercises in convalescent burn patients can maintain and improve body mass, augment incorporation of amino acids into muscle proteins, and increase muscle strength and ability to walk distances by about 50%.[61] It has been demonstrated that resistance exercising can be safely accomplished

in pediatric burn patients without exercise-related hyperpyrexia due to inability to dissipate the generated heat.[62,63] In a recent study one group participated in a 12-week in-hospital physical rehabilitation program supplemented with an individualized and supervised exercise training program while the other group participated in a 12-week, home-based physical rehabilitation program without individualization and supervision of exercise. The results showed a significant improvement in muscle strength, power, and lean body mass in the hospital-supervised exercise group (Figure 31.9).[62]

Prevention of infection, excision, and early closure of burn wound

Early excision and grafting

Of all the changes over the last few decades in burns treatment it is the introduction of expeditious removal of full-thickness burn wounds that has had the greatest impact on survival and outcome. Conservative treatment of large full-thickness burn wounds followed by skin grafting is a lengthy process associated with a not inconsiderable burden of pain and suffering, severe metabolic derangement, and increased septic episodes, and results in an increased length of hospital stay. Several studies have shown attenuation of the hypermetabolic response in patients of all ages.[64,65] Early excision together with aggressive enteral feeding has also been shown to be effective in reducing muscle catabolism and improving infectious outcomes in pediatric patients.[66]

Studies have shown that when a large burn wound (>50% TBSA) is excised and covered with autograft, cadaver skin or bio-engineered skin substitute within the first 72 hours following injury, the patient's resting metabolic rate will be 40% less than a patient whose wound is not excised and covered until 7 days post injury.[16] Cross-leg nitrogen studies have shown an increase of 230% in net protein losses when comparing those patients who were excised and covered within 72 hours and those who received delayed primary reconstruction at 10–21 days (Figure 31.10).

Another study involving pediatric burns patients revealed that those admitted early whose burn eschar was removed

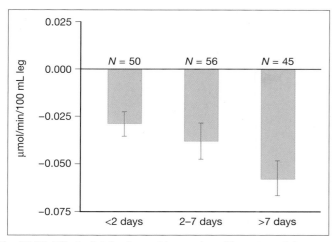

Fig. 31.10 Effect of delay to excision and grafting on protein catabolism. (Reproduced with permission from Hart et al. Ann Surg 2000; 232(4):455–465.[16])

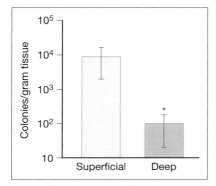

Fig. 31.11 Indicating that burn wound excision significantly reduced bacterial colonization among patients in the early excision group. *$p < 0.05$ (paired t test), deep versus superficial biopsies. (Reproduced with permisson from: Barret JP. Plast Reconstr Surg 2003; 111(2):744–750.)

within 48 hours of initial injury had reduced incidence of infection and graft loss when compared to those admitted late for delayed excision (day 7). In the same study greater bacterial colonization and higher rates of infection were correlated with topical treatment and late excision (Figures 31.11 and 31.12).

Early excision and prompt coverage is also associated with decreased mortality, reduced length of hospital stay,[65] less operative blood loss[67] and fewer septic complications[68] in children and young adults when compared to conservative serial debridement.

Prompt removal of burn eschar is of paramount importance for the invasively infected burn wound in patients with severe burns and should be performed as early as possible to reduce an increased release of inflammatory mediators and to control the hypermetabolic response during sepsis. A significant reduction in interleukin-6 (IL-6), interleukin-8 (IL-8), tumor necrosis factor-alpha (TNF-α) and lipopolysaccharide (LPS) has been shown in those patients following the thorough debridement of infected burn tissue.[69] In a more recent study we were able to show a reduction in C-reactive protein (CRP), C3 complement, IL-6 and serum TNF-α (Figure 31.13).[70]

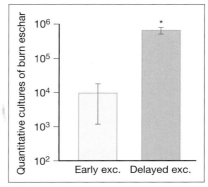

Fig. 31.12 Indicating that patients treated conservatively for 1 week (Delayed exc.) demonstrated greater bacterial colonization than did patients treated with early excision (Early exc.). *$p < 0.05$, delayed excision group versus early excision group. (Reproduced with permission from: Barret JP. Plast Reconstr Surg 2003; 111(2):744–750.)

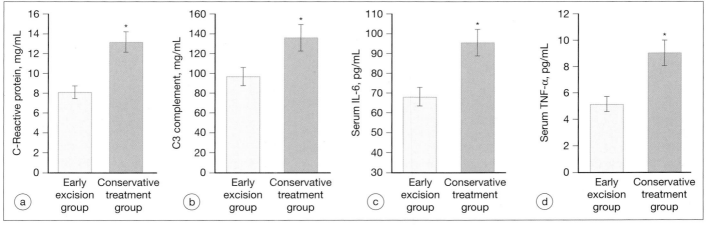

Fig. 31.13 Patients treated conservatively had higher serum levels of C-reactive protein (a) and C3 complement (b) compared with patients in the early burn wound excision group on day 5 postoperatively. Asterisk indicates $p < 0.05$ (unpaired t test) for the early excision group vs. the conservative treatment group. Serum levels of IL-6 (c) and TNF-α (d) were higher in patients treated conservatively 5 days after the injury. Levels of IL-1β and IL-10 were similar in both patient groups. Asterisk indicates $p < 0.05$ (unpaired t test) for the early excision group vs. the conservative treatment group. (Reproduced with permission from Barret and Herndon.[70] Copyright © 2003 American Medical Association. All right reserved.)

TABLE 31.5 DEFINITIONS OF SEPSIS

Burn sepsis	Modified AACP/SCCM sepsis
At least 3 of the following:	At least 2 of the following:
T > 38.5 or <36.5°C	T >38.5 or <36.5°C
Progressive tachycardia	HR >20% above NL for age
Progressive tachypnea	RR >20% above NL for age
WBC >12000 or <4000 cells/mm³	or $PaCO_2$ < 32 mmHg
Refactory hypotension	WBC >12000 or <4000
Thrombocytopenia	*and*
Hyperglycemia	Bacteremia or fungeremia
Enteral feeding intolerance	Pathological, tissue source
and	identified
Pathological tissue source identified	

Reproduced from Hart DW et al. Ann Surg 2000; 232(4):455–465.[16]

Effect of sepsis on metabolic response

Sepsis raises the metabolic response to burn by 40% when compared to non-septic patients with burns of a comparable size. This increase in catabolism is seen throughout the acute stay and well into rehabilitation. Consequently, prevention and/ or aggressive treatment of sepsis is important in reducing the ensuing mortality and morbidity of increased protein loss. Within the burns setting it is difficult to determine sepsis according to standard protocols. Table 31.5 shows modified scoring systems based upon the American Academy of Chest Physicians (AACP) and the Society of Critical Care Medicine (SCCM) score. Together with an experienced burn clinician, a diagnosis of sepsis can be reached and acted upon (Table 31.5).

Pharmacological modulation

The hypermetabolic response to severe burns leads to a shift in protein kinetics such that there is a marked increase in protein breakdown and a concomitant decrease in protein synthesis. The drop in protein synthesis is sufficient to fall below the rate of protein degradation and so lead to a net loss of protein. The anabolic phase during rehabilitation following a burn injury is due to protein synthetic rates rising above protein degradation.[71] This is an important finding as it shows us that an anabolic state can be achieved during persistent hypermetabolism. Analgesia and sedatives help to ameliorate the pain and anxiety associated with such injuries and hence prevent a rise in the metabolic rate that would otherwise be seen. Pharmacotherapy specific for the hypermetabolic response includes anabolic hormones such as recombinant human growth hormone, insulin, insulin-like growth factor-I (IGF-I), IGF-I and insulin-like growth factor binding protein-3 (IGFBP-3) in combination; anabolic steroids such as testosterone or its synthetic analogue oxandrolone; and adrenergic antagonists such as propranolol or metoprolol.

Analgesia

The metabolic rate of the patient is adversely affected by activity, anxiety and pain secondary to increases in sympathetic nervous system activity. Day-to-day burn care including range of motion exercises, debridement, dressing changes and application of topical antimicrobials, increases the otherwise almost unbearable pain levels still further. Therefore, prodigious quantities of narcotics and sedatives as well as supportive psychotherapy are helpful in reducing these effects.

Anabolic hormones
Recombinant human growth hormone

rhGH administered via injection at a dose of 0.2 mg/kg during the acute admission resulted in reduced donor site healing time by 25%, reduced length of stay in hospital from 0.80 days/ %TBSA to 0.54 days/%TBSA[72] and led to improved quality of wound healing with no rise in scarring.[73] The growth retardation also typically seen following severe burns in pediatric patients was prevented during administration of rhGH during hospital admission.[74] A favorable attenuation of the hepatic acute phase response[75] was also seen, with increased concentrations of IGF-I (the secondary mediator of rhGH) and increased albumin production.[76] When given at a dose of 0.05 mg/kg/day for the first year following burn injury, improvements in height, lean body mass, and bone mineral content were seen. These improvements remained after cessation of the treatment. Additionally, rhGH has a positive effect on immune function by reducing T-helper-2 and enhancing T-helper-1 cytokine production.[77]

The benefits of rhGH are not without some side effects, most notably hyperglycemia during the acute admission.[78] An increased mortality rate seen in non-burned critical care patients[79] is not present in burned pediatric patients.[76] Improved wound healing, reduced tissue wastage, and length of stay in hospital are all major benefits that will improve both the physiological and psychological rehabilitation of the patient. Currently the drawbacks for rhGH are the side effects and mode of delivery. Ongoing investigations are addressing these points, along with trials incorporating beta-blocking agents.

Insulin

Recently it has been restated that severe hyperglycemia in patients suffering from massive burns is associated with an increase in muscle protein catabolism,[29] reduced graft take, and an increase in mortality.[80] Euglycemia, maintained using insulin for non-burned, surgical critical care patients, significantly reduced incidence of infection and mortality.[81] The use of insulin has been shown to significantly reduce donor site healing time from 6.51 (± 0.95) days to 4.71(± 2.3) days.[82] A continuous infusion used in burn patients prevents muscle catabolism and conserves lean body mass in the absence of increased hepatic triglyceride production.[83] Submaximal doses (3 mU/kg/min) of insulin administered via infusion to burns patients resulted in net protein muscle anabolism without the need for large doses of carbohydrate.[84] Insulin has been shown to attenuate the inflammatory response by decreasing the pro-inflammatory and increasing the anti-inflammatory cascade, thus restoring systemic homeostasis and reducing the drive of the hypermetabolic response.[85] Continuous intravenous insulin infusions at doses that will maintain euglycemia (glucose between 100 and 140 mg/mL) after severe burns down-regulates acute phase protein levels[86] and attenuates muscle catabolism, preserving lean muscle mass.[87] Recently, insulin administered to burned children was shown to blunt the increase in C-reactive protein, IL-1β, and TNF-α levels after injury,[88,89] in the absence of normoglycemia. In another recent study involving pediatric patients in whom the glucose levels were maintained at between 90 and 120 mg/mL, intensive insulin therapy was shown to be safe and effective, reducing infection rates and improving survival.[90] The mechanisms are unclear for this response; however, it is likely to be caused by inhibition of NF-κB with stimulation of I-κB in monocytes.[91] This would result in reduced length and severity of infections and attenuate multiorgan dysfunction associated with burn shock. Although pharmacological doses of insulin have been shown to increase glucose uptake into tissue and this uptake is accompanied by increased amino acid uptake and increased lactate release,[92] the exact mechanisms are still unclear. Proposed pathways include activation of sodium-dependent transport systems, initiation of protein translation, and direct regulation of proteolytic activities. Metformin may also be used to attenuate hyperglycemia in patients with severe burns, thereby increasing muscle protein synthesis.[93,94] Other antihyperglycemic agents such as dichloroacetate may also show beneficial results in reduction of postburn hyperglycemia.[95]

Anabolic steroids

Oxandrolone is a synthetic testosterone analogue that can be taken orally, is inexpensive and has only 5% of the virilizing action seen in testosterone. Use of oxandrolone in the burns setting at a dose of 0.1 mg/kg bd increases protein synthetic efficiency,[96] anabolic gene expression in muscle,[97] and improves lean body mass by increasing net muscle protein synthesis,[98] thereby attenuating muscle wasting.[99,100] In severely burned children treated during acute hospitalization, oxandrolone significantly improved net protein synthesis, lean body mass, bone mineral content, synthesis of the hepatic constitutive proteins such as albumin and prealbumin, and attenuated the acute phase reactive protein levels.[96,101,102] Oxandrolone improved body composition and strength in severely burned children during the 12 months of treatment. Its effect on height and weight continued after treatment was discontinued (Figure 31.14).[103]

Due to the ability of this treatment option to increase lean body mass in an outpatient setting together with the enteral route of administration makes it an ideal medication in the postburn rehabilitation of children. Bone mineral content was also shown to be improved following long term treatment with oxandrolone versus unburned controls.[96]

Catecholamine antagonists

Propranolol has been used successfully to block the effects of endogenous catecholamines that have been implicated as primary mediators of the hypermetabolic response.[104] In the initial stages after burn, levels of catecholamines show a 10-fold increase.[1,105] The resulting hyperdynamic circulation, increased basal energy expenditure, and catabolism of skeletal muscle proteins are all deleterious for the patient. As described at the beginning of the chapter, catecholamines stimulate lipolysis via the β_2 adrenoceptor. The effects of propranolol in the burn patient include reduced thermogenesis,[106] tachycardia,[107] cardiac work, and resting energy expenditure.[104] The dose used is different for each patient; however, a reduction of heart rate by 20% is seen to produce reduced cardiac work

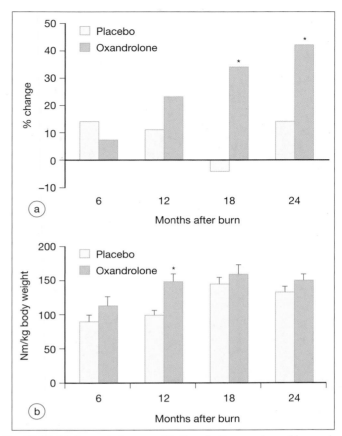

Fig. 31.14 (a) Percent change with time in the number of burned children in the >25th percentile/total for height when compared with values obtained at hospital discharge. *Significant changes in height were observed 6–12 months after oxandrolone was discontinued, $p < 0.05$.[103] (b) Muscle strength was significantly improved with oxandrolone 12 months after burn. Normal values for healthy children: 182 Nm/kg body weight (SD 40). Data are presented as mean ± SEM. *Significant difference between oxandrolone and placebo at $p < 0.05$. Reproduced with permission from Przkora R. Ann Surg 2005; 242(3):384–391.[103]

load and fatty infiltration (secondary to reducing peripheral lipolysis and hepatic blood flow) (Figure 31.15).[108]

Propranolol is shown to enhance intracellular recycling of free amino acids, leading to reduced skeletal muscle wasting and increased lean body mass.[109] The exact mechanisms for the beneficial changes seen in the burns patient following administration of this mixed β_1/β_2 adrenoceptor antagonist remain to be found.

Possible future pharmacotherapeutic options

IGF-I

The beneficial effects of rhGH are derived through IGF-I and IGFBP-3, the levels of which are raised by 100% during treatment, relative to healthy individuals. Therefore an infusion of equimolar doses of IGF-I and IGFBP-3 has been shown to improve protein metabolism in both adult and pediatric burns patients with significantly less hyperglycemia than rhGH alone.[110] Interestingly there was no additional benefit seen

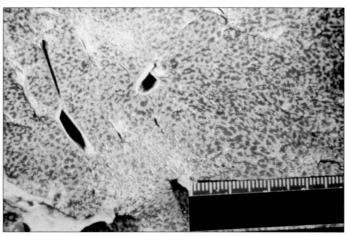

Fig. 31.15 Fatty infiltration of the liver following severe thermal injury. (Reprinted with permission from Barret JP, Herndon DN, eds. Color atlas of burn care. London: WB Saunders; 2001:133, Plate 8.39.)

with higher doses of the infusion; using 1 mg/kg/day was sufficient to achieve the desired effect. Attenuation of the type I and II acute phase response was seen following infusion, leading to reduced acute phase protein production and increased constitutive protein production by the liver.[111,112] Another potential beneficial effect of an infusion of IGF-I/IGFBP-3 has been shown in a human model where there was a partial reversal of the detrimental change in Th1/Th2 cytokine profile.[113] Typically, following massive thermal injury, there is a shift to a predominant Th2 cytokine response,[114,115] resulting in increases in lymphocyte production of IL-4 and

IL-10, together with decreased production of IL-2 and interferon-? (IFN-?). However this combination drug has yet to become commercially available and therefore further studies are required.

Ketoconazole

Ketoconazole is an imidazole antifungal agent. As with other imidazoles, it has a five-membered ring structure containing two nitrogen atoms. Ketoconazole has oral tablet, cream and dandruff shampoo formulations. The oral formulation has been available in the USA since 1981. Like all azole antifungal agents, ketoconazole works principally by inhibition of cytochrome P450 14α-demethylase (P45014DM) an enzyme in the sterol biosynthesis pathway that leads from lanosterol to ergosterol.[116] Ketoconazole inhibits the 11β-hydroxylation and 18-hydroxylation reactions in the final steps during the synthesis of adrenocorticosteroids[117] and may even function as a glucocorticoid receptor antagonist.[118]

Gene profiling for the future

Ongoing studies to correlate genomic and proteomic changes induced by burn with phenotypic changes and clinical outcomes are being conducted by the Inflammation and the Host Response to Injury Large-Scale Collaborative Research Program. Recent experiments demonstrate that dramatic, tissue-specific alterations in genomic expression patterns occur in a temporal fashion in blood leukocytes, skin, muscle, and fat. Further experiments will elucidate the genomic and proteomic differences in adults who survive a burn versus those who do not. Additional information (data and publications) can be found at www.gluegrant.org.

References

1. Goodall M, Stone C, Haynes BW Jr. Urinary output of adrenaline and noradrenaline in severe thermal burns. Ann Surg 1957; 145(4):479–487.
2. Kinney JM, Long CL, Gump FE, et al. Tissue composition of weight loss in surgical patients. I. Elective operation. Ann Surg 1968; 168(3):459–474.
3. Long CL, Spencer JL, Kinney JM, et al. Carbohydrate metabolism in man: effect of elective operations and major injury. J Appl Physiol 1971; 31(1):110–116.
4. Farrell K, Bradley S. Estimation of nitrogen requirements in patients with burns. J Burn Care Rehabil 1994; 15(2):174.
5. Hart DW, Wolf SE, Mlcak R, et al. Persistence of muscle catabolism after severe burn. Surgery 2000; 128(2):312–319.
6. Asch MJ, Feldman RJ, Walker HL, et al. Systemic and pulmonary hemodynamic changes accompanying thermal injury. Ann Surg 1973; 178(2):218–221.
7. Yu YM, Tompkins RG, Ryan CM, et al. The metabolic basis of the increase of the increase in energy expenditure in severely burned patients. JPEN 1999; 23(3):160–168.
8. Reiss E, Pearson E, Artz CP. The metabolic response to burns. J Clin Invest 1956; 35(1):62–77.
9. Turner WW Jr, Ireton CS, Hunt JL, et al. Predicting energy expenditures in burned patients. J Trauma 1985; 25(1):11–16.
10. Jahoor F, Herndon DN, Wolfe RR. Role of insulin and glucagon in the response of glucose and alanine kinetics in burn-injured patients. J Clin Invest 1986; 78(3):807–814.
11. Wolfe RR, Herndon DN, Peters EJ, et al. Regulation of lipolysis in severely burned children. Ann Surg 1987; 206(2):214–221.
12. Newsome TW, Mason AD Jr, Pruitt BA Jr. Weight loss following thermal injury. Ann Surg 1973; 178(2):215–217.
13. Bessey PQ, Jiang ZM, Johnson DJ, et al. Posttraumatic skeletal muscle proteolysis: the role of the hormonal environment. World J Surg 1989; 13(4):465–470; discussion 471.
14. Wolfe RR, Klein S, Herndon DN, et al. Substrate cycling in thermogenesis and amplification of net substrate flux in human volunteers and burned patients. J Trauma 1990; 30(12 Suppl): S6–S9.
15. Newsholme EA, Crabtree B. Substrate cycles in metabolic regulation and in heat generation. Biochem Soc Symp 1976; 41:61–109.
16. Hart DW, Wolf SE, Chinkes DL, et al. Determinants of skeletal muscle catabolism after severe burn. Ann Surg 2000; 232(4): 455–465.
17. Sheridan RL. A great constitutional disturbance. N Engl J Med 2001; 345(17):1271–1272.
18. Chance WT, Dayal R, Friend LA, et al. Possible role of CRF peptides in burn-induced hypermetabolism. Life Sci 2006; 78(7):694–703.
19. Chai J, Wu Y, Sheng ZZ. Role of ubiquitin-proteasome pathway in skeletal muscle wasting in rats with endotoxemia. Crit Care Med 2003; 31(6):1802–1807.
20. Chau V, Tobias JW, Bachmair A, et al. A multiubiquitin chain is confined to specific lysine in a targeted short-lived protein. Science 1989; 243(4898):1576–1583.
21. Deng L, Wang C, Spencer E, et al. Activation of the IkappaB kinase complex by TRAF6 requires a dimeric ubiquitin-conjugating enzyme complex and a unique polyubiquitin chain. Cell 2000; 103(2):351–361.
22. Wertz IE, O'Rourke KM, Zhou H, et al. De-ubiquitination and ubiquitin ligase domains of A20 downregulate NF-kappaB signalling. Nature 2004; 430(7000):694–699.

23. Spence J, Sadis S, Haas AL, et al. A ubiquitin mutant with specific defects in DNA repair and multiubiquitination. Mol Cell Biol 1995; 15(3):1265–1273.

24. Arnason T, Ellison MJ. Stress resistance in Saccharomyces cerevisiae is strongly correlated with assembly of a novel type of multiubiquitin chain. Mol Cell Biol 1994; 14(12):7876–7883.

25. Wing SS. Control of ubiquitination in skeletal muscle wasting. Int J Biochem Cell Biol 2005; 37(10):2075–2087.

26. Wolfe RR. Regulation of skeletal muscle protein metabolism in catabolic states. Curr Opin Clin Nutr Metab Care 2005; 8(1):61–65.

27. Biolo G, Fleming RY, Maggi SP, et al. Inverse regulation of protein turnover and amino acid transport in skeletal muscle of hypercatabolic patients. J Clin Endocrinol Metab 2002; 87(7):3378–3384.

28. Barret JP, Jeschke MG, Herndon DN. Fatty infiltration of the liver in severely burned pediatric patients: autopsy findings and clinical implications. J Trauma 2001; 51(4):736–739.

29. Gore DC, Chinkes DL, Hart DW, et al. Hyperglycemia exacerbates muscle protein catabolism in burn-injured patients. Crit Care Med 2002; 30(11):2438–2442.

30. Flakoll PJ, Hill JO, Abumrad NN. Acute hyperglycemia enhances proteolysis in normal man. Am J Physiol 1993; 265(5 Pt 1): E715–E721.

31. Moore FA, Feliciano DV, Andrassy RJ, et al. Early enteral feeding, compared with parenteral, reduces postoperative septic complications. The results of a meta-analysis. Ann Surg 1992; 216(2):172–183.

32. Herndon DN, Stein MD, Rutan TC, et al. Failure of TPN supplementation to improve liver function, immunity, and mortality in thermally injured patients. J Trauma 1987; 27(2):195–204.

33. Herndon DN, Barrow RE, Stein M, et al. Increased mortality with intravenous supplemental feeding in severely burned patients. J Burn Care Rehabil 1989; 10(4):309–313.

34. Moss G. Maintenance of gastrointestinal function after bowel surgery and immediate enteral full nutrition. II. Clinical experience, with objective demonstration of intestinal absorption and motility. JPEN J Parenter Enteral Nutr 1981; 5(3):215–220.

35. Tinckler LF. Surgery and intestinal motility. Br J Surg 1965; 52:140–150.

36. McDonald WS, Sharp CW Jr, Deitch EA. Immediate enteral feeding in burn patients is safe and effective. Ann Surg 1991; 213(2):177–183.

37. Mochizuki H, Trocki O, Dominioni L, et al. Reduction of postburn hypermetabolism by early enteral feeding. Curr Surg 1985; 42(2):121–125.

38. Selby AM, McCauley JC, Schell DN, et al. Indirect calorimetry in mechanically ventilated children: a new technique that overcomes the problem of endotracheal tube leak. Crit Care Med 1995; 23(2):365–370.

39. McArthur CD. Metabolic measurement using indirect calorimetry during mechanical ventilation – 2004: revision & update. Respir Care 2004; 49(9):1073–1079.

40. Goran MI, Peters EJ, Herndon DN, et al. Total energy expenditure in burned children using the doubly labeled water technique. Am J Physiol 1990; 259(4 Pt 1):E576–E585.

41. Hart DW, Wolf SE, Herndon DN, et al. Energy expenditure and caloric balance after burn: increased feeding leads to fat rather than lean mass accretion. Ann Surg 2002; 235(1):152–161.

42. Liusuwan RA, Palmieri TL, Kinoshita L, et al. Comparison of measured resting energy expenditure versus predictive equations in pediatric burn patients. J Burn Care Rehabil 2005; 26(6):464–470.

43. Curreri PW, Richmond D, Marvin J, et al. Dietary requirements of patients with major burns. J Am Diet Assoc 1974; 65(4):415–417.

44. Gore DC, Rutan RL, Hildreth M, et al. Comparison of resting energy expenditures and caloric intake in children with severe burns. J Burn Care Rehabil 1990; 11(5):400–404.

45. Wolfe RR, Goodenough RD, Burke JF, et al. Response of protein and urea kinetics in burn patients to different levels of protein intake. Ann Surg 1983; 197(2):163–171.

46. Patterson BW, Nguyen T, Pierre E, et al. Urea and protein metabolism in burned children: effect of dietary protein intake. Metabolism 1997; 46(5):573–578.

47. Crozier SJ, Kimball SR, Emmert SW, et al. Oral leucine administration stimulates protein synthesis in rat skeletal muscle. J Nutr 2005; 135(3):376–382.

48. Lynch CJ, Hutson SM, Patson BJ, et al. Tissue-specific effects of chronic dietary leucine and norleucine supplementation on protein synthesis in rats. Am J Physiol Endocrinol Metab 2002; 283(4): E824–E835.

49. Garrel D, Patenaude J, Nedelec B, et al. Decreased mortality and infectious morbidity in adult burn patients given enteral glutamine supplements: a prospective, controlled, randomized clinical trial. Crit Care Med 2003; 31(10):2444–2449.

50. Gadek JE, DeMichele SJ, Karlstad MD, et al. Effect of enteral feeding with eicosapentaenoic acid, gamma-linolenic acid, and antioxidants in patients with acute respiratory distress syndrome. Enteral Nutrition in ARDS Study Group. Crit Care Med 1999; 27(8):1409–1420.

51. Nelson JL, DeMichele SJ, Pacht ER, et al. Effect of enteral feeding with eicosapentaenoic acid, gamma-linolenic acid, and antioxidants on antioxidant status in patients with acute respiratory distress syndrome. JPEN J Parenter Enteral Nutr 2003; 27(2): 98–104.

52. Shakespeare PG. Studies on the serum levels of iron, copper and zinc and the urinary excretion of zinc after burn injury. Burns Incl Therm Inj 1982; 8(5):358–364.

53. Shenkin A. Trace elements and inflammatory response: implications for nutritional support. Nutrition 1995; 11(1 Suppl):100–105.

54. Berger MM, Cavadini C, Bart A, et al. Cutaneous copper and zinc losses in burns. Burns 1992; 18(5):373–380.

55. Gosling P, Rothe HM, Sheehan TM, et al. Serum copper and zinc concentrations in patients with burns in relation to burn surface area. J Burn Care Rehabil 1995; 16(5):481–486.

56. Boosalis MG SR, Talwalker R, McClain CJ. Topical silver sulfadiazine decreases plasma copper and ceruloplasmin in a rat model of thermal injury. J Trace Elem Exp Med 1994; (7): 119–124.

57. Berger MM, Shenkin A. Trace elements in trauma and burns. Curr Opin Clin Nutr Metab Care 1998; 1(6):513–517.

58. Saitoh D, Okada Y, Ookawara T, et al. Prevention of ongoing lipid peroxidation by wound excision and superoxide dismutase treatment in the burned rat. Am J Emerg Med 1994; 12(2): 142–146.

59. Bang RL, Dashti H. Keloid and hypertrophic scars: trace element alteration. Nutrition 1995; 11(5 Suppl):527–531.

60. Wilmore DW, Mason AD Jr, Johnson DW, et al. Effect of ambient temperature on heat production and heat loss in burn patients. J Appl Physiol 1975; 38(4):593–597.

61. Mlcak RP, Desai MH, Robinson E, et al. Temperature changes during exercise stress testing in children with burns. J Burn Care Rehabil 1993; 14(4):427–430.

62. Suman OE, Spies RJ, Celis MM, et al. Effects of a 12-wk resistance exercise program on skeletal muscle strength in children with burn injuries. J Appl Physiol 2001; 91(3):1168–1175.

63. McEntire SJ, Herndon DN, Sanford AP, et al. Thermoregulation during exercise in severely burned children. Pediatr Rehabil 2006; 9(1):57–64.

64. Muller MJ, Herndon DN. The challenge of burns. Lancet 1994; 343(8891):216–220.

65. Herndon DN, Barrow RE, Rutan RL, et al. A comparison of conservative versus early excision. Therapies in severely burned patients. Ann Surg 1989; 209(5):547–552; discussion 552–553.

66. Hart DW, Wolf SE, Chinkes DL, et al. Effects of early excision and aggressive enteral feeding on hypermetabolism, catabolism, and sepsis after severe burn. J Trauma 2003; 54(4):755–761; discussion 761–764.

67. Desai MH, Herndon DN, Broemeling L, et al. Early burn wound excision significantly reduces blood loss. Ann Surg 1990; 211(6):753–759; discussion 759–762.

68. Gray DT, Pine RW, Harnar TJ, et al. Early surgical excision versus conventional therapy in patients with 20 to 40 percent burns. A comparative study. Am J Surg 1982; 144(1):76–80.

69. Chai J, Sheng Z, Diao L, et al. Effect of extensive excision of burn wound with invasive infection on hypermetabolism in burn patients with sepsis. Zhonghua Wai Ke Za Zhi 2000; 38(6): 405–408.

70. Barret JP, Herndon DN. Modulation of inflammatory and catabolic responses in severely burned children by early burn wound excision in the first 24 hours. Arch Surg 2003; 138(2): 127–132.

71. Jahoor F, Desai M, Herndon DN, et al. Dynamics of the protein metabolic response to burn injury. Metabolism 1988; 37(4): 330–337.

72. Herndon DN, Barrow RE, Kunkel KR, et al. Effects of recombinant human growth hormone on donor-site healing in severely burned children. Ann Surg 1990; 212(4):424–429; discussion 430–431.

73. Barret JP, Dziewulski P, Jeschke MG, et al. Effects of recombinant human growth hormone on the development of burn scarring. Plast Reconstr Surg 1999; 104(3):726–729.

74. Aili Low JF, Barrow RE, Mittendorfer B, et al. The effect of short-term growth hormone treatment on growth and energy expenditure in burned children. Burns 2001; 27(5):447–452.

75. Jeschke MG, Herndon DN, Wolf SE, et al. Recombinant human growth hormone alters acute phase reactant proteins, cytokine expression, and liver morphology in burned rats. J Surg Res 1999; 83(2):122–129.

76. Ramirez RJ, Wolf SE, Barrow RE, et al. Growth hormone treatment in pediatric burns: a safe therapeutic approach. Ann Surg 1998; 228(4):439–448.

77. Takagi K, Suzuki F, Barrow RE, et al. Recombinant human growth hormone modulates Th1 and Th2 cytokine response in burned mice. Ann Surg 1998; 228(1):106–111.

78. Singh KP, Prasad R, Chari PS, et al. Effect of growth hormone therapy in burn patients on conservative treatment. Burns 1998; 24(8):733–738.

79. Takala J, Ruokonen E, Webster NR, et al. Increased mortality associated with growth hormone treatment in critically ill adults. N Engl J Med 1999; 341(11):785–792.

80. Gore DC, Chinkes D, Heggers J, et al. Association of hyperglycemia with increased mortality after severe burn injury. J Trauma 2001; 51(3):540–544.

81. Van den Berghe G, Wouters PJ, Bouillon R, et al. Outcome benefit of intensive insulin therapy in the critically ill: insulin dose versus glycemic control. Crit Care Med 2003; 31(2):359–366.

82. Pierre EJ, Barrow RE, Hawkins HK, et al. Effects of insulin on wound healing. J Trauma 1998; 44(2):342–345.

83. Aarsland A, Chinkes DL, Sakurai Y, et al. Insulin therapy in burn patients does not contribute to hepatic triglyceride production. J Clin Invest 1998; 101(10):2233–2239.

84. Ferrando AA, Chinkes DL, Wolf SE, et al. A submaximal dose of insulin promotes net skeletal muscle protein synthesis in patients with severe burns. Ann Surg 1999; 229(1):11–18.

85. Jeschke MG, Klein D, Herndon DN. Insulin treatment improves the systemic inflammatory reaction to severe trauma. Ann Surg 2004; 239(4):553–560.

86. Wu X, Thomas SJ, Herndon DN, et al. Insulin decreases hepatic acute phase protein levels in severely burned children. Surgery 2004; 135(2):196–202.

87. Thomas SJ, Morimoto K, Herndon DN, et al. The effect of prolonged euglycemic hyperinsulinemia on lean body mass after severe burn. Surgery 2002; 132(2):341–347.

88. Jeschke MG, Klein D, Bolder U, et al. Insulin attenuates the systemic inflammatory response in endotoxemic rats. Endocrinology 2004; 145(9):4084–4093.

89. Hansen TK, Thiel S, Wouters PJ, et al. Intensive insulin therapy exerts antiinflammatory effects in critically ill patients and counteracts the adverse effect of low mannose-binding lectin levels. J Clin Endocrinol Metab 2003; 88(3):1082–1088.

90. Pham TN, Warren AJ, Phan HH, et al. Impact of tight glycemic control in severely burned children. J Trauma 2005; 59(5):1148–1154.

91. Dandona P, Aljada A, Mohanty P, et al. Insulin inhibits intranuclear nuclear factor kappaB and stimulates IkappaB in mononuclear cells in obese subjects: evidence for an anti-inflammatory effect? J Clin Endocrinol Metab 2001; 86(7):3257–3265.

92. Sakurai Y, Aarsland A, Herndon DN, et al. Stimulation of muscle protein synthesis by long-term insulin infusion in severely burned patients. Ann Surg 1995; 222(3):283–294; 294–297.

93. Gore DC, Wolf SE, Sanford A, et al. Influence of metformin on glucose intolerance and muscle catabolism following severe burn injury. Ann Surg 2005; 241(2):334–342.

94. Gore DC, Wolf SE, Herndon DN, Wolfe RR. Metformin blunts stress-induced hyperglycemia after thermal injury. J Trauma 2003; 54(3):555–561.

95. Ferrando AA, Chinkes DL, Wolf SE, et al. Acute dichloroacetate administration increases skeletal muscle free glutamine concentrations after burn injury. Ann Surg 1998; 228(2):249–256.

96. Hart DW, Wolf SE, Ramzy PI, et al. Anabolic effects of oxandrolone after severe burn. Ann Surg 2001; 233(4):556–564.

97. Barrow RE, Dasu MR, Ferrando AA, et al. Gene expression patterns in skeletal muscle of thermally injured children treated with oxandrolone. Ann Surg 2003; 237(3):422–428.

98. Wolf SE, Thomas SJ, Dasu MR, et al. Improved net protein balance, lean mass, and gene expression changes with oxandrolone treatment in the severely burned. Ann Surg 2003; 237(6):801–10; discussion 810–811.

99. Demling RH, DeSanti L. Oxandrolone, an anabolic steroid, significantly increases the rate of weight gain in the recovery phase after major burns. J Trauma 1997; 43(1):47–51.

100. Berger JR, Pall L, Hall CD, et al. Oxandrolone in AIDS-wasting myopathy. Aids 1996; 10(14):1657–1662.

101. Thomas S, Wolf SE, Murphy KD, et al. The long-term effect of oxandrolone on hepatic acute phase proteins in severely burned children. J Trauma 2004; 56(1):37–44.

102. Murphy KD, Thomas S, Mlcak RP, et al. Effects of long-term oxandrolone administration in severely burned children. Surgery 2004; 136(2):219–224.

103. Przkora R, Jeschke MG, Barrow RE, et al. Metabolic and hormonal changes of severely burned children receiving long-term oxandrolone treatment. Ann Surg 2005; 242(3):384–349, discussion 390–391.

104. Wilmore DW, Long JM, Mason AD Jr, et al. Catecholamines: mediator of the hypermetabolic response to thermal injury. Ann Surg 1974; 180(4):653–669.

105. Wilmore DW, Aulick LH. Metabolic changes in burned patients. Surg Clin North Am 1978; 58(6):1173–1187.

106. Honeycutt D, Barrow R, Herndon D. Cold stress response in patients with severe burns after beta-blockade. J Burn Care Rehabil 1992; 13(2 Pt 1):181–186.

107. Minifee PK, Barrow RE, Abston S, et al. Improved myocardial oxygen utilization following propranolol infusion in adolescents with postburn hypermetabolism. J Pediatr Surg 1989; 24(8):806–810; discussion 810–811.

108. Barrow RE, Wolfe RR, Dasu MR, et al. The use of beta-adrenergic blockade in preventing trauma-induced hepatomegaly. Ann Surg 2006; 243(1):115–120.

109. Herndon DN, Hart DW, Wolf SE, et al. Reversal of catabolism by beta-blockade after severe burns. N Engl J Med 2001; 345(17):1223–1229.

110. Herndon DN, Ramzy PI, DebRoy MA, et al. Muscle protein catabolism after severe burn: effects of IGF-1/IGFBP-3 treatment. Ann Surg 1999; 229(5):713–720; discussion 720–722.

111. Jeschke MG, Barrow RE, Herndon DN. Insulinlike growth factor I plus insulinlike growth factor binding protein 3 attenuates the proinflammatory acute phase response in severely burned children. Ann Surg 2000; 231(2):246–252.

112. Spies M, Wolf SE, Barrow RE, et al. Modulation of types I and II acute phase reactants with insulin-like growth factor-1/binding protein-3 complex in severely burned children. Crit Care Med 2002; 30(1):83–88.

113. Wolf SE, Woodside KJ, Ramirez RJ, et al. Insulin-like growth factor-I/insulin-like growth factor binding protein-3 alters lym-

phocyte responsiveness following severe burn. J Surg Res 2004; 117(2):255–261.

114. Matsuo R, Herndon DN, Kobayashi M, et al. CD4- CD8- TCR alpha/beta+ suppressor T cells demonstrated in mice 1 day after thermal injury. J Trauma 1997; 42(4):635–640.

115. Zedler S, Faist E, Ostermeier B, et al. Postburn constitutional changes in T-cell reactivity occur in CD8+ rather than in CD4+ cells. J Trauma 1997; 42(5):872–880; discussion 880–881.

116. Lyman CA, Walsh TJ. Systemically administered antifungal agents. A review of their clinical pharmacology and therapeutic applications. Drugs 1992; 44(1):9–35.

117. Engelhardt D, Dorr G, Jaspers C, et al. Ketoconazole blocks cortisol secretion in man by inhibition of adrenal 11 beta-hydroxylase. Klin Wochenschr 1985; 63(13):607–612.

118. Loose DS, Stover EP, Feldman D. Ketoconazole binds to glucocorticoid receptors and exhibits glucocorticoid antagonist activity in cultured cells. J Clin Invest 1983; 72(1):404–408.

Chapter 32

Etiology and prevention of multisystem organ failure

Robert L. Sheridan and Ronald G. Tompkins

Chapter contents

> The cure of many diseases remains unknown.
> Socrates, circa 400 BC

Introduction

Despite its common occurrence in critically ill burn patients, our understanding of the multisystem organ failure syndrome remains fragmented and incomplete. The cascade of organ dysfunctions which typify the multisystem organ failure syndrome is driven by an unregulated inflammatory state, often, but not always, associated with uncontrolled infection.[1] Other potential 'engines' driving this cascade of organ dysfunctions are an impaired gastrointestinal barrier,[2,3] the open burn wound,[4] and inadequate delivery of oxygen to peripheral tissues.[5] The line between organ dysfunction and failure is admittedly unclear, but a set of organ-specific definitions of failure is helpful and has been developed (Box 32.1).[6] Approximately 15% of patients admitted to surgical intensive care units have multisystem organ failure,[7] and perhaps 8% of burn patients ultimately develop the syndrome.[8]

The sequence of failures often follows a predictable course, although the cascade can be modified by various treatments, such as the prophylactic use of H_2 receptor blockers. In burn patients, two cascades have been described.[8] An early cascade characterized by resuscitation failure, adult respiratory distress syndrome, hemodynamic failure, renal failure, liver failure, gut failure, and infection, and a late cascade typified by pulmonary failure, hemodynamic instability, renal failure, gut failure, and liver failure. Frequently, vasomotor failure and death is seen at the end of both cascades. Mortality increases with increasing numbers of failed organ systems. When three organs have failed, mortality has been reported as 100%, although survival is sometimes seen in patients with even more failed organ systems.[9] An understanding of the progression of the syndrome aids in prognostication and facilitates decisions regarding termination of futile efforts.[10,11] The management of specific organ failures will be presented in the next chapter. The purpose of this chapter is to discuss the etiology and prevention of the syndrome.

Etiology

The etiology of multisystem organ failure remains a mystery under intense investigation. All patients seem to share characteristics associated with an uncontrolled inflammatory state, and there are several proposed 'engines' which drive this uncontrolled inflammation, including sepsis, the open burn wound, the gut, and hypoperfusion.

Sepsis is clearly the most common initiator of the syndrome, and was recognized early on as the primary cause.[1] One single overwhelming infection is not required, as small repetitive infections may initiate the cascade,[12] perhaps by priming immune cells, making them react more intensely to each subsequent stimulus.[12] It was recognized later that many patients with multisystem organ failure did not have infection,[13] and this led the search for other 'engines'. Endotoxin liberated from the walls of Gram-negative bacteria is a major, but not the only, intermediary,[14] as Gram-positive bacteria cause similar aberrations in oxygen transport and hemodynamics,[15] via similar cascades of mediators.[16]

In burn patients the wound may also be a source of the inflammatory mediators leading to multiple organ failure. Certainly, an infected wound will do this, but wound sepsis is decreasing in incidence with the advent of early burn wound excision[17] and most infectious deaths in burn patients today are caused by pneumonia rather than wound sepsis.[18] Complete wound closure, without donor sites, decreases oxygen consumption[19] and presumably ameliorates the inflammatory response to the open wound. Incomplete wound closure does not have this effect.[20] Increased levels of circulating mediators such as interleukin-6 (IL-6), IL-8, and tumor necrosis factor (TNF) have been shown to originate from the burn wound[21] and contribute to the hypermetabolic and inflammatory state seen in burn patients. Interleukin-8 has been demonstrated to be upregulated in the lung after burn injury[21] and the stimulus for this upregulation, which is associated with pulmonary dysfunction, may come from the wound.[21]

Intensive recent work has demonstrated the importance of gut barrier function and the relation of gut barrier failure to the development of multisystem organ failure.[22] Normal barrier function prevents the movement of bacteria and their products

---

BOX 32.1 Organ-specific definitions of failure (OSF)

If the patient had one or more of the following during a 24-hour period (regardless of the values), OSF existed on that day.

CARDIOVASCULAR FAILURE (PRESENCE OF *ONE OR MORE* OF THE FOLLOWING):

- Heart rate ≤54 beats/min
- Mean arterial blood pressure ≤49 mmHg
- Occurrence of ventricular tachycardia and/or ventricular fibrillation
- Serum pH ≤7.24 with a $PaCO_2$ of ≤49 mmHg

RESPIRATORY FAILURE (PRESENCE OF *ONE OR MORE* OF THE FOLLOWING):

- Respiratory rate ≤5 beats/min or ≥40 beats/min
- $PaCO_2$ ≥50 mmHg
- $AaDO_2$ ≥350 mmHg ($AaDO_2 = 713\ FIO_2 - PaCO_2 - PaO_2$)
- Dependent on ventilator on the fourth day of OSF, e.g. *not* applicable for the initial 72 hours of OSF

RENAL FAILURE (PRESENCE OF *ONE OR MORE* OF THE FOLLOWING):*

- Urine output ≤479 mL/24 h or ≤159 mL/8 h
- Serum BUN ≥100 mg/dL
- Serum creatinine ≥3.5 mg/dL

HEMATOLOGICAL FAILURE (PRESENCE OF *ONE OR MORE* OF THE FOLLOWING):

- WBC ≤1000 cells/mm³
- Platelets ≤20 000 cells/mm³
- Hematocrit ≤20%

NEUROLOGICAL FAILURE

- Glasgow Coma Score ≤6 (in absence of sedation at any one point in day)
- Glasgow Coma Score: sum of best eye opening, best verbal, and best motor responses. Scoring of responses as follows: (points)

Eye

Open: spontaneously (4), to verbal command (3), to pain (2), no response (1)

Motor

Obeys verbal command (6); response to painful stimuli: localizes pain (5), flexion-withdrawal (4), decorticate rigidity (3), decerebrate rigidity (2); no response (1); movement without any control (4)

Verbal

Oriented and converses (5), disoriented and converses (4), inappropriate words (3), incomprehensible sounds (2), no response (1). If intubated, use clinical judgment for verbal responses as follows: patient generally unresponsive (1), patient's ability to converse in question (3), patient appears able to converse (5)

*Excluding patients on chronic dialysis before hospital admission.
Reproduced from Knaus et al., Ann Surg 1985; 202:685–693.[6] with permission.

---

a tribute to normal barrier function. Although not seen immediately after trauma,[24] several insults have been shown to result in increased translocation of bacteria and their products into the portal and lymphatic circulations. Hemorrhagic shock,[25] endotoxin administration,[26] burns,[27] and burn wound sepsis[28] have each been shown to result in increased translocation of bacteria from the gut. Gut permeability to macromolecules, such as endotoxin, has been shown to increase with increasing burn wound size using polyethylene glycol 3350 as a tracer.[29] Smaller molecules, with lactulose as the tracer, have also been shown to pass more readily through the gastrointestinal membrane after injury.[30] The exact mechanism by which bacteria and their products pass through the gastrointestinal barrier is not clear. Both intra- and transcellular processes may be involved.[31,32] The consequences of loss of the gastrointestinal barrier are profound. Translocating whole bacteria can be a direct source of sepsis or can activate Kupffer cells[2,3] and promulgate an inflammatory response in conjunction with bacterial products such as endotoxin.

Cellular dysfunction, caused by inadequate oxidative metabolism secondary to hypoperfusion, is another potential 'engine' resulting in multisystem organ failure. In ischemia-reperfusion models, oxygen radicals are generated, resulting in peroxidation of cell membrane lipids and accumulation of activated neutrophils,[33] with progressive cellular and whole-organ dysfunction. It has been proposed that critically ill patients suffer from supply-dependent oxygen consumption because of defects in cellular oxygen extraction and utilization.[34,35] This results in inadequate aerobic metabolism unless supranormal levels of oxygen are supplied.[36] The reality of this proposal is still actively debated.[37,38] Certainly, a grossly inadequate amount of oxygen available to cells dependent on aerobic metabolism can lead to cellular dysfunction, and this may be followed by organ failures.[5] Maintaining oxygen delivery at at least normal, and possibly supranormal, levels should help maintain cellular homeostasis and minimize the risk of multiple organ failure.[39] Although the requirement for a supranormal level of tissue oxygenation in critical illness is controversial and our ability to predict organ-specific oxygen delivery and consumption from whole-body data is poor,[40] careful attention to whole-body hemodynamics is an integral part of the management of any critically ill patient.

Common ground: mediators

Sepsis, open burn wounds, impaired gut barrier function, and hypoperfusion are all associated with multiorgan failure. The similarity in the response to these differing events implies that there is some common ground. These processes all probably impact on individual organs via a number of mediators, whose complex interactions are still very poorly understood,[41] but are being unraveled by investigators using blocking antibodies, soluble receptors, and receptor antagonists.[42] At this point, these mediators, including endotoxin, arachidonic acid metabolites, cytokines, platelet activating factor, activated neutrophils and adherence molecules, nitric oxide, complement, and oxygen free radicals will be reviewed briefly.

Endotoxin, a lipopolysaccharide component of Gram-negative bacterial cell walls, induces many of the symptoms associated with sepsis, including fever, hypotension, the release of

from the gut lumen into the portal and lymphatic circulations. Bacterial densities range from near 0 in the stomach, to $10^4–10^5$ in the distal small bowel, to $10^{11}–10^{12}$/g of stool in the normal colon.[23] That the normal gut can carry this bacterial load, without the frequent occurrence of Gram-negative infection, is acute phase proteins, and the production of multiple cytokines including TNF and IL-1.[43] Endotoxin also activates complement,[44] causes activation of the coagulation cascade,[45] and results in the release of platelet activating factor.[46] Potential sources of endotoxin include both Gram-negative bacteria in foci of infection and Gram-negative bacteria within the gut when the gut barrier fails.

Arachidonic acid makes up approximately 20% of cell membranes, is released from these membranes in response to a multitude of stimuli which activate phospholipases A_2 and C, and is then metabolized by one of two major enzyme systems (Figure 32.1).

The cyclooxygenase pathway results in production of prostaglandins and thromboxanes, and the lipoxygenase pathway results in the production of leukotrienes.[47] The prostaglandins and leukotrienes interact with other mediators in a complex fashion, and are later degraded by enzyme systems, which are dispersed throughout the body.[48]

Arachidonic acid, which is metabolized via the cyclooxygenase pathway, results in the formation of prostaglandins and thromboxanes. Prostacyclin inhibits platelet aggregation, thrombis formation, and gastric secretion.[49] Thromboxane A_2 (TXA_2) causes platelet aggregation, has profound vasoconstricting effects on both the splanchnic and pulmonary microvasculature, and causes bronchoconstriction and increased membrane permeability.[50] It is studied via its longer-lived but inactive metabolite, TXB_2. Aspirin has its physiological effects by inhibiting thromboxane synthetase.[51]

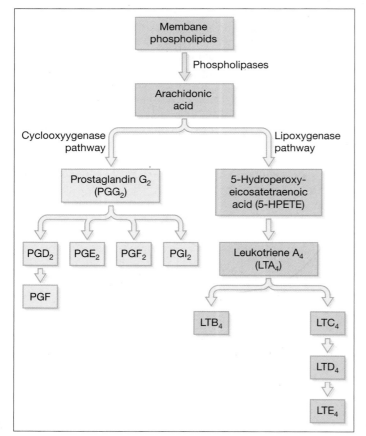

Fig. 32.1 The cyclooxygenase and lipoxygenase pathways of arachidonic acid metabolism.

Arachidonic acid metabolized via the lipoxygenase pathway results in the formation of leukotrienes. There are two types based on their metabolism after the action of 5-lipoxygenase, leukotrienes (LT) C_4, D_4, and E_4 (the sulfidopeptide group) and LTB_4.[52] Leukotrienes are generated in response to multiple stimuli by several cell types, including neutrophils, macrophages, and monocytes.[53] Vessel walls are also capable of generating leukotrienes.[54] Leukotrienes C_4, D_4, and E_4 have variable actions on vascular tone depending on the presence or absence of other mediators such as cyclooxygenase product.[55] In addition to their variable effects in redirecting blood flow, LTC_4, LTD_4, and LTE_4 also increase vascular permeability,[56] and have been described as being elevated immediately prior to the development of pulmonary failure.[57] The major effect of LTB_4 is an enhancement of neutrophil chemotaxis.[58] Thus, leukotrienes as a group may be involved in the edema formation and pulmonary and systemic vascular changes that are seen in the multisystem organ failure syndrome.

Cytokines are regulatory proteins that are secreted by immune cells and have multiple paracrine and endocrine effects. There are six major classes,[59] including interleukins, TNF, interferons, colony-stimulating factors, chemotactic factors, and growth factors. Those which have been most extensively characterized are IL-1, IL-6, and TNF.

Interleukin-1 and IL-6 are elevated in septic states, and high levels are associated with a fatal outcome[60] and predict systemic infection.[61] Interleukin-1β causes hypotension and decreased systemic vascular resistance, which may be synergistic with the effects of TNF.[62] Even better characterized is TNF, the administration of which causes hypotension, cardiac depression, and pulmonary dysfunction in animals.[63–65] When administered to humans, TNF causes fever, hypotension, decreased systemic vascular resistance, increased protein turnover, elevation of stress hormone levels,[66,67] and activation of the coagulation cascade.[68]

Platelet activating factor is a nonprotein phospholipid that is secreted by many cells including platelets, endothelial cells, and inflammatory cells,[69] and is a major mediator of the pulmonary[70] and hemodynamic[71] effects of endotoxin. The major effects of platelet activating factor are vasodilation, cardiac depression, and enhancement of capillary leak. Its complex interactions with other mediators are still poorly understood.

Although tissue injury can occur in the absence of neutrophils,[72] the inflammatory process results in local accumulation of activated inflammatory cells which release various local toxins such as oxygen radicals, proteases, eicosanoids, platelet activating factor, and other substances. When unregulated, such accumulations of activated cells can cause tissue injury.[73] The initial attachment of neutrophils to the vascular endothelium at an inflammatory site is facilitated by the interaction of adherence molecules on the neutrophil and endothelial cell surfaces.[74]

These neutrophil adherence receptors are induced by numerous stimuli but, interestingly, are reduced after major thermal and nonthermal injury,[75] perhaps explaining in part the increased incidence of infection in such patients. The importance of this adherence mechanism can be seen in patients who are deficient in one of the integrin class of neutrophil adherence receptors, CD-18, who suffer from frequent bacterial infections.[76] The biology of the transmembrane polypeptides that govern these complex cell-to-cell interactions is an active area of research[77] and holds promise for therapeutic interventions in the future.

Oxygen radicals, such as hydrogen peroxide and superoxide anion, are released by activated neutrophils in response to a variety of stimuli.[78] They are also released when xanthine oxidase is activated after reperfusion in ischemia-reperfusion models. These highly reactive products cause cell membrane dysfunction, increased vascular permeability, and release of eicosanoids.

Nitric oxide, released when citrulline is formed from arginine (Figure 32.2), was only identified as an endothelial product in the middle 1980s.[79] Its half-life is only a few seconds, as it is quickly oxidized, but it has profound local microvascular effects. Nitric oxide synthesis is stimulated by various cytokines, endotoxin, thrombin, and by injury to the vascular endothelium. It is a potent vasodilator,[80] but its actions vary depending on the vascular bed and presence of other mediators.[81] Nitric oxide is one of the major mediators of the hypotensive response to sepsis.[82,83]

Antigen–antibody complexes activate the complement cascade, and complement fragments thus generated can interact with other cytokines to promulgate the inflammatory response.[84] Diminished levels of a natural inhibitor of C5a have been demonstrated in patients with adult respiratory distress syndrome (ARDS)[85] and administration of anti-C5a antibody diminishes hypotension in an animal model of endotoxemia.[86] Complement fragments may be involved in the development of burn wound edema.[87]

Obviously, our understanding of the incredibly complex cellular and subcellular biology, of which multisystem organ failure is but one manifestation, is poorly understood at the present time. This dim understanding highlights the important role that prevention plays in managing the syndrome.

Prevention of multisystem organ failure

Once established, multisystem organ failure is very difficult to reverse, emphasizing the importance of prevention.[88] Prevention is based on our crude knowledge of the 'engines' that drive the process — sepsis, the gut, the wound, and inadequate perfusion (Table 32.1). Dealing with these issues is far more practical than dealing with an incompletely understood complex web of mediators. Also, this complex cascade evolved in numerous species over thousands of generations and interference in the network may do more harm than good. The discussion that follows will address prevention of sepsis via proper wound management and attention to unusual causes of sepsis, support of the gut, and prevention of inadequate oxygen delivery. Subsequently, the potential role of nutritional and specific immunomodulators will be addressed.

Prevention of sepsis

In the burn patient, prevention of multisystem organ failure is greatly facilitated by prevention of wound sepsis via an aggressive surgical approach to deep wounds. The increasing survival of burn patients has paralleled the evolution of this approach to the burn wound.[89–91] Not only is overt wound sepsis prevented by early removal of devitalized tissue, but multiple smaller septic insults are also prevented, as manipulation of heavily colonized burn wounds is a frequent source of

TABLE 32.1 MULTIPLE ORGAN FAILURE ETIOLOGY AND ESTABLISHED PREVENTIVE MEASURES

Etiology	Prevention
Sepsis	Early excision and biologic closure of deep wounds. Anticipation and early treatment of occult septic foci
Gut barrier failure	Optimize whole-body hemodynamics. +/– Early enteral feedings
Inadequate organ perfusion	Optimize whole-body hemodynamics. +/– Enhanced oxygen delivery

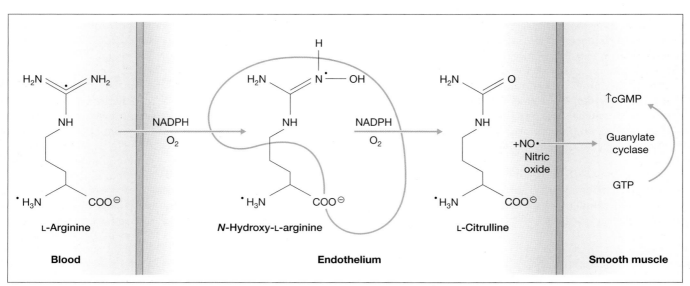

Fig. 32.2 Nitric oxide metabolism. (From Cobb et al.,[189] with permission.)

transient bacteremia.[92,93] Such multiple occult bacteremias occurring during frequent manipulation of heavily colonized wounds could contribute to the development of multisystem organ failure by priming immune cells, making them react more intensively to each subsequent insult.[12] The role of perioperative antibiotics in minimizing bacteremias in the perioperative period has yet to be defined clearly. However, they are clearly beneficial in patients with injuries greater than 60% of body surface and in any other patient in whom the probability of bacteremia with wound manipulation is felt to be high.[94] Appropriate perioperative antibiotics are guided by surface cultures. Burn patients are prone to a large number of unusual and often occult infectious complications[95] which can result in sepsis and potentially contribute to the development of multiorgan failure. Rapid diagnoses and treatment are facilitated by a high index of suspicion.

Intravascular infections such as suppurative thrombophlebitis and endocarditis typically present in burn patients with fever and bacteremia without localizing signs. Burn patients with endocarditis develop a new murmur in only 9% of cases,[96] and only 10% have been reported to present antemortem.[97] Of those with septic thrombophlebitis, 68% have no localizing signs and present with fever and positive blood cultures only.[98] The diagnosis is made in patients without localizing signs only by thorough examination of all sites of prior cannulation, with surgical exposure of any suspicious sites and complete excision of any involved veins.[99] Vigilant care and scheduled replacement of intravascular devices will minimize the occurrence of catheter-related sepsis. Occult intracompartmental sepsis can also present with fever and bacteremia without localizing signs, and is diagnosed only by careful examination and exploration of suspicious compartments.[100]

Pneumonia, seen in approximately 35% of patients with inhalation injury, adds between 20 and 60% to the expected mortality of burn patients.[101] Although a difficult diagnosis to make in critically ill patients, pneumonia should be vigilantly anticipated and aggressively treated with appropriate endobronchial toilet and specific antibiotics. The incidence of nosocomial pneumonia increases with longer durations of intubation,[102] emphasizing the importance of judicious use of mechanical ventilation.

Suppurative sinusitis is being recognized with increasing frequency in the intensive care unit, and may be more frequent in patients who are nasotracheally intubated.[103] Diagnosis may require examination and culture of material obtained by antral puncture, in addition to plain radiographs and computed tomography. Although there is some controversy about the role of the nasotracheal tube in causing sinusitis,[104] treatment involves removing all nasotracheal devices, topical decongestants, and appropriate antibiotics. Surgical drainage is reserved for recalcitrant cases.

Acalculous cholecystitis often presents with generalized sepsis without localizing signs in the burn patient, and, like intravascular infection, is a very difficult diagnosis to make.[105] Recently, bedside placement of percutaneous cholecystostomy tubes under ultrasonic guidance has become an option in the management of suspected cholecystitis in critically ill patients.[106] This technique allows an accurate diagnosis to be made and the condition to be temporarily treated in patients too unstable for immediate operation.

Sepsis accounts for at least half of cases of multisystem organ failure. In perhaps no other area can the vigilance of the burn team have a greater impact in multisystem organ failure prevention than in the early detection and aggressive treatment of occult septic foci.

Support of the gut

Bacteria and their products released when the gut barrier fails may fuel the multiorgan failure syndrome. Gut mucosal integrity suffers when mesenteric flow is inadequate and gut blood flow is decreased after burn injury, a response exacerbated by the release of TXA_2.[107] Thus, support of splanchnic blood flow is an important aspect of multisystem organ failure prevention,[108] and this is best done by careful attention to whole-body hemodynamics. There is no substitute for a carefully monitored burn resuscitation.

The enterocyte may be better supported by intraluminal, rather than parenteral feedings, as gut deprived of intraluminal feedings develops mucosal atrophy.[109] Early enteral feedings are tolerated in the burn patients,[110] and may reduce the magnitude of the hypermetabolic response to the injury.[111] Parenteral feedings do not prevent gut mucosal atrophy as well as isocaloric and isonitrogenous intraluminal feeds,[112] although convincing human data are not available to support the clinical significance of this point.

The value of specific nutrients to support the enterocyte is far less clear than the value of providing adequate mesenteric blood flow and perhaps intraluminal nutrition. However, this is an exciting and active area of research. Glutamine, a nonessential amino acid, is the preferred fuel of the small bowel enterocyte[113] as well as other rapidly dividing cells. Sepsis has been shown to decrease glutamine uptake by the small bowel enterocyte, which may result in barrier failure,[114] and the addition of glutamine to the nutritional regimen has been theorized to improve barrier function. Glutamine is not a component of commercial parenteral nutritional formulas because of its short shelf life, although the dipeptide is well tolerated parenterally, and has a longer shelf life.[115] Although supplemental glutamine may improve protein balance in surgical patients,[115] and may partially reverse gut atrophy,[116] it has not been shown to improve gut barrier function when given parenterally.[117]

The role of specific nutrients in support of the large intestinal mucosa is less clear, but butyrate, a fatty acid liberated by fiber fermentation, is a favored fuel of the colonic mucosal cell.[118] Enteral pectin may help support the colonic mucosa, but the value of such support in the hypermetabolic burn patient is as yet unclear. Limited work has been done suggesting possible benefit of probiotics for gut barrier support.[119]

A decontaminated gut lumen might diminish the impact of gastrointestinal barrier failure. Attempts have been made to access the impact of selective decontamination of the gut[120] and coating enteric bacteria to inhibit their ability to attach to the intestinal mucosa and translocate.[121] Although there is a suggestion that the rate of pneumonia may be decreased by such maneuvers, there is no apparent impact on mortality.

Support of the gut in an effort to prevent multisystem organ failure is certain to have real value. Maintenance of adequate mesenteric perfusion via careful attention to whole-body hemodynamics is crucial. There are some data to support the contention that enteral feedings have beneficial effects on outcome in injured patients when compared with parenteral feedings, possibly via an enhancement of gastrointestinal barrier integrity.[122] However, these data require confirmation prior to general application. Data supporting the administration of specific mucosal substrates or gut decontamination are less convincing, but further research in these important areas may show such benefit.

Insuring adequate oxygen delivery

The normal intracellular partial pressure of oxygen is 0.5 mmHg, and this small amount of mitochrondial oxygen allows for the aerobic generation of most of the cell's adenosine triphosphate (ATP). When cells have to adapt to a lower oxygen tension, ATP generation continues at a lower rate by anaerobic channels,[123] possibly triggered by the build-up of adenosine diphosphate (ADP). As outlined by Gutierrez, the anaerobic reactions which generate ATP are glycolysis, the creatine kinase reaction, and the adenylate kinase reaction.[123] Glycolysis describes the conversion of glucose to lactate with the generation of two ATP molecules. The creatine kinase reaction is the breakdown of the high-energy phosphate storage molecule, phosphocreatine, with the generation of ATP and creatine. The adenylate kinase reaction describes the combination of nucleotides to form ATP and AMP which, although generating ATP, depletes the cells of adenine nucleotides. In conjunction with this conversion to anaerobic ATP generation, the intracellular concentration of hydrogen ion increases, the amount of adenine nucleotides within the cell decreases, and intracellular calcium levels increase with decreased function of the ATP-driven sodium–calcium pump.[124] There also may be an increase in the liberation of intracellular oxygen free radicals with the activation of xanthine oxidase.[125] If low oxygen tensions continue, membrane phospholipids may be degraded by the combined effects of elevated calcium, oxygen free radicals, and the decreased synthetic capabilities coincident with decreased levels of ATP.[126] These effects may be magnified if there is also systemic sepsis as cellular oxygen extraction may be impaired. That such cellular hypoxic dysfunction is involved in the development of organ dysfunction is implied by the fact that cocarboxylase, which enhances ATP generation by ischemic cells, ameliorates some of the metabolic and hemodynamic consequences of endotoxic shock in an animal model.[127]

An understanding of progressive cell destruction and dysfunction which is caused by low intracellular oxygen tensions, coupled with the perception of oxygen extraction abnormalities associated with sepsis, has led to an intense interest in the delivery of supranormal amounts of oxygen to prevent organ dysfunction, as clinical data suggest that inadequate oxygen delivery is associated with the development of multisystem organ failure.[128] Clinically, it is somewhat cumbersome to measure and follow oxygen delivery, and other markers of the adequacy of tissue oxygenation have been tried, including the use of lactate and the lactate/pyruvate ratio, base deficit, mixed venous oxygen tension and pH, and gut tonometry. However, none of these secondary markers of oxygen delivery have proven to be as reliable as the direct determination of oxygen delivery and consumption by the reverse Fick technique.

Normal physiological oxygen supply dependency is different than the pathological supply dependency seen in septic states. In this circumstance, supranormal oxygen delivery is said to be required, as extraction is decreased.[129] The exact reasons for this pathological supply dependency are unclear, but may involve microcirculatory shunting or aberrations of intracellular physiology. It has been proposed that the purposeful delivery of supranormal amounts of oxygen is associated with a decreased incidence of multiple organ failure and increased survival.[130] The reality of the proposal is still controversial, with data showing no increase in oxygen consumption with transfusion of critically ill children[131] and the absence of a consumption plateau in patients with ARDS.[132] Also, regional blood flow is poorly predicted by whole-body oxygen delivery and consumption data,[133] implying that whole-body delivery and consumption data may be of no value even if pathological supply dependency was real. Normally, oxygen consumption is approximately 25% of oxygen delivery, and delivery can be maximized by optimizing the hemoglobin, partial pressure of oxygen, and cardiac output, which are the major determinants of oxygen delivery, although total flow may be more important than the blood's oxygen-carrying capacity.[134]

Inadequate oxygen delivery clearly leads to organ dysfunction. At a minimum, the clinician should insure that injured patients are resuscitated to the conventional clinical endpoints of appropriate urine output, skin perfusion, blood pressure, and sensorium. In selected critically ill patients, invasive monitoring is justified to document oxygen delivery and consumption, extraction ratio, and the possible presence of supply dependency in which circumstance supranormal levels of oxygen delivery with plateau of oxygen consumption is an appropriate resuscitation endpoint.

The potential role of nutritional and specific immunomodulators

The holy grail of those who study the complex biology of the multisystem organ failure syndrome is an ability to modulate the common pathways that lead to organ dysfunction and death. The three general approaches to this goal are nutritional, nonspecific, and specific immunomodulation.

Nutritional immunomodulation

Three categories of substances show some promise as potential nutritional immunomodulators in burn patients: long-chain fatty acids; arginine, glutamine, and branched-chain amino acids; and nucleotides. Short- and medium-chain fatty acids are commonly utilized for energy, whereas long-chain fatty acids are important constituents of cell membranes and can profoundly influence cell function.[135] Omega-3 long-chain fatty acids play a particularly important role in the membranes of immunocompetent cells.[136] There are animal data suggesting that supplementation of the diet with ω-3 fatty acids may improve immune function after burn injury;[137] however, there are no clear clinical data yet available to support the routine administration of ω-3 fatty acids as a dietary supplement in injured patients.

The potential immunostimulating effects of specific amino acids, particularly arginine, glutamine, and the branched-chain amino acids leucine, isoleucine, and valine, are an active area of research. Arginine is a nonessential amino acid with important functions in the urea cycle and in the generation of nitric oxide.[138] It also may have important effects in insuring immune cell competence.[139,140] Although there are some animal data suggesting improved immunocompetence and outcome after burn with supplementation of arginine,[141–143] human data are not yet adequate to support its routine administration to burn patients. Glutamine, the most common amino acid in the body, and a preferred fuel of rapidly dividing cells, may be conditionally essential in hypermetabolic patients,[113,114] and its administration has been proposed as a method to support the gut barrier, thereby abrogating the consequences of barrier failure. Early human data suggest that administration of supplemental glutamine may improve amino acid protein economy in stressed surgical patients,[115] but there are inadequate data as yet to support the routine administration of glutamine as an immune stimulant.

The branched-chain amino acids leucine, isoleucine, and valine are important energy sources in stressed surgical patients. Although there was an early enthusiasm for the supplemental administration of these substrates, subsequent data have suggested that the supplemental administration of branched-chain amino acids does not benefit stressed surgical patients.[144]

Based on limited animal and human data it has been suggested that the administration of adenine nucleotides may have beneficial effects on immune function in stressed patients.[145] Again, at the present time there is inadequate human data to support the routine use of supplemental nucleotides.

The concept of nutritional immunomodulation via supplementation of specific substances is exciting. However, despite preliminary human studies suggesting a beneficial effect of supplemental arginine and ω-3 fatty acids,[146] with additional nucleotides,[145] and glutamine,[115] there do not yet exist adequate data to support nutritional immunomodulation as a routine maneuver in the management of burned patients.

Non-specific and specific immunomodulation

It seems intuitively unlikely that there exists a magic immunomodulating bullet that will prevent the development of multisystem organ failure in critically ill surgical patients, particularly if sepsis is uncontrolled, the integrity of the gut barrier is compromised, burn wounds are unaddressed, or patients are inadequately supported hemodynamically. However, such efforts have tremendous potential to facilitate our understanding of cellular and subcellular biology and may, in time, provide a clinical dividend. Efforts at nonspecific immunomodulation have included the use of steroids,[147] immunoglobulin G,[148] and naloxone[149] with no significant impact on patient outcomes. With the exception of steroids for those with suspected adrenal insufficiency[150] and naloxone for those with opiate intoxication, there is no role for these substances in critically ill burn patients.

Although there have been efforts to absorb lipopolysaccharide,[151] and to prevent endotoxemia with prophylactic polymyxin B in burn patients,[152] the greatest efforts at specific immunomodulation have been applied to the development of anti-endotoxin antibodies. The earliest clinical efforts used human serum with anti-J5 activity and demonstrated an enhanced survival in patients with Gram-negative septic shock.[153] Later, two monoclonal IgMs were developed, and

human trials were completed. The first was anti-E5, a murine monoclonal antibody. Clinical trials suggested a benefit in septic patients without refractory shock.[154] Large numbers of treated patients developed antibodies to the murine monoclonal, and although these patients were not retreated, attention turned more toward a human product. A subsequent effort with this murine monoclonal did not show statistically significant improvements in outcome.[155]

HA-1A, a human monoclonal IgM, was trailed in a large multicenter effort without statistically significant improvement in outcome, except in a subgroup of patients that had Gram-negative bacteremia and shock.[156] Multiple confounding factors made these marginally beneficial results suspect, leaving the ultimate utility of HA-1A still unclear.

Anti-endotoxin monoclonal therapy, which may have potential to be beneficial if significantly refined, has also been criticized for its expense. It is estimated that it would cost $24 100 per year of life saved should this technology be used widely.[157] Integrating such advanced and expensive technology into common practice poses tremendous practical problems, and is therefore very unlikely to happen soon when one considers its lack of clear efficacy and high expense.

Significant efforts have also been made toward modifying the actions of arachidonic acid metabolites or eicosanoids, both cyclooxygenase and lipoxygenase products. Numerous animal models of sepsis and endotoxemia exist, and cyclooxygenase pathway blockade with nonsteroidal anti-inflammatory agents has demonstrated improved survival,[158,159] improved pulmonary hemodynamics,[160] and improved mesenteric blood flow.[161] There has been little work documenting outcome improvement in human patients, but it has been suggested that nonsteroidal anti-inflammatory agents improve symptoms associated with endotoxin infusion in normal volunteers[162] and septic patients,[163] and may improve immune function after surgical trauma.[164] In an animal model, infusion of the vasodilating arachidonic acid metabolite, prostacyclin, ameliorates the pulmonary dysfunction associated with endotoxin infusion.[165] Less work has been done with lipoxygenase pathway inhibitors. Survival is enhanced in a murine model of endotoxin infusion with lipoxygenase pathway blockade.[166] Endotoxin-associated pulmonary dysfunction is diminished in sheep[167] and pigs[168] when this pathway is blocked. The ultimate role of lipoxygenase blockade in human remains uninvestigated.

Cytokines are difficult to measure accurately and their complex interactions are poorly understood. The production of IL-1 receptor antagonist is increased in human endotoxemia,[169] and, in an animal model, its administration enhances survival.[170] However, infusion of IL-1 may improve immune function in humans.[171] Clearly our understanding of the complex functions of this cytokine are inadequate to allow intelligent intervention.

Tumor necrosis factor is produced by macrophages and other inflammatory cells when stimulated by endotoxin.[172] In animal models, the physiological effects of both endotoxin infusion and Gram-negative sepsis[173,174] are attenuated by TNF blockade with monoclonal antibodies. Circulating levels of TNF are high immediately after sepsis begins and then fall, implying that only anti-TNF pretreatment would be beneficial.[175] However, even anti-TNF administration prior to experimental sepsis[176] and endotoxemia[177] has variable effects, at best, on survival. Again, our incomplete understanding precludes effective intervention.

Interference with the effects of platelet activating factor (PAF) has been shown to decrease neutrophil priming by human burn serum,[178] to improve endotoxin-induced pulmonary dysfunction,[179] to decrease eicosanoid release,[180] and to attenuate thromboxane release and improve survival[181] in various animal models of endotoxemia. These exciting initial results, and the availability of several blockers and receptor antagonists, portend a future use for PAF modification.

Efforts to modulate both the adherence and function of inflammatory cells are an exciting area of research, as activated neutrophils clearly play an important role in the development of multiple organ failure. Blockade of neutrophil adhesion receptors with monoclonal antibodies enhances survival in animal models of endotoxic and hemorrhagic shock.[182,183] Again, our basic understanding is not yet adequate to intelligently modify such important processes.

Oxygen free radicals generated by activated neutrophils or xanthine oxidase may oxidize membrane lipids, forming lipid peroxides, resulting in membrane dysfunction.[184] Native antioxidant systems do exist, but can be overwhelmed. Circulating levels of vitamin E, a natural antioxidant, are low in patients with ARDS.[185] Efforts to modify oxidant activity have included blockade of free radical generation, addition of free radical scavengers, augmentation of host antioxidant defenses, and prevention of amplification of tissue damage by neutrophils.[184] Particularly exciting are free radical scavengers such as superoxide dismutase[186] and spin-trapping nitrones[187] which improve survival in animal models of endotoxic and hemorrhagic shock. But, despite such encouraging initial animal work, such therapy is not yet appropriate in human patients.

The continuous synthesis of nitric oxide (Figure 32.2) plays an important role in the regulation of pulmonary and systemic vascular tone in sepsis[188] and this presents potential opportunities for intervention.[189] Aerosolized nitric oxide has been shown to be useful in reversing the pulmonary hypertension associated with ARDS[190] and nitric oxide synthesis blockade may improve the hypotension and renal dysfunction associated with sepsis. However, its complex interactions with other cytokines and variable effects on different vascular beds render any nitric oxide-based interventions investigational at the present time.

Recently, recombinant activated protein C (rAPC) has been shown to have a favorable influence in patients with sepsis-induced multiple organ failure, after it demonstrated a 6% absolute reduction in mortality in a large multicenter trial.[191] Institutional criteria for administration of rAPC infusion vary, but generally include those patients with vasopressor-dependent septic shock and multiple organ failure of recent onset. Its major complication is bleeding, which has precluded its general use in septic shock in burn patients. However, it may ultimately have a role in septic shock associated with isolated inhalation injury.[192]

Most patients who die in the burn unit after surviving resuscitation succumb to multiple organ failure.[193] Although modification of the cascade of events leading to multiorgan failure at the cellular and subcellular level is an enticing possibility, our fragmented understanding of these processes mitigates against such therapy in human patients at the present time. That TNF enhances the ability of neutrophils to kill invading bacteria[194] and of rats to survive Gram-negative sepsis;[195] that cyclooxygenase inhibition increases TNF production after burn;[196] that PGE_2 is important in renal autoregulation;[197] and that cytokine levels vary significantly over the course of critical illness[198] makes one loath to interfere in such complex, and poorly understood processes. Vigilant clinical care in the intensive care unit, with the prevention of sepsis, proper management of burn wounds, support of the gut barrier, and careful attention to whole-body hemodynamics is a much more fruitful area in which a vigilant clinician can make a difference. On the near horizon is an exciting new understanding of the molecular mechanisms of critical illness that is likely to lead to effective targeted interventions.[199]

References

1. Fry DE, Pearlstein L, Fulton RL, et al. Multiple system organ failure. The role of uncontrolled infection. Arch Surg 1980; 115:136–140.
2. Biffi WL, Moore EE, Moore FA, et al. Interleukin-6 potentiates neutrophil priming with platelet-activating factor. Arch Surg 1994; 129(11):1131–1136.
3. Saadia R, Schein M, McFarlane C, et al. Gut barrier function and the surgeon. Br J Surg 1990; 77:487–492.
4. Echinard CE, Sajdel-Sulkowska E, et al. The beneficial effect of early excision on clinical response and thymic activity after burn injury. J Trauma 1982; 22:560–565.
5. Schumacker PT, Samsel RW. Oxygen delivery and uptake by peripheral tissues: physiology and pathophysiology. Crit Care Clin 1989; 5:255–269.
6. Knaus WA, Droper EA, Wagner DP, Zimmerman JE. Prognosis in acute organ-system failure. Ann Surg 1985; 202:685–693.
7. Duke G, Santamaria J, Shann E, et al. Outcome-based clinical indicators for intensive care medicine. Anaesth Intensive Care 2005; 33(3):303–310.
8. Goodwin CW. Multiple organ failure: clinical overview of the syndrome. J Trauma 1990; 30:S163–S165.
9. Huanag YS, Yang ZC, Liu XS, et al. Serial experimental and clinical studies on the pathogenesis of multiple organ dysfunction syndrome (MODS) in severe burns. Burns 1998; 24(8):706–716.
10. Meisel A, Jernigan JC, Younger SJ. Prosecutors and end-of-life decision making. Arch Intern Med 1999; 159(10):1089–1095.
11. Poulton B, Ridley S, Mackenzie-Ross R, et al. Variation in end-of-life decision making between critical care consultants. Anaesthesia 2005; 60(11):1101–1105.
12. Meakins JL. Etiology of multiple organ failure. J Trauma 1990; 30:S165–S168.
13. Bone RC, Fisher CJ Jr, Clemmer TP, et al. Sepsis syndrome: a valid clinical entity. Crit Care Med 1989; 17:389–393.
14. Suffredini AF, Fromm RE, Parker MM, et al. The cardiovascular response of normal humans to the administration of endotoxin. N Engl J Med 1989; 321:280–287.
15. Ahmed AJ, Kruse JA, Haupt MT, et al. Hemodynamic responses to Gram-positive versus Gram-negative sepsis in critically ill patients with and without circulatory shock. Crit Care Med 1991; 19:1520–1525.
16. Wakabayashi G, Gelfand JA, Jung WK, et al. Staphylococcus epidermidis induces complement activation, tumor necrosis factor

and interleukin-1, a shock-like state and tissue injury in rabbits without endotoxemia. Comparison to Escherichia coli. J Clin Invest 1991; 87:1925–1935.

17. Merrell SW, Saffle JR, Larson CM, et al. The declining incidence of fatal sepsis following thermal injury. J Trauma 1989; 29:1362–1366.

18. Peck MD, Heimbach DM. Does early excision of burn wounds change the pattern of mortality? J Burn Care Rehabil 1989; 10:7–10.

19. Lalonde C, Demling RH. The effect of complete burn wound excision and closure on postburn oxygen consumption. Surgery 1987; 102:862–868.

20. Demling RH, Lalonde C. Effect of partial burn excision and closure on postburn oxygen consumption. Surgery 1988; 104:846–852.

21. Rodriguez JL, Miller CG, Garner WL, et al. Correlation of the local and systemic cytokine response with clinical outcome following thermal injury. J Trauma 1993; 34:684–694.

22. Deitch EA. The role of intestinal barrier failure and bacterial translocation in the development of systemic infection and multiple organ failure. Arch Surg 1990; 125:403–404.

23. Schaedler RW, Goldstein F. Bacterial populations of the gut in health and disease; basic microbiologic aspects. In: Brochus HL, Beck JE, Haubrich WS, et al., eds. Gastroenterology. Philadelphia: WB Saunders; 1976:147–149.

24. Magnotti LJ, Deitch EA. Burns, bacterial translocation, gut barrier function, and failure. J Burn Care Rehabil 2005; 26(5):383–391.

25. Baker JW, Deitch EA, Li M, et al. Hemorrhagic shock induces bacterial translocation from the gut. J Trauma 1988; 28:896–906.

26. Deitch EA, Berg R, Specian R. Endotoxin promotes the translocation of bacterial from the gut. Arch Surg 1987; 122:185–190.

27. Deitch EA, Winterton J, Berg R. Thermal injury promotes bacterial translocation from the gastrointestinal tract in mice with impaired T-cell-mediated immunity. Arch Surg 1986; 121:97–101.

28. Jones WG, Minei JP, Barber AE, et al. Bacterial translocation and intestinal atrophy after thermal injury and burn wound sepsis. Ann Surg 1990; 211:399–405.

29. Ryan CM, Yarmush ML, Burke JF, et al. Increased gut permeability early after burns correlates with the extent of burn injury. Crit Care Med 1992; 20:1508–1512.

30. Deitch EA. Intestinal permeability is increased in burn patients shortly after injury. Surgery 1990; 107:411–506.

31. Chang JX, Chen S, Ma LP, et al. Functional and morphological changes of the gut barrier during the restitution process after hemorrhagic shock. World J Gastroenterol 2005; 11(35):5485–5491.

32. Gosain A, Gamelli RL. Role of the gastrointestinal tract in burn sepsis. J Burn Care Rehabil 2005; 26(1):85–91.

33. Schoenberg MH, Beger HG. Reperfusion injury after intestinal ischemia. Crit Care Med 1993; 21:1376–1386.

34. Bihari D, Smithies M, Gimson A, et al. The effects of vasodilation with prostacyclin on oxygen delivery and uptake in critically ill patients. N Engl J Med 1987; 317:397–403.

35. Poeze M, Solberg BC, Greve JW, et al. Monitoring global volume-related hemodynamic or regional variables after initial resuscitation: What is a better predictor of outcome in critically ill septic patients? Crit Care Med 2005; 33(11):2494–2500.

36. Mira JP, Fabre JE, Baigorri F, et al. Lack of oxygen supply dependency in patients with severe sepsis. A study of oxygen delivery increased by military antishock trouser and dobutamine. Chest 1994; 106(5):1524–1531.

37. Barone JE, Lowenfels AB. Maximization of oxygen delivery: a plea for moderation. J Trauma 1992; 33:651–653.

38. Hotchkiss RS, Karl IE. Reevaluation of the role of cellular hypoxia and bioenergetic failure in sepsis. JAMA 1992; 267:1503–1510.

39. Shoemaker WC, Kram HB, Appel PL, et al. The efficacy of central venous and pulmonary artery catheters and therapy based upon them in reducing mortality and morbidity. Arch Surg 1990; 125:1332–1337.

40. Kvarstein G, Mirtaheri P, Tonnessen TI. Detection of organ ischemia during hemorrhagic shock. Acta Anaesthesiol Scand 2003; 47(6):675–686.

41. Cerra FB. The systemic septic response: concepts of pathogenesis. J Trauma 1990; 30:S169–S174.

42. Dinarello CA. The proinflammatory cytokines interleukin-1 and tumor necrosis factor and treatment of the septic shock syndrome. J Infect Dis 1991; 163:1177–1784.

43. Fukushima R, Alexander JW, Gianotti L, et al. Bacterial translocation-related mortality may be associated with neutrophil-mediated organ damage. Shock 1995; 3(5):323–328.

44. Morrison DC, Kline LF. Activation of the classical and the properdin pathways of complement by bacterial lipopolysaccharides (LPS). J Immunol 1977; 118:362–368.

45. Gorbet MB, Sefton MV. Endotoxin: the uninvited guest. Biomaterials 2005; 26(34):6811–6817.

46. Chang SW, Fedderson CO, Henson PM, et al. Platelet-activating factor mediates hemodynamic changes and lung injury in endotoxin-treated rats. J Clin Invest 1987; 79:1498–1509.

47. Ramwell PW, Leovey EM, Sintetos AL. Regulation of arachidonic acid cascade. Biol Reprod 1977; 16:70–87.

48. Henderson WR Jr. Eicosanoids and lung inflammation. Am Rev Respir Dis 1987; 135:1176–1185.

49. Whittle BJ, Moncada S. Pharmacological interactions between prostacyclin and thromboxanes. Br Med Bull 1983; 39:232–238.

50. Ogletree ML. Overview of physiological and pathophysiological effects of thromboxane A_2. Fed Proc 1987; 46:133–138.

51. Fitzgerald GA, Reilly IA, Pedersen AK. The biochemical pharmacology of thromboxane synthase inhibition in man. Circulation 1985; 72:1194–1201.

52. Sprague RS, Stephenson AH, Dahms TE, et al. Proposed role for leukotrienes in the pathophysiology of multiple systems organ failure. Crit Care Clin 1989; 5:315–329.

53. Lewis RA, Austen KF. The biologically active leukotrienes. Biosynthesis, metabolism, receptors, functions, and pharmacology. J Clin Invest 1984; 73:889–897.

54. Leite MS, Pacheco P, Gomes RN, et al. Mechanisms of increased survival after lipopolysaccharide-induced endotoxic shock in mice consuming olive oil-enriched diet. Shock 2005; 23(2):173–178.

55. Pfister RR, Haddox JL, Sommers CL. Injection of chemoattractants into normal cornea: a model of inflammation after alkali injury. Invest Ophthalmol Vis Sci 1998; 39(9):1744–1750.

56. Hedqvist P, Dahlen SE, Bjork J. Pulmonary and vascular actions of leukotrienes. Adv Prostaglandin Thromboxane Leukot Res 1982; 9:187–200.

57. Davis JM, Meyer JD, Barie PS, et al. Elevated production of neutrophil leukotriene B_4 precedes pulmonary failure in critically ill surgical patients. Surg Gynecol Obstet 1990; 170:495–500.

58. Goetzl EJ, Pickett WC. The human PMN leukocyte chemotactic activity of complex hydroxy-eicosatetraenoic acids (HETEs). J Immunol 1980; 125:1789–1791.

59. Arai KI, Lee F, Miyajima A, et al. Cytokines: coordinators of immune and inflammatory responses. Annu Rev Biochem 1990; 59:783–836.

60. Carrol ED, Thomson AP, Jones AP, et al. A predominantly anti-inflammatory cytokine profile is associated with disease severity in meningococcal sepsis. Intensive Care Med 2005; 31(10):1415–1419.

61. Fassbender K, Pargger H, Muller W, et al. Interleukin-6 and acute-phase protein concentrations in surgical intensive care unit patients: diagnostic signs in nosocomial infection. Crit Care Med 1993; 21:1175–1180.

62. Okusawa S, Gelfand J, Ikejima T, et al. Interleukin-1 induces a shock-like state in rabbits. Synergism with tumor necrosis factor and the effect of cyclooxygenase inhibition. J Clin Invest 1988; 81:1162–1172.

63. Zhange B, Huang YH, Chen Y, et al. Plasma tumor necrosis factor-alpha, its soluble receptors and interleukin-1beta levels in critically burned patients. Burns 1998; 24(7):599–603.

64. Hollenberg SM, Cunnion RE, Parrillo JE. The effect of tumor necrosis factor on vascular smooth muscle. In vitro studies using rat aortic rings. Chest 1991; 100:1133–1137.

65. Takeyoshi I, Yoshinari D, Kobayashi M, et al. A dual inhibitor of TNF-alpha and IL-1 mitigates liver and kidney dysfunction and improves survival in rat endotoxemia. Hepatogastroenterology 2005; 52(65):1507–1510.

66. Lozano FS, Rodriguez JM, Garcia-Criado FJ, et al. Postoperative evolution of inflammatory response in a model of suprarenal aortic cross-clamping with and without hemorrhagic shock. Systemic and local reactions. World J Surg 2005; 29(10): 1248–1258.

67. Carrol ED, Thomson AP, Jones AP, et al. A predominantly anti-inflammatory cytokine profile is associated with disease severity in meningococcal sepsis. Intensive Care Med 2005; 31(10): 1415–1419.

68. van der Poll T, Buller HR, ten Cate H, et al. Activation of coagulation after administration of tumor necrosis factor to normal subjects. N Engl J Med 1990; 322:1622–1627.

69. Anderson BO, Bensard DD, Harken AH. The role of platelet activating factor and its antagonists in shock, sepsis and multiple organ failure. Surg Gynecol Obstet 1991; 172:415–424.

70. Rabinovici R, Esser KM, Lysko PG, et al. Priming by platelet-activating factor of endotoxin-induced lung injury and cardiovascular shock. Circ Res 1991; 69:12–25.

71. Qi M, Jones SB. Contribution of platelet activating factor to hemodynamic and sympathetic responses to bacterial endotoxin in conscious rats. Circ Shock 1990; 32:153–163.

72. Pawlik MT, Schreyer AG, Ittner KP, et al. Early treatment with pentoxifylline reduces lung injury induced by acid aspiration in rats. Chest 2005; 127(2):613–621.

73. Weiss SJ. Tissue destruction by neutrophils. N Engl J Med 1989; 320:365–376.

74. Horgan MJ, Ge M, Gu J, et al. Role of ICAM-1 in neutrophil-mediated lung vascular injury after occlusion and reperfusion. Am J Physiol 1991; 261:H1578–H1584.

75. White-Owen C, Alexander JW, Babcock GF. Reduced expression of neutrophil CD11b and CD16 after severe traumatic injury. J Surg Res 1992; 52:22–26.

76. Anderson DC, Springer TA. Leukocyte adhesion deficiency: an inherited defect in the Mac-1, LFA-1, and p150, 95 glycoproteins. Annu Rev Med 1987; 38:175–194.

77. Benton LD, Khan M, Greco RS. Integrins, adhesion molecules, and surgical research. Surg Gynecol Obstet 1993; 177:311–327.

78. Bautista AP, Shuler A, Spolarics Z, et al. Tumor necrosis factor-α stimulates superoxide anion generation by perfused rat liver and Kupffer cells. Am J Physiol 1991; 261:G891–G895.

79. Palmer RM, Ferrige AG, Moncada S. Nitric oxide release accounts for the biological activity of endothelium-derived relaxing factor. Nature 1987; 327:524–526.

80. Thatcher GR. An introduction to NO-related therapeutic agents. Curr Top Med Chem 2005; 5(7):597–601.

81. Bernard C, Szekely B, Philip I, et al. Activated macrophages depress the contractility of rabbit carotids via an L-arginine/nitric oxide-dependent effector mechanism. Connection with amplified cytokine release. J Clin Invest 1992; 89:851–860.

82. Nava E, Palmer RM, Moncada S. Inhibition of nitric oxide synthesis in septic shock: how much is beneficial? Lancet 1991; 338: 1555–1557.

83. Mathru M, Lang JD. Endothelial dysfunction in trauma patients: a preliminary communication. Shock 2005; 24(3):210–213.

84. Harkin DW, Marron CD, Rother RP, et al. C5 complement inhibition attenuates shock and acute lung injury in an experimental model of ruptured abdominal aortic aneurysm. Br J Surg 2005; 92(10):1227–1234.

85. Allen JN, Pacht ER, Gadek JE, et al. Acute eosinophilic pneumonia as a reversible cause of noninfectious respiratory failure. N Engl J Med 1989; 321:569–574.

86. Smedegard G, Cui LX, Hugli TE. Endotoxin-induced shock in the rat. A role for C5a. Am J Pathol 1989; 135:489–497.

87. Friedl HP, Till GO, Trentz O, et al. Roles of histamine, complement and xanthine oxidase in thermal injury of skin. Am J Pathol 1989; 135:203–217.

88. Livingston DH. Management of the surgical patients with multiple system organ failure. Am J Surg 1993; 165:8S–13S.

89. Tompkins RG, Burke JF, Schoenfeld DA, et al. Prompt eschar excision: a treatment system contributing to reduced burn mortality. A statistical evaluation of burn care at the Massachusetts General Hospital (1974–1984). Ann Surg 1986; 204:272–281.

90. Sheridan RL, Remensnyder JP, Schnitzer JJ, et al. Current expectations for survival in pediatric burns. Arch Pediatr Adolesc Med 2000; 154(3):245–249.

91. Herndon DN, Barrow RE, Rutan RL, et al. A comparison of conservative versus early excision. Therapies in severely burned patients. Ann Surg 1989; 209:547–552.

92. Sasaki TM, Welch GW, Herndon DN, et al. Burn wound manipulation-induced bacteremia. J Trauma 1979; 19:46–48.

93. Beard CH, Ribeiro CD, Jones DM. The bacteraemia associated with burns surgery. Br J Surg 1975; 62:638–641.

94. Piel P, Scarnati S, Goldfarb IW, et al. Antibiotic prophylaxis in patients undergoing burn wound excision. J Burn Care Rehabil 1985; 6:422–424.

95. Luterman A, Dacso CC, Curreri PW. Infections in burn patients. Am J Med 1986; 81(1A):45–52.

96. Apple J, Hunt JL, Wait M, et al. Delayed presentations of aortic valve endocarditis in patients with thermal injury. J Trauma 2002; 52(2):406–409.

97. Srivastava RF, MacMillan BG. Cardiac infection in acute burned patients. Burns 1979; 6:48–54.

98. Pruitt BA Jr, Stein JM, Foley FD, et al. Intravenous therapy in burn patients. Suppurative thrombophlebitis and other life threatening complications. Arch Surg 1970; 100:399–404.

99. Pruitt BA Jr, McManus WF, Kim SH, et al. Diagnosis and treatment of cannula-related intravenous sepsis in burn patients. Ann Surg 1980; 191:546–154.

100. Sheridan RL, Tompkins RG, McManus WF, Pruitt BA Jr. Intracompartmental sepsis in burn patients. J Trauma 1994; 36:301–305.

101. Shirani KZ, Pruitt BA, Jr, Mason AD Jr. The influence of inhalation injury and pneumonia on burn mortality. Ann Surg 1987; 205:82–87.

102. Silvestri L, van Saene HK, de la Cal MA, et al. Adult hospital and ventilator-associated pneumonia guidelines: eminence- rather than evidence-based. Am J Respir Crit Care Med. 2006; 173(1): 131–133

103. Deutschman CS, Wilton P, Sinow J, et al. Paranasal sinusitis associated with nasotracheal intubation: a frequently unrecognized and treatable source of sepsis. Crit Care Med 1986; 14: 111–114.

104. Fourrier F, Dubois D, Pronnier P, et al. PIRAD Study Group. Effect of gingival and dental plaque antiseptic decontamination on nosocomial infections acquired in the intensive care unit: a double-blind placebo-controlled multicenter study. Crit Care Med 2005; 33(8):1728–1735.

105. Slater H, Goldfarb IW. Acute septic cholecystitis in patients with burn injuries. J Burn Care Rehabil 1989; 10:445–447.

106. Vauthey JN, Lerut J, Martini M, et al. Indications and limitations of percutaneous cholecystostomy for acute cholecystitis. Surg Gynecol Obstet 1993; 176:49–54.

107. Chung DH, Herndon DN. Multiple converging mechanisms for postburn intestinal barrier dysfunction. Crit Care Med 2004; 32(8):1803–1804.

108. Herndon DN, Lal S. Is bacterial translocation a clinically relevant phenomenon in burns? Crit Care Med 2000; 28(5): 1682–1683.

109. Johnson LR, Copeland EM, Dudrick SJ, et al. Structural and hormonal alterations in the gastrointestinal tract of parenterally fed rats. Gastroenterology 1975; 68:1177–1183.

110. McDonald WS, Sharp CW, Deitch EA. Immediate enteral feeding in burn patients is safe and effective. Ann Surg 1991; 213:177–183.

111. Heyland DK, Dhaliwal R, Drover JW, et al. Canadian Critical Care Clinical Practice Guidelines Committee. Canadian clinical practice guidelines for nutrition support in mechanically ventilated, critically ill adult patients. JPEN J Parenter Enteral Nutr 2003; 27(5):355–373.

112. De-Souza DA, Greene LJ. Intestinal permeability and systemic infections in critically ill patients: effect of glutamine. Crit Care Med 2005; 33(5):1125–1135.

113. Sheridan RL, Prelack K, Yu YM, et al. Short-term enteral glutamine does not enhance protein accretion in burned children: a stable isotope study. Surgery 2004; 135(6):671–678.

114. Souba WW, Herskowitz K, Klimberg VS, et al. The effects of sepsis and endotoxemia on gut glutamine metabolism. Ann Surg 1990; 211:543–549.

115. Mittendorfer B, Gore DC, Herndon DN, et al. Accelerated glutamine synthesis in critically ill patients cannot maintain normal intramuscular free glutamine concentration. JPEN J Parenter Enteral Nutr 1999; 23(5):243–250.

116. Wischmeyer PE. Can glutamine turn off the motor that drives systemic inflammation? Crit Care Med 2005; 33(5):1175–1178.

117. Spaeth G, Gottwald T, Haas W, et al. Glutamine peptide does not improve gut barrier function and mucosal integrity in total parenteral nutrition. JPEN J Parenter Enteral Nutr 1993; 17:317–323.

118. Roediger WE. Utilization of nutrients by isolated epithelial cells of the rat colon. Gastroenterology 1982; 83:424–429.

119. Fedorak RN, Madsen KL. Probiotics and prebiotics in gastrointestinal disorders. Curr Opin Gastroenterol 2004; 20(2):146–155.

120. Gastinne H, Wolff M, Delatour F, et al. A controlled trial in intensive care units of selective decontamination of the digestive tract with nonabsorbable antibiotics. The French Study Group on Selective Decontamination of the Digestive Tract. N Engl J Med 1992; 326:594–599.

121. Wang X, Andersson R, Soltesz V, et al. Water-soluble ethylhydroxyethyl cellulose prevents bacterial translocation induced by major liver resection in the rat. Ann Surg 1993; 217:155–167.

122. Gupta R, Patel K, Calder PC, et al. A randomised clinical trial to assess the effect of total enteral and total parenteral nutritional support on metabolic, inflammatory and oxidative markers in patients with predicted severe acute pancreatitis (APACHE II > or = 6). Pancreatology 2003;3(5):406–413.

123. Gutierrez G. Cellular energy metabolism during hypoxia. Crit Care Med 1991; 19:619–626.

124. Dixon IM, Elyolfson DA, Ohalla NS. Sarcolemmal Na^+-Ca^{2+} exchange activity in hearts subjected to hypoxia reoxygenation. Am J Physiol 1987; 253:H1026–H1034.

125. Crimi E, Sica V, Williams-Ignarro S, et al. The role of oxidative stress in adult critical care. Free Radic Biol Med 2006; 40(3):398–406.

126. Das DK, Engelman RM, Rousou JA, et al. Role of membrane phospholipids in myocardial injury induced by ischemia and reperfusion. Am J Physiol 1986; 251:H71–H79.

127. Lopez-Neblina F, Toledo AH, Toledo-Pereyra LH. Molecular biology of apoptosis in ischemia and reperfusion. J Invest Surg 2005; 18(6):335–350.

128. Shoemaker WC, Appel PL, Kram HB. Role of oxygen debt in the development of organ failure sepsis, and death in high risk surgical patients. Chest 1992; 102:208–215.

129. Cain SM. Supply dependancy of oxygen uptake in ARDS: myth or reality? Am J Med Sci 1984; 288:119–124.

130. Dellinger RP, Carlet JM, Masur H, et al. Surviving Sepsis Campaign Management Guidelines Committee. Surviving sepsis campaign guidelines for management of severe sepsis and septic shock. Crit Care Med 2004; 32(3):858–873.

131. Mink RB, Pollack MM. Effect of blood transfusion on oxygen consumption in pediatric septic shock. Crit Care Med 1990; 18:1087–1091.

132. Clarke C, Edwards JD, Nightingale P, et al. Persistence of supply dependency of oxygen uptake at high levels of delivery in adult respiratory distress syndrome. Crit Care Med 1991; 19:497–502.

133. Ruokonen E, Takala J, Kori A, et al. Regional blood flow and oxygen transport in septic shock. Crit Care Med 1993; 21:1296–1303.

134. Schultz MJ, Gajic O. Transfusion and mechanical ventilation: two interrelated causes of acute lung injury? Crit Care Med 2005; 33(12):2857–2858.

135. Heyland D, Dhaliwal R. Immunonutrition in the critically ill: from old approaches to new paradigms. Intensive Care Med 2005; 31(4):501–503.

136. Barton RG, Wells CL, Carlson A, et al. Dietary omega-3 fatty acids decrease mortality and Kupffer cell prostaglandin E_2 production in a rat model of chronic sepsis. J Trauma 1991; 31:768–773.

137. Hasselmann M, Reimund JM. Lipids in the nutritional support of the critically ill patients. Curr Opin Crit Care 2004; 10(6):449–450.

138. Singer P, Cohen JD. From immune-enhancing diets back to nutritional-enhancing diets. Nutrition 2005; 21(2):282–283.

139. Sacks GS, Genton L, Kudsk KA. Controversy of immunonutrition for surgical critical-illness patients. Curr Opin Crit Care 2003; 9(4):300–305.

140. Kieft H, Roos AN, van Drunen JD, et al. Clinical outcome of immunonutrition in a heterogeneous intensive care population. Intensive Care Med 2005; 31(4):524–532.

141. Hurt RT, Matheson PJ, Mays MP, et al. Immune-enhancing diet and cytokine expression during chronic sepsis: an immune-enhancing diet containing L-arginine, fish oil, and RNA fragments promotes intestinal cytokine expression during chronic sepsis in rats. J Gastrointest Surg 2006; 10(1):46–53.

142. Shang HF, Hsu CS, Yeh CL, et al. Effects of arginine supplementation on splenocyte cytokine mRNA expression in rats with gut-derived sepsis. World J Gastroenterol 2005; 11(45):7091–7096.

143. Saito H, Trocki O, Wang SL, et al. Metabolic and immune effects of dietary arginine supplementation after burn. Arch Surg 1987; 122:784–789.

144. Yu YM, Wagner DA, Walesreswski JC, et al. A kinetic study of leucine metabolism in severely burned patients. Comparison between a conventional and a branched-chain amino acid-enriched nutritional therapy. Ann Surg 1988; 207:421–429.

145. Daly JM, Lieberman MD, Goldfine J, et al. Enteral nutrition with supplemental arginine, RNA, and omega$_3$-fatty acids in patients after operation: immunologic, metabolic, and clinical outcome. Surgery 1992; 112:56–67.

146. Gottschlich MM, Jenkins M, Warden GD, et al. Differential effects of three enteral dietary regimens on selected outcome variables in burn patients. JPEN J Parenter Enteral Nutr 1990; 14:225–236.

147. Meduri GU, Chrousos GP. Effectiveness of prolonged glucocorticoid treatment in acute respiratory distress syndrome: the right drug, the right way? Crit Care Med 2006; 34(1):236–238.

148. Jolles S, Sewell WA, Misbah SA. Clinical uses of intravenous immunoglobulin. Clin Exp Immunol 2005; 142(1):1–11.

149. Hackshaw KV, Parker GA, Roberts JW. Naloxone in septic shock. Crit Care Med 1990; 18:47–51.

150. Siraux V, De Backer D, Yalavatti G, et al.Relative adrenal insufficiency in patients with septic shock: comparison of low-dose and conventional corticotropin tests. Crit Care Med 2005; 33(11):2479–2486.

151. McCune S, Short BL, Miller MK, et al. Extracorporeal membrane oxygenation therapy in neonates with septic shock. J Pediatr Surg 1990; 25:479–482.

152. Munster AM, Xiao GX, Guo Y, et al. Control of endotoxemia in burn patients by use of polymyxin B. J Burn Care Rehabil 1989; 10:327–330.

153. Ziegler EJ, McCutchan JA, Fierer J, et al. Treatment of gram-negative bacteremia and shock with human antiserum to a mutant Escherichia coli. N Engl J Med 1982; 307:1225–1230.

154. Greenman RL, Schein RM, Martin MA, et al. A controlled clinical trial of E5 murine monoclonal IgM antibody to endotoxin in the treatment of gram-negative sepsis. JAMA 1991; 266:1097–102.

155. Wentzel RP. Anti-endotoxin monoclonal antibodies — a second look. N Engl J Med 1992; 326:1151–1153.

156. Zeigler EJ, Fisher CJ Jr, Sprung CL, et al. Treatment of gram-negative bacteremia and septic shock with HA-1A human monoclonal antibody against endotoxin. A randomized, double blind, placebo-controlled trial. N Engl J Med 1991; 324:429–436.

157. Panacek EA, Marshall JC, Albertson TE, et al. Monoclonal anti-TNF: a randomized controlled sepsis study investigation. Efficacy and safety of the monoclonal anti-tumor necrosis factor antibody F(ab')2 fragment afelimomab in patients with severe sepsis and elevated interleukin-6 levels. Crit Care Med 2004; 32(11):2173–2182.

158. Wise WC, Cook JA, Eller T, et al. Ibuprofen improves survival from endotoxic shock in the rat. J Pharmacol Exp Ther 1980; 215:160–164.

159. Rice TW, Bernard GR. Therapeutic intervention and targets for sepsis. Annu Rev Med 2005; 56:225–248.

160. Virdis A, Colucci R, Fornai M, et al. Cyclooxygenase-2 inhibition improves vascular endothelial dysfunction in a rat model of endo-

toxic shock: role of inducible nitric-oxide synthase and oxidative stress. J Pharmacol Exp Ther 2005; 312(3):945–953.

161. Temple GE, Cook JA, Wise WC, et al. Improvement in organ blood flow by inhibition of thromboxane synthetase during experimental endotoxic shock in the rat. J Cardiovasc Pharmacol 1986; 8:514–519.

162. Revhaug A, Michie HR, Manson JM, et al. Inhibition of cyclooxygenase attenuates the metabolic response to endotoxin in humans. Arch Surg 1988; 123:162–170.

163. Bernard GR, Reines HD, Halushka PV, et al. Prostacyclin and thromboxane A₂ formation is increased in human sepsis syndrome. Effects of cyclooxygenase inhibition. Am Rev Respir Dis 1991; 144:1095–1101.

164. Virdis A, Colucci R, Fornai M, et al. Cyclooxygenase-2 inhibition improves vascular endothelial dysfunction in a rat model of endotoxic shock: role of inducible nitric-oxide synthase and oxidative stress. J Pharmacol Exp Ther 2005; 312(3):945–953.

165. Demling RH, Smith M, Gunther R, et al. The effect of prostacyclin infusion on endotoxin-induced lung injury. Surgery 1981; 89:257–263.

166. Schutzer KM, Haglund U, Falk A. Cardiopulmonary dysfunction in a feline septic shock model: possible role of leukotrienes. Circ Shock 1989; 29(1):13–25.

167. Coggeshall JW, Christman BW, Lefferts PL, et al. Effect of inhibition of 5-lipooxygenase metabolism of arachidonic acid on response to endotoxemia in sheep. J Appl Physiol 1988; 65:1351–1359.

168. Patel JP, Beck LD, Briglia FA, et al. Beneficial effects of combined thromboxane and leukotriene receptor antagonism in hemorrhagic shock. Crit Care Med 1995; 23(2):231–237.

169. Granowitz EV, Santos AA, Poutsiaka DD, et al. Production of interleukin-1 receptor antagonist during experimental endotoxaemia. Lancet 1991; 338:1423–1424.

170. Ohlsson K, Bjork P, Bergenfeldt M, et al. Interleukin-1 receptor antagonist reduces mortality from endotoxin shock. Nature 1990; 348:550–552.

171. Watters JM, Bessey PQ, Dinarello CA, et al. The induction of interleukin-1 in humans and its metabolic effects. Surgery 1985; 98:298–305.

172. Beutler BA, Milsark IW, Cerami A. Cachectin/tumor necrosis factor: production, distribution, metabolic fate in vivo. J Immunol 1985; 135:3972–3977.

173. Tracey KJ, Fong Y, Hesse DG, et al. Anti-cachectin/TNF monoclonal antibodies prevent septic shock during lethal bacteremia. Nature 1987; 330:662–664.

174. Hinshaw LB, Tekamp-Olson P, Chang AC, et al. Survival of primates in LD₁₀₀ septic shock following therapy with antibody to tumor necrosis factor. Circ Shock 1990; 30:279–292.

175. Marks JD, Marks CB, Luce JM, et al. Plasma tumor necrosis factor in patients with septic shock. Mortality rate, incidence of adult respiratory distress syndrome, and effects of methylprednisolone administration. Am Rev Respir Dis 1990; 141:94–97.

176. Gallagher J, Fisher C, Sherman B, et al. A multicenter, open-label, prospective, randomized, dose-ranging pharmacokinetic study of the anti-TNF-alpha antibody afelimomab in patients with sepsis syndrome. Intensive Care Med 2001; 27(7):1169–1178.

177. Eskandari MK, Bolgos G, Miller C, et al. Anti-tumor necrosis factor antibody therapy fails to prevent lethality after cecal ligation and puncture or endotoxemia. J Immunol 1992; 148:2724–2730.

178. Pitman JM 3rd, Thurman GW, Anderson BO, et al. WEB2170, a specific platelet-activating factor antagonist, attenuates neutrophil priming by human serum after clinical burn injury: the 1991 Moyer Award. J Burn Care Rehabil 1991; 12:411–509.

179. Chang S-W, Fernyak S, Voelkel NF. Beneficial effect of a platelet-activating factor antagonist, WEB 2086, on endotoxin-induced lung injury. Am J Physiol 1990; 258:H153–H158.

180. Fletcher JR, DiSimone AG, Earnest MA. Platelet activating factor receptor antagonist improves survival and attenuates eicosanoid release in severe endotoxemia. Ann Surg 1990; 211:312–316.

181. Iwase M, Yokota M, Kitaichi K, et al. Cardiac functional and structural alterations induced by endotoxin in rats: importance of platelet-activating factor. Crit Care Med 2001; 29(3):609–617.

182. Eichacker PQ, Farese A, Hoffman WD, et al. Leukocyte CD1 1b/18 antigen-directed monoclonal antibody improves early survival and decreases hypoxemia in dogs challenged with tumor necrosis factor. Am Rev Respir Dis 1992; 145:1023–1029.

183. Van Amersfoort ES, Van Berkel TJ, Kuiper J. Receptors, mediators, and mechanisms involved in bacterial sepsis and septic shock. Clin Microbiol Rev 2003; 16(3):379–414.

184. Levy RJ, Stern WB, Minger KI, et al. Evaluation of tissue saturation as a noninvasive measure of mixed venous saturation in children. Pediatr Crit Care Med 2005; 6(6):671–675.

185. Richard C, Lemonnier F, Thibault M, et al. Vitamin E deficiency and lipoperoxidation during adult respiratory distress syndrome. Crit Care Med 1990; 18:4–9.

186. Bayir H. Reactive oxygen species. Crit Care Med 2005; 33(12 Suppl):S498–S501.

187. Novelli GP. Oxygen radicals in experimental shock: effects of spin-trapping nitrones in ameliorating shock pathophysiology. Crit Care Med 1992; 20:499–507.

188. Hauser B, Bracht H, Matejovic M, et al. Nitric oxide synthase inhibition in sepsis? Lessons learned from large-animal studies. Anesth Analg 2005; 101(2):488–498.

189. Cobb JP, Cunnian RE, Donner RL. Nitric oxide as a target for therapy in septic shock. Crit Care Med 1993; 21:1261–1263.

190. Pepke-Zaba J, Higenbottam TW, Dinh-Xuan AT, et al. Inhaled nitric oxide as a cause of selective pulmonary vasodilatation in pulmonary hypertension. Lancet 1991; 338:1173–1174.

191. Dellinger RP, Carlet JM, Masur H, et al. Surviving Sepsis Campaign guidelines for management of severe sepsis and septic shock. Crit Care Med 2004; 32:858–873.

192. Wong SS, Sun NN, Hyde JD, et al. Drotrecogin alfa (activated) prevents smoke-induced increases in pulmonary microvascular permeability and proinflammatory cytokine IL-1beta in rats. Lung 2004; 182(6):319–330.

193. Saffle JR, Sullivan JJ, Tuohig GM, et al. Multiple organ failure in patients with thermal injury. Crit Care Med 1993; 21:1673–1683.

194. Honma K, Udono H, Kohno T, et al. Interferon regulatory factor 4 negatively regulates the production of proinflammatory cytokines by macrophages in response to LPS. Proc Natl Acad Sci USA 2005; 102(44):16001–16006.

195. Alexander HR, Sheppard BC, Jensen JC, et al. Treatment with recombinant human tumor necrosis factor-alpha protects rats against the lethality, hypotension, and hypothermia of gram-negative sepsis. J Clin Invest 1991; 88:34–39.

196. Dong YL, Herndon DN, Yan TZ, et al. Blockade of prostaglandin products augments macrophage and neutrophil tumor necrosis factor synthesis in burn injury. J Surg Res 1993; 54:480–485.

197. Md S, Moochhala SM, Siew Yang KL, et al. The role of selective nitric oxide synthase inhibitor on nitric oxide and PGE₂ levels in refractory hemorrhagic-shocked rats. J Surg Res 2005; 123(2):206–214.

198. Cabioglu N, Bilgic S, Deniz G, et al. Decreased cytokine expression in peripheral blood leukocytes of patients with severe sepsis. Arch Surg 2002; 137(9):1037–1043.

199. Cobb JP, Mindrinos MN, Miller-Graziano C, et al. Inflammation and host response to injury large-scale collaborative research program. Application of genome-wide expression analysis to human health and disease. Proc Natl Acad Sci 2005; 102(13):4801–4806.

Chapter 33

Renal failure in association with thermal injuries

Shawn P. Fagan

Chapter contents

Introduction

Acute renal dysfunction is a major complication affecting the thermally injured individual and is commonly associated with a high mortality rate. Currently, the incidence of acute renal failure in burn patients varies between 0.5 and 30% with a reported mortality rate between 73 and 100%.[1–4] Prior to 1965, there were no reported survivors from acute renal failure following burns.[5] While advances have been made in the understanding of the etiology of acute renal failure in association with thermal injury, little has been accomplished with the actual treatment. The application of dialysis as a treatment modality has not significantly changed the mortality rate of individuals suffering from acute renal failure.[6] Therefore, the best treatment for acute renal dysfunction is prevention by understanding the pathophysiology of renal dysfunction in the thermally injured individual. This chapter will review the definition, the etiology, the pathophysiology, the diagnosis, and the treatment of acute renal failure in association with thermal injury (Figure 33.1).

Definition

Historically, acute renal failure has been defined as an abrupt and sustained decrease in renal function. Unfortunately, there is no consensus regarding an absolute definition for acute renal failure. This is exemplified by more than 30 different definitions having been used in the literature creating much confusion and making comparisons between studies impossible.[7] Although the definitions are numerous, the common theme of all definitions in the literature is an abrupt decline in glomerular filtration rate with the inability of the kidneys to appropriately regulate fluid, electrolytes, and acid–base homeostasis. In an effort to standardize the definition of renal dysfunction, the International Acute Dialysis Quality Initiative group has developed the RIFLE criteria (Table 33.1). The RIFLE criteria

is a classification system that utilizes the glomerular filtration rate (GFR) and urine output to define increasing levels of renal dysfunction. Patients are classified into one of five categories:

1. *r*enal dysfunction,
2. *i*njury to kidney,
3. *f*ailure of kidney,
4. *l*oss of kidney function, and
5. *e*nd-stage kidney disease

RIFLE is based on the worst value between glomerular filtration rate (GFR) or urine output and the need for sustained renal replacement therapy. The classification system has been clinically validated, with increasing severity grades of acute renal failure corresponded with increasing mortality.[8] This new classification system should aid in future experimental designs and allow for relative comparisons between studies investigating acute renal failure associated with thermal injuries.

Etiology of acute renal failure

Burn-related renal insufficiency is most commonly observed during the period of initial resuscitation after burn injury or as a component of the multi-organ dysfunction associated with severe sepsis.

The major etiological factors associated with the development of early acute renal dysfunction in the burn individual are hypovolemia or an ineffective perfusion gradient between the glomerulus and Bowman's space. The principal driving force for glomerular pressure/filtration is effective renal blood flow that is controlled by the relative resistance between the afferent and efferent renal arterioles. During early burn resuscitation, decreased glomerular filtration rate can be due to:

- hypovolemia,
- depressed myocardium (cardiac output),
- extrinsic compression via abdominal compartment syndrome, or
- denatured proteins.

Hypovolemia

The most common cause of early renal dysfunction in the thermally injured patient is hypovolemia secondary to extravascular fluid loss from the burn injury. Burns affecting more than 20% total body surface area are of sufficient size to induce decreased renal blood flow from extravascular fluid loss.[9,10] This concept is supported by the observations of Kim et al. that burn size is an independent predictor of acute renal failure in the burn population.[11] The depressed renal blood flow results in ischemia and cell death. The ischemic insult is known to produce oxygen free radicals that cause direct tubular cellular damage, disruption of tight junctions between cells resulting in obstructing casts which further reduces the effective glomerular filtration rate. Thus, the time the kidneys are ischemic is critically important to the development of acute renal insufficiency. Nguyen et al. found initial management of the burn individual to be critically important to overall survival. Fluid replacement therapy was demonstrated to have a protective affect against acute renal failure.[12] Similarly, the Shriners Burn Institute for Children, Galveston observed that time to initiation of resuscitative fluids was directly related to the incidence of renal dysfunction and overall mortality.[13] They concluded that early aggressive fluid resuscitation lessens kidney damage, thus preventing renal dysfunction and hence improving overall outcome.

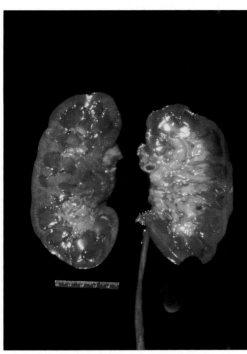

Fig. 33.1 Autopsy specimen from a patient with acute tubular necrosis and renal failure. Note the edema and the alteration of medullar pyramids. Acute renal failure in burn patients carries a high mortality.

Cardiac dysfunction

Cardiac dysfunction is known to result in reduced renal blood flow and thus induces renal insufficiency. While diminished cardiac output following thermal injury has been attributed to decreased preload or hypovolemia, there is increasing evidence of direct myocardial suppression. Myocardial dysfunction after thermal injury is commonly overlooked by physicians due to the concentrated effort to correct the overwhelming state of hypovolemic shock and electrolyte abnormalities.[14] However, an effective burn surgeon must re-establish adequate renal blood flow early by correcting the diminished preload state but be aware of the impact of the burn injury on the entire cardiovascular system. Patients suffering burns larger than 50% total body surface area are subject to decreased cardiac output, increased myocardial workload, myocardial ischemia, and acute cardiac infection from the large area of wounded skin.[15–19] Several authors have suggested theories to explain the decreased cardiac output associated with thermal injury:

- increased sympathetic activity with impaired adrenal response,
- hypovolemia resulting in myocardial ischemia, and
- direct myocardial suppression.[16–18,20–22]

Of the potential theories, direct myocardial suppression by tumor necrosis factor (i.e. myocardial depressant factor) has gained substantial interest. Tumor necrosis factor is known to be released by myocytes stimulated by endotoxin or direct thermal injury.[23–28] The effects of tumor necrosis factor on cardiac function include reversible biventricular dilatation, decreased ejection fraction, and decreased stimulation to catecholamines (Figure 33.2).[25,29–31] While most early cardiac dysfunction caused by tumor necrosis factor can be reversed by inotropic support, the key is early diagnosis to prevent ineffective renal perfusion and thus prevent the morbidity and mortality associated with renal insufficiency.

Extrinsic compression via abdominal compartment

Burns larger than 20% total body surface area generally require intravenous resuscitative efforts. During resuscitation of a thermally injured patient, the initial volume of fluids utilized should be proportional to the area of burn injury. Despite a physician's greatest effort to monitor endpoints of resuscitation, obligatory intercompartmental fluid shifts will occur during resuscitation.[32] These intercompartmental fluid shifts can be specifically hazardous if they occur into fascial bond

TABLE 33.1 THE RIFLE CRITERIA		
	GFR	Urine output
Risk of renal dysfunction	Serum creatinine ×1.5	<0.5 mL/kg/h × 6 h
Injury to the kidney	Serum creatinine ×2.0	<0.5 mL/kg/h × 12 h
Failure of kidney function	Serum creatinine ×3.0 or creatinine >4 mg/dL when there was an acute increase of >0.5 mg/dL	<0.5 mL/kg/h × 24 h or anuria × 12 h
Loss of kidney function	Persistent ARF ≥ 4 weeks	
End-stage kidney disease	Persistent ARR ≥ 3 months	

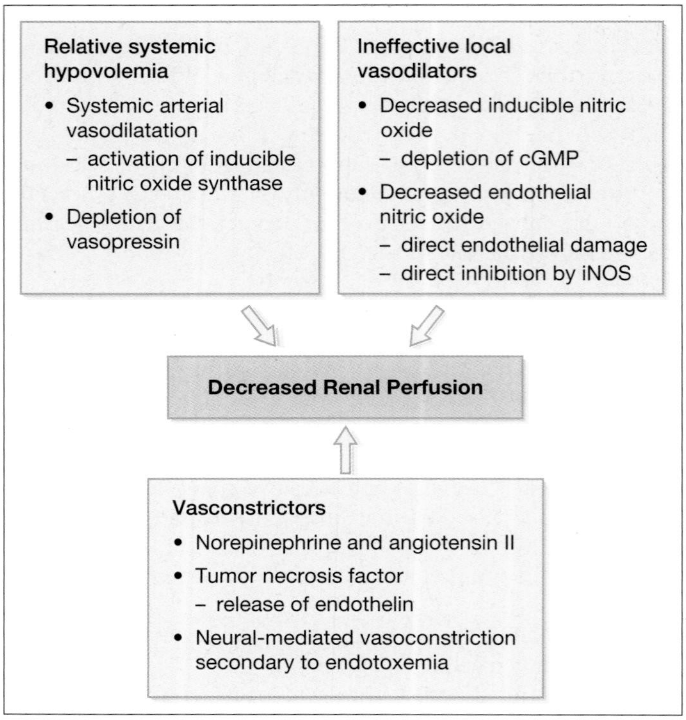

Fig. 33.2 Multifactorial etiology of sepsis-induced acute renal failure.

TABLE 33.2 RENAL FAILURE DYSFUNCTION AND SEPSIS			
	Sepsis	Severe sepsis*	Septic shock†
Acute renal dysfunction	19%	23%	51%

*Sepsis associated with lactic acidosis or altered mental status.
†Sepsis associated with hypotension.

compartments such as the peritoneal cavity. Numerous studies from the trauma literature have described the adverse physiological effects of increasing intra-abdominal pressure on visceral perfusion.[33–35] Abdominal compartment hypertension is a known pathological process that occurs during initial burn resuscitation as defined by intraperitoneal pressures greater than 25 mmHg.[32,36–38] However, the exact incidence of abdominal compartment syndrome, the point of decreased visceral perfusion, is currently unknown during burn shock resuscitation.[32] O'Mara et al. demonstrated that the volume and type of fluid resuscitation affects the development of abdominal compartment syndrome in the burn patient. It has been suggested that fluid resuscitation with crystalloid greater than 25 L/kg alerts the clinician to possible abdominal compartment hypertension and to monitor for decreased cardiac output, decreased lung compliance, or decreased renal perfusion — abdominal compartment syndrome.

Denatured proteins

Rhabdomyolysis and free hemoglobin have both been implicated in the development of acute renal failure.[39] Of the two, rhabdomyolysis has been implicated to cause renal insufficiency to a greater extent following thermal injury. Rhabdomyolysis can arise secondary to direct thermal affect, compartment syndrome, or following electrical injury. The release of myoglobin or unconjugated hemoglobin into the systemic circulation results in blockage of renal tubules, constriction of afferent arterioles, and the generation of oxygen free radicals.[40] The generation of oxygen free radicals directly injures the renal tubular cells, contributing to the renal insufficiency. The extent of renal injury is directly related to the amount of iron-containing molecules released and the state of hydration and degree of acidosis.[41] Fortunately, the incidence of denatured proteins causing burn-associated acute renal insufficiency is low and the overall prognosis is favorable if the pathological source is identified early and appropriate treatment is initiated.[42]

Sepsis

There have been significant advances made in the treatment of burn injuries since 1965. Early aggressive resuscitation and excision have significantly influenced the course of acute renal failure immediately associated with thermal injury.[43,44] However, acute renal dysfunction associated with the septic syndrome continues to cause significant mortality.[45]

Sepsis and septic shock are the most common causes of death in the intensive care unit (ICU) and are responsible for approximately 35–50% of the cases of acute renal dysfunction within the ICU. Several authors have found the degree of sepsis to be directly related to the incidence of acute renal dysfunction[46,47](Table 33.2). The key to treatment is a basic understanding of the pathophysiology of acute renal failure associated with sepsis. The basis of the physiological changes associated with sepsis-induced acute renal dysfunction is multifactorial in nature but begins clinically with a generalized arterial vasodilatation secondary to a decreased systemic vascular resistance (Figure 33.2). Initially, bacteria or their products activate sepsis-associated mediators (cytokines) locally at the site of direct invasion. In sepsis, the homeostatic balance between production and inactivation of these mediators is altered, allowing for release of these mediators systemically. The systemic effect of this imbalance is a procoagulant state with direct damage to the endothelium and vasoparalysis. It has been theorized that acute renal insufficiency associated with sepsis is the result of each of these pathological processes. The vasoparalysis seen in sepsis results in a relative or profound state of hypotension that activates the neurohumoral axis. The sympathetic nervous system and renin–angiotensin–aldosterone axis responds to the hypotension by increasing the cardiac output to maintain the systemic arterial circulation. However, this systemic response may actually worsen renal perfusion and therefore function by inducing a prerenal state by direct renal arteriole vasoconstriction.[45] This pathological process is aided by other direct vasoconstrictors (tumor necrosis factor — endothelin) known to be released during sepsis, and the inabilities of locally secreted vasodilators (endothelial and inducible nitric oxide) to counterbalance these sepsis-associated vasoconstrictors.[45,48] Finally, as mentioned previously, sepsis induces a procoagulant state by affecting the expression of complement and the fibrinolytic cascade.[49–51] This alteration in the homeostasis of coagulation may result in a state of disseminated intravascular coagulation with direct injury to the kidney by glomeruli microthrombi.[52] The net result is a lack of perfusion to the kidneys during sepsis that will ultimately culminate in acute tubular necrosis secondary to ischemia.

Diagnosis of acute renal insufficiency

The key to the diagnosis of acute renal injury following thermal injury is to have a strong fund of knowledge in the pathophysiology affecting the burned patient throughout their treatment course. Significant renal injury may be present despite normal urine output or significant changes in the biochemical markers of renal injury; therefore, a physician must constantly review the global physiological state of a thermally injured patient and anticipate conditions that may affect the renal system so that a stepwise approach to the diagnosis and treatment may be initiated.

Of the physiological parameters of renal function, altered urine output is probably the first and most recognized sign of renal dysfunction. Urine output has been demonstrated to be a very specific but unfortunately not a very sensitive measure of renal function.[53] Most clinicians regard urinary output of little diagnostic value in the evaluation of renal dysfunction since severe renal injury may exist with any pattern of urinary output. The variability is due to the fact that urinary output is not determined by the GFR alone, but by the difference between the GFR and tubular reabsorption. The one clinical scenario in which urinary output may be diagnostic is the presence of anuria (<50 mL/day) or complete cessation of GFR.[54] The most common cause of anuria, excluding postrenal obstruction, is a severe prerenal condition. While it is true that other conditions (acute cortical necrosis, bilateral arterial occlusion and rapidly progressive acute glomerulonephritis) may cause anuria, their incidence is low and the diagnosis is usually readily apparent due to additional clinical signs.

Although urinary output is commonly non-diagnostic regarding the type of renal injury, both microscopic and biochemical analysis may aid in the diagnosis of acute renal injury and thus guide treatment options.[55] Microscopic examination of the urinary sediment is an easy and inexpensive initial evaluation of acute renal injury to determine the underlying renal pathology. The combination of normal urinary sediment and oliguric/anuric urinary output would suggest a prerenal condition, whereas the presence of epithelial casts and abundant tubular epilethial cells is pathognomonic for acute tubular necrosis. Similarly, the identification of pigmented casts on microscopic evaluation signifies the diagnosis of myoglobinuria most likely secondary to rhabdomyolysis. If, however, the microscopic evaluation is non-diagnostic, urinary electrolytes will allow for the evaluation of the renal response to the individual's physiological state.

The main goal in evaluating urinary electrolytes of a thermally injured individual is to differentiate between the prerenal and renal forms of acute renal failure. It has been well established that a prerenal state in the presence of a functional nephron is associated with an enhanced absorption of sodium or a low fractional excretion of sodium. The fractional excretion of sodium (FeNa) is defined as:

$$FeNa = \frac{(\text{urine sodium} \times \text{plasma creatinine})}{(\text{plasma sodium} \times \text{urinary creatinine})}$$

with a value <1% associated with a prerenal condition and a value >1% associated with a renal condition.[56] While this is the accepted rule, there are conditions that affect renal absorption of sodium and thus have been shown to affect the calculated value (Table 33.3). Additionally, chronic renal insufficiency has been demonstrated to be associated with altered sodium homeostasis and therefore the interpretation of the FeNa in the setting of renal insufficiency is difficult. In this situation, an alternative agent such as urea may be appropriate. Recently, fractional excretion of urea (<35) was suggested to be more specific and sensitive than sodium in distinguishing between prerenal and renal forms of acute renal failure.[57] The prerenal state does not just affect the homeostasis of sodium and urea; several additional indexes can be utilized to differentiate between the two forms of acute renal failure (Table 33.4).

Ideally, we would have a biochemical marker of acute renal injury that would:

- allow early detection of renal injury,
- identify the nephron segment affected,
- reflect improvement and worsening of renal function, and
- be easily and rapidly measured.[58]

Currently, no such 'ideal' biomedical filtration marker exists. However, creatinine has been utilized as the standard marker for determining the glomerular filtration rate. Serum creatinine is freely filtered across the glomerulus and neither absorbed nor metabolized by the kidney. However, the amount of creatinine excreted is approximately 10–20% greater than the amount filtered. Therefore, the calculated creatinine clear-

TABLE 33.3 FACTORS THAT AFFECT FRACTIONAL SECRETION OF SODIUM

Condition	Effect on fractional sodium excretion
Glycosuria	Increase
Diuretics	Increase
Mannitol	Increase
Dopamine	Increase
Myoglobinuria	Decrease
Radiocontrast media	Decrease

TABLE 33.4 DIFFERENTIAL DIAGNOSIS OF ACUTE RENAL FAILURE

Urinary index	Prerenal	Renal
U_{osm} (mOsmol/L)	>500	<350
U_{Na} (mEq/L)	<20	>40
Specific gravity	1.020	1.010
U_{creat}/P_{creat}	>40	<20
Fractional excretion of sodium	<1	>2
Fractional excretion of urea	<35	>50

ance by definition overestimates the true GRF during normal steady-state conditions.[59] Creatinine is thus not an 'ideal' marker but a 'reasonable' marker of GRF in a normal host.

The impact of illness appears to have a significant affect on utilizing creatinine as a marker of GFR due to the non-steady-state environment. Plasma creatinine is not only dependent on its urinary clearance but also on its production and volume of distribution within the body. Several studies have demonstrated the impact of illness on each of these parameters[53,60] (Table 33.5). In critically ill patients, serum creatinine appears to be an inaccurate absolute determinant of GFR. In fact, serum creatinine has been demonstrated to often lag behind the true degree of progressive renal dysfunction and renal recovery.[53] Therefore, in these conditions, serum creatinine should be viewed by the degree of change over time, which in turn should grossly reflect the degree of GFR change over time.

Moran and Myers demonstrated the importance of understanding the degree of creatinine change over time.[61] They investigated creatinine kinetics following ischemic postoperative acute renal failure. Based on their observations, they developed hypothetical profiles of acute renal failure and recovery focusing on changes in GFRs and their corresponding changes in serum creatinine. Their work suggested that the two variables are often not inversely related but may often dissociate during acute renal failure and recovery: i.e. a rising serum creatinine is not always indicative of worsening GFR and a decreasing serum creatinine is not always indicative of an improving GFR. What did appear to be prognostic in acute renal failure is the number of days the plasma creatinine continued to rise after the initial ischemic insult. Post-insult day 4 appeared to be significant in determining the state of recovery. An abrupt insult followed by immediate recovery caused the serum creatinine to peak around post-insult day 4. However, if serum creatinine continued to rise beyond post-insult day 4, this indicated that renal recovery had not begun and this was followed by a severe protracted course of acute renal insufficiency. While this study was not conducted in a burn population, the underlying pathophysiology (ischemic) is germane to the burn population, especially after initial resuscitation.

A clinician should understand the limitations of any marker used to calculate or follow GRF during renal injury. While not an 'ideal marker,' creatinine is the gold standard for this calculation. GFR calculations based on creatinine clearance should be made over short time intervals with the serum cre-

atinine value reflecting the mean of the values obtained at the beginning and end of the collection interval.

Treatment of acute renal failure

The key to the treatment of acute renal failure is prompt diagnosis coupled with a rapid reversal of the underlying pathophysiology while preventing iatrogenic injury. If the process is progressive despite initial therapeutic maneuvers, early continuous renal replacement is indicated. This section will focus on the prevention of early and late acute renal injury and the current theories behind renal replacement.

As stated previously, early acute renal failure is secondary to ineffective renal perfusion. Several authors have demonstrated that the timing of initiation of resuscitative fluids is directly related to the incidence of renal dysfunction.[12,13] Therefore, resuscitative efforts should be begun immediately to re-establish effective renal perfusion. Several resuscitative formulas have been established based on multivariate logistic regression analysis (Table 33.6). Which formula to utilize is unimportant, but the clinician should recognize that these formulas are estimates of volumes of fluids needed over a period of time. The true amount is directly dependent on the patient's own physiological status and degree of injury. A clinician should continuously monitor endpoints of resuscitation to guide fluid therapy and prevent over-resuscitation. If the true volume status (preload) or ability to assess effective renal perfusion is difficult, one should initiate monitoring of central pressures or global volume-related variables (extravascular lung water volume, intrathoracic blood volume). Currently, the best means to measure the degree of resuscitation is unknown; however, recent data suggest monitoring of regional perfusion variables as a more reliable means of correlating the degree of resuscitation than monitoring any single pressure- or volume-related variable.[62] While establishing an effective circulating volume is of prime importance, an astute clinician should also carefully assess myocardial contractility in every patient to exclude myocardial dysfunction as a contributing factor to ineffective renal perfusion. The universal goal is to reestablish effective renal perfusion through a well thought

TABLE 33.5 FACTORS AFFECTING SERUM CREATININE

Factors	Effect on serum creatinine
Liver insufficiency	Decreased production
Decreased muscle mass: deconditioning aging	Decreased production Decreased production
Trauma	Increased production
Fever	Increased production
Immobilization	Increased production

TABLE 33.6 BURN FORMULAS FOR ESTIMATING INITIAL RESUSCITATION

	Crystalloid	Colloid
Colloid: Evans	NS 1 mL/kg/%burn	1 mL/kg/%burn
Crystalloid: Parkland Modified Brooke	4 mL/kg/%burn 2 mL/kg/%burn	
Pediatric formulas: Cincinnati Shriners Institute for Burn Children	4 mL/kg/%burn + 1500 mL/m^2 TBSA	
Galveston Shriners Institute for Burn Children	5000 mL/m^2 BSA + 2000 mL/m^2 TBSA	

TBSA = total body surface area. BSA = burn surface area.

out resuscitation plan based on proven resuscitation formulas and modified by variables correlated with the degree of resuscitation.

The etiology of late renal dysfunction is directly related to the development of sepsis and is multifactorial in nature. Thus the most effective therapy is prevention or early recognition of the septic state (Box 33.1). Every thermally injured patient should be continuously monitored for early markers of sepsis (feeding intolerance, increasing insulin resistance, elevation of acute phase reactants) so that early therapy may be initiated. Once a clinically significant infectious organism is identified, early goal-directed therapy should be initiated. Rivers et al. demonstrated a significant reduction in mortality if early goal-directed therapy is applied to the septic patient.[63] This work has recently been acknowledged and summarized in the Surviving Sepsis Campaign published as a consortium agreement of several different governing bodies.[64] The principle is simple:

- establish early source control while providing effective antibiotic therapy and maximizing global perfusion and thus renal perfusion.

The strategy is effective and important since no renal protective pharmacological agent has been demonstrated to prevent or limit renal dysfunction. The importance of infectious surveillance to minimize the affects of a variety of known pathogens that infect the thermally injured patient cannot be overstated. The goal is to effectively treat local infections and prevent systemic dissemination to avoid the morbidity and mortality of septic shock.

Fortunately due to major advances in burn care resuscitation and the treatment of sepsis, renal failure requiring renal replacement therapy is a rare event.[65] The reported incidence is approximately 1%, but the overall mortality associated with acute renal failure requiring renal replacement therapy approaches 80%.[2,3] Burn patients with renal insufficiency are at particular risk for renal replacement therapy due to the large positive fluid balances associated with the initial resuscitation therapy, enhanced catabolism leading to elevated urea levels, and need for substantial nutritional support to maintain a positive nitrogen balance.[65] Previously, renal replacement therapy has been successfully performed utilizing peritoneal dialysis.[66] However, this form of therapy has been limited by its clearance rates and the need for catheter insertion through the abdominal wall, which is a common donor site or thermally injured area. Over the past two decades, continuous hemofiltration has become the standard renal replacement therapy for critically ill patients. The technique provides a smooth and continuous control of volume stasis without inducing hemodynamic instability. It is a proven therapy in the burn population; however, the incidence of bleeding complications is higher compared to traditional renal replacement therapies.[65]

An additional theoretical benefit of continuous hemofiltration is the removal of proinflammatory mediators, which may be associated with the development of multiple organ failure.[67] The experimental and clinical data suggest that the rate of hemofiltration and biological nature of the filters affect the overall results.[68] Currently, there is insufficient data to recommend continuous hemofiltration solely on the basis of removal of inflammatory mediators. Future randomized prospective studies will hopefully resolve this theoretical benefit.

Major advances in the treatment of the thermally injured individuals have been accomplished over the past four decades. Early aggressive resuscitation coupled with early excision has significantly reduced the early complications of burn injury including renal insufficiency. This is exemplified by the fact that prior to 1965 there were no reported survivors from acute renal failure following burn injury. While the incidence of acute renal insufficiency following burn injury has been reduced, the disorder is still clinically significant after prolonged delayed initial resuscitation and following the development of sepsis. Therefore, a physician must constantly review the global physiological state of a thermally injured patient and anticipate conditions that may affect the renal system so that a stepwise approach to the diagnosis and treatment may be initiated. Currently, there are no pharmacological agents that prevent or treat acute renal insufficiency. Therefore, the best treatment option is prevention. However, if renal insufficiency develops requiring renal replacement therapy, the therapy should be initiated early to prevent an edematous state and allow for early nutritional support. The future of acute renal injury lies in the development of 'early markers' of acute renal insufficiency to allow for early aggressive treatment of the disorder by maximizing renal perfusion while minimizing nephrotoxic agents.

BOX 33.1 Definition of SIRS/sepsis

Documentation of confirmed infectious source
Heart rate >90 beats per minute
Body temperature <36°C or >38°C
Hyperventilation: respiratory rate >20 breaths per minute or $PaCO_2$ less than 32 mmHg
White blood cell count <4000 cell/mm^3 or >12 000 cells/mm^3 or >10% immature neutrophils

---

References

1. Marshall VC. Acute renal failure in surgical patients. Br J Surg 1970; 58(1):17–21.
2. Cameron JS, Miller-Jones CM. Renal function and renal failure in badly burned patients. Br J Surg 1967; 54(2):132–141.
3. Davies DM, Pusey CD, Rainford DJ, et al. Acute renal failure in burns. Scand J Plast Reconstr Surg 1979; 13(1):189–192.
4. Schiavon M, Di Landro D, Baldo M, et al. A study of renal damage in seriously burned patients. Burns Incl Therm Inj 1988; 14(2)107–114.
5. Davies MP, Evans J, McGonigle RJ. The dialysis debate: acute renal failure in burns patients. Burns 1994; 20(1):71–73.
6. Star RA. Treatment of acute renal failure. Kidney Int 1998; 54(6):1817–1831.
7. Kellum JA, Levin N, Bouman C, et al. Developing a consensus classification system for acute renal failure. Curr Opin Crit Care 2002 8(6); 509–514.
8. Hoste E, Clermont G, Kersten A, et al. Clinical evaluation of the new Rifle criteria for acute renal failure. Crit Care 2004; 8(Suppl 1):160.

9. Holliday MA. Extravascular fluid and its proteins: dehydration, shock and recovery. Pediatr Nephrol 1999; 13(9):989–995.

10. Boswich JA Jr, Thompson JD, Kershner CJ. Critical care of the burned patient. Anesthesiology 1977; 47(2):164–170.

11. Kim GH, Oh KH, Yoon JW, et al. Impact of burn size and initial serum albumin level on acute renal failure occurring in major burn. Am J Nephrol 2003; 23(1):55–60.

12. Nguyen NL, Gun RT, Sparnon AL, et al. The importance of initial management: a case series of childhood burns in Vietnam. Burns 2002; 28(2):167–172.

13. Jeschke MG, Barrow RE, Wolf SE, et al. Mortality in burned children with acute renal failure. Arch Surg 1998; 133(7):752–756.

14. Mukherjee GD, Basu PG, Roy S, et al. Cardiomegaly following extensive burns. Ann Plast Surg 1987; 19(4):378–380.

15. Munster AM. Alterations of the host defense mechanism in burns. Surg Clin N Am 1970; 50(6):1217–1225.

16. Merriam TW Jr. Myocardial function following thermal injury. Circ Res 1962; 11:669–673.

17. Fozzard HA. Myocardial injury in burn shock. Ann Surg 1961; 154:113–119.

18. Baxter CR, Cook WA, Shires GT. Serum myocardial depressant factor of burn shock. Surg Form 1966; 17:1–2.

19. Fang RH, Chen JS, Lin JT, et al. A modified formula of GIK (glucose-insulin-potassium) therapy for treatment of extensive burn injury in dogs. J Trauma 1989; 29(3):344–349.

20. Leffler JN, Litvin Y, Barenholz Y, et al. Proteolysis in formation of a myocardial depressant factor during shock. Am J Physiol 1967; 213:492–498.

21. Lefer AM, Cowgill R, Marshall FF, et al. Characterization of a myocardial depressant factor present in hemorrhage shock. Am J Physiol 1967; 213(2):492–498.

22. Reilly JM, Cunnion RE, Burch-Whitman C, et al. A circulating myocardial depressant substance is associated with cardiac dysfunction and peripheral hypoperfusion (lactic acidemia) in patient with septic shock. Chest 1989; 95(5):1502–1503.

23. Giroir BP, Horton JW, White DJ, et al. Inhibition of tumor necrosis factor (TNF) prevents myocardial dysfunction during burn shock. Am J Physiol 1994; 267(1 pt 2):H118–H124.

24. Herbertson MJ, Werner HA, Goddard CM, et al. Anti-tumor necrosis factor-alpha prevents decreased ventricular contractility in endotoxemic pigs. Am J Resp Circ Care Med 1995; 152(2):480–488.

25. Bryant D, Becker L, Richardson J, et al. Cardiac failure in transgenic mice with myocardial expression of tumor necrosis factor-alpha. Circulation 1998; 97(14):1375–1381.

26. Odeh M. Tumor necrosis factor-alpha as a myocardial depressant substance. Int J Cardiol 1993; 42(3):231–238.

27. Kapadia S, Lee J, Torre-Amiore G, et al. Tumor necrosis factor-alpha gene and protein expression in adult feline myocardium after endotoxin administration. J Clin Invest 1995; 96(2):1042–1052.

28. Torre-Amiore G, Kapadia S, Lee J, et al. Tumor necrosis factor-alpha and tumor necrosis factor receptors in the failing human heart. Circulation 1996; 93(4):704–711.

29. Kumar A, Haery C, Parrillo JE. Myocardial dysfunction in septic shock. Crit Care Clin 2000; 16(2):251–287.

30. Hegewisch S, Weh HJ, Hossfeld DK. TNF-induced cardiomyopathy. Lancet 1990; 335(8684):294–295.

31. Habib FM, Springall DR, Davies GJ, et al. Tumor necrosis factor and inducible nitric oxide synthase in dilated cardiomyopathy. Lancet 1996; 347(9009):1151–1155.

32. Hobson KG, Young KM, Ciraulo A, et al. Release of abdominal compartment syndrome improves survival in patients with burn injury. J Trauma 2002; 53(6):1129–1134.

33. Richardson JD, Trinkle JK. Hemodynamic and respiratory alterations with increased intra-abdominal pressure. J Surg Res 1976; 20(5):401–404.

34. Kashtan J, Green JF, Parsons EQ, et al. Hemodynamic effect of increased abdominal pressure. J Surg Res 1981; 30(3):249–255

35. Harman PK, Kron IL, McLachlan HD, et al. Elevated intra-abdominal pressure and renal function. Ann Surg 1982; 196(5):594–597.

36. O'Mara MS, Slater H, Goldfarb IW, et al. A prospective, randomized study of intra-abdominal pressure with crystalloid and colloid resuscitation in burn patients. J Trauma 2005; 58(5):1011–1018.

37. Greenhalgh DG, Warden GD. The importance of intra-abdominal pressure measurements in burn children. J Trauma 1994; 36(5):685–690.

38. Ivy ME, Atweh NA, Palmer J, et al. Intra-abdominal hypertension and abdominal compartment syndrome. J Trauma 2000; 49(3):387–391.

39. Lazarus D, Hudson DA. Fatal rhabdomyolysis in a flame burn patient. Burns 1997; 23(5):446–450.

40. Sharp LS, Rozycki GS, Feliciano DV. Rhabdomyolysis and secondary renal failure in critically ill surgical patients. Am J Surg 2004; 188(6):801–806

41. Morris JA Jr, Mucha P Jr, Ross SE, et al. Acute posttraumatic renal failure: a multicenter perspective. J Trauma 1991; 31(12):1584–1590.

42. Rosen CL, Adler JN, Rabban JT, et al. Early predictors of myoglobinuria and acute renal failure following electrical injury. J Emerg Med 1999; 17(5):783–789.

43. Jeschke MG, Barrow RE, Wolf SE, et al. Mortality in burned children with acute renal failure. Arch Surg 1998; 133(7):752–756.

44. Chrysopoulo MT, Jeschke MG, Dziewulski P, et al. Acute renal dysfunction in severely burned adults. J Trauma 1999; 46(1):141–144.

45. Schrier RW, Wang W. Acute renal failure and sepsis. N Engl J Med 2004; 351(2):159–169.

46. Riedemann NC, Guo RF, Ward PA. The enigma of sepsis. J Clin Invest 2003; 112(4):460–467.

47. Rangel-Frausto MS, Pittet D, Costigan M, et al. The natural history of the systemic inflammatory response syndrome (SIRS): a prospective study. JAMA 1995; 273(2):117–123.

48. Hohlfeld T, Klemm P, Thiemermann C, et al. The contribution of tumor necrosis factor-alpha and endothelin-1 to the increase of coronary resistance in hearts from rats treated with endotoxin. Br J Pharmacol 1995; 116(8):3309–3315.

49. Riedemann NC, Guo RF, Neff TA, et al. Increased C5a receptor expression in sepsis. J Clin Invest 2002; 110(1):101–108.

50. Huber-Lang MS, Riedeman NC, Sarma JV, et al. Protection of innate immunity by C5aR antagonist in septic mice. FASEB J 2002; 16(12):1567–1574.

51. Czermak BJ, Sarma V, Pierson CI, et al. Protective effects of C5a blockade in sepsis. Nat Med 1999; 5(7):788–792.

52. Reinhart K, Bayer O, Brunkhorst R, et al. Markers of endothelial damage in organ dysfunction and sepsis. Crit Care Med 2002; 30(5 Suppl):S302–S312.

53. Lameire N, Hoste E. Reflections on the definition, classification, and diagnostic evaluation of acute renal failure. Curr Opin Crit Care 2004; 10(6):468–475.

54. Miller PD, Krebs RA, Neal BJ, et al. Polyuric prerenal failure. Arch Intern Med 1980; 140(7):907–909.

55. Anderson RJ, Barry DW. Clinical and laboratory diagnosis of acute renal failure. Best Pract Res Clin Anaesthesiol 2004; 18(1):1–20.

56. Steiner RW. Interpreting the fractional excretion of sodium. Am J Med 1984; 77(4):699–702.

57. Carvounis CP, Nisar S, Guro-Razuman S. Significance of the fractional excretion of urea in the differential diagnosis of acute renal failure. Kidney Int 2002; 62(6):2223–2229.

58. Han WK, Bonventre JV. Biological markers for the early detection of acute kidney injury. Curr Opin Crit Care 2004; 10(6):476–482.

59. Doolan PD, Alpen EL, Theil GB. A clinical appraisal of the plasma concentration and endogenous clearance of creatinine. Am J Med 1962; 32:65–72.

60. Clark WR, Mueller BA, Kraus MA, et al. Quantification of creatinine kinetic parameters in patients with acute renal failure. Kidney Int 1998; 54(2):554–560.

61. Moran SM, Myers BD. Course of acute renal failure studied by a model of creatinine kinetics. Kidney Int 1985; 27(6):928–937.

62. Poeze M, Solberg BC, Greve JW, et al. Monitoring global volume-related hemodynamic or regional variables after initial resuscitation: What is a better predictor of outcome in critically ill septic patients? Crit Care Med 2005; 33(11):2494–2500.

63. Rivers E, Nguyen B, Havstad S, et al. Early goal directed therapy in the treatment of severe sepsis and septic shock. N Engl J Med 2001; 345(19):1368–1377.

64. Dellinger RP, Carlet JM, Masur H, et al. Surviving Sepsis Campaign guidelines for management of severe sepsis and septic shock. Crit Care Med 2004; 32(3):858–873.

65. Leblanc M, Thibeault Y, Querin S. Continuous haemofiltration and haemodiafiltration for acute renal failure in severely burned patients. Burns 1997; 23(2):160–165.

66. Pomeranz A, Reichenberg Y, Schurr D, et al. Acute renal failure in a burn patient: the advantages of continuous peritoneal dialysis. Burns 1985; 11(5):367–370.

67. Vincent JL, Tielemans C. Continuous hemofiltration in severe sepsis: is it beneficial? J Crit Care 1995; 10(1):27–32.

68. Cheung AK. Membrane biocompatibility. In Nissenson AR, Fine RN, Gentile DE, eds. Clinical dialysis. East Norwalk, CT: Appleton and Lange; 1990:69–96.

Chapter 34

Critical care in the severely burned: organ support and management of complications

Steven E. Wolf

Chapter contents

Introduction

About 500 000 people are burned and seek medical care in the USA every year, most of whom have minor injuries and are treated in the outpatient setting. However, approximately 50 000 burns per year in the USA are moderate to severe and require hospitalization for treatment. Some of these will require critical care for at least part of their hospitalization, and some will require it for months. About 4000 die from complications related to the burn.[1] Burn deaths generally occur in a bimodal distribution, either immediately after the injury, or weeks later due to multiple organ failure, a pattern similar to all trauma-related deaths.

Morbidity and mortality from burns are decreasing in incidence. Recent reports revealed a 50% decline in burn-related deaths and hospital admissions in the USA over the last 20 years.[1] This rate of decline was similar for all burned patients seeking medical care. The declines were likely most affected by prevention efforts causing a decreased number of patients with potentially fatal burns, and improved critical care and wound management for those who sustain severe burns. In 1949, Bull and Fisher reported 50% mortality rates for children aged 0–14 years with burns of 49% of the total body surface area (TBSA), 46% TBSA for patients aged 15–44, 27% TBSA for those aged between 45 and 64, and 10% TBSA for those 65 and older.[2] These dismal statistics have improved, with the latest studies reporting a 50% mortality for 98% TBSA burns in children 14 years and under, and 75% TBSA

burns in other young age groups.[3] Therefore, a healthy young patient with almost any size burn should be expected to survive using modern wound treatment and critical care techniques.

Burned patients generally die from two causes: 'burn shock' resulting in early deaths, and multiple organ failure and sepsis, leading to late deaths. With the advent of vigorous fluid resuscitation protocols in the severely burned, irreversible burn shock has been replaced by sepsis and subsequent multiple organ failure as the leading cause of death associated with burns in those who do not die at the scene. Those who do not die precipitously with any risk for mortality will require what is termed *critical care*, a service performed in specialized units containing the equipment, supplies, and personnel required for intensive monitoring and life-sustaining organ support to encourage recovery.

Critical illness in burned patients has typically been equated to sepsis. In a pediatric burn population with massive burns over 80% TBSA, 17.5% of the children developed sepsis, defined as bacteremia with clinical signs of sepsis.[4] The mortality rate in the whole group was 33%, most of whom succumbed to multiple organ failure. Some of the patients who died were bacteremic and 'septic', but the majority were not. These findings highlight the observation that the development of severe critical illness and multiple organ failure is often associated with infectious sepsis, but it is by no means required to develop this syndrome. What is required is an inflammatory focus, which in severe burns is the massive skin injury that requires inflammation to heal.

It has been postulated that the progression of patients to multiple organ failure exists in a continuum with the systemic inflammatory response syndrome (SIRS).[5] Nearly all burn patients meet the criteria for SIRS as defined by the consensus conference of the American College of Chest Physicians and the Society of Critical Care Medicine.[6] It is therefore not surprising that severe critical illness and multiple organ failure are common in burned patients.

Patients who develop dysfunction of various organs, such as the cardiopulmonary system, renal system, and gastrointestinal system, can be supported to maintain homeostasis until the organs repair themselves or a chronic support system can be established. Critical care may be defined loosely as the process of high-frequency physiological monitoring coupled with short response times for pharmacological, ventilatory, and procedural interventions. This chapter will describe the organization of specialized burn intensive care units (BICUs), including requirements for personnel and equipment. The techniques used in BICUs will be described, and then organ-specific management will be addressed.

Burn intensive care unit organization

Physical plant

Optimally, a BICU should exist within a designated burn center in conjunction with a recognized trauma center, thus providing the capability to treat thermal and non-thermal injuries. This unit, however, need not be physically located in the same space as that designated for non-burned trauma patients. In fact, the requirements for the care of wounds in burned patients necessitates additional equipment such as shower tables and overhead warmers, and thus separate space dedicated to the severely burned is optimal. This space may be located in a separate hospital with established guidelines for transfer to the facility.[7]

The number of beds required in the unit may be calculated by the incidence of moderate to severe burns in the referral area, which in the USA is approximately 20 per 100 000 people per year. The Committee on Trauma of the American College of Surgeons recommends that 100 or more patients should be admitted to this facility yearly, with an average daily census of three or more patients to maintain sufficient experience and acceptable access to specialized care.[7]

Most moderate to severe burns requiring admission will require intensive monitoring for at least the day of admission during the resuscitative phase. Thereafter, approximately 20% will require prolonged cardiopulmonary monitoring for inhalation injury, burn shock, cardiopulmonary compromise, renal dysfunction, and the development of SIRS and multiple organ dysfunction syndrome (MODS). In these severely burned patients, the average length of stay in the BICU is approximately 1 day per % TBSA burned. Using an average of 25 days admission for a severely burned patient and 2 days for those not so severely injured, this will require approximately 130–150 BICU inpatient days per 100 000 population. An eight-bed BICU can then serve a population of 1 000 000 sufficiently. Space provided should be at least 3000 ft[2], including patient beds and support space for nursing/charting areas, office space, wound care areas, and storage.

Personnel

A BICU functions best using a team approach between surgeons/intensivists, nurses, laboratory support staff, respiratory therapists, occupational and physical therapists, mental health professionals, dietitians, and pharmacists (Box 34.1). The unit should have a designated medical director who is a burn surgeon, to coordinate and supervise personnel, quality management, and resource utilization. The burn surgeon will usually work with other qualified surgical staff to provide sufficient care for the patients. It is recommended that medical directors and each of their associates be well versed in critical care techniques, and care for at least 50 patients per year to maintain skills.[7] In teaching hospitals, two to three residents or other medical providers should be assigned to the eight-bed unit described above. A coverage schedule should be devised to provide 24-hour prompt coverage.

BOX 34.1 Assigned burn unit personnel

- Experienced burn surgeons (burn unit director and qualified surgeons)
- Dedicated nursing personnel
- Physical and occupational therapists
- Social workers
- Dietitians
- Pharmacists
- Respiratory therapists
- Psychiatrists and clinical psychologists
- Prosthetists

BOX 34.2 Consultants for the BICU

General surgery	Pediatrics
Plastic surgery	Psychiatry
Anesthesiology	Cardiology
Cardiothoracic surgery	Gastroenterology
Neurosurgery	Hematology
Obstetrics/gynecology	Pulmonology
Ophthalmology	Nephrology
Orthopedic surgery	Neurology
Otolaryngology	Pathology
Urology	Infectious disease
Radiology	

Nursing personnel should consist of a nurse manager with at least 2 years of intensive care and acute burn care experience, and 6 months of management responsibilities. The rest of the nursing staff in the BICU should have documented competencies specific to the care of burned patients, including critical care and wound care.[7] Owing to the high intensity of burn intensive care, at least two full-time equivalents are required per ICU bed to provide sufficient 24-hour care. Additional personnel are required for respiratory care, occupational and physical therapy, and other support. A dedicated respiratory therapist for the burn unit is optimal.

Owing to the nature of critical illness in burned patients, complications may arise that are best treated by specialists not generally in the field of burn care (Box 34.2). For these reasons, these specialists should be available for consultation should the need arise.

Equipment

The equipment that must be present or available in the BICU are those items which are common for all ICUs, and some which are specialized to the BICU (Box 34.3). Each BICU bed must be equipped with monitors to measure heart rate, continuous electrocardiography, noninvasive blood pressure, invasive arterial and venous blood pressures, and right heart cardiac output using either dye dilution or thermal dilution techniques. Continuous arterial blood oxygen saturation measurement is also required, while continuous mixed venous saturation monitoring is optional. Equipment to measure weight and body temperature should also be standard. Oxygen availability and at least two vacuum pumps must be present for each bed.

Ventilatory equipment too must be available for all beds. The availability of a number of types of ventilators is optimal, including conventional ventilators with the capability to deliver both volume-targeted and pressure-targeted breaths as well as high-frequency ventilators that are oscillatory and/or percussive in design. An emergency cardiac cart containing advanced cardiac life support (ACLS) medications and a battery-powered electrocardiograph/defibrillator must be present on the unit should the need arise. Infusion pumps to deliver continuous medications and intravenous/intra-arterial fluids must also be readily available. A laboratory providing blood gas analysis, hematology, and blood chemistry must be located on site. Microbiological support to complete frequent, routine bacterial cultures should also be present.

Specialty equipment to be available includes various sizes of fiberoptic bronchoscopes for the diagnosis and treatment of pulmonary disorders, including personnel versed in these techniques. Fiberoptic gastroscopes and colonoscopes for gastrointestinal complications are also necessary. For renal support, equipment to provide peritoneal dialysis and both intermittent and continuous hemodialysis and hemofiltration should be available. Portable radiographic equipment for standard chest/abdominal/extremity radiographs must be immediately available. Equipment for computed tomography, fluoroscopy, and angiography should be available in other parts of the hospital. Indirect calorimeters to measure metabolic rate are preferable. Overhead warmers and central heating with individualized ambient temperature controls must be available for each room.

Hemodynamic monitoring in the burn intensive care unit

Most burned patients follow an anticipated course of recovery, which is 'monitored' in the ICU by measuring physiological parameters. Experienced clinicians assess these physiological measures in a repeated and sequential fashion to discern when potential interventions may be initiated to improve outcomes. Oftentimes, no intervention will be required, as the patient is following the anticipated course. At other times, this is not the case and procedural or pharmacological intervention is necessary. Physiological monitoring is then used further to determine the adequacy of the interventions. The following is a survey of monitoring techniques used in the BICU.

Cardiovascular monitoring
Arterial lines

Hemodynamic monitoring is directed at assessing the results of resuscitation and maintaining organ and tissue perfusion. Currently used measures are only estimates of tissue perfusion, as the measurement of oxygen and nutrient transfer to cells cannot be made directly at the bedside. Instead, global physiological measures of central pressures serve as the principal guides.

Measurement of arterial blood pressure is the mainstay for the assessment of tissue perfusion. In critical illness, this measurement can be made using cuff sphyngomanometers; however, in practice this technique is not useful because the measurement is episodic, and placement of these cuffs on burned extremities is problematic. In addition, blood pressure can be increased in the extremity from the inflation and deflation of the cuff. Diastolic pressures can also be artificially elevated in the elderly and obese. Instead, continuous monitoring for hemodynamic instability through the use of intra-arterial catheters is generally preferable. Lines are typically placed in either the radial or femoral artery. The radial artery is the preferred site for most critically ill patients, because of safety with the dual arterial supply to the hand should a complication occur. However, it has been shown that radial artery catheters are inaccurate in the measurement of central blood pressure when vasopressors are used,[9] and are notoriously inaccurate in children because of greater vascular reactivity.[10] For these reasons, we recommend femoral arterial blood pressure measurement in burned patients.

In arterial catheters, systolic, diastolic, and mean arterial pressures should be displayed continuously on the monitor screen. Either systolic or mean arterial pressure can be used to determine adequacy of pressure, although a mean arterial pressure of greater than 70 mmHg is considered a more accurate description of normal tissue perfusion. The mean pressure is a more accurate description of central arterial pressure, because as the arterial pressure wave traverses proximally to distally, the systolic pressure gradually increases, while the diastolic pressure decreases. The mean pressure determined by integrating areas under the curve, however, remains constant. The adequacy of the waveform must also be determined, with a diminished waveform indicative of catheter dampening, requiring catheter replacement. Care must be taken to insure that the diminished waveform is not true hypotension, which can be determined using a manual or cycling sphygomanometer placed on the arm or leg. Exaggerated waveforms with elevated systolic pressure and additional peaks in the waveform (generally only two are found) may be a phenomenon referred to as 'catheter whipping', which is the result of excessive movement of the catheter within the artery. Typically, this problem is self-limited, but care must be taken not to interpret typically normal systolic blood pressure values with evidence of catheter whipping as normal, as the effect generally overestimates pressures. Again, use of mean arterial pressures as the principal guideline for the assessment of blood pressure is optimal as the effects of catheter whipping are then diminished.

Complications associated with arterial catheters include distal ischemia associated with vasospasm and thromboembolism, catheter infection, and arterial damage/pseudoaneurysm during insertion and removal. Although these complications are uncommon, the results can be devastating. Physical evidence of ischemia in the distal hand or foot should prompt removal of the catheter and elevation of the extremity. If improvement in ischemic symptoms is not seen in 1–2 hours, angiography should be considered. Should thromboembolism be found, the clot can be removed with operative embolectomy or clot lysis at the discretion of the treating physician. If during angiography, extensive arterial damage is found with ischemia, operative repair will be necessary.

Catheter infection as evidenced by purulence and surrounding erythema should instigate removal of the catheter, which will often suffice. With continued evidence of infection, antibiotics and incision and drainage of the site should be entertained. Great caution must be exercised if an incision is made over the catheter site to avoid arterial bleeding. If a pseudoaneurysm is encountered after arterial catheterization and removal without signs of distal ischemia, compression with a vascular ultrasound device until no further flow is seen in the pseudoaneurysm will often alleviate the problem without operative intervention.[11]

Pulmonary artery catheters

Pulmonary artery catheters placed percutaneously through a central vein (internal jugular, subclavian, or femoral vein) and 'floated' into the pulmonary artery through the right heart have been used extensively in hemodynamic monitoring in ICUs. By measuring the back pressure through the distal catheter tip 'wedged' into an end-pulmonary branch, an estimate of left atrial pressure can be made. In addition, dyes or isotonic solutions injected into a proximal port can be used to determine cardiac output from the right heart. These data are used to estimate preload delivery to the heart, cardiac contractility, and afterload against which the heart must pump, which then directs therapy at restoration of hemodynamics. These catheters are used in ICUs under conditions of unexplained shock, hypoxemia, renal failure, and monitoring of high-risk patients.

Pulmonary artery catheters, while used widely in critical care settings, have come under scrutiny from reports indicating no benefit with their use. A study of 5735 critically ill adults in medical and surgical ICUs showed an increase in mortality and use of resources when pulmonary artery catheters were used. Most of these patients had medical conditions. The authors of this report suggested that their results should prompt a critical evaluation of the use of pulmonary artery catheters under all conditions.[12] An accompanying editorial went so far as to suggest an FDA-mandated moratorium on pulmonary artery catheters until further data were forthcoming.[13] While this suggestion may be somewhat draconian, it should certainly cause the clinician to question whether using a pulmonary catheter would be of benefit in the particular situation.

Several reports exist in the literature regarding the use of pulmonary artery catheters in burned patients, most in regards to parameters of resuscitation immediately after the injury. The first report in 1978 on pulmonary artery catheterization in 39 patients concluded that pulmonary wedge pressure was a more reliable indicator of circulating volume than central venous pressures. These authors also noted a consistent depression in myocardial function in the early phase of injury.[14] Other authors have noted similar findings in terms of heart dysfunction using pulmonary artery catheters in children. They concluded that routine use of pulmonary artery catheters is useful in directing therapy during resuscitation, including modifying resuscitation volumes and the use of inotropes.[15] Another report indicated that use of values generated from the pulmonary artery catheter during resuscitation to hyperdynamic endpoints improved survival in severely burned patients.[16] Furthermore, they found that if patients were unable to reach the hyperdynamic parameters measured by the pulmonary artery catheter, they were more likely to die.[17] These studies used historical controls, and their conclusions must be held in this light. In spite of the above findings, pulmonary artery catheters are rarely used during resuscitation in most burn centers, and their use is primarily limited to patients with unresponsive hemodynamic problems.

As mentioned above, the values derived from the pulmonary artery catheter can be used to drive heart function to supranormal levels with intravascular volume and inotropic support under defined protocols to improve oxygen consumption and presumably improve outcomes.[18] While this approach received enthusiasm after the initial report, other studies have not found any benefit with the use of pulmonary artery catheters in the critically ill, and some have found them to be detrimental.[19] The only study in burns is mentioned above, which found improved survival using the technique.[17] Regardless, no well-designed prospective trial investigating whether pulmonary artery catheter-guided supraphysiological resuscitation parameters improve outcomes has been performed in burns, and this practice cannot be widely espoused.

Newly designed pulmonary artery catheters with sensors providing additional data have been used in critically ill patients other than burns. One of these catheters contains an oxygen saturation monitor on its tip, allowing the continuous measure of mixed venous oxygen saturation. The potential benefits of such a measure would be to give earlier notice of cardiogenic compromise, and allow for a more direct measure of whole-body resuscitation. Problems with calibration and position sensitivity, however, have limited its use. Another of these catheters has an implanted rapid response thermistor, and when combined with a electrocardiographic lead measuring P–R interval on a beat-to-beat basis, can give a reasonable estimate of right heart ejection fraction and thus heart function on a frequent basis.[20] Another variant of this is a catheter with an implanted heating filament and sensor that uses thermodilution to measure cardiac output every 30 seconds. The accuracy of both these catheters has been verified in clinical studies, but neither has been widely accepted for use.[21]

Base deficit

The base deficit is a value calculated using the Henderson–Hasselbalch equation based on the relationship between pH, pCO_2, and serum bicarbonate:

$$pH = 6.1 + \log (HCO_3^-)/(pCO_2)(0.03)$$

The base deficit is the stoichiometric equivalent of base required to return the pH to 7.40. Base deficit is routinely calculated on blood gas analysis, and provides a reasonable estimate of the degree of tissue anoxia and shock at the whole body level, particularly in hemorrhagic shock. A rising base deficit indicates increasing metabolic acidosis, and may stratify mortality in patients after major trauma.[22] The same can be said for the use of base deficit in burn resuscitation.[4,23] These studies showed a correlation of higher base deficit and increased mortality, and some have suggested this value is a better monitor of resuscitation than the time-honored monitors of urine output and arterial blood pressure.[24] Despite its utility as an indicator of shock, base deficit is a nonspecific indicator of metabolic acidosis, and may be elevated with alcohol, cocaine, and methamphetamine use. Interpretation may be difficult under these circumstances.

Transesophageal echocardiography

Transesophageal echocardiography has been used for a number of years as an intraoperative monitor in high-risk cardiovascular patients. It has not been used extensively in other critically ill patients because of the lack of available expertise and paucity of equipment. Since this device can be used as a diagnostic tool for the evaluation of hemodynamic function, it serves to reason that it could be used as a monitor in critically ill severely burned patients. A report documented the use of transesophageal Doppler measurements of cardiac output in a series of severely burned patients undergoing early escharotomy, and found that while it was able to detect changes in cardiac performance, its variation was dampened in comparison to measurements made with a pulmonary artery catheter.[25] Another report used it during resuscitation of a child with a 30% TBSA burn, which was successful.[26] Another more remote study used transesophageal echocardiography to measure cardiac function after burn, revealing the typical depression in left ventricular function documented using other means.[27] Others have found using the same technique that intravascular volume and cardiac contractility are significantly diminished the first day after burn in spite of high-volume resuscitation.[28] No study has been done to date investigating whether transesophageal echocardiography is of clear benefit in monitoring hemodynamics in burned subjects.

Arterial hemodilution and intrathoracic blood volume

Cardiac output can also be measured using a transpulmonary approach with a thermistor inserted into an arterial port that can measure thermodilution injected into a central venous line. One report showed reasonable agreement between this technique and standard pulmonary artery thermodilution measurements in severely burned patients.[29] The same group of authors showed that measurement of intrathoracic blood volume using a double indicator dilution technique as a measurement of adequate preload in severely burned patients might be a better indicator of adequate resuscitation compared to traditional techniques of urine output and blood pressure. Interestingly, they showed that the volumes given for resuscitation with this method were much higher than those predicted by the Parkland formula, but that no significant increases in extravascular lung water were seen.[30]

Mechanical ventilation

The use of mechanical ventilation is central to the function of the BICU. Burned patients are at risk for airway compromise, necessitating endotracheal intubation and mechanical ventilation for a number of reasons. Inhalation of smoke causing damage to the upper airway, development of massive whole-body edema restricting the airway, and hypoxia occur relatively frequently during the initial resuscitation, all of which may require endotracheal intubation and mechanical ventilation. Thereafter, acute lung injury and acute respiratory distress syndrome may intervene, necessitating pulmonary support with ventilators. This section will deal briefly with indications for intubation, common ventilator strategies, and monitoring of mechanical ventilation.

Indications for intubation

Intubation entails passing an endotracheal tube from either the nose or the mouth through the pharynx into the trachea. This tube is then connected to a mechanical ventilator to cause inspiration and passive exhalation through the lungs. Indications for intubation in burned patients are in general to improve oxygenation and ventilation, or to maintain gas exchange during clinical conditions expected to compromise the airway. These indications are as follows (see also Table 34.1):

- Respiratory distress indicated by:
  - tachypnea
  - hypoxia
- Impending need for airway maintenance:
  - initial management of smoke inhalation injury
  - expected massive whole-body edema after resuscitation for a major burn.

Ventilatory modes

The complexity of mechanical ventilators has increased dramatically since the first generation of volume cycle ventilators used in the 1960s. The development of positive end-expiratory pressure (PEEP) to maintain functional residual capacity was followed by development of modes using partial ventilatory support, such as intermittent mandatory ventilation in the 1970s. Efficient microprocessors were then developed that permitted modes of ventilation such as pressure support ventilation, time-cycled pressure control ventilation, and inverse

TABLE 34.1 CLINICAL INDICATIONS FOR INTUBATION

Criteria	Value
PaO$_2$ (mmHg)	<60
PaCO$_2$ (mmHg)	>50 (acutely)
P/F ratio	<200
Respiratory rate	<40
Respiratory/ventilatory failure	Impending
Upper airway edema	Severe

ratio ventilation. Most recently, new processors have been used to combine modes of ventilation, such as pressure support and time-cycled pressure control ventilation, and open lung strategies such as airway pressure-release ventilation to some success. However, even with these new developments, the function of mechanical ventilators remains identical to those first used. Whether these new ventilators have had any appreciable effect on mortality remains to be fully elucidated.

The principal difference in mechanical ventilation from spontaneous ventilation, that each of us does every minute of the day, is the effect of positive pressure as opposed to normal physiological negative pressure. The use of positive pressure improves gas exchange by recruiting alveoli and increasing functional residual capacity (i.e. the number and volume of open alveoli at the end of expiration), thus improving ventilation perfusion mismatching and decreasing intrapulmonary shunting of blood past nonventilated lung areas (Figure 34.1). Adverse effects of positive pressure ventilation lie in its propensity to produce trauma to the airways (barotrauma) and its effects on intrathoracic pressure which can impede venous return to the heart and decrease cardiac output.

Control and assist control ventilation

The volume control modes are volume-cycled settings that deliver a preset tidal volume at a minimum respiratory rate and inspiratory flow rate regardless of the patient's own respiratory efforts (Figure 34.2). Of the two, the control mode will not trigger with patient effort. This mode is typically very uncomfortable for patients due to ventilator–patient dyssynchrony, with use limited to patients under general anesthesia. The assist control mode differs in that a breath will be delivered regularly according to a prescribed rate, but it will also deliver a breath upon patient negative pressure effort to open a flow valve, at which time the ventilator will fire allowing the patient to control his or her own ventilatory rate with a preset minimum rate as a back-up. This mode is typically used in heavily sedated patients who cannot generate enough tidal volume under pressure support modes or intermittent mandatory ventilation mode, or in those patients that the clinician wishes to minimize the work of breathing. It must be noted, however, that the work of breathing can be increased dramatically in patients with excessive ventilator triggering. Increasing the minimum number of breaths to match the patient's effort can minimize this effect. When using this mode of ventilation, it is important to monitor lung compliance by measuring serial peak and plateau pressures for diagnostic purposes as well as minimization of barotrauma.

Time-cycled pressure control ventilation

Volume-cycled ventilation delivers a set volume of air regardless of pressure required. In the case of poor lung compliance, such as in acute respiratory distress syndrome (ARDS), the mode could lead to excessive ventilatory pressures leading to significant airway injury. For this reason, time-cycled pressure control ventilation was developed that delivers inspiration at a given flow rate to a preset pressure. The breath is terminated at a set cycle time, not on the basis of volume of flow as is the case with volume-controlled ventilation. Therefore, pressure control has the advantage of limiting inspiratory pressure despite changes in compliance. It also has the disad-

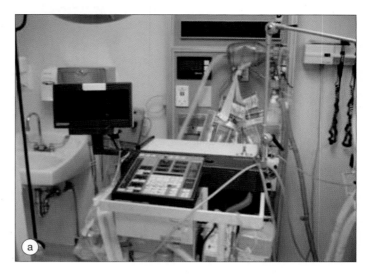

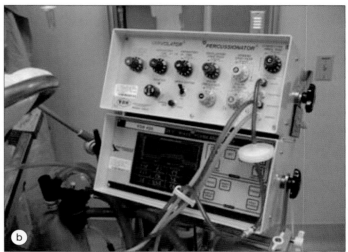

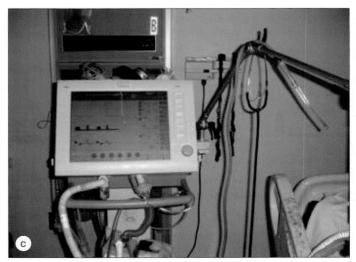

Fig. 34.1 Photos of different ventilators commonly used in burn units in the USA. (a) The most commonly used is the 'servo' type ventilator, which can be set to give volume- or pressure-regulated breaths with or without pressure support or PEEP. The I:E ratios can also be reversed. (b) The second type is the VDR ventilator, which delivers HFPV or CPAP. (c) The third type is the APRV ventilator, which can be set to all the servo settings as well as APRV.

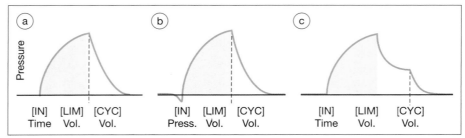

Fig. 34.2 Airway pressure curves illustrating the three mechanical functions: IN, initiation of the cycle; LIM, the preset limit (i.e. pressure or volume) imposed on the positive pressure cycle; CYC, the function (i.e. time or volume) ending the cycle. Each mechanical function is governed by one of four physical factors: volume, pressure, flow, and time. (a) A time-initiated, volume-limited mode. (b) A pressure-initiated (sub-baseline pressure produced by the patient's effort to breathe), volume-limited mode. (c) A time-initiated, volume-limited, time-cycled mode that extends inspiration beyond the time that the volume is delivered. A plateau is reached after flow has stopped but before the ventilator cycles into exhalation. (Reprinted with permission from Shapiro et al.[128])

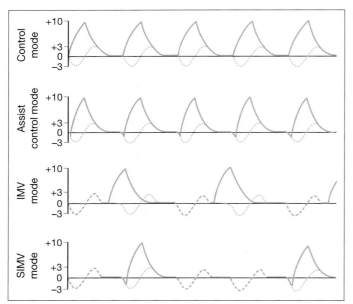

Fig. 34.3 Airway pressure tracings of four volume-cycled modes. The thick solid lines represent ventilator breaths. The thick dotted lines are spontaneous breaths. The thin dotted lines illustrate the spontaneous breathing pattern in the absence of ventilator breaths. IMV, intermittent mandatory ventilation; SIMV, synchronized intermittent mandatory ventilation. (Reprinted with permission from Shapiro et al.[128])

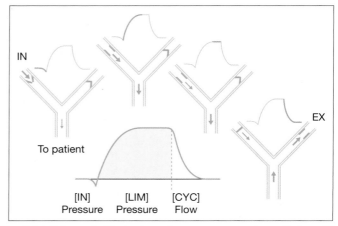

Fig. 34.4 Schematic illustration of pressure support ventilation. IN, initiation by spontaneous breath; LIM limit (pressure); CYC, cycle (derived from decreasing inspiratory flow); EX, expiration. (Reprinted with permission from Shapiro et al.[128])

vantage of a variable tidal volume during dynamic changes in lung compliance which can lead to inadequate excessive minute ventilation if compliance worsens or improves respectively. This puts the onus on the provider to monitor changes in compliance to make appropriate changes in the preset pressure to compensate. This differs from the volume-cycled mode that requires monitoring of peak and plateau pressures. Another disadvantage is that this mode is not as well tolerated by awake patients as other modes.

Intermittent mandatory ventilation

Intermittent mandatory ventilation (IMV) was developed to allow spontaneous ventilation interspersed with volume-cycled or time-cycled pressure control mechanical ventilation. It was developed initially as a method to wean patients from the ventilator by depending more and more on patient effort

for ventilation. The addition of a synchronized mode (SIMV) to avoid placing a mechanical breath on top of a spontaneous patient breath greatly improved this mode of ventilation. This mode has the advantage of maintaining some patient work in breathing to preserve respiratory strength when mechanical ventilation is required, and as a weaning tool to progressively increase patient effort while decreasing mechanical support in preparation for discontinuing mechanical ventilation. This method can be problematic in patients with low pulmonary compliance, and the IMV mode may not allow for sufficient spontaneous tidal volumes due to extremely limited inspiratory capacity. The addition of pressure support to augment spontaneous ventilatory efforts can be used (Figure 34.3).

Pressure support ventilation

Pressure support ventilation is a patient-triggered, pressure-limited, flow-cycled ventilatory mode (Figure 34.4). Each pressure support breath is triggered by patient negative pressure effort, at which time a valve opens producing a high-flow, pressure-limited breath. The breath ends when the patient's inspiratory demand falls below a preset limit, allowing spontaneous respiration and complete patient control. It also differs from the other modes in that it is flow-cycled as opposed to volume- or pressure-cycled. Because this mode is triggered and completed entirely from patient response, it cannot be used in patients with decreased respiratory drive, such as paralyzed patients and those who are heavily sedated. This mode has a number of advantages because of improved synchrony with patient effort. It can be used to provide full ventilatory support by setting a flow and pressure such that an adequate tidal volume is delivered. It can also be used effectively during weaning by decreasing the pressure incrementally to allow for progressively greater patient effort. Caution must be exercised when decreasing ventilatory support such that a sufficient tidal volume is still delivered to maintain adequate ventilation.

Inverse ratio ventilation

Inverse ratio ventilation is a mode of ventilation which is designed to improve oxygenation at a given level of inspired oxygen. Conventional ventilation uses the times of inspiration and expiration in a ratio of 1:4 or 1:2, giving a longer time for expiration, which is generally a passive process. Inverse ratio ventilation reverses this ratio to give a longer inspiratory time (1:1 or 2:1) by using rapid inspiratory flow rates and decelerating flow patterns during the inspiratory phase. The effect of inverse ratio ventilation is to increase mean airway pressures and thus recruit alveoli in an effect similar to PEEP. Secondly, in severe lung disease, ventilation in the lung is unequal due to peribronchial narrowing. Thus, some underventilated alveoli that are actually open are not able to exchange gases efficiently, increasing the intrapulmonary shunt and decreasing arterial oxygenation. Inverse ratio ventilation can improve this by selective air-trapping, or intrinsic PEEP, in these compromised air spaces. Inverse ratio ventilation can be done either in a volume-cycled or time-cycled pressure ventilation mode, but it is most commonly used with pressure-controlled ventilation to decrease peak airway pressures.

The beneficial effects of inverse ratio ventilation are questionable. It may be that the same effect can be gained by just increasing peak airway pressures with PEEP or peak inspiratory pressures. In fact, studies have showed no benefit of inverse ratio ventilation compared to conventional volume ventilation in terms of oxygenation.[31] These studies did show some slight improvements in ventilation ($PaCO_2$). Other studies have shown that functional residual capacity is indeed not improved with inverse ratio ventilation, and in fact is detrimental to cardiac function because of increased intrathoracic pressures.[32] For these reasons, inverse ratio ventilation cannot be recommended except in the setting of ARDS refractory to other therapies.

High-frequency oscillatory ventilation

High-frequency oscillatory ventilation (HFOV) is a new mode of ventilation which combines features of conventional ventilation with jet ventilation. It delivers subtidal, high-frequency oscillatory breaths at a constant mean-airway pressure (mPAW). It is thought to maintain open alveoli by recruiting collapsed portions of diseased lung by applying the equivalent of continuous positive airway pressure used during conventional ventilation. Optimizing mean airway pressure limits peak pressure, thereby making this a 'lung protective' mode. A recent randomized prospective trial in adult patients with ARDS demonstrated that HFOV resulted in brief improvement in oxygenation while mortality difference or complication rates were not different.[33] In burned patients, one center reported early success reversing profound hypoxemia in patients with ARDS while facilitating early excision and grafting with intraoperative use.[34] HFOV, where available, should be given consideration in burned patients with severe hypoxemia.

High-frequency percussive ventilation

High-frequency percussive ventilation (HFPV) is a pressure-limited, time-cycled mode of ventilation that delivers subtidal pressure-limited breaths at a high frequency (400–800 beats/min) superimposed on a conventional inspiratory and expiratory pressure-controlled cycle (10–30 breaths/min). The purported advantages are to loosen airway exudate and casts for better pulmonary toilet, and to provide adequate gas exchange at lower airway pressures. This method of ventilation has been tested primarily in burned patients with inhalation injury, and was first reported in 1989.[35] In this study, HFPV was used as a salvage therapy in patients with inhalation injury and as primary therapy in another group. Improvements in oxygenation and a lower rate of pneumonia were seen. Another study documented an improvement in mortality in burned patients with inhalation injury treated with high-frequency percussive ventilation compared to historical controls.[36] Other studies have shown significant decreases in the work of breathing, and lower inspiratory pressures in addition to improvements in oxygenation and the rate of pneumonia.[36,37] In fact, the use of this mode of ventilation in burned patients has been extended to non-burned patients in some ICUs with salvage of many patients.[38] This method of ventilation seems to be particularly efficacious in the treatment of inhalation injury.

Airway pressure-release ventilation

Airway pressure-release ventilation (APRV) is a mode which delivers continuous positive airway pressure with a time-cycled pressure-release phase (to allow for expiration). Advantages of APRV include optimization of mean airway pressure, limitation of peak inspiratory pressures, and integration of spontaneous breathing independent of the ventilatory cycle. These characteristics allow for an open lung with optimal alveolar recruitment and, as a result, improved ventilator-perfusion mismatching. This mode is best utilized in patients who are permitted to spontaneously breathe with negative pressure induced by diaphragmatic contraction that aids in lung recruitment of areas that were previously atelectatic. This is in contrast to conventional positive pressure ventilation where positive pressure from within the bronchus through the volume of air is preferentially distributed down the path of least resistance to areas of the lung that are already well aerated predisposing them to overdistention and barotrauma. Theoretically, this mode of ventilation is thought to be the ideal lung protective strategy. APRV gained popularity in the late 1990s, and is becoming the preferred mode of ventilation in many centers. Small prospective trials have suggested that APRV is associated with fewer ventilator days, improved gas exchange, improved hemodynamic performance, and less need for sedation when compared to conventional modes.[39] This mode is being increasingly used in burn units around the world, but to date no trials have been reported in this population.

Inhaled nitric oxide

Nitric oxide is a short-lived gaseous product of endothelial cells that is a powerful local vasodilator. Because it is a gas, this product can be delivered through the endotracheal tube to areas of ventilated lung where it can provide localized pulmonary vasodilation. Thus, areas of ventilated lung can receive more blood flow to decrease intrapulmonary shunting and improve oxygenation. This gas has been used extensively in neonates and children[40] with hypoxemic respiratory failure with beneficial effect. It has also been used in ventilated burned children to improve oxygenation.[41] Although nitric oxide therapy has received considerable attention as a potential therapeutic option in severe pulmonary disease, no reports to date have documented improved mortality in spite of improvements in oxygenation. For this reason, its use cannot be recommended outside of a clinical trial.

Limiting barotrauma

Barotrauma is a common complication of mechanical ventilation and results in pneumothorax, pneumomediastinum, subcutaneous emphysema, interstitial emphysema, and pneumatoceles. In a volume-cycled mode, elevated peak and plateau pressures have been implicated in inducing barotrauma. Thus, it is conceivable that limiting airway pressures may decrease morbidity. Early reports showed no clear benefit of pressure-limited ventilation,[42,43] which was accomplished by giving lower tidal volumes more frequently to maintain minute ventilation, and to accept a higher $PaCO_2$ value and lower arterial pH, which is termed permissive hypercapnia. Criticism of these trials lay in their low enrollment and lack of power to show differences. A recent large multicenter trial, however, documented improved survival and increased ventilator-free days in the first 28 days in the ICU in patients with ARDS treated with low-tidal volumes (6 mL/kg predicted body weight) versus traditional tidal volumes (12 mL/kg predicted body weight) In fact, this study was stopped early by the data safety committee because of the benefits incurred to the treated group.[44] Suspected reasons for the improvements seen

in this trial contrary to the earlier trials was the number of subjects enrolled as well as the defined protocol to limit plateau pressures <30 cmH_2O. Theoretically, the low-tidal volume strategy prescribes to the theory of ARDS which dictates that small healthy areas of lung exist adjacent to diseased and collapsed areas. In the conventionally treated group, higher tidal volumes and pressure are only distributed to open healthy alveoli; therefore the barotrauma of high pressures is delivered to this 'healthy' lung, thus increasing the damage there and thus worsening outcomes.[45] In burned patients, decreased chest wall compliance, presence of smoke inhalation injury to the upper airways, and massive fluid requirements are just a few variables that make effective gas exchange challenging while optimally minimizing barotrauma. Prospective trials comparing modes of ventilation to minimize barotrauma are lacking in the burn literature, making it difficult to determine which approach is best suited in this population. One recent study showed no statistically significant differences were found between a pressure-limited strategy and a conventional strategy in 61 burned patients for mortality, pulmonary complications, or incidence of pneumothoraces.[46] It serves to reason, however, that pressure-limited ventilation strategies might be of benefit in burned patients in sufficiently powered studies, although the merits have not been sufficiently tested.

Weaning from mechanical ventilation

Regardless of the mode of ventilation, almost all patients surviving the initial insult requiring mechanical ventilation will arrive at a stage to be weaned off the ventilator. Clinicians continue to debate the advantages of weaning patients with various forms of mechanical ventilation. Some clinicians prefer to use pressure support ventilation (PSV) with or without SIMV because of the ease with which the level can gradually be reduced. Others maintain that intermittent trials with abrupt cessation of ventilator support while maintaining endotracheal intubation ('t-tube trials') result in more rapid weaning (Figure 34.5).[47] It must be noted that weaning from ventilation depends upon the rate at which the patient recovers

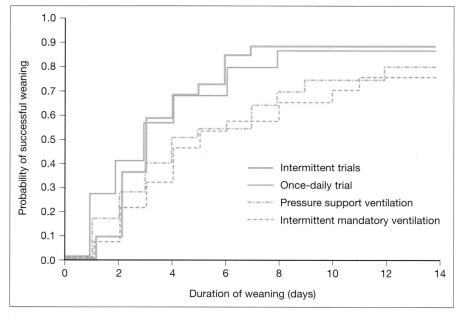

Fig. 34.5 The probability of successful weaning with intermittent mandatory ventilation, pressure support ventilation, intermittent trials of spontaneous breathing, and once-daily trials of spontaneous breathing (Kaplan–Meier curves). After adjustments for baseline characteristics (Cox proportional hazards model), the rate of successful weaning with a once-daily trial of spontaneous breathing was 2.83 times higher than that with intermittent mandatory ventilation ($p < 0.006$) and 2.05 times higher than that with pressure support ventilation ($p < 0.04$). (Reprinted with permission from Esteban et al. N Engl J Med 1995; 332–350. Copyright Massachusetts Medical Society.[47])

from the condition causing mechanical ventilation and the aggression of the clinician driving the weaning process. In practice, either method of weaning from the ventilator (gradual weaning with pressure support or intermittent t-tube trials) will be successful. What will certainly prolong the process is random changes in ventilation parameters without a directed plan.

Monitoring of mechanical ventilation

For patients on mechanical ventilation, the normal physiological regulation of ventilation and oxygenation are often impaired by sedatives and paralytics required for the presence of the endotracheal tube, or due the pathophysiological condition requiring mechanical ventilation. For these reasons, monitoring of ventilation and oxygenation by the clinician is required.

Ventilation

Arterial CO_2 tension remains the most accurate means of assessing ventilation. This is typically measured on blood gas analysis. After assessment of the pCO_2, ventilatory settings to adjust minute ventilation can be made to reach the desired level. Another method that has received attention of late is expiratory end-tidal CO_2 monitoring through infrared measurement of CO_2. This technique allows for continuous online determination of end-tidal CO_2, which is an estimate of arterial $PaCO_2$. For end-tidal CO_2 to equate with $PaCO_2$, an assumption of a low alveolar–arterial gradient must be made. In patients with healthy lungs, this gradient is only 2–3 mmHg. In certain trauma patients, particularly those with head injuries, the gradient remains low, and may be used for continuous $PaCO_2$ monitoring. However, in other critically ill patients, the alveolar–arterial gradient may be in a state of flux, calling into question values received from an end-tidal CO_2 monitor. Factors affecting the alveolar–arterial gradient include cardiac output, airway dead space, airway resistance, and metabolic rate. Each of these may change in a severely burned patient, particularly patients with inhalation injury. For these reasons, end-tidal CO_2 monitoring is not recommended in burned patients for the estimation of $PaCO_2$.

In general, $PaCO_2$ varies indirectly with minute ventilation, and thus, this value must be considered when making ventilator adjustments to alter $PaCO_2$. Minute ventilation is equal to tidal volume multiplied by respiratory rate. Therefore, $PaCO_2$ can be adjusted downward by either increasing tidal volume or respiratory rate. In general, respiratory rate should be set between 10 and 20 breaths and tidal volume at 6 mL/kg for the initial settings. Adjustments can then be made in minute ventilation to optimize $PaCO_2$, which is usually 40 mmHg. When making these adjustments, it should be noted that the respiratory rate cannot be increased above 40 breaths/min, and tidal volume should be minimized to avert barotrauma.

When plateau airway pressures are greater than 30 mmHg, the ventilated lung is relatively noncompliant, indicative of ARDS or pulmonary edema. In this situation, 'permissive hypercapnia' is a strategy that may be used to decrease barotrauma. This strategy seeks to limit peak and plateau airway pressures by decreasing tidal volumes to allow for respiratory acidosis ($PaCO_2 > 45$ mmHg, arterial pH < 7.30). This strategy was used to some extent in the trial investigating the efficacy of pressure-limited ventilation on improving outcomes in critically ill ventilated patients.[48]

Oxygenation

As with the determination of the adequacy of ventilation, oxygenation has been classically determined using the partial pressure of O_2 in arterial blood. In general, a pO_2 value of 60 mmHg has been considered sufficient. Another frequently used monitor is pulse oximetry, which is an optical measurement of oxygenated hemoglobin in pulsatile vessels. Using differences in absorption of red and infrared light, the percentage of oxygenated hemoglobin in the arteries can be calculated. Shortcomings of this technique are that methemoglobin and carboxyhemoglobin are falsely measured as oxygen saturated hemoglobin, which is common initially in patients with smoke inhalation injury. Otherwise, this is a very accurate technique for the determination of oxygen content in arterial blood, as 97% of oxygen is carried to the tissues via hemoglobin. This assertion has been corroborated by in vitro studies,[49] which showed the accuracy of pulse oximetry to within 2–3% of oxyhemoglobin levels. The major limitations of this technique lie in the insensitivity to changes in pulmonary gas exchange. Because of the shape of the oxyhemoglobin dissociation curve, when the SaO_2 exceeds 90% and the PaO_2 is greater than 60 mmHg, the curve is flat and changes in PaO_2 can change considerably with little change in SaO_2. Regardless, it is assumed that an SaO_2 value greater than 92% is indicative of adequate oxygenation. An advantage to oxygen saturation measurements that should not be overlooked is that it is a continuous measure that is immediately available, while blood gas measurement of PaO_2 is by nature intermittent.

Initial ventilator settings to assure adequate oxygenation are usually 40% oxygen in the inspired gas with 5 mmHg PEEP. This amount of PEEP is used to mimic the normal physiological pressures in nonintubated subjects. When oxygenation begins to decline, initial maneuvers are to increase the fractional inspired oxygen (FiO_2) to greater than 40% and possibly to 100%. Concentrations of oxygen greater than 60% are considered toxic to airway epithelium, and other means to increase oxygenation should be employed. This should consist initially of increasing the level of PEEP incrementally until the desired level of oxygenation is reached while keeping the FiO_2 to less than 60%. Once a level of 15–20 mmHg of PEEP is reached, other means of increasing oxygenation will need to be employed. These consist of inverse ratio ventilation, HFOV, HFPV, APRV with and without inhaled nitric oxide, etc., which are described above.

Organ system failure and management

Etiology and pathophysiology

As stated earlier, it has been hypothesized that organ dysfunction commonly seen in the critically ill exists in a continuum with SIRS. Certain patients with SIRS will go on to develop MODS, which is characterized by nonfatal signs of organ system dysfunction, such as renal insufficiency or ventilator dependence. A subset of these patients will go on to develop frank organ failure, termed multiple system organ failure (MSOF), which often leads to death (Figure 34.6).[5,6] What is

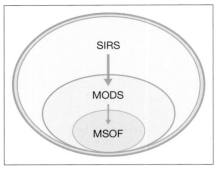

Fig. 34.6 Progression to multiple organ failure. All severely burned patients have the systemic inflammatory response syndrome (SIRS). A subset of these will develop signs and symptoms of multiple organ dysfunction syndrome (MODS). Still fewer will go on to develop multiple system organ failure (MSOF).

BOX 34.4 Theories for the development of multiple organ failure

- Infectious causes
- Macrophage theory
- Microcirculatory hypothesis
- Endothelial–leukocyte interactions
- Gut hypothesis
- Two-hit theory

---

required for the development of SIRS is inflammation, which in the severely burned emanates primarily from the burn wound. Factors associated with progression from the systemic inflammatory response syndrome to multiple organ failure are not well explained, although *some* of the responsible mechanisms in *some* patients are recognized. Occasionally, failure of the gut barrier, with penetration of organisms into the systemic circulation, may incite a similar reaction. However, this phenomenon has only been demonstrated in animal models, and it remains to be seen if this is a cause of human disease.

A number of theories have been developed to explain the progression to multiple organ failure (Box 34.4). One of these is the infection theory that incriminates uncontrolled infection as the major cause. In the severely burned patient, these infectious sources most likely emanate from invasive wound infection, or from lung infections (pneumonias). As organisms proliferate out of control, endotoxins are liberated from Gram-negative bacterial walls, and exotoxins from Gram-positive and Gram-negative bacteria are released.[50] Their release causes the initiation of a cascade of inflammatory mediators called cytokines, as well as the recruitment of inflammatory cells that can result, if unchecked, in organ damage and progression toward organ failure. Cytokines are a group of signaling proteins produced by a variety of cells that are thought to be important for host defense, wound healing, and other essential host functions. Although cytokines in low physiological concentrations preserve homeostasis, excessive production may lead to widespread tissue injury and organ dysfunction. Four of these cytokines – tumor necrosis factor alpha (TNF-α), interleukin 1 beta (IL-1β), interleukin 6 (IL-6), and interleukin 8 (IL-8) – have been most strongly associated with sepsis and multiple organ failure. The primary detraction to this theory is that many patients, including burned patients, can develop multiple organ failure without identified infection. It seems that inflammation from the presence of necrotic tissue and open wounds can incite a similar inflammatory mediator response to that seen with endotoxin. The mechanism by which this occurs, however, is not well understood. Regardless, it is known that a cascade of systemic events is set in motion either by invasive organisms or from open wounds that initiates the systemic inflammatory syndrome, which may progress to multiple organ failure.

Another theory implicates macrophages and their activity in the development of multiple organ failure. Macrophages activated by inflammation release excessive levels of cytokines and inflammatory mediators into the systemic circulation which cause end-organ damage, and incite further inflammation and macrophage activation. Elevated circulating and bronchoalveolar fluid cytokine levels have been associated with increased risk for SIRS/MODS; however, trials investigating the efficacy of cytokine blockade in patients with multiple organ failure have not improved survival rates in very large studies.

Yet another theory implicates prolonged tissue hypoxia and the generation of toxic free radicals during reperfusion as the primary mediator of end-organ damage. Deficits in resuscitation then would lead to areas of the microcirculation throughout the body that receive inadequate nutrients, and shift to anaerobic metabolism and formation of superoxides from ATP metabolites. The effects of the toxic products of oxygen free radical formation are only now being elucidated. From *in vitro* models and *in vivo* animal models, we know that tissues that initially were in shock and are then reperfused produce oxygen free radicals that are known to damage a number of cellular metabolism processes. This process occurs throughout the body during burn resuscitation, but the significance of these free radicals in human burn injury is unknown. It was found that free radical scavengers such as superoxide dismutase improve survival in animal models; however, these results were not established in patients.[51] Oxygen free radicals oxidize membrane lipids, resulting in cellular dysfunction. Endogenous natural antioxidants, such as vitamins C and E, are low in patients with burns, suggesting that therapeutic interventions may be beneficial.[52] Serum nitrate levels correlate well with multiple organ failure scores in critically ill patients, implying a role for this constellation of events in SIRS/MODS.

The role of vascular endothelium and leukocyte interactions to cause the changes seen in multiple organ failure has also been suggested. Cytokines and oxidants can convert endothelial cells to a proinflammatory state with upregulation of adhesion molecule expression, leading to leukocyte adherence and neutrophil-mediated tissue damage. Inhibition of this association with monoclonal antibodies has been shown to reduce tissue damage and organ injury in animal models of hemorrhagic shock, and was shown to attenuate skin injury when used during burn resuscitation.[53] The relevance of this model to the generation and maintenance of organ failure is yet to be established.

The last two theories revolve around the role of the gut in the generation of organ failure, and the 'two-hit' theory of multiple organ failure. For years, investigators have implicated the gut as the 'engine' of organ failure, which is associated with loss of gut barrier function and translocation of enteric bacteria and their toxic metabolites. Bacterial translocation has been shown to occur in animal models after burn,[54] as well as in humans.[55] These bacteria and their products then activate the inflammatory cells described above, culminating in organ failure. The relevance of gut-mediated bacterial translocation to human disease, however, has been hotly debated. No clear studies have shown whether bacterial translocation is the cause of SIRS/MODS, probably because investigators have been unable to control bacterial translocation effectively during shock in humans, and thus a cause and effect relationship cannot be established. The 'two-hit' theory ascribes a summation of insults to the development of organ failure. Each of the insults alone is inadequate to cause the response, but one or more of these insults can 'prime' the inflammatory response system such that another normally insignificant injury causes the release of toxic mediators that end in multiple organ failure.

Prevention

This brief outline of the potential pathophysiology and causes of burn-induced critical illness and multiple organ failure demonstrates the complexity of the problem. Since different cascade systems are involved in the pathogenesis, it is so far impossible to pinpoint a single mediator that initiates the event. Thus, since the mechanisms of progression are not well known and thus specific treatments cannot be accurately devised, it seems that prevention is likely the best solution. The current recommendations are to prevent the development of organ dysfunction, and to provide optimal support to avoid conditions which promote the onset.

Course of organ failure

Even with the best efforts at prevention, the presence of the systemic inflammatory syndrome that is ubiquitous in burn patients may progress to organ failure. Experience with the severely burned dictates that virtually all burned patients will display the signs and symptoms of SIRS, including tachycardia, tachypnea, increased white blood cell count, etc. Thereafter, various organ systems may begin to show signs of dysfunction. Generally, these will begin in the renal and/or pulmonary systems and progress through the liver, gut, hematological system, and central nervous system in a systematic fashion. The development of multiple organ failure does not preclude mortality, however, and efforts to support the organs until they heal is justified.

Renal system

Pathophysiology

Acute renal failure (ARF) is a potentially lethal complication of burns. Despite substantial technical developments in dialysis to replace the function of the kidneys, mortality meets or exceeds 50% for all critically ill patients who develop acute renal failure.[56] Interestingly, mortality associated with ARF requiring dialysis in the critically ill has not improved significantly for over 30 years. The same can be said for renal failure

requiring dialysis in the severely burned specifically.[57] The causes of death in these critically ill patients is not uremia because of advances in dialysis, but primarily sepsis and cardiovascular and pulmonary dysfunction.

With the advent of early aggressive resuscitation after burn, the incidence of renal failure coincident with the initial phases of recovery has diminished significantly in severely burned patients.[57] However, a second period of risk for the development of renal failure 2–14 days after resuscitation is still present, and is probably related to the development of sepsis.

Acute renal failure, usually in the form of acute tubular necrosis (ATN), is characterized by deterioration of renal function over a period of hours to days, resulting in the failure of the kidney to excrete nitrogenous waste products and to maintain fluid and electrolyte homeostasis. It may be caused by a number of factors interfering with glomerular filtration and tubular resorption. In burned patients, the causes can be generally narrowed to renal hypoperfusion, or nephrotoxic insults from pharmacological treatments (e.g. aminoglycosides or intravenous contrast agents) or sepsis (Figure 34.7).

Ischemic renal failure is the more common of the two causes, and is induced by hypoperfusion from an imbalance between vasoconstrictive and vasodilatory factors acting on the small renal vessels during low-flow states. Decreased flow to the renal cells directly alters endothelial cell function, decreasing the production of and response to vasodilatory substances. The renal medulla is the most sensitive portion of the kidney to hypoxia, and the damage is initially to the renal tubular cells. The outer medulla and proximal tubules have high oxygen requirements, and the resulting ischemia causes swelling of tubular and endothelial cells with necrosis, apoptosis, and inflammation evident on histological examination.[58] These changes lead to further vascular congestion and decreased blood flow, leading to more cell loss and further decrements in renal function.

Structural changes in the tubular cells include loss of polarity and the integrity of the tight junctions.[59] Integrins are redistributed to the apical surface, resulting in live and dead cells sloughing into the tubular lumen, causing cast formation. The casts then cause increased intratubular pressure and reduced glomerular filtration rate. Loss of epithelial cell barrier and the tight junctions between viable cells causes back-leakage of the glomerular filtrate, further reducing the effective glomerular filtration rate. Arg-Gly-Asp peptides, which prevent adhesion between cells in the tubular lumen and thus decrease cast formation, prevent increases in proximal tubular pressure and mitigate ischemic renal failure in experimental animals.[60]

After the initiating event, tubular function and the glomerular filtration rate decrease to reduce urine production. The progression of ARF is commonly divided into three phases – initiation, maintenance, and recovery – and can be oliguric (urine output <400 mL/day) or nonoliguric (urine output >400 mL/day) in nature. Patients with nonoliguric ARF have a better prognosis that those with oliguric renal failure, probably due in large measure to the decreased severity of the insult and the fact that many have drug-associated nephrotoxicity or interstitial nephritis. The percentage of critically ill patients with ARF who require dialysis ranges from 20 to 60%. Among the subgroup who survive initial dialysis, less

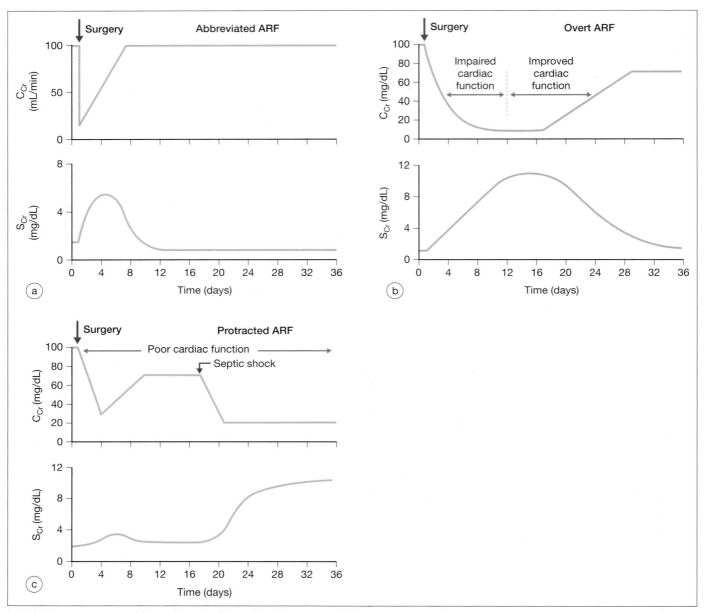

Fig. 34.7 Three patterns of hemodynamically mediated acute renal failure (ARF) occur after major burn. (a) Abbreviated ARF consists of an acute reduction in creatinine clearance (C_{Cr}) with prompt recovery. Serum creatinine (S_{Cr}) may increase even as C_{Cr} is recovering. (b) Overt ARF consists of concurrent mirror image increases in C_{Cr} and S_{Cr} in association with compromised cardiac function followed by recovery. (c) Protracted ARF develops as a consequence of prolonged hemodynamic compromise often complicated by systemic sepsis. (Reproduced with permission from Myers and Moran. N Engl J Med 1986; 314:97–105. Copyright Massachusetts Medical Society.[129])

than 25% require long-term dialysis, demonstrating the potential reversibility of the syndrome.[61]

Once ARF is established, pharmacological improvement of renal blood flow will not reverse the injury. Agents such as dopamine, which dilates renal arterioles and increases renal blood flow and creatinine clearance in normal animals,[62] improves creatinine clearance and the fractional excretion of sodium in stable, critically ill patients for 24 hours, after which the effect diminishes. At 48 hours, no effect remains.[63] Other investigators have shown no efficacy of dopamine treatment in preventing acute renal failure in septic, oliguric patients.[64] Other agents such as calcium channel blockers have been shown to improve vascular tone, and decrease vasoconstric-

tion associated with radiocontrast agents,[65] but to date, no studies have been done to document their usefulness in acute renal failure induced by hypoperfusion. Natriuretic peptides also have conceivable benefit, and were shown to improve renal function for up to 24 hours in a group of patients with either ischemic or toxic acute renal failure, including a reduced requirement for dialysis in the treated group.[66] Another trial showed an improvement in dialysis-free survival in a subgroup of patients with oliguric ATN.[67] These results, however, were not borne out in other studies.[68] Recently, the potent dopamine-1 receptor agonist fenoldopam has garnered some interest as an agent to improve renal perfusion. A recent randomized controlled trial demonstrated that low-dose fenoldopam may have some prophylactic benefit when used in septic patients in a mixed ICU population.[69]

Diuretic therapies, such as mannitol and loop diuretics, have been used extensively in patients with acute renal failure to increase urine flow, and protect the kidney from further ischemic damage. Mannitol can decrease cellular swelling in the proximal tubule and increase intratubular flow, thus potentially decreasing intratubular obstruction and further renal dysfunction. Mannitol is recommended along with vigorous volume replacement and sodium bicarbonate for the treatment of early myoglobinuric acute renal failure. Loop diuretics also increase intratubular flow rates, and can convert an oliguric state to a nonoliguric state, thus making clinical management of renal failure easier. Although nonoliguric renal failure is generally associated with a lower mortality rate, there is no evidence that conversion from an oliguric to a nonoliguric state improves mortality. It is likely that those patients who respond to diuretics have less severe renal damage at the outset of treatment; thus the outcomes are better.

Treatment

The initial care of patients with ARF is focused on reversing the underlying cause, and correcting fluid and electrolyte imbalances. Renal failure is heralded by a decrease in urinary output. Volumes of urine less than 1 mL/kg/h may indicate the onset of ARF. This failure may be due to prerenal causes, which is typically decreased renal blood flow from hypoperfusion, or intrinsic renal causes, which are associated with medications or sepsis. Differentiation between these etiologies can be made with laboratory examinations (Table 34.2). Prerenal etiologies are associated with concentrated urine (urine osmolality >400 mOsmol/kg), decreased urinary sodium concentrations, and decreased fractional excretion of sodium. Intrinsic renal causes will be associated with more dilute urine with higher sodium concentrations. These tests should be performed before diuretics are used, as this treatment will increase urinary sodium and decrease urine osmolality even in prerenal conditions. In general, urine osmolality and urinary sodium concentrations are primarily used for these determinations because of the ease of measurement.

Should these tests reveal a prerenal cause, volume replacement should ensue to prevent further renal ischemia. The physical exam and invasive monitoring if deemed appropriate should guide this volume replacement. The decision to administer or remove fluids may prove difficult, however, since both strategies have detrimental consequences if followed inappro-

priately. Although volume replacement is ineffective in restoring renal function once tubular necrosis is established, it remains our most effective prophylactic strategy, and is generally the place to start with the onset of renal failure.

Once renal failure begins, serum creatinine will begin to increase with the decrease in glomerular filtration. However, up to 70% of renal function must be lost prior to significant increases in serum creatinine concentrations, making its use as a screening examination for renal failure suspect. Increases in serum creatinine may also be masked by increased plasma volume associated with aggressive volume resuscitation. Because renal failure is treated best by prevention with early detection, the use of a clinical measure of glomerular filtration rate, such as creatinine clearance (C_{cr}), may be of greater clinical utility early in the course of failure. Creatinine clearance can be measured effectively over short-time periods (2-hour collections), with the only caveat for an overestimation of glomerular filtration rate when compared to inulin. Nonetheless, serial measurements to examine changes in creatinine clearance will improve monitoring for acute renal failure.

After assuring adequate volume status, every effort should be made to prevent other causes of renal injury. All nephrotoxins should be discontinued or avoided. Hyperkalemia that may develop can be treated with resins, glucose and insulin, and sodium bicarbonate in the presence of metabolic acidosis. Medications eliminated through the kidney should be adjusted. Once the diagnosis of ARF is established, consideration can be given for diuretic therapy, especially if it is determined that the patient is volume overloaded. Decreasing the volume of fluid given can also alleviate volume overload in burned patients. These patients have increased insensible losses from the wounds which can be roughly calculated at 3750 mL/m² TBSA wound plus 1500 mL/m² TBSA total. Decreasing the infused volume of intravenous fluids and enteral feedings below the expected insensate losses may alleviate some of these problems. Decreasing potassium administration in the enteral feedings and giving oral bicarbonate solutions can minimize electrolyte abnormalities. Almost invariably, severely burned patients require exogenous potassium because of the heightened aldosterone response which results in potassium wasting; therefore, hyperkalemia is rare even with some renal insufficiency.

Intermittent dialysis remains the standard replacement therapy for severe ARF in the hemodynamically normal ICU patient. The indications for dialysis are edema and volume overload or electrolyte abnormalities not amenable to other treatments. In recent years, continuous renal replacement therapies have emerged as yet another option for critically ill patients with ARF[70] (Figure 34.8). The advantages of continuous treatment over intermittent include more precise fluid and metabolic control, decreased hemodynamic stability, and the enhanced ability to remove injurious cytokines.[71] Disadvantages include the need for anticoagulation and heightened surveillance. Bleeding problems are particularly prevalent in burned patients during anticoagulation.[72] Nonetheless, trials to date have not shown any benefit of continuous hemodialysis over traditional intermittent dialysis.

Peritoneal dialysis is another option for burned patients with severe acute renal failure.[73] Catheters can be placed at the bedside with near continuous exchanges to improve

---

TABLE 34.2 LABORATORY TESTS TO DISTINGUISH PRERENAL FROM INTRINSIC RENAL FAILURE

Examination	Prerenal	Intrinsic renal
Urine osmolality (mOsmol/kg)	>400	<400
Urinary sodium (mEq/dL)	<20	>40
FE$_{Na}$ (%)*	<1	>2

*FE$_{Na}$, fractional excretion of sodium, calculated as $(U/P_{Na} / U/P_{Cr}) \times 100$, where U is urinary concentration, and P is plasma concentration. Na is sodium and Cr is creatinine.

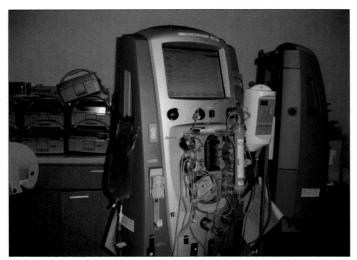

Fig. 34.8 Photograph of a new model dialysis machine that can deliver either intermittent or continuous renal replacement therapy.

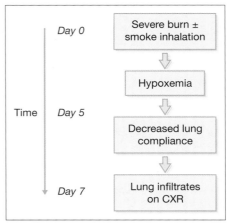

Fig. 34.9 Typical timeline for progression to ARDS. Patients are typically intubated for airway compromise and operative intervention. At day 4 or 5 after severe burn, oxygenation will deteriorate, requiring higher inspired concentrations of oxygen. These measures will soon fail with the introduction of decreased lung compliance requiring higher inspired airway pressures. Only then will infiltrates begin to appear on the chest x-ray (CXR).

BOX 34.5 Definitions of acute lung injury and acute respiratory distress syndrome

- Acute onset
- Bilateral infiltrates on chest radiography
- Pulmonary artery wedge pressure <18 mmHg
- Acute lung injury (ALI) if P_aO_2/F_iO_2 is <30 but >200
- Acute respiratory distress syndrome (ARDS) if P_aO_2/F_iO_2 is <200

---

electrolyte and volume overload problems. The capital required for this treatment is minimal. Hypertonic solutions are used to remove fluid volume, and the concentrations of potassium and bicarbonate are modified to produce the desired results. The dwell time is usually 30 minutes followed by drainage for 30 minutes. This treatment can be repeated in cycles until the problem is resolved. For maintenance, 4–6 such cycles a day with prolonged dwell times (1 hour) is usually sufficient during the acute phase.

After beginning dialysis, renal function will likely return in survivors, especially in those patients that maintain some urine output. Therefore, patients requiring such treatment may not require lifelong dialysis. It is a clinical observation that whatever urine output was present will decrease once dialysis is begun, but it may return in several days to weeks once the acute process of closing the burn wound nears completion.

Pulmonary system

Mechanical ventilation in the severely burned generally takes place for three reasons:
- airway control during the resuscitative phase,
- airway management for smoke inhalation, and
- for the development of acute lung injury and ARDS.

The first is for airway control early in the course with the development of massive whole-body edema associated with the great resuscitative volumes required to maintain euvolemia. In this situation, the need for mechanical ventilation is not due to lung failure, *per se*, but instead to maintain the airway until the whole-body edema resolves. Once this occurs, usually 2–3 days into the course, extubation can be accomplished. Ventilator management during this phase is routine.

The second primary reason for mechanical ventilation is for airway management early in the course of smoke inhalation. Another chapter in the book will deal specifically with this issue.

The third is the development of hypoxemia. Severe burns are known to be associated with hypoxemia and the development of acute lung injury (ALI) and its more severe counter-part, ARDS. The clinical manifestations are dyspnea, severe hypoxemia, and decreased lung compliance with radiographic evidence of diffuse bilateral pulmonary infiltrates (Figure 34.9). These conditions exist as a continuum from ALI, which is a mild form, to its most severe form, which is dense ARDS. These conditions have been defined by the American–European Consensus Conference Committee, and are listed in Box 34.5. These definitions are relatively simple, and are used in other critically ill populations. The rest of the discussion will be related to ALI and ARDS.

Epidemiology and pathophysiology

ALI and ARDS occur as a result of injury to the lung, which can be direct through smoke inhalation or pneumonia, or indirect through mediators associated with sepsis. Until recently, most studies of ALI and ARDS reported mortality rates between 40 and 60%.[74] The majority of deaths were attributable to sepsis or multiorgan dysfunction.

Recently, two reports suggest that mortality in ARDS has been decreasing, with a group from Seattle reporting a 67% decrease in mortality for 1987–1993 compared to a period from 1983 to 1987. Another group in the United Kingdom reported a 50% decline in mortality over a similar time period. Explanations include more effective treatment of sepsis, changes in methods of mechanical ventilation, and improved support of the critically ill. No reports of improved mortality have been forthcoming in the severely burned with ARDS.

ALI and ARDS occur because of damage to the endothelium and lung epithelium. It is speculated that the products of inflammation, such as cytokines, endotoxin, complement, and coagulation system products, induce the changes that are characteristic of ALI and ARDS. The acute phase of ALI is characterized by influx of protein-rich edema fluid into the air spaces as a consequence of increased permeability of the alveolar–capillary barrier. The importance of endothelial injury and increased vascular permeability to the formation of pulmonary edema is well established.[74] Epithelial injury is also of great importance. In fact, the degree of alveolar epithelial injury is an important predictor of outcome.

The normal alveolar epithelium is composed of two cell types. Flat type I cells make up 90% of the alveolar surface, and these cells are easily injured. Cuboidal type II cells make up the remaining 10%, and are more resistant to injury. Type I cells function to move gases from the interstitium to the alveoli. Type II cells function to produce surfactant, participate in ion transfer and fluid movement, and proliferate/differentiate to type I cells after injury.

Loss of epithelial integrity has a number of consequences. Under normal conditions, the epithelial barrier is much less permeable than the endothelial barrier; therefore its loss contributes to alveolar flooding. Also, loss of type II cells disrupts epithelial fluid transport, impairing the removal of edema from the alveolar space. Lastly, loss of type II cells reduces the turnover and production of surfactant, causing a loss of surface tension in the alveoli and contributing to alveolar collapse.

Neutrophils are likely to play a role in the pathogenesis of ALI. Histological studies of lung specimens obtained early in the course demonstrate marked accumulation of neutrophils in the alveolar fluid.[75] These neutrophils can be recovered from bronchoalveolar lavage fluid from affected patients,[76] demonstrating a clear association between neutrophil accumulation and lung injury. However, it must be stated that ALI and ARDS develop in patients with profound neutropenia,[77] and some animals models of ARDS are neutrophil independent, intimating that neutrophils may be nothing more than bystanders in the inflammatory process.

The effects of ventilator injury on the development and progression of ALI and ARDS are just now coming to light. Previous studies focused on the potential damaging effects of high oxygen concentrations on lung epithelium.[78] Recent evidence suggests that mechanical ventilation at high pressures can injure the lung,[44] causing increased pulmonary edema in the uninjured lung and enhanced edema in the injured lung.[79] Alveolar overdistention and cyclic opening and closing of alveoli associated with high ventilatory pressures is also potentially damaging to the lung.

After the development of ALI and ARDS, some patients have a rapid recovery over a few days.[80] Others progress to fibrotic lung injury, which is observed as early as 5–7 days into the course of the disease.[75] The alveolar space becomes filled with mesenchymal cells, extracellular proteins, and new blood vessels.[81] The finding of fibrosis on histological analysis correlates with increased mortality.[82]

In the nonfatal cases of ARDS, the lung heals by proliferation of type II epithelial cells, which begin to cover the denuded basement membrane and differentiate into type I epithelial cells, thus restoring normal alveolar architecture and increasing the fluid transport capacity of the alveolar epithelium. This proliferation is associated with a keratinocyte growth factor and an hepatocyte growth factor.[74] Alveolar edema is resolved by active transport of sodium from the distal airspace into the interstitium by intact alveoli.[83] Soluble protein is removed primarily by diffusion between alveolar cells, and insoluble protein is eliminated by endocytosis and transcytosis by alveolar epithelial cells and phagocytosis by macrophages.[84]

The severely burned are unique among patients that develop ALI and ARDS. Because direct injury to the lung from smoke inhalation is common, oftentimes patients will present with respiratory insufficiency and relative hypoxia caused by increased capillary permeability, ciliary dysfunction, and interstitial edema associated with the chemical injury of smoke. A few days later, the damaged and necrotic respiratory mucosa begins to slough, causing bronchial plugging and atelectasis, further worsening the clinical condition. However, it is not usually until 4–8 days into the course of injury that severe hypoxemia and ARDS develop in burned patients, a scenario not unlike other types of patients who develop ALI and ARDS, such as after abdominal sepsis or multiple blunt trauma. It serves to reason that smoke inhalation is associated with the development of ARDS, but perhaps this association is related to the inflammation associated with the injury in addition to that rendered by the burn wound. In fact, it was recently shown that the degree of inhalation injury was not associated with the development of ARDS in burned patients.[85] It may be, then, that smoke inhalation and ALI/ARDS are two separate conditions which are inter-related.

Treatment

The treatment of ALI and ARDS is largely supportive until the healing processes described above can be accomplished. A careful search for potential underlying causes should ensue, including attention to potentially treatable causes such as intra-abdominal infections, pneumonia, line sepsis, and invasive burn wound infection. An improved understanding of the pathogenesis of ALI has led to the assessment of several novel treatment strategies,[74] including changes in mechanical ventilation strategies, fluid management, surfactant therapy, nitric oxide treatments, and anti-inflammatory strategies.

Potential treatments

The most appropriate method of mechanical ventilation for ALI and ARDS has been controversial for some time. Older strategies recommended supraphysiological tidal volumes of 12–15 mL/kg, which, as stated previously, may contribute to further alveolar damage. This was recognized in the 1970s, which led to studies of extracorporeal membrane oxygenation to reduce tidal volumes to 8 mL/kg. However, this strategy failed to decrease mortality.[86] Similar studies have been performed in severely burned patients, with no effect on mortality.[87] Recently, a National Institutes of Health (NIH) study group reported a 22% decline in mortality in patients with ALI and ARDS treated with tidal volumes of 6 mL/kg compared to those treated with conventional volumes of 12 mL/kg. In this study, peak airway pressures could not exceed 30 cmH$_2$O in the lower tidal volume group, and a detailed protocol was used to adjust the fraction of inspired oxygen and PEEP.[44]

These results were different from previous smaller studies showing no improvement with pressure-limited ventilation.[43] Potential reasons for the discrepancy between the NIH study and the others are as follows:

- the NIH study had the lowest tidal volume of the three studies,
- respiratory acidosis was allowed in the NIH study with sodium bicarbonate treatment if necessary to maintain homeostasis, and
- the NIH study had more patients, and thus may have been more sufficiently powered to show differences between treatment groups.[74]

Positive end-expiratory pressure has clearly been shown to benefit patients with ALI and ARDS;[88] however, the most optimum level has been controversial. The best documented effect of PEEP is to increase functional residual capacity, or the number of open alveoli at the end of expiration.[89] However, the use of prophylactic PEEP therapy in patients at risk for ALI showed no benefit for the treatment group compared to controls.[90]

A more recent study of PEEP therapy aimed at raising the level of PEEP above the lower inflection point on pressure–volume curves to prevent alveolar closure in addition to low tidal volumes and pressure-controlled inverse ratio ventilation showed improved mortality compared to a control group managed with conventional ventilation.[91] Drawbacks to this study were the unusually high mortality (71%) in the control group, and improvements in mortality for the treatment group compared to controls could only be determined at hospital day 28, which was not appreciated at hospital discharge. Nonetheless, the potentials for benefit of this therapy have warranted further studies, which are underway.

Surfactant therapy has been suggested for patients with ALI and ARDS, which should decrease alveolar surface tension, and maintain open alveoli. This therapy was proved effective in neonates with respiratory distress;[92] however, a study done in adults with ARDS showed no effect on oxygenation, duration of mechanical ventilation, or survival.[93] Newer preparations of surfactant with recombinant proteins and new approaches to instillation such as bronchoalveolar lavage and tracheal administration are being evaluated in clinical trials.

Inhaled nitric oxide is an effective pulmonary vasodilator with effects localized to ventilated areas of the lung, thus directing more blood to the functional areas of the lung. The conceivable effect, then, is to diminish the fraction of blood shunted through the lungs without oxygenation, thus improving pulmonary venous oxygenation. Observational studies suggest that inhaled nitric oxide might be beneficial in the treatment of ARDS by improving oxygenation without increased ventilatory pressures and reducing barotrauma. However, randomized trials testing this hypothesis have been disappointing. In a recent study, inhaled nitric oxide therapy did not reduce mortality or decrease the duration of mechanical ventilation. Improvements in oxygenation were seen; however, the effects were not sustained.[94] Treatment with less selective pulmonary vasodilators such as sodium nitroprusside,[95] and alprostadil (prostaglandin E_1)[96] have not been shown to be beneficial.

Glucocorticoids have been used in the treatment of ARDS because of the inflammatory nature of the disease. However, these agents were not shown to be of any benefit when given at the onset of the condition.[97] More recently, glucocorticoids have been used in the later fibroproliferative phases of the disease to good effect.[98] Preliminary studies in a small population have shown improved oxygenation, decreased ventilator dependence, and decreased mortality with no increased risk of sepsis in nonburned patients.[99] This type of therapy may be treacherous in burned patients at risk for invasive burn wound infection, but might be considered upon complete burn wound closure.

Cardiovascular system

Principles

Treatment of cardiovascular responses after burn requires an understanding of cardiovascular physiology and the effects of treatment. One of the hallmarks of serious illness is the direct link between cardiac performance and patient performance. The four determinants of cardiac function and thus tissue perfusion of blood at the whole-body level are the following:

- ventricular preload or end-diastolic muscle fiber length;
- myocardial contractility or strength of the heart muscle;
- ventricular afterload, or the degree of resistance against which the heart must pump; and
- heart rate and rhythm.

A thorough comprehension of the effects of each of these components on heart function is required in order to initiate effective treatments for burned patients with cardiovascular abnormalities.

Preload

Preload is defined as the force that stretches the cardiac muscle prior to contraction. This force is composed of volume that fills the heart from venous return. Because of the molecular arrangement of actin and myosin in muscle, the more the muscle is stretched with incoming venous volume, the further it will contract. This is best demonstrated on a Frank–Starling curve (Figure 34.10), which was first described by Otto Frank

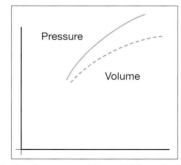

Fig. 34.10 Frank–Starling curve. The solid line depicts the pressure–volume relationship of the heart, showing that as pressure to the heart (preload) increases, the volume pumped by the heart increases. Immediately after burn, contractility diminishes, shifting the curve downward (dashed line). It still must be noted that with this change, the volume pumped by the heart still increases with increased pressure (preload), validating the use of increased atrial pressure as a means of increasing cardiac output after severe burn.

in a frog heart preparation in 1884; Ernest Starling extended this observation in the mammalian heart in 1914. The relationship demonstrated in the Frank–Starling curve justifies the use of preload augmentation by volume resuscitation to increase cardiac performance. However, when the end-diastolic volume becomes excessive, cardiac function can decrease, probably by overstretch of the muscle fibers such that the contractile fibers are pulled past each other, thus reducing the contact required for contractile force. The preload required to decrease cardiac function in experimental settings is in excess of 60 mmHg, which is rarely encountered in patients.

Preload is measured clinically by either central venous pressure or by pulmonary artery wedge pressure obtained with a pulmonary artery catheter. Of these, the pulmonary artery wedge pressure is the best estimate since it assesses the left side of the heart.

Cardiac contractility

The force with which the heart contracts is referred to as cardiac contractility. It is directly related to the number of fibers contracting, and will be diminished in patients with vascular occlusive disease of the myocardium who lose muscle fibers from infarction and ischemia, and in burned patients during the acute resuscitation.[100] Calculating the left ventricular stroke work from pulmonary artery catheter-derived values provides the best estimate of cardiac contractility, and can be calculated with the following formula:

$$LVSW = SV (MAP - PCWP) \times 0.0136$$

where LVSW is left ventricular stroke work, SV is the stroke volume (cardiac index / heart rate), MAP is mean arterial pressure, and PCWP is pulmonary capillary wedge pressure.

Afterload

Afterload is the force that impedes or opposes ventricular contraction. This force is equivalent to the tension developed across the wall of the ventricle during systole. Afterload is measured clinically by arterial resistance as an estimate of arterial compliance. Arterial resistance is measured as the difference between inflow pressure (mean arterial) and outflow pressure (venous) divided by the flow rate (cardiac output):

$$SVR = (MAP - CVP)/CO$$

where SVR is systemic vascular resistance, MAP is mean arterial pressure, CVP is central venous pressure, and CO is cardiac output.

Heart rate and rhythm

For the heart to function properly, the electrical conduction system must be intact, so as to provide rhythmic efficient contractions to develop sufficient force to propel blood through the circulatory system. For example, if the heart rate approaches 200 beats/min, the heart will not have time to fill completely, thus decreasing myocardial fiber stretch and decreasing heart function. Also, if frequent premature ventricular contractions are present, the heart will not perform as well for similar reasons. Heart rate and rhythm are monitored continuously as a routine in all critically ill patients using electrocardiography.

Effects of burn on cardiac performance

Severe burns affect cardiac performance in a number of ways. The first is to reduce preload to the heart through volume loss into the burned and nonburned tissues. It is for this reason that volumes predicted by resuscitation formulas must be used to maintain blood pressure and maintain hemodynamics. In addition, severe burn induces myocardial depression characterized by a decrease in tension development and velocities of contraction and relaxation.[101] Cardiac output is then reduced. These effects are most evident early in the course of injury; however, they are followed shortly thereafter by a hyperdynamic phase of increased cardiac output caused primarily by a decrease in afterload through vasodilation and an increase in heart rate. Deficits in myocardial contractility are for the most part maintained.

Hemodynamic therapy: preload augmentation

When hypotension or other signs of inadequate cardiac function (i.e. decreased urine output) are encountered, the usual response is to augment preload by increasing intravascular volume. This is a sound physiological approach based on the Frank–Starling principle, and should be the first therapy for any patient in shock. Intravascular volume can be increased with either crystalloid or colloid to increase the central venous pressure and pulmonary capillary wedge pressure to a value between 10 and 20 mmHg. The adequacy of this therapy can be monitored by the restoration of arterial blood pressure, a decrease in tachycardia, and a urine output greater than 0.5 mL/kg/h.

Some caution must be exercised when augmenting preload for hemodynamic benefit in burned patients. Excessive volume administration may lead to significant interstitial edema and volume overload with the development of peripheral and pulmonary edema. These changes can lead to conversion of partial-thickness burns to full-thickness injuries in the periphery, and can cause significant respiratory problems. Judicious use of fluid administration after hemodynamics are restored with spontaneous diuresis will usually alleviate this problem; however, at times, pharmacological diuresis will be required.

Hemodynamic therapy: inotropes

If volume replacement is insufficient to improve hemodynamics in burned patients in shock, inotropes may be required. These inotropes generally consist of adrenergic receptor agonists, although phosphodiesterase inhibitors that increase intracellular cAMP levels to increase myocyte Ca^{2+} levels or digoxin that acts to increase myocyte Ca^{2+} levels by inhibiting the Na^+/K^+ pump can also be used to improve myocardial contractility.

Dopamine is a commonly used inotropic agent which has both α-adrenergic and β-adrenergic properties. The α effects are seen primarily at higher doses (10–20 μg/kg/min), while the β effects are seen at all doses. Therefore, dopamine can be thought of as an 'inoconstrictor', because it has both intropic and vasoconstrictive properties. Other inotropes in this class include epinephrine and norepinephrine. One caveat to the use of these inoconstrictors is that myocardial oxygen consumption increases, which may affect areas of the heart that are ischemic.

At low doses, dopamine also produces splanchnic and renal vasodilation through specific dopamine receptors. It is thought that these vasodilatory effects can be used to optimize renal function through antagonism of α-receptor-induced vasoconstriction. However, this practice has recently been questioned. Dopamine has also been used in burned patients to increase left ventricular stroke work during myocardial depression seen during resuscitation.[14]

Dobutamine is another commonly used inotrope which has effects limited to β-adrenergic stimulation; thus, cardiac contractility is increased without vasoconstriction. The effect is to improve cardiac output generally without specific splanchnic or renal effects.

Agents with primary effects on the α-adrenergic receptor can be used to induce vasoconstriction and increase blood pressure. These agents consist of norepinephrine and phenylephrine, and can be used effectively during septic shock or neurogenic shock to increase vascular tone. In burned patients, it is felt that these agents will cause vasoconstriction of the skin circulation and the splanchnic circulation to preserve blood flow to major organs such as the heart and brain. This redistribution in blood flow can cause conversion of partial-thickness skin injuries to full-thickness and result in ischemic injury to the gut. The use of specific vasoconstrictors must be weighed against these effects.

Another vasoconstrictive agent that is being used with more popularity is vasopressin, which is a very potent vasoconstrictor mediated through its own receptor independent of the adrenergic receptors. Levels of vasopressin have been shown to be low in septic shock and physiological replacement at 0.02 mg/kg without titration is used in some units to increase mean arterial pressure to good effect.

Effects of β-blockade on cardiac performance after severe burn

One of the responses to severe burn is a dramatic increase in catecholamine production that has been linked to a number of metabolic abnormalities, including increased resting energy expenditure,[102] muscle catabolism, and altered thermoregulation.[103] The effects of this sustained catecholamine surge on the cardiac system are to increase heart rate and therefore myocardial work. Propranolol, as a nonspecific β-blocker, has been used to decrease heart rate and myocardial work in severe burns.[104] Propranolol can be given through both the intravenous and oral routes to equal effect on heart rate and myocardial work without detrimental effect on cardiac output or response to stress.[105] Propranolol administration also decreases peripheral lipolysis[106] and muscle catabolism,[107] which are additional beneficial effects. Consideration should be given to further trials with the use of propranolol to improve outcomes in burned patients.

Gastrointestinal system

Pathophysiological changes in the gut after cutaneous burn

The gastrointestinal response to burn is highlighted by mucosal atrophy, changes in digestive absorption, and increased intestinal permeability. Atrophy of the small bowel mucosa occurs within 12 hours of injury in proportion to the burn size,[108] and is related to increased epithelial cell death by apoptosis.[109] The cytoskeleton of the mucosal brush border undergoes atrophic changes associated with vesiculation of microvilli and disruption of the terminal web actin filaments. These findings were most pronounced 18 hours after injury,[54] which suggests changes in the cytoskeleton, such as those associated with cell death by apoptosis, are processes involved in the changed gut mucosa. Burn also causes reduced uptake of glucose and amino acids,[110] decreased absorption of fatty acids, and reduction in brush border lipase activity. These changes peak in the first several hours after burn, and return to normal at 48–72 hours after injury, a timing that parallels mucosal atrophy.

Intestinal permeability to macromolecules that are normally repelled by an intact mucosal barrier increases after burn.[111] Intestinal permeability to polyethylene glycol 3350, lactulose, and mannitol increases after injury, which correlates to the extent of the burn. Gut permeability increases even further when burn wounds become infected.[112] A study using fluorescent dextrans showed that larger molecules appeared to cross the mucosa between the cells, while the smaller molecules traversed the mucosa through the epithelial cells, presumably by pinocytosis and vesiculation.[113]

Changes in gut blood flow are related to changes in permeability (Figure 34.11). Intestinal blood flow was shown to decrease in non-resuscitated animals, a change that was associated with increased gut permeability at 5 hours after burn.[114] This effect was abolished at 24 hours. Systolic hypotension has been shown to occur in the first hours after burn in animals with a 40% TBSA full-thickness injury. These animals showed an inverse correlation between blood flow and permeability to intact *Candida albicans*.[115]

Clinical changes in the gut after burn

Given the changes in the gut to burn described above, it is common to see some evidence of gut dysfunction after burn evidenced by feeding intolerance,[116] and mucosal ulceration and bleeding particularly in the stomach and duodenum. Enteral feeding is one of the most important means of providing nutrition to burned patients and has led to a decrease in mortality,[117] but at times the gut will not cooperate. Reduced motility and ileus are common, at times requiring parenteral nutrition to meet caloric needs. At the present time, there is no specific treatment for burn-induced ileus, but it seems that early enteral feeding will prevent some of these potential complications.

Stress ulceration of the stomach and duodenum, on the other hand, can be prevented effectively with antacid therapy. In the 1970s stress ulceration leading to life-threatening hemorrhage was common. The mechanism of injury is related to an imbalance between protective factors such as mucus production, protective prostaglandin output, and bicarbonate secretion, and injurious factors such as decreased blood flow and acid production. Gastric ulcers develop in the watershed zones between capillary beds which are worsened by gastric acid-induced injury.

Antacid therapies and early enteral feeding have dramatically decreased the incidence of gastrointestinal ulceration and life-threatening hemorrhage after severe burn,[118] such that this complication is very rare in modern burn units. A number

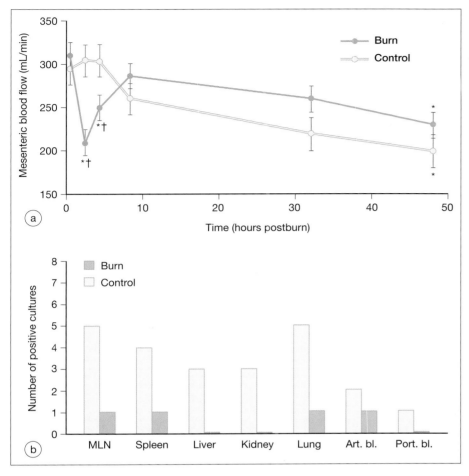

Fig. 34.11 (a) After a severe burn in pigs, superior mesenteric blood flow (solid line) decreased abruptly, then recovered with resuscitation. *$p = 0.05$ vs. baseline, †$p = 0.05$ vs. unburned controls (dotted line). (b) Bacterial tissue culture results from mesenteric lymph nodes (MLN), spleen, liver, kidney, lung, arterial blood (Art. bl.), and portal blood (Port. bl.) after sham injury (open bars) and severe burn (solid bars). (Reprinted with permission from Tokyay et al. J Appl Physiol 1993; 74:1521–1527. with permission. Copyright American Physiological Society.[130])

of types of therapies including gastric antacids, cimetidine, ranitidine, and sucralfate have been tested in various combinations or alone, all of which are equally effective. Some have even suggested that early enteral nutrition alone is sufficient.[119] A survey of critical care physicians found that most use histamine-2 antagonists such as ranitidine for stress ulceration prophylaxis, followed by sucralfate.[120] Regardless, it can be concluded that some type of prophylaxis against gastrointestinal hemorrhage is required in the severely burned, and will be very effective in preventing this complication.

Endocrinopathies

Hyperglycemia and insulin resistance are common in the critically ill, and the burned patient is no exception. In 2001, Greet van den Berghe reported in a landmark trial that intensive insulin treatment with continuous infusions of insulin aimed at normalizing blood glucose levels between 80 and 110 mg/dL improved mortality, and decreased bloodstream infections and acute renal failure.[121] Even more recently, she showed again that this treatment reduced renal insufficiency, ventilator requirement, intensive care unit length of stay, and mortality in those in the ICU for more than 3 days.[122] These studies are among the first to show some benefit of a treatment for all critically ill patients. Other investigators have shown the benefit of insulin treatment in burned patients,[123] particularly in terms of muscle mass.[124] Further evidence is accumulating for other beneficial

effects, and it has become the standard of care to avoid hyperglycemia in burned patients in the ICU with continuous insulin therapy. It remains to be seen whether the effects are mediated directly through insulin activity, if the effect is indirect through the avoidance of hyperglycemia, or both.

In another landmark trial, cortisol levels were found to be low in many critically ill patients and a mortality benefit accrued with physiological replacement with hydrocortisone.[125] This was followed by a trial of hydrocortisone in all critically ill patients with ARDS, and a mortality benefit was again seen.[126] These studies highlight that hypocortisolemia is at least associated with septic shock and hypotension, and that replacement with hydrocortisone at 50 mg every 6 hours improves outcomes. The same was seen in burned patients in the ICU.[127] It must be noted, however, that the benefits seem to be limited to those with relative adrenal insufficiency assessed by corticotropin stimulation. Regardless, in the case of hypotension not related to hypovolemia in burned patients, cortisol levels and adrenal stimulation should be performed to determine if relative adrenal insufficiency exists, and treatment with hydrocortisone should ensue.

Summary

Improved critical care of the severely burned has decreased mortality over the past two to three decades. This has been in part through the development of specialized units for care of burned patients which are equipped with the personnel and equipment to deliver state-of-the-art care. Better understanding of the processes of critical illness and multiple organ failure has led to effective prevention strategies and treatment modalities. Further advances in the understanding of mechanisms of the progression from SIRS to multiple organ failure will engender new breakthroughs that can be expected to further improve the outcomes of burned patients.

References

1. Brigham PA, McLoughlin E. Burn incidence and medical care in the United States: estimates, trends, and data sources. J Burn Care Rehabil 1996; 17:95–107.
2. Bull JP, Fisher AJ. A study in mortality in a burn unit: standards for the evaluation for alternative methods of treatment. Ann Surg 1949; 130:160–173.
3. Herndon DN, Gore DC, Cole M, et al. Determinants of mortality in pediatric patients with greater than 70% full thickness total body surface area treated by early excision and grafting. J Trauma 1987; 27:208–212.
4. Wolf SE, Rose JK, Desai MH, et al. Mortality determinants in massive pediatric burns: an analysis of 103 children with greater than 80% TBSA burns (70% full-thickness). Ann Surg 1997; 225:554–569.
5. Baue AE, Durham R, Faist E. Systemic inflammatory response syndrome (SIRS), multiple organ dysfunction syndrome (MODS), multiple organ failure (MOF): are we winning the battle? Shock 1998; 10:79–89.
6. Muckart DJ, Bhagwanjee S. American College of Chest Physicians/Society of Critical Care Medicine Consensus Conference definitions of the systemic inflammatory response syndrome and allied disorders in relation to critically injured patients. Crit Care Med 1997; 25:1789–1795.
7. Committee on Trauma of the American College of Surgeons. Guidelines for the operation of burn units. In: Resources for the optimal care of the injured patient. CTACS 1999:55–62.
8. Bruner JMR, Krewis LJ, Kunsman JM, et al. Comparison of direct and indirect methods of measuring arterial blood pressure. Med Instr 1981; 15:11–21.
9. Dorman T, Breslow MJ, Lipsett PA, et al. Radial artery pressure monitoring underestimates central arterial pressure during vasopressor therapy in critically ill surgical patients. Crit Care Med 1998; 26:1646–1649.
10. Park MK, Robotham JL, German VF. Systolic amplification in pedal arteries of children. Crit Care Med 2000; 11:286–289.
11. Chatterjee T, Do DD, Mahler F, et al. A prospective randomized evaluation of nonsurgical closure of femoral pseudoaneurysm by compression device with and without ultrasound guidance. Catheter Cardiovasc Interv 1999; 47:304–309.
12. Connors AF, Speroff T, Dawson NV, et al. The effectiveness of right heart catheterization in the initial care of critically ill patients. JAMA 1996; 276:889–897.
13. Dalen JE, Bone RC. Is it time to pull the pulmonary artery catheter? JAMA 1996; 276:916–919.
14. Aikawa N, Martyn JA, Burke JF. Pulmonary artery catheterization and thermodilution cardiac output determination in the management of critically burned patients. Am J Surg 1978; 135:811–817.
15. Reynolds EM, Ryan DP, Sheridan RL, et al. Left ventricular failure complicating severe pediatric burn injuries. J Pediatr Surg 1995; 30:264–269.
16. Schiller WR, Bay RC, Garren RL, et al. Hyperdynamic resuscitation improves survival in patients with life-threatening burns. J Burn Care Rehabil 1997; 18:10–16.
17. Schiller WR, Bay RC, Mclachlan JG, et al. Survival in major burn injuries is predicted by early response to Swan-Ganz-guided resuscitation. Am J Surg 1995; 170:696–699.
18. Shoemaker WC, Appel PL, Kram HB, et al. Prospective trial of supranormal values of survivors as therapeutic goals in high-risk surgical patients. Chest 1988; 94:1176–1186.
19. Gattinoni L, Brazzi L, Pelosi P, et al. A trial of goal-oriented hemodynamic therapy in critically ill patients. SvO$_2$ Collaborative Group. N Engl J Med 1995; 333:1025–1032.
20. Vincent JL, Thirion M, Brimioulle S, et al. Thermodilution measurement of right ventricular ejection fraction with a modified pulmonary artery catheter. Intensive Care Med 1986; 12:33–38.
21. Haller M, Zollner C, Briegel J, et al. Evaluation of a new continuous thermodilution cardiac output monitor in critically ill patients: a prospective criterion standard study. Crit Care Med 1995; 23:860–866.
22. Rutherford EJ, Morris JA Jr, Reed GW, et al. Base deficit stratifies mortality and determines therapy. J Trauma 1992; 33:417–423.
23. Kaups KL, Davis JW, Dominic WJ. Base deficit as an indicator or resuscitation needs in patients with burn injuries. J Burn Care Rehabil 1998; 19:346–348.
24. Jeng JC, Lee K, Jablonski K, et al. Serum lactate and base deficit suggest inadequate resuscitation of patients with burn injuries: application of a point-of-care laboratory instrument. J Burn Care Rehabil 1997; 18:402–405.
25. Kim K, Kwok I, Chang H, et al. Comparison of cardiac outputs of major burn patients undergoing extensive early escharectomy: esophageal Doppler monitor versus thermodilution pulmonary artery catheter. J Trauma 2005; 59:506–507.
26. Gueugniaud PY, David JS, Petit P. Early hemodynamic variations assessed by an echo-Doppler aortic blood flow device in a severely burned infant: correlation with the circulating cytokines. Pediatr Emerg Care 1998; 14: 282–284.
27. Kuwagata Y, Sugimoto H, Yoshioka T, et al. Left ventricular performance in patients with thermal injury or multiple trauma: a clinical study with echocardiography. J Trauma 1992; 32: 158–164.
28. Papp A, Uusaro A, Parviainen I, et al. Myocardial function and haemodynamics in extensive burn trauma: evaluation by clinical signs, invasive monitoring, echocardiography and cytokine concentrations. A prospective clinical study. Acta Anaesthesiol Scand 2003; 10:1257–1263.
29. Holm C, Melcer B, Horbrand F, et al. Arterial thermodilution: an alternative to pulmonary artery catheter for cardiac output assessment in burn patients. Burns 2001; 27:161–166.
30. Holm C, Melcer B, Horbrand F, et al. Intrathoracic blood volume as an end point in resuscitation of the severely burned: an observational study of 24 patients. J Trauma 2000; 48:728–734.
31. Zavala E, Ferrer M, Polese G, et al. Effect of inverse I:E ratio ventilation on pulmonary gas exchange in acute respiratory distress syndrome. Anesthesiology 1998; 88:35–42.
32. Ludwigs U, Klingstedt C, Baehrendtz S, et al. A comparison of pressure- and volume-controlled ventilation at different inspiratory to expiratory ratios. Acta Anaesthesiol Scand 1997; 41:71–77.
33. Derdak S, Mehta S, Stewart T, et al. High frequency oscillatory ventilation for acute respiratory distress syndrome: a randomized controlled trial. Am J Respir Crit Care Med 2002; 166:801–808.
34. Cartotto R, Ellis S, Gomez M, et al. High frequency oscillatory ventilation in burned patients with acute respiratory distress syndrome. Burns 2004; 30:453–463.
35. Cioffi WG, Graves TA, McManus WF, et al. High-frequency percussive ventilation in patients with inhalation injury. J Trauma 1989; 29:350–354.
36. Cortiella J, Mlcak R, Herndon D. High frequency percussive ventilation in pediatric patients with inhalation injury. J Burn Care Rehabil 1999; 20:232–235.
37. Mlcak R, Cortiella J, Desai M, et al. Lung compliance, airway resistance, and work of breathing in children after inhalation injury. J Burn Care Rehabil 1997; 18:531–534.
38. Paulsen SM, Killyon GW, Barillo DJ. High frequency percussive ventilation as a salvage modality in adult respiratory distress syndrome; a preliminary study. Am Surg 2002; 68:852–856.

39. Patel S, Sandu R, Miller K, et al. Evaluation of airway pressure release ventilation compared to low tidal volume ventilation in ALI: prospective randomized pilot study. Crit Care Med 2004; 32: A117.

40. Ream RS, Hauver JF, Lynch RE, et al. Low-dose inhaled nitric oxide improves the oxygenation and ventilation of infants and children with acute, hypoxemic respiratory failure. Crit Care Med 1999; 27:989–996.

41. Sheridan RL, Zapol WM, Ritz RH, et al. Low-dose inhaled nitric oxide in acutely burned children with profound respiratory failure. Surgery 1999; 126:856–862.

42. Brower RG, Shanholtz CB, Fessler HE, et al. Prospective, randomized, controlled clinical trial comparing traditional versus reduced tidal volume ventilation in acute respiratory distress syndrome patients. Crit Care Med 1999; 27:1492–1498.

43. Brochard L, Roudot-Thoraval F, Roupie E, et al. Tidal volume reduction for prevention of ventilator-induced lung injury in acute respiratory distress syndrome. The Multicenter Trial Group on Tidal Volume Reduction in ARDS. Am J Respir Crit Care Med 1998; 158:1831–1838.

44. The Acute Respiratory Distress Syndrome Network. Ventilation with lower tidal volumes as compared with traditional tidal volumes for acute lung injury and acute respiratory distress syndrome. N Engl J Med 2000; 342:1301–1308.

45. Gattinoni L, Bombino M, Pelosi P, et al. Lung structure and function in different stages of severe adult respiratory distress syndrome. JAMA 1994; 271:1772–1779.

46. Wolter TP, Fuchs PC, Horvat N, et al. Is high PEEP low volume ventilation in burned patients beneficial? A retrospective study of 61 patients. Burns 2004; 30:368–373.

47. Esteban A, Frutos F, Tobin MJ, et al. A comparison of four methods of weaning patients from mechanical ventilation. N Engl J Med 1995; 332:345–350.

48. Habashi NM. Other approaches to open-lung ventilation: airway pressure release ventilation. Crit Care Med 2005; 33:S228–S240.

49. Tremper KK, Barker SJ. Pulse oximetry. Anesthesiology 1989; 70:98–108.

50. Tanaka H, Mituo T, Yukioka T, et al. Comparison of hemodynamic changes resulting from toxic shock syndrome toxin-1-producing Staphylococcus aureus sepsis and endotoxin-producing gram-negative rod sepsis in patients with severe burns. J Burn Care Rehabil 1995; 16:616–621.

51. Rhee P, Waxman K, Clark L, et al. Superoxide dismutase polyethylene glycol improves survival in hemorrhagic shock. Am Surg 1991; 57:747–750.

52. Schiller HJ, Reilly PM, Bulkley GB. Tissue perfusion in critical illnesses. Antioxidant therapy. Crit Care Med 1993; 21: S92–S102.

53. Mileski WJ, Winn RK, Vedder NB, et al. Inhibition of CD18-dependent neutrophil adherence reduces organ injury after hemorrhagic shock in primates. Surgery 1990; 108:206–212.

54. Carter EA, Gonnella A, Tompkins RG. Increased transcellular permeability of rat small intestine after thermal injury. Burns 1992; 18:117–120.

55. Deitch EA. Intestinal permeability is increased in burn patients shortly after injury. Surgery 1990; 107:411–416.

56. Chertow GM, Christiansen CL, Cleary PD, et al. Prognostic stratification in critically ill patients with acute renal failure requiring dialysis. Arch Intern Med 1995; 155:1505–1511.

57. Jeschke MG, Wolf SE, Barrow RE, et al. Mortality in burned children with acute renal failure. Arch Surg 1998; 134:752–756.

58. Conger JD, Robinette JB, Hammond WS. Differences in vascular reactivity in models of ischemic acute renal failure. Kidney Int 1991; 39:1087–1097.

59. Kellerman PS, Clark RA, Hoilien CA, et al. Role of microfilaments in maintenance of proximal tubule structural and functional integrity. Am J Physiol 1990; 259:F279–F285.

60. Goligorsky MS, DiBona GF. Pathogenic role of Arg-Gly-Asp recognizing integrins in acute renal failure. Proc Natl Acad Sci USA 1993; 90:5700–5704.

61. Pascual M, Orofino L, Liano F, et al. Prognosis of acute renal failure among elderly patients. J Am Geriatr Soc 1991; 39:102–103.

62. Lindner A, Cutler RE, Goodman G. Synergism of dopamine plus furosemide in preventing acute renal failure in the dog. Kidney Int 1979; 16:158–166.

63. Ichai C, Passeron C, Carles M, et al. Prolonged low-dose dopamine infusion induces a transient improvement in renal function in hemodynamically stable, critically ill patients: a single-blind, prospective, controlled study. Crit Care Med 2000; 28:1329–1335.

64. Marik PE, Iglesias J. Low-dose dopamine does not prevent acute renal failure in patients with septic shock and oliguria. NORASEPT II Study Investigators. Am J Med 1999; 107:387–390.

65. Neumayer HH, Junge W, Kufner A, et al. Prevention of radiocontrast media induced nephrotoxicity by the calcium channel blocker nitrendipine: a prospective randomized clinical trial. Nephrol Dial Transplant 1989; 4:1030–1036.

66. Rahman SN, Kim GE, Mathew AS, et al. Effects of atrial natriuretic peptide in clinical acute renal failure. Kidney Int 1994; 45:1731–1738.

67. Allgren RL, Marbury TC, Rahman SN, et al. Anaritide in acute tubular necrosis. Auriculin Anaritide Acute Renal Failure Study Group. N Engl J Med 1997; 336:828–834.

68. Lewis J, Salem MM, Weisburg et al. Atrial natriuretic factor in oliguric acute renal failure. Anaritide Acute Renal Failure Study Group. Am J Kidney Dis 2001; 37:454–465.

69. Morelli A, Ricci Z, Bellomo R. Prophylactic fenoldopam for renal protection in sepsis: a randomized double-blind placebo controlled pilot trial. Crit Care Med 2005; 33:2451–2456.

70. Bellomo R, Parkin G, Love J, et al. A prospective comparative study of continuous arteriovenous hemofiltration and continuous venovenous hemodiafiltration in critically ill patients. Am J Kidney Dis 1993; 21:400–404.

71. Bellomo R, Tipping P, Boyne N. Continuous veno-venous hemofiltration with dialysis removes cytokines from the circulation of septic patients. Crit Care Med 1993; 21:522–526.

72. Leblanc M, Thibeault Y, Querin S. Continuous haemofiltration and haemodiafiltration for acute renal failure in severely burned patients. Burns 1997; 23:160–165.

73. Pomeranz A, Reichenberg Y, Schurr D, et al. Acute renal failure in a burn patient: the advantages of continuous peritoneal dialysis. Burns Incl Therm Inj 1985; 11:367–370.

74. Ware LB, Matthay MA. The acute respiratory distress syndrome. N Engl J Med 2000; 342:1334–1349.

75. Bachofen M, Weibel ER. Structural alterations of lung parenchyma in the adult respiratory distress syndrome. Clin Chest Med 1982; 3:35–56.

76. Ware LB, Matthay MA. Maximal alveolar epithelial fluid clearance in clinical acute lung injury: an excellent predictor of survival and the duration of mechanical ventilation. Am J Respir Crit Care Med 1999; 159:Suppl: A694. abstract.

77. Laufe MD, Simon RH, Flint A, et al. Adult respiratory distress syndrome in neutropenic patients. Am J Med 1986; 80:1022–1026.

78. Pratt PC, Vollmer RT, Shelburne JD, et al. Pulmonary morphology in a multihospital collaborative extracorporeal membrane oxygenation project. Am J Pathol 1979; 95:191–214.

79. Dreyfuss D, Soler P, Basset G, et al. High inflation pressure pulmonary edema: respective effects of high airway pressure, high tidal volume, and positive end-expiratory pressure. Am Rev Respir Dis 2000; 137:1159–1164.

80. Ware LB, Golden JA, Finkbeiner WE, et al. Alveolar epithelial fluid transport capacity in reperfusion lung injury after lung transplantation. Am J Respir Crit Care Med 1999; 159:980–988.

81. Fukuda Y, Ishizaki M, Masuda Y, et al. The role of intraalveolar fibrosis in the process of pulmonary structural remodeling in patients with diffuse alveolar damage. Am J Pathol 1992; 126:171–182.

82. Martin C, Papazian L, Payan MJ, et al. Pulmonary fibrosis correlates with outcome in adult respiratory distress syndrome: a study in mechanically ventilated patients. Chest 1995; 107:196–200.

83. Matthay MA, Folkesson HG, Verkman AS. Salt and water transport across alveolar and distal airway epithelia in the adult lung. Am J Physiol 1996; 270:L487–L503.

84. Folkesson HG, Matthay MA, Westrom BR, et al. Alveolar epithelial clearance of protein. J Appl Physiol 1996; 80:1431–1435.

85. Liffner G, Bak Z, Reske A, et al. Inhalation injury assessed by score does not contribute to the development of acute respiratory distress syndrome in burned victims. Burns 2005; 31:263–268.

86. Morris AH, Wallace CJ, Menlove RL, et al. Randomized clinical trial of pressure-controlled inverse ratio ventilation and extracorporeal CO₂ removal for adult respiratory distress syndrome. Am J Respir Crit Care Med 2000; 149:295–305.

87. Pierre EJ, Zwischenberger JB, Angel C, et al. Extracorporeal membrane oxygenation in the treatment of respiratory failure in pediatric patients with burns. J Burn Care Rehabil 1998; 19:131–134.

88. Falke KJ, Pontappidan H, Kumar A, et al. Ventilation with end-expiratory pressure in acute lung disease. J Clin Invest 1972; 51:2315–2323.

89. Gattinoni L, Presenti A, Bombino M, et al. Relationships between lung computed tomographic density, gas exchange, and PEEP in acute respiratory failure. Anesthesiology 1988; 69:824–832.

90. Pepe PE, Hudson LD, Carrico CJ. Early application of positive end expiratory pressure in patients at risk from adult respiratory distress syndrome. N Engl J Med 1984; 311:281–286.

91. Amato MB, Barbas CS, Medeiros DM, et al. Effect of a protective ventilation strategy on mortality in acute respiratory distress syndrome. N Engl J Med 1998; 338:347–354.

92. Long W, Thompson T, Sundell H, et al. Effects of two rescue doses of a synthetic surfactant on mortality rate and survival without bronchopulmonary dysplasia in 700 to 1350 gram infants with respiratory distress syndrome. J Pediatr 1991; 118:595–605.

93. Anzueto A, Baughman RP, Guntupalli KK, et al. Aerosolized surfactant in adults with sepsis induced acute respiratory distress syndrome. N Engl J Med 1996; 334:1417–1421.

94. Dellinger RP, Zimmerman JL, Taylor RW, et al. Effects of inhaled nitric oxide in patients with acute respiratory failure: results of a randomized phase II trial. Crit Care Med 1998; 26:15–23.

95. Prewitt RM, Wood LDH. Effect of sodium nitroprusside on cardiovascular function and pulmonary shunt in canine oleic acid pulmonary edema. Anesthesiology 1981; 55:537–541.

96. Abraham E, Baughman R, Fletcher E, et al. Liposomal prostaglandin E₁ (TLC C-53) in acute respiratory distress syndrome: a controlled, randomized, double-blind, multicenter trial. Crit Care Med 1999; 27:1478–1485.

97. Bernard GR, Luce JM, Sprung CL, et al. High-dose corticosteroids in patients with adult respiratory distress syndrome. N Engl J Med 1987; 317:1565–1570.

98. Meduri GU, Chinn AJ, Leeper KV, et al. Corticosteroid rescue treatment of progressive fibroproliferation in late ARDS. Patterns of response and predictors of outcome. Chest 1994; 105: 1516–1527.

99. Meduri GU, Headley AS, Golden E, et al. Effect of prolonged methylprednisolone therapy in unresolving acute respiratory distress syndrome: a randomized controlled trial. JAMA 1998; 280:159–165.

100. Suzuki K, Nishina M, Ogino R, et al. Left ventricular contractility and diastolic properties in anesthetized dogs after severe burns. Am J Physiol 1991; 260:H1433–H1442.

101. Cioffi WG, DeMeules JE, Gamelli RL. The effects of burn injury and fluid resuscitation on cardiac function in vitro. J Trauma 1986; 26:638–642.

102. Breitenstein E, Chiolero RL, Jequier E, et al. Effects of beta-blockade on energy metabolism following burns. Burns 1990; 16:259–264.

103. Wilmore DW, Long JM, Mason AD, et al. Catecholamines: mediators of the hypermetabolic response in thermally burned patients. Ann Surg 1974; 180:280–290.

104. Baron PW, Barrow RE, Pierre EJ, et al. Prolonged use of propranolol safely decreases cardiac work in burned children. J Burn Care Rehabil 1997; 18:223–227.

105. Honeycutt D, Barrow RE, Herndon DN. Cold stress response in patients with severe burns after beta blockade. J Burn Care Rehabil 1992; 13:181–186.

106. Aarsland AA, Chinkes DL, Wolfe RR, et al. Beta-blockade lowers peripheral lipolysis in burn patients receiving growth hormone.

107. Herndon DN, Hart DW, Wolf SE, et al. Propranolol decreases muscle catabolism associated with severe burn. N Engl J Med 2001; 345:1223–1229.

Rate of hepatic very low density lipoprotein triglyceride secretion remains unchanged. Ann Surg 1996; 223:777–789.

108. Chung DH, Evers BM, Townsend CM, et al. Role of polyamine biosynthesis during gut mucosal adaptation after burn injury. Am J Surg 1993; 165:144–149.

109. Wolf SE, Ikeda H, Matin S, et al. Cutaneous burn increases apoptosis in the gut epithelium of mice. J Am Coll Surg 1999; 188:10–16.

110. Carter EA, Udall JN, Kirkham SE, et al. Thermal injury and gastrointestinal function. I. Small intestinal nutrient absorption and DNA synthesis. J Burn Care Rehabil 1986; 7:469–474.

111. Carter EA, Tompkins RG, Schiffrin E, et al. Cutaneous thermal injury alters macromolecular permeability of rat small intestine. Surgery 1990; 107:335–341.

112. Ryan CM, Bailey SH, Carter EA, et al. Additive effects of thermal injury and infection on gut permeability. Arch Surg 1994; 129:325–328.

113. Berthiaume F, Ezzell RM, Toner M, et al. Transport of fluorescent dextrans across the rat ileum after cutaneous thermal injury. Crit Care Med 1994; 22:455–464.

114. Horton JW. Bacterial translocation after burn injury: the contribution of ischemia and permeability changes. Shock 1994; 1:286–290.

115. Gianotti L, Alexander JW, Fukushima R, et al. Translocation of Candida albicans is related to the blood flow of individual intestinal villi. Circ Shock 1993; 40:250–257.

116. Wolf SE, Jeschke MG, Rose JK, et al. Enteral feeding intolerance: an indicator of sepsis associated mortality in burned children. Arch Surg 1997; 132:1310–1314.

117. Herndon DN, Barrow RE, Stein M, et al. Increased mortality with intravenous supplemental feeding in severely burned patients. J Burn Care Rehabil 1989; 10:309–313.

118. Moscona R, Kaufman T, Jacobs R, et al. Prevention of gastrointestinal bleeding in burns: the effects of cimetidine or antacids combined with early enteral feeding. Burns Incl Therm Inj 1985; 12:65–67.

119. Raff T, Germann G, Hartmann B. The value of early enteral nutrition in the prophylaxis of stress ulceration in the severely burned patient. Burns 1997; 23:313–318.

120. Lam NP, Le PD, Crawford SY, Patel S. National survey of stress ulcer prophylaxis. Crit Care Med 1999; 27:98–103.

121. van den Berghe G, Wouters P, Weekers F, et al. Intensive insulin therapy in the critically ill patients. N Engl J Med 2001; 345:1359–1367.

122. Van den Berghe G, Wilmer A, Hermans G, et al. Intensive insulin therapy in the medical ICU. N Engl J Med 2006; 354:449–461.

123. Pham TN, Warren AJ, Phan HH, et al. Impact of tight glycemic control in severely burned children. J Trauma 2005; 59: 1148–1154.

124. Thomas SJ, Morimoto K, Herndon DN, et al. The effect of prolonged euglycemic hyperinsulinemia on lean body mass after severe burn. Surgery 2002; 132:341–347.

125. Annane D, Sebille V, Charpentier C, et al. Effect of treatment with low doses of hydrocortisone and fludrocortisone on mortality in patients with septic shock. JAMA 2002; 288:862–871.

126. Annane D, Sebille V, Bellissant E, Ger-Inf-05 Study Group. Effect of low doses of corticosteroids in septic shock patients with or without early acute respiratory distress syndrome. Crit Care Med 2006; 34:236–238.

127. Winter W, Kamolz L, Donner A, et al. Hydrocortisone improved haemodynamics and fluid requirement in surviving but not non-surviving of severely burned patients. Burns 2003; 29:717–720.

128. Shapiro BA, Lacmak RM, Care RD, et al. Clinical application of respiratory care. St Louis, MO: Mosby Year Book; 1991.

129. Myers BD, Moran SM. Hemodynamically mediated renal failure. N Engl J Med 1986; 314:97–105.

130. Tokyay R, Zeigler ST, Traber DL, et al. Post-burn gastrointestinal vasoconstriction increases bacterial and endotoxin translocation. J Appl Physiol 1993; 74:1521–1527.

Chapter 35

Burn nursing

Mary Gordon and Janet Marvin

Acute care

Healthcare continues to change. It is described as rapid, overwhelming, chaotic, and problematic. Thus, some models of healthcare service are creating a flattening of the traditional organizational pyramid. It is replaced by decen-tralized decision-making and professional autonomy at the bedside. These changes require different skill sets to address the needs of facilitating and advancing clinical work. It requires a more professional and emotional maturity from practitioners regarding their relationship to their own work and their willingness to change their practices.

There are new issues in nursing practice today: clinical judgment and evidence-based practice. Nurses operate in an age of accountability where quality and cost issues drive healthcare. The public demands high-quality results (better outcomes). Evidence-based practice integrates providers' clinical expertise with the best evidence. It helps nurses structure how to make accurate and timely decisions. It improves the odds of doing the right thing at the right time for the patient. Closing the gap between research and practice affects all aspects of medical care. Workplaces must support the use of evidence-based practice (EBP) by creating structures and processes, building the infrastructure to support EBP.

Practicing nurses today need strong and effective clinical leadership. In today's settings, every nurse is a leader, using knowledge and skills to make decisions, and accepting accountability for competent care and safe patient outcomes. Transformational leadership is well suited to nursing in the clinical environment. It repositions staff nurses from the bottom of the organization pyramid to the center. Each nurse emerges as a leader when the clinical situation demands. Power is not given away, but rather partnerships develop between nurses at the bedside and management. Management becomes a partner and resource as opposed to a controlling force. Attractive work environments for professional people recognize the contributions of each individual and value the power necessary for each partner to participate fully.

Introduction

The care of the burn patient is most challenging for the nurse. Care begins with the immediate resuscitation of the patient in the emergency department and continues until the patient is completely rehabilitated. During the intitial resuscitation the role of the nurse is to assess and monitor the patient's hemodynamic alterations. Fluid resuscitation and nursing management of fluid resuscitation are adequately discussed in Chapter 9 in this book. Therefore this chapter will cover other areas where the nurse's care and management are crucial.

Pulmonary priorities

Inhalation injury continues to be the most serious and life-threatening complication of burn injury today. Early diagnosis and treatment greatly impact the outcome of care.

Impaired gas exchange is a potential problem for patients who have face and neck burns and/or inhalation injury. Inhalation injury may include carbon monoxide poisoning, upper airway injury (heat injury above the glottis), lower airway injury (chemical injury to lung parenchyma), and restrictive defects (circumferential third-degree burn around the chest). Upper airway edema causes respiratory distress and is the primary concern during the initial 24–48 hours postburn phase. Tracheobronchitis, atelectasis, bronchorrhea, pneumonia, and adult respiratory distress syndrome (ARDS) may occur during the acute, postburn stage either related or unrelated to inhalation injury.

Nursing care of a patient with inhalation injury begins with a detailed history of the accident. Inhalation injury is suspected when the accident occurred in a closed space. Close observation of the patient and frequent respiratory assessments are made throughout the initial and acute phase postburn. Initially, the patient is observed for hoarseness and stridor, which indicate narrowed airways. Emergency equipment is placed at the bedside to facilitate intubation if necessary. Observing the frequency of cough, carbonaceous sputum, and increased inability to handle secretions may indicate possible inhalation injury and the potential for impaired gas exchange. Other important observations include respiratory rate, breath sounds, use of accessory muscles to aid in respiratory effort, nasal flaring, sternal retractions, increased anxiety, and complaint of shortness of breath. Disorientation, obtundation, and coma may be due to significant exposure to smoke toxins such as carbon monoxide or cyanide. These conditions are managed emergently with 100% oxygen.

Bronchoscopy may be done early to diagnose inhalation injury as well as facilitate airway clearance. Humidified oxygen should be readily available and applied to patients who have evidence of impaired gas exchange (especially pediatric patients). Aggressive nasotracheal suction may be indicated if the patient has difficulty with managing secretions either because of the increased amount of secretions and/or the decreased effectiveness of the cough. In addition, aggressive pulmonary toilet, including turning, coughing, and deep breathing, up and out-of-bed rocking in mother's arms may be done regularly and frequently. Elevation of the head of the bed, unless contraindicated, will also support and possibly improve ventilation. Trends and changes should be correlated with laboratory results and shared with the team.

Another complication is circumferential third-degree burns around the chest and neck, which often cause restrictive defects. The increased amount of edema combined with decreased chest excursion may greatly decrease tidal volume. This condition may progress and can become life-threatening, in which case chest escharotomy may be necessary to release the constricting eschar. The procedure may be done at the bedside or in the operating room. Equipment includes sterile drapes, scalpel, and Bovie (to control bleeding).

Intubation and mechanical ventilation may be required to improve gas exchange. Tube placement should be checked and documented frequently and verified daily by x-ray. Securing the endotracheal tube requires a standard technique for stabilization and prevention of pressure necrosis. Adequate humidity is necessary to prevent secretions from drying and causing mucous plugging. Remember to provide pre/post-suctioning hyperoxygenation. Sterile technique is used when suctioning to prevent infection. Attention to the details of oral hygiene will provide comfort for the patient and may reduce the occurrence of ventilator-associated pneumonia related to colongation in the the oral pharynx.[1]

Criteria for extubation depend on why the tube was inserted initially, but, overall, stable vital signs and hemodynamic parameters will support the plan for extubation. The patient should be awake and alert in order to protect the airway; therefore, pain medications may be reduced before extubation. Ventilatory measurements and blood gas analysis should be within normal limits.

Immediately following extubation, the nurse must be alert for signs and symptoms of respiratory distress, administer suction as needed, monitor blood gas measurements, provide optimal positioning for ventilation, as well as provide reassurance and support to decrease anxiety.

Age, burn size, and the presence of inhalation injury and pneumonia have been identified as major contributors to mortality.[2] Thus, vigilant nursing care (frequent nursing assessments, aggressive pulmonary toilet, etc.) combined with anticipating potential problems and being prepared to deal with the problems will add to the team effort and possibly improve the patient outcome.

Burn wound care

The primary goal for burn wound management is to close the wound as soon as possible. Prompt surgical excisions of the eschar and skin grafting have contributed to reduced morbidity and mortality in severely burned patients.[3–5]

Wound care in the burn unit has become an art of burn nursing practice. It can be extremely challenging and complicated and, for a new nurse, it can be the most difficult and misunderstood part of burn nursing. The complexity exists because there are many different wounds that require different interventions in relation to time postburn or time postoperative. Wound assessment and care is a learned skill that develops over time. The expert burn nurse must teach these skills to new burn nurses in the hydrotherapy area, and operating room, and at the bedside.

Wounds may consist of eschar, pseudoeschar, skin buds, autograft, donor sites, hypermature granulating tissue, blisters, and exposed bone and tendons. Besides the many kinds of possible wounds, there are many topical antibacterial agents available for managing wounds. These choices raise many decisions for the team to address. Topical antimicrobial creams and ointments include mafenide acetate, silver nitrate, silver sulfadiazine, petroleum and mineral oil-based antibacterial products, and Mycostatin powder. Wounds may be treated in the open fashion (topicals without dressings) or closed fashion (topicals with dressings or soaks). Also there are many, many techniques for applying dressings to every area of the body to withstand exercise, ambulation, and moving around in bed. Biological dressings such as homograft or heterograft may be used as temporary wound coverage. Dressings may also be synthetic or biosynthetic or silver impregnated. Selection is based on the present condition of the wound and the expected outcome.

Secondary goals of wound care are to promote healing and to maintain function of the affected body part. These goals are accomplished by preventing wound infection, treating wound infection, preventing graft loss and tissue necrosis, providing personal hygiene, and maintaining correct positioning and splinting throughout hospitalization. To prevent burn wound infection, the burn nurse must use clean technique: cleanse the wound with soap and water; debride the wound of loose necrotic tissue, crusts, dried blood, and exudate; and apply topicals and/or dressings and change as often as ordered. The nurse must inspect the wound for evidence of infection: cellulitis, odor, increased wound exudate, and/or change in exudate; change in wound appearance; and increased pain in the wound. The physician should be notified so that changes in wound care can be made. Cultures and biopsies may be ordered to identify the type and count of organisms and treat with a specific systemic antibiotic and/or topical dressing and/or soak. The wound is often the source of sepsis in the bloodstream. The five cardinal signs of sepsis are: hyperventilation, thrombocytopenia, hyperglycemia, disorientation, and hypothermia.[6]

Preventing graft loss is another wound care challenge for nursing. Usually the patient returns from the operating room in a position that is maintained for 3 or 4 days. Any interaction with the patient during this time of graft immobilization requires creativity and care in order to prevent shearing of the graft. Postoperative dressings on the thighs and back are protected with polymycin, fine-mesh gauze to prevent soiling by feces and to minimize cleanup. The dressings are continuously monitored for increased drainage and odor, which would indicate possible wound infection. If infection is suspected, then the postoperative dressings may be removed early for a closer inspection of the wound.

Donor sites will also require additional care to prevent infection. Of course, the care postoperatively depends on the coverage of the donor site. If the donor site is covered with fine-mesh gauze, the initial care is to ensure homeostasis and adherence of the gauze to the wound. Therefore the post-op pressure dressing remains intact for 6–12 hours and is then removed. The focus of managing the donor site is to keep the wound dry. If grafts/donor sites are on the back or backs of the legs, the patient is placed in a Clinitron bed for 4–5 days to promote drying. If the donor site remains wet, additional drying techniques (hair dryers, external heaters) may be used periodically during the day.[7]

If the donor site is covered with a synthetic or biological dressing, the same principles apply. Basically, apply a pressure dressing to ensure adherence to the wound for a short period of time postoperative and then expose to the air to support drying of the wound. A bed cradle is used to keep bed linen from contacting the wounds. The location of the graft, donor site, and eschar may all be on the same extremity, which again requires creativity to accomplish all three interventions of care.

Nurses today must accept the challenge of preventing pressure ulcers in major burn patients. No longer is it OK to treat the ulcer as though it is a burn wound. We need evidence to support our nursing practices to prevent pressure ulcers in burn patients because they have many risk factors that predispose to the development of pressure ulcers. Initially, hypovolemic shock with blood flow shunted away from the skin to preserve vital organ function is a factor. Additional injuries may add to the increased risk for pressure ulcers, such as: inhalation injury, which may require intubation and use of paralytic agents to manage the airway. As fluid resuscitation is begun, massive edema in both burned and unburned areas may occur. The edema is maximized at about 2–3 days postburn, which also decreases the blood flow to the skin and adds weight to all parts of the body.

Maintaining systemic hydration can continue to be a problem long after the patient has received adequate resuscitation for burn shock. Continued fluid therapy to replace fluid loss through the burn wound is essential. If systemic hydration is not maintained, even normal skin may be at risk. To complicate this situation, the quantity of fluid lost through the burn wound may increase the moisture on normal skin adjacent to the burn wound. This moisture may cause the normal skin to break down and predispose the skin to further compromise.

Many burn-injured patients will make repeated trips to the operating room for surgical excision of the burn wound and grafting, with graft taken from unburned areas. These procedures may require the patient to be anesthetized for long periods of time. Patients are at risk for pressure ulcers in the operating room, which necessitates the use of pressure-reducing devices. Likewise during these operative procedures the patient may loose large quantities of blood and/or may develop septic shock, resulting in decreased tissue perfusion. Vasopressors, antibiotics, and fluid resuscitation are the usual treatment for septic shock. The low-flow states and the use of vasopressors may also result in decreased tissue perfusion and increased risk of pressure sore formation.

Post surgery the patient is often immobilized with large bulky dressings and splints to protect the graft. These dressings need to be put on with enough pressure to stop the bleeding from the grafted wound and the donor site. But if the dressings are applied too tightly, or if edema develops after dressing application, this pressure may cause increased pressure on the skin.

Throughout the acute phase of care the burn patient is predisposed to pain and anxiety. Pain in the burn wound and fear of pain causes patients to try not to move. Careful titration of anxiolytics and narcotics can result in an alert patient that is relatively pain free but requires intense attention to detail from the nursing staff.

To prevent wound bed desiccation, soaks are used to maintain moisture in the grafted wound and to aid in decreasing wound colonization with bacteria. This moisture, when in contact with adjacent normal skin, may increase the risk of tissue breakdown.

Inadequate nutrition prior to or after the burn injury is potentially a significant problem. The hypermetabolic response in the burn-injured patient leads to protein malnutrition if caloric intake is compromised. To reduce the risks of systemic infection and to promote wound healing, enteral hyperalimentation is most frequently used and the patient is fed by nasogastric or nasojejunal tubes.

In summary, the physiology of the burn injury combined with many of the therapies and treatments during hospitalization impacts the burn patient's risk for pressure ulcers. Burn patients are among the high-risk populations for pressure ulcer development.

All patients, except those with skin grafts postoperatively, will benefit from a bath or shower. Large acute burns are placed on a shower cart and the wounds are gently showered with warm water. The overhead heater is on and the room temperature is 85°F (29°C) or above. Large acute burns are not immersed in a tub of water, so as to prevent autocontamination and electrolyte imbalance.[8] Time in the hydrotherapy area can be used for careful observation of the wound as well as personal hygiene such as shampoo, mouth care, face care, and perineal care.

The hydrotherapy area affords an excellent opportunity for teaching the patient and family about wound care and dressing application. As the patient gets closer to discharge, families are required to do more of the care. The trend for earlier release from the hospital poses additional challenges for nursing since it reduces the time available to prepare the patient for discharge. The better the patient and families are educated, the better the outcome will be. Early involvement with patient and family helps identify potential obstacles at discharge and facilitates care coordination in the discharge process.

Metabolic and nutritional support

Hypermetabolism, or metabolic stress, is the direct response to a burn injury. The amount of stress increases proportionally to the extent of the injury and strongly influences a patient's nutritional requirements. This response can magnify the normal metabolic rate by 200%. Malnutrition, starvation, and delayed wound healing will result if calories are not provided consistently to meet nutritional requirements. Children require more calorie and protein replacement than adults, because they have additional nutritional demands to support growth and development.

Monitoring output and managing nutritional intake are among nursing's primary responsibilities. An accurate record of intake and output is critical to patient care because potential problems can be detected early and alternate options of care can be individualized to help the patient achieve his/her goals. Accurate weights, daily or as ordered, are also important. Remember to record whether dressings, splints, or linens are included in the weight. Obviously, including additional elements does not reflect an accurate weight, but trends in weight either up or down may be identified and may be helpful in the overall management of the patient.

Typically, when patients cannot consume enough calories by mouth, then enteral feedings are begun. Sometimes enteral feedings are started before the patient is given the option of eating because the amount of calories is so great and/or the condition of the patient is unstable. Parenteral nutrition is used when enteral fails. The goal is to provide adequate nutrients, calories, and protein. A nasogastric tube is inserted initially and used to decompress the stomach until bowel sounds return. Then tube feedings are started at a very low volume per hour to act as a buffer against ulcer formation. The nasogastric tube allows for checking hourly gastric residuals, gastric pH, and guaiac. If the gastric pH falls below 5, or if the guaiac is positive, Maalox and Amphagel are given every 2 hours, alternately every hour.

Aspiration of stomach contents is a potential complication and always a concern. Gastric residuals are checked before suctioning to prevent the patient from vomiting and possibly causing aspiration. Another precaution is to keep the head of the bed elevated somewhat. A Dobhoff tube is also inserted initially, and feedings are begun as soon as 6 hours postburn. The rate starts slow and is advanced as tolerated to meet the calculated amount of nutritional replacement. Tube feedings continue until the patient can take the required amount of calories by mouth.

Another potential problem with both tubes is dislocation; therefore, it is important to check placement periodically throughout the day. When gastric residuals start climbing, it may be because the Dobhoff tube has slipped into the stomach or the patient is septic. Because tube feedings may become the source of contamination, routine care should include sterilization of the blender and limiting to 4 hours the amount of time that tube feedings can be hung at the bedside. The tubing and container should be changed every 4 hours (Mary Jaco, personal communication, 2004).

Sometimes when patients are encouraged to begin taking food by mouth, it will help to stop the tube feedings during the day and feed only at night. Not scheduling painful activities around meal-time and providing frequent mouth care will also contribute to improved oral intake.

Regular bowel patterns are expected in the postburn period. Patients are given many medications during hospitalization that may contribute to either diarrhea or constipation. Patients are expected to have at least one bowel movement per day. If not, then a bowel evacuation regimen should be initiated. If diarrhea is the problem and the volume exceeds 1500 mL/day, then bulking agents and/or antidiarrhea medication may be useful to promote routine bowel elimination.

The importance of monitoring and documenting the many parameters of intake and output cannot be overemphasized. Established clinical protocols and guidelines facilitate the implementation and evaluation of the nutritional program.

Other strategies to support the hypermetabolic phenomenon of the burn patient are to keep the room temperature above 85°F (29°C) and to keep the room door closed to prevent drafts across the room. Also frequent rest periods must be provided during the day. Nursing generally makes the schedule of activities for the day, so including frequent rest periods is just as important as anything else that needs to be done during the day. Adequate sleep during the night is also very important: it oftentimes is what makes the difference between a good day and a bad day. A quiet comfortable environment without sensory overload (lights and noise) is essential for the patient to sleep.

Nurses are the grand communicators of progress and/or problems. Nurses work closely with dietitians, physicians, patients, and families to ensure that optimal metabolic and nutritional support is achieved during the postburn period.

Pain and anxiety assessment and management

The expected outcome for pain and anxiety management is for the patient to achieve a balance between successful participation in activities of daily living and therapies and being comfortable enough to rest and sleep as needed. The ultimate goal is for the patient to be satisfied with the pain management plan as it is implemented. Assessment of pain and anxiety provides a baseline for evaluation of pain and anxiety relief measures. Pain and anxiety scales are essential to quantify painful episodes and to evaluate effectiveness of medication. Knowing when and how much to intervene is guided by knowing the baseline pain and anxiety rating for the individual. Patients and families should be given information upon admission on how to use the assessment scales and to identify an acceptable level of pain and anxiety. The assessment scales should be age appropriate. Common pain assessment scales include the visual analog scale, color scale, adjective scales, and faces scale. A pain history may provide valuable insight into how to individualize the pain management plan. Assessment of pain in the pre-verbal child (0–3 years of age) includes crying, irritability, lethargy, depression, facial grimacing and tensing, increased heart rate and blood pressure, abnormal sleep/wake patterns, and withdrawal of a body part when touched.

Intravenous administration of opioids and anxiolytic agents is essential to manage pain and anxiety during the initial stage of injury due to the altered absorption and circulation volume following a major burn injury. A PCA (patient-controlled analgesia) pump is useful on children older than 5 years of age and adults. It is important to manage background pain as well as procedural pain for which medication should be given 15–30 minutes prior to a painful procedure. Constipation is frequently a complication of pain management; thus, a bowel management program should be instituted at the same time. Relaxation, guided imagery, music therapy, hypnosis, and therapeutic touch are adjunct techniques to complement analgesia and reduce anxiety.[9] Emotional support and patient and family education decrease fear and anxiety, thereby enhancing the pain management plan.[10]

Patient/family education

In order for nurses to be competent teachers, they must be competent practitioners with solid theoretical foundations. Continuing education is key to maintaining competency of a staff as educators of patients and families. Reinforcement of the educational process (assess, plan, implement, evaluate, and document), characteristics of patient population, updates on educational strategies, age-appropriate interventions, and ways to evaluate learning are topics that will sharpen educator competency.

Discharge planning and education begins upon admission. It begins with a thorough assessment of the patient's life prior to the injury. Identifying knowledge deficits and barriers to education, prioritizing strategies for education, providing supplemental educational handouts and/or classes as well as developing a plan for evaluating the effectiveness of the teaching opportunity are integral parts of the educational process.

Assessment provides essential information for planning an educational program to meet the specific individual needs of each patient and family. It is also done periodically during different stages of the educational process to determine if the plan remains valid or changes need to be made.

The assessment findings become part of the educational plan, in that the plan is tailored to meet the needs and concerns of the patient and family. The plan includes the learning objectives, the strategies for education, and the learning materials. All of these parts of the educational goal are agreed upon by the patient/family and the educator.

Implementation of the plan is the next step, followed by a thorough evaluation of the effectiveness of learning and/or determination of whether the education goal is being accomplished. Alterations in the original plan may be needed any time during the educational process depending on unforeseen situations or changes in conditions that were not anticipated.

The plan and how it was implemented and evaluated are documented on a multidisciplinary education documentation form. All disciplines document the educational encounters on the same form (required by JCAHO).[11] The benefits are many. This process ensures communication of educational topics among the team members, provides a historical account of education, and documents progress and/or changes in the plan. It benefits the patient and family by making them competent in their role as care provider when discharged from the hospital. Knowledge allays anxiety about the unknown and aids in compliance with recommended care after discharge, improving the long-term outcomes.[12] Patients and families can be empowered to become active participants in the burn care team early in the postburn course through a well-structured educational plan.

Rehabilitation of the burn-injured patient

A major burn is one of the most devastating injuries, both physically and emotionally, known to man. After weeks of being an invalid, undergoing repeated surgeries, fighting infection, having the body ravaged by the metabolic consequences of injury, and enduring pain and anxiety, the patient now faces months of continued physical therapy to regain the level of function that they had known before the injury. Most patients who have sustained a major burn will continue to have a higher than normal metabolic rate and find that they do not have the stamina to easily regain their lifestyle.[13] In children, bone metabolism is affected and these children are more prone to fractures.[14] Although these patients must continue to exercise to prevent contractures, they may not have the physical strength to actively participate in such programs. Likewise, these patients frequently become depressed, as they face an altered self-image and fear that they will not be able to return to a normal life. For the adult, the concerns of whether they will be able to return to work or have to change their occupation is also a factor. What is the role of the nurse at this phase of treatment? Although nurses have been very involved in the care of the patient in the early phases of care, many nurses do not see how they can continue to be involved. The transition from the hospital to home care is often difficult for both the patient and family. It is important prior to discharge that the patient and family be educated in the care of wounds and healed skin before they leave the hospital. They also need information about the normal depression that occurs posthospitalization and resources in their home community to which they have access. This is where the nurse case manager becomes an integral part of the patient care team. Nurse case managers that are hospital based can begin to work with the patient and family soon after admission to assess the patient's future needs and coordinate these with outside agencies to ensure that the transition goes smoothly. Often case managers from workman's compensation carriers or health maintenance organizations (HMOs) are involved during the early phase as well. Coordination of activities between case managers is important to provide seamless care. With children, it is important for the nurse case manager to begin working with the school nurse or community health nurses to provide for this seamless transition in care.

Although the rehabilitation therapist plays an important role in providing referrals to community therapists and psychologists, and social workers frequently make referrals to community mental health providers, the nurse case manager should be involved in the overall coordination of these and other services to foster a unified approach. The free flow of communication between all providers is necessary for optimal rehabilitation of the patient.

Work-hardening programs for adults

Work-hardening programs have been shown in adults to more rapidly return the patient to their optimum level of functioning.[15]

These programs may be available through community rehabilitation facilities, vocational rehabilitation agencies, HMOs hospitals or health centers with cardiac rehabilitation programs or through Workmen's Compensation carriers. The major concern for the nurse case manager and the burn team is which patients need these programs and at what point the patient will benefit the most from such intensive programs.

Assessment

Burn patients, like those recovering from coronary heart disease and surgery, find themselves deconditioned. Even 3 weeks of bedrest in a healthy subject can result in a 25% decrease in maximal oxygen consumption. Thus, burn patients who are hospitalized for 2 or more weeks may need to be considered for such programs. Burn patients should be first assessed for risk factors associated with coronary heart disease. Such risk factors include:

- age and sex,
- elevated blood lipids,
- hypertension,
- cigarette smoking,
- physical inactivity,
- obesity,
- diabetes mellitus,
- diet,
- heredity,
- personality and behavior patterns,
- high uric acid levels,
- pulmonary function abnormalities,
- ethnic race,
- electrocardiographic abnormalities during rest and exercise,
- tension and stress.

Cardiac stress testing is usually recommended prior to beginning an exercise program. If the patient has several risk factors, the exercise program can be tailored to fit the patient's needs.[16]

Planning

What is available? Often the major issue is what is available and who will pay for this care. When an adult is injured on the job, this is often arranged and paid for by the compensation carrier, since they have a vested interest in returning the patient to work as soon as possible.

Implementation

Once the details are worked out the next hurdle is to get buy-in from the patient and family. Some programs require the patient to be in a facility some distance from their home; this may present issues for both the patient and family. Similarly, if the program is in the local community, daily visits to the rehabilitation facility may pose transportation issues, especially if the patient is unable to transport him or herself. These details can usually be worked out with cooperation of all caregivers and the family involved. Motivation and determination are often the most difficult factors to overcome. This is especially true if the patient is suffering from depression. The nurse case manager can be very instrumental in rallying the burn team and caregivers in the community to help the patient and family to see this as a way to return the patient to more normal function.

Evaluation

Success in such programs requires that all involved have the same goals and that these goals result in measurable outcomes. The goal of such programs is not only to increase the patients tolerance to exercise but also to improve their psychological and social functioning and to return the patient to work or to the same level of functioning pre-injury.

Extensive exercise in children

Children may suffer from the same deconditioning as adults, especially if they have suffered 40% or greater burns. Cucuzzo et al. have shown that children with greater than 40% burns have bone demineralization.[17] Treatment of these patients with long-term anabolic steroids and intensive exercise programs can return the patient's metabolic status and bone remineralization to normal much sooner.

Assessment

Children seem to do better if they are at least 4 years old when they begin this exercise program. The best time to start such a program is approximately 6–9 months postburn. With most patients this is after they have had 2–3 months away from the hospital after discharge from their initial injury. Like adults, individualized programs considering their current general state of health is necessary. When children enter these intensive exercise programs it is important for the parent or a responsible adult member of the family to be involved. This may be a significant factor in when the patient is able to start such a program. Similar results can be obtained in younger children through active play and exercise accompanied by music therapy. The use of activities set to music can increase stamina and actively stretch scar tissue and increase joint mobility.

Planning

Although cardiac rehabilitation programs and the like may be readily available in most major towns and cities in this country, often they do not take children. Children's hospitals often have rehabilitation units or outpatient programs for children that can offer similar programs to the adult cardiac programs. Children's hospitals are usually found in major cities; thus, these programs may not be as accessible as programs for adults. In some communities, school-age children may be able to obtain help within the school sport programs, especially if they have qualified athletic trainers. Children aged 4–6 may have more difficulty finding programs outside of children's hospitals. Some early childhood intervention and pre-kindergarten program may be available for younger children.

Another question is who pays for this care? Unlike the adult with insurance or workman's compensation insurance, children are often without funding for this rehabilitative care. State programs for children with special need (i.e. Title V programs) are one avenue to explore. Other sources of funding may come from private or public charities, school-mandated programs, or vocational rehabilitation programs for the older teenager.

Implementation

Motivating the child and parent can be a major task. Often the parent and child have spent weeks or months during the acute phase of care away from home. If there are other children in the home or if the parent normally works outside the home, the parent may not feel that he/she can be away from home an additional 2–3 months. The child may also not want to leave the safety of the home environment. Thus motivating the child and parent is often difficult. Helping the parent see this as a valuable program will require the whole burn team to work together with the patient and family.

Evaluation

The outcome of these programs for the child can be measured in increased exercise tolerance and improved psychological and social adjustment. A major function of these programs is to convince the child and parent that the patient is a normal child and can succeed mentally and physically. If the child returns home and can keep up with his/her peers, this alone improves the child's self-esteem.

Reconstructive surgery

Assessment

The role of the nurse in the reconstructive surgery phase is to be an advocate for the patient and family. Education of the patient and family throughout the course of burn care is an important nursing function. Many people have unrealistic expectations for reconstructive surgery. The nurse's role in the outpatient clinic or physician's office is to listen to the patient and family and to understand their hopes and expectations. Often when the surgeon discusses what should or could be done to improve the patient's appearance or function, the patient and family member are reticent to ask questions or to describe what they want. Patient's priorities are often different from the surgeons and this leads to dissatisfaction. Most surgeons prefer to wait until the scar has matured to begin reconstructive surgery. Occasionally, if the scar tissue is interfering with function, correction of the scar will be attempted. This is especially true in children where scar tissue may cause bone deformity if left until it has matured. In children, some reconstructive procedures are best postponed until the child has matured. Usually, surgery is best accepted by the child at the beginning of high school or just prior to starting further education. Although it is difficult to continue to be supportive of the patient and family during the scar maturation process, the nurse's role is one of education, support, and encouraging the patient to continue with exercise, splints, and pressure garments, if ordered.

Planning

Once again, the nurse case manager can be instrumental in helping the family find the funding and resources to provide reconstructive surgery for the patient. If the patient is working or in school planning, the procedures should accommodate the patient's school or work schedule as much as possible. For children, funding through Services for Children with Special Needs may be available. Working with insurance companies and HMOs can be tricky if the surgery is presented as cosmetic rather than corrective surgery.

Implementation

Preparing the patient for surgery is the responsibility of the nurse and physician. Providing the patient with realistic expectations is often difficult. Many times, immediately after the surgery, the area will look worse and the patient may feel dissatisfied and depressed. Preoperative preparation of the patient and family may allay some of these issues. Surgery, itself, is frightening enough for the patient and family. In children, this can be especially frightening because it may bring up memories of their original burn treatment and the pain associated with this treatment. Postoperatively, the nurse should teach the patient and family how to care for the wound to prevent infection and further scarring.

Evaluation

Whose body is it anyway! A line from a famous play actually sums up the evaluative process for reconstructive surgery. As professionals, we may see great improvement in the patient's condition after surgery. But if the patient is not satisfied with his or her appearance, little has been gained by the surgery. This is the reason that the patient and family must have realistic expectations prior to surgery.

Further Reading

1. Hixon S, Sole M, Kir T. Nursing strategies to prevent ventilator associated pneumonia. AACN Clinical Issues 1998; 9(1):1–15.
2. Shirani KZ, Pruitt BA Jr, Mason AD. The influence of inhalation injury and pneumonia on burn mortality. Ann Surg 1987; 205: 82–87.
3. Tompkins RG, Burke JF, Schoenfield DA, et al. Prompt eschar excision: a treatment system contributing to reduced burn mortality. Ann Surg 1986; 204:272–281.
4. Herndon DN, Gore D, Cole M, et al. Determinants of mortality in pediatric patients with greater than 70% full thickness total body surface areas thermal injury treated by early total excision and grafting. J Trauma 1987; 27:208–212.
5. Tompkins RG, Remensnyder JP, Burke JF, et al. Significant reductions in mortality for children with burn injuries through the use of prompt eschar excision. Ann Surg 1988; 208:577–585.
6. Ramzy PI. Infections in burns. In: Wolf SE, Herndon DN, eds. Burn care. Austin, TX: Landes Bioscience; 1999:73–80.
7. Dziewulski P, Barret J. Assessment, operative planning and surgery for burn wound closure. In: Wolf SE, Herndon DN, eds. Burn care. Austin, TX: Landes Bioscience; 1999:19–51.
8. Carrougher G, Gretchen G. Burn wound assessment and topical treatment. In: Carrougher G, ed. Burn care and therapy. St Louis: Mosby; 1998:133–165.
9. Patterson DR. Non-opioid based approaches to burn pain. J Burn Care Rehabil 1995; 16:372–376.
10. Marvin JN. Pain assessment versus measurement. J Burn Care Rehabil 1995; 16:348–357.
11. Iacono J, Campbell A, eds. Patient and family education the compliance guide to the JCAHO standards. Marblehead, MA: Opus Communications; 2000.
12. Falvo DR, Donna R. Effective patient education. Gaithersburg, MD: Aspen; 1994.
13. Hart DW, Herndon DN, Klein G, et al. Attenuation of posttraumatic muscle catabolism and osteopenia by long-term growth hormone. Ann Surg 2001; 233:827–834.
14. Klein GL. Bone loss in children following severe burns: increase risk for fractures in osteoporosis. Osteoporosis Update 1999. Xian, PR, China: Proceedings of the Third International Congress on Osteoporosis:63–68.
15. Zeller J, Strum G, Cruse C. Patients with burns are successful in work hardening programs. J Burn Care Rehabil 1993; 14:189–196.
16. Adams RB, Tribble GC, Tafel AC, et al. Cardiovascular rehabilitation of patients with burns. J Burn Care Rehabil 1990; 11:246–255.
17. Cucuzzo N, Ferrando A, Herndon D. The effects of exercise programming vs traditional outpatient therapy in the rehabilitation of severely burned children. J Burn Care Rehabil 2001; 22:214–220.

Further reading

Baxter CR. Fluid volume and electrolyte changes in the early postburn period. Clin Plast Surg 1974; 1(4):693–703.

Carleton SC, Tomassoni AJ, Alexander JK. The cardiovascular effects of environmental trauma. Cardiol Clin 1997; 13(2):257–262.

Demling RH. Fluid replacement in burned patients. Surg Clin North Am 1987; 67(1):15–30.

Demling RH. Pathophysiologic changes after cutaneous burns and approaches to initial resuscitation. In: Martyn JAJ, ed. Acute management of the burn patient. Philadelphia: WB Saunders; 1990.

Gordon MD, Gottschlich M, Helvig EL, et al. Review of evidence-based practice for the prevention of pressure sores in burn patients. J Burn Care Rehabil 2004; 25:388–410.

Chapter 36

The pediatric burned patient

Jong O. Lee and David N. Herndon

Chapter contents

Introduction

Burn injuries are the third most common injury causing death in children, following motor vehicle crash and drowning accidents.[1] Burn injuries have the greatest length of stay (average of 7.8 days) for all hospital admissions due to injuries.[2] Approximately 1.25 million people are burned in the United States every year. Fortunately, most burns do not require hospitalizations; however, 60 000 to 80 000 patients sustain severe enough burns to demand hospital admission.[3,4] Of those, 40% are children younger than 15 years.[5] About 5500 burn patients die each year,[3] and approximately 2500 of them are children.

House fires injure or kill over 10 000 people per year. House fires are among the leading causes of burn-related deaths in children at a rate of 12%; they are the leading cause of injury-related deaths for black children between the ages of 1 and 9 years. Children between 0 and 5 years of age are at a greater risk as a disproportionate number of fire deaths occur in homes. Deaths among preschool children are at a rate of more that twice the national average (29.6 deaths/million children) or an average of 20% of the total percentage of all home fire deaths.

Scalds are another common burn injury in children 2 years and under. Scald injuries may be due to household accidents or deliberate abuse. These may include spilling hot coffee or water, children reaching up to counter tops pulling pot handles or cords attached to cooking appliances and spilling the contents onto themselves, unknowingly putting body parts under a hot water faucet or climbing into a hot tub without realizing the water was too hot, and intentionally or unintentionally being placed into or brought in contact with a hot substance by another individual.

Great improvements have been made in the reduction of mortality related to thermal injuries over the past few decades. Advances in fluid resuscitation, early surgical excision and grafting of the burn wound, infection control, treatment of inhalation injury, nutritional support, and support of hypermetabolic response to injury have contributed to a 50% decline in burn-related deaths and hospital admissions in the United States.[3] This overall improvement in mortality is most perceptible in the pediatric population. In 1949, Bull and Fisher reported the expected 50% mortality rate for 49% total body surface area (TBSA) burn size in children aged 0 to 14.[6] This has improved to 50% expected mortality in 98% TBSA burn in the same population group.[7]

The burn injury produces overwhelming physiological and psychological challenges to a child. The unique anatomical and physiological attributes of the child require the attention of physicians and nurses who are trained not only in burn care but also in the specifics of pediatric care. The most obvious differences between adults and children are in size and body proportion. Shorter lengths, tighter angles, and smaller diameters of various anatomical structures and spaces make certain manipulations more difficult. These differences also require the provision of special equipment and supplies, which reflect the configurations of pediatric anatomy. In addition to anatomical differences there are also many physiological differences between children and adults, which must be considered and will be discussed concerning the treatment of the pediatric burn patient.

Initial evaluation

A patient must be immediately removed from the source of burn and clothing and jewelry removed immediately as these burning items can prolong the burning process. Pouring cool water to minimize the depth of the burn can cause hypothermia in large burns and should be avoided. After the burning process is stopped, the patient should be kept warm by wrapping with a sterile sheet or blanket, if available, or clean sheet or blanket. If the burn involves chemical burns, the patient should be removed from the chemical immediately and the wound irrigated with copious amount of water at least for 30 minutes to dilute the chemicals.

Burn patients should be treated as a trauma patient and any other traumatic injuries diligently ruled out. Any potential life-threatening injuries should be identified and treated.

The airway should be assessed first: 100% oxygen should be administered and oxygen saturation monitored using pulse oximetry. Arterial blood gas and carboxyhemoglobin are obtained when appropriate. A full-thickness circumferential chest burn can interfere with ventilation. Chest expansion should be observed to ensure equal air movement. If the patient is on a ventilator, airway pressure and P_{CO_2} should be monitored. If ventilation is compromised, escharotomy of the chest should be performed to allow better chest movement and improve ventilation. Wheezing, tachypnea, stridor, and hoarseness indicate an impending airway problem due to inhalation injury or edema, and immediate attention is required.

A cuff blood pressure measurement may be difficult in patients with burned extremities. These patients may need an arterial line to monitor their blood pressure especially if they require a long transfer. A radial arterial line may not be reliable in patients with extremity burns and may be difficult to secure. A femoral line may be more reliable and easy to secure. These should be secured with sutures. Persistent tachycardia should alert a practitioner for a missed injury. Accurate and rapid determination of burn depth is vital to the proper management of burn injury.

A nasogastric tube is placed in all patients with major burns, as the majority of children develop gastric distension or ileus. A bladder drainage catheter is placed to monitor urine output accurately as a measure of successful resuscitation.

Resuscitation

In the hours after a serious burn, there is a systemic capillary leak that increases with burn size. Capillary usually regains competence after 18–24 hours if resuscitation has been successful. Intravenous (IV) access should be established immediately for the administration of resuscitative fluid. Increased times to beginning resuscitation of burned patients results in poorer outcomes, and delays should be minimized.[8] It is crucial that venous access be obtained early postburn, even though such access may be extremely difficult to obtain. Due to the small circulating volume, delays in resuscitation for periods as short as 30 minutes can result in profound shock. Peripheral IV access is preferred and may need to go through burned skin if necessary. When peripheral IV is not available due to extremity burns, a central venous line may be secured. Either subclavian or femoral line can be obtained but femoral venous access may be easier to obtain in edematous patients. Small-bore catheters limit the rates at which fluid can be administered; therefore, children with large burns require two large-bore IVs so that sufficient fluid can be given. The presence of two IVs also provides a safety margin if one infiltrates to allow continued resuscitation while the 'safety' line is re-established.

When vascular access is unobtainable in small children (less than 6 years old), the intraosseous route is a viable option and it is relatively easy to obtain. Children can be administered fluid volumes in excess of 100 mL/h directly into the bone marrow.[9] Intramedullary access can be utilized in the proximal tibia until IV access is accomplished. There is a very rare incidence of embolic complications with this procedure. A 16–18 gauge bone marrow aspiration needle can be used to cannulate the bone marrow compartment, although spinal needles and even butterfly needles can be pushed through the soft bone of a child. Although previously advocated only for children younger than 3 years of age, intraosseous fluid administration can be safely performed in children under 6 years of age, if the bone is sufficiently soft to allow needle penetration.[10] The anterior tibial plateau, medial malleolus, anterior iliac crest, and the distal femur are preferred sites for intraosseous infusion. The needle should be introduced into the bone, taking care to avoid the epiphysis, either perpendicular to the bone or at a 60° angle with the bevel facing the greater length of bone (Figure 36.1). The needle has been properly inserted when bone marrow can be freely aspirated. Fluid should be allowed to infuse by gravity drip. The needle should be well secured to prevent inadvertent removal. The use of pumps should be discouraged in case the needle is dislodged from the marrow compartment.

Due to their small body weight to body surface area ratio, fluid losses are proportionally greater in children. Normal blood volume in children is approximately 80 mL/kg body weight and neonates, 85–90 mL/kg, compared to the adult whose normal blood volume is 70 mL/kg. Evaporative water losses in a 20% TBSA burn in a 10 kg child are 475 mL or 60% of the circulating volume, while the same size burn in a 70 kg adult causes the loss of 1100 mL or only 25% of the blood volume. Although fluid losses after a burn injury are directly proportional to the burned surface area, the commonly used

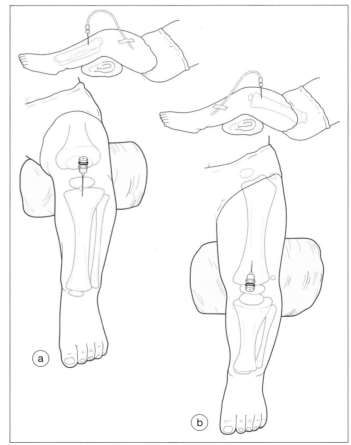

Fig. 36.1 Intraosseous line placement in the proximal tibia (a) and distal femur (b). (Redrawn with permission from Fleisher and Ludwig.[60])

'rule of nines', useful in adults, adequate in adolescents, does not accurately reflect the surface area of children under 15 years of age (Figure 36.2). The standard relationships between surface area and weight in adults do not hold true in children, as infants possess a larger cranial surface area with less area in the extremities than adults. Most routinely used resuscitation formulas were developed using adult patients and are almost exclusively weight-based. Since the linear relationship between weight and surface area does not exist in children (surface area varies to weight as a 2/3 function), use of these formulas in children results in under- or over-resuscitation (Table 36.1).

Therefore pediatric burned patients should be resuscitated using formulas based on body surface area, which can be calculated from height and weight using a standard nomogram (Figure 36.3) or formulas (Table 36.2). The most commonly

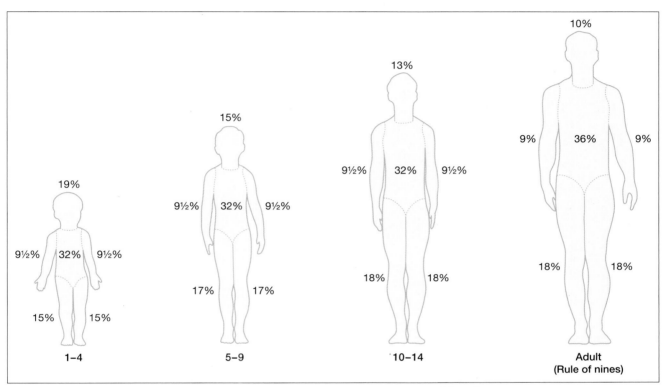

Fig. 36.2 The 'rule of nines' altered for the anthropomorphic differences of infancy and childhood.

TABLE 36.1 RESUSCITATION BY THE PARKLAND FORMULA ONLY COMPARED TO MAINTENANCE FLUID REQUIREMENTS ALONE					
		Calculated needs		**Replacement burn loss**	
Example	% Burn	Resuscitation*	Maintenance†	mL	mL/kg/%
1 year old	15	600	800	−200	−1.33
10 kg	30	1 200	800	400	1.33
0.48 m² BSA	60	2 400	800	1 600	2.67
	90	3 600	800	2 800	3.11
4 years old	15	990	1 200	−210	−0.85
16.5 kg	30	1 980	1 200	780	1.58
0.68 m² BSA	60	3 900	1 200	2 760	2.79
	90	5 940	1 200	4 940	3.33
12 years old	15	2 400	2 250	1 150	1.92
40 kg	30	4 800	2 550	2 550	2.12
1.13 m² BSA	60	9 600	2 250	7 350	3.06
	90	14 400	2 250	12 150	3.38
*4 mL/kg/% burn. †2000 mL/m² BSA.					

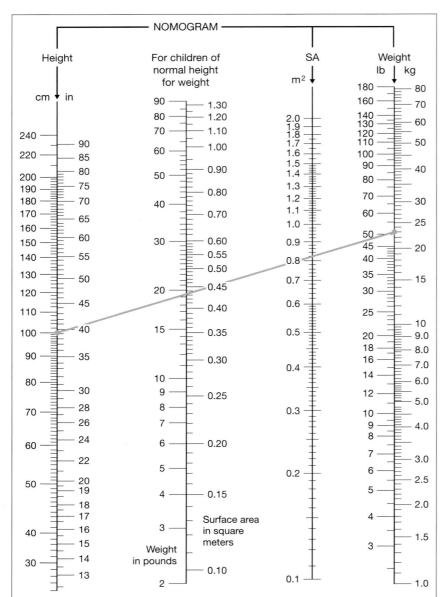

┌─ NOMOGRAM ─┐

Height · For children of normal height for weight · SA m² · Weight lb | kg

Fig. 36.3 Standard nomogram for the determination of body surface area based on height and weight. The example depicted is for a child of 100 cm in height and 23 kg in weight. (Reprinted with permission from Eichelberger.[61])

TABLE 36.2 FORMULAS FOR CALCULATING BODY SURFACE AREA (BSA)	
Dubois formula	BSA (m²) = ht (cm)$^{0.725}$ × wt (kg)$^{0.425}$ × 0.007184
Jacobson formula	BSA (m²) = [ht (cm) + wt (kg) − 60]/100

used resuscitation formula in pediatric patients calls for the administration of 5000 mL/m² total body surface area (TBSA) burned plus 2000 mL/m² TBSA for maintenance fluid given over the first 24 hours after burn, with half the volume administered during the first 8 hours and the second half given over the following 16 hours.[11] The subsequent 24 hours, and for the rest of the time their burn is open, call for 3750 mL/m² TBSA burned or remaining open area (for evaporation from wound) plus 1500 mL/m² TBSA (for maintenance requirements). This need decreases as a patient achieves more wound coverage and

healing. As in the adult patient, resuscitation formulas offer a guide to the initial starting point for the amount of fluid necessary for replacing lost volume in children and the amount of fluid should be titrated according to effects.

Loss of renal medullary concentrating capacity is usual secondary to washout of the medulla during resuscitation and immature kidneys' inherent inability to concentrate. Hyponatremia is a frequently observed complication in pediatric patients after the first 48 hours post-injury. Frequent monitoring of serum sodium is necessary to guide appropriate salt or water supplementation. Children of less than 1 year of age may require more sodium supplementation due to higher urinary sodium losses. Further, potassium losses should usually be replaced with oral potassium phosphate rather than potassium chloride as hypophosphatemia is frequently observed in this population.[12] Calcium and magnesium losses must also be supplemented.

An indwelling urinary catheter is essential for burns greater than 20%. During the early phase of resuscitation urine output should be assessed as frequently as every 15 minutes and titrated appropriately. Fluid administration should be titrated to achieve a urine output of 1 mL/kg/h in children and 2 mL/kg/h for infants. If the patient is making more than that, IV fluid should be titrated down. Other endpoints should also be followed, such as mental status, heart rate, blood pressure, and capillary refills. One can also follow the trend of either lactic acid or base deficit and see the resolution. Initial fluid boluses should be administered in amounts appropriate for the size of the child and should represent no more than 25% of the total circulating volume (10 mL/kg). If urine output is less than minimal, it may be more appropriate to increase the rate of IV fluid rather than giving bolus.

Intravenous resuscitation fluid should be isotonic and replace lost electrolytes. Lactated Ringer's (LR) is the most commonly used solution for the first 24 hours postburn. Electrolyte loss in the wound correlates better with LR. Children less than 1 year of age should also receive maintenance fluid containing dextrose solution to prevent hypoglycemia as their glycogen stores are limited.

Mortality

In a review of 103 children with >80% TBSA burns over a 15-year period, it was found that 69 survived with an overall mortality of 33%. Mortality was greatest in children under 2 years of age and in burns >95% TBSA (Figures 36.4 and 36.5).[8] Another major predictor in mortality was the length of time to intravenous access (Figure 36.6). Burns that received resuscitation fluids within the first hour had a significantly higher chance of survival.[8] The mortality rate also increases significantly with smoke inhalation injury. In no pediatric patient, no matter how large the burn, how young or with what type of inhalation injury could it be accurately predicted whether they would live or die at the time of admission.[8]

Assessment of resuscitation

Evaluation of the efficacy of resuscitation is difficult in children. The routine clinical signs of hypovolemia for the adult burn patients – low blood pressure and decreased urine output – are late manifestations of shock in the pediatric patient and tachycardia is omnipresent. Children have remarkable cardiopulmonary reserve, often not exhibiting clinical signs of hypovolemia until more than 25% of the circulating volume has been lost and complete cardiovascular decompensation is imminent. Mental status, pulse pressures, arterial blood gases, distal extremity color, capillary refill, and body temperature reflect volume status. Capillary refill is a good indicator of volume status in burned children. Decreased capillary refill should warn a practitioner of imminent danger. A child with normal blood pressure and acceptable heart rate, but with cool clammy extremities, obtundation, and a delayed

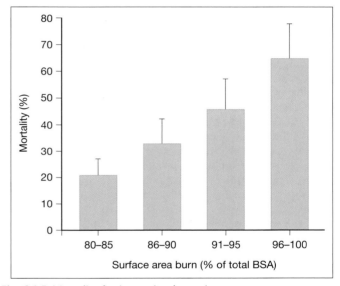

Fig. 36.5 Mortality for increasing burn size.

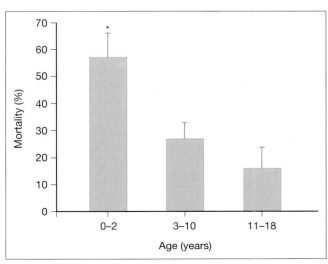

Fig. 36.4 Mortality in burns >80% total body surface area for various ages.

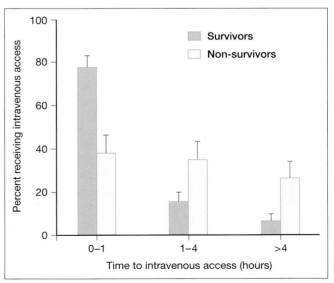

Fig. 36.6 Time to intravenous access in survivors and non-survivors. Mortality increases with delays in starting an intravenous line and instituting volume resuscitation.

TABLE 36.3 NORMAL PEDIATRIC VITAL SIGNS

Age	Minimum heart rate (beats/min)	Systolic BP (mmHg)	Respirations (breaths/min)	Minimal hemoglobin (g/dL)	Minimal hematocrit (%)
<2 years of age	100–160	60	30–40	11.0	33.0
2–5 years of age	80–140	70	20–30	11.0	33.0
6–12 years of age	70–120	80	18–25	11.5	34.5
>12 years of age	60–110	90	16–20	12.0	36.0

capillary refill, is a child in dire danger. Measurement of arterial blood pH with attention to base deficit or lactic acid is of particular importance in this age group, reflecting decreased tissue perfusion.

Children frequently develop a reflex tachycardia after even the most trivial injury due to an overexuberant catecholamine response to the trauma or anxiety. Systolic blood pressures of less than 100 mmHg are common in children younger than 5 years of age (Table 36.3). Young children with immature kidneys have less tubular concentrating ability than adults, and urine production may continue in spite of hypovolemia. Arterial pH, lactic acid, or base deficit can be followed to assist resuscitation.

Volume overload must be avoided. Volume overload can lead to pulmonary edema, right heart failure, abdominal deep muscle compartment syndromes, and cerebral edema in burn patients. Although children possess a large cardiopulmonary reserve, the young heart is less compliant, and stroke volumes plateau at relatively low filling pressures, shifting the Starling curve to the left. Cardiac output is almost completely dependent upon heart rate, and the immature heart is more sensitive to volume and pressure overload. Cardiac output can be measured using a PiCCO monitor, which is less invasive than a Swan–Ganz catheter and only requires an arterial line and a central venous line. Transthoracic or transesophageal echocardiograms should be utilized early to assess the cardiac function in patients who are failing or not responding to the conventional therapy. Children are particularly prone to the development of edema from both vasogenic and hydrostatic sources. Vasogenic edema occurs within the early postburn period when vascular integrity is impaired. Of particular concern is the development of cerebral edema. Care should be taken in order to maintain head of bed elevation, particularly during the initial 24–48 hours postburn and avoid hypercarbia. The maintenance of intravascular osmotic pressures decreases the likelihood of edema development. Salt-poor albumin can be expected to remain in the intravascular space if administered after 8 hours postburn in amounts necessary to maintain serum albumin levels at more than 2.5 g/dL. Albumin deficit can be calculated using the formula:

$$[2.5\,\text{g/dL} - \text{current serum albumin (g/dL)}] \times [\text{wt (kg)} \times 3]$$

The deficit can be administered as 25% albumin and given in three divided doses gradually.

Evaluation and management of airways

The smaller aperture of the pediatric trachea predisposes it to obstruction. Equal amounts of airway edema in pediatric and adult airway results in significantly disproportionate increases in amounts of resistance and decreases in cross-sectional area. A 1 mm increase in tissue thickness of a 4 mm diameter pediatric trachea results in a 16-fold increase in resistance with a 75% decrease in cross-sectional area. The same edema in an adult airway would increase the airway resistance threefold and reduce airway area by 44%.[13] Therefore early intubation is advocated. As edema develops promptly following injury, airway evaluation and management must be given priority in pediatric patients. During emergent conditions when edema is present, inability to secure the airway with an endotracheal tube is a clear indication of the need for surgical airway control.

Potential hemorrhage and edema formation make emergency intubation difficult. Early intubation should be considered when a long transfer is anticipated or a patient has a large burn which likely will develop airway edema with a large amount of fluid resuscitation. Concurrent placement of an endotracheal tube over the bronchoscope should be considered at the time of bronchoscopy. A readily available estimate of airway diameter is the width of the patient's little finger, an age-based formula (age + 16)/4 or the use of Broselow tape.

Following placement of the ET tube, it must be adequately secured. With a child, oozing wounds and moist dressings, this can be a difficult task. One successful approach is to attach the ET tube with tape around the back of the head both above and below the ears. An additional piece of tape over the top of the head, secured to the tape behind the head, will prevent accidental extubation in most children.[14]

Inhalation injury

Inhalation injury, and its sequelae of infection and pulmonary failure, are major determinants of mortality after burn injury.

The mortality rate of children with isolated thermal burns is 1–2%, but it increases to approximately 40% in the presence of in-halation injury.[15,16] Carbon monoxide poisoning coupled with hypoxia is the most frequent cause of death due to 'smoke inhalation'. Any flame-related injury, particularly if it is confined in closed space, should be evaluated for an inhalation component. If inhalation injury is suspected, arterial blood gas and carboxyhemoglobin level should be obtained and the patient placed on 100% oxygen. Children may be spared some of the overt signs of inhalation injury due to their short stature and proximity to the floor-level cool air. As with adults, the only definitive method to diagnose an inhalation injury is through direct visualization of the airway and early examination of arterial carboxyhemoglobin level. Signs of potential inhalation injury include facial burns, singed nasal hairs, carbonaceous sputum, abnormal mental status (agitation or stupor), respiratory distress (dyspnea, wheezing, stridor, hoarseness), or elevated carboxyhemoglobin level >10%.[17] Carboxyhemoglobin levels must be calculated from the time drawn, back to the time of the accident or for O_2 given as described in the chapter on this subject. A carboxyhemoglobin level >60% has more than 50% chance of mortality (Table 36.4).

Common treatment modalities for inhalation injury include airway maintenance, clearance, and pharmacological management (Table 36.5). A recent study has shown that a group of children treated with a regimen of nebulized heparin and acetylcysteine had a significant decrease in reintubation rates, atelectasis, and mortality when compared to a control group.[18]

Hypermetabolism

Children with burn injury demonstrate a remarkable increase in metabolic rate. No other disease state produces as dramatic an effect on the metabolic rate as burn injury.[19,20] This hypermetabolism is thought to slow wound healing and prolong generalized weakness. This prolonged metabolic dysfunction can lead to loss of lean body mass and increase morbidity. Marked wasting of lean body mass occurs within a few weeks of injury.

The hypermetabolic response increases with increasing burn size. There is an upregulation of catabolic agents, such as cortisol, catecholamine, and glucagons,[21] which induces a hyperdynamic cardiovascular response, an increased oxygen consumption, energy expenditure, proteolysis, lipolysis, and glycogenolysis, loss of lean body mass and body weight, delayed wound healing, and immune depression.[22,23]

Pharmacological agents have been used to attenuate catabolism and to stimulate growth in burn injury. To further minimize erosion of lean body mass, administration of anabolic hormones such as growth hormone, insulin, insulin-like growth factor-1 (IGF-1)/IGF-binding protein-3 (IGFBP-3), oxandrolone or testosterone and catecholamine antagonists such as propranolol have been used in pediatric burns. These agents contribute to maintenance of lean body mass and promote wound healing.[24–29]

Thermoregulation

Core body temperature is consistently elevated after a major burn. A hypothalamic reset induced by various inflammatory cytokines and pain causes this elevation even in the absence of infection. The temperature reset is thought to be an adaptive mechanism to bolster host defense against potential pathogens. Burned patients strive for temperatures of about 38°C. Depressed or 'normal' temperatures are more likely indicative of overwhelming sepsis or exhausted physiological capabilities to maintain temperature and should be viewed as an ominous sign. After major thermal injuries, routine methods of heat conservation are inadequate due to the extensive heat loss through convection and evaporation. Infants and toddlers, with their increased surface area/volume ratios, less insulating fat, and lower muscle mass for shivering, are particularly susceptible to hypothermia.

Hypothermia produces numerous consequences. The heart is particularly sensitive to temperature, and ventricular arrhythmias are not uncommon. Hypothermia also increases the susceptibility of the myocardium to changes in electrolyte concentrations. The oxyhemoglobin dissociation curve is shifted to the left by lowered body temperature, impairing peripheral oxygenation. In extreme cases, hypothermia

TABLE 36.4 CARBON MONOXIDE POISONING

Carboxyhemoglobin (%)	Symptoms
0–10	Normal
10–20	Headache, confusion
20–40	Disorientation, fatigue, nausea, visual changes
40–60	Hallucination, combativeness, convulsion, coma, shock state
60–70	Coma, convulsions, weak respiration and pulse
70–80	Decreasing respiration and stopping
80–90	Death in less than 1 hour
90–100	Death within a few minutes

TABLE 36.5 AIRWAY MAINTENANCE, CLEARANCE, AND PHARMACOLOGICAL MANAGEMENT

Turn side to side	q 2 h
Sitting or rocked in chair	As soon as physiologically stable
Ambulation	Early
Chest physiotherapy	q 2 h
Suctioning and lavage (nasal/oral tracheal)	q 2 h
Bronchodilators	q 2 h
Aerosolized heparin/acetylcysteine	q 2 h alternating
	Heparin 5000–10 000 units with 3 mL NS q 4 h
	Alternated with acetylcysteine 20% 3 mL q 4 h

produces central nervous system and respiratory depression, coagulopathies, and loss of peripheral vasomotor tone.

Every effort should be made to reduce the heat loss experienced by pediatric patients. Ambient temperatures and humidity should be maintained at 30–33°C and 80%, respectively, in order to decrease energy demands and evaporative water losses. Wet dressings should be avoided or at least wrapped, and wet bedding promptly changed so as to decrease evaporative or conductive cooling. The patient should be positioned so that drafts are avoided, including the inlets and outlets for air-conditioning and heating ducts. Bathing or showering should be expeditiously completed, avoiding undue environmental exposure.

Nutritional support

Nutritional support of the hypermetabolic response in severely burned patients is best accomplished by early enteral nutrition. Early institution of enteral feeding can abate the hypermetabolic response to burn.[30,31] Patients with smaller burns are immediately placed on a high-protein, high-caloric diet to support their metabolic response. Those with larger burns (>30%) are placed on enteral feedings.

Almost immediate enteral nutrition can be initiated via a transpyloric feeding tube. Most children will tolerate enteral feedings as early as 1–2 hours postburn, if not immediately. Several studies have demonstrated the efficacy of early alimentation and the additional salutary effects.[32,33] Enteral feedings can be given through a flexible Silastic duodenal feeding tube, bypassing the stomach, which may be experiencing decreased peristaltic action.

Early enteral feeding preserves gut mucosal integrity and improves intestinal blood flow and motility.[30]

Milk has been demonstrated to be one of the least expensive and best tolerated of all enteral formulas. Additionally, it is palatable and easily recognized by children when they are able to take oral feedings. Because of the low sodium content of milk, sodium supplementation may be necessary. Hyperosmolar feedings, commercially available, should be diluted because of the high incidence of subsequent diarrhea if used full strength. It is diluted to $1/2$ or $3/4$ strength. Diarrhea is particularly troublesome in children because of their increased sensitivity to volume deficits.

Several formulas are available to estimate caloric requirement in burn patients. Since caloric demands are related to burn size, caloric support should be given in amounts calculated based on body surface area. A series of different formulas based on body surface area have been developed at Shriners Hospitals for Children, Galveston to meet the differing requirements of the various age groups.[34–36] The Curreri formula has likewise been amended to reflect the differing demands of the pediatric group (Table 36.6).

Growth

Hypermetabolism and muscle protein catabolism persist long after the wound is closed.[37] Protein breakdown continues 6–9 months after severe burn. There is almost a complete lack of bone growth for 2 years after injury. This results in long-term osteopenia, which may adversely affect peak bone mass accumulation in children.[38,39] Severely burned children with a burn size of >80% have a linear growth delay for years after injury.[40]

TABLE 36.6 NUTRITIONAL REQUIREMENTS FOR CHILDREN

	Galveston	Modified Curreri
Infant	2100 kcal/m² + 1000 kcal/m² burn	BMR + 15 kcal/% burn
Toddler		BMR + 25 kcal/% burn
Child	1800 kcal/m² + 1300 kcal/m² burn	BMR + 40 kcal/% burn
Adolescent	1500 kcal/m² + 1500 kcal/m² burn	

In severely burned patients, nail and hair growth are attenuated during the acute postburn period, and bone growth is slowed.[41–43] Dampened height and weight gain velocities have been documented in children during the first 3 years postburn, thereby rendering these burned children slighter and shorter than their age-matched peers.[44]

Nutritional support of acute burn patients becomes an essential part of treatment during their hospitalization.

Wound closure

One of the more important advances in the last 20 years has been the development of early excision and early wound closure. Improvements in the treatment of burn wounds and utilization of antimicrobial dressings have dramatically decreased the incidence of fatal sepsis in burned patients.[45] Two decades ago third-degree burns were treated by removing small amounts of eschar at a time, approximately 10–15%, followed by grafting. Commonly, eschar was allowed to separate with lysis by bacterial enzymes. This led to a high incidence of invasive infection and wound sepsis and prolonged length of hospital stay with increased mortality. Today massive excision can be easily managed in children, providing results of decreased mortality and decreased length of hospital stay.[46,47] Early excision even in the first 24 hours is safe and effective.[48] Performing early excision within the first 48 hours can significantly reduce blood loss.[49] By using skin substitutes such as allograft skin, xenograft, and Integra (Figure 36.7), the burn wound can be covered and protected for many weeks until enough donor site is available for grafting (repeat autografting is performed when the donor site is healed for reharvesting). Cultured epidermal autografts (CEA) is available for massive burn injuries (Figure 36.8). Although it is an effective way to cover large burns with limited donor sites, it may not be the most cost-effective approach. A group of patients treated with CEA had greater hospital costs, a longer length of stay, and more reconstructive admissions than conventional treatment with meshed autograft skin.[46] Cultured skin substitute (CSS) is currently undergoing investigative study and holds promise. CSS, consisting of autologous cultured keratinocytes and fibroblasts attached to collagen-based sponges, may reduce the requirement for donor skin and number of autograftings in massive burns.

Scald burns in young children are best managed with delayed treatment. Unless the wound is clearly third degree, the scald injury should be conservatively managed for approximately 2 weeks to allow the wound to heal or demarcate (Figures

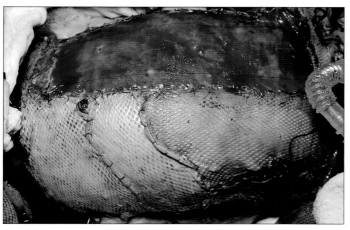

Fig. 36.7 Dermal and skin substitutes can be used as temporary cover for severe burns. Integra, a bilaminar skin substitute, can replace homografts as temporary cover. The Silastic superficial layer can be removed after 3 weeks and a super-then autograft then placed on top. The entire wound can be covered with Integra, which is subsequently autografted when donor sites are available. (Reprinted with permission from Barret J, Herndon DN, eds. Color atlas of burn care. London: WB Saunders; 2001: 107, Plate 6.95.)

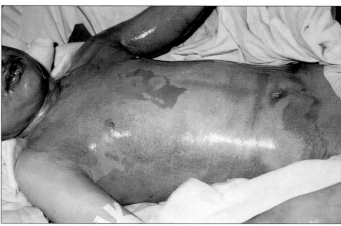

Fig. 36.9 Superficial and small areas of deep second-degree scald burns before topical treatment: 25% total body surface area. (Reprinted with permission from Barret J, Herndon DN, eds. Color atlas of burn care. London: WB Saunders; 2001: 79, Plate 5.39.)

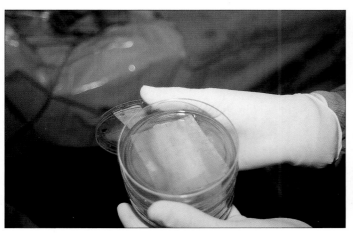

Fig. 36.8 The cultured epidermal autografts are ready to use 18–21 days later. Extreme care with handling is needed because of the fragility of the cultured cells. (Reprinted with permission from Barret J, Herndon DN, eds. Color atlas of burn care. London: WB Saunders; 2001: 106, Plate 6.89.)

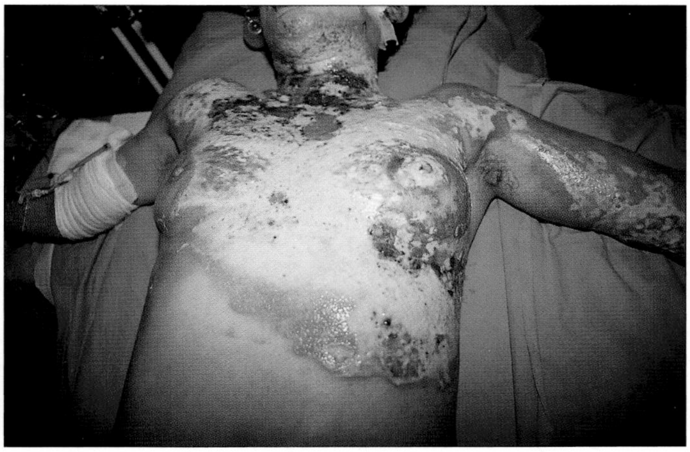

Fig. 36.10 Deep second-degree burns treated for 10 days with silver sulfadiazine. Note that the edges are regenerating. Pseudo-eschar challenges the evaluation of the wounds. Foul smell, discoloration, surrounding cellulitis, and eschar separation are signs of infection. (Reprinted with permission from Barret J, Herndon DN, eds. Color atlas of burn care. London: WB Saunders; 2001: 77, Plate 5.31.)

36.9 and 36.10). This conservative treatment results in less wound excised, less blood loss, and less apparent scarring.[50] Treatment methods for the conservative care of scald burns were analyzed. Scald injuries greater the 20% TBSA (mean 31%) were randomized to treatment with allograft skin versus topical antimicrobial therapy. Treatment with allograft led to decreased time to healing and decreased pain.[51] In another study, patients greater than 40% TBSA burn (mean 65%) were randomized to allograft skin or topical antimicrobial. Patients who received treatment with allograft skin had a significantly decreased length of stay.[52] The current recommended treatment for second-degree burns, primarily scalds less than 30% TBSA, is immediate application of Biobrane. Biobrane can be safely used in children, even in infants less than 2 years of age. When applied within 48 hours of injury there is no

difference in infection between Biobrane and topical antimicrobials. Further, application of Biobrane versus topical antimicrobials leads to decreased pain, decreased length of hospitalization, and decreased healing time.[53,54]

Pain management

Children do not always express their pain in the same way as adults.[55] Children may display pain through behaviors of fear, anxiety, agitation, anger, aggression, tantrums, depression, withdrawal, and regression.[56,57] How the child's experience of pain from the burn injury and anxiety from the hospitalization are clinically managed will have lasting psychological effects for many months and years to follow. A severe burn injury brings many weeks of surgeries, dressing changes, and exercises that can cause intense pain. Pain can also exist as a constant state throughout the hospitalization. Morphine sulfate is the most commonly used analgesia. It should be given intravenously, and not intramuscularly. Fentanyl can be also used. Fentanyl Oralet can be used successfully for dressing changes (10 μg per kg). Most outpatients are treated with hydrocodone/acetaminophen.

Rehabilitation

Rehabilitation is a key component to success of burn treatment and starts at the time of the admission. During the acute phase of burn care, splints are used to minimize joint deformities and contractures. Splints are used continuously except during a therapy session. They are fabricated to each patient's needs and used from day 1 of hospitalization. Bedside therapy, including passive and active range of motion, is started early. Early mobilization should be practiced. Early ambulation after the grafts has taken and early physical and occupational therapies are important to success of rehabilitation of burned children. Patients with leg grafting are kept bedrest after the operation, but on postoperative day 4, they are gotten out of bed and started on ambulation. Early therapy and ambulation are keys to success of long-term rehabilitation of burned children. When patients are discharged from their acute care hospitalization, they undergo rigorous therapies, including stretching, and range of motion and strengthening exercises.

In general, deep partial-thickness burn wounds requiring 3 or more weeks to heal will likely produce hypertrophic scars. The longer it takes to heal, the more likely are scars. Using dressings that exert constant pressure on the healing wound and pressure garments exerting constant pressure on the healed wound are the most effective ways of decreasing the incidence of hypertrophic scar formation. Pressure garments may be worn up to 2 years or until scars mature.

Prevention

Prevention remains the single best way to manage pediatric burn injuries. National prevention and education efforts have positively impacted the number of pediatric burns each year. Lowering the temperature set point on hot water heaters and teaching families to check the bath water temperature before placing a child in the bath has decreased hot water scald injuries. Prevention groups have worked with gas hot water heater companies and the Consumer Product Safety Commission (CPSC) to provide education to raise gas water heaters 12 inches off the ground, which significantly reduces the risk of accidental explosions and fires.[58]

Much work still needs to be done in the area of 'child fire play'. Three-fourths of 'child fire play' involves matches or lighters. All matches and other ignition sources must be placed out of reach of children. A positive step toward prevention occurred in 1994 when CPSC placed into effect a child-resistant lighter to protect children under 5 years of age. The importance of placing smoke detectors in multiple areas in a house has received much public education over the last several years. Current prevention education focuses on children, and especially infants that are not able to remove themselves from a fire. Since the CPSC has reduced flammability standards on children's sleepwear in 1997, there has been an increased incidence of sleepwear-related burn injuries in children.[59] One way to protect infants and children is to dress them in fire-resistant sleepwear and clothing to protect them from a burn injury if a fire does occur.

Children have no idea of the dangerous situations they place themselves in. Educating children as early as possible that fire is dangerous is imperative. Providing safe environments for our children and providing appropriate education to them is the responsibility of healthcare providers, the adults that care for them, and the community at large.

References

1. National Vital Statistics System. Deaths. Final data for 1997. Centers for Disease Control and Prevention 1999; 47(19):1–105.
2. National Center for Health Statistics. Hospitalizations for injury, United States 1996. Centers for Disease Control and Prevention 1996; (318):1–10.
3. Brigham PA, McLoughlin E. Burn incidence and medical care in the United States: estimates, trends, and data sources. J Burn Care Rehabil 1996; 17:95–107.
4. Pruitt BA, Goodwin CW, Mason AD Jr. Epidemiologic, demographic, and outcome characteristics of burn injury. In: Herndon DN, ed. Total burn care. London: WB Saunders; 2002:16–30.
5. Barillo DJ, Goode R. Fire fatality study: demographics of fire victims. Burns 1996; 22:85–88.
6. Bull JP, Fisher AJ. A study in mortality in a burn unit: standards for the evaluation for alternative methods of treatment. Ann Surg 1949; 130:160–173.
7. Herndon DN, Gore DC, Cole M, et al. Determinants of mortality in pediatric patients with greater than 70% full thickness total body surface area treated by early excision and grafting. J Trauma 1987; 27:208–212.
8. Wolf SE, Rose JK, Desai MH, et al. Mortality determinants in massive pediatric burns: an analysis of 103 children with 80% TBSA burns (70% full thickness). Ann Surg 1997; 225(5):554–569.
9. Tocantins LM, O'Neill JF. Infusions of blood and other fluids into the general circulation via the bone marrow. Surg Gynecol Obstet 1941; 73:281–287.
10. Fiser DH. Intraosseous infusion. N Engl J Med 1990; 322:1579–1581.
11. Caravajal HF. A physiologic approach to fluid therapy in severely burned children. Surg Gynecol Obstet 1980; 150:379–384.
12. Kruesser W, Ritz E. The phosphate depletion syndrome. Contrib Nephrol 1978; 14:162–166.
13. Ryan JF, Todres ID, Cotes CJ, et al., eds. A practice of anesthesia for infants and children. New York: Grune & Stratton; 1986:39.
14. Mlcak R, Cortiella J, Desai MH, et al. Emergency management of pediatric burn victims. Pediatr Emerg Care 1998; 14(1):51–54.
15. Herndon DN, Thompson PB, Traber DL. Pulmonary injury in burned patients. Crit Care Clin 1985; 1:79–96.
16. Thompson PB, Herndon DN, Traber DL, et al. Effect on mortality of inhalation injury. J Trauma 1986; 26:163–165.
17. Bennett JDC, Milner SM, Gheranrdini G, et al. Burn inhalation injury. Emerg Med 1997; 12(17):22–24, 31, 32.
18. Desai MH, Mlcak R, Richardson J, et al. Reduction in mortality in pediatric patients with inhalation injury with aerosolized heparin/N-acetylcysteine therapy. J Burn Care Rehabil 1998; 19(3):210–212.

19. Yarborough MF, Herndon DN, Curreri PW. Nutritional management of the severely injured patient: (1) thermal injury. Contemp Surg 1978; 13:15–20.

20. Wilmore DW. Nutrition and metabolism following thermal injury. Clin Plast Surg 1974; 1:603–619.

21. Fleming RYD, Rutan RL, Jahoor F, et al. Effects of recombinant human growth hormone on catabolic hormones and free fatty acids following thermal injury. J Trauma 1992; 32:698–702.

22. Lee JO, Herndon DN. Modulation of the post-burn hypermetabolic state. In: Cynober L, Moore FA, eds. Nutrition and critical care. Switzerland: Nestec; 2003(8):39–56.

23. Herndon DN. Mediators of metabolism. J Trauma 1981; 21:701–705.

24. Pierre E, Barrow R, Hawkins H, et al. Effects of insulin on wound healing. J Trauma 1998; 44:342–345.

25. Wolf SE, Barrow RE, Herndon DN. Growth hormone and IGF-I therapy in the hypercatabolic patient. Baillières Clin Endocrinol Metabol 1996; 10:447–463.

26. Herndon DN, Ramzy PI, DebRoy MA, et al. Muscle protein catabolism after severe burn: effect of IGF-1/IGFBP-3 treatment. Ann Surg 1999; 229:713–720.

27. Hart DW, Wolf SE, Ramzy PI, et al. Anabolic effects of oxandrolone after severe burn. Ann Surg 2001; 233:556–564.

28. Ferrando AA, Sheffield-Moore M, Wolf SE, et al. Testosterone administration in severe burns ameliorates muscle catabolism. Crit Care Med 2001; 29:1936–1942.

29. Herndon DN, Hart DW, Wolf SE, et al. Reversal of catabolism by beta-blockade after severe burns. N Engl J Med 2001; 345:1223–1229.

30. Mochizuki H, Trocki O, Dominioni L, et al. Mechanism of prevention of postburn hypermetabolism and catabolism by early enteral feeding. Ann Surg 1984; 200:297–310.

31. Dominioini L, Trocki O, Fang CH, et al. Enteral feeding in burn hypermetabolism: nutritional and metabolic effects at different levels of calorie and protein intake. JPEN J Parenter Enteral Nutr 1985; 9(3):269–279.

32. Enzi G, Casadei A, Sergi G, et al. Metabolic and hormonal effects of early nutritional supplementation after surgery in burn patients. Crit Care Med 1990; 18:719–721.

33. McDonald WS, Sharp CW, Deitch EA. Immediate enteral feeding in burn patients is safe and effective. Ann Surg 1991; 213:177–183.

34. Hildreth MA, Herndon DN, Desai MH, et al. Caloric requirements of patients with burns under 1 year of age. J Burn Care Rehabil 1993; 14(1):108–112.

35. Hildreth MA, Herndon DN, Desai MH, et al. Caloric needs of adolescent patients with burns. J Burn Care Rehabil 1989; 10(6):523–526.

36. Hildreth MA, Herndon DN, Desai MH, et al. Current treatment reduces calories required to maintain weight in pediatric patients with burns. J Burn Care Rehabil 1990; 11(5):405–409.

37. Hart DW, Wolf SE, Mlcak RP, et al. Persistence of muscle catabolism after severe burn. Surgery 2000; 128:312–319.

38. Klein GL, Herndon DN, Langman CB, et al. Long-term reduction in bone mass after severe burn injury in children. J Pediatr 1995; 126:252–256.

39. Klein GL, Wolf SE, Goodman WG, et al. The management of acute bone loss in severe catabolism due to burn injury. Horm Res 1997; 48:83–87.

40. Rutan RL, Herndon DN. Growth delay in postburn pediatric patients. Arch Surg 1990; 125:392–395.

41. Artz CP, Moncrief JA. Treatment of burns, 3rd edn. Philadelphia: WB Saunders; 1974.

42. Artz LP, Stern PJ, Wurick JD. Skeletal changes after burn injuries in an animal model. J Burn Care Rehabil 1988; 9:148–151.

43. Klein GL, Herndon DN, Rutan TC, et al. Bone disease in burn patients. J Bone Miner Res 1993; 8(3):337–345.

44. Rutan RL, Herndon DN. Growth delay in postburn pediatric patients. Arch Surg 1990; 125:392–395.

45. Merrell SW, Saffle JR, Larson CM, et al. The declining incidence of fatal sepsis following thermal injury. J Trauma 1989; 29:1362–1366.

46. Herndon DN, Parks DH. Comparison of serial debridement and autografting and early massive excision with cadaver skin overlay in the treatment of large burns in children. J Trauma 1986; 26(2):149–152.

47. Thompson P, Herndon DN, Abston S, et al. Effect of early excision on patients with major thermal injury. J Trauma 1987; 27(2):205–207.

48. Barret JP, Wolf SE, Desai M, et al. Total burn wound excision of massive paediatric burns in the first 24 hours post-injury. Ann Burns Fire Disasters 1999; XIII(1):25–27.

49. Herndon DN, Barrow RE, Rutan RL, et al. A comparison of conservative versus early excision therapies in severely burned patients. Ann Surg 1989; 209(5):547–553.

50. Desai MH, Rutan RL, Herndon DN. Conservative treatment of scald burns is superior to early excision. J Burn Care Rehabil 1991; 12:482–484.

51. Rose JK, Desai MH, Mlakar JM, et al. Allograft is superior to topical antimicrobial therapy in the treatment of partial-thickness scald burns in children. J Burn Care Rehabil 1997; 18(4):338–341.

52. Lal SO, Barrow RE, Heggers JP, et al. Biobrane, a synthetic skin substitute, improves wound healing without increased risk of infection. Surgical Infection Society, April 2000 (Abstract 33).

53. Barret JP, Dziewulski P, Ramzy PI, et al. Biobrane versus 1% silver sulfadiazine in second-degree pediatric burns. Plast Reconstr Surg 2000; 105(1):62–65.

54. Naoum JJ. The use of homograft compared to topical antimicrobial therapy in the treatment of second-degree burns of more than 40% total body surface area. American College of Surgeons Committee on Trauma, October 2000 (Abstract).

55. Schecter N, Allen DA, Hanson K. Status of pediatric pain control: a comparison of hospital analgesic usage in children and adults. Pediatrics 1986; 77:11–15.

56. Stevens B, Hunsberger M, Browne G. Pain in children: theoretical research and practice dilemmas. J Pediatr Nurs 1987; 2:154–166.

57. Staddard FJ. Coping with pain: a developmental approach to treatment of burned children. Am J Psychiatry 1982; 139:736–740.

58. Benjamin D, Herndon D. Successful prevention programs for gas hot water heater burn injuries. J Burn Care Rehabil 2000; 21(1 part 2):S152.

59. Benjamin DA, Tompkins RG, Warden GD, et al. Increasing incidence in sleepwear related burns. J Burn Care Rehabil 2001; 21(2): S67.

60. Fleisher G, Ludwig S, eds. Textbook of pediatric emergency medicine, 2nd edn. Baltimore: Williams & Wilkins; 1988:268.

61. Eichelberger MR, ed. Pediatric trauma: prevention, acute care and rehabilitation. St Louis: Mosby Year Book; 1993:572.

Chapter 37

Care of geriatric patients

Robert H. Demling, Clifford T. Pereira, and David N. Herndon

Chapter contents

Introduction

The geriatric patient, usually defined as over 65 years of age, now constitute about 10% of the major burn population, with an anticipated progressive rise as the geriatric population in the United States continues to increase. Improvements in the quality of life over the past 50 years in developed countries have increased the average life span by nearly 30 years.[1] The proportion of the population in the United States over 65 years of age is expected to increase from 12.4% in 2000 to 19.4% in 2030, with a projected increase from 420 million to 973 million elderly citizens.[2] This trend presents a special challenge since the elderly will constitute an ever-growing segment of the average surgeon's practice and will influence clinical and ethical decisions along with healthcare costs. The elderly and the very young pediatric population are most likely to succumb to severe burns.[3–6] It has been reported that nearly 12 deaths per day result from residential fires with infants, toddlers, and the elderly representing the high-mortality population.[4,5] Children less than 5 years of age and adults over 65 years of age have a mortality from burns that is six times the national average.[6] Treatment of the elderly burned patient remains a greater challenge compared with middle-aged and younger patients, due to lower physiological reserves, higher underlying co-morbidities, reducing the margin for error.[7] The number of elderly people seeking medical attention for minor burns is also increasing, making the recognition of the physiological and metabolic changes which occur with age even more important for the burn care professional.[8–10]

Epidemiology

Contact with flame is the main (65%) cause of burn injury, while one-third of injuries are due to cooking accidents — scalds in 15% and contact with hot objects close to 15%.[8–11] The latter cause is much more prevalent in the elderly, reflecting increasing psychological and physical disability. This fact is also reflected in the statistic that the rate of fire-related deaths in an individual over 75 years of age is four times the national average. The male to female ratio is nearly even compared to the 5 to 1 male to female ratio for the young adult burn victim. This ratio is explained by the fact that 95% of burns in elderly people occur in the home compared to less than half for the younger adult. Prevention therefore must be focused on the home. Prevention should also focus on the fact that 30% of geriatric patients are the victims of self-neglect and at least 10% are the victims of elder abuse.[11]

Outcome

As expected, mortality and morbidity is higher for the geriatric patient with a burn.[1–5] Mortality in a young adult with a burn 80% total body surface area (TBSA) is 50%; in a person aged 60–70 years a burn 35% TBSA has a 50% mortality and in a person over 70 years old, a 20% TBSA burn will have a 50% mortality.[9,12] Pereira et al.[13] analyzed 1674 patients admitted to the Shriners Burn Hospital, Galveston, Texas, between 1989 and 2005 as well as 179 autopsies conducted during this period, to study mortality trends and primary causes of death in the entire spectrum of age over time. The data demonstrated that mortality has indeed reduced in all age groups over the last decade, including the elderly (>65 years) group. Gender dimorphism was noted in mortality in patients over 65 years of age. Lung injury and sepsis was the commonest primary cause of death noted at autopsy. Increase in weights of heart, lung, spleen, and liver were noted in all age groups postmortem. These data indicate that chronological age alone is not an independent cause of mortality and morbidity after severe burns.

Furthermore, the long-term disability is much greater in the geriatric patient. Approximately 50% of elderly patients with a major burn return to a home environment within the first year[8,9,14] compared to nearly 90% for the younger adult. The increased risk factors present in this population explain these outcome statistics. It is also possible that the increased complications seen in the elderly burns result from a more cautious and less-aggressive treatment regimen. This is due to existing beliefs among clinicians that elderly burn patients tolerate eschar excision less than their younger counterparts, resulting in a greater delay in excision of burned tissue.[15] However, it is important to recognize that despite these risk factors the elderly burn patient has been repeatedly demonstrated to tolerate multiple and early surgical procedures, and early wound closure corresponds to a better outcome.[16-18]

Risk factors

There are a number of well-recognized risk factors, present in elderly people, which will lead to increased morbidity after a burn. Some of the more prominent factors are shown in Box 37.1.

Decreased cardiopulmonary reserve

Aging is known to decrease pulmonary reserve for both gas exchange and lung mechanics.[19] Elderly people are more prone to pulmonary failure, which is the major cause of death in all burns. The presence of atherosclerosis, coronary artery disease, and previous myocardial infarcts are also common.

Chronic illness including malnutrition

A number of disease states are commonly seen, such as adult-onset diabetes and a previous or current cancer. Some degree of protein-energy malnutrition is found in over 50% of elderly burn patients on admission. Malnutrition increases morbidity and mortality after a burn and may well increase the elder's risk for burn injury.[20-22] Micronutrient deficiency is particularly prevalent. A well-recognized alteration in the gastrointestinal tract is a decrease in the ability to breakdown whole proteins and to tolerate a carbohydrate load, which leads to inadequate calories and protein.[21] Daily protein requirements are higher in the elderly than in the younger population.[21]

Decreased lean body mass

There is a progressive decrease in lean body mass with aging.[23] The lean mass or body protein compartment is responsible for all the physiological and metabolic activity needed for survival, and any significant decrease is detrimental since a burn injury characteristically leads to catabolism-induced loss of lean mass. Any pre-existing loss will result in increased morbidity, especially the early onset of immune deficiency, weakness, and impaired healing.[22,24,25] The cause of the loss is multifactorial. Impaired nutrition, decreased activity, and a decrease in levels of the endogenous anabolic hormones, human growth hormone, and testosterone with age are all causative.[19,22]

Decreased anabolic activity leads to a longer recovery time as well as causing the restoration of muscle to be very slow. Of importance is the fact that elderly people respond to exogenous anabolic stimuli such as testosterone analogs, human growth hormone, and resistant exercise in a similar fashion to the younger population. Therefore, exercise, high protein nutrition, and anabolic agents are essential for recovery.[26-28]

Aging skin and wound healing

There are significant changes in the skin with aging which are responsible for the greater percent of deep burns in the elderly, even after scalds, compared to a younger patient.[29-31] A 50% decrease in the turnover rate of the epidermis is present after age 65, as well as a flattening of the rete pegs and fewer epidermal-lined skin appendages. These properties will significantly decrease the healing rate of a partial-thickness burn.[29-31]

In addition, there is a progressive thinning of the dermis and a decrease in both collagen content and matrix, especially glycosaminoglycan. The latter is responsible for loss of skin turgor. In addition, there is a decrease in vascularity and in the key resident cells, i.e. macrophages and fibroblasts. The thinner dermis with less blood flow explains the greater amount of deep burn, and the decreased cellularity explains a decrease in all phases of healing[29-31] (Box 37.2).

Treatment

In general, treatment is identical to that for the younger patient except for the fact that massive burns are more commonly managed expectantly.

Initial resuscitation

In general, more fluid is required to resuscitate the same burn size to avoid hypovolemia.[32] The reason is likely the decreased skin turgor which decreases the resistance to fluid accumulation or edema production. Another possible factor is some impairment in cardiac function. Early ventilatory support is more commonly required due to decreased lung reserve and earlier fatigue.

Wound management

The same aggressive approach at wound closure used in the younger patient applies to the elderly. Removal of the burn wound is essential to survival.[16-18] Since older patients do

---

BOX 37.1 Risk factors in elderly people

- Chronic illness, e.g. adult diabetes
- Cardiovascular disease, e.g. previous infarct
- Pulmonary reserve decreased with age
- Unintentional weight loss
- Decrease in lean body mass
- Impaired nutrition with presence of deficiency states in energy, protein, and macronutrients
- Decreased endogenous anabolic hormones
- Skin aging (thin, decreased synthesis)

BOX 37.2 Aging of skin

- Decreased epidermal turnover
- Decrease in skin appendages
- Thinning of dermis
- Decreased vascularity
- Decreased collagen and matrix
- Decreased fibroblasts, macrophages

tolerate operative procedures, a conservative approach is not warranted. However, thinner skin grafts are necessary due to the thinner dermis, and a longer healing time is expected.[29]

Metabolic and nutritional support

Although elderly patients do not generate the degree of hypermetabolism seen with younger patients, the catabolic response is comparable, necessitating a 1.5 g/kg/day protein intake.[33,34] Since many older patients already have a lean mass deficit evidenced by prior weight loss,[13] the goal of nutritional support must not be 'maintenance' alone, but rather replacement therapy, especially of protein and micronutrients, as pre-existing deficiency states are common.[22,23] Nutrient supplements are invariably required. As most supplements are protein hydrolysates, the gut is more capable of absorbing the peptides and amino acids compared to the breakdown of whole proteins in food.[35,36] Anabolic agents can be valuable adjuncts to optimal nutrition.[37,38]

Anabolic agents such as insulin and oxandrolone have been studied in improving postburn hypercatabolism in the pediatric population and their use could be extended to the elderly considering the reduction in endogenous anabolic hormones in this group post-injury.[45] Continuous infusions of the anabolic peptide insulin, with tight euglycemic control, in victims of major thermal injury prevents muscle catabolism and preserves lean body mass, without increasing hepatic triglyceride production.[39,40] Lower dose infusions at 9–10 U/h, promotes substantial muscle anabolism without the need for additional large doses of carbohydrate.[41] Maintenance of euglycemia with insulin for non-burned patients in surgical critical care units, substantially diminished infection and the mortality rate and is a critical hormonal manipulation in the acute setting.[42] Insulin infusions are suited to the closely monitored environment of the burn intensive care unit but are impractical in the rehabilitative outpatient setting. Testosterone restoration is an effective therapeutic maneuver in both male and female burn victims. However oxandrolone, a synthetic analog, is preferable since it possesses only 5% of testosterone's virilizing androgenic effects and has a per oral formulation available. Oxandrolone improved net muscle protein synthesis in healthy young men[45] and was later found to effectively improve lean body mass in burned patients, especially emaciated subjects whose treatment had been delayed.[37,43] The effects were independent of age.[44] Treatment of acute pediatric burn patients with oral oxandrolone (0.1 mg/kg twice daily) enhances efficiency of protein synthesis, increases anabolic gene expression in muscle, and significantly increases lean body mass at 6, 9, and 12 months after burn and bone mineral content 12 months after injury versus unburned controls.[40] Recombinant human growth hormone has been successfully used in pediatric patients; however, has several adverse side effects, particularly during acute care in burned patients, most notably hyperglycemia, and has shown an increased mortality rate in critically ill, non-burned adults in Europe.[46,47] We therefore do not recommend its use in the elderly.

Pain, sedation, and comfort care

There is increasing evidence that the geriatric burn patient is undertreated for pain due to the misconception that there is less pain with age.[48] Both pain and anxiety further increase catecholamine levels, which is deleterious. Management of standard drug therapy is affected by the decreased clearance of many of these agents with aging, requiring decreased dosages[49] (Table 37.1). Evidence from investigations of experimental pain suggests that there is an increased response in the elderly to high-intensity stimuli and a reduced pain tolerance to high-intensity stimuli.[50] Undertreated postoperative pain in the elderly does seem to increase the incidence of delirium.[51] Also, although the initial burn injury and sepsis-related complications principally determine the extent of the metabolic response in burn victims, obligatory activity, background and procedural related pain, and anxiety also greatly increase metabolic rates. Judicious maximal narcotics support, appropriate sedation, and supportive psychotherapy are mandatory to minimize their effects.[52] Another area of potential benefit is the use of a proactive geriatrics consultation team. Involving the geriatrician early reduced the perioperative incidence of delirium by one-third due to targeted recommendations based on predefined areas of high risk. Comfort care only measures need to be strongly considered for elderly patients with likely fatal burns. Age, burn size, and pre-existing health problems dictate which patients should have comfort care. Since these factors are evident very early, this approach should not be delayed to avoid excessive suffering by patient and family.[53]

Perioperative optimization

Aging leads to many changes in the cardiovascular system that makes hemodynamic stability more difficult to achieve, leading to increased adverse outcomes. Coronary artery disease is prevalent and is estimated to exceed 80% in patients over 80 years.[54] The incidence of congestive heart failure may be as high as 10% in the elderly.[55] The revised cardiac risk index helps stratify patients into risk groups and helps to identify those in whom additional cardiac evaluation might be indicated.[56] Patients at risk for a perioperative myocardial event either by the revised cardiac risk index or who have other risk factors (e.g. peripheral vascular disease, unexplained chest pain, diabetes, ECG abnormalities, etc.) should undergo further evaluation. For patients unable to exercise at all, pharmaco-

TABLE 37.1 COMMONLY USED DRUGS REQUIRING DECREASED DOSES IN ELDERLY PATIENTS*

Drug	Comments
Barbiturates (should be avoided in elderly)	Paradoxical pharmacological response often leading to restlessness, agitation, or psychosis: decreased rate of elimination
Benzodiazepines	Increased sensitivity to pharmacological effect; some benzodiazepines may be metabolized more slowly
Narcotic analgesics	Increased sensitivity to analgesic effects: possibly impaired clearance
Tricyclic antidepressants	Increased incidence of cardiac and hemodynamic adverse effects; urinary retention and other anticholinergic effects; decreased drug clearance

*Decreased dose in part due to decreased renal function in the elderly.

logical stress perfusion imaging using dipyridamole, adenosine or dobutamine provides comparable prognostic information compared with exercise perfusion imaging. A normal stress perfusion scan or a normal stress echocardiogram is associated with <1% combined perioperative death or infarction rate. Patients with minor perfusion abnormalities undergoing lower-risk operations may not require catheterization, but should be considered for prophylactic β-blockers and aspirin before operation. High-risk subgroups of patients based on clinical risk factors and individuals with positive non-invasive tests should undergo cardiac catheterization. Patients with significant cardiac lesions should have definitive coronary revascularization via angioplasty before large body surface area burns are excised. Increasingly the potential benefits of using β-adrenergic blocking agents in the perioperative period are being studied.[57–59] The rationale is that perioperative ischemic events are related to an exaggerated postoperative sympathetic response leading to increases in heart rate.[57,58,60,61] β-blockade has an added advantage in the burn patient. Severe thermal injury is associated with persistent hypermetabolism that can last for up to 9–12 months post injury,[62] with deleterious consequences in the acute and the convalescent phase. The resting metabolic rates in burn patients increase from near normal for burns less than 10% TBSA to twice normal in >40% TBSA involvement.[60] Previous studies have demonstrated that catecholamines play a key role in the initiation of the various cascades leading to postburn hypermetabolism.[66,67] Once initiated, these cascades, their mediators and their by-products appear to stimulate the persistent and increased metabolic rate seen after severe burn injury. Blocking the triggering of these cascades at the onset by blocking the action of catecholamines at the receptor level attenuates this response and decreases supraphysiological thermogenesis,[63] tachycardia, cardiac work[64] and resting energy expenditure.[66] Severely burned subjects treated with propranolol titrated to produce 20% reductions in baseline heart rates, diminished obligatory thermogenesis, tachycardia, cardiac work, resting energy expenditure, reduced fatty infiltration of the liver and increased muscle–protein balance.[64] However no study has directly focused on the geriatric patient. Furthermore, the drawback of β-blockade in the elderly is that the aging cardiovascular system has a decreased response to β-receptor stimulation. This decrease together with anesthetic agents may have additive effects in the setting of prophylactic β-blockade administration and lead to deleterious and profound hypotension intraoperatively. Despite being well tolerated, as demonstrated by Mangano et al.,[57] many practitioners still withhold β-blockers in the elderly for fear of drug-related complications. Individualized dosing of β-blockers as suggested by Raby et al.[61] to control myocardial ischemia postoperatively may be more beneficial due to different coronary anatomy and ischemic thresholds among patients. This target-based approach may decrease the incidence of drug-related side effects. Further investigations will be necessary to evaluate the most appropriate therapeutic regimen that will reduce perioperative ischemia, cardiac morbidity, and postburn hypermetabolic response in the elderly burn survivors.

Pulmonary complications are more strongly linked to coexisting comorbidities than to chronological age.[68] Because of the prevalence and importance of chronic obstructive pulmonary disease (COPD) and asthma in the elderly, physicians need to have a high index of suspicion for these conditions during the perioperative evaluation. Perioperative chest x-rays should be ordered selectively. The value of pulmonary function tests remains controversial. With the appropriate diagnosis, aggressive pulmonary rehabilitation including exercise training, patient education, nutritional counseling, smoking cessation, and optimization of medication have been shown to be effective for the elderly patient.[68] Aggressive use of antibiotics, judicious use of bronchodilators, adequate hydration and postural drainage and chest physiotherapy are also liable to reduce the incidence of pneumonia.

Rehabilitation

The elderly patient needs to be aggressively managed in the rehabilitation phase to avoid any further loss of function or strength, which will be difficult to recover. As previously described, the geriatric patient is capable of restoring muscle strength with resistance exercise and therefore should not be managed conservatively.[69] As with children, providing support and guidance for family or caretakers is an integral part of care. The patient will depend on these individuals for their well-being on discharge.[70,71]

Intentional burns in the elderly

Identifying elder abuse is harder than identifying child abuse. Children cannot legally live alone and must attend school, whereas the elderly often live alone, interacting predominantly or exclusively, with the very family or carers who enact their abuse.[72] The abused elderly may collude with their abusers (unwittingly or purposefully), keeping their abuse secret due to shame or guilt, especially if children are responsible, or fear of reprisal if they are dependent on the abuser.[73,74] There is evidence that 80% of elder abuse comes to light only when someone other than the victim or a relative becomes involved.[75] Most forms of intentionally inflicted burns have a higher associated morbidity and mortality than equivalent accidental burns, in part due to comorbidity from other physical or substance abuse or from psychological problems that pre-existed and contributed to the inflicted burn or that result from it. Unlike with children, in dealing with elder mistreatment the duties of a doctor to report suspected abuse may produce ethical difficulties with respect to confidentiality, when competent elderly victims of abuse do not want it reported. The initial priority of the examining doctor is to identify life-threatening conditions and treat them, and thereafter, to identify and promptly and completely record symptoms and signs of abuse or neglect (including photographs). A deliberately inflicted burn on another human being represents a criminal act and as such must be reported. Intentionally inflicted burn injuries are not simply physical injuries and are best managed within a multidisciplinary team of specially interested and prepared healthcare, social service and legal professionals.

Conclusion

Surgical decision-making in the burned elderly patient requires consideration of the patient's physiological age, preburn functional status, degree of impairment from comorbid conditions, and clear treatment goals. No patient should be denied an operation on the basis of age alone, since decline in organ function with aging is predictable for the population as a whole but less so for an individual. Currently, no 'score' can improve decisions based upon sound clinical judgment after a thorough evaluation and discussion with the patient and the family.

Favorable outcomes in the elderly burned patient should pertain more to relief of suffering and maintaining independence and quality of life rather than expanding life span. And finally, clear and repeated communication between the burn team and patients or their surrogates remains a critical aspect for guidance of therapy and the achievement of acceptable outcomes.

References

1. Thompson JC. Gifts from surgical research. Contributions to patients and to surgeons. J Am Coll Surg 2000; 190(5):509–521.
2. US Department of Census. 65+ in the United States. Washington, DC: US Bureau of the Census; 1996.
3. Saffle JR, Davis B, Williams P. Recent outcomes in the treatment of burn injury in the United States: a report from the American Burn Association Patient Registry. J Burn Care Rehabil 1995; 16(3 Pt 1):219–232.
4. Herndon DN, Gore D, Cole M, et al. Determinants of mortality in pediatric patients with greater than 70% full-thickness total body surface area thermal injury treated by early total excision and grafting. J Trauma 1987; 27(2):208–212.
5. Jeschke MD, Barrow RE, Herndon DN. Recombinant human growth hormone treatment in pediatric burn patients and its role during the hepatic acute phase response. Cri Care Med 2000; 28(5):1578–1583.
6. Colebrook L, Colebrook V. The prevention of burns and scalds. Lancet 1949; 11:181–188.
7. Feller I, Crane KH. National Burn Information Exchange. Surg Clin North Am 1970; 50(6):1425–1436.
8. O'Neill A, Rabbits A, Hamel H, et al. Burns in the elderly; our burn centers' experience with patients over 75 years old. J Burn Care Rehabil 2000; 21:183.
9. McGill V, Kowal-Vern A, Gainelli R. Outcome for older burn patients. Arch Surg 2000; 135:320–325.
10. Rossignol AM, Locke JA, Boyle CM, et al. Consumer products and hospitalized burn injuries among elderly Massachusetts residents. J Am Geriatr Soc 1985; 33:768–772.
11. Bird P, Narrington D, Bavillo D, et al. Elder abuse: a call to action. J Burn Care Rehabil 1998; 19:522–527.
12. Saffle JR, Davis B, Williams P. Recent outcomes in the treatment of burn injury in the United States: a report from the American Burn Association Patient Registry. J Burn Care Rehabil 1995; 16;219–232.
13. Pereira CT, Barrow RE, Sterns AM, et al. Age-dependent differences in survival after severe burns: a unicentric review of 1674 patients and 179 autopsies over 15 years. J Am Coll Surg 2006; 202:536–548.
14. Larson C, Soffle J, Sullivan J. Lifestyle adjustments in elderly patients after burn injury. Burn Care Rehabil 1992; 13:48–52.
15. Stern M. Comparison of methods of predicting burn mortality. Burns 1978; 6:119–123.
16. Frye K, Luterman A. Management of the burn wound requiring excision. Geriatric Patients 2000; 21:200.
17. Kirn D, Luce E. Early excision and grafting versus conservative management of burns in the elderly. Plast Reconstr Surg 1998; 102:1013–1017.
18. Burdge JJ, Katz B, Edwards R, et al. Surgical treatment of burns in elderly patients. J Trauma 1988; 28:214–217.
19. Koupil J, Brychta P, Rehova H. Special features of burn injuries in elderly patients. Acta Chir Plast 2001; 43;57–66.
20. Demling RH. The incidence and impact of pre-existing protein energy malnutrition on outcome in the elderly burn patient population. J Burn Care Rehabil 2005; 26;94–100.
21. Ausman L, Russell R. Nutrition and the elderly. In: Linden M, ed. Nutritional biochemical and metabolism. New York: Elsevier; 1991;120.
22. Kagansky N, Berner Y, Levy S. Poor nutritional habits are predictors of poor outcome in very old hospitalized patients. Am J Clin Nutr 2005; 82;784–791.
23. Forbes G. Body composition: influence of nutrition, disease growth and aging. In: Shils M, ed. Modern nutrition in health and disease. Philadelphia: Lea and Febiger; 1994:781.
24. Kotler P. Magnitude of cell body mass depletion and timing of death from wasting. Am J Clin Nutr 1989; 50:440–447.
25. Darby E, Anawalt B. Male hypogonadism: an update on diagnosis and treatment. Treat Endocrinol 2005; 4:293–309.
26. Demling RH, DeSanti L. The beneficial effects of the anabolic steroid oxandrolone in the geriatric burn population. Wounds – A compendium of Clinical Research and Practice. 2003; 15:34–58.
27. Rudman P, Fillor A. Effect of growth hormone on body composition in elderly men. Horm Res 1991; 36:73–81.
28. Fralarone M, O'Neil E. Exercise training and nutritional supplements for physical frailty in very elderly people. N Engl J Med 1994; 330:1769–1775.
29. Goodson W, Hunt T. Wound healing and aging. J Invest Dermatol 1979; 73:88–91.
30. Jacobsen R, Flowers F. Skin changes with aging and disease. Wound Rep Reg 1996; 4:311–315.
31. Walter J, Maibach H. Age and skin structure and function, a quantitative approach: blood flow pH, thickness and ultrasound echogenicity. Skin Res Technol 2005; 11:221–235.
32. Bowser-Wallace BH, Cone JB, Caldwell FT. Hypertonic lactated saline resuscitation of severely burned patients over 60 years of age. J Trauma 1985; 25(1):22–26.
33. Wolfe R. Relation of metabolic studies to clinical nutrition: the example of burn injury. Am J Clin Nutr 1996; 64:800–808.
34. Bessy J. Stress response to injury: endocrinologic and metabolic response. In: Greenfield L, ed. Current practice of surgery. New York: Churchill Livingstone; 1995:1–12.
35. Lupschitz D. Approaches to the nutritional support of the older patient. Clinic Geriatr Med 1995; 11:715–725.
36. Larsson J, Masson M. Effect of a dietary supplement on nutritional status and clinical outcome: a randomized geriatric study. Clin Nutr 1990; 9:179–184.
37. Demling R, DeSanti L. Oxandrolone, an anabolic steroid, significantly increases the rate of weight gain in the recovery phase after major burns. J Trauma 1997; 43:47–51.
38. Ziegler T. Growth hormone administration during nutritional support: what is to be gained. New Horizons 1999; 2:249–256.
39. Sakurai Y, Aarsland A, Herndon DN, et al. Stimulation of muscle protein synthesis by long-term insulin infusion in severely burned patients. Ann Surg 1995; 222(3):283–297.
40. Aarsland A, Chinkes DL, Sakurai Y, et al. Insulin therapy in burn patients does not contribute to hepatic triglyceride production. J Clin Invest 1998; 101(10):2233–2239.
41. Ferrando AA, Chinkes DL, Wolf SE, et al. Submaximal dose of insulin promotes skeletal muscle protein synthesis in patients with severe burns. Ann Surg 1999; 229(1):11–18.
42. Van den Berghe G, Wouters PJ, Bouillon R, et al. Outcome benefit of intensive insulin therapy in the critically ill: insulin dose versus glycemic control. Crit Care Med 2003; 31(2):359–366.
43. Wolf SE, Thomas SJ, Dasu MR, et al. Improved net protein balance, lean mass, and gene expression changes with oxandrolone treatment in the severely burned. Ann Surg 2003; 237(6):801–810.
44. Demling RH, DeSanti L. The rate of restoration of body weight after burn injury, using the anabolic agent oxandrolone, is not age dependent. Burns 2001; 27(1):46–51.
45. Sheffield-Moore M, Urban RJ, Wolf SE, et al. Short-term oxandrolone administration stimulates muscle protein synthesis

in young men. J Clin Endocrinol Metabol 1999; 84(8):2705–2711.

46. Singh KP, Prasad R, Chari PS, et al. Effect of growth hormone therapy in burn patients on conservative treatment. Burns 1998; 24(8):733–738.

47. Takala J, Ruokonen E, Webster NR, et al. Increased mortality associated with growth hormone treatment in critically ill adults. N Engl J Med 1999; 341(11):785–792.

48. Honari S, Patterson D, Gibbons J, et al. Comparison of pain control medication in three age groups of elderly patients. J Burn Care Rehabil 1997; 18:500–504.

49. Tsujimoto G, Hashimoto K, Hoffman B. Pharmacokinetic and pharmacodynamic principles of drug therapy in old age. Clin Pharmacol Ther Toxicol 1989; 27:13–26.

50. Gibson S, Helme R. Age-related differences in pain perception and report. Clin Geriatr Med 2001; 17(3) v–vi:433–456.

51. Lynch EP, Lazor MA, Gellis JE, et al. The impact of postoperative pain on the development of postoperative delirium. Anesth Analg 1998; 86(4):781–785.

52. Murphy KD, Lee JO, Herndon DN. Current pharmacotherapy for the treatment of severe burns. Exp Opin Pharmacother 2003; 4(3): 369–384.

53. Stassen N, Lukan J, Mizuguchi N, et al. Thermal injury in the elderly: when is comfort care the right choice? Am Surg 2001; 67:704–708.

54. Mangano DT. Perioperative cardiac morbidity. Anesthesiology 1990; 72(1):153–184.

55. Kannel WB, Belanger AJ. Epidemiology of heart failure. Am Heart J 1991; 121(3 Pt 1):951–957.

56. Lee TH, Marcantonio ER, Mangione CM, et al. Derivation and prospective validation of a simple index for prediction of cardiac risk of major noncardiac surgery. Circulation 1999; 100(10):1043–1049.

57. Mangano DT, Layug EL, Wallace A, et al. Effect of atenolol on mortality and cardiovascular morbidity after noncardiac surgery. Multicenter Study of Perioperative Ischemia Research Group. N Engl J Med 1996; 335:1713–1720.

58. Wallace A, Layug B, Tateo I, et al. Prophylactic atenolol reduces postoperative myocardial ischemia. Anesthesiology 1998; 88(1):7–17.

59. Poldermans D, Boersma E, Bax JJ, et al. The effect of bisoprolol on perioperative mortality and myocardial infarction in high-risk patients undergoing vascular surgery. Dutch Echocardiographic Cardiac Risk Evaluation Applying Stress Echocardiography Study Group. N Engl J Med 1999; 341(24):1789–1794.

60. Mangano DT, Hollenberg M, Fegert G, et al. Perioperative myocardial ischemia in patients undergoing noncardiac surgery – Incidence and severity during the 4 day perioperative period. The Study of Perioperative Ischemia (SPI) Research Group. J Am Coll Cardiol 1991; 17(4):843–850.

61. Raby KE, Brull SJ, Timimi F, et al. The effect of heart rate control on myocardial ischemia among high-risk patients after vascular surgery. Anesth Analg 1999; 88(3):477–482.

62. Hart DW, Wolf SE, Mlcak R, et al. Persistence of muscle catabolism after severe burn. Surgery 2000; 128(2):312–319.

63. Herndon DN, Barrow RE, Rutan TC, et al. Effect of propranolol administration on hemodynamic and metabolic responses of burned pediatric patients. Ann Surg 1988; 208(4):484–492.

64. Baron PW, Barrow RE, Pierre EJ, et al. Prolonged use of propranolol safely decreases cardiac work in burned children. J Burn Care Rehabil 1997; 18(3):223–227.

65. Breitenstein E, Chiolero RL, Jequier E, et al. Effects of beta-blockade on energy metabolism following burns. Burns 1990; 16(4):259–264.

66. Goodall MC, Stone C, Haynes BW Jr. Urinary Output of adrenaline and nonadrenaline in severe thermal burns. Ann Surg 1957; 145:479.

67. Aprille JR, Aikawa N, Bell TC, et al. Adenylate cyclase after burn injury: resistance to desensitization by catecholamines. J Trauma 1979; 19(11):812–818.

68. Couser JI Jr, Guthmann R, Hamadeh MA, et al. Pulmonary rehabilitation improves exercise capacity in older elderly patients with COPD. Chest 1995; 107(3):730–734.

69. Franberg W, Meredith C, O'Reilly K, et al. Strength conditioning in older men: skeletal muscle hypertrophy and improved function. J Appl Physiol 1988; 64:1038–1044.

70. Manktelow A, Meyer AA, Herzog SR, et al. Analysis of life expectancy and living status of elderly patients surviving a burn injury. J Trauma 1989; 29:203–207.

71. Suter-Gut D, Metcalf AM, Donnelly MA, et al. Post-discharge care planning and rehabilitation of the elderly surgical patient. Clin Geriatr Med 1990; 6(3):69–83.

72. Brogden M, Nijhar P. Crime, abuse and the elderly, 1st edn. Uffculme: Willan; 2000.

73. Prichard J. Dispelling some myths. J Elder Abuse Neglect 1993; 52(2):27–36.

74. O'Connor F. Granny bashing — abuse of the elderly. New York: Human Sciences Press; 1989.

75. Plwell S, Berg R. When the elderly are abused. Educ Gerontol 1987; 13(1):71–83.

Chapter 38

Surgical management of complications of burn injury

Elizabeth A. Beierle and Dai H. Chung

Introduction

A multitude of surgical complications can occur in burn patients depending on the size and depth of burn injury. Burns, sustained as a result of concomitant blunt trauma (e.g., vehicle explosion), can present with multiple organ system injuries, requiring thorough systemic assessment and management according to the Advanced Trauma Life Support (ATLS) guidelines. Patients with large total body surface area (TBSA) burns generally require prolonged hospital stay with numerous debridement and skin grafting procedures and are at risk for potential surgical complications involving various organ systems. The gastrointestinal (GI) tract complications include stress gastritis and ulceration, acalculous cholecystitis, superior mesenteric artery (SMA) syndrome, and pancreatitis. Additionally, despite pharmacological advances in prevention of stress gastritis and ulceration, it remains as the most common cause of GI tract bleeding in burn patients. Burn injury-induced enterocolitis as a result of transient ischemia-reperfusion injury to the gut is a serious GI tract complication, which can progress to full-thickness necrosis of involved segment. Abdominal compartment syndrome can also occur during acute phase of massive fluid resuscitation in large TBSA burned patients. Moreover, burn patients are susceptible to common GI tract pathology such as appendicitis and intussusception (in toddlers) during their prolonged hospitalization. Other potential complications include conditions associated with vascular access procedures, which are frequently performed in large TBSA burn patients. Major burn injury significantly affects hemodynamic status, requiring central venous as well as arterial pressure monitoring. Various catheter-related complications are frequently encountered in burn intensive care units. A variety of non-thermal surgical problems can occur in burned patients.[1,2] The cause for occult systemic sepsis is frequently attributed to GI tract pathology such as ischemic bowel, acute cholecystitis, abscess and gastric perforation resulting in significant morbidity and mortality, especially with delay in diagnosis and treatment. In our own experience at Shriners Hospital for Children at Galveston, common surgical problems encountered were enterocolitis, gastroduodenal ulceration, septic thrombophlebitis, mesenteric ischemia with bowel necrosis, small bowel obstruction, and arterial vascular injury with distal limb ischemia. These secondary and sometimes fatal complications in burn-injured patients deserve immediate recognition and treatment. Major burn patients need diligent care and attention throughout their hospital course to avoid complications arising from other organ systems. This chapter reviews the frequently encountered general surgical problems in burned patients with respect to diagnosis and management.

Burns and multiple traumas

Blunt trauma

Burn injury in association with multiple trauma poses an unusual and often vexing challenge for the surgeon. There are few published data pertaining to this topic, primarily due to the regionalization of burn care in areas not commonly associated with trauma centers. Approximately 24% of military burn casualties and 2–7% of civilian burns are associated with other traumatic injuries.[3–5] Mortality is obviously related to burn size and depth, but is also directly related to the number and severity of associated multiple organ injuries. Of 2914 major burn patients admitted over a period of 10 years to Los Angeles County and University of Southern California burn center, combined injuries accounted for approximately 5% of admissions with an overall mortality of 13%, nearly twice that of burns without associated trauma. In addition, the presence of inhalation injury further compromised the prognosis, carrying a mortality of 41% in the group of patients with major burns, multiple trauma and smoke inhalation.[6]

Knowledge of the mechanism of the burn injury aids in predicting the full scope of concomitant traumatic injuries. For example, motor vehicle crashes account for the majority of multiple injured burned patients. Industrial accidents and attempts to escape house fires, explosions, and electrical burns with falls account for the other majority of victims. One group found that 88% of burned patients injured in motorcycle crashes and 36% of those injured in other motor vehicles crashes have additional injuries other than burns.[5] Motor vehicle crash victims that require extrication from the vehicle and those that are ejected typically have the most severe injuries. Those trapped or unconscious in or near a burning vehicle are obviously in danger of severe inhalation injury. The most frequently encountered organ system injuries in motor vehicle crash victims in order of frequency are musculoskeletal, head and neck, abdominal, thoracic, and genitourinary system. Attempts to escape from the building during a fire commonly lead to falls resulting blunt trauma with potential multiple organ injuries. The median lethal height for this mechanism of injury is 40 feet (four building floors) and spinal injuries may be overlooked.[6] Spinal cord lesions are seldom complete and they may not necessarily present with obvious evidence of associated vertebral fractures.[7,8] High-voltage electrical burns rarely occur at ground level and are, therefore, often accompanied by falls, resulting in multiple injuries. In addition, tetanic contractures resulting in fractures, massive neurovascular, orthopedic and soft-tissue destruction are frequently seen with major electrical burn injury.

Primary assessment

In burned patients with multiple organ injuries, the spectacular appearance of the burn injury may unduly shift the caregiver's attention away from the seemingly underwhelming associated injuries, resulting in delay of diagnosis and subsequent increased morbidity and mortality. The initial assessment of patients with combined thermal and non-thermal injuries should focus on airway, breathing, and circulation, as recommended by the ATLS guidelines from the Committee on Trauma of the American College of Surgeons. The burn injury itself is usually not immediately life threatening, but rather asphyxia, airway obstruction, impaired breathing from neurological injury, exsanguination, tension pneumothorax or cardiac tamponade pose more ominous threats. Thoracic injuries such as rib fractures, pneumothorax and hemothorax should be managed as in any other trauma patients with blunt thoracic injury. Thoracostomy tubes, if possible, are placed away from burned skin to decrease the risk of infectious complications such as empyema. Although rare, empyema with loculated fibrous thoracic collections is best handled with minimally invasive thoracoscopic approach. Pericardial tamponade resulting from heavy impact to anterior chest wall can be detected by focused assessment with sonography for trauma (FAST) exam and managed with pericardiocentesis or a pericardial window.

Associated injuries

Approximately 5% of civilian combined injury patients have associated intraabdominal trauma.[6,9] The diagnosis of intraabdominal injury may prove difficult, as the abdominal examination is often unreliable in the face of a severe burn. In addition, the usual practice of monitoring changes in vital signs and hemoglobin to detect intra-abdominal injury may be unreliable since these changes may be significantly affected by the intravascular volume shift from severe burn. Tools such as diagnostic peritoneal lavage (DPL), computed tomography (CT) scan or ultrasonography (FAST exam) that are currently used to evaluate trauma patients with blunt or penetrating mechanisms should also be considered when evaluating a burned patient with suspected intra-abdominal injury. In a prospective, randomized study, the sensitivity, specificity and accuracy of these diagnostic modalities in victims of blunt abdominal trauma were similar and the diagnostic studies

were actually complementary in minimizing the incidence of missed injuries.[10] It is imperative to avoid 'negative' celiotomies, while promptly detecting all significant intra-abdominal injuries that could compromise the overall outcome of the patient. However, once the decision has been made for surgical abdomen, extreme care must be taken to avoid abdominal wall complications such as dehiscence and infection. Dehiscence of abdominal wounds in burned patients is frequent, independent of whether or not the burn wound was traversed.[11] If abdominal wall closure demonstrates significant tension, retention sutures should be utilized. Occasionally, a temporary abdominal closure using silo sheet or organ bag may be required due to massive bowel edema for delayed abdominal wall closure. Although DPL is now rarely used due to advances in CT imaging, when necessary, closed rather than open technique for DPL should be used. Diagnostic laparoscopy can be a helpful, non-invasive method to accurately determine injuries such as bowel perforation or ischemia that are difficult to diagnose with CT alone. However, adequate intra-abdominal insufflation for laparoscopy is often difficult to achieve in patients with eschar in the trunk area.

Vascular injuries may be difficult to diagnose due to the appearance of the burned skin, soft tissue edema, compartment syndrome, or hypotension. Although angiography continues to be the gold standard in the diagnosis of major vascular injuries, the invasive nature of the exam and necessity of moving patients to the angiography suite pose a significant burden and risks. On the other hand, ankle-brachial index (ABI) and a Doppler ultrasound are non-invasive bedside techniques to assess adequacy of arterial blood flow; however, the results can be difficult to interpret, especially for ABI when extremities are burned full-thickness. Although extremely rare to face significant vascular injury requiring graft placement, potential problems with contamination of either autologous or synthetic grafts need to be weighed, and the liberal use of prophylactic muscle flaps for graft coverage has proven to be helpful. As is standard in all trauma patients, the cervical spine should be considered unstable until a complete evaluation has been performed. True unstable cervical spine fractures should be treated with traction via halo or tongs, which may be placed through the burn, if accompanied with compulsive site care and early burn wound excision. When necessary, intracranial pressure monitoring via a bolt placed through healthy skin is preferred over a ventriculostomy. If a neurosurgical procedure is required, debridement of the scalp and non-viable tissue is completed at the same time as the craniotomy. Orthopedic injuries, primarily fractures, are the most common associated injuries in thermally injured patients. The burn surgeon and the orthopedist make decisions regarding the optimal management of these patients jointly. Therapeutic decisions are based upon the following considerations:

* stability of the fracture,
* need for excision and grafting of the burn,
* access required for adequate burn wound care, and
* early aggressive physical therapy after the injury.

Although fractures away from the burns may be managed with reduction and casting, in cases where fractures are associated with severe soft-tissue damage, internal fixation should be carried out prior to bacterial colonization of the wound (within 24–48 hours). In a review of 101 thermally injured patients with orthopedic injuries, 75% of the patients had definitive orthopedic procedures within 24 hours of their injuries. Early, aggressive fracture treatment has resulted in decreased orthopedic complications without additional risks of infection, poor fracture healing, or amputation.[9,12–15] All open fractures must have incision and drainage in the operating room within 24 hours of the injury. Skeletal traction is used infrequently due to resultant patient immobility; however, it may be a good option in patients with severe hemodynamic instability. Antibiotic coverage is provided as deemed appropriate to the orthopedic injury. A majority of dislocations may be managed with closed reduction but when open reduction through a burn wound is inevitable, the wound is closed to the level of the fascia without drains.[14,16]

Child abuse

A mechanism of injury of particular interest is that of non-accidental trauma, as seen in cases of abuse and assault. Assault-provoked burn injuries carry a 7–16% risk of other associated injuries. Burn injury is found in 10–25% of documented cases of child abuse and most occur in children under 3 years.[17] Inconsistent history involving the burns, delay in seeking medical attention, history of previous trauma and specific patterns of the lesions (bilateral stocking glove pattern, sharply delineated edges of the burn, dependent location, tide or splash marks, and marks left by cigarettes, irons, heaters and curling devices) should alert the healthcare giver to possible child abuse.[18] A skeletal survey may confirm the presence of old fractures of ribs and long bones also suggestive of non-accidental trauma. In children with an altered state of consciousness or developmental delay, head CT scan is a reliable diagnostic tool to detect abusive head injury. In addition, an ophthalmological examination may reveal retinal hemorrhages, typical of the 'shaken baby syndrome.'[19] This topic is extensively discussed in Chapter 61.

Gastrointestinal pathology

Pathophysiology

Burn wounds of sufficient size (>30% TBSA burns in adults) initiate a generalized physiological response, which affects other organ systems, including the GI tract. The GI tract has long been recognized as an internal target of systemic shock and disruption of gut mucosal integrity is thought to be the initiating focus for sepsis in burn patients. These physiological changes include splanchnic hypoperfusion due to massive intravascular fluid loss along with vasoactive hormones, hypermetabolism leading to profound catabolic state and malnutrition, and immunosuppression with a breakdown of mucosal barriers to bacterial invasion in the GI tract. Combinations of these derangements initiate various organ system dysfunctions, resulting in non-thermal complications of burn injury. Massive burn injury results in diffuse capillary leak, hypovolemia, and release of vasoconstrictive agents, which cause selective decrease in splanchnic blood flow[20,21] (Figure 38.1). The splanchnic hypoperfusion shown to occur in the early postburn period[22,23] along with inadequate fluid resuscitation contribute to significant tissue hypoxia. In the GI tract, burn injury can result in decreased blood flow to the gut by

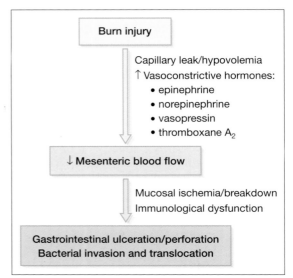

Fig. 38.1 Pathogenesis of mucosal barrier disruption. Massive burn injury induces diffuse capillary leak syndrome leading to decrease in intravascular volume along with outpouring of vasoconstrictive hormones. Subsequent decreased splanchnic circulation contributes to mesenteric ischemia, mucosal atrophy, enterocolitis and intestinal necrosis. Gut mucosal barrier disruption along with immunological dysfunction can lead to systemic inflammatory response.

one-third despite maintaining adequate cardiac output with fluid resuscitation.[22] A 40% flame-burned pig model showed an early reduction in superior mesenteric blood flow associated with intestinal mucosal hypoxia, acidosis and increased bacterial translocation despite adequate fluid resuscitation.[24] Sepsis and burn injury have additive effects on intestinal integrity.[25] Multiple factors can influence intestinal blood flow and this may be improved by enteral feeding.[23] Further, an increased plasma level of thromboxane B_2, a vasoactive inflammatory mediator, has been noted both in the acute phase (3 days postburn) and during sepsis.[26] A selective reduction in blood flow to liver, small intestine and kidney during massive burns contributes to surgical complications. Hypoperfusion with ischemia insult to gallbladder can result in bile stasis, leading to acalculous cholecystitis.[27] Ischemia-induced injury to GI tract mucosa can produce ulcer formation (Curling's ulcer) and enterocolitis severe enough to cause full-thickness necrosis and even intestinal perforation.[28] Poor perfusion to kidney and liver can also result in organ dysfunction and failure. In addition to complications involving GI tract organs, decreased perfusion to burn wounds results in poor wound healing and increased incidence of wound infection.

The hypermetabolic response to burn injury altering immunological function also significantly contributes to non-thermal complications in burned patients. The hypermetabolic response causes a profound catabolic state, deterring wound healing and immunological function. The activation of the hypothalamic–pituitary axis, sympathetic outflow, and the acute phase response take place, resulting in fat and protein breakdown and increase in gluconeogenesis.[29] Defective fibroblast function also contributes to impaired wound healing. Leukocyte dysfunction and reduced cellular immunity cause immunological compromise. Blunting this hypermetabolic response has been thought to be critical to improve the overall recovery of burn patients.[30–33] Growth hormone administration, which blunts hypermetabolic response in burn patients, has recently been reported to enhance small bowel homeostasis during burns by significantly increasing gut mucosal villus height and cell number.[34] Early enteral feeding has been shown to blunt hypermetabolic response.[31,32,35] The combination of transient mesenteric hypoperfusion along with hypermetabolic response to burns has been shown to contribute to breakdown of gut mucosal barrier, subsequently leading to bacterial translocation from the gut, initiating systemic inflammatory response and, ultimately, sepsis. Numerous studies have demonstrated the link between massive cutaneous burn injury and bacterial translocation.[36–40] Early mucosal atrophy that occurs after burn injury has been found to be a major contributing factor for impaired gut barrier function. An increase in intestinal epithelial cell turnover in mice has been shown to result from both apoptosis and proliferation of gut epithelial cells.[41] Furthermore, an increase in intestinal apoptosis that occurs after cutaneous burn injury does not appear to be the result of mesenteric hypoperfusion alone, but is speculated to be related to pro-inflammatory mediators produced by the burn wound.[42] Intervention aimed at preventing splanchnic hypoperfusion along with hypermetabolic response to burn injury may prevent immunological dysfunction and GI tract complications that are associated with severe burns.

Stress gastritis

The decreasing trend of stress gastritis and/or gastroduodenal ulceration in burned patients reflects both improvement in the treatment of acutely burned patients and the success of specific prophylactic measures. The incidence of acute gastroduodenal disease was previously reported to be as high as 86%, depending on the method of diagnosis (routine endoscopic evaluation, presence of gastrointestinal bleeding, postmortem).[43] Since the introduction of aggressive fluid resuscitation, antacid, early enteral feeding and proton pump inhibitors, the incidence of clinically significant gastroduodenal ulcer disease in burned patients (Curling's ulcer) has significantly decreased, fallen below 2%,[44] with a mortality of less than 0.2%.[45] The exact pathogenesis of Curling's ulcer remains unknown; however, reduced mucosal blood flow along with production of deleterious prostaglandins is thought to contribute to ulcer formation.[46] These lesions tend to be encountered more frequently in patients with larger burns and in the presence of sepsis.[47] Gastric ulcers are characteristically multifocal, and duodenal ulcers are usually solitary, with 15% of patients having combination of both gastric and duodenal ulcerations. Hemorrhage is the predominant presenting sign, and is often massive. Perforation is less common and is seen in about 12% of the patients.

A significant number of patients with major burn injury may develop mucosal changes within 72 hours of the burn, and with subsequent septic episodes and hypoxemia it may progress to ulceration. Multiple factors are implicated as potential causes of stress ulcers in burned patients,[47] including mucosal ischemia, increased acid production, increased acid back-diffusion, energy depletion, bile reflux, and direct mucosal injury due to the presence of intraluminal tubes. The state of mucosal perfusion is dependent upon a complex interplay of local and systemic factors, and inadequate perfusion may contribute to breakdown of mucosal barrier function to acids. The prevention of stress ulcers in thermally injured patients requires eliminating or minimizing these factors. Aggressive fluid resuscitation aids in maintaining adequate mucosal blood flow. The administration of H_2 receptor antagonists or proton pump inhibitor is also important in reducing stress ulcer formation. Although these pharmacological agents have been shown to be effective against ulcers,[45] early enteral feeding is the most effective approach in the prevention of stress hemorrhage in burn patients.[48]

Proper treatment of established stress ulcers includes those measures currently in use for prevention. More aggressive medical therapy includes combinations of intravenous (IV) vasopressin, somatostatin, and/or endoscopic cautery. Surgical options should be utilized early in order to prevent the profound effects of bleeding and hypotension on a maximally stressed burned patient. Specific surgical indications include massive bleeding (>2.5 liters in adult, >50% blood volume in child), ongoing uncontrolled blood loss, and evidence of a perforated viscus. If operative repair is necessary, vagotomy with antrectomy is considered as the operation of choice.[47] The overall mortality for patients requiring operative intervention remains significant at 50%. Although Curling's ulcers are far less frequent than in the past, they remain a potential hazard to all burn-injured patients. The current low incidence of stress ulceration is due to successful aggressive burn injury management and the use of specific preventive measures, especially early enteral feeding.

Acalculous cholecystitis

Acute acalculous cholecystitis is a rare complication of burn injury, as it is typically identified searching for source of sepsis in critically ill patients. The incidence is estimated at 0.4–3.5% in burned patients.[49,50] Predisposing factors for acalculous cholecystitis include extensive burns (>40% TBSA burn), multiple transfusions, sepsis, a history of total parenteral nutrition, and a history of narcotics usage.[49] It is associated with high mortality, and the appropriate treatment depends on the patient's overall stability. Proposed etiologies are bile stasis, altered bile composition, acute gallbladder hypoperfusion due to third space fluid loss, and systemic sepsis.[49,51] The lack of enteral feeding, resulting in decreased cholecystokinin level, along with narcotic use contributes to bile stasis. Multiple blood transfusions that are frequently required in major burned patients alter the composition of bile. Systemic sepsis with the resultant effects of circulating vasoactive mediators upon local tissue perfusion also leads to local ischemia of the gallbladder wall, inflammation, gangrene, and even perforation in unrecognized cases. The common histological finding in acalculous cholecystitis consists of intense injury to blood vessels within the muscularis and serosa.

Acute acalculous cholecystitis commonly presents with fever, right upper quadrant abdominal tenderness, leukocytosis, and elevated liver enzymes. These findings also commonly pre-exist in severely burned patients; therefore, a high index of suspicion is required for prompt diagnosis. The significant rates of gangrenous gallbladder and perforation are noted to be 33–100% and 12%, respectively.[52] Ultrasound exam is the preferred diagnostic study demonstrating thickened gallbladder wall, pericholecystic fluid, and intraluminal sludge. A positive cholecystoscintigraphy (HIDA scan) can also confirm the diagnosis but is often unavailable and may be difficult to obtain for critically ill patients. Once the diagnosis of acalculous cholecystitis is confirmed, cholecystectomy via laparoscopic approach should be considered for burned patients.[50] Patients who are extremely ill may be considered for ultrasound-guided percutaneous cholecystostomy placement.[53] Clinical response rates with this technique range from 56 to 100%.[53,54] In a recent review of 163 patients who underwent percutaneous cholecystostomy, over 80% of patients were able to undergo removal of the cholecystostomy tube and did not require a cholecystectomy.[55] Caution must be employed when utilizing this technique, as the incidence of gangrenous cholecystitis is significant in thermally injured patients, and a lack of clinical response after percutaneous cholecystostomy should prompt the surgeon to proceed with a cholecystectomy.

Superior mesenteric artery syndrome

Superior mesenteric artery (SMA) syndrome occurs when the third part of duodenum is extrinsically compressed by the superior mesenteric vascular pedicle. SMA syndrome is usually precipitated by rapid and substantial weight loss, leading to a loss of retroperitoneal fat. In burned patients, weight loss through malnutrition, loss of abdominal wall muscles, and a recombinant position contribute to the severity of the duodenal compression. With aggressive immediate early enteral feeding, SMA syndrome is now rarely encountered in acute burn patients. Bilious emesis and intolerance to tube or oral feedings are common at presentation. The diagnosis is established by an upper gastrointestinal series demonstrating a dilated stomach and proximal duodenum with extrinsic compression of the third portion of the duodenum. Management of SMA syndrome is primarily medical, by enhancing caloric intake by utilizing a nasojejunal enteral feeding or parenteral nutrition. Surgical procedures are rarely indicated, but when they are necessary, the operative goal should be bypassing the point of obstruction caused by superior mesenteric vascular pedicle. In a reported series of 37 of 3536 patients treated for SMA syndrome over a 12-year period, 18 patients were successfully managed medically with nasogastric decompression and intravenous nutrition.[56] Operative intervention (side-to-side duodenojejunostomy) was necessary in 30%, either for failed medical therapy or perforated ulcer. There were 3 postoperative deaths and 8 deaths following medical therapy alone for an overall mortality rate of 27%. A more recent report found that the average burn size for pediatric patients experiencing SMA syndrome was 64% TBSA and weight loss ranged from 10 to 30%.[57] The decrease in the incidence of SMA syndrome in recent years is attributed to more aggressive enteral nutritional support limiting weight loss to less than 5% of pre-burn weight. In general, enteral feeding, beyond the point of obstruction utilizing a fluoroscopically or endoscopically placed nasojejunal enteral feeding tube, should be administered as initial line of therapy.[58] Recently, a minimally invasive laparoscopic approach has been used to relieve the duodenal obstruction in patients with SMA syndrome.[59]

Enterocolitis

Splanchnic hypoperfusion occurs as a result of hypovolemia and circulating vasoactive mediators and the degree of intestinal insult is a product of the severity and duration of ischemia along with reperfusion by resuscitative efforts. Complications of intestinal injury span from mucosal barrier breakdown with subsequent bacterial translocation to full-thickness intestinal necrosis with perforation. The pathogenesis of enterocolitis is multifactorial. Ischemia-reperfusion injury to the gut as well as the presence of virulent bacteria and fungi in the immunocompromised state contribute to intestinal complications. Desai et al.[28] reported a series of burned patients with both clinically recognized ischemic intestinal complications (incidence 1%) and those identified only at autopsy (incidence 55%) with an overall survival of 30%. Children actually faired better with a survival rate twice that of their adult counterparts. When intestinal ischemic injury occurs, multiple operations are frequently required, with one series reporting up to 41 interventions for 16 patients.[28,60] These patients also commonly experience systemic sepsis. Nearly 75% of burned patients with bowel ischemia at autopsy had documented sepsis at the time of their death.[28] These results show both the high incidence of sepsis and mortality associated with intestinal ischemic complications in burned patients.

Ten of 2114 patients with burn injury have been shown to experience ischemic necrotic bowel disease in one study.[61] The patients with ischemic bowel disease had a higher mean TBSA burn (53%) compared to that of the patients with other GI tract problems (22%). The patients with ischemic bowel disease typically demonstrated dilated bowel loops, intolerance to tube feedings, high gastric residual volumes, and even radiological evidence of pneumatosis intestinalis. Severity of thermal injury, the presence of systemic infection, and altered intestinal flora secondary to systemic antibiotic therapy contributed to increased ischemic intestinal complications.[61] Although the overall incidence of clinically recognized intestinal ischemic complications in thermally injured patients is low (1–3%), early recognition and intervention requires a high index of suspicion. Signs and symptoms may be falsely attributed to the burn wound and lead to a delay in recognizing intra-abdominal pathology. Thermally injured patients who develop sepsis and intolerance of enteral feedings should be treated immediately with bowel rest and broad-spectrum antibiotic coverage. Abdominal radiographs frequently demonstrate massively dilated multiple bowel loops without organized pattern (Figure 38.2). Persistent, relatively fixed dilated bowel loops is an ominous sign for necrotic intestine. Failure to respond to conservative treatment mandates surgical intervention. At operation, frank necrotic intestinal segments should be resected (Figure 38.3); however, indeterminate areas of necrosis, particularly when they involve extensive lengths, should be reexamined at a second-look operation within 24–48 hours. The primary goal of surgical intervention is to eliminate obviously non-viable bowel, while preserving as much intestine as possible to avoid risks of developing short bowel syndrome.

Pseudomembranous colitis is caused by the overgrowth of toxigenic strains of *Clostridium difficile*, which derives its virulence from an alteration of the intestinal bacterial flora.

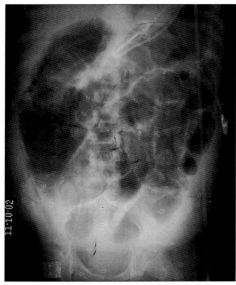

Fig. 38.2 Diffuse distention of multiple loops of bowel. Relatively-fixed dilated appearance of bowel loops over time suggests progression of intestinal complication to involve an ischemic segment.

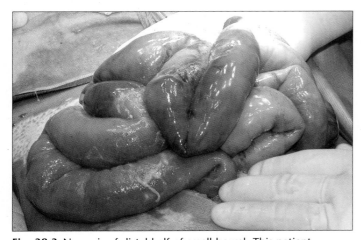

Fig. 38.3 Necrosis of distal half of small bowel. This patient underwent resection of necrotic bowel with exteriorization of proximal small bowel as ileostomy, which was later reversed uneventfully.

In a reported series of 112 thermally injured patients, the overall incidence of *C. difficile* colitis was 8% with mean burn size in these patients of 47% TBSA.[62] Pseudomembranous colitis occurs most commonly as a result of systemic antibiotic therapy, although oral or even topical administration of antibiotics has also been linked to development of pseudomembranous colitis and toxic megacolon. Topical silver sulfadiazine, used commonly in all burned patients, has been shown to cause toxic megacolon, which may then progress to colonic perforation.[63] The clinical features of colitis, such as fever and

leukocytosis with abdominal pain, distention, and diarrhea, must be promptly recognized. Major burned patients are at high risk for pseudomembranous colitis since they are frequently treated with multiple antibiotics for documented systemic infections and for prophylaxis during excision and grafting. The presence of heme-positive or grossly bloody stools should immediately alert one to further investigate an overgrowth of *C. difficile* with a toxin assay. Eliminating unnecessary systemic antibiotic therapy is the key to prevention of this disease; however, when it occurs, oral vancomycin or metronidazole is the appropriate treatment. Metronidazole can also be administered intravenously as effective therapy.

Ileus

Sepsis, electrolyte imbalance, narcotics, and renal failure are common causes for generalized ileus in burn patients. In the presence of ileus, management of enteral feeding becomes a delicate issue to avoid intestinal complication. Patients will obviously experience abdominal distention and pain; this can also be further complicated by the overuse of narcotics in an attempt to alleviate pain. In particular, intestinal ileus may represent as an early indicator of systemic sepsis in burn patients and, therefore, the etiology for ileus should be carefully explored. In addition to small intestinal ileus, pseudo-obstruction of the colon (Ogilvie's syndrome) is commonly encountered in burn patients.[64] Presenting symptoms include abdominal distention with constipation or diarrhea. Diagnosis is established by a plain abdominal radiograph, which typically shows massive colonic distention. Signs and symptoms are usually minimal or attributable to the burns. Optimal therapy should be based on the degree of cecal distention. Distention <10 cm in its greatest diameter is treated conservatively with saline enemas, rectal tube decompression; colonoscopy-assisted decompression is the preferred option for persistently dilated cecum lasting more than 3 days or distention >10 cm. However, a special consideration must be used to appropriately adjust the 'acceptable' size of cecal distention based on patient's size and weight, especially in pediatric patients. An operative intervention is rarely necessary with the creation of a cecostomy or occasionally with resection accompanied by diversion.

Pancreatitis

Acute pancreatitis can occur in burned patients. The pathogenesis is usually idiopathic but may be attributable to ischemia, sepsis, and medications. The diagnosis may be difficult and masked by overwhelming burn injuries. Symptoms of epigastric abdominal pain along with hyperamylasemia confirm the diagnosis. Treatment is similar to pancreatitis in non-burn patients, consisting of supportive care such as bowel rest, fluid resuscitation, and IV nutrition. The exact roles of enteral versus parental nutrition as well as use of antibiotics remain greatly debated. Abdominal ultrasound examination of the biliary tract should be performed to determine presence of gallstone. Occasionally, detailed work-up with abdominal CT scan is necessary to identify complications such as pseudocyst formation, pancreatic necrosis, and pancreatic abscess. Operative intervention is rarely indicated unless infective complications occur.

Feeding tubes

The importance of enteral nutrition in critically ill patients, including burns, has been clearly established. Parenteral nutrition is associated with increased risks for complication such as line sepsis, intestinal atrophy and bacterial overgrowth. However, the excessive caloric intake required in a burned patient, coupled with appetite suppression and/or inability to consume oral intake, necessitates alternative means of delivering calories than the simple oral route. Nasogastric, nasojejunal, gastrostomy, and jejunostomy tubes can all deliver enteral nutrition but each of these options has its own unique advantages and disadvantages. Selecting the inappropriate enteral formula can also cause diarrhea and malabsorption, which complicates wound healing and local wound care, especially in the areas of perineum. An advantage of the nasogastric tube is avoidance of potential complications associated with a procedure (i.e. endoscopic or open abdominal approach). Nasogastric feeding tubes are soft, thin, and pliable, and they avoid the gastric, pulmonary, and nasal complications of large decompression nasogastric tubes. However, these tubes are difficult to maintain, and can inadvertently be displaced or migrate into the pulmonary tree, resulting in potentially serious complications of aspiration. A nasoduodenal or nasojejunal feeding tube placed under fluoroscopic guidance with its tip well beyond the pylorus has become a standard practice for many burn centers. This method is especially useful in major burn patients, who frequently experience gastric ileus during immediate postburn period. Immediate enteral feedings are initiated at the same time the gastric decompression is accomplished with the nasogastric tube. However, these feeding tubes require careful titration of formula volume to avoid abdominal distention, diarrhea or discomfort.

A surgically placed gastrostomy tube can be maintained for long periods and requires minimal experience to manage;[65] however, the surgical site care may be complicated by the presence of burn wound. In addition to high risk for burned wound breakdown at the gastrostomy, a lack of subcutaneous tissue makes them more susceptible to complications such as gastric prolapse (Figure 38.4). Although alternate techniques

of placement such as percutaneous endoscopic[66] and laparoscopic assisted[67] methods are now available to minimize the morbidity associated with surgically placed gastrostomy, it still requires diligent care to avoid complications related to the gastrostomy tube itself. In general, laparoscopy-assisted feeding tube placement has become a standard approach for pediatric patients. However, relatively non-compliant abdominal wall due to full-thickness burns in the torso area can create difficulty achieving adequate insufflation of the abdominal cavity. Further, a gastrostomy tube is not an adequate method for effective gastric decompression. Although jejunostomy feeding can eliminate a risk of gastroesophageal reflux associated with gastric tube feedings, it also carries the disadvantage of requiring an operative procedure. The pathophysiology of diarrhea in tube-fed burn patients has been extensively examined. In one study, tube feeding osmolality, anti-stress ulcer medication or hypoalbumenia did not have an adverse effect on intestinal absorption. A low-fat (<20% of caloric intake), vitamin A-enriched (>10 000 IU/day), early enteral support program maximizes conditions to promote tube feeding tolerance.[68] Increased incidence of diarrhea occurred in older patients, >40% TBSA burns, patients receiving antibiotic treatment, or late initiation of tube feedings (>48 hours postburn). Given these findings, enteral feeding should be initiated early after burn injury, specifically formulated to avoid diarrhea. Even in pediatric patients who required laparotomy for abdominal compartment syndrome, surgical intervention did not preclude the safe postoperative delivery and advancement of enteral feedings.[69]

Others

Massively burned patients generally require prolonged hospital stay; therefore, they are also susceptible to common GI tract pathology such as appendicitis. The limited ability to discern history and abdominal exam findings may create some difficulty for prompt diagnosis. Imaging modalities such as ultrasound and CT scan are readily used to ensure accuracy of diagnosis. Although laparoscopic appendectomy has become a standard approach, restrictive abdominal cavity to gas insufflation in burns patients with major burns to the trunk area prohibits minimally invasive approach. In pediatric burn patients, bleeding per rectum, especially in toddlers 1–3 years of age, should alert the possibility of ileocolic intussusception. Ultrasound exam can frequently identify this condition; however, non-operative enema reduction may be more difficult to attempt for this group of patients. At operation, intussusception is manually reduced, appendectomy is performed, and the viability of involved bowel segment thoroughly assessed (Figure 38.5). A critical nature of prompt diagnosis to prevent, necrosis or perforation was also emphasized in a recent case report of an 18-month-old infant with intussusception.[70]

Vascular access complications

Adequate venous access is imperative to administer aggressive fluid resuscitation during the critical acute postburn period. Although peripheral venous access with large-bore catheters is the preferred route for resuscitating trauma patients, the placement of peripheral venous lines can be extremely difficult

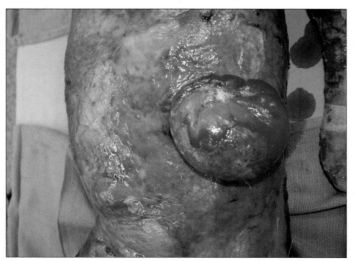

Fig. 38.4 Gastric prolapse at gastrostomy site. Gastrostomy through the area of full thickness burns is at high risk for gastric prolapse.

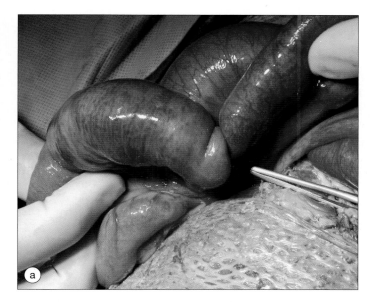

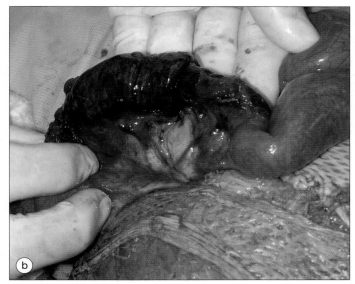

Fig. 38.5 Ileo-ileal intussusception in a burn patient. Persistent intolerance of enteral feedings with high gastric residuals along with 'current' jelly-like stool was noted in a 19-month-old infant. (a) Ileo-ileal intussusception at mid-ileum. (b) Manual reduction revealed necrotic ileal segment requiring resection with primary anastomosis.

in major burns involving the extremities. Therefore, central venous lines have become the standard practice in major burn patients to provide secure vascular access for administration of fluid and blood products as well as perioperative monitoring of intravascular volume status. However, central venous line placement is associated with potentially serious complications. A particular attention should be given to the use of various available cannulation sites depending on the size of the patient, as well as taking into consideration clinical conditions of burn wounds. Arterial monitoring is frequently necessary in critically ill burn patients. At Shriners Hospital for Children at Galveston, femoral arterial catheterization has become routine for hemodynamic monitoring in major burn patients. The potential risks for complications from femoral arterial access are obviously far greater than for radial and/or pedal arterial catheterization.

Suppurative thrombophlebitis

The incidence of suppurative thrombophebolic complications in burn patients has been estimated to range from 0.4% to 7% with significant risk in patients with >20% TBSA burns.[71–74] A review of 2103 patients over 10-year period showed that 25 patients (1.2%), with a mean age of 40 years and 49% TBSA burns, were found to having significant pulmonary thromboembolism.[71] An increasing experience with catheter-related septic central venous thrombosis has been reported. Not all of these infections occur in association with venous thrombosis, and specific risk factors for developing suppurative thrombophlebitis include both burn injury and prolonged intravenous catheterization. Factors such as prolonged catheterization (>72 hours), concentrated IV solutions, venous cut-down, lower extremity catheters, emergency IV access have all been associated with increased risk for septic thrombophlebitis.[75] The presentation of suppurative thrombophlebitis is often occult with approximately 20% of patients showing no local clinical signs.[75] In burned patients, occult suppurative thrombophlebitis is most frequent; only 36% of patients was reported to exhibit local signs in one study.[73] Burned patients frequently display a positive blood culture and clinical sepsis without obvious source. Thorough examination of all catheter sites must be performed to identify catheter-related sepsis. The absence of pus at the site or within the vein does not necessarily rule out suppurative thrombophlebitis.[75] Proper exploration of an infected vein requires surgical cut-down and expression of vein contents. If pus or clot is found, the vein segment should be excised to a normal-appearing vein (usually at the first uninvolved tributary). If exploration is negative at one site, then sequential exploration of other sites is necessary until the source of infection is identified. Aside from surgical excision, systemic IV antibiotics must be administered. The most commonly found organisms in infected veins in burned patients reflect those cultured from a burn wound.[73] In non-burned patients, *Staphylococcus*, *Klebsiella*, and *Candida* are found in descending order of frequency.[75] Catheter-related septic central venous thrombosis has increasingly been recognized in the burn population as it parallels the increased use of central venous catheters in these patients. Typically, patients with septic central venous thrombosis demonstrate positive catheter tip culture, blood culture, and ongoing bacteremia after catheter removal. The majority of patients also show local evidence of disease manifested by ipsilateral upper extremity swelling.[76] Catheter-related thrombosis can be managed by removal of catheter alone; however, if significant obstruction of flow is present, full systemic heparinization may be required. Surgical intervention is rarely required. In order to minimize the incidence of these catheter-related complications of thrombosis or infection, the current standard practice for central venous access at Shriners Hospital for Children at Galveston consists of meticulous aseptic care at the catheter insertion site along with regularly scheduled catheter site change. Central venous catheters are changed over a guidewire placed through an existing catheter every 3 days and a new central venous cannula on a fresh site is placed every 6 days.

Thoracic complications

With frequent use of central venous access in major burn patients, the risk for potential thoracic complications associated with placement of central venous lines must be recognized. Although the overall incidence is quite small (1–4%), any thoracic complications can potentially lead to life-threatening conditions. Pneumothorax is caused by lung parenchyma injury during venipuncture of central veins, and can be treated with observation or small chest tube placement. However, if unrecognized, especially in patients receiving positive ventilatory pressure support, it can rapidly progress to tension pneumothorax with hemodynamic compromise. In order to reduce the risk of puncturing the lung parenchyma during attempted central venous line placement, it is crucial to be familiar with the central venous anatomy in the neck and chest areas. Especially in small pediatric patients, percutaneous access to subclavian veins may require a more acute cephalad angle of approach under the clavicle due to its venous anatomical differences when compared to adults.[77,78] Proper shoulder roll should be placed to maximally enhance the space between the first rib and the clavicle for easier access to subclavian veins. A patient should be adequately sedated and given sufficient pain medication to avoid any movement during the procedure.

Bleeding related to placement of central venous catheters varies in location and can be local, mediastinal, intrathoracic, or pericardial. Local hemorrhage occurs typically in patients with a coagulopathy but should be controlled with local pressure. Hemorrhage into the thoracic space can occur at the time of catheter insertion or after the catheter has been in place, from erosion through the vein wall. Blood may accumulate into the mediastinum, pleural space or pericardium. The most common situation leading to venous wall perforation occurs during an insertion of a percutaneous introducer sheath over a guide wire. As the sheath is introduced, it can fail to negotiate a path of a vein and traumatize the vein wall. If the injury is small, it can resolve on its own with thrombosis formation; however, in cases of larger venous tear, rapid bleeding into thoracic cavity can occur and emergent thoracotomy may be necessary. In order to reduce the risk of bleeding complication, many burn centers rely on guidance of fluoroscopy and/or ultrasound during the insertion of central venous lines. Pericardial tamponade can also occur with high mortality. Bleeding or infusion of fluid into pericardial space can rapidly compromise the cardiac function and results in hemodynamic collapse. Patients typically manifest hypotension, muffled heart sounds, and distended neck veins (Beck's triad). However, the classic triad of symptoms is rarely all present and a physician must have a high index of suspicion in order to recognize this condition early. Echocardiograms can confirm the clinical suspicion and pericardiocentesis or pericardial window can return the cardiac function to baseline.

Distal limb ischemia

Arterial monitoring is frequently required in patients with major burns, especially during the perioperative period. Although radial and pedal arterial cannulas are routinely placed without significant complications, they can be associated with problems such as hematoma and pain. Occasionally, a larger and more proximal femoral artery is considered for access, but this site should only be used with extreme caution due to potentially serious complications that can occur. Especially in pediatric burn patients, the femoral artery can be very small and a catheter within the vessel can result in near complete occlusion of blood flow to distal aspect of the limb. If this occurs, the catheter should be immediately removed and a Doppler flow study should be obtained to assess for the presence of intimal flap. Recently, magnetic resonance arteriography has been utilized as a diagnostic tool with excellent yield. Conservative treatment, with optimizing hemodynamics and occasional systemic heparinization, are usually adequate to restore blood flow. Surgical intervention is rarely necessary and can potentially result in further compromise of the integrity of arterial blood flow. Most importantly, arterial cannulas should be removed as soon as its potential benefit of invasive monitoring is no longer present for the care of major burn patients.

Summary

Surgical problems secondary to burn injury can cause devastating physiological responses. Physicians must have a high index of suspicion to identify any associated nonthermal injuries when evaluating patients with major burn injury. When presented with patients with multiple organ injuries, the protocols for ATLS should be followed, ensuring the airway, breathing, and circulation. Injuries to other organ system should be handled in a systemic fashion with involvement of appropriate consultant surgeons. A multitude of gastrointestinal complications can occur during the course of prolonged hospitalization for major burn patients. Ulcers and other complications must be prevented when possible and detected and treated when present. Finally, medical professionals must be constantly on the alert for problems related to intravenous catheters and tube feedings, as related infections and complications can be fatal.

References

1. Counce JS, Cone JB, McAlister L, et al. Surgical complications of thermal injury. Am J Surg 1988; 156(6):556–557.
2. Marzek PA, Miller FB, Cryer HM, et al. Nonthermal surgical complications in burn patients. South Med J 1991; 84(6):689–691.
3. Brandt CP, Yowler CJ, Fratianne RB. Burns with multiple trauma. Am Surg 2002; 68(3):240–243; discussion 243–244.
4. Pruitt BA Jr. Management of burns in the multiple inury patient. Surg Clin North Am 1970; 50(6):1283–1300.
5. Purdue GF, Hunt JL. Multiple trauma and the burn patient. Am J Surg 1989; 158(6):536–539.
6. Dougherty W, Waxman K. The complexities of managing severe burns with associated trauma. Surg Clin North Am 1996; 76(4):923–958.
7. Briggs D, Kirwin M, Morrison KM. Severe occupational traumatic injuries. Prim Care 1994; 21(2):349–366.
8. Baxter CR. Present concepts in the management of major electrical injury. Surg Clin North Am 1970; 50(6):1401–1418.
9. Purdue GF, Hunt JL, Layton TR, et al. Burns in motor vehicle accidents. J Trauma 1985; 25(3):216–219.
10. Liu M, Lee CH, P'Eng FK. Prospective comparison of diagnostic peritoneal lavage, computed tomographic scanning, and ultraso-

nography for the diagnosis of blunt abdominal trauma. J Trauma 1993; 35(2):267–270.

11. Goodwin CW Jr, McManus WF, Mason AD Jr, et al. Management of abdominal wounds in thermally injured patients. J Trauma 1982; 22(2):92–97.

12. Wong L, Grande CM, Munster AM. Burns and associated nonthermal trauma: an analysis of management, outcome, and relation to the Injury Severity Score. J Burn Care Rehabil 1989; 10(6):512–516.

13. Dossett AB, Hunt JL, Purdue GF, et al. Early orthopedic intervention in burn patients with major fractures. J Trauma 1991; 31(7):888–892; discussion 892–883.

14. Saffle JR, Schnelby A, Hofmann A, et al. The management of fractures in thermally injured patients. J Trauma 1983; 23(10):902–910.

15. Curtis MJ, Clarke JA. Skeletal injury in thermal trauma: a review of management. Injury 1989; 20(6):333–336.

16. Frye KE, Luterman A. Burns and fractures. Orthop Nurs 1999; 18(1):30–35.

17. Hornor G. Physical abuse: recognition and reporting. J Pediatr Health Care 2005; 19(1):4–11.

18. Peck MD, Priolo-Kapel D. Child abuse by burning: a review of the literature and an algorithm for medical investigations. J Trauma 2002; 53(5):1013–1022.

19. Listman DA, Bechtel K. Accidental and abusive head injury in young children. Curr Opin Pediatr 2003; 15(3):299–303.

20. Banks RO, Gallavan RH Jr, Zinner MH, et al. Vasoactive agents in control of the mesenteric circulation. Fed Proc 1985; 44(12):2743–2749.

21. Hilton JG, Marullo DS. Trauma induced increases in plasma vasopressin and angiotensin II. Life Sci 1987; 41(19):2195–2200.

22. Jones WG 2nd, Minei JP, Barber AE, et al. Splanchnic vasoconstriction and bacterial translocation after thermal injury. Am J Physiol 1991; 261(4 Pt 2):H1190–H1196.

23. Inoue S, Lukes S, Alexander JW, et al. Increased gut blood flow with early enteral feeding in burned guinea pigs. J Burn Care Rehabil 1989; 10(4):300–308.

24. Tokyay R, Zeigler ST, Traber DL, et al. Postburn gastrointestinal vasoconstriction increases bacterial and endotoxin translocation. J Appl Physiol 1993; 74(4):1521–1527.

25. Jones WG 2nd, Minei JP, Barber AE, et al. Additive effects of thermal injury and infection on the small bowel. Surgery 1990; 108(1):63–70.

26. Herndon DN, Abston S, Stein MD. Increased thromboxane B_2 levels in the plasma of burned and septic burned patients. Surg Gynecol Obstet 1984; 159(3):210–213.

27. Slater H, Goldfarb IW. Acute septic cholecystitis in patients with burn injuries. J Burn Care Rehabil 1989; 10(5):445–447.

28. Desai MH, Herndon DN, Rutan RL, et al. Ischemic intestinal complications in patients with burns. Surg Gynecol Obstet 1991; 172(4):257–261.

29. Kupper TS, Deitch EA, Baker CC, et al. The human burn wound as a primary source of interleukin-1 activity. Surgery 1986; 100(2):409–415.

30. Herndon DN, Barrow RE, Rutan TC, et al. Effect of propranolol administration on hemodynamic and metabolic responses of burned pediatric patients. Ann Surg 1988; 208(4):484–492.

31. McArdle AH, Palmason C, Brown RA, et al. Early enteral feeding of patients with major burns: prevention of catabolism. Ann Plast Surg 1984; 13(5):396–401.

32. Sologub VK, Zaets TL, Tarasov AV, et al. Enteral hyperalimentation of burned patients: the possibility of correcting metabolic disorders by the early administration of prolonged high calorie evenly distributed tube feeds. Burns 1992; 18(3):245–249.

33. Fleming RY, Rutan RL, Jahoor F, et al. Effect of recombinant human growth hormone on catabolic hormones and free fatty acids following thermal injury. J Trauma 1992; 32(6):698–702; discussion 702–693.

34. Jeschke MG, Herndon DN, Finnerty CC, et al. The effect of growth hormone on gut mucosal homeostasis and cellular mediators after severe trauma. J Surg Res 2005; 127(2):183–189.

35. Mochizuki H, Trocki O, Dominioni L, et al. Mechanism of prevention of postburn hypermetabolism and catabolism by early enteral feeding. Ann Surg 1984; 200(3):297–310.

36. Jones WG 2nd, Minei JP, Barber AE, et al. Bacterial translocation and intestinal atrophy after thermal injury and burn wound sepsis. Ann Surg 1990; 211(4):399–405.

37. Carter EA, Tompkins RG, Schiffrin E, et al. Cutaneous thermal injury alters macromolecular permeability of rat small intestine. Surgery 1990; 107(3):335–341.

38. LeVoyer T, Cioffi WG Jr, Pratt L, et al. Alterations in intestinal permeability after thermal injury. Arch Surg 1992; 127(1):26–29; discussion 29–30.

39. Magnotti LJ, Deitch EA, Burns, bacterial translocation, gut barrier function, and failure. J Burn Care Rehabil 2005; 26(5):383–391.

40. Gosain A, Gamelli RL. Role of the gastrointestinal tract in burn sepsis. J Burn Care Rehabil 2005; 26(1):85–91.

41. Wolf SE, Ikeda H, Matin S, et al. Cutaneous burn increases apoptosis in the gut epithelium of mice. J Am Coll Surg 1999; 188(1):10–16.

42. Ramzy PI, Wolf SE, Irtun O, et al. Gut epithelial apoptosis after severe burn: effects of gut hypoperfusion. J Am Coll Surg 2000; 190(3):281–287.

43. Czaja AJ, McAlhany JC, Pruitt BA Jr. Acute gastroduodenal disease after thermal injury. An endoscopic evaluation of incidence and natural history. N Engl J Med 1974; 291(18):925–929.

44. Moscona R, Kaufman T, Jacobs R, et al. Prevention of gastrointestinal bleeding in burns: the effects of cimetidine or antacids combined with early enteral feeding. Burns Incl Therm Inj 1985; 12(1):65–67.

45. Prasad JK, Thomson PD, Feller I. Gastrointestinal haemorrhage in burn patients. Burns Incl Therm Inj 1987; 13(3):194–197.

46. Battal MN, Hata Y, Matsuka K, et al. Effect of a prostaglandin I_2 analogue, beraprost sodium, on burn-induced gastric mucosal injury in rats. Burns 1997; 23(3):232–237.

47. Pruitt BA Jr, Goodwin CW Jr. Stress ulcer disease in the burned patient. World J Surg 1981; 5(2):209–222.

48. Raff T, Germann G, Hartmann B. The value of early enteral nutrition in the prophylaxis of stress ulceration in the severely burned patient. Burns 1997; 23(4):313–318.

49. Ross DC, Lee KC, Peters WJ, et al. Acalculous cholecystitis in association with major burns. Burns Incl Therm Inj 1987; 13(6):488–491.

50. McClain T, Gilmore BT, Peetz M. Laparoscopic cholecystectomy in the treatment of acalculos cholecystitis in patients after thermal injury. J Burn Care Rehabil 1997; 18(2):141–146.

51. Glenn F, Becker CG. Acute acalculous cholecystitis. An increasing entity. Ann Surg 1982; 195(2):131–136.

52. Still J, Scheirer R, Law E. Acute cholecystectomy performed through cultured epithelial autografts in a patient with burn injuries: a case report. J Burn Care Rehabil 1996; 17(5):429–431.

53. Sosna J, Copel L, Kane RA, et al. Ultrasound-guided percutaneous cholecystostomy: update on technique and clinical applications. Surg Technol Int 2003; 11:135–139.

54. Boland GW, Lee MJ, Leung J, et al. Percutaneous cholecystostomy in critically ill patients: early response and final outcome in 82 patients. AJR Am J Roentgenol 1994; 163(2):339–342.

55. Wise JN, Gervais DA, Akman A, et al. Percutaneous cholecystostomy catheter removal and incidence of clinically significant bile leaks: a clinical approach to catheter management. AJR Am J Roentgenol 2005; 184(5):1647–1651.

56. Lescher TJ, Sirinek KR, Pruitt BA Jr. Superior mesenteric artery syndrome in thermally injured patients. J Trauma 1979; 19(8):567–571.

57. Ogbuokiri CG, Law EJ, MacMillan BG. Superior mesenteric artery syndrome in burned children. Am J Surg 1972; 124(1):75–79.

58. Milner EA, Cioffi WG, McManus WF, et al. Superior mesenteric artery syndrome in a burn patient. Nutr Clin Pract 1993; 8(6):264–266.

59. Kingham TP, Shen R, Ren C. Laparoscopic treatment of superior mesenteric artery syndrome. JSLS 2004; 8(4):376–379.

60. Wilson MD, Dziewulski P. Severe gastrointestinal haemorrhage and ischaemic necrosis of the small bowel in a child with

70% full-thickness burns: a case report. Burns 2001; 27(7): 763–766.

61. Kowal-Vern A, McGill V, Gamelli RL. Ischemic necrotic bowel disease in thermal injury. Arch Surg 1997; 132(4):440–443.

62. Grube BJ, Heimbach DM, Marvin JA. Clostridium difficile diarrhea in critically ill burned patients. Arch Surg 1987; 122(6):655–661.

63. Jennings LJ, Hanumadass M. Silver sulfadiazine induced Clostridium difficile toxic megacolon in a burn patient: case report. Burns 1998; 24(7):676–679.

64. Kadesky K, Purdue GF, Hunt JL. Acute pseudo-obstruction in critically ill patients with burns. J Burn Care Rehabil 1995; 16(2 Pt 1):132–135.

65. Gauderer MW, Stellato TA. Gastrostomies: evolution, techniques, indications, and complications. Curr Probl Surg 1986; 23(9):657–719.

66. Grant JP. Comparison of percutaneous endoscopic gastrostomy with Stamm gastrostomy. Ann Surg 1988; 207(5):598–603.

67. Chung DH, Georgeson KE. Fundoplication and gastrostomy. Semin Pediatr Surg 1998; 7(4):213–219.

68. Gottschlich MM, Warden GD, Michel M, et al. Diarrhea in tube-fed burn patients: incidence, etiology, nutritional impact, and prevention. JPEN J Parenter Enteral Nutr 1988; 12(4):338–345.

69. Mayes T, Gottschlich MM, Warden GD. Nutrition intervention in pediatric patients with thermal injuries who require laparotomy. J Burn Care Rehabil 2000; 21(5):451–456; discussion 450–451.

70. Kincaid MS, Vavilala MS, Faucher L, et al. Feeding intolerance as a result of small-intestine intussusception in a child with major burns. J Burn Care Rehabil 2004; 25(2):212–214; discussion 211.

71. Rue LW 3rd, Cioffi WG Jr, Rush R, et al. Thromboembolic complications in thermally injured patients. World J Surg 1992; 16(6):1151–1154; discussion 1155.

72. Pruitt BA Jr, McManus AT. The changing epidemiology of infection in burn patients. World J Surg 1992; 16(1):57–67.

73. Pruitt BA Jr, McManus WF, Kim SH, et al. Diagnosis and treatment of cannula-related intravenous sepsis in burn patients. Ann Surg 1980; 191(5):546–554.

74. Pruitt BA Jr, Stein JM, Foley FD, et al. Intravenous therapy in burn patients. Suppurative thrombophlebitis and other life-threatening complications. Arch Surg 1970; 100(4):399–404.

75. Golueke PJ, Zinner MJ. Management of septic thrombophlebitis. In: Ernst CB, Stanley JC, eds. Current therapy in vascular surgery. Philadelphia: BC Decker; 1991:1014–1019.

76. Kaufman J, Demas C, Stark K, et al. Catheter-related septic central venous thrombosis – current therapeutic options. West J Med 1986; 145(2):200–203.

77. Cobb LM, Vinocur CD, Wagner CW, et al. The central venous anatomy in infants. Surg Gynecol Obstet 1987; 165(3):230–234.

78. Chung DH, Ziegler MM. Vascular access procedures. In: Ziegler MM, Azizkhan RG, Weber TR, eds. Operative pediatric surgery. New York: McGraw-Hill; 2003:85–93.

Chapter 39

Electrical injuries

Gary F. Purdue, Brett D. Arnoldo, and John L. Hunt

Chapter contents

Electrical burns

Introduction

Electricity is now an indispensable part of civilization, invisible and often taken for granted. Unfortunately, electrical burns are the most devastating of all thermal injuries on a size for size basis, usually involving both the skin and deeper tissues. They primarily affect young, working males, often have legal involvement and are the most frequent cause of amputations on the Burn Service. In addition to power company linemen and electricians, construction workers, laborers and crane operators are at special risk.[1]

Electrical burns have multiple acute and chronic manifestations not seen with other types of thermal injury. Morbidity, length of hospital stay and number of operations are much higher than expected, based on burn size alone.

Pathophysiology

Electrical burn severity is determined by voltage, current (amperage), type of current (alternating or direct), path of current flow, duration of contact, resistance at the point of contact and individual susceptibility. Electrical burns are classified as low-voltage (<1000 volts) and high-voltage injuries (1000 volts and higher). Low voltage burns are generally localized to the area immediately surrounding the injury while at high voltage, the cutaneous burn is associated with deep, underlying tissue damage very closely resembling a crush injury.[2] Nearly all burns occurring indoors, except in specialized industrial settings, are of the low-voltage type. While the victim or witness(es) often knows the voltage involved, the amount of current is unknown, with current flow related to voltage by Ohm's Law:

$$\text{Current (I)} = \text{Voltage (E)} / \text{Resistance (R)}$$

Animal experiments have demonstrated that resistance varies continuously with time, initially dropping slowly, then much more rapidly until arcing occurs at the contact sites. Resistance then rises to infinity and current flow ceases.[3] Temperature measurements, taken simultaneously, showed that rate of temperature rise parallels changes in amperage. Tissue temperature was the critical factor in the magnitude of tissue damage. Interestingly, there was no increase in temperature distal to the contact points.

In North America, more than 90% of all electrical burns are caused by 60 cycle-per-second commercial alternating current, which reverses its polarity 120 times per second. Only an occasional low- or high-frequency industrial injury is encountered. With one half of the time spent positive with respect to ground and one half spent negative, the verbiage 'entrance' and 'exit' wounds are archaic, as one does not know whether a given point on the body contacted the wire or the ground. These terms should be replaced by 'contact points.' A descriptive term such as blow-out type injury describes concentration of current and not its causation (Figure 39.1).

The path of current makes a significant difference in prehospital fatalities, but in patients reaching the hospital alive, current path determinations are often less than precise and meaningful. The patient may have no, one, or many visible contact points and an untold number of invisible contacts. An example of this is the surgical electrocautery where the large grounding pad contact site is not visible (hopefully). Despite some misconceptions, the term 'electrocution' does not apply to these living patients, as electrocution is defined as 'to kill by electric shock.'[4]

Alternating current causes tetanic muscle contractions, which may either throw victims away from the contact or draw them into continued contact with the electrical source creating the potential for continually increasing severity. Altered levels of consciousness, reported in about one half of high voltage victims, also contribute to prolonged periods of contact.[5] Resistance at the point of contact varies from very low values for sweat-soaked hands or skin in the summer to more than 100000 ohms for heavily calloused hands or feet during very dry winter weather. Individual susceptibility is a non-quantifiable term to explain why two or more individuals exposed to the same situation have extremely varied injuries.

The burn injury has the potential to cause three different components: the true electrical injury caused by current flow, an arc injury resulting from the electrical arc generated as the current passes from the source to an object, and a flame injury caused by ignition of clothing and/or surroundings. Electricity arcs at temperatures of up to 4000°C create a flash-type injury,[6] most often seen in electricians working with metal objects in

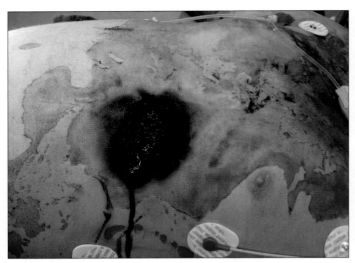

Fig. 39.1 High-voltage contact point with a blow-out type injury of the chest wall.

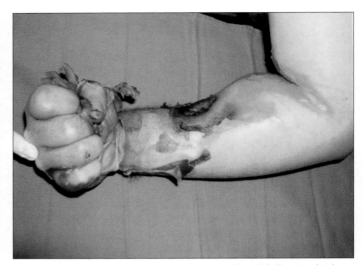

Fig. 39.2 Characteristic contracted arm and hand following high-voltage contact to the hand with extensive myonecrosis to the entire forearm.

close proximity to an electrical source. These injuries, when occurring without actual current flow through the victim, are treated and classified in the same manner as any flash burn.

The exact mechanism of electrical injury continues to be the subject of much research, very often appearing clinically to be a multifactorial combination of both thermal and non-thermal causes. Electricity flowing through tissue generates heat, much as it does flowing through the wire of a toaster, with Joule's law defining the amount of power (heat) delivered to an object:

$$\text{Power (J-Joule)} = I^2 \text{ (Current)} \times R \text{ (Resistance)}$$

Tissue resistance (from lowest to highest) is nerve, blood vessels, muscle, skin, tendon, fat, and bone. Theoretically, current flow would be distributed in proportion to resistance, with tissues having the highest resistance generating the most heat. However, in the animal model, the body acts as a single uniform resistance rather than a collection of different resistances; i.e. it behaves as a volume conductor.[3] Deep tissues appear to retain heat so that the peri-osseous tissues, especially between two bones (i.e. tibia–fibula, radius–ulna) often sustain a more severe injury than superficial tissue. The associated macro- and microscopic vascular injury appears to occur nearly immediately and is not reversible.[7]

Direct and indirect electrical destruction of cells also play a role in tissue injury. This appears to be especially important for nervous system cells as their injury is not well explained by heating alone. Cells maintaining their integrity with a sodium-potassium-ATPase pump operating at −90 millivolts direct current, certainly have the potential for disruption with high voltage alternating current. Breakdown of cell membranes is one of the mechanisms by which cell damage can occur.[8] This process of electroporation of cellular membranes may explain the injury not apparently caused by heat.[9]

Acute care

Severity of injury is inversely proportional to the cross-sectional area of tissue able to carry current. Thus the most severe

injuries are seen at the wrists and ankles, with decreasing severity proximally. In hand-foot current flow, 30% of the resistance is in the ankle and 25% in the wrist.[10] The extremities are the most frequently injured body parts, with severe injury often occurring in the arm and hand (Figure 39.2) As current follows the path of least resistance, it may generate small deep arc injuries in the axilla, groin, popliteal and antecubital fossae as seen here.

Electrocardiographic monitoring

While ventricular fibrillation is the most common cause of death at the scene of injury, virtually any cardiac arrhythmia can be precipitated by an electrical injury. Arrhythmias are treated using the same indications and modalities as for medical causes. In the authors' experience, new-onset atrial fibrillation has been the most common arrhythmia seen in patients reaching the hospital alive. All have responded to appropriate medical management.

Direct myocardial injury may also result. This injury behaves more like a traumatic myocardial contusion than a true myocardial infarction, not having the hemodynamic or recurrence consequences of atherosclerotic myocardial infarctions. Housinger et al. have shown that creatine kinase (CK) and MB-creatine kinase (MB-CK) levels are poor indicators of myocardial injury in the absence of ECG finding of myocardial damage, especially in the presence of significant skeletal muscle injury.[11–13] Myocardial damage and arrhythmias are manifested very soon after injury.[14] All patients should be monitored during transport and in the emergency room. Rather than a policy of more prolonged cardiac monitoring for all patients, a selective policy makes most efficient use of expensive medical resources, without patient risk.[1,14]

Indications for cardiac monitoring

- Documented cardiac arrest
- Cardiac arrhythmia on transport or in ER
- Abnormal EKG in ER (other than sinus brady- or tachycardia)
- Burn size or patient age would require monitoring.

Myoglobinuria

The presence of pigmented (darker than light pink) urine in a patient with an electrical burn indicates significant muscle damage. Myoglobin and hemoglobin pigments present risk of acute renal failure and must be cleared promptly. While low levels are of little clinical concern, grossly visible urinary pigmentation requires rapid response to minimize tubular obstruction (Figure 39.3). The urine dipstick is too sensitive for both pigment and hematuria to serve as a guide for treatment. Evaluation of the serum to differentiate myoglobin from hemoglobin depends on the fact that the smaller myoglobin complex is cleared by the kidney at a threshold below visibility, while hemoglobin as a polymer bound to albumin, has a much higher renal threshold. Differentiating between the two is of little clinical significance, however, as both require prompt clearance and must be treated. Urine with a color darker than light pink is promptly treated with two ampules of mannitol (25 g) given IV push, followed immediately by two ampules of sodium bicarbonate, also given IV push. Ringer's lactate is administered at a rate sufficient to grossly clear the urine of pigment. The rationale of this protocol is to create a rapid, osmotic diuresis with initial alkalinization to minimize pigment precipitation in the renal tubules. If adequate organ perfusion is maintained, repeat administration of mannitol and bicarbonate is not required. Loop diuretics are not as efficient as mannitol. The required urinary output is generally very high for several hours following injury, followed by significant reduction in urine requirements, as venous return from the injured part to the central circulation is thrombosed. Using this protocol, the authors have had a zero incidence of acute renal failure in 187 consecutive patients with grossly visible urinary pigment.

Resuscitation

The hidden injury associated with an electrical burn makes the use of burn resuscitation formulas based on body surface area burned inaccurate, except to establish a minimum volume required. In the absence of gross myo/hemoglobinuria, the goal of resuscitation is to maintain normal vital signs and a urine output of 30–50 mL/h with Ringer's lactate whose rate is adjusted on an hourly basis to achieve those goals.

Traumatic injuries

Approximately 15% of electrical burn victims sustain traumatic injuries in addition to their burn, a rate nearly double that of other burn patients. Most of these injuries are caused

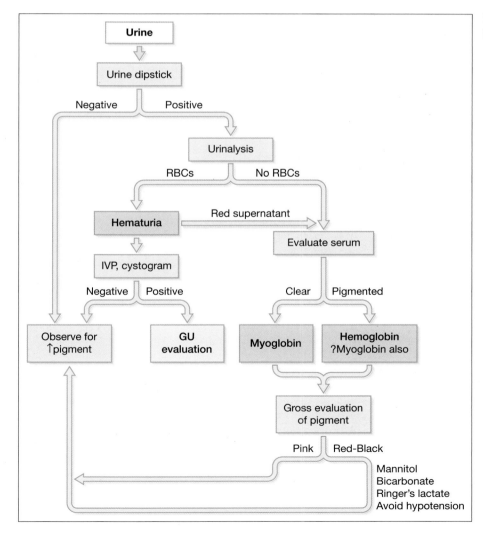

Fig. 39.3 Work-up and treatment of pigmented urine.

by falls from a height or being thrown against an object, with some resulting from the tetanic muscle contractions associated with the electrical shock itself; forces strong enough to cause compression fractures.[15] A careful history and physical examination should select those patients who require a full trauma evaluation.

Compartment syndrome

Patients with high-voltage electrical injuries of the extremities are at risk for development of compartment syndromes during the first 48 hours post injury. Damaged muscle, swelling within the investing fascia of the extremity, may increase pressures to the point where muscle blood flow is compromised. Loss of pulses is one of the last signs of a compartment syndrome, unlike the early loss of pulses occurring in a circumferentially burned extremity requiring an escharotomy. A high index of suspicion is paramount for the early diagnosis (either by serial examinations of the affected extremities or repeated measurements of compartment pressures) and prompt treatment of these increased compartment pressures. While a very aggressive approach to fasciotomies has been advocated in the past, significant morbidity attends a fasciotomy and its closure. Mann et al. has made a convincing argument for a conservative course regarding the indications for fasciotomies, that is for the usual clinical signs of compartment syndrome, progressive nerve dysfunction or failure of resuscitation with other patients undergoing exploration and aggressive debridement on the third to fifth postburn day.[16] Elevated CK levels have been correlated to the extent of muscle damage, with the authors advocating early decompression and aggressive surgical managements in patients with strongly elevated CK levels.[17]

Four compartment fasciotomies of the lower leg and anterior/posterior fasciotomies[18] of the upper extremity are performed in the operating room under general anesthesia. Rarely, medial and lateral fasciotomies of the thigh and upper arm are required to completely release all damaged areas. Incisions can be made with either a knife or electrocautery, with care taken to assure complete release of all affected muscle groups. Coverage of the ensuing wound is with a biologic dressing such as porcine heterograft[19] and the extremity is kept elevated to hasten resolution of edema. At this initial operation, we place a silk suture in the muscle at the proximal limit of gross necrosis in order to determine progression of visible damage. While a great deal of discussion concerns the progressive nature of electrical burns, ultimate division of the muscle is seldom more than 1 cm proximal to that seen at a careful initial evaluation. The initial operation is followed by a second look operation in 24–48 hours with debridement/amputation and the earliest possible closure. Fasciotomy wound closure is facilitated by use of traction on the affected skin edges by carefully placed sutures, vessel loop tensioning[20] or commercially available tensioning devices. Skin grafting is minimized if fasciotomy closure is appropriately planned. In order to minimize operating time and blood loss at the initial operation primary amputations are not generally performed, except to remove mummified, contracted extremities.

Wound care

Local burn care is performed using mafenide acetate (Sulfamylon®) on the thick eschar of the contact points, because of its excellent penetration. Silver sulfadiazine is used for microbial control on the deep flash/flame components and a biologic dressing used on more superficial areas. Surgical excision is begun 2–3 days postburn either as a second look operation following fasciotomy or as the first procedure in patients not requiring fasciotomies. All obviously necrotic tissue is removed, while tissues of questionable viability are retained and re-evaluated every 2–3 days until wound closure can be achieved. A very conservative course of tissue removal and wound closure with a combination of skin grafts and/or flaps for soft tissue coverage gives the best functional results. An ongoing program of physical therapy and functional splinting is begun the day of admission and continued throughout the hospital stay. Serial neuromuscular examinations are performed to document neurological status. Regional anesthesia is best avoided to minimize medicolegal complications should late neurological dysfunction arise.

Diagnosis

Multiple diagnostic modalities have been investigated attempting to speed up the process of identifying the extent of deep tissue necrosis. Radionuclide scanning with xenon-133[21] and technetium pyrophosphate[22,23] have been shown to be accurate predictors of tissue damage. Hammond showed that scanning did not decrease hospital stay or number of operations required.[23] Magnetic resonance imaging provides poor sensitivity for evaluation of muscle damage in non-perfused areas. Gadolinium-enhanced MR imaging demonstrates potential viability in zones of tissue edema and good correlation with histopathology.[24-26] While very sensitive and specific, diagnostic scans often add little to direct clinical evaluation and create logistical problems of their own. For all practical purposes, the use of the above cited techniques are expensive and unnecessary.

Problem areas

Contact points on the scalp, chest, and abdomen provide additional specific management problems. The scalp must be carefully searched for these lesions as scalp burns are rarely painful and are easily missed on cursory physical examinations (Figure 39.4). Scalp burns which spare the galea are managed by excision and skin grafting directly onto the galea, while wounds that penetrate to the outer table of the skull or deeper require a different approach. Exposure of non-viable calvaria has historically been approached by providing a viable wound bed after removing the dead bone with an osteotome or a dental-type burr. Drilling multiple holes in a close set pattern, deep enough to cause bleeding from viable cancellous bone is another method to develop granulation tissue which eventually covers the entire area. The latter method is still useful in situations where a patient's advanced age or large burn size precludes more aggressive approaches to wound closure. All of the above methods require weeks to months of wound care before the wound is ready for autograft coverage. The best and most expedient approach to these deep skull burns is a rotation scalp flap(s) over the burned area. Split-thickness skin grafts cover the resulting adjacent defect. This provides rapid closure and is associated with minimal morbidity (Figure 39.5).[27] Skin expansion of the hair-bearing area can be performed 12–18 months later to obliterate the areas of alopecia.

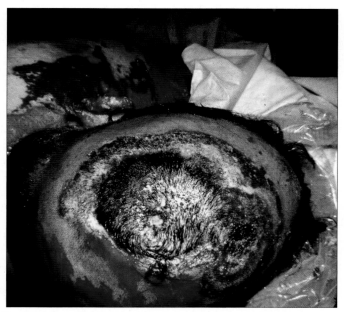

Fig. 39.4 Contact point on scalp with deep necrosis through galea. Patient had no complaints of pain.

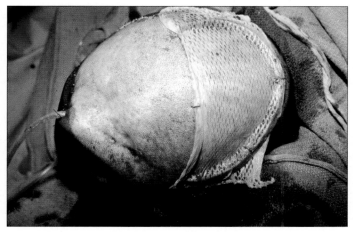

Fig. 39.5 Rotation scalp flap to cover deep necrotic contact point.

Larger scalp defects are closed with free flaps anastomosed to appropriate vessels lying outside the zone of injury.

In addition to the myocardial effects of electricity enumerated above, thoracic injury to the deep structures including the phrenic nerve and direct thermal injury to the heart may occur. Chest wall injuries present special closure problems (adjacent or remote soft tissue flaps) for coverage of exposed bone and cartilage. Costal chondritis is the most frequent complication of deep chest wall burns, becoming a source of long-term morbidity, requiring multiple debridements.

Abdominal wounds provide the potential for internal injuries both directly under contact points and remotely as the result of late ischemic necrosis.[28,29] Patients must be frequently evaluated for changes in their abdominal examination and/or feeding tolerance. Deterioration mandates laparotomy. Repair of large abdominal wall wounds requires careful planning and often a multidisciplinary team for optimal results.

Lightning injury

Approximately 100 000 thunderstorms occur in the USA each year with lightning killing more people than any other weather phenomena, causing about 80 fatalities per year with Florida and Texas having the most deaths.[30–32] While lightning strikes involve millions of volts of electricity, the spectrum of burn injury is extremely varied, from minimal cutaneous burn to significant burns equal in depth to commercial high voltage electricity. Major cutaneous injury is rare unless a nearby object is turned incandescent, causing a flash/flame-type injury, as when a bag of golf clubs on the victim's back is struck. The pathognomonic cutaneous sign of a lightning strike is a dendritic, arborescent or fern-like branching erythematous pattern on the skin (Lichtenberg figure) which appears within an hour of injury and fades rapidly, much like a wheal and flare reaction.[33] Full-thickness isolated burns on the tips of the toes has also been reported as being characteristic. Both findings are useful in determining the cause of injury in the patient found down under uncertain circumstances.[34]

Lightning may cause both respiratory and cardiac standstill for which CPR is especially effective when promptly initiated.[35] The ears should be carefully examined as injuries are frequent, ranging from ruptured tympanic membranes (most common) to middle and inner ear destruction.[36]

Neurological complications are relatively common and include unconsciousness, seizures, paresthesias and paralysis which may develop over several days after injury. The term keraunoparalysis has been used to describe the latter symptom complex and is associated with vasomotor disorders. Fortunately these are usually transient. Surgically treatable lesions including epidural, subdural and intracerebral hematomas may occur, mandating a high index of suspicion for an altered level of consciousness.[31] The prognosis of many lightning-caused neurological injuries are generally better than for other types of traumatic causes, although subtle neurological changes may persist, suggesting a very conservative, watchful waiting and supportive approach with serial neurological examinations after an initial CT scan to rule out correctable causes. A recent study by Muehlberger et al. with follow-up to 12.3 years after injury showed that none of their 10 patients had long-term neurological or psychological deficits.[37] Differences in long-term outcomes may be more related to effectiveness of CPR than the injury itself.

Low-voltage burns

Low-voltage direct current causes both direct injury and thermal injuries most often due to the heating effect of electricity turning a ring, wristwatch, bracelet or necklace incandescent resulting in a deep circumferential thermal burn. These are treated in the same manner as other thermal burns.[38] Mechanics and persons working on automobiles are at greatest risk for this injury as automotive electrical systems are the most common source of low-voltage–high-amperage electricity.

Low-voltage alternating current injury is usually localized to the points of contact, although with prolonged contact, tissue damage may extend into deep tissues with little lateral extension as seen in high-voltage wounds. These wounds are treated by excision to viable tissue and appropriate coverage based on wound depth and location.

Burns of the oral cavity are the most common type of serious electrical burn in young children.[39] Most of these injuries result from the child chewing on an electrical cord or on the male–female plug interface between two cords. Injuries involving only the oral commissure are initially treated very conservatively as the extent of injury is difficult to predict (Figure 39.6). Simple wound care is performed as an outpatient.[40,41] The most serious complication is bleeding from the labial artery, occurring 10–14 days after injury. Families are instructed to digitally compress the labial artery if bleeding occurs and return to the ER. Following healing, treatment varies by the severity of injury. Gentle stretching and the use of oral splints give good cosmetic and functional results in most patients, with reconstructive surgery being reserved for the remainder. Severe mircostomia is corrected by mucosal advancement flaps. Burns of the mid-portions of mouth heal very poorly and require a much more aggressive surgical approach with carefully planned reconstruction.[42,43]

Complications

The primary early complications of electrical injury include renal, septic, cardiac, neurological, and ocular manifestations. Renal failure and sepsis are preventable by adequate resuscitation and rapid removal of necrotic tissue, while cardiac damage is recognized and treated on admission. Neurological deficits may be present on admission or develop days to weeks after injury.

Cataract formation is the most frequent ocular complication of electrical injury, although ocular manifestations may affect all portions of the eye.[44,45] The exact pathophysiology appears to be unknown, but ocular changes may affect as many as 5–20% of patients with true electrical burns. Saffle reported on seven patients with 13 cataracts, noting a high rate of bilaterality and little association with voltage or location of contact points, although often thought of as being more frequently associated with contact points of the head, neck and upper trunk.[46] Seventy-seven percent eventually progressed to the point where surgical therapy was necessary, the results of which were uniformly good. Lag time before appearance may be as short as 3 weeks and as long as 11 years after injury.[47]

Neurological complications are protean in their diversity and may present either early or late (occurring up to 2 years after injury). Neuromuscular defects including paresis, paralysis, Guillain–Barré syndrome, transverse myelitis or amyotrophic lateral sclerosis can be caused by electrical injury.[48] A study by Grube puts the incidence into perspective.[5] Of 64 patients with high-voltage burns, 67% developed immediate central or peripheral neurological symptoms. One third had peripheral neuropathies with one third of those persistent. Twelve percent had delayed onset of peripheral neuropathy with 50% of those resolving. They reported no late onset, central neuropathies. Ko reported on 13 patients with delayed onset of spinal cord injuries postulating on a vascular cause of the deficit.[49] The most common peripheral defect is a peripheral neuropathy, with weakness being the most commonly found clinical finding.[50] In general, resolution of early-onset lesions is much better than for late onset, spasticity is more frequent than flaccidity, and function is affected more than sensation. Sympathetic overactivity with changes in bowel habits, urinary and sexual function is the primary autonomic complex complication. Although the exact mechanism of nerve injury has not been explained, both direct injury by electrical current and/or a vascular cause receive the most attention. To date, imaging studies, including angiography and MR imaging, have not been helpful in either predicting or evaluating the extent of deficit. Very often, neuropsychological status is abnormal. In a study comparing electrical burn patients with non-burned electricians, Pliskin showed significantly higher cognitive, physical and emotional complaints not related to injury or litigation status.[51] A full neurological examination must be performed on admission, documenting initial presentation. Consistent long-term follow-up with careful neuromus-

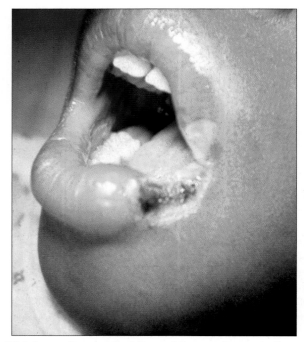

Fig. 39.6 Low-voltage contact burn of the mouth, most often involving the commissure.

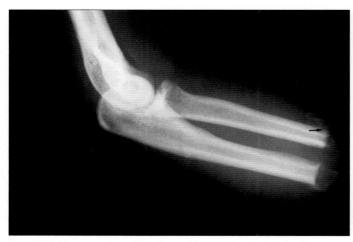

Fig. 39.7 Heterotopic ossification arising at the cut ends of a forearm amputation and requiring excision.

cular examinations becomes an important part of patient care. Electrodiagnostic evaluation may be helpful in delineating the defect. Early involvement of an experienced, interested physiatrist is important in assessing long-term needs and participating in the creation of a therapy plan.

Heterotopic ossification occurring at the cut ends of amputation sites is unique to the electrically burned patient. This occurs in about 80% of patients with long bone amputations, but not in patients with disarticulations or small bone amputa-

tions. Ossification was severe enough to require surgical revision of the bone end in 28% (Figure 39.7).[52] This is easily accomplished by opening the stump incision and using a bone ronguer to remove the soft heterotopic bone and reclosing the stump.

Although electrical burns are only about 3% of all burn injuries, they consume enormous amounts of resources, requiring a carefully planned team approach for optimal care.

References

1. Arnoldo BD, Purdue GF, Kowalske K, et al. Electrical injuries: a 20-year review. J Burn Care Rehabil 2004; 25:479–484.
2. Artz CP. Electrical injury simulates crush injury. Surg Gynecol Obstet 1967; 125:1316–1317.
3. Hunt JL, Mason AD, Masterson TS, et al. The pathophysiology of acute electric burns. J Trauma 1976; 16:335–340.
4. Merriam-Webster's Collegiate Dictionary, 10th edn. Springfield, MA: Merriam-Webster; 2000:371.
5. Grube BJ, Heimbach DM, Engrav LH, et al. Neurologic consequences of electrical burns. J Trauma 1990; 30:254–258.
6. Nichter LS, Bryant CA, Kenney JG, et al. Injuries due to commercial electric current. J Burn Care Rehabil 1984; 5:124–137.
7. Hunt JL, McManus WF, Haney WP, et al. Vascular lesions in acute electric injuries. J Trauma 1974; 14:461–473.
8. Lee RC, Kolodney SB. Electrical injury mechanisms: electrical breakdown of cell membranes. Plast Reconstr Surg 1987; 80:672–680.
9. Lee RC, Canaday DJ, Hammer SM. Transient and stable ionic permeabilization of isolated skeletal muscle cells after electrical shock. J Burn Care Rehabil 1993; 14:528–540.
10. Freiberger H. The electrical resistance of the human body to commercial direct and alternating currents. (Der elektrische widerstand des menschilichen Koepers gegen technischen gleich und wechselstrom.) Berlin. Elertrizitatswirtschaft 1933; 2:442–446.
11. Housinger TA, Green L, Shahangian S, et al. A prospective study of myocardial damage in electrical injuries. J Trauma 1985; 25:122–124.
12. McBride JW, Labrosse KR, McCoy HG, et al. Is serum creatine kinase-MB in electrically injured patients predictive of myocardial injury? JAMA 1986; 255:764–768.
13. Dilworth D, Hasan D, Alford P, et al. Evaluation of myocardial injury in electrical burn patients. J Burn Care Rehabil 1998; 19 (Pt 2): S239.
14. Purdue GF, Hunt JL. Electrocardiographic monitoring after electrical injury: necessity or luxury. J Trauma 1986; 26:166–167.
15. Layton TR, McMurtry JM, McClain EJ, et al. Multiple spine fractures from electric injury. J Burn Care Rehabil 1984; 5:373–375.
16. Mann R, Gibran N, Engrav L, et al. Is immediate decompression of high voltage electrical injuries to the upper extremity always necessary? J Trauma 1996; 40:584–589.
17. Koop J, Loos B, Spilker G, et al. Correlation between serum creatinine kinase levels and extent of muscle damage in electrical burns. Burns 2004; 30:680–683.
18. Fazi B, Raves JJ, Young JC, et al. Fasciotomy of the upper extremity in the patient with trauma. Surg Gyn Obstet 1987; 165:447–448.
19. Parshley P, Kilgore J, Pulito J, et al. Aggressive approach to the extremity damaged by electric current. Am J Surg 1985; 150:78–82.
20. Berman SS, Schilling JD, McIntyre KE, et al. Shoelace technique for delayed primary closure of fasciotomies. Am J Surg 1994; 167:435–436.
21. Clayton JM, Hayes AC, Hammel J, et al. Xenon-133 determination of muscle blood flow in electrical injury. J Trauma 1977; 17:293–298.
22. Hunt J, Lewis S, Parkey R, Baxter C. The use of technetium-99m stannous pyrophosphate scintigraphy to identify muscle damage in acute electric burns. J Trauma 1979; 19:409–413.
23. Hammond J, Ward CG. The use of technetium-99 pyrophosphate scanning in management of high voltage electrical injuries. Am Surg 1994; 68:886–888.
24. Fleckenstein JL, Chason DP, Bonte FJ, et al. High-voltage electric injury: assessment of muscle viability with MR imaging and Tc-99m pyrophosphate scintigraphy. Radiology 1993; 195:205–210.
25. Ohashi M, Koizumi J, Hosoda Y, et al. Correlation between magnetic resonance imaging and histopathology of an amputated forearm after electrical injury. Burns 1998; 24:362–368.
26. Lee RC. Injury by electrical forces: pathophysiology, manifestations, and therapy. Curr Probl Surg 1997; 34:738–740.
27. Hunt J, Purdue G, Spicer T. Management of full-thickness burns of the scalp and skull. Arch Surg 1983; 118:621–625.
28. Newsome TW, Curreri PW, Kurenius K. Visceral injuries – an unusual complication of an electrical burn. Arch Surg 1972; 105:494–497.
29. Reilley AF, Rees R, Kelton P, et al. Abdominal arotic occlusion following electric injury. J Burn Care Rehabil 1985; 6:226–229.
30. Lightning-Associated deaths – United States, 1980–1995. MMWR 1998; 19:391–394.
31. Hiestand D, Colice GL. Lightning-strike injury. J Intensive Care 1988; 3:303–314.
32. Tribble CG, Persing JA, Morgan RF, et al. Lightning injury. Curr Concept Trauma Care 1984; Spring:5–10.
33. ten Duis HJ, Klasen HJ, Nijsten MWN. Superficial lightning injuries – their 'fractal' shape and origin. Burns 1987;13:141–146.
34. Fahmy FS, Brinsden MD, Smith J, et al. Lightning: the multisystem group injuries. J Trauma 1999; 46:937–940.
35. Moran KT, Thupari JN, Munster AM. Electric- and lightning-induced cardiac arrest reversed by prompt cardiopulmonary resuscitation. JAMA 1986; 255:2157.
36. Bergstrom L, Neblett LM, Sando I, et al. The lightning-damaged ear. Arch Otolaryngol 1974; 100:117–121.
37. Muehlberger T, Vogt PM, Munster AM. The long-term consequences of lightning injuries. Burns 2001; 27:829–833.
38. Manstein CM, Manstein ME, Manstein G. Circumferential electric burns of the ring finger. J Hand Surg 1987; 12A:808.
39. Rai J, Jeschke MG, Barrow RE, et al. Electrical injuries: a 30-year review. J Trauma 1999; 46:933–936.
40. Leake JE, Curtin JW. Electrical burns of the mouth in children. Clin Plast Surg 1984; 11:669–683.
41. D'Italia JG, Hulnick SJ. Outpatient management of electric burns of the lip. J Burn Care Rehabil 1984; 5: 465–466.
42. Sadove AM, Jones JE, Lynch TR, et al. Appliance therapy for perioral electrical burns: a conservative approach. J Burn Care Rehabil 1988; 9:391–395.
43. Pensler JM, Rosenthal A. Reconstruction of the oral commissure after an electrical burn. J Burn Care Rehabil 1990; 11: 50–53.
44. Johnson EV, Klein LB, Skalka HW. Electrical cataracts: a case report and review of the literature. Ophthalmic Surg 1987; 18:283–285.
45. Boozalis GT, Purdue GF, Hunt JP, et al. Ocular changes from electrical burn injuries: a literature review and report of cases. J Burn Care Rehabil 1991; 5:458–462.

46. Saffle JR, Crandall A, Warden GD. Cataracts: a long-term complication of electrical injury. J Trauma 1985; 25:17–21.

47. Mutlu FM, Duman H, Cli Y. Early-onset unilateral electric cataract: a rare clinical entity. J Burn Care Rehabil 2004; 25:363–365.

48. Petty PG, Parkin G. Electrical injury to the central nervous system. Neurosurgery 1986; 19:282–284.

49. Ko SH, Chun W, Kim HC. Delayed spinal cord injury following electrical burns: a 7-year experience. Burns 2004; 30:691–695.

50. Haberal MA, Gureu S, Akman N, et al. Persistent peripheral nerve pathologies in patients with electric burns. J Burn Care Rehabil 1996; 17:147–149.

51. Pliskin NH, Capelli-Schellpfeffer M, Law RT, et al. Neuropsychological symptom presentation after electrical injury. J Trauma 1998; 44:709–715.

52. Helm PA, Walker SC. New bone formation at amputation in electrically burn-injured patients. Arch Phys Med Rehabil 1987; 68:284–286.

Suggested reading

Andrews CJ, Cooper MA, Darveniza M, et al. Lightning injuries: electrical, medical and legal aspects. Boca Raton: CRC; 1992.

Kurtz EB, Shoemaker TM. The lineman's and cablemans's handbook, 7th edn. New York: McGraw-Hill; 1985.

Chapter 40

Electrical injury: reconstructive problems

Peter M. Vogt, Andreas D. Niederbichler, Marcus Spies, and Thomas Muehlberger

Chapter contents

Introduction

> Severe cases (of electrical injury) coming for reconstruction present a formidable problem of flexion contracture and loss of many tendons and nerves, new pedicled skin and grafted-in tendons and nerves usually being necessary. One encounters inside the limb the same type of destruction and cicatrix as is found after any severe infection.
>
> Sterling Bunnell, 1948

This chapter will focus on the multitude of surgical and reconstructive problems that result from electrical injury. The spectrum of electrical injuries is complex due to various factors determining manifestation, severity, and distribution of the resulting tissue damage. In common with other types of trauma, especially burn injuries, the consequences of electrical injuries may affect a wide range of physiological functions. Its distinct features warrant a differentiated approach to this unique kind of trauma. The resulting tissue loss and the damage to essential structures of the involved body areas often require extensive plastic-reconstructive procedures.

Although the incidence of low-voltage burns steadily declined over the last decades, most probably due to progress made in the field of home and occupational safety education and equipment, electrical injuries still account for 3–5% of all admissions to major burn centers.[1,2] Electrical fatalities are relatively uncommon and most of them occur accidentally. Advances in reconstructive operative techniques resulting in higher rates of limb salvage in other causes of trauma so far have not achieved similar results in electrical injuries. Therefore, although earlier reported limb amputation rates of up to 71% decreased over the last decades with the increasing ability to reconstruct anatomic parts and restore function, limb salvage remains a surgical challenge.[3,4]

Diagnosis and acute treatment

Diagnosis and acute treatment of electrical injury have been described in Chapter 39. However, several important characteristics need to be emphasized.

Assessment of tissue damage

The correct assessment of the extent of tissue damage is difficult. The percentage of burned body surface area grossly underestimates the injury to underlying tissue. Electrical burns may appear as mere pinpoint marks. In contrast, fatal electrocution may even take place without any visible skin burns in case of a large contact area. In a series of 59 patients with high-voltage injuries, the extent of visible burns showed no correlation to any other complications or sequelae.[5] The actual cutaneous resistance depends on contact size, pressure applied during contact, the magnitude and duration of the current, and the moisture status of the skin (Table 40.1).

In contrast to thermal burns, deposition of metallic iron and copper is found on the epidermis after electrical injuries as electrolysis occurs in the extracellular fluid of the skin. These metal condensations produce a black coating of the skin resembling an eschar.

Clinical determination of tissue viability is based on inspection and the demonstration of muscle contractility. As yet, there are no other diagnostic tools available to accurately assess the extent of tissue damage in the early phase following electrical injuries. The value of magnetic resonance imaging (MRI) for the detection of non-perfused non-edematous muscle is debated.[6,7] Serial measurement of skin temperature, muscle perfusion scintigraphy, Xe-133 clearance test, and radionuclide arteriography with labeled microspheres show no significant advantages.[8] Angiography, although not providing information on tissue viability, demonstrates the absence of tissue perfusion, and may lead to an early indication of limb amputation.[9]

Rhabdomyolysis and myoglobinuria

Rhabdomyolysis leads to hyperkalemia, calcium deposition in damaged muscle cells, release of intracellular phosphate and eventually hypocalcemia. Destroyed muscle cells release myoglobin, resulting in myoglobinemia. Hemolysis also often occurs with electrical injury, resulting in concurrent hemoglobinemia. Thus urine measurements of hemochromogens cannot be used as a guide to adequate therapy.[10,11] Serum levels of creatinine and creatinine phosphokinase (CPK) are used as indicators of rhabdomyolysis. It is important to note that the

TABLE 40.1 DEPENDENCY OF CUTANEOUS RESISTANCE ON SKIN MOISTURE[6]

	Resistance
Dry skin	100 000 Ω
Wet skin	2 500 Ω
Skin immersion	1 500 Ω
Rubber soles	70 000 Ω
Reproduced from Ohashi et al. Burns 1998; 24:362–368.	

TABLE 40.2 RECOMMENDATION FOR CARDIAC MONITORING IN THE ABSENCE OF OTHER INJURIES

Admission and cardiac monitoring	Discharge
Loss of consciousness[36]	Asymptomatic patient[37]
Extensive burns[32]	Normal initial ECG[38]
Current passing through the thorax[34]	Uneventful 4-hour observation[39]
Cardiac dysrhythmias[36]	Voltage less than 240/260 in adults[37,38]
	Voltage less than 120/240 in children[30,39]PP. 1257–1259 (PC65)

destruction of 2 g of skeletal muscle can already yield a 10-fold increase of the normal CPK level. After a muscle injury the CPK level will peak by 24 hours and return to baseline within 48–72 hours. This diminishes the diagnostic value of serum and urine chemistry testing.[11,12]

Renal failure

Myoglobinuria has traditionally been considered a major risk factor for the development of acute renal failure. Recently, patients with electrical injuries have been shown to have a surprisingly low risk for renal failure.[13] In 162 patients, only 14% had myoglobinuria and none developed renal failure. Suggested criteria to evaluate the risk of acute renal failure after electrical injury include: prehospital cardiac arrest, full-thickness burns, compartment syndrome, and high-voltage injury. Presence of at least two criteria should instigate immediate treatment, as the time-frame to prevent the progression to acute renal failure is limited to a few hours postinjury. Renal complications after low-voltage injuries are rare.

Cardiac monitoring

Among the estimated 1300 deaths that occur annually in the United States from electrical injury (including lightning strike), 30% of the patients present with cardiac complications. The complex mechanisms of cardiac tissue affection by electrical current implicate a wide range of cardiac complications of electrical injury. The majority of ECG abnormalities are sinus tachycardia and non-specific changes in the ST-segment and the T-wave.[14] Death from electric injury most commonly results from current-induced cardiac arrest.

Various degrees of heat generation, direct cellular destruction (electroporation) and effects on excitation–contraction coupling mechanisms such as ion shifting make predictions of the clinical course difficult. Keeping that and the wide range of possible trauma mechanisms in mind (low/high-voltage injury, current flow direction through the body, duration of exposure, pre-existing comorbidities, etc.) it is clear that algorithms for cardiac monitoring of electrically injured patients need to be critically discussed and are best viewed as an orientation for the physician.

However, the current literature review allows the following recommendations: if an initial ECG shows no abnormalities, the delayed development of cardiac problems is very unlikely, irrespective whether the patients sustained high- or low-voltage injuries.[15–17]

Conversely, the presence of dysrhythmias or conduction abnormalities on initial presentation, electrical injury in children, or if the projected path of the current flow crosses the thorax on initial presentation, warrants prolonged cardiac monitoring.[18–21] Depending on the nature of the current-induced arrhythmia, pharmacotherapeutic and/or invasive interventions may be necessary to prevent life-threatening arrhythmias and re-establish normorhythmia. Table 40.2 outlines recommendations for cardiac monitoring of electrically injured patients based on central clinical findings and specific features of the trauma mechanism.

Apart from specific therapeutic measures of cardiac complications, acute treatment of patients with electrical injuries adheres to guidelines of ABLS®, ATLS®, and current practice of intensive care medicine. This includes the maintenance of a patent airway, effective ventilation, and systemic circulation to provide adequate tissue perfusion and oxygenation. The reduced extent of visible skin burns may lead to underestimation of resuscitation fluid requirements. The patients must be continuously monitored for signs of neurovascular compromise, and deranged tissue perfusion and oxygenation. Pulse oximetry may be useful for this purpose.

Surgical debridement

In the last decades, the concept of progressive tissue necrosis has led to the treatment strategy of early debridement and fasciotomy, followed by serial debridement and delayed wound closure. However, extensive studies have failed to support the notion that electrical injury causes progressive ischemia secondary to electrically induced endothelial damage.[22–24] In serial arterial angiograms of electrically injured extremities no vascular changes could be found.[25] The observed changes may more likely be explained by vascular changes similar to ischemia–reperfusion injury with immediate cessation of capillary blood flow in response to current passage. This event is followed by vascular spasms lasting for extended time, with subsequent vasodilatation and restoration of flow.[26,27] Although still controversial, these findings may shift the acute treatment paradigm.

While there is little discussion about the early time point of debridement, several recent studies question the need of extensive and total necrectomy and advocate the approach of delayed soft tissue coverage. 'Conservative debridement' consisting of removal of charred and obviously necrotic tissue has been promoted in a study on 40 patients.[28] In this study partially damaged tendons, muscles, and nerves were preserved, and wound closure was achieved by immediate flap coverage. Patients treated in this manner with immediate soft tissue coverage had a significantly better outcome compared with a control group who underwent serial debridement procedures. Similar results were found in a study using early free-flap coverage for electrical injuries, suggesting that careful limited initial debridement is an adequate measure.[29] According to this study overly extensive and repeated debridement to ensure viability of all remaining tissue appears not only unnecessary but also quite likely harmful. It appears safe to abandon these strategies and to perform an early extensive, but selective debridement in order to preserve continuity of functionally important structures (Figure 40.1). Available options for wound closure encompass the total range of plastic reconstructive procedures, from skin grafts and local flaps to free tissue transfer.[30] Limb salvage with functional preservation of vital structures should be attempted and may require revascularization using segmental vein grafts or segmental cable grafting of nerves. Pedicled flaps should be considered in cases of suspected arterial compromise.

Despite the encouraging results of the studies recommending early soft tissue reconstruction by all means it should be noted that for the extent of electrical injury no scoring system has been established so far. Therefore, the comparison of different studies using both aggressive debridement alone or selective debridement and early soft tissue coverage is difficult with respect to the severity of tissue damage treated. Alternative approaches to salvage upper extremity function such as the temporary ectopic implantation of an undamaged hand have been reported, but cannot be considered standard of care.[31]

The condition of the individual patient and the level of tissue destruction varies considerably and determines the available therapeutic options.

Compartment syndrome

Muscle compartment pressure should be monitored clinically and by invasive pressure measurements. In contrast to blunt trauma, pain is not a reliable indicator of increased compartment pressure due to the high incidence of electrical nerve injury. When compartment pressures exceed 30 mmHg, surgical decompression by open fasciotomy becomes necessary to prevent ischemic muscle injury. In case of lower compartment pressure, progression may be prevented by administration of nonsteroidal anti-inflammatory drugs (NSAIDs) and antioxidants, protective splinting, and rest without elevation of the affected extremities. However, general operative decompression in high-voltage injuries of extremities appears not to be warranted. In a cohort study, Mann et al. found an increased amputation rate of 45% with immediate operative decompression compared with patients undergoing selective fasciotomy, and they recommend fasciotomy only in case of progressive peripheral nerve dysfunction, manifested compartment syndrome, or other major injuries.[22] With a fixed neurological deficit, however, surgical decompression shows no influence on outcome.[32] If the clinical situation remains doubtful, however, the performance of open fasciotomy with early debridement may be preferred (Figures 40.2 and 40.3).

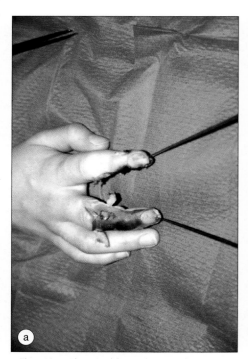
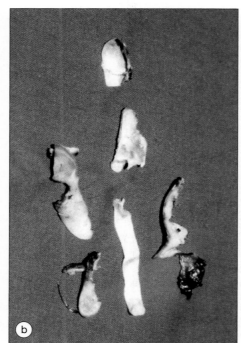
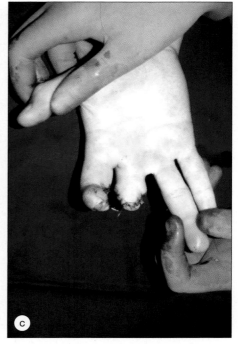

Fig. 40.1 Electrical burn from a domestic water heater (220V). The 13-year-old girl manipulated the device while being immersed in the bathtub. She sustained third- and fourth-degree burns of the digits (a). Debridement revealed full-thickness injuries involving tendons, nerves, and phalangeal bones (b), which necessitated primary amputation (c).

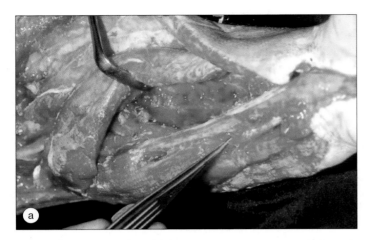

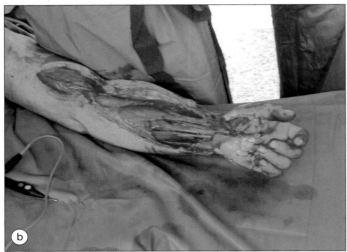

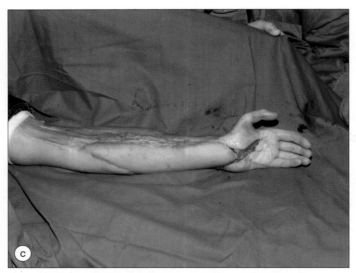

Fig. 40.2 High-voltage injury from an overhead power line (30 000V). The teenager climbed a train and was struck by an arc without touching the power line. The spectrum of injury included third- and fourth-degree burns and deep tissue necrosis of the forearm (a). After fasciotomy due to impending compartment syndrome (b). Coverage with free latissimus dorsi flap after 'conservative' debridement. Significant functional deficits after 4 years (c).

Reconstructive challenges

When treating a patient with severe electrical injury the plastic reconstructive surgeon encounters many surgical challenges. The anatomic regions most often concerned are the head and the extremities, especially the upper extremities. Bearing that in mind the appropriate reconstruction is of utmost importance for the functional outcome and the resulting quality of life of the injured person.

Head: scalp, skull, and mouth

The head is a common injury site in electric burns. The resulting injury usually appears as a circular area with a central full-thickness damage of the scalp, often reaching through galea, periosteum, and sometimes bone. Exposure and necrosis of bone may consequently lead to osteomyelitis and even an epidural abscess. Treatment strategies depend on the extent of the injury to the bone. In case of only a partial necrosis of the bone the outer table of the skull can be tangentially removed with a high-speed bone drill and the viable diploic cavity exposed. In case of sufficient vascularization the exposed bone can be grafted immediately or, when blood supply is questionable, grafted when suitable granulation tissue has developed.[33] A vacuum sealing system of the wound may be of significant efficiency in growing adequate amounts of granulation tissue. When the initial wound debridement is delayed, necrotic and infected bone might become the source of a full-thickness skull defect. However, with grafting of skin on partially debrided viable bone the lack of a subcutaneous or galea layer often causes long-term problems such as ulceration and scar formation. Full-thickness injury of the skull theoretically requires a complete excision of the necrotic bone to prevent infectious complications. However, this poses the patient at risk for a neurosurgical procedure and requires coverage of the excised area by a rotation flap or even a microvascular graft. Another approach suggested is the partial debridement followed by definitive flap coverage of the exposed bone. This, however, requires early debridement and the prevention of localized bacterial colonization and infection.[34,35] Fortunately, involvement of the dura occurs rarely. This usually requires an extensive free flap procedure.[36] We preferably use the latissimus flap connected to cervical vessels, occasionally using interpositional vein grafts. This reduces the risk of perfusion problems considerably. When these options are not available, the use of acellular human dermis to reconstruct the dural defect followed by split-thickness skin grafting after vascularization may be an option.[37]

In children, especially in toddlers, common sites of low-tension injury include the mouth and occur usually in the area of the oral commissure, affecting the commissure, the lips, and the tongue. The injury happens when the child bites into a cord or a light switch, or touches the male end of an improperly connected cord. The injury usually results in a localized partial necrosis of the lips and the commissure, the subsequent contracture results in microstomia. The treatment strategies, conservative versus early surgical intervention, are debated. The more aggressive early approach of excision and reconstruction results in faster healing, shorter length of hospital stay, and

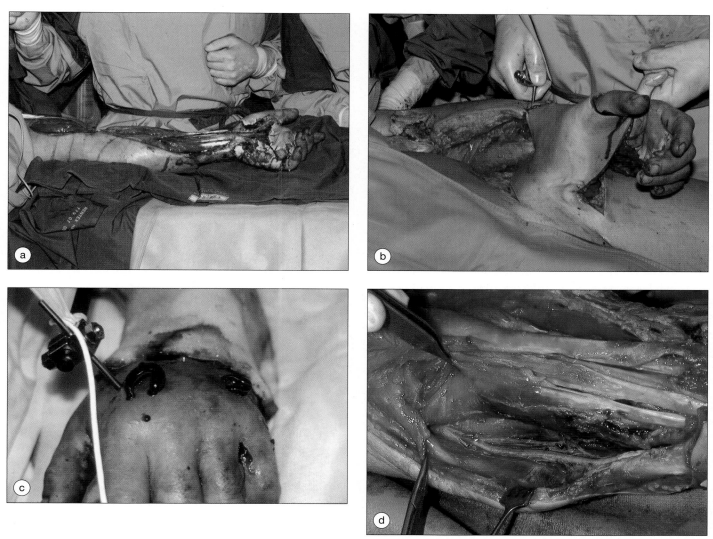

Fig. 40.3 High-voltage injury from a power line (50000V). Presentation with primary loss of perfusion, loss of function, and compartment syndrome. Initial operation with fasciotomy, revascularization of the radial artery and necrectomies. On the following days adequate perfusion with a patent radial artery without coexisting veins. Coverage with groin flap on day 6. Venous congestion and subsequent malperfusion was temporarily treated with leeches. Secondary amputation on day 10 due to late occlusion of the radial artery.

fewer surgical procedures.[38,39] However, in this sensitive age group, early excision and reconstruction may also result in a tightened lower lip, and consequent inhibition of normal mandible growth.[40,41] The conservative management, which is favored by us, performs the reconstructive procedure after maturation of the burn wound scar. Thus the extent of the damage is more apparent and the reconstruction can be performed electively.[42] Oral splinting has been advocated during the initial healing period to decrease the need for reconstructive surgery. However, this more likely reduces scar contractures, so the planned reconstructive procedure can be performed after scar maturation.[43–45] The risk of acute hemorrhage by erosion of the oral arteries after sloughing of the

necrotic tissue appears low in our patient population. With adequate caution and education to the patient, this does not prohibit the conservative approach.

Thorax and abdomen

Electrical injury to the trunk commonly is of minor concern. However, high-tension injuries can cause damage to underlying parenchymatous organs such as the lung. Clinically this may lead to atelectasis and edema, requiring aggressive ventilator support. Intra-abdominal injuries are uncommon, but may require treatment like penetrating injury. When exploration during escharectomy and debridement reveals necrotic underlying muscle and fascia, exploratory laparotomy may be indicated. Potential bowel injury may require segmental bowel resection. Reconstructive options for the closure of chest or abdominal wall defects include direct closure or placement of a synthetic mesh covered by local fasciocutaneous or musculocutaneus flaps. However, the potential negative effects of direct closure on intra-abdominal pressure with subsequent development of an abdominal compartment syndrome or compromise of respiratory function must be considered.

Extremities

Electrical injuries to the extremities, especially to the arms and hand, are more common in adult members of the workforce. The actual effects and the sequelae depend on the current, the path of the current, and the patient's medical condition. Often the electrical source is grasped by the hand, leading to entry wounds at the hands and upper extremities and exit wounds at the lower extremities. As the resistance and thus the local energy production are dependent on the tissue mass and the cross-sectional diameter of the injured body part, high-tension injuries often lead to extensive tissue damage and loss of the involved extremity. Despite aggressive treatment strategies with early debridement and decompression of neurovascular structures, the likelihood of amputation is high.[22–24,46] Even if amputation can be avoided, the resulting outcome may be a non-functioning extremity. With the phenomenon of kissing lesions, extensive tissue damage may occur with resulting thermal necrosis of muscle, tendon, nerves, and blood vessel. The superficial injury may appear innocuous, but the operative debridement shows deep tissue destruction often mandating limb amputation. The role of initial debridement cannot be overstated as remaining non-viable tissue leads to infection and tissue loss. In our view the early debridement of non-viable tissue prevents this fatal development. Imminent or suspected compartment syndrome should always trigger open fasciotomy to prevent further compromise to the involved extremity. With involvement of the hand and the wrist region in form of an 'arcing phenomenon' release of the Guyon canal and the carpal tunnel, in addition to fasciotomy of the forearm, appears necessary. The reconstruction and coverage at this injury site may require microvascular reconstruction using nerve cable grafts for the median or ulnar nerve and vein grafts for reconstruction of the radial and ulnar artery in combination with coverage by free flaps. However, these options require sufficient soft tissue coverage and absence of any infection. If in doubt, it appears wise to perform a simple skin grafting procedure followed by elective secondary flap coverage and nerve cable grafting. Other regions of selective destruction in the upper extremity are elbow and axilla. The visible amount of tissue damage does not correlate with the destruction found on exploration. The underlying neuro-vascular structures, such as brachial artery, median and ulnar nerve or the brachial plexus in the axilla, are at risk. Debridement often leaves a vast tissue defect, which may be covered by rotation flaps from anterior or posterior chest wall in the axilla. Microvascular free flaps at the level of the elbow are rarely used. For extensive defects on the hand and forearm, pedicled groin flaps provide good coverage providing independent blood supply. The groin flap also avoids a vascular 'steal phenomenon' as it can be seen after microvascular free flaps in such severely injured extremity.

Despite all surgical options available, when exploration and initial debridement yield vast irreversible destruction of vital structure, the decision for amputation is justified and should be made early.

Amputations

Although distressing to the patient, amputation often remains the only option. The main objective for the surgical procedure is the achievement of a stably covered stump, allowing early fitting and adaptation of prosthetic devices. The optimal level of amputation is determined by the extent of remaining viable tissue and the intention to create sufficient stump length for function and cosmetic appearance of a prosthesis. In electrical injury involving the lower extremity this often requires higher amputation than initially anticipated in order to achieve sufficient stability of the stump and thus allow early prosthetic fitting and ambulation. The local situation often is similar to peripheral vascular disease and the amputation techniques should be appropriately chosen. However, open (guillotine) amputation should be avoided whenever possible. Split-thickness skin grafting onto open stumps is an additional but less preferable approach as breakdown of the skin occurs more often in grafted areas, especially at graft borders or at point where grafts adhere to underlying bone and further surgical interventions will be required. However, if valuable stump length can be maintained by skin grafting it should be attempted since secondary plastic surgical correction and specific prosthetic fitting are available.

In the upper extremity more length should be preserved, as the resulting weight bearing load to the stump is less compared to the lower extremity. This allows for better control of the prosthesis by the patient and thus enhanced functionality. In the forearm the muscle length of the flexor–extensor system should be preserved to improve function. In long forearm stumps atraumatic handling of tendons and muscles is necessary to preserve pronation and supination. Upper arm amputations should be made to preserve as much length as possible as this eases subsequent kineplastic procedures for a functional prosthesis. As in the forearm, muscular length of the flexor–extensor system is maintained by joining them over the bone end. Although it is technically feasible to maintain extremity length by coverage with a free flap this appears only useful in upper extremity amputation where the functional implications warrant such large-scale operation and the load on the stump is reduced.

Despite the availability of sophisticated modern myoelectric prostheses the old techniques of surgical rehabilitation should be kept in mind. This includes the Sauerbruch kinematomyoplasty of the biceps humeri muscle and the Krukenberg plasty of the forearm, which provides sensible chopstick-like stumps. Especially, for upper arm amputations distraction-osteogenesis procedures (Ilizarov technique) provide valuable options to lengthen a short amputation stump.

Peripheral nerve injury

Peripheral nerves are very sensitive to electric alterations, and even minor injury may cause transient dysfunction. Clinical findings may be anesthesia, paresthesia, or dysesthesia of usually short-term duration. In rare cases minor electrical injury may cause temporary autonomic dysfunction and trigger a complex regional pain syndrome (sympathetic reflex dystrophy). Treatment for reflex sympathetic dystrophy should be initiated early and include elevation of the extremity to reduce edema formation, active exercise, non-steroidal anti-inflammatory drugs, and adequate pain relief. The autonomic dysfunction may be influenced by α-adrenergic antagonists, Ca-channel blockers, and low-dose diazepam medication, or may require intravenous regional blocks and sympathetic ganglion blockade.[47]

Electrical injury of the upper extremity commonly results in peripheral nerve injury of median and ulnar nerve. The clinical findings may resemble upper extremity compression syndromes or peripheral neuropathy.[48,49] Nerve lesions may be caused by secondary factors such as incorrect positioning and splinting, constricting dressing, or delayed inadequate escharotomy or fasciotomy. Due to the accompanying severe muscle loss and scarring, the extent of pure nerve damage is sometimes difficult to determine.

Direct damage to peripheral nerves occurs following the before-mentioned mechanisms of local heat production depending on cross-sectional resistance or the proximity of peripheral nerves to underlying bone. The local thermal effect affects vascularity and perfusion perineural tissue by producing thrombosis, necrosis or hemorrhage of epineural vessels. Delayed development of fibrosis and therefore a delayed onset of symptoms are not uncommon. Other mechanisms of nerve injury are development of focal axonal degeneration following axonal excitation,[50] or electroporation, which more likely affects myelinated axons.[51,52]

Complications

Central nervous system

Approximately 60% of all patients with high-voltage injury present with immediate neurological complications, loss of consciousness being the predominant symptom.[53] The involvement of the spinal cord has been described in 2–27% of patients with an entry point of the current located in the head region.[54–56] The incidence of a delayed paralysis progressing to tetraplegia followed by partial remission has been described.[57] However, the cause and mechanism of this phenomenon remain unclear.

The neuropsychological effects of electrical injury have been described, mainly in case reports and retrospective studies. Typical consequences and complaints are related to physical, cognitive, and emotional changes.[58,59] The existing problems could not be directly attributed to physical manifestations of injury, and are similar to problems associated with prolonged stress, sleep deprivation, or after blunt head injury. In a study on 481 professional electricians, 97% reported having experienced an electrical shock at some point in their career.[60] The low incidence of neuropsychological dysfunction in this study differed from other findings about the nature and progression of a characteristic neuropsychological syndrome

of electrical injury.[59,61] Although the development of transient and progressive neuropsychiatric complications is possible and undisputed, the actual specific effects of electrical injury are difficult to determine. Other confounding factors such as the posttraumatic stress disorder, the grief reaction to disfigurement or extremity loss, and the disposition of the individual, all influence systematic evaluation.

Cataracts

An increased incidence of cataract formation has been described after electrical injury. The incidence in different reports varies from 1% to 8%.[62,63] Patients with head and neck wounds appear to be most at risk. However, the path of the current and the location of the entry point were not related to the development of ocular sequelae. Cataracts may also occur without injury to the head and appear even years after injury. Common initial complaints are blurred vision or diminished visual acuity.[64]

Skeletal injury

Besides direct tissue destruction through electrical energy, additional trauma can be indirectly inflicted by electric current. Fractures occur due to secondary falls or with forceful tetanic muscle contractions. These are mostly seen in the shoulder,[65] wrists,[66] femurs,[67] and the spine,[68] and may require open reduction and internal fixation. Late sequelae of electrical injury similar to severe thermal burns include major joint contractures and limited function of the extremities.

Another common late complication of electrical burns is heterotopic calcification in periarticular tissue of large joints, especially elbows. Causative factors include forced passive mobilization, secondary articular bleeding, and calcium precipitation and deposition in damaged or degenerating muscle and connective tissue. Particularly for electrical injury, heterotopic bone formation also occurs in amputation stumps of long bones. This, as well as the common formation of bone cysts in the amputation stump, may lead to secondary skin erosion, inflammation, and difficult adjustment of prosthesis. In both situations surgical excision and wound closure may provide adequate therapy.[69]

Summary

Electrical injuries result in deceptively large tissue loss, often leading to amputation of involved extremities. After initial resuscitation, early debridement, necessary decompression of neurovascular structures, and early wound closure are essential to successful restoration of function. Extensive surgical procedures including free soft-tissue transfer may be necessary to achieve wound closure, and to save and restore limb function. Sometimes, however, early amputation may provide easier and earlier recovery and reintegration into daily life. Long-term complications such as central nervous sequelae, cataracts, and heterotopic ossification must be considered and addressed early in the rehabilitation process.

References

1. Rai J, Jeschke MG, Barrow RE, et al. Electrical injuries: a 30-year review. J Trauma 1999; 46:933–936.

2. Tredget EE, Shankowsky HA, Tilley WA. Electrical injuries in Canadian burn care. Ann N Y Acad Sci 1999; 888:75–87.

3. Rouge RG, Dimick AR. The treatment of electrical injury compared to burn injury: a review of patholphysiology and comparison of patient management protocols. J Trauma 1978; 18:43.

4. Edlich RF, Farinholt HM, Winters KL, et al. Modern concepts of treatment and prevention of electrical burns. J Long Term Eff Med Implants 2005; 15(5):511–532.

5. Ferreiro I, Melendez J, Ragalado J, et al. Factors influencing the sequelae of high-tension electrical injuries. Burns 1998; 24:649–653.

6. Ohashi M, Koizumi J, Hosoda Y, et al. Correlation between magnetic resonance imaging and histopathology of an amputated forearm after an electrical injury. Burns 1998; 24:362–368.

7. Fleckenstein JL, Chason DP, Bonte FJ, et al. High voltage electric injury: assessment of muscle viability with MR imaging and Tc-99m pyrophosphate scintigraphy. Radiology 1995; 195:205–210.

8. Sayman HB, Urgancioglu I, Uslu I, et al. Prediction of muscle viability after electrical burn necrosis. Burns 1998; 24:649–653.

9. Vedung S, Arturson G, Wadin K, et al. Angiographic findings and need for amputation in high tension electrical injuries. Scand J Plast Reconstr Surg Hand Surg 1990; 24(3):225–231.

10. Brumback RA, Feedback DL, Leech RW. Rhabdomyolysis following electrical injury. Semin Neurol 1995; 15:329–334.

11. Feinfeld DA, Cheng JT, Beysolow TD, et al. A prospective study of urine and serum myoglobin levels in patients with acute rhabdomyolysis. Clin Nephrol 1992; 38:193–195.

12. Grossmann RA, Hamilton RW, Morse BM, et al. Nontraumatic rhabdomyolysis and acute renal failure. N Engl J Med 1974; 291:807–811.

13. Rosen CL, Adler JN, Rabban JT, et al. Early predictors of myoglobinuria and acute renal failure following electrical injury. J Emerg Med 1999; 17:783–789.

14. Cooper MA. Emergent care of lightning and electrical injuries. Semin Neurol 1995; (15):268–278.

15. Bailey B, Gaudreault P, Thivierge RL, et al. Cardiac monitoring of children with household electrical injuries. Ann Emerg Med 1995; 25:612–617.

16. Arrowsmith J, Usgaocar RP, Dickson WA. Electrical injury and the frequency of cardiac complications. Burns 1997; 23:576–578.

17. Fish RM. Electric injury, part III: cardiac monitoring indication, the pregnant patient, and lightning. J Emerg Med 2000; 18:181–187.

18. Purdue GF, Hunt JL. Electrocardiographic monitoring after electrical injury: necessity or luxury. J Trauma 1986; 26:166–167.

19. Cunningham PA. The need for cardiac monitoring after electrical injury. Med J Aust 1991; 154:765–766.

20. Guinard JP, Chiolero R, Buchser E, et al. Myocardial injury after electrical burns: short and long term study. Scand J Plast Reconstr Hand Surg 1987; 21:301–302.

21. Wilson CM, Fatovich DM. Do children need to be monitored after electric shocks? J Paediatr Child Health 1998; 34:474–476.

22. Mann R, Gibran N, Engrav L, et al. Is immediate decompression of high-voltage electrical injuries to the upper extremities always necessary? J Trauma 1996; 40:584–587.

23. Luce EA, Gottlieb SE. 'True' high-tension electrical injuries. Ann Plast Surg 1984; 12:321–325.

24. Garcia C, Smith GA, Cohen DM, et al. Electrical injuries in a pediatric emergency department. Ann Emerg Med 1995; 26:604–608

25. Jaffe RH, Willis D, Bachem A. The effect of electric currents on the arteries. Arch Pathol 1929; 7:244–249.

26. Hussmann J, Zamboni WA, Russell RC, et al. A model for recording the microcirculatory changes associated with standardized electrical injury of skeletal muscle. J Surg Res 1995; 59:725–732.

27. Ponten B, Erikson U, Johansson SH, et al. New observations on tissue changes along the pathway of the current in an electrical injury. Scand J Plast Reconstr Surg 1970; 4:75–82.

28. Zhi-Xiang Z, Yuan-Tie Z, Xu-Yuan L, et al. Urgent repair of electrical injuries: analysis of 40 cases. Acta Chir Plast 1990; 32:142–151.

29. Chick LR, Lister GD, Sowder L. Early free-flap coverage of electrical and thermal burns. Plast Reconstr Surg 1992; 89:1013–1019.

30. Yang JY, Noordhoff MS. Early adipofascial flap coverage of deep electrical burn wounds of upper extremities. Plast Reconstr Surg 1993; 91:819–825.

31. Godina M, Bajec J, Baraga A. Salvage of the mutilated upper extremity with temporary ectopic implantation of the undamaged part. Plast Reconstr Surg 1986; 78:295–299.

32. Engrav LH, Gottlieb JR, Walkinshaw MD, et al. Outcome and treatment of electrical injury with immediate median and ulnar nerve palsy at the wrist: a retrospective review and a survey of members of the American Burn Association. Ann Plast Surg 1990; 25:166–168.

33. Sheridan RL, Choucair RJ, Donclean MB. Management of massive calvarial exposure in young children. J Burn Care Rehabil 1998; 19:29–32.

34. Luce EA, Hoopes JE. Electrical burns of the scalp and the skull. Plast Reconstr Surg 1974; 54:359.

35. Bizhkol P, Slesarenko SV. Operative treatment of deep burns of the scalp and skull. Burns 1992; 18:220–223.

36. Miyamoto Y, Harada K, Kodama Y, et al. Cranial coverage involving scalp, bone and dura using free inferior epigastric flap. Br J Plast Surg 1986; 39:483–490.

37. Barret JP, Dziewulski P, McCauley RL, et al. Dural reconstruction of a class IV calvarial burn with decellularized human dermis. Burns 1999; 25:459–462.

38. Zarem HA, Greer DM. Tongue flap for reconstruction of the lip after electrical burns. Plast Reconstr Surg 1974; 53:310.

39. DeLaPlaza R, Quetgals A, Rodriguez E. Treatment of electrical burns of the mouth. Burns 1983; 10:49.

40. Hartford CD, Kealy GP, Lavelle WE, et al. An appliance to prevent and treat microstomia from burns. J Trauma 1975; 15:356.

41. Ortiz-Monasterio F, Factor R. Early definitive treatment of electric burns of the mouth. Plast Reconstr Surg 1980; 65:169.

42. Pensler JM, Rosenthal A. Reconstruction of the oral commissure after an electrical burn. J Burn Care Rehabil 1990; 11:50–53.

43. Leake JE, Curtin JW. Electrical burns of the mouth in children. Clin Plast Surg 1984; 11:669.

44. Dado DV, Polley W, Kernahan DA. Splinting of oral commissure electrical burns in children. J Pediatr 1985; 107:92.

45. Silverglade D, Ruberg RL. Nonsurgical management of burns to the lips and commissures. Clin Plast Surg 1986; 13:87.

46. Luce EA, Dowden WL, Su CT, et al. High tension electrical injury of the upper extremity. Surg Gynecol Obstet 1978; 147:38.

47. Gellman H, Nichols D. Reflex sympathetic dystrophy in the upper extremity. J Am Acad Orthop Surg 1997; 5:313–322.

48. Still JM, Law EJ, Duncan W, et al. Long thoracic nerve injury due to an electric burn. J Burn Care Rehabil 1996; 17:562–564.

49. Haberal MA, Gürer S, Akman N, et al. Persistent peripheral nerve pathologies in patients with electric burns. J Burn Care Rehabil 1996; 17:147–149.

50. Agnew WF, McCreery DB, Yuen TG, et al. Local anaesthetic block protects against electrically induced damage in peripheral nerve. J Biomed Eng 1990; 12:301–308.

51. Abramov GS, Bier M, Capelli-Schellpfeffer M, et al. Alteration in sensory nerve function following electrical shock. Burns 1996; 22:602–606.

52. Gaylor DC, Prakah-Asante K, Lee RC. Significance of cell size and tissue structure in electrical trauma. J Theoret Biol 1988; 133:223–237.

53. Grube BJ, Heimbach DM, Engrav LH, et al. Neurologic consequences of electrical burns. J Trauma 1990; 30:254–257.

54. Koller J, Orsagh J. Delayed neurological sequelae of high tension electrical burns. Burns 1989; 15:175–178.

55. Varghese G, Mani H, Redford SH. Spinal cord injuries following electric accident. Paraplegia 1986; 24:159–162.

56. Levine NS, Atkins A, McKeel DW, et al. Spinal cord injury following electrical accidents: case reports. J Trauma 1975; 15:459–463.

57. Breugem CC, van Hertum W, Groenevelt F. High voltage electrical injury leading to a delayed onset tetraplegia, with recovery. Ann N Y Acad Sci 1999; 888:131–136.

58. Janus TJ, Barrash J. Neurologic and neurobehavioural effects of electric and lightning injuries. J Burn Care Rehabil 1996; 17:409–415.

59. Pliskin NH, Capelli-Schellpfeffer M, Law RT, et al. Neuropsychological symptom presentation after electrical injury. J Trauma 1998; 44:709–715.

60. Tkachenko TA, Kelley KM, Pliskin NH, et al. Electrical injury through the eyes of professional electricians. Ann N Y Acad Sci 1999; 888:42–59.

61. Pliskin NH, Fink J, Malina A, et al. The neuropsychological effects of electrical injury. Ann N Y Acad Sci 1999; 888:140–149.

62. Boozalis GT, Purdue GF, Hunt JL, et al. Ocular changes from electrical burn injuries: a literature review and report of cases. J Burn Care Rehabil 1991; 12:458–462.

63. Solem L, Fisher R, Strate R. The natural history of electrical injury. J Trauma 1977; 17:487–492.

64. Saffle JR, Crandall A, Warden GD. Cataracts: a long-term complication of electrical injury. J Trauma 1985; 25:17.

65. Dumas JL, Walker N. Bilateral scapular fractures secondary to electrical shock. Arch Orthop Trauma Surg 1992; 111:287–288.

66. Adams AJ, Beckett MW. Bilateral wrist fractures from accidental electric shock. Injury 1997; 28:227–228.

67. Tompkins GS, Henderson RC, Peterson HD. Bilateral simultaneous fractures of the femoral neck: case report. J Trauma 1990; 30:1415–1416.

68. van den Brink WA, van Leeuwen O. Lumbar burst fracture due to low voltage shock. A case report. Acta Orthop Scand 1995; 66:374–375.

69. Helm PA, Walker SC. New bone formation at amputation in electrically burn-injured patients. Arch Phys Med Rehabil 1987; 68:284–286.

Chapter 41

Cold-induced injury: frostbite

Stephen E. Morris

Chapter contents

Frostbite is a traumatic injury that is caused by the failure of the normal protective mechanisms against the thermal environment that classically results in localized tissue temperatures falling below freezing, although cold-induced injury can result from non-freezing environmental insults. Cold-induced injury continues to be a relatively frequent injury in the United States due to increasing interest in out-of-door winter recreational activities as well as the high prevalence of homeless and socioeconomically disadvantaged individuals in large urban centers.[1,2]

One of the earliest cases of frostbite has been found in a pre-Columbian Chilean mummy from about 3000 BC.[3] Much knowledge about the incidence and circumstances surrounding this injury has been derived from the extensive military experiences of the past.[4] Hannibal lost nearly half of his army of 46 000 soldiers during a 2-week crossing of the Pyrenean Alps due to frostbite injury. During the Revolutionary War, it is recorded in 1778 that Washington lost 10% of his army to cold-related casualties during a single winter.[5]

The first modern published report of cold-induced injury did not occur until 1805,[6] and Baron Larrey produced the first systematic medical observations of frostbite during the Russian campaign of 1812–1813.[7] As Surgeon General of Napoleon's forces in Russia, Dominique Larrey was able to produce classic descriptions of frostbite and trench foot, and to identify the severe effects of refreezing that occurred with bonfire thawing and subsequent marching in frigid conditions. With this information, Larrey made therapeutic recommendations that were adhered to for more than 150 years of military medicine. This included the use of friction massage with snow or ice rather than rapid thawing over an open fire as he had seen more severe injuries subjected to such freezethaw-freeze conditions. He also noted that the number of cold-induced injuries was much greater during periods of wet, near-freezing conditions as opposed to similar periods when conditions were dry, but below freezing. He described the loss of all but 360 troops

due to cold in a division of 12 000 men. Larrey reported essentially the total loss of one-quarter million troops within a 6-month period due to cold and starvation. Over the past century, military medical experience has only been somewhat better. It is estimated that World Wars I and II and the Korean conflict included one million frostbite injuries. The United States Army reported 90 000 cold injuries during World War II. German troops underwent 15 000 amputations during the winter of 1942,[8] and Greek troops 25 000 amputations due to frostbite alone during the course of the war.[9] High-altitude bomber crews suffered from frostbite more than any other injury.[10] Modern military cold-induced injury data continue to accrue.[11–16] Interestingly, the Vietnam War and other military conflicts fought in tropical climates produced substantial non-freezing cold injuries in soldiers exposed to wet environments in the temperature range of 35–40°F (1.6–4.4°C).[10,17,18] Although there has been little epidemiological data in the civilian population, significant numbers have accumulated in relatively few series.[19,20] This significant body of military and emerging civilian data stimulated first basic laboratory investigations, starting with Merryman[21–23] and, subsequently, clinical research that has taken us from the empiric recommendations of Larrey to the rapid rewarming[24] recommendations of Mills[25,26] and others.[27] Such efforts have paved the way to more systematic investigation and eventually to refinement of patient care practices.

Physiology of temperature regulation

In the human, temperature regulation is achieved through a complex interaction of heat production, loss, and conservation mechanisms that require both autonomic and voluntary functions. Normal body temperature ranges from 36.2 to 37.7°C. Any impairment of autonomic or voluntary behavioral functions may result in dysregulation of thermal homeostasis. Control of thermal homeostasis resides in the central nervous system. Core blood cooling will result in hypothalamic–pituitary axis stimulation of catecholamine release, peripheral vasoconstriction, and inhibition of sweating to conserve heat as well as thyroid hormone release with upregulation of oxidative metabolism and shivering for an increase in heat production. Core temperature, which may be measured by rectal thermometer, is generally expected to be 0.5°C higher than surface temperatures, which may be measured orally or tympanically. Peripheral extremity skin temperature is expected to fluctuate much more widely. In a warm environment, temperature of the distal extremities may substantially exceed core temperature, while the reverse may be true in the heat conservation mode in a cold environment.[28] Acral blood flow may vary from 0.5 to 100 mL/min/100 g of tissue.[29] When blood flow falls below this range, eventual tissue necrosis may occur. With environmental conditioning the maximal blood flow may exceed 100–122 mL/min/100 g of tissue. Such range in peripheral blood flow response affords the core body temperature substantial thermal homeostasis at a relatively cheap metabolic price, but the cost is at the expense of the extremities. The primary function of this response is to maintain core blood temperature. Sir Thomas Lewis described a vasomotor response in cold environments and termed it the 'hunting reaction'.[30–33] In this response, vasoconstriction alternates with vasodilation in 5–10-minute cycles. The cycling is somewhat irregular and results in non-uniform changes in peripheral temperature, but this cycling both conserves core heat and allows extremity viability. The hunting reaction is more pronounced in people indigenous to colder climates. There appears to be maintenance of higher extremity temperature with more rapid cycling and rewarming.[31] Voluntary behaviors may be important in protection of extremities from cold injury and, as such, mental status impairment can constitute a substantial risk for frostbite in the cold environment.[34] Consequently, alcohol and drug intoxication have been roundly implicated among the risk factors for cold-induced injury.[35–39]

Pathophysiology of cold-induced injury

A number of factors have been associated with the development of frostbite. One well-recognized factor is that of ethanol consumption. Valnicek et al. reviewed their 12-year experience in Saskatchewan with patients admitted for frostbite and identified ethanol use in 46%, psychiatric disorders in 17%, vehicular trauma in 19%, vehicular failure in 15%, and drug abuse in 4% of patients.[38] Overt or covert manifestation of psychiatric disease[39] as well as neurovascular factors such as smoking and diabetes mellitus, homelessness, fatigue, improper clothing, previous cold weather injury, high altitude, extremes of age, and male gender,[19,40] have all been cited in cold injury. A number of physical factors appear to play a role in the development of frostbite. The duration and efficiency of tissue cooling understandably have a marked effect on the extent of cold injury. Moist or wet skin is substantially more susceptible to frostbite than dry skin.[41] Efficiency of thermal conduction is important as evidenced by the effectiveness of metal contact as opposed to fabric or wood contact. Windchill is a principle of physiological importance that was demonstrated by Paul Siple who was well-known for his physiological observations with the Antarctic Byrd expeditions.[42] He developed formulas, taking into account the effects of temperature and wind speed on tissue cooling, that are a basis for the wind chill charts published by the US Air Force. Thus, exposed skin may suffer similar injuries exposed to air at 0°F in calm conditions or to a 15 mile-per-hour breeze at 25°F.[26] Although high-altitude conditions have been associated with cold injury, there has been no independent risk factor associated with this environment.[41] The physical state of skin can have an effect on the development of cold injury. Water in the stratum corneum can predispose to water crystallization in the skin and deeper tissue.[43] This may explain recommendations of using oil or ointment on exposed skin at risk for frostbite and the practice of polar explorers to avoid washing during expeditions. The nature of clothing also plays a significant role. Mills[25] documented the association of ill-fitting boots and the development of frostbite. Similarly, some authors have touted the relationship of snug-fitting or damp clothing and cold-induced injury, reporting the effect of clothing on circulation or the thermal conduction of moisture compared to dry air by a factor of 25.[44] Cigarette smoking is cited as a cause of local circulatory compromise. This has been demonstrated with smoking nude models as well as random skin flaps.[45,46] Chronic smoking does not appear to have an effect on cold-induced injury. Lastly, a history of previous cold injury places the patient at substantial risk for frostbite:[47,48] not only the incidence of injury but also the extent may be increased with previous exposure.[44] There is no real evidence of tolerance or indigenous adaptation to the cold environment that is intrinsically protective against frostbite.[16,49]

The injury associated with frostbite is attributed to two broad mechanistic categories: the first is that of direct cellular damage and death due to the cold insult, and the second is the more delayed process mediated by progressive tissue ischemia.[50–56] The immediate effects of frostbite are evidenced by formation of extracellular ice crystals. These crystals cause direct injury to the cell membrane, resulting in cellular dehydration due to a change in the osmotic gradient.[22,57] The rate of cooling is reported to have an effect on the development of extracellular or intracellular ice crystals.[58] Rapid cooling results in intracellular freezing, which causes more severe cellular damage and cell death, while a slower rate of cooling produces extracellular ice crystals. This slower process, nevertheless, results in transmembrane osmotic shift that drives water from within the cell and produces intracellular dehydration. This dehydration causes changes in protein[59,60] and lipid conformation, as well as changes in pH and other biochemical processes such as electrolyte concentration that are deleterious to intracellular homeostasis.[61–64] As temperature continues to fall, intracellular crystals develop regardless of cooling rate[20,65] with a loss of the linear relationship of temperature to metabolism,[31,66] decreased DNA synthesis[67] and the vascular response that has been called the 'triple response of Lewis', which is characterized by localized reddening of the wheal and may indicate release of histamine from injured cells.[68]

Microvascular pathophysiology may be even more important in outcome than the direct thermal injury to the cell. This was suggested by studies showing survival of full-thickness skin subjected to freezing and thawing that progressed to necrosis when left in situ but survived when transplanted to a normal, uninjured recipient site.[50] Zacarian identified a number of processes that may play a role in the microcirculatory changes of frostbite. There appears to be a transient vasoconstriction of both arterioles and venules with subsequent resumption of capillary blood flow. Concomitantly there have been microemboli observed.[65] With thawing, the capillaries demonstrate restoration of blood flow, but this diminished within minutes. Complete cessation of blood flow is often seen within 20 minutes after rewarming of frozen tissue. Such similar changes have been seen with random skin flap models after reperfusion which has suggested reactive oxygen species as mediators of injury.[69] Within 72 hours there is a significant de-epithelialization in the capillary bed and deposition of fibrin. Examination of the endothelial ultrastructure has shown swelling, fluid extravasation, vascular endothelial cell dilation and significant projection of the cell into the vascular lumen prior to cell lysis.[70] There is regional variation in the extent of injury with venules being most profoundly affected,[71] with the hypothesis that, as evidenced by lower flow, stasis must play a role in this pathophysiological process.

Pathobiochemistry of frostbite has been closely compared to the inflammatory response in the burn wound.[27,72] Inflammatory mediators such as eicosanoids in burns,[73–76] in burn blister fluid,[77,78] as well as bradykinin[79] and histamine[80] draw parallels with findings in cold-induced injury. This has prompted investigators to hypothesize a model similar to that of Jackson including zones of necrosis and stasis.[81] Similar to their burn blister analysis, Robson and Heggers examined the fluid in frostbite blisters and found high levels of prostaglandin F_2 and thromboxane B_2. These agents or their precursors have been implicated in vasoconstriction and leukocyte adherence.[72] The inhibition of these eicosanoids has had a salubrious effect in animal models.[82,83] Clinical efficacy has been suggested by the use of thromboxane inhibition.[20] It appears that this process is significantly different than the previously proposed mechanism of vasospasm, thrombosis, and fibrin deposition.[2] Much about this mechanism has yet to be elucidated, including the nature of microemboli that have been observed.[84]

Signs and symptoms of frostbite injury

Most frequently, the patient is basically unaware that frostbite injury is occurring. The association of hypothermia and the use of substances known to alter mental status may contribute to this problem. Typical distribution in 90% of patients is acral, with others suffering injuries to ears, nose, cheeks and penis.[13,19,38,40] The patient may note insensitivity and clumsiness of the affected part. This complex of symptoms rapidly reverses upon rewarming. Insensitivity is rapidly replaced by severe pain during and immediately after the rewarming process. The pain is often described as throbbing in character, sometimes requiring parenteral opioids for relief. Pain symptoms increase for the first few days and gradually abate during the following 3 weeks. Assessment of injury must be deferred until rewarming of the affected part is complete.

A condition often termed 'frostnip' may be present in which there is not true tissue injury; the condition may be manifested by numbness and pallor of exposed skin. This will often affect skiers and others exposed to cold winds for brief periods of time. Rewarming results in near-complete resolution of symptoms and physical findings, with the possible exception of some hyperemia, edema, and tingling in the region. The nonfreezing manifestation of mild cold injury is often termed chilblains, pernio, kibes or cold urticaria. These are often chronic in nature with itching and erythema as more prominent findings. True frostbite, on the other hand, always involves some degree of tissue injury. Classification of severity of cold injury can be helpful in planning medical management. It must be emphasized that clinical appearance will evolve over a period of time after rewarming. Even after rewarming, the initial appearance is often deceptive.[11,19] Most injuries appear hyperemic after rewarming regardless of the degree of involvement. The development of skin blebs is a time-dependent process that often requires many hours to days. Sensation returns during this period, which is often replaced by bothersome tingling and pain. This may develop into severe neuropathic pain that can be aggravated by warm environments and dependent position of the injured member. After 12–24 hours the character of the blebs becomes apparent and an assessment of the degree of involvement may be helpful in planning management of the injury. Traditional classification is similar to that of the burn injury. First-degree injury is superficial without formation of vesicles or blebs. There may initially be an area of pallor with surrounding erythema that evolves into general edema and erythema without long-term sequelae. Second-degree injury has associated light-colored blisters and subsequent peeling. This often correlates with dermal involvement but has a generally favorable prognosis. Third-degree frostbite typically has dark or hemorrhagic blisters that evolve into thick, black eschar over 1–2 weeks. Fourth-degree injury involves bone, tendon or muscle and will result in definite tissue loss. Exactness in depth of injury cannot be expected and some favor more general classification of superficial (first- and second-degree injury) or deep (third- and fourth-degree) frostbite injury. Poor prognostic findings include hemorrhagic blisters and a woody or nondeforming tissue consistency. Preservation of pinprick sensation and light-colored and large blebs predict less risk of tissue loss. Long-term symptoms include hypersensitivity to cold, sensory deficits, chronic pain, and hyperhidrosis.[1] Growth abnormalities and heterotopic calcification have also been described as long-term complications of frostbite.[33,85]

Diagnostic methods and management

The time-dependent evolution of the clinical manifestations of frostbite and the inability to assess tissue involvement deep to the skin are significant limitations in the prompt management of this injury. A number of imaging methods have been explored in an attempt to decrease the duration of disability and the length of stay in hospitals. Plain radiographs can demonstrate soft-tissue swelling or, as time progresses, tissue loss, bone demineralization or periosteal inflammation. Arteriography has constituted the traditional method for assessment of distal perfusion, but its usefulness is limited by the same factors as clinical assessment in the early phases of injury.[2] The usefulness of laser Doppler flowmetry in frostbite injury is presently unknown. Radioisotope scintigraphy has emerged as an early diagnostic modality.[86–89] Magnetic resonance imaging is now being proposed as a method to evaluate even individual vessel status and as a means to identify a line of demarcation earlier in the clinical course.[90]

Only a few general principles of frostbite care are generally accepted. Larrey's methods of rubbing the affected area with snow or with vigorous massage have only recently fallen out of usage in the main medical community. Mills and others at the Arctic Aeromedical Laboratory have documented the results of thawing and refreezing with the resultant worsening of outcome.[48] Thus it is recommended that partial or slow rewarming during transport should be avoided. Rapid rewarming means warming at the temperature of 40°C with a protocol such as that based upon the work of McCauley et al.[27]

Frostbite care protocol

- Admit frostbite patient to a specialized treatment unit.
- Transfer of acute frostbite patient should be avoided unless necessary for specialized care with great care to protect patient from further cold exposure.
- Immediate rapid rewarming should be performed at a temperature of 40–42°C for 15–30 minutes or until rewarming is complete.

After complete rewarming:

- White blisters are debrided and topical treatment with *Aloe vera* (Dermaide aloe) q6h is initiated.
- Hemorrhagic blisters are left intact.
- Injured parts are elevated and splinted as required.
- Tetanus prophylaxis is followed.
- Appropriate analgesia is administered.
- Ibuprofen 400 mg PO q12h is administered.
- Antibiotic prophylaxis is administered as appropriate.
- Hydrotherapy or gentle wound care is provided daily.
- Photodocumentation is essential upon admission, at 24 hours, and at every 2–3 days during hospitalization.
- Outpatient care must be tailored to patient situation to maintain adequate wound care and appropriate medical follow-up.

A number of adjunctive therapeutic modalities have been suggested with some experimental rationale, but there is minimal clinical evidence in support of the therapies. Sympathectomy has been examined with mixed results.[91,92] The series by Taylor is of interest with favorable outcomes in a small number of patients. Although suggestive of more rapid resolution of edema and possibly decreased tissue loss, there is no randomized controlled study to answer this question. As is suggested by basic science investigation, the use of anticoagulation does not appear to have any clinical application in frostbite.[49]

Dextran has been thought to have some theoretical utility because of the appearance of microemboli in this disease process. These have been poorly characterized, but basic animal experiments have demonstrated some decrease in tissue loss with the administration of dextrans.[50] Again, this has not been examined in a rigorous fashion clinically.

Vasodilators have been used widely in the past. Intra-arterial reserpine has been used successfully for vasospasm but there are no clinical data to recommend its use for frostbite at the present time. Other efforts to improve tissue oxygenation such as hyperbaric oxygen have likewise been inconclusive and no substantial clinical or laboratory investigation has been produced recently.

In the past decade, the use of thrombolytic agents has been examined in a collected series of patients[93] as well as in an animal model.[94] A multicenter trial will be necessary to measure the effects in a controlled fashion.

Surgical intervention is often required with frostbite injury, but as the adage has been often repeated, 'Frostbite in January, amputate in July',[95] a conservative approach is needed in the present management scheme. Mills described the need for early escharotomy or fasciotomy in certain individuals, but this is indeed rare.[26] He likewise suggested that skin grafting after development of healthy granulation tissue may decrease the amount of postfrostbite pain. Meticulous debridement and gentle but thorough wound care is important in the maintenance of the frostbitten part which is an effort to allow complete demarcation prior to amputation. This is not always possible and surgical intervention may be needed for control of infection as well as wound closure after clinical wound demarcation or as guided by technetium scintigraphy. The need for improved treatment of frostbite has become widespread, with this disease being seen more frequently in the general population over the past few decades. There has been some fascinating progress in the understanding of this injury process, but clinical investigations are presently lacking in most aspects of care for the frostbite injury. Biochemical intervention and improved imaging methods can help to speed the recovery and enhance the ultimate functionality of these patients.

References

1. Edlich R, Chang D, Birk K, et al. Cold injuries. Compr Ther 1989; 15:13–21.
2. Purdue G, Hunt J. Cold injury: a collective review. J Burn Care Rehabil 1986; 7:331–342.
3. Post PW, Donner DD. Frostbite in a pre-Columbian mummy. Am J Phys Anthropol 1972; 37:187–191.
4. Schechter D, Sarot L. Historical accounts of injuries due to cold. Surgery 1968; 63:527–535.
5. Smith D, Robson M, Heggers J. Frostbite and other cold-induced injuries. In: Puerbach P, Geehr E, eds. Management of wilderness and environmental emergencies. St Louis: CV Mosby; 1989:101–118.
6. Zingg W. The management of accidental hypothermia. Can Med Assoc J 1967; 96:214.
7. Larrey D. Memoirs of military surgery. Baltimore: Joseph Cushing, 1814; (5):156–164.
8. Vaughn P. Local cold injury — menace to military operations. A review. Military Med 1980; 145:305.
9. Katsas A, Agnantis J, Smyrnis S. Carcinoma on old frostbites. Am J Surg 1977; 133:377–378.
10. Dembert M, Dean L, Noddin E. Cold weather morbidity among US Navy and Marine Corps personnel. Military Med 1981; 146:771–775.
11. Orr K, Fainer D. Cold injuries in Korea during the winter of 1950–1951. Medicine 1952; 31:177–184.
12. Taylor M, Kulungowski M, Hamelink J. Frostbite injuries during winter maneuvers: a long-term disability. Military Med 1989; 154:411–413.
13. Lehmuskallio E, Lindholm H, Koskenvuo K, et al. Frostbite of the face and ears: epidemiological study of risk factors in Finnish conscripts. Br Med J 1995; 311:1661–1663.
14. Marsh A. A short but distant war: the Falklands campaign. J R Soc Med 1983; 76:972–982.
15. Groom A, Coull J. Army amputees from the Falklands: review. J R Army Med Corps 1984; 130:114–116.
16. Candler WH, Ivey H. Cold weather injuries among US soldier in Alaska: a five-year review. Military Med 1997; 162:788–791.
17. Allen A. Tropical immersion foot. Lancet 1983; 1:1185–1189.
18. Hanifin J, Cuetter A. In patients with immersion type of cold injury diminished nerve conduction velocity. Electromyogr Clin Neurophysiol 1974; 14:173–178.
19. Boswick J, Thompson J, Jonas R. The epidemiology of cold injuries. Surg Gynecol Obstet 1979; 149:326.
20. Heggers J, Robson M, Manavalen K. Experimental and clinical observations on frostbite. Ann Emerg Med 1987; 16:1056.

21. Kulka J. Histopathologic studies in frostbitten rabbits. In: Ferrer M, ed. Cold injury. New York: Josiah Macy Jr. Foundation, 1956:94–151.

22. Merryman H. Mechanics of freezing in living cells and tissue. Science 1956; 124:515–521.

23. Merryman H. Tissue freezing and local cold injury. Physiol Rev 1957; 37:233–251.

24. Mills W, Whaley R, Fish W. Frostbite: experience with rapid rewarming and ultrasonic therapy. Alaska Med 1961; 3:28.

25. Mills W. Out in the cold. Emerg Med 1976; 18:134.

26. Mills W. Summary of treatment of the cold injured patient. Frostbite. Alaska Med 1983; 35:61–66.

27. McCauley R, Hing D, Robson M. Frostbite injuries: a rational approach based on the pathophysiology. J Trauma 1983; 23:143–147.

28. Holm P, Vanggard L. Frostbite. Plast Reconstr Surg 1974; 54:544–551.

29. Barton A. Physiology of cutaneous circulation, thermoregulatory functions. In: Rothman S, ed. The human integument. Washington, DC: American Association for the Advancement of Science, 1959.

30. Lewis T. Observations upon the reactions of the vessels of the human skin to cold. Heart 1930; 15:177–208.

31. Dana A, Rex I, Samitz M. The hunting reflex. Arch Dermatol 1969; 99:441–450.

32. Adams T, Smith R. Effect of chronic local cold exposure on finger temperature responses. J Appl Physiol 1962; 17:317–322.

33. Britt L, Dascombe W, Rodriguez A. New horizons in management of hypothermia and frostbite injury. Surg Clin N Am 1991; 71:345–370.

34. Cold hypersensitivity [editorial]. Br Med J 1975; 1:643–644.

35. Hashmi M, Rashid M, Haleem A, et al. Frostbite: epidemiology at high altitude in the Karakoram mountains. Ann R Coll Surg Engl 1998; 80:91–95.

36. Kyosola K. Clinical experiences in the management of cold injuries: a study of 110 cases. J Trauma 1974; 14:32–36.

37. Urschel J. Frostbite. Predisposing factors and predictors of poor outcome. J Trauma 1990; 30:340–342.

38. Valnicek S, Chasmir L, Clapson J. Frostbite in the prairies: a 12-year review. Plast Reconstr Surg 1993; 92:633–641.

39. Pinzur M, Weaver F. Is urban frostbite a psychiatric disorder? Orthopedics 1997; 20:43–45.

40. Hermann G, Schecter D, Owens J. The problem of frostbite in civilian medical practice. Clin North Am 1963; 43:519–536.

41. Washburn B. Frostbite — what it is — how to prevent it — emergency treatment. N Engl J Med 1962; 266:974–989.

42. Siple PA, Passel CF. Measurements of dry atmospheric cooling in sub-freezing temperatures. Proc Am Phil Soc 1945; 89:177–199.

43. Lewis T. Observations on some normal and injurious effects of cold upon the skin and underlying tissues: III. Frostbite. Br Med J 1941; 2:869.

44. Knize D. Cold injury in reconstructive plastic surgery. In: Conversen J, McCarthy J, Littler J, eds. General principles. Philadelphia: WB Saunders, 1977:(1)516–530.

45. Lawrence WT, Murphy RC, Robson MC. The detrimental effect of cigarette smoking on flap survival: an experimental study on the rat. Br J Plast Surg 1984; 87:216.

46. Reus WF, Robson MC, Zachary L. Acute effects of tobacco smoking on blood flow in the cutaneous micro-circulation. Br J Plast Surg 1984; 37:213.

47. Whayne TJ, DeBakey MF. Cold injury, ground type. Washington, DC: US Government; 1958.

48. Mills WJ, Whaley R. Frostbite: a method of management. Proceedings of the symposium on Arctic biology and medicine: IV, frostbite. Fort Wainwright, Alaska: Arctic Aeromedical Laboratory; 1964.

49. McCauley RL, Smith DJ, Robson MC, et al. Frostbite and other cold-induced injuries. In: Auerback PS, ed. Wilderness medicine. St Louis: Mosby; 1995:129–145.

50. Weatherly-White R, Sjostrom B, Paton B. Experimental studies in cold injury II: the pathogenesis of frostbite. J Surg Res 1964; 4:17–22.

51. Weatherly-White R, Paton B, Sjostrom B. Experimental studies in cold injury III: observations on the treatment of frostbite. Plast Reconstr Surg 1965; 36:10–18.

52. Quintanilla R, Krusen F, Essex H. Studies on frostbite with special reference to treatment and effect on minute blood vessels. Am J Physiol 1947; 149:149–161.

53. Eubanks R. Heat and cold injuries. J Arkansas Med Soc 1974; 71:53–58.

54. Furhman F, Crismon J. Studies on gangrene following cold injury, II. General course of events in rabbit feet and ears following untreated cold injury. J Clin Invest 1947; 47:236–244.

55. Rasmussen D, Zook E. Frostbite: a review of pathophysiology and newest treatments. J Indiana State Med Assoc 1972; 65:1237–1241.

56. Welch G. Frostbite. Practitioner 1974; 213:801–804.

57. Moran T. Critical temperature of freezing living muscle. Proc R Soc B 1929; 105:107.

58. Merryman HT. The exceeding of a minimum tolerable cell volume in hypertonic suspension as a cause of freezing injury. In: Walstenholme G, O'Conner M, eds. The Frozen cell. London: Churchill; 1970:51.

59. Shikama K, Yamazaki I. Denaturation of catalase by freezing and thawing. Nature 1961; 190.

60. Marhert C. Lactate dehydrogenase isozymes: dissociation and recombination of subunits. Science 1963; 140:1629.

61. Lovelock JE. Physical instability in thermal shock in red blood cells. Nature 1954; 173:659.

62. Lovelock JE. The denaturation of lipid–protein complexes as a cause of damage by freezing. Proc R Soc Biol 1957; 147:427.

63. Mazur P. Studies in rapidly frozen suspension of yeast cells by differential thermal analysis and conductometry. Biophys J 1963; 3:323.

64. Mazur P. Causes of injury in frozen and thawed cells. Fed Proc 1965; 24(Suppl 14–15):5.

65. Zacarian SA. Cryogenics: the cryolesion and the pathogenesis of cryonecrosis. In: Stone D, Clater H, eds. Cryosurgery for skin and cutaneous disorders. St Louis: CV Mosby; 1985:(7)27.

66. Vanggaard L. Arteriovenous anastomoses in temperature regulation. Acta Physiol Scand 1969; 76:13A.

67. Johnson BE, Daniels F Jr. Enzyme studies in experimental cryosurgery of the skin. Cryobiology 1974; 11:22.

68. Lewis T. The blood vessels of the human skin and their responses. London: Shaw; 1927:147–150.

69. Bulkley GB. The role of oxygen free radicals in human disease processes. Surgery 1983; 94:407.

70. Rabb JM, Renaud ML, Brandt PA. Effect of freezing and thawing on the microcirculation and capillary endothelium of the hamster cheek pouch. Cryobiology 197; 11:508.

71. Zacarian SA, Stone D, Clater H. Effects of cryogenic temperatures on the microcirculation in the golden hamster cheek pouch. Cryobiology 1970; 7:27–39.

72. Robson MC, Heggers JP. Evaluation of hand frostbite blister fluid as a clue to pathogenesis. J Hand Surg [Am] 1981; 6:43–47.

73. Nakae H, Endo S, Inada K. Plasma concentrations of type II phospholipase A_2, cytokines and eicosanoids in patients with burns. Burns 1995; 21:422–426.

74. Huribal M. Endothelin-1 and prostaglandin E_2 levels increase in patients with burns. J Am Coll Surg 1995; 180:318–322.

75. Harms BA, Bodai BI, Smith M, et al. Prostaglandin release and altered microvascular integrity after burn injury. J Surg Res 1981; 31:274–280.

76. Robson MC, Del Beccaro EJ, Heggers JP. The effect of prostaglandins on the dermal microcirculation after burning, and the inhibition of the effect by specific pharmacological agents. Plast Reconstr Surg 1979; 63:781–787.

77. Heggers JP, Ko F, Robson MC, et al. Evaluation of burn blister fluid. Plast Reconstr Surg 1980; 65:798–804.

78. Heggers JP, Loy GL, Robson MC, et al. Histological demonstration of prostaglandins and thromboxanes in burned tissue. J Surg Res 1980; 28:110–117.

79. Back N, Jainchill J, Wilkens HJ, Ambrus JL. Effect of inhibitors of plasmin, kallikrein and kinin on mortality from scalding in mice. Med Pharmacol Exp Int J Exp Med 1966; 15:597–602.

80. Tanaka H, Wada T, Simazaki S. Effects of cimetidine on fluid requirement during resuscitation of third-degree burns. J Burn Care Rehabil 1991; 12:425–429.

81. Jackson DM. The diagnosis of the depth of burning. Br J Surg 1953; 40:588–596.

82. Raine TJ, London MD, Goluch L. Antiprostaglandins and antithromboxanes for treatment of frostbite. Surg Forum 1980; 31:557.

83. Bourne MH, Piepcorn MW, Clayton F. Analysis of microvascular changes in frostbite injury. J Surg Res 1986; 40:26.

84. Zook N, Hussmann J, Brown R. Microcirculatory studies of frostbite injury. Ann Plast Surg 1998; 40:246–253.

85. Reed MH. Growth disturbances in the hands following thermal injuries in children, II. frostbite. Can Assoc Radiol J 1988; 39:95–99.

86. Cauchy E, Chetaille E, Lefevre M, et al. The role of bone scanning in severe frostbite of the extremities: a retrospective study of 88 cases. Eur J Nucl Med 2000; 27:497–502.

87. Greenwald D, Cooper B, Gottlieb L. An algorithm for early aggressive treatment of frostbite with limb salvage directed by triple-phase scanning. Plast Reconstr Surg 1998; 102:1069–1074.

88. Kenney A III, Vyas P. Frostbite injury: appearance on three-phase bone scan. Clin Nucl Med 1998; 23:188.

89. Sarikaya I, Aygit AC, Candan L, et al. Assessment of tissue viability after frostbite injury by technetium-99m-sestamibi scintigraphy in an experimental rabbit model. Eur J Nucl Med 2000; 27:41–45.

90. Barker JR, Haws MJ, Brown RE, et al. Magnetic resonance imaging of severe frostbite. Ann Plast Surg 1997; 38:275–279.

91. Taylor MS. Lumbar epidural sympathectomy for frostbite injuries of the feet. Mil Med 1999; 164:566–567.

92. Boumand DL, Morrison S, Lucas CE. Early sympathetic blockade for frostbite: is it of value? J Surg Res 1980; 20:744–747.

93. Salimi Z, Wolverson MK, Herbold DR, et al. Treatment of frostbite with streptokinase: an experimental study in rabbits. AJR Am J Roentgenol 1987; 149:773–776.

94. Skolnick AA. Early data suggest clot-dissolving drugs may help save frostbitten limbs from amputation. JAMA 1992; 267:2008–2010.

95. Erikson U, Ponten B. The possible value of arteriography supplemented by a vasodilator agent in the early assessment of tissue viability in frostbite. Injury 1974; 6:150–153.

Chemical burns

Arthur P. Sanford

Introduction

We live in an increasingly dependent world on chemical agents. Our cars are powered by petroleum distillates in the combustion chambers of the engine and chemical reactions in the batteries, our gardens are fertilized by specially enriched products, and our houses are kept clean by powerful agents to dissolve and remove. This makes chemical burns more commonplace in the household, yet industrial applications to provide these chemicals are also expanding. Whenever the news of an armed conflict with a country not armed with nuclear weapons is broadcast, the possibility of chemical weapons is included. The variety of chemical exposures is so vast, that a short chapter cannot describe all of the agents and their treatments, but this chapter can provide general principles for the treatment of chemical injuries (Figures 42.1 and 42.2). The importance of understanding these principles is underscored by the fact that while only 3% of all burns are due to chemical exposures, approximately 30% of burn deaths are due to chemical injuries.[1]

Pathophysiology

All burn wounds, whether due to chemical or thermal sources, have in common the denaturation of proteins. The structure of biological proteins involves not only a specific amino acid sequence, but also a three-dimensional structure dependent on weak forces, such as hydrogen bonding or Van der Waals' forces. These three-dimensional structures impart the biological activity on the proteins, and are easily disrupted by outside influences. Heat energy breaks these weak bonds to unfold and denature proteins, just as changes in pH or dissolution of surrounding lipids that may stabilize a protein disrupt its function. Direct chemical effects on a reactive group in a protein will similarly render it ineffective. In addition, chemical agents may act in a systemic fashion as their elements are circulated throughout the victim, with potential metabolic toxicity.

Severity of a chemical burn injury is determined by several factors:
- strength (concentration),
- quantity of burning agent,
- manner and duration of skin contact (progression),
- penetration, and
- mechanism of action.

Broadly classified, there are six mechanisms of action for chemical agents in biological systems:[2]

- *Reduction*: Reducing agents act by binding free electrons in tissue proteins. Examples include hydrochloric acid, nitric acid, and alkyl mercuric agents.
- *Oxidation*: Oxidizing agents are oxidized on contact with tissue proteins. The byproducts are also often toxic and continue to react with the surrounding tissue. Examples of oxidizing agents are sodium hypochlorite (Clorox, Dakin's solution), potassium permanganate, and chromic acid.
- *Corrosive agents*: Corrosive substances denature tissue proteins on contact. Typically, eschar formation and a shallow ulcer represent their injury. Examples of corrosive agents include phenols and cresols, white phosphorus, dichromate salts, sodium metals, and the lyes.
- *Protoplasmic poisons*: These agents produce their effects by binding or inhibiting calcium or other organic ions necessary for tissue viability and function. Examples of protoplasmic poisons include 'alkaloidal' acids, acetic acid, formic acid, and metabolic competitors/inhibitors such as oxalic and hydrofluoric acid.
- *Vesicants*: Vesicant agents produce ischemia with anoxic necrosis at the site of contact. For example, substances such as cantharides (Spanish Fly), dimethyl sulfoxide (DMSO), mustard gas, and Lewisite.
- *Desiccants*: These substances cause damage by dehydrating tissues and at the same time are involved in exothermic reactions to release heat into the tissue. Examples here include sulfuric and muriatic (concentrated hydrochloric) acid.

Within these groups, there are different categories of compounds, each with their own characteristics. This method of describing burn injuries as acid or alkali is less accurate than describing the classes by how they coagulate proteins. Although the mechanisms of action for individual acids or alkali may differ, the resulting wounds are similar enough to warrant consideration as separate groups.[3] Acids act as proton donors in the biological system, and strong acids have a pH < 2. The best predictor of ability of an acid to cause injury,

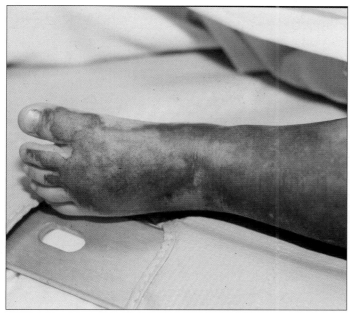

Fig. 42.1 Acid burn to foot illustrating coagulation of blood vessels ('coagulative necrosis').

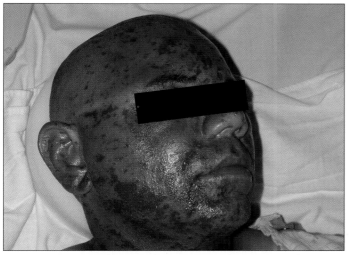

Fig. 42.2 Alkali splash burn to face.

however, is the amount of neutralizing material to correct the pH of the acid to neutral.[4] Alkali, or basic material, capable of producing injury typically has a pH > 11.5.[5] In general alkaline material causes more injury than acidic compounds because acids cause coagulation necrosis with precipitation of protein, while the reaction to alkali is 'liquefaction' necrosis allowing the alkali to penetrate deeper into the injured tissue.[6] The alkalis dissolve and unite with the proteins of the tissues to form alkaline proteinates, which are soluble and contain OH ions, allowing further reactions deeper into the tissues.[7] Organic solutions will tend to dissolve the lipid membrane of cell walls and cause disruption of cellular architecture as their mechanism of action. Inorganic solutions would tend more to remain on the exterior of cells, but may act as vehicles to carry the above-mentioned agents that denature proteins or form

salts with proteins themselves. It is important to consider that the introduction of a chemical agent into a biological system does not result in a simple organic chemistry reaction, but a complex variety of chemical changes across the spectrum of substrates present in a human cell.

General principles of management

The most important aspects of first aid for chemical burn victims involve removal of the offending agent from contact with the patient. This requires removal of all potentially contaminated clothing and copious irrigation. Important principles in the irrigation of chemical burn patients involve protection of healthcare providers to prevent additional injuries. Further, the wounds should not be irrigated by placing the patient into a tub, thereby containing the chemical and spreading the injurious material. Irrigation should be large volume, and 'to the floor' or out an appropriate drain. Lavage of chemical injuries is meant to dilute the agent already in contact with the skin, and prevent additional agent from being exposed to the skin. Early, copious lavage has been shown to reduce the extent and depth of full-thickness injury.[8] No measure of adequacy of lavage has been developed, but monitoring of the pH from the effluent can provide quantifiable information as to adequacy of lavage, but quite often after a period of 30 minutes to 2 hours of lavage may be necessary, and clinically the input of the patient is important to tell that the symptoms of the injury have been reduced signal the end of lavage. The adage 'dilution as the solution to the pollution' applies.

Material Safety Data Sheets (MSDS) are mandated to be available for all chemicals present in the workplace. These can be valuable resources for potential systemic toxicity and side effects of an agent. Plant safety officers should be available at all times to provide this information in cases of industrial accidents. Further assistance is available from regional poison control centers for household chemicals or unidentified agents.

One of the most controversial areas of chemical burn treatment involves the use of neutralizing agents. In theory, they should effectively remove the active chemical form in a wound and provide relief from further injury. However, because of the wide range of chemicals potentially involved, their correct use cannot be assured, so they are generally discouraged. The practical problems encountered with their use are exothermic reactions (i.e. when an acid is used to neutralize an alkali solution, the resulting reaction may liberate a large amount of heat), causing further thermal damage on top of the pre-existing chemical injury. When the burning agent is known and an appriate antidote is known, there is some benefit demonstrated in its use.[9] Despite this, no agent has been found to be more effective than plain water for irrigation.[10]

General principles of trauma management are followed (the ABCs). Airway patency is assured, followed by adequate air movement, and maintenance of hemodynamics. Despite the increasing awareness of chemical burns, no one center has undertaken a study of the resuscitative needs of a chemical burn victim, and hence we rely on the conventional thermal burn formulas for resuscitation. Monitoring of urine output remains paramount to assessment of adequacy of end-organ perfusion and hence resuscitation. Systemic disturbances of pH are potential complications and must be monitored until electrolyte trends are stabilized.

The typical large-volume lavage required to adequately dilute chemical exposures puts the victim at potential risk for hypothermia, both from evaporative cooling losses and the use of unwarmed lavage fluid. First aid performed in outdoor decontamination areas can compound the possibility of hypothermia. Recognition of these risks can prevent added complications.

Principles of wound care for chemical burns are typically the same as for thermal injuries. Early excision and grafting of obvious non-viable tissue is advocated, particularly in light of the observation that chemical burns tend to heal more slowly than thermal burns. Topical application of antimicrobials can be useful for partial thickness injuries. With the development of temporary wound coverings, such as Biobrane™, it is tempting to use this technology in the setting of chemical injuries, but there is no significant experience to support this use.

Specific agents

Acetic acid

Table vinegar, a dilute solution of acetic acid is usually harmless. Glacial or nearly 100% pure acetic acid acts as a metabolite by forming esters with proteins of metabolic pathways.

Strong alkali

Lime, sodium hydroxide and potassium hydroxide are common alkali agents that burn. They are present in many household cleaning solutions, and have historically been commonly ingested as well as causing cutaneous burns.

Dry residues of alkali (e.g. lime) must be brushed away to reduce the total amount of alkali present; then copious irrigation is undertaken. Attempts to neutralize alkali are not recommended.

Alkali injury to the eye is particularly devastating. These compounds penetrate the cornea quickly causing scarring, opacification of the cornea, and perforation.[11]

Assorted acids

Acids tend to cause hard, dry eschars on contact with skin, sparing deeper tissue. In fact, tannic acid has been described as a treatment for thermal injury,[12] and even Native Americans have used unrefined products in the treatment of burns since pre-history. Many of these compounds are absorbed as protoplasmic poisons and are renal and hepatic toxins.

Alkyl mercuric compounds

Skin reaction with these substances releases free mercury, which can be found in blister fluid. With time, this mercury is absorbed, which can cause systemic effects. After blisters are debrided, repeat washing to lavage the blister fluid contents away is necessary.

Cantharides

'Spanish Fly' is used as an aphrodisiac that acts as a vesicant upon contact with the skin. This leads to the formation of multiple, small blisters.

Cement

Cement acts both as a desiccant and an alkali. It penetrates clothing and combines with sweat, causing an exothermic reaction. The dry powder is very hygroscopic and will cause desiccation injury if not hydrated or washed away. Cement is calcium oxide, which becomes calcium hydroxide upon exposure to water. Injury results from the action of the hydroxyl ion.[13]

Chromic acid

Contact with chromic acid, a powerful oxidizing agent used to clean other metals, will cause protein coagulation. The lethal dose for ingestion is between 5 and 10 g, and results in gastroenteritis, followed by vertigo, muscle cramps, peripheral vascular collapse, and coma. Water lavage is again the primary treatment for exposure, but in an industrial setting where this acid is used; washing with a dilute solution of sodium hyposulfite, followed by rinsing in a buffered phosphate solution may be a more specific antidote. Dimercaprol may be used at 4 mg/kg IM every 4 hours for 2 days followed by 2–4 mg/kg/day for 7 days total to treat the systemic effects.

Dichromate salts

A highly corrosive substance with similar symptoms of systemic toxicity as chromic acid. Lethal dose is 50–100 mg/kg. Emergency treatment is by lavage, but more specific treatments include lavage with 2% hyposulfite solution or a buffer of 7% potassium dihydrogen phosphate and 18% disodium hydrogen phosphate.

Dimethyl sulfoxide (DMSO)

This is a powerful organic solvent, with the ability to carry non-lipid soluble compounds quickly across cell membranes. It is used commonly in 'alternative medicine' as a relief for joint pain itself, but commonly is the vehicle for other agents. If implicated in a cutaneous injury, it is likely the dissolved substance, rather than the DMSO itself causing injury.

Formic acid

All patients injured by formic acid should be hospitalized due to multiple systemic effects of this metabolic poisoning agent. These problems include metabolic acidosis, intravascular hemolysis with hemoglobinuria, renal failure, pulmonary complications, and abdominal pain with necrotizing pancreatitis and vomiting.[14]

Hydrocarbons

Prolonged contact with petroleum distillates results in dissolution of lipid cell membranes and resulting cell death.[15] These burns tend to be superficial and heal spontaneously.[16] Systemic toxicity includes respiratory depression and, when lead additives were present, systemic lead poisoning was common. The present epidemic of 'huffing' or inhaling volatile hydrocarbons has produced a syndrome of neurological damage as well.

Hydrochloric acid/muriatic acid

Muriatic acid is the commercial grade of concentrated hydrochloric acid. Once in contact with the skin, it denatures proteins into their chloride salts. Most significantly, hydrochloric acid fumes can cause inhalation injury with a sudden-onset pulmonary edema.

Hydrofluoric acid

Hydrofluoric acid (HF) is a commonly used acid with industrial applications. It is used as a cleaning agent in the petroleum industry and glass etching. It is also one of the strongest inorganic acids known. Hydrofluoric acid is particularly lethal due to its properties both as an acid and as a metabolic poison. The acid component causes coagulation necrosis and cellular death. Fluoride ion then gains a portal of entry that then chelates the positively charged ions like calcium and magnesium.[17] This causes an efflux of intracellular calcium with resultant cell death. The fluoride ion remains active until it is completely neutralized by the bivalent cations, including penetration to bone. This may exceed the body's ability to mobilize calcium and magnesium rapidly enough and muscle contraction and cellular function, dependent on these cations, will become dysfunctional. Fluoride ion is also a metabolic poison and inhibits the Na-K ATPase, allowing efflux of potassium as well.[18] These electrolyte shifts at nerve endings are thought to be the cause of the extreme pain associated with HF burns.[19]

HF burns are classified based on the concentration of the exposure according to a system developed by the National Institutes of Health-Division of Industrial Hygiene.[20] Concentrations greater than 50% cause immediate tissue destruction and pain. Concentrations of 20–50% result in a burn becoming apparent within several hours of exposure. Injuries from concentrations less than 20% may take up to 24 hours to become apparent. Studies on the protective properties of skin correlate well with this scheme, as there was noted to be some protection for a period at all acid concentrations; then the still undefined barrier broke down, allowing the HF to penetrate.[21] Interestingly, the barrier was disrupted by nicks in the skin and organic solvents, suggesting that some lipid element is lost as the wound turns from superficial to full thickness.

The systemic symptoms typical of hypocalcemia or hypomagnesemia are generally absent. Serum calcium levels and electrocardiogram are important monitors of patient status.[22] Once the cardiac dysrhythmias develop, they are hard to restore to a normal rhythm.[23] Compounding the problem of hypocalcemia, the fluoride ion may be acting as a metabolic poison in the myocardium to promote the irritability. The typical electrocardiographic change is Q–T interval prolongation. The fluoride ions can be removed by hemodialysis or cation exchange resins.[24,25]

Treatments of HF exposure are designed to neutralize the fluoride ion and prevent systemic toxicity. Topical calcium gluconate gel (3.5 g of 2.5% calcium gluconate mixed with 5 oz of water-soluble lubricant is applied to the wound 4–6 times each day for 3–4 days) can be used after the wounds have been copiously irrigated.[26] Calcium gluconate injections into the area of the wound (0.5 cc/cm² of 10% calcium gluconate) have also been used with good success.[27] Pain relief with these treatments is often swift, and it is felt that return of symptoms indicate need for repeat treatment. Calcium chloride delivers more milliequivalents per cc of solution, but is contraindicated in subcutaneous injection due to its tissue irritating properties. Burns to the hand with HF are common in workplace accidents, and present special problems; how to deliver large amounts of calcium to limited areas. Palmar fasciotomy may be needed to relieve the pressure after tissue injections.[28] Another option is intra-arterial injections of dilute calcium salts (10 cc of 10% calcium gluconate or calcium chloride in 40 cc of 5% dextrose) into the radial artery that would supply the injured area.[29] Infusion continues until the patient is symptom free of pain in the injured extremity. This technique is commonly described, but there is not wide clinical acceptance, owing to the difficulty and risk of peripheral arterial cannulation while infusing an agent potentially causing distal ischemia. Injury to eyes by HF is treated with copious irrigation with water or saline, not calcium chloride, which is associated with increased corneal ulceration.[30] After the acute period is over, the eye may irrigate with 1% calcium gluconate every 2–3 hours and recovery usually occurs in 4–5 days. Pulmonary reaction to HF vapor may persist for up to 3 weeks after exposure. Nebulized solutions of calcium gluconate and intermittent positive pressure breathing device support are recommended.[31]

Hypochlorite solutions

These are potent oxidizers delivered in alkaline solution used as bleaches and household cleaners. Commonly available solutions are 4–6% and are lethal only when a large surface area is involved; however, exposure to 30 cc of 15% solution is potentially fatal. Systemic manifestations of toxicity include vomiting, dyspnea, and edema of the airway, confusion, cardiovascular collapse, cyanosis and coma.[32]

Nitric acid

A strong acid that can combine with organic proteins to produce organonitrates which act as metabolic poisons.

Oxalic acid

This is a potent metabolic poison that combines with calcium to limit its bioavailability. After exposure, serum calcium should be monitored closely, as well as signs of cardiac or respiratory muscle dysfunction: 0.5 g oxalic acid exposure or ingestion may be fatal.

Phenol (carbolic acid)

This substance was originally used as an antiseptic, but its use declined after serious side effects were noted. It is bound irreversibly to albumin after exposure and ingestion of as little as 1 g may cause death. Cardiovascular effects include ventricular arrhythmias,[33] and skin necrosis also results from prolonged contact.

Industrial use of this compound and its derivatives (resorcinol or 1,3-dihydroxybenzene) has shown the most common adverse effects to be dermatitis and depigmentation of the skin.[34] Acute poisonings are potentially fatal, so prompt action is necessary with copious irrigation to decontaminate the wounds.[35] Polyethylene glycol (PEG molecular weight 300 or 400) has been shown to be of potential benefit,[36,37] but large-volume lavage should not be delayed while PEG application is begun.

Reports in the literature indicate intravenous sodium bicarbonate may be of use to prevent some of the systemic effects of phenol.[38] The mechanism is not clear, as phenol is not dissociated from the albumin by this treatment.

Phosphoric acid

An industrial acid used in strong concentrations. Lavage followed by electrolyte monitoring (phosphorus is a strong calcium binder) is the treatment of choice.

Phosphorus

Phosphorus has both military and civilian uses. It is an incendiary agent found in hand grenades, artillery shells, fireworks and fertilizers.[39] White phosphorus ignites in the presence of air and burns until the entire agent is oxidized or the oxygen source is removed (for example, as with immersion in water). The wounds are irrigated with water, the easily identifiable pieces of phosphorus are removed from the wound, and soaked dressings are applied for transport. Ultraviolet light can be used to identify embedded particles through phosphorescence, or a solution of 0.5% copper sulfate can be applied which will impede oxidation and turn the particles black to aid in their identification and removal. Hypocalcemia, hyperphosphatemia, and cardiac arrhythmias have been reported with phosphorus burns.[40]

Potassium permanganate

This is an oxidizing agent that is highly corrosive in dry, crystalline form. It is poorly absorbed, so systemic effects are rare.

Sulfuric acid

Sulfuric acid and its precursor sulphur trioxide are strong acids and desiccants with many industrial applications. Copious irrigation and early excision are the treatments of choice.[41]

Vesicant chemical warfare agents (lewisite, nitrogen mustard)

These agents were historically used during the trench warfare of World War I. They affect all epithelial tissues, including skin, eyes, and respiratory epithelium. Symptoms described after exposure to mustard gas include burning eyes and a feeling of suffocation associated with a burning throat.[42] This is followed by erythema of the skin in 4 hours with blisters developing in 12–48 hours. Severe pruritis develops, particularly in the moist areas, such as the axilla and perineum. When the blisters rupture, they leave painful, shallow ulcers. Exposure to larger quantities of these agents produces coagulative necrosis of the skin with either no blistering or 'doughnut blisters' surrounding a central necrotic zone.[43] Secondary respiratory infection and bone marrow suppression often lead to death. Lewisite (2-chlorovinyl-dichloroarsine) is the best known arsine. It is more powerful than the mustards and the symptoms occur sooner. Phosgene oxime is another common agent in chemical warfare. It is the most widely used halogenated oxime and has the immediate effect of stinging, likened to contact with a stinging needle.[44] Affected areas quickly become swollen with blister formation, and eschars develop over the next week, but wound healing is slow (over 2 months). Eye involvement is extremely painful and can result in permanent blindness. Inhalation leads to hypersecretion and pulmonary edema.

Treatment primarily includes prophylaxis against exposure, and those administering aid to victims should be suitably protected with respirator, butyl rubber gloves, and boots. Clothing is removed from the victims and large-volume lavage of the skin is undertaken. Eyes are irrigated with water or 'balanced salt solution.' Symptomatic relief of itch is provided with benzodiazepines, antihistamines, or phenothiazines. Blisters are debrided and dressed with topical antimicrobials (but silver sulfadiazine neutralizes dimercaprol). Dimercaprol is a chelating agent that is an antidote for lewisite poisoning, available as an ointment, eyedrops or intramuscular preparation. There is no specific antidote for nitrogen mustard, but sodium thiosulfate and cysteine may be helpful to reduce the effects if administered early.[45] Early excision and grafting has not been shown to be of benefit with nitrogen mustard burns, but the deeper lesions seen with the other agents seem best suited to treatment as if they were full-thickness thermal burns. The blister fluid from nitrogen mustard injuries does not contain active agent and is hence harmless.[46] Symptomatic treatment of ocular and respiratory complications is undertaken. Agranulocytosis or aplastic anemia can result from exposure to these agents, as was seen in Iranian casualties from the Iran–Iraq war.[47] Transfusion of blood products was not helpful,[48] and in the appropriate setting, bone marrow transplantation may be considered. Other marrow stimulators (e.g. granulocyte maturation colony-stimulating factor of lithium carbonate) have not been tried.

Ingestions of caustic substances are common in young children as they begin to explore their environment and get into the household chemicals, or in adults as a suicide gesture. In a 15-year review of chemical burn injuries at our institution, we identified 154 chemical burn injuries, with 26 patients involved with ingestion injuries (17% incidence), but significantly 14 patients under age 4 years (unpublished data). Management of these injuries is not necessarily undertaken in a specialized burn unit, but can be handled by a general surgeon, or foregut surgery specialist. Similar principles apply, with neutralization, lavage, and avoidance of vomiting which might re-expose tissue to the offending agent. Early endoscopic evaluation of the oral pharynx, esophagus and stomach/proximal duodenum with endoscopy will help to define extent of injury before scarring eliminates access to these structures. Particularly vulnerable areas include compromise of the upper airway due to the concentrated exposure in this area and subsequent risk requiring intubation. In general, endoscopic gastrostomy tubes should be considered early in the course of treatment to provide feeding access to the stomach and a guide string should be left in the lumen of the esophagus. The reader is referred to an appropriate general surgery text for the current management of this problem.

References

1. Luterman A, Curreri P. Chemical burn injury. In: Jurkiewcz M, Krizek T, Mathes S, eds. Plastic surgery: principles and practice. St. Louis: CV Mosby; 1990:1355–1440.
2. Jelenko C. Chemicals that burn. J Trauma 1974; 14(1):65–72.
3. Moriarty R. Corrosive chemicals: acids and alkali. Drug Therapy 1979; (3):89.
4. Mozingo DW, Smith AA, McManus WF, Pruitt BA Jr, Mason AD Jr. Chemical burns. J Trauma 1988; 28(5):642–647.
5. Leonard LG, Scheulen JJ, Munster AM. Chemical burns: effect of prompt first aid. J Trauma 1982; 22(5):420–423.
6. Yano K, Hata Y, Matsuka K, Ito O, Matsuda H. Effects of washing with a neutralizing agent on alkaline skin injuries in an experimental model. Burns 1994; 20(1):36–39.

7. Milner S, Nguyen TT, Herndon DN, et al. Chemical injury. In: Herndon D, ed. Total burn care. Philadelphia: WB Saunders: 1996:415–424.

8. Pfister RR. Chemical injuries of the eye. Ophthalmology 1983; 90(10):1246–1253.

9. Cope Z. General treatment of burns. Medical history of the Second World War: surgery. London: HMSO; 1953:288–312.

10. Pike J, Patterson A Jr, Arons MS. Chemistry of cement burns: pathogenesis and treatment. J Burn Care Rehabil 1988; 9(3):258–260.

11. Naik RB, Stephens WP, Wilson DJ, Walker A, Lee HA. Ingestion of formic acid-containing agents – report of three fatal cases. Postgrad Med J 1980; 56(656):451–456.

12. Hunter GA. Chemical burns of the skin after contact with petrol. Br J Plast Surg 1968; 21(4):337–341.

13. Mistry DG, Wainwright DJ. Hydrofluoric acid burns. Am Fam Physician 1992; 45(4):1748–1754.

14. McIvor ME. Delayed fatal hyperkalemia in a patient with acute fluoride intoxication. Ann Emerg Med 1987; 16(10):1165–1167.

15. Klauder J, Shelanski L, Gabriel K. Industrial uses of compounds of fluorine and oxalic acid. AMA Arch Ind Health 1955; 12:412–419.

16. Division of Industrial Hygeine, National Institutes of Health, Hydrofluoric acid burns. Int Med 1943; 12:634.

17. Noonan T, Carter EJ, Edelman PA, Zawacki BE. Epidermal lipids and the natural history of hydrofluoric acid (HF) injury. Burns 1994; 20(3):202–206.

18. Mayer TG, Gross PL. Fatal systemic fluorosis due to hydrofluoric acid burns. Ann Emerg Med 1985; 14(2):149–153.

19. McIvor ME, Cummings CE, Mower MM, et al. Sudden cardiac death from acute fluoride intoxication: the role of potassium. Ann Emerg Med 1987; 16(7):777–781.

20. Yolken R, Konecny P, McCarthy P. Acute fluoride poisoning. Pediatrics 1976. 58(1):90–93.

21. Dibbell DG, Iverson RE, Jones W, et al. Hydrofluoric acid burns of the hand. J Bone Joint Surg Am 1970; 52(5):931–936.

22. Anderson WJ, Anderson JR. Hydrofluoric acid burns of the hand: mechanism of injury and treatment. J Hand Surg Am 1988; 13(1):52–57.

23. Vance MV, Curry SC, Kunkel DB, Ryan DJ, Ruggeri SB. Digital hydrofluoric acid burns: treatment with intraarterial calcium infusion. Ann Emerg Med 1986; 15(8):890–896.

24. McCulley JP, Whiting DW, Petitt MG, Lauber SE. Hydrofluoric acid burns of the eye. J Occup Med 1983; 25(6):447–450.

25. Caravati EM. Acute hydrofluoric acid exposure. Am J Emerg Med 1988; 6(2):143–150.

26. Miller F. Poisoning by phenol. Can Med Assoc J 1942; 46:615.

27. Saunders A, Geddes L, Elliott P. Are phenolic disinfectants toxic to staff members? Aust Nurses J 1988; 17(10):25–26.

28. Abbate C, Polito I, Puglisi A, et al. Dermatosis from resorcinal in tyre makers. Br J Ind Med 1989; 46(3):212–214.

29. Schutz W. Phenoldermatosen. Berufsdermatosen 1959; 7:266.

30. Brown VKH, Box VL, Simpson BL. Decontamination procedures for skin exposed to phenolic substances. Arch Environ Health 1975; 30(1):1–6.

31. Bennett I, James D, Golden A. Severe acidosis due to phenol poisoning. Report of two cases. Ann Intern Med 1959; 32:214.

32. Summerlin WT, Walder AI, Moncrief J. White phosphorus burns and massive hemolysis. J Trauma 1967; 7(3):476–484.

33. Bowen TE, Whelan TJ Jr, Nelson TG. Sudden death after phosphorus burns: experimental observations of hypocalcemia, hyperphosphatemia and electrocardiographic abnormalities following production of a standard white phosphorus burn. Ann Surg 1971; 174(5):779–784.

34. Sawhney CP, Kaushish R. Acid and alkali burns: considerations in management. Burns 1989; 15(2):132–134.

35. Willems J. Clinical management of mustard gas casualties. Ann Med Milit (Belg) 1989; 3(Suppl):1–61.

36. Papirmeister B, Feister AJ, Robinson SI, et al. The sulfur mustard injury: description of lesions and resulting incapacitation. In: Medical defence against mustard gas. Florida: CRC; 1990:13–42.

37. Vesicants. In: NATO handbook on the medical effects of NBC defensive operations. AMedP-6 Part III-Chemical. Amended final draft. (NATO Unclassified).

38. Parpmeister B, Feister AJ, Robinson SI, et al. Pretreatments and therapies. In: Medical defense against mustard gas. Florida: CRC; 1990.

39. Sultzberger M, Katz J. The absence of skin irritants in the contents of vesicles. US Navy Med Bull 1943; 43:1258–1262.

40. Vedder E. The medical aspects of chemical warfare. Baltimore: Williams and Wilkins; 1925.

Chapter 43

Radiation injuries, vesicant burns, and mass casualties

Stephen M. Milner

Introduction

In the aftermath of 9/11, with the threat of constant and unrelenting terrorism, the possibility of employment of nuclear weapons, crude nuclear devices, attacks on nuclear facilities and use of chemical agents cannot be ignored. Such attacks may result in types of injuries in previously unimaginable numbers. Given the devastating medical consequences that would follow the use of such weapons, the training of medical personnel will be a crucial factor in the effective management of such casualties, should the unthinkable ever occur.

Only 4 months after Roentgen reported the discovery of x-rays, Dr John Daniel observed that irradiation of his colleague's skull caused hair loss. Since this finding was reported in 1896, many biomedical effects of radiation have been described.[1] Knowledge of nuclear physics was rapidly amassed in the early part of the 20th century, leading eventually to the Manhattan project and the development of the atomic bomb. The last 50 years has also seen widespread deployment of energy-generating nuclear reactors, and the expanding use of radioactive isotopes in industry, science, and healthcare.[2] More recently, major industrial accidents of note at Three Mile Island in Pennsylvania, Chernobyl in the Ukraine and at Goiania, Brazil have resulted in potential or real radiation injuries to hundreds of people.

Exposure to ionizing radiation can follow one of three patterns:

1. small-scale accidents, as might occur in a laboratory or from an x-ray device in a hospital setting;
2. large industrial accidents (such as those mentioned above), stretching the need for treatment beyond available resources; and

3. detonation of a nuclear device in a military conflict where resources are totally overwhelmed or unavailable and associated multiple and combined injuries also exist.

This chapter first describes the terminology used in standard measurement of radiation exposure and discusses the frequency of radiation accidents, injuries and fatalities. The effects of exposure to ionizing radiation and triage and care protocols are considered according to known and projected prognostic factors. The complications that arise specifically with this injury and the supportive measures that need to be taken will be addressed.

Vesicant agents are characterized by their ability to produce cutaneous blisters resembling 'burns.' Although most physicians are unlikely to encounter casualties of chemical weapons, the proliferation of these agents has increased the risk to both military and civilian populations. They are likely to require expertise found in burn centers and for this reason an account of the management of these injuries is included in this text. Finally, the problem of mass casualties is examined, and recommendations for management are made.

Radiation injuries

Terminology

Damage to biological tissue by ionizing radiation is mediated by energy transference. This can be the result of exposure to electromagnetic radiation (e.g. x-rays and gamma rays) or particulate radiation (e.g. alpha and beta particles or neutrons). The severity of tissue damage is determined by the energy deposited per unit track length, known as linear energy transfer (LET).[3] Electromagnetic radiation passes through tissue almost unimpeded by the skin and are called low LET since little energy is left behind. In contrast, neutron exposure has high-LET, resulting in significant energy absorption within the first few centimeters of the body. Alpha and low-energy beta particles do not penetrate the skin, and represent a hazard only when internalized by inhalation, ingestion or absorption through a wound.

Radiation dosing can be expressed in several ways (Table 43.1):

- The roentgen (R) is the unit of exposure and is related to the ability of x-rays to ionize air. It is defined as the quantity of low-energy x-rays or gamma rays required to produce 1.61×10^{15} ion pairs per kilogram of air.
- The curie (Ci) or becquerel (Bq) is the unit of activity (rate of decay) of a radioactive material. One curie

TABLE 43.1 RADIATION UNITS AND CONVERSION FACTORS

Old unit	New unit	Conversion factor
Rad (rad)	Gray (Gy)	1 Gy = 100 rad
Rem (rem)	Sievert (Sv)	1 Sv = 100 rem
Curie (Ci)	Becquerel (Bq)	1 Bq = 2.7×10^{-11} Ci

TABLE 43.2 MAJOR RADIATION ACCIDENTS: HUMAN EXPERIENCE 1944 — MARCH 2005

Location	No. of accidents	No. of persons involved	Significant exposures*	Fatalities*
US	252	1347	799	30
Non-US	176	132457	2251	104
Total	428	133804	3050	134
*FSU Registry Data (not in totals — data incomplete)				
	(137)	(507)	(278)	(35)

Source: REAC/TS Registry.
**DOE/NRC dose criteria.

equals 3.7×10^{10} decays per second, a definition originally based on the rate of decay of 1g of radium.[4] The becquerel is a smaller but more basic unit and equals one decay per second.

- The rad is the unit of absorbed dose of radiation and corresponds to an energy absorption of 100 ergs/g. A newer international unit, the gray (Gy), is now in use and is defined as 1 Joule (J) of energy deposited in each kg of absorbing material, and is equal to 100 rads.[5]

Not all radiation is equally effective in causing biological damage, although it may cause the same energy deposition in tissue. For example, 1 Gy of neutron radiation will not have the same effect as 1 Gy of gamma or x-radiation. For this reason, a unit of dose equivalence was derived that allows radiations with different LET values to be compared. One such unit is the rem (acronym of roentgen equivalent man). The dose in rem is equal to the dose in rads multiplied by a quality factor (QF).[6] The QF takes into account the linear energy transfer and has a different value for different radiations; for x-rays it is 1.0, for neutrons 10. The international unit, now more widely in use, is the sievert (Sv). One sievert equals 100 rem; 1 rem equals 10 mSv. This allows radiations with different LET values to be compared, since 1 Sv of neutron radiation has the same biological effect as 1 Sv of low LET gamma or x radiation.

Incidence

A significant radiation accident is one in which an individual exceeds at least one of the following criteria:[7]

- Whole body doses equal to or exceeding 25 rem (0.25 Sv).
- Skin doses equal to or exceeding 600 rem (6 Sv).
- Absorbed dose equal to or greater than 75 rem (0.75 Sv) to other tissues or organs from an external source.
- Internal contamination equal to or exceeding one-half the maximum permissible body burden (MPBB) as defined by the International Commission on Radiological Protection (this number is different for each radionuclide).
- Medical misadministrations provided they result in a dose or burden equal to or greater than the criteria already listed above.

Radiation accidents within the United States should be reported to the federally funded Radiation Emergency Assistance Center/Training Site (REAC/TS). This is operated by Oak Ridge Institute for Science and Education (ORISE) at Oak Ridge, Tennessee and can be contacted by calling (865) 576–

1005. A radiological emergency response team of physicians, nurses, health physicists, and support personnel provides consultative assistance on a 24-hour basis and has the capability of providing medical treatment, whenever a radiation accident occurs. REAC/TS also maintains a Radiation Accident Registry System.

The number of accidents, number of persons involved, as well as the number of fatalities, in the United States and worldwide is shown in Tables 43.2 and 43.3. There have been a total of 134 fatalities recorded by the Registry worldwide.[7] The majority of the radiation deaths occurred as a result of the Chernobyl accident in 1986 (>40). The classification of radiation accident by device for the period 1944 until March 2005 and their frequency distribution is illustrated in Table 43.4 and Figure 43.1.[7] The majority of radiation accidents are due to radiation devices. This may be an accelerator; however, most devices involved in accidents are encapsulated, highly radioactive sources used for industrial radiography. Next most frequent accidents are radioisotope accidents that involve radioactive materials, which are unsealed such as tritium, fission products, radium and free isotopes used for diagnosis and therapy. Uncommon criticality accidents occur when enough fissionable material, such as enriched uranium is brought together to produce a neutron flux so high that the material undergoes a nuclear reaction (becomes critical).

The most devastating radiation injuries and fatalities yet seen, however, resulted from detonation of nuclear weapons at Hiroshima and Nagasaki during World War II. Since 1945 nuclear weapon technology has developed enormously and current strategic thermonuclear warheads dwarf those weapons used in Japan.[8]

Perhaps a more likely weapon of terrorism will involve the use of a radiological dispersal device (RDD). The term dirty bomb generally refers to conventional explosive packaged with radioactive material that is scattered over a wide area when detonated. It is believed that these devices would probably elicit more harm by public fear and panic than by serious injury.[9] Perhaps a greater threat might be the use of radioactive material placed in a public place without use of explosives, as illustrated by the event in Goiania, Brazil where 249 people were affected by radiation when cesium-137 was unwittingly released by scrap metal workers.

TABLE 43.3 MAJOR RADIATION ACCIDENTS WORLDWIDE 1944 — MARCH 2005: ACUTE, ASSOCIATED, AND NON-RADIATION DEATHS

United States		Other	
New Mexico	3	Algeria	2
Ohio	10	Argentina	1
Oklahoma	1	Belarus	1
Pennsylvania	1	Brazil	4
Rhode Island	1	Bulgaria	1
Texas	9	China (PR)	6
Wisconsin	1	Costa Rica	7
Total US	**26**	Egypt	2
		El Salvador	1
		Estonia	1
		Israel	1
		Italy	1
		Japan	2
		Marshall Islands	1
		Mexico	5
		Morocco	8
		Norway	1
		Panama	5
		Russia	5
		Spain	10
		Thailand	3
		USSR	29
		UK	2
		Yugoslavia	1
		Total Non-US	**100**
Non-radiation deaths			
Canada	1		
Idaho	3		
USSR	3		
Washington	1		
Total	**8**		

Pathophysiology

The detonation of a nuclear device over a population center will produce an extremely hot, luminous fireball, which emits intense thermal radiation capable of causing burns and starting fires at considerable distance. This is accompanied by a destructive blast wave moving away from the fireball at supersonic speed and the emission of irradiation, mainly gamma rays and neutrons.[10] The result of a combination of thermal and radiation injuries is said to have a synergistic effect on the outcome. Several animal experiments have demonstrated a significant increase in mortality when a standard burn wound model is irradiated, over and above that expected from either injury alone.[11,12]

Thermal effects

Exact information about the cause of fatalities in a nuclear blast is not available, but from the nuclear attack on Japan, it has been estimated that 50% of deaths were due to burns and

TABLE 43.4 MAJOR RADIATION ACCIDENTS WORLDWIDE (1944–MARCH 2005): 'CLASSIFICATION BY DEVICE'

Radiation devices	**316**
Sealed sources	208
x-ray devices	82
Accelerators	25
Radar generators	1
Radioisotopes	**93**
Diagnosis and therapy	38
Transuranics	28
Fission products	11
Tritium	2
Radium spills	1
Other	13
Criticalities	**19**
Critical assemblies	7
Reactors	6
Chemical operations	6
Total	**428**

Source: REAC/TS Registries.

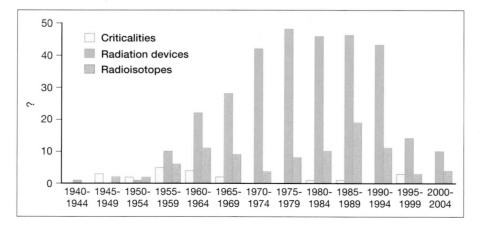

Fig. 43.1 Frequency distribution of major radiation accidents (by device) worldwide 1944—March 2005

some 20–30% was flash burns.[13] The clinical picture may range from an erythema of the exposed areas (most commonly face, hands, arms and legs), to a charring of the superficial layers of the skin. Secondary flame burns may be present following the ignition of the victim's clothing or environment. The physicians at Hiroshima and Nagasaki observed that the 'flame' burn wound seemed to heal at first. However, between 1 and 2 weeks later, a serious relapse occurred. Wound infection set in; there was a disorder in granulation tissue formation; a gray, greasy coating would form on the wounds. Thrombocytopenia resulted in spontaneous bleeding both into the wound and elsewhere. Histologically, the normal collection of leukocytes delineating a necrotic area were found to be absent due to agranulocytosis and gross bacterial invasion was evident;[14] both these changes obviously affecting the prognosis of these otherwise relatively small injuries.

Radiation effect

Damage to biological tissue by ionizing radiation is mediated by energy transference. The transference of this energy can damage critical parts of the cell directly or indirectly by formation of free radicals (such as the hydroxyl radical). The primary targets are cellular and nuclear membranes and DNA.[15]

The morbidity of radiation is dependent on its dose, the dose rate and the sensitivity of the cell exposed. Cells are most sensitive when undergoing mitosis so that those that divide rapidly such as bone marrow, skin and the gastrointestinal tract are more susceptible to radiation damage. Radiation to an organ such as brain or liver, which has parenchymal cells with a slow turnover rate, results in damage to the more sensitive connective tissue and microcirculation.

The overall effect on the organism depends on the extent of the body surface involved, duration of exposure and homogeneity of the radiation field. It is convenient to consider radiation injuries as localized or whole body (acute radiation syndrome).

Localized injury

In a localized injury a relatively small part of the body is affected without significant systemic effects.[16] The skin and subcutaneous tissue alone may be involved following exposure to low-energy radiation. Exposure to high-energy radiation may injure deeper structures.

Radiation damage depends on the dose of exposure and several progressive features are observed in skin: erythema is equivalent to a first-degree thermal burn and occurs in two stages. Mild erythema appears within minutes or hours following the initial exposure and subsides in 2–3 days. The second onset of erythema occurs 2–3 weeks after exposure and is accompanied by dry desquamation of the epidermal keratinocytes. Epilation (loss of hair) may occur as soon as 7 days post injury. It is usually temporary with doses less than 5 Gy but may be permanent with higher doses.

Moist desquamation is equivalent to a second-degree thermal burn and develops after a latent period of about 3 weeks with a dose of 12 to 20 Gy. The latency period may be shorter with higher doses. Blisters form, which are susceptible to infection if not treated.

Full-thickness skin ulceration and necrosis are caused by doses in excess of about 25 Gy. Onset varies from a few weeks to a few months after exposure. Blood vessels become telangiectatic and deeper vessels occluded. Obliterating endarteritis results in fibrosis, atrophy and necrosis. Skin cancers may be evident after months or years.

The acute radiation syndrome

The physiological effects of whole-body radiation are described as the acute radiation syndrome (ARS). The clinical course usually begins within hours of exposure. Prodromal symptoms include nausea, vomiting, diarrhea, fatigue, fever and headache. There then follows a latent period, the duration of which is related to the dose. Haematopoietic and gastrointestinal complications follow this. The ARS can be subdivided into three overlapping subsyndromes, which are related to the dose exposure.

Haematopoietic syndrome

This may occur after an exposure of between 1 and 4 Gy. The bone marrow is the most sensitive and pancytopenia develops. Opportunistic infections result from the granulocytopenia and spontaneous bleeding results from thrombocytopenia. Hemorrhage and infection is the usual cause of death.

Gastrointestinal syndrome

This requires a larger dose exposure usually in the range of 10 to 12 Gy. Severe nausea and vomiting associated with bowel cramps and watery diarrhea occurs within hours of irradiation. There is a shorter latent period of 5–7 days, which reflects the turnover time of the gut epithelium (3–5 days). The epithelial damage results in loss of transport capability, bacterial translocation with sepsis, bowel ischemia and bloody diarrhea. Large fluid imbalances can result in hypovolemia, acute renal failure and anemia from both bleeding and the loss of erythropoiesis. Critical exposure will lead to rapid deterioration with unrelenting bloody diarrhea, fever, refractive hypovolemic shock, sepsis and death.

Neurovascular syndrome

An exposure to a dose of 15–30 Gy or greater can cause an immediate total collapse of the vascular system superimposed on the aforementioned syndromes. This may be due to the massive release of mediator substances, nitric oxide abnormalities or destruction of endothelium.[11] This syndrome can progress rapidly with variable neurological symptoms, respiratory distress, cardiovascular collapse and death.

Triage

Triage is the initial classification of casualties into priority groups for treatment and is essential in the management of large numbers of casualties. Those patients unlikely to survive should not be allowed to overwhelm available resources, so that adequate treatment reaches those most likely to survive. In most circumstances, ionizing radiation is not immediately life threatening and any associated injury should be treated first. Once lifesaving measures has been carried out and the patient stabilized, assessment of radiation exposure can proceed.

If large-scale casualties are encountered, triage may, of necessity, seem to be draconian. In conventional warfare with limited medical resources, 50% of soldiers with thermal injuries of up to 70% TBSA will be expected to survive (Table 43.5). This survival rate should be bettered in a smaller civilian major accident. Thus burns alone over 70% TBSA should receive expectant treatment and those under 20% can have their treatment delayed. If there has been a significant exposure to radiation as well as a thermal injury, individuals with over 30% TBSA burns are unlikely to survive without the use of major resources.[17]

Treatment

The treatment of any burn requires massive support from a dedicated team. This will be available for small accidents. With larger accidents or a nuclear attack, the number of victims could swamp the services; treatment facilities may be destroyed; normal supply channels would be drastically reduced, if present at all; production, distribution and transportation of supplies may be greatly impaired and local care workers may also be the victims.[18]

First aid

The victims must be evacuated from the source of radiation in order to limit the exposure. Normal resuscitation procedures must be followed (i.e. airway, breathing, circulation, etc.). Contaminated clothing must be removed and the skin wounds decontaminated by copious but gentle irrigation with water or saline. The goal of decontamination is to dilute and neutralize particles without spreading them to unexposed areas. Thus patients should not be immersed in tubs. Irrigation should be continued until a dosimeter such as a Geiger–Muller counter indicates a steady state or minimum radiation count has been reached.

Intact skin may also be irrigated with a soft brush or surgical sponge preferably under a stream of warm tap water. If this is inadequate, a second scrubbing with mild soap or detergent (pH 7) for 3–4 minutes is recommended. This is followed by application of povidone-iodine solution or hexachlorophene soap, which is then rinsed again for 2–3 minutes and dried. If the patient is known to have had less than 100 rem he/she can be followed as an outpatient. Exposures greater than 100 rem require full evaluation in hospital. Patients with exposures over 200 rem or who have symptoms of ARS should preferably be sent to specialist centers with facilities to treat bone marrow failure.[19]

TABLE 43.5 SURVIVAL RATES WITH MAJOR RESOURCES AVAILABLE		
Burn alone	<70% TBSA	50% survival
Burn alone	>70% TBSA	Probably fatal
Burn plus radiation	<30% TBSA	May survive
Burn plus radiation	>30% TBSA	Probably fatal
TBSA, total body surface area.		

Assessment

The assessment of thermal injury has been covered in preceding chapters. Exposure to radiation can be estimated clinically, by noting the onset of symptoms of ARS, supported by biological parameters. A complete blood count, including platelets and differential count, should be performed immediately and repeated at 12–24 hours if indicated by a change in the absolute lymphocyte count. If the patient sustains a fall in lymphocyte count of 50% or a count less than 1×10^9/liter in a time period of 48 hours post exposure, a moderate dose of radiation has been encountered.[20] Levels of serum amylase and diamine oxidase (produced by intestinal villi) may be useful biological dosimeters of the future. Amylase levels are only reliable when the salivary glands have been exposed and diamine oxidase has not yet been fully assessed in humans. Lymphocyte chromosomal analysis allows very accurate measurement even at low levels of exposure. However, the need for the test to be performed in cell cultures in laboratories over 48 hour incubation would render this test impractical with large numbers of casualties.[21]

General care of the irradiated patient

Where possible a history should be obtained from the patient or others. Factors such as age, concurrent medical problems, smoke inhalation and multiple trauma will affect the prognosis. With this in mind a full physical examination is carried out to exclude other injuries. Victims of radiation exposure may not appear to differ clinically from the thermally injured and should receive the same care. Those exposed to lethal doses of radiation will exhibit early signs of radiation sickness and should be triaged accordingly.

All patients should be given adequate analgesia. Opiates or opioids are the drugs of choice. They must be titrated to effect and administered by the intravenous route. Early nausea and vomiting will be distressing and must be treated with available antiemetic drugs. Prochlorperazine has to be given by intramuscular injection but the newer agent, ondansetron, may prove successful as it is used against the similar symptoms encountered in radiotherapy and chemotherapy. It can also be used in children.

Patients with thermal burns in excess of 40% TBSA or with associated inhalation or major trauma should be treated expectantly in the mass casualty situation. They should be made comfortable, given adequate analgesia and/or sedatives if available and thought appropriate. Resuscitation should be the same as that for an uncomplicated thermal injury. Any resuscitation formula can be used, but it must be closely monitored and altered as necessary to maintain an adequate urine output. The fluid requirement will be increased as fluid is sequestered into damaged internal organs especially the gut. Fluid losses from diarrhea and vomiting may also be excessive and need to be replaced. Intravenous fluids may be limited and the victims may be advised to take oral fluids consisting of balanced salt solutions and maintain a large urine output. A number of oral fluid replacement formulas exist although the best known, Moyer's solution, can be readily formulated by mixing a teaspoon (5 mL) of sodium chloride and a teaspoonful of sodium bicarbonate in a liter of tap water.

Care of the burn wound

The patient is bathed gently to remove loose non-viable skin, the remnants of burnt clothing and any other external debris, which may be contaminated with radioactive material. After the patient has been cleaned, decontaminated and debrided, the extent of any thermal burn and its depth can be ascertained more accurately. The major problems that will be experienced with a radiation burn and/or thermal injuries are those associated with sepsis, fluid balance and the non-healing wound. Mild erythema may require little treatment; however, it is important to avoid further irritation of the skin by exposure to abrasive decontamination, irritating solutions and sunlight. With a slightly higher radiation dose causing dry desquamation, a bland lotion and loose clothing to alleviate itching may be all that is required. Deeper burns with moist desquamation are treated like conventional thermal injuries. Topical chemotherapeutic agents can be used and regularly applied as described elsewhere. Burns are best treated closed because of the high risk of sepsis in immunosuppressed patients whose wounds are susceptible to dehydration, colonization and portal entry of organisms. Early tangential excision and split skin grafting provides early wound closure, decreased burn wound colonization and sepsis and shortened hospital stay.[22,23] This technique is recommended by the authors and probably has advantages where the potential to develop septic wounds is great. Information regarding the grafting of radiation burns is not yet available but is probably best delayed. Dubos et al.[24] performing early excision and grafting of burns in irradiated monkeys have shown that healing occurred fully by the end of the second week, although histologically there was a slight delay in the healing process. The procedure however is not without risks. Blood loss in excess of 300 mL per %TBSA excised presents an increased anesthetic hazard. In irradiated tissue that is severely injured, definitive management usually involves resection of damaged tissue and replacement with well-vascularized non-radiated tissue, usually from a distant site.

Hyperbaric oxygen therapy (HBO) may be combined with surgical treatment potentially to enhance wound healing in irradiated tissue. The mechanism of action is not certain but appears to be related to the creation of a high oxygen gradient across the irradiated tissues, which stimulates capillary ingrowth. Hyperbaric oxygen treatments have been devised using an empirical approach.[25] A single treatment or 'dive' consists of 90 minutes in the chamber breathing an oxygen-rich mixture at 2.4 ATA (atmosphere absolute). Soft-tissue defects are usually treated with 30 dives. When combined with surgery a '20/10 protocol' is used in which the operative procedure is 'sandwiched' between 20 preoperative and 10 postoperative dives.

Treatment of complications
Hematological

Blood and platelets are administered to maintain an adequate hemoglobin concentration and a platelet level of 20×10^9 per liter. If surgery is contemplated this level should be raised to 75×10^9 per liter. All blood products should be irradiated to avoid graft versus host disease.

Bone marrow transplantation is the treatment of choice following total body irradiation. It should be performed between 3 and 5 days post exposure as the immunosuppression is at its peak.

An important goal of medical treatment is to stimulate the proliferation and differentiation of residual hematopoietic stem and progenitor cells (HSPC). Administration of anti-apoptotic cytokine combinations such as stem cell factor, Flt-3 ligand, thrombopoietin, and interleukin-3, may assist recovery, if administered early.[26] Moreover, hematopoietic growth factors such as granulocyte colony-stimulating factor (G-CSF) and granulocyte–macrophage colony-stimulating factor (GM-CSF) have also been recommended[27,28] based on demonstration of improved survival in irradiated primates and reduced neutropenia in humans following accidental irradiation.

Infection

The immunosuppression associated with irradiation makes the victim susceptible to exogenous and endogenous pathogens. Exogenous infection can be limited by adequate aseptic technique and nursing the patient in a sterile environment. Monitoring the patient adequately will allow the early diagnosis of sepsis and its treatment before it becomes well established. The antibiotic chosen should reflect the current pattern of susceptibility and nosocomial infections in that particular unit at that time. Combination therapy will be required where there is a profound neutropenia. With the large fluid losses and shifts, gentamicin is not recommended unless there is no other choice. Therapeutic levels will be difficult to obtain without risking toxicity and there are now safer broad-spectrum antibiotics (imipenem, ceftazidime and ciprofloxacin). If Gram-positive infection is suspected, vancomycin or the newer and safer teicoplanin should be administered. If there is an inadequate response, an antifungal agent must be added. The use of fresh frozen plasma, gamma globulin solutions and monoclonal antibodies is at present speculative, but if resources allow and the patient's condition is not stabilizing, these agents should be considered.

Cardiovascular collapse

This complication may occur due to the exposure, sepsis, fluid loss or hemorrhage. The patient should be given adequate fluid resuscitation, the airway must be protected and oxygen therapy instituted. Sedation and mechanical ventilation will decrease the oxygen debt that will inevitably occur. Inotropic support may become necessary and should be started as early as possible accompanied by the relevant cardiovascular monitoring. Invasive cardiovascular monitoring will aid in the treatment of volume replacement, but invasive intravenous lines must be inserted in aseptic conditions, kept meticulously clean, changed regularly and removed when no longer indicated. Agents that manipulate the release of nitric oxide may become available in the near future and may turn out to be the agents of choice in the treatment of septic shock.

Occupational exposure

In clinical practice there are concerns that relatively low levels of radiation delivered over a long period of time might induce cancer and/or exert genetic or teratogenetic effects. The radiation dose can be limited by reducing the duration of exposure or by increasing the distance from the source of radiation. Since distance and radiation intensity obey the inverse square law, the latter is particularly effective. While the efficacy of shielding devices will be determined by the type and thickness of the material and the energy and type of radiation, Table 43.6 illustrates the effectiveness of these devices when used at diagnostic x-ray energies. It should be noted that the bodies of others provide very effective shielding.

Cumulative doses of radiation can be recorded on radiation badges containing photographic emulsion. The personnel dosimeter is relatively cheap and accurate but has limitations. The smallest exposure that can be measured is 10 millirem; film badges can be exposed by heat, giving false readings, and they are analyzed only at monthly intervals.

Summary

Treatment of radiation injury, whether or not it is combined with other injuries, requires specialized knowledge and resources. The combination of radiation injury with associated injuries appears to have a synergistic effect on outcome. Significant increases in mortality occur because of immunosuppression secondary to radiation exposure in patients already vulnerable to infections. For localized radiation injury, it is often difficult to assess the level of severity quickly and with accuracy, because of the delay between exposure and appearances of lesions, and because of hidden lesions in underlying tissues. Medical treatment deals with inflammation, moist desquamation, and chronic pain; the most favorable time for surgical intervention is difficult to specify. Full intensive care support is needed for whole-body irradiation causing ARS, and is available only if small numbers are involved. Those that survive and show signs of regeneration of tissues will warrant late surgical intervention. Aplastic anemia, immunosuppression, hemorrhage, and sepsis will be major problems for survivors. The improving therapy of bone marrow transplantation is the treatment of choice. Large numbers of casualties will necessitate expectant treatment only. Evacuation of survivors will take days and a natural selection will take place.

Vesicant burns

Vesicant agents are characterized by their ability to produce cutaneous blisters resembling 'burns.' They have posed a major military threat since the use of sulfur mustard [bis (2-chloroethyl) sulfide] in the trenches of World War I. Since this time various nations have deployed chemical weapons and terrorist organizations have used it in public places.[29] More recently, the conflict between Iraq and Iran in the 1980s displayed the most open and widespread use of chemical weapons

on a battlefield in recent decades. Chemical weapons were believed to have been deployed by Iraq in the 1990 Persian Gulf War when nerve gas and blister agent were detected in the theater of operations.[30,31] Although sulfur and nitrogen mustard is the most important vesicant militarily, the vesicant category includes other agents, such as lewisite and phosgene oxime. These compounds affect not only skin but all epithelial tissue with which they come into contact, particularly the eyes and respiratory tract. Although most physicians are unlikely to encounter casualties of chemical weapons, the proliferation of these agents has increased the risk to both military and civilian populations. They are likely to require expertise found in burn centers and for this reason an account of the management of these injuries is included in this text.

Mechanisms of action

The mechanism of action of mustard has eluded identification; however, most of the toxic effects are believed to be related to alkylation of DNA and critical target molecules. The DNA cross-links, which prevent replication and repair of DNA ultimately, lead to cell death. The dermal epidermal separation, which causes the skin lesions, is believed to be due to release of proteases and other enzymes. Breakage of anchoring filaments connecting the basal cell layer to the basement membrane results in a blister with the basement membrane on its dermal side. There are three main hypotheses to explain the biochemical processes leading to enzyme release.

The first proposes that strand breaks in the DNA activate the nuclear DNA repair enzyme poly (ADP-ribose) polymerase. This initiates a cascade of reactions in which cellular stores of nicotinamide adenine dinucleotide (NAD) are depleted, glycolysis is inhibited, and the hexose monophosphate shunt is stimulated. This is thought to lead to induction and secretion of proteases.[32]

The second hypothesis proposes a mechanism based on an interaction between mustard and the intracellular scavenger glutathione (GSH).[33] This is thought to inactivate thiol proteins, including calcium and magnesium adenosine triphosphatases, which regulate calcium levels. Elevation of cytosolic calcium concentration activates production of proteases, phospholipases and endonucleases, which break down membranes, cytoskeleton and DNA leading to cell death. A separate consequence of depleted GSH could also be lipid peroxidation with the formation of lipid peroxides toxic to cell membranes.[34]

The third hypothesis involves lipid peroxidation where the principal toxic consequence of GSH depletion is the formation of toxic lipid peroxides with resulting cell membrane disruption.

The exact mechanism of action of the other agents is unknown although lewisite has been shown to inhibit several important enzyme systems, such as the pyruvate dehydrogenase complex.

Clinical features

Early symptoms ascribed to mustard gas include an ocular burning sensation and a feeling of suffocation associated with a burning throat.[35] After 4 hours, erythema is seen; in 12–48 hours, blistering appears accompanied by severe pruritus which has a predilection for moist areas such as the axilla and

TABLE 43.6 THE EFFECTIVENESS OF SHIELDING DEVICES	
Device	Transmission
Lead apron	<10%
Thyroid shield	<10%
Leaded glasses	<10%
Unleaded glasses	50%
Human body	1%
Human body wearing lead apron	0.1%
Portable lead shields	<1%

perineum. The blisters tend to rupture, discharging an amber serous fluid and leaving painful shallow ulcers. Greater exposure produces coagulative necrosis of skin, with either no blistering or 'doughnut blisters' surrounding a central necrotic zone.[36] This will be accompanied by severe conjunctivitis, corneal erosion and necrotizing bronchitis. A secondary respiratory infection may develop over the next few days which coupled with associated marrow suppression could prove fatal. Following absorption of large amounts of mustard other systems may be affected. Severe stem cell suppression may lead to pancytopenia and involvement of the gastrointestinal tract can have effects ranging from nausea and vomiting to severe hemorrhagic diarrhea. Excitation of the CNS, resulting in convulsions, has been reported.[37] Mustard may also affect other organs, but rarely do these produce clinical effects

Lewisite (2-chlorovinyl-dichlorarsine) is the best known arsine. It is more powerful than the mustards and symptoms occur sooner. Eye irritation is produced immediately and sneezing, salivation and lacrimation occur sooner. Non-lethal chronic exposure may lead to arsenical poisoning.

Exposure to phosgene oxime, the commonest halogenated oxime, has the immediate effect of stinging, and is likened to that on contact with a stinging nettle.[38] Within a minute, the affected area becomes swollen and solid lesions resembling urticaria are seen. An eschar will form after 1 week, but healing is often delayed beyond 2 months. Contamination of the eyes is extremely painful and may result in permanent blindness. Inhalation causes irritation and coughing, hypersecretion, and pulmonary edema.

Treatment for exposure to a vesicant agent

The only prophylaxis against these agents is butyl rubber gloves, boots and a respirator. The clothing of a victim must either be removed or decontaminated with Fuller's earth powder. Eyes can be irrigated with water but, if available, 1.26% sodium bicarbonate solution or 0.9% saline should be used. Upon reaching a treatment facility, patients must have all their clothing removed if this has not already been done, and all the exposed areas must be cleansed with copious water lavage. Attendants should also be suitably protected and contaminated clothing must be placed in special bags.

Current treatment of vesicant agents centers around symptomatic relief. Itching can be treated with sedatives (benzodiazepines or phenothiazines), and antipruritic agents. Dimercaprol (British antilewisite), a chelating agent, is a specific antidote for lewisite poisoning. It is of note that it is incompatible with silver sulfadiazine. It is available as an ointment for skin lesions, as drops for eye applications (5–10% in oil), and in an intramuscular preparation for systemic toxicity. Other chelating agents are:

- DMSA – mesodimercaptosuccinic acid,
- DMPS – 2,3-dimercapto-1 propanesulfonic acid sodium, and
- DMPA – N-(2,3-dimercaptopropyl) phthalamidic acid.

These have a higher therapeutic index, are water soluble, and are effective orally. There is no specific antidote to mustard poisoning and no pretreatments or treatments exist that provide practical or effective protection against mustard toxicity.[39]

There are also no standardized methods for the treatment of mustard injury. For patients experiencing cutaneous injuries, erythema requiring more than 5% TBSA in non-critical areas (face, hands, perineum) require hospitalization. The systemic fluid derangement is less than that seen with thermal burns; however, patients should be carefully monitored. Fluid requirements in Iranian casualties during the Iran–Iraq war appeared to have been relatively independent of TBSA.

Blisters should be deroofed and dressed with topical antimicrobials. The mustard blister fluid is harmless.[40]

Favorable outcomes have now been demonstrated in the pig model by use of various debriding techniques and resurfacing with split-thickness skin grafts. Such methods have included laser,[41] dermabrasion,[42] sharp surgical excision,[43] and enzymatic debridement.[44]

Proposed strategies for the development of improved therapies have been discussed in detail by Graham et al.[45]

Affected eyes should be irrigated, treated with antibiotics, and inspected at the earliest time by an ophthalmologist. Respiratory injury requires symptomatic treatment according to its severity. Inhalation of high-dose steroids is controversial at present. Severe exposure will lead to agranulocytosis or aplastic anemia.[46] The pancytopenia seen after 7 days with the Iranian casualties did not appear to be helped by transfusion of relevant blood products. Bone marrow transplantation may prove useful, although of little practical value with large numbers of casualties. The effect of bone marrow stimulants such as oxymethalone and lithium carbonate is unknown but may be considered. Fluid replacement may be carried out dynamically with adequate cardiovascular monitoring. The maximum fluid loss occurs during blister formation and not necessarily in the first 24 hours.

Long-term effects of acute exposure

Individuals who sustain mustard injury may experience difficulties even after the initial effects of the injury have subsided. Destruction of melanocytes leaves hypopigmented areas, otherwise hyperpigmentation tends to predominate. Acute and severe exposure can also lead to chronic skin ulceration, scar formation and the development of skin cancer.

Recurrent or persistent corneal ulceration can occur after latent periods of 10–25 years. Chronic conjunctivitis and corneal clouding may accompany this delayed keratopathy.[47]

Clinical follow-ups on 200 Iranian soldiers who suffered injuries from mustard during the Iran–Iraq War indicate that about one third had experienced varied respiratory ailments, such as chronic bronchitis, asthma, recurrent pneumonia, bronchiectasis and even tracheobronchial stenosis, more than 2 years after exposure. Some 12% of all British soldiers exposed to mustard in World War I were awarded disability compensation for respiratory disorders believed to have been due to mustard exposures during combat.[48]

Summary

The vesicant agents are perhaps poorly named since they have the ability to affect all epithelial surfaces, particularly the eyes and respiratory surfaces, and not just the skin. The most important vesicant is sulfur mustard, which acts as an alkylating agent, causing a series of clinical reactions ranging from vesicles to severe skin necrosis. Systemic effects are seen with high doses and the combination of depressed bone marrow activity and respiratory involvement often proves fatal. There is no effective antidote, and treatment depends on prevention of contact and local therapy to achieve wound healing, which tends to be slow. There is no risk to the caregiver from the blister fluid which contains no active agent.

Mass burn casualties

Burn-injured patients should ideally be managed individually with treatment tailored to their personal needs. However with mass casualties, following monumental disasters, whether natural or otherwise, lack of experienced staff, paucity of equipment and insufficient time to perform all relevant tasks, may make this an impossible goal. Nevertheless, every medical facility should be prepared at a moment's notice to cope with such situations. The handling of mass casualties is not confined to hospitals and the success of medical support will depend on adequate planning. It is informative to consider past disasters where mass casualties have involved large numbers of burned patients.[49] These have fared badly over the last 30 years and have included the circus fires in Niteroi, Brazil[50] in 1961 and at Bangalore[51] in 1981, and the camping ground explosion in 1978 at Los Alfaques[52] where more than 400, 100, and 200 victims died, respectively. European disasters have been smaller but have included the Bradford Football Stand fire[53] in 1985, and the Ramstein Air Show disaster[54] in 1988. Clinical management must continue throughout the chain of evacuation and can be divided for descriptive purposes into that occurring at the site of injury, the receiving (trauma or accident and emergency) center and the specialist burns unit. At each site the overall management of large-scale burn disasters revolves around the three principles of triage, treatment and transport.

Principles of triage

Triage is the process by which casualties are sorted on the basis of treatment priorities. It must first facilitate the application of maneuvers that are lifesaving.[55] The ABCs of trauma management are carefully followed so that a patient with an airway or breathing problem takes priority over a patient with a circulatory disability. Remember, the overall severity of the injury is determined by the combined effect of different injuries. For instance, the priority of a 40% burn will be increased if there is an associated fracture which may contribute to overall fluid loss. In a mass casualty situation, the patient with the most severe injury or greatest threat to life is not necessarily the patient that receives first priority. Consideration must be given to likelihood of survival, to optimize available resources. Furthermore, if patients' needs exceed available resources (equipment and personnel) they may be given a lower priority for triage until the necessary resources are secured. It is important to note that the triage should be performed by the person with the greatest experience of the types of injuries expected.

Management

Clinical management must continue throughout the chain of evacuation and can be divided for descriptive purposes into

that occurring at the site of injury, the receiving (trauma or accident and emergency) center, and the specialist burns unit. At each site the overall management of large-scale burn disasters revolves around the three principles of triage, treatment and transport.

On site
Triage

Casualties at the site of the accident are triaged according to:

- The general condition of each patient, the extent and depth of the burn injuries and a patient's ambulatory status.
- Availability of facilities and personnel in the adjacent hospitals.

All patients undergoing triage must be adequately labeled. This will enable them to be identified according to their group. Large colored labels that are waterproof should be attached to each victim. The label will denote the triage group, treatment, drugs administered, and time given. Cases can be graded as follows:[56]

A. Ambulant patients with less then 10% burns — wounds are dressed and treatment is continued as an outpatient unless there is a reason for admission, i.e. extremes of age, deep burns requiring surgery, areas requiring special nursing.

B. 10–30% burns — after first aid these patients can be moved to distant hospitals initially, so as not to overload burn centers.

C. Serious burns involving 30–50% TBSA — these patients may be saved by energetic measures and should be transferred immediately to specialist centers for optimum treatment of shock and respiratory problems.

D. Patients with more than 50% TBSA burns, especially those with respiratory burns and the elderly, are unlikely to survive. These patients should be transferred to the nearest hospital but admitted to a separate ward.

In any disaster it is advisable to group similar injured casualties in the same installations. Certain hospitals near the disaster should be designated as 'burn centers' and all cases requiring immediate and intensive care should be sent to these institutions.

Treatment

At this level, treatment of casualties may be limited to maintenance of airway, management of respiratory problems, commencement of intravenous infusions, protection of the burn wound, and analgesia. Escharotomy should be carried out for full-thickness circumferential burns, and antitetanus prophylaxis given.

Transport

The transportation of the burned patient between the site of injury and the receiving hospital is known as primary transport. The initial call will reveal the location; the number of injuries; the approximate time of the incident. This information will aid in decisions regarding the personnel, vehicles, equipment, and protective clothing that must be sent. On arrival at the scene, vehicles must be parked where they are out of danger and not blocking essential access or exits.

Most burn patients can be safely transported provided that they are properly stabilized and accompanied by competent medical personnel. The patient's physiology should be monitored throughout the journey.[57] Treatment including additional analgesia must be continued en route as necessary. Transfer itself can exacerbate the existing deleterious physiological changes. The parameters that should be monitored continually during transfer are listed in Box 43.1.

Accepting hospital

Triage

Cases greater than 70% TBSA probably will not survive in the mass casualty situation. They should be made comfortable with adequate analgesia and sedation if thought necessary. They should be treated after patients in the more salvageable groups (see above).

Treatment

Mass nuclear casualties have been dealt with previously. When supplies and facilities are overloaded, compromises will be necessary. These are:

- Plasma and blood products are reserved for cases with associated trauma. Electrolyte solutions are effective in uncomplicated burns for the first 24 hours.
- Local wound care. Exposure method may be useful in this situation.
- Grafting. Lack of operating space may be a problem. Patients whose wounds can be covered by a single grafting procedure take priority to allow early discharge.

With larger burns temporary biological cover may be necessary until space becomes available.

Away from the site of the disaster, opportunity is taken to carry out the 'secondary survey', a full examination from head to foot. A full history is recorded and an assessment of the extent of the burn and associated injuries is included. A respiratory evaluation based clinically, together with arterial blood gases and fiberoptic bronchoscopy (if practical), enables an early decision on whether patients require intubation and ventilation. This decision can be made by analysis of frequent arterial PO_2 measurements on a constant FiO_2 to detect early shunting. A pulse oximeter may provide a more practical substitute for arterial catheterization.

If the casualty is unconscious, attention must be paid to the possibility of associated head and neck injury, pneumothorax

---

Box 43.1 Parameters to be monitored continually during patient transfer

- Respiratory rate and pattern
- Heart rhythm and rate
- Capillary refill time
- Blood pressure
- Level of consciousness
- Blood and fluid Loss
- Oxygen saturation
- Drugs and fluids administered

---

and carbon monoxide poisoning.[58] The burn wounds are then cleaned with a mild antiseptic solution and debrided. The extent and depth of burns are then estimated, which, together with the weight of the patient, can be used to guide intravenous fluid resuscitation along well-established formulas. Success is measured by careful cardiovascular monitoring, aiming to produce a urine output in the range of 0.5 mL/kg/h in adults and 1.0 mL/kg/h in children.

Ideally each patient should have their fluid requirements calculated on an individual basis. However, when large numbers of casualties are involved, problems can occur in applying the standard formulas.[59] To obviate this problem the Burns Calculator has been developed[60] to assist non-experienced personnel to prescribe fluid to adults and children over the first 8 hours.

Transport

Transfer from the receiving hospital to the burns unit is known as secondary transport; it is established that full assessment and resuscitation before moving the patient is invaluable in preventing cardiovascular and respiratory disasters.[61,62] A full examination may reveal other injuries, e.g. ruptured spleen, that could prove fatal if not diagnosed. Biochemical and hematological parameters are optimized. For example, abnormal potassium predisposes to arrhythmias. Equally, transferring a hypoxic patient increases the morbidity and mortality. Airway problems need managing definitively before transport. Any suggestion of airway involvement must alert the need for intubation. There is no place for intubated patients breathing spontaneously during transfer. Adequate analgesia, sedation, and muscle relaxation should be given so that pain, anxiety, or restlessness does not interfere with the clinical picture. Attention must be paid to the wound, the immobilization of fractures and need for escharotomy before transport is commenced. All the necessary drugs and equipment needed during transfer must be available. It is wise to assume that the journey time will be twice that normally encountered so that enough drugs and oxygen are available in case of delays. All documents, including drugs and fluids administered, must be taken with the patient. A contemporaneous record of events during the journey must be kept.

Tertiary referral center

At the burn center, the patient is reassessed. Physiological stabilization is obtained and those with lesser injuries may be transferred to peripheral hospitals with their treatment plan so as to reduce the strain on the facilities of the burn center. Similarly, cases found to require grafting at a later date can be sent back to the unit so that a two-way traffic is established. It is important that only those needing the tertiary center remain there. Transportation between tertiary referral centers is very similar to that already mentioned.[63]

Summary

In mass casualty situations involving burns, local resources may not be able to cope with the large and unexpected number of victims. The system is therefore so stressed that treatment must be prioritized. Patients with the most urgent needs are given the earliest care. This may differ from non-mass casualty situations in that the most critically injured may be placed in an expectant category, to allow resources to be distributed to as many victims as possible. The objective is to provide a protocol for assessment of injured patients, and transportation to appropriate hospital facilities.

Conclusion

Planning for mass casualties is important. Well-trained personnel, preset protocols, specialized transport, and adequate supplies of documents, drugs and equipment will ensure minimal mortality and proper use of facilities. Paradoxically, the threat of chemical and thermonuclear injury is heightened by the breakup of the Soviet Union, producing a glut of weapons specialists on the world employment market. Also small chemical industries can produce dangerous chemicals with ease and minimal cost. Healthcare workers serving a civilian population or military force have the obligation to learn the basics of management of radiation and chemical injury to achieve the greatest good for the greatest number of injured.

References

1. Daniel J. The x-rays. Science 1896; 3:562–563.
2. Hirsch EF, Bowers GJ. Irradiated trauma victims: the impact of ionizing radiation on surgical consideration following a surgical mishap. World J Surg 1992; 16:918.
3. Rubin P, Casarett GW. Clinical radiation pathology. Philadelphia: WB Saunders; 1968:15.
4. Luckett LW, Vesper BE. Radiological considerations in medical operations. In: Walker RI, Cerveny TJ, eds. Textbook of military medicine — medical consequences of nuclear warfare. Virginia: TMM, Office of The Surgeon General; 1989:227–244.
5. Hall EJ. Physics and chemistry of radiation absorption. In: Radiobiology for the radiologist. Maryland: Harper & Rowe; 1994:2–13.
6. Mettler FA, Kelsey CA. Fundamentals of radiation accidents. In: Mettler FA, Kelsey CA, Ricks RC, eds. Medical management of radiation accidents. Boca Raton: CRC; 1990:2.
7. DOE/REAC/TS Radiation Accident Registries, personal communication and unpublished data, November 2005.
8. Eisman B, Bond V. Surgical care of nuclear casualties. Surg Gynecolo Obstet 1978; 146:877–883.
9. A. Zimmerman PD. Dirty bombs: the threat revisited. Def Hor 2004; 38:1–11.
10. Lewis KN. The prompt and delayed effect of nuclear war. Sci Am 1979; 241(1):35–47.
11. Kelleher D. Acute effects of ionizing radiation. In: United States Navy, Royal Navy workshop on nuclear warfare combat casualty care. US Navy 1983:71–80.
12. Brooks JW, Evans EI, Han WT, et al. The influence of external body radiation on mortality from thermal burns. Ann Surg 1953; 136(3):533–534.
13. Glasstone S, Dolan PJ. The effects of nuclear weapons. United States Department of Defense and the United States Department of Energy; 1977:541–628.
14. Oughterson AW, Warren S. Medical effects of the atomic bomb in Japan. New York: McGraw-Hill; 1956.
15. Need JV. Update on the genetic effects of ionizing radiation. JAMA 1991; 32:698.
16. Nenot JC. Medical and surgical management for localized radiation injuries. Int J Radiat Biol 1990; 57:784.
17. Becker WK, Buescher TM, Cioffi WG, et al. Combined radiation and thermal injury after nuclear attack. In: Browne D, Weiss JF, MacVittie, et al., eds. Treatment of radiation injuries. New York: Plenum; 1990:10.
18. Hirsch EF, Bowers GJ. Irradiated trauma victims: the impact of ionizing radiation on surgical considerations following a nuclear mishap. World J Surg 1992; 16:918.
19. Radiation Injury. American Burn Association advanced burn life support course. provider's manual. Chicago, American College of Surgeons 1999:(Appendix 1)66.
20. Browne D, Weiss JF, MacVittie, et al. eds. Consensus summary: treatment of radiation injuries. New York: Plenum; 1990.
21. Walden TL, Farzaneh MS. Biological assessment of radiation damage. In: Walker RI, Cerveny TJ, eds. Textbook of military medicine — medical consequences of nuclear warfare. Virginia: TMM, Office of The Surgeon General; 1989:85–104.
22. Burke JF, Bondoc CC, Quinby WC. Primary burn excision and immediate grafting: a method shortening illness. J Trauma 1974; 14:389–395.
23. Gray D, Pine R, Harnar T, et al. Early surgical excision versus conventional therapy in patients with 20 to 40 percent burns. Am J Surg 1982; 189:147–151.
24. Dubos M, Neveux Y, Monpeyssin M, et al. Impact of ionizing radiation on response to thermal and surgical trauma. In: Walker RI, Gruber DF, MacVittie TJ, et al. eds. The pathophysiology of combined injury and trauma. Baltimore: University Park Press 1985: 19–25.
25. Kindwall EP. Hyperbaric oxygen's effect on radiation necrosis. Clin Plast Surg 1993; 20:473–483.
26. Herodin F, Drouet M. Cytokine-based treatment of accidentally irradiated victims and new approaches. Exp Hematol 2005; 33:1071–1080.
27. Waselenko JK, MacVittie TJ, Blakely WF, et al. Medical management of the acute radiation syndrome: recommendations of the Strategic National Stockpile Radiation Working Group. Ann Intern Med 2004; 140(12):1037–1051.
28. Dainiak N, Waselenlso JK, Armitage JO, et al. The hematologist and radiation casualties. Hematol 2003; 1:473–95 Online. Available at: http://www.asheducationbook.org/cgi/content/full/2003/1/473. Accessed March 15, 2005.
29. Sidell FR, Urbanetti JS, Smith WJ, et al. Vesicants. In: Zajtchuk R, Bellamy RF, eds. Textbook of military medicine — medical aspects of chemical and biological warfare. Washington DC: Office of The Surgeon General, Department of the Army; 1997: 197–228.
30. New York Times News service. 20 000 troops may have faced gas. The Sun 23 Oct 1996: A-1.
31. Eddington PG. Gassed in the Gulf, xiii pp. Washington: Insignia; 1997:72–82.
32. Papirmeister B, Feister AJ, Robinson SI, et al. Molecular mechanisms of cytotoxity. In: Medical defense against mustard gas: toxic mechanisms and pharmacological implications. Boca Raton: CRC; 1990:155–197.
33. Orrenius S, McConkey DJ, Nicotera P. Biochemical mechanisms of cytotoxity. Trends Pharmacol Sci Fest Suppl 1985; 15:18–20.
34. Somani SM. Toxicokinetics and toxicodynamics of mustard. In: Somani SM, ed. Chemical warfare. San Diego: Academic Press; 1992:13–45.
35. Willems JL. Clinical management of mustard gas casualties. Ann Med Milit (Belg) 1989; 3(Suppl):1–61.
36. Papirmeister B, Feister AJ, Robinson SI, et al. The sulfur mustard injury: description of lesions and resulting incapacitation. In: Medical defense against mustard gas: toxic mechanisms and pharmacological implications. Boca Raton: CRC; 1990:13–34.
37. Vesicants (blister agents), mustard and nitrogen mustards. In: NATO handbook on the medical aspects of NBS defensive operations. US. Washington DC: US Army, US Navy, US Air Force; 1984:3:12–15.
38. McManus J, Huebner K. Vesicants. Crit Care Clin 2005; 21(4):707–718.

39. Papirmeister B, Feister AJ, Robinson SI, et al. Pretreatments and therapies. In: Medical defense against mustard gas: toxic mechanisms and pharmacological implications. Boca Raton: CRC; 1990:243–287.

40. Sultzberger MB, Katz JH. The absence of skin irritants in the contents of vesicles. US Navy Med Bull 1943; 43:1258–1262.

41. Graham JS, Schomacker KT, Glatter RD, et al. Efficacy of laser debridement with autologous split-thickness skin grafting in promoting improved healing of deep cutaneous sulfur mustard burns. Burns 2002; 28(8):719–730.

42. Rice P. The use of dermabrasion to accelerate the naturally slow rate of epidermal healing mustard injuries in pigs. Proceedings of the 1995 NATO Research Study Group-3 Meeting on Prophylaxis and Therapy against Chemical Agents. CTC No. AD-B209142. Porton Down, Salisbury England: Chemical and Biological Defense Establishment; 1995.

43. Graham JS, Schomacker KT, Glatter RD, et al. Bioengineering methods employed in the study of wound healing of sulfur mustard burns. Skin Res Technol 2002; 8(1):57–59.

44. Eldad A, Weinberg A, Breitman S, et al. Early nonsurgical removal of chemically injured tissue enhances wound healing in partial-thickness burns. Burns 1988; 24(2):166–172.

45. Chilcott RP, Rice P, Milner SM, et al. Wound healing of cutaneous sulfur mustard injuries: strategies for the development of improved therapies. J Burns Wounds [serial line] 2005; 4(1):1. Online. Available at: url://www.journalofburnsandwounds.com

46. Anslow WP, Houck CR. Systemic pharmacology and pathology of sulfur and nitrogen mustards. In: Chemical warfare agents and related chemical problems. DTIC No AD-234–249. Summary technical report of division 9. Washington DC: National Defense Research Committee of the Office of Scientific Research and Development; 1946:Pts 3–4.

47. Blodi FC. Mustard gas keratopathy. Int Ophtalmol Clin 1971; 2:1.

48. Gilchrist HL. A comparative study of world war casualties from gas and other weapons. Washington DC: Government Printing Office; 1928.

49. Barclay TL. Planning for mass burns casualties. Royal Society of Medicine Services. Round Table series No 3. In: Wood C, ed. Accident and emergency burns: lessons from the Bradford disaster. Oxford: Alden; 1986:81–88.

50. Pitanguy I. Treatment of victims from the great catastrophe of the Gran Circus at Niteroi (Brazil). In: Wallace AB, Wilkinson AW, eds. Research in burns. Edinburgh: E & S Livingstone; 1966:216–221.

51. Das RAP. Circus fire at Bangalore. Burns 1983; 10:17–29.

52. Arturson G. The Los Alfaques disaster: a boiling liquid expanding vapour explosion. Burns 1981; 7:233–251.

53. Sharpe DT, Roberts AHN, Barclay TL, et al. Treatment of burns casualties after fire at Bradford City Football Club ground. Br Med J 1985; 291:945–949.

54. Seletz JM. Flugstag-88 (Ramstein Air Show Disaster): an Army response to a MASCAL. Mil Med 1990; 155:153–155.

55. Advanced Trauma Life Support for Doctors. Student course manual, 6th edn. Chicago: American College of Surgeons; 1997.

56. Low Chee AW. Mass casualty organisation in burn disasters. Med J Malaysia 1977; 31:349–352.

57. Edbrooke DL, John RE, Murray RJ. Transportation. In: Rylah LTA, ed. Critical care of the burned patient. Cambridge: Cambridge University Press; 1992.

58. Safar P, Pretto EA, Bircher NG. Resuscitation medicine involving the management of severe trauma. In: Baskett P, Weller R, eds. Medicine for disasters. London: John Wright; 1988:36–87.

59. Milner SM, Rylah LTA. Burn casualties in war: a simplified resuscitation protocol. Br J Hosp Med 1993; 50:163–167.

60. Milner SM, Hodgetts TJ, Rylah LTA. The Burns Calculator: a simple proposed guide for fluid resuscitation. Lancet 1993; 341:1089–1091.

61. Bion JF, Edlin SA, Ramsey G, et al. Validation of a prognostic score in critically ill patients undergoing transport. Brit Med J 1985; 291:432–434.

62. Ehrenworth J, Sorbo S, Hackel A. Transport of critically ill adults. Crit Care Med 1986; 14:534–537.

63. Ellis A, Rylah LTA. Transfer of the thermally injured patient. Br J Hosp Med 1990; 44:206–208.

Chapter 44

Exfoliative and necrotizing diseases of the skin

*Shawn Fagan, Marcus Spies, Maureen Hollyoak, Michael J. Muller,
Cleon W. Goodwin, and David N. Herndon*

Introduction

Acute, severe exfoliative, and necrotizing diseases of skin and underlying structures may cause significant morbidity in the afflicted patient. The problems associated with these diseases, such as wound infection, sepsis, adequate nutrition, and pain, are similar to those seen in patients with major burns. Burn centers provide expertise in the treatment and management of critically ill patients with skin loss from all causes, not solely from thermal injury. This chapter describes the pathophysiological processes of severe exfoliative skin disorders, their diagnosis, and the specialized treatment offered by burn units.

Severe exfoliative disorders

Erythema multiforme minor (EM), Stevens–Johnson syndrome (SJS), and toxic epidermal necrolysis (TEN) are severe exfoliative diseases of skin and mucous membranes. There is great controversy on the classification of these exfoliative skin disorders and the terminology is confusing. Erythema multiforme minor is characterized by skin lesions isolated to no more than one mucosal surface. Erythema multiforme major involves two of more mucous membranes and may affect internal organs with systemic symptoms. However, most authors consider erythema multiforme major, SJS, and TEN to be the same disease entity, differing only by the area of involved skin. In this classification, SJS is considered to affect less than 10% total body surface area (TBSA), whereas TEN covers greater than 30% TSBA, leaving a zone of overlap between 10 and 30% TBSA, which is referred to as SJS/TEN.[1,2] The most common characteristics of these disease entities are defined in Table 44.1.[3,4] The incidence of TEN is estimated at 0.4–1.2 cases per million persons per year. The incidence of SJS has been reported to be 1–7 cases per million persons per year.[5–9] These exfoliative disorders occur in all age groups; however, the incidence is increased in the elderly and females.[3,10–13] In addition, TEN is seen more often in patients with HIV infection[14] and in bone marrow transplant recipients.[15] Mortality of TEN ranges from 25 to 80%. However, reports are variable and usually based only on small patient populations.[16–18] Death may occur early in the course of the disease, with sepsis being the most frequent cause. *Pseudomonas aeruginosa* and *Staphylococcus aureus* are the predominant organisms involved.[16] Pulmonary embolism and gastrointestinal hemorrhage are other causes of death.[10,16] The prognosis of SJS/TEN is worse than that of a burn victim with the same extent of skin loss.[16] Mortality is increased significantly in those patients at the extremes of age, and in relation to the percentage of denuded skin and serum urea nitrogen levels.[16,19] SJS is associated with a mortality rate of 0–38%.[11,20] Erythema multiforme rarely causes death.[20]

Etiology

TEN and SJS both appear to be caused by immunological reactions to foreign antigens. TEN, as the more severe entity, has a much higher percentage associated with antecedent drug therapy. Drugs are implicated in 77–94% of cases of TEN.[6,21] Antibacterials and antifungals (36%), anticonvulsants (24%), analgesics and nonsteroidal anti-inflammatory agents (38%), and even corticosteroids (14%) have been implicated.[21,22] Attempts to identify drugs suspected of having caused exfoliative necrolysis by skin test and laboratory tests seldom have been rewarding.[16] Upper respiratory tract infections, pharyngitis, otitis media, or viral illness are frequently reported.[10–12,23–25] *Mycoplasma pneumoniae* and herpes viruses (cytomegalovirus, Epstein–Barr virus, herpes simplex, and varicella zoster) have been implicated in the cause of EM and SJS, but not TEN.[11,26,27] It can be difficult to differentiate some prodomal symptoms as due to viral or other infectious agents, or due to the primary disease process. Recently, the incidence of HIV infection in patients with toxic epidermal necrolysis has risen.[14,28] Whether this increase is due to their immunocompromised state or to the increased prescription of high-risk drugs, particularly sulfonamides, is debated. No history of drug ingestion or preceeding illness may be noted in these patients. Many of these cases may actually suffer from lack of patient recall of current medication because of the severity of the underlying disease or the patient's age. Idiopathic cases, not related to drugs, accounted for only 3–4% of TEN.[6,7]

Morphology/histopathology

An early skin biopsy is essential for diagnosis. Skin manifestations vary from patient to patient and with the age of the lesion (Figure 44.1). Skin lesions may evolve to different stages of development with recurrent attacks of EM in a single patient.[29]

TABLE 44.1 CHARACTERISTICS OF ERYTHEMA MULTIFORME, SJS, AND TEN

	Erythema multiforme	Stevens–Johnson syndrome	Toxic epidermal necrolysis
Prodrome	Absent	High fever, malaise	High fever, malaise
Acute phase	4–8 days	4–8 days Sensation of skin burning or tenderness	Sudden onset, 1–2 days Sensation of skin burning or tenderness
Skin lesions	Symmetrical, primarily located on the extremities, some target lesions without blisters	Variable distribution, individual vesicles on an erythematous base <10% TBSA Nikolsky's positive	Diffuse generalized epidermal detachment, absence of target lesions, large confluent plaques >30% TBSA Nikolsky's positive
Mucosal involvement	Limited to one surface, usually oral	Severe, two or more surfaces involved	Severe, two or more surfaces involved
Histopathology	Dermoepidermal separation, mononuclear perivascular cell infiltrate, small areas of epidermal detachment associated with target lesions	Dermoepidermal separation, more intense dermal infiltrate, areas of epidermal detachment	Epidermal necrosis, dermoepidermal separation, minimal dermal inflammatory infiltrate, large areas of epidermal detachment
Recovery	1–4 weeks	1–6 weeks	1–6 weeks
Mortality	0%	0–38%	25–80%

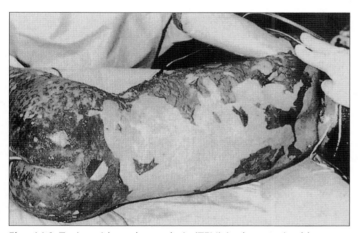

Fig. 44.1 Toxic epidermal necrolysis (TEN) is characterized by massive sloughing of the epidermal tissue.

Advancing edges of the target lesions show scattered necrotic keratinocytes in the epidermis and only mild dermal inflammation. In older lesions and central zones of target lesions, the dusky appearance corresponds to areas of extensive keratinocyte necrosis, often with the formation of subepidermal bullae and dermoepidermal separation. The surrounding erythematous zone shows papillary dermal edema, vascular dilation with endothelial cell swelling, and perivascular mononuclear cell infiltrate.[13] Extravasated erythrocytes may be seen in the surrounding papillary dermis. The reticular dermis is normal.

Epidermal and dermoepidermal suppressor/cytotoxic T-lymphocytes in addition to dermal infiltrates of helper T-lymphocytes have been demonstrated.[30–32] Hertl has confirmed that these epidermal cells are cytotoxic T-cells.[33] Langerhans cells appear to be reduced in the epidermis, although numerous dermal macrophages are observed.[34] A more intense dermal cell infiltrate is present in SJS, especially in postherpetic cases.[26,30] Dendritic lymphoid cells are observed, opposed to damaged dermal macrophages and necrotic keratinocytes. Further, at the point where the cytoplasmic processes contact the keratinocyte, the plasma membrane of the keratinocyte is absent.[34] Aberrant expression of HLA-DR on keratinocytes has been observed, a phenomenon which has been observed in many other inflammatory skin disorders.[31,35]

Immunofluorescence microscopy has demonstrated IgM and C3 along the dermoepidermal junction and dermal vessels in cases of postherpetic SJS and EM.[26,30] There have been only two reports of basal cell immunofluroscence in TEN.[34,36] The pathogenesis of TEN is not completely understood. Type IV delayed hypersensitivity reaction, type II cytotoxic reaction, keratinocyte cytotoxicity mediated by lymphocytes, drug-related nonimmunological mechanisms, and keratinocyte apoptosis mediated by receptors of the TNF superfamily are possible mechanisms which amplify predisposing factors of infection and genetic susceptibility.[14,37–39] Positive patch tests in patients with TEN have been used to support the delayed hypersensitivity hypothesis.[32] This view is somewhat at odds with the fact that HIV patients display increased frequency of TEN.[14,40]

Suppression/cytotoxic T-cell infiltrates are observed in the epidermis in TEN[32,34] and graft versus host disease.[41] It is hypothesized that cytotoxic T-cells recognize drug metabolites which are complexed with the MHC-I molecule on the surface of keratinocytes, migrate into the epidermis, react with keratinocytes, and cause epidermal necrolysis. The occurrence of sicca syndromes in patients with TEN and graft versus host disease further supports the autoimmune theory.[42] The observation of blebbing of the keratinocyte plasma membrane in TEN is considered a reliable morphological finding of cytotoxic T-lymphocyte cytolysis.[34] Further, the observation that cyclophosphamide aids TEN patients supports this theory, as cyclophosphamide is known to inhibit cytotoxic T-lymphocyte activity.[34] Type II cytotoxic reactions involve the binding of either IgG or IgM antibodies to a cell-bound antigen. The antigen–antibody complex then activates the complement cascade and results in the cell destruction. This mechanism is not generally supported since nuclear fragmentation, common to keratinocytes of toxic epidermal necrolysis patients, is not a consequence of complement-mediated cytolysis.[34,36,43] Keratinocyte apoptosis as the primary mechanism in the pathogenesis of TEN has been favored recently.[38] This event is thought to be mediated by ligand/receptor interaction of the tumor necrosis factor (TNF) superfamily (as TNFα/TNFreceptor or FasL/Fas interaction).[38,44] In SJS, keratinocyte DNA fragmentation has been found in about 90% of cases associated with dermal perforin-positive lymphocytes.[39] Nonimmunological mechanisms include keratinocyte injury by either drug, drug metabolite, or toxic products derived from a drug in the epidermis.[14,28,45]

Clinical features

A prodromal phase of TEN/SJS is identified frequently and usually consists of low-grade fever, malaise, and cough, all of which may suggest a respiratory tract infection. These symptoms may precede any cutaneous manifestation by 1–21 days, but usually last for 2–3 days.[2,11] Additionally, patients may present with conjunctivitis, sore throat, and generalized, tender erythema. This may evolve from morbilliform eruptions or discrete erythematous or purpuric macules.[37] Later, vesicles and large bullae emerge from areas of erythema. Patients may exhibit diffuse red erythema immediately followed by epidermolysis.[16] On light digital pressure, the epidermis desquamates in sheets: Nikolsky's sign is positive (Figure 44.2). Generally, a lag period of 1–3 weeks is observed from initiation of drug until skin eruption, which may be shorter on reexposure of a previously sensitized individual.[1,2]

Two or more areas of mucosa involvement are typical of SJS or TEN. Mucosal involvement precedes skin lesions by 1–3 days in one-third of cases.[13,46] Several sites are usually affected, in the following order of frequency: oropharynx, ocular, genitalia, and anus. Most TEN patients have multiple mucosal lesions, and they generally persist longer than cutaneous lesions.[16]

Complications

Toxic epidermal necrolysis is frequently associated with serious complications. The skin re-epithelializes from the dermal elements without scarring. Some patients experience hemodynamic instability and shock, and secondary full-thickness necrosis of the skin may develop; however, abnormal pigmentation is common (Figure 44.3). Nail plates are frequently lost and nail regrowth may be abnormal or absent.[13] Mucosal membrane erosions may result in cicatricial lesions causing phimosis in men and vaginal synechiae in women. Oropharyngeal involvement is common and often results in severe dysphagia[47] (Figure 44.4). Although mucocutaneous erosions are the most common features of TEN/SJS, the disease may present with multisystem involvement. The onset of intestinal symptoms generally occurs concurrently with the cutaneous lesions.[48] Epidermal and epithelial sloughing may extend into the gastro-

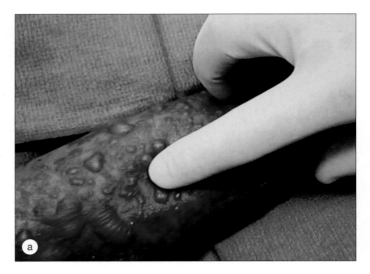

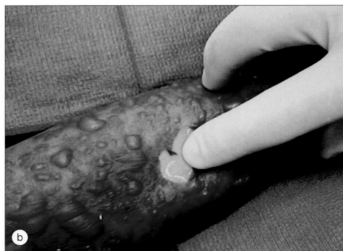

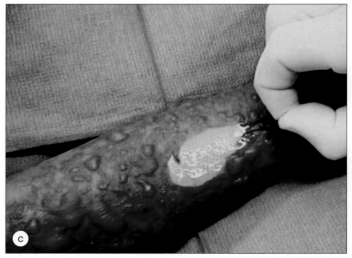

Fig. 44.2 (a–c) Nikolsky's sign. Epidermal separation induced by gentle pressure on the skin surface.

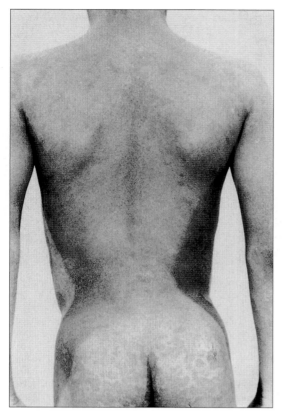

Fig. 44.3 One-year post-TEN, wounds are completely closed with minimum of residual scarring but with abnormal pigmentation.

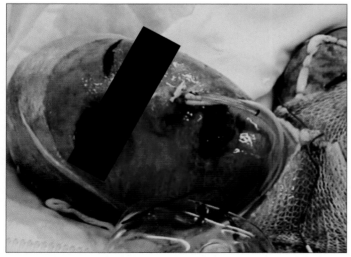

Fig. 44.4 TEN patient demonstrating significant oropharangeal involvement. (Arrows demonstrate membraneous conjunctivitis.)

intestinal mucosa, and may induce esophagitis with frequent subsequent stricture formation.[45] Gastrointestinal erosions macroscopically resemble ulcerative or pseudomembranous colitis and massive hemorrhage requiring resection has been reported.[10,16,23] Intestinal involvement worsens the prognosis.[16,48] Respiratory tract involvement occurs and is associated

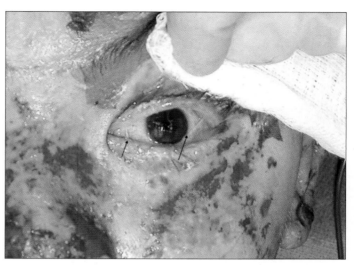

Fig. 44.5 Ocular involvement in TEN is common and can lead to blindness. Early and aggressive ocular care must be intiated to prevent pseudomembranes.

with increased mortality.[47,49] These complications include diffuse erythema to extensive confluent tracheal and bronchial erosion covered by fibrinous exudate.[37,47] Epiglottal swelling, necessitating intubation, has been reported.[47] Desquamation of alveolar lining cells also has been reported and these patients require frequent tracheobronchial toilet.[48] Subclinical interstitial edema is often noticed and 30% of cases progress to frank pulmonary edema and respiratory decompensation.[13,50] Bronchopneumonia was found to be the most frequent complication, occurring in 50% of patients.[20,23,49] Pulmonary embolism is an important cause of death in patients with TEN.[16] Renal manifestations like glomerulonephritis and acute tubular necrosis,[51] as well as hepatitis and hepatocellular necrosis, have been described.[13,37] Hypoalbuminemia, increased erythrocyte sedimentation rate, leukocytosis, thrombocytopenia, and normochromic and normocytic anemia are common.[20,47] Leukopenia is a frequent and poor prognostic sign.[12,13,16,23] This is due, in part, to depletion of the T-helper/inducer lymphocyte population (CD4+).[52] Ocular sequelae are the most severe long-term complications and occur in half of the survivors. Pseudomembranous or membranous conjunctivitis resulting from coalesced fibrin and necrotic debris can lead to opacification, secondary infection, and blindness[4] (Figure 44.5). Conjunctival scarring may result in lacrimal duct destruction, leading to reduced tear production and keratoconjunctivitis siccal, a Sjögren-like syndrome. Ectropion, entropion, trichiasis, and symblepharon can also occur.[11,42]

Management

Toxic epidermal necrolysis is a life-threatening disease and such a patient is best managed in an intensive care burn unit where vigorous fluid resuscitation, nutritional support, wound care, physical therapy, and social services are provided routinely in a multidisciplinary team approach.[10,12,17,18,23,24,37]

Surgical approach

Debridement of necrotic epidermis and coverage of the large wound surface with biological or synthetic dressings are essential.[10,53–55] Sloughed epidermis should be removed in order to reduce bacterial growth and the risk for infection. The exposed and tender dermis should be covered. Debridement is best undertaken under general anesthesia as soon as diagnosis by histology is established. Blood loss associated with debridement is minimal, so over-resuscitation must be avoided. Synthetic dressings, such as Biobrane™, and biological dressings, such as homograft (cadaver allograft) and porcine xenograft skin, greatly reduce the pain, decrease fluid loss, promote healing, and reduce the risk of wound infection and sepsis (Figure 44.6).[10,53–56] Biobrane™ is readily available as a commercial shelf product; however, in our own experience it is associated with increased local infection when covering greater than 40% TBSA wound areas (Figure 44.7). Porcine xenograft adheres well to the skin and is commercially available in large quantities.[54,55] Homograft is more likely to become vascularized and therefore reduces the number of graft changes.[10,57] However, this must be weighed against the potential poor cosmetic results of vascularized homograft (Figure 44.8). Grafted areas must be immobilized and protected from shear forces. In children, Steinmann pins to suspend extremities may be useful.[54] In both adults and children, continuous rotation or air fluidized (Clinitron) beds frequently are used.

Topical therapy

As separation occurs at the dermal–epidermal junction, varying depths of viable dermis remain. If this dermis can be protected from toxic detergents, desiccation, mechanical trauma, and wound infection, then rapid re-epithelialization by proliferation of basal keratinocytes from the skin appendages will occur.[53] However, bacterial proliferation on the unprotected wound surface with invasive infection leads to full-thickness skin necrosis. Hydrotherapy and topical antimicrobials provide debridement and infection control which should be initiated early in the course of the disease.[11,25] Effective topical antimicrobial agents include silver sulfadiazine cream,[29] silver nitrate solution,[13,23,25] chlorhexidine gluconate solution,[13] and polymyxin-bacitracin ointment.[11] Silver sulfadiazine is widely used but may exacerbate the disease process

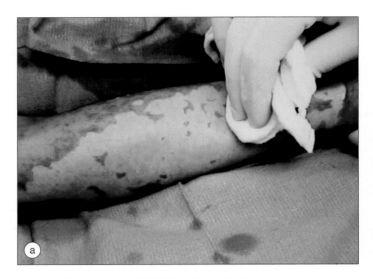

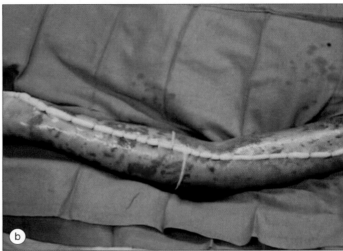

Fig. 44.7 Application of Biobrane™ to left upper extremity after debridement of TEN patient.

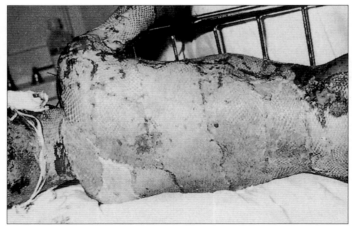

Fig. 44.6 As with many partial-thickness wounds, biological dressings do much to encourage re-epithelialization and reduce the pain associated with these wounds.

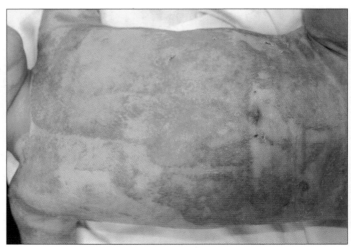

Fig. 44.8 Homograft vascularization occurring over a second-degree thermal injury, resulting in a poor cosmetic result.

due to its sulfonamide component. Additionally, an inhibitory effect on epithelialization and leukopenia requiring discontinuation has been observed. Silver nitrate solution does not contribute to the ongoing drug reaction, and epithelialization is not inhibited. However, silver nitrate solutions are hyponatremic, and thus associated with approximately 350 mmoles of sodium loss per day per meter square treated. Therefore, serum electrolytes and osmolarity must be carefully monitored. For patients with contaminated wounds due to delayed initiation of treatment, silver nitrate soaks can reduce contamination and prepare the wound for eventual biological dressing. Chlorhexidine gluconate and polymyxin ointment are effective against Gram-negative organisms, including *P. aeruginosa*, with low incidence of sensitivity. Moreover, chlorhexidine gluconate also shows bactericidal effects against Gram-positive organisms.

Immunomodulation therapy

As mentioned previously, the pathophysiology of TEN appears to be initiationally immunologic. Therefore it is logical to consider immunosuppressive therapy as an early treatment modality for TEN. The following sections will briefly review the literature with regards to use of corticosteroids, cyclosporine A, intravenous immunoglobins, and thalidomide.

Corticosteroid therapy

Corticosteroid treatment of toxic epidermal necrolysis has promoted much controversy. In regard to the delayed hypersensitivity reaction or antibody-dependent cytotoxicity theories of pathogenesis, corticosteroids would seem to be an appropriate form of medical therapy.[37,58] However, the practice of administering continuous high-dose corticosteroid in an attempt to stop the progression of the disease is widely rejected.[11–13,37,41,45,59,60] Rational assessment of the benefit of corticosteroids administration is not possible due to the lack of randomized, controlled, prospective trials. Many authors feel that steroids enhance the risk of sepsis,[23,54] increase protein catabolism, delay wound healing,[16] cause severe gastrointestinal bleeding,[16,23] prolong hospitalization,[60] and increase mortality.[12,23,61] Lyell states that the indication for the use of steroids in the treatment of toxic epidermal necrolysis is vague.[45]

One study found no decrease in the progression of SJS with steroids, but instead found significant morbidity.[61] In a prospective, although not randomized, study, increased survival (66%) was seen in matched patients who did not receive steroids compared to only 33% survival in those who did receive steroids.[23] Pediatric SJS patients treated with steroids had a longer hospital stay and a complication rate of 74% compared to 28% in those without steroids.[60] Another study demonstrated 80% mortality associated with steroid therapy, which was reduced to 20% when steroids were withheld.[12] In several studies, patients with antecedent glucocorticoid therapy before the onset of TEN showed no significant survival benefit,[62,63] and corticosteroid use itself has been linked to an increased risk for developing TEN.[22] Currently, the body of evidence suggests that the treatment of TEN with corticosteroids has no significant benefit and may in fact be detrimental.[59,64] Therefore corticosteroids cannot be recommended in the treatment of TEN.

Cyclosporin A

Cyclosporin A is an agent that has the properties of both being a powerful immunosuppressant and antiapoptotic. The mechanism of action is inhibition of the synthesis of interleukin-2 by selective inhibition of calcineurin, thus arresting the proliferation of T helper cells. To date, there have been nine individual cases and one case series of the use of cyclosporin A in the treatment of TEN.[65] In the only case series, Arevalo et al. observed a significantly shorter time to disease arrest (24–36 hours) and time to re-epithelialization when compared to historical controls.[65] Although intriguing, the currently published studies do not have similar methodologies, varying with regards to the dosage administered, route of administration, and duration of therapy. Furthermore, cyclosporin A therapy has been associated with a septicemia rate of 55%.[64] Therefore; a well-performed prospective clinical trail is warranted prior to advocating the use of cyclosporin A in the treatment of TEN.

Intravenous immunoglobulin

It has been suggested that the Fas-Fas ligand interaction may be responsible for the apoptosis seen in TEN.[66] Through a series of experiments, Viard et al. observed, *in vitro*, that TEN patients expressed lytically active Fas ligand and that the action of this ligand could be blocked by both a monoclonal antibody and human immunoglobins.[67] These observations suggest that human immunoglobins may contain a Fas blocking antibody and therefore may be useful in the treatment of TEN. Unfortunately, clinical data are less impressive, with some case series suggesting a benefit while others demonstrate less encouraging results.[66–70] As in the case with cyclosporin A, a controlled multicenter clinical trail is required prior to advocating the use of human immunoglobins routinely in the treatment of TEN.

Thalidomide

The primary mechanism in the pathogenesis of TEN is keratinocyte apoptosis. Accordingly, tumor necrosis factor A has been implicated in the pathogenesis of TEN. Thalidomide, a potent inhibitor of tumor necrosis factor A, would appear to be a logical therapeutic agent in the treatment of TEN. Unfortunately, Wolkenstein et al. had to prematurely terminate a randomized clinical trail of thalidomide versus placebo in the treatment of TEN due to excess mortality in the treatment group. Ten of 12 patients expired in the thalidomide group compared to 3 of 10 in the control group. The authors theorized that thalidomide may have paradoxically increased the production of tumor necrosis factor in the treatment group, a previously reported phenomenon of thalidomide administration. Therefore, thalidomide as a treatment for TEN should not be initiated, owing to the detrimental effects, but does demonstrate the usefulness of randomized, double-blinded, placebo-controlled clinical trails.

Until these treatment modalities have proven their efficacy in controlled trials, the gold standard of treatment for TEN patients consists of a multidisciplinary approach, such as used in severe burns, focusing on wound care, infection control, and prevention of complications. The specific requirements of these patients are best met in an intensive burn care unit, so early referral to a burn center is strongly recommended. Guidelines for the transfer decision may rely on the referral criteria for severe burn injury established by the American Burn Association (see also algorithm in Figure 44.9). The multidisciplinary burn team for specialized treatment of patients with extensive skin loss with trained critical care physicians, surgeons, critical care nursing specialists, respiratory therapists, and physical and occupational therapists is able to provide the best acute care as well as early and adequate rehabilitation.

General management

Drugs suspected of having initiated the disease should be discontinued immediately. Administration of pain medication is of high priority and antipyretic agents may be required. The empirical use of broad-spectrum antibiotics may be necessary if neutropenia exists, as these patients are prone to septic complications. The white blood cell count generally returns to normal levels after 2–5 days. The cause of this immunosuppression is unclear; it may be part of the primary disease or a secondary event.[58] Neutropenia is the only complication in which 'prophylactic' antibiotics are indicated. Otherwise, systemic antibiotics only should be used for documented infections or suspected sepsis. Oral nystatin prevents intestinal overgrowth of *Candida* and decreases the risk of *Candida* sepsis.[23,58] Frequent monitoring of urinary tract, respiratory tract, skin, and catheters allows early detection of systemic infection and identification of organisms.

Intravenous replacement of fluid losses through the exposed body surface is required. However, as patients do not develop the massive edema and fluid losses evident in burn patients, fluid resuscitation formulas commonly employed in the management of thermal injuries overestimate the actual need.[13,37,53–55] Ringer's lactate solution is given at a rate determined by close monitoring of the patient's condition and urine output. Once wound coverage is accomplished, fluid requirements usually decrease. Central line placement should be avoided, if possible, to reduce the risk of infection and sepsis.

To further minimize this risk, lines should be placed in areas of uninvolved skin. Invasive devices are removed as soon as possible, and oral and nasogastric routes are utilized at earliest convenience. Environmental temperature should be raised to 30–32°C to reduce metabolic energy expenditure. Heat shield and infrared lamps are beneficial in patients' rooms, bathrooms, and operating rooms.

Stress ulceration prophylaxis is advisable. Mouth erosion, resulting in severe dysphagia, can be alleviated by the use of viscous lidocaine or cocaine rinses, and thus ease oral administration of nutrients and fluids. Oral debris should be removed and the mouth sprayed with antiseptic several times a day.[59] Pulmonary involvement requires close supervision, with careful toileting including bronchoscopy, incentive spirometry, mobilization, and coughing to prevent infections and complications. If mechanical ventilatory support is necessary, the prevention of bronchopulmonary infection gains even more importance. Daily monitoring by blood assessment, including blood gas analysis, chest x-ray, and bacteriological culture, are required to initiate timely antibiotic therapy or ventilatory support. Measures to prevent thromboembolism, such as low-dose or low-molecular-weight administration of heparin, should be instituted on admission.

Ocular involvement should be assessed daily by an ophthalmologist. Conjunctival crusting can be minimized by the application of saline eye drops every hour. Any adhesions should be broken using a blunt instrument, and bland eye drops or ointment applied frequently.[11,53] Documented ocular infections are treated with organism-specific antibiotic therapy. After recovery, special ophthalmological follow-up is needed to prevent and address ocular long-term sequelae. Lacrimal duct obstruction may be detected early by performing Schirmer's test.[11,59]

During hospitalization, patients with TEN and SJS may demonstrate limitations in mobility, decreased strength, postural and gait deviation, contractures, and impaired coordination. Therefore, patients should be treated and closely followed throughout the course of the disease by a physiotherapist.[64]

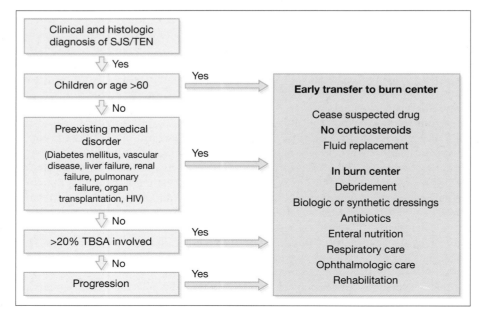

Fig. 44.9 Algorithm for management of SJS/TEN.

Nutritional support

Enteral nutrition should be started on admission. Due to the frequent presence of oral mucosal ulcerations, patients may be reluctant to take nutrition orally, and thus require a nasogastric tube placement. Unlike burned patients who have significantly elevated metabolic rate, these patients appear to have metabolic rates only slightly above basal requirements.[53,58] Weight stabilization and a positive nitrogen balance have been achieved in adults with 2500 kcal/day.[53] If gastrointestinal function becomes impaired or sepsis intervenes, requirements may increase. Total parenteral nutrition should be avoided, but initiated if enteral intolerance persists.

Skin and soft-tissue infections

Staphylococcal scalded skin syndrome, necrotizing fasciitis, and purpura fulminans are examples of a group of conditions characterized by extensive soft-tissue loss, rapid onset of critical illness, and death. Early, accurate diagnosis is essential to initiate appropriate action, such as extensive surgical excision in the case of necrotizing fasciitis or crepitant soft-tissue infections. Burn care centers with their acute and reconstructive capacities have much to offer these patients with extensive skin loss.

Staphylococcal scalded skin syndrome

Staphylococcal scalded skin syndrome is the severe condition caused by exfoliative staphylococcal toxins and is characterized by systemic signs and symptoms and generalized involvement of the skin (Figure 44.10). It is important to make a diagnosis early, particularly to differentiate it from TEN, which has a different management and much greater mortality. Staphylococcal scalded skin syndrome is predominantly a disease of infancy (Ritter's disease) and early childhood, with most cases occurring before the age of 5 years.[71] Newborn nurseries are often the sites of outbreaks. Attendant staff may be infected or colonized with *Staphylococcus aureus* strains producing epidermolytic toxin, thus emphasizing the importance of standard hygienic measures. Adult staphylococcal scalded skin syndrome is rare and usually associated with compromised renal function. Mortality is generally only 4%, but can be much higher in adults (40%) depending on underlying diseases.[71,72]

Two distinct epidermolytic toxins (ETA and ETB), are responsible for the blistering in staphylococcal scalded skin syndrome.[45] ETA is heat-stabile, whereas ETB is heat-labile and encoded by a bacterial plasmid. Most toxigenic strains of *S. aureus* are identified as group 2 phage.[73] The exfoliative toxin is metabolized and excreted by the kidneys, leading to a predisposition of patients with renal immaturity (children) or renal compromise. The exfoliative toxins produce blistering by disrupting the epidermal granular cell layers through interdesmosomal splittings but without epidermal necrosis and with very few inflammatory cells. The exact mechanism of action of the toxins has not been determined, although it is felt that the toxins directly affect desmosomes. One might be proteolytic disruption of desmosomes with the toxin or part of its sequence acting as a serine protease.[71,74,75]

Diagnosis of staphylococcal scalded skin syndrome can be made rapidly with a skin biopsy. The characteristic intraepi-

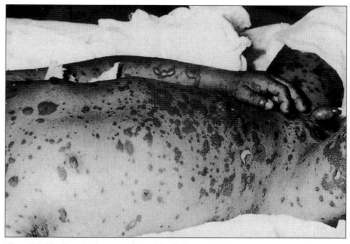

Fig. 44.10 Staphylococcal scalded skin syndrome is characterized by diffuse, erythematous lesions with bullae formation (see left forearm). Epidermis is shed in sheets with minimal abrasion. The wounds are partial-thickness and heal without surgical intervention.

dermal level of splitting is seen, with the split occurring at the granular layer level (stratum granulosum) with no epidermal necrosis or inflammatory cells in the corium.[73] Immunofluorescent studies of the skin are negative.[73] A Tzanck preparation from a scraping of the base of a freshly denuded area will reveal the affected cell population, i.e. acanthocytic keratinocytes.[73] Bullae, denuded skin and blood are usually sterile, however, and staphylococci can usually be cultured from nares, conjunctiva, or pharynx.[76]

Management

Onset may be marked by fever, malaise, and irritability. Scarlatiniform erythema is often accentuated in flexural and periorificial areas.[71] The skin is generally tender to touch, and sheets of skin may peel away in response to minor trauma (Nikolsky's sign). Blisters appear within 24–48 hours of rupture, leaving a characteristic moist erythematous epidermal base. Severe mucosal involvement is not a typical feature. With diagnosis antibiotics should be started, and semisynthetic penicillinase-resistant penicillin analogs are indicated (e.g. methicillin or oxacillin), since the majority of group 2 staphylococci show resistance to penicillin. Administration of steroids to these patients is contraindicated.[73] After screening for colonization, decontamination of colonized areas, especially the nasopharyngeal region in patients and nursing staff, may be advisable to prevent further spread. Fluid resuscitation is usually required at a lesser volume compared to a burn patient with a similar involved body surface area. Fluid substitution should be guided by urine output, hemodynamic parameters, electrolyte, and colloid status.

Until skin barrier function is restored, patients should receive appropriate wound dressings to prevent secondary wound infection. Topical agents are soothing and bacteriostatic. It needs to be pointed out that the wound initially is not colonized or infected, so alternatively, large areas can be more effectively managed with biological or synthetic dressings. They have the advantage of eliminating the need for frequent dressing changes which can be particularly traumatic for young children. Mortality usually is low, but may occur in very young and adult patients, usually from sepsis or electrolyte imbalance on the basis of underlying disease.[73] Complete wound healing is usually observed within 7 days, and scarring and altered pigmentation are not common.

Necrotizing fasciitis and bacterial myonecrosis

Necrotizing fasciitis is a soft-tissue infection which is characterized by widespread necrosis of fascia and subcutaneous tissue which may progress to muscle and skin necrosis. Overall mortality may still be as high as 50%.[72,77] Most cases of necrotizing fasciitis are due to polymicrobial infection including both anaerobic Gram-positive cocci and Gram-negative bacilli.[77] *Streptococcus, Staphylococcus, Enterococcus*, and *Bacteroides* are commonly found. Infection with many bacterial species may result in bacterial myonecrosis. However, gas gangrene by *Clostridia* spp. results in severe systemic toxicity and higher mortality than necrotizing fasciitis. A deep contaminated wound frequently preceeds the severe soft-tissue infection. Streptococcal myositis has a mortality rate of between 80 and 100%.[78] Risk factors for both necrotizing fasciitis and bacterial myonecrosis have been identified as diabetes mellitus, intravenous drug use, age greater than 50 years, hypertension, and malnutrition/obesity. The presence of three or more of these risk factors was found to give a predictive mortality rate of 50%[79] (see Figure 44.11).

Diagnosis

Early diagnosis is of extreme importance and consequence. Initial presentation is deceptive as the findings may be localized pain and edema without discoloration of the skin. Later, induration and erythema may be evident. Paresthesia of overlying skin and eventual dusky discoloration and local blistering may occur in the later course. Severe toxemia may develop, usually out of proportion to the local signs. Severe systemic alterations are characteristic of myonecrosis. Gas inclusion may be evident in subcutaneous tissues on x-ray. CT and MRI may help in the diagnosis and provide information on the nature and extent of the infection.[80] Frozen section biopsies may provide early histological evidence of infection.[81] Gram stains and microbiological testing are very important diagnostic tools and guide antibiotic treatment. However, a definite distinction between necrotizing fasciitis, myonecrosis, and other soft-tissue infections often can only be established during surgery.

Management

The key to successful management of necrotizing infections is early diagnosis and radical surgical intervention. Surgical exploration involves complete excision of all necrotic tissues. If more than one operation for debridement of infected necrotic tissue is needed, mortality increases from 43 to 71%; this outcome drastically highlights the importance of adequate initial necrosectomy.[82] In patients with many risk factors, early amputation of the extremity, especially in cases of myonecro-

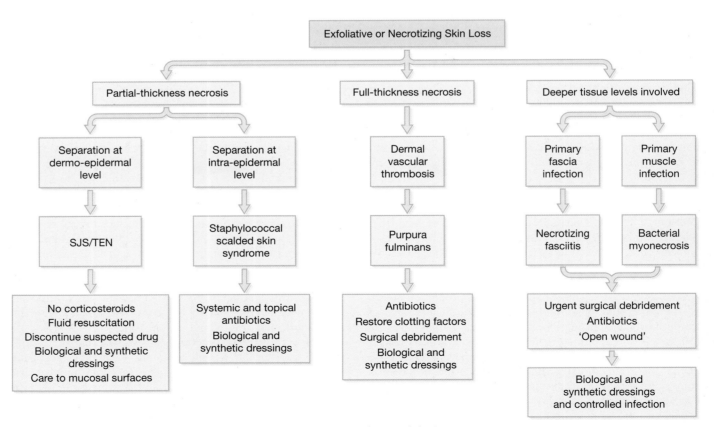

Fig. 44.11 Flowchart of management of exfoliative and necrotizing conditions of the integument.

sis, should be considered. Broad-spectrum antibiotics are started preoperatively, although high-dose penicillin is appropriate for clostridial infections. However, antibiotic treatment is no substitution for surgical intervention. Adequate fluid resuscitation and nutritional support are also required. Wounds are packed open with antiseptic-soaked dressings, which need to be changed frequently. Kaiser and Cerra have reported unsatisfactory results with either early application of porcine xenografts or burn wound topical antimicrobials.[83] Complete control of local and systemic infection is required before wound closure is addressed.

As in burns, secondary infections must be prevented by proper wound management, Biological or synthetic dressings offer the advantages of decreased pain, decreased fluid loss, and prevention of secondary infection. Frequently, large areas of skin and soft-tissue loss result from this disease and will eventually require extensive surgery to achieve adequate closure. Some authors advocate the use of hyperbaric oxygen and claim that it results in decreased mortality and reduced need for debridement; however, most of these reports are case reports or uncontrolled trials and adequate prospective controlled trials in patients are still lacking.[84,85] In animals, hyperbaric oxygen therapy alone did not improve survival or bacterial colonization, but did show adjuvant effects to antibiotic treatment.[86] In summary, hyperbaric oxygen therapy, if available, should not delay radical surgical debridement and should be used as an adjunct to radical surgery and antibiotic therapy.[85,87]

Purpura fulminans

Purpura fulminans is a term that describes an acute syndrome of rapidly progressive hemorrhagic necrosis of the skin due to dermal vascular thrombosis associated with vascular collapse and disseminated intravascular coagulation (DIC).[88] It may occur in individuals with dysfunction of the protein C anticoagulant system, with acute severe infection, or idiopathically without any coagulation dysfunction or infection.

It has been associated with systemic infection by *Meningococcus*, Gram-negative bacilli, *Staphylococcus*, *Streptococcus*,

and *Rickettsia* organisms. Skin necrosis begins in a region of dermal discomfort, which rapidly progresses to evanescent flush, followed by petechiae. Hemorrhagic bullae progress to frank skin necrosis. The process generally involves the skin and subcutaneous tissues, without involvement of muscle. Skin involvement is frequently an early manifestation of the disease process. Skin biopsy will, therefore, allow an earlier diagnosis.[88] Mortality in the acute phase is 18–40%.[89]

Management is directed at halting progression of the underlying infectious disease, preventing secondary infections, and removing non-viable tissue. Early heparin administration and replacement of clotting factors have proven useful to stop intravascular clotting.[89] Shock from blood extravasation and sepsis require extensive volume replacement. Limb vascular and compartmental pressure should be monitored closely to enable early escharotomy and/or fasciotomy, when needed. Skin lesions resulting only in blisters should be treated with topical antimicrobials (e.g. silver sulfadiazine) to prevent secondary infection. Non-viable tissue should be removed as soon as the patient's condition allows. Small areas can be covered with autografts but, as large areas are frequently involved, allograft or xenograft skin coverage may be required. Limb amputations may be frequently required due to vascular compromise, as well as revisions for progression of disease.[90] Isolation of the affected patient, as well as monitoring and prophylactic treatment of patients and staff, may be necessary to prevent further spread and outbreaks of the disease, especially in case of meningococcal infection.

Conclusion

Inflammatory and infectious conditions of the skin and underlying tissues represent a major diagnostic and therapeutic challenge. The team approach to their care is essential, and wound management is paramount. Burn units are ideally suited to deal with patients with these conditions and should be considered as the appropriate site of referral for these critically ill patients.

References

1. Rasmussen JE. Erythema multiforme. Should anyone care about the standards of care? Arch Dermatol 1995; 131:726–729.
2. Becker DS. Toxic epidermal necrolysis. Lancet 1998; 351: 1417–1420.
3. Patterson R, Dykewicz MS, Gonzales A, et al. Erythema multiforme and Stevens–Johnson syndrome: descriptive and therapeutic controversy. Chest 1990; 98:331–336.
4. Wilkins J, Morrison L, White CR. Oculocutaneous manifestations of the erythema multiforme/Stevens–Johnson syndrome/toxic epidermal necrolysis spectrum. Dermatol Clin 1992; 10:571–582.
5. Chan HC, Stern RS, Arndt KA, et al. The incidence of erythema multiforme, Stevens–Johnson syndrome and toxic epidermal necrolysis. Arch Dermatol 1990; 126:43–47.
6. Roujeau JC, Guillaume JC, Fabre JP, et al. Toxic epidermal necrolysis (Lyell syndrome): incidence and drug etiology in France, 1981–1985. Arch Dermatol 1990; 126:37–42.
7. Schoepf E, Stuehmer A, Rzany B, et al. Toxic epidermal necrolysis and Stevens–Johnson syndrome: an epidemiologic study from West Germany. Arch Dermatol 1991; 127:839–842.
8. Naldi L, Locasti F, Marchesi, et al. Incidence of toxic epidermal necrolysis in Italy. Arch Dermatol 1990; 126:1103–1104.
9. Strom BL, Carson JL, Halpern AC, et al. A population-based study of Stevens–Johnson syndrome: incidence and antecedent drug exposures. Arch Dermatol 1991; 127:831–838.
10. Halebian P, Corder V, Herndon D, et al. A burn center experience with toxic epidermal necrolysis. J Burn Care Rehabil 1983; 4:176–183.
11. Prendiville JS, Hebert AA, Greenwald MJ, et al. Management of Stevens–Johnson syndrome and toxic epidermal necrolysis in children. J Pediatr 1987; 115:881–887.
12. Kim PS, Goldfarb IW, Gaisford JC, et al. Stevens–Johnson syndrome and toxic epidermal necrolysis: a pathophysiologic review with recommendations for a treatment protocol. J Burn Care Rehabil 1983; 4:91–100.
13. Roujeau JC, Chosidow O, Saiag P, et al. Toxic epidermal necrolysis (Lyell syndrome). J Am Acad Dermatol 1990; 23:1039–1058.
14. Saiag P, Caumes E, Chosidow O, et al. Drug-induced toxic epidermal necrolysis (Lyell syndrome) in patients infected with the human immunodeficiency virus. J Am Acad Dermatol 1990; 26:567–574.
15. Villada G, Roujeau J, Cordonnier C, et al. Toxic epidermal necrolysis after bone marrow transplantation: study of nine cases. J Am Acad Dermatol 1990; 23:870–875.

16. Revuz J, Penson D, Roujeau JC, et al. Toxic epidermal necrolysis: clinical findings and prognostic factors in 87 patients. Arch Dermatol 1987; 123:1160–1166.

17. Murphy JT, Purdue GF, Hunt JL. Toxic epidermal necrolysis. J Burn Care Rehabil 1997; 18:417–420.

18. McGee T, Munster A. Toxic epidermal necrolysis syndrome: mortality rate reduced with early referral to regional burn center. Plast Reconstr Surg 1998; 102:1018–1022.

19. Scully MC, Frieden IJ. Toxic epidermal necrolysis in early infancy. J Am Acad Dermatol 1992; 27:340–344.

20. Ruiz-Maldonado R. Acute disseminated epidermal necrosis type 1, 2 and 3: study of sixty cases. J Am Acad Dermatol 1985; 13:623–635.

21. Guillaume JC, Roujeau JC, Revuz J, et al. The culprit drugs in 87 cases of toxic epidermal necrolysis (Lyell syndrome). Arch Dermatol 1987; 123:1166–1170.

22. Roujeau JC, Kelly JP, Naldi L, et al. Medication use and the risk of Stevens–Johnson syndrome or toxic epidermal necrolysis. N Engl J Med 1995; 333:1600–1607.

23. Halebian PH, Madden MR, Finkestein JL, et al. Improved burn center survival of patients with toxic epidermal necrolysis managed without corticosteroids. Ann Surg 1986; 204:503–511.

24. Adzick NS, Kim SH, Bondoc CC, et al. Management of toxic epidermal necrolysis in a pediatric burn center. Am J Dis Child 1985; 139:499–502.

25. Yetin J, Bianchini JR, Owens JA. Etiological factors in Stevens–Johnson syndrome. South Med J 1980; 73:599–602.

26. Howland WW, Golitz LE, Weston WL, et al. Erythema multiforme: clinical histopathologic, and immunologic study. J Am Acad Dermatol 1984; 10:438–446.

27. Avakian R, Flowers FP, Araulo OE, et al. Toxic epidermal necrolysis: a review. J Am Acad Dermatol 1991; 25:69–79.

28. Goldstein SM, Wintroub BW, Elias PM, et al. Toxic epidermal necrolysis: unmuddying the waters. Arch Dermatol 1987; 123:1153–1155.

29. Huff JC, Weston WL, Tonnesen MG. Erythema multiforme: a critical review of characteristics, diagnostic criteria and causes. J Am Acad Dermatol 1983; 8:763–775.

30. Merot Y, Gravallese E, Guillen FJ, et al. Lymphocyte subsets and Langerhans' cells in toxic epidermal necrolysis. Arch Dermatol 1986; 122:455–458.

31. Villada G, Roujeau JC, Clerici T, et al. Immunopathology of toxic epidermal necrolysis. Keratinocytes, HLA-DR expression, Langerhans cells and mononuclear cells: an immunopathologic study of five cases. Arch Dermatol 1992; 128:50–53.

32. Miyauchi H, Hosokawa H, Akaeda T, et al. T-cell subsets in drug-induced toxic epidermal necrolysis. Arch Dermatol 1991; 127:851–855.

33. Hertl M, Merk HF, Bohlen H. T-cell subsets in drug-induced toxic epidermal necrolysis. Arch Dermatol 1992; 128:272.

34. Heng MC, Allen SG. Efficiency of cyclophosphamides in toxic epidermal necrolysis: clinical and pathophysiologic aspects. J Am Acad Dermatol 1991; 25:778–786.

35. Roujeau JC, Huynh TN, Bracq C, et al. Genetic susceptibility to toxic epidermal necrolysis. Arch Dermatol 1987; 123:1171–1173.

36. Stein KM, Schlappner OL, Heaton CL, et al. Demonstration of basal cell immunofluorescence in drug-induced toxic epidermal necrolysis. Br J Dermatol 1972; 86:246–252.

37. Parson JM. Toxic epidermal necrolysis. Int J Dermatol 1992; 31:749–768.

38. Paul C, Wolkenstein P, Adle H, et al. Apoptosis as a mechanism of keratinocyte death in toxic epidermal necrolysis and Stevens–Johnson syndrome. Br J Dermatol 1996; 134:710–714.

39. Inachi S, Muizutani H, Shimuzu M. Epidermal apoptotic cell death in erythema multiforme and Stevens–Johnson syndrome. Contribution of perforin positive cell infiltration. Arch Dermatol 1997; 133:845–849.

40. Correia O, Chosidow O, Saiag P, et al. Evolving pattern of drug-induced toxic epidermal necrolysis. Dermatology 1993; 186:32–37.

41. Paller AS, Nelson A, Steffen L, et al. T-lymphocyte subset in the lesional skin of allogenic and autologous bone marrow transplant patients. Arch Dematol 1988; 124:1795–801.

42. Roujeau JC, Philippoteau C, Koso M, et al. Sjögren-like syndrome following toxic epidermal necrolysis. Lancet 1985; 1:609–611.

43. Hensen EJ, Claas FHJ, Vermeer BJ. Drug-dependent binding of circulating antibodies in drug-induced toxic epidermal necrolysis. Lancet 1981; 2:151–152.

44. Haake AR, Polaskowska RR. Cell death by apoptosis and epidermal biology. J Invest Dermatol 1993; 101:107–112.

45. Lyell A. Toxic epidermal necrolysis (the scalded skin syndrome): a reappraisal. Br J Dermatol 1979; 100:69–86.

46. Rasmussen J. Toxic epidermal necrolysis. Med Clin N Am 1980; 64:901–920.

47. Wahle D, Beste D, Conley SF. Laryngeal involvement in toxic epidermal necrolysis. Otolaryngol Head Neck Surg 1992; 6:796–799.

48. Chosidow O, Delchier JC, Chaumette MT. Intestinal involvement in drug-induced toxic epidermal necrolysis. Lancet 1991; 337:928.

49. Lebargy F, Wolkenstein P, Gisselbrecht M, et al. Pulmonary complications in toxic epidermal necrolysis: A prospective clinical study. Intensive Care Med 1997; 23:1237–1244.

50. Mclvor R, Zaidi J, Peters W, et al. Acute and chronic respiratory complications of toxic epidermal necrolysis. J Burn Care Rehabil 1996; 17:237–240.

51. Krumlovsky F, Del Greco F, Herdson P, et al. Renal disease associated with toxic epidermal necrolysis (Lyell's disease). 1975; 57:817–825.

52. Roujeau JC, Moritz S, Guillaume JC, et al. Lymphopenia and abnormal balance of T-lymphocyte subpopulation in toxic epidermal necrolysis. Arch Dermatol Res 1985; 277:24–27.

53. Heimbach DM, Engrav LH, Marvin JA, et al. Toxic epidermal necrolysis: a step forward in treatment. JAMA 1987; 257:2171–2175.

54. Marvin JA, Heimbach DM, Engrav LH, et al. Improved treatment of the Stevens–Johnson syndrome. Arch Surg 1984; 119:601–605.

55. Taylor JA, Grube B, Heimbach DM, et al. Toxic epidermal necrolysis: a comprehensive approach. Clin Pediatr 1989; 28:404–407.

56. Sowder LL. Biobrane wound dressing used in the treatment of toxic epidermal necrolysis: a case report. J Burn Care Rehabil 1990; 11:237–239.

57. Birchall N, Langdon R, Cuono C, et al. Toxic epidermal necrolysis: an approach to management using cryopreserved allograft skin. J Am Acad Dermatol 1987; 16:368–372.

58. Halebian PH, Shires GT. Burn unit treatment of acute, severe exfoliating disorders. Ann Rev Med 1989; 40:137–147.

59. Revuz J, Roujeau JC, Guillaume JC, et al. Treatment of toxic epidermal necrolysis: Creteil's experience. Arch Dermatol 1987; 123:1156–1158.

60. Ginsburg CM. Stevens–Johnson syndrome in children. Pediatr Infect Dis 1982; 1:155–158.

61. Rasmussen JE. Cause, prognosis and management of toxic epidermal necrolysis. Compr Ther 1990; 16:3–6.

62. Rzany B, Schmitt H, Schoepf E. Toxic epidermal necrolysis in patients receiving glucocorticosteroids. Acta Derm Venereol 1991; 71:171–172.

63. Guibal F, Bastuji-Garin S, Chosidow O, et al. Characteristics of toxic epidermal necrolysis in patients undergoing long-term glucocorticoid therapy. Arch Dermatol 1995; 131:669–672.

64. Chave TA, Mortimer NJ, Sladden MJ, et al. Toxic epidermal necrolysis: current evidence, practical management and future directions. Br J Dermatol 2005; 153(2):241–253.

65. Arevalo JM, Lorente JA, Gonazlez-Herrada C, et al. Treatment of toxic epidermal necrolysis with cyclosporin A. J Trauma 2000; 48(3):473–478.

66. Bachot N, Revuz J, Roujeau JC. Intravenous immunoglobulin treatment for Stevens–Johnson syndrome and toxic epidermal necrolysis: a prospective noncomparative study showing no benefit on mortality or progression. Arch Dermatol 2003; 139(1):33–36.

67. Viard I, Wehrli P, Bullani R, et al. Inhibition of toxic epidermal necrolysis by blockade of CD95 with human intravenous immunoglobulin. Science 1998; 282(16):490–493.

68. Shortt R, Gomez M, Mittman N, et al. Intravenous immunoglobulin does not improve outcome in toxic epidermal necrolysis. J Burn Care Rehabil 2004; 25(3):246–255.

69. Stella M, Cassano P, Bollero D, et al. Toxic epidermal necrolysis treated with intravenous high-dose immunoglobulins: our experience. Dermatology 2001; 203(1):45–49.

70. Prins C, Vittorio C, Padilla RS, et al. Effect of high-dose intravenous immunoglobulin therapy in Stevens–Johnson syndrome: a retrospective , multicenter study. Dermatology 2003; 207(1):96–99.

71. Resnick SD. Staphylococcal toxin-mediated syndromes in childhood. Semin Dermatol 1992; 11:11–18.

72. Canoso JJ, Barza M. Soft tissue infections. Rheum Dis Clin North Am 1993; 15:235–239.

73. Elias PM, Fritsch P, Epstein EH. Staphylococcal scalded skin syndrome: clinical features, pathogenesis, and recent microbiological and biochemical developments. Arch Dermatol 1977; 113: 207–219.

74. Dancer SJ, Garratt R, Sanhanha J, et al. The epidermolytic toxins are serine proteases. FEBS Lett 1990; 268:129–132.

75. Vath GM, Earhart CA, Rago JV, et al. The structure of the superantigen exfoliative toxin A suggests a novel regulation as a serine protease. Biochemistry 1997; 36:1559–1566.

76. Itani O, Crump R, Minouni F, et al. Ritter's disease (neonatal staphylococcal scalded skin syndrome). Am J Dis Child 1992; 146:425–426.

77. Patino JF, Castro D. Necrotizing lesions of soft tissue: a review. World J Surg 1991; 15:235–239.

78. Steven DL. Invasive group A streptococcal infections. Clin Infect Dis 1992; 14:2–13.

79. Francis KR, Lamaute HR, Davis JM, et al. Implications of risk factors in necrotizing fasciitis. Am J Surg 1993; 59:304–308.

80. Sharif HS, Clark DC, Aabed MY, et al. MR imaging of thoracic and abdominal wall infections: comparison with other imaging procedures. AJR Am J Roentgenol 1990; 154:989–995.

81. Stamenkovic I, Lew PD. Early recognition of potentially fatal necrotizing fasciitis: the use of frozen-section biopsy. N Engl J Med 1984; 310:1689–1693.

82. Freischlag JA, Ajalat G, Busuttil RW. Treatment of necrotizing soft tissue infection: the need for a new approach. Am J Surg 1985; 149:751–757.

83. Kaiser RE, Cerra FB. Progressive necrotizing surgical infections: a unified approach. J Trauma 1981; 24:349–352.

84. Risemann JA, Zamboni WA, Curtis A, et al. Hyperbaric oxygen therapy for necrotizing fasciitis reduces mortality and the need for debridement. Surgery 1990; 108:847–850.

85. Green RJ, Dafoe DC, Raffin TA. Necrotizing fasciitis. Chest 1996; 110:219–229.

86. Zamboni WA, Mazolewski PJ, Erdmann D, et al. Evaluation of penicillin and hyperbaric oxygen in the treatment of streptococcal myositis. Ann Plast Surg 1997; 39:131–136.

87. McHenry CR, Piotrowski JJ, Petrinic D, et al. Determinants of mortality for necrotizing soft-tissue infections. Ann Surg 1995; 221:558–565.

88. Adcock DM, Hicks MJ. Dermatopathology of skin necrosis associated with purpura fulminans. Semin Thromb Hemost 1990; 16:283–292.

89. Chasan PE, Hansbrough JF, Cooper ML. Management of cutaneous manifestations of extensive purpura fulminans in a burn unit. J Burn Care Rehabil 1992; 13:410–413.

90. Genoff MC, Hoffer MM, Achauer B, et al. Extremity amputation in meningococcemia induced purpura fulminans. Plast Reconstr Surg 1992; 89:878–881.

Chapter 45

The burn problem: a pathologist's perspective

Hal K. Hawkins and Hugo A. Linares

Introduction

'Burns are not a simple injury, but a very complicated disease.' This statement, published by J Long in 1840 and cited by Dr Linares in the first edition of this book, holds true with additional force in 2006.[1] Massive destruction of viable tissue, which occurs in burn injury, and injury to the airways by inhalation of toxic products of combustion, stimulate complex reactions which are only beginning to be understood. Burn injury is frequently complicated by malfunction of every organ system. The nature of this malfunction is often clarified by examination of the body after death. Postmortem examination also has the potential to reveal adverse effects of therapy, which might not be clear during life. An important example of this is that the treatment of burned skin with tannic acid was popular until degeneration of the liver was described in autopsies of burned patients treated with tannic acid. The causative link was later confirmed experimentally.[2] In addition, every death after burn injury has medicolegal implications. Postmortem examination often contributes substantial evidence in this regard. The process of analysis of an entire case from the point of view of pathogenesis often clarifies the nature of the patient's most significant problems. This chapter systematically reviews the observations made at autopsy in patients who have died after burn injury. Where possible, hypothetical interpretations of the mechanisms of disease are suggested. Often the interpretation includes comparison of autopsy findings with results of animal experiments. To quote

Dr Linares on this method, 'Pathology combines anatomy, physiology, and theories of disease, and it is a point of convergence for medicine and the biological disciplines.' The observations reviewed here include our experience of approximately 300 autopsies performed on burned children at the Shriners Burns Hospital in Galveston from 1966 to the present.

To introduce the sections that follow, the major medical problems that complicate burn injury are summarized here. The degree of disruption of normal physiological processes after burn injury is extreme. Immediately after burn injury, massive loss of intravascular fluid into the burned tissue begins to occur.[3,4] Unless this fluid loss is replaced by the physician very promptly and carefully, serious *hypovolemia* develops.[5–7] The consequences of hypovolemia often include the death of neurons in the brain, focal necrosis of the intestinal epithelium, and necrosis of the proximal tubules of the kidneys. The neural and endocrine responses to the traumatic injury may lead to recognizable lesions in the stomach and in the heart. Thermal injury to skeletal muscle, or lack of perfusion of muscle, may lead to local exudation of fluid and development of such high pressure in muscle compartments that arterial perfusion is prevented. This 'compartment syndrome,' unless relieved by prompt surgical intervention, leads to necrosis of muscle throughout the compartment.[8] The consequences of massive necrosis of muscle often include secondary injury to the lungs, due to release of reactive oxygen species, and myoglobinuria, with secondary renal damage.[9] At the time of injury, patients frequently inhale sufficient carbon monoxide to compromise the oxygen-carrying capacity of the blood. The resultant tissue *hypoxia* can cause death at the scene, and if the patient survives, it can be sufficient to lead to irreversible neuronal injury and brain death. Hypoxia, sometimes related to carbon monoxide intoxication, also contributes to cardiac and renal injury. In addition, when fires occur in closed spaces, the 'flashover' process consumes all available oxygen, so that the patient's environment may contain too little oxygen to sustain life. Occasionally a burn victim is found without pulse or respiratory effort, probably as a consequence of hypoxia, and is revived by cardiopulmonary resuscitation. In such cases ischemic and hypoxic injury may be profound in multiple organs, and there may be significant 'ischemia/reperfusion injury' to the lungs after resuscitation. Patients injured in house fires often suffer injury to the respiratory tract caused by inhalation of toxic products of combustion.[10] This *smoke inhalation* injury stimulates an intense inflammatory reaction, which can lead to obstruction of airways and further tissue injury. This problem is discussed below in the section on the respiratory system. *Infection* is the next major risk experienced by patients after burn injury. Necrotic skin provides an excellent environment for proliferation of bacteria and fungi, and as long as necrotic tissue remains, the risk of infection remains high. Injury to the intestinal epithelium by hypoxia or ischemia leads to translocation of intestinal bacteria into the portal circulation. In addition, patients all experience substantial immunosuppression, partly as a result of excessive secretion of endogenous glucocorticoids and release of cytokines into the circulation, which leads to ineffective host defense. *Coagulopathy* may be a very serious complication of burn injury. It may lead directly to tissue ischemia, or the resultant hemorrhage may lead to secondary hypovolemia. Patients often require transfusion of very large quantities of blood products during their treatment.

Disease processes involving multiple organ systems

Hypoxia and ischemia

All cells require a constant supply of oxygen and metabolic substrates, such as glucose, to remain viable. This is largely because animal cells exist in a state of dynamic equilibrium that requires membrane transport to maintain integrity. In hypoxia, when the supply of oxygen is insufficient, cells generate a limited amount of metabolic energy by anaerobic glycolysis, releasing lactic acid. With ischemia, when the flow of blood is insufficient, this metabolic perturbation is complicated by a lack of supply of glucose and other fuels, and the extracellular fluid composition may change dramatically. Tissues vary greatly in their sensitivity to injury by hypoxia or ischemia. In general, tissues with the greatest metabolic activity are the first to lose viability under conditions of hypoxia and ischemia. These tissues include the neurons of the central nervous system, the myocytes of the heart, the epithelial cells of the small intestine, and the proximal tubular cells of the kidney. The location and extent of necrosis in these organs depends on the severity and duration of the ischemic or hypoxic injury.

After ischemia and hypoxia have led to irreversible injury and death of selected cell types or whole segments of organs (infarcts), responses are initiated that may lead to further injury of remote organs. Cellular necrosis stimulates an intense acute inflammatory reaction, probably initiated by activation of the complement cascade, degranulation of mast cells, and other processes. This reaction surrounds an infarct, or proceeds throughout a region of tissue injury if the local circulation is sufficient. Monocytes recruited to the regions of injury secrete cytokines in large quantities, and polymorphonuclear neutrophils activate their antibacterial mechanisms. Cytokines have effects throughout the body, and superoxide released by neutrophils has important distant effects. In addition, in endothelial cells injured by hypoxia, the enzyme xanthine dehydrogenase is converted to xanthine oxidase, which releases superoxide during degradation of adenosine, which in turn is released by necrotic cells.[11,12] Superoxide, released into the circulation by this metabolic process and by neutrophils, can injure the lung by damaging both endothelial and epithelial cells and allowing protein-rich fluid to exude into alveoli. The inflammatory reaction to thermal tissue injury also stimulates an intense influx of neutrophils, which undoubtedly contributes to this injury by releasing superoxide. In experimental models of burn injury, as well as in models of ischemia–reperfusion injury, the lungs have been shown to be injured by these processes.[13] Endogenous antioxidants such as glutathione are depleted, and conjugated dienes appear, indicating that cell membrane injury due to lipid peroxidation has occurred in the lung.[14]

Infection and sepsis

The skin normally provides a highly effective barrier against invasion of tissues by infectious agents. Necrotic tissue provides an excellent culture medium, and the body surface is inevitably exposed to multiple potential pathogens. Patients who are treated for deep burn injury with traditional debridement and washing for several days generally arrive at this institution with large quantities of multiple microorganisms growing in the necrotic skin. The bacteria appear to proliferate initially in areas that have insufficient circulation to develop a significant inflammatory response. As large numbers of bacteria accumulate, those with high pathogenic capacity invade the adjacent viable tissue, produce further necrosis, and gain access to the circulation. This is the condition of burn wound sepsis, which historically has been the leading cause of death in burn patients. In Dr Linares' published series of 115 autopsies, sepsis was present in 73%, as documented by positive blood cultures and demonstration of invasive infection of viable tissue.[15,16] In 80% of these fatal cases of sepsis, the burn wound was the source of the infection. The pathogens that were most important were *Pseudomonas aeruginosa*, *Staphylococcus aureus*, *Klebsiella pneumoniae*, *Escherichia coli*, *Enterobacter*, and *Candida* species. Burn wound sepsis is suspected clinically when a burn wound is the site of proliferating microorganisms exceeding 10^5/g of tissue, and there is histological evidence of active invasion of subjacent unburned tissue.[17] In our institution, the wounds of burn patients, especially the open areas, are routinely sampled for quantitative culture and for histological study when excision and grafting procedures are done, and whenever clinical examination suggests the possibility of tissue infection. The histological classification used and its rationale are discussed below under the integumentary system. Once septicemia occurs, there is a generalized reaction that often includes hypotension, tachycardia, increased hyperthermia or hypothermia, and poor perfusion of the intestines and other viscera.[18] In the case of Gram-negative bacteria, endotoxin stimulates monocytes via their CD14 receptors to become activated and set up a cascade of release of proinflammatory and anti-inflammatory mediators that affect all organs and tissues in the body.[19–21] Coagulopathy is another important complication of sepsis.[22] Once bacteria gain entrance to the general circulation, it becomes possible for foci of tissue infection to develop at distant sites. This is most likely to occur in sites of tissue necrosis or on cardiac valves, or in the lungs. Abscesses in distant organs can allow the infection to resist eradication by specific antibiotics, and thus allow sepsis to develop again after initially effective therapy. The risk of infection is proportional to the severity of the burn, the time before the initiation of fluid therapy, the presence of metabolic alterations, the development of immunological deficiency, the concurrence of trauma, the local evolution of wounds, and the age of a patient.

An infection may begin in a burn wound, the respiratory system, the gastrointestinal tract, the urinary tract, the blood vessels, or from localized infection in any other area of the body. Although most serious infections in burn patients appear to be due to endogenous flora, and many derive from wound infections present at the time of admission, nosocomial infection is a constant hazard.[23,24]

The problem of burn wound sepsis is amenable to therapy. The strategy of excision of the potentially infected burn wound as early as possible, together with judicious administration of effective antibiotics, has greatly reduced the number of deaths due to infection. Coincident with the institution of early excision and grafting of burn patients in our institution, the incidence of burn wound sepsis as a cause of death declined dramatically.[25] The problem of sepsis has not disappeared, however. Certain organisms can evade the best current efforts at management, and have caused death in recent cases, including bacteria resistant to nearly all available antibiotics, and invasive fungi. Those patients who are referred for therapy more than 1 week after burn injury often have extensive invasive wound infection and sepsis, which may be difficult or impossible to eradicate.

Coagulopathy

The burn wound has procoagulant effects, and may induce coagulation throughout the circulation (DIC, disseminated intravascular coagulation).[26,27] Tissue necrosis, particularly lethal injury to endothelial cells, with exposure of subendothelial collagen, and release of tissue thromboplastin, can activate coagulation and lead to coagulopathy. Generation of thrombin within the circulation not only leads to generation of fibrin peptides but also stimulates acute inflammatory reactions including increased vascular permeability and upregulation of adhesion molecules on neutrophils and endothelial cells.[28] Generation of fibrin degradation products may be sufficient to interfere with normal thrombosis, and thrombocytopenia can develop in response to abnormal intravascular fibrin generation.[29] Activation of the kinin system can stimulate further abnormal vascular permeability and hypotension.[21] Consumption of coagulation factors can lead to abnormal bleeding, which can cause extensive tissue injury secondarily. It is important to note that the acute phase response to burn injury includes increased synthesis of fibrinogen and factor VIII. During the first 3–10 days after burn injury, patients often have greater than normal clotting activity. This may increase their susceptibility to development of DIC, especially if sepsis supervenes. It also implies that laboratory testing of levels of fibrinogen and factor VIII may yield normal values even in the presence of abnormal consumption of these factors. When disseminated intravascular coagulation occurs in the patient's terminal course, as was the case in a majority of the autopsies reviewed by Dr Linares, microscopic fibrin thrombi are seen in many organs at the time of autopsy. These microthrombi are seen most commonly in the lungs, the skin, the kidneys, and the gastrointestinal tract.[15,30]

Integumentary system

The skin is the site of initial injury in burn patients, and many of the events that lead to dysfunction or failure of other organs begin in the skin. Thermal injury rapidly produces irreversible injury and cell death in epidermal keratinocytes, in the epidermal appendages including hair follicles and their attached sebaceous glands and sweat glands, and in the connective tissue cells of the dermis. In many cases, the burn wound excised within 48 hours of injury shows that the entire dermis and all of the hair follicles are necrotic, but that much of the subcutaneous adipose tissue remains viable. It appears that the greater insulating capacity of adipose tissue protects it to some extent. In some cases, of course, necrosis due to the initial thermal injury may extend deep into the subcutaneous tissue. In extreme cases, the underlying skeletal muscle may become necrotic as a result of thermal injury. Necrosis of skeletal muscle is especially prominent in some cases of electrical injury, in which more heat may be generated adjacent to bone than near the body surface. An interesting observation is that there is often a band-like infiltrate of degenerating polymorphonuclear neutrophils in the midst of a totally necrotic dermis. This suggests that the boundary between necrotic and viable tissue may have extended deeper after the initial burn injury and its inflammatory response. There is experimental evidence that burn wounds often evolve from an initial level of necrosis to a deeper level of necrosis, even from second to third degree, as a result of poor perfusion of the tissue immediately deep to the initial burn injury.[31] This process of vascular stasis deep to the burn is undoubtedly due in part to the rapid loss of intravascular fluid from the damaged capillaries and venules just below the necrotic burn wound. In addition, there is evidence that neutrophils contribute to this process of burn wound extension, most likely by adhering to endothelium and to each other, with resulting obstruction of the microvasculature.[32]

It is important to assess the presence and extent of infection within the burn wound, both in the excised wound during therapeutic procedures, and by biopsy of suspicious areas in open foci after grafting procedures. A high index of suspicion serves the burn patient well. Biopsy and excision specimens in our institution are routinely sampled and studied histologically with stains for bacteria (Brown and Hopps) and fungi (methenamine silver). Within large excision specimens, samples are taken from sites of especially deep tissue injury and sites that show abnormal discoloration of dermal or subcutaneous tissue. When infectious microorganisms are found, it is important to determine their location with respect to the boundary between living and necrotic tissue. This boundary may be irregular. It is generally distinct and marked by inflammation in wounds several days old, but may be indistinct in very fresh specimens, as karyolysis takes several days to develop in burn wounds. As noted above, wound infections generally begin with colonization of the skin surface and proliferation of organisms on the surface, often with extension into hair follicles, followed by growth within the necrotic tissue. Both the coagulum on the surface and the necrotic epidermis and dermis are considered part of the burn eschar. Growth within necrotic tissue is considered evidence of tissue infection, however, and potentially more dangerous than growth on the surface of necrotic skin. Even when quantitative cultures show more than 10^5 bacteria per gram of tissue, when careful histological study shows that the organisms are limited to the skin surface or the superficial necrotic tissue, the risk of sepsis appears to be low. Such growth on or in necrotic tissue, however, does set the stage for invasion of viable tissue. The finding of clusters of bacteria or fungi within viable tissue does imply a serious risk of sepsis and further tissue invasion. As a rule, bacterial invasion of viable tissue is readily apparent by histological study of appropriate tissue samples, and often includes a zone of tissue necrosis surrounded by intact tissue (Figure 45.1a). Invasive fungal infection presents a somewhat different pattern, in that there is often a wavefront of necrosis that accompanies fungal invasion. Thus fungal infection that extends to a boundary between necrotic and viable tissue is considered evidence of fungal invasion of viable tissue (Figure 45.1b). On this basis, infections identified within burn wounds are reported as surface colonization, invasion of necrotic tissue, which may be superficial or deep, and invasion of viable

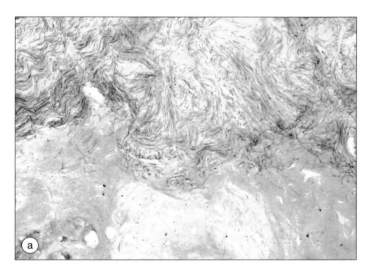

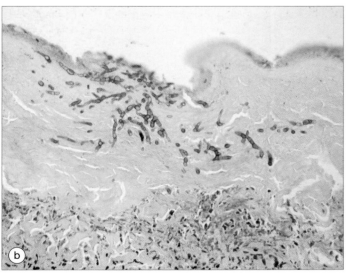

Fig. 45.1 (a) This micrograph of Gram-stained tissue shows a dense aggregate of filamentous Gram-negative rods in the wall of a vein in the chest skin of a patient who presented with severe wound infection due to *Pseudomonas aeruginosa*. (b) This micrograph of tissue stained with the periodic acid Schiff stain (PAS) shows a portion of a burn wound of the skin in a patient who presented with focal fungal invasion of viable tissue. Branching fungal hyphae extend near the border of the viable tissue.

tissue. The responsible surgeon is called immediately when invasion of viable tissue is found. If the level of clinical suspicion is especially high, frozen sections have been found useful for this determination, using a tape transfer device to facilitate handling of these difficult specimens, with confirmation of the results with routine sections on the following day.

Respiratory system

In recent years respiratory failure, defined as inability to maintain adequate oxygen saturation while administering 100% oxygen by ventilator, has been the most common immediate cause of death in patients at the Shriners Burns Hospital in Galveston. The causes and mechanisms of respiratory failure are multiple, and will be addressed separately, although more than one mechanism operates in many cases. Direct thermal injury to the trachea and bronchi probably does not occur, except in cases of burn injury due to exposure to large quantities of steam. Patients also may develop problems related to the airways such as pneumothorax or interstitial emphysema, aspiration of gastric contents, pulmonary embolism, and non-specific pulmonary edema due to increased venous pressure. In Dr Linares' series of 115 burn autopsies, every patient had severe lung lesions of various kinds.[33]

Infection

In most patients who die with respiratory failure, postmortem cultures of lung tissue are sterile. However, in those patients who have sepsis at the time of death, extensive infection of the lungs is commonly present, and it may represent a terminal event. As is true of sepsis in general, fatal pneumonia is most often seen as a consequence of infection with a highly resistant bacterial strain, an invasive fungal infection, or in a further compromised host with renal failure or some other additional cause of immunodeficiency. Virulent and antibiotic-resistant strains of *Pseudomonas* may produce an angioinvasive infection in the lung, with massive proliferation of bacteria within the walls of pulmonary arteries and ischemic necrosis of segments of lung tissue (Figure 45.2)[34] This pattern is similar to that of ecthyma gangrenosum of the skin.[35,36] A similar angioinvasive pattern of pulmonary infection can be seen with generalized infection due to *Aspergillus* or similar filamentous fungi.

Diffuse alveolar damage

This process affects the pulmonary parenchyma in all lobes and segments, and begins with exudation of protein-rich fluid into alveolar spaces. This proteinaceous exudate, representing the exudative phase of the acute inflammatory reaction, is a consequence of damage or increased permeability of both capillary endothelial cells and the epithelial type I cells of the alveolar lining. Within hours, the exudates form the hyaline membranes that are a histological hallmark of this disease process (Figure 45.3a). Within a few days, the exudate begins to undergo organization by spindle-shaped fibroblasts, and collagenous fibrosis develops, which obliterates alveoli and greatly thickens the septa between alveoli (Figure 45.3b). Macrophages accumulate within alveoli, and alveolar epithelial type II cells multiply. In the late stages, there is severe interstitial fibrosis.

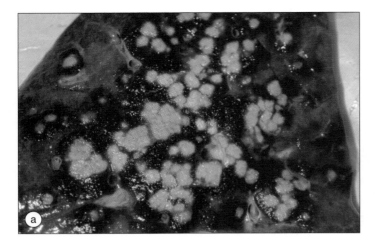

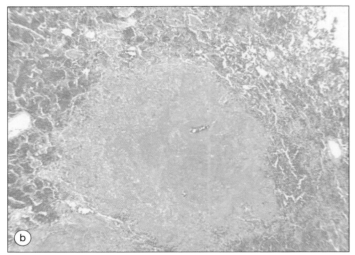

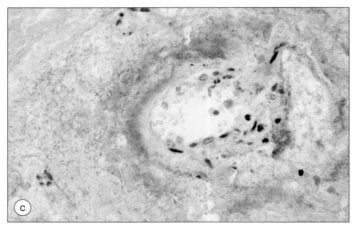

Fig. 45.2 (a) This photograph of a slice of lung tissue taken at autopsy shows numerous round light tan nodules of firm necrotic tissue scattered on a dark red background. This was a patient who developed disseminated infection from burn wounds infected with multiple antibiotic-resistant *Pseudomonas aeruginosa.* (b) This low-magnification micrograph of tissue stained with hematoxylin and eosin (H&E) shows a typical round nodule of necrotic tissue surrounded by intact tissue with congestion and hemorrhage and a minimal acute inflammatory reaction. (c). The tissue Gram stain reveals numerous long Gram-negative rods occupying the muscular wall of a pulmonary artery branch.

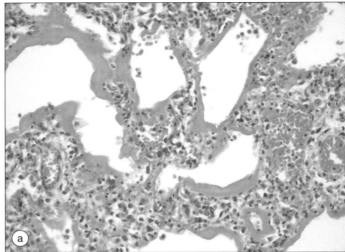

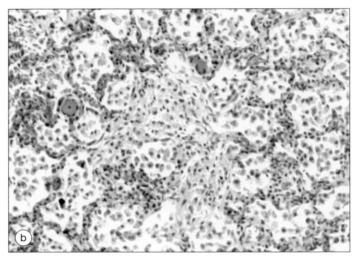

Fig. 45.3 (a) This micrograph shows prominent hyaline membranes in H&E-stained lung tissue from a 2-year-old patient who died 8 days after a large scald burn. This represents the exudative phase of the acute respiratory distress syndrome (ARDS). (b) This micrograph shows proliferation of fibroblasts within alveolar spaces, representing the proliferative phase of ARDS. The patient survived 1 month after a large flame burn with clinical evidence of smoke inhalation injury.

There are multiple pathogenetic mechanisms that may be responsible for this process, but it is not clear which of these are most significant in patients with burn injury.[37,38] The burn injury itself stimulates activation of complement, liberating peptides including C5a and C3a, which could, in spite of their short half-lives, directly stimulate vascular leakage in the pulmonary bed. More likely, these and many other peptides activate circulating neutrophils, which produce secondary injury to the vascular and epithelial membranes in the lung.[39,40] Conversion of xanthine dehydrogenase to xanthine oxidase in the burn wound, muscles or other tissues can cause release of superoxide into the venous circulation, stimulating endothelial injury and oxidative stress in the lung.[11] The neutrophils reacting to the burn wound also undergo an oxidative burst, contributing to the release of superoxide into the circulation. This process is greatly enhanced if the patient's course is complicated by ischemic injury of muscle compartments, limbs or other organs. Lipid peroxidation is a recognized consequence of burn injury. Superoxide can also react with nitric oxide, produced in the lung, to form peroxynitrite, a highly toxic substance.[41] Thrombin peptides, released during thrombosis of blood vessels in the wound, can also activate neutrophils.[42] The kinin system can be activated during thermal injury, with its systemic consequences. When patients develop sepsis, additional pulmonary damage can be produced by release of proinflammatory cytokines and augmentation of the processes that lead to inflammatory injury of the lung.[15,43] Neuropeptides including substance P may have a role in increasing vascular permeability in the airways.[44,45] Finally, the presence of oxygen in high concentration within the lung can itself lead to injury, and this injury can be manifest in the form of diffuse alveolar damage.[46–48] Despite this plethora of mechanisms that can lead to pulmonary injury in burn patients, many patients with massive burn injury do not develop clinically apparent respiratory difficulty. The conditions most strongly associated with this form of pulmonary injury are delayed fluid resuscitation, limb ischemia, and, of course, sepsis.

Smoke inhalation injury

Patients often inhale products of combustion in house fires, and the toxic effects of these gases and fumes directly injure tissues with the lung. These patients are recognized clinically during bronchoscopy by observing prominent hyperemia of the tracheobronchial mucosa, and small particles of carbonaceous soot within the airways. Associated findings include facial burns and singed nasal hairs. These patients usually do not require ventilator therapy for several days, but are at high risk of developing respiratory failure later, which responds poorly to ventilator therapy and may prove fatal even when the burn injury is small. The mortality of burn injury has been found to be increased substantially when inhalation injury is present as well.[49–53] Experimental studies in sheep and dogs have partially clarified the mechanisms of smoke inhalation injury.[54–57] The immediate reaction to inhalation of toxic smoke, in animals, includes detachment of numerous ciliated columnar cells from the tracheobronchial epithelium, secretion of stored mucus by airway secretory cells and glands, and a dramatic increase (10-fold or greater) in tracheobronchial blood flow.[58–60] Within a few hours, an intense acute inflammatory reaction develops, with exudation of numerous neutrophils into the airways (Figure 45.4a), and release of protein-rich fluid that may coagulate within airways, forming occlusive 'casts' containing mucus and desquamated cells. After 48 hours, the exudate of neutrophils, which is most intense in the trachea at earlier times, fills many terminal bronchioles (Figure 45.4b), and begins to extend into the lung parenchyma, together with mucus. This inflammatory reaction resolves in the experimental animal, and the epithelium slowly regenerates. However, autopsy evidence suggests that in human patients, exudation of neutrophils, protein and mucus into the airways may persist for more than a week (Figure 45.4c). The lost airway epithelium does not regenerate for long periods of time. Perhaps because of failure of the mucociliary escalator, mucus can be seen to accumulate around terminal bronchioles focally. This lesion is illustrated in Figure 45.4d.

Multiple mechanisms may be responsible for the respiratory disease evoked by inhalation of toxic smoke.[61] As in the case of diffuse alveolar damage, the available evidence indicates that neutrophils may be responsible for much of the injury, but the locus of injury appears to be different, centered on the airways rather than the pulmonary parenchyma. Factors that may be likely to lead to selective damage to the airways include local release of neuropeptides by afferent C-fibers in the airways, and activation of proinflammatory processes in reaction to injury to the airway mucosa, including local production of interleukin-8.[62–65] Local production of nitric oxide and other reactive nitrogen species apparently has significant deleterious effects in this form of acute lung injury.[66,67] Local activation of thrombin during the formation of fibrin clots, and local production of endothelin-1 may further enhance the inflammatory reaction in the airways.[68,69] Secretory cells appear to be especially sensitive to smoke inhalation injury. Recent experimental studies in sheep have demonstrated that activation of poly-adenosyl-ribose polymerase contributes to lung injury after burn and smoke inhalation injury.[70] Obstruction of small bronchi and bronchioles is thought to lead to failure of ventilation of multiple small segments of lung tissue, and inappropriate vasodilation in these poorly ventilated segments may well lead to shunting of flow through unventilated lung tissue and contribute to the failure of adequate oxygenation.[71] Treatment with either nebulized heparin or tissue plasminogen activator has been found to reduce the degree of injury in the ovine model, demonstrating the importance of fibrin formation in this model.[72,73] Segmental atelectasis and prominent vasodilation in focal areas are features of smoke inhalation injury seen in experimental animals, and also in patients examined at autopsy after burn injury and smoke inhalation injury. Obstruction of bronchi and bronchioles by mucus, fibrin and cell debris contributes to respiratory malfunction in experimental animals, and similar obstructive material is seen in human lung tissue at autopsy.[71,74,75] As is the case with diffuse alveolar damage, the toxic effects of high concentrations of oxygen may complicate the reaction to injury.

Cardiovascular system

Despite the tachycardia and increased cardiac output common to patients with burn injury, structural lesions of the heart have been uncommon in our autopsies done on a pediatric population. Cardiac dilation and clinical evidence of poor myocardial contractility do develop in some patients after burn injury. Cardiac hypertrophy is common, probably in reaction to tachycardia and catecholamine stimulation. Bacterial endocarditis occurs in occasional patients with sepsis complicating burn injury. Non-bacterial thrombotic endocarditis (marantic endocarditis) has also been seen, and also may give rise to embolic complications (Figure 45.5a and b). This lesion has been seen more often in patients who had extensive wound infection and clinical signs of sepsis due to *Acinetobacter* species. When the endocardial region of the left ventricle is examined at autopsy, small foci of necrosis associated with local hemorrhage are observed in some cases. Contraction band necrosis is often the only evidence of myocardial injury (Figure 45.5c). These lesions may reflect poor perfusion of a

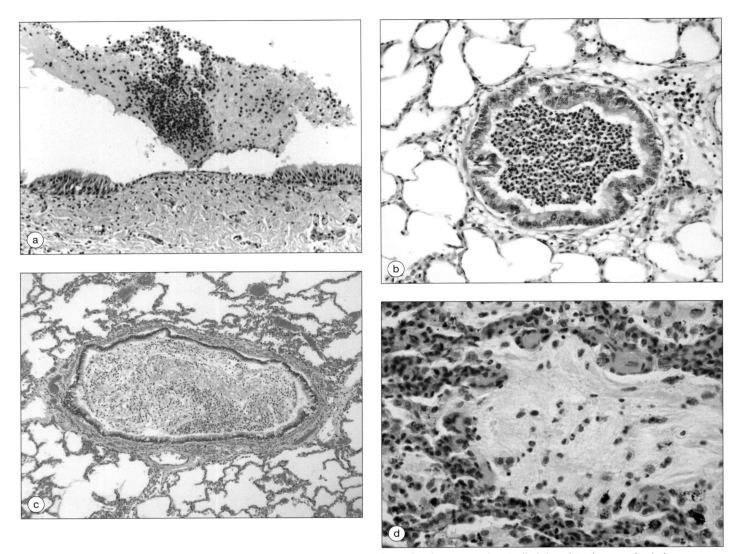

Fig. 45.4 (a) This micrograph shows an H&E-stained section of the trachea of a sheep experimentally injured under anesthesia by insufflation of cooled cotton smoke through a tracheostomy 3 hours prior to sacrifice. Numerous polymorphonuclear neutrophils are flowing into the trachea through a gap in the epithelial lining. (b) This micrograph shows neutrophils largely obstructing a small bronchiole in a sheep 48 hours after smoke inhalation injury. (c) This micrograph shows obstructive material in a bronchiole in an autopsy sample from a human patient who lived for 7 days after a large flame burn. (d) This micrograph shows mucus and neutrophils in lung parenchyma in an autopsy specimen from a patient who lived 5 days after a flame burn associated with smoke inhalation injury. Upper airway mucus is frequently seen in terminal airways and adjacent parenchyma in the lungs of burn patients who have had ventilator treatment.

tissue with high metabolic demand during terminal episodes of hypotension. In some cases, they may represent the effects of endogenous or exogenous adrenergic stimulation. Rona and his associates have demonstrated that β-adrenergic agents, at high doses, stimulate development of small foci of myocyte necrosis and hemorrhage in the subendocardial region of the heart.[76,77]

Urinary system

Patients with extensive burn injury, if resuscitated adequately during the first few hours after injury, may have normal renal function throughout their hospital course. It is not uncommon, however, for renal failure to develop, especially when the initial fluid resuscitation was not optimal, or when patients have episodes of sepsis. In such cases, the autopsy frequently reveals evidence of acute tubular necrosis, the morphological expression of which depends upon the timing of the injury.[78] In Dr Linares' autopsy series, evidence of acute tubular necrosis was present in 86% of the cases, and all of these patients had clinical evidence of renal failure.[33] The morphological features of acute tubular necrosis include edema of the entire kidney with substantial increase in weight, and necrosis of proximal tubular cells with karyolysis, karyorrhexis and sloughing of the injured cells from the tubular basal lamina. Within 48 hours, these events are followed by regeneration of surviving renal tubular cells, which flatten, become basophilic, and undergo mitosis as they migrate to reconstitute the epi-

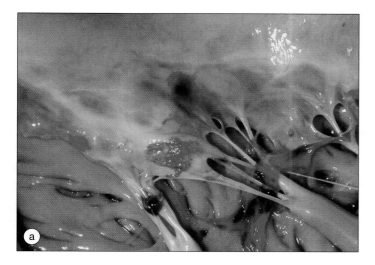

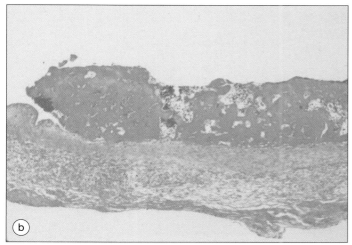

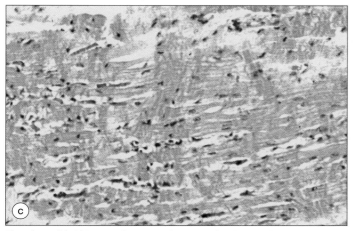

Fig. 45.5 (a) This is a close-up photograph of a small lesion on the tricuspid valve of the heart in a patient with non-bacterial thrombotic endocarditis who died of sepsis. (b) An H&E-stained section of this lesion shows that it is composed of fibrin. (c) This micrograph shows acute contraction band necrosis in heart muscle cells in a small area in the left ventricular subendocardial region.

thelial lining. Renal failure was an independent factor associated with increased mortality in the analysis of prognosis in patients with greater than 80% TBSA burns in our institution.[79] Patients with renal failure seem to be at especially high risk for the infectious complications of burn injury.

Digestive system, hepatobiliary tract, and pancreas

The association of duodenal ulcers with burn injury, described by Curling, is a classical lesion that still occurs in patients with burn injury.[80] In a pediatric population treated prophylactically with inhibitors of gastric acid secretion, these lesions are distinctly uncommon. Local mucosal necrosis and hemorrhage, early manifestations of this process, are seen with some frequency. Such defects in the mucosa are often multiple, typically small and round, and can be associated with significant hemorrhage from the exposed blood vessels deep to the lesions. They heal rapidly and rarely lead to serious complications.

The intestinal tract is especially susceptible to ischemic and hypoxic injury, and lesions related to poor perfusion are often found at the time of autopsy. Decreased blood flow in the splanchnic circulation is a well-established physiological consequence of endotoxemia.[17,81] Thus sepsis is associated with an increased risk of intestinal injury. Hypoxic or ischemic injury of the intestinal epithelium, which may be very limited, can lead to translocation of intestinal flora into the mesenteric lymphatic circulation and into the portal venous circulation.[82–85] Additional factors favoring the escape of bacteria from the intestine include alterations in the bacterial ecology of the gut.[86] Hypotension and hypoxia, then, can also be causes of sepsis. In our autopsy experience, formation of abscesses or foci of tissue infection in the intestinal tract was uncommon, except when many organs including the skin were heavily infected in patients with generalized sepsis. The intestinal lesion most commonly seen at autopsy consists of transverse streaks of hemorrhage in the small intestine in a 'ladder' pattern, associated with focal necrosis of folds of mucosa. This lesion is called superficial hemorrhagic necrosis.[87] Perhaps surprisingly, perforation of the intestinal tract is an uncommon occurrence in patients with burn injury. Pseudomembranous colitis does occur occasionally (Figure 45.6a).

The liver is enlarged at the time of autopsy in most children who succumb to burn injury, often to double or triple its normal weight. The increase in liver weight is rather consistent as a function of time after injury.[88] Occasionally such hepatomegaly is thought to compromise ventilation. The lesions often seen in the liver at autopsy include steatosis, with deposition of large and small lipid droplets in hepatocytes (Figure 45.6b) and congestion, often with centrilobular necrosis. This pattern of central necrosis may be a consequence of reduced splanchnic blood flow in patients with sepsis. Intracellular cholestasis is commonly observed in patients with burn injury. The basis for this abnormality is not clear, although multiple physiological derangements could be expected to lead to cholestasis.[89–91]

Pancreatitis is a frequent complication of burn injury in children. The lesions most often seen at autopsy are focal necrosis of pancreatic tissue, focal hemorrhage and focal fat necrosis (Figure 45.6c). This abnormality is clinically silent in

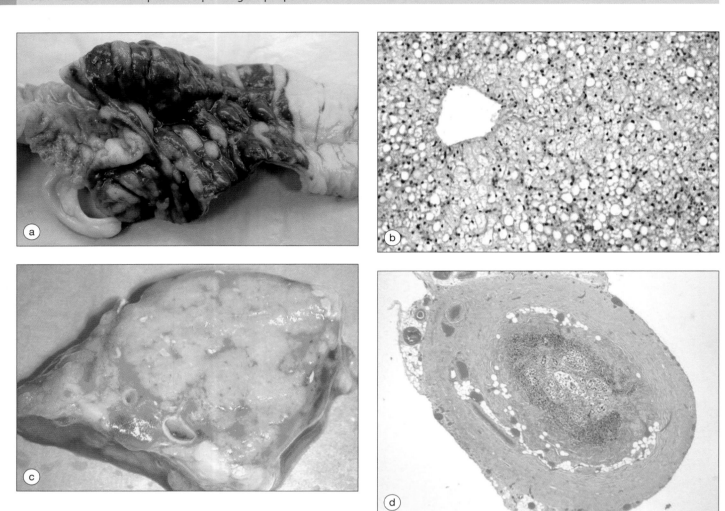

Fig. 45.6 (a) This autopsy photograph illustrates pseudomembranous colitis in the cecum. (b) This micrograph of H&E-stained liver tissue shows moderate steatosis in a 6-year-old patient who lived for 1 month after a large burn and whose liver was 2.2 times heavier than normal. (c) This cross-section of a patient's pancreas at autopsy shows foci of hemorrhage and several small bright yellow foci of fat necrosis. The patient succumbed to disseminated bacterial infection. (d) This is a micrograph at low magnification showing the extensive loss of lymphoid tissue in the appendix that is typical of children hospitalized for burns who live more than 1 week.

most cases, but is associated with transient elevations in amylase and lipase.

Lymphoid system

Depletion of lymphocytes from lymphoid tissues throughout the body is a consistent feature seen at autopsy in patients with burn injury. The abnormalities were well described by Dr Linares in 1978.[92] The thymus is consistently very small, even in young children. The lymph nodes often lack germinal centers, and may be strikingly depleted of lymphocytes. Sinus histiocytosis is often present, and pyroninophilic cells resembling plasma cells are often prominent, in the portions of the node normally occupied by B cells. The splenic white pulp is deficient, sometimes strikingly so. The gastrointestinal lymphoid tissue of the terminal ileum is generally atrophic, in spite of its normal prominence in children, and the appendix often shows a striking lack of normal lymphoid tissue in its wall (Figure 45.6d). These abnormalities of lymphoid tissue corre-late with the deficient immune responsiveness typical of patients with extensive burn injury. To some extent they may represent the effects of high levels of endogenous glucocorticoids in burn patients.

Musculoskeletal system

Lesions of skeletal muscle are uncommon in burn patients, but are ominous when they occur. Occasionally, direct thermal injury extends into deep muscle, and at times this injury can be so severe that adequate debridement is not practical. Electrical injury often is associated with extensive necrosis of muscle. When invasive bacterial or fungal infection extends into muscle, again, it may not be feasible to treat adequately by excision of the infected tissue, and the infection may be resistant to antibiotic therapy and likely to disseminate. Atrophy of skeletal muscle occurs as part of the catabolic state of burn patients, and represents a challenge for those involved in rehabilitative efforts.

Central nervous system

When the brain and spinal cord are examined carefully at autopsy, abnormalities can be found in the great majority of patients who die after burn injury. The commonest lesion is degeneration or loss of neurons in the portions of the cortex most susceptible to hypoxic and ischemic injury. These lesions can be a result of hypovolemia during resuscitation, shock developing as part of the syndrome of sepsis, or as a consequence of respiratory failure. Of course, extensive hypoxic brain injury may occur in patients who are asphyxiated during the initial burn injury. Some patients who require cardiopulmonary resuscitation at the scene of injury develop massive cerebral edema and brain death several days after the initial injury, reflecting the response to extensive hypoxic–ischemic injury in the brain. Severe hypoxic brain injury also can occur in burn patients who are deprived of oxygen during the progress of a house fire, or who are poisoned by carbon monoxide at the scene of the burn. Occasionally prolonged delay in fluid resuscitation of a patient with a large burn is associated with hypoxic–ischemic brain injury and brain death. Another special case is the patient who has direct thermal injury to the brain. Such lesions, which occur occasionally in young children, can be detected by radiological imaging studies, and are represented at autopsy by small foci of tissue necrosis on the cortical surface, surrounded by a hyperemic reaction.

The burn autopsy

As long as patients continue to develop complications of burn injury that are difficult to manage, and as long as the pathogenesis of these complications remains uncertain, careful postmortem examination of patients who do not survive will continue to contribute to patient care. There is a paradox here. Tissue injury occurs due to elevated temperature, a very simple physical alteration. However, there is no disease with more complex clinical and physiopathological derangements than an extensive burn. Observations made at the time of autopsy often clarify the nature of the problems that led to the patient's demise. Sometimes the findings lead to suggestions for changes in procedure that may lead to improved patient safety. Often a causal sequence of events can be reconstructed by including the clinical evidence and the autopsy findings. Infectious processes, for example, often can be traced from their sites of origin, in the skin or elsewhere, to the fatal conclusion. The emergence of unusually resistant bacterial strains can be traced. The autopsy should always be approached from the point of view of using both clinical and autopsy evidence to better understand the reactions of the patient to the burn injury and to the treatments provided. In other words, the burn autopsy can provide not only an appropriate morphological analysis but also a dynamic interpretation of the pathogenesis of the disease processes of importance in an individual patient. When approached in this way, investigation of patient deaths becomes a valuable learning experience for all those who participate in it. Not infrequently, unexpected lesions are found which were likely to have been significant in the patient's course. Of course, the circumstances of burn injury may have legal implications, and documentation of the patient's injuries and careful interpretation of the hospital course can have the beneficial effect of providing factual evidence where only supposition would be available otherwise. We advocate a policy of carrying out complete autopsies on all patients who die after burn injury, whenever possible, including microscopic study and consultation with specialists, in collaboration with the local medical examiner or coroner.

References

1. Long J. Post-mortem appearances found after burns. London Medical Gazzette 1840; 25:743–750.
2. McClure RD, Lam CR, Romence H. Tannic acid and the treatment of burns: an obsequy. Ann Surg 1944; 120:387–398.
3. Harkins HN. Experimental burns. I. The rate of fluid shift and its relation to the onset of shock in severe burns. Arch Surg 1935; 31:71–85.
4. Underhill FP, Kapsinow R, Fisk M. Studies on the mechanism of water exchange in the animal organism. Am J Physiol 1930; 95:302–314.
5. Cope O, Moore FD. The redistribution of body water and the fluid therapy of the burned patient. Ann Surg 1947; 126:1010–1045.
6. Evans EI, Purnell OJ, Robinett PW, et al. Fluid and electrolyte requirements in severe burns. Ann Surg 1952; 135:804–817.
7. Demling RH. Fluid replacement in burned patients. Surg Clin North Am 1987; 67:15–30.
8. Justis DL, Law EJ, MacMillan BG. Tibial compartment syndromes in burn patients. A report of four cases. Arch Surg 1976; 111:1004–1008.
9. Rosen CL, Adler JN, Rabban JT, et al. Early predictors of myoglobinuria and acute renal failure following electrical injury. J Emerg Med 1999; 17:783–789.
10. Aub JC, Beecher HK, Cannon B, et al. Management of the Coconut Grove burns at the Massachusetts General Hospital. Philadelphia: Lippincott; 1943.
11. Horton JW. Free radicals and lipid peroxidation mediated injury in burn trauma: the role of antioxidant therapy. Toxicology 2003; 189:75–88.
12. Meneshian A, Bulkley GB. The physiology of endothelial xanthine oxidase: from urate catabolism to reperfusion injury to inflammatory signal transduction. Microcirculation. 2002; 9:161–175.
13. Sakano T, Okerberg CV, Shippee RL, et al. A rabbit model of inhalation injury. J Trauma 1993; 34:411–416.
14. Clements NC Jr, Habib MP. The early pattern of conjugated dienes in liver and lung after endotoxin exposure. Am J Respir Crit Care Med 1995; 151:780–784.
15. Linares HA. Sepsis, disseminated intravascular coagulation and multiorgan failure: catastrophic events in severe burns. In: Schlag G, Redl H, Siegel JH, et al., eds. Shock, sepsis, and organ failure. Berlin: Springer-Verlag; 1991:370–398.
16. Linares HA. A report of 115 consecutive autopsies in burned children: 1966–80. Burns 1981; 8:263–270.
17. Teplitz C. The pathology of burns and the fundamentals of burn wound sepsis. In: Atrz CL, Moncrief JA, Pruitt BA, eds. Burns: a team approach. Philadelphia: WB Saunders; 1979:45.
18. Bone RC, Sibbald WJ, Sprung CL. The ACCP-SCCM consensus conference on sepsis and organ failure. Chest 1992; 101:1481–1482.
19. Fredholm B, Hagermark O. Studies on histamine release from skin and from peritoneal mast cells of the rat induced by heat. Acta Derm Venereol 1970; 50:273–277.
20. Horakova Z, Beaven MA. Time course of histamine release and edema formation in the rat paw after thermal injury. Eur J Pharmacol 1974; 27:305–312.
21. Olsson P. Clinical views on the kinin system. Scand J Clin Lab Invest 1969; 24:123–124.

22. Effeney DJ, Blaisdell FW, McIntyre KE, et al. The relationship between sepsis and disseminated intravascular coagulation. J Trauma 1978; 18:689–695.

23. Wisplinghoff H, Perbix W, Seifert H. Risk factors for nosocomial bloodstream infections due to Acinetobacter baumannii: a case-control study of adult burn patients. Clin Infect Dis 1999; 28:59–66.

24. Wurtz R, Karajovic M, Dacumos E, et al. Nosocomial infections in a burn intensive care unit. Burns 1995; 21:181–184.

25. Hawkins HK, Linares H, Desai MH, et al. Declining incidence of burn wound sepsis at autopsy. J Burn Care Rehabil 1999; 20(1 pt 2):211.

26. Curreri PW, Kak AF, Dotin LN, et al. Coagulation abnormalities in the thermally injured patient. In: Skinner DB, Ebert PA, eds. Current topics in surgical research. New York: Academic Press; 1970:401.

27. McManus WF, Eurenius K, Pruitt BA. Disseminated intravascular coagulation in burned patients. J Trauma 1973; 13:416–422.

28. Alkjaersig N, Fletcher AP, Peden JC, et al. Fibrinogen catabolism in burned patients. J Trauma 1980; 20:154–159.

29. Bick R. Disseminated intravascular coagulation and related syndromes: a clinical review. Semin Thromb Hemost 1988; 14:299–337.

30. Watanabe T, Imamura T, Nakagaki K, et al. Diseminated intravascular coagulation in autopsy cases: its incidence and clinico-pathologic significance. Pathol Res Pract 1979; 165:311–322.

31. Papp A, Kiraly K, Harma M, et al. The progression of burn depth in experimental burns: a histological and methodological study. Burns 2004; 30:684–690.

32. Mileski WJ, Borgstrom D, Lightfoot E, et al. Inhibition of leukocyte-endothelial adherence following thermal injury. J Surg Res 1992; 52:334–339.

33. Linares HA. Autopsy findings in burned children. In: Carvajal HF, Parks DH, eds. Burns in children. Chicago: Year Book Medical; 1988.

34. Teplitz C, Davis D, Mason AD, et al. Pseudomonas burn wound sepsis. 1. Pathogenesis of experimental pseudomonas burn wound sepsis. J Surg Res 1964; 4:200–222.

35. Eldridge JP, Baldridge ED, MacMillan BG. Ecthyma gangrenosum in a burned child. Burns Incl Therm Inj 1986; 12:578–585.

36. Jones SG, Olver WJ, Boswell TC, et al. Ecthyma gangrenosum. Eur J Haematol 2002; 69:324.

37. Demling RH, Wong C, Jin LJ, et al. Early lung dysfunction after major burns: role of edema and vasoactive mediators. J Trauma 1985; 25:959–966.

38. Clowes GHA, Zuschneid W, Dragacevic S, et al. The nonspecific pulmonary inflammatory reactions leading to respiratory failure after shock, gangrene and sepsis. J Trauma 1968; 8:899–914.

39. Swank DW, Moore SB. Roles of the neutrophil and other mediators in adult respiratory distress syndrome. Mayo Clin Proc 1989; 64:1118–1132.

40. Mulligan MS, Smith CW, Anderson DC, et al. Role of leukocyte adhesion molecules in complement-induced lung injury. J Immunol 1993; 150:2401–2406.

41. Huie RE, Padmaja S. The reaction of NO with superoxide. Free Radic Res Commun 1993; 18:195–199.

42. Cooper JA, Solano SJ, Bizios R, et al. Pulmonary neutrophil kinetics after thrombin-induced intravascular coagulation. J Appl Physiol 1984; 57:826–832.

43. Lentz LA, Ziegler ST, Cox CS, et al. Cytokine response to thermal injury, shock sepsis and organ failure. The Second Wiggers Bernard Conference. In: Schlag G, Redl H, Siegel JH, et al., eds. New York: Springer-Verlag; 1993:245–264.

44. Lin YS, Kou YR. Acute neurogenic airway plasma exudation and edema induced by inhaled wood smoke in guinea pigs: role of tachykinins and hydroxyl radical. Eur J Pharmacol 2000; 394:139–148.

45. Siney L, Brain SD. Involvement of sensory neuropeptides in the development of plasma extravasation in rat dorsal skin following thermal injury. Br J Pharmacol 1996; 117:1065–1070.

46. Fukushima M, King LS, Kang KH, et al. Lung mechanics and airway reactivity in sheep during development of oxygen toxicity. J Appl Physiol 1990; 69:1779–1785.

47. Moran JF, Robinson LA, Lowe JE, et al. Effects of oxygen toxicity on regional ventilation and perfusion in the primate lung. Surgery 1981; 89:575–581.

48. Barazzone C, Horowitz S, Donati YR, et al. Oxygen toxicity in mouse lung: pathways to cell death. Am J Respir Cell Mol Biol 1998; 19:573–581.

49. Barrow RE, Spies M, Barrow LN, et al. Influence of demographics and inhalation injury on burn mortality in children. Burns 2004; 30:72–77.

50. Kobayashi K, Ikeda H, Higuchi R, et al. Epidemiological and outcome characteristics of major burns in Tokyo. Burns 2005; 31 (Suppl 1):S3–S11.

51. Muller MJ, Pegg SP, Rule MR. Determinants of death following burn injury. Br J Surg 2001; 88:583–587.

52. Suzuki M, Aikawa N, Kobayashi K, et al. Prognostic implications of inhalation injury in burn patients in Tokyo. Burns 2005; 31:331–336.

53. Tredget EE, Shankowsky HA, Taerum TV, et al. The role of inhalation injury in burn trauma. A Canadian experience. Ann Surg 1990; 212:720–727.

54. Linares HA, Herndon DN, Traber DL. Sequence of morphologic events in experimental smoke inhalation. J Burn Care Rehabil 1989; 10:27–37.

55. Herndon DN, Traber DL, Niehaus GD, et al. The pathophysiology of smoke inhalation injury in a sheep model. J Trauma 1984; 24:1044–1051.

56. Murakami K, Traber DL. Pathophysiological basis of smoke inhalation injury. News Physiol Sci 2003; 18:125–129.

57. Soejima K, Schmalstieg FC, Sakurai H, et al. Pathophysiological analysis of combined burn and smoke inhalation injuries in sheep. Am J Physiol Lung Cell Mol Physiol 2001; 280:L1233–L1241.

58. Abdi S, Evans MJ, Cox RA, et al. Inhalation injury to tracheal epithelium in an ovine model of cotton smoke exposure. Early phase (30 minutes). Am Rev Respir Dis 1990; 142:1436–1439.

59. Abdi S, Herndon DN, McGuire J, et al. Time course of alterations in lung lymph and bronchial blood flows after inhalation injury. J Burn Care Rehabil 1990; 11:510–515.

60. Stothert JC Jr, Ashley KD, Kramer GC, et al. Intrapulmonary distribution of bronchial blood flow after moderate smoke inhalation. J Appl Physiol 1990; 69:1734–1739.

61. Enkhbaatar P, Traber DL. Pathophysiology of acute lung injury in combined burn and smoke inhalation injury. Clin Sci (Lond) 2004; 107:137–143.

62. Veronesi B, Carter JD, Devlin RB, et al. Neuropeptides and capsaicin stimulate the release of inflammatory cytokines in a human bronchial epithelial cell line. Neuropeptides 1999; 33:447–456.

63. Zimmerman BJ, Anderson DC, Granger DN. Neuropeptides promote neutrophil adherence to endothelial cell monolayers. Am J Physiol 1992; 263:G678–G682.

64. Lentz CW, Abdi S, Traber LD. The role of sensory neuropeptides in inhalation injury. Proc Am Burn Assoc 1992; 24:A18.

65. Kunkel SL, Standiford TJ, Kasahara K, et al. Interleukin-8 (IL-8): the major neutrophil chemotactic factor in the lung. Exp Lung Res 1991; 17:17–23.

66. Enkhbaatar P, Murakami K, Shimoda K, et al. Inhibition of neuronal nitric oxide synthase by 7-nitroindazole attenuates acute lung injury in an ovine model. Am J Physiol Regul Integr Comp Physiol 2003; 285:R366–R372.

67. Enkhbaatar P, Murakami K, Shimoda K, et al. The inducible nitric oxide synthase inhibitor BBS-2 prevents acute lung injury in sheep after burn and smoke inhalation injury. Am J Respir Crit Care Med 2003; 167:1021–1026.

68. Cox RA, Soejima K, Burke AS, et al. Enhanced pulmonary expression of endothelin-1 in an ovine model of smoke inhalation injury. J Burn Care Rehabil 2001; 22:375–383.

69. Cox RA, Enkhabaatar P, Burke AS, et al. Effects of a dual endothelin-1 receptor antagonist on airway obstruction and acute lung injury in sheep following smoke inhalation and burn injury. Clin Sci (Lond) 2005; 108:265–272.

70. Shimoda K, Murakami K, Enkhbaatar P, et al. Effect of poly(ADP ribose) synthetase inhibition on burn and smoke inhalation injury

in sheep. Am J Physiol Lung Cell Mol Physiol 2003; 285: L240–L249.

71. Cox RA, Burke AS, Kazutaka S, et al. Airway obstruction in sheep with burn and smoke inhalation injuries. Am J Respir Cell Mol Biol 2003; 29:295–302.

72. Murakami K, McGuire R, Cox RA, et al. Recombinant antithrombin attenuates pulmonary inflammation following smoke inhalation and pneumonia in sheep. Crit Care Med 2003; 31:577–583.

73. Murakami K, McGuire R, Cox RA, et al. Heparin nebulization attenuates acute lung injury in sepsis following smoke inhalation in sheep. Shock 2002; 18:236–241.

74. Enkhbaatar P, Traber DL. Pathophysiology of acute lung injury in combined burn and smoke inhalation injury. Clin Sci (Lond) 2004; 107:137–143.

75. Murakami K, Traber DL. Pathophysiological basis of smoke inhalation injury. News Physiol Sci 2003; 18:125–129.

76. Rona G, Boutet M, Huttner I, et al. Pathogenesis of isoproterenol-induced myocardial alterations: functional and morphological correlates. Recent Adv Stud Cardiac Struct Metab 1973; 3:507–525.

77. Kahn DS, Rona G, Chappel CI. Isoproterenol-induced cardiac necrosis. Ann NY Acad Sci 1969; 156:285–293.

78. Martineau PP, Hartman FW. The renal lesions in extensive cutaneous burns. JAMA 1947; 134:429–436.

79. Wolf SE, Rose JK, Desai MH, et al. Mortality determinants in massive pediatric burns. An analysis of 103 children with ≥80% TBSA burns (≥70% full-thickness). Ann Surg 1997; 225:554–565.

80. Curling TB. On acute ulceration of duodenum in cases of burn. Trans R Med Chir Soc Lond 1842; 25:260–281.

81. Fronek K, Zweifach BW. Changes of splanchnic hemodynamics in hemorrhagic hypotension and endotoxemia. J Surg Res 1971; 11:232–237.

82. Berg RD, Garlington AW. Translocation of certain indigenous bacteria from the gastrointstinal tract to the mesenteric lymph nodes and other organs in a gnotobiotic mouse model. Infect Immun 1979; 23:403–411.

83. Deitch EA, Berg R. Bacterial translocation from the gut: a mechanism of infection. J Burn Care Rehabil 1987; 8:475–482.

84. Wells CL, Maddaus MA, Simmons RL. Proposed mechanisms for the translocation of intestinal bacteria. Rev Infect Dis 1988; 10:958–979.

85. Baker JW, Deitch EA, Berg RD, et al. Hemorrhagic shock induces bacterial translocation from the gut. J Trauma 1988; 28:896–906.

86. Berg RD, Wommack E, Deitch EA. Immunosuppression and intestinal bacterial overgrowth synegistically promote bacterial translocation. Arch Surg 1988; 123:1359–1364.

87. Ahren C, Haglund V. Mucosal lesions in the small intestine of the cat during low flow. Acta Physiol Scand 1973; 88:541–550.

88. Barrow RE, Mlcak R, Barrow LN, et al. Increased liver weights in severely burned children: comparison of ultrasound and autopsy measurements. Burns 2004; 30:565–568.

89. Hurd T, Lysz T, Dikdan G, et al. Hepatic cellular dysfunction in sepsis: an ischemic phenomenon? Curr Surg 1988; 45:114–119.

90. Cano N, Gerolami A. Intrahepatic cholestasis during total parenteral nutrition. Lancet 1983; 1:985.

91. Barrow RE, Hawkins HK, Aarsland A, et al. Identification of factors contributing to hepatomegaly in severely burned children. Shock 2005; 24:523–528.

92. Linares HA, Beathard GA, Larson DL. Morphological changes of lymph nodes of children following acute thermal burns. Burns 1978; 4:165–170.

Chapter 46

Wound healing

David G. Greenhalgh

Introduction

The ultimate goals of all burn team members are to heal the patient's wounds with the least scarring and to maximize the functional and cosmetic outcome. The management of the burn wound depends on the depth and extent of the injury. Those wounds that are superficial need to re-epithelialize. Smaller but deep wounds heal by scar formation and contraction. These processes are beneficial at times but detrimental at other times. Understanding how these wounds heal will help with choosing an appropriate treatment. Larger wounds require grafting. By understanding how a graft heals, one can optimize the outcome. It is clear that all patients with burns greater than 20–25% total body surface area (TBSA) develop systemic changes that influence their survival. The burn wound is a major source of inflammatory mediators that lead to hypermetabolism, muscle wasting and, potentially, dysfunction of multiple organ systems. The best way to treat these systemic problems is to eliminate the source of the inflammatory mediators by expeditiously removing the source of the mediators and covering the wound. The strategies for covering these massive wounds will be discussed in this chapter. The factors that influence wound healing will also be described. Finally, much of our time is devoted to the management of scars. While relatively little is known about reducing scar formation, more options are available to us compared to the past. Hopefully, we will gain further insights into the control of scar formation in the future.

There are several basic principles that the burn team must remember when treating a wound:

1. The goal is to maximize the functional and cosmetic outcome of the burn.
2. Optimizing initial wound care will minimize the need for scar management and reconstructive surgery. (Do it right from the start.)
3. If a burn heals within 2 weeks, then scarring is minimal. If the wound has not healed within 2 weeks, then grafting is probably indicated.
4. Topical agents do heal a wound but, instead, reduce infection risks. In addition, they do not eliminate bacteria. Target the topical agent for the wound type and the likely bacterial flora.
5. Make treatment simple (especially in the outpatient setting):
   - Sterile techniques are unnecessary. Use clean techniques.
   - The patient may get into the shower or tub.
   - Caregivers should wash their hands and use clean barriers (gowns, gloves) in the inpatient setting.
   - At home, barrier techniques are probably not indicated. Hand washing is still important.
   - Try to minimize pain.

The goal of this chapter is to describe the types of wound healing in order to develop better principles of wound management that will lead to the best possible outcome for burn patients.

Types of burns

In order to optimally treat burn wounds, one must first know the types of burn injuries that exist. The type of healing that is involved in each type of wound changes depending on wound depth. Skin can be simply considered to consist of two major components, the epidermis and dermis (Figure 46.1). The major function of the *epidermis* is to keep invading organisms 'out' and keep water 'in.' At the base of the epidermis are the basal cells, which are the only keratinocytes of the epidermis that can proliferate and migrate. These cells are attached to a basement membrane that separates the epidermis from the dermis. The basal cells differentiate as they leave the basement membrane and eventually die and slough in the more superficial layers of the epithelium. The detachment, migration away from the basement membrane, differentiation, and sloughing is the normal life cycle of the keratinocytes. The *dermis* adds the strength to the skin, since it is made of collagen and other extracellular matrix (ECM) proteins. The dermis also contains a vascular and neural plexus. The vascular plexus

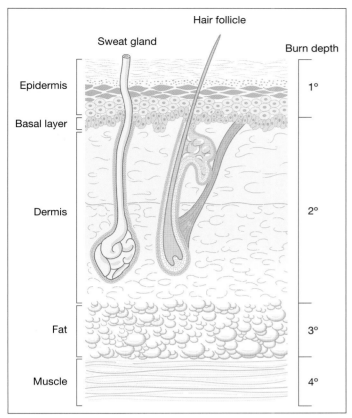

Fig. 46.1 This drawing demonstrates the major layers of the skin. The epidermis has a basal cell layer of keratinocytes that have the potential to migrate and proliferate to cover a wound. The dermis contains adnexa (hair follicles, oil glands) that contain epithelial cells that migrate on to the open wound and re-epithelialize it. The type of healing that occurs after a burn depends on which layers of the skin are damaged. A 1° burn does not extend deeper than the basal layer of the epidermis. A 2° burn involves the dermis and a 3° burn extends beneath the dermis and into the fat. A 4° burn involves tissue beneath the fat.

is vital for temperature control, and the neural plexus gives the skin the ability to sense the environment. The neural network also produces the sharp pain that results from superficial burns. The dermis also contains the skin adnexa (hair follicles, oil glands, sweat glands) which are lined by epithelial cells. These adnexa are essential for the healing of superficial burns.

The depth of burn has traditionally been divided into first degree (1°), second degree (2°), third degree (3°) and fourth degree (4°) (Figure 46.1). A 1° burn does not extend below the basal cell layer of the epidermis. These burns are dry, red and painful. The 2° burn extends into the dermis and is characterized by being moist, painful and red with blanching. The wound is moist because of the loss of the barrier function of the epidermis. The pain and blanching redness exist because the dermal nerves and blood supply persist. A 3° burn extends completely through the dermis and into the subdermal fat. These burns are dry, less painful and do not blanch because the dermal nerves and blood supply are destroyed. These burns can be almost any color (white, tan, black, brown, red) and tend to be leathery as result of the 'eschar' produced from

the coagulated proteins that result from the burn. The eschar should not be confused with the 'scab' that develops over time on a 2° burn. This scab is the result of fibrin and cellular deposition from the exuding wound fluid. Finally, a 4° burn is one that extends to fascia, bone, tendon, muscle or other tissue beneath the subcutaneous fat.

Types of tissue repair

Re-epithelialization

Since 1° and 2° burns leave behind remnants of epithelium the major form of healing for these types of wounds is re-epithelialization. For 1° burns, such as sun burns, the basal cell layer of keratinocytes persists. The basal cell layer simply differentiates to recreate the multiple layers of the epidermis. This process is usually complete within 3–4 days. Little treatment is needed to manage these wounds other than possibly a moisturizer.

Once the burn extends into the dermis (2°), then the entire epidermis has to be reconstructed from the skin adnexa. Fortunately, the skin adnexa (hair follicles, sweat glands, oil glands and others) are lined with epithelial cells. There are several stimuli for the basal keratinocytes at the wound edge and the adnexal epithelial cells to migrate on to the surface of the wound.[1] First, the loss of basal cell–cell contact leads to signals for the keratinocytes to migrate. In addition, growth factors that target epithelial cell growth and migration are released from the wound to stimulate migration. Growth factors that specifically target epithelial cells include epidermal growth factor (EGF), transforming growth factor-α (TGF-α), keratinocyte growth factors-1 and -2 (KGF-1 and KGF-2).[2-6] Other growth factors stimulate keratinocyte growth and migration either directly or indirectly in addition to having other wound healing activities (transforming growth factor-β [TGF-β] and interleukin-1 [IL-1]).[6,7] Finally, if keratinocytes come in contact with specific proteins, then they are stimulated to migrate. For instance, basal cells are content to stay put if they are in contact with proteins that are in the basement membrane (such as laminin or collagen type IV). When they come in contact with proteins found in the wound, such as fibrin, fibronectin, or collagen type I, then they are stimulated to migrate.[8] All of these stimuli are produced in a 2° burn or split-thickness skin graft (STSG) donor site.

Keratinocytes migrate from the original wound edge and from the skin adnexa, and travel over the viable wound bed (Figure 46.2). If there is a moist and viable surface, then the cells can migrate most rapidly. As the epithelial cells march up from the adnexa, whitish dots (epithelial buds) appear on the reddish background of the wound (Figure 46.3). When the cells regain contact with other migrating keratinocytes (covering the wound), then they differentiate and form all of the layers of the epidermis. The wounds with the highest concentration of skin adnexa heal the fastest. This is why the scalp heals within 4–5 days while areas lacking hair, such as the lower legs in older people, take longer to re-epithelialize. If the wound dries and forms a 'scab' (composed of fibrin, dead neutrophils and other debris), then the keratinocytes have to 'cut' their way along the viable surface by releasing proteases and other enzymes. If a thick scab does develop, then light

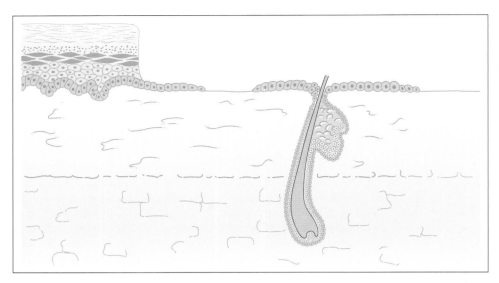

Fig. 46.2 A diagram of re-epithelialization. Basal cells of the epidermal edge migrate across the viable wound bed. In addition, skin adnexa, such as hair follicles, also contain epithelial cells that migrate onto the surface and participate in the resurfacing. If the surface is moist and free of fibrinous exudate, then re-epithelialization proceeds faster.

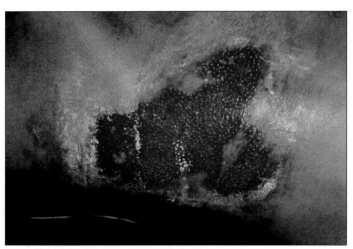

Fig. 46.3 Epithelial buds are the white dots in the middle of the red wound in this superficial burn that is re-epithelializing.

debridement will assist with healing. One must be careful, however, to avoid pulling off the new epithelium.

It has been shown that maintaining a moist environment leads to more rapid re-epithelialization than if the wound is allowed to dry. Many ointments and dressings have been designed to assist with optimizing healing of these superficial wounds. For instance, an ointment such as bacitracin prevents drying while at the same time decreasing Gram-positive organisms. Dressings have also been designed to maintain the moist environment. These 'biologic dressings' are designed to cover the wound and maintain the optimal environment until re-epithelialization is completed. Transparent polyurethane dressings were designed with this in mind. Other dressings are designed to stick to the wound and allow for healing. Biobrane™, which has a layer of type I collagen, sticks to the wound until re-epithelialization is complete. TransCyte™ uses the same principle but has fibroblasts in the dressing that release a variety of growth factors. Other biologics have been used to improve wound healing in chronic ulcers. Derma-

graft™, a 'three-dimensional, allogeneic, human neonatal dermal fibroblast culture grown on a biodegradable scaffold that is cryopreserved', and Graftskin™, a 'living skin equivalent' consisting of a dermis (with fibroblasts) and keratinocytes, have been used to treat diabetic ulcers with success. Some of the older biologic dressings are porcine skin and human allograft. All of these biologic dressings have many advantages as well of disadvantages. These agents stick to the wound and allow for protected re-epithelialization under the dressing. The biologic dressings that contain live cells also have the advantage of releasing growth factors and other agents that may accelerate healing. One problem is the cost of using these new technologies. Some of the viable biologics can cost thousands of dollars just to cover a relatively small area. These costs must be balanced with the advantages of each dressing. A jar of bacitracin may reduce costs by a factor approaching hundreds to a thousand times less.

Another approach to accelerating healing of superficial burn wounds and STSG donor sites has been to apply exogenous growth factors. At one time there was a great deal of interest in applying these cytokines to a wound to accelerate re-epithelialization. Many animal studies have demonstrated accelerated healing of superficial wounds.[2–6] Several controlled, randomized, prospective and double-blinded clinical trials have been performed using different growth factors.[9–11] Most of the trials were performed using small donor sites on opposite sides of the body and revealed that a statistically significant improvement in tissue repair was found. Unfortunately, what proved to be statistically significant was not clinically relevant. Wounds would heal a day or two faster compared to the control. Since the healing of small donor sites does not impact length of stay, the benefit did not justify the cost. It is difficult to greatly accelerate healing of small donor sites. The healing of donor sites in massive burns, however, often appears to be slower than that of small wounds. Herndon's group has treated children with relatively large burns (>40%) with systemic human recombinant growth hormone and found that the time to reharvesting of donor sites was significantly shortened.[12] With the requirement for multiple reharvests, the length of stay per percent burn was also significantly shortened. The decreased length of stay more than counteracts the increased cost of the recombinant protein.

While discussing re-epithelialization one must also consider repigmentation. Melanocytes reside in the basal cell layer of the epithelium. After a 2° burn pigment is lost. This is also true for split-thickness donor sites (which heal by the same re-epithelialization process). Like keratinocytes, melanocytes reside in the adnexa of the dermis. After re-epithelialization one will notice that brown dots of repigmentation will gradually appear. The sizes of the pigmentation areas gradually enlarge and coalesce to repigment the area. With deeper burns melanocytes are eliminated and pigment can be lost. This can be a significant problem for people with increased skin color. There is also a tendency for skin grafts to hyperpigment while donor sites frequently will not match the surrounding skin. Unfortunately, we do not have very good options for treating pigmentation problems. There are quinolone creams that may lighten color but they are difficult to control and often do not match the surrounding areas. People have tried to replace pigment with tattoos with poor outcomes. There are those who will dermibrade an area and then regraft the area for return of pigment. This technique may also lead to other scarring problems.

Scar formation

A second form of healing involves re-creating the 'tough' component of the tissue. For skin, the body attempts to form a 'new dermis.' During this process new connective tissue (the ECM) that gives tissue its strength is created. In simpler forms of life, and in the fetus, skin and other tissues can be regenerated. In mammals (at least after birth), wounds close by creating a less than perfect scar. No one knows why mammals scar instead of regenerating the original tissue but one can guess that in our contaminated world that more expeditious closure at the expense of regeneration may have been an evolutionary compromise for controlling bacterial invasion. Scar formation is both essential (to prevent dehiscence) and a hindrance in that excessive fibrosis is an ultimate complication of many disease processes (contractures, hypertrophic scars, keloids, pulmonary fibrosis, cirrhosis, arthritis, plus more). Investigators are trying to understand the controls of these processes. Much more is known about the factors that turn on the process than is known about what turns off the process. These factors will be discussed in this section.

Scar formation is usually divided into three phases. The three phases were originally determined by measuring the tensile strength of incisions over time (Figure 46.4). During the first 4–5 days after closing an incision, little change in wound strength is noted. During this time, inflammatory cells invade the incision, so it is called the *inflammatory* or *lag phase*. After this period, there is a rapid increase in collagen content in the incision that is associated with a rapid increase in tensile strength. This phase is called the *proliferative* or *collagen phase*. Two key events occur during this phase, the deposition of the ECM and the ingrowth of new vessels. Finally, there is a prolonged phase where the incision continues to gain strength (up to approximately 80% of the original skin) but there is no increase in collagen content. Also during

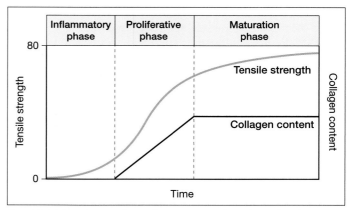

Fig. 46.4 The phases of scar formation are based on the changes of tensile strength and collagen deposition in an incision. For the first 4–5 days after closing an incision, there is little increase in strength. During this *inflammatory phase*, inflammatory cells prepare the wound for the arrival of fibroblasts. Once the fibroblasts arrive in the *proliferative phase*, there is a rapid increase in tensile strength as collagen content increases. After 2–3 weeks, there is no more increase in collagen content but the incision strength continues to increase in the *maturation phase*.

this *maturation phase*, the wound tends to become less cellular and vascular until a quiescent, white scar is formed.

The inflammatory phase prepares the wound for the subsequent repair process. The main role of this phase is to eliminate invading organisms and remove foreign tissue. The inflammatory phase is divided into vascular and cellular components. All of the components of healing are controlled by the release of local and systemic mediators. In the *vascular response*, there is a release of local catecholamines that induce vasoconstriction in an attempt to control bleeding. In addition, when platelets and coagulation factors are exposed to proteins outside the vessels (collagen type I, thrombin, tissue factor, Hageman factor) hemostasis is initiated. After bleeding is controlled, different mediators (histamine, serotonin, kinins, nitric oxide, prostaglandins and leukotrienes) induce vasodilation and increased permeability. The increase in permeability allows for the leakage of serum proteins and water into the local wound area. When the wound is large enough, such as after a burn that is greater than 20% TBSA, then the mediators 'spill over' into the systemic circulation and cause the total body edema that we are familiar with in major burns.

In the *cellular response*, multiple signals are released to attract inflammatory cells to the wound. Platelets contain multiple growth factors in their alpha granules that attract the cells. Other factors such as complement (C3a and C5a) and clotting factors (thrombin and fibrin) are chemotactic for inflammatory cells. The first cells to arrive in the wound are neutrophils. These cells are mainly responsible for killing invading organisms. They release many mediators, such as proteases and oxygen radicals, that can be destructive to tissues if produced in excessive amounts. Several investigators also implicate an excessive neutrophil response that is responsible for the 'systemic inflammatory response syndrome' (SIRS). Studies that were performed in the 1970s, however, suggest that neutrophils are not essential for the healing process.[13]

Macrophages (and monocytes) have been found to be the major regulators of the healing process.[14–17] When these cells were eliminated from a wound, very little tissue repair took place. Macrophages release multiple cytokines and growth factors that stimulate the migration and proliferation of fibroblasts, keratinocytes, endothelial cells and other cells involved in tissue repair. The list of growth factors released by these cells has become quite large and is best reviewed in other publications.[17] Macrophages are found in the wound in relatively high numbers after 3–4 days. In the incision, fibroblasts follow very soon after the arrival of macrophages. The role of lymphocytes in the healing process is less clear. Lymphocytes release multiple cytokines that influence macrophages.[18,19] Tissue repair is not greatly affected, however, in mice with severe-combined immunodeficiency (lacking lymphocytes).[20] As discussed below, lymphocytes do release interferons (IFNs) that appear to have antifibrotic tendencies.

Once fibroblasts arrive in the wound, the proliferative phase begins. Two events occur in the proliferative phase: the *synthesis of the extracellular matrix* (ECM: collagens and other matrices) and *re-creation of a blood supply* (angiogenesis, vasculogenesis and arteriogenesis). Fibroblasts are the cells that produce the majority of the ECM. Since collagen is the major strength of tissues, its biosynthesis has been well studied and will only be briefly mentioned here. There are excellent reviews that describe the details of collagen production.[21,22] There are at least 19 types of collagen. All collagens can be divided into fibril-forming and non-fibrillar collagens. All collagens have at least some component of amino acid triplet repeats of 'glycine-X-Y,' with the 'X' often being proline and the 'Y' frequently being hydroxyproline or hydroxylysine. The peptide chains then form into a triple helix that gives collagen its strength. One of the most important biochemical reactions in the biosynthesis of collagen is the hydroxylation of proline or lysine. The enzyme 'protocollagen hydroxylase' required for

this reaction requires oxygen, iron (Fe^{++}), α-ketoglutarate, and most importantly vitamin C. In vitamin C deficiency (scurvy), hydroxylation does not occur and the triple helix fails to form. The malformed collagen collects within the fibroblasts and healing is markedly impaired. There are many other steps in the biosynthesis of collagen where abnormalities can occur. Another key stage is during the creation of inter-collagenous bonds that help bind fibrils of collagen together. Lysyl oxidase, the enzyme required for this process, can be blocked by such agents as penicillamine and β-aminopropionitrile (BAPN). The role of these agents and the other steps in collagen synthesis are reviewed elsewhere.[23–25] The deposition of the other ECM components also is essential for normal healing. The role of these other proteins includes glycosaminoglycans (GAGs) and elastins. Their synthesis will not be covered here.

In order to create the ECM, fibroblasts require oxygen and nutrients. In order for healing to continue, a new blood supply must be created. A great deal has been learned about the creation of a new blood supply, and the process has become quite complex. Three processes occur in the creation of a new blood supply: vasculogenesis, angiogenesis, and arteriogenesis. In addition, vascular myogenesis (recruiting the smooth muscle cells to surround the vessels) must also occur. Excellent reviews give more detail.[26–28] Most of new vessel development involves angiogenesis and arteriogenesis. With *vasculogenesis*, undifferentiated precursor stem cells to endothelial cells (angioblasts) arrive in the site of injury and differentiate to form new vessels. This type of vessel development is important in embryogenesis but does not appear to be as involved after birth. The stem cells do persist into adulthood and thus there is a potential for vasculogenesis to occur.

Angiogenesis involves sprouting of endothelial cells from postcapillary venules (Figure 46.5). Several stimuli can acti-

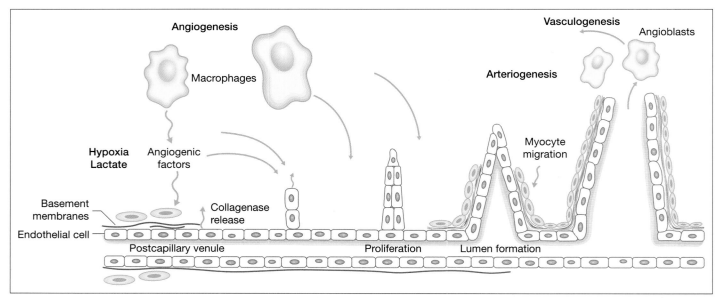

Fig. 46.5 Neovascularization of a wound involves three components. *Angiogenesis* involves the release of angiogenic factors from cells (macrophages) in a hypoxic environment. These angiogenic factors stimulate endothelial cells to release collagenases and proteases that digest the basement membrane. Endothelial cells then migrate towards the angiogenic stimuli. The migrating endothelial cells eventually form a lumen at the original vessel. During *arteriogenesis,* smooth muscle cells migrate along the newly formed vessel to recreate the muscle layer. A third type of process is called *vasculogenesis.* This process of angioblasts migrating into a tissue to initiate new blood vessel formation dominates embryonic development but appears to play a lesser role in adults.

vate the process. Low oxygen levels and lactic acid are two stimuli that can induce the process.[29,30] In addition, there are multiple angiogenic factors (such as fibroblast growth factor-2 [FGF-2] and vascular endothelial growth factor [VEGF]) that stimulate endothelial migration and proliferation.[31–34] After an injury, hypoxia and lactic acid are commonly present. In addition, macrophages release angiogenic growth factors in response to the hypoxic environment. The endothelial cells lining the postcapillary venules release proteases that digest the basement membrane. The endothelial cells then migrate towards the chemotactic signals (the concentration gradient of growth factors). As the endothelial cells migrate, endothelial cells in the original venule proliferate to replace those that have migrated away. As the sprout migrates towards the stimulus a lumen is formed to create a new vascular pathway. Recent data also suggest that angiogenesis involves other methods to modify the primitive vascular complex by causing the sprout to divide by intussusception or creating transendothelial cell bridges..

For larger vessels, *arteriogenesis* completes the process by adding the smooth muscle wall of the vessel. The process of *vascular myogenesis* involves the migration of smooth muscle cells along the perimeter of the endothelial sprout. Growth factors, such as platelet-derived growth factor-BB (PDGF-BB), are involved in this process. The smooth muscle cells stabilize the new vessel and at the same time limit its growth.

The process of neovascularization is important for other fields besides wound healing. Many tumors produce increased angiogenic factors or have mutated angiogenic receptors. A great deal of research is being performed to understand this process. Investigators have also found inhibitors of the angiogenic process (such as angiostatin)[35,36] that may be useful for cancer chemotherapy and possibly scar control.

The final phase of scar formation is *maturation*. During this phase, in an incision, there is no net increase in collagen content, despite an increase in tensile strength. When studying these wounds, collagen synthesis is occurring but there is an equal rate of collagen breakdown by collagenases. Collagen tends to be broken down where it is not needed and it is increased along lines of stress. In essence, fibroblasts are attempting to reorganize the scar to the most efficient configuration possible. In addition, intermolecular bonds are formed between collagen fibrils which tend to increase the strength of the protein (especially collagen type I, the most common collagen in the scar). Lysyl oxidase is the key enzyme that is required for this process. Any inhibition of the enzyme will lead to a weaker scar. If there is an imbalance between collagen synthesis and breakdown, then pathological healing occurs. If there is too little synthesis or excessive collagenase activity, then healing can fail, wounds weaken or chronic wounds develop. Studies have demonstrated that there is both a decrease in growth factor synthesis and increased collagenase activity in chronic, non-healing ulcers.[37–40] On the opposite extreme, if the balance is shifted to excessive collagen deposition, then hypertrophic scarring or keloids may form. Unfortunately, the controls of the collagen synthesis/breakdown balance are not well understood and are the topics of many investigations.

During the maturation process, the wound goes from being highly cellular and vascular to one that is relatively acellular

and avascular. For burn patients, we know that the burn wound tends to get redder and more raised before it matures. The duration of the maturation process can vary depending on how long the wound remains open. Wounds that heal rapidly, such as a sunburn, tend to remain red for a very short time. Those that are open for weeks tend to require 1–2 years to fade out and flatten. The controls of the maturation process are just starting to become known and are discussed below.

The wounds that the burn team handles do not follow the simplified healing of an incision. With large wounds, all three phases tend to blend together (Figure 46.6). If one examines the histology of a 10-day open wound, the center is full of inflammatory cells. The original wound edge tends to be less cellular and has a great deal of collagen deposition. At the edge of the migrating epithelium, there appears to be a transition between inflammation and wound maturation. In essence, all of the three phases of healing are blended together with the edge of the migrating epithelium being the center of transition. In the center, where the wound is exposed to chronic bacterial invasion, there is a persistent stimulus for inflammation (thus the presence of the inflammatory phase). This tissue is full of inflammatory cells, immature vessels and collagen. When the inflammatory response is not eliminated, the tissue becomes the moist, red and raised 'granulation tissue' that we are familiar with. Once the epithelium marches across the wound, then the inflammatory stimuli are eliminated and fibroblasts tend to predominate. In addition, there appears to be a signal from the epithelial cells that induces apoptosis in the nearby inflammatory cells[41,42] As one follows the wound farther behind the migrating epithelium there appears to be fewer and fewer fibroblasts. In essence, the wound covered with an epithelium appears to be going through a maturation phase.

The relationship between wound coverage and maturation has been known for a while. Deitch, et al. noted that wounds that healed within 2–3 weeks tended not to scar.[43] If exposure persisted for longer periods, then the wounds tended to develop hypertrophic scarring (Figure 46.7). Other investigators have demonstrated that the apoptosis was induced in fibroblasts

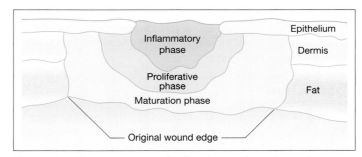

Fig. 46.6 In large open wounds, the phases of scar formation blend together. In the middle of the open wound there is a continuous inflammatory stimulus. Inflammatory cells persist in this area. When the epithelium covers the wound, the inflammatory cells undergo apoptosis and disappear. Fibroblasts dominate this part of the wound, which resembles the proliferative phase in an incision. Farthest from the center and nearest to the original wound edge, maturation of the wound is evident with a less cellular and more organized collagen pattern being found.

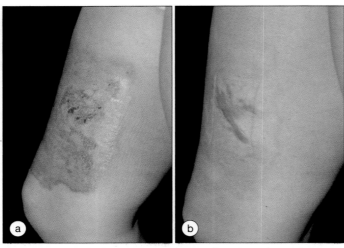

Fig. 46.7 Wounds that stay open longer than 2 weeks tend to develop hypertrophic scarring. As an example, the central area remains open at 2 weeks after a scald burn (a). The same area ultimately developed hypertrophic scarring (b).

after epithelial closure[41,42,44] or coverage of a wound with a flap.[45] Apparently, the epithelium has signals that regulate the amount of scar formation. If the wound is left open for too long, then the usual controls that prevent an excessive scar are lost. Several investigators have demonstrated that TGF-β is a likely candidate for a factor that is involved in excessive scar formation.[46–49] Tredgett's group has demonstrated that patients with hypertrophic scars tend to have increased serum levels of TGF-β1.[48,49] He and others have demonstrated that different isoforms of interferon (IFN) may reverse the effects of TGF-β1.[50–52] Others have found that elimination of TGF-β1 (by knockout technology) leads to the eventual death of the animal from overwhelming inflammation.[53,54] The lymphocytes are involved in the regulation since elimination of both TGF-β1 and lymphocytes leads to the elimination of the inflammatory response.[20] One hypothesis is that in its attempt to control inflammation and at the same time wall off the inflammatory source by inducing fibrosis, TGF-β1 regulation may be lost.[41] Interestingly, Ferguson's group has shown that only the TGF-β1 and TGF-β2 isoforms appear to induce scarring, while TGF-β3 has antiscarring effects.[55] Eventually, we will be able to understand the controls of collagen deposition enough to greatly reduce excessive scar formation. More on this topic is covered later in this chapter.

Contraction

The final type of healing is *contraction*. This process must be differentiated from contracture, which is the pathological result of the long-term shrinkage of a scar. Contraction is the relatively rapid, mechanical reduction in size of a wound.[56,57] The classical example of contraction occurs in open wounds in rodents. If one creates a sizeable open wound in a mouse, the wound edges 'pull' together to heal the wound within 10–14 days. An open wound will actually contract to 80–90% of the original wound size. The rest of the wound closure occurs by creation of a new scar and re-epithelialization. Most likely, the process of contraction evolved as a rapid and efficient way

to close an open wound. It certainly makes more sense for a wound to shrink rapidly than for it to regenerate over a much longer period.

Contraction also occurs on wounds in people. The wounds that contract the most are those that tend to be surrounded by loose skin. Small, open wounds on the buttocks (as for the small but deep electric burns) are amenable to contraction. The elderly, with their much looser skin, also can have wounds that can be left to contract. In areas where the skin is tight, such as over the dorsal fingers or ankles, wounds tend to resist contraction. These wounds tend to take much longer to heal and lead to scarring problems.

There are three phases of contraction, just as there are for scar formation. Initially, there is a 'lag period' while waiting for new fibroblasts to enter the wound. Then there is a phase of rapid contraction that is followed by a slower and more drawn-out contraction phase. The contraction of the wound is the result of specialized fibroblasts that contract to shrink the wound. These fibroblasts express α-actin, one of the key components of muscle, so they are called 'myofibroblasts.' There is considerable debate as to whether these cells are just a different phenotype of fibroblasts or whether they are a different type of cell. That debate is not essential for this chapter. As fibroblasts synthesize their collagen, they maintain contact so that millions of cells are intertwined with the new matrix. As the cells contract through an actin/myosin interaction process, the ECM which is attached to the wound edge also contracts.

Scar contracture is a more gradual process, which to some extent involves the same process. Contracture occurs over months as opposed to weeks for contraction. Scar maturation involves the continual remodeling of collagen. During the synthesis of the new collagen along lines of stress, fibroblasts probably contract in an attempt to continually shrink the wound. If there is little resistance, as for those patients who do not participate in a therapy program, then the scar contractures can be profound. Lips can be pulled to the chest and fingers extended to the forearm. Fortunately, the forces of contracture can be counteracted with stretching and massage. Compliant patients may end up with little functional abnormality. The ability of something to splint the contraction also applies to thicker grafts. Thin grafts have little resistance to shrinkage while thicker grafts shrink less. The splinting ability also applies to the surrounding tissue. Areas where the skin is tight, such as over the forehead tend not to shrink. When a graft is placed on looser skin, then the contraction process is more noticeable. While there is a great interest in the control of the contracture process, relatively little is known at this time. Hopefully, the future will bring better preventive treatments.

Types of wound coverage

Different strategies are required for closing different-sized wounds. The goal should always be to obtain the most cosmetic and functional wound closure the first time. Small and clean wounds may be treated by *primary closure*. A small burn wound or scar can be excised and re-approximated with sutures or staples. This closure tends to lead to relatively narrow scars. The limitation on this type of closure is the tension of the wound and whether it is relatively free of contamination. If there is a concern about the bacterial load, a *delayed primary closure* can be performed. These wounds are left open and treated with dressing changes for 4–5 days and then closed. Since this period is during the inflammatory (lag) phase, then little inhibition in wound strength occurs. For larger wounds, the tension of a closure can lead to a scar that widens over time. Placement of tissue expanders beneath nearby healthy skin may be used as a strategy for 'stretching' the healthy skin to accommodate a larger wound. The best example of this technique is for the removal of burn alopecia (baldness) from the scalp. Surgeons can cover the scalp with as little as one-third of the hair-bearing skin. If a wound is too large or dirty to be closed, then a *secondary closure* is an option. This term is a euphemism for 'allowing the wound to heal on its own.' This strategy is useful for relatively large burns in older patients (with loose skin) and those who could not tolerate an operative treatment. Sizeable areas on the trunk or thighs heal amazingly well in these high-risk patients.

There are many other strategies for covering larger areas of skin loss. Burn caregivers routinely deal with these types of wounds. Open wounds that need to be closed can be closed with a skin graft. Areas that are functionally important (such as fingers and hands) or cosmetically important are best treated with a sheet graft. If possible, the thickest graft (full-thickness skin graft [FTSG]) should be used if the skin is readily available.[58] As stated before, the thicker the graft, the less the contraction. One must balance the need for a thick graft with the potential scar that a donor site may make. One strategy is to use the thickest skin for split-thickness skin graft (STSG) donor sites. The back has very thick skin and tends to scar less than other areas.[59] Another strategy is to use the scalp for a donor site. The scalp matches the color of the face nicely and if not taken too thickly will not transfer hair. The scalp heals extremely rapidly and the hair hides the donor site. It is important to know that many donor sites leave a mark and many produce hypertrophic scars. One strategy is to harvest skin from areas that are relatively hidden with clothes.[60] Instead of harvesting skin down the length of a thigh one can harvest skin circumferentially around the upper thigh so that shorts would cover the region. If possible, one should avoid harvesting skin from the upper back and chest since these areas are often exposed when wearing normal clothing, especially for women.

There are three phases of skin graft healing.[61] Initially, the graft survives by diffusion of nutrients from the wound bed. Since the skin 'imbibes' nutrients from the wound bed, this phase is called the *phase of imbibition*. If any barrier forms between the wound bed and the graft (such as a hematoma, a seroma, pus, or non-viable tissue from inadequate excision), then the graft dies. Since the graft is only held in place by the natural fibrin, there is little resistance to shear, so staples, sutures, fibrin glue or complete immobilization are required. After 2–3 days, blood vessels invade the graft in the *phase of neovascularization*. New blood vessels invade the graft by angiogenesis (as described above) and by a process of 'inosculation,' where old capillaries in the wound bed are said to 'hook up' with those in the graft. Any shear at this time leads to hematoma formation and loss of the graft. Gradually, new

collagen bridges form between the wound bed and the graft in the final *phase of maturation*. This process takes months, with the graft tending to get thicker and more vascular for 3–4 months before finally fading out over the ensuing months (Figure 46.8). This maturation process parallels the maturation phase described earlier and can take 1–2 years for completion.

Since grafts require a viable wound bed, flap techniques have been developed to cover difficult wound beds where exposed bone or tendon exist. A flap contains its own blood supply and thus does not depend on the 'imbibition' from the wound bed. Flaps also have the benefit of being thicker than skin grafts and thus tend to prevent contraction. One must remember that a flap leaves a defect that must be closed. A local flap involves transfer of a nearby tissue by rotation, advancement or transposition. Part of the skin must stay attached to the original donor site until a new blood supply develops from the recipient site. A 'random' flap has its blood supply maintained by the dermal plexus. Other flaps, such as a groin flap, have an axial vessel that 'travels' with the tissue. Myocutaneous flaps utilize the underlying muscle in transfer since the skin derives its blood from that muscle. Finally, free flaps are myocutaneous flaps that have their main vessels separated and re-attached to distant vessels. For a more detailed review of flaps, check plastic surgery textbooks.

Cosmetically and functionally, sheet grafts are the best type of skin graft for covering large areas of the body.[62] One must remember that the seams between sheets of skin behave like incisions and thus leave linear scars. One should try to place seams so that scarring is minimized. For instance, placing a seam across the flexion surface of a joint will increase the tendency to develop a contracture. One can also break up seams by creating 'darts' that lead to a zig-zag seam instead of a linear one.[63] The goal should be to minimize all seams. This can be done by using newer dermatomes that harvest 6 inch wide skin or harvesting long and curved pieces of skin that allow for a graft to 'wrapped' around the face, for instance. By reharvesting donor sites, relatively large areas can be covered with sheets of skin without significant donor site morbidity. The author has covered as much as 55% TBSA of a patient with sheet grafts. Unfortunately, as wounds cover more of the body surface area, different strategies are required for wound coverage. *Meshing* skin grafts has become the standard method for covering large areas. The size of the mesh can be increased to cover larger and larger areas. Healing of the mesh graft requires not only skin graft 'take' but also the interstices must heal by scar formation, contraction and re-epithelialization. These grafts lead to a permanent mesh pattern, because of this required interstice healing.

Once massive wounds are encountered, then new strategies are required. It is clear that the large burn wound leads to a massive and continuous systemic inflammatory response syndrome (SIRS) that is a major contributor to patient mortality. Most burn surgeons believe that the source of the inflammatory stimulus should be expeditiously excised and covered with some type of permanent or temporary material which functions as skin. Some feel that the wound should be closed within hours while others feel that the wound should be closed within days. Most cover the wound with as much autograft as possible and then they use some other form of coverage. The

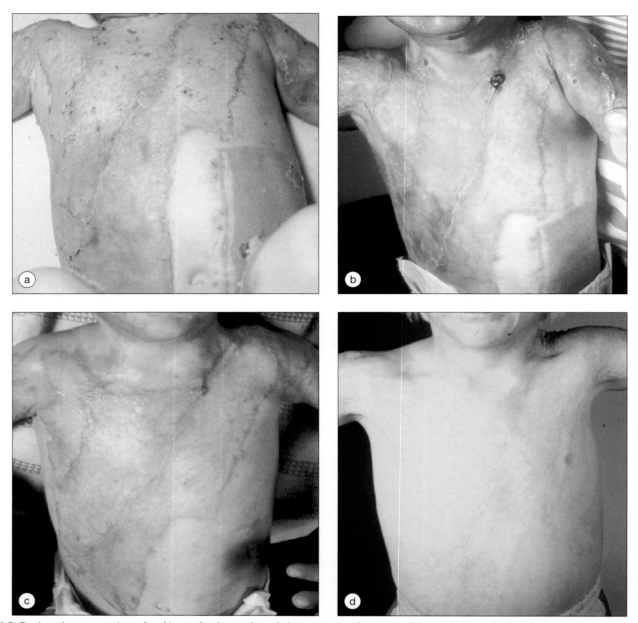

Fig. 46.8 During the maturation of a skin graft, the graft and donor site tend to get redder and thicker before fading into the more supple and naturally colored mature wound. At 5 days after grafting (a) both the graft and donor site are pink and dry. At 4 months (b), the wound has become thicker, tighter and redder. If the patient continues therapy and massage, the wounds begin to smooth out and become less red at 8 months (c). The mature wound becomes flat, supple and loses its redness (d).

'gold standard' has been to use allograft (cadaver skin) as a temporary wound cover. If fresh skin is available, then the skin will 'take' as a viable skin transplant until the body rejects. Patients with massive burns, however, are significantly immunosuppressed, so rejection may take several weeks to months. During that time, the donor sites can be recropped as they heal to gradually replace the allograft.

Other strategies have been developed. Cultured epithelial autografts can be grown from the patient's skin and massively expanded to cover the entire body.[64] Unfortunately, the lack of a dermis leads to prolonged fragility and significant scarring, so most believe that a 'dermis' is required along with an epithelium.[65] One strategy has been to place allograft and, then, when the cultured epithelium has been prepared, apply

it to the dermal allograft.[66] Since it has been found that the epithelium is the major source of the immune reaction, and not the dermis, this technique is possible.

Others have developed dermal substitutes that can be used with very thin autografts.[67–69] One of the most commonly used dermal substitutes is Integra™, which is a dermis that is created from collagen type I and chondroitin-6-sulfate. The dermis is covered with a silicone 'epithelium' that reduces water loss and bacterial invasion. The dermal substitute is applied to the excised wound and allowed to vascularize. After 2–4 weeks, the silicone can be removed and a thin, meshed autograft is applied over the surface. More recent reports have described placing Integra™ on harder-to-heal areas such as bone and tendon with at least some success.[70] Other dermal substitutes exist. AlloDerm™ is a freeze-dried human dermis that can be applied beneath a thin autograft. This product has been used to create a 'thicker' dermis with less donor site morbidity. The advantage of this product over Integra™ is that the thin autograft can be applied at the same time as the initial grafting. There is some risk of having less 'take' in this situation. TransCyte™ is silicone/nylon membrane that has allogeneic neonatal fibroblasts cultured in its ECM. This material is sold as both a dermis and as a temporary dressing that releases growth factors and thus can accelerate healing of superficial burns. It has not been used as a dermal substitute very often and is usually applied as a biologic dressing to accelerate epithelial healing.

Several others have described developing composite skins that are composed of a viable dermis (often containing fibroblasts) and cultured keratinocytes.[71–73] These 'skins' are available on the market as allogeneic products (Apligraf™), while investigators are using biopsies from patients to grow a new composite skin. Recent reports suggest that there are excellent graft takes with some types of composite skin.[74] There is an entire chapter devoted to the use of skin substitutes. All of these 'skin substitutes' do have the problems of being expensive and have lower resistance to infection than autografts. Great progress has occurred and, someday, autografting may be a procedure of the past.

Factors affecting wound healing

Age

The basic components of tissue repair do not change throughout the life of an individual. There are some relatively minor differences that are dependent upon age but for the most part healing occurs efficiently throughout life. The most profound differences of tissue repair occur before birth. In the 1980s, surgeons began to experiment with trying to operate on fetuses to treat congenital abnormalities such as diaphragmatic hernias. They discovered that incisions produced in the fetuses healed without a noticeable scar. Soon, many investigators were studying fetal healing in an attempt to determine the factors that were involved in 'scarless' tissue repair.[75,76] It became clear that there was a period when healing transformed from scarless to 'scar forming.' That gestational time was consistent for each species and occurred before birth. Prior to that period, an incision would regenerate to the normal 'scarless' architecture of the surrounding tissue. It was discovered that TGF-β was lacking during scarless healing but was present later during the creation of a scar. In addition, there appeared to be a paucity of inflammatory cells with scarless healing, but increased inflammation during the creation of a scar. Another finding in the early fetal wound was a higher concentration of hyaluronic acid than that which was found in the more mature animals. Teleologically, these findings make sense. During the period of fetal organ growth and differentiation, the animal exists in an environment of minimal risk from outside invasion. The fetus can afford to 'take the time' to regenerate that tissue. If a wound developed later in life, then that organism needs to be ready for fighting outside invaders. The development of an inflammatory response is essential to survival. Unfortunately, in order to rapidly close a wound and fight invasion, the body sacrifices regeneration for a more expeditious but less than perfect scar. There is a great deal of research on fetal wound healing that cannot be covered here but many reviews exist for those interested.[75,76]

There is feeling among many burn team members that the very young child heals differently than the adult. I have heard several physicians state that younger children tend to take longer to mature their wounds than adults. To examine the question of whether scar maturation was different in younger children versus teenagers, the time to maturation was followed for different ages in children.[77] We found that there was no difference in scar maturation in the very young when compared with teenagers. I have also heard that therapy is of no assistance in the prevention of scar contractures in children. While different strategies are necessary for children, their scars can be modified by occupational and physical therapy. Wounds in children can mature very nicely. One problem with children is that their bones tend to grow faster than their scars do. They must be followed as they grow since they may develop contractures that may need reconstructive surgery later in their teen years. One difference does exist, however: the thickness of the skin is thinner for the very young child. Strategies to utilize thicker skin, such as from the back, do help with avoiding donor site scarring.[58]

At the other extreme, the very elderly patient tends to have looser and thinner skin. Any experienced burn caregiver will know that a burn that appears to be superficial in an elderly person will often tend to 'convert' to third degree. The burn does not 'convert' but, instead, the skin is much thinner and thus the wound is deeper from the start. Another problem with the elderly is that the blood supply to some areas of the skin decreases. Along with the decrease in vascularity, the same area will often have decreased hair and other skin adnexa. (The classic signs of vascular insufficiency to an extremity are decreased hair density, and thinner, more fragile skin.) These changes, along with relative hypoxia, lead to delayed healing. The thinner skin in the elderly must be kept in mind when planning grafting procedures. It is not uncommon for the recipient site to have excellent graft take but to have the donor site fail to heal. Donor sites should be harvested as thinly as possible. In addition, using dermal substitutes that allow for the use of ultra-thin donor sites should be of benefit. It is covered elsewhere in this text, but one must also be aware that the elderly patient has much less ability to survive larger burns when compared with younger patients. Relatively small burns often lead to multiple organ failure and critical illness that impairs tissue repair. Many elderly burn patients are treated non-operatively since their operative risks are prohibitive.

Not all healing is impaired in the elderly. The older patient does have looser skin that allows for contraction of larger wounds. Larger wounds can be allowed to contract with less disfigurement. For example, I have treated a 90-year-old woman with a tea spill to the thigh without grafting. A large open area on the anterior thigh healed over months without range of motion problems. Her family was taught care and she was discharged in their care within days of admission. The ultimate treatment of any elderly patient does require different strategies when compared to the younger patient.

Nutrition

The importance of adequate nutrition for the healing of wounds has been known for over a century. Studies at the beginning of the last century proved that healing was impaired with either total protein-calorie or just isolated protein malnutrition.[78,79] These studies have been repeated hundreds of times.[80,81] The aggressive nutritional support of burn patients has contributed to not only improved healing but also improved survival. While growth factors potentially may improve healing during malnutrition, there is no substitute for aggressive nutritional support. One should assess the nutritional state of the patient prior to the injury. Those patients who were malnourished prior to their burn will be at higher risk for complications and death.

There have been many investigations to determine whether the addition of specific nutrients may improve healing. Certain amino acids have been given in excess to animals to determine whether healing could be augmented. Several amino acids (methionine, cysteine, arginine) have provided statistically significant improvements in tissue repair, but whether their addition leads to clinical improvement is not clear.[82,83] Arginine has been shown to improve collagen deposition and tensile strength.[84] In addition, it stimulates the immune system and thus may benefit the patient. Several 'immune-stimulating' tube feeding formulas include arginine. Glutamine is another nutrient that has been found to protect the enterocytes of the gut. The amino acid has not been proven to improve tissue repair.[85]

Other nutrients such as vitamins and trace elements are essential for wound healing. The importance of vitamin C has already been discussed. Without vitamin C, collagen synthesis is impaired at the same time as collagen breakdown continues.[86] Since the balance between collagen synthesis and breakdown is lost, old incisions may break down. The other important vitamin for tissue repair is vitamin A. Vitamin A has been found to accelerate tissue repair and even may reverse the healing deficit after radiation or steroid treatment.[87,88] The vitamin is pro-inflammatory and stimulates fibroblast function. Some of the B vitamins may also improve some aspects of wound healing.[89] The one vitamin that is commonly felt to improve healing but has no studies to support that contention is vitamin E — at least one study has demonstrated that vitamin E fails to accelerate tissue repair.[90] While it may not have profound effects on healing, vitamin E is essential for other aspects of burn treatment.

Trace elements are also known to improve healing. Zinc is the most notable mineral that has been found to reverse healing defects.[91] The mineral is essential for many enzymes that are involved in tissue repair. The commonly used Unna boot contains zinc oxide. Zinc deficiency also leads to impaired tissue repair. Copper is essential for lysyl oxidase, the enzyme that is required for crosslinks between collagen molecules.[92] A recent report suggests that a copper deficiency led to impaired healing in a burned patient.[93] Other trace elements may play a lesser role in tissue repair. Most burn centers supplement patients with extra vitamins and minerals. Whether the extra supplements help burn patients has not been proven. It does appear that extra vitamin C may be helpful for reducing fluid requirements during resuscitation.[94]

Infection

It is well known that infection has profound effects on tissue repair. Surprisingly, infection does not *always* lead to impaired healing but some studies have demonstrated that contaminating a wound with bacteria does lead to impaired tissue repair.[95–97] However, others attempted similar experiments but found that tissue repair was improved.[98–100] It appears that if minor contamination occurs, then inflammation is augmented and the result is improved healing. If, on the other hand, large amounts of virulent bacteria are present then the host is overwhelmed and the infection is destructive. The same may be true for skin graft take. Robson has stated that if a wound bed has greater than 10^5 bacteria, then a graft will not take.[101] Lesser numbers tend not to have an effect.

The systemic effects of infection also affect tissue repair. An abscess distant from the wound has been found to impair tensile strength.[102] However, at least a portion of the decrease was attributed to impaired nutritional intake. But on the whole, it is most likely that sepsis does lead to altered tissue repair. Experience suggests that donor sites heal poorly and graft take is decreased in profound sepsis. Just the burden of a large burn wound appears to decrease the rate of donor site closure.

Associated illnesses

There are several systemic problems that have adverse affects on tissue repair. The most recognized disease affecting healing is *diabetes mellitus*.[103–105] Diabetes can affect healing by several causes:

- First, the disease leads to both macrovascular and microvascular disease. The altered perfusion may lead to impaired nutrient and oxygen delivery.
- Secondly, the peripheral neuropathy of diabetes mellitus contributes to the tendency to develop ulcers. Insensate feet will not feel minor injury so that a minor irritation may turn into a more serious wound. Loss of the normal reflexes of the muscles that maintain the arch of the foot may lead to increased pressure areas, especially over the second metatarsal.
- Finally, the wounds in diabetic patients tend to have a higher propensity to become infected. A minor wound frequently becomes infected and more extensive. Diabetic patients tend to have a higher risk for amputation when compared to patients without the problem.

Fortunately, there is a growth factor (Regranex™ [PDGF-BB]) available to treat these wounds and which does appear to help healing.[106]

Other diseases do affect healing:

- Obviously, any vascular abnormality that leads to tissue hypoxia has adverse effects.[29,30,107]
- In addition, uremia[108] and liver failure[109] have adverse affects on tissue repair.
- Malignancy has been known for a long time to have adverse affects on wound healing.[110,111] It is likely that the body shunts nutrients away from the wound and to the cancer. In addition, cancer patients tend to have anorexia and weight loss, both of which contribute to impaired wound closure.

Any other disease that impairs nutrition will predispose the patient to altered healing.

Cytotoxic treatments (steroids, chemotherapy, radiation)

Any agent that impairs cellular proliferation will lead to some impairment in tissue repair:

- Steroids are the most notable class of drug that leads to altered healing.[112,113] Steroids decrease the inflammatory response and decrease collagen production. The inhibition of collagen production is occasionally used as a strategy to decrease scar formation in those patients with a tendency towards hypertrophic scarring. Its efficacy varies from patient to patient; however, growth factors have been found to reverse some of the adverse affects of steroids.[114–116]
- Most chemotherapy agents lead to impaired healing.[117,118] These agents are designed to kill rapidly proliferating cells. Unfortunately, the cells required for tissue repair must also grow rapidly. The agents affect healing if given systemically and can lead to chronic non-healing ulcers if they extravasate into the subcutaneous tissues. Growth factors have had some beneficial effects in animal studies.[119]
- Finally, radiation leads to similar problems as for chemotherapy agents.[120,121] The effects can also be improved with topical growth factors.[122]

Other drugs may have effects on healing but are not of major clinical importance.

Methods of stimulating wound healing

For years people have been trying to stimulate wound healing. Most of the time healing progresses at a reasonable rate and does not need to be accelerated. Healthy people rarely have healing problems and do very well without factors that stimulate healing. Those patients, however, with impairments such as diabetes, malnutrition, infection, treatment with cytotoxic agents are the ones who would benefit from a wound that heals more rapidly.[123]

There have been literally thousands of publications that have studied agents that improve healing in animals. Very few have made it past the preclinical studies to become therapeutic agents for augmenting tissue repair. (See the nutrition section above, describing the studies relating to the addition of nutritional factors.)

Growth factors

The major thrust of improving healing has been through the addition of growth factors. Growth factors are natural cytokines that attract cells into the wound, stimulate their proliferation and induce the production of extracellular matrix.

Recombinant proteins

Initial studies involved harvesting growth factors from patients' own cells. Platelet releasates were the most common source for growth factors.[124] With the development of the ability to mass-manufacture any protein, recombinant growth factors were produced. Currently, Regranex™ (recombinant human PDGF-BB) is available and has been proved to be efficacious for diabetic ulcers.[106]

The use of this growth factor for clinical wound healing stimulation has not been very extensive. Recombinant proteins are expensive and have not been embraced by clinicians.

Gene therapy

A current focus for inducing growth factor activity in the wound has been through gene therapy. There have been numerous studies that utilized different vectors for delivering a gene (usually a growth factor) into a wound.[125–136] Most known growth factor genes have been delivered to wounds and have been found to stimulate tissue repair in animal models.

There have also been clinical trials that utilize gene therapy for treating many diseases. One recent review suggested that there were hundreds of gene transfer protocols.[137] There have, however, been major setbacks in the use of gene therapy for human disease. In 2003, there were two publications that revealed that gene therapy techniques have the potential for major complications. In one study, two children developed lymphoproliferative disorders after retroviral gene transfer to their hematopoietic stem cells.[138] In the most disturbing case, an 18-year-old patient died from a systemic inflammatory response syndrome and ultimately, multiple organ failure after gene transfer for ornithine transcarbamylase deficiency.[139] Despite these setbacks trials are proceeding. There are two publications that describe the use of adenoviral-mediated gene overexpression of PDGF-BB to treat diabetic foot ulcers and venous stasis ulcers in clinical trials.[140,141] The results of the clinical trials have not been published so we will have to wait to determine whether this technology will lead to a new way of accelerating wound healing.

Combined gene therapy and skin substitute technologies

Another strategy for stimulating healing in the burn wound is to combine gene therapy and skin substitute technologies.[142–144] Since autogenous skin substitutes must be initiated from a biopsy and then cells must be grown in culture, there is ample opportunity to transfect them to augment or reduce a specific gene. There are studies that have used cultured keratinocytes or fibroblasts to increase production of PDGF-A, FGF-7, or KGF. This technology would allow for the skin substitute to release pharmacological doses of growth factors and stimulate angiogenesis, keratinocyte migration or collagen deposition. It would also be conceivable that a skin substitute would allow for the production of a factor that would minimize hypertrophic scarring.

Stem cells

The most recent interest in research has been the investigation of the role of stem cells in many areas of medicine. Wound healing in burns using stem cells has also been investigated.[145] In a recent publication from Lancet, fetal skin constructs have been reported to improve healing.[146] They utilized a bank of fetal skin cells from one donor and placed them on native horse collagen. The constructs were applied to eight patients for each dressing change for 1–3 weeks. They had complete healing with minimal hypertrophy. One must wonder, however, whether this application is really an elaborate way of delivering growth factors to a wound. It can be imagined that the cost of such a treatment would make its use unlikely.

A group from Russia has described using bone marrow mesenchymal stem cells in a similar type of treatment.[147] Both reports lead to the speculation that stem cell research to improve healing in burns is a feasible treatment for the future.

Scar control

A great deal of knowledge has been gained about the factors that accelerate healing. Growth factors and other agents have been developed to reverse healing abnormalities of all kinds.

The factors that 'turn off' the healing process have not been well elucidated. Failure to control healing leads to excessive scarring that affects other organs beside the skin. The same processes lead to impaired cardiac function after a myocardial infarction, pulmonary fibrosis, cirrhosis, arthritis and many other fibrotic diseases. If one were able to control scar formation, then a great number of diseases would have better outcomes.

The mechanisms involved in 'turning off' of scar formation are starting to be elucidated (Figure 46.9). In order to stop the

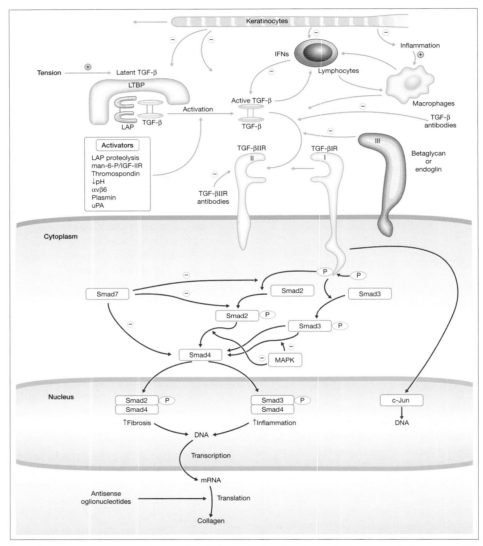

Fig. 46.9 The extent of scar formation appears to be regulated through the signaling of a key growth factor — TGF-β. Multiple factors affect signaling of this growth factor. First, there are signals that emanate from the migrating epithelium that inhibit the signals that induce scarring. TGF-β activity is highly regulated through multiple checks and feedback loops. There are different stimuli that up-regulate or down-regulate its activity. Once TGF-β is synthesized, the protein exists in a latent form as a proprotein. In addition, the latent TGF-β is 'protected' by latent TGF-β-binding protein (LTBP). Several factors have the potential to activate TGF-β: decreased pH, proteolysis (plasmin, urokinase), thrombospondin, αvβ6, or binding by the IGF-II/mannose-6-phosphate (man-6-P) receptor. Inflammation tends to increase TGF-β activity through signaling through leukocytes such as macrophages. Lymphocytes produce interferons (IFNs) that inhibit the effects of TGF-β. TGF-β signaling may be inhibited by proteins or antibodies that interfere with receptor binding. There is also a type III receptor (betaglycan or endoglin) that binds some isoforms of TGF-β without inducing a signal. Once bound to the active receptors (TGF-βIIR which then interacts with TGF-βIR), intracellular serine kinases are phosphorylated. Signaling then proceeds with Smad2 or Smad 3 becoming phosphorylated. Smad2 or Smad3 then bind with Smad 4. Smad2 may be more involved with fibrosis while Smad3 may be more essential for the control of inflammation. The Smad2/3-Smad4 combination then enters the nucleus for binding to specific binding sites on the DNA. Ultimately, binding to these genes leads to transcription and translation of new proteins. One may also block collagen synthesis by providing antisense oligonucleotides that interfere with translation from mRNA to protein. Finally, there are inhibitory Smad proteins (particularly Smad7 for TGF-β) that block Smad signaling.

healing process, inflammation must stop. It is clear that covering a wound with an epithelium is required to begin stopping the inflammatory response. As long as there is exposure to foreign antigens and organisms the body will continue to 'try to protect' the organism with an inflammatory response. Studies have demonstrated that the epithelium induces apoptosis (programmed cell death) in inflammatory cells as it marches across a wound.[41,42] In addition, as a wound is covered with a graft or flap, apoptosis is induced in fibroblasts and other inflammatory cells.[45] The signal produced by the covering epithelium has not yet been elucidated but studies suggest that factors that affect apoptosis are produced in the migrating keratinocytes.[148] More studies are needed to understand how the epithelium influences the ultimate scar.

We do know that if a wound is left open for too long, then it has a tendency to develop hypertrophic scarring.[43] Several investigators have demonstrated that TGF-β plays a role in the extent of scar formation (Figure 46.9).[46–49] Those patients with a greater tendency to scar have higher serum levels of TGF-β1.[48,49] One study has revealed that antibodies to TGF-β1 can reduce the amount of scarring that is present in a rat wound.[55] Interestingly, TGF-β3 may have antiscarring effects.[55] In addition, interferons may reverse the tendency towards hypertrophic scarring. Both interferon-γ and interferon-α2b have been found to reverse some of the scarring tendencies in patients.[50–52] Also, tension that is produced in a scar contracture increases TGF-β1 and collagen production. Reducing the tension in a scar band by performing a release will decrease TGF-β1 expression.[149]

Newer techniques have been developed to counteract TGF-β1 signaling (Figure 46.9).[150] Using an antibody against the protein is one strategy that might be effective. As stated before, an antibody to TGF-β1 has been shown to reduce the extent of collagen deposition in a rat.[55]

Instead of interfering with the protein, another strategy is to inhibit TGF-β1 activity at the receptor.[151] One study has examined the possibility of inhibiting scar formation by adenovirus-mediated overexpression truncated TGF-β receptor II. The publication suggested that overexpression of a nonfunctional receptor to bind TGF-β did inhibit scar formation.

Other studies suggest that hypertrophic scar cells have an impaired ability to undergo apoptosis.[152,153] Strategies are being promoted to develop technologies to induce apoptosis in these cells. One interesting strategy has been to treat wounds with antisense oligonucleotides that actually inhibit mRNA signaling.[154–157] Antisense oligonucleotides bind to mRNA and prevent translation of that specific protein. The antisense technology has been used to block collagen, TGF-β and other proteins to inhibit collagen synthesis.

Other strategies use agents that block key proteins in the cell cycle. A couple of publications have shown the potential of blocking p21 to inhibit healing.[158,159]

Research has now gone past the role of growth factors and has studied the role of cell signaling in scar control. Nice studies from Ashcroft have revealed that intracellular proteins involved in signaling of TGF-β1 are related to scar control.[160] After binding to the TGF-β receptor, signaling occurs through a family of proteins called Smads. There are two potential proteins, Smad3 or Smad2, that can be used for signaling. If Smad3 is eliminated then there are signs of good healing but less inflammation.[161,162] It appears that signaling through Smad3 tends to increase fibrosis while signaling through Smad2 induces an inflammatory response. The relative amount of signaling between Smad2 and Smad3 may ultimately influence the extent of scarring. It is conceivable that therapies that direct intracellular signaling could lead to better scar control.

Another intracellular protein, Smad7 acts as an inhibitor of TGF-β signaling.[163,164] Up-regulation of this protein could lead to improved control of hypertrophic scarring after burns. Hopefully, more therapeutic agents will be available in the future.

Despite these advances there are only a few current clinical modalities used for scar control in patients. Scar massage and stretching (therapy) appear to very efficacious. Patients who are compliant with a therapy program do much better than those who are not.

Silicone is another product that is available for the treatment of scarring. The exact mechanisms of how silicone works are not clear.[165,166] Providing pressure on to the scar through hard materials or stretchy cloth (garments) has been used for decades to reduce hypertrophic scarring. There are some studies being published that suggest that pressure garments are not effective, but there are also many years of experience that suggest that they are very helpful. Hopefully, third-party support for garments is not lost before well-controlled studies are completed to answer the question of their efficacy.

Conclusion

Understanding the principles of wound healing is essential to the adequate treatment of burn patients. The skin is the first barrier to the outside world. If enough of the skin is lost, then any other defense will be overwhelmed. In addition, we now know that the wound is not an isolated event that affects only the local tissues. An open wound leads to a profound systemic response that, if large enough, will lead to major systemic changes and potentially the ultimate failure of the organism (through multiple organ failure). Our job as caregivers of the burn patient is to heal the wound as expeditiously as possible, while at the same time maintaining the best cosmetic and functional outcomes as possible. The best way to succeed in completing that goal is to have as good an understanding of tissue repair as possible.

References

1. Woodley DT, O'Keefe EJ, Prunieras M. Cutaneous wound healing: a model for cell-matrix interactions. J Am Acad Dermatol 1985; 12:420–433.

2. Barrandon Y, Green H. Cell migration is essential for sustained growth of keratinocyte colonies: the roles of transforming growth factor-α and epidermal growth factor. Cell 1987; 50:1131–1137.

3. Cooper ML, Hansbrough JF, Foreman TJ, et al. The effects of epidermal growth factor and basic fibroblast growth factor on epithelialization of meshed skin graft interstices. Prog Clin Biol Res 1991; 365:429–442.

4. Staiano-Coico L, Kreuger JG, Rubin JS, et al. Human keratinocyte growth factor effects in a porcine model of epidermal wound healing. J Exp Med 1993; 178:865–878.

5. Jimenez PA, Rampy MA. Keratinocyte growth factor-2 accelerates wound healing in incisional wounds. J Surg Res 1999; 81:238–242.

6. Hebda PA. Stimulatory effects of transforming growth factor-beta and epidermal growth factor on epidermal growth factor from porcine skin explant cultures. J Invest Dermatol 1988; 91:440–445.

7. Chen JD, Lapierre J-C, Suder D, et al. Interleukin-1 alpha stimulates keratinocyte migration through an EGF/TGF-alpha independent pathway. J Invest Dermatol 1995; 104:729–733.

8. Woodley DT, Wynn KC, O'Keefe EJ. Type IV collagen and fibronectin enhance human keratinocyte thymidine incorporation and spreading in the absence of soluble growth factors. J Invest Dermatol 1990; 94:139–143.

9. Falanga V, Eaglstein WH, Bucalo B, et al. Topical use of human recombinant epidermal growth factor (h-EGF) in venous ulcers. J Dermatol Surg Oncol 1992; 18:604–610.

10. Brown GL, Nanney LB, Griffin J, et al. Enhancement of wound healing by topical treatment with epidermal growth factor. N Engl J Med 1989; 321:76–83.

11. Greenhalgh DG, Rieman M. Effects of basic fibroblast growth factor on the healing of partial-thickness donor sites: a prospective, randomized, double-blinded trial. Wound Repair Regen 1994; 2:113–121.

12. Herndon DN, Barrow RE, Kunkel KR, et al. Effects of human growth hormone on donor-site healing in severely burned children. Ann Surg 1990; 212:424–432.

13. Simpson DM, Ross R. The neutrophilic leukocyte in wound repair: a study with antineutrophil serum. J Clin Invest 1972; 51:2009–2023.

14. Leibovich SJ, Ross R. The role of the macrophage in wound repair. a study with hydrocortisone and antimacrophage serum. Am J Pathol 1975; 78:71–100.

15. Korn JH, Halushka PV, LeRoy EC. Mononuclear cell modulation of connective tissue function. J Clin Invest 1980; 65:543–554.

16. Diegelmann RF, Cohen IK, Kaplan AM. The role of macrophages in wound repair: a review. Plast Reconstr Surg 1981; 68:107–113.

17. Riches DWH. Macrophage involvement in wound repair, remodeling, and fibrosis. In: Clark RAF, ed. The molecular and cellular biology of wound repair, 2nd edn. New York: Plenum; 1996:95–141.

18. Wahl SM, Wahl LM, McCarthy JB. Lymphocyte-mediated activation of fibroblast proliferation and collagen production. J Immunol 1978; 121:942–946.

19. Barbul A. Role of T cell-dependent immune system in wound healing. Prog Clin Biol Res 1988; 266:161–175.

20. Crowe MJ, Doetschman TC, Greenhalgh DG. Expression of TGF-β isoform mRNAs during wound healing in immunodeficient TGF-β1 knockout mice. J Invest Dermatol 2000; 115:3–11.

21. Prockop DJ. The biosynthesis of collagen and its disorders. Part I. N Engl J Med 1979; 301:13–23.

22. Prockop DJ. The biosynthesis of collagen and its disorders. Part II. N Engl J Med 1979; 301:77–85.

23. Fuller GC, Cutroneo KR. Pharmacological interventions. In: Cohen IK, Diegelmann RF, Lindblad WJ, eds. Wound healing. biochemical and clinical aspects. Philadelphia: WB Saunders; 1992:311–313.

24. Bamert W, Stojan B, Wiedman V. D-penicillamine and wound healing in patients with rheumatoid arthritis. Z Rheumatol 1980; 39:9–13.

25. Arem AJ, Misiorowski R, Chvapil M. Effects of low-dose BAPN on wound healing. J Surg Res 1979; 27:228–232.

26. Carmeliet P. Mechanisms of angiogenesis and arteriogenesis. Nature Med 2000; 6:389–395.

27. Folkman J. Towards an understanding of angiogenesis: search and discovery. Perspect Biol Med 1985; 29:10–36.

28. Carmielet P. Angiogenesis in life, disease and medicine. Nature 2005; 438:932–936.

29. Hunt TK, Pai MP. The effect of varying ambient oxygen tensions on wound metabolism and collagen synthesis. Surg Gynecol Obstet 1972; 135:561–567.

30. LaVan FB, Hunt TK. Oxygen and wound healing. Clin Plast Surg 1990; 17:463–472.

31. Roesel JF, Nanney LB. Assessment of differential cytokine effects on angiogenesis using an in vivo model of cutaneous wound repair. J Surg Res 1995; 58: 449–459.

32. Roberts AB, Sporn MB, Assoian RK, et al. Transforming growth factor type beta: rapid induction of fibrosis and angiogenesis in vivo and stimulation of collagen formation in vitro. Proc Natl Acad Sci USA 1986; 83:4167–4171.

33. Davidson JM, Benn SI. Regulation of angiogenesis and wound repair. Interactive role of the matrix and growth factors. In: Sirica AE, ed. Cellular and molecular pathogenesis. Philadelphia: Lippincott-Raven; 1996:79–106.

34. Folkman J, Klagsbrun M. Angiogenic factors. Science 1987; 235:442–447.

35. Crum R, Szabo S, Folkman J. A new class of steroids inhibits angiogenesis in the presence of heparin or a heparin fragment. Science 1985; 230:1375–1378.

36. Brem H, Gresser I, Grosfeld J, et al. The combination of antiangiogenic agents to inhibit primary tumor growth and metastasis. J Pediatr Surg 1993; 28:1253–1257.

37. Werner S, Breeden M, Greenhalgh DG, et al. Induction of keratinocyte growth factor is reduced and delayed during wound healing in the genetically diabetic mouse. J Invest Dermatol 1994; 103:469–472.

38. Frank S, Hubner G, Breier G, et al. Regulation of vascular endothelial growth factor expression in cultured keratinocytes. J Biol Chem 1995; 270:12607–12613.

39. Brown DL, Kane CD, Chernausek SD, et al. Differential expression and localization of IGF-I and IGF-II in cutaneous wounds of diabetic versus nondiabetic mice. Am J Pathol 1997; 151: 715–724.

40. Trengove NJ, Stacey MC, MacAuley S, et al. Analysis of the acute and chronic wound environments: the role of proteases and their inhibitors. Wound Repair Regen 1999; 7:442–452.

41. Greenhalgh DG. The role of apoptosis in wound healing. Int J Biochem Cell Biol 1998; 30:1019–1030.

42. Brown DL, Kao WW-Y, Greenhalgh DG. Apoptosis down-regulates inflammation under the advancing epithelial wound edge: delayed patterns in diabetes and improvement with topical growth factors. Surgery 1997; 121:372–380.

43. Deitch EA, Wheelahan TM, Rose MP, et al. Hypertrophic scars: analysis of variables. J Trauma 1983; 23:895–898.

44. Desmouliere A, Redard M, Darby I, et al. Apoptosis mediates the decrease in cellularity during the transition between granulation tissue and scar. Am J Pathol 1995; 146: 56–66.

45. Garbin S, Pittet B, Montandon D, et al. Covering by a flap induces apoptosis of granulation tissue myofibroblasts and vascular cells. Wound Repair Regen 1996; 4:244–251.

46. Bettinger DA, Yager DR, Diegelmann RF, et al. The effect of TGF-β on keloid fibroblast proliferation and collagen synthesis. Plast Reconstr Surg 1995; 98:827–833.

47. Lin RY, Sullivan KM, Argenta PA, et al. Exogenous transforming growth factor-beta amplifies its own expression and induces scar formation in a model of human fetal skin repair. Ann Surg 1995; 222:146–154.

48. Ghahary A, Shen YJ, Scott PG, et al. Enhanced expression of mRNA for transforming growth factor-beta, type I and type III procollagen in human post-burn hypertrophic scar tissues. J Lab Clin Med 1993; 122:465–473.

49. Wang R, Ghahary A, Shen Q, et al. Hypertrophic scar tissues and fibroblasts produce more transforming growth factor-β1 mRNA and protein than normal skin and cells. Wound Repair Regen 2000; 8:128–137.

50. Harrop AR, Ghahary A, Scott PG, et al. Regulation of collagen synthesis and mRNA expression in normal and hypertrophic scar fibroblasts in vitro by interferon-γ. J Surg Res 1995; 58:471–477.

51. Granstein RD, Rook A, Flotte TJ, et al. A controlled trial of intra-lesional recombinant interferon-gamma in the treatment of keloidal scarring. Arch Dermatol 1990; 126:1295–1301.

52. Tredget EE, Shen YJ, Liu G, et al. Regulation of collagen synthesis and messenger RNA levels in normal and hypertrophic scar fibroblasts in vitro by interferon alfa-2b. Wound Repair Regen 1993; 1:156–165.

53. Shull MM, Ormsby I, Kier AB, et al. Targeted disruption of the mouse transforming growth factor-1 gene results in multifocal inflammatory disease. Nature 1992; 35:693–699.

54. Brown RL, Ormsby I, Doetschman TC, et al. Wound healing in the transforming growth factor-1-deficient mouse. Wound Repair Regen 1995; 3:25–36.

55. Shah M, Foreman DM, Ferguson WJ. Neutralization of TGF-β1 and TGF-β2 or exogenous addition of TGF-β3 to cutaneous rat wounds reduces scarring. J Cell Sci 1995; 108:985–1002.

56. Montandon D, D'Andiran G, Gabbiani G. The mechanism of wound contraction and epithelialization. Clin Plast Surg 1977; 4:325–346.

57. Tranquillo RT, Murray JD. Mechanistic model of wound contraction. J Surg Res 1993; 55:233–247.

58. Schwanholt C, Greenhalgh DG, Warden GD. A comparison of full-thickness versus partial-thickness autografts for the coverage of deep palm burns in the very young pediatric patient. J Burn Care Rehabil 1993; 14:29–33.

59. Greenhalgh DG, Barthel PP, Warden GD. Comparison of back versus thigh donor sites in pediatric burn patients. J Burn Care Rehabil 1993; 14:21–25.

60. Greenhalgh DG. Frontiers in wound healing. Prob Gen Surg 2003; 20:70–79.

61. Greenhalgh DG, Staley MJ. Burn wound healing. In Richard RL, Staley MJ, eds. Burn care and rehabilitation: principles and practice. Philadelphia: FA Davis; 1994:70–102.

62. Archer SB, Henke A, Greenhalgh DG, et al. The use of sheet autografts to cover patients with extensive burns. J Burn Care Rehabil 1998; 19:33–38.

63. Greenhalgh DG, Palmieri TL. Zigzag seams for the prevention of scar bands after sheet split-thickness skin grafting. Surgery 2003; 133:586–587.

64. Gallico GG, O'Connner NE, Compton CC, et al. Permanent coverage of large burn wounds with autologous cultured human epithelium. N Engl J Med 1984; 311:448–511.

65. Rue LW, Cioffi WG, McManus WF, et al. Wound closure and outcome in extensively burned patients with cultured autologous keratinocytes. J Trauma 1993; 34:662–668.

66. Cuono C, Langdon R, McGuire J. Use of cultured epidermal autografts and dermal allografts as skin replacement after burn injury. Lancet 1986; 1:1123–1124.

67. Heimbach D, Luterman A, Burke J, et al. Artificial dermis for major burns. A multi-center randomized clinical trial. Ann Surg 1988; 208:313–320.

68. Hansbrough JF, Dore C, Hansbrough WB. Clinical trials of a dermal tissue replacement placed beneath meshed, split-thickness skin grafts on excised burn wounds. J Burn Care Rehabil 1992; 13:519–529.

69. Wainwright DJ. Use of an acellular allograft dermal matrix (AlloDerm) in the management of full-thickness burns. Burns 1995; 21:243–248.

70. Komorowska-Timek E, Gabriel A, Bennett DC, et al. Artificial dermis as an alternative for coverage of complex scalp defects following excision of malignant tumors. Plast Reconstr Surg 2005; 115:1010–1017.

71. Hansbrough JF, Boyce ST, Cooper ML, et al. Burn wound closure with cultured autologous keratinocytes and fibroblasts attached to collagen-glycosaminoglycan substrate. JAMA 1989; 262:2125–2130.

72. Boyce ST, Goretsky MJ, Greenhalgh DG, et al. Comparative assessment of cultured skin substitutes and native skin autograft for the treatment of full-thickness burns. Ann Surg 1995; 222:743–752.

73. Hansbrough JF, Morgan JL, Greenleaf GE, et al. Composite grafts of human keratinocytes grown on a polyglactin mesh-cultured fibroblast dermal substitute as a bilayer skin replacement in full-thickness wounds in thymic mice. J Burn Care Rehabil 1993; 14:485–494.

74. McCallion RL, Ferguson MWJ. Fetal wound healing and the development of antiscarring therapies for adult wound healing. In: Clark RAF, ed. The molecular and cellular biology of wound repair, 2nd edn. New York: Plenum; 1996:561–599.

75. Boyce ST, Kagan RJ, Yakuboff KP, et al. Cultured skin substitutes reduce donor skin harvesting for closure of excised, full-thickness burns. Ann Surgery 2002; 235:269–279.

76. Mast BA, Nelson JM, Krummel TM. Tissue repair in the mammalian fetus. In: Cohen IK, Diegelmann RF, Lindblad WJ, eds. Wound healing. Biochemical and clinical aspects. Philadelphia: WB Saunders; 1992:326–343.

77. Schwanholt CA, Ridgway CA, Greenhalgh DG, et al. A prospective study of burn scar maturation in pediatrics: does age matter? J Burn Care Rehabil 1994; 15:416–420.

78. Howes EL, Briggs H, Shea R, et al. Effect of complete and partial starvation on the rate of fibroplasia in the healing wound. Arch Surg 1993; 26:846–858.

79. Rhoads JE, Fliegelman MT, Panzer LM. The mechanism of delayed wound healing in the presence of hypoproteinemia. JAMA 1942; 118:21–25.

80. Daly JM, Vars HM, Dudvich SJ. Effects of protein depletion on strength of colonic anastomoses. Surg Gynecol Obstet 1972; 134:15–21.

81. Irvin TT. Effects of malnutrition and hyperalimentation on wound healing. Surg Gynecol Obstet 1978; 146:33–37.

82. Localio SA, Morgan ME, Hinton JW. The biological chemistry of wound healing. The effect of methionine on the healing of wounds in protein-depleted animals. Surg Gynecol Obstet 1948; 86:582–589.

83. Williamson MB, Fromm HJ. The incorporation of sulphur amino aids into proteins of regenerating wound tissue. J Biol Chem 1955; 212:705–712.

84. Seifter E, Rettura G, Barbul A, et al. Arginine: an essential amino acid for injured rats. Surgery 1978; 84:224–230.

85. McCauley R, Platell MB, Hall J, et al. Effects of glutamine infusion on colonic anastomotic strength in the rat. JPEN J Parenter Enteral Nutr 1991; 15:437–439.

86. Bartlett MK, Jones CM, Ryan AE. Vitamin C and wound healing. I. Experimental wounds in guinea pigs. N Engl J Med 1942; 226:469–473.

87. Ehrlich HP, Hunt TK. Effects of cortisone and vitamin A on wound healing. Ann Surg 1968; 167:324–328.

88. Levenson SM, Gruber CA, Rettura G, et al. Supplemental vitamin A prevents the acute radiation-induced defect in wound healing. Ann Surg 1984; 200:494–512.

89. Alvarez OM, Gilbreath RL. Thiamine influence on collagen during the granulation of skin wounds. J Surg Res 1982; 32:24–31.

90. Ehrlich HP, Tarver H, Hunt TK. Inhibitory effects of vitamin E on collagen synthesis and wound repair. Ann Surg 1972; 175:235–240.

91. Pories WJ. Acceleration of healing with zinc oxide. Ann Surg 1967; 165:432–436.

92. Pinnell SR, Martin GR. The cross linking of collagen and elastin. Proc Natl Acad Sci USA 1968; 61:708–714.

93. Liusuwan RA, Palmieri T, Warden N, et al. Impaired healing due to copper deficiency in a pediatric burn: a case report. J Trauma 2006; 51:in press.

94. Tanaka H, Hanumadass M, Matsuda H, et al. Hemodynamic effects of delayed initiation of antioxidant therapy (beginning two hours after burn) in extensive third-degree burns. J Burn Care Rehabil 1995; 16:610–615.

95. Smith M, Enquist IF. A quantitative study of impaired healing resulting from infection. Surg Gynecol Obstet 1967; 125:965–973.

96. Irvin TT. Collagen metabolism in infected colonic anastomoses. Surg Gynecol Obstet 1976; 143:220–224.

97. Bucknall TE. The effect of local infection upon wound healing. Br J Surg 1980; 67:851–855.

98. Tenorio A, Jindrak K, Weiner M, et al. Accelerated healing in infected wounds. Surg Gynecol Obstet 1976; 142:537–543.

99. Raju DR, Jindrak K, Weiner M, et al. A study of the critical bacterial inoculum to cause a stimulus to wound healing. Surg Gynecol Obstet 1977; 144:347–350.

100. Levenson SM. Wound healing accelerated by Staphylococcus aureus. Arch Surg 1983; 118:310–320.

101. Krizek TJ, Robson MC, Kho E. Bacterial growth and skin graft survival. Surg Forum 1967; 18:518–519.

102. Greenhalgh DG, Gamelli RL. Is impaired wound healing caused by infection or nutritional depletion? Surgery 1987; 102:306–312.

103. McMurry JF Jr. Wound healing with diabetes mellitus. Surg Clin North Am 1984; 64:769–778.

104. Goodson WH, III, Hunt TK. Wound healing and the diabetic patient. Surg Gynecol Obstet 1979; 149:600–608.

105. Greenhalgh DG. Wound healing and diabetes mellitus. Clin Plast Surg 2003; 30:37–45.

106. Steed DL, The Diabetic Study Group. Clinical evaluation of recombinant human platelet-derived growth factor for the treatment of lower extremity diabetic ulcers. J Vasc Surg 1995; 21:71–77.

107. Wu L, Mustoe TA. Effect of ischemia on growth factor enhancement of incisional wound healing. Surgery 1995; 117:570–576.

108. Yue DK, McLennan S, Marsh M, et al. Effects of experimental diabetes, uremia, and malnutrition on wound healing. Diabetes 1987; 36:295–299.

109. Bayer I, Ellis HL. Effect of obstructive jaundice on wound healing. Br J Surg 1976; 63:392–396.

110. Devereux DF, Thistlewaite PA, Thibault LF, et al. Effects of tumor bearing and protein depletion on wound breaking strengths in the rat. J Surg Res 1979; 27:233–238.

111. Weinzweig J. Supplemental vitamin A prevents the tumor-induced defect in wound healing. Ann Surg 1990; 211:269–276.

112. Howes EL, Plotz CM, Blunt JW, et al. Retardation of wound healing by cortisone. Surgery 1950; 28:177–181.

113. Sandberg N. Time relationship between administration of cortisone and wound healing in rats. Acta Chir Scand 1964; 127:446–455.

114. Laato M, Heino J, Kahari VM, et al. Epidermal growth factor (EGF) prevents methylprednisolone-induced inhibition of wound healing. J Surg Res 1989; 47:354–359.

115. Pierce GF, Mustoe TA, Lingelbach J, et al. Transforming growth factor β reverses the glucocorticoid-induced wound healing deficit in rats: possible regulation in macrophages by platelet-derived growth factor. Proc Natl Acad Sci USA 1989; 86:2229–2233.

116. Beck LS, DeGuzman L, Lee WP, et al. TGF-β1 accelerates wound healing: reversal of steroid-impaired healing in rats and rabbits. Growth Factors 1991; 5:295–300.

117. Ferguson MK. The effects of antineoplastic agents on wound healing. Surg Gynecol Obstet 1982; 154:421–429.

118. Falcone RE, Napp JF. Chemotherapy and wound healing. Surg Clin North Am 1984; 64:779–795.

119. Lawrence WT, Sporn MB, Gorschboth C, et al. The reversal of an Adriamycin induced healing impairment with chemoattractants and growth factors. Ann Surg 1986; 203:142–147.

120. Reinisch JF, Puckett CL. Management of radiation wounds. Surg Clin North Am 1984; 64:795–802.

121. Luce EA. The irradiated wound. Surg Clin North Am 1984; 64:821–829.

122. Mustoe TA, Purdy J, Gramates P, et al. Reversal of impaired wound healing in irradiated rats by platelet-derived growth factor-BB. Am J Surg 1989; 158:345–350.

123. Greenhalgh DG. The role of growth factors and wound healing. J Trauma 1996; 41:159–167.

124. Knighton DR, Fiegel VD, Austin LL, et al. Classification and treatment of chronic nonhealing wounds: successful treatment with autologous platelet-derived wound healing factors (PDWHF). Ann Surg 1986; 204:322–330.

125. Crombleholme TM. Adenoviral-mediated gene transfer in wound healing. Wound Repair Regen 2000; 8:460–472.

126. Liechty KW, Sablich TJ, Adzick NS, et al. Recombinant adenoviral mediated gene transfer in ischemic impaired wound healing. Wound Repair Regen 1999; 7:148–153.

127. Liechty KW, Nesbit M, Herlyn M, et al. Adenoviral-mediated overexpression of platelet-derived growth factor-B corrects ischemic impaired wound healing. J Invest Dermatol 1999; 113:375–383.

128. Sun L, Xu L, Chang H, et al. Transfection with aFGF cDNA improves wound healing. J Invest Dermatol 1997; 108:313–318.

129. Jeschke MG, Barrow RE, Hawkins HK, et al. IGF-I gene transfer in thermally injured rats. Gene Ther 1999; 6:1015–1020.

130. Chandler LA, Doukas J, Gonzalez AM, et al. FGF2-targeted adenovirus encoding platelet-derived growth factor-B enhances de novo tissue formation. Mol Ther 2000; 2:153–160.

131. Tyrone JW, Mogford JE, Chandler LA, et al. Collagen-embedded platelet-derived growth factor DNA plasmid promotes wound healing in a dermal ulcer model. J Surg Res 2000; 93:230–236.

132. Ailawadi M, Lee JM, Lee S, et al. Adenovirus vector-mediated transfer of the vascular endothelial growth factor cDNA to healing abdominal fascia enhances vascularity and bursting strength in mice with normal and impaired wound healing. Surgery 2002; 131:219–227.

133. Deodato B, Arsic N, Zentilin L, et al. Recombinant AAV vector encoding human VEGF165 enhances wound healing. Gene Ther 2002; 9:777–785.

134. Jeschke MG, Richter G, Hofstadter F, et al. Non-viral liposomal keratinocyte growth factor (KGF) cDNA gene transfer improves dermal and epidermal regeneration through stimulation of epithelial and mesenchymal factors. Gene Ther 2002; 9:1065–1074.

135. Chesnoy S, Lee PY, Huang L. Intradermal injection of transforming growth factor-beta1 gene enhances wound healing in genetically diabetic mice. Pharm Res 2003; 20:345–350.

136. Galeano M, Deodato B, Altavila D, et al. Effect of recombinant adeno-associated virus vector-mediated vascular endothelial growth factor gene transfer on wound healing after burn injury. Crit Care Med 2003; 31:1017–1025.

137. Raper SE. Gene therapy: the good, the bad, and the ugly. Surgery 2005; 137:487–492.

138. Hacein-Bey-Urbina S, Von Kalle C, Schmidt M, et al. LMO2-associated clonal T cell proliferation in two patients after gene therapy for SCID-X1. Science 2003; 302:415–419.

139. Raper S, Chirmule N, Lee F, et al. Fatal systemic inflammatory response syndrome in a ornithine transcarbamylase deficient patient following adenoviral gene transfer. Mol Genet Metab 2003; 80:148–158.

140. Margolis DJ, Crombleholme T, Herlyn M. Clinical protocol: phase I trial to evaluate the safety of H5.020CMV.PDGF-B for the treatment of a diabetic insensate foot ulcer. Wound Repair Regen 2000; 8:480–493.

141. Margolis DJ, Crombleholme T, Herlyn M, et al. Clinical protocol: phase I trial to evaluate the safety of H5.020CMV.PDGF-b and limb compression bandage for the treatment of venous leg ulcer: trial A. Hum Gene Ther 2004; 15:1003–1019.

142. Supp DM, Bell SM, Morgan JR, et al. Genetic modification of cultured skin substitutes by transduction of human keratinocytes and fibroblasts with platelet-derived growth factor-A. Wound Repair Regen 2000; 8:26–35.

143. Erdag G, Medalie DA, Rakhorst H, et al. FGF-7 expression enhances the performance of bioengineered skin. Mol Ther 2004; 10:76–85.

144. Kopp J, Wang GY, Kulmburg P, et al. Accelerated wound healing by in vivo application of keratinocytes overexpressing KGF. Mol Ther 2004; 10:86–96.

145. Shumakov VI, Onishechenko NA, Rasulov MF, et al. Mesenchymal bone marrow stem cells more effectively stimulate regeneration of deep burn wounds than embryonic fibroblasts. Bull Exp Biol Med 2003; 136:192–195.

146. Hohfeld J, de Buys Roessingh A, Hirt-Burri N, et al. Tissue engineered fetal skin constructs for paediatric burns. Lancet 2005; 366:840–842.

147. Rasulov MF, Vasilchenkov AV, Onishchenko NA, et al. First experience of the use of bone marrow mesenchymal stem cells for the treatment of a patient with deep skin burns. Bull Exp Biol Med 2005; 139:141–144.

148. Kane CD, Greenhalgh DG. Expression and localization of p53 and bcl-2 in healing wounds in diabetic and nondiabetic mice. Wound Repair Regen 2000; 8:45–58.

149. Grinnell F, Zhu M, Carlson MA, et al. Release of mechanical tension triggers apoptosis of human fibroblasts in a model of regressing granulation tissue. Exp Med Res 1999; 248:608–619.

150. Scott PG, Ghahary A, Tredget EE. Molecular and cellular aspects of fibrosis following thermal injury. Hand Clin 2000; 16:271–287.

151. Liu W, Chau C, Wu X, et al. Inhibiting scar formation in rat wounds by adenovirus-mediated overexpression of truncated TGF-β receptor II. Plast Reconstr Surg 2005; 115:860–870.

152. Chodon T, Sugihara T, Igawa HH, et al. Keloid-derived fibroblasts are refractory to Fas-mediated apoptosis and neutralization of autocrine transforming growth factor-beta1 can abrogate this resistance. Am J Pathol 2000; 157:1661–1669.

153. Linge C, Richardson J, Vigor C, et al. Hypertrophic scar cells fail to undergo a form of apoptosis specific to contractile collagen — the role of tissue transglutaminase. J Invest Dermatol 2005; 125:72–82.

154. Cutroneo KR, Chiu JF. Sense oligonucleotide competition for gene promoter binding and activation. Int J Biochem Cell Biol 2003; 35:32–38.

155. Cordeiro MF, Mead A, Ali RR, et al. Novel antisense oligonucleotides targeting TGF-beta inhibit in vivo scarring and improve surgical outcome. Gene Ther 2003; 10:59–71.

156. Wolff RA, Ryomoto M Stark VE, et al. Antisense to transforming growth factor-beta1 messenger RNA reduces vein graft intimal hyperplasia and monocyte chemotactic protein 1. J Vasc Surg 2005; 41:498–508.

157. Wang Z, Inokuchi T, Nemoto TK, et al. Antisense oligonucleotide against collagen-specific molecular chaperone 47-kDa heat shock protein suppresses scar formation in rat wounds. Plast Reconstr Surg 2003; 111:1980–1987.

158. Gu D, Atencio I, Kang DW, et al. Recombinant adenovirus-p21 attenuates proliferative responses associated with excessive scarring. Wound Repair Regen 2005; 13:480–490.

159. Perkins TW, Faha B, Ni M, et al. Adenovirus-mediated gene therapy using human p21WAF-1/Cip-1 to prevent wound healing in a rabbit model of glaucoma filtration surgery. Arch Ophthalmol 2002; 120:941–949.

160. Ashcroft J, Yang X, Glick AB, et al. Mice lacking Smad3 show accelerated wound healing and an impaired local inflammatory response. Nature Cell Biol 1999; 1:260–266.

161. Flanders KC, Major CD, Arabshahi A, et al. Interference with transforming growth factor-beta/Smad3 signaling results in accelerated healing of wounds in previously irradiated skin. Am J Pathol 2003; 163:2247–2257.

162. Sumiyoshi K, Nakao A, Setoguchi Y, et al. Exogenous Smad3 accelerates wound healing in a rabbit dermal ulcer model. J Invest Dermatol 2004; 123:229–236.

163. Saika S, Ikeda K, Yamanaka O, et al. Expression of Smad7 in mouse eyes accelerates healing of corneal tissue after exposure to alkali. Am J Pathol 2005; 166:1405–1418.

164. Saika S, Ikeda K, Yamanaka O, et al. Transient adenoviral gene transfer of Smad7 prevents injury-induced epithelial-mesenchymal transition of lens epithelium in mice. Lab Invest 2004; 84:1259–1270.

165. Perkins K, Davey R, Wallis KA. Silicone gel: a new treatment for burn scars and contractures. Burns 1982; 9:201–204.

166. Ahn ST, Monafo WW, Mustoe TA. Topical silicone gel for the prevention and the treatment of hypertrophic scar. Arch Surg 1991; 126:499–504.

Chapter 47

Molecular and cellular basis of hypertrophic scarring

Paul G. Scott, Aziz Ghahary, JianFei Wang, and Edward E. Tredget

Chapter contents

Introduction

The postburn hypertrophic scar presents as a raised, erythematous, pruritic and inelastic mass of tissue. If left untreated the collagen within its dermal matrix may undergo a reorganization leading to the development of contractures, and thus adding functional impairment to the discomfort and cosmetic problems already suffered by the recovering burn patient (Figure 47.1). The undesirable physical properties of hypertrophic scar tissue can be attributed to the presence of a large amount of extracellular matrix that is of altered composition and organization, compared to normal dermis or mature scar. This matrix is the product of a dense population of fibroblasts (and other cell types) maintained in a hyperactive state by inflammatory cytokines such as transforming growth factor-β (TGF-β) and other factors, some of which may be physical in origin. Eventually most hypertrophic scars undergo at least some degree of spontaneous resolution: a process that may have led to some of the conflicting descriptions of the histology, cell biology or chemistry of hypertrophic scar that have appeared in the literature from time to time. This chapter will review what is known about the molecular and cellular characteristics of the postburn hypertrophic scar and how these help to explain its development and properties, drawing comparisons with normal wound healing and mature scars. While it would be misleading to suggest that the etiology of this debilitating condition is completely understood, it is nevertheless our hope that the better understanding of its pathogenesis that is now emerging will lead eventually to more rational and successful, non-surgical treatments.

Chemical composition and organization of the extracellular matrix

Collagen

Collagen is the predominant extracellular matrix protein in both normal dermis and hypertrophic scar, where it is responsible for the tensile strength of the tissue. However collagen constitutes a smaller proportion (about 30% less of the dry weight) of hypertrophic scars because there are greater increases in other components such as the proteoglycans and glycoproteins[1] (see below). The major genetic form of collagen in skin and scars is type I, which characteristically assembles into thick fibrils, fibers and fiber-bundles. In normal dermis there are smaller amounts of type III (10–15% of the total) and very small amounts of type V and type VI collagens. Pure types III and V collagens assemble *in vitro* into thin fibrils[2–4] but are found in tissues mainly in heterotypic fibrils mixed with larger amounts of type I collagen.[5–7] Both types III and V collagens are considered to reduce the diameters of the collagen fibrils of which they form part. Hypertrophic scars generally contain thinner collagen fibrils than normal dermis (averaging around 60 nm in diameter compared to 100 nm).[8] This difference might be explained by the higher proportions of types III and V collagens, reported to be about 33%[9,10] and 10%,[11] respectively. Type III collagen appears in healing wounds within a few days after injury[12] and its persistence at high levels in hypertrophic scars is probably a reflection of their biological immaturity. Type VI collagen does not assemble into fibrils, but rather into thin beaded filaments, 5–20 nm wide, that are seen to run perpendicular to the fibrils and possibly to link them together.[13] These may constitute the interfibrillar elements that have been described in hypertrophic scar.[14]

In the light microscope, it can be seen that much of the collagen in hypertrophic scars is arranged in 'whorls' or 'nodules,' rather than the thick fibers or fiber-bundles that are characteristically oriented parallel to the surface in normal dermis.[8] In some specimens (e.g. Figure 47.2) there are extensive regions of almost hyaline appearance where little organization of the fine-fibered collagen is apparent. In the electron microscope the narrow collagen fibrils in these regions are seen to be more widely spaced than in normal dermis or mature scar and to be ovoid or irregular in cross-section.[14] The interfibrillar space in fibrous connective tissues is occupied mainly by

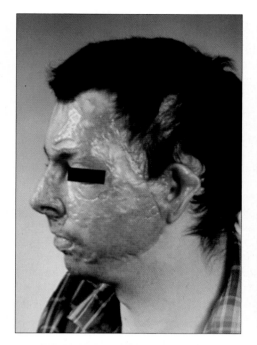

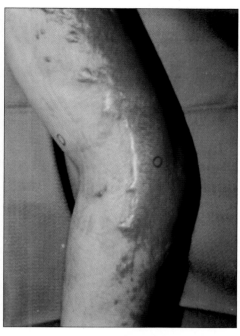

Fig. 47.1 Hypertrophic scarring in a 34-year-old white man, 8 months following a 60% total body surface area burn involving the face, upper extremities and hands. (From Scott et al.,[36] with permission.)

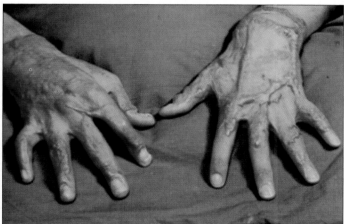

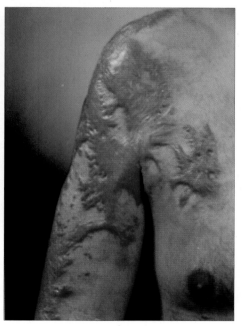

matrix macromolecules of two other classes: the proteoglycans and glycoproteins.

Proteoglycans and glycoproteins

Proteoglycans influence physical properties of connective tissues such as turgor, resilience and resistance to compression, while glycoproteins such as fibronectin and tenascin are involved in cell-matrix adhesion and have effects on cell behavior mainly through this mechanism. Proteoglycans also influence cellular activity, but through a variety of mechanisms including both positive and negative modulation of growth factor activity. The morphology of collagen fibrils and

their organization are profoundly affected by the nature and amounts of proteoglycans present in the connective tissue.

Proteoglycans consist of one or more glycosaminoglycan chains, which are linear polymers of anionic disaccharides, covalently attached to a protein core. In the most common glycosaminoglycans (dermatan sulfate, chondroitin sulfate, heparan sulfate and hyaluronic acid), one unit of the repeating disaccharide is a uronic acid. Early chemical analyses of hypertrophic scars revealed elevated concentrations of uronic acid (and hence glycosaminoglycans).[15] Since it is the anionic polysaccharide glycosaminoglycan chains that are mainly responsible for the water-holding capacity of connective tissues,[16] it

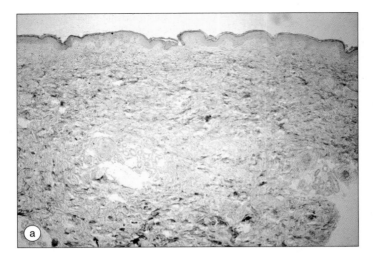

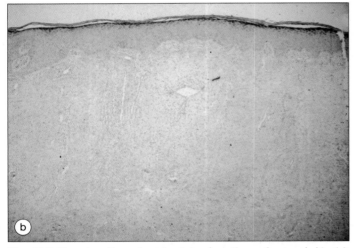

Fig. 47.2 Hematoxylin and eosin-stained sections of normal skin (a) and a hypertrophic scar containing a nodule (b) (original magnification ×10).

is not surprising that hypertrophic scars are hyperhydrated relative to normal dermis or mature scars. However, the 2.4-fold increase in glycosaminoglycan content (and presumably osmotic pressure) is disproportionately high relative to the 12% increase in water content.[1] Since the collagen fibers normally restrict swelling of connective tissues, it may be proposed that the high concentration of glycosaminoglycans in hypertrophic scars is responsible for their enhanced turgor.

Following the initial analyses of total glycosaminoglycan content in hypertrophic scars, it was reported that the nodular areas were virtually devoid of dermatan sulfate (the major glycosaminoglycan in normal dermis) and contained instead chondroitin sulfate, which is usually only a minor component.[17] The corresponding changes in the proteoglycans were defined more recently, when it was reported that hypertrophic scars contain on average only 25% of the amount of the small dermatan sulfate proteoglycan decorin (the major proteoglycan found in normal dermis) and 6-fold higher concentrations of a large proteoglycan resembling versican.[1] This latter proteoglycan, which carries 12–30 chondroitin sulfate chains, is normally present only in the proliferating zone of the epider-

mis and in association with elastin in the dermis.[18] Decorin and versican, as detected by immunohistochemistry, show a strikingly inverse distribution in the nodules,[19] thus explaining the earlier observations on the distribution of the glycosaminoglycans: dermatan and chondroitin sulfates.

Decorin is implicated in the regulation of collagen fibril formation and in the organization of fibrils into fibers and fiber-bundles.[20,21] In the decorin-null mouse, collagen fibrils were found to be variable in diameter and irregular in outline.[22] This latter characteristic was earlier described for the collagen fibrils in the nodules of hypertrophic scar[8] and may be explained by the virtual absence of the decorin that normally defines and delimits the fibril surface. A second small proteoglycan, biglycan, present in lesser amounts than decorin in normal dermis, is found at elevated levels in postburn hypertrophic scars.[1,19] In most connective tissues biglycan is found close to the cell surface[23] but in hypertrophic scars it is associated with the collagen in the extracellular matrix,[19] possibly because there is little decorin to compete for the restricted number of proteoglycan core protein binding sites on the collagen fibrils.[24]

The differences in proteoglycan proportions and distributions between normal dermis and hypertrophic scars could in principle result either from altered biosynthesis or altered degradation. There is evidence for the former mechanism, since fibroblasts cultured from postburn hypertrophic scar contain less decorin mRNA and synthesize less of the protein than do normal fibroblasts.[25] It was shown by *in situ* hybridization that there are relatively few cells expressing mRNA for decorin in healing burn scars until about 12 months after injury.[26] Surprisingly, in fibroblasts cultured from hypertrophic scars there were no differences in contents of mRNAs for versican or biglycan, suggesting that other factors such as transforming growth factor-β (see below) were influencing fibroblast behavior and responsible for the elevated amounts of these two proteoglycans in the scars.[25]

As hypertrophic scars mature, the collagen fibrils become coarser and better organized and there is an increase in immunohistochemically detectable decorin (Figure 47.3). At about 12 months after injury, a time when many scars start to resolve spontaneously,[27] there is a large increase in numbers of cells expressing decorin, suggesting that this proteoglycan may play an active role in the resolution.[26] Mature scars show contents of collagen, proteoglycans and water that are indistinguishable from those in normal dermis.[1]

The results of early chemical analyses of hexose and sialic acid contents[15] showed that hypertrophic scars contained elevated concentrations of glycoproteins, at least part of which is fibronectin.[28] This extracellular matrix macromolecule has effects on cell attachment and activity (reviewed in Hynes[29]) that could be important in the development and organization of hypertrophic scar but its role does not appear to have been investigated directly.

The hypertrophic scar fibroblast phenotype

Many laboratory investigations have been based on the premise that the fibroblasts that can be grown from tissue explants retain the hypertrophic scar phenotype in culture. This is at least partly justified since these cells show characteristics that

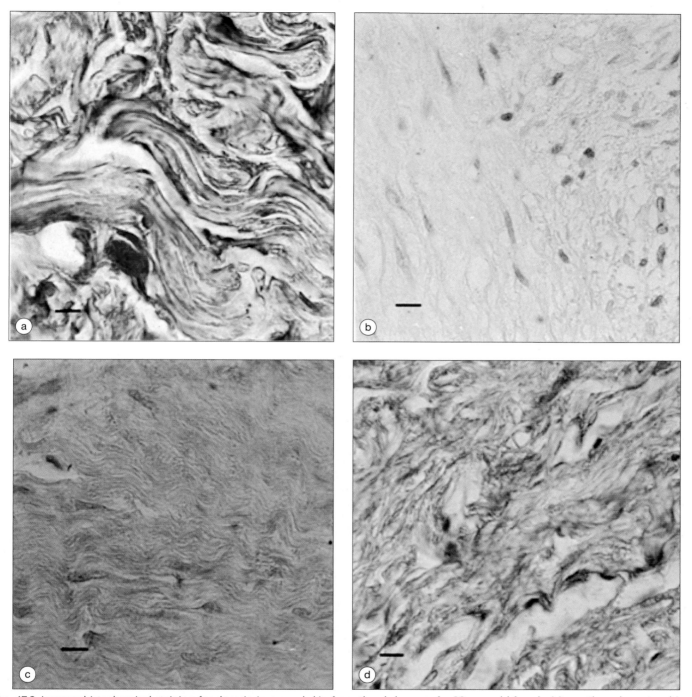

Fig. 47.3 Immunohistochemical staining for decorin in normal skin from the abdomen of a 39-year-old female (a), postburn hypertrophic scar from the neck of a 4-year-old male, 5 months (b) and 12 months (c) after burn injury and postburn mature scar from the neck of a 22-year-old female, 216 months after burn injury (d). Bars = 10 μm. (From Sayani et al., Histopathology 2000; 36:262–272.[26] with permission.)

would be predicted from what is known about the tissue. Some strains of hypertrophic scar fibroblast synthesize more collagen[30] and fibronectin[31] than do normal dermal fibroblasts and all strains investigated make less decorin,[25] collagenase[32,33] and nitric oxide.[34] Rather less consistent are the reports of altered cell replication rates *in vitro*. Since hypertrophic scars have a greater density of fibroblast-like cells than normal dermis or mature scar,[26] it might be predicted that these cells

would divide more rapidly in culture but the consensus is that population doubling times are unchanged or slightly longer.[31,35,36] Possible explanations for this apparent anomaly are the absence *in vitro* of stimulatory cytokines, such as transforming growth factor-β (see below), that are present in the tissue,[19,37] or that the cells that grow out of the explants are approaching the end of their replicative life span. There have been reports of enhanced incorporation of bromodeoxyuridine into hypertrophic scar fibroblasts *in vitro*[38] but labeling with tritiated thymidine led Oku and colleagues to conclude that most fibroblasts in hypertrophic scar are dormant, although there may be a small population of more rapidly proliferating cells.[39]

Myofibroblasts and delayed apoptosis in hypertrophic scars

The presence of myofibroblasts, cells characterized by an indented nuclear envelope and well-developed stress-fibers, has been considered pathognomonic for fibrous tissue that is prone to undergo contracture.[40] Hypertrophic scar tissue contains elevated numbers of cells identified as myofibroblasts on morphological criteria.[41] Myofibroblasts are now usually identified by their positive staining for α-smooth muscle actin,[42] and such cells are especially prominent in palmar fascia in Dupuytren's disease[43] and in hypertrophic scar but not in keloid.[44] All fibroblasts probably have contractile ability, as seen in experimental model systems such as the fibroblast-populated collagen lattice where myofibroblasts do not appear until contraction is complete.[45] Moreover, cells with the morphological characteristics of myofibroblasts can be induced in skin by the application of tension in the absence of wounding.[46] Nevertheless, electroinjected antibodies against α-smooth muscle actin block the contraction of the fibroblast-populated collagen lattice,[47] indicating that this minor actin isoform (normally accounting for about 14% of the total actin in fibroblasts) is an integral component of the contractile apparatus.

The reduction in cellularity that accompanies the conversion of granulation tissue into scar tissue, or of hypertrophic scar into mature scar, is associated with induction of apoptosis (programmed cell death).[48] (See Perl et al.[49] for a brief review of this complex process.) The myofibroblast has been suggested to be a terminally differentiated pre-apoptotic cell.[40] However, this suggestion appears inconsistent with reports that organization of α-smooth muscle actin into stress fibers protects fibroblasts against the induction of apoptosis,[50] and with the different distributions of α-smooth muscle actin staining and apoptotic cells in skin wounds in guinea pigs treated with interferon-α2b.[51] The prevalence of myofibroblasts in hypertrophic scar may actually be a sign of a delay in the normal onset of apoptosis in the healing wound and this delay may be responsible at least in part for the hypercellularity.

Influence of extracellular matrix on fibroblast survival

The extent and strength of interactions between attachment-dependent cells such as fibroblasts and epithelial cells and the underlying extracellular matrix are important factors determining cell survival. Detachment of such cells often leads to apoptosis, a phenomenon for which the term 'anoikis' (Greek for homelessness) was coined.[52] In this context the high concentration of fibronectin in hypertrophic scars might be important, since binding of the α5β1 integrin to this adhesive glycoprotein has been shown to inhibit Chinese hamster ovary (CHO) cells from undergoing apoptosis.[53] Results obtained with the fibroblast-populated collagen lattice model *in vitro* also support the paradigm that the extracellular matrix regulates fibroblast behavior in healing wounds ('outside-in signaling'). In the anchored lattice, which resists deformation in all

but the short vertical dimension, fibroblasts continue to proliferate, while in floating or stress-relaxed collagen lattices that are rapidly reorganized, they are triggered to undergo apoptosis.[54,55] The overabundant glycosaminoglycans in postburn hypertrophic scars, through their contribution to tissue osmotic pressure and turgor, might inhibit reorganization of the collagen matrix by the fibroblasts.[55] Alternatively (or additionally), reorganization of the matrix may be impaired as a result of its chemical stabilization (cross-linking) by tissue transglutaminase, an enzyme that is expressed in greater amounts by hypertrophic scar than by normal dermal fibroblasts.[56] Either mechanism could delay the onset of apoptosis. Treatment of hypertrophic scars with pressure therapy has been used for many years and is generally considered beneficial. It has been shown that such treatment promotes the reorganization of postburn scar tissue and the disappearance of α-smooth actin staining myofibroblasts, probably by accelerating the onset of apoptosis.[57] A similar phenomenon is seen in the scars of burn patients treated with systemically injected interferon α2b.[58]

Modulation of fibroblast behavior by fibrogenic and antifibrogenic cytokines

Two general mechanisms might be suggested to account for the altered phenotype of fibroblasts in hypertrophic scars. The first, and simplest, is that thermal injury selectively destroys certain cells, for example those in the superficial dermis, while the second, and more extensively investigated possibility, is that the proliferation and/or activities of certain subsets of fibroblasts are affected by fibrogenic cytokines present in the wounds. These two mechanisms are not mutually exclusive. Some of the activities of the cytokines in healing wounds are shown in Figure 47.4.

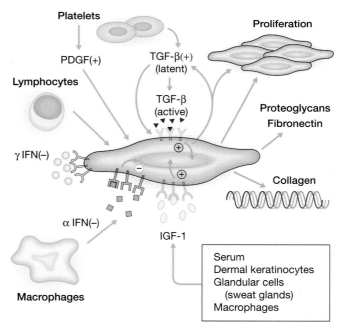

Fig. 47.4 The fibrogenic and antifibrogenic factors that modulate fibroblast function during wound healing. (From Tredget EE, Nedelec B, Scott PG, Ghahary A. Hypertrophic scars, keloids and molecular basis for therapy. Surg Clin North Am 1997; 77:701–730, with permission.)

Transforming growth factor-β

The best-characterized fibrogenic cytokine is transforming growth factor-β (TGF-β), actually a family of (in mammals) three closely related proteins (for review see Roberts and Sporn[59]). Cellular sources of this cytokine include degranulating platelets, macrophages, T-lymphocytes, endothelial cells, smooth muscle cells, epithelial cells and fibroblasts, i.e. all the major cell types participating in wound healing.[59] Transforming growth factor-β1 is a potent chemoattractant for monocytes[60] and fibroblasts.[61] It stimulates fibroblasts to synthesize collagen, fibronectin, and glycosaminoglycans,[62–64] down-regulates decorin synthesis while up-regulating production of versican and biglycan,[65] enhances neovascularization[66] and modulates production of a variety of proteinases and their inhibitors.[67,68] Subcutaneous injection of TGF-β1 into newborn mice stimulates formation of granulation tissue[66] and accelerates healing of incisional wounds in rats.[69] Many of the effects of TGF-β1 on mesenchymal cells may be mediated by connective tissue growth factor. This protein, which stimulates the proliferation of fibroblasts and synthesis of extracellular matrix proteins,[70] is coordinately expressed with TGF-β in several fibrotic conditions.[71]

Transforming growth factor-β stimulates the expression of α-smooth muscle actin in fibroblasts and may delay the onset of apoptosis by this pathway.[50] Fibroblasts cultured from hypertrophic scar synthesize more TGF-β1 than do normal dermal fibroblasts[72] and the protein has been detected in the scar by immunohistochemistry.[19,37] The serum of recovering burn patients contains levels of TGF-β1 about twice those in control patients.[73] All these observations, and evidence implicating it in other fibrotic conditions (reviewed in Ghahary et al.[74]), point to the probable involvement of TGF-β in postburn hypertrophic scarring.

The activity of TGF-β in connective tissue may be modified by interaction with components of the extracellular matrix, such as the proteoglycans. Decorin has been shown to bind to TGF-β and to neutralize at least some of its activities[75,76] and mature postburn scars stain intensely for TGF-β that appears to be co-distributed with the decorin.[19] Consequently we suggest that decorin, which is massively re-expressed in healing burn wounds starting around 12 months after injury,[26] down-regulates TGF-β activity and promotes the natural resolution of hypertrophic scarring.

Insulin-like growth factor-1

Other cytokines that may play a role in hypertrophic scarring include insulin-like growth factor-1 (IGF-1). Like TGF-β1, IGF-1 is expressed locally in response to tissue injury,[77,78] including postburn hypertrophic scar tissue.[79] Insulin-like growth factor-1 is mitogenic for fibroblasts and endothelial cells, stimulates collagen production by osteoblasts,[80] lung[81] and dermal[82] fibroblasts and in growth plate chondrocytes,[83] and reduces expression of collagenase by dermal fibroblasts.[33] The remarkable similarity in activities of IGF-1 and TGF-β1 can be explained by the observation that IGF-1 induces transcription of the gene for TGF-β1, so that at least some of its actions on fibroblasts might be mediated through this indirect mechanism.[84] Expression of IGF-1 in uninjured skin seems to be restricted to epidermis, sweat and sebaceous glands[85] but in a healing burn wound these elements are disrupted and epithelial cells migrating towards the wound surface could possibly secrete IGF-1 in proximity to fibroblasts and affect their activity.

Interferons

The interferons (IFNs) are naturally occurring cytokines that were originally detected as proteins expressed in response to viral infection[86] but which may have therapeutic application in the treatment of hypertrophic scars and keloids. There are two main classes of interferon: type I comprising IFNs-α and -β (produced by leukocytes and fibroblasts, respectively), and type II (IFN-γ, produced by activated T-lymphocytes). They are distinguished by the degree of their amino acid sequence similarity and by their receptors and intracellular signaling pathways.[86] Treatment of fibroblasts in vitro with either type of interferon inhibits cell proliferation and reduces expression of type I and III collagens,[87,88] fibronectin[89] and TGF-β.[73] Interferon-α2b, but not IFN-γ, also induces the expression of collagenase, suggesting that it may possibly be of greater benefit than the latter in the treatment of fibroproliferative disorders where an excessive amount of collagen is present.[90] Treatment of fibroblasts in vitro with IFNs reduces the rate of contraction of collagen lattices,[91,92] probably by down-regulating the expression of the genes for the major β and γ isoforms of actin.[93] Administration of IFN-α2b to guinea pigs through osmotic mini-pumps reduces the rate of wound closure and the frequency of α-smooth muscle actin-positive cells, and increases the frequency of apoptotic cells in healing wounds at late stages.[51]

Although keloids in patients treated with IFN-α2b showed only limited improvement,[94,95] early (phase II) trials in postburn hypertrophic scar patients have shown promising results, associated with a reduction in scar height, increase in scar suppleness and reduced levels of circulating methylhistamine and TGF-β.[73] In these same patients there was an increased frequency of apoptotic cells following treatment with IFN-α2b.[96] Induction or augmentation of apoptosis by IFNs has been demonstrated in activated T cells, squamous cell carcinoma cells and non-myeloma skin cancer cells.[97–99] It does not appear to have been previously shown in fibroblasts but is consistent with the report that IFN-γ down-regulates α-smooth muscle actin.[100]

Given the evidence, reviewed above, that interferons can modify fibroblast behavior both in vivo and in vitro, the question naturally arises of whether depressed intrinsic levels of these cytokines might play a role in the pathogenesis of aberrant scarring. McCauley et al. isolated peripheral blood mononuclear cells (PBMC) from black keloid patients and from a control group of patients who had suffered equivalent trauma but not developed keloids.[101] After appropriate stimulation, PBMC from the keloid patients secreted less IFN-α and IFN-γ but more IFN-β. Cytokine production by T-cell clones that could be grown from active hypertrophic scar tissue and scars undergoing remission, were compared by Bernabei et al.[102] In both cases clones producing IFN-γ predominated but the amounts of this cytokine released were 4–6 times lower in clones from scars undergoing remission. It was suggested that the IFN-γ, a potent pro-inflammatory cytokine, was responsible for the prolonged inflammation in active hypertrophic scars.

The T-helper-2 cell response to burn injury

It has long been recognized that hypertrophic scars are heavily infiltrated with lymphocytes, often forming perivascular cuffs.[8] These cells are surrounded by a proteoglycan-rich matrix that they may have secreted themselves.[103] The largest population of lymphocytes in hypertrophic scars is activated (CD4+) T-helper cells, found especially in the subpapillary dermis but also in the epidermis and reticular dermis.[104] There are also increased numbers of macrophages and Langerhans' cells but B-lymphocytes are not seen. Two subsets of T-helper cells (Th1 and Th2) can be differentiated by the cytokines that they synthesize.[105] Th1 cells secrete IFN-γ, interleukin-2 (IL-2) and tumor necrosis factor-β (TNF-β) and are principally involved in cell-mediated immunity, whereas Th2 cells secrete IL-4, IL-5 and IL-10 and induce antibody production. The activation of naïve mouse CD4+ T-lymphocytes to secrete TGF-β is promoted by the Th2 cytokine IL-10 and the amounts of TGF-β secreted are greater in T-cell populations from IFN-γ null mice and lower in IL-4 null mice.[106] For an extensive review of the evidence linking the type of T-cell response to the development and mechanism of fibrosis, see Wynn.[107] In burned mice there is depletion of splenocytes synthesizing IFN-γ and IL-2 (Th1 cytokines) and an increase in synthesis of IL-5 (a Th2 cytokine).[108] There is evidence for a similar 'Th2 response' in human burn victims. Stimulated PBMC from patients with 25–90% surface area burns showed diminished production of IL-2.[109] Increased production of IL-4, accompanied by decreased IFN-γ, was subsequently reported in a group of burn and major trauma patients.[110] Interleukin-4 has been reported to be even more potent than TGF-β at promot-ing collagen synthesis by fibroblasts.[111] A link between the type of Th response to injury and the severity of fibrosis has been demonstrated: hepatic fibrosis is much more severe in BALB/c mice, which show a Th2 response to chemically induced liver injury, than in C57BL/6 mice, which respond with a Th1 cytokine profile.[112] Moreover, shifting the Th2 response toward a Th1 response by treatment with a neutralizing antibody to IL-4, or with IFN-γ, ameliorated fibrosis in the BALB/c mice. Intradermal administration of IFN-α2b has been reported to be ineffective in preventing the recurrence of resected keloids[113] and this treatment might therefore be expected to be minimally effective for the treatment of hypertrophic scarring. It is nevertheless possible that systemic administration of IFN-α2b to recovering burn patients does affect the T-helper cell phenotype and that its beneficial effects are mediated in part through this mechanism.[73,114] We have recently reported results of a longitudinal study on recovering burn patients that supports the hypothesis that there is 'locked on Th2 response' to burn injury.[115] Cytokine synthesis by T-cells was assessed from the time of injury to 1 year after injury, during which time many burn patients develop hypertrophic scarring. Within 1 month of injury, few interferon-γ (IFN-γ) positive T cells (Th1) were found in association with low serum IL-12 levels (Figure 47.5a,b) and no detectable serum IFN-γ. By 2 months, IL-4 positive Th2 cells were significantly increased as compared to normal controls (Figure 47.5c). In burn patients who later developed hypertrophic

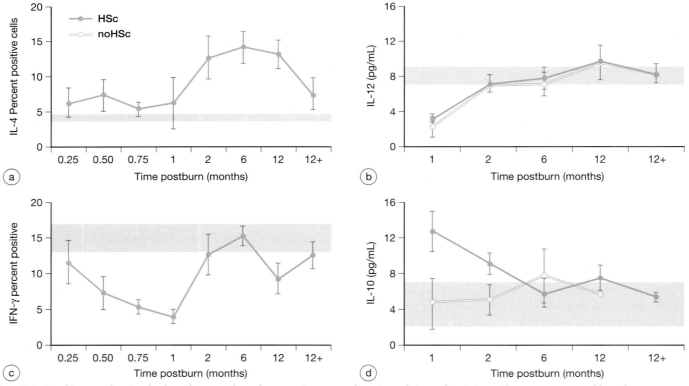

Fig. 47.5 Cytokine production by lymphocytes from burn patients as a function of time after injury. The percentages of lymphocytes producing IFN-γ (a) or IL-4 (c) were estimated by flow cytometry analysis of cells stained for intracellular cytokines using fluorescent-labeled antibodies (n = 22). (b,d) Time course of IL-12 (b) and IL-10 (d) production by peripheral blood mononuclear cells (PBMC) cultured from burn patients who developed hypertrophic scar (HSc) and those who did not (noHSc), measured by ELISA (n = 16). The values measured for cells from normal human volunteers are shown in the shaded boxes (mean ± SD). (From Tredget et al., Interferon Cytokine Res 2006; in press[115] with permission.)

scarring, serum IL-10 (Figure 47.5d) and TGF-β levels were also significantly increased early after injury, as compared to normal volunteers and to a subset of burn patients who did not develop hypertrophic scarring. These elevated levels of IL-10 and TGF-β returned to normal after 6 months. Activated peripheral blood mononuclear cells (PBMC) contained mRNA for IFN-γ only in normal volunteers or patients without hypertrophic scarring, whereas IL-4 mRNA levels were increased in the PBMC of burn patients with hypertrophic scarring. In tissues, IL-4 mRNA was increased in the hypertrophic scars, whereas IFN-γ mRNA was reduced, as compared to normal skin and mature scar. Increased numbers of CD3+ and CD4+ cells were present in hypertrophic scar tissues as compared to normal skin, together with increased staining for the fibrogenic cytokine TGF-β. These longitudinal studies in human burn patients strongly suggest that hypertrophic scarring is associated with a polarized Th2 systemic response.

Fibrocytes

Blood-borne cells that are rapidly recruited into wound chambers in mice, adopt a spindle shape and synthesize collagen, were identified in 1994 and termed 'fibrocytes'.[116] These cells, believed to constitute 0.1–0.5% of peripheral blood leukocytes, exhibit characteristics of both fibroblasts and monocytes. They synthesize extracellular matrix molecules such as collagen types I and III and fibronectin, while expressing certain surface antigens, such as CD11b, CD34, and CD45, that are characteristic of cells derived from the bone marrow (for a review see Metz[117]). In addition to possibly forming some of the extracellular matrix in healing wounds, fibrocytes may be involved in antigen presentation,[118] cytokine production[119] and the stimulation of angiogenesis.[120] They may also be a source of myofibroblasts and contribute to wound closure.[121,122]

Fibrocytes, identified by their staining for CD34, have been reported in various experimental and naturally occurring fibrotic conditions, including bleomycin-induced pulmonary fibrosis,[123,124] renal fibrosis,[125] and liver fibrosis.[119]

Fibrocytes may contribute to the pathogenesis of postburn hypertrophic scarring. Adherent, spindle-shaped cells, synthesizing type I collagen, can be cultured with higher efficiency from the peripheral blood mononuclear cell population of burn patients than from normal subjects.[126] These cells develop in culture from adherent CD14+ leukocytes under the influence of transforming growth factor-β (TGF-β), and possibly other cytokines, secreted by non-adherent CD14− lymphocytes. The efficiency with which they develop is positively correlated with the serum level of TGF-β in the donor,[126] and this cytokine has been found to be persistently elevated in burn patients.[73] During culture these fibrocytes lose cell surface proteins such as CD34 (which is also expressed by other cell types including vascular endothelial cells). Therefore to detect and quantify fibrocytes in tissue, a more stable and specific marker is desirable. Both adherent ('fibrocyte precursor') and non-adherent lymphocytes contain LSP-1 (leukocyte-specific protein-1, formerly known as 'lymphocyte-specific protein-1') but this particular cytoskeleton-associated protein is upregulated in fibrocytes from burn patients and completely absent from fibroblasts.[127] Moreover, LSP-1 is expressed by cultured fibrocytes for at least 28 days (unpublished data), during which time 80% of the cells lose CD34 expression.[123] Fibrocytes in human scar tissue can therefore be identified, and distinguished from other lymphocytes and from fibroblasts, by dual staining with antibodies directed against LSP-1 and procollagen type I (Figure 47.6). Although such cells probably constitute only a small proportion of the collagen-producing cells in hypertrophic scar, they are more abundant than in mature scar and none were seen in normal dermis.[127] Recent work in our laboratory (unpublished data) has shown that fibrocytes from

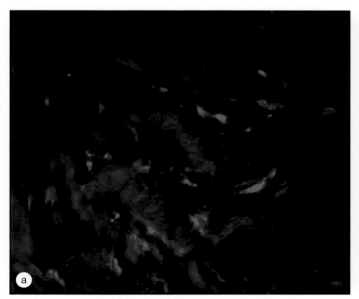
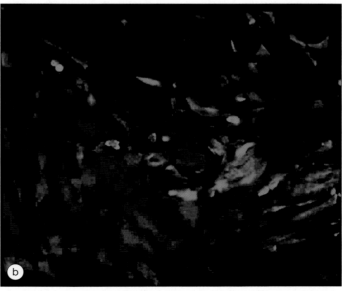

Fig. 47.6 Dual immunofluorescent labeling of fibrocytes in scar tissue. Cryosections of hypertrophic scar (a–c) and mature scar (d–f) were stained with antibodies to leukocyte-specific protein-1 (LSP-1) (green color) and the N-terminal propeptide of type I procollagen (red color). In double-exposure photomicrographs fibrocytes (arrowed in c) are visualized in hypertrophic scar by the colocalization of LSP-1 and procollagen (yellow color). (From Yang et al., Wound Rep Reg 2005; 13:398–404.[127] with permission.)

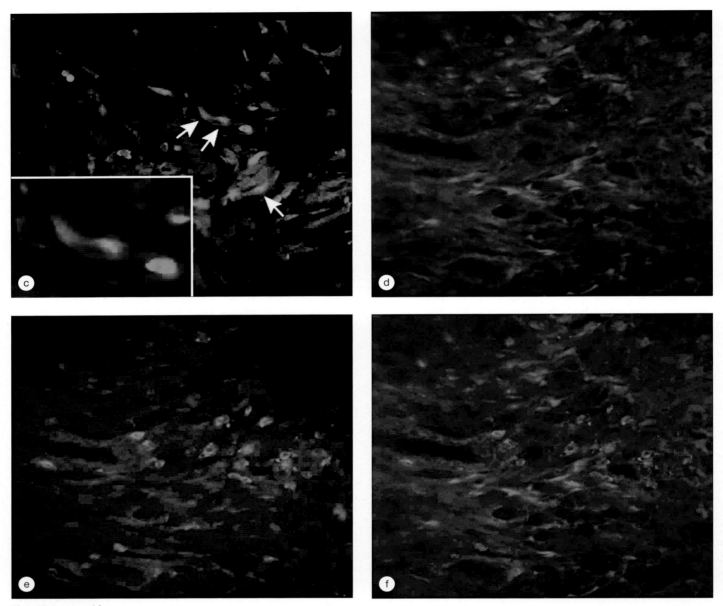

Fig. 47.6 – cont'd.

burn patients, but not those from normal subjects, can secrete factors stimulating the proliferation, migration and contractility of normal dermal fibroblasts. Fibrocytes may therefore play an important, albeit indirect, role in the pathogenesis of postburn hypertrophic scar.

Summary

The postburn hypertrophic scar consists of a mass of hypercellular and disorganized connective tissue overlain with a thickened epidermis. Within the connective tissue much of the collagen is arranged in whorls and nodules, rather than the thick fibers and fiber-bundles running parallel to the surface that are characteristic of normal dermis. This derangement of the collagen, together with the very high content of glycosaminoglycans, accounts for the inelasticity and turgor of the tissue which might be further stabilized by cross-linking by tissue transglutaminase. The hypercellularity characteristic of hypertrophic scar probably results from a blockade in the induction of the programmed cell death (apoptosis) that normally accompanies scar maturation, consequent upon altered cytokine profiles and signals from the extracellular matrix. Abnormalities in the extracellular matrix may themselves result from the selection and stimulation of subpopulations of fibroblasts, synthesizing increased amounts and altered proportions of specific types of collagen and proteoglycan, and reduced amounts of proteolytic enzymes (for example collagenase), that are normally responsible for the remodeling phase of wound healing. A polarized T-helper-2 cell response to burn injury, leading to increased levels of circulating and local fibrogenic cytokines, such as transforming growth factor-β, and decreased antifibrogenic cytokines such as the interferons, may mediate these shifts in phenotype. A recently recognized blood-borne cell, the fibrocyte, may accumulate in hypertrophic scar and modulate the activity of the many fibroblasts within it.

References

1. Scott PG, Dodd CM, Tredget EE, et al. Chemical characterization and quantification of proteoglycans in human postburn hypertrophic and mature scars. Clin Sci 1996; 90:417–425.
2. Adachi E, Hayashi T. In vitro formation of hybrid fibrils of type V collagen and type I collagen. Limited growth of type I collagen into thick fibrils by type V collagen. Connect Tissue Res 1986; 14:257–266.
3. Lapiere CM, Nusgens B, Pierard GE. Interaction between collagen type I and type III in conditioning bundles organization. Connect Tissue Res 1977; 5:21–29.
4. Birk DE, Fitch JM, Babiarz JP, et al. Collagen fibrillogenesis in vitro: interaction of types I and V collagen regulates fibril diameter. J Cell Sci 1990; 95:649–657.
5. Henkel W, Glanville RW. Covalent crosslinking between molecules of type I and type III collagen. The involvement of the N-terminal, nonhelical regions of the α 1 (I) and α 1 (III) chains in the formation of intermolecular crosslinks. Eur J Biochem 1982; 122:205–213.
6. Keene DR, Sakai LY, Bachinger HP, et al. Type III collagen can be present on banded collagen fibrils regardless of fibril diameter. J Cell Biol 1987; 105:2393–2302.
7. Birk DE, Fitch JM, Babiarz JP, et al. Collagen type I and type V are present in the same fibril in the avian corneal stroma. J Cell Biol 1988; 106:999–1008.
8. Linares HA, Kischer CW, Dobrkovsky M, et al. The histiotypic organization of the hypertrophic scar in humans. J Invest Dermatol 1972; 59:323–331.
9. Bailey AJ, Bazin S, Sims TJ, et al. Characterization of the collagen of human hypertrophic and normal scars. Biochim Biophys Acta 1975; 405:412–421.
10. Hayakawa T, Hashimoto Y, Myokei Y, et al. Changes in type of collagen during the development of human postburn hypertrophic scars. Clin Chim Acta 1979; 93:119–125.
11. Ehrlich HP, White BS. The identification of αA and αB collagen chains in hypertrophic scar. Exp Mol Pathol 1981; 34:1–8.
12. Gay S, Viljanto J, Raekallio H, et al. Collagen types in early phases of wound healing in children. Acta Chir Scand 1978; 144:205–211.
13. Engel J, Furthmayr H, Odermatt E, et al. Structure and macromolecular organization of type VI collagen. Ann N Y Acad Sci 1985; 460:25–37.
14. Kischer CW. Collagen and dermal patterns in the hypertrophic scar. Anat Rec 1974; 179:137–145.
15. Shetlar MR, Dobrkovsky M, Linares L, et al. The hypertrophic scar. Glycoprotein and collagen components of burn scars. Proc Soc Exp Biol Med 1971; 138:298–300.
16. Ogston AG. In: Balazs EA, ed. Chemistry and molecular biology of the intercellular matrix. New York: Academic Press; 1970: 1231–1240.
17. Shetlar MR, Shetlar CL, Linares HA. The hypertrophic scar: location of glycosaminoglycans within scars. Burns 1977; 4:14–19.
18. Zimmerman DR, Dours-Zimmerman NT, Schubert M, et al. Versican is expressed in the proliferating zone in the epidermis and in association with the elastic network of the dermis. J Cell Biol 1994; 124:817–825.
19. Scott PG, Dodd CM, Tredget EE, et al. Immunohistochemical localization of the proteoglycans decorin, biglycan and versican and transforming growth factor-β in human postburn hypertrophic and mature scars. Histopathology 1995; 26:423–431.
20. Scott JE, Orford CR, Hughes EW. Proteoglycan-collagen arrangements in developing rat tail tendon. Biochem J 1981; 195: 573–581.
21. Scott JE. Proteoglycan-fibrillar collagen interactions in tissues: dermatan sulphate proteoglycan as a tissue organizer. In: Scott JE, ed. Dermatan sulphate proteoglycans: chemistry, biology, chemical pathology. London: Portland; 1993:165–182.
22. Danielson KG, Baribault H, Holmes DF, et al. Targeted disruption of decorin leads to abnormal collagen fibril morphology and skin fragility. J Cell Biol 1997; 136:729–743.
23. Bianco P, Fisher LW, Young MF, et al. Expression and localization of the two small proteoglycans biglycan and decorin in developing human skeletal and non-skeletal tissues. J Histochem Cytochem 1990; 38:1549–1563.
24. Brown DC, Vogel KG. Characteristics of the in vitro interaction of a small proteoglycan (PGII) of bovine tendon with type I collagen. Matrix 1989; 9:468–478.
25. Scott PG, Dodd CM, Ghahary A, et al. Fibroblasts from postburn hypertrophic scar tissue synthesize less decorin than normal dermal fibroblasts. Clin Sci 1998; 94:541–547.
26. Sayani K, Dodd CM, Nedelec B, et al. Delayed appearance of decorin in healing burn scars. Histopathology 2000; 36:262–272.
27. Reid WH, Evans JH, Naismith RS, et al. Hypertrophic scarring and pressure therapy. Burns 1987; 13:S29–S32.
28. Kischer CW, Hendrix MJC. Fibronectin (FN) in hypertrophic scars and keloids. Cell Tissue Res 1983; 231:29–37.
29. Hynes RO. Fibronectins. New York: Springer-Verlag; 1990.
30. Ghahary A, Scott PG, Malhotra SK, et al. Differential expression of type I and type III procollagen mRNA in human hypertrophic burn fibroblasts. Biomed Letts 1992; 47:169–184.
31. Kischer CW, Wagner HN, Pindur J, et al. Increased fibronectin production by cell lines from hypertrophic scar and keloid. Connect Tissue Res 1989; 23:279–288.
32. Arakawa M, Hatamochi A, Mori Y, et al. Reduced collagenase gene expression in fibroblasts from hypertrophic scar tissue. Br J Dermatol 1996; 134:863–868.
33. Ghahary A, Shen YJ, Nedelec B, et al. Collagenase production is lower in postburn hypertrophic scar fibroblasts than normal fibroblasts and is down-regulated by insulin-like growth factor-1. J Invest Dermatol 1996; 106:476–481.
34. Wang R, Ghahary A, Shen YJ, et al. Nitric oxide synthase expression and nitric oxide production are reduced in hypertrophic scar tissue and fibroblasts. J Invest Dermatol 1997; 108:438–444.
35. Savage K, Swann DA. A comparison of glycosaminoglycan synthesis by human fibroblasts from normal skin, normal scar, and hypertrophic scar. J Invest Dermatol 1985; 84:521–526.
36. Scott PG, Ghahary A, Chambers MM, et al. Biological basis of hypertrophic scarring. In: Malhotra SK, ed. Advances in structural biology. Greenwich, Connecticut: JAI; 1994:(3)157–202.
37. Ghahary A, Shen YJ, Scott PG, et al. Immunolocalization of transforming growth factor-β1 in human hypertrophic and normal dermal tissue. Cytokine 1995; 7:184–190.
38. Zhou LJ, Ono I, Kaneko F. Role of transforming growth factor-β1 in fibroblasts derived from normal and hypertrophic scarred skin. Arch Dermatol Res 1997; 289:646–652.
39. Oku T, Takigawa M, Fukamizu H, et al. Growth kinetics of fibroblasts derived from normal skin and hypertrophic scar. Acta Derm Venereol 1987; 67:526–528.
40. Desmouliere A, Gabbiani G. The role of the myofibroblast in wound healing and fibrocontractive diseases. In: Clark RAF, ed. The molecular and cell biology of wound repair, 2nd edn. New York: Plenum; 1996:391–423.
41. Baur PS, Larson DL, Stacey TR. The observation of myofibroblasts in hypertrophic scars. Surg Gynecol Obstet 1975; 141:22–26.
42. Skalli O, Ropraz P, Trzeciak A, et al. A monoclonal antibody against α-smooth muscle actin: a new probe for smooth muscle differentiation. J Cell Biol 1986; 103:2787–2796.
43. Skalli O, Schurch W, Seemayer T, et al. Myofibroblasts from diverse pathological settings are heterogeneous in their content of

actin isoforms and intermediate filament proteins. Lab Invest 1989; 60:275–285.

44. Ehrlich HP, Desmouliere A, Diegelmann RF, et al. Morphological and immunochemical differences between keloid and hypertrophic scar. Am J Pathol 1994; 145:105–113.

45. Ehrlich HP, Rajaratnam JB. Cell locomotion forces versus cell contraction forces for collagen lattice contraction: an in vitro model of wound contraction. Tissue Cell 1990; 22:407–417.

46. Squier CA. The effect of stretching on formation of myofibroblasts in mouse skin. Cell Tiss Res 1981; 220:325–335.

47. Arora PD, McCulloch CAG. Dependence of collagen remodelling on α-smooth muscle actin expression by fibroblasts. J Cell Physiol 1994; 159:161–175.

48. Desmouliere A, Redard M, Darby I, et al. Apoptosis mediates the decrease in cellularity during the transition between granulation tissue and scar. Am J Pathol 1995; 146:56–66.

49. Perl M, Chung C-S, Ayala A. Apoptosis. Crit Care Med 2005; 33: S526–S529.

50. Arora PD, McCulloch CAG. The deletion of transforming growth factor-β-induced myofibroblasts depends on growth conditions and actin organization. Am J Pathol 1999; 155:2087–2099.

51. Nedelec B, Dodd CM, Scott PG, et al. Effect of interferon-α2b on guinea pig wound closure and the expression of cytoskeletal proteins in vivo. Wound Repair Regen 1998; 6:202–212.

52. Frisch SM, Francis H. Disruption of epithelial cell-matrix interactions induces apoptosis. J Cell Biol 1994; 124:619–626.

53. Zhang Z, Vuori K, Reed JC, et al. The α5β1 integrin supports survival of cells on fibronectin and up-regulates Bcl-2 expression. Proc Natl Acad Sci USA 1995; 92:6161–6165.

54. Varedi M. The effects of reorganization of cytoskeleton and matrix on gene expression, growth and apoptosis of dermal fibroblasts. Ph.D. Thesis, University of Alberta, 1997.

55. Varedi M, Tredget EE, Ghahary A, et al. Stress-relaxation and contraction of a collagen matrix induces expression of TGF-β and triggers apoptosis in dermal fibroblasts. Biochem Cell Biol 2000; 78:427–436.

56. Linge C, Richardson J, Vigor C, et al. Hypertrophic scar cells fail to undergo a form of apoptosis specific to contractile collagen — the role of tissue transglutaminase. J Invest Dermatol 2005; 125:72–82.

57. Costa AM, Peyrol S, Porto LC, et al. Mechanical forces induce scar remodeling. Study in non-pressure-treated versus pressure-treated hypertrophic scars. Am J Pathol 1999; 155:1671–1679.

58. Nedelec B, Shankowsky H, Scott PG, et al. Myofibroblasts and apoptosis in human hypertrophic scars: the effect of interferon-α2b. Surgery 2001; 130:798–808.

59. Roberts A, Sporn MB. Transforming growth factor-β. In: Clark RAF, ed. The molecular and cell biology of wound repair, 2nd edn. New York: Plenum; 1996:275–308.

60. Wakefield LM, Smith DM, Masui T, et al. Distribution and modulation of the cellular receptor for transforming growth factor-β. J Cell Biol 1987; 105:965–975.

61. Postlethwaite AE, Keski-Oja J, Moses HL, et al. Stimulation of the chemotactic migration of human fibroblasts by transforming growth factor-β. J Exp Med 1987; 165:251–256.

62. Ignotz RA, Massague J. Transforming growth factor-β stimulates the expression of fibronectin and collagen and their incorporation into the extracellular matrix. J Biol Chem 1986; 261:4337–4345.

63. Sporn MB, Roberts AB, Wakefield LM, et al. Some recent advances in the chemistry and biology of transforming growth factor-β. J Cell Biol 1987; 105:1039–1045.

64. Varga J, Rosenbloom J, Jimenez SA. Transforming growth factor β causes a persistent increase in steady state amounts of type I and type III collagen and fibronectin mRNAs in normal human dermal fibroblasts. Biochem J 1987; 247:597–604.

65. Kahari V-M, Larjava H, Uitto J. Differential regulation of extracellular matrix proteoglycan (PG) gene expression. J Biol Chem 1991; 266:10608–10615.

66. Roberts AB, Sporn MB. In: Sporn MB, Roberts AB, eds. Peptide growth factors and their receptors. New York: Springer-Verlag; 1990:421.

67. Edwards DR, Murphy G, Reynolds JJ, et al. Transforming growth factor-β stimulates the expression of collagenase and metalloproteinase inhibitor. EMBO J 1987; 6:1899–1904.

68. Overall C, Wrana, JL, Sodek J. Independent regulation of collagenase, 72 kDa progelatinase, and metalloendoproteinase inhibitor expression in human fibroblasts by transforming growth factor-β. J Biol Chem 1989; 264:1860–1869.

69. Mustoe TA, Pierce GF, Thomason A, et al. Accelerated healing of incisional wounds in rats induced by transforming growth factor-β. Science 1987; 237:1333–1336.

70. Grotendorst GR. Connective tissue growth factor: a mediator of TGF-β action on fibroblasts. Cytokine Growth Factor Rev 1997; 8:171–179.

71. Igarashi A, Nashiro K, Kikuchi K, et al. Connective tissue growth factor gene expression in tissue sections from localized scleroderma, keloid and other fibrotic skin disorders. J Invest Dermatol 1996; 106:729–733.

72. Wang R, Ghahary A, Shen Q, et al. Hypertrophic scar tissue and fibroblasts produce more TGF-β1 mRNA and protein than normal skin and cells. Wound Repair Regen 2000; 8:128–137.

73. Tredget EE, Shankowsky HA, Pannu R, et al. Transforming growth factor-β in thermally injured patients with hypertrophic scars: effects of interferon-α2b. Plast Reconstr Surg 1998; 102:1317–1328.

74. Ghahary A, Pannu R, Tredget EE. Fibrogenic and anti-fibrogenic factors in wound repair. In: Malhotra SK, ed. Advances in structural biology. London: JAI; 1996:(4)197–232.

75. Yamaguchi Y, Mann DM, Ruoslahti E. Negative regulation of transforming growth factor-β by the proteoglycan decorin. Nature 1990; 346:282–284.

76. Hausser H, Groning A, Hasilik A, et al. Selective inactivity of TGF-β/decorin complexes. FEBS Letts 1994; 353:243–245.

77. Blatti SP, Foster DN, Ranganathan G, et al. Induction of fibronectin gene transcription and mRNA is a primary response to growth-factor stimulation of AKR-2B cells. Proc Natl Acad Sci USA 1988; 85:1119–1123.

78. Edwall D, Schalling M, Jennische E, et al. Induction of insulin-like growth factor-1 messenger ribonucleic acid during regeneration of rat skeletal muscle. Endocrinology 1989; 124:820–825.

79. Ghahary A, Shen YJ, Nedelec B, et al. Enhanced expression of mRNA for insulin-like growth factor-1 in post burn hypertrophic scar tissue and its fibrogenic role by dermal fibroblasts. Mol Cell Biochem 1995; 148:25–32.

80. McCarthy TL, Centrella M, Canalis E. Regulatory effects of insulin-like growth factor I and II on bone collagen synthesis in rat calvarial cultures. Endocrinology 1989; 124:301–309.

81. Goldstein RH, Poliks CF, Pilch PF, et al. Stimulation of collagen formation by insulin and insulin-like growth factor I in cultures of human lung fibroblasts. Endocrinology 1989; 124:964–970.

82. Bird JL, Tyler JA. Dexamethasone potentiates the stimulatory effect of insulin-like growth factor-1 on collagen production in cultured human fibroblasts. J Endocrinol 1994; 142:571–579.

83. Hill DJ, Logan A, McGarry M, et al. Control of protein and matrix-molecule synthesis in isolated bovine fetal growth-plate chondrocytes by the interactions of basic fibroblast growth factor, insulin-like growth factor-I and II, insulin and transforming growth factor-β1. J Endocrinol 1992; 133:363–373.

84. Ghahary A, Shen Q, Shen YJ, et al. Induction of transforming growth factor-β1 by insulin-like growth factor-1 in dermal fibroblasts. J Cell Physiol 1998; 174:301–309.

85. Ghahary A, Shen YJ, Wang R, et al. Expression and localization of insulin-like growth factor-1 in normal and postburn hypertrophic scar tissue in human. Mol Cell Biochem 1998; 183:1–9.

86. Sen GC, Lengyel P. The interferon system. A bird's eye view of its biochemistry. J Biol Chem 1992; 267:5017–5020.

87. Harrop AR, Ghahary A, Scott PG, et al. Effect of γ-interferon on cell proliferation, collagen production and procollagen mRNA expression in hypertrophic scar fibroblasts in vitro. J Surg Res 1995; 58:471–477.

88. Tredget EE, Shen YJ, Liu G, et al. Regulation of collagen synthesis and mRNA levels in normal and hypertrophic scar fibroblasts in vitro by interferon-α2b. Wound Repair Regen 1993; 1:156–165.

89. Ghahary A, Shen YJ, Scott PG, et al. Expression of fibronectin messenger RNA in hypertrophic and normal dermis tissues and in vitro regulation by interferon-α2b. Wound Repair Regen 1993; 1:166–174.

90. Ghahary A, Shen YJ, Nedelec B, et al. Interferons γ and α2b differentially regulate the expression of collagenase and tissue inhibitor of metalloproteinase-1 messenger RNA in human hypertrophic and normal dermal fibroblasts. Wound Repair Regen 1995; 3:176–184.

91. Sahara K, Kucukcelebi A, Ko F, et al. Suppression of in vitro proliferative scar fibroblast contraction by interferon-α2b. Wound Repair Regen 1993; 1:22–27.

92. Dans MJ, Isseroff R. Inhibition of collagen lattice contraction by pentoxifylline and interferon-α, -β and -γ. J Invest Dermatol 1994; 102:118–121.

93. Nedelec B, Shen YJ, Ghahary A, et al. The effect of interferon-α2b on the expression of cytoskeletal proteins in an in vitro model of wound contraction. J Lab Clin Med 1995; 126:474–484.

94. Al-Khawajah MM. Failure of interferon-α2b in the treatment of mature keloids. Int J Dermatol 1996; 35:515–517.

95. Wong TW, Chiu HC, Yip KM. Intralesional interferon-α2b has no effect in the treatment of keloids [letter]. Br J Dermatol 1994; 130:683.

96. Nedelec B, Shankowsky H, Scott PG, et al. Myofibroblasts and apoptosis in human hypertrophic scars: the effect of interferon-α2b. Surgery 2001; 130:798–808.

97. Dao T, Ariyasu T, Holan V, et al. Natural human interferon-α augments apoptosis in activated T cell line. Cell Immunol 1994; 155:304–311.

98. Egle A, Villunger A, Kos M, et al. Modulation of Apo-1/Fas (CD95)-induced programmed cell death in myeloma cells by interferon-α2. Eur J Immunol 1996; 26:3119–3126.

99. Rodriguez-Villanueva J, McDonnell TJ. Induction of apoptotic cell death in non-melanoma skin cancer by interferon-α. Int J Cancer 1995; 61:110–114.

100. Desmouliere A, Rubbia-Brandt L, Abdiu A, et al. α-smooth muscle actin is expressed in a subpopulation of cultured and cloned fibroblasts and is modulated by γ-interferon. Exp Cell Res 1992; 201:64–73.

101. McCauley RL, Chopra V, Li Y-Y, et al. Altered cytokine production in black patients with keloids. J Clin Immunol 1992; 12: 300–308.

102. Bernabei P, Rigamonti L, Ariotti S, et al. Functional analysis of T lymphocytes infiltrating the dermis and epidermis of postburn hypertrophic scar tissues. Burns 1999; 25:43–48.

103. Linares HA. Proteoglycan–lymphocyte association in the development of hypertrophic scars. Burns 1990; 16:21–24.

104. Castagnoli C, Trombotto C, Ondei S, et al. Characterization of T-cell subsets infiltrating postburn hypertrophic scar tissues. Burns 1997; 23:565–572.

105. Mosmann TR, Coffman RL. Th 1 and Th2 cells: different patterns of lymphokine secretion lead to different functional properties. Annu Rev Immunol 1989; 7:145–173.

106. Seder RA, Marth T, Sieve MC, et al. Factors involved in the differentiation of TGF-β-producing cells from naïve CD4+ T cells: II-4 and IFN-γ have opposing effects while TGF-β positively regulates its own production. J Immunol 1998; 160:5719–5728.

107. Wynn TA, Fibrotic disease and the Th1/Th2 paradigm. Nature Rev Immunol 2004; 4:583–594.

108. Hunt JP, Hunter CT, Brownstein MR, et al. The effector component of the cytotoxic T-lymphocyte response has a biphasic pattern after burn injury. J Surg Res 1998; 80:243–251.

109. Horgan AF, Mendez MV, O'Riordain DS, et al. Altered gene transcription after burn injury results in depressed T-lymphocyte activation. Ann Surg 1994; 220:342–351.

110. O'Sullivan ST, Lederer JA, Horgan AF, et al. Major injury leads to predominance of the T helper-2 lymphocyte phenotype and diminished interleukin-12 production associated with decreased resistance to infection. Ann Surg 1995; 222:482–90.

111. Fertin C, Nicolas JF, Gillery P, et al. Interleukin-4 stimulates collagen synthesis by normal and scleroderma fibroblasts in dermal equivalents. Cell Mol Biol 1991; 37:823–829.

112. Shi Z, Wakil AE, Rockey DC. Strain-specific differences in mouse hepatic wound healing are mediated by divergent T helper cytokine responses. Proc Natl Acad Sci USA 1997; 94:10663–10668.

113. Davison SP, Mess S, Kauffman LC, et al. Ineffective treatment of keloids with interferon α2b. Plast Reconstr Surg 2006; 117:247–252.

114. Tredget EE, Wang R, Shen Q, et al. Transforming growth factor-β mRNA and protein in hypertrophic scar tissues and fibroblasts: antagonism by IFN-α and IFN-γ in vitro and in vivo. J Interferon Cytokine Res 2000; 20:143–151.

115. Tredget EE, Yang L, Delehanty M, et al. J Interferon Cytokine Res 2006; in press.

116. Bucala R, Spiegel LA, Chesney J, et al. Circulating fibrocytes define a new leukocyte subpopulation that mediates tissue repair. Mol Med 1994; 1:71–81.

117. Metz CN. Fibrocytes: a unique cell population implicated in wound healing. Cell Mol Life Sci 2003; 60:1342–1350.

118. Chesney J, Bacher M, Bender A, et al. The peripheral blood fibrocyte is a potent antigen-presenting cell capable of priming naïve T cells in situ. Proc Natl Acad Sci USA 1997; 94:6307–6312.

119. Chesney J, Metz C, Stavitsky AB, et al. Regulated production of type I collagen and inflammatory cytokines by peripheral blood fibrocytes. J Immunol 1998; 160:419–425.

120. Hartlapp I, Abe R, Saeed RW, et al. Fibrocytes induce an angiogenic phenotype in cultured endothelial cells and promote angiogenesis in vivo. FASEB J 2001; 15:2215–2224.

121. Abe R, Donnelly SC, Peng T, et al. Peripheral blood fibrocytes: differentiation pathway and migration to wound sites. J Immunol 2001; 166:7556–7562.

122. Mori L, Bellini A, Stacy MA, et al. Fibrocytes contribute to the myofibroblast population in wounded skin and originate from the bone marrow. Exp Cell Res 2005; 304:81–90.

123. Phillips RJ, Burdick MD, Hong K, et al. Circulating fibrocytes traffic to the lungs in response to CXCL12 and mediate fibrosis. J Clin Invest 2004; 114:319–321.

124. Hashimoto N, Jin H, Liu T, et al. Bone marrow-derived progenitor cells in pulmonary fibrosis. J Clin Invest 2004; 113:243–252.

125. Okada H, Kalluri R. Cellular and molecular pathways that lead to progression and regression of renal fibrogenesis. Curr Mol Med 2005; 5:467–474.

126. Yang L, Scott PG, Giuffre J, et al. Peripheral blood fibrocytes from burn patients: identification and quantification of fibrocytes in adherent cells cultured from peripheral blood mononuclear cells. Lab Invest 2002; 82:1183–1192.

127. Yang L, Scott PG, Dodd CM, et al. Identification of fibrocytes in postburn hypertrophic scar. Wound Repair Regen 2005; 13:398–404.

Chapter 48

Pathophysiology of the burn scar

Hal K. Hawkins and Clifford T. Pereira

Chapter contents

Introduction

Scarring secondary to burns leads to a multitude of adverse medical consequences including loss of function, restriction of joint mobility, restriction of growth, altered appearance and adverse psychological effects. Studies have begun to reveal the processes of intercellular communication via peptides, such as cytokines and growth factors, that initiate and regulate the process of wound healing. This chapter reviews current knowledge of the process of wound healing in humans and animals, with special emphasis on abnormal long-term responses to thermal injury.

Prehistoric and historic perspectives

Wounds due to combat, hunting injuries, accidents and thermal injuries undoubtedly were the leading causes of death in humans for millennia. On the other hand, prolonged survival of large full-thickness wounds is a recent phenomenon. Several complex biological responses to injury to the skin have evolved over time, but there has been no evolutionary pressure to evolve appropriate responses to very large wounds. There are records of human attempts to improve wound healing in the most ancient texts from Mesopotamia and Egypt. When the prophet Jeremiah asked 'Is there no balm in Gilead? Is there no physician there?' (Jeremiah 8:16, King James Bible) he bemoaned the absence of the expected skill in treatment of open wounds about 2600 years ago. Guido Majno, in his excel-

lent book 'The healing hand: man and wound in the ancient world,' has explored what can be learned from archeology and paleontology regarding wounds and their treatment in ancient times, and has even gone on to do experimental studies of the beneficial properties of substances such as honey that were widely used to treat wounds.[1] He also provided a very accurate brief description of the process of wound healing in lay terms (pp. 1–6), and this elegant overview:

> . . . long before the birth of anything that could be called experimental medicine, wounds also functioned as natural experiments, multiplied millions of times. They were treated with dressings, and in the long run the better dressings stood out. In this permanent battle between man and bacteria, it is thrilling to watch the birth of the first antiseptics . . . (preface, p. viii)

In the development of modern medicine, the advances in wound treatment advocated by Ambroise Paré (1510–1590) stand out, together with the campaign for antisepsis of Joseph Lister (1827–1912), and the development of antibiotics as well as the development of the modern methods of treatment described in this book.

Incisional wounds with primary closure

The essential components of wound healing are easily understood, and represent the simultaneous activation in the wound of tissue repair by fibroblasts and small blood vessels, and an inflammatory response initiated by vascular leakage and entry into the wound of circulating polymorphonuclear neutrophils, lymphocytes and monocytes.[2] When a sharp incision is closed while still sterile, there is only minimal vascular leakage and inflammation, and the predominant reaction to injury occurs in the fibroblasts present in the dermis and subcutaneous tissue. These resting connective tissue cells are rapidly activated to secrete collagen, which quickly bridges the small remaining gap to restore the resistance of the skin to tearing. Vascular continuity is restored by budding and remodeling of blood vessels, and the basal keratinocytes of the epidermis divide briefly to restore the complete structure of the epidermal barrier. All that remains to indicate the site of injury is a linear ribbon of dense collagen with little flexibility that marks the site of the incision, as well as some small scars that mark the sites where sutures were inserted. This process of incisional wound healing was well described in humans by Russell Ross and his colleagues in Seattle.[3,4]

Delayed wound closure by second intention and wound contraction

If the epidermis and dermis are incised or removed and the edges of the wound remain separated, inflammatory and reparative events are much more prominent. Extensive leakage of blood plasma by damaged small blood vessels maintains an outward flow that serves to keep the wound clean, but causes deposition of coagulated fibrin and other dessicated proteins on the wound surface. Conversion of fibrinogen into fibrin fills the gap in the epidermis and provides a gelatinous matrix capable of sustaining migrating cells. Thrombin stimulates expression of interleukin-6 in connective tissue cells as well as production of important cytokines by infiltrating cells.[5-7] Degranulation of platelets during the process of coagulation releases platelet-derived growth factor (PDGF), as well as several other proinflammatory cytokines.[8] Degradation of fibrin releases peptides that stimulate fibroblast proliferation and secretion and division of vascular endothelial cells, and production of cytokines by other cells.[9,10] The resting fibroblasts of the dermis, together with circulating stem cells, divide rapidly in the wound bed and secrete large quantities of collagen and proteoglycans, particularly those typically present in skin during fetal life, with predominance of type III collagen.[11,12] Simultaneously, the endothelial cells of small blood vessels proliferate rapidly and form numerous small capillary loops that extend upward toward the surface. Together, these cells form a mass of granulation tissue that covers the wound. All these activities of fibroblasts and endothelial cells are stimulated by cytokines and other peptides secreted by monocytes and lymphoid cells that infiltrate the wound bed. Certain proteins and peptides that are normally present in blood plasma also stimulate and enable formation of the wound matrix, notably fibronectin and vitronectin.[13-15] Numerous polymorphonuclear neutrophils also enter the wound bed, where they phagocytize and kill bacteria and fungi, which are always present in the outside world and gain entry to the dermis and subcutis through the open wound. Next, the fibroblasts develop interconnections among themselves and produce contractile machinery of actin and myosin within the cytoplasm of each cell.[16] Then these interconnected myofibroblasts contract to shrink the size of the open wound, pulling adjacent intact skin to cover the wound bed. This process of wound contraction is more dramatic in experimental wounds of rodents than in human wounds. The effects of wound contracture in applying tension to surrounding tissues, however, are sometimes very clear in humans as well. Simultaneously with these processes, the basal keratinocytes of the cut edges of the epidermis change to a migratory and secretory phenotype, and begin to invade the wound bed between the granulation tissue layer and the scab of dried proteins on the surface.[17] Cell division of keratinocytes occurs near the cut edge of the wound to supply cells for this migration. Once they make contact to seal the center of the wound, the migrating keratinocytes change their phenotype again and restore the normal laminated structure of the epidermis and produce a new basal lamina.[18,19] Melanocytes also seem to develop migratory properties during healing of large wounds, since they establish a degree of pigmentation in the healed wound that approximates the pigmentation of the uninjured skin. It should be noted that only the epidermis regenerates to resemble the normal structure. Hair follicles, sweat glands and other epidermal appendages do not regenerate. Thus the part of the wound that was closed by epithelial migration remains dry, hairless and flat. The restored dermis in a fully healed scar is composed of collagen type I fibers running in straight lines adjacent to one another parallel to the surface, providing good strength (though somewhat less than the native skin) but far less elasticity and flexibility than the connective tissue of the normal dermis.

The pathophysiology of burn wound healing

The biophysics of thermal injury

Cells of human skin are susceptible to killing when their temperature is increased, largely because of the sensitivity of the cell surface membrane to disruption outside fairly narrow limits of temperature. Burns also can lead to pyrolysis and disruption and oxidation of tissues. Among the various cell types present in the skin, some are likely to be more sensitive to killing by elevated temperature than others. The degree of temperature elevation at a given site in the skin also depends on the rate of heat transfer within the tissue. The thermal conductivity of the dermis is greater than that of the subcutis, since fat is a good insulator. Perhaps for this reason, thermal injury often leads to necrosis of the entire dermis with little cell death in the subcutis, as seen in wound biopsies. Hair follicles in some sites typically extend well beyond the dermis into the adipose tissue of the upper subcutis, and eccrine sweat glands are also seen in the subcutaneous fat (Figure 48.1). Despite the presence of adipose tissue around them, often hair follicles are entirely destroyed by burns even though there is little or no apparent necrosis in the upper subcutis. In the most severe burns, however, the entire subcutis may become necrotic, and cell death may occur in the underlying fascia and skeletal muscle or even in underlying internal organs.

First-degree or superficial injury of skin

Superficial burn wounds are those in which part or all of the epidermis is lost, but the epidermal basal lamina remains intact and the dermis is uninjured. In these areas, only epidermal regeneration is required, hair follicles and sweat glands remain intact, and healing can occur with little or no disfigurement.[20]

Second-degree or partial-thickness injury

In partial-thickness wounds, the entire epidermis and the upper part of the dermis become necrotic. If the wound is left intact, the presence of a large quantity of devitalized tissue requires prolonged activity of macrophages to clear the necrotic debris. Granulation tissue forms underneath the necrotic dermal tissue, and epidermal migration occurs under the eschar formed by dead tissue, leading to restoration of the epidermis, and production of dermal connective tissue in the form of a thin scar. The deep portions of the hair follicles remain viable, and the keratinocytes lining the hair follicles become migratory and undergo mitosis behind the migrating cells, eventually covering the surface with new epidermis.[17,21] In severe cases, loss of hair follicles may lead to insufficient regenerative activity to cover the surface.[22-24]

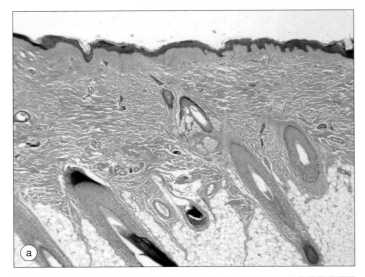

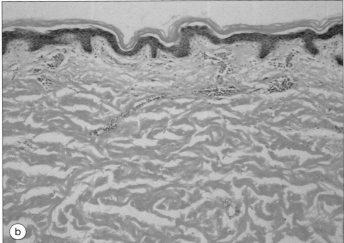

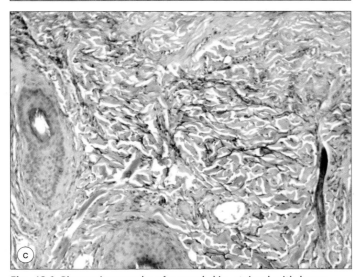

Fig. 48.1 Photomicrographs of normal skin, stained with hematoxylin and eosin. (a) The hair follicles often extend through the dermis into the subcutaneous adipose tissue. The epidermis forms irregular rete ridges at its base. (b) The reticular dermis of normal skin has an orderly arrangement of collagen fibers with no preferred orientation. (c) With the Movat pentachrome stain, normal collagen fibers stain yellow-orange, and delicate interconnecting black elastin fibers are present between collagen fibers.

Third-degree or full-thickness injury

In full-thickness burns, thermal injury extends deep enough to destroy the entire hair follicle including its root, and some of the upper subcutaneous tissue may also become necrotic. In this case regeneration of the epidermis from hair follicles is not possible, and the wound can develop an epidermal covering only slowly as the epidermis lateral to the wound spreads out over the entire wound surface.[2] During this time, the necrotic tissue in the wound bed is at risk of infection, and extensive activity of tissue macrophages is required to remove it.

Changes in vascular permeability

In order to review current understanding of the processes important in wound healing, each process will be considered separately. Changes in local blood vessels are the earliest component of the response to injury, and are essential for the succeeding steps. Plasma exudation is due in part to increased permeability of venules to proteins due to local release of substance P from local sensory nerve endings and histamine from mast cells. In burn injury, there is an added component of plasma leakage that occurs for a few hours throughout the body in response to unknown stimuli. Of course, both plasma and red blood cells enter the wound through broken or necrotic blood vessels. Infection triggers further plasma exudation by constantly stimulating and prolonging the vascular phase of acute inflammation. In addition, the newly formed capillaries of granulation tissue allow passage of plasma proteins and fluid until they mature. Certain plasma proteins, notably fibronectin and vitronectin, are important in stimulating reparative responses in the wound.

Granulation tissue and the proliferative phase of wound healing

Massive proliferation of fibroblasts and vascular endothelial cells is characteristic of the early phase of wound healing. These cells, the fine fibrils of collagen, and the gel provided by multiple mucopolysaccharides and proteoglycans, make up the granulation tissue that is a major feature of all wounds that remain open. The most important of many peptides that stimulate fibroblast growth appear to be transforming growth factor beta (TGF-β) and basic fibroblast growth factor (FGF-2), while the most important peptide that stimulates growth of endothelial cells appears to be vascular endothelial growth factor (VEGF).[25–31] In order for wound contraction to occur, it is important for fibroblasts to form networks within the dermis that allow the wound to contract. As Donald Ingber has pointed out, interactions between the extracellular matrix and the cellular cytoskeleton are important in controlling cellular differention and function.[32–34] Apparently, when wound healing is abnormal and hypertrophic scars develop, there is disruption of this process of interlinking of fibroblasts to form a meshwork that supports tension parallel to the surface, since nodules of collagen develop.

Influx of circulating inflammatory cells and stem cells

Many circulating cells actively migrate into wound beds and play important roles in defense against bacteria and fungi, clearance of devitalized tissue components, and stimulation of later phases of healing of the dermis and epidermis. Based on experiments with partially selective ablation of individual cell types, the cells most important in stimulating and maintaining tissue repair appear to be the T lymphocytes and monocytes.[35] Monocytes, which differentiate into tissue macrophages, are responsible for synthesis and release of many of the cytokines important in wound healing, together with connective tissue cells and epithelial cells. In addition, recent research has shown that circulating stem cells enter healing wounds, where they can differentiate to form fibroblasts and other connective tissue cells needed to restore tissue integrity.[36,37]

Migration of keratinocytes to cover the wound (epiboly)

When the epidermis is transected, changes take place rapidly in the basal cells of the epidermis adjacent to the wound. The signals that induce these changes are not clear and may include responses to changes in mechanical stresses. The process of epidermal regeneration has been well studied and clarified by the studies of Kenneth Stenn and his colleagues.[17,38,39] Altered basal keratinocytes send out thin sheets and undergo ameboid motion over the wound bed, but under the non-viable eschar and/or scab, secreting a provisional matrix as they go.[40,41] Development of this migratory phenotype is stimulated by the plasma protein vitronectin, and requires the presence of albumin as a cofactor.[17,39,42] Cell division occurs to support this migration, not among migratory cells, but among their precursors in the residual epidermis. Similar processes stimulate migration and replacement of epithelial cells from hair follicles in partial-thickness wounds. After a complete sheet of epithelial cells is established over the entire wound surface, the keratinocytes that previously migrated over the surface begin to divide and eventually create a multilayered stratified squamous epithelium with a granular layer and keratinization. Epidermal cells secrete substantial quantities of interleukin-1 beta (IL-1β) and other cytokines.[43,44] The new proliferative epidermal basal cells also secrete a new basal lamina composed of laminin, type IV collagen and bullous pemphigoid antigen, adhere tightly to that basal lamina, and develop attachments of type VII collagen between the basal lamina and the underlying fibers of type I collagen in the scarred dermis. Just after the newly formed epithelial layer completely covers the wound, the phenotype of the connective tissue cells in the matrix undergoes a series of changes, and much less fibronectin is found in the wound matrix.[18] The stimuli responsible for these changes in the dermal wound matrix are still unclear.

Collagen matrix formation and maturation

As shown by the work of many researchers, scars gradually increase in their strength, as measured by their resistance to tearing, but scars never reach the strength of normal dermis. During this process, the delicate fibers of newly secreted collagens I and III are replaced by large collagen I fibers that are oriented parallel to each other and the skin surface (Figure 48.2). Maturation of collagen fibers is largely a chemical process of remodeling that involves covalent crosslinking of adjacent polypeptide chains. Collagen fibers normally form and are degraded continuously in normal skin as well as in scars, but the processes that control the rates of formation and

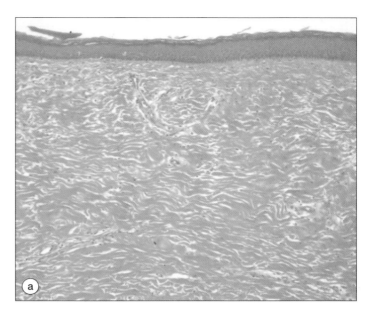

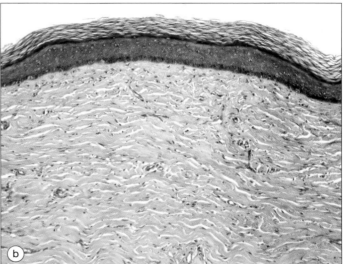

Fig. 48.2 (a) In a normal flat scar, the epidermis is flat and does not have any rete ridges, and the dermis is replaced by collagen fibers that are oriented parallel to the skin surface. (b) A Movat pentachrome stain of a normal scar shows mature collagen fibers stained yellow-orange, and does not demonstrate any elastin fibers.

degradation and the orientation of the mature fibers are not fully understood.

Cytokines and other peptides

Many short polypeptides, mostly cytokines and growth factors, are responsible for the changes in cells that lead to wound healing and the termination of wound healing processes, and the formation and organization of a scar. Among the most important are the transforming growth factor beta family (TGF-β), basic fibroblast growth factor (FGF-2), platelet-derived growth factor (PDGF), and vascular endothelial growth factor (VEGF).[45–52] Frequently, the response of a particular cell type to a particular peptide depends not only upon binding of cell surface receptors by the right peptide but also upon simultaneous signals from other cellular receptors. Thus the network of peptide signaling is complex, and the range of possible cellular responses is large enough to allow generation of complex structures with considerable fine-tuning.[48,53] There are also many opportunities for reparative processes to go wrong, to proceed in an unbalanced fashion, or to fail to complete an appropriate cycle of activation and regression.

Factors that may alter normal wound healing

Changes in blood supply and perfusion

Development of methods to study local blood supply by ultrasonic measurement has led to the discovery that there is usually a zone of greatly increased blood flow below a burn wound, which is not surprising as part of a local inflammatory response to tissue injury. Above this zone of hyperemia is a zone of tissue ischemia in which blood flow is less than normal. Remarkably, during the first 24 hours after a burn wound, the zone of ischemia typically becomes deeper, indicating that ischemic injury actually leads to an increased depth of tissue necrosis compared to that produced by the immediate thermal injury.[54] Experiments in animals have shown that neutrophils are involved in this process of ischemic injury deep to a burn wound.[55] Altered blood flow may lead to vascular thrombosis in a burn wound, also contributing to the risk of ischemic tissue injury. In normal skin, there is a plexus of arteries and veins immediately below the dermis in the upper layer of subcutaneous adipose tissue. This subdermal plexus is at risk of thrombosis in deep partial-thickness burns and in full-thickness burns, and it is vulnerable to damage in the process of tangential wound excision, with further loss of blood supply to the wound.

Compromised wound healing and requirements for optimal wound healing

Long clinical experience has demonstrated that wound healing is greatly slowed and impaired when essential ingredients for construction of the scar, or an adequate energy supply, are not available. Vitamin C deficiency and protein-calorie malnutrition are characterized by deficient wound healing, and provision of sufficient calories and reversal of the usual protein catabolism are major goals of general burn care. Diabetic vasculopathy is associated with deficient wound healing, demonstrating the importance of an adequate microcirculation. Heart failure similarly compromises wound healing. Radiation, cigarette smoking, and hypoxemia also have been associated with delayed wound healing.[54] Advanced age is associated with increased mortality from large burns, but does not in itself prevent good wound healing.[20,56]

Biological responses to wound excision and grafting

The current standard of treatment in our institution is early excision of the burn wound, normally within 24 hours of admission, with removal of all necrotic tissue, using either tangential excision to leave most of the subcutaneous fat, or fascial excision which removes the entire subcutis. The wound is initially covered with meshed cadaver skin from the skin bank. Within a few days autografting is done using meshed partial-thickness grafts from unburned regions. Over the face and the hands, unmeshed sheet autografts are often used to obtain the best cosmetic results. The epidermis of the cadaveric homograft slowly degenerates, but the dermal matrix often is incorporated into the healing wound. The interstices of the autograft fill with granulation tissue derived partly from the underlying fibrous or adipose tissue, and partly by migration of fibroblasts from the strands of autograft. The epidermis of the autograft migrates over the granulation tissue matrix and under the fibrin layer, and reconstitutes the epidermis, but without any follicles or other epidermal appendages. The pattern of the meshed grafts is usually visible in the healed wound. The incorporation of dermal connective tissue elements from the donor site may enhance the pliability of the final scar. Occasionally, epidermal inclusion cysts develop within grafted burn wounds, which may grow and rupture. These cysts could develop from residual hair roots that had lost their connection to the surface, from aberrant migration of epidermal cells during wound resurfacing, or from compression of residual hair follicles within the autograft by expanding connective tissue. Tiny bits of hair shaft are sometimes encountered in burn scars, associated with giant cell foreign body reactions, perhaps representing hairs left behind after necrosis of the hair follicles that produced them.

Wound infection

Bacterial infection frequently complicates wound healing, despite the presence of migrating neutrophils and macrophages that work to kill bacteria within the wound. The risk is increased in burn patients, since large amounts of necrotic tissue and cell debris are present in the wound, providing a good culture medium for bacteria. When infection occurs, the inflammatory component of wound healing is amplified, and the processes of conversion of granulation tissue to a dense scaffolding of collagen, wound contraction, and regeneration of the epidermis are delayed. Frequently the wound suppurates, oozing creamy yellow pus. Some bacteria cause additional tissue necrosis, and some bacteria can invade into normal tissues, leading to enlargement and deepening of the original wound. In response to the bacterial infection and the enhanced inflammatory reaction, the cytokine mileu of the wound is altered.[57-59] Grafts placed over wounds with residual infected tissue typically do not take, and when large numbers of bacteria are present deep in the wound bed there is always the hazard that the bacteria may enter the bloodstream, incite septicemia, and colonize and invade remote tissues. These processes, which were common in the era before antibiotics and before the practice of early wound excision became common, are now being seen again in cases of infection with highly antibiotic-resistant strains of bacteria, particularly *Pseudomonas* and *Acinetobacter*.

Hypertrophic scarring

Hypertrophic healing

In most patients with large burns in our institution, healing of the burn wounds is complicated in some areas by development of elevated, thick, firm, reddish scars that itch constantly. These occur more commonly in wounds that had become infected or took longer than usual to become fully covered. They may cover large areas, but generally do not extend beyond the original burn wound. These abnormal wounds also are associated with more severe wound contraction. There are often abnormalities of skin pigmentation, either depigmentation or hyperpigmentation (Figure 48.3). In the majority of affected cases, these hypertrophic scars enlarge for a period of months, then gradually regress over a period of a few years, eventually becoming flat scars with no further symptoms. Special problems associated with scars of the head and neck are discussed in Chapters 54 and 55. The largest hypertrophic scars are surgically excised, often with creation of Z-plasties or sheet grafting to release scar contractures. Usually, new hypertrophic scars do not occur after excision of the original hypertrophic scar. Many of the patients at our institution are Mexican nationals with predominantly Native American ethnicity. However, in our experience this type of hypertrophic scarring occurs in about 75% of Caucasian patients as well as in African-American and Hispanic patients.[60]

Clearly, this experience is quite different from that described in the literature with keloids, which have been described as frequently occurring spontaneously or in response to puncture wounds or clean incisions that were closed primarily.[61-63] They extend beyond the initial site of injury, respond poorly to medical therapy, persist for many years, and usually recur after surgical excision. There is often a positive family history of keloidal scarring, and keloids are 10–15 times more common in dark-skinned people of African ancestry than in northern Europeans and their descendants. Elaborate patterns of raised scars are a symbol of status in many African tribes, leading one to wonder whether this practice may have exerted selective pressure during human evolution.

Histological features of hypertrophic scars

Numerous hypertrophic scars have been examined histologically in our laboratory, including scars removed during plastic surgical procedures to release wound contractures, and also samples taken for research purposes. The abnormal elevated scars consistently show several distinct differences from uncomplicated flat scars. The most striking is the presence of rounded whorls of immature collagen that consist of delicate thin collagen fibrils, rich in type III collagen, small blood vessels, and plentiful acidic mucopolysaccharide. These nodules are often sharply demarcated from the surrounding scar tissue, which may be composed of similar material or of mature thick collagen fibers that are oriented parallel to each other and to the wound surface, typical of mature scars. Although they are clearly visible with routine H&E staining, these dermal nodules are most distinctly seen with the Movat stain, which stains mucopolysaccharides blue-green and mature collagen fibers yellow-orange (Figures 48.4 and 48.5). The nodules of hypertrophic scars vary in size from 0.5 mm to more than 1 cm in diameter, and appear to be sometimes spherical and sometimes ovoid or cylindrical in shape. The abnormal dermal tissue is very firm, almost like cartilage in its firmness and cutting properties, and may reach a thickness of several centimeters. Both normal and hypertrophic scars are characterized by lack of elastin, which is also visible using the Movat stain. However, there are often residual elastin fibers in the deepest part of the dermis below zones of

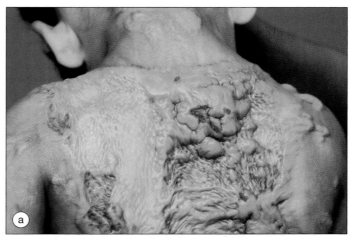

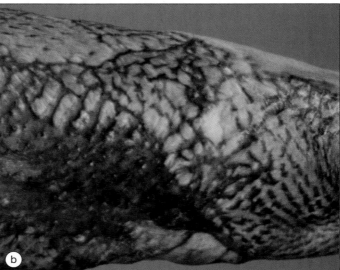

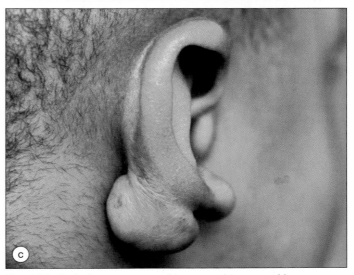

Fig. 48.3 Typical appearances of hypertrophic scars of burn patients. (a) The hypertrophic scar is raised above the surrounding normal skin, has sharp borders, and is very firm to the touch. This scar recurred after complete excision. (b) Hypertrophic scars often have patterns corresponding to meshed grafts, and often are hyperpigmented, as shown here, or hypopigmented. (c) This round firm lesion developed from a minor burn on the patient's ear. It did not recur after excision.

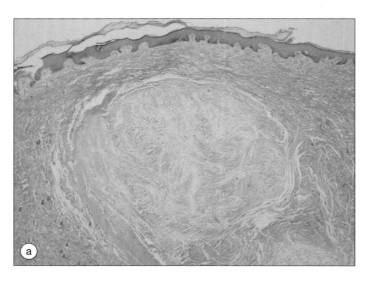

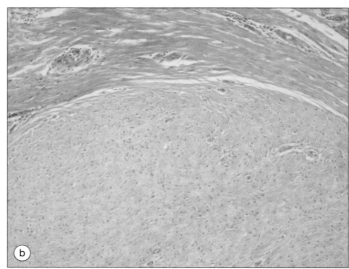

Fig. 48.4 Photomicrographs of hypertrophic scars. (a) Within the dermis there is a rounded nodule of collagen that has a sharp border and is distinct from the surrounding scar tissue. (b) The border of a collagenous nodule in a hypertrophic scar. In the surrounding scar tissue, collagen fibers are oriented parallel to the skin surface. Within the nodule, collagen fibers are very thin and are oriented circumferentially.

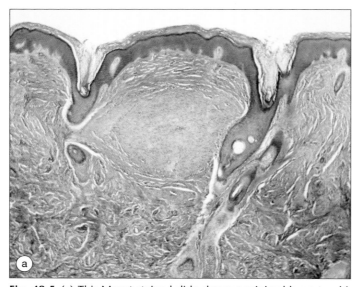

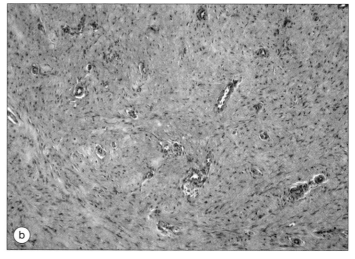

Fig. 48.5 (a) This Movat-stained slide shows a minimal hypertrophic scar consisting of a single round nodule between hair follicles. The nodule stains light green, in contrast to the yellow-orange color of the surrounding mature collagen fibers. The greenish color reflects a larger quantity of sulfated proteoglycans within the collagen nodule. (b) At higher magnification, numerous small blood vessels can be seen within a large, green-staining nodule from a hypertrophic scar.

hypertrophic scarring, and sometimes there is a narrow zone of normal elastin fibers above the hypertrophic scar, perhaps derived from the applied skin grafts. Occasionally, small rounded nodules of hypertrophic scar tissue are seen scattered between intact hair follicles (Figure 48.5a). It is not unusual to see residual eccrine sweat glands in the adipose tissue beneath a large hypertrophic scar, suggesting that hypertrophic scars may often originate in deep partial-thickness burns. In addition, in a minority of these abnormal scars, an additional histological feature is seen, consisting of very broad, hypereosinophilic collagen fibers oriented parallel to each

other, but at varying angles with the skin surface. In some cases such broad, dense fibers dominate the wound. Generally, they are surrounded by whorls of circularly oriented, immature collagen typical of hypertrophic scars (Figure 48.6). These are the features that have been described as typical of the histology of keloids. However, in our patient population, typical keloids are distinctly unusual, and there is no evidence to suggest that the patients with these thick, eosinophilic collagen fibers have a worse prognosis or a delayed course of maturation of their hypertrophic scars than other patients with abnormal scars. Thus, in our experience with the histology of

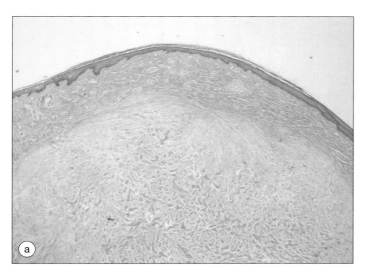
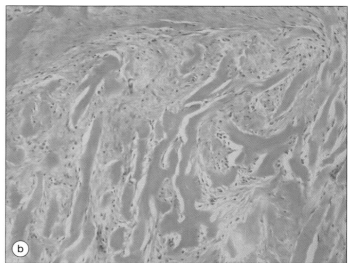

Fig. 48.6 (a) Some otherwise typical dermal nodules in hypertrophic scars contain very broad, hypereosinophilic collagen fibers similar to those typical of keloids. This specimen is from the patient shown in Figure 48.3c. (b) The typical appearance of the thick, dense collagen fibers that stain intensely with eosin can be seen at higher magnification.

scars from large burns in children, the histological features typical of keloids are seen as part of the spectrum of hypertrophic scarring.

The distinction between hypertrophic scars and keloids was first made by Mancini and Quaife in 1962, and was further described by Peacock et al. in 1970.[64,65] The thick, hypereosinophilic collagen fibers typical of keloids were first described by Blackburn and Cosman in 1966, and subsequently by Ehrlich in 1970 and many others.[66,67] The features typical of hypertrophic scars were first described by these authors and by Linares, Kischer and others.[68–71] All of these authors noted that there was considerable overlap in the histological appearances of hypertrophic scars and keloids, and no claim was made that the histological features were diagnostical. Since both hypertrophic scars and keloids represent abnormal reactions to injury in the skin, characterized by abnormal regulation of the processes involved in wound healing, it has been suggested by many authors that they might share common mechanisms, yet the groups of affected patients are quite distinct. The literature on hypertrophic scars and keloids was thoroughly reviewed in 1999 by Niessen.[72]

Multiple concepts have been proposed to explain the origin and development of hypertrophic scars and keloids. For purposes of this discussion, it may be best to assume that the etiology and pathogenesis of hypertrophic scars is different from that of keloids, and to limit our discussion to hypertrophic scars. It is sometimes difficult to be certain in reviewing the literature which findings really pertain to which group, since the clinical characteristics of the patients who were the sources of the experimental material are often not given in detail. At this institution, our experience is much more extensive with hypertrophic scarring than with keloids.

A number of differences have been described between normal scars and hypertrophic scars. Hypertrophic scars contain more type III collagen, more fibronectin, and more hyaluronic acid, all characteristic of the early phases of wound repair, than normal flat scars. They appear more vascular, and studies of cutaneous blood flow by Doppler sonography have shown consistently higher flows in hypertrophic scars. Hypertrophic scars contain significantly more T cells and macrophages than normal scars. Larger numbers of mast cells have been found in hypertrophic scars, and indeed a clinical history of atopy and higher levels of circulating IgE have been found in patients with hypertrophic scars. Recently, larger numbers of epidermal Langerhans cells have been identified in association with hypertrophic scars.[73,74]

Immunohistochemical staining has demonstrated additional striking differences between hypertrophic scars and normal scars. Staining for α-smooth-muscle actin has consistently demonstrated this contractile protein within fibrocytic cells in the characteristic collagen nodules of hypertrophic scars. The sulfated proteoglycans of hypertrophic scars are quite different from those of normal scars, in that much less decorin is present, and versican is predominant in the rounded nodules. More immunostaining for VEGF is seen in hypertrophic scars. Larger numbers of small nerve fibers have been identified by immunostaining in hypertrophic scars. Recently, studies have been done in which bone marrow-derived stem cells have been identified in fibroblasts and other tissue components of healing wounds in animals. Thus far, these stem cells have not been described in human hypertrophic scars. These findings may provide important clues as to the pathogenesis of hypertrophic scarring, but at this time they are difficult to incorporate into a single hypothesis. Study of the biology of hypertrophic scars has been complicated by the lack of a suitable animal model, and by the scarcity of relevant material from human scars, as well as by confusion as to the proper identification of cases of hypertrophic scarring. However, study of cell culture models has yielded important information on biological processes that may be important in human hypertrophic scars, and potential animal models are being developed.

Experimental models of hypertrophic healing

The first animal model of keloids was described in 1959, based on immunization of experimental animals with autologous skin, followed by induction of wounds.[75] Extensive work has been done with implantation of human scar tissue into the athymic nude mouse, a model that allows testing of potential therapies and modification of the biological mileu *in vivo*.[76–79] It is even possible to irradiate the mouse and transplant human bone marrow to study interactions between immune reactions involving human cells and the human skin grafts. Adult horses have been described as having abnormal wounds clinically similar to hypertrophic scars, but these lack the typical histological features of hypertrophic scars in humans. Recently, Engrav and his colleagues in Seattle have developed a model in the female red Duroc pig that seems to mimic most of the features of human hypertrophic scarring.[80–83] It will be of great interest to test interventions that might modify the development of hypertrophic scars in that model.

Phenotypic abnormalities of hypertrophic scars

There have been many studies of the functions and molecular biology of fibroblasts derived from hypertrophic scars and keloids in tissue culture. It does appear from these studies that there is a significantly different phenotype of fibroblasts from hypertrophic scars that persists in culture. Hypertrophic scar fibroblasts have been found to secrete collagen more rapidly than fibroblasts derived from normal skin or normal mature scars. More secretion of TGF-β has also been described.[84] Several groups have described abnormal control of proliferation, collagen secretion or peptide secretion in fibroblasts derived from keloids in response to cytokine stimulation or treatment with glucocorticoids. However, in most of these studies the regulatory responses of hypertrophic scar fibroblasts were similar to those of fibroblasts from normal skin.

The reduction in cellularity that accompanies the conversion of granulation tissue into scar tissue during normal wound healing is due to apoptosis (programmed cell death). Studies have demonstrated that the advancing edge of epithelium induces apoptosis in fibroblasts and other inflammatory cells by an as yet unknown signal.[84] Even the epithelium of a graft or flap used to cover wounds acts similarly.[85] Hence the presence of excessive myofibroblasts in postburn hypertrophic scars may indicate a delay or reduction in the normal onset of apoptosis. This delay has been reflected in the differential expression of apoptosis-modulating proteins, i.e. an increase in antiapoptotic proteins such as bcl-2 and c-jun and absence of antiproliferative proteins such as p53.[86]

Genotypic abnormalities of hypertrophic scars

DNA microarray technology has enabled us to look more broadly at patterns of gene expression and to explore relationships in gene expression in hypertrophic scars.[87,88] Preliminary results from these studies suggest that there may be common patterns of gene expression in hypertrophic scars compared with normal skin. Forty-four genes were found to be overexpressed and 124 were underexpressed in a study of hypertrophic scars compared with normal scars.[87] Some notable genes that have consistently shown more than 2-fold increases in gene expression in hypertrophic scars include collagen types

X and XVI, thrombospondin-4 and matrix metalloproteinase 16 (MMP-16). In a recent study from our institution, cultured fibroblasts from hypertrophic scars showed a greatly reduced response to IL-6 compared to fibroblasts from adjacent normal skin, suggesting that decreased receptor activation might be a factor in hypertrophic scarring.[89] Better appreciation of altered patterns of gene expression in hypertrophic scars could lead to better delineation of its causes, and help to develop future therapy directed at specific gene targets.

Possible implications for future modes of therapy

Our ability to control hypertrophic scar formation is limited, and no available therapy has been consistently effective. Therapeutic induction of apoptosis is currently being researched as an antifibrogenic therapy for rheumatoid arthritis and lung fibrosis, and might find a place in treatment of hypertrophic scarring. Apoptotic agents such as bcl-2, FLIP, recombinant TRAIL, FasL and C2-Ceramide are now in or on the brink of human clinical trials,[90] and could be utilized in postburn hypertrophic scar modulation. Recent developments in wound healing research are beginning to unveil the mechanisms behind fetal scarless wound healing. In fetal wound healing there are prominent differences in cytokine profile, specially that of transforming growth factor beta (TGF-β). This cytokine has three isoforms, TGF-β1, TGF-β2 and TGF-β3. While TGF-β1 and TGF-β2 have been shown to produce fibrotic scarring, TGF-β3 has been shown to produce scarless healing.[91] Thus manipulating the level of cytokines at the time of injury or immediately after injury could affect the type of scar formation. This could be achieved using any of several techniques, including application of recombinant proteins or neutralizing antibodies or transient gene therapy.

Pathogenic concepts and gaps in knowledge

Understanding of the biology of hypertrophic scarring has been hampered by multiple factors, including problems in gaining consensus on the definition of the lesion and the lack of a suitable animal model. As a consequence, it has not been possible to test hypotheses by altering the course of the disease. Multiple concepts of pathogenesis have been proposed. None has yet gained wide acceptance, and none has been experimentally excluded. It does seem clear that development of a hypertrophic scar represents an abnormality in control of the normal processes of wound healing. The abnormality may occur early, as Dr Linares suggested, or late.[60] The normal processes that limit collagen secretion and begin to restore a connective tissue matrix apparently fail in hypertrophic scars. One might suppose that the normal processes by which tensions in the matrix signal cellular responses have become defective in hypertrophic scars.[32,34] Myofibroblasts are more prominent in hypertrophic scars than in normal or mature scars, and they are thought to play an important role in excessive wound contraction. These myofibroblasts may derive from resting dermal fibroblasts, or they might arise from pre-existing pericytes, as suggested by Kischer.[92] They also might represent bone marrow-derived fibrocytes in increased numbers.[37] The fibrous nodules of hypertrophic scars might represent persistence and uncontrolled growth of a separate population of connective tissue cells, perhaps related to the perifollicular cells that normally express versican. Since burn patients have higher circulating levels of glucocorticoids and interleukin-6 than normal individuals, a selection process might operate that would tend to allow proliferation of cells resistant to the usual effects of these agents to suppress fibroblast proliferation. A recent suggestion was made that less vitamin D_3 is made in patients with strongly pigmented skin.[93] Finally, abnormal macromolecular expression by the covering epithelium may lead to abnormal development of the dermal scar, or fail to suppress inappropriate fibroblast functions.[94] Clearly, it continues to be important to develop and test many hypotheses until the problem of hypertrophic scarring is finally solved.

Summary

Healing of burn wounds requires activation of several host processes, including fibrin clotting and lysis, deposition of an immature connective tissue matrix and its reorganization into a mature scar, and epithelial outgrowth and interaction between the epidermis and the dermal matrix. In many burn patients, excessive scar tissue forms, with adverse consequences. Continued study of this problem will continue to be important until more effective modes of treatment are developed.

References

1. Majno G. The healing hand — man and wound in the ancient world. Cambridge: Harvard University Press; 1975.
2. Clark RA. Basics of cutaneous wound repair. J Dermatol Surg Oncol 1993; 19:693–706.
3. Ross R. Wound healing. Sci Am 1969; 220:40–50.
4. Ross R, Odland G. Human wound repair. II. Inflammatory cells, epithelial–mesenchymal interrelations, and fibrogenesis. J Cell Biol 1968; 39:152–168.
5. Sower LE, Froelich CJ, Carney DH, et al. Thrombin induces IL-6 production in fibroblasts and epithelial cells. Evidence for the involvement of the seven-transmembrane domain (STD) receptor for alpha-thrombin. J Immunol 1995; 155:895–901.
6. Naldini A, Pucci A, Carney DH, et al. Thrombin enhancement of interleukin-1 expression in mononuclear cells: involvement of proteinase-activated receptor-1. Cytokine 2002; 20:191–199.
7. Naldini A, Carney DH, Bocci V, et al. Thrombin enhances T cell proliferative responses and cytokine production. Cell Immunol 1993; 147:367–377.
8. Ross R, Bowen-Pope DF, Raines EW. Platelet-derived growth factor: its potential roles in wound healing, atherosclerosis, neoplasia, and growth and development. Ciba Found Symp 1985; 116:98–112.
9. Lorenzet R, Sobel JH, Bini A, et al. Low molecular weight fibrinogen degradation products stimulate the release of growth factors from endothelial cells. Thromb Haemost 1992; 68:357–363.
10. Drew AF, Liu H, Davidson JM, et al. Wound-healing defects in mice lacking fibrinogen. Blood 2001; 97:3691–3698.
11. Clark RA. Biology of dermal wound repair. Dermatol Clin 1993; 11:647–666.
12. Clark RA. Fibrin and wound healing. Ann NY Acad Sci 2001; 936:355–367.
13. Grinnell F. Fibronectin and wound healing. Am J Dermatopathol 1982; 4:185–188.
14. Greiling D, Clark RA. Fibronectin provides a conduit for fibroblast transmigration from collagenous stroma into fibrin clot provisional matrix. J Cell Sci 1997; 110(Pt 7):861–870.
15. Swerlick RA, Brown EJ, Xu J, et al. Expression and modulation of the vitronectin receptor on human dermal microvascular endothelial cells. J Invest Dermatol 1992; 99:715–722.
16. Gabbiani G, Ryan GD, Majno G. Presence of modified fibroblasts in granulation tissue and their possible role in wound contraction. Experientia 1971; 27:549–550.
17. Stenn KS, Depalma L. Re-epithelialization. In: Clark RAF, ed. The molecular and cellular biology of wound repair. New York: Plenum; 1996:321–335.
18. Clark RA. Fibronectin matrix deposition and fibronectin receptor expression in healing and normal skin. J Invest Dermatol 1990; 94:128S–134S.
19. Staiano-Coico L, Carano K, Allan VM, et al. PAI-1 gene expression is growth state-regulated in cultured human epidermal keratinocytes during progression to confluence and postwounding. Exp Cell Res 1996; 227:123–134.
20. Gamelli RL, He LK. Incisional wound healing. Model and analysis of wound breaking strength. Methods Mol Med 2003; 78:37–54.
21. Daly TJ. The repair phase of wound healing — re-epithelialization and contraction. In: Kloth LC, McCullough J, Feedar JA, eds. Wound healing. Philadelphia: FA Davis; 1990:14–30.
22. Barret JP, Dziewulski P, Wolf SE, et al. Outcome of scalp donor sites in 450 consecutive pediatric burn patients. Plast Reconstr Surg 1999; 103:1139–1142.
23. Chang LY, Yang JY, Chuang SS, et al. Use of the scalp as a donor site for large burn wound coverage: review of 150 patients. World J Surg 1998; 22:296–299.
24. McCauley RL, Oliphant JR, Robson MC. Tissue expansion in the correction of burn alopecia: classification and methods of correction. Ann Plast Surg 1990; 25:103–115.
25. Schultz GS, Rotatori DS, Clark W. EGF and TGF-alpha in wound healing and repair. J Cell Biochem 1991; 45:346–352.
26. Spindler KP, Murray MM, Detwiler KB, et al. The biomechanical response to doses of TGF-beta 2 in the healing rabbit medial collateral ligament. J Orthop Res 2003; 21:245–249.
27. Broadley KN, Aquino AM, Hicks B, et al. Growth factors bFGF and TGF beta accelerate the rate of wound repair in normal and in diabetic rats. Int J Tissue React 1988; 10:345–353.
28. Bennett NT, Schultz GS. Growth factors and wound healing: Part II. Role in normal and chronic wound healing. Am J Surg 1993; 166:74–81.
29. Broadley KN, Aquino AM, Woodward SC, et al. Monospecific antibodies implicate basic fibroblast growth factor in normal wound repair. Lab Invest 1989; 61:571–575.
30. Davidson JM, Broadley KN. Manipulation of the wound-healing process with basic fibroblast growth factor. Ann NY Acad Sci 1991; 638:306–315.
31. Falanga V. Growth factors and wound healing. J Dermatol Surg Oncol 1993; 19:711–714.
32. Ingber DE. Cellular tensegrity: defining new rules of biological design that govern the cytoskeleton. J Cell Sci 1993; 104:613–627.
33. Ingber DE. Mechanical control of tissue growth: function follows form. Proc Natl Acad Sci USA 2005; 102:11571–11572.
34. Huang S, Ingber DE. The structural and mechanical complexity of cell-growth control. Nat Cell Biol 1999; 1:E131–E138.
35. Barbul A, Breslin RJ, Woodyard JP, et al. The effect of in vivo T helper and T suppressor lymphocyte depletion on wound healing. Ann Surg 1989; 209:479–483.
36. Quan TE, Cowper S, Wu SP, et al. Circulating fibrocytes: collagen-secreting cells of the peripheral blood. Int J Biochem Cell Biol 2004; 36:598–606.
37. Mori L, Bellini A, Stacey MA, et al. Fibrocytes contribute to the myofibroblast population in wounded skin and originate from the bone marrow. Exp Cell Res 2005; 304:81–90.
38. Stenn KS. The role of serum in the epithelial outgrowth of mouse skin explants. Br J Dermatol 1978; 98:411–416.

39. Stenn KS. Epibolin: a protein of human plasma that supports epithelial cell movement. Proc Natl Acad Sci USA 1981; 78:6907–6911.

40. Kubo M, Van de WL, Plantefaber LC, et al. Fibrinogen and fibrin are anti-adhesive for keratinocytes: a mechanism for fibrin eschar slough during wound repair. J Invest Dermatol 2001; 117:1369–1381.

41. Stenn KS, Madri JA, Roll FJ. Migrating epidermis produces AB2 collagen and requires continued collagen synthesis for movement. Nature 1979; 277:229–232.

42. Stenn KS. Coepibolin, the activity of human serum that enhances the cell spreading properties of epibolin, associates with albumin. J Invest Dermatol 1987; 89:59–63.

43. Qwarnstrom EE, Jarvelainen HT, Kinsella MG, et al. Interleukin-1β regulation of fibroblast proteoglycan synthesis involves a decrease in versican steady state mRNA levels. Biochem J 1993; 294:613–620.

44. Niessen FB, Andriessen MP, Schalkwijk J, et al. Keratinocyte-derived growth factors play a role in the formation of hypertrophic scars. J Pathol 2001; 194:207–216.

45. Karr BP, Bubak PJ, Sprugel KH, et al. Platelet-derived growth factor and wound contraction in the rat. J Surg Res 1995; 59:739–742.

46. Savage K, Siebert E, Swann D. The effect of platelet-derived growth factor on cell division and glycosaminoglycan synthesis by human skin and scar fibroblasts. J Invest Dermatol 1987; 89:93–99.

47. Tredget EE. Pathophysiology and treatment of fibroproliferative disorders following thermal injury. Ann NY Acad Sci 1999; 888:165–182.

48. Scott PG, Ghahary A, Tredget EE. Molecular and cellular aspects of fibrosis following thermal injury. Hand Clin 2000; 16:271–287.

49. Tran KT, Griffith L, Wells A. Extracellular matrix signaling through growth factor receptors during wound healing. Wound Repair Regen 2004; 12:262–268.

50. Younai S, Venters G, Vu S, et al. Role of growth factors in scar contraction: an in vitro analysis. Ann Plast Surg 1996; 36:495–501.

51. Tonnesen MG, Feng X, Clark RA. Angiogenesis in wound healing. J Invest Dermatol Symp Proc 2000; 5:40–46.

52. Grinnell F. Fibroblasts, myofibroblasts, and wound contraction. J Cell Biol 1994; 124:401–404.

53. Roberts AB. The ever-increasing complexity of TGF-beta signaling. Cytokine Growth Factor Rev 2002; 13:3–5.

54. Burns JL, Mancoll JS, Phillips LG. Impairments to wound healing. Clin Plast Surg 2003; 30:47–56.

55. Mileski WJ, Borgstrom D, Lightfoot E, et al. Inhibition of leukocyte-endothelial adherence following thermal injury. J Surg Res 1992; 52:334–339.

56. Ono I. The effects of basic fibroblast growth factor (bFGF) on the breaking strength of acute incisional wounds. J Dermatol Sci 2002; 29:104–113.

57. Hunt TK, Hopf H, Hussain Z. Physiology of wound healing. Adv Skin Wound Care 2000; 13:6–11.

58. Thornton FJ, Schaffer MR, Barbul A. Wound healing in sepsis and trauma. Shock 1997; 8:391–401.

59. van den Boom R, Wilmink JM, O'Kane S, et al. Transforming growth factor-beta levels during second-intention healing are related to the different course of wound contraction in horses and ponies. Wound Repair Regen 2002; 10:188–194.

60. Linares HA, Larson DL. Early differential diagnosis between hypertrophic and nonhypertrophic healing. J Invest Dermatol 1974; 62, 514–516. Abstract.

61. Burd A, Huang L. Hypertrophic response and keloid diathesis: two very different forms of scar. Plast Reconstr Surg 2005; 116:150e–157e.

62. Ketchum LD, Cohen IK, Masters FW. Hypertrophic scars and keloids. A collective review. Plast Reconstr Surg 1974; 53: 140–154.

63. Murray JC, Pollack SV, Pinnell SR. Keloids: a review. J Am Acad Dermatol 1981; 4:461–470.

64. Mancini RE, Quaife JV. Histogenesis of experimentally produced keloids. J Invest Dermatol 1962; 38:143–181.

65. Peacock EE Jr, Madden JW, Trier WC. Biologic basis for the treatment of keloids and hypertrophic scars. South Med J 1970; 63:755–760.

66. Blackburn WR, Cosman B. Histologic basis of keloid and hypertrophic scar differentiation. Arch Pathol 1966; 82:65–71.

67. Ehrlich HP, Desmouliere A, Diegelmann RF, et al. Morphological and immunochemical differences between keloid and hypertrophic scar. Am J Pathol 1994; 145:105–113.

68. Linares HA, Kischer CW, Dobrkosky M, et al. On the origin of the hypertrophic scar. J Trauma 1973; 13:70–75.

69. Linares HA, Kischer CW, Dobrkosky M, et al. The histiotypic organization of the hypertrophic scar in humans. J Invest Dermatol 1972; 59:323–331.

70. Kischer CW. Collagen and dermal patterns in the hypertrophic scar. Anat Rec 1974; 179:137–145.

71. Kischer CW, Shetlar MR, Chvapil M. Hypertrophic scars and keloids: a review and new concept concerning their origin. Scan Electron Microsc 1982:1699–1713.

72. Niessen FB, Spauwen PH, Schalkwijk J, et al. On the nature of hypertrophic scars and keloids: a review. Plast Reconstr Surg 1999; 104:1435–1458.

73. Niessen FB, Schalkwijk J, Vos H, et al. Hypertrophic scar formation is associated with an increased number of epidermal Langerhans cells. J Pathol 2004; 202:121–129.

74. Cracco C, Stella M, Alasia ST, et al. Comparative study of Langerhans cells in normal and pathological human scars. II. Hypertrophic scars. Eur J Histochem 1992; 36:53–65.

75. Chytilova M, Kulhankek V, Horn V. Experimental production of keloids after immunization with autologous skin. Acta Chir Plast 1959; 1:72–79.

76. Shetlar MR, Shetlar CL, Hendricks L, et al. The use of athymic nude mice for the study of human keloids. Proc Soc Exp Biol Med 1985; 179:549–552.

77. Kischer CW, Sheridan D, Pindur J. Use of nude (athymic) mice for the study of hypertrophic scars and keloids: vascular continuity between mouse and implants. Anat Rec 1989; 225:189–196.

78. Kischer CW, Pindur J, Shetlar MR, et al. Implants of hypertrophic scars and keloids into the nude (athymic) mouse: viability and morphology. J Trauma 1989; 29:672–677.

79. Barbul A, Shawe T, Rotter SM, et al. Wound healing in nude mice: a study on the regulatory role of lymphocytes in fibroplasia. Surgery 1989; 105:764–769.

80. Zhu KQ, Engrav LH, Armendariz R, et al. Changes in VEGF and nitric oxide after deep dermal injury in the female, red Duroc pig-further similarities between female, Duroc scar and human hypertrophic scar. Burns 2005; 31:5–10.

81. Zhu KQ, Engrav LH, Tamura RN, et al. Further similarities between cutaneous scarring in the female, red Duroc pig and human hypertrophic scarring. Burns 2004; 30:518–530.

82. Liang Z, Engrav LH, Muangman P, et al. Nerve quantification in female red Duroc pig (FRDP) scar compared to human hypertrophic scar. Burns 2004; 30:57–64.

83. Zhu KQ, Engrav LH, Gibran NS, et al. The female, red Duroc pig as an animal model of hypertrophic scarring and the potential role of the cones of skin. Burns 2003; 29:649–664.

84. Brown DL, Kao WW, Greenhalgh DG. Apoptosis down-regulates inflammation under the advancing epithelial wound edge: delayed patterns in diabetes and improvement with topical growth factors. Surgery 1997; 121:372–380.

85. Garbin S, Pittet B, Montandon D, et al. Covering by a flap induces apoptosis of granulation tissue myofibroblasts and vascular cells. Wound Repair Regen 1996; 4:244–251.

86. Wassermann RJ, Polo M, Smith P, et al. Differential production of apoptosis-modulating proteins in patients with hypertrophic burn scar. J Surg Res 1998; 75:74–80.

87. Tsou R, Cole JK, Nathens AB, et al. Analysis of hypertrophic and normal scar gene expression with cDNA microarrays. J Burn Care Rehabil 2000; 21:541–550.

88. Paddock HN, Schultz GS, Baker HV, et al. Analysis of gene expression patterns in human postburn hypertrophic scars. J Burn Care Rehabil 2003; 24:371–377.

89. Dasu MR, Hawkins HK, Barrow RE, et al. Gene expression profiles from hypertrophic scar fibroblasts before and after IL-6 stimulation. J Pathol 2004; 202:476–485.

90. Nicholson DW. From bench to clinic with apoptosis-based therapeutic agents. Nature 2000; 407:810–816.

91. Ferguson MW, O'Kane S. Scar-free healing: from embryonic mechanisms to adult therapeutic intervention. Philos Trans R Soc Lond B Biol Sci 2004; 359:839–850.

92. Kischer CW, Thies AC, Chvapil M. Perivascular myofibroblasts and microvascular occlusion in hypertrophic scars and keloids. Hum Pathol 1982; 13:819–824.

93. Cooke GL, Chien A, Brodsky A, et al. Incidence of hypertrophic scars among African Americans linked to vitamin D-3 metabolism? J Natl Med Assoc 2005; 97:1004–1009.

94. Andriessen MP, Niessen FB, Van de Kerkhof PC, et al. Hypertrophic scarring is associated with epidermal abnormalities: an immunohistochemical study. J Pathol 1998; 186:192–200.

Chapter 49

Comprehensive rehabilitation of the burn patient

Michael A. Serghiou, Sheila Ott, Scott Farmer, Dan Morgan, Pam Gibson and Oscar E. Suman

Chapter contents

With severe burn injuries, as perhaps with any other order of trauma, there is an urgent need for immediate and aggressive initiation of patient-specific rehabilitation programs. The distribution and depth of the burn clearly predict the patterns of deformity and joint contractures and mandate the establishment of therapeutic goals and the initiation of treatment as soon as possible. The more extensive the burn is, the greater the rehabilitation challenge becomes. A seriously burned extremity in an otherwise modestly burned patient is much easier to restore to function than an extremity similarly burned in a patient with full-thickness burns involving multiple sites. Among seriously burned patients, the immediate and primary focus will always be preservation of life and wound coverage. Basic treatment priorities, however, do not preclude the development and implementation of an aggressive rehabilitation program.

The short-term rehabilitation goal is to preserve the patient's range of motion and functional ability. Long-term rehabilitation goals include the return of the patient to independent living and to train patients on how to compensate for any functional loss suffered as a result of the burn.

This chapter addresses positioning, splinting, casting, skeletal suspension, traction, prosthetics and orthotics, scar management, exercise, performance of activities of daily living (ADL) and patient and caregiver education utilized in burn rehabilitation along the continuum of care.

Positioning and splinting of the burned patient for the prevention of contractures and deformities

Positioning of the burned patient is vital in bringing about the best functional outcomes in burn rehabilitation. Positioning programs should begin immediately upon admission to the burn center and continue throughout the rehabilitative process. The role of the burn therapist is invaluable in designing a positioning program, which counteracts all contractile forces without compromising function. In planning and implementing an effective patient-specific positioning program the therapist should be aware of the patient's total body surface area (TBSA) of burns, the depth of all injuries, respiratory status and associated injuries such as exposed tendons/joints or fractures. Individualized positioning programs are monitored closely for any necessary adjustments depending on the patient's medical status. The quote that 'the position of comfort is the position of deformity' applies to every burned patient who sustained a serious injury.

Anti-deformity positioning can be achieved through multiple means. Splinting, mechanical traction, cut out foam troughs and mattresses, pillows, strapping mechanisms, serial casting and in some cases through surgical application of pins. The burn therapist needs to be aware of physician-specific protocols and work closely with the entire burn team to design the most effective positioning program. Orthotics and splinting devices are vital in burn rehabilitation as they are utilized extensively to obtain appropriate positioning of the entire body and to counteract the contractile forces that lead to deformity. No matter how the burn therapist approaches splinting (material choice, design, and application schedules) the goal is to achieve the best functional outcome at the completion of rehabilitation. When fabricating a splint or an orthosis the burn therapist must be aware of the anatomy and kinesiology of the body surface to be splinted. Also, the therapist should be well aware of all mechanical principles of splinting as they relate to pressure, mechanical advantage, torque, rotational forces, first-class levers, friction, reciprocal parallel forces and material strength.[1]

Positioning and splinting must be designed in a way to:
- Allow for edema reduction.
- Maintain joint alignment.
- Support, protect and immobilize joints.
- Maintain and/or increase range of motion.
- Maintain tissues elongated.
- Remodel joint and tendon adhesions.
- Promote wound healing.
- Relieve pressure points.
- Protect newly operated sites (grafts/flaps).
- Stabilize and/or position one or more joints, enabling other joints to function correctly.
- Assist weak muscles to counteract the effects of gravity and assist in functional activity.
- Strengthen weak muscles by exercising against springs or rubber bands.[1]

All devices should:
- Not cause pain.
- Be designed with function in mind.
- Be cosmetically appealing.
- Be easy to apply and remove.
- Be lightweight and low profile.
- Be constructed out of appropriate materials.
- Allow for ventilation in preventing skin/wound maceration.[1]

Head

In aiding with facial edema reduction, the head may be positioned by elevating the head of the bed at 30–45° if the patient's hips are not involved. In cases where the hips are burned the entire bed may be elevated at the head of the bed with the use of shock blocks (wooden blocks 12–16 inches high with recessed slots for bed legs). This will avoid positioning the hips in the flexion contracture position (Figure 49.1). In the cases where the ears are burned they may be protected from wrapping on pillows with ear cups made of thermoplastic materials or foam.[2] An ear conformer may be constructed to prevent the rim of the ear from contracting toward the head. Internal ear canal splints may also be fabricated and serially adjusted as the circumference of the canal increases. A nasal obturator may be required to maintain the nostrils open. These obturators may be serially adjusted as the circumference of the nostril increases. Mouth splints are utilized for the prevention of oral microstomia. These devices are custom-made by the therapist or they may be obtained commercially. Mouth splints may be fabricated static or dynamic for the horizontal or vertical opening of the mouth.[3–6] In cases of severe microstomia where compliance is an issue, an orthodontic commissure appliance which attaches to the teeth may be fabricated by an orthodontist.[7] The use of stacked tongue blades is an acceptable technique to aid in reversing oral microstomia. Ongoing research looks at the development of a microstomia device that circumferentially opens the mouth according to its anatomy (Figure 49.2). Facial scar hypertrophy may require fabricating a high thermoplastic transparent mask such as the Uvex™ and W-clear™ masks or a silicone elastomer face mask.[8–10] A semi-rigid low thermoplastic opaque

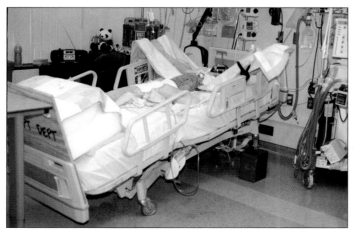

Fig. 49.1 Wooden blocks are utilized to place the bed on an incline to help with edema reduction and prevent hip contractures.

mask may also be fabricated depending on the state of scar maturation.

Neck

The neck is positioned in neutral or in slight extension of approximately 15° without any rotation. The amount of neck extension must not be so great that traction on the chin causes the mouth to open. Positioning may be achieved with a short mattress supine, a rolled towel or foam cushion placed behind the upper back on the scapular line. Pillows should be avoided in the cases of anterior neck burns as they may lead to flexion contractures. In the case of anterior neck burns a conforming custom thermoplastic collar may be fabricated (Figure 49.3).[11] A soft neck collar or a Watusi-type collar may also be fabricated.[10,12,13] It has been observed that in some cases acute patients rotate or laterally flex their neck on one side, which may lead to a lateral neck contracture (torticollis). If the patient is to remain in bed for a while, a dynamic head strap mechanism may be fabricated to counteract the lateral neck contractile forces and bring the neck in the neutral position. For the prevention of torticollis the therapist may fabricate a lateral neck splint which conforms to the head of the patient, the lateral neck and anterior/posterior shoulder (Figure 49.4).

Spine

Contracture resulting from unilateral or asymmetric burns of the neck, axilla, trunk and groin will cause lateral curvature of the spine (scoliosis). The level and amplitude of curvature will vary with the site and severity of the contracture. In addition, pelvic obliquity accompanying asymmetric hip or knee flexion contracture will impose a lateral lumbar curve. As long as the patient is recumbent, lateral curvature can be prevented by maintaining straight alignment of the trunk and neck (Figure 49.5). However, the curve is often insidious in onset and will not be recognized until the patient begins to walk. Trunk list observed early in the ambulation period can be simply a transient accommodation to pain and wound tightness, but a persistent list may herald the development of scoliosis. Other subtle signs of spinal curvature are asymmetry of shoulder levels, scapular asymmetry, asymmetry of dependent upper extremity alignment to the trunk and asymmetry of pelvic rim levels. Once there is an established asymmetric contracture it is difficult by therapeutic means to stretch it out, so it is probably better to deal surgically with a deforming scar early than to permit even minor scoliosis to persist.

Exaggerated thoracic kyphosis secondary to anterior chest and neck burn is difficult to prevent because the recumbent position cradles the back and encourages protraction of the scapulae. The two-plane contracture extending from chin and neck to thorax and from shoulder to shoulder anteriorly pulls the chin down, flexes the neck and pulls the scapulae forward. Protraction of the scapulae alone may cause a normal thoracic kyphosis to appear to be exaggerated. However, if the protraction posture is not corrected, it tends to become habitual, and the final result features a prominent and rounded thoracic spine (Figure 49.6). As this spinal deformity in its genesis is linked to neck and shoulder contractures, the measures for its prevention and correction are discussed in the section dealing with neck and shoulders.

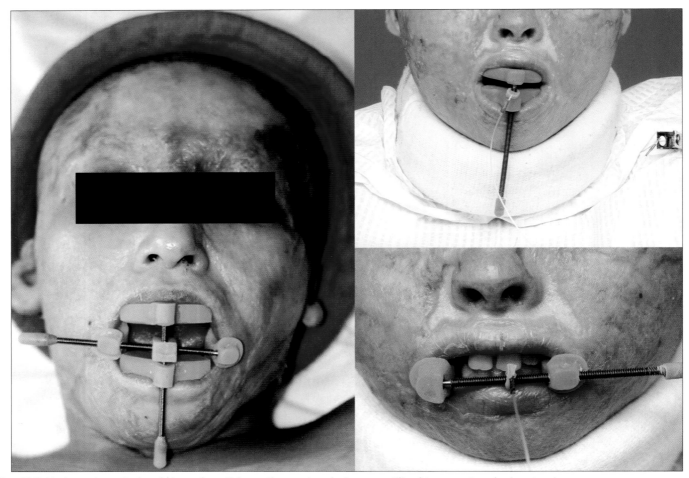

Fig. 49.2 Horizontal, vertical and circumferential mouth-opening devices are utilized to correct oral microstomia.

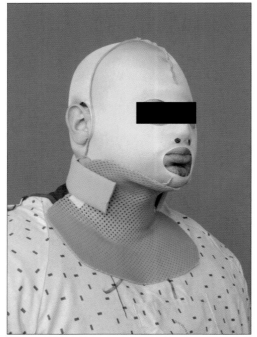

Fig. 49.3 An anterior neck conformer helps prevent neck flexion contractures.

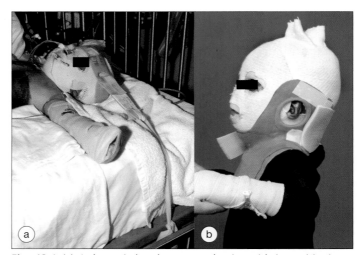

Fig. 49.4 (a) A dynamic head strap mechanism aids in positioning the neck in neutral position during a prolonged ICU bed confinement. (b) A lateral neck splint is utilized to prevent lateral neck flexion contractures (torticollis).

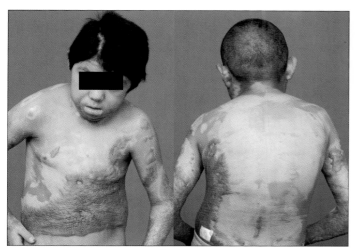

Fig. 49.5 Scoliosis resulting from a left chest, abdomen and left lateral trunk injury.

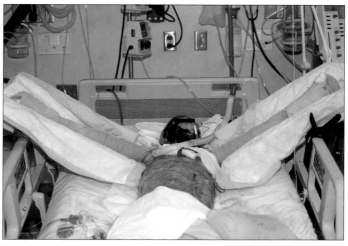

Fig. 49.7 Foam arm troughs are utilized for positioning the shoulders in bed.

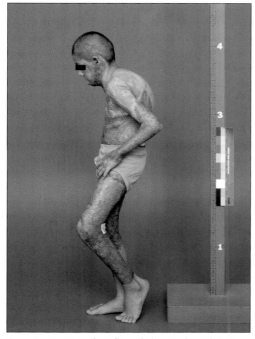

Fig. 49.6 Scar contracture has flexed the neck and protracted the scapulae. A full-thickness injury to the anterior neck, chest and shoulders resulted in thoracic kyphosis due to a neck flexion contracture, and scapular protraction.

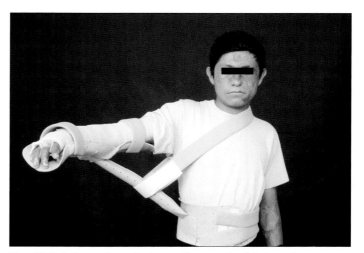

Fig. 49.8 A three-piece airplane splint may be fabricated to accommodate wound dressings and promote healing while maintaining the shoulder abducted.

Exaggeration of spinal lumbar lordosis is rarely related to overlying burn of the back. On the other hand, full-thickness burns of the abdomen are occasionally deep enough to compromise or even eliminate abdominal muscle function. In this circumstance the pelvis, for lack of support of anterior motors, will roll forward and lumbar lordosis will increase. The hamstring and gluteus maximus muscles, though strong posterior stabilizers of the pelvis, cannot compensate for loss of abdominal muscle power. If all abdominal muscles are lost, viscera will protrude, shifting the center of gravity forward. To compensate and achieve balance the patient must lean backwards, further increasing the lumbar lordosis. There is no way to prevent this sequence if abdominal muscle function is lost and, since surgical correction often is not practical, the only treatment recourse may be sturdy external abdominal support to relieve the burden of protruding viscera.

Shoulder girdle/axilla

Elevation of the arms should be in the corono-sagittal plane with the glenoid humeral joint at approximately 15–20° of horizontal flexion. Abduction in the coronal plane places the glenohumeral joint in relative extension and uncovers the head of the humerus, rendering it more prone to anterior subluxation if the position is chronically maintained. Also, abduction in the coronal plane may cause excessive tension to the brachial plexus over time, resulting in a neuropathy such as radial nerve palsy. Positioning may be achieved with splints, pillows, bedside tables, foam arm troughs and thermoplastic slings suspended from an overhead trapeze mechanism (Figure 49.7). Airplane splints are custom fabricated or obtained commercially for the prevention of axillary contractures. To accommodate wound dressings and promote healing, a three-piece airplane splint may be fabricated (Figure 49.8). This splint positions the patient's arm in abduction by connecting the elbow and the lateral trunk troughs with a thermoplastic custom-made rod. Commercially available airplane splints come equipped with a mechanism that allows for adjustments depending on available shoulder abduction ranges.[10,11,13] A figure-of-eight axillary wrap may be fabricated during the rehabilitative phase of recovery to provide pressure and stretch the axillary skin surfaces (Figure 49.9).

Elbow/forearm

Severe burns involving the elbow may result in flexion contracture and threaten posterior exposure of the joint. Full extension is the protecting position for the elbow. If the joint is exposed posteriorly, extension may need to be rigidly maintained for several weeks. If the joint is not exposed, mobilization into increasing flexion range can begin very soon after the burn. The elbow is integral to the so-called delivery system for the hand, and elbow range to full or near-full flexion is more important for overall function than range to full or near-full extension.

Radial head rotation for pronation and supination is less often affected by the burn injury than flexion and extension. The pronators and supinators are frequently injured in electrical accidents where bone, being a poor conductor, heats destroying the muscles closest to it. Forearm rotation is essential for accurate hand placement and the rehabilitative program must seriously address that function. Depending on the location and severity of the injury the forearm may be positioned in neutral or in slight supination. Static elbow splints may be soft or custom-fabricated of thermoplastic materials. An anterior elbow conformer may be fabricated over the burn dressing or a 3-point elbow extension splint which avoids contact with wounds or fresh grafts/flaps may be constructed. Dynamic elbow extension or flexion splints may be utilized to provide prolonged gentle sustained stretch and aid in the correction of contractures.[14] Forearm dynamic pronation/supination splints may be custom-fabricated or obtained commercially for the correction of contractures.[10,11,13]

Wrist/hand

The usual posture of the unsupported burned hand is wrist flexion, metacarpophalangeal (MCP) extension, interphalangeal (IP) flexion and first metacarpal extension and adduction. MCP extension is imposed to some degree by dorsal swelling of the hand and the overall posture may be the position of greatest comfort. If the hand rests unsupported on the bed, all features of the deformity may be positionally reinforced with the first metacarpal being pushed farther into extension and adduction. The overall appearance is that of an intrinsic minus or claw deformity (Figure 49.10).

If, in the acute burn phase, the wrist is securely supported in extension, the metacarpophalangeal joints of digits 2 through 5 will tend to fall into flexion because of gravity if the forearm is pronated or the hand elevated and because of the reciprocal tendering action between digital flexors and extensors. The first metacarpal will likewise fall forward into flexion. Wrist extension is, thus, basic to control of hand and digit position and to prevention of hand and wrist deformity.

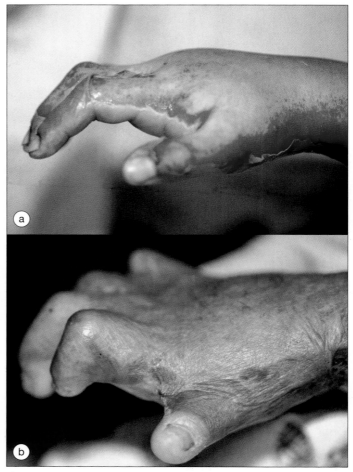

Fig. 49.10 (a) Edema following a full-thickness burn of the dorsum of the hand — imposed metacarpophalangeal extension and interphalangeal flexion. (b) The deformity resulting from the persistence of this position is that of a claw hand.

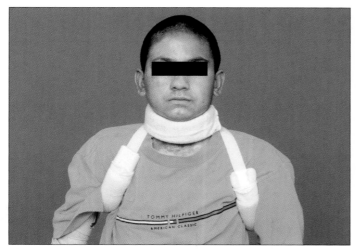

Fig. 49.9 A figure-of-eight axillary wrap provides a constant stretch of the axillary skin surfaces.

Among the digits, the second and fifth most easily drift into MCP extension because each has a proper extensor and has relative functional freedom from the third and fourth digits. The fifth is occasionally pulled into extreme abduction and extension by scar contracture. The thumb may become similarly displaced and to a lesser degree the index finger. The severe displacement of these digits gives a grotesque, but characteristic deformity (Figure 49.11).

For adults, adolescents and older children preventive static positioning with a custom thermoplastic splint can be relatively efficient. There are, however, two common faults in custom splints that are designed to gain MCP flexion and to position the thumb in flexion and abduction. If the transverse fold of the splint is not proximal to the MCP joints of digits 2 through 5, the splint will impede rather than favor MCP flexion. If the thumb component of the splint applies volar rather than medial pressure the MCP joint will extend and the metacarpal will become correspondingly more adducted. The first MCP joint should be maintained in slight flexion and pressure from the splint should be applied just to the medial surface of the digit. Any degree of first metacarpal adduction contracture increases the likelihood that the proximal phalanx will be pushed into hyperextension and eventually into subluxation by the splint. The optimal position for the burned hand and wrist includes 0–15° wrist extension, 50–70° MCP joint flexion and neutral IP joint position. The thumb should be positioned in a combination of palmar and radial abduction with the first MCP joint slightly flexed as mentioned above. This positioning, which resembles the intrinsic plus position of the hand, is achieved through a burn hand splint fabricated by the therapist (Figure 49.12). Superficial hand burns should not be splinted in order to allow for frequent movement and the freedom to function independently. In the case of circumferential hand burns, a hand extension splint may also be fabricated to prevent flexion contractures and cupping of the palm. The flexion and extension splints are alternated depending on the burn center's protocols. A 'sandwich' hand splint may be fabricated which includes the volar burn hand splint with a dorsal platform over the IP joints in order to prevent flexion

of the digits. The splint may be secured with an elastic bandage or with Velcro® strapping (Figure 49.13).[15] Individual static finger splints may include a gutter splint for the prevention of flexion contractures or a boutonnière deformity, a thumb c-bar for the prevention of syndactyly in the first web space, a figure-of-eight digit splint for the prevention/correction of swan neck deformity and a distal IP joint extension splint for the prevention of mallet finger deformity. Dynamic splinting of the hand may include MCP extension or flexion splints, proximal/distal IP flexion or extension splints, thumb outriggers, digital knuckle benders or flexion/extension spring-loaded splints (Figure 49.14). The therapist must monitor dynamic splinting closely and make frequent adjustments to the outriggers in maintaining a 90° angle of pull at all times. Wrist splints may be fabricated dorsally, volarly or in the cases of a deviation contracture they may be constructed on the medial or lateral aspect of the joint. The therapist should design these splints having in mind the importance of the wrist

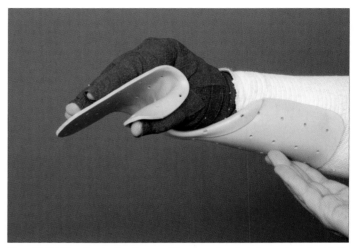

Fig. 49.12 The intrinsic plus position hand splint (burn hand splint) positions the hand appropriately to prevent contractures and preserve function.

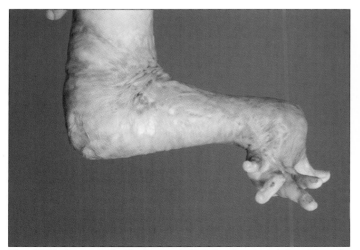

Fig. 49.11 Severe wrist flexion and digital extension deformities of the right upper extremity.

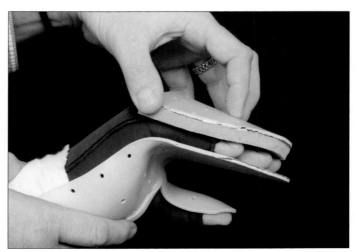

Fig. 49.13 The 'sandwich' hand splint prevents PIP flexion contractures.

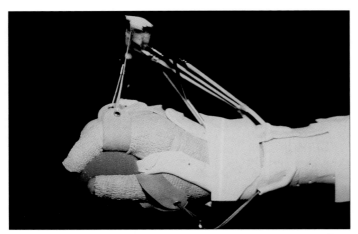

Fig. 49.14 A dynamic MCP extension splint promotes functional use of the hand.

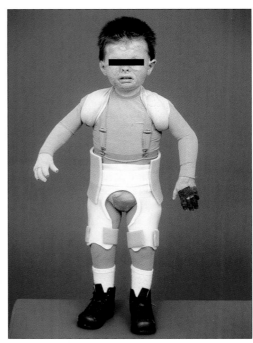

Fig. 49.15 An anterior hip spica splint is utilized to prevent anterior hip flexion contractures.

joint in the performance of activities of daily living. A dynamic wrist splint may be utilized which provides a prolonged stretch in counteracting any contractile forces. In treating the edematous hand, it is important to position the hand above the heart level at all times, to aid edema reduction. Elevation should not compromise the vascular supply to the hand.[10,11,13]

Hip

When anterior burns extend from the abdomen to the thigh, hip flexion is the position of comfort. If the hip is fixed in any degree of flexion, posture will be modified. Bilateral symmetric contractures impose increased lumbar lordosis or knee flexion or both. Asymmetric contracture will cause pelvic obliquity and scoliosis. In adults and older children thighs are more likely to be held in adduction than in abduction, whereas in pre-ambulatory infants the secondary component of the contracture is abduction. Thus, for the hips the preventive position is full extension, 0° rotation and symmetric abduction of 15–20°. If elevation of the upper body is needed for edema reduction then the entire frame of the bed is elevated with the use of wooden shock blocks placed at the head of the bed. Soft mattresses should be avoided as they may promote hip flexion. Hip positioning is accomplished with the use of abduction pillows and other strapping mechanisms eliminating hip rotation. If the patient wears bilateral foot splints then connector bars may be utilized on the splints to bring about the desired bilateral hip positioning stated above. Hip flexion contractures may be serially corrected with an anterior hip spica or with a 3-point hip extension splint (Figure 49.15).[10,11,13] Subtle hip flexion contractures can be easily overlooked when the patient stands, there being only a slight increase in lumbar lordosis or forward or lateral shift of the trunk. If established hip flexion contractures are not surgically corrected, body posture is likely to be permanently altered with scoliosis or exaggerated lordosis.

Knee

Burn injury to the anterior or posterior surface of the lower extremity that crosses over the knee joint may result in knee flexion. Deep anterior burns may expose the joint, occasionally destroying the patellar tendon. Deep posterior burns result in bridging scar formation. The appropriate position for the knee is full extension to be maintained by splint or skeletal traction until there is efficient quadriceps function and the patient is ambulatory. Thereafter, night splints must be used until scar contracture is no longer a threat. Knee splints may include a posterior custom-made thermoplastic knee conformer or a soft knee immobilizer.

Persisting bilateral knee flexion contractures will impose hip flexion. Persisting unilateral contractures may impose pelvic obliquity and scoliosis. As with the hip, posture alteration may be so subtle as to be overlooked. Correction of even a slight contracture should be a surgical priority as should elimination of a soft bridging scar band that does not prevent complete willful knee extension but causes the patient habitually to hold the knee in slight flexion.

Foot/ankle

Ankle equinus is the most frequently occurring deformity involving the foot. Initially it is related more to gravity and failure to support the foot at neutral at the talotibial joint than to the early effect of the burn. Loss of deep and superficial peroneal nerve function will compound the problem by encouraging the foot to drift into inversion as well as equinus because of loss of dorsiflexion and eversion motors. In the end, the total deformity for the unsupported foot may be ankle equinus, hind-foot inversion, and forefoot varus and equinus. Ankle equinus quickly becomes a resistant deformity so that within a few days or even hours the foot can no longer be positioned at 90° of dorsiflexion in the neutral ankle position. Eventually the contractures of scar, muscle and capsular structures combine to fix the deformity.

Equinus deformity and the attending inversion and forefoot varus can be prevented by accurate and unyielding support of the foot in neutral alignment or slight dorsiflexion. If the patient must be nursed prone, the feet must be allowed to fall free from the mattress. Static splinting if not performed correctly by an experienced therapist is often unsuccessful because of the patient's desire and tendency to plantarflex strongly, displacing the splint and leading to ulcers of the heel, malleoli, toes and where the splint edges touch the skin. A stable footboard may be effective if the feet are kept securely and totally against it. For large burns and particularly for circumferential burns of the lower extremities, skeletal suspension incorporating calcaneal traction will support the foot at neutral if the traction pin is placed in the calcaneus well behind the axis of ankle motion. A balanced traction system demands that the knees be supported in flexion with tibial pins at the level of the tibial tubercle. Calcaneal pins will not prevent forefoot equinus. If traction must be employed for several weeks, proximal pull dorsal pins in the first or first and second metatarsals may be required for support of the forefoot. Transmetatarsal pins are useful as well when calcaneal traction alone is not sufficient to correct equinus.

Minor established equinus deformity can be corrected with a standing and walking program. At the outset graduated heel lifts may be used to accommodate to the deformity. If the patient must be bed confined, skeletal traction through the calcaneus may be the quickest and most efficient way to correct the deformity. Traction is effective even if scar contracture contributes to the deformity. Serial corrective casts or posterior splints alone are useful mainly for minor contractures. For the treatment of circumferential foot/ankle burns anterior foot splints are also fabricated and their application is alternated with the posterior foot splints in preventing plantar or dorsal foot contractures.[10,11,13] The Multi Podus® System foot splints may be utilized for the positioning of the burn foot/ankle as they relieve heel pressure in preventing pressure ulcers (Figure 49.16). For fixed, unyielding deformity, scar release combined with tendoachillis lengthening with or without posterior capsulotomy is a standard surgical procedure that yields inconsistent results. The correction achieved is often just to neutral or to slight dorsiflexion. The Ilizarov technique has been used

with generally satisfactory immediate results in severe cases.[16] No matter how correction is achieved, if there are no dorsiflexion motors and if the range of ankle motion is only a few degrees, ankle fusion may in the end yield the best functional result.

The most common intrinsic deformity of the foot is extreme extension of the toes due to dorsal scar contracture. This deformity is insidious in onset and is difficult to prevent as there is no type of non-skeletal splinting that will hold the toes flexed. In its extreme, the deformity includes dorsal metatarsophalangeal (MTP) subluxation which may involve one or all toes depending on the location of the scar. The metatarsal heads become prominent on the plantar surface and walking may be painful. Correction of the deformity requires dorsal surgical release of the contracture, manual correction of the deformity and in severe cases intrinsic or extrinsic pinning of the digit or digits in an overcorrected position, i.e. MTP and interphalangeal flexion. The deformity will commonly if not inevitably recur to some degree unless the patient, after the operation, is able to achieve in all digits active MTP flexion.

Dorsal scar contractures extending from leg to foot to toes may pull the foot into marked inversion if the scar is medial or into eversion if the scar is lateral. The fifth and first toes may be separately displaced by the same scar bands. These contractures must always be surgically corrected. Their persistence will lead to bone deformity in a growing child and will permanently adversely affect foot and ankle function. Even slight inversion, whether imposed by scar contracture or motor weakness, will increase pressure on the lateral border of the foot, leading to callous formation and a painful inefficient gait. Occasionally, the base of the fifth metatarsal is so offensive as to require partial surgical osteotomy.

When there is both anterior and posterior scar contracture, the talus will remain aligned with the calcaneus in a relatively plantar flexed position as the midfoot and forefoot are pulled into dorsiflexion. The result is so-called rocker bottom foot with the head of the talus being the principal weight-bearing feature. This deformity once established defies correction by usual surgical means because of the shortage of soft tissue and because vessels and nerves cannot be stretched to accommodate to the corrected position. The Ilizarov technique may offer a partial solution to the problem. Removal of the head of the talus may give a reasonable weight-bearing surface. With chronic painful ulceration, amputation is the best treatment.[16]

A Unna boot may be applied at time of skin grafting to the lower extremity and contribute to early patient ambulation. The Unna boot is a bandage impregnated with calamine lotion and zinc oxide which, when applied over the grafted lower extremity (6 layers), hardens to a semi-rigid dressing resembling a plaster cast. This cast-like total contact dressing provides uniform support to the fresh skin graft and when reinforced with a thermoplastic or plaster splint is facilitates early ambulation. A Unna boot may be applied for up to 7 days post grafting although it could be removed earlier for the inspection of the skin graft. If removed, a new Unna boot needs to be fabricated depending on the burn center's lower extremity postoperative immobilization protocol.[17]

Typical burn care positioning protocols describe the supine position in great detail. More emphasis is now being placed on

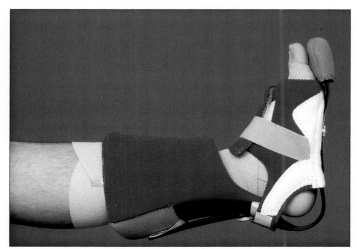

Fig. 49.16 The Multi Podus splint is utilized to position the burned feet appropriately and prevent heel and malleoli skin breakdown.

the use of side-lying and prone positioning for patients with large burns who must be immobilized for extended periods of time due to newer grafting techniques that cover larger areas with fragile skin substitutes. When designing a program for these patients the traditional joint angles are maintained, and the supporting surfaces are modified to maximize surface area while protecting bony prominences.

Side-lying may be used on a rotating basis for patients at risk for sacral or scapular skin breakdown. In a preventive program, the rotation is right side to supine to left side. The order is then reversed on a 1- to 2-hour schedule. Full side-lying at 90° from supine should not be allowed for any significant length of time due to excessive pressure over the greater trochanter. A more appropriate position for side-lying is approximately 30–40° from the supine position, which distributes pressure more evenly between the head of the femur and the lateral portion of the sacrum.

The mechanics of a side-lying position can be accomplished using pillows or wedges made of foam or wood. Pillows are typically used to prop up a patient in side-lying and require direct handling of the patient. The advantage of foam or wooden wedges is that they can be placed directly under the mattress with less manipulation of the patient. As the rotation schedule is completed the wedge can either be removed for the supine position or transferred to the opposite side of the mattress to achieve side-lying on the opposite surface.

Prone positioning systems are usually the position of last resort (Figure 49.17). They are reserved for patients who are not successfully being managed in supine or side-lying. There may be non-healing grafts or wounds in the rectal region that increase the risk of sepsis due to the introduction of fecal matter. Other common candidates for this protocol include those with sacral pressure ulcers or posterior trunk grafts that are not healing.

There are a host of issues that must be considered when instituting a prone program. Airway is always the first issue that must be considered when designing a prone positioning mattress. The supporting surface is cut from a solid open-cell foam mattress that is placed on a wire mesh bed frame. Airway concerns are addressed first and the patient is evaluated for mode of respiration. Nasal and tracheal intubation are issues

to consider, but are not contraindications for the prone position. A trough should be provided so that direct access can be obtained for routine airway care and if breaths are needed using an Ambu-bag. If the airway becomes compromised the prone position should be abandoned immediately until proper respiration is established.

The facial opening should be cut in a manner that maximizes weight distribution without allowing the head to enter into the opening. Using this protocol places direct weight-bearing pressure on the brow ridge, zygomatic arches, and the anterior mandible. These structures should be monitored closely and the patient should be educated that breakdown is likely to occur due to the limited subcutaneous tissue protecting the face. If burn scars are encroaching on the eyelids then the corneas should be evaluated as well. Corneal abrasion can be avoided with due diligence and prevention of the foam from contacting the unprotected eye. Countersinking a gel cushion into the upper portion of the foam mattress can protect the forehead and brow-ridge.

The sternum, pelvic region, and patellae are protected with the use of an air-cell mattress that is inserted into the mattress in a length-wise manner. The air-cell segments are typically supplied in standard lengths and may not reach from the sternum to the ankles. If there is an unsupported area between the distal portion of the air-cell mattress and the dorsum of the foot, then the area can be supported with open cell egg-crate type foam. The feet are supported at the distal end of the mattress with a foam footboard. Extra precautions should be taken to evaluate the elevation of the great toe from the supporting bed frame.

In the prone position all of the traditional joint alignment suggestions are maintained with the possible exception of the elbows. Shoulder mobility dictates the style of mattress that can be made for the individual burn patient. If the patient has greater than 115° of abduction, then the mattress is modified to horizontally adduct and externally rotate the shoulder while flexing the elbow to allow for elevation of the hands. This minimizes edema in the hands and allows for greater function once the prone position is no longer needed. If the shoulders have limited abduction then a 'butterfly' cut is used to allow for horizontal adduction of the shoulder to protect the brachial plexus with the hands remaining slightly dependent. This will result in some hand edema, which can be addressed with pressure wrapping (Coban™ glove) and active exercise.

Serial casting

Serial casting is frequently utilized in burn rehabilitation for the correction of significant contractures. Joints with over 30° of contracture respond well to casting. The applied cast provides total contact with circumferential and evenly distributed pressure. The prolonged gentle sustained stretch provided by the cast aids in tissue elongation without causing microtrauma to the surfaces targeted for the correction of contractures (Figure 49.18). Casting is a relatively simple, fast and painless intervention and provides an alternative to dynamic splinting when patient compliance is an issue (i.e. pediatrics).

Plaster casting bandages come in different widths and may also be cut in strips by the therapist prior to casting a patient. Plaster casts are inexpensive, lightweight, easy to fabricate and allow for ventilation down to the skin surface (plaster is porous when cured), thus avoiding skin/wound maceration.

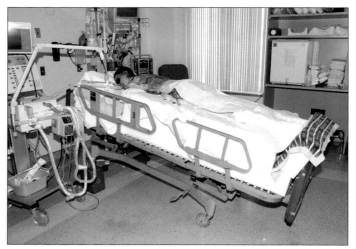

Fig. 49.17 Patients may be positioned in prone in order to protect posterior grafts from shearing.

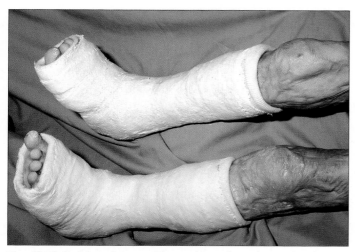

Fig. 49.18 Serial casting provides prolonged gentle sustained stretch and aids in tissue elongation and correction of contractures without pain.

Plaster is fast setting when reacting with warm water. Disadvantages of this technique include the decreased water resistance of plaster and breakage if not constructed strongly enough to withstand the patient's own muscle strength.

Fiberglass casts are an alternative technique to plaster casts. Fiberglass bandages are fast setting when reacting with water, they are lightweight and the casts are stronger (mostly preferred for lower extremity walking casts). Because of fiberglass's abrasive properties, therapists must wear gloves prior to handling it.

Recently, non-latex polyester materials such as Delta-Cast™ are utilized as alternatives to plaster and fiberglass. These materials, which resemble fiberglass, are very lightweight, flexible and because of their elastic properties they conform very well. They may be univalve so they can be applied and removed for cleaning and exercise.[18]

A light dressing and padding on the bony prominences should be applied prior to either casting technique. Prior to casting the therapist should consider therapeutic heat, massage and stretching of the joints about to receive a cast. When casting is completed the patient should feel a gentle but not painful stretch. The first cast should be removed at approximately 24 hours and thereafter depending on the patient's tolerance it could be applied up to a week at a time. In cases of casting over wounds the cast should be removed at 1–2 days in order to avoid complications in wound healing.[19,20]

Skeletal suspension and traction

Skeletal suspension and traction systems have been used to a limited extent in burn management for a number of years. The early reports of Larson[21] and Evans[22–24] described the use of skeletal suspension for positioning and for extremity elevation for open wound management and of skeletal traction for prevention and correction of contractures. The later reports of Harnar[25] and Youel[26] deal mainly with the management of hand burns with the skeletally anchored digital traction splints bearing the names banjo, halo, and hay rake (Figure 49.19).

The adaptation of skeletal suspension and traction systems to burn management grew out of earlier experience with traction to correct the elbow and knee contractures of patients

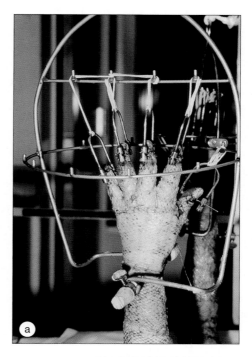

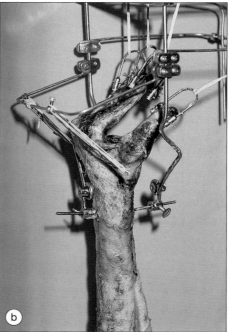

Fig. 49.19 (a) Banjo external fixator. (b) Functional position external fixator.

with rheumatoid disease and of traction and suspension as definitive means for treating certain extremity fractures. In its earliest application to burn management, skeletal suspension was used for extremity elevation only to facilitate wound care. From this experience evolved better-defined traction systems, including those expressly designed for hands and feet. Rehabilitation therapists may remove the patient from the traction apparatus as indicated for exercises and ambulation and reapply the traction at the completion of treatment. Positioning within the traction is often changed by nurses and therapists by altering the amount of the traction weights, thus preventing the affected joints from being locked into one position over time (Figure 49.20).

In the suspension mode for both upper and lower extremities, distal weight is such as to maintain desired position of the extremity when the patient is asleep or inactive, but is not so great as to prevent active motion or functional exercise. In the traction mode, weight must be sufficient for constant uniform pull to correct a contracture or to maintain surgically gained positioning. With lower extremity suspension or traction, a proximal tibial pin is always required to control rotation of the extremity and to prevent hyperextension of the knee. In the management of a patient with extensive burns, lower extremity weights for the proximal tibia and calcaneus can be alternately increased or decreased to favor flexion or extension of the knee. In the upper extremity, elbow flexion can be gained just by decreasing the distal weight. Occasionally when there is an elbow extension contracture, it is necessary to insert an olecranon pin for traction to gain elbow flexion.

Prosthetic and orthotic intervention

The prosthetist's role

To date, little has been published regarding prosthetics relating to thermal injury, yet patients with burn injuries can present interesting problems which are simultaneously the same as with other patients and yet unique. Patients who have suffered severe burns have complex, long-term problems and considerable self-care to provide. The challenge to the orthotist and prosthetist is to design a device which is maximally useful to a patient who may have multiple limitations. To be useful, a device must be as easy to use as possible. Simplicity often determines whether the device is successful or discarded by a patient.

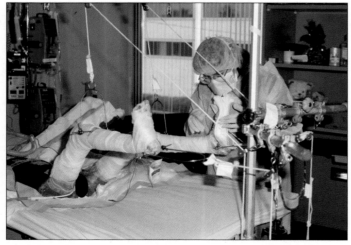

Fig. 49.20 Skeletal traction is utilized for positioning of extensive burns and for the protection of delicate grafts through suspension. Rehabilitation therapists may remove the traction and ambulate or exercise patients as needed. Traction weights may be changed to achieve different positions within the traction system and help shift the weight of patients in bed.

Planning for function

Prosthetic rehabilitation begins with surgery and progresses to splinting, exercise therapy, preparatory, and then definitive prosthetics. Surgeons performing amputations must be familiar with optimal levels for function and growth. Consultation with rehabilitation team members prior to surgery regarding the planned surgical level, weight-bearing areas and alternatives can provide useful information in providing a patient with optimum function while using a prosthesis.

Additional multiple involvement

Many burned patients have severe limitations in the function of intact extremities which affect their ability to utilize a prosthesis. Their limitations and strengths are important considerations when planning treatment. For example, functional status has been improved in patients with considerable knee instability secondary to burn trauma by performing transtibial rather than above-knee amputation, stabilizing the knee with prosthetic components, and allowing knee stability to improve over time with the formation of scar tissue. Salvaging part of the forearm where there is an active elbow flexor and no extensor, or even extremely limited range of motion, can provide increased function both with and without a prosthesis compared to a higher amputation level with better skin coverage. Limited function of the contralateral extremity, especially the hand, will affect decisions regarding amputation, amputation level, and reconstructive surgery. Severely burned patients may need to use their remaining functioning extremities differently than patients without total body involvement. Prosthetic rehabilitation should enhance adaptations.

Prosthetic components

Standard prosthetic texts are useful in providing broad basic information and explanation of the many components available and their use.[27,28] Components for various regions are described below.

Hand

Improved techniques of plastic surgery of the partial hand have greatly reduced the need for partial hand prostheses other than those for cosmesis. On the other hand, opposition posts can be useful for patients awaiting further surgical improvement.

Transradial

- Wrist flexion units, especially when there is contralateral upper extremity involvement.
- Distal cushions in below-elbow sockets.
- Padding — which can be attached to a harness ring so as to distribute pressure from straps.
- Rapid adjust buckles for donning and doffing for patients with limited range of motion at the glenohumeral joint.
- Cross-chest straps for patients with protracted scapulae and/or scarring and poor definition in the deltopectoral area.
- Utilization of 'preflexion' of the forearm relative to the socket or wrist flexion units at the mid forearm to compensate for limited range of motion (Figure 49.21).
- Transhumeral and shoulder level.

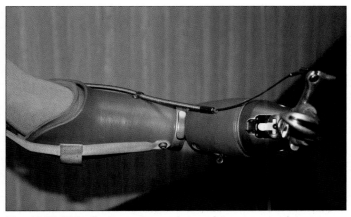

Fig. 49.21 Wrist flexion units can be used to accommodate upper extremity range of motion limitations. The prostheses can provide wrist flexion and rotation. A secondary flexion unit can be applied at mid forearm for increased flexion.

- A flexible thermoplastic inner socket provides reduction in shear stress at trim lines and enhanced adjustability and socket replacement.
- For extremely short transhumeral and shoulder level cases, chest expansion is rarely useful for activating the elbow lock. Other means, such as attaching the elbow lock cable to a waistband, may be necessary.
- Electronics have been used rarely due to physiological and environmental factors.

Lower extremity

Choice of prosthetic components for the lower extremity is based on a patient's functional ability and physiology pertaining to the maintenance of skin integrity. When these criteria are satisfied, cosmesis is addressed. Severely burned patients may exhibit muscle weakness not usually seen at the same amputation levels in the non-burn patient. These should be noted and compensation such as increasing stability of a prosthetic knee through alignment or components should be provided.

Transtibial

Proximal weight-bearing components, such as knee joints/thigh lacer or ischial-gluteal weight-bearing brims can be helpful with patients who have problems tolerating full weight bearing on the amputation stump or who have the sagittal plane leverage which a below-knee residual limb can provide but lack the frontal plane stability at the knee. They also assist a patient with diminished strength. For partial feet, several types of prostheses have been utilized. Pressure, especially for dorsal foot burns, should be incorporated into the prosthesis or the shoe so as to inhibit hypertrophic burn scar formation. Where bony overgrowth and bone spurs occur, the use of extra socket depth with replaceable distal cushions is helpful. Use of suspension sleeves with and without suction valves has been rewarding.

Above the knee

Neoprene-type suspension belts are well tolerated. Suction, especially suction using 'hypobaric sheaths,' can work if no excessively deep scarring is present. Where scarring is present, the sockets are contoured to the shape presented. Ischial con-

tainment with utilization of large surface areas, increased stump to socket stability, and flexible inner sockets are routinely prescribed.

Socket fitting

With early fitting, some skin problems will be encountered, but these have not been of major significance. Silicone gel or urethane socket inserts have been used successfully, for mature skin/burn scar but they create extra bulk, weight, and replacement expense (especially with still-growing pediatric patients). They are used when other methods are unsuccessful. Distal cushions made from the usual prosthetic materials such as silicone foam are used. On occasion, patients have removed the distal cushions on their own, and no distal edema problems have been noted.

Initial prosthetics

Initial and early prosthetic treatment of an upper extremity amputee includes splinting for the prevention of contracture. A splint may be extended past the distal end of a residual limb to match the length of the whole limb, thus assisting a patient in retaining the concept of length. This is especially useful for patients whose active participation in a rehabilitation program is delayed. A preparatory prosthesis is provided when early definitive fitting is not prudent, e.g. when reduction of stump volume is anticipated or when fitting over a bulky dressing is necessary. For young children, a socket with harness/cable and PVC tube extension has been used.[29] The distal tube is filled with plastic resin, drilled, and tapped to accept a prosthetic device. Friction is provided through a set screw on the side of the distal tube. Wrist flexion units can be added, but they add weight and require maintenance, as well as careful training by an occupational therapist. Unless this component significantly increases a patient's function, it may be more of an irritant than an aid. Standard figure-of-eight harnessing can be used to attach a prosthesis. To distribute pressure, pads are placed under the harness from C7 to the distal scapular area and extend laterally the width of the back.

Preparatory weight-bearing treatment is provided through an air bag system, utilizing air bags designed for stabilization of a lower extremity. Containers have been fabricated from laminated plastics or polypropylene, using neoprene on the distal end or a solid ankle cushion heal foot with adapters built into the containers (Figure 49.22). Treatment usually begins on a tilt table, progressing to standing and then ambulation in the parallel bars. Most below-knee prosthetic devices are self-suspending. A belt with straps attached to the containers (when fabricated) has been used for above-knee cases. When a patient experiences hypersensitivity at the amputated sites and the skin at those sites is very fragile, a hybridized prosthesis/orthosis (prosthesis) may be fabricated. This allows for early ambulation by having patients shift their weight from side to side (Figure 49.23). In the cases where bilateral amputations occur above the knee, an Ilizarov external fixator may be applied to lengthen the femoral bones bilaterally and prevent hip contractures. A 2–3-inch gain bilaterally will eventually make the fitting of prosthesis much easier. Prosthetic pylons may be attached to the orthotic fixators in order to allow for some weight bearing before the lengthening and healing of the bones is completed (Figure 49.24).

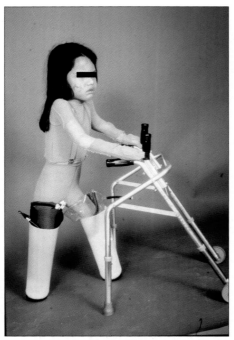

Fig. 49.22 This girl is walking on a set of preparatory temporary prostheses which employ air bags surrounding the partially healed residual limbs. These air bag prostheses allow the patient to begin weight bearing and practice walking before full healing has occurred.

Definitive prosthetics

Knowledge about a patient's prosthetic ability, work, and recreational activities will have been accrued by the time of definitive fitting. Most patients welcome the opportunity to provide feedback regarding changes in components or changes for function and fit with the definitive prosthesis. Information is provided to a patient regarding available options. Some patients will sacrifice cosmesis for hi-tech, maximum function such as a thermoplastic socket with a frame for a hydraulic knee and energy return foot with no cosmetic covering. Others will part with some function in order to achieve a desired level of cosmesis. The current array of the available prosthetic socket/weight-bearing and suspension combination, as well as application and use of the many component combinations, is beyond the scope of this chapter. In general, the simplest system which provides the most functional–cosmetic level is accepted by the amputee as the best choice.

Some patients will continue to use their preparatory prosthesis for extended periods of time while other areas of the body are treated. Prior to definitive fitting, body weight, residual limb volume, wear and use patterns should be stable in order to optimize the long-term result with the definitive prosthesis. Return clinic visits should include prosthetic evaluation. Children may require length adjustments even prior to definitive fitting. Other patients may leave the hospital with the prosthetic knee locked and may need additional therapy and prosthetic alignment for improved ambulation with swing phase knee flexion. The overall process of prosthetic evaluation and fitting is described in Figure 49.25.

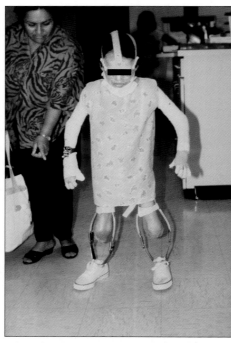

Fig. 49.23 When the skin at the residual limb is too fragile to permit weight bearing, a special prosthetic/orthotic device such as this can allow a patient to begin walking by shifting their weight to a proximal site (in this case the ischium) when it cannot be borne distally.

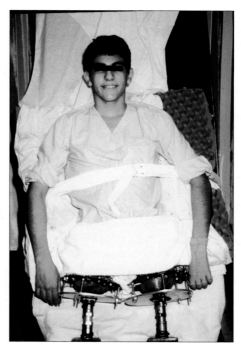

Fig. 49.24 When a bilateral amputation occurs at the proximal femoral level a prosthesis cannot readily be fitted. An orthotic external fixator can be used to lengthen the bones and reduce contractures. In this case, prosthetic pylons were attached to the orthotic fixators in order to allow some weight bearing before the lengthening and healing process were complete.

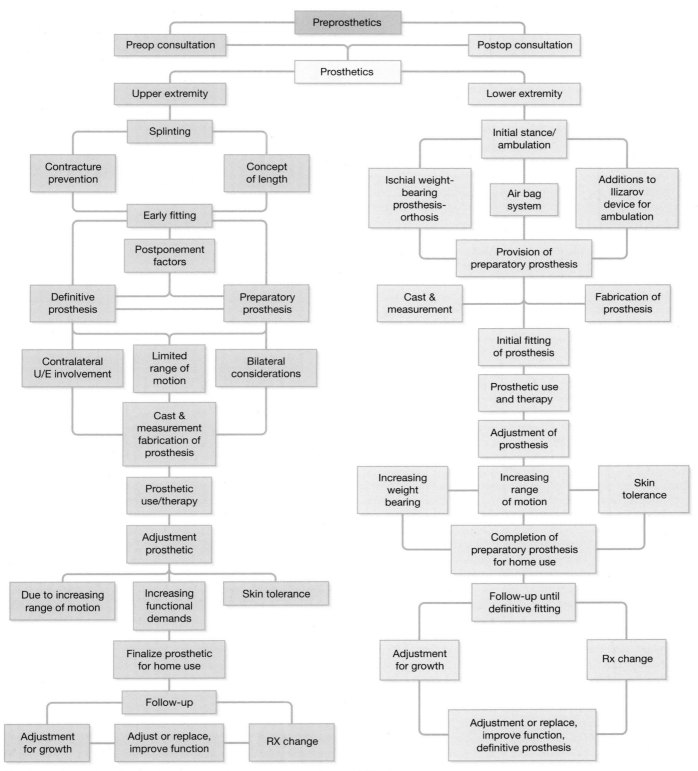

Fig. 49.25 Algorithm showing the process of prosthetic evaluation and fitting.

The orthotist's role

The role of the orthotist in treating the burn patient is similar to treating any other patient with orthopedic deficits. Soft-tissue deformities involving structural and mechanical properties are addressed by the same forces which are harnessed and applied to any orthotic user. Treating the burn patient for his orthotic needs may, however, pose a significant challenge to the orthotist in the cases where fitting of an orthosis may be complicated by poor skin integrity, fragile and/or sensitive skin, and fluctuation in the volume of the extremity to be treated. Additional factors which may have an influence on the type of the orthosis used may include the patient's neurological status, pressure points due to pressure garment presence, projected duration of the orthotic utilization, geographic location or a patient's proximity to a clinic for follow-up visits and orthotic modifications, and language/cultural barriers which may affect the compliance with an orthosis.

Orthotic treatment of the lower extremity

The approach of the orthotist in treating the injured foot depends on the extent of the burn injury. Orthotic shoes, which are the fundamental component of most lower extremity orthotics, may be utilized with some modifications in correcting deformities of the burned foot. Modifications of these shoes may include arch pads, molded foot thermoplastics, tongue pads, and metatarsal bars. The orthotic shoes should distribute all forces to the foot appropriately and should reduce pressure on sensitive or deformed structures and encourage total surface weight bearing along the plantar aspect of the foot. Inserts for plantar foot support such as the University of California Biomechanical Laboratory (UCBL) type may be utilized as indicated.

During the preambulation stage the patient may be fitted with those orthoses; if properly utilized, they can position the ankle joint appropriately, and assist in preventing or correcting plantar/dorsal contractures and inversion/eversion of the foot.

Leg length discrepancies are seen frequently in the cases of severe lower extremity burn injuries and they should be addressed with a shoe lift. The ankle–foot complex is difficult to address, especially in the case of a severe thermal injury. In most cases, the resultant deformity is the equinovarus foot. Both conventional and thermoplastic systems may be designed to treat the equinovarus or equinovalgus foot. Such systems may include a metal ankle–foot orthosis (AFO), polypropylene plastic posterior AFO (solid ankle or with an articulation), an AFO with stirrup attachment, an AFO with stirrups and patellar tendon support. A dorsiflexion spring assist may be incorporated in the AFO to aid weak ankle motion. Different straps such as a valgus correction strap may be attached to the AFO for the correction of specific problems. Interface materials, such as silicone, Plastizote® and Aliplast®, can be incorporated into an AFO to provide protection of the soft tissue, provide for total surface weight bearing, and to accommodate any anatomical anomalies that may be present (Figure 49.26). In the event that a return of range of motion is anticipated, an AFO could be fabricated that can be modified as the patient progresses. The ankle joints can be incorporated into the AFO, however, left solid and articulated at a later date.

During more complicated cases, and depending on the anatomy and function of the lower extremities, a knee–ankle–foot orthosis, hip–knee–ankle–foot orthosis or a trunk–knee–ankle–foot orthosis may also be designed for the best functional outcome.[30]

Burn scar management

History

The burn wound like any other wound heals by the formation of scar at the injured site in order to replace the destroyed

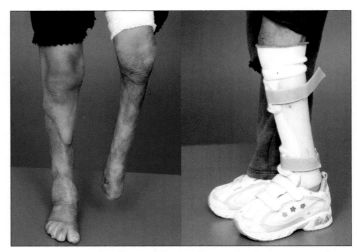

Fig. 49.26 Specialized materials may be required to accommodate anatomical anomalies that may be present. Standard ankle–foot orthoses can be fabricated utilizing silicone materials to accommodate excessive scarring and limb loss.

tissues. Scar is defined as the fibrous tissue replacing normal tissues destroyed by injury or disease.[31] In the case of a burn injury the scars, if not managed appropriately, have the potential of becoming thick and raised, resulting in scar hypertrophy. Hypertrophic scars are not cosmetically appealing and if they cross any joints they may restrict function. Pressure therapy for scar management is a very old and established component of a recovering burn patient's continuing rehabilitation program. Extensive historical notes on the earliest references to scarring are provided by Linares and colleagues who attribute the first full medical description of scars to Petz in 1790.[32] They also state that the first medical reference to the use of pressure for treatment was written by Johnson in 1678 referring to the work of Ambroise Paré in the 16th century.[32] Other historical events noted by Linares et al. are: first known accounts of the use of pressure for treatment of children in 1859; use of elastic bandages in 1860; adhesive plaster for pressure in 1881; and use of traction to treat scars in 1902. Linares' review includes descriptions of Nason's work in 1942 in which he noted that ischemia produced by pressure arrests the overproduction of scar tissue, 'where the imprint of the elastic of an undergarment or a belt may be seen — no keloid is present.'[32] Another historical review by Ward[33] reveals that Blair in 1924 reported the positive influence of pressure on healing wounds. Nason's application of the 'constant pressure' principle included developing a type of neck splint made of a piece of dental impression compound or a piece of heavy felt strapped tightly over the scar for 6–8 weeks and possibly longer. Later, various splints were developed utilizing pressure and immobilization.[34] In the 1960s Drs Silverstein and Larson observed the influence of pressure on healing burns. Their observations led to the manufacture of customized pressure garments that revolutionized scar management in the 1970s which continues to date with some modifications.[32,33]

The scar

As the burn wound progresses toward healing, or after skin grafting operations take place, scars begin to form. Generally, the deeper the burns are the higher the risk is for the development of hypertrophic scars. Also, the longer a wound remains open the higher the chances for hypertrophic scar formation are.[34,35] As the wound begins the healing process, collagen fibers develop to bridge the wound, forming an immature (active) scar which appears as a red, raised and rigid mass.[36–39] Abston reported that pressure therapy during maturation led to a flatter, softer and a more devascularized scar.[40] Burn scars may take up to 2 years or longer to mature. Factors contributing to the formation of hypertrophic scars may include: wound infection, genetics, immunological factors, repeated harvesting of donor sites, altered ground substance, age, chronic inflammatory process, location of the injury, and tension.[41] Scar hypertrophy may be evident at 8–12 weeks after wound closure.[42]

Scar assessment

In order to better study the process of scar maturation, ongoing research is looking at alternative techniques in assessing the state of scars. Hambleton and colleagues studied the thickness of scars with ultrasonic scanning. This method, which is completely non-invasive, allows for a comparison of the thickness of dermal tissue in the traumatized area with that in the normal skin at regular intervals following initial healing.[43] Darvey et al. described a technique for the objective assessment of scars utilizing a video camera image on a computer and quantitatively analyzing the color of the scars using a custom-written computer program.[44] Esposito used a modified tonometer to measure skin tone which correlates to skin pliability and tension.[45] Bartell and co-workers used the elastometer properties of normal vs. injured skin. In his study Bartell showed that scars, if left untreated, will show improvement over time.[46] The Vancouver Burn Scar Assessment developed by Sullivan and colleagues is a subjective way of rating the burn scar pigmentation, vascularity, pliability and height.[47] Hosoda utilized laser flowmetry to determine the perfusion of hypertrophic scars vs. non-hypertrophic scars.[48] Other studies suggest that laser Doppler flowmetry and monitoring of transcutaneous oxygen tension may in the future be ways of determining scar maturation.[49]

Treatment of hypertrophic scars

To this date hypertrophic scars remain very problematic and difficult to manage. Even though the mechanism of scar maturation is not yet well understood, clinically the accepted protocol to treat hypertrophic scars includes the use of pressure therapy, which should be instituted early on in the maturation process of the burn scar. Means of pressure therapy include pressure garments, inserts, and conforming orthotics. Once the skin has healed enough to withstand sheering, massage and heat modalities may be utilized as an adjunct in scar management. The use of pressure in effectively depressing scars was well documented by Drs Silverstein and Larson in the 1970s; their observations and studies sparked the near-universal use of pressure garments. When an active scar is compressed, it blanches, which indicates decreased blood flow in the area.[50] Less blood leads to decreased oxygen in the tissues, which in turns leads into decreased collagen production, which brings a balance between collagen synthesis and collagen breakdown (lysis). When a balance in the production

and breakdown of collagen is established, the resultant scar appears flatter.[51] Kealey et al. conducted a prospective randomized study to compare efficacy of pressure garment therapy in patients with burns. Patients were randomly assigned to receive either pressure garment therapy or no pressure garment therapy. Assessment of the maturity of scar included use of the Vancouver Burn Scar Assessment Scale. The results on 113 patients studied in the follow-up revealed no significant differences between groups when age, body surface area burned, length of hospital stay or time to wound maturation were compared.[52] In addition to this study, other studies have reported problems related to lack of adherence and discomfort, blistering, ulceration or scar breakdown, swelling of extremities and skeletal and dental deformity due to excessive pressures which often leads to stoppage of treatment, significant side effects and deformity.[52–58]

On the other hand, studies have also reported benefits of pressure garments.[59–61] The reader is referred to various recent excellent review articles on the efficacy or lack of efficacy of pressure garments in the management of hypertrophic burn scars.[62,63] Reasons for the absence of unequivocal evidence is that garments must be worn continuously for a least 23 hours a day, making compliance or adherence difficult.[55,64,63] In addition, the optimal pressure that must be applied to the scar for treatment is not known.[55,65–67] Thus, the studies and debates continue, and, at least until more evidence is gathered, pressure therapy with the familiar elastic garments is still prescribed. Patients and families would no doubt feel relieved if the data eventually show that pressure does not make a significant difference in long-term outcomes. However, it should be noted that the studies thus far include neither the examination of burns over joints nor do they include burns of the hands, neck and face. In addition, none of the studies to date address the use of pressure in the form of splints, another source of discomfort and tension for burned children and their families.

None of the known studies yet have broached the face with an attempt to determine the efficacy of pressure versus no pressure. Facial pressure garments in children may pose problems due to interference with growth.[68,69] We recommend that these patients should be closely monitored for normal facial and dental development by physicians including dental specialists. The elastic hood and underlying silicone face pad present special problems for patients, and some extreme challenges for the adults trying to assist a burned child or adolescent. The elastic mask and hood, covering head, face, and hair, effectively hides the identity of the person wearing it. It is perceived by children as sinister, associated with 'bad men' or monsters, and most children who have worn this garment can relay stories of being ridiculed by strangers who did not know the purpose of the garment. Emotional expressiveness, usually apparent in facial movements, is hidden by the hood. More than one child has explained non-adherence with the prescribed wearing of the elastic mask with a statement similar to 'I want my friends to see me laugh.' A study by Groce et al. compared the elastic mask and hood with silicone pad to the transparent silicone face mask and found no significant differences between the amount of pressure applied by each to the forehead, cheeks, and chin.[70] Many children have expressed a preference for, and seem to wear more readily, the transparent mask. This study should make it easier for them to be granted their choice — an important event during a time when so much is happening to them outside of their control. Please see text on Reconstruction for further details.

Pressure therapy

As long as the scars are active they may be influenced by pressure therapy. However, not all burn scars require pressure. Patients with burn wounds which heal within 7–14 days do not need pressure therapy. Those patients whose wounds heal within 14–21 days are closely monitored for pressure therapy needs and may be generally advised to use pressure garments prophylactically. A wound that heals after 21 days will require the use of pressure garments.[51] The correct amount of pressure in suppressing the hypertrophic scar has not yet been determined. Pressure of as little as 10 mmHg may be effective in remodeling the scar tissue over time. Pressures over 40 mmHg, however, may be destructive to tissues and cause paresthesias.[42] Early forms of pressure therapy include the use of elastic bandages directly applied on the newly healed skin or on top of the burn dressings. The use of conforming thermoplastics along with elastic bandages may also be utilized as means of early pressure therapy.[71] Once the wounds are almost or completely closed, tubular elastic bandages such as Tubigrip™ may be utilized. These tubular bandages are offered in different sizes and accommodate all anatomical circumferences. Care should be taken in applying these tubular bandages so that the fragile skin or the freshly applied skin grafts do not sheer, or the minimal dressing underneath is not disturbed. The burn therapist should be aware that these tubular bandages are materials made of a single elastic thread spiraling through the weave of the fabric, and disturbance of the continuous elastic by cutting holes into it will alter the pressure gradient provided by these materials. The tubular elastic bandages should be doubled over the skin surface area treated in order to provide adequate pressure.[72] Early pressure application over the hand and digits can be accomplished by the use of thin, elastic and self-adherent wraps such as Coban™ (Figure 49.27). This form of pressure is excellent for adult and pediatric patients for controlling edema and aids in the early scar management of hands when the shearing forces of a glove cannot be tolerated. Small children are excellent candidates for Coban™ gloves vs. a garment glove because of compliance issues, comprehension of instructions in assisting with the application of a custom glove and difficulties in obtaining accurate measurements for a custom glove. Coban™ may be applied over the burn dressings or directly onto the healed digits. The burn therapist needs to be aware that if Coban™ is wrapped too tight it may deform the interosseous structures of the healing hand. However, if Coban™ is wrapped too lose it may encourage swelling of the hands when used in combination with arm elastic garments. Coban™ strips are pre-cut approximately twice the length of the digits to be wrapped. Each strip is wrapped in a spiral fashion beginning at the nail bed of each digit, overlapping half of the Coban™ width and ending in the adjacent web space. Each fingertip needs to be exposed so that blood circulation can be monitored at all times. The Coban™ is stretched from 0–25% of the entire elasticity of each strip. Once all web spaces are covered, the rest of the hand is wrapped with Coban™, extending approxi-

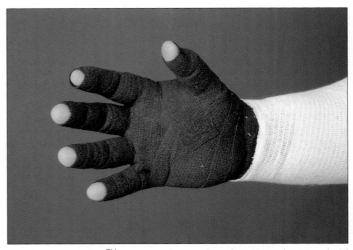

Fig. 49.27 A Coban™ wrap can be used to decrease edema and aid in the effective management of hand scar hypertrophy.

mately 1 inch past the wrist joint. No skin areas should be visible once the Coban™ glove is completed. If small hand areas remain uncovered, a small piece of Coban™ is stretched over the area and adheres to the rest of the Coban™. When the glove is completed, the therapist should very superficially lubricate the entire glove with lotion in order to eliminate the adherent effect of the Coban™ and allow for the functional use of the hand. Coban™ should be removed on a daily basis by the therapist or the caregiver. Removal of Coban™ should be done carefully by cutting off or unwrapping each digit strip individually to avoid disturbing any small wound healing. The use of prefabricated interim pressure garments is widely accepted and utilized in burn rehabilitation. These garments are available commercially by different companies and they include pieces for the entire body. Interim garments which are made of softer materials introduce the burn patient to circumferential pressure and protect the newly healed skin. Another reason for using these garments prior to ordering custom-made garments is to allow for the patient's weight to stabilize (post acute hospitalization) and any remaining edema to subside. In some cases where obtaining custom-made garments on regular intervals (approximately 12 weeks) is not an option the recommendation should be that interim garments should be the choice for long-term pressure therapy. Once the patient's weight has stabilized, edema has subsided and the skin is able to withstand some shearing (approximately 3–4 weeks post wound closure), measurements are taken for the fabrication of custom-made pressure garments (Figure 49.28). Today several companies specialize in the fabrication of these garments. Clinically, custom therapeutic pressure for the prevention, control and correction of scar hypertrophy averages 24–28 mmHg, which is approximately equal and opposing to the capillary pressure (25 mmHg). At this pressure level, many researchers believe that scars may be altered.[73] In order for pressure therapy to be effective, pressure garments need to be worn at all times, day and night. They should only be removed for bathing and on occasion during exercises should they interfere with movements. Each order is duplicated so one set of garments can be worn while the other is being washed. Today,

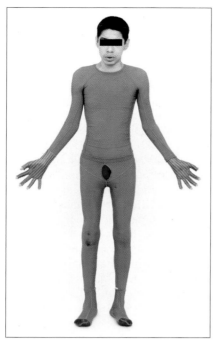

Fig. 49.28 Custom-made pressure garments may be fabricated for the entire body.

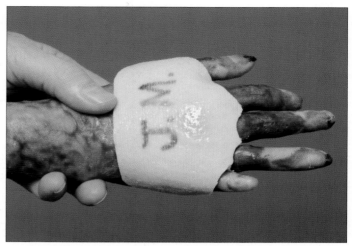

Fig. 49.29 Silicone elastomer inserts for the dorsum of the hand and web spaces are utilized for the prevention of syndactyly and depression on scar tissue.

pressure garment companies offer multiple colors of materials and for the pediatric population cartoon characters may be sewed on the garments to make them cosmetically appealing and improve the patients' compliance.[74] The burn therapist should choose a reputable company that provides excellent service and support for the patient and the therapist. The company's willingness and flexibility to manufacture non-standard garments, availability of special options, cost and turnaround time should be taken into consideration when selecting the burn center's pressure garment provider.[75]

Inserts

Inserts are widely utilized in burn rehabilitation as an adjunct to achieving effective pressure over certain anatomical locations where pressure garments do not provide adequate pressure. These locations include concave body areas such as the face, neck, antecubital fossae, sternum, palm of the hands, web spaces, upper back and arches of the feet. These materials come commercially prefabricated or may be custom-made by the burn therapist or the medical sculpture technician. Inserts come in different forms such as silicone gels, elastomers, putties mixed with a silicone catalyst, skin care silastic pads, foam and even in the form of hard thermoplastic materials contouring to different anatomical locations. The experienced burn therapist chooses the appropriate insert material best suitable for the patient according to the stage of scar maturation and skin sensitivity. Generally, pressure therapy begins with a soft, thin and elastic insert and progresses to a more rigid insert in depressing the more unyielding burn scar. Inserts need to be worn underneath pressure garments, starting with a few hours of application and progressing as tolerated, toward a 24-hour application. They should be removed frequently for cleaning (warm water and soap), drying and application of

cornstarch to avoid scar maceration and skin breakdown. Patients may be allergic to certain insert materials so the burn therapist may try different inserts until one is found to be best tolerated by the patient's skin. In cases of scar maceration, blisters, skin breakdown, contact dermatitis and a rash or an allergic reaction, inserts should be removed until healing occurs. Silicone, a polymer based on the element silicon, appears to be the trend in the treatment of hypertrophic scars. To date, the mechanism of how silicone affects the burn scar is not known. Clinically, silicone has been observed to depress the height of hypertrophic scars, prevent shrinking of fresh skin grafts (hard elastomer silicone pads vs. silicone gel pads), and increase the pliability of a scar, thus allowing for increase in the range of motion of affected joints. Patients report that silicone is soothing to the skin and aids in decreasing pain. Silicone, being occlusive, may cause the collection of excessive moisture and cause skin maceration if not removed frequently for cleaning and drying. Its disadvantages are that it is very expensive and short-lived.[76-78] The therapist should look for silicone gel pads with a non-shearing protective medium on the non-skin surface in order for the gel to last longer. Also, buying larger-size gel pads and cutting them to fit the patient's need may be a cost-effective method for today's shrinking clinic budgets.

Other insert materials include liquid silicone elastomer, which when mixed with a catalyst form a solid but elastic insert (Figure 49.29). The experienced therapist could create custom inserts for difficult anatomical locations such as the face and web spaces using this technique. Prosthetic Foam™ is a liquid-based silicone elastomer which, when mixed with a catalyst, solidifies in the form of a very pliable foam insert that works best for the palm of the hands where function needs to be preserved while pressure is applied. These foam inserts also work best for applying pressure to contour surfaces on the face (around eyes, mouth, nose) while protecting these sensitive areas from excess and rigid pressure. Elastomer putties such as Otoform K™ or Rolyan Ezemix® form semi-rigid but still elastic inserts for different areas of the body where the scar can tolerate more pressure such as in the web spaces to prevent syndactyly.[77] Early on in scar management, a soft foam such as Plastizote®, Velfoam™ or Betapile™ may be utilized to apply gentle pressure to the very fragile and sensitive scar.

High thermoplastic transparent masks were developed in 1968 by Padewski to be applied directly to the face to prevent, control and reverse scar hypertrophy. These masks require the moulaging of the patient in creating a negative facial mold. A positive mold of the face is fabricated with the use of plaster. The patient's positive facial mold is then 'sculptured' in an attempt to recreate the patient's non-burned face. A high thermoplastic material such as Uvex™ or W-Clear™ is then pulled over the positive mold in order to create the hard plastic mask (Figure 49.30a). Holes for the eyes, nose and mouth are cut. The mask is worn under pressure garments or with a head strapping mechanism. In cases of significant scar hypertrophy on the face, the positive mold is 'sculptured' sequentially over a period of time in order to avoid excessive pressure over facial scar leading to skin breakdown. A silicone elastomer face mask may be created utilizing the existing positive facial mold and is worn under facial pressure garments (Figure 49.30b). The use of the clear and silastic masks is preferred over the use of just a facial garment as they provide conforming pressure around facial openings (eyes, nose, and mouth). Frequently, the burn therapist manufactures the clear mask to be worn during the day and the silastic mask along with the facial garment to be worn at night.[32,79–81]

Burn scar massage

Once the burn scars have matured enough to tolerate sheering forces, massage may be incorporated into the scar management regimen. Scar massage is an effective modality for maintaining joint mobility in the case of contractures. It aids in softening or remodeling the scar tissues by freeing adhering fibrous bands, allowing the scars to become more elastic and stretchy, thus improving joint mobility. Initially, the therapist may utilize a non-frictional massage applying mostly stationary pressure to skin blanching and mobilizing the skin surface

without friction. Utilization of lubricants during this massage technique should be avoided. As the skin begins to tolerate frictional massage, the scar tissue is manipulated in rotary, parallel and perpendicular motions, using a lubricant and pressing the skin to blanching. Clinically, massage is found to alleviate itching. It is also used for desensitization purposes. An electrical massager with a heat attachment may be used along with lubrication, as heat and massage in combination may increase scar pliability. Massage should be performed at least twice daily (3–5 times preferred) for 5–10 minutes on each treated body surface. The burn therapist should frequently assess the skin condition in avoiding further injuries. The patient and/or family are instructed on home massage techniques and electrical massagers may be issued for home use. Other therapeutic modalities for scar management may include the use of heat. Heat relaxes tissues and makes them pliable in preparation for mobilization. Heat modalities may include hot packs, paraffin wax, fluidotherapy and ultrasound. Even though the use of therapeutic heat as an adjunct to rehabilitation is well documented, therapeutic heat modalities are infrequently being utilized in burn rehabilitation.[82,83]

Burn scar management is a complicated and lengthy process and for it to be successfully completed the patient and caregivers should be committed to follow the therapist's recommendations. Extensive training should take place addressing the use and care of pressure garments, inserts, lubrication and other therapeutic scar management procedures to be performed by the patients and their caregivers. Lubricants which do not contain perfume and other skin irritants should be selected and applied at least (2–3 times daily) to the healing skin. Lubricants with sun protection factor (SPF) of at least 15 are recommended.[84] Written instructions with pictures and diagrams along with videos addressing scar management should accompany the patient home upon discharge from the hospital. Follow-up visits to the burn or rehabilitation clinic for the assessment of overall recovery to include garments, inserts and other home therapeutic interventions are needed for the patient to successfully complete his/her burn rehabilitation. The therapists' knowledge, creativity and continuing research in improving the currently existing scar management techniques may be the key to positive outcomes in pressure therapy.

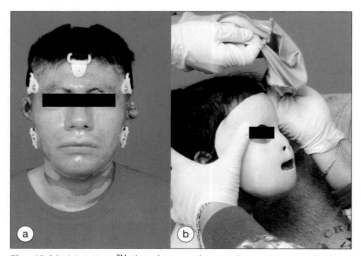

Fig. 49.30 (a) A Uvex™ clear face mask provides pressure to the face so as to prevent scar hypertrophy and to preserve facial features. (b) A silicone elastomer face mask provides pressure to the face in preventing facial scar hypertrophy and preserving facial features.

Therapeutic exercise

Therapeutic exercise is motion of the body or its parts to relieve symptoms or to improve function.[85] The need for therapeutic exercise to enhance mobility of the burn patient begins acutely and continues throughout the months of healing. Even though painful and extensive therapy is required during the long rehabilitation process, the results are for the most part dependent on the patients' and families understanding, involvement and dedication to the treatment.[82]

The goals of therapeutic exercise in burn rehabilitation are to:
* reduce the effects of edema and immobilization;
* maintain functional joint motion and muscle strength;
* stretch the scar tissue;
* return the patient to optimal level of function.

Exercise for the patient

Exercise sessions depend upon the patient's physical, psychological, and medical status. In the conservative treatment of burn wounds, a vigorous physical therapy program is instituted immediately so as to maintain function.[86] Postoperatively, exercises involving autografted skin over joints are usually discontinued for 4–5 days. Escharotomies, fasciotomies, heterografts, and synthetic dressings are not contraindications for exercise.[87] Early mobilization to decrease edema, proper exercise techniques, and accurate documentation of function are more important than the type of wound closure.[86]

Scar contracture and joint mobility limitations are the result of the shortening of immature connective tissue. Therapy aims to prevent deformity and the subsequent limitation of movement. In circumferential burns, both the flexor and extensor surfaces are at risk of contracture. Therapeutic exercise in conjunction with splinting should promote agonist and antagonist movements around those joints in order to maintain mobility.[88] Treatments are tailored to each individual patient, with independent living being the ultimate goal throughout the rehabilitation continuum.

Exercise activities can typically be divided into four categories: stretching, strengthening, cardiovascular, and functional activity exercises.

'Stretching' exercises are performed with a slow, prolonged force. Gentle, sustained stretch is more effective than multiple repetitive movements in gaining length of burned tissues. An indication of effective stretching is that the scar tissue blanches. If scars extend across more than one joint, each joint should be stretched individually, and then the skin stretched as a whole unit across the involved joints. 'Passive' exercise is a form of stretching exercise which is performed without voluntary muscle contraction. It is a slow, gentle stretch provided by an outside force with the prime result being the stretching of tissue. The use of a continuous passive motion (CPM) device has been documented to be an effective modality for improving joint range of motion.[87] Rehabilitation advances have shown CPM treatment to be a viable option because of its benefits to soft tissue remodeling, joint nutrition, wound healing, and venous dynamics.[89,90] Active and active-assistive exercises should become the focus of the session in lieu of passive stretch once the patient has achieved full range of motion. All passive exercise should be performed cautiously when there is evidence of bone or tendon exposure.

'Strengthening' exercise improves the muscle's ability to perform work. 'Active' exercise is performed independently by a patient. This is the form of exercise most recommended because it stretches healing skin and provides strength-inducing benefits. Frequent exercise performed actively (with voluntary muscle contribution) by a patient promotes the greatest increase in movement. 'Active-assistive' exercises utilize the same principles; however, a patient is 'assisted' by an outside force (therapist or assistive device) to achieve the full range of motion. A patient will achieve improvements in strength and range of motion, but not equal to those provided by active exercise. Active-assistive exercises are suggested for those patients who are too weak to perform a full range of motion exercise independently. In 'resistive' exercises, manual or mechanical resistance is applied to a movement. A variety of modalities offer resistance, ranging from traditional weights to innovative combinations of rubber bands. Resistive exercises can begin in an 'assistive' fashion with minimal resistance and assistance provided to complete the range of motion.

'Cardiovascular' exercises are designed to improve a patient's overall endurance level. These activities are performed for prolonged periods of time with minimum resistance and can be designed to involve activities which are enjoyable for the patient.

'Functional' exercises include those activities which incorporate all types of the above-mentioned exercises. They are designed to improve the coordination and performance of patients in tasks which are relevant to activities of daily living. For example, feeding requires both coordination and strength as well as stretching to take the hand to the mouth. Performing functional activities is generally rewarding to patients. The goal(s) and purpose of these activities are clearly defined and understood. Completion of these tasks requires concentration and appears to distract a patient from the pain of movement. Functional tasks also seem to provide a feeling of accomplishment and encouragement to a patient who wants to regain independence.

Therapeutic exercise begins immediately after the burn. For a patient being treated conservatively, movement helps maintain strength and range of motion, and aids in circulation and healing. For a patient who has been grafted, isometric exercises can be performed during the immobilization period. The benefit of isometric exercise is that a patient does not 'forget' how to contract the muscle, a common phenomenon with periods of prolonged immobilization. Isometric exercise also helps in maintaining muscle strength. When skin grafts have become stable, active exercise may begin. Active exercise is initially performed by allowing a patient to limit the intensity by pain. It is followed by passive stretching exercise and strengthening to maintain mobility.

Exercise can be performed with dressing and wraps in place. Care should be taken when dressings are applied so that joint range of motion is not restricted. Dressings which have been correctly applied will minimize discomfort and promote movement, while dressings applied too tightly will limit mobility, increase pain, and may create pressure-induced neuropathies. Exercise can also be performed while the patient is in the tub, where the buoyancy of the water and the absence of confining dressings can make exercise less painful. Exercise is initially painful and the very first repetition is often the most difficult. Discomfort is due to stretching skin which has lost its natural lubricating mechanism and has become dry and tight. Movement itself decreases pain. Each subsequent repetition will be easier as the skin stretches, and the muscle pumping action of active movement helps resolve edema, thus significantly reducing pain.

Specific movements can be targeted to prevent burn scar contracture. We find that the patients tend to position themselves in a comfortable position, which most frequently is the position of contracture. Based on knowledge about typical contractures, the following movements are encouraged: neck extension and lateral flexion, shoulder abduction and flexion, elbow extension and supination, metacarpophalangeal flexion, interphalangeal extension, wrist extension, knee extension, ankle dorsiflexion, and metatarsophalangeal flexion. Exercise sessions may be indicated three to four times daily for more involved areas. Patients should be encouraged to exercise between therapy sessions.

To walk or ambulate again following a severe burn is an important goal shared by patients of all ages. However, we believe ambulation should happen on the fourth day after every operation.

The benefits of ambulation include:

- maintenance of range of motion;
- maintenance of strength in the lower extremities;
- prevention of thromboemboli;
- maintenance of bone density via weight bearing;
- promotion of independence in functional activities.[88]

Ambulation exercises may also help prevent decubiti, provide mild, cardiovascular conditioning, and increase appetite. In addition, ambulatory patients have fewer problems with lower extremity contractures and physical endurance.[87]

All wounds must have the proper dressings prior to ambulation. Lower extremity burn wounds should be wrapped with elastic bandages in order to facilitate capillary support. Wrapping will decrease edema and therefore decrease pain and promote healing. The extremities should be wrapped distal to proximal from the toes to the groin crease. The foot should always be included to avoid distal edema. Those extremities that have had skin grafting generally have less graft loss when there is a second elastic wrap to provide further support. Lower extremity donor sites are less painful when wrapped with elastic bandages. Wrapping which incorporates the figure-of-eight pattern has been reported to provide better pressure than the spiral wrap, perhaps due to increased vascular support.[91]

As with other exercise, proper positioning facilitates proper gait.[88] The patient who has been allowed to assume a position of comfort will have difficulty extending the hips and knees during ambulation. The ankle may be tight, limiting plantigrade position when in the upright position. If the joints are in the normal alignment, the amount of pain and energy are greatly reduced.

In preparing for ambulation, therapists may use a tilt table with patients who lack the capacity to stand and mobilize their lower extremities (Figure 49.31).[91–94] There are a variety of reasons why erect positioning may prove difficult. For example, prolonged bedrest, which influences blood pressure or ankle tightness, may inhibit plantigrade position. However, therapists should keep in mind that a tilt table represents a mostly passive introduction of gravity to the body and does not promote proper alignment of the musculoskeletal system. Creative efforts and aggressive techniques are sometimes necessary to encourage ambulation in patients that first appear incapable or unprepared to begin erect weight-bearing exercise.

Patients that present with fragile tissue over the terminal end of a lower extremity amputation site may initially appear incapable of walking for fear of damage to the weight-bearing surface by compressive or shear forces. This issue can be resolved with the use of a bypass orthosis that shifts the force of weight bearing to the ischium by using a quadrilateral ischial containment socket with metal uprights that connect directly to a foot mechanism. This protocol can be introduced

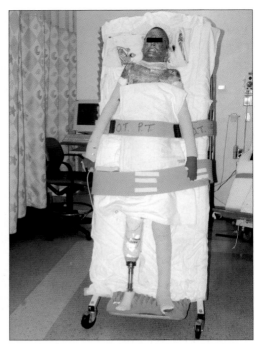

Fig. 49.31 The tilt table may be utilized prior to ambulation for those patients who may have difficulty assuming the upright position.

on a tilt table and then progressed to a walking program as the individual's condition warrants.

Patients tend to perform much better when given an achievable goal such as walking a specific distance or to a certain place. Children do well when provided with a desired incentive such as a toy or a game. Frequent rest periods may be necessary secondary to decreased endurance levels or pain. Patients should be encouraged to ambulate further distances each day. Care should be taken to avoid prolonged periods of standing so that hypotension does not develop. The lower extremities, even when properly wrapped for support, will show signs of venous insufficiency when dependent for too long a period of time. The use of assistive devices, i.e. crutches or walkers, is discouraged because the legs need the muscle pumping action to prevent edema.[90] Exercise and ambulation are integral parts of the rehabilitation of burn patients. Both allow a patient to resume a lifestyle as active and independent as possible.

Exercise for the outpatient

This section describes methodology used in designing an exercise-training program for persons with severe burns that have been discharged from the hospital. Exercise training is defined here as 'a planned, structured and repetitive body movement done to improve or maintain one or more components of physical fitness.'[95,96] The evidence for the use of exercise in the outpatient setting and the methodology presented here is based primarily on the outpatient exercise program that is implemented in severely burned children at Shriners Hospitals for Children in Galveston, Texas and in some severely burned adults.[97] This exercise program is supplemented by physical and occupational therapy. The program has proven beneficial in children 7–18 years of age.[97–99] Recently, effects of a music- and movement-based exercise program on children younger than 7 years of age has been assessed in a pilot study at Shriners Burns Hospital in Galveston, Texas. The effects include increases, as well as maintenance, of range of motion in children that participated in a movement and music program versus those that did not. The principles in designing an exercise program in children and adults with severe burns is based largely on guidelines offered to healthy, non-burned children and adults (Figure 49.32).[95,96,100–104]

Exercise evaluation

It is important to perform an initial evaluation of risks factors and/or symptoms for various chronic conditions concomitant to the burn. These include pre-existing conditions such as chronic cardiovascular, pulmonary and metabolic diseases. The objective of the exercise evaluations is to obtain information to optimize safety during exercise testing and training and also to develop a sound and effective exercise rehabilitation program.

Health screening before exercise evaluation should begin with the collection of subjective data. This should include evaluation of exercise or sports interests, objectives, level of activity prior to burn, functional limitations (e.g. loss of digits, lower body bilateral amputee), and other pertinent information. To our knowledge, there are no burn-specific physical activity questionnaires. However, simple questionnaires for assessing pre-burn physical activity exist and can be modified to fit a specific given population.[105–107] This evaluation can consist of muscle strength, cardiopulmonary and muscle joint flexibility testing. The information gathered during the subjective and objective evaluations can then be used to design a structured exercise program or plan to be carried out at home or at an exercise facility. Finally, a plan to periodically re-evaluate subjective and objective data, and the exercise program should be incorporated.

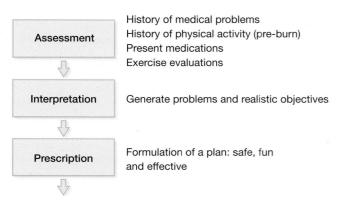

- Intensity: 45% to 95% of HRR
- Duration: 20 to 60 minutes
- Frequency: 3-5 days per week
- Mode: Involves large muscle groups, rhythmic, sustained
- Progression: Variable, based on goals, pain tolerance

Fig. 49.32 Basic diagram depicting various components involved in the design of an exercise program.

Subjective data: Characterization of limitations or problems of a patient should be done. Obtaining a history of pre-burn physical activity or habits, present medical complaints, symptoms and limitations is crucial to develop a sound exercise program. Symptoms or limitations which may affect exercise tolerance may include pain during ambulation, weakness in ambulation, itching, joint contractures, amputations, shortness of breath, or ease of fatigability. In addition, you should note present medications and note possible effects of these. Following the evaluation of subjective data, an exercise evaluation to gather objective data on the patient's exercise or physical capacity should be performed.

Objective data: Assessment of objective data includes age, height and weight, percent TBSA burn, and percent full-thickness burn. Variables before, during, and after a cardiopulmonary exercise test (CPET) should be obtained if possible. These include heart rate, blood pressure, Borg's rated perceived exertion (RPE), basic electrocardiogram (ECG), and spirometry.[108,109] However, if a CPET is not possible, an exercise program that is effective can also be designed. Assessment of upper and lower body muscle strength should also be done. This includes assessment of peak strength levels (if possible), as well as determining the loads or weights that will be used during the resistive component of the exercise program. The assessment of peak muscle strength can be accomplished during knee or elbow extension but can also be accomplished during a handgrip.[97,110,111] These tests involve peak-to-maximal efforts and good communication between patient and tester must exist. In addition, there is a developmental mental maturity that must exist in order for many of these objective data to be maximally helpful. We recommend a chronological age of 7 years and above, though children as young as 3–4 have also been tested successfully.[112] Finally, major muscle/joint flexibility should be assessed using measures such as sit-and-reach or goniometry for range of motion. Other types of tests may include neuromuscular tests such as gait analysis, balance time or reaction time. Finally, assessment of functional performance can also be done such as sit-and-stand scores, timed walk/jog and or lifting. The results of these evaluations will be used to identify major problem areas, to write an exercise prescription or to design the exercise program, and to assess progress during and after an exercise program.

Components of an exercise program

An exercise program typically consists of a warm-up phase, an endurance phase, recreational activities (optional), and a cool-down phase. While aerobic training activities should be done 3–5 days per week, complementary flexibility and resistance exercises may be performed at a lower frequency (2–3 days per week).[113] Flexibility exercises can be included as part of the warm-up or cool-down, or done at a separate time. Resistive training is often performed on alternate days as aerobic training; however, both types of activities can be combined into the same workout session. Typically the warm-up period will be of approximately 5–10 minutes, though it can be longer. This will be followed by a stimulus or endurance phase of 20–60 minutes, and a cool-down period of approximately 5–10 minutes. Aerobic and resistance training should be prescribed in specific terms of intensity, duration, frequency, and mode of exercise. Each of these terms will be discussed in greater detail later. An optional recreational game may occasionally substitute the endurance phase. However, because of potential difficulties in setting an appropriate intensity for an appropriate length of time, it is suggested that it be done as a complement to the endurance phase. If a recreational activity is added to the endurance phase, then the shortening of the endurance phase should be carefully considered though maintaining a minimum of 20 minutes.

Warm-up stage

Prior to the endurance phase, a variety of very light exercises, low-intensity calisthenics, should be done to improve the transition from rest to the endurance phase of the exercise session. The emphasis at the onset of an exercise session is to gradually increase the level of activity until the proper intensity is reached to begin the endurance phase. Stretching exercises to increase the range of motion of the joints involved in the activity were previously included in the warm-up. However, recently, evidence has been introduced to contraindicate the inclusion of stretching during the warm-up period.[114,115]

In fact, evidence suggests that a pre-exercise warm-up that consists of only light aerobic exercise to increase body temperature is adequate for increasing flexibility before an exercise session.[96] For example, patients might walk moderately fast during the endurance phase, but might conclude the warm-up period with slow, easy walking. However, a moderate walk (e.g. 3.5 mph) can be a warm-up for a patient that jogs at 5.5 mph during the endurance phase. Heart rate may be monitored or assessed if needed to ensure that the warm-up activity is not too strenuous.

Endurance stage

The endurance phase develops cardiorespiratory or aerobic fitness and includes 20–60 minutes of continuous or intermittent (minimum of 10-minute bouts accumulated throughout the day) aerobic activity. Duration depends on the intensity of the activity; thus, moderate-intensity activity should be conducted over a longer period of time (30 minutes or more), and, conversely, individuals training at higher levels of intensity (i.e. vigorous exercise) should train for at least 20 minutes or more.[113] The most effective exercises for the endurance phase employ large muscle groups in activities that are rhythmic or dynamic in nature. Sports such as soccer, basketball or tennis also have aerobic conditioning potential if a sufficient amount of time for inducing aerobic improvement is achieved (minimum of 20 minutes total). On the other hand, activities like golf and bowling are unlikely to elicit a cardiovascular training effect, but are enjoyable and may yield health-related, as well as psychosocial, benefits.

Recreational activities

The inclusion of enjoyable recreational activities during (or immediately after) the endurance phase often enhances compliance with the exercise program. Rules of the games may need to be modified to adjust skill level requirements, competition, and to ensure safety. The outcome of the game (winning or losing) should be of lesser importance than the safety, participation and enjoyment of the patient. It is important to remember that recreational activities complement the endurance phase and should not consistently replace it. Recreational activities may also promote development or improvements in psychosocial health, by increasing the amount of social interaction.

Cool-down stage

At the end of the activity session, about 2–5 minutes of cool-down activities – slow walking and stretching exercises – are recommended to gradually return HR and BP toward resting levels. This period includes exercises of diminishing intensities; for example, slower walking or jogging, calisthenics and stretching exercises. This part of the exercise session is viewed as important in reducing the chance of a hypotensive episode after the exercise session, as well as other cardiovascular complications.[116]

Exercise prescription

Some basic exercise physiology principles should be kept in mind when designing an exercise program for burned patients. Two such principles are: the progressive overload principle, and the specificity principle. The progressive overload principle refers to the observation that a body system must be exercised at a level above which it is presently accustomed in order for a training effect to occur.[95] The system or tissue gradually adapts to this overload. The typical variables that comprise the overload include the intensity, duration and frequency (days per week) of exercise. The principle of specificity refers to the concept that the training effect is specific to the muscle fibers involved in the activity. Specificity also refers to the types of training in a very specific manner to produce a very specific adaptation or outcome. If a muscle is engaged in endurance types of exercise, the primary adaptations are in the capillary and mitochondrial number, which increase the aerobic capacity of the muscle. These principles are applicable to burned patients; however, it must be noted that a high intensity of exercise is not needed (low to moderate intensity) to achieve health-related benefits. On the other hand, to achieve athletic performance or competitive-related goals, moderate to high levels of intensity will be required. Another consideration that should be kept in mind when designing an exercise program is the age of the population. Prepubescent children are very different in their physiological and mental response to exercise training than postpubescent children. Older adults also have different health and physical problems than younger adults. It is for these reasons that medical exams, as well as exercise evaluations, are strongly recommended prior to starting an exercise program. It is beyond the scope of this chapter to address these differences and/or problems. However, general guidelines for both children are adults are offered and it is suggested to the reader to seek additional information for population-specific recommendations or position stands on exercise and physical activity, from associations such as the American College of Sports Medicine (http://www.acsm.org/publications/positionStands.htm), the American Academy of Pediatrics (http://www.aap.org/), the American Medical Association (http://www.ama-assn.org/) or the American Heart Association (http://www.americanheart.org/).

Aerobic training

Intensity: To improve aerobic fitness, generally the intensity of exercise should be between 65% and 95% of the peak heart rate or between 45% and 85% of the heart rate reserve (HRR).[117] The heart rate reserve is the difference between peak heart rate obtained during a CPET and resting heart rate. The range of heart rate values associated with the exercise intensity needed to induce an improvement in cardiovascular fitness is termed the 'target heart rate zone.'

The peak heart rate (HR$_{peak}$) is obtained from the CPET. However, when this not possible, one simple method to estimate HR$_{peak}$ is to use the formula (220 minus age).[95]

The rating of perceived exertion or (RPE) scale can also be used as a guideline in setting the intensity of exercise.[118] The RPE is a valuable and reliable indicator of exercise tolerance, but also intensity. This method of monitoring exercise intensity is useful when it is impossible to obtain a HR$_{peak}$ or if patients are on medications which affect heart rate such as β-blockers.

There are currently two RPE scales that are commonly used: the original or category scale, which rates exercise intensity on a scale of 6–20 and the revised or category-ratio scale of 0–10. It is reported that the category-ratio scale uses terminology better understood by the subject, thereby providing the tester with more valid information. It has been found that an aerobic training effect and the threshold for the start of anaerobic training are achieved at a rating of 'somewhat hard' to 'hard,' which approximates a rating of 12–16 on the category scale or 4–5 on the category-ratio scale.[119]

Finally, if a patient cannot use the heart rate method or the RPE method, the 'Talk Test' can also be used as a highly consistent method to set and monitor intensity of exercise.[120]

The 'Talk Test', or the point where speech first becomes difficult, approximates exercise intensity almost exactly equivalent to the ventilatory threshold. One could advise the patient to exercise at an intensity where speech is comfortable. When speech becomes uncomfortable, one can assume, based on previous studies, that exercise intensity is consistently above ventilatory threshold or above the desired intensity of exercise needed for general improvements in fitness.[120] It must be noted that when setting the exercise intensity, safety and effectiveness are linked. An appropriate intensity should also be well suited to result in a long-term, active lifestyle.

Duration: The duration of an aerobic exercise session is closely linked to the intensity of the activity: i.e. a longer duration of low-intensity exercise can be accomplished than a high-intensity exercise. In general, the duration of exercise for burned patients once discharged, should be from 5 to 20 minutes the first week. This will depend on the functional status of the patient and also pain tolerance.

If the patient tolerates up to 20 minutes, then this duration is appropriate. The objective should be to exercise 20–60 minutes of aerobic activity. This can be accomplished continuously or intermittently throughout the day, with a minimum of 10-minute bouts. Typically a duration of 20–30 minutes at between 40% and 50% to 85% of the heart rate reserve (excluding time for warm-up and cool-down) should induce health and fitness improvements.[113,121]

In burned patients with extremely low aerobic capacity or endurance, four to six; 5-minute bouts with rest periods between bouts would be a program that would induce benefits. The duration of the exercise sessions (or bouts) can be progressively increased over time. However, as mentioned before, a high intensity of exercise or very long duration of exercise are not needed to achieve health-related benefits, particularly during the initial stages of outpatient exercise rehabilitation.

Frequency: It is reported that deconditioned persons may improve cardiorespiratory fitness with only twice-weekly exercise.[113] However, it is generally agreed that optimal training frequency appears to be achieved with 3–5 workouts per week. The additional benefits of more frequent training appear to be minimal, whereas the incidence of lower extremity injuries increases abruptly. For those exercising at 60–80% HRR, an exercise frequency of 3 days per week is sufficient to improve or maintain VO$_{2peak}$. When exercising at the lower end of the intensity continuum, exercising more than 3 days per week is not deleterious. Patients with extremely low functional capacities may benefit from multiple, short (5 days per week) exercise sessions. Clearly, the number of exercise sessions per week will vary depending on the patient's limitations, but also by the patient and caregiver's lifestyle.

Mode: The most important consideration in choosing the mode of exercise for the endurance phase of the sessions is to engage large muscle groups in activities that are rhythmic or dynamic. The greatest improvements in aerobic fitness result when exercise involves the use of large muscle groups over appropriate periods of time (Figure 49.33). The mode of exercises includes treadmill walking/running, rowing or cycling. If no treadmill is available, then walk/jog at a track or field is appropriate. Swimming is also an appropriate mode of exercise, though closure of burn wounds should be ensured to minimize infection of wound or the contamination of others. Endurance games are also appropriate modes of exercise.

In the development of the exercise prescription for burned patients, it is suggested that the exercise begins with walking, or cycling. These two activities are easy to tolerate, are safe, intensity is easily set and gives the trainer a better ability to monitor progress for the first few weeks. In contrast, other individuals might progress at a faster rate through walking, jogging and cycling programs because of the nature of the burn, but also because of personality, previous athletic experience or psychosocial health. The risk of injury associated with high-impact activities or high-intensity weight training must also be considered when prescribing exercise modalities, especially for the burned individual. This is particularly important if the patient is overweight or novice. It may be desirable to have the patient participate in different exercise activities (cross-train) to reduce repetitive orthopedic stresses.

Progression of exercise

We recommend starting slowly and safely progressing in duration and intensity, but also in transitioning from early activities to activities that are more difficult to perform. This method of progression decreases the potential for inducing excessive muscle soreness, causing new injuries or aggravating old injuries. The emphasis on slow-to-moderate walking as the primary activity early in the fitness program is consistent with this recommendation, and the participant must be educated to not move too quickly into the more demanding activities. For example, if the individual can walk about 1–2 miles without

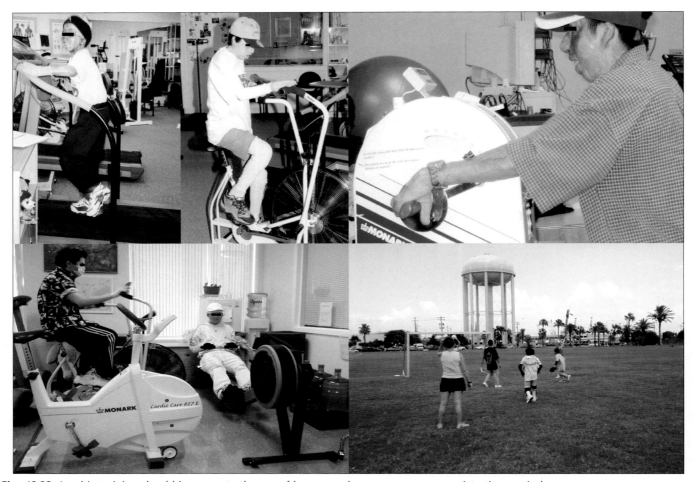

Fig. 49.33 Aerobic training should incorporate the use of large muscle groups over appropriate time periods.

fatigue, then the progression to a walk-jog or jogging program is a reasonable recommendation.

The recommended rate of progression in an exercise conditioning program depends on the functional capacity, medical and health status, pain tolerance, location of burns, age, individual activity preferences and goals, and an individual's tolerance to the current level of training. For burned patients, the endurance aspect of the exercise prescription can be divided into three stages of progression: initial, improvement, and maintenance.[96]

Initial conditioning stage

The initial stage should include light and moderate muscular endurance activities (for example, 40–60% of HRR). These exercises typically have a low potential for injury, and induce minimal muscle soreness and pain. Exercise adherence may be compromised if the level or intensity of exercises in the program is initiated too aggressively. The amount of time spent in this stage varies depending on the individual's adaptation to the exercise program. We recommend at least 4 weeks of initial conditioning. The duration of the exercise session during the initial stage may begin with approximately 15–20 minutes and progress up to 30 minutes, at least 3 times per week. Deconditioned individuals should be allowed more time for adaptation at each stage of conditioning. Age of the individual should also be taken into account when progressions are recommended, as adaptation to conditioning likely takes longer in older individuals, but also in extremely debilitated individuals.[113]

Improvement stage

The goal of the improvement stage of training is to provide a progressive increase in the overall exercise stimulus, which will allow for significant improvements in aerobic fitness. The improvement stage of the exercise-conditioning program differs from the initial stage in that the participant is progressed at a more rapid rate. This stage is reported to usually last from 4 to 5 months, during which intensity is progressively increased within the upper half of the target range of 50–85% of HRR. However, our experience in a 12-week training program in children 7–18 years of age indicates that after 3–4 weeks of initial conditioning, some patients are able to start the improvement stage. In this stage, duration may be increased consistently every 2–3 weeks until participants are able to exercise at a moderate-to-vigorous intensity for 20–30 minutes continuously. During this stage, interval training may also be beneficial, provided the total time engaged in moderate to vigorous exercise is at least 20 minutes.

Maintenance stage

The goal of this stage of training is the long-term maintenance of the cardiopulmonary fitness level developed during the improvement stage. This stage of the exercise program may begin at any time the participant has reached previously agreed objectives. During this stage, the individual may no longer be interested in continually increasing the conditioning stimulus. Also, in this stage, further improvement may be none to minimal, but continuing the same workout routine enables individuals to maintain their fitness levels, as well as develop the healthy exercise habit. At this point, it is suggested that goals of the program be re-examined and new goals or objectives set.

Resistive training

Strength is defined as the ability to produce force, and the ability to produce force over an extended period of time is referred to as muscular endurance. Both muscle strength and endurance impact activities of daily living (ADL) because ADL require a percentage of an individual's muscular capacity to perform these everyday tasks. Severe burns result in extensive and prolonged loss of muscle mass; therefore, resistance training, which increases LBM, should be part of an exercise rehabilitation program for burned individuals.[97,99]

Similarly to designing the aerobic portion of an exercise program, the resistive training portion of an exercise program follows similar principles of training. Both the overload principle and specificity principle are applicable. Strict rules of proper technique and safety must be observed to reduce potential for injury or accidents. A normal breathing pattern should be maintained, with breath holding avoided. Breath holding during lifting can induce excessive increases in blood pressure, which in individuals with hypertension, diabetes or other medical risks can be dangerous.

Similarly to the aerobic exercise program, testing or evaluation of muscle function precedes the resistive exercise program. This helps individuals identify problem areas, areas in need of required improvement, goal setting and tracking progress of individuals. In addition, muscle strength tests have value in determining back to work status.[122] Some of these tests involve peak to maximal muscular efforts. These tests can be done on weight machines or using dumbbells.

Typically these tests are done at 100% of one-repetition maximum (1RM), but can also be done at 3RM. For extremely deconditioned individuals or for very young children, modification of these guidelines can involve testing using 3RM up to 12RM if needed. An important point to remember is that safety of the individual is crucial. Therefore, correct technique during all testing and training must be observed. The order of exercises or muscle tested is also important. It is recommended that large muscle groups are tested first and alternate between upper body and lower body. For example, a 3RM test may be done in the following order of exercises: bench press, leg press (or squats), shoulder press, leg extension, biceps curl, leg curl, and triceps curl. The three repetitions maximum (3RM) load can be determined as follows. After an instruction period on correct weight-lifting technique, the patient or individual warms up with lever arm and bar (or wooden dowel) and is allowed to become familiar with the movement. After this, the patient lifts a weight that allows successful completion of four repetitions. If the fourth repetition is achieved successfully and with correct technique, a 1-minute resting period is allowed. After the resting period, a progressively increased amount of weight or load is instructed to be lifted at least four times. If the patient lifts a weight that allows successful completion of three repetitions, with the fourth repetition not being volitionally possible, because of fatigue or inability to maintain correct technique, the test is terminated and the amount of weight lifted from the successful set is recorded as their individual 3RM. This weight is then used to determine the amount of weight or load that will be used during the first 1–2 weeks (of for example, a 12-week program) as baseline loads.

Exercise type: There are many resistance-training exercises. However these can be divided into core exercises or assistance exercises. Core exercises recruit one or more large muscle group (for example, chest, shoulder and back). Assistance exercises typically recruit smaller muscle groups such as biceps, triceps, calves. A good program should typically involve both types of exercises.

Training frequency: The number of days to train varies according to the individual's training status. For severely burned individuals, we recommend 2–3 days per week of resistance training.

Type of contraction: Resistance exercise programs or exercises that emphasize accentuated lengthening or contractions (eccentric) are not recommended for severely burned individuals. These types of contractions have a high potential for acute delayed onset of muscle soreness, while having similar outcomes as concentric or isometric muscle contractions. The muscle soreness if severe enough has the potential for discouraging further participation in exercise activities. The movements during weightlifting should be rhythmic, done at moderate repetition duration.

Amount of load lifted: Commonly, a certain percentage of the 1RM or 3RM is used as guideline for choosing a training load. The amount of load lifted can be as much as 100% of 1RM or as little as lifting no load. We recommend initially during the first week of training, allowing the individual to become familiarized with the exercise equipment and to be instructed on proper weight-lifting techniques. Initially, the weight or load the subjects will lift should be set at 50–60% of their individual 3RM for 12–15 repetitions for the first 1–2 weeks. Thereafter, the load lifted can be increased to 70–75% (8–10 repetitions) of their individual 3 RM and continued for weeks 2 or 3 to week 6. After this, the training intensity can be increased to 75–85% (8–12 repetitions) of the 3RM and implemented from weeks 7–12 or longer. We must note that these are guidelines to provide an estimate of training load and have some limitations.[123] Another method of determining training load is to perform multiple RM based on the number of repetitions planned for the specific exercise. For example, if 8 repetitions were desired for biceps curl, then one would test the individual by having him or her perform 8RM testing sets.

Number of repetitions: It is believed that muscle strength and endurance can be obtained simultaneously by performing a specific number of repetitions within a certain range (for example 6–10 repetitions). The number of repetitions will depend on load lifted (% of 1RM) and also the objective or goals set at the start of the exercise program. However, we recommend 8–12 repetitions, at a moderate to high intensity to improve both muscle strength and endurance.[97]

Number of sets: There are very limited data in children as to whether 3 sets or 1 set is required to increase muscle strength and hypertrophy. Much of the adult-based literature supports similar responses of muscle strength, muscle endurance, hypertrophy between single and multiple set resistance training programs.[113,124–127] Finally, it is important to stress two points: (1), the difference in strength gains is typically more pronounced in trained individuals; and (2), both single and multiple training increased strength. The first point is usually not the case with burned patients, and the second point stresses the fact that an increase in strength is expected with resistance training compared to the standard of care in burned individuals.

Exercise order: There are many methods of ordering resistance exercises. One of these is to arrange core exercises, then assistance exercises.[128] Another method is to arrange large muscle groups and then small muscle groups.[129–131] Yet another method, which allows the individual to recover more fully between exercises, is to alternate upper body with lower body exercises. This is especially well suited for deconditioned individuals or untrained individuals.[129,130] For example, we have successfully implemented in severely burned children, the following order of resistive exercises: bench press, leg press or squats, shoulder press, leg extension, biceps curl, leg curl, triceps curl, and toe raises. These exercises can be done on variable resistance machines or free weights.[97] Both free weights, bands or variable resistance machines are appropriate for burned individuals wishing to participate in an exercise program (Figure 49.34).

Rest periods: As a general rule, it is important to allow enough time between exercises to perform the next exercise in proper form. The rest period also varies depending on the individual's training status and also specific training objectives.

Progressive overload: In order for improvements to continue over time, it is important to carefully monitor and chart the individual's workouts or loads lifted. Progressive overload can be applied in a variety of ways, such as increasing the weight lifted, increasing the repetitions while keeping load constant,

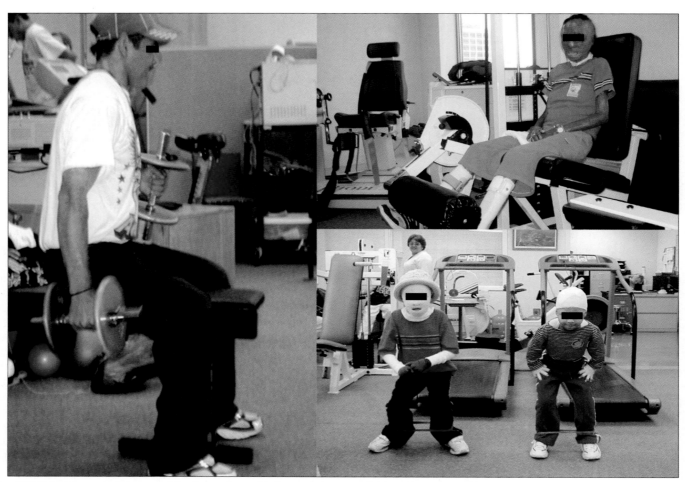

Fig. 49.34 Resistance training consists of exercises with free weights or variable resistance machines.

or decreasing rest periods. A conservative method termed '2-for-2 rule' is suggested. This rule states 'if an individual can perform two or more repetitions above his or her assigned repetitions goal in the last set, for two consecutive workouts for a specific exercise, then weight or load should be added to that specific exercise for the next training session.'[131] For example, if the assigned number of sets and repetitions is 3 sets of 8–12 reps in the chest press machine, and the individual performs 12 reps in all 3 sets, after several workout sessions (the specific number of sessions depends on many factors), the individual is able to complete 12 reps in the third set (i.e. the last set) for two consecutive workouts sessions, then in the following training session, the load for that exercise should be increased. The amount of weight (load) that should be added depends on factors such as the physical condition of the individual (strong or weak) and the body area (upper body or lower body). In general, an increase of 1–2 kilograms for a less trained, weaker individual is suggested for upper body exercises, while an increment of 2–4 kilograms is suggested for lower body exercises.[123]

Example of an exercise program

An example of our exercise rehabilitation program is described below (Table 49.1). The results of this program are published.[97–99] This program has been successfully implemented at discharge from hospital, but also at 6 months post burn.

Final considerations

- The ultimate goal of an exercise rehabilitation program should be to improve physical function. However, the way or the means in which this is achieved are also important. An exercise program should be challenging, effective, but also must be safe and fun. It should also promote lifelong healthy habits. This will maximize compliance with the exercise program.
- The American College of Sports Medicine (ACSM) has an extensive list of absolute and relative contraindications to exercise and exercise testing that should be carefully considered when designing an exercise program for adults or children. These contraindications will also pertain to individuals with severe burns.
- Individual goals should be established early in the exercise program. Whenever possible, they should be developed by the participant with the guidance of an exercise professional. The goals or objectives must be realistic, and an intrinsic or extrinsic rewards system should be implemented at that time.
- It is recommended that exercise professionals work together with an occupational and/or physical therapist to avoid duplication of services, as well as to identify areas in need of special attention.
- Based on our clinical experience with children and adolescent patients, individuals with severe burns should participate, as soon as possible after hospital discharge, in a structured exercise program. This program should be supervised and if possible conducted in the presence of a trained professional. However, if this is not possible, the exercise program, with some commonsense guidelines, should offer a choice for safe and effective participation.

TABLE 49.1 BRIEF DESCRIPTION OF THE SHRINERS HOSPITALS FOR CHILDREN-GALVESTON HOSPITAL OUTPATIENT EXERCISE REHABILITATION PROGRAM	
Aerobic workout	
Intensity	70–85% of each individual's previously determined individual peak aerobic capacity. However, heart rate and rated perceived exertion is obtained at regular intervals during aerobic exercise
Duration	20–40 minutes
Frequency	3–5 days per week
Mode	Aerobic exercise on treadmills, cycle ergometers, arm ergometers, rowing machines, and outdoor activities such as soccer or kickball
Resistance workout	
Exercise type	Upper and lower body of core and assistance exercises
Amount of load lifted and number of repetitions	The weight or load lifted set at approximately 50–60% of each individual 3RM and lifted for 4–10 repetitions for three sets. During the second week, the lifting load, increased to 70–75% (3 sets, 4–10 repetitions) of their individual 3RM and continued for weeks 2–6. After this, training intensity is increased to 80–85% (3 sets, 8–12 repetitions) of the 3RM and implemented from weeks 7–12
Number of sets	3 sets
Exercise order	Bench press, leg press or squats, shoulder press, biceps curl, leg curl, triceps curl, toe raises, and abdominals
Type of exercises	Eight basic resistance exercises done using variable-resistance machines or free weights: 4 for upper body, 3 for lower body, and abdominals
Rest period	A rest interval of approximately 1 minute between sets

Note: Each exercise training session consisted of resistance and aerobic exercises, with aerobic exercise preceding resistance exercise. This outpatient exercise program is supplemented with outpatient physical and occupational therapy.

- For adults, a careful medical and exercise evaluation should be conducted prior to starting an exercise program. Cardiovascular or pulmonary problems, as well as other conditions, such as diabetes, must be identified prior to starting an exercise program to avoid potential fatal or near-fatal complications.
- It is important to get the burned individual started with an exercise program or a more active lifestyle as soon as possible, but it is never too late to get started, regardless of the time post burn.
- When beginning the exercise program, it is better to start slowly and build up gradually, than to start too fast and risk injury.
- For children, avoid using very intense or maximal (1RM) resistance training or testing. Gradual progression is of utmost importance to avoid injury and to promote exercise adherence.
- The individual should 'listen' to his or her body. During and after workouts, the individual (and supervisor) should be alert to signs of a potential health problem as a result of overexertion. Signs may include pain, shortness of breath, dizziness or nausea.
- Be flexible and allow individuals to be flexible. Don't rigidly stick to a schedule if the patient doesn't feel up to it. If he or she is overly tired or under the weather, allow them to take a day or two off.
- Monitor the individual's progress. Reassess fitness every 6 weeks. You may notice that you need to increase the amount of time you exercise in order to continue improving (if part of the original goals).
- The exercise professional or individual should keep an exercise diary or logbook to help chart progress.
- If the patient loses motivation, try setting new goals or try a new activity (or activities). Sometimes, bringing a friend or family member into the program may help in motivation. Incorporate variety into the exercise routine.
- Lastly, work on conveying to the patient or client that a fun and safe exercise program can result in maintenance of lifelong physical, as well as psychosocial, healthy habits (Figure 49.35).

Patient and/or caregiver education

When patients are being discharged from the acute hospital stay, it is vital that they leave with an individualized home exercise program. In addition, splinting and positioning exercises, activity or daily living performance, scar control measures, and psychosocial issues should be addressed. This

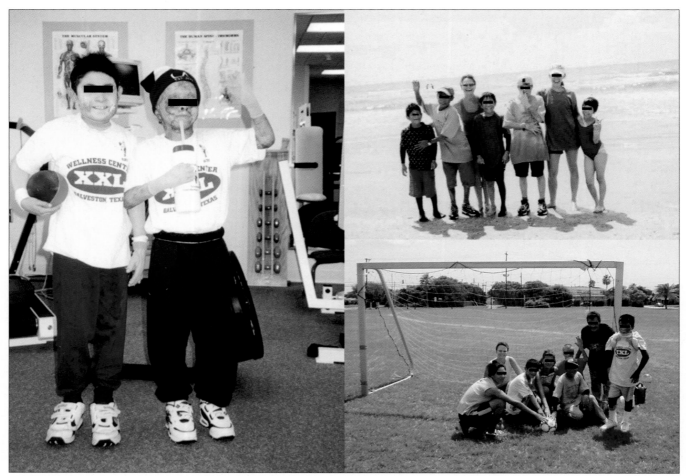

Fig. 49.35 Overall long-term burn rehabilitation should result in lifelong physical as well as psychosocial healthy habits and improvements in quality of life.

program can then be updated and upgraded to allow for progression during the ever-changing phases that the burned individual goes through, in what may be in excess of a 2-year recovery period. During follow-up visits, screening and monitoring of the patient's progress regarding the above categories is performed and the necessary changes are completed. This detailed knowledge of the patient's status will allow the burn team to coordinate the care for the patient so that recommendations can be followed through. Providing the patients with a checklist is a valuable tool to enable patients to assume some control of the rehabilitation process, enable them to track their progress and encourage their continuation of the program. Many patients and their caregivers are often overwhelmed by the rehabilitation program. It takes an extraordinary amount of time and energy to plan and participate in a home exercise/instruction program. Continuous communication among the patient, caregiver and the burn team will ease the patient's transition into recovery.

One way of helping patients with the exercise program is to establish communication with a community-based exercise center, such as a commercial or hospital-based facility. Often, direct and constant communication between a burn hospital's physical therapist, exercise physiologists and/or physician and the community-based exercise facility will maximize the potential for adherence to and the efficacy of such 'home' exercise programs, by adding supervision and structure.

Summary

The rehabilitation after a severe burn, although challenging, can be rewarding to the rehabilitation team. The medical staff must continuously evaluate the interventions provided to ensure each patient's maximum functional outcome. Through experience, education and research, the production of therapeutic interventions that will enhance each patient's recovery and will provide them with a more meaningful, productive life will be made possible.

References

1. Fess EE, Philips CA. Hand splinting — principles and methods, 2nd edn. St Louis: CV Mosby; 1987:125–254.
2. Harries CA, Pegg SP. Foam ear protectors for burned ears. J Burn Care Rehabil 1989; 10:183–184.
3. Ridgway CL, Warden GD. Evaluation of a vertical mouth stretching orthosis: two case reports. J Burn Care Rehabil 1995; 16.1:74–78.
4. Taylor LB, Walker J. A review of selected microstomia prevention appliances. Pediatr Dent 1997; 19:413–418.
5. Heinle JA, Kealey GP, Cram AE, et al. The microstomia prevention appliance: 14 years of clinical experience. J Burn Care Rehabil 1988; 9.1:90–91.
6. Maragakis GM, Tempone MG. Microstomia following facial burns. J Clin Pediatr Dent 1999; 23:69–73.
7. Sykes L. Scar traction appliance for a patient with microstomia: a clinical report. J Prosthet Dent 1996; 76(1):464–465.
8. Rivers, et al. The transparent face mask. Am J Occup Ther 1979; 33:108–113.
9. Linares HA, Larson DL, Willis-Galstraun B. Historical notes on the use of pressure in the treatment of hypertrophic scar and keloids. Burns 1993; 19(1):17–21.
10. Malick MH, Carr JA. Manual on management of the burned patient, including splinting, mold and pressure techniques. Pittsburgh: Harmarville Rehabilitation Center; 1982.
11. Leman CJ. Splints and accessories following burn reconstruction. Clin Plast Surg 1992; 19(3):721–731.
12. Walters CJ. Splinting the burn patient. Laurel, Maryland: RAMSCO; 1987.
13. Richard R, Stalay M. Burn care and rehabilitation principles and practice. Philadelphia: FA Davis; 1994:Ch 11, 242–323.
14. Richard RL. Use of the dynasplint to correct elbow flexion contracture: a case report. J Burn Care Rehabil 1986; 7:151–152.
15. Ward RS, Schnebly WA, Kravitz M, et al. Have you tried the sandwich splint? A method of preventing hand deformities in children. J Burn Care Rehabil 1989; 10:83–85.
16. Calhoun JH, Evans EB, Herndon DN. Techniques for the management of burn contractures with the Ilizarov fixator. Clin Orthop Rel Res 1993; 280:117–124.
17. Harnar T, Engrav L, Marvin J, et al. Dr Paul Unna's boot and early ambulation after skin grafting of the leg. Plast Reconstr Surg 1982; 69:359–360.
18. Delta Cast: M Daugherty-Vancouver 04.
19. Bennett GB. Serial casting: a method of treating burn contractures. J Burn Care Rehabil 1989; 10(6):543–545.
20. Ridgway CL, Daugherty MB, Warden GD. Serial casting as a technique to correct burn scar contractures: a case report. J Burn Care Rehabil 1991; 12:67–72.
21. Larson DL, Evans EB, Abston S, et al. Skeletal suspension and traction in the treatment of burns. Ann Surg 1986; 168(6):981–985.
22. Evans EB. Orthopedic measures in the treatment of severe burns. J Bone Joint Surg Am 1966; 48:643–669.
23. Evans EB, Larson DL, Abston S, et al. Prevention and correction of deformity after severe burns. Surg Clin North Am 1979; 50(6):136–175.
24. Evans EB, Larson DL, Yates S. Preservation and restoration of joint function in patients with severe burns. JAMA 1968; 204:843–848.
25. Harnar T, Engrav L, Heimbach D, et al. Experience with skeletal immobilization after excision and grafting of the severely burned hands. J Trauma 1985; 25:299–302.
26. Youel L, Evans EB, Heare TC, et al. Skeletal suspension in the management of severe burns in children. J Bone Joint Surg Am 1986; 68:1375–1379.
27. Bowker JH. In: Michael JWM, ed. Atlas of limb prosthetics: surgical prosthetic and rehabilitation principles. St Louis, MO: CV Mosby; 1992.
28. Pritham CH. Cumulative volume of clinical orthotics and prosthetics. Alexandria, VA: The American Academy of Orthotists and Prosthetists; 1988:8(3)–12(3).
29. Fletchall S, Tran T, Ungarao V, et al. Updating upper extremity temporary prosthetics. Thermoplastics. J Burn Care Rehabil 1992; 13:584–6.
30. O'Sullivan SB, Schmitz TJ. Physical rehabilitation assessment and treatment, 3rd edn. Orthotic assessment and management. Philadelphia: FA Davis; 1994:Ch 30, 655–684.
31. Stedman's medical dictionary, 23rd edn. Baltimore: Williams and Wilkins; 1976.
32. Linares HA, Larson DL, Willis-Galstraun B. Historical notes on the use of pressure in the treatment of hypertrophic scars and keloids. Burns 1993; 19(2):17–21.
33. Ward RS. Pressure therapy for the control of hypertrophic scar formation after burn injury, a history and review. J Burn Care Rehabil 1991; 12(3):257–262.
34. Linares HA. Hypertrophic healing: controversies and etiopathogenic review. In: Carvajal HF, Parks DH, eds. Burns in children: pediatric burn management. Chicago: Yearbook Medical; 1988:305–323.
35. Shakespeare PG, Renterghem L. Some observations on the surface structure of collagen in hypertrophic scars. Burns 1985; 11:175:180.
36. Hayakawa T, Hino M, Fuyamada H, et al. Lysyl oxidase activity in human normal skins and post-burn scars. Clin Chim Acta 1976; 7:245–250.

37. Hayakawa T, Hino M, Fuyamada H, et al. Prolyl hydroxylase activity in human normal skins and post-burn scars. Clin Chim Acta 1977; 75:137–142.

38. Hayakawa T, Hashimoto Y, Myokei Y, et al. Changes in type of collagen during the development of human post-burn hypertrophic scars. Clin Chim Acta 1979; 93:119–125.

39. Hayakawa T, Hashimoto Y, Myokei Y, et al. The effects of skin grafts on the ratio of collagen types in human post-burn wound tissues. Connect Tissue Res 1982; 9:249–252.

40. Abston S. Scar reaction after thermal injury and prevention of scars and contractures. In: Boswick JA, ed. The art and science of burn care. Rockville: Aspen; 1987; 360–361.

41. Staley M, Richard R. Burn care and rehabilitation principles and practice. Philadelphia: FA Davis; 1994:Ch 14, 380–418.

42. Reid WH, Evans JH, Naismith RS, et al. Hypertrophic scarring and pressure therapy. Burns 1987; 13 (Suppl):S29.

43. Hambleton J, Shakespeare PG, Pratt BJ. The progress of hypertrophic scars monitored by ultrasound measurements of thickness. Burns 1992; 18(4):301–307.

44. Darvey RB, Sprod RT, Neild TO. Computerized colour: a technique for the assessment of burn scar hypertrophy. A preliminary report. Burns 1999; 25(3):207–213.

45. Esposito G, Ziccardi P, Scioli M, et al. The use of a modified tonometer in burn scar therapy. J Burn Care Rehabil 1990; 11:86–90.

46. Bartell TH, Monafo WW, Mustoe TA. A new instrument for serial measurement of elasticity in hypertrophic scar. J Burn Care Rehabil 1988; 9:657–660.

47. Sullivan T, Smith J, Kermode J, et al. Rating the burn scar. J Burn Care Rehabil 1990; 11:256–260.

48. Hosoda G, Holloway GA, Heimback DM. Laser Doppler flowmetry for the early detection of hypertrophic burn scars. J Burn Care Rehabil 1986; 7:490–497.

49. Berry RB, Tan OT, Cooke ED, et al. Transcutaneous oxygen tension as an index of maturity in hypertrophic scars treated by compression. Br J Plast Surg 1985; 38:163–173.

50. Reid WH, Evans JH, Naismith RS, et al. Hypertrophic scarring and pressure therapy. Burns 1987; 13(Suppl):S29.

51. McDonald WS, Deitch EA. Hypertrophic skin grafts in burn patients: a prospective analysis of variables. J Trauma 1987; 27:147–150.

52. Kealey GP, Jensen KL, Laubenthal KN, et al. Prospective randomized comparison of two types of pressure therapy garments. J Burn Care Rehabil 1990; 11:334–336.

53. Hubbard M, Masters IB, Williams GR, et al. Severe obstructive sleep apnoea secondary to pressure garments used in the treatment of hypertrophic burn scars. Eur Respir J 2000; 16:1205–1207.

54. Sawada Y. A method of recording and objective assessment of hypertrophic burn scars. Burns 1994; 20:76–78.

55. Cheng JC, Evans JH, Leung KS, et al. Pressure therapy in the treatment of post-burn hypertrophic scar — a critical look into its usefulness and fallacies by pressure monitoring. Burns Incl Therm Inj 1984; 10:154–163.

56. Leung KS, Cheng JC, Ma GF, et al. Complications of pressure therapy for post-burn hypertrophic scars. Biomechanical analysis based on 5 patients. Burns Incl Therm Inj 1984; 10:434–438.

57. Reid WH, Evans JH, Naismith RS, et al. Hypertrophic scarring and pressure therapy. Burns Incl Therm Inj 1987; 13(Suppl): S29–S32.

58. Stewart R, Bhagwanjee AM, Mbakaza Y, et al. Pressure garment adherence in adult patients with burn injuries: an analysis of patient and clinician perceptions. Am J Occup Ther 2000; 54:598–606.

59. Perkins K, Davey RB, Wallis K. Current materials and techniques used in burn scar management program. Burns Incl Therm Inj 1987; 13:406–410.

60. Staley MJ, Richard RL. Use of pressure to treat hypertrophic burn scars. Adv Wound Care 1997; 10:44–46.

61. Van den Kerckhove E, Stappaerts K, Fieuws S, et al. The assessment of erythema and thickness on burn related scars during pressure garment therapy as a preventative measure for hypertrophic scarring. Burns 2005; 31:696–702.

62. Macintyre L, Baird M. Pressure garments for use in the treatment of hypertrophic scars — a review of the problems associated with their use. Burns 2006; 32:10–15.

63. Puzey G. The use of pressure garments on hypertrophic scars. J Tissue Viability 2002; 12:11–15.

64. Linares HA, Larson DL, Willis-Galstaun BA. Historical notes on the use of pressure in the treatment of hypertrophic scars or keloids. Burns 1993; 19:17–21.

65. Giele HP, Liddiard K, Currie K, et al. Direct measurement of cutaneous pressures generated by pressure garments. Burns 1997; 23:137–141.

66. Larson DL, Abston S, Willis B, et al. Contracture and scar formation in the burn patient. Clin Plast Surg 1974; 1:653–656.

67. Robertson JC, Hodgson B, Druett JE, et al. Pressure therapy for hypertrophic scarring: preliminary communication. J R Soc Med 1980; 73:348–354.

68. Fricke NB, Omnell ML, Dutcher KA, et al. Skeletal and dental disturbances after facial burns and pressure garments use: a 4 year follow-up. J Burn Care Rehabil 1999; 20:239–249.

69. Fricke NB, Omnell ML, Dutcher KA, et al. Skeletal and dental disturbances in children after facial burns and pressure garments. J Burn Care Rehabil 1996; 17:338–345.

70. Groce A, Meyers-Paal R, Herndon DH, et al. Are your thoughts of facial pressure transparent? J Burn Care Rehabil 1999; 20:478–481.

71. Engrav LH, et al. Do splinting and pressure devices damage new grafts? J Burn Care Rehabil 1983; 4:107–108.

72. Rose MP, Deitch GA. The effective use of a tubular compression bandage, Tubigrip, for burn scar therapy in the growing child. J Burn Care Rehabil 1983; 4:197–201.

73. Cheng, JCY, Evans JH, Leung KS, et al. Pressure therapy in the treatment of post-burn hypertrophic scar — a critical look into its usefulness and fallacies by pressure monitoring. Burns Incl Therm Inj 1984; 10:154–163.

74. Thompson R, Summers S, Rampey-Dobbs R, et al. Color pressure garments vs traditional beige pressure garments: perceptions from the public. J Burn Care Rehabil 1992; 13:590–596.

75. Ward RS. Reasons for the selection of burn-scar-support suppliers by burn centers in the United States: a survey. J Burn Care Rehabil 1993; 14(3):360–367.

76. Van den Kerckhove E, Boechx W, Kochreyt A. Silicone patches as a supplement for pressure therapy to control hypertrophic scarring. J Burn Care Rehabil 1991; 12(4):361–369.

77. McNee S. The use of silicone gel in the control of hypertrophic scarring. Physiotherapy 1990; 76:194–197.

78. Quinn KJ. Silicone gel in scar treatment. Burns 1987; 13:533–540.

79. Derwin-Baruch L. UVA therapists meet the challenge of scar management. OT Week 1993; April 15:15–17.

80. Rivers EA, Strate RG, Solem LD. The transparent facemask. Am J Occup Ther 1979; 33:108–113.

81. Gallagher J, Goldfarb W, Slater H, et al. Survey of treatment modalities for the prevention and treatment of hypertrophic burn scars. J Burn Care Rehabil 1990; 11(2):118–120.

82. Miles WK, Grigsby de Linde L. Remodeling of scar tissue in the burned hand. In: Hunter JM, et al. eds. Rehabilitation of the hand, 4th edn. St. Louis, CV: Mosby; 1995:Vol II, 1267–1294.

83. Wood EC. Beard's massage: principles and techniques, 2nd edn. Philadelphia: WB Saunders; 1974:48–59.

84. Huruitz S. The sun and sunscreen protection: recommendations for children. J Dermatol Surg Oncol 1988; 14(6):657–660.

85. Licht S. History. In: Baasmajian JV, ed. Therapeutic exercise, 4th edn. Baltimore, MD: Williams & Wilkins; 1984:Ch 1.

86. Johnson CL. The role of physical therapy. In: Boswick JA, ed. The art and science of burn care. Rockville: Aspen; 1987:Ch 34, 304.

87. Robson MC, Smith DJ, VanderZee AJ, et al. Making the burned hand functional. Clin Plast Surg 1992; 19(3):663–671.

88. Fisher SV, Helm PA. Rehabilitation of the patient with burns. In: DeLisa, Gans, Currie, et al. eds Rehabilitation medicine principles and practice, 2nd edn. Philadelphia: JB Lippincott; 1993:Ch 53.

89. Salter RB, Hamilton HW, Wedge JH, et al. Clinical application of basic research on continuous passive motion for disorders and injuries of synovial joints: a preliminary report. J Orthop Res 1983; 1(3):325–342.

90. Lynch JA. Continuous passive motion: a prophylaxis for deep vein thrombosis following total knee replacement. Orthop Trans 1984; 8(3):400.

91. Harden NG, Luster SH. Rehabilitation considerations in the care of the acute burn patient. Crit Care Nurs Clin North Am 1991; 3(2):245–253.

92. Pessina MA, Ellis SM. Burn management. Rehabilitation. Nurs Clin North Am 1997; 32(2):365–374.

93. Trees DW, Ketelsen CA, Hobbs JA. Use of a modified tilt table for preambulation strength training as an adjunct to burn rehabilitation: a case series. J Burn Care Rehabil 2003; 24(2):97–103.

94. Chang AT, Boots R, Hodges PW, et al. Standing with assistance of a tilt table in intensive care: a survey of Australian physiotherapy practice. Aust J Physiother 2004; 50(1):51–54.

95. Franklin BA. General principles of exercise prescription. ACSM's guidelines for exercise testing and prescription. Philadelphia: Lippincott Williams & Wilkins; 2006.

96. Wallace J, Kaminsky LA. Principles of cardiorespiratory endurance programming. ACSM's resource manual for guidelines for exercise testing and prescription. Philadelphia: Lippincott Williams & Wilkins; 2006:336–349.

97. Suman OE, Spies RJ, Celis MM, et al. Effects of a 12-wk resistance exercise program on skeletal muscle strength in children with burn injuries. J Appl Physiol 2001; 91(3):1168–1175.

98. Suman OE, Mlcak RP, Herndon DN. Effect of exercise training on pulmonary function in children with thermal injury.' J Burn Care Rehabil 2002; 23(4):288–293; discussion 287.

99. Suman OE, Thomas SJ, Wilkins JP, et al. Effect of exogenous growth hormone and exercise on lean mass and muscle function in children with burns. J Appl Physiol 2003; 94(6):2273–2281.

100. The American Academy of Pediatrics. Strength training by children and adolescents. Pediatrics 2001; 107(6):1470–1472.

101. America Academy of Pediatrics Committee on Sports Medicine. Risks in distance running for children. Pediatrics 1990; 86(5): 799–800.

102. Baechle TR, Earle RW, Wathen D, eds. Resistance training in essentials of strength training and conditioning; National Strength and Conditioning Association. Hong Kong: Human Kinetics; 2000; 395–425.

103. Baechle TR, Earle RW. Resistance training. Essentials of strength training and conditioning. Hong Kong: Human Kinetics; 2000: 395–425.

104. Adams RB, Tribble GC, Tafel AC, et al. Cardiovascular rehabilitation of patients with burns. J Burn Care Rehabil 1990; 11(3):246–255.

105. Physical activity readiness questionnaire (Par-Q) and you. Gloucester, Ontario: Canadian Society for Exercise Physiology; 1994:1–2.

106. Kriska AM, Caspersen CJ. Introduction to a collection of physical activity questionnaires. Medicine Sci Sports Exerc 1997; 29(6)Suppl:29(26):25–29.

107. Sallis JF, Strikmiller PK, Harsha DW, et al. Validation of interviewer- and self-administered physical activity checklists for fifth grade students. Med Sci Sports Exerc 1996; 28(7):840–851.

108. Noble BJ, Borg GA, Jacobs I, et al. A category-ration perceived exertion scale: relationship to blood and muscle lactates and heart rate. Med Sci Sports Exerc 1983; 15(6):523–528.

109. Borg G. Borg's perceived exertion and pain scales. Champaign: Human Kinetics; 1998.

110. Cucuzzo NA, Ferrando A, Herndon DN. The effects of exercise programming vs traditional outpatient therapy in the rehabilitation of severely burned children. J Burn Care Rehabil 2001; 22(3):2120–2124.

111. Roberts L, Alvarado MI, McElroy K, et al. Longitudinal hand grip and pinch strength recovery in the child with burns. J Burn Care Rehabil 1993; 14(1):99–101.

112. Rowland TW. Aerobic exercise testing protocols. In: Rowland TW, ed. Pediatric laboratory exercise testing: clinical guidelines. Champaign: Human Kinetics; 1993:19–42.

113. American College of Sports Medicine Position Stand. The recommended quantity and quality of exercise for developing and maintaining cardiorespiratory and muscular fitness, and flexibility in healthy adults. Med Sci Sports Exerc 1998; 30(6):975–991.

114. Kokkonen J, Nelson AG, Cornwell A. Acute muscle stretching inhibits maximal strength performance. Res Q Exerc Sport 1998; 69(4):411–415.

115. Behm DG, Button DC, Butt JC. Factors affecting force loss with prolonged stretching. Can J Appl Physiol 2000; (3):261–272.

116. Haskell WL. Cardiovascular complications during exercise training of cardiac patients. Circulation 1978; 57(5):920–924.

117. Howley ET. Type of activity: resistance, aerobic and leisure versus occupational physical activity. Med Sci Sports Exerc 2001; 33(6 Suppl):S364–S369; discussion S419–S420.

118. Borg G, Hassmen P, Langerstrom M. Perceived exertion related to heart rate and blood lactate during arm and leg exercise. Eur J Appl Physiol Occup Physiol 1987; 56(6):679–685.

119. Foster C, Florhaug JA, Franklin J, et al. A new approach to monitoring exercise training. J Strength Cond Res 2001; 15(1):109–115.

120. Persinger R, Foster C, Gibson M, et al. Consistency of the talk test for exercise prescription. Med Sci Sports Exerc 2004; 36(9): 1632–1636.

121. Welsch MA, Pollock ML, Brechue WF, et al. Using the exercise test to develop the exercise prescription in health and disease. Prim Care 1994; 21(3):589–609.

122. Cronan T, Hammond J, Ward CG. The value of isokinetic exercise and testing in burn rehabilitation and determination of back-to-work status. J Burn Care Rehabil 1990; 11(3):224–227.

123. Baechle TR, Earle RW, Wathen D, et al. Resistance training. Essentials of strength training and conditioning. Hong Kong: Human Kinetics; 2000:395–425.

124. Stone MH, Fleck, SJ, Triplett NT, et al. Health- and performance-related potential of resistance training. Sports Med 1991; 11(4): 210–231.

125. Carpinelli RN, Otto RM. Strength training. Single versus multiple sets. Sports Med 1998; 26(2):73–84.

126. Faigenbaum AD, Pollock ML. Prescription for resistance training in health and disease. Med Sci Sports Exerc 1999; 31:38–45.

127. Hass CJ, Garzarella L, de Hoyos D, et al. Single versus multiple sets in long-term recreational weightlifters. Med Sci Sports Exerc 2000; 32(1):235–242.

128. Stone MH, Wilson GD. Resistive training and selected effects. Med Clin North Am 1985; 69(1):109–122.

129. Pauletto B. Choice and order of exercise. NSCA J 1986; 8(2):71–73.

130. Fleck SJ, Kraemer WJ. Designing resistance training programs. Champaign: Human Kinetics; 1997.

131. Baechle TR, Groves BR. Weight training: steps to success. Champaign: Human Kinetics; 1998.

Chapter 50

Musculoskeletal changes secondary to thermal burns

E. Burke Evans

Among trauma states the burn is alone in the ability and tendency of its wound, even as it heals, to create major musculoskeletal deformity. In addition, the protracted burn illness which accompanies severe burns may result in other skeletal change. Box 50.1 presents a classification of musculoskeletal changes secondary to burns; from that, the most commonly occurring and clinically significant alterations have been selected for discussion in detail.

Changes confined to bone

Osteoporosis

Osteoporosis is the most frequently occurring postburn change involving the bone. In Shiele's radiographic study of patients with burns confined to the upper extremities, osteoporosis was found in 24 of 70 patients.[1] Klein's ongoing studies suggest that, among persons with serious burns, reduction of bone mass density is pervasive.[2] Stated causes of osteoporosis in thermal burns are bed confinement, immobilization, hyperemia,[3] reflex vasomotor phenomena,[4] and adrenocortical hyperactivity.[5] In Chapter 27 of this book, Klein thoroughly reviews the effects of burn injury on bone metabolism.[2,6] In this section only what is clinically apparent will be discussed.

The more extensive the burn and the greater the number of complications, the longer the patient will be bed confined and relatively immobile. It is easy to understand that the onset of osteoporosis might be accelerated and its intensity more marked in the burn illness which features a hypermetabolic state. If a single extremity of an otherwise normal person is immobilized for a long period of time because of local trauma, as with a fracture, the bones of that extremity will lose mineral to a degree that loss of density can be easily seen in a plain radiograph. So with burns isolated to the extremities, the bones of the affected extremities become osteoporotic; and, in persons with generalized burns, the bones of deeply burned

extremities may show more profound mineral loss than is observed in non-burned extremities or in the axial skeleton (Figure 50.1). Van Der Wiel et al.[7] found in an x-ray absorptiometry study of 16 adults with fractures of one tibia that there was eventual loss of bone mineral density in the contralateral femur and in the lumbar spine, but to a lesser degree than in the ipsilateral femur. These findings, though not strictly analogous to those observed in burns, nevertheless point to the occurrence of generalized osteoporosis in other trauma states and the difference in loss of bone density relative to local factors. In fractures or in burns, impaired mobility and local hyperemia could account for this difference.

Another characteristic of the osteoporosis of burns that seems to set it apart is its persistence, not just until restoration of the anabolic state, but for months and years after the burn has healed (Figure 50.2). This phenomenon may be most clearly observed in patients who have survived 90% burns, but Klein records less than normal bone among even moderately burned children as long as 17 months after injury.[2] It seems obvious that muscle atrophy and/or the failure or inability of the person to return to the preburn level of physical activity surely account in part for this protracted state of reduced bone mineralization.

Probably there is no way to prevent osteoporosis in any patient whose burn is of such severity as to require an extended period of bed confinement. On the other hand, the advance of bone atrophy can at least be favorably modified even among patients with large burns if mobilization and active exercise are initiated soon after the burn. The bones of the axial skeleton, the pelvis, and the lower extremities are most efficiently stressed by weight bearing. Thus, standing is a priority measure. Muscle contraction alone may help to forestall bone atrophy and bone is better stressed if the contraction is resisted. Incrementally increasing resistance during motion or at the termination of an arc of motion or to muscle contraction in an extremity which may not be moved can be supplied by anyone who attends the patient. Isometric muscle contraction can be exacted from even seriously burned patients and is important for bone stress, for maintaining muscle tone and bulk, and for the patient's continuing ready identification of the affected extremity. Passive motion has little or no effect on bone and thus does not figure in the prevention of osteoporosis. Other preventive measures, e.g. closure of the wound and maintenance of nutrition, are routine in critical burn care. Treatment of established osteoporosis involves the more aggressive employment of measures for prevention. There are no long-term studies, however, which persuasively measure the

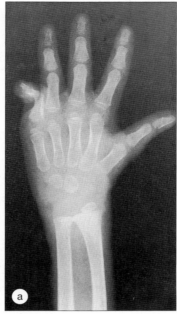 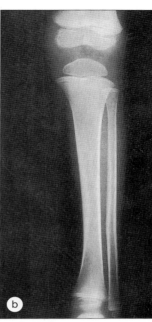

Fig. 50.1 (a) Six months after injury there is the coarsened trabeculation of marked osteoporosis of bones of the left hand and forearm of a 4-year-old male whose 70% full-thickness burn involved head, chest, and both upper extremities. (b) A roentgenogram of the left tibia and fibula obtained on the same date as that of the hand shows minimal atrophy.

effectiveness of exercise, diet, medication, or modality in the treatment of osteoporosis in any state.

Osteomyelitis

In burns, bones can become infected by exposure of bone by the burn; by an open fracture accompanying the burn; by extension of infection from a septic joint, introduction of organisms along traction pins, internal fracture fixation devices; or by blood-borne organisms of bacteremia. Considering the apparent great liability of seriously burned patients for developing osteomyelitis, it is surprising that it does not regularly occur. As it turns out, clinically significant osteomyelitis in burned patients is rare. Antibiotics given for the general state may prevent seeding of the bone or may repress any small focus of bone infection.

The cortex of long bones is a good barrier to surface organisms. Even exposure of cortex will have little adverse effects if the blood supply of the bone remains intact. Prolonged exposure will kill the outer layer of the cortex, which will in time sequestrate, separating at a well-defined cleft between dead and living bone. With minor or moderate exposure, the bone will usually survive long enough for bordering granulation tissue to cover it. For larger defects, it is common practice to drill closely spaced holes through the exposed cortex so as to encourage buds of granulation tissue to emerge from the still vascular medullary canal. Another way to encourage granulation tissue formation over exposed bone is with decortication with an osteotome or burr to expose the capillaries of the inner cortex. With these practices, there seems to be little risk of infecting the bone, no matter how contaminated the rest of the limb. It may be that there is sufficient centripetal pressure to discourage the invasion of organisms when the holes are fresh and that the holes are rapidly sealed by blood clot and advancing tissue. There are no reports of deep bone infection related to cortex drilling.

With open fractures which remain at the base of part of a major soft tissue burn wound, bone infection is probaby inevitable. Even so, the infection tends to remain at the fracture site and not to involve the rest of the bone, so that local dedridement and stabilization of the soft tissue wound are all that are required for treatment. Dowling reported osteomyelitis of the tibia related to an open bimalleolar fracture in an extensively burned extremity.[8] On the other hand, osteomyelitis developed in neither of the two open fractures reported separately by Choctaw[9] and Wang.[10] Three patients have been treated in whom open fractures of the femur complicated thigh burns. Each case required aggressive and repeated debridement. One fracture was treated in traction, while the other two were treated with external fixators. In one of the patients

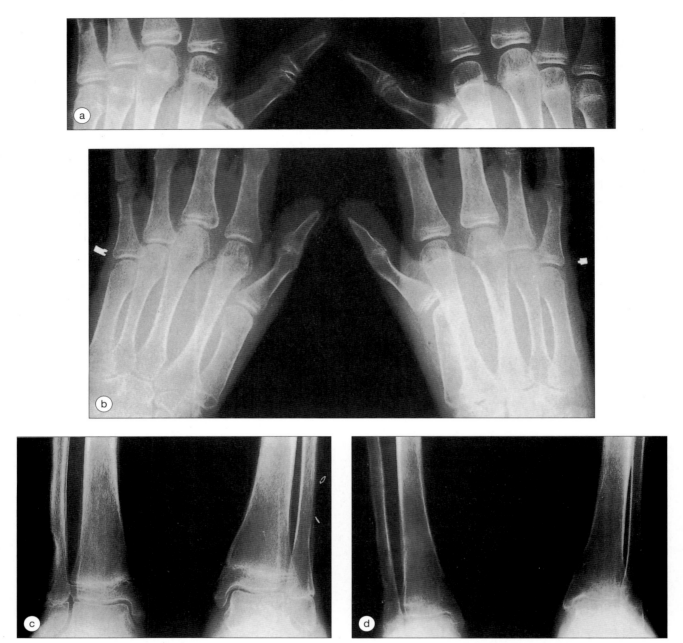

Fig. 50.2 (a) Advanced osteoporosis in the hands of a 14-year-old male 9 months after 100% TBSA burn. All growth plates are open. (b) Twenty-four months after injury, osteoporosis persists and there is irregular closure of metacarpal and phalangeal growth plates. (c) Eight months after injury, growth plates of distal tibiae and fibulae remain open. (d) Twenty-four months after injury, distal growth plates of tibiae and fibulae are closed. Other major growth plates remain open. Osteoporosis is unchanged.

who was admitted 8 months after acute burn, there was established osteomyelitis of the femur in relation to the exposed fracture. Osteomyelitis did not develop in either of the other patients; in the end, all three had sound femurs.

When traction pins are directed through burned skin for the treatment of fractures or for suspension of a burned extremity, the factors favoring development of infection along the pin track and the formation of cigarette sequestra are:

- the introduction or migration of organisms from the burn wound;
- linear pressure of the traction pin;
- prolonged traction;
- excessive movement of the extremity leading to loosening of the pin;
- sealing of the pin sites.

For traction or suspension, pins may be inserted through acutely burned skin, through eschar, through granulation tissue, or later through ischemic burn scar which may be colonized with uncommon and antibiotic-resistant organisms. No amount of local cleaning is likely to sterilize the surface through which the pin must pass, yet it seems that organisms in sufficient numbers to colonize are rarely introduced in this manner.

Local low-grade infections usually resolve when pins are removed if the pin sites are vigorously curetted of granulation tissue. In one case in which a four-pin custom external fixator was used in the treatment of an open infection of the elbow, there resulted diffuse osteomyelitis of humerus and radius. The infection was controlled with antibiotics and without surgery after the pins were removed. This case was included in Barret's report of skeletal pinning in 41 severely burned children.[11] In experience with the use of the Ilizarov system for correction of skeletal deformity in burns, one patient developed a pin track infection of such severity as to require removal of the pin, curettage, and intravenous antibiotics for control of methicillin-resistant staphylococcus.[12]

Hematogenous osteomyelitis and that due to spread from an infected joint are rare. The literature entertains no report of the occurrence of either entity in association with burns. Were bone infection of this sort to be recognized, effective treatment would depend upon the identification of the offending organisms for organism-specific antibiotic regimen.

Fractures

Pathological fractures were at one time common in burn management because of the practices of delayed excision of eschar and of keeping patients in bed until wounds were completely covered. During that time, fractures occurred because of bone collapse when patients first stood or walked after a prolonged period of bed confinement or when stiff joints were manipulated[13] (Figure 50.3). The bones most commonly affected were the femur at its distal metaphysis and the tibia at its proximal

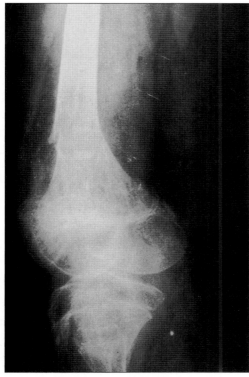

Fig. 50.3 Pathological fracture of the osteoporotic femur of a 9-year-old girl sustained on the first day she stood after 5 weeks of confinement for 40% TBSA burn.

one. The only treatment required was support of the extremity until the fracture consolidated, usually in 4–6 weeks. Children were more often affected than adults and the fractures usually compressed one cortex, producing an angular deformity which rapidly corrected with growth. More currently, Klein's[2] study strongly suggests that fractures occur more frequently in burned children than in a matched normal population even months after the acute burn. Now, however, in acute burn management the most frequently seen fractures are those occurring at the time of, or in association with, the burn injury. Falls or violent trauma account for many of the fractures, and the sites are those common to the causes, bearing no relation to the burn itself.

Although fractures complicate burn treatment and occasionally delay mobilization of patients, their management need not be complex. Fractures in extremities not burned can be treated in a routine manner by manipulative reduction and plaster immobilization, by open reduction and internal fixation, with an external fixator, or with skeletal traction (Figure 50.4). Fractures in extremities with first-degree or superficial second-degree burns can be managed in the same way. Deep second-degree and third-degree burns present a different problem only with respect to the early bacterial colonization of third-degree burns and the degradation of deep second-degree burns to full-thickness burns which will, in turn, become colonized. There is thus, a precious window of time when fractures requiring open reduction and internal fixation can be definitively treated without increased risk of infecting the bone; however, fracture reduction and stabilization are so important in the functional management of a severely burned patient that the risk of bone infection should be acknowledged and shouldered at any postburn stage. Skeletal traction can often be the management choice, particularly in children and adolescents, even if the treatment protocol requires that the patient be moved from bed for tubbing, dressing change, or additional surgery. The disadvantages of skeletal traction are the confinement to bed and the imposed relatively fixed position of the affected extremity. External fixators, now in common use, have made it possible to align and stabilize fractures in burned extremities without open operation. In fact, external fixation may be the treatment of choice for open fractures in burns, as it often is for open fractures not associated with burns. There is the added functional advantage of patient mobility. Brooker's extensive favorable experience supports this concept.[14] With both skeletal traction and external fixation, there is an added risk of bone infection because of the path from surface to bone provided by the pins. This is a risk worth taking, and it is minimized by scrupulous pin site care and by removal and replacement of any loosening pin. Frye recognized and discussed the specific and continuous difficulties encountered in the management of fractures and burns.[15]

When casts are used for stabilization of fractures in burned extremities, the wound is made inaccessible and there is an abiding fear that the unattended wound will seriously degrade or at best not improve. Those fears may be well founded; however, Wang[10] showed that a bivalved circular cast could be used effectively for an open comminuted fracture of a proximal tibia with overlying deep burns, and Choctaw[9] reported successful use of a cast for immobilization of an open comminuted fracture after immediate postburn grafting of the

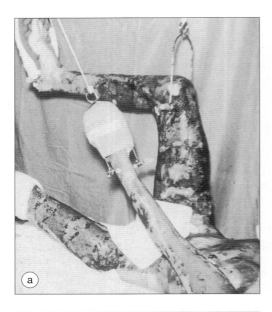

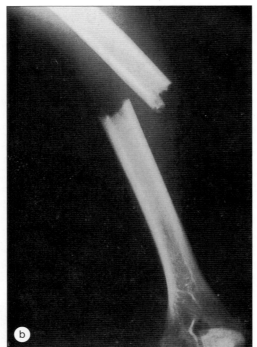

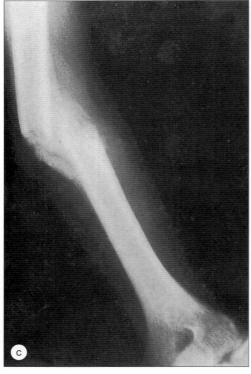

Fig. 50.4 (a) This 15-year-old male sustained closed fractures of the right femur, left tibia and left humerus at the time of a 46% TBSA burn involving mainly trunk and right lower extremity. The femur and humerus fractures were treated in skeletal traction. Suspension of the right lower extremity aided management of circumferential deep burns of that extremity. Lesser burns of the left leg made it possible to treat the minimally displaced fracture of the left tibia in a circular cast. All fractures consolidated in 6 weeks in satisfactory alignment. (b) Fracture of the left humerus as it appeared at the time of admission to the hospital. (c) Five weeks after injury, the fracture showed maturing callus. Traction was discontinued at 6 weeks.

affected extremity. Common sense should dictate which fractures can be treated with circular or bivalved casts or with splints. If a reduced or moderately displaced but aligned fracture is so stable as to require external support only for maintenance of alignment, then cast or splint immobilization should be all that is needed. On the other hand, if a fracture because of instability requires for maintenance of reduction, three-point pressure or molding of the cast material, then it will be better treated by other means.

Dowling[8] reported osteomyelitis resulting from open bimalleolar fracture in an extremity with extensive deep burns. In neither of the cases reported by Wang and Choctaw did the

bone become infected. There were also no infections among Saffle's[42] fractures, nine of which were treated by open reduction and internal fixation.[17] With two fractures of the femur, each of which was exposed at the base of a deep chronic burn, aggressive debridement of the wounds and the fracture ends was followed by treatment with skeletal traction in one and by external fixation with the Ilizarov system in the other. Both fractures healed without further complication.

Fractures in burned patients heal quickly. There is no recorded experience which suggests that healing is delayed by the burn. Neither is there any record of failure of union. Callus formation may be abundant.

Among severely burned patients, non-displaced or minimally displaced fractures may not be detected until unusual local pain in an affected extremity prompts radiographic examination or when a radiograph obtained for other reasons reveals the fracture as an incidental finding. These fractures are usually of no functional significance. Modest angular deformity near a joint may be a problem in adults, though not in children. On the other hand, undetected transphyseal fractures in children can be a major functional threat.

Changes involving pericapsular structures

Heterotopic bone

Heterotopic bone formation is a rare but functionally important complication of thermal burns. The incidence in a general burn population is reported to be somewhere between 1 and 3%.[1,18–21] In select populations, the incidence may be higher as it will be if patients with periarticular calcification are included in the statistics. For example, Tepperman et al. reported a 35.3% incidence among patients referred to a tertiary care center for rehabilitation.[22] Jackson made the observation that the incidence of heterotopic bone could be expected to be less in institutions which admit patients with minor burns.[23] Munster's[24] radiographic survey of 88 adult and teenage patients with 160 burned upper extremities yielded a 16% incidence of pericapsular calcification; and the 23% incidence reported by Schiele et al.[1] included both heterotopic ossification and calcification. In the early routine radiographic study reported by Evans[13] periarticular calcification which did not progress to heterotopic bone was excluded from the final calculation of an incidence of 2%. The 3.3% incidence recorded by Kolar and Vrabec[25] included patients with pericapsular calcification. Even if heterotopic bone occurs infrequently in thermal burns, it remains that once it develops, it often compromises joint motion and is difficult to treat. In addition, its pathogenesis is still incompletely understood; and, thus, protocols for prevention may in fact miss the mark.

Pathogenesis

The metabolic changes occurring after thermal burn are increased metabolic rate; protein catabolism; ureagenesis; fat mobilization; glucogenolysis; gluconeogenesis; elevated glucose flow; and eventual total body weight loss.[26,27] There is an accompanying suppression of the immune system which favors wound infection, but, at the same time, favors survival of skin allografts. Infection, failure of skin graft take or anything which delays closure of a burn wound will extend the altered metabolic state. Though it might be assumed that there occurs, along with the metabolic upheaval, an adverse change in connective tissue milieu, the exact nature of such a change is not known. It is also not known what the metabolic changes have to do with the development of heterotopic bone, but it is clear that the burn disease is necessary to its formation. Other factors to be considered in the genesis of heterotopic bone are percentage of burn, location of burn, period of confinement, osteoporosis, superimposed trauma and genetic predisposition. These factors, though identifiable, are not easy to implicate.

Percentage of burn

Most reported cases of heterotopic bone have had a 20% or greater total body surface area burn; however, heterotopic bone has been found in patients with as little as 10% third-degree burn.[13] Peterson et al.,[28] Munster et al.,[24] and Elledge et al.[20] have reported affected patients with total body surface burns of 8%, 14%, and 12% respectively. In addition, with the now extensive experience with salvage of patients with 80% or greater burns, it is clear that heterotopic bone occurs no more frequently among these patients at the other end of the percentage spectrum than in the general burn population. It cannot be said, thus, that the percentage of burn is a determining factor.

Location of burn

A high percentage, but by no means all, of the reported heterotopic bone has occurred in joints with overlying deep burn. In their initial report, Evans and Smith described heterotopic bone occurring a distance from any third-degree burn involvment.[29] Johnston, in his early report, noted that in one of his three patients, the skin overlying one affected joint was not even superficially burned.[30] If it be assumed that degradation of connective tissue milieu in burns is a total body phenomenon, it follows that heterotopic bone formation need not be burn-site dependent. Thus, the location of the burn cannot alone be a determining factor.

Period of confinement

Evans and Smith expressed the belief that length of bed confinement was perhaps the most important factor in the development of heterotopic bone.[29] At the time of that report, patients with even moderate burns might be kept in bed for several weeks. The consequences of prolonged confinement were loss of active range of joint motion and bone demineralization; it was thought that each of these adverse changes might contribute to the formation of heterotopic bone. Thus, any maloccurrence which necessitated longer confinement could be a factor in the pathogenesis. Kolar implicated wound sepsis as such an independent factor along with the length of confinement.[25] Other investigators have not addressed the period of confinement as specifically as Kolar, and there have been no studies of comparative groups of confined and non-confined patients. Thus, it may never be determined whether or not current aggressive practice of early mobilization of patients will have an effect on the incidence of heterotopic bone.

Osteoporosis

Only Schiele et al. have reported a relationship between heterotopic bone formation and osteoporosis.[1] We have noted previously that among their group of 70 adults with burns confined to the upper extremities, 11 of the 16 who developed heterotopic bone had radiographically identifiable osteoporosis. In their series of patients, there were 24 who had osteoporosis. Thus, fewer than one-half of these developed heterotopic bone and there were two in the group that developed heterotopic bone who did not have osteoporosis. If the findings in that study are not altogether persuasive, the matter is further confused by the knowledge that the survivors of extensive total body surface burns who may develop profound osteoporosis seem to have no greater liability to the formation of heterotopic bone than the general burn population.

Superimposed trauma

In one of the patients reported by Evans and Smith, the elbow of the more often used and minimallly burned right upper extremity developed heterotopic bone, whereas the elbow of the less used but more seriously burned left upper extremity did not.[29] In the same patient, the right hip spontaneously dislocated. After reduction, that hip developed extensive heterotopic bone in the planes of the rectus femoris and iliopsoas, the muscles stressed by the posterior displacement. The opposite hip developed only a small spicule of heterotopic bone anteriorly at the joint line. Experience with this one patient reinforced the authors' belief that there occurred with burns a general compromise of connective tissue which rendered it particularly susceptible to superimposed trauma and that it was this liability to injury which accounted for the appearance of heterotopic bone at sites of repeated stretching of soft tissue, as at the minimally burned elbow or at sites of recognized abrupt excessive stretching as at the dislocated hip. According to all reports, the elbow is the most common site of heterotopic bone formation in adults and children.[20,21,25,31–38] Perhaps it is the regular use of this joint which accounts for that orientation. Jackson has pointed out that the elbows are subjected to pressure posteriorly and medially when they are used for leverage or are simply in contact with the bed.[23] He suggests with this observation that external pressure is a factor in the orientation of heterotopic bone to the elbow. There may be other factors as well that favor the elbow. Commonly, the elbow is splinted in extension to prevent flexion contracture. If flexion range is lost, passive stretch and encouragement of active flexion are part of the rehabilitation effort. The posterior structures most affected by this effort are those attached to the olecranon. Thus, it is not surprising that heterotopic bone develops medially in line with and deep to the medial fibers of the triceps. If a flexion contracture develops, the heterotopic bone is commonly in the line of brachialis or biceps attachments to coronoid process and biceps tubercle. And if there is loss of pronation and supination range, stretching may cause heterotopic bone to form in line with the proximal radioulnar ligaments and interosseous membrane. There is an implication here that both the quality and timing of postburn exercise may be important. Gentle passive and active motion should cause less tissue disruption than abrupt passive or active or even chronically repeated motion, and the effect of any mobilization effort must vary with the relative stiffness of the joint and the intrinsic resistance of soft tissue. Thus, the longer a joint is limited in its motion, the stiffer it will become and the greater will be the soft tissue damage with any forced manipulation.

The concept of superimposed trauma as a cause of heterotopic bone is supported by the experimental work of Evans[39] and of Michelsson and Rauschning.[40] Evans found that all burned and non-burned rabbits given a single necrotizing injection of alcohol in one quadriceps muscle readily healed the lesions, whereas rabbits, burned or non-burned, which were given a second same-site injection 7 days after the first, uniformly developed well-defined and histologically identifiable ossicles of heterotopic bone. In this experiment, it was clear that, in susceptible animals, it was not the burn which made the difference, but the chronicity of the wound. Michelsson and Rauschning determined that forceful or regular active remobilization of rabbit knees, which had been immobilized for 1–5 weeks, resulted in the development of heterotopic calcification and ossification in the muscles which were stretched. The response was more consistent in the quadriceps of the knees immobilized in extension than in the hamstrings of those immobilized in flexion. The longer the period of immobilization and the more vigorous the remobilization, the greater the response. Muscle necrosis was a prominent histological finding.

Superimposed trauma is implicated in the development of heterotopic bone in head-injured patients or those with post-traumatic or infectious transverse myelitis.[41–43] In these patients, it is assumed that tissue media are altered by injury to the central nervous system. The secondary injury, as in burns, is periarticular. In post-traumatic myositis ossificans, the development of heterotopic bone depends upon persistence of the muscle lesion and local necrosis and, thus, at least by inference, upon repeated insults to the affected muscle.

The development of heterotopic bone in burns has been associated with the agitation of patients and their resistance to physical therapy.[29,44] Two affected adults and one affected child in a 10-year study resisted physical therapy programming.[39] One adult refused to move and the other was extremely apprehensive. The child was likewise apprehensive and refused to cooperate with the therapist. The development in all three of posterior heterotopic bone in both elbows could have been ascribed both to the difficulty encountered in mobilizing the elbows and to the continual pressure on the elbows in bed.

Genetic predisposition

It is difficult to explain the low incidence of heterotopic bone among great numbers of patients similarly burned except on the basis of some, as yet unidentified, inherited factor. It is known that persons with proliferative non-inflammatory arthritis of the hip are more likely to develop heterotopic bone after total hip replacement than persons who have hips replaced for other reasons. In this instance, the predisposing inherited abnormality is identifiable. Though heterotopic bone formation may occur more regularly among spinal cord-injured and head-injured patients than among burned ones, by no means do all persons with head and spinal cord injuries develop heterotopic bone. The total burn experience at the University of Texas Medical Branch has yielded only two similarly affected siblings. Twin brothers who had 19% and 20% total body surface burns and who were mobile throughout much of their treatment and recovery period developed near identical heterotopic bone of both elbows.[45] There is, however, no scientific proof that genetic predisposition has anything to do with the formation of heterotopic bone in burns. Nor is there any literature to support the idea that a person who develops heterotopic bone when burned will be liable to develop it if he or she sustains head or spinal cord injury. Vrbicky,[46] in a comprehensive review of postburn heterotopic bone formation, suggests that a key for the genetic predisposition may be in the human leukocyte antigen (HLA), reporting that a HLA B27 survey showed a 7% HLA distribution in the normal population compared with 70% in a population with heterotopic bone.

Characteristics and behavior

Heterotopic bone associated with burns has been reported to occur about all major joints. The joints most commonly affected are elbow, shoulder, and hip, in that order of frequency. The early manifestations are joint swelling and tenderness not unlike any acute inflammatory process. The patient may call attention to the process by a reluctance to move the affected joint. Onset may be as early as 1 month and as late as 3 months or more after the burn, but it is more likely to be associated with the acute recovery phase of treatment than later. Crawford et al. reported that the clinical diagnosis was made in advance of radiographic changes in 9 of his 12 patients.[31] Tepperman et al.[22] and Peterson et al.[21] found that bone scans could help to make a diagnosis before there were radiographic changes. The earliest radiographic alteration is local periarticular increase in soft tissue density. There follows diffuse stippled calcification in the same distribution in or about the capsule of the joint. It is at this point that the process may reverse itself, perhaps due to the improved state of the patient. Because of this change in course, there may be many patients whose periarticular calcification is never detected. If the calcification persists, it may be assumed that bone will develop by either the intramembranous or the enchondral route or both as it does in animal models.

The flecks of calcification appear radiographically to lie within the capsule, whereas heterotopic bone may involve not only capsular structures but may extend as well into the planes of muscles and tendons. At each major joint there is a more or less characteristic distribution of heterotopic bone which is similar to that associated with patients with head and spinal cord injury. At the elbow, posteriorly, disposed bone extends from the olecranon to the medial epicondylar ridge of the humerus in line with the medial border of the triceps muscle (Figure 50.5a,b). At the joint, it may extend medially to bridge the ulnar groove.[16,47] The medial, rather than lateral, orientation of the heterotopic bone may be related to the medial position of the olecranon and the greater tension on soft tissue on that side. As Jackson points out, the contact area of the elbow is medial, and continual pressure in this area may have something to do with the orientation.[23] Heterotopic bone on the anterior surface of the elbow develops in the planes of the brachialis and biceps muscles extending from humerus to coronoid process or biceps tubercle. Occasionally, a bridge of heterotopic bone develops between the radius and ulna just distal to the joint. More rarely, bone has been found to fill the olecranon fossa and even to ensheath the entire joint. At the shoulder, bone has been found to extend from the acromion to the humerus in the line of the rotator muscles or deep to the deltoid (Figure 50.5c), to lie anteriorly in the plane of the pectoralis major, and, more deeply, to parallel the subscapularis. Hoffer et al.[48] reported that heterotopic bone at the shoulder lay anteriorly in the plane of the capsule. At the hip heterotopic bone may extend from pelvis to femur in the planes of rectus or iliopsoas anteriorly or in the plane of the gluteal muscles laterally. Jackson has reported heterotopic bone in the plane of the quadratus femoris.[23] Like the shoulder, the hip may be ensheathed anteriorly with heterotopic bone which appears to originate in the capsule.

When heterotopic bone bridges a joint, it becomes part of the skeleton and may, if loaded, increase in dimension as fully developed ossicles with mature cortex and medullary cavity. If the bone does not bridge a joint, it will, in children, gradually disappear when the burn wound has healed and the child is healthy. In recovering adults, non-bridging bone will, in time, diminish in size, but it may never completely disappear. The same tendency for heterotopic bone to regress after resolution of disease was noted by Lorber, who reported on two patients with paraplegia secondary to tuberculosis in whom deposits of heterotopic bone diminished in size, after return of motor function.[41] Bottu and Van Noyen[49] reported a similar experience with a patient who had transient viral meningoencephalitis, and Jacobs reported almost complete resorption of large bilateral deposits of heterotopic bone in a patient who recovered from paralytic measles encephalomyelitis.[42]

Serum levels of calcium, phosphorus, and alkaline phosphatase have been reported by most authors to be normal or, at best, insignificantly higher in burned patients who have developed heterotopic bone.[18,24,29,50,51] In addition, there is no convincing evidence that calcium intake affects heterotopic bone formation one way or the other. Evans and Smith's limited routine studies of affected and unaffected patients led the authors to believe that the values of serum calcium, phosphorus, and alkaline phosphatase were so consistently normal as to make further investigation unnecessary.[29] One interesting observation was that of Koepke, whose early, but incomplete, studies suggested that those patients who were susceptible had elevation of serum alkaline phosphatase before development of heterotopic bone, but not afterwards.[19]

Prevention and treatment

The incidence of heterotopic bone in burns is so low as to make it impractical to administer aspirin or indometacin or other non-steroidal anti-inflammatory drugs which are currently used for patients at risk for development of heterotopic bone after major hip surgery. Rather, the thrust in prevention should be toward reducing the period of bed confinement and the duration of the postburn hypermetabolic state. The now prevailing practice of early wound excision and grafting may, in fact, address both of these problems as nearly as it is possible to do so. Even patients with extensive total body surface burns may be out of bed and walking within the first postburn week. Extremity motion is begun as soon as graft and wound stability permit. With this programming, the incidence and intensity of osteoporosis should be reduced as well.

If certain patients are predisposed to the development of heterotopic bone, then the quality and timing of joint mobilization for those patients may be critical. Stretching edematous pericapsular structures in the early postburn period may very well be hazardous if additional tissue damage is the result; however, maintenance of joint motion and muscle function is part of the early excision and grafting program, and it is certain that the longer joint motion is restricted the more likely it is that pericapsular structures will be damaged by stretching. We should like to think that any secondary injury to soft tissue could be avoided by controlled and assisted active motion, gentle terminal stretch, and terminal resistance.

When a patient is reluctant to move a joint previously moved with relative ease, and certainly when there is evidence of unusual swelling about the joint, radiographs should be obtained to determine if there is pericapsular calcification or

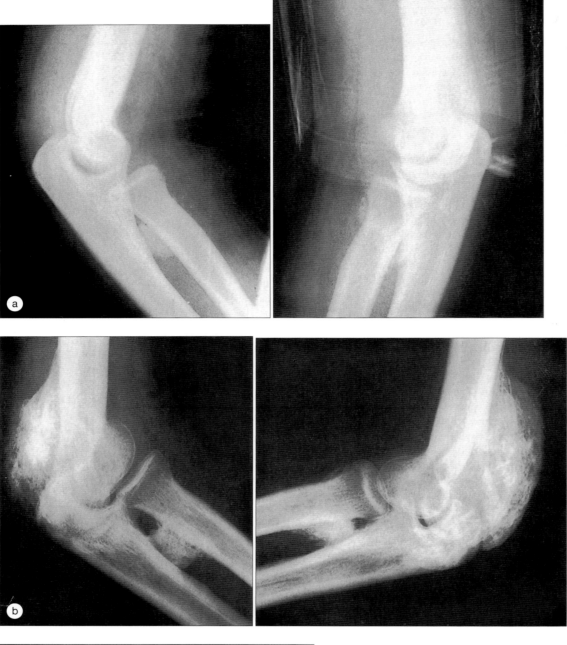

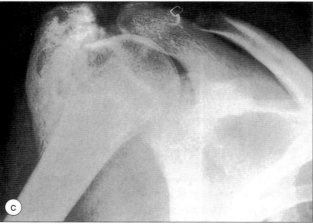

Fig. 50.5 (a) Three months after 94% TBSA burn of a 16-year-old male, resistance to motion, local swelling, and pain of both elbows prompted obtaining roentgenograms, each of which showed spotty linear soft-tissue calcification and ossification along the distal humerus and between the radius and ulna at the level of the biceps tubercle. (b) Six months after burn, elbow flexion and extension were reduced to 10° on the left and to less than 5° on the right. Bridges of immature heterotopic bone extended from the medial epicondylar ridges to the olecranons. Forearm rotation was 0% due to interosseous bridges of heterotopic bone at the level of the bicipital tuberosities. Prognosis for restoring functional range of motion in the elbows is poor. (c) At 6 months postburn, glenohumeral motion on the right was limited to a few degrees by heterotopic bone underlying the deltoid. At the same time, a lesser deposit of heterotopic at the left hip did not limit motion.

ossification. Once heterotopic bone or calcification is recognized, joint exercise should be restricted to gentle passive and assisted active motion only. Crawford et al.[31] observed that ossification progressed to complete ankylosis in all patients who persisted in moving an affected joint beyond the pain-free range. They concluded that active range of motion exercises and stretching were contraindicated if heterotopic bone or calcification was suspected, but that active range of motion could be safely resumed within pain-free range once the diagnosis had been confirmed. In the series of Peterson et al.,[21] patients suspected of having heterotopic bone had active range of motion exercises only. Ten regained functional range of motion and eight developed ankylosis.

Surgical excision of heterotopic bone is indicated when joint motion is lost or significantly compromised by bridging bone or exostoses. Evans has suggested that surgery be postponed until the burn wound has healed, scars are soft and associated with no inflammatory response, the patient is healthy, and the offensive bone is radiographically mature, i.e. well defined and not increasing in dimension[13] (Figure 50.6). This position makes sense considering the behavior of heterotopic bone: i.e. proliferation while there are open burn wounds or active scars and regression with wound healing and scar softening. For removal of heterotopic bone, surgical exposures should be planned with extensible incisions so as to facilitate total excision. When there is a bridge of bone, each end of the bridge should be slightly excavated. When there is attachment at only one end, the cartilaginous or fibrous extension should be removed along with the bone. Capsular sheets of bone should be removed completely. If bridging heterotopic bone is incompletely excised, the bridge is likely to recur. When a joint is bridged by bone in only one plane, removal of the offending bone will usually restore functional motion and the likelihood of recurrence of the bridge is small. When a joint is bridged in more than one plane, recurrence is more likely and the chance for restoration of functional range of motion is correspondingly diminished. When the local inflammatory process has caused intra-articular synovial proliferation and cartilage destruction, the joint is most likely destined for ankylosis. Removal of the heterotopic bone about a joint so affected may allow more functional positioning of the joint, but it is not likely to arrest the process. On the other hand, extra-articular arthrodesis by a bridge of heterotopic bone may preserve the joint. This is particularly the case at the elbow when there is only one posterior bridge of bone from olecranon to medial epicondylar ridge of the humerus. In this situation, the olecranon is fixed in the trochlea, but the radiocapitellar and radioulnar joints remain functional. In Evans' experience with removal of single bridges at the elbow, joint cartilage was found to be healthy as long as 5 years after ankylosis. Preservation of pronation and supination was credited with maintaining the synovial bath to provide nutrition for the humeroulnar cartilage. Indeed, when pronation and supination additionally are blocked by bridging bone, cartilage degradation is certain. Evans' further experience with long-term survival of glenohumeral cartilage after ankylosis by bridging bone from acromion to humerus is not as easily explained.

Reported experience with excision of heterotopic bone in burns has not been uniformly favorable. Dias,[51] Hoffer et al.,[48] and Peterson et al.[21] reported restoration of functional range of motion in most of their patients with timely excision of heterotopic bone. Gaur et al.[32] reported good functional return

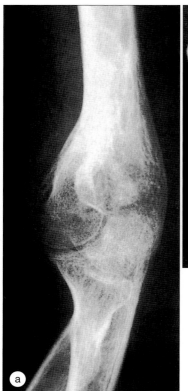
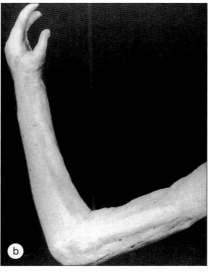
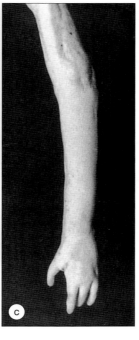

Fig. 50.6 (a) A mature sheet of heterotopic bone extends from humerus to olecranon, obliterating the olecranon fossa 11 months after 53% TBSA burn in a 13-year-old female. Elbow flexion and extension range was less than 10%. Pronation and supination were near normal range. (b), (c) Three months after excision of heterotopic bone, the patient had attained 90° of elbow motion and a continuing increase to functional (hand to mouth) range was predicted. Now the patient can extend the elbow and can flex it to 90°.

in 7 burned children with 9 affected elbows. Ring and Jupiter[33] reported good results in a varied population, and Chung et al.[34] reported good results with early excision a mean of 9 months after the burn. Other surgeons have reported less satisfactory results. In our own experience, results have varied, as anticipated, with severity of affliction. We have learned that if heterotopic bone recurs after excision, it is worthwhile to excise again if the joint affected remains structurally identifiable. For the most part, however, attempts to improve joint function with second operations have failed. We believe that ultimate failure can be predicted at the time of initial surgery; we are convinced that the single most important factor in successful initial excision is in timing surgery to coincide with the patient's return to good health.

Changes involving the joint

Dislocation

Luxations and subluxations of joints in burned patients may occur as a result of direct destruction by the burn of ligaments and capsules, loss of articular cartilage due to infection, faulty positioning, and eventually scar contracture. In all phases of management, but particularly in the acute phase, positioning is of prime importance in the prevention of joint deformity. The preferred positions, listed in Table 50.1, serve as a guide for the prevention of dislocation of joints and of malposition secondary to scar contracture.

The joints most liable to structural compromise due to exposure by the burn and loss of soft tissue support are knee, elbow, proximal interphalangeal joints of the hand, and metacarpophalangeal joints. These hinge joints have in common a subcutaneous dorsal surface, accounting for their ready exposure.

The elbow, for its trochlear architecture, is more intrinsically stable than the other joints in this group. It requires loss of collateral support to render it easily displaceable. The knee, on the other hand, is immediately in danger of subluxation if there is loss of continuity of its central slip, the patellar tendon, even if the retinacula remain intact. In this circumstance, gravity alone will displace the tibia posteriorly in relation to the femur if the patient is recumbent. The hamstring muscles contribute to the displacement force regardless of the position of the extremity. Loss of collateral ligaments compounds the problem, but loss of collateral ligament stability in the presence of an intact patellar tendon and functioning quadriceps constitutes far less a threat than loss of patellar tendon. For the lower extremity, persistent posterior translation of the tibia beneath the femur with inefficient quadriceps pull is potentially a functional disaster.

For both the elbow and the knee the protecting position is extension. These two joints are rarely at risk for articular displacement from contracture alone and, if there is no ligament or tendon loss, extension resting splints will give adequate positional support. When there is soft tissue disruption, splinting may not adequately protect either joint. An external fixator with two pin, four cortex fixation above and below the joint will provide stability and will permit access to the wound. For the elbow, it allows fine adjustment to the normal carrying angle as well. If the knee is accurately reducible at the time of application of the fixator, there is a good possibility that the reduction can be maintained. If the tibia cannot be brought forward completely by manual manipulation, it may be necessary to suspend the tibia through a transverse pin at the level of the tibial tubercle. For static vertical traction, the extremity must be elevated from the bed. For dynamic traction, enough weight must be used to accomplish the same elevation. If the tibia can be brought forward by this means, an external fixator will likely hold the reduction. For the knee to remain stable with the tibia forward, the patellar tendon must be reattached and quadriceps integrity reestablished; otherwise, when the fixator is removed, the tibia will once again begin an incremental posterior shift toward its own point of stability. No amount of external splinting or bracing is likely to prevent that shift.

The proximal interphalangeal joints of the hands are more frequently exposed by burn than any others. If the central extensor slip remains intact, there is less risk of subluxation of the joint. Even if there is loss of continuity of the central slip but preservation of the lateral bands, subluxation is easily prevented if the joint is maintained in extension while soft tissue cover is being achieved. It is with loss of the support of lateral bands and collateral ligaments that the joints become liable to dislocation. With the metacarpophalangeal joints, the tendency to displacement or subluxation may be greater because these joints are functionally multiplaner, while the interphalangeal joints are uniplaner. Happily, the metacarpophalangeal joints are less often exposed than the interphalangeal ones.

The protecting position for the proximal interphalangeal joints is full extension. If only the central slip is lost, the position may be held with an external splint. In states of greater instability it may be necessary to use intramedullary transarticular Kirschner wires to hold the position. The wires, though

TABLE 50.1 PREFERRED POSITIONS FOR MAJOR JOINTS	
Joint	Preferred position
Neck	Midline in neutral or slight extension
Shoulders	Scapulothoracic retraction and depression 85° of glenohumeral elevation with 20–25° of horizontal flexion
Elbows	Extension
Wrists	Slight extension
Metacarpophalangeal joints 2–5	80–90° of flexion
Fingers	Proximal and distal interphalangeal extension
Thumbs	Carpometacarpal flexion and abduction, metacarpophalangeal flexion 5–10°, interphalangeal extension
Spine	Extension with no lateral deviation
Hips	Extension and slight external rotation in 15° of symmetric abduction
Knees	Extension
Ankles	Neutral
Feet	Neutral

reasonably efficient, do not control rotation, and they carry with them a risk of post-treatment joint stiffness. In small children it is impossible to introduce the Kirschner wires through the distal phalanx; thus, it is better, with the distal phalanx flexed to 90 degrees, to place the wire through the corresponding metacarpal head into the proximal and middle phalanges. The short-term transfixation of the joint does not harm the joint, and metacarpal phalangeal flexion is the favored position for functional restoration. Pin traction through the distal phalanges in a skeletally stabilized metal splint is another method for maintaining extension of threatened digital joints.[52,53] It has the advantages of patient comfort and mobility, secure positioning of hand and upper extremity, easy maintenance of elevation, and easy access for dressings, for additional surgery, and for exercise of lesser affected joints. The system likewise makes it possible to keep digits separated, thus facilitating local care. Traction should not be used if collateral ligaments are not intact. By whatever means attained, the corrected position must be maintained until the joint is covered with graft. Protection should continue with a standard splint or brace until the joint is sound.

The two joints most likely to dislocate because of faulty positioning are the shoulder and the hip. These two ball and socket multiplaner joints sacrifice stability in favor of mobility. This is particularly true of the shoulder, where the shallow glenoid contains at any one time only one-third of the head of the humerus. In burns, the head of the humerus may begin to subluxate forward if, during prone positioning for management of back and buttock wounds, the arms are maintained in full abduction in the coronal plane. In this position the arms are in at least 15–20 degrees of extension from the more secure neutral position in line with the scapulae and the humeral heads are forced forward against the anterior capsule. Even when the patient is supine, full abduction and extension of the arms should be avoided. For short-term management, particularly when the patient gets out of bed every day, this position probably does not threaten the joint. But if the patient is to be bed confined and the position unrelieved for days or weeks, the head of the humerus may begin to subluxate forward. In the extreme situation, the head of the humerus will dislocate to a medial subcoracoid position. In patients with deep burns extending from chin to axillae to chest, the common posture of elevation and protraction of the scapulae may be associated with upward subluxation of the humeral heads. With one patient in whom the right clavicle was sacrificed distally because of the depth of the burn, the head of the right humerus moved forward and then upward because of loss of anterior stabilizers.

The head of the humerus is most secure in the glenoid fossa when the arm is adducted to neutral and internally rotated, a position which is incompatible with wound management of burns of the trunk, neck, and upper extremities. The protecting position which accommodates the need for abduction for axillary burns is elevation of the arms in line with the scapulae. The arm is then approximately 20 degrees forward of the coronal plane or in 20 degrees of horizontal flexion. When the patient is prone, the protecting position can be gained only if the chest is supported on a chest width mattress, folded blankets or towels, or a foam rubber pad, any of which will allow the arms to drop forward. When the patient is positioned this way, whether supine or prone, the forearms will be pronated and the arms will be in sufficient internal rotation to favor seating of the head of the humerus in the glenoid.

The hip will tend to subluxate posteriorly if the thigh is persistently allowed to remain flexed, adducted and internally rotated during the acute burn phase. For the most part, however, the protecting position of extension to neutral or 180 degrees and 15–20 degrees of symmetric abduction is easy to attain and maintain and is, in fact, the most desirable position for wound management.

If dislocation of the head of humerus or femur is undetected or if reduction is delayed for other reasons, open reduction will likely be required. Reduction of a chronically displaced head of humerus in one seriously burned patient using the Ilizarov technique was hampered by the fragility of the bone. Another head of humerus that had been dislocated anteriorly for several weeks was found at the time of open reduction to have extensive erosion of the articular cartilage.

Infection of a joint may result in its subluxation or dislocation. Hip displacement because of apparent spontaneous dissolution has been described by Evans and Smith.[29] Eszter and Istvan[54] and Cristallo and Dell'Orto[55] reported similar cases. In none of these cases, however, could it be determined that the joint destruction was due to infection.

Septic arthritis

A joint exposed by a burn or by removal of burn eschar is presumed to be infected. The joints most frequently exposed are the knee, the elbow, the proximal interphalangeal joints of the hand, and the metacarpophalangeal joints, all on the subcutaneous dorsal surfaces. Wrist and ankle are less often affected and other joints rarely. Treatment requires stable positioning of the joint for maximum reduction of wound size so as to facilitate soft tissue closure or grafting and to allow aggressive daily lavage. The position for all of the joints listed except the ankle is extension. The ankle is positioned in neutral. External fixation, intramedullary pinning, or skeletal traction may be required to secure the position. To maintain ankle position it is sometimes appropriate to insert a large vertical Steinmann pin through calcaneus and talus into the tibia. The position should be maintained until the exposed joint is covered with epithelialized granulation tissue or skin graft. Exposed adjacent bone can be shaved or drilled, as previously described, to encourage surface granulation. Drilling is particularly useful at the elbow where the olecranon is regularly exposed. Often, however, granulation tissue will quickly extend the wound margins and effectively close the wound so as to allow split-thickness skin grafting. If the burn is isolated to the joint or if the extremity is not otherwise seriously burned, a local muscle, skin or compound flap may be used to close the joint. Free vascularized flaps are useful and should always be considered if it is anticipated that nerve graft or tendon graft or transfer at the site will be required in the future. Incremental remobilization of the joint may proceed when wound closure is sound. Culture of material from an exposed joint will likely yield a variety of organisms consistent with those of the general burn wound, thus requiring broad-spectrum antibiotic management.

The incidence of hematogenous septic arthritis is obscured by its frequent association with severe burns and because there are rarely separable clinical signs such as local heat and swelling, elevation of temperature, and elevation of sedimentation rate. Local tenderness and greater than usual pain with motion may focus attention on the affected joint. Aspiration of the joint will confirm a diagnosis. A radiograph is helpful, but in the early phases of infection will show only local cellulitis as increased periarticular soft tissue density. If a patient has been receiving broad-spectrum antibiotics, material aspirated from the affected joint may not grow an organism in culture. Clearly, without organism identification and sensitivity determinations, specific antibiotic therapy cannot be initiated.

We have been of the opinion that debridement and exteriorization of the joint and regular vigorous lavage are as important as antibiotics in the treatment of closed infected joints. We believe now that arthroscopic debridement and closed irrigation should be considered as an alternative method of management whether or not skin over the affected joint is burned. Rarely in burns, a joint may become infected from adjacent metaphyseal osteomyelitis. In this situation joint preservation is the treatment priority, and measures are the same as for septic arthritis of strictly hematogenous origin.[45] In children most infected joints can be salvaged. Adult joints are less resilient. Persistent joint infection will destroy cartilage and lead to ankylosis.[28,56] All chronically infected joints are liable to dislocation because of surface destruction and capsular laxity.

Amputations

In burns, major amputations are most often performed because of non-viability of the extremity or because a surviving extremity is rendered useless by scar, deformity or insensitivity. Occasionally, in an extensive burn, a severely burned extremity which might be salvaged in part is sacrificed to reduce the extent of the burn or as a lifesaving measure.

In thermal burns, the level of extremity amputation is determined by the viability of muscles and tendons. The more distal the site the better, and it is important to retain joints even if motion will be restricted. For example, if a forearm or leg must be sacrificed, the elbow or knee should be spared if the more proximal muscles controlling that joint are intact, if the bone bleeds, and if there is the possibility that the remaining tissue of the stump has sufficient blood supply to produce granulations for grafting. Aside from affording a better functional prospect, sparing the joint will provide the surgeon opportunity at a later time to choose an appropriate revision level if the joint does not function. The patient will at that time be healthier and stump closure will be routine. Jackson suggests that it may be technically feasible to cover even non-viable bone with a free flap in order to maintain extremity length.[23]

Prostheses can be easily fitted over stumps covered with split-thickness grafts. Ridges of hypertrophic scar will break down if there is friction within the socket of the prosthesis. A scar often softens and flattens because of the constant even pressure of a well-fitted socket; prostheses fitted early over grafted stumps may prevent scar thickening. Breakdown may occur at points where the graft is adherent to bone. This problem may necessitate surgical freeing of the adherent graft and reshaping of the bone. Minor hip and knee flexion con-

tractures complicate the fitting and function of a prosthesis; thus, every effort should be made to maintain full extension of these joints. Late revisions of amputations in children are required when the bone overgrows in length and when offensive terminal exostoses develop. The overgrowing bone can be shortened and the exostoses removed.

It is important, in the early management of upper extremity amputations in infants and young children, to supply temporary prosthetic extensions. This provides functional orientation to a prosthesis, maintains muscle bulk and tone, and encourages continuing bimanual activity at normal extremity length until a prosthesis with appropriate terminal device can be applied. Children quickly acquire prehension and transfer skills if they have an opposable stump and they may reject prostheses if they are not applied early. It is equally important to restore bipedal function as soon as possible. If delay of healing or ulceration of a lower extremity stump prevents early prosthetic fitting, an ischial weight-bearing device which suspends the stump will permit the child to walk in advance of prosthetic fitting. Inflatable plastic air bags provide both even pressure and accurate fit for weight bearing in container sockets. Early prosthetic fitting is desirable in teenagers and adults as well, but is not as critical as it is in children. As in non-burned persons, an upper extremity prosthesis may be rejected at any age if the opposite extremity is fully functional.[57]

Alterations in growth

In 1959, Evans and Smith[29] reported that a patient who was 24 years of age when burned had a subsequent 1½ inch increase in height. It was suggested that one explanation for this growth spurt might be local change in hemodynamics with stasis, passive hyperemia, and chronic inflammation. We have not since documented height changes in burned adults, but we have observed children whose growth after burn has seemed to be retarded. If growth plates remain open, it is difficult to explain overall growth retardation except on an endocrine or humoral basis. It is easy, however, to explain extremity length differences on the basis of premature closure of growth plates due to direct involvement of the bone or to severity of overlying burn. Frantz reported lower limb length discrepancy in four patients with foot and ankle burns.[58] Growth plates closed prematurely in only two of the cases. Jackson described two patients with digital and lower extremity deformity, respectively, due to partial closure of growth plates.[23] In Ritsila's case, contracture alone was apparently the cause of growth retardation in an upper extremity.[59] It seems reasonable, though hard to prove, that growth in a severely burned extremity would be retarded because of functional impairment. One patient, a 3-year-old boy with 80% total body surface burn and sufficiently deep burns of the right upper extremity to require mid-humerus amputation, demonstrated, 4 years after the burn, failure of development of the right shoulder girdle. The factors operant in this case could be premature closure of growth plates of scapula and clavicle, restrictive scar, and disuse atrophy.

There is yet another confusing aspect of premature closure of growth plates in that within an extremity with total full-thickness burn, only a few of the growth plates will close prematurely. The explanation for this capricious selectivity is at best obscure. Evans and Calhoun recorded an example of spotty closure of growth plates in a 14-year-old male with 90% total body surface burn.[12] There was complete closure of distal tibial and fibular epiphyses 1 year after burn together with closure of all digital epiphyses in the feet and of several digital epiphyses in the hands. Other major epiphyses were spared (Figure 50.2).

In early experience, abnormal growth plate closure was observed in a 6-year-old girl with 50% third-degree burn which did not involve legs or ankles.[60] Rapidly destructive septic arthritis of one ankle resulted in closure of the adjacent tibial growth plate.

Only occasionally can growth changes be anticipated because of obvious affection of the bone. More often the changes are subtle. It seems clear, thus, that among seriously burned children, regular height and extremity length measure-ments must be part of ongoing postburn assessment until it is determined that the extremities and trunk are developing symmetrically and on schedule. Extremity and trunk align-ment must likewise be part of the assessment as subtle angular deformity can occur because of partial closure of a growth plate. Jackson's report addresses this problem.[23]

So-called growth arrest lines seen in the radiographs of non-burned children, who have serious illness or major trauma other than burns, are commonly observed in burned children. In burns, as in other conditions, these transverse markers of relatively increased mineralization represent normal recovery from an insult to enchondral bone formation due to serious stress. They are of no clinical or functional significance. They are more related to total burn than to involvement of select burned extremities as all major long bones are affected. There is no evidence that growth arrest lines *per se* have any effect on growth.

References

1. Schiele HP, Hubbard RB, Bruck HM. Radiographic changes in burns of the upper extremity. Diagn Radiol 1972; 104:13–17.
2. Klein G, Herndon H, Rutan T, et al. Long term reduction in bone mass after severe burn injury in children. J Pediatr 1995; 126(2):252–256.
3. Owens N. Osteoporosis following burns. Br J Plast Surg 1949; 1:245–256.
4. Colson P, Stagnara P, Houot H. L-osteoporose chez les brules des membres. Lyon Chir 1953; 48:950–956.
5. Artz CP, Reiss E. The treatment of burns, 1st edn. Philadelphia: WB Saunders; 1957.
6. Klein G, Herndon D, Rutan T, et al. Bone disease in burn patients. J Bone Miner Res 1993; 8(3):337–345.
7. Van Der Wiel H, Lips P, Naura J, et al. Loss of bone in the proximal part of the femur following unstable fractures of the leg. J Bone Joint Surg Am 1994; 76:230–236.
8. Dowling JA, Omer E, Moncrief JA. Treatment of fractures in burn patients. J Trauma 1968; 8:465–474.
9. Choctaw WT, Zawacki BE, Dorr L. Primary excision and grafting of burns located over an open fracture. Arch Surg 1979; 114:1141–1142.
10. Wang Xue-wei, Zhang Zhong-ning. The successful treatment of a patient with extensive deep burns and an open comminuted frac-ture of a lower extremity. Burns 1984; 10:339–343.
11. Barret JP, Desai MH, Herndon DN. Osteomyelitis in burn patients requiring skeletal fixation. Burns 2000; 26:487–489.
12. Evans EB, Calhoun JH. Musculoskeletal changes complicating burns. In: Epps CH Jr, ed. Complications in orthopaedic surgery. Philadelphia: JB Lippincott; 1994:(2)1239–1278.
13. Evans EB. Orthopaedic measures in the treatment of severe burns. J Bone Joint Surg Am 1966; 48:643.
14. Brooker AF. The use of external fixation in the treatment of burn patients with fractures. In: Brooker AF, Edwards CC, eds. Fracture fixation: the current state of the art. J Pediatr 1995; 126(2):252–256.
15. Frye KE, Luterman A. When burn injury and skeletal trauma are two components of the multiple trauma. Orthop Nurs 1999; 18(1):30–35.
16. Cope R. Heterotopic ossification. South Med J 1990; 83(9):1058.
17. Saffle JR, Schnelby A, Hoffmann A, et al. The management of fracture in thermally injured patients. J Trauma 1983; 23:902–910.
18. Boyd BM, Robers WM, Miller GR. Periarticular ossification follow-ing burns. South Med J 1959; 52:1048.
19. Koepke GD. Personal communication, 1964.
20. Elledge ES, Smith AA, McManus WF, et al. Heterotopic bone for-mation in burned patients. J Trauma 1988; 28:684–687.
21. Peterson SI, Mani MM, Crawford CM, et al. Postburn heterotopic ossification: insights for management decision making. J Trauma 1989; 29:365.
22. Tepperman PS, Hilbert L, Peters WJ, et al. Heterotopic ossification in burns. J Burn Care Rehabil 1984; 5:283.
23. Jackson D, Mac G. Destructive burns: some orthopaedic complica-tions. Burns 1979; 7:105–122.
24. Munster AM, Bruck HM, John LA, et al. Heterotopic calcification following burns: a prospective study. J Trauma 1972; 12:1071–1074.
25. Kolar J, Vrabec R. Periarticular soft-tissue changes as a late consequence of burns. J Bone Joint Surg Am 1959; 41:103–111.
26. Heggers JP, Heggers R, Robson MC. Biochemical abnormalities in the thermally injured. J Am Med Technol 1981; 43:333.
27. Herndon D. Mediators of metabolism. J Trauma 1981; 12:701.
28. Evans EB, Larson DL, Abston S, et al. Prevention and correction of deformity after severe burns. Surg Clin North Am 1970; 50:1361–1375.
29. Evans EB, Smith JR. Bone and joint changes following burn. J Bone Joint Surg Am 1959; 41:785.
30. Johnston JTH. Atypical myositis ossificans. J Bone Joint Surg Am 1957; 39:189–194.
31. Crawford CM, Varghese G, Mani MM, et al. Heterotopic ossifica-tion: are range of motion exercises contraindicated? J Burn Care Rehabil 1986; 7:323–327.
32. Gaur A, Sinclair M, Caruso E, et al. Heterotopic ossification around the elbow following burns in children: results after excision. J Bone Joint Surg Am 2003; 85:1538–1543.
33. Ring D, Jupiter JB. Operative release of complete ankylosis of the elbow due to heterotopic bone in patients without severe injury of the central nervous system. J Bone Joint Surg Am 2003; 85:849–857.
34. Chung D, Hatfield S, Dougherty ME, et al. Heterotopic ossification of the elbow in burn patients: results after early surgical treatment. Proceedings of the 38th Annual Meeting of the American Burn Association. Las Vegas, NV: American Burn Association; 2006: April 4–7.
35. Djurickovic S, Meek RN, Snelling CF, et al. Range of motion and complications after postburn heterotopic bone excision about the elbow. J Trauma 1996; 41(5):825–830.
36. Tsionos I, Leclercq C, Rochet JM. Heterotopic ossification of the elbow in patients with burns. J Bone Joint Surg Br 2004; 86(3):396–403.

37. Holguin PH, Rico AA, Garcia JP, et al. Elbow anchylosis due to postburn heterotopic ossification. J Burn Care Rehabil 1996; 17(2):150–154.

38. Vorenkamp SE, Nelson RL. Ulnar nerve entrapment due to heterotopic bone formation after a severe burn. J Hand Surg Am 1987; 12(3):378–380.

39. Evans EB. Heterotopic bone formation in thermal burns. Clin Orthop 1991; 263:94–101.

40. Michelsson JE, Rauschning W. Pathogenesis of experimental heterotopic bone formation following temporary forcible exercising of immobilized limbs. Clin Orthop Rel Res 1983; 176:265–272.

41. Lorber J. Ectopic ossification in tuberculous meningitis. Arch Dis Child 1953; 28:98.

42. Jacobs P. Reversible ectopic soft tissue ossification following measles encephalomyelitis. Arch Dis Child 1962; 37:90.

43. Garland DE, Blum CE, Waters RL. Periarticular heterotopic ossification in head-injured adults. J Bone Joint Surg Am 1985; 62:1261.

44. VanLaeken N, Snelling CT, Meek RN, et al. Heterotopic bone formation in the patient with burn injuries. A retrospective assessment of contributing factors and methods of investigation. J Burn Care Rehabil 1989; 10:331.

45. Evans EB. Musculoskeletal changes complicating burns. In: Epps CH Jr, ed. Complications in orthopaedic surgery. Philadelphia: JB Lippincott; 1978:(2)1133–1158.

46. Vrbicky B. Post-burn heterotopic joint ossifications. Annals of Burns and Fire Disasters 1991; 4(3):161–164.

47. Peters WJ. Heterotopic ossification: can early surgery be performed, with a positive bone scan? J Burn Care Rehabil 1978; 11(4):318.

48. Hoffer M, Brody G, Ferlic F. Excision of heterotopic ossification about elbows in patients with thermal injury. J Trauma 1978; 18:667–670.

49. Bottu Y, Van Noyen G. Un cas d'ossification reversible des tissus mous chez une petite patiente paraplegique. Acta Paediatr Belg 1963; 17:223.

50. Proulz R, Dupuis M. Ossifications et calcifications para-articulaires à la suite de brulures: revue de la literature et présentation de 3 cas. Union Med Can 1972; 101:282–293.

51. Dias D. Heterotopic para-articular ossification of the elbow with soft tissue contracture in burns. Burns 1982; 9:128–134.

52. Harnar T, Engrav L, Heimbach D, et al. Experience with skeletal immobilization after excision and grafting of the severely burned hands. J Trauma 1985; 25:299–302.

53. Youel L, Evans E, Heare TC, et al. Skeletal suspension in the management of severe burns in children. J Bone Joint Surg Am 1986; 68:1375–1379.

54. Eszter V, Istvan S. Atipusos septicus arthritisek spontan luxatiok egesi serulteken. Orv Hetil 1972; 113:48.

55. Cristallo V, Dell'Orto R. Pathological dislocation of the hip. Arch Ortop 1966; 79:57–61.

56. Jackson D, Mac G. Burns into joints. Burns 1976; 2:90–106.

57. Malone JM, Fleming LL, Roberson J, et al. Immediate, early and late postsurgical management of upper-limb amputation. J Rehabil Res Dev 1984; 21:33–41.

58. Frantz CH, Delgado S. Limb-length discrepancy after third-degree burns about the foot and ankle. J Bone Joint Surg Am 1966; 48:443–450.

59. Ritsila V, Sundell B, Alhopura S. Severe growth retardation of the upper extremity resulting from burn contracture and its full recovery after release of the contracture. Br J Plast Surg 1976; 29:53–55.

60. Evans EB, Larson L, Yates S. Preservation and restoration of joint function in patients with severe burns. JAMA 1968; 204: 843–848.

Chapter 51

Mitigation of the burn-induced hypermetabolic response during convalescence

Oscar E. Suman, Rene Przkora, Patricia Blakeney, and David N. Herndon

Background

Management of burns in children remains a major challenge to medical science, not only in terms of mortality, but in discovering ways to improve their recoveries. The ultimate goal is for young burn survivors to grow into active, self-supporting, happy adults, thereby achieving an optimal quality of life. Though advances in burn care have reduced the high mortality associated with massive burns in children, burn team scientists and clinicians have barely begun to gain knowledge into what the long-term quality of life for these survivors can be.[1–4] Rehabilitative challenges with such children are numerous, and the best methods of achieving good outcomes for children with severe burns are still being developed.[5]

Treatment of pediatric burns is similar in many ways to that of adults. However, pediatric injuries present unique challenges, both at the time of acute treatment and throughout rehabilitation. Increased experience and new data, gathered in large part from courageous young survivors, have allowed burn team clinicians and scientists to identify many long-term problems associated with large burns. A major problem during convalescence is the prolonged hypermetabolic and catabolic response.

This hypermetabolic response appears to play an early and central role in many of the long-lasting difficulties for children with severe burns. In response to a severe burn, afferent stimuli are activated causing a hypothalamic thermoregulatory re-setting to occur. This results in increased heat production, a faster heart rate and a greater cardiac output, in addition to an exaggerated increase in resting energy expenditure.[6] The stress response to a severe burn is characterized by a cascade of hormones such as catecholamines, cortisol and glucagon that results in a hypercatabolic state.[7] The effects of this hypermetabolic, hypercatabolic state are rapid muscle breakdown[8] and reduced bone formation, resulting in severe osteopenia or osteoporosis[9] as well as linear growth retardation.[10–12]

One can think of this physical state as the body running at almost twice its normal rate even though the individual is at rest. The patient requires enormous amounts of nutritional intake to keep up with the energy expenditure. Even with adequate caloric intake, individuals in this state lose muscle mass and bone density. Conventional thinking has been that this state should dissipate with full healing of the burn wound. However, in clinical work, we observed that the children fail to develop muscle, to grow, and to gain weight for a period of time extending far beyond wound healing.

Only a few years ago were we able to follow systematically 25 severely burned children for 1 year to ascertain the duration of the hypermetabolic–catabolic state.[13] Stable isotope metabolic and body composition studies were performed during acute hospitalization, at initial hospital discharge, and at 6, 9, and 12 months postburn. The resting energy expenditure of these children peaked at 1-week post-injury with a metabolic rate of 180% of normal and progressively declined with time. At the 12-month exit from the study, their resting energy expenditure remained 15% above basal metabolic rate. Catabolism persisted for at least 9 months, which was 7 months after complete wound healing.

Knowledge of the duration and extensive harm resulting from the catabolic effects of trauma has also led to efforts to better delineate mechanisms of catabolism[14] and to a vigilant pursuit of early interventions that could attenuate the effects of the hypermetabolic–catabolic response. Factors affecting the convalescence of severely burned children are shown in Figure 51.1. The effect of the hypermetabolic–catabolic response 6 months after burn is displayed in Figure 51.2. Such long-lasting deleterious effects upon the recovery of severely burned children demand that we develop strategies to attenuate the hypermetabolic–catabolic response during and after discharge from acute hospitalization. For most of the issues evolving from massive burn, we are still in the early stages of this process; we are still learning about problems and devising methods of improving treatments. Our progress in developing such strategies is the subject of this chapter.

Growth delay

In 1990, Rutan and Herndon demonstrated a dampened growth curve for both height and weight in male and female pediatric patients who had sustained major thermal injury.[10] The growth velocities were delayed up to 3 years after burn injury. Even

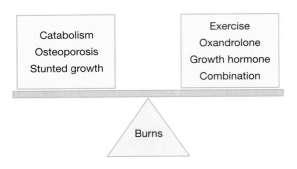

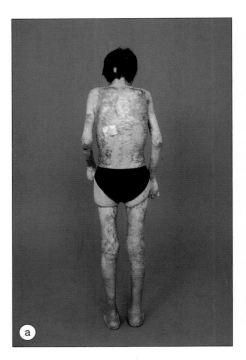

Fig. 51.1 Various burn-induced problems that afflict many severely burned survivors (left side of balance). These problems can last up to 2 years. On the right side are strategies to attenuate these problems.

after the return to normal growth velocities, the burned patients lagged behind age- and sex-matched peers.

Normal linear growth and weight gain in children are dependent upon a number of factors. The prenatal environment, adequate nutritional intake, and an emotionally nurturing household environment are crucial. Long hospitalizations alone have been known to produce profound arrests in growth and development in children. The management of massively burned children includes multiple operations and prolonged hospitalization. In cases of fascial excision, subcutaneous fat layers in the injured area are also removed. Fat stores are further depleted in providing energy for the process of gluconeogenesis from existing protein stores for dietary supply. All the reasons for the growth delay following severe burns are not currently known. However, plasma growth hormone (GH) levels have been shown to decrease in severely burned adults,[15] and it is likely that children experience a similar decrease. Administration of an anabolic agent such as recombinant

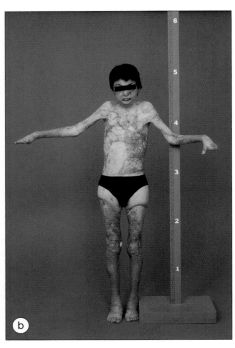

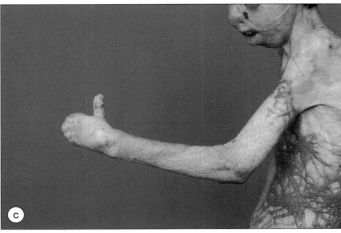

Fig. 51.2 The ravaging effects of a severe burn are illustrated in these photos (a, b, c). The body is in a hypermetabolic and catabolic state. This results in loss of muscle mass and bone mass, and is worsened by prolonged inactivity. In addition, there are physical limitations sometimes caused by the loss of digits or extremities and of burn scar contractures.

human growth hormone (rhGH) during the acute treatment of severely burned children has been demonstrated to be extremely beneficial in promoting healing and health.[7] Studies of GH demonstrate that it can be given safely to severely burned children,[16] and that it accelerates wound healing[17] and reduces tissue wasting commonly seen in the catabolic patient.[18] Using rhGH in the acute treatment of children with severe thermal injuries has been shown to improve net muscle protein synthesis[18] as well as to accelerate wound healing and reduce length of hospital stay.[17,19] Knowledge gained from such studies suggests improved treatment approaches that can be evaluated. Improvement in each of these areas could contribute to improved growth and weight gain; therefore, administration of GH was perceived as a probable advantageous tool in the management of pediatric burn patients toward normal growth.

Low et al.[20] tested the hypothesis that rhGH would ameliorate the growth delay by following, for 3 years, 49 children in a prospective, randomized, masked study. Twenty-six children received 0.2 mg/kg GH during their acute hospitalizations; 23 children received 0.9% saline as placebo during the same time periods of acute hospitalization. Children who were treated with GH during their acute care maintained stature (height for age percentile and height-velocity), whereas untreated children who were not in a growth spurt at the time of burn remained delayed in linear growth at the end of the study 3 years post-injury. Continuing with this study, Low et al. found that the differences in height percentiles had nearly resolved at 5 years postburn.[21] Short-term (average of 6 weeks) administration of GH did not attenuate the hypermetabolic state; resting energy expenditures remained elevated for both groups of children during the time they were being treated acutely. However, the administration of GH apparently made up for a deficit that commonly occurs following severe burn injury. Children burned during a growth spurt are thought to have the advantage of higher levels of growth hormone available and thus can maintain normal growth without exogenous hormone.

Catabolism

As mentioned previously, the catabolic response decreases lean mass and muscle strength. Lean mass and strength are essential for normal daily activities. Several treatment options have been investigated at our institution.

Exercise

Resistance exercise has an established influence on muscle strengthening and muscle protein synthesis. The beneficial effects of resistance training have been well documented in healthy adults, adolescents, and older children.[22-26] Ferrando et al. demonstrated in healthy adults that moderate resistance exercise is capable of ameliorating the decreases in skeletal muscle protein synthesis and strength that accompany inactivity.[27] The acute stimulatory effects of resistance exercise may last up to 48 hours.[28] In burns, resistance exercise alone is also capable of inducing increases in lean mass and muscle strength. Suman et al. demonstrated in severely burned children and adolescents that a 12-week exercise program of resistive and aerobic exercise significantly improved lean mass and muscle

strength relative to standard of care treatment (Figure 51.3).[29]

Anabolic agents

Recently, Przkora et al. studied the effects of administering 0.05 mg per kg per day of GH from hospital discharge to 12 months after burn to children. The investigators showed that growth and bone mass as well as lean mass were significantly increased in patients receiving GH compared to the placebo group. Furthermore, not only lean mass but also muscle strength was significantly improved in the treatment group. The observed beneficial effects on body composition were associated with significant elevations in anabolic hormones such as insulin-like growth factor-1 (IGF-1). Additionally, serum cortisol, a catabolic hormone, was significantly lower with GH treatment when compared to placebo. The enrolled patients were followed for an additional year and the authors demonstrated a persisting effect on growth and on bone mass in the former GH group 1 year after the treatment was discontinued. No rebound phenomena on body composition or on

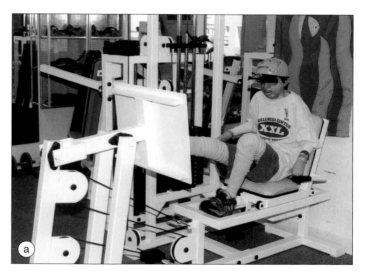

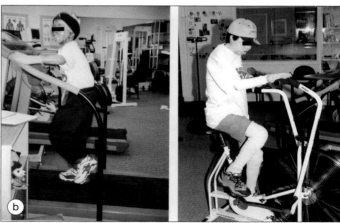

Fig. 51.3 (a, b) A structured and supervised program of resistance and aerobic exercises has been shown to be beneficial in attenuating loss of muscle mass and muscle function, as well as improving aerobic capacity in burned victims.

hormone metabolism were noted during the year following cessation of GH.

A difficulty confronted in this study is that GH is administered via daily injections. Although these injections are relatively painless (the investigators have first given them to themselves to be sure of this), they present a daily source of irritation and tension to parent and child. Therefore, we searched for a less-intrusive means to improve body composition. Oxandrolone is an anabolic steroid that has been used in catabolic situations such as hepatitis and AIDS patients and can be administered orally, thus eliminating one source of stress for children and families.[30] In a randomized trial Przkora et al. treated severely burned children with oxandrolone (0.1 mg/kg twice daily *per os*) or placebo from hospital discharge up to 12 months after trauma. They found a significant improvement in body composition, including linear growth, bone density, and lean mass. Muscle strength was also significantly improved with oxandrolone. As with long-term GH treatment, no adverse side effects were observed in the year following treatment. Beneficial effects on growth were noted even 1 year after treatment.[31] Other anabolic agents are likely to have similar benefits. Herndon et al.[32] have demonstrated that propranolol attenuates catabolism and hypermetabolism during the acute hospitalization of severely burned children. This finding suggests that long-term administration of propranolol may be beneficial in ways similar to those of growth hormone and oxandrolone and offers possible benefits for mitigating symptoms of post-traumatic stress disorder as well.[33]

Exercise in combination with anabolic agents

Because of the positive results obtained with exercise intervention alone and with GH alone, we rationalized that an exercise program that included resistance exercise in combination with GH would provide for a synergistic effect on skeletal muscle protein synthesis by addressing separate stimulatory mechanisms for an extended period of time. Suman et al. studied 44 severely burned children and adolescents who received GH (0.05 mg per kg per day) or placebo for 9 months and either participated in a 12-week exercise program or received standard of care treatment (daily physical and occupational therapy).[34] In this study, the mean percent change in lean body mass after 12 weeks was similar for the groups of participants receiving GH alone, exercise alone, or the combination of both. On the other hand, the mean percent change in muscle strength was significantly greater only in the groups receiving exercise, independent of GH. Preliminary results using a higher dose of GH (0.1 mg per kg per day) also yielded similar results; lean mass increased by GH alone, exercise alone, or the combination. However, similar to low-dose GH, muscle strength was only increased via exercise. It is presently unknown what are the effects of higher doses of GH on muscle mass of severely burned children.

We have begun studying effects of oxandrolone in conjunction with the exercise program, and results of preliminary data analyses are very exciting in their promise of enhanced overall well-being for survivors of very large and severe burn injuries. Oxandrolone in combination with exercise increased lean mass significantly more than either the drug or exercise treatment alone. Muscle strength and functional improvement were significantly improved with the combination of oxandrolone

and exercise as well as with oxandrolone or exercise alone. A planned future study will introduce propranolol instead of GH or oxandrolone and follow the same design.

Exercise and young children: because of the difficulties with having young children (i.e. under 7 years of age) use the exercise equipment or cooperate in obtaining certain measures, the exercise studies described above were conducted with children ages 7–18. However, as exercise treatment has proven so beneficial, we have now begun a program using music and movement for young children. Movements are chosen to increase strength, flexibility, and endurance. Children enjoy this 'play,' and preliminary data indicate the program to be beneficial to overall development and specifically to maintaining or improving joint range of motion beyond standard of care (prescribed occupational–physical therapy exercises).[35,36]

Long-term outcomes of children with massive burns

Contrary to what many people expect, long-term outcomes studies indicate that most children who survive severe burns do well. For the past 20 years, doctors at Shriners Burns Hospital in Galveston have followed, longitudinally, children who survived massive injuries, assessing physical and psychosocial adaptation on an annual basis with standardized measures when available. In 1986, assessments of 12 survivors of such massive injuries were reported.[37] Of the 12, eight (66%) were found to be well adjusted; four were described as regressed with excessive fear, neurotic symptoms, and somatic complaints. A later follow-up report of eight of the children found satisfactory adjustment in six (75%) and two who were not doing well.[38] Four years later, we reported the results of psychosocial assessments of 25 children with 80% total body surface area (TBSA) burned in which the burned children appeared, as a group, to have no more behavioral problems than their age-matched cohorts in a normative reference group.[39] The burned children also had positive self-esteem, equal to and sometimes surpassing, that of the non-burned reference group. Examining the impact of physical impairment upon the psychosocial competence of 19 survivors of massive burns, we found the competence scores of the burned children, as reported by both the parents of the children and the children themselves, to be equal to those of the normal, age-matched reference group.[40] Physical impairment was related to competence only in the area of activity, and not in academic or social competence. Perhaps most surprising to us was that two of the 19 children had ratings of 'no physical impairment' based upon range of motion measurements according to AMA guidelines. We concluded that severe childhood burn injury does not necessarily induce onerous physical impairment, and even severe impairment does not necessarily lead to poor psychosocial adjustment.

In a more recent examination of the psychological and behavioral adjustment of 74 of our survivors of massive injury (80% TBSA = 70% full-thickness), we found that 70% of the children and young adults had no significant difficulty; most were doing well and described themselves as being 'happy'. Most were still in school. Three young adults had married or were living with a committed partner and had become parents.[41]

Of 41 who were also assessed for physical functioning, 32 patients were independent with completion of age-appropriate activities of daily living skills. Only the amputation of fingers seemed to impede the self-sufficiency of these individuals.[42] Although some, like those with finger amputations, required adaptive devices and compensations such as extra time to achieve successful performance, most of these survivors of massive injury had managed the skills required to meet developmental milestones, to develop appropriate autonomy, and to achieve psychological and social well-being.

In a study conducted at our sister institution, the Shriners Hospital in Boston, 80 survivors of burns involving >70% TBSA were evaluated almost 15 years following their injuries.[43] The investigators used a quality of life assessment tool to measure achievement in several domains, including general health, psychological health, family function, physical function, and physical role. The scores of these young people were similar to those of the normal population with the exception of physical functioning and physical role. In these areas, the scores were more than 2 standard deviations below the age- and gender-matched norms, indicating that some had continuing serious physical disabilities. Thus, while some children surviving severe burns had, as young adults, lingering physical disabilities, most reported having accomplished a satisfying quality of life.

Another outcomes study of 100 young adults with severe burns treated at the Galveston Hospital also reports that on the standardized self-report measures[44] and on the assessment of physical impairment,[45,46] young survivors appeared to be doing well; however, measures that prodded more intensely into their psychological/emotional lives revealed that many of them suffered from difficulties, most often anxieties that were at times debilitating.[47] It would seem that while burned children may harbor fear, anxiety, and sadness at a private level, at a public level, most of them, even those most severely burned, perform well. In terms of achievement in school, occupationally, and socially, most burn survivors are judged by outside observers to be doing well with only 20–30% having behavioral difficulties significant enough to warrant further clinical attention.[39–46]

The children in these outcomes studies did not have the benefits of the strategies we now use to deal with the hypermetabolism and catabolism occurring in response to large burns, which makes their achievements even more remarkable. Psychosocial difficulties related to the hypermetabolic response are numerous; fatigue, stunted linear growth, diminished muscle mass and weakness, and bone fragility limit the child's ability to fully participate in many ordinary childhood activities for a prolonged period after returning home even though their wounds were closed. Not only did the children miss many physical benefits of such activities, but they also missed the social interactions and the feeling of 'belonging' that accompany participation. Thus children who already felt stigmatized because of their burn scars and disfigurement, felt increasingly isolated from their peers. For psychosocial reasons, we pushed children to return to school quickly upon return home; but that meant that children with severe burns were attending school during the months when they fatigued quickly and so were hampered in their ability to concentrate and learn. Thus, they were at risk for feeling (and being stigmatized) as academically incompetent. If arrangements for shortened school days or special considerations were made to assist a child, the child often had to be classified as a 'special education' student — again stigmatizing and further isolating the child.

Decreasing the physical impact of hypermetabolism–catabolism also improves the opportunities for successful psychosocial adaptation following severe burn injury. The young survivors who participate in the 3-month, in-house exercise program also are able to receive regular psychological and psychiatric treatment by our burn team during that time. They and their parents receive regular individual psychotherapy for minimally 1 hour per week. During these sessions, many issues are addressed, e.g. bereavement for others lost in the fire, sadness at losing one's former self, pain, anger, social anxiety, preparing to return to their homes and communities. The children participate in age-matched groups for art therapy and for play activities. Similarly they receive schooling within the hospital school, again matched with other burned children of similar age and educational level for classroom participation. All of these experiences also allow the children to share with each other and to support each other in their difficult work of recovery and rehabilitation. Parents likewise benefit from the support and comfort of other parents who are in similar situations, and parents are well educated about how to assist their children before returning home. Tasks of treatment and issues addressed are essentially the same as described in more detail in Chapter 66. The major differences for the children and families who participate in the in-house program are the regularity with which they are scheduled to see a helping expert and the number and diversity of experts easily available to help on a non-scheduled basis.

For all children surviving massive burn injuries, whether having the advantage of 3 months of special attention or not,

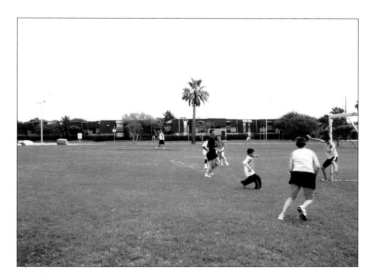

Fig. 51.4 The ultimate objective of strategies to attenuate catabolism, hypermetabolism, and other burn-induced problems should be to improve the quality of life in burn victims. This may be accomplished by offering the burn victims physical and psychosocial rehabilitation strategies to enhance the potential to a full and effective re-incorporation into society.

recognition that many of the difficulties of the first year post-burn are part of the illness of severe burns removes some of the strife from the process of rehabilitation. In the past, burn care professionals and patients and their families, all feeling frustrated, have alternated between blaming themselves and blaming each other for their failures during this first terrible year post-injury. With the evidence that this extraordinary physical disruption continues for most of that first year, the informed team can teach the family about this part of the illness and assist them in planning to manage this phase just as they have managed the acute phase. Successful management of the hypermetabolic response diminishes the extent and severity of psychosocial obstacles burned children and their families must overcome. Knowledge that many former survivors, in spite of their impediments, have successfully met their challenges to become participating members of their communities allows us to hope for even happier futures for our current patients (Figure 51.4).

References

1. Herndon DN, Parks DH. Comparison of serial debridement and autografting and early massive excision with cadaver skin overlay in the treatment of large burns in children. J Trauma 1986; 26(2):149–152.
2. Herndon DN, Barrow RE, Rutan RL, et al. A comparison of conservative versus early excision. Therapies in severely burned patients. Ann Surg 1989; 209(5):547–552; discussion 552–553.
3. Wolf SE, Rose JK, Desai MH, et al. Mortality determinants in massive pediatric burns. An analysis of 103 children with ≥80% TBSA burns (≥70% full-thickness). Ann Surg 1997; 225(5):554–565; discussion 565–569.
4. Herndon DN, LeMaster J, Beard S, et al. The quality of life after major thermal injury in children: an analysis of 12 survivors with greater than or equal to 80% total body, 70% third-degree burns. J Trauma 1986; 26(7):609–619.
5. Constable JD. The state of burn care: past, present and future. Burns 1994; 20(4):316–324.
6. Wolfe RR, Herndon DN, Jahoor F, et al. Effect of severe burn injury on substrate cycling by glucose and fatty acids. N Engl J Med 1987; 317(7):403–408.
7. Ramirez RJ, Wolf SE, Herndon DN. Is there a role for growth hormone in the clinical management of burn injuries? Growth Horm IGF Res 1998; 8(Suppl B):99–105.
8. Sakurai Y, Aarsland A, Herndon DN, et al. Stimulation of muscle protein synthesis by long-term insulin infusion in severely burned patients. Ann Surg 1995; 222(3):283–294; 294–297.
9. Klein GL, Herndon DN, Goodman WG, et al. Histomorphometric and biochemical characterization of bone following acute severe burns in children. Bone 1995; 17(5):455–460.
10. Rutan RL, Herndon DN. Growth delay in postburn pediatric patients. Arch Surg 1990; 125(3):392–395.
11. Klein GL, Herndon DN, Rutan TC, et al. Bone disease in burn patients. J Bone Miner Res 1993; 8(3):337–345.
12. Klein GL, Herndon DN, Langman CB, et al. Long-term reduction in bone mass after severe burn injury in children. J Pediatr 1995; 126(2):252–256.
13. Hart DW, Wolf SE, Mlcak R, et al. Persistence of muscle catabolism after severe burn. Surgery 2000; 128(2):312–319.
14. Hart DW, Wolf SE, Chinkes DL, et al. Determinants of skeletal muscle catabolism after severe burn. Ann Surg 2000; 232(4):455–465.
15. Jeffries MK, Vance ML. Growth hormone and cortisol secretion in patients with burn injury. J Burn Care Rehabil 1992; 13(4):391–395.
16. Ramirez RJ, Wolf SE, Barrow RE, et al. Growth hormone treatment in pediatric burns: a safe therapeutic approach. Ann Surg 1998; 228(4):439–448.
17. Gilpin DA, Barrow RE, Rutan RL, et al. Recombinant human growth hormone accelerates wound healing in children with large cutaneous burns. Ann Surg 1994; 220(1):19–24.
18. Gore DC, Honeycutt D, Jahoor F, et al. Effect of exogenous growth hormone on whole-body and isolated-limb protein kinetics in burned patients. Arch Surg 1991; 126(1):38–43.
19. Herndon DN, Barrow RE, Kunkel KR, et al. Effects of recombinant human growth hormone on donor-site healing in severely burned children. Ann Surg 1990; 212(4):424–429; discussion 430–431.
20. Low JF, Herndon DN, Barrow RE. Effect of growth hormone on growth delay in burned children: a 3-year follow-up study. Lancet 1999; 354(9192):1789.
21. Aili Low JF, Barrow RE, Mittendorfer B, et al. The effect of short-term growth hormone treatment on growth and energy expenditure in burned children. Burns 2001; 27(5):447–452.
22. Biolo G, Maggi SP, Williams BD, et al. Increased rates of muscle protein turnover and amino acid transport after resistance exercise in humans. Am J Physiol 1995; 268(3 Pt 1):E514–E520.
23. Chesley A, MacDougall JD, Tarnopolsky MA, et al. Changes in human muscle protein synthesis after resistance exercise. J Appl Physiol 1992; 73(4):1383–1388.
24. MacDougall JD, Gibala MJ, Tarnopolsky MA, et al. The time course for elevated muscle protein synthesis following heavy resistance exercise. Can J Appl Physiol 1995; 20(4):480–486.
25. Blimkie CJ. Resistance training during pre- and early puberty: efficacy, trainability, mechanisms, and persistence. Can J Sport Sci 1992; 17(4):264–279.
26. Ramsay JA, Blimkie CJ, Smith K, et al. Strength training effects in prepubescent boys. Med Sci Sports Exerc 1990; 22(5):605–614.
27. Ferrando AA, Tipton KD, Bamman MM, et al. Resistance exercise maintains skeletal muscle protein synthesis during bed rest. J Appl Physiol 1997; 82(3):807–810.
28. Phillips SM, Tipton KD, Aarsland A, et al. Mixed muscle protein synthesis and breakdown after resistance exercise in humans. Am J Physiol 1997; 273(1 Pt 1):E99–E107.
29. Suman OE, Spies RJ, Celis MM, et al. Effects of a 12-wk resistance exercise program on skeletal muscle strength in children with burn injuries. J Appl Physiol 2001; 91(3):1168–1175.
30. Hart DW, Wolf SE, Ramzy PI, et al. Anabolic effects of oxandrolone after severe burn. Ann Surg 2001; 233(4):556–564.
31. Przkora R, Jeschke MG, Barrow RE, et al. Metabolic and hormonal changes of severely burned children receiving long-term oxandrolone treatment. Ann Surg 2005; 242(3):384–389, discussion 390–391.
32. Herndon DN, Hart DW, Wolf SE, et al. Reversal of beta-blockade after severe burns. N Engl J Med 201; 345(17):1223–1229.
33. Vaiva G, Ducrocq F, Jezequel K, et al. Immediate treatment with propranolol decreases posttraumatic stress disorder two months after trauma. Biol Psychiatry 2003; 54(9):947–949.
34. Suman OE, Thomas SJ, Wilkins JP, et al. Effect of exogenous growth hormone and exercise on lean mass and muscle function in children with burns. J Appl Physiol 2003; 94(6):2273–2281.
35. Neugebauer CT, Serghiou M, Marvin J. A comprehensive 8–12 week group music & movement program for severely burned children. Proceedings of the American Burn Association. J Burn Care Rehabil 2005; 26(2):Abstract 79:S85.
36. Neugebauer CT, Serghiou M, Herndon DN, et al. Follow-up range of motion in a music and movement-based exercise with rehabilitation program versus standard of care in very young children with severe burns. Proceedings of the American Burn Association. J Burn Care Rehabil 2006; 27(2):Abstract 140:S119.
37. Herndon DN, LeMaster J, Beard S, et al. The quality of life after major thermal injury in children: an analysis of 12 survivors with greater than or equal to 80% total body, 70% third-degree burns. J Trauma 1986; 26(7):609–619.

38. Beard SA, Herndon DN, Desai M. Adaptation of self-image in burn-disfigured children. J Burn Care Rehabil 1989; 10(6): 550–554.

39. Blakeney P, Meyer W, Moore P, et al. Psychosocial sequelae of pediatric burns involving 80% or greater total body surface area. J Burn Care Rehabil 1993; 14(6):684–689.

40. Moore P, Moore M, Blakeney P, et al. Competence and physical impairment of pediatric survivors of burns of more than 80% total body surface area. J Burn Care Rehabil 1996; 17(6)(Pt 1):547–551.

41. Blakeney P, Meyer W 3rd, Robert R, et al. Long-term psychosocial adaptation of children who survive burns involving 80% or greater total body surface area. J Trauma 1998; 44(4):625–632; discussion 633–634.

42. Meyers-Paal R, Blakeney P, Robert R, et al. Physical and psychologic rehabilitation outcomes for pediatric patients who suffer 80% or more TBSA, 70% or more third degree burns. J Burn Care Rehabil 2000; 21(1)(Pt 1):43–49.

43. Sheridan RL, Hinson MI, Liang MH, et al. Long-term outcome of children surviving massive burns. JAMA 2000; 283(1):69–73.

44. Meyer WJ III, Blakeney P, Russell W, et al. Psychological problems reported by young adults who were burned as children. J Burn Care Rehabil 2004; 25:98–106.

45. C Baker, W Meyer, III. Self-care skills in young adults burned as children. Poster presented at ISBI 11th Quadrennial Congress in Seattle, WA, 2002; APTA Combined Sections Meeting in Boston, MA, 2002, and at the 2001 TPTA Annual Conference in Arlington, TX.

46. Meyer WJ, Russell W, Robert RS, et al. Incidence of major psychiatric illness in young adults who were burned as children. Submitted for publication, 2005.

Chapter 52

Overview of burn reconstruction

Ted Huang

Chapter contents

Burn injuries are a systemic illness of trauma in etiology. The severity of 'illness' is usually assessed, if not by patient survival, by the consequence of burn injuries; i.e. scar hyperplasia/hypertrophy, scar contracture, and structural deformities due to loss of bodily components. Since the bodily deformity is closely related to the magnitude of injuries, restorative procedures are seldom indicated if the depth of injury is superficial and the burned area limited (Figures 52.1 and 51.2).

The possibility of surviving burn injuries has changed dramatically over the past 20 years attributable singularly to an aggressive approach in surgical treatment of burn wounds; i.e. early wound debridement and wound coverage.[1–3] It is ironic that the success attained in burn treatment has resulted in a higher number of patients who will need to undergo reconstruction because of an aggressive 'lifesaving' surgical treatment.

Formation of scar tissues at a wound site and contraction of the scar tissues are the normal consequence of an injury. Although the exact mechanisms accounting for the sequential changes in wound healing and scar formation remain incompletely understood, wounds with infection and/or allowed to heal spontaneously, for instances, tend to form scars that are thickened and contracted circumferentially; an observation suggestive of various fibrogenic cytokines such as transforming growth factor β could play an important role in the pathogenesis of these otherwise clinically undesirable consequences.[4,5]

The thickened and contracted scar tissues, the changes that are 'normal' and 'expected' consequences of the wound healing processes, are microscopically found to be composed of collagen arranged in whorls and nodules. The changes may be observed as early as 3–4 weeks following the injury and they are cosmetically unsightly and functionally disturbing (Figure 52.3).

Reconstruction of burn deformities

General principles

Burn injuries are a traumatic illness affecting every physiological system of the body. In short, each and every physiological process of the body is altered because of thermal destruction of the skin. The altered physiological processes will affect not only the healing of the original burn wounds but also healing processes of the secondary surgical procedures aiming to restore the consequence of the original injuries. The treatment, under an aberrant physiological circumstance, should aim to repair the burn wounds first. Attempts to restore deformities should be delayed until recovery from the initial phase of injury is complete.[6]

An early treatment of deformity

Of the consequences of burn injuries, hyperplasia and contracture of resultant scars at the wound sites and the contraction of mobile bodily parts (i.e. eyelids, neck, axilla, elbow, hands–fingers, groin, knee and ankle–foot) are two of the most common problems that are in need of attention. The regimen of applying pressure upon scar tissues and of immobilizing joint structures has been advocated to minimize the undesirable consequences of scarring and scar contracture (Figure 52.4).

Although the true efficacy of a non-surgical regimen to control the deformities has not been established, the frequency of secondary joint release among individuals who had 'endured' the morbidities associated with proper joint splinting for a period of no less than 6 months[7,8] has been noted. The use of pressure dressing, especially in the areas such as upper and lower limbs, with proper splinting of the hand and fingers, is strongly recommended soon following the injury. The regimen of non-surgical management of burn deformity must include daily physiotherapy and exercise to maintain joint mobility and to prevent muscle wasting.

Reconstruction of burn deformities

Objective assessment of deformities by the patients themselves is neither physically nor psychologically possible soon after the accident and while they are recovering from injury. Instead, restoration of physical changes resulting from the injury, in addition to the need to obtain relief of pain and discomfort, are the only concerns of the patient. Medical assessment of physical problems caused by scarring and scar contracture, in this sense, will require detailed understanding of the extent of the original injury and the precise treatment approach used to manage the burned wound. Formulating a realistic plan to restore physical problems and to alleviate pain and discomfort in the area of injury similarly requires in-depth analysis of the physical deformities and psychological disturbance sustained by the patient. Psychiatric, psychosocial, and physiotherapeu-

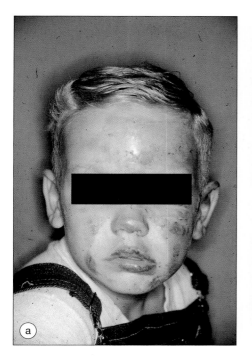
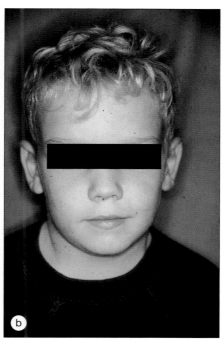

Fig. 52.1 (a) A 3-year-old boy sustained flash flame burns of the face. The depth of injury was judged to be superficial. (b) The wounds healed spontaneously and the scar formed was judged to be minimal.

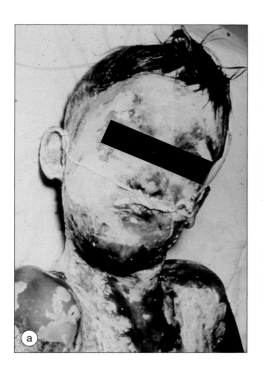
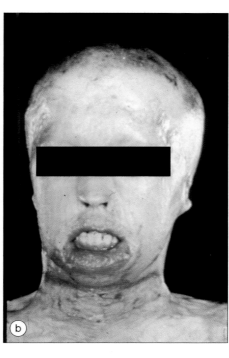

Fig. 52.2 (a) A 9-year-old boy sustained flame burns involving 60% of his total body surface. (b) The injury was found to be extensive, requiring staged debridement and skin grafting.

tic cares, in this sense, must be continued while a surgical treatment plan is instituted.

Indication and timing of surgical intervention

For a surgeon, making a decision *how* to operate on a patient with burn deformities is quite simple. In contrast, deciding *when* to operate on a patient with burn deformities can be difficult. The dilemma, however, may be alleviated if a basic principle is understood and followed:

- restoring bodily deformities that impose functional difficulties must precede any surgical effort to restore the appearance.

In short, a surgeon's effort must be concentrated upon restoring the deformed bodily parts essential for physical functions if not for patient survival. An exposed skull or a calvarial defect, contracted eyelids, constricted nares, contracted major joints, and a urethral and/or anal stricture in individuals with severe perineal burns are the prime indications for an early surgical

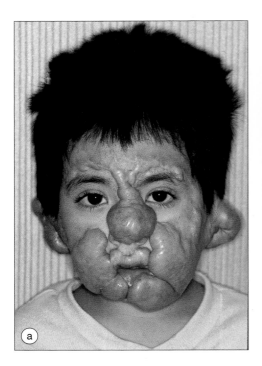 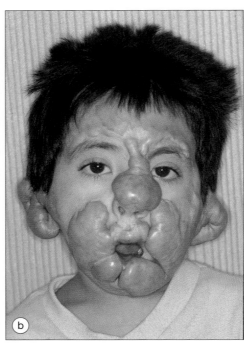

Fig. 52.3 (a) Scars formed around the injured site can become hypertrophic as quickly as in 3–4 weeks following injuries. (b) The scar was so tight as to interfere with mouth opening.

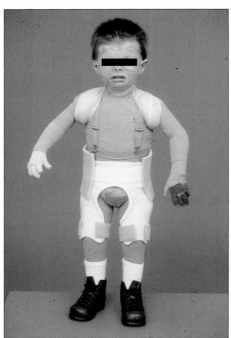

Fig. 52.4 The use of splints over the mobile joints and pressure garment is an essential component of patient management.

intervention. In contrast, restoration of deformed bodily parts in general, can be delayed. In fact, reconstruction of the nose and the ear, for instance, should not be initiated until its growth pattern has reached the growth peak at 6–8 years of age.

Although the exact scientific basis remains unclear, it is advocated that attempts at reconstructing burn deformities should be delayed for at least 2 years (the time needed for scar maturation). During the interim, the use of pressure garments and splinting is recommended to facilitate scar maturation and to minimize joint contracture. The true efficacy of a pressure garment in facilitating scar maturation remains undefined. Lack of a reliable method in determining various stages of scar maturation and personal difference in assessing scar appearance could account for the controversy. Splinting a joint imbedded in burned scars with an external device to maintain a proper joint angulation, on the other hand, was found to be effective in reducing the need for reoperation to achieve joint function. However, this was possible only if the patient would have worn the splint faithfully for more than a minimal period of 6 months. A physical exercise regimen to provide vigorous movements of a burned joint was found to be similarly effective in reducing the need for surgical intervention.

The 2-year moratorium on early burn reconstruction, in some instances, is justifiable. Operating on an immature scar characterized by redness and induration is technically more cumbersome; hemostatic control of the wound is difficult and inelasticity and lack of tensile strength, noted in scar tissues, render tissue manipulation more difficult. A high rate of contracture, noted in instances where a piece of partial-thickness skin graft is used for releasing a wound showing active inflammatory processes, may further support the advocacy of 2 years of delay in initiating burn reconstruction.[9]

Our recent change in handling individuals who were in need of reconstruction showed that contracted bodily parts can be effectively reconstructed if a skin flap, fasciocutaneous flap or musculocutaneous flap technique is used. The reconstruction is initiated as early as 3–6 months following the initial injury. This approach is well suited for those encountering functional difficulties because of scarring and scar contracture.[10]

The techniques of reconstruction

There are several techniques routinely used to reconstruct bodily deformities common to burn injuries; i.e. unsightly scar, scar contracture, and joint contracture. Principally, they are:

- primary closure technique,
- closure with a piece of free skin grafting technique with or without the use of dermal template,
- closure with an adjacent skin flap technique,
- closure with an adjacent fasciocutaneous (FC) flap technique,
- closure with an adjacent musculocutaneous (MC) flap technique, and
- closure with a distant skin, fasciocutaneous (FC) flap, or musculocutaneous (MC) flap via microsurgical technique.

Primary wound closure technique:

Excision of the unsightly scar with layered closure of the resultant wound is the simplest and the most direct approach in burn reconstruction. The technique is also useful in handling scars that are hyperesthetic and pruritic.

The margins of the scar requiring excision are marked. It is important to determine the amount of scar tissue that can be removed so that the resultant defect can be closed directly. 'Pinching' the edge of a scar at three or four different sites along the length of the scar to determine the mobility of the wound edges is the simplest yet most reliable method of determining the amount of scar tissue that can be removed safely. Leaving a rim of scar tissue is generally necessary, unless the size of the scar is so small that removal and direct closure of the resultant wound would not lead to contour deformity. A circumferential incision is made in the line marked and is carried through the full thickness of the scar down to the subcutaneous fatty layer. While the outer layer of the scarred tissue is excised, 4–5 mm of the collagen layer is left attached to the base. The conventional approach of wedged scar excision will result in a depression along the site of the scar excision, an iatrogenic consequence that could be difficult to amend secondarily. In order to minimize vascular supply interference along the wound edges, undermining of the scar edge should be kept to a minimum. Synthetic sutures are preferred for wound closure (Figure 52.5).

Skin grafting technique:

Free skin graft without incorporating a dermal template — Covering an open wound with a piece of skin graft harvested at a various thickness is the conventional approach of wound closure. Whole components of the skin removed as an intact unit – i.e. epidermis and dermis – is defined as a full-thickness skin graft, and a piece of skin cut at a thickness varying between 8/1000 of an inch (0.196 mm) and 18/1000 of an inch (0.441 mm) is considered to be a partial- or a split-thickness skin graft. The thickness of a full-thickness skin graft is quite variable depending upon the body site. A full-thickness skin graft harvested from the back, for instance, will be 160/1000 of an inch (4 mm) in thickness while the one harvested from the upper eyelid will be around 35/1000 of an inch (0.8 mm). The difference is attributable to the difference in the thickness of the dermis.

While a power-driven dermatome is usually used to harvest a piece of partial (split)-thickness skin graft, a free hand knife could be used to cut a piece of full-thickness skin graft. A paper template may be made to determine the size of the skin graft needed to close a wound. The skin graft is laid down to

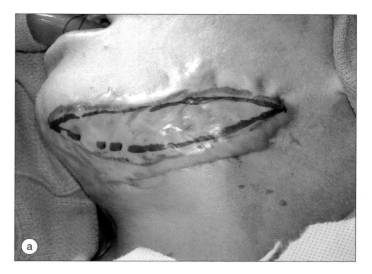

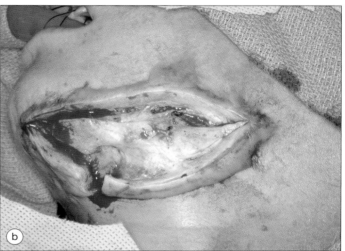

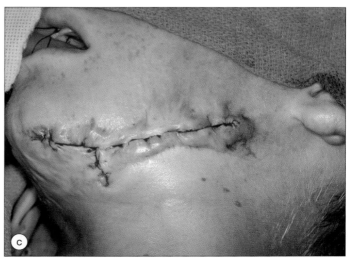

Fig. 52.5 (a) The scar formed in the left submental area was pruritic and unsightly. The extent of the excision was marked and the area was infiltrated with 0.25% lidocaine containing 1:400 000 epinephrine to achieve hemostasis. (b) The epidermal layer was sharply excised, leaving the dermal layer intact. (c) The wound edges were closed primarily in layers using nylon sutures.

the wound, colloquially termed as 'wound bed,' and is anchored into place by suturing the graft to the wound edge to edge at various sites. An apposition of the skin graft with the 'wound bed' is essential to ensure an in-growth of a vascular network in the graft within 3–5 days for graft survival as any mechanical barriers – i.e. blood clot or pool of serous or purulent fluid – will restrain the vascularizing processes, leading to graft loss. A gauze or cotton bolster tied over a graft has been the traditional technique to anchor and to prevent fluid accumulating underneath a graft even though there has been no objective evidence to support the efficacy of this maneuver. A quilting technique, instead of the bolstering technique, has been found to be more effective in immobilizing a skin graft and is associated with lesser morbidities (Figure 52.6).

The basis for using a free skin graft of various thicknesses to close all wounds is not entirely clear. It is, however, clear that the use of a thin graft is more appropriate for closing wounds with unstable vascular supplies, particularly if the skin graft donor site is scarce. Although the exact reasons remain undefined, the quality and the presence of dermis could influence the extent of wound contraction. That is, the extent of contraction noted in a 'wound bed' is more if a piece of skin graft with minimal dermal inclusion – i.e. a thin partial-thickness skin graft – is used. By inference, the presence of a dermal structure in the 'wound bed' could affect wound contracture.

Free skin graft with prior incorporation of a dermal regenerative template — For the past several years, artificial dermal substitutes have been manufactured from alloplastic or xenographic materials; e.g. AlloDerm™, Integra™ (the manufacturing processes was initially described by Yannis and Burke in 1980); these are biosynthetic two-layered membranes composed of a three-dimensional porous matrix of fibers and cross-linked with bovine tendons and glycosaminoglycan (chondroitin-6-sulfate). This material, when implanted over an open wound, has been found to form a layer of parenchymal structures resembling a dermis, thus providing wound coverage with an autologous skin graft in situations where, previously, immediate closure was not possible. However, the need

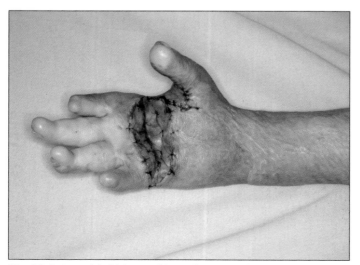

Fig. 52.6 A partial-thickness skin graft was used to cover an open wound that had resulted from releasing a contracted wound.

for a staged approach to graft a wound using this technique is considered cumbrous (Figure 52.7).

Skin flap technique:

The approach using a segment of skin with its intrinsic structural components attached to restore a destroyed and/or missed bodily part follows the fundamental principle of reconstructive surgery. This technique, however, will not only cause skin scarring in the flap donor site but also a donor site contour alteration that may be considered cosmetically unsightly. The loss of the skin flap, more commonly encountered in burn patients because of altered vascular supplies to the skin attributable to injuries and surgical treatment, could render this technique unsuitable. Despite the drawbacks, the approach to restore a destructed bodily part with a piece of like tissue is technically sound and the procedure can provide restored bodily function and contour. The recent technical innovation of incorporating a muscle and/or facial layer in the skin flap design, especially in a burned area, further expanded the scope of burn reconstruction as more burned tissues could be used for flap fabrication.

The axial skin flap — The skin in many areas is nourished directly by known cutaneous arteries. A skin flap without regard to its length-to-width ratio requisite may be fabricated if the vascular trees are included in the flap pattern (Figure 52.8)

The z-plasty technique — This technique, in short, is based upon the principle of mobilizing a full segment of skin with its vascular supplies undisturbed, from an area adjacent to the site needing tissue replacement. This is conventionally achieved by interposing two skin flaps of an equilateral triangle – i.e. 60° – that has a common limb drawn in the midst of the scarred area. A scarred and contracted area is released as the flaps are interposed in an opposite direction. Any space defect due to skin and underlying tissue movement is made up for by mobilizing tissues from an adjacent area (Figure 52.9).

The modified z-plasty technique; alias 3/4 z-plasty technique — Two flaps are, unlike in the conventional z-plasty technique, of a right-angled triangle; i.e. one internal 90° angle and the other with a 45° angle. The angle for the triangular flap has decreased from a conventional 60° to 45°; hence the 3/4 z-plasty technique. The limb of the 90° triangle is made in the scarred area resulting from the tissue loss. The second limb of the triangle is made perpendicular to the first one. The angle formed by the second limb of the right-angled triangle and the hypotenuse of the second right-angled triangle is 45°. A triangular skin flap fabricated in this manner is rotated to fill the tissue defect formed by the surgical releasing of the contracted scarred area. The procedure is a variant of the conventional rotational/interpositional skin flap technique by rotating the 45° triangular skin flap singularly to make up the defect (Figure 52.10)

Despite its geometric advantage in flap design, fabricating a skin flap or skin flaps for z-plastic reconstruction burn deformities is not infrequently plagued with skin necrosis. Aberrant vascular supplies to the skin attributable to the original injury and/or surgical treatment could be the factor responsible for the problems. In recent years, the use of a skin flap designed

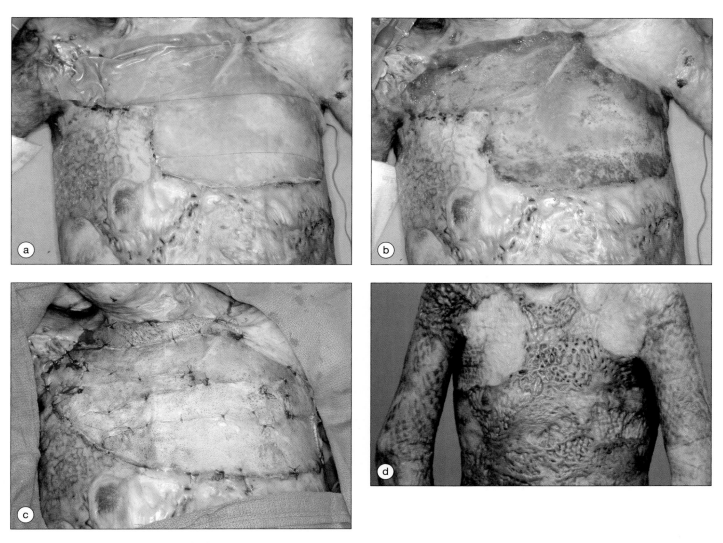

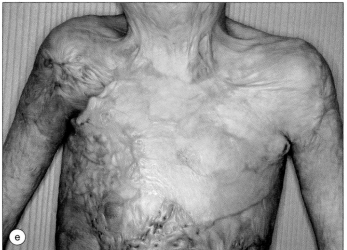

Fig. 52.7 (a) A piece of Integra™ was used to cover the wound. (b) Erythematous changes noted in the wound indicated satisfactory capillary in-growth. (c) A partial-thickness skin graft of $^8/_{1000}$ of an inch in thickness was harvested for wound coverage. (d) The scarred chest area required surgical treatment because of pruritis. (e) The appearance of wound 12 months following the re-grafting procedure using the dermal template + STSG technique. The scar was noted to be soft and pliable.

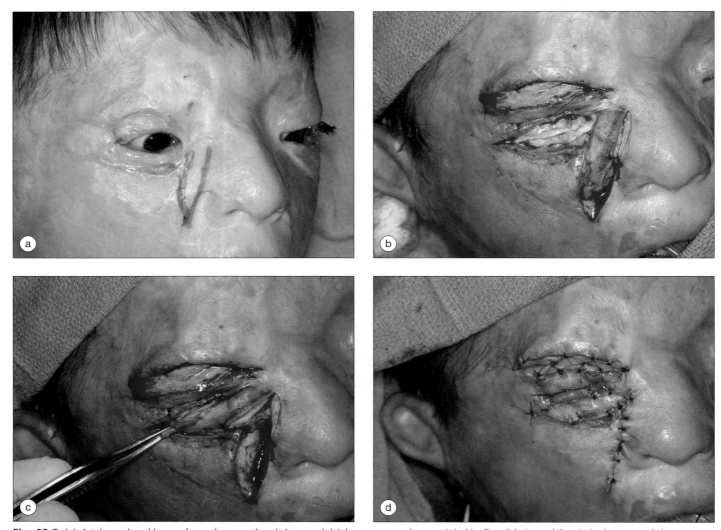

Fig. 52.8 (a) A triangular skin mark made over the right nasolabial area to mark an axial skin flap fabricated for right lower eyelid reconstruction. (b) The size of skin flap was equal to the size of lower eyelid defect. (c) The triangular flap was rotated cephalad and laterally to fill the right lower eyelid tissue defect. (d) The wounds were closed with dissolvable sutures.

to include muscle or fascia underneath has expanded further the usefulness of conventional z-plasty and the ³/4 z-plasty technique in burn reconstruction.

Musculocutaneous (MC) or fasciocutaneous (FC) flap technique:

Inclusion of not only the skin but also the subcutaneous tissues and the fascia and the muscle is necessary to fabricate a skin flap to reconstruct a tissue defect in individuals with deep burn injuries. That is, fabricating a flap in a burned area is possible if the underlying muscle or the fascia is included in the design.

Musculocutaneous z-plasty technique — While the skin pattern is identical to the conventional z-plasty technique, the muscle underneath must be included in the flap fabrication. Although physical characteristics of the normal skin – i.e. the skin pliability and expandability – are absent if scarred skin

is included in the flap design, a 'scarred-skin' MC or FC flap could be safely elevated and transferred to close an open wound. In practice, an MC z-plasty technique is useful in the neck release and in the eyelid because of the underlying muscle; i.e. platysma and orbicularis oculi muscles are thin, pliable, and easily movable (Figure 52.11).

Fasciocutaneous z-plasty technique — This is a technical modification of the MC z-plasty technique by including the muscular fascia only. Separation of the skin and its subcutaneous tissues from the underlying fascia must be avoided in order not to impair the blood supply to the flap. In practice, the technique is useful in reconstructing contractural deformities around the knee and ankle areas.

³/4 Fasciocutaneous z-plasty technique — A 45° triangular FC flap that includes the fascial layer may be fabricated anywhere in the body. The flap is elevated and then turned 90° to cover a tissue defect resulting from releasing a contracted

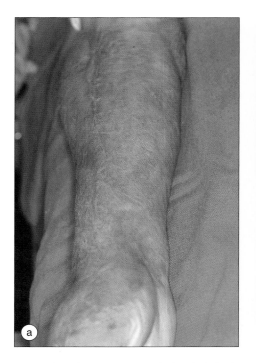

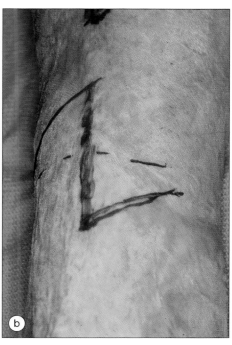

Fig. 52.9 (a) A tight scar band was noted over the forearm. (b) Two equilateral triangles were marked into a 'z.' (c) Incisions were made to free up two triangle skin flaps. (d) Two flaps were interposed to achieved the release.

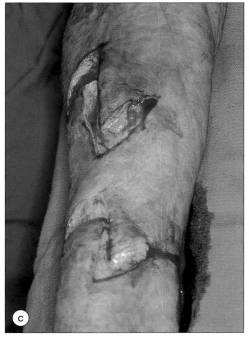

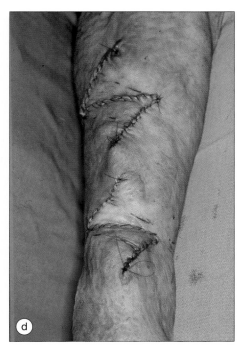

wound. Although unburned skin, when used to fabricate a triangular flap, is more versatile, scarred skin with or without subcutaneous tissues may be used for flap fabrication. Suturing the fascia to the skin edge is a useful maneuver to avoid impairing vascular supplies to the dermal structures by accidental separation of the fascia from the overlying skin (Figure 52.12).

Paratenocutaneous z-plasty and ³/₄ paratenocutaneous z-plasty techniques — In instances where fabrication of a composite skin flap is indicated in the distal section of the upper

and lower extremities – i.e. wrist and ankle, the paratenon – a fascial extension of the voluntary musculatures should be included in the flap design and fabrication (Figure 52.13).

Tissue expansion technique:

An extreme stretching of the integument is quite commonly observed in human bodies. The tissue expansion technique follows the same principle except it is carried out intentionally with an inflatable device; i.e. a tissue expander. Because of the excessively active scarring processes more frequently observed

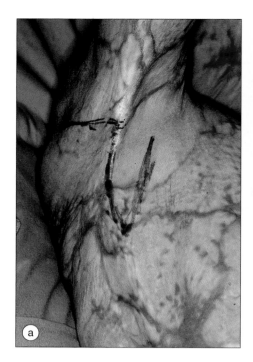

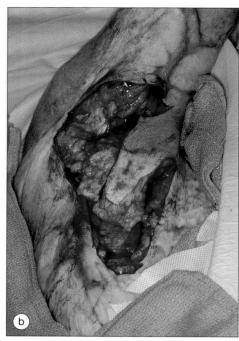

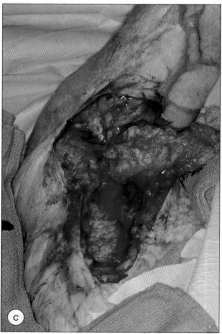

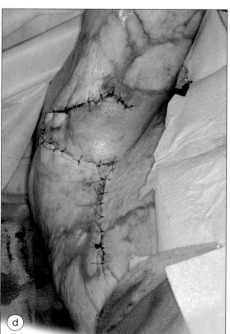

Fig. 52.10 (a) A right-angled triangle with the cathetus marked along the line of contracture and perpendicular to the line of release. (b) Incisions were made to release the contracture and to fabricate a triangular skin flap. (c) The right-angled triangle skin flap was elevated and rotated anteriorly. (d) The triangular flap was rotated 90° to fill the tissue defect that had resulted from the release.

in burn victims, especially during the period soon following the accident, timing of the initiation of the procedure could be difficult and its use may be limited because of the pain and discomfort associated with expansion (Figure 52.14).

Free composite tissue transfer via microsurgical technique:

With the advent of microsurgical techniques, transplanting a composite tissue can be carried out with minimal morbidities. The regimen, in caring for burn victims, however, may be limited because of a paucity of donor materials. It is ironic that

burn patients with suitable donor sites seldom require such an elaborate treatment. Those who are in need of microsurgical tissue transplantation are inevitably without appropriate donor sites because of extensive tissue destruction.

Comments

The regimen of burn treatment has changed drastically over the past 50 years. The center of burn treatment moved from understanding the pathophysiology of burn injuries and mastering the patient resuscitation in the 1950s to learning how to cover a burn wound in the 1960s, even though the principle

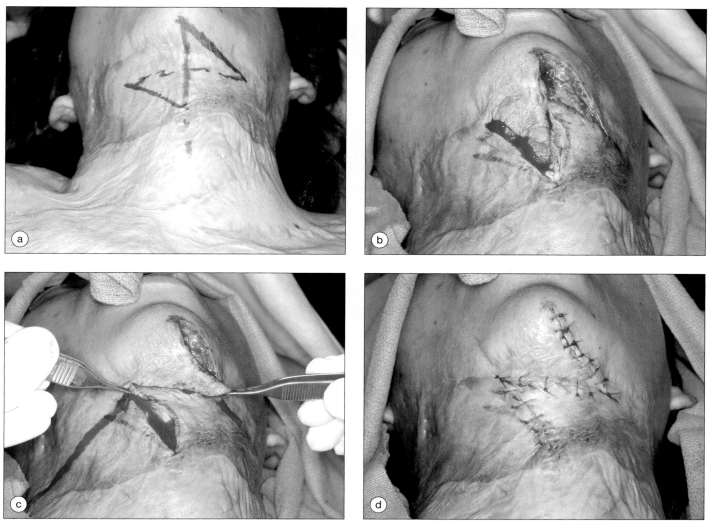

Fig. 52.11 (a) Two equilateral triangles were marked over the anterior surface of the neck with scar contracture. (b) The skin flap was fabricated to include the platysma muscle underneath the scarred neck skin. (c) Two MC flaps were interposed to achieve the release. (d) The appearance of the neck area indicated satisfactory release.

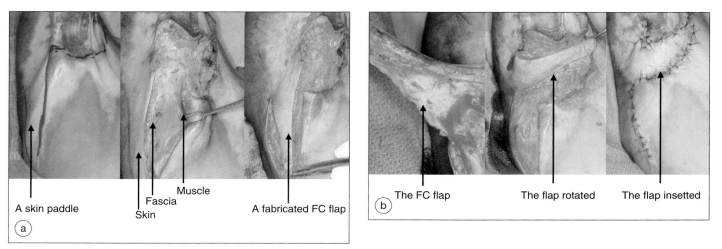

Fig. 52.12 (a) (Left) A transverse skin marking was made in the right axilla to release a tight scar band located anteriorly in the chest. A vertical line – i.e. a limb of the triangle – was drawn perpendicular to the line of scar release. (Center) The dissection was carried down to expose the fascial layer and the muscle. (Right) An FC flap was fabricated. The inner angle of the right-angled triangle is about 30–35°. (b) (Left) A fascia inclusion indicated an FC flap fabrication. (Center) The flap was rotated 90° to make up the tissue defect resulting from release. (Right) The flap insetted and the wound closed.

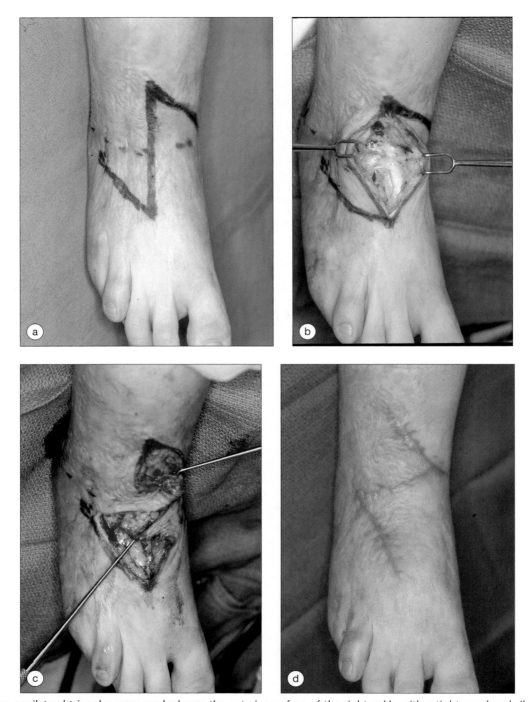

Fig. 52.13 (a) Two equilateral triangles were marked over the anterior surface of the right ankle with a tight scar band. (b) The skin flap was fabricated to include the paratenon underneath, forming a paratenocutaneous (PC) flap. (c) Two PC flaps were interposed to achieve the release. (d) The appearance of the ankle area indicated satisfactory healing of the wound and release of the joint contracture.

of early debridement of the burn wound was clear to the physicians. Reconstructive efforts offered to those who had survived the trauma were mostly limited to the restoration of lost bodily functions and cosmetic reconstruction was simply not offered. The treatment outcome, however, was in most instances, suboptimal because of excessive scarring and scar contracture, the two consequences that limited the outcome of burn reconstruction.

A more aggressive approach in managing burned wounds came in the 1980s. Various pharmacological agents used to control aberrant metabolic processes induced by the trauma, the control of infectious consequences, and safer anesthetic agents, for examples, have contributed substantially to the survival of burn victims. The regimen of an early debridement and wound coverage, initially with biological dressing and later with autologous skin grafts, had further enhanced the

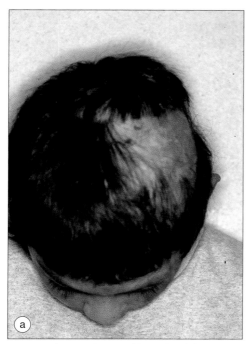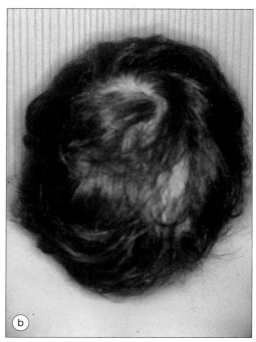

Fig. 52.14 (a) A tissue expander was inserted into the right temporoparietal scalp. The hair-bearing scalp would be expanded to cover an alopecia deformity on the left side. (b) The appearance of the scalp 9 months following the removal of the tissue expander. The alopecia was removed and the defect was covered with expanded hair-bearing scalp mobilized from the right side.

survival rate. It is, however, ironic that this improvement in survival rate has caused an increase of patients in need of reconstruction. That is to say that everyone who now survives burns that would result in scarring and scar contration needs reconstruction, functional or otherwise.

Unsightly hypertrophic scar, scar contracture, affecting particularly the joint structures, and missing bodily parts are still the most common sequelae of burn injuries today. Although the use of skin grafting and skin flap techniques remain the mainstay of burn reconstruction, the outcomes can still be suboptimal because sometimes these techniques are not effective enough to achieve the desired therapeutic objectives (the correcting of the three sequelae listed above).

The exact timing of initiating reconstruction of burn deformities remains uncertain. Difficulty in obtaining suitable tissues for replacement, the risks associated with surgical procedures that involve scar tissues that are active, and the inability to assure outcomes could account for the uncertainty.

The predicament associated with the timing of intervention, on the other hand, could be due to the techniques used. For instance, the use of flap techniques, particularly the use of techniques such as 3/4 fasciocutaneous z-plasty and/or 3/4 paratenocutaneous z-plasty, enable us to reconstruct contractural deformities that involve the major joints as well as eyelid deformities as early as 4–6 months following the injuries.

Questions concerning the ideal approach in managing burn deformities remain unanswered. Although surgery has been the mainstay of the reconstructive approach for the past half century, these problems, perhaps, should be handled completely non-surgically or with limited use of surgical means. For example, reducing the inflammatory phase following injury and controlling the level of various fibrogenic cytokines could be useful in forming scar tissues considered to be physiomechanically sound yet cosmetically pleasant. The know-how of tissue engineering could lead to the formation of bodily parts that may be used to replace missing body components.

Summary

Reconstruction of bodily deformities due to burns is difficult if not impossible. The difficulty is largely due to a lack of understanding of the pathomechanism of wound healing and scar tissue formation. Furthermore, technical limitations on replacing a missing bodily part further fuels the psychological frustrations of reconstructive surgeons.

The use of a musculocutaneous flap and/or a fasciocutaneous flap, particularly modified to follow the principles of z-plasty or 3/4 z-plasty, has been found to be effective in restoring bodily functions lost because of scarring and scar contracture. Furthermore, it is conceivable that refinement in microsurgical tissue transfer technique in conjunction with advances made in tissue engineering/body parts formation would render the task of reconstructing burn deformities easy and simple.

References

1. Tomkins RG, Burke JF, Schoenfeld DA. Prompt eschgar excision: a treatment system contributing to reduced burn mortality. Ann Surg 1986; 204:272–281.

2. Munster AM, Smith-Meek M, Sharkey P. The effect of early surgical intervention in mortality and cost-effectiveness in burn care. Burns 1994; 20:61–64.

3. Brigham PA, McLoughlin E. Burn incidence and medical care use in the United States: estimates, trends, and date sources. J Burn Care Rehabil 1996; 17:95–107.

4. Larson DL, Abston S, Willis B, et al. Contracture and scar formation in the burn patient. Clin Plast Surg 1974; 1:653–656.

5. Scott PG, Ghahary A, Tredget EE. Molecular and cellular basis of hypertrophic scarring. In: Herndon D, ed. Total burn care. Philadelphia: WB Saunders; 2002:Ch 43.

6. Brou J, Robson MC, McCauley, RL. Inventory of potential reconstructive needs in the patients with burns. J Burn Care Rehabil 1989; 10:556–560.

7. Huang T, Larson DL, Lewis SR. Burned hands. Plast Reconstr Surg 1975; 56:21–28.

8. Celis MM, Suman OE, Huang T, et al. Effect of a supervised exercise and physiotherapy program on surgical intervention in children with thermal injury. J Burn Care Rehabil 2003; 24:57–61.

9. Robson MC, Barnett RA, Leitch IOW, et al. Prevention and treatment of postburn scars and contracture. World J Surg 1992; 16:87–96.

10. Huang T, Herndon D. The early burn reconstruction in burned patients. Presented at the annual meeting,. San Antonio, Texas: Texas Surgical Society; 2005:April 1.

Chapter 53

Reconstruction of the burned hand

Nora Nugent, Joseph M. Mlakar, William R. Dougherty, and Ted Huang

Introduction

Although the hand accounts for only 2.5–3% of the total body surface area, it is involved in up to 80% of treated burn injuries.[1,2] The hand may be burned as an isolated injury, or in conjunction with other body areas, and is rarely spared in burns greater than 60% TBSA. Many hand burns occur at the workplace.[3,4] Injuries that occur on the work site are more likely to be flame burns or electrical burns. Injuries that occur at home are more likely to be due to scalds, explosions or open flames. Contact burns to the hand and scald injuries are common in small children.[5]

The function of the hand depends upon stability, sensibility, mobility, dexterity and controllable power. The hand requires stable coverage, an adaptable skeletal framework and a gliding balance of multiple tendinous/muscular forces. The function of an individual is very dependent on the use of their hands. Loss of hand function negatively impacts on occupation, activities of living, and social interaction.[6] Thumb loss alone accounts for a 50% function loss of the whole hand.[7] Our hands are also an important aesthetic feature of the human form. Many patients, who sustain hand burns, are self-conscious about the resulting deformity.

Management of the burned hand provides many challenges to the treating physician. The priority is to maximize the functional outcome for the patient. The final outcome is dependent on the initial severity of the injury, including surface area involved and depth of burn injury, and avoidance of complications such as ischemia secondary to edema, infection and burn scar contractures.

Acute management of the burned hand

Initial assessment

Before focusing on the hand injury, basic trauma principles should be followed. A primary survey of the injured patient, followed by a secondary survey needs to be completed, as the hand burn often is not an isolated injury but part of a larger thermal injury. Once the more emergent needs of the patient, such as airway, breathing and circulatory problems, have been identified and treated appropriately, the burn wound, as a whole, and the burnt hand need to be evaluated.[2,3]

A history of the mechanism of injury and surrounding circumstances is very helpful. The injuring agent should be established – for example, flame, grease, chemical, water or electrical – and duration of contact. This will impact the depth of the injury, as certain agents retain heat longer such as grease, and chemical agents can continue to penetrate the skin if not properly irrigated (Figure 53.1). Neuromuscular damage and remote injuries, as well as systemic problems such as arrhythmias and renal failure, need to be considered in electrical injuries. Some chemical agents require specific therapies: notably hydrofluoric acid, which can rapidly cause fatal hypocalcemia. Calcium gluconate needs to be administered locally or intravascularly in this scenario.[3] Any first-aid measures undertaken, such as cooling the burn, should be enquired about. Additional trauma, for example a crush injury, also needs to be outruled. A combination of a burn and crush injury can have more severe consequences than either alone. Tetanus status, hand dominance, occupation, and past medical history are also important.[8]

Physical examination of the hand should include an assessment of the area of burn and the depth of burn. Circumferential areas need to be documented. While the extremes of burn depth – superficial/superficial partial thickness and full thickness – are usually easy to distinguish, it can be difficult to determine the depth of deeper partial-thickness burns. Briefly, superficial/first-degree and superficial partial-thickness/second-degree burns are usually erythematous, painful and blistering. They blanch readily with pressure (Figures 53.2, 53.3, and 53.4). Deeper partial-thickness/second-degree wounds can be pale or erythematous. They are often mottled, and usually blanch on pressure, although this may not be as obvious as with the more superficial burns. Nerve endings are present,

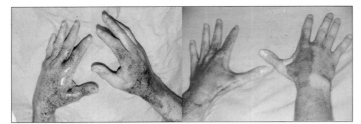

Fig. 53.1 Tar burns to both hands. Acute injury on the left, healed hands on the right.

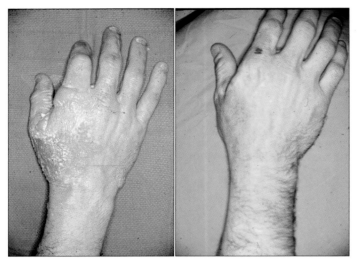

Fig. 53.2 Superficial burns to the hand. Acute injury on the left, healed hand on right.

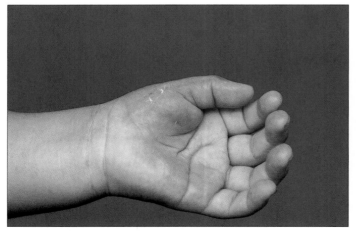

Fig. 53.3 First-degree burn to palmar surface of a child.

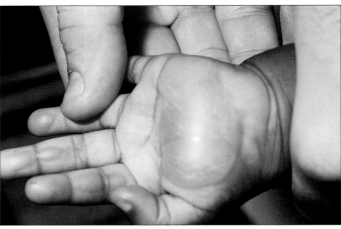

Fig. 53.4 Second-degree burn to palm of child with blistering from contact burn.

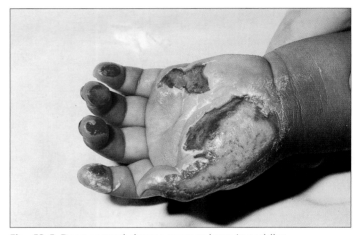

Fig. 53.5 Deep second-degree contact burn in toddler.

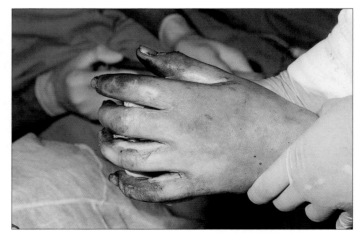

Fig. 53.6 Superficial second-degree burn to dorsum of hand.

but may be damaged; hence pain is present but variable in severity (Figures 53.5, 53.6, and 53.7). Full-thickness/third-degree areas are pale to brown in appearance and often leathery. Nerve endings are destroyed; thus the eschar is anesthetic. Coagulated blood vessels may be visible[2,8] (Figure 53.8). Fourth-degree wounds occur when the underlying soft tissue and/or bone is involved. However, depth classification rarely falls into such clear categories. Depth determination often

proceeds by serial observation of progression of healing (Figure 53.9).

The hand is especially prone to thermal injury. The hand is the only appendage that operates outside of a two-foot circle from our central axis. The dorsal hand has non-glabellar skin,

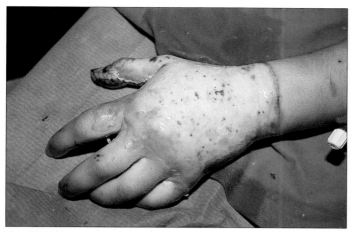

Fig. 53.7 Deep second-degree burn to dorsum of hand.

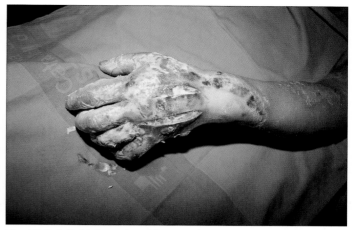

Fig. 53.8 Full-thickness hand burn with dorsal escharotomies.

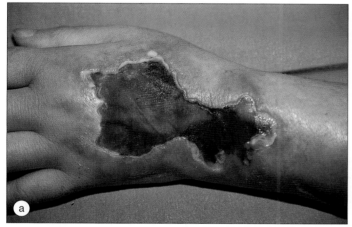

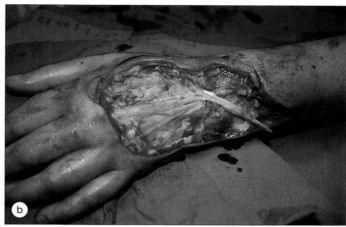

Fig. 53.9 (a) Extravasation injury from antineoplastic agent. (b) Extravasation injury from antineoplastic agent post debridement; the extensor tendons are severely damaged.

which is thin and mobile, allowing for individual joint motions. There is thin areolar tissue coverage overlying the tendons and overlying the surface of the joints. The separation between skin and tendon gets extremely thin, especially over the joints, making extensor tendon and dorsal hood involvement more likely. The palmer aspect has a glabrous, thick, hairless skin-bearing surface. There is minimal mobility, allowing for extreme stability and a high concentration of sensory receptors. Palm skin is heavily anchored to underlying fascia by fibrous septae.[3] Thus the extensor apparatus on the dorsum of the hand is more vulnerable to injury than the flexor mechanism volarly. Children have thinner skin, so it requires less burn depth to produce a full-thickness injury.[5] Soft tissue swelling and circulation of the hand and individual digits should be evaluated. If the hand is very edematous and tense or there is evidence of circulatory compromise, such as coolness, poor capillary refill, anesthesia or increasing pain/severe pain on passive motion in the presence of a circumferential or significant burn to the hand, esharotomies plus or minus release of the fascial compartments need to be considered.[2] A full motor and sensory neurological examination should be documented.[3]

Initial care and wound management

After the preliminary evaluation, if escharotomies are indicated, these should be carried out without delay. Subeschar and muscular compartmental pressures can be measured using a needle; however, if clinically indicated, escharotomies are generally completed. Escharotomies can be carried out at the bedside using either cautery or a scalpel. Cautery carries an advantage in that hemostatic control is easier. Full-thickness incisions in the medial and lateral midaxial lines should be made, which should extend just beyond the area of full-thickness burn. The superficial branch of the radial nerve is vulnerable to damage at the wrist. Digital escharotomies can be made in the midaxial line between the neurovascular bundle and the extensor apparatus. This is usually done radially in the thumb and ulnarly in the index, middle and ring fingers to allow preservation of the opposing sides of a pinch grip. In the little finger, the medial escharotomy can be continued down the ulnar side of the finger, or this can be preserved to protect ulnar sensation as it is a border digit, and the radial side released.[2] Intrinsic musculature is extremely sensitive to the effects of soft-tissue ischemia. Shortening and fibrosis of the intrinsic muscles creates a tendon imbalance and additional clawing, which is very difficult to correct in the burn-injured hand. Incisions can be made longitudinally in the spaces between the 2nd, 3rd, and 4th metacarpals on the dorsum of the hand and extended into the webspaces (Figures 53.10, 53.11, and 53.12). If decompression is still inadequate, the fascial compartments can be released here. An artery forceps can be passed through the fascia between the metacarpals and spread longitudinally to release this compartment.[2] Carpal tunnel releases may also be necessary to achieve full decompression of the hand (Figure 53.13). Electrical and crush injuries require a much lower threshold for full decompression. Due to small cross-sectional diameters, children are more prone to compartmental syndromes and digital tip necrosis. However, digital escharotomies are somewhat controversial in children, and not always performed due to concerns about damaging the neurovascular bundle.[5]

The wound should be cleaned and debrided if necessary. Very superficial wounds only require moisturization and can undergo immediate mobilization. Dressings should be comfortable, prevent desiccation and protect against infection. In the hand, they should also allow mobilization. Superficial

partial-thickness wounds that are clean and present early for treatment may have dressings such as Biobrane™, a bilaminate, semipermeable silicone membrane bound to a layer of nylon and containing porcine dermal collagen. It is available in a glove form, and once adherent to the burn wound, no

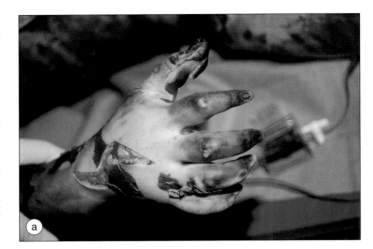

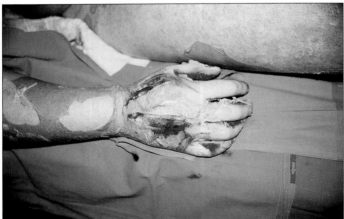

Fig. 53.10 Full-thickness forearm and hand burns. Dorsal escharotomies are visible.

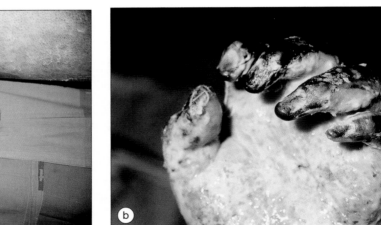

Fig. 53.12 (a) Inadequate escharotomies resulting in necrosis of the fingers. (b) Necrosis of the fingers.

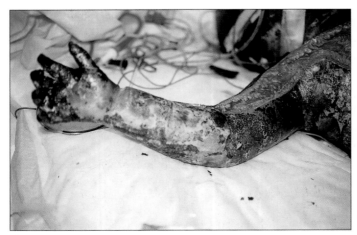

Fig. 53.11 Third- and fourth-degree forearm and hand burns. Escharotomies have been done.

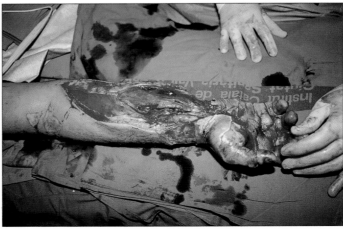

Fig. 53.13 Upper limb fasciotomies. The carpal tunnel has also been released.

dressing changes are required. After application, for the first 24–48 hours, it needs to be monitored for adherence and any signs of infection. If non-adherent or infected, it needs to be removed. Other options include Mefix™, or topical ointments such as silver sulfadiazine or mafenide acetate. Ointments may be applied within a glove for ease of movement. The wound should be cleaned between applications. Indeterminate depth and deeper wounds are usually treated with topical ointments, such as silver sulfadiazine, until healing is complete or surgery is scheduled.[2,6]

Elevation of the affected limb is crucial to control the development of edema and to reduce that already developed. Inpatients can have the arm suspended in a sling from an IV pole or bed frame. Outpatients should be provided with a sling and clear instructions.[3] Less severe or superficial hand burns may be treated on an outpatient basis. If it is unclear whether or not surgery will be required, often the patient can be treated as an outpatient and readmitted if necessary for surgery. However it is essential to have a compliant patient with regard to elevation of the hand, wound care, physical therapy, and follow-up. Adequate arrangements also need to be in place for dressing changes and analgesia.

Surgical management

If wounds are not healing in a timely manner (2 weeks) with dressings, or it is clearly a third-degree burn, debridement and skin grafting should take place. In the patient with an isolated hand burn or a relatively small total body surface area burnt, definitive wound coverage can take place as soon as the decision for surgical management is taken. However in larger burns with limited donor site availability, survival of the acute burn patient takes precedence over hand function. Initial grafting is generally performed to maximize surface wound coverage of large areas of the massively burned patient. This expedites wound closure and increases probability of survival. Delay in healing results in hypertrophic scars, contracture formation, limitations in motion, decreased strength and endurance and poor overall outcome. In general, deeper burns are managed by surgical intervention as soon as practical, to minimize immobility and to decrease duration of both illness and discomfort. Traditionally, maximization of hand function is the second priority after survival. Therefore, hands take high priority.[2,3] If the hands are not grafted as part of the early surgical plan, it is imperative to maintain range of motion and good hand position.

The burn should be tangentially excised to healthy, bleeding tissue, with preservation of as much viable tissue as possible, i.e dermis in partial-thickness burns and dorsal veins and paratenon in full-thickness areas. In the case of electrical and crush injuries, a second-look procedure may be advisable as more debridement than initially thought may be necessary. For the dorsum of the hand, sheet split-thickness autograft provides a good cosmetic result, although good results have also been achieved with 1:1 and 1.5:1 meshed split-thickness grafts.[2,3,5,6] Meticulous hemostasis is necessary, especially when sheet grafts are used, and these should also be inspected frequently in the first 48 hours for hematomas and seromas (Figure 53.14). With the advent of synthetic dermal and skin substitutes, e.g. Integra™, it is possible to excise the hand early

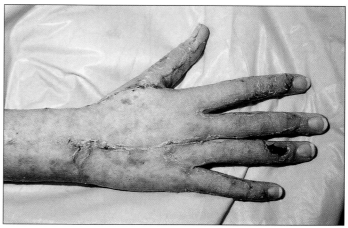

Fig. 53.14 Sheet autograft on the dorsum of the hand.

in large burns and cover the area with the dermal substitute. When neovascularization of the dermal component (a cross-linked collagen and chondroitin-6-sulfate layer) takes place, the silicone top layer can be removed and a thin autograft placed on top approximately 2–3 weeks later.[9] AlloDerm™, an inert human cadaver Dermis with the cellular elements removed, can also be used.[6] If these substitutes are not available the excised area can be covered temporarily with porcine or cadaver skin.

The palmar skin is thicker and as a result recovers from burn injury more frequently than the thinner dorsal skin. Conservative management is often continued for 2–3 weeks longer because of this. When it is necessary to surgically treat these burns, the same principles of preservation of as much viable tissue as possible apply. In the large burn, split-thickness grafts may be the only option for wound closure. However in smaller burns, some centers use full-thickness skin grafts to resurface the palm as they give a good cosmetic result and contract less.[10] Others have not found a significant difference in outcome with the two methods.[11] Glabrous skin grafts from both plantar and palmar surfaces have also been used with good aesthetic and functional results.[12]

Over the dorsum of the fingers with debridement, the extensor tendons and joints are easily exposed. It may be necessary to stabilize the joints in extension with Kirschner wires (K-wires), until stable wound coverage is achieved.[2] In fourth-degree wounds, it may be necessary to debride tendons and amputate non-viable digits. Again, maintenance of any potentially viable tissue is advised. Tendon and bone are frequently exposed in the wound in these scenarios. The interphalangeal joints may again need stabilization with pins. The wound can be allowed to granulate and then grafted, or flap coverage can be used. For small areas, local flaps such as the cross-finger flap or dorsal metacarpal flaps can be used; larger areas will need distant flaps, such as the reverse radial forearm flap, the ulnar forearm flap or the two-stage pedicled groin flap, although this can be bulky.[2,6] Alternatively, the crane principle can be used, where a flap is transposed to cover a defect. At the time of division, the flap is then split into two lamina, with the skin and outer lamina being returned to the original site and the soft tissue now adherent to the wound providing for a stable platform for skin grafting.[3] The radial forearm flap can be used as a fasciocutaneous or a fascial flap. Using this flap or the ulnar-based flap sacrifices a major vessel to the already traumatized hand. Free tissue transfer can also be used; however, this is usually reserved for when other options are unavailable in this scenario. In patients with extensive burns, flaps may not be available, or may sacrifice valuable donor sites. The patient also needs to be medically stable enough to withstand a prolonged procedure.

Hand therapy and splinting

For acute injuries, initial management consists of a simple program of elevation to decrease both edema and pain.[2] Edema of the hand results in a loss of joint and dorsal skin laxity and impairs flexion at the metacarpal-phalangeal (MCP) joints. Protective splinting may be required to maintain joint and hand posture. Prevention of hand deformities is better than the subsequent treatment. Because the dorsal skin has a great propensity for swelling, edema naturally drives the MCP joints into an extended posture. However, if the hand remains in this posture for too long, the collateral ligaments shorten and tighten. Once the hand gets stiff with an MCP extended posture, the contractual forces of the shortened collateral ligaments can be tough to overcome. In addition, with the MCP joints in extension, increased tension on the balance of the extrinsic and intrinsic tendons drives the IP (interphalangeal) joints of the digits into acute flexion. The hand is naturally moved to a posture of MCP extension/IP flexion during the course of scar contracture and healing. If unchecked, end-stage contracture disease of the burned hand results, called the claw-hand deformity. This deformity is defined by wrist flexion, MCP joint hyperextension, PIP flexion, boutonnière's deformities of the digits (PIP flexion and slight DIP extension), and a thumb adduction contracture.[13] Active and passive range of motion exercises are begun as soon as possible. Splinting should be done in a position of protection, which places the hand in the best position to help overcome the imbalance of tendon forces working on the hand during the edema phase. The position of protection keeps the collateral ligaments of the MCP joint in a flexed position at 70–90°. When the joint is in full flexion, the collateral ligaments are tight. Wrist extension is maintained at 20–30°, IP joints are held in full extension, and the thumb is kept abducted and slightly opposed.[1] The ideal posture of the thumb is to separate the first metacarpal and second metacarpal heads at a maximum distance. This occurs when the first metacarpal is about 45° from both the plane of the palm and 45° from a line drawn along the first ray extending into the radius. In a severely burned hand, the position of the thumb is very difficult to maintain (Figure 53.15).

A temporary pre-manufactured splint can be placed on the patient with the initial dressing and first assessment. A customized manufactured splint can then be made over the first 1–2 days. Pre-manufactured splints sometimes create pressure points in the hand. Most therapy programs recommend removal of the splints for range of motion activities at least twice a day. Some units have used continuous passive motion as an adjunct.[13,15] All splinting and ranging programs are designed to maximize active use of the hand, maintaining function and

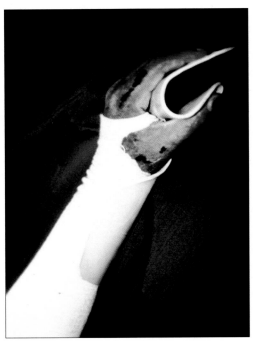

Fig. 53.15 Hand splint showing protective position of wrist, MCP, and IP joints.

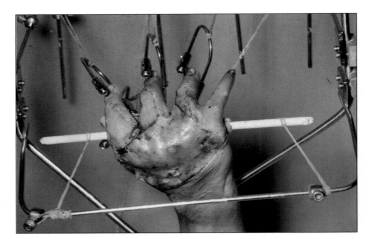

Fig. 53.16 External skeletal fixation holding a grafted hand in position.

protecting posture. Patients should be encouraged to use the hands for self-care activities as this speeds return to functional activities.[3] Static splinting is used mainly to hold position between therapy sessions, or if active participation with the range of motion program is not possible. Due to their small size, it can be difficult to maintain position when splinting pediatric hands. However, they are less prone to stiffness following immobilization periods.

Postoperatively, the hand is usually splinted in the protective position until graft review at 4–5 days. K-wires or skeletal traction, using a Steinmann pin through the radius and attaching hayrake or banjo splints, has also been used[6] (Figure 53.16). Then the program of active and passive movement is recommended. However, when the dorsum of the hand is grafted, maximum surface length is achieved when the hand is in the fist position; all joints flexed. Split-thickness skin grafts contract as the scar matures up to 50%, and if a lesser area of skin is grafted (as in the safe or protective position of the hand), this may manifest itself as a greater contractural deformity than might otherwise occur. While the majority of surgeons favor the protective position, the fist position has been used without adverse consequences for the initial immobilization post grafting, with resumption of standard rehabilitation after graft take.[14] When the palm is grafted, it can be splinted with the hand joints in extension until the graft has taken and hand therapy can resume.[2]

Pressure garments are usually fitted following significant burn injury to the hand. Their purpose is to try to control scar formation, but they can also help in controlling/decreasing edema and improving skin conditioning.[13] Coban wraps can also be used to help with edema. Desensitization programmes may also be necessary if hypersensitivity of the burned area develops.[16]

Reconstruction of established hand deformities postburn

General principles

In spite of early splinting, adequate therapy, and vigilant treatment, postburn hand deformities commonly develop. It is important to remember that for the majority of reconstructive procedures in the hand, the priority is to restore or improve function rather than appearance. The timing of these procedures should be decided on an individual basis, and in order of priority, as several procedures may be needed in some cases. The burned hand may not be an isolated injury for the patient, who may wish or need an alternative deformity to be addressed first, e.g. facial deformities. The hand reconstructive surgeon should coordinate care with the rest of the team looking after the patient and with the patient to develop the individual's reconstructive plan in a way that maximizes use of resources and benefits the patient the most. The choice of reconstructive method may also be affected by the patient's other needs, as use of one area as a donor site for a skin graft or flap may prevent its use in the future for another reconstructive purpose.[16]

For the isolated hand deformity, these concerns are less. Nevertheless, patient and procedure selection are still important. Many patients simply adapt to their boutonnière fingers or slight contractures, and are tired of the surgical process following recovery from their acute injury. Other patients are not compliant with their hand therapy and, therefore, will not be good candidates for completing complex reconstructive maneuvers.

The timing of surgery also needs consideration. Traditional teaching was that reconstructive procedures should wait until scar maturation had occurred, at least 6 months and up to 2 years post injury. Many centers now undertake reconstructive procedures once stable wound coverage has been achieved, if there is a clear impairment that can benefit from early intervention.[2] The surgeon should also take into consideration schooling and work commitments when scheduling surgery. In children, body growth may outstrip that of scarred tissue, and

procedures may need to be repeated as the child grows and deformities redevelop.[16]

The key to the plan is an ability to communicate between surgeon and patient. Patients need to understand from the surgeon what is possible and what is realistic. Surgeons need to listen to the patients to determine exactly what they need and what they desire. For some patients, the loss of self-image associated with the burn of the hand or with other burns is so devastating that they may not want additional deformity, but opt for another treatment regardless of advantages or expected gains. For example, a patient who has lost multiple fingers may opt for a metacarpal stacking as opposed to a toe-to-hand transfer simply because the feet are still normal.[16]

In formulating the plan for the reconstruction of the burned hand, it is important to take into account the rest of the extremity. In the upper extremity, function of the elbow is critical to adequate positioning of the hand. Given deformity at all three levels, it is often appropriate to do releases of wrist, elbow and axilla, and complete large motion reconstructions prior to attempting finer motion reconstruction of the hand. However, it is also possible to complete all of the releases at a single setting.

Reconstructive methods commonly used

Reconstructive methods range from the very simple excision of a scar and primary closure to complex tendon transfers and microvascular free tissue transfers. The repertoire used depends on the complexity of the deformity and surgeon preference. Deformities involving skin only are easier to reconstruct and carry a higher chance of full functional recovery than those with neurological, tendon and/or bony defects.[17] Principles for reconstruction of burn scar contractures include:

- Incisional release of scars at each joint level to allow for maximum restoration of movement.
- Excisional removal of hypertrophic scars when feasible.
- Restoration of transverse and longitudinal hand arches.
- Release or lengthening of deep tissue contractures, including but not limited to extensor tendons, lateral bands and/or accessory collateral ligaments.
- Stabilization of bones and joints in positions of function with either internal K-wires, external splints or external skeletal fixation.
- Resurfacing of hand and digits with thin pliable acceptable tissues, skin grafts if tendons are protected — flaps if joints or tendons are apparent.
- Use of flaps whenever feasible for reconstruction of web spaces.

Here we will briefly discuss some of the more common techniques. Individual deformities that require a more tailored approach will be discussed in the next section.

- Primary closure: This technique can be used for excision of unsightly/hypertrophic scars or scars that are pruritic or hypersensitive. Unless the area is small, it may require serial excision to achieve closure. If part of the base of the scar is left in the wound, it can avoid contour deformities that are sometimes seen when the entire scar is excised.
- Skin grafting: Here the choice lies between split-thickness and full-thickness grafts. Full-thickness grafts

give a better cosmetic result and contract less, however donor site availability and size limit use. Split-thickness grafts can be utilized with or without a dermal template such as Integra[TM18] or AlloDerm[TM]. Skin grafts can be used to resurface the defect created from contracture release. Bolster or quilting techniques can be used to immobilize the graft, as can splinting, until graft take at 4–7 days.

- Skin flaps: A segment of skin with its vascular supply in the subcutaneous tissue intact is transferred from its original location to resurface a defect following release of contracture. Flaps can be used over surfaces unsuitable for grafting, e.g exposed tendon or bone. They can however be bulky, and if the vascular supply is inadequately preserved, can necrose. The donor site will have a scar. Some examples include:
  - Axial skin flap: the blood supply is known and included in the flap design.
  - Z-plasty: two skin flaps from the area adjacent to the site in question, forming an equilateral triangle (60° angles) with a common limb in the scarred area are interposed. This technique is most suited for isolated linear scars.[17]
  - Modified z-plasty/3/4 z-plasty: the scar is released and the defect forms the base of a right-angled triangle, the second limb being perpendicular to the scar release. A second triangular flap is designed with a 45° angle at the tip, using the perpendicular limb of the first triangle as one of its limbs. Its base contains the blood supply and is adjacent to the scar defect. This flap is elevated and then transposed 90° into the defect.
- Musculocutaneous (MC) and fasciocutaneous (FC) flaps: in these flaps, the skin, subcutaneous tissue, fascia plus/minus muscle is raised. Skin grafting may be required to close the donor if the flap is large. Care must be taken when elevating to avoid separating the subcutaneous tissue from the fascia and disrupting vascular supply. Scarred skin can be incorporated into these flaps, if the muscle and fascia are included. Some of the many suitable flaps are:
  - Pedicled flaps: examples include reverse radial or ulnar forearm flaps. These can sometimes be taken as fascial flaps alone, and then a skin graft placed over the fascia, to minimize donor site morbidity. A major vessel is sacrificed going into the hand if these flaps are used. They are thin, pliable, close to the site of coverage and extremely versatile in their use. Other suitable flaps include reverse digital artery flaps, first and second metacarpal flaps, and the dorsal ulnar artery flap which does not sacrifice the ulnar artery.
  - Distant pedicled flaps: the groin flap is the most commonly used. This involves a two- to three-stage procedure. First, attachment, then separation 3 weeks later, plus or minus separation of digits at a later stage, depending on the area resurfaced.
- Free composite tissue transfer: this technique involves microsurgical techniques. Use of free flaps requires presence of satisfactory recipient vessels, which must be documented in postburn hand injuries. Suitable donor sites may be in short supply in the extensively burned patient. Typically, a segment of vessel is chosen for an anastomosis, which is close to the reconstruction but outside the zone of injury. In the burned hand, flaps can be connected into the radial artery and the cephalic vein in the anatomic snuffbox. The most commonly used flaps are:
  - Free radial forearm flap: this can cover entire surface of hand and digits and is thin and supple. It can be innervated if medial and lateral antebrachial nerves included.
  - Dorsalis pedis free flap: this can be harvested with tendons, portions of second metatarsal and superficial peroneal nerve if needed, but is not large enough to cover the entire surface of the hand.
  - Temporoparietal fascial flap: this can cover the entire surface of the hand, and is thin and pliable. It is covered with a skin graft. Donor site morbidity is minimal, but the venous outflow is variable.
  - Lateral arm flap: for small defects it has similar advantages to the radial forearm flap, but with less donor site morbidity. It can be sensate if the posterior brachial nerve is included.
- Capsulotomy: release of the capsular ligaments around a joint. Used when the joint has been contracted so long that release of the skin contracture alone is not enough to release the contracture as the ligaments have shortened. If the appropriate postoperative hand therapy is not followed, the capsulotomy will result in increased scarring and poor functional outcome.[16]
- Arthrodesis: fusion of the joint. The angle of fusion varies depending on the joint involved. It is fused in the position of maximum function. In general, the angle of fusion increases from radial to ulnar, and proximal to distal from MCP and PIP joints, with the index and middle orientated to oppose the thumb, and the ring and little more flexed. They can be fixed using K-wires or other methods of bony fixation.[2]
- Amputation: if other reconstructive methods have been exhausted, or the patient is unwilling to undergo several procedures or the postoperative rehabilitation, amputation may sometimes be the best option, e.g. an abducted, contracted fifth digit.[16]

Reconstruction of phalangeal deformities

- *Flexion deformities:* (Figure 53.17) Usually the flexor tendons are deep enough that release of the band still leaves paratenon intact. Isolated bands of scar on the volar surface of the digits may be treated by z-plasties.[2,8] Alternatively, the scar band can be excised, and the defect resurfaced with a split- or full-thickness skin graft. These areas may also recontract however. V-V advancement in combination with z-plasties, similar to the trident or 'jumping man' flap, has also been described for linear flexion contractures.[19] Local skin flaps from adjacent fingers, such as the cross-finger flap,[2,8] or the dorsal webspace, may be suitable to cover small defects.[20] This method of coverage recontracts less. Periarticular structures, such as the volar plate,

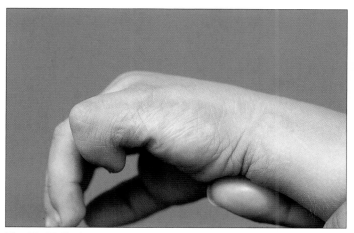

Fig. 53.17 Flexion contracture of the little finger.

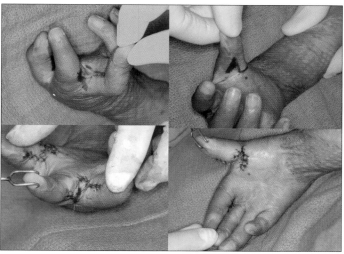

Fig. 53.19 Release of webspace contractures using z-plasties. Clockwise from the top left.

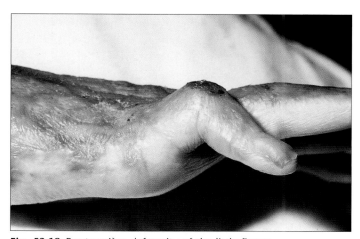

Fig. 53.18 Boutonnière deformity of the little finger.

joint capsule and collateral ligaments may also require release. Care is needed to avoid injury to the neuro-vascular bundles, which can become displaced by the pull of the scar band. As the vessels may have also contracted in chronic contractures, it is important to monitor for signs of ischemia as the vessels may spasm as they stretch, when releasing the contractures.[2] The finger will need to be splinted or held with a K-wire into extension postoperatively.

- *Boutonnière deformity* (Figure 53.18): This is a deformity resulting from the destruction or weakening of the central extensor slip, which allows the lateral bands to migrate volar to the axis of motion in the proximal IP (PIP) joint. In this position, they flex the PIP joint and extend the distal IP (DIP) joint. If in this position chronically, the PIP joint collateral ligaments and volar plate become tight, and the position is very difficult to correct. Attempts at repairing the central slip can be made, by interweaving segments from the lateral bands to form a neocentral slip, or by rotating back some of the distal central slip and securing it. The PIP joint may not fully correct if flexed for a long period. Also, there is usually poor-quality skin

coverage following the burn injury, so the results of these repairs are poor. Tendon plasty using palmaris longus and a groin flap for coverage, after achieving full range of motion in the joints, has been described with success in one series.[21] Often the best result for the patient is to fuse the joint at an angle of 25–50°, with the angle increasing toward the ulnar digits.[2,8]

- *Mallet finger deformity*: If there is a burn over the dorsum of the DIP joint, which damages the extensor tendon, this deformity results. Acutely, the joint can be splinted or held in extension by a K-wire until fibrosis of the tendon occurs. If this is not feasible due to the chronicity of the problem, the joint can be fused in slight flexion.[2]

- *Webspace contractures*: These are extremely common contractures following hand burns. Numerous techniques have been described for their release. Dorsal hooding is the most common problem. This can be released using a variety of local flaps, such as Y-V advancement, z-plasty, 3/4 z-plasty or the trident or 'jumping man' combination and many other variations[2,22] (Figures 53.19, 53.20, 53.21, and 53.22). As some further web creep may occur, if it is possible mild overcorrection should be done. Contracture of the first webspace, bringing the thumb into adduction, is the most symptomatic of the webspace contractures. For mild cases, especially if there is an isolated scar band, z-plasty or 'jumping man' local flaps work well. More severe defects require full release plus or minus release of fascia or adductor policis from its insertion (it then needs to be reinserted more proximally on the thumb metacarpal). The defect is usually grafted; however, flap coverage, either local or distant, has been described, particularly if the carpometacarpal joint is exposed.[2,8,23] The release should be maintained postoperatively. A C-bar splint is commonly used. An external skeletal distractor can also be used to gradually stretch out the webspace over 2–4 weeks.

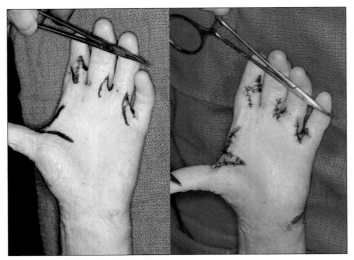

Fig. 53.20 Release of webspace contractures using ³/4 z-plasties.

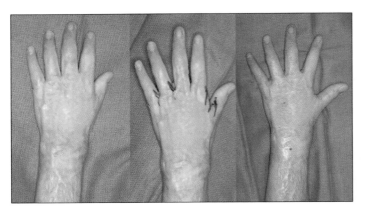

Fig. 53.21 Release of webspace contractures using z-plasties. Preoperative on the left, postoperative on the right.

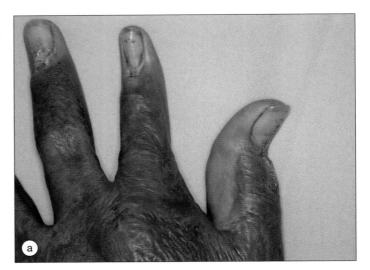

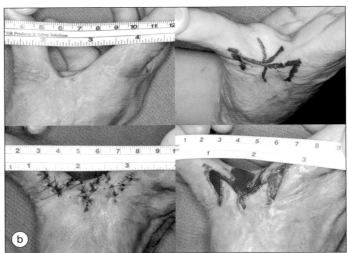

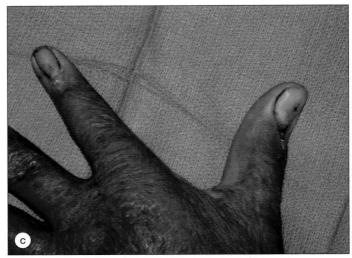

Fig. 53.22 (a) First webspace contracture. (b) Release of previous first webspace contracture using trident flap. Clockwise from top left. (c) Postoperative from release of first webspace contracture.

- *Syndactyly*: This condition can be treated by surgical separation of the digits. The resulting webspace defect can be filled by local transposition flaps, e.g. from the dorsum of the adjacent finger, with grafting of their donor sites, as the defect is usually too large to allow primary closure. If local tissue is not available for transposition flaps, the defect should be grafted with a split- or full-thickness skin graft.[23]
- *Thumb reconstruction*: Options for thumb reconstruction include metacarpal stacking, distraction osteogenesis and pedicle flaps, pollicization, or toe-to-hand transfers.[7] The goal in all of these is to provide for pinch or key grip. All are useful and workable, but need to be adapted by the patient's desires and the state of the postburn hand at the time of reconstruction. Partial thumb reconstruction can be completed using island pedicle flaps taken from other digits to provide for a sensate stable pad. This is done, however, with loss of sensation to the donor digit. Free tissue transfer options for simple soft tissue reconstruction of the thumb include wraparound flaps, first webspace flaps taken from the foot for base reconstruction, and

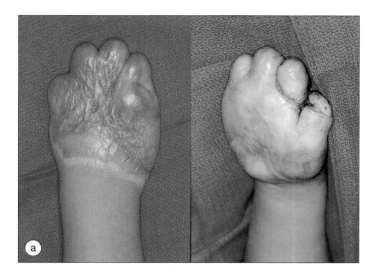

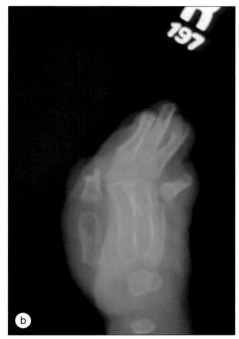

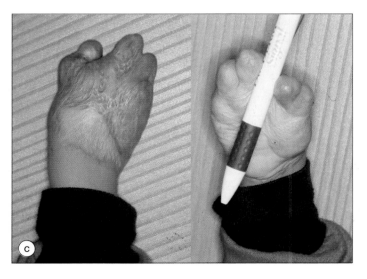

Fig. 53.23 (a) Hand preoperative dorsum and volar surfaces. (b) Preoperative x-ray of the hand in (a). (c) Postoperative view of the same hand as (a) and (b) after thumb stacking procedure.

toe pulp flaps to rebuild a sensate digital tip. All of these are useful for coverage of finger defects as neurosensory flaps and are based upon the first dorsal metatarsal artery and plantar digital nerves. Metacarpal stacking has shown great utility in reconstruction of the first burned hand by providing a viable, accomplishable pinch-grip and even some of the most devastated multiple amputation hands (Figure 53.23). In this procedure, the remnant of the index finger is transferred on to the remnant of the thumb and fixed with K-wires. Flexor tendons and the neurovascular bundle are transferred with the bony remnant.[24] This procedure was first used by Littler in multiple digital reconstruction, and repeated in burn patients. Metacarpal stacking provides for a stable vascularized osteocutaneous transfer with concomitant deepening of a first web. Distraction osteogenesis and pedicled flaps do provide for a stable post with coverage. However, their usefulness is limited due to poor sensation and less mobility than with either pollicization or toe-to-hand transfers. Pollicization is most commonly done for congenital deficiencies of the hand where forearm musculature is deficient and nerve and functional retraining occurs at a younger age. Free toe-thumb transfer can provide a good alternative to provide a prehensile digit if other options are not available. Adequate soft tissue cover must be in place first to sufficiently cover vital structures and the thumb web.[7] Digital transfers in the hand allow for re-establishment of a functioning sensate thumb and provide an opportunity for maximum recovery of thumb function. It requires, however, an intelligent cooperative patient for retraining and the availability of an experienced microvascular team.

Reconstruction of dorsal hand deformities

- *MCP joint hyperextension*: This deformity usually arises from a relative deficit of skin on the dorsal surface of the hand as the skin grafts contract. In severe cases, the MCP joints are subluxed. Once the scar is released or excised, if there is not sufficient gain in flexion, it may be necessary to do dorsal capsulotomies to fully release a tight joint. Aggressive physiotherapy and splinting is required postoperatively.[23] The defect can be skin grafted, or if sufficient unburnt skin is available nearby a 3/4 z-plasty flap can provide coverage. Other options include regional or distant flap coverage (Figures 53.24, 53.25, and 53.26).
- *Wrist hyperextension*: The deformity here is also as a result of contracture of the dorsal skin cover. After release, the defect can be resurfaced by skin grafting, or if unburnt skin is available nearby, by using a 3/4 z-plasty which can incorporate paratenon if necessary.

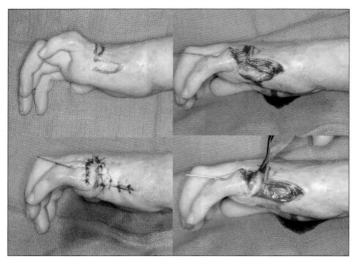

Fig. 53.24 MCP joint hyperextension of fifth digit, released by 3/4 z-plasty. Clockwise from top left.

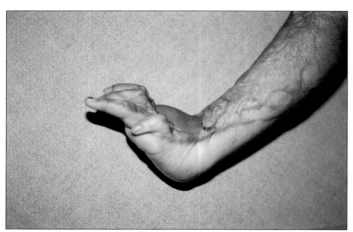

Fig. 53.25 Dorsal hand and wrist contracture.

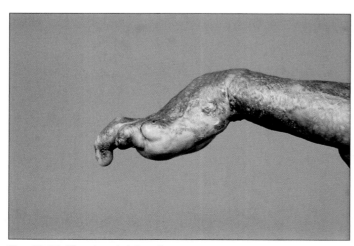

Fig. 53.26 Claw hand deformity.

Isolated linear scar bands may be suitable to z-plasty release. If tendons are exposed post release without a paratenon cover, a flap will be required for coverage (Figures 53.27 and 53.28).

• *Tendon reconstruction*: Isolated extensor tendons can be reconstructed by attaching the remnant of tendon, if there is one, to the adjacent finger's extensor tendon, or the extensor digiti minimi tendon from the little finger and/or the extensor indicis propris tendon can be used,

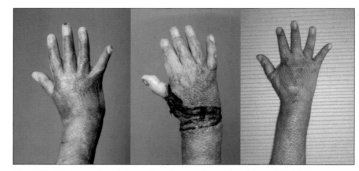

Fig. 53.27 Dorsal wrist contracture released with split-thickness skin graft.

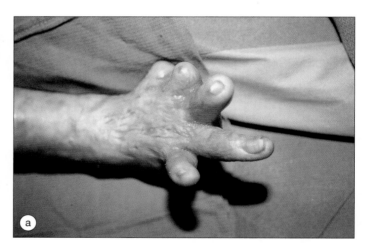

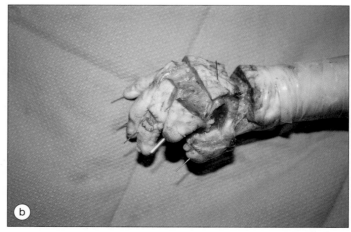

Fig. 53.28 (a) Dorsal wrist and MCP joint contractures. (b) Dorsal wrist and MCP joint contractures of the hand in Figure 53.25a released with split-thickness skin graft and open capsulotomies. K-wires hold the MCP joints in position.

as these fingers have two extensor tendons.

If more complex repair is required, palmaris longus or extensor tendons from the foot can be used. Surface coverage will be required postoperatively, and in the burn case, this usually requires a flap. The reverse forearm flaps are suitable. A free dorsalis pedis can also be used, and this has the advantage in that the pedal extensor tendons can be harvested as part of this flap.

Reconstruction of volar hand deformities

- *Palmar contracture*: During release of palmar contractures, it is important not to excise any palmar skin, as this affords the best protection and function for the palm. The scar should be incised and released. Many recommend using a full-thickness skin graft to resurface the defect, citing increased durability and decreased rate of recontraction as the benefits. Not all studies have found this to be so, and one study has not found any significant long-term difference between full- and split-thickness grafts[11] (Figure 53.29). The dorsal neurocutaneous island flap has also been used for palmar contractures with good results.[25]

- *Wrist flexion contracture*: The scar contracture may be released, and the defect skin grafted. Again, if unburnt skin is available adjacent to the defect, a 3/4 z-plasty flap may be used. If tendons are exposed, flap coverage may be required. However, if the paratenon is preserved, a skin graft will take. Reverse forearm flaps may be suitable to reconstruct the defect over exposed tendons. Abduction and adduction should also be assessed when releasing.

Reconstruction of the neurologically impaired hand

Reconstruction of the hand with neurological injury, such as can occur with crush or electrical injuries, may require the use of nerve and tendon grafts. The sural nerve can be used as a donor graft and palmaris longus, the extensor tendons of the foot and plantaris can be used as free tendon grafts. Flap coverage is required to afford protection to the grafts if inadequate local soft tissue is available.[26] Tendon transfers may be necessary in some cases.

Vitiligo

Skin grafting can also be extremely useful for treatment of hypopigmentation of the hand. Hypopigmentation areas can be treated by dermabrasion and epithelial sheet graft application[27] (Figure 53.30).

Comment

Success in hand reconstructive surgery relies not only on the surgeon but also on patient compliance with the rehabilitation postoperatively. It is also imperative that splinting and mobilization begin early in the acute phase of the injury. Sensitivity to the needs of the burned hand may often be overlooked in the face of other, more overwhelming, burn injuries. However, neglect of the hand during the acute stage makes reconstruction more difficult. In the burned hand, timing of return to work is a very useful indication of early hand care outcome. Early restoration of function aids the return of the patient to society.

All patients with significant hand burns will have some setbacks and delays in the course of their rehabilitation and retraining. Commonly, despite excellent care and state-of-the-art wound dressings, wound excision and skin resurfacing, patients will continue to be plagued with a number of postburn sequelae and less than optimal outcomes related to the depth of their original injury. These include problems with wound healing and development of deformities. Furthermore, patients who suffer from burns of the hand also can develop significant bouts of depression and post-traumatic stress disorders, which impair the burned survivor's ability to participate fully with the rehabilitation progress.

Summary

Reconstruction of the burned hand begins with acute care. Early therapy, control of edema and adequate positioning are

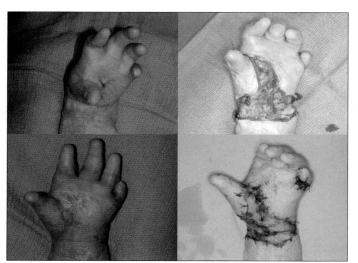

Fig. 53.29 Release of palmar contracture with split-thickness skin graft. Clockwise from top left.

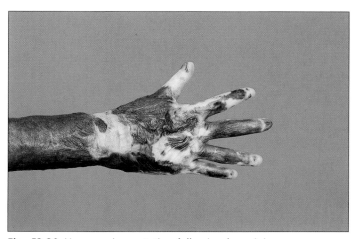

Fig. 53.30 Uneven pigmentation following burn injury.

integral to the successful outcome of the burned hand. Acute soft tissue coverage is chosen based on limitations versus needs. Successful outcomes require cooperation of patient, surgeon and therapist in formulating an acceptable plan for maximum rehabilitation and recovery of the burned person. Despite adequate care in the initial period, a number of postburn sequelae and contractures still occur. Digital and hand reconstruction require formulation of a well-thought-out plan.

Options include skin grafts, local and distant flaps, and joint capsulotomies. Microvascular transfer of thin, soft-tissue substitutes provides further options for postburn reconstruction. Postoperative rehabilitation is vital for success of hand reconstructive procedures. Outcome of burned hand treatment is related to function and appearance as determined by return to work, quality of daily living and patient self-acceptance.

References

1. Luce EA. The acute and subacute management of the burned hand. Clin Plast Surg 2000; 27(1):49–63.
2. Smith MA, Munster AM, Spence RJ. Burns of the hand and upper limb – a review. Burns 1998; 24:493–505.
3. Tredget EE. Management of the acutely burned upper extremity. Hand Clin 2000; 16(2):187–203.
4. Baack BR, Osler T, Nachbar J, et al. Steam press burns of the hand. Ann Plast Surg 1993; 30:345–349.
5. Greenhalgh DG. Management of acute burn injuries of the upper extremity in the pediatric population. Hand Clin 2000; 16(2):175–186.
6. Heimbach DM, Logsetty S. Modern techniques for wound coverage of the thermally injured upper extremity. Hand Clin 2000; 16(2):205–214.
7. Kurtzman LC, Stern PJ, Yakuboff KP. Reconstruction of the burned thumb. Hand Clin 1992; 8(1):107–119.
8. Belliappa PP, McCabe SJ. The burned hand. Hand Clin 1993; 9(2):313–324.
9. Dantzer E, Queruel P, Salinier L, et al. Dermal regeneration template for deep hand burns: clinical utility for both early grafting and reconstructive surgery. Br J Plast Surg 2003; 56:764–774.
10. Pham TN, Hanley C, Palmieri T, et al. Results of early excision and full-thickness grafting of deep palm burns in children. J Burn Care Rehabil 2001; 22:54–57.
11. Pensler JM, Steward R, Lewis SR, et al. Reconstruction of the burned palm: full-thickness versus split-thickness skin grafts – long-term follow up. Plast Reconstr Surg 1988; 81(1):46–49.
12. Wu LC, Gottlieb LJ. Glabrous skin grafting: a 12-year experience with the functional and aesthetic restoration of palmar and plantar skin defects. Plast Reconstr Surg 2005; 116:1679–1685.
13. Leman CJ. Splints and accessories following burn reconstruction. Clin Plast Surg 1992; 19(3):721–731.
14. Burm JS, Chung CH, Oh SJ. Fist position for skin grafting on the dorsal hand: I. Analysis of length of the dorsal hand surface in various positions. Plast Reconstr Surg 1999; 104:1350–1355.
15. Harrison DH, Parkhouse N. Experience with upper extremity burns. The Mount Vernon experience. Hand Clin 1990; 6(2):191–209.
16. Salisbury RE. Reconstruction of the burned hand. Clin Plast Surg 2000; 27(1):65–69.
17. Peterson HD, Elton R. Reconstruction of the thermally injured upper extremity. In: Salisbury RE, Pruitt BA, eds. Burns of the upper extremity. Philadelphia, PA: WB Saunders; 1976.
18. Dantzer E, Braye FM. Reconstructive surgery using artificial dermis (Integra): results with 39 grafts. Br J Plast Surg 2001; 54:659–664.
19. Peker F, Celebiler O. Y-V advancement with z-plasty: an effective combined model for the release of postburn flexion contractures of the fingers. Burns 2003; 29:479–482.
20. Gozu A, Genc B, Ozsoy Z, et al. A new flap design for the repair of proximal phalanx base defects in flexion contractures of adjacent fingers. Ann Plast Surg 2005; 54:33–38.
21. Grishkevich V. Surgical treatment of postburn boutonniere deformity. Plast Reconstr Surg 1996; 97:126–132.
22. Scott Hultman C, Teotia S, Calvert C, et al. STARplasty for reconstruction of the burned web space. Introduction of an alternative for the correction of dorsal neosyndactyly. Ann Plast Surg 2005; 54:281–287.
23. Kurzman LC, Stern PJ. Upper extremity burn contractures. Hand Clin 1990; 6(2):261–279.
24. Ward JW, Pensler JM, Parry SW. Pollicization for thumb reconstruction in severe pediatric hand burns. Plast Reconstr Surg 1985; 76(6):927–932.
25. Ulkur E, Acikel C, Eren F, et al. Use of dorsal ulnar neurocutaneous island flap in the treatment of chronic postburn palmar contractures. Burns 2005; 31:99–104.
26. Fleegler EJ, Yetman RJ. Rehabilitation after upper extremity burns. Orthop Clin North Am 1983; 14(4):699–718.
27. Kahn AM, Cohen MJ. Vitiligo: treatment by dermabrasion and epithelial sheet grafting. J Am Acad Dermatol 1995; 33:646–648.

Chapter 54

Reconstruction of the head and neck

Matthias B. Donelan

Chapter contents

Introduction

Reconstruction of the head and neck following burn injuries presents great challenges and great opportunities. Successful treatment requires sound surgical judgment and technical expertise, as well as a thorough understanding of the pathophysiology of the burn wound and contractures. Many disciplines are required to successfully care for patients with burns of the head and neck. These include skilled nursing, experienced occupational and physical therapy, and psychological and social support systems. The surgeon must also have familiarity and expertise with non-surgical treatment modalities such as pressure therapy, steroids, and laser therapy. Realistic expectations on the part of both patients and surgeons are essential to achieve successful treatment outcomes. Burns to the head and neck of a serious nature result in tissue injury with scarring and complete removal of scars is not possible. A scar can only be modified or exchanged for a scar or scars of a different variety. Despite this fundamental limitation, reconstruction of the burned face and neck creates great opportunities for plastic surgery to significantly improve functional and aesthetic deformities resulting in profound improvement for this large group of challenging patients.

Burn injuries constrict and deform the face, distorting its features, proportions and expression.[1] Burns also alter the surface of the facial mask by causing scars and altering texture and pigmentation. The changes to the surface of the skin are deforming but are much less important to facial appearance than are the changes in proportion, features, and expression. The removal of scars should not be the primary goal of facial burn reconstruction. A normal looking face with scars is always better looking than an even slightly grotesque looking face with fewer scars. Mature scars that result from burn injury will often be less conspicuous than surgically created scars or surgically transferred flaps or grafts. The subtle and gradual transition between unburned skin and burn scar is an excellent example of nature's camouflage and can render scarring remarkably inconspicuous. The principal goal of facial burn reconstruction should be the restoration of a pleasing and tension-free facial appearance with appropriate animation and expression.[2] If this goal is kept in mind and pursued with persistence and determination, the amount of improvement that can result after severe facial burn injury can be remarkable. Ignoring this basic principle can result in iatrogenic catastrophes during reconstructive surgery of the head and neck following burn injury.

Successful reconstruction of burn deformities of the head and neck requires a well-functioning and extensive team.[3] Major burn deformities in this area can be intimidating and overwhelming. Experience and a specialized infrastructure are required to take care of these patients comfortably and successfully. Familiarity with their unique problems and a firm commitment to correcting their challenging deformities is required from all members of the reconstructive team. The care of a patient from the onset of a major burn involving the head and neck to a successful reconstructive outcome requires skill, patience, determination, and enthusiasm from all who are involved.

Acute management

Although the main focus of this chapter is the reconstruction of established facial burn deformities, an understanding of the acute care of facial burn injuries is necessary in order for the surgeon to have an accurate perspective. Excision and grafting of deep second-degree and full-thickness burns has become the standard of care since it was first proposed in 1947.[4–6] It remains controversial whether this is the optimum treatment for facial burn injuries. Early excision and grafting of the face is problematic because of the difficulty in diagnosing the depth of the facial burn and accurately predicting an individual patient's long-term prognosis both functionally and aesthetically. The overwhelming majority of facial burns treated conservatively with a moist regimen of topical antibiotics will be healed within 3 weeks. Burns which are clearly full-thickness are best treated by early excision and grafting within 7–10 days to promote early wound closure and minimize contractile forces (Figure 54.1). The problem cases are those where healing has not occurred by 2–4 weeks or longer. Early

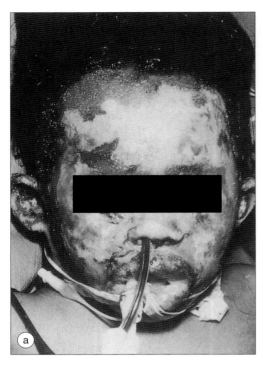

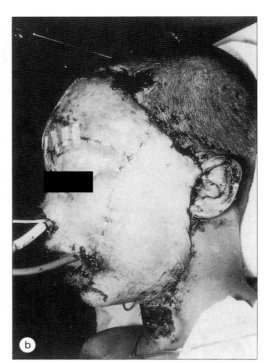

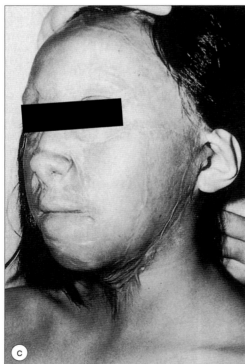

Fig. 54.1 (a) Five-year-old Native American girl 3 days after deep second- and third-degree burns to her face. (b) Tangential excision and split-thickness autografting were performed on the 10th postburn day. (c) Five years after facial excision and grafting. She has had a subsequent nasal reconstruction.

tangential excision and grafting has been proposed for these patients in order to achieve more favorable healing with less eventual contracture deformities.[7] Proponents of conservative therapy argue that early excision and grafting may result in a patient with a grafted face who would otherwise have healed favorably by successfully epithelializing their partial-thickness burn from skin appendages.[8] Conservative management has been facilitated by the myriad ancillary techniques currently available to favorably influence the healing of facial burns such as pressure, silicone, silicone-lined computer-generated face masks, topical and interlesional steroids, vitamin E, massage, and treatment with the pulsed-dye laser. Impressive results have been obtained by advocates for early excision and grafting.[9] Very good outcomes, however, can also be achieved by being more conservative with this difficult group of patients (Figure 54.2). The majority of acute facial burns are treated conservatively in most burn centers, with early excision and grafting limited to those cases where it is clear that a full-thickness burn injury has occurred.

Pathogenesis

Superficial second-degree burns usually heal without scarring or pigmentary changes. Medium-thickness second-degree burns which epithelialize in 10–14 days usually heal without scarring, although there can be long-term changes in skin texture and pigmentation. Deep second-degree burns which epithelialize in 14–28 days or longer must be carefully managed for they have a propensity to develop severe late hypertrophic scarring (Figure 54.3). These patients should be closely monitored after initial healing and at the first sign of hypertrophy must be managed with all available ancillary treatment modalities. Pressure garments have been shown over several decades to be effective in suppressing and reversing hypertrophic scarring. Adding silicone to pressure therapy seems to increase its efficacy. Computer-generated clear face masks lined with sili-

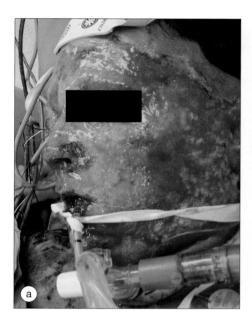
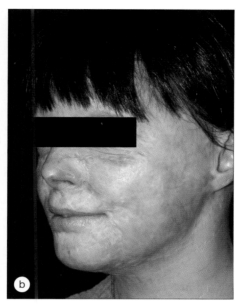

Fig. 54.2 (a) Ungrafted facial burn injury 30 days following 85% burn in a 34-year-old electrician. Wound closure was obtained with split-thickness grafts at 5 weeks. (b) Four years following burn injury. Lower lids and alar lobules have been released and grafted.

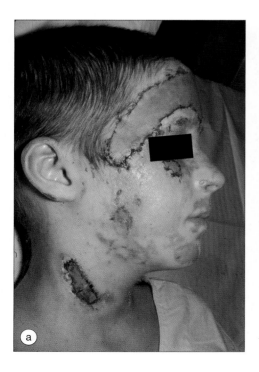
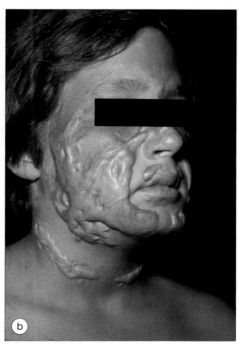

Fig. 54.3 (a) One month following a flash burn, the right cheek is epithelialized. (b) Ten months later there is massive hypertrophy. Pressure therapy was inconsistent. No steroids were used.

cone have improved the ability to deliver pressure to facial hypertrophic scars and are better tolerated by patients (Figure 54.4). When tension plays a role in the development of early hypertrophic scarring, relief of the tension with either focal z-plasty or judicious release and grafting can be very helpful. Full-thickness facial burns should usually be excised and grafted unless focal and small.

Evaluation of facial burn deformities

Facial burn reconstruction should be based on an overall strategy and a clear understanding of the fundamental problems. Many reconstructive techniques have been described in the literature and most can be successful if the strategic goals are appropriate.[10–12] The best reconstructive plan is usually a judicious combination of contracture releases by z-plasty, grafts, and flaps, followed by appropriate scar revision.[2]

Deep second- and third-degree burns heal by contraction and epithelialization. The more severe the burn injury, the more contraction takes place during the healing process. The changes in facial appearance following a deep second-degree burn injury are dramatically demonstrated in Figure 54.5. Three weeks following a deep second-degree burn, the patient's facial features and proportions remain essentially normal. Six months later, contractile forces have deformed the facies in a pattern that is repeated to a variable degree in virtually all severe facial burns. These changes make up the stigmata of facial burn injury and are listed in Box 54.1. The eyelids are distorted with ectropion, the nose is foreshortened with ala flaring, the upper lip is shortened and retruded with loss of philtral contour, the lower lip is everted and inferiorly displaced, the lower lip is wider than the upper lip in anterior view. The tissues of the face and neck are drawn into the same

plane with loss of jawline definition. The severity of these changes is proportional to the severity of the injury.

Fortunately, the majority of facial burn injuries are not severe and do not involve the entire face. A relatively small number of patients sustain injuries which deeply involve the entire face such as shown in Figure 54.5. It can be helpful to separate patients with facial burn deformities into two funda-

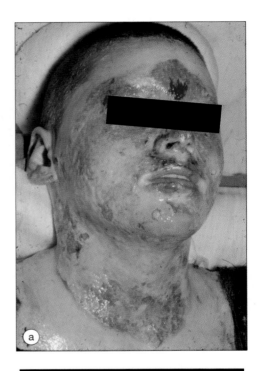

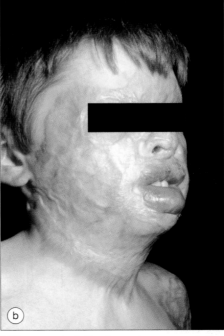

Fig. 54.5 (a) Three weeks following a deep second-degree burn with essentially normal facial features and proportions. (b) Six months later, contraction and hypertrophy have created facial burn stigmata.

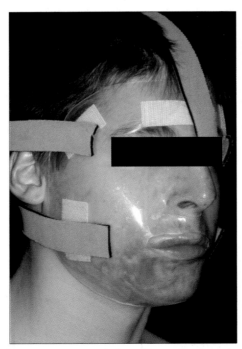

Fig. 54.4 Computer-generated clear silicone-lined masks are well tolerated and more efficacious than previous devices.

BOX 54.1 Stigmata of facial burns

- Lower eyelid ectropion
- Short nose with ala flaring
- Short retruded upper lip
- Lower lip eversion
- Lower lip inferior displacement
- Flat facial features
- Loss of jawline definition

BOX 54.2 Facial burn categories

TYPE I:

Essentially normal faces with focal or diffuse burn scarring with or without contractures

TYPE II:

Pan-facial burn deformities with some or all of the stigmata of facial burns

---

mentally different categories as described in Box 54.2. Type I deformities consist of essentially normal faces that have focal or diffuse scarring from their burns and may have associated contractures. Type II deformities make up a much smaller number of patients who have 'pan-facial' burn deformities with some or even all of the facial burn stigmata. Although these categories are not rigidly defined and there are some patients who do not fit neatly into one or the other, understanding the fundamental difference between these two groups of patients can help define treatment goals. It can also aid in selecting the most appropriate methods for reconstructive surgery.

Patients with type I deformities have an essentially normal facial appearance despite scars from their burns. In these patients, one must be certain that surgical intervention does not adversely alter normal facial features or create distortion from iatrogenically induced tension. Overall facial appearance should not be sacrificed in an effort to 'excise scars.' The best reconstructive options for patients with type I facial burn deformities are usually scar release and revision with z-plasties, full-thickness skin grafts, or tissue rearrangement with local flaps. The pulsed-dye laser can be helpful for decreasing post-burn erythema and treating persistently erythematous burn scars. Full-thickness skin grafts are excellent for focal contractures. Z-plasties in combination with the pulsed-dye laser can be a powerful scar-improving combination (Figure 54.6). Excision of scars and resurfacing operations in aesthetic units and major flap transpositions with or without tissue expansion are rarely indicated.

The much less frequently encountered group of patients with type II facial burn deformities presents a completely different clinical situation. Examples of patients falling into the type II category are shown in Figure 54.7. The surgical goals for this group of patients should be the restoration of normal facial proportion and as much as possible the restoration of the position and shape of normal facial features. The intrinsic and extrinsic contractures that exist in these patients require large amounts of skin. The correction of these contractures should be carried out in a carefully planned and staged fashion. The sequence of operations is usually the following: eyelids, lower lip and chin, upper lip, cheeks, nose, and then other residual deformities. As each area is reconstructed, the addition of skin results in the relief of tension, which benefits other areas of the face. Excision of normal skin or elastic healed second-degree burned skin is almost never indicated. After facial proportion has been achieved and facial features have been restored to their normal location and shape without tension, scar revision can be carried out to smooth and blend the remaining junctional scars (Figure 54.8).

Normal faces are a mosaic of colors, textures, wrinkles and irregularities. In a face which has undergone major burn injury, a mosaic appearance of scars, grafts, pigmentary abnormalities and other flaws can be attractive as long as the facial features are restored to a normal location and are sufficiently loose and mobile for normal and appropriate facial expression. Cosmetics can be useful for blending and camouflaging areas of pigmentary and texture abnormalities, particularly in females.

Fundamental principles and techniques

Contractures

Burn injuries result in open wounds which heal by either contraction and epithelialization or are closed by skin grafting. Contractures result from both of these forms of wound healing. Contractures are either intrinsic or extrinsic. Intrinsic contractures result from loss of tissue in the injured area with subsequent distortion of the involved anatomic part. Extrinsic contractures are those in which the loss of tissue is at a distance from the affected area but the distorted structures such as eyelids or lips are not injured themselves. Corrective measures should be directed at the cause of the contracture in order to provide optimal benefit and prevent iatrogenic deformities. It is helpful to minimize the amount of skin and scar which is excised when correcting facial contractures. When tension is released, many scars will mature favorably and become inconspicuous. Even long-standing scars will respond to a change in their environment. Healed second-degree burns under tension may be unattractive but when restored to a tension-free state can be superior in function and appearance to any replacement tissue. Minimizing excision also decreases the amount of new skin which must be provided in the reconstruction. Every effort should be made to relieve tension from the face when performing burn reconstruction. Tight faces are never attractive. Tight scars are always hypertrophic and erythematous. Relaxed scars are happy scars.

Aesthetic units

The concept of facial aesthetic units has profoundly affected plastic surgical thinking since its introduction by Gonzalez-Ulloa.[13] Initially conceived as the ideal approach for resurfacing the face following burn injury, this important concept has been emphasized in virtually all subsequent writings about facial burns. It is important to keep facial aesthetic units in mind during burn reconstruction but the desire to adhere to this concept should not supersede common sense. When small

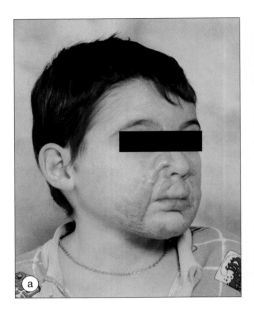

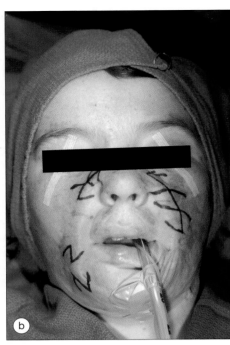

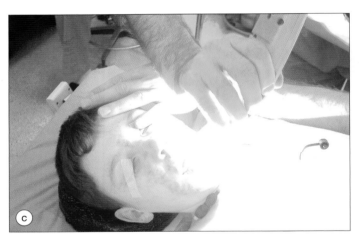

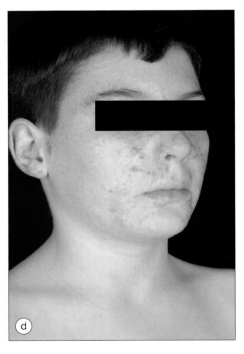

Fig. 54.6 (a) Hypertrophic scarring of both cheeks, lips and chin 6 months following flame burn. (b) Multiple z-plasties release tension on facial scars. (c) Pulsed-dye laser therapy can be used to decrease erythema. (d) Improved appearance 3 years following burn. No scars have been excised.

unburned and unimportant islands of skin are in an aesthetic unit that is being resurfaced, they can be sacrificed. Otherwise, the excision of normal facial skin is rarely indicated in burn reconstruction. All burned faces to some degree are mosaic. Scar revision with z-plasties is an excellent technique to camouflage scars in a burned face. Mosaic faces which are proportional, tension free, and normally expressive appear much better in real life than they do in images.

Z-plasty

The z-plasty operation is a powerful tool in the surgeon's armamentarium for facial burn reconstruction. The z-plasty has been used for over 150 years to lengthen linear scars by recruiting lax adjacent lateral tissue.[14] Z-plasty can also cause a profound beneficial influence on the physiology of scar tissue when it is carried out within the scarred tissues rather than after excising them.[15] The physiology of this phenomenon is related to the immediate and continuing breakdown of collagen which occurs in hypertrophic scars following the relief of tension.[16] Z-plasty also narrows scars at the same time that it lengthens them. In addition, the z-plasty adds to scar camouflage by making the borders of the scar more irregular. In order for z-plasties to lengthen a burn scar and restore elasticity, the lateral limbs of the z-plasty must extend beyond the

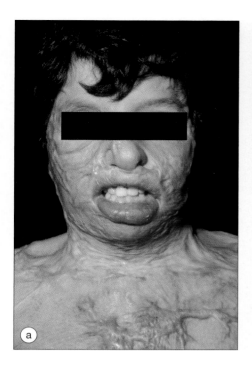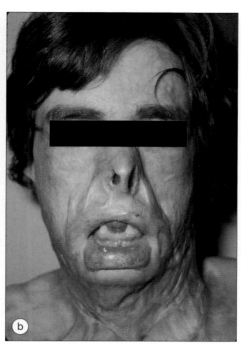

Fig. 54.7 (a, b) Typical examples of patients with 'pan-facial' burns resulting in type II facial deformities.

margins of the scar. The improvement in the appearance of facial scars following z-plasty and without any scar excision can be dramatic, particularly when combined with pulsed-dye laser treatment (Figure 54.6).

Grafts

Skin grafts are an essential part of facial burn reconstruction. Surgical decisions regarding donor site selection, the use of split-thickness versus full-thickness grafts, the timing of intervention and the postoperative management of grafts often determine the success or failure of facial burn reconstruction. Split-thickness skin grafts contract more than full-thickness grafts, wrinkle more, and always remain shiny with a 'glossy finish' look. Split-thickness skin grafts should be used primarily in the periphery of the face unless the limited availability of donor sites requires their use in more prominent areas. Split-thickness skin grafts can be excellent for upper eyelid releasing and resurfacing. Hyperpigmentation of split-thickness grafts on the face is a frequently occurring problem in dark-skinned patients, particularly of African descent.

The full-thickness skin graft is a reliable workhorse in facial burn reconstruction. The broad, central, conspicuous areas of the face such as the cheeks, upper and lower lips, and dorsum of the nose are excellent sites for the use of full-thickness grafts. The missing or damaged parts in the vast majority of even severe facial thermal burns are the epidermis and the dermis and that is what full-thickness skin grafts provide. After facial burns, the subcutaneous fat may be compressed or distorted by contractures but it is rare that it is lost or injured. Adequate skin must be provided when doing definitive resurfacing operations with full-thickness grafts. Contractures must be overcorrected and postoperative management with conformers and pressure is essential. Full-thickness skin grafts are very reliable when used electively in the face for reconstruction after burns.[17]

Flaps

Flaps can be useful for facial burn reconstruction but they must be used judiciously and skillfully, recognizing their problems and limitations. The thickness of skin flaps from all distant donor sites is greater than that of the normal facial skin. The face is tight following burn injury and flaps tend to contract when transferred. They can, therefore, compress or obscure underlying tissue contours. Transposing or advancing flaps from the neck and chest up to the face can easily create extrinsic contractures that adversely affect facial appearance. When flaps have been enlarged by tissue expansion, they are even more dangerous in this regard. Contractures with a downward vector create a 'sad' facial appearance that is distressing to patients. Cervicopectoral flaps provide the best color match in color and texture to facial skin. Distant flaps, whether transferred by traditional technique or microsurgery, share the common flaw of poor match in terms of color and texture.

Tissue expansion

Tissue expanders must be used with caution in the reconstruction of the head and neck. The underlying theme of almost all burn deformities is tension secondary to tissue deficiency. Stretching adjacent tissue in order to carry out scar excision can easily result in an increase in tension and, therefore, create iatrogenic contour abnormalities. The complication rate of tissue expansion in the head and neck area following burn injury is high.[18-20] As noted before, care must be taken when advancing or transposing expanded flaps from the cervicopectoral area to the face as it can create extrinsic contractures with a downward vector.

Timing of reconstructive surgery

The timing of reconstructive plastic surgery following facial burn injury falls into three separate phases: acute, intermediate, and late. Specialized burn centers create an ideal patient-care environment where acute care and reconstructive surgery

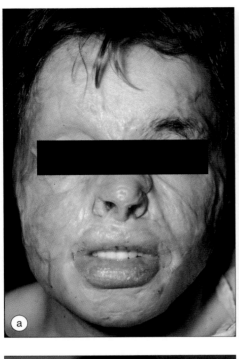

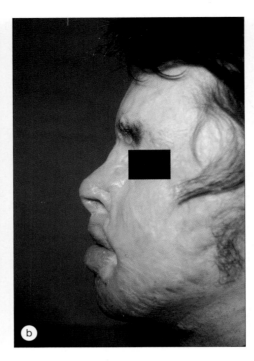

Fig. 54.8 (a, b) Twenty-nine-year-old firefighter with 'pan-facial' burn deformity causing facial burn stigmata. (c, d) Seven years later following the reconstructive sequence outlined in the text. Facial features and proportion have been restored. Note philtril reconstruction with composite graft from ear triangular fossa.

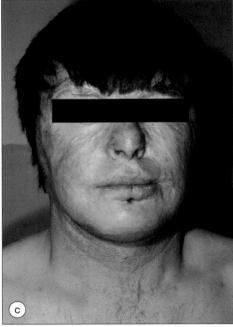

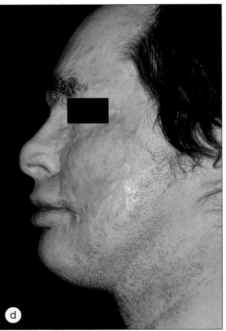

can be planned and carried out in optimal circumstances with collaboration among acute and reconstructive physicians and surgeons. The reconstruction of facial burn injuries to the head and neck should optimally begin with the acute care.

Acute reconstructive surgery occurs during the first months following the burn injury and includes urgent procedures which are required to facilitate patient care or to prevent acute contractures from causing permanent secondary damage. Acute reconstructive intervention is most frequently indicated in the eyelid, perioral, and cervical areas. Intermediate reconstructive surgery takes place during the months to years after wounds are closed and the scar maturation process is proceeding. During this phase of recovery, some patients will present

to the reconstructive surgeon after having received their acute burn care at another facility. Timely intervention when indicated is important in this group of patients as it can positively influence further maturation of scars and grafts. Late-phase reconstructive patients present to the reconstructive surgeon with established facial burn deformities many years following their acute injury.

Acute-phase reconstruction
Eyelids

Upper and lower eyelid ectropion can occur from burn injuries to the periorbital region (intrinsic contracture) or may arise secondarily as a result of the contracture of open wounds and skin grafts at more distant sites (extrinsic contracture). With severe ectropion such as shown in Figure 54.9a, early intervention is mandatory in order to prevent irreversible injury to the cornea. Conservative measures to protect the cornea, such as temporary sutures or contact lenses, are often ineffective. Tarsorrhaphy can cause irreversible iatrogenic injury and should not be used. The best treatment is early intervention with release of contracture and resurfacing with split-thickness skin grafts (Figure 54.9b). Release of even extreme contractures with grafting can be done in the presence of open wounds and effectively restores protective eyelid function.

Perioral deformities

Microstomia occurs from circumferential scarring at the junction between lips and cheek. Perioral scarring from either open wounds or contraction of skin graft suture lines can act as a pursestring, resulting in diminished oral opening (Figure 54.10). This can compromise alimentation and airway access. Microstomia is best addressed by the acute release of the oral commissures taking care to avoid extensive transverse releasing incisions in the aesthetic units of the cheek. Overcorrection can easily result in macrostomia. As soon as adequate oral opening is achieved for feeding and airway access, definitive reconstruction is best left for the post-acute period.

Macrostomia is caused by rapid contraction of open wounds or grafts in the cheek and perioral region, resulting in eversion of the upper and lower lips and lateral movement of the oral commissures (Figure 54.11). The loss of an effective oral sphincter causes drooling and desiccation of the oral mucosa, and can result in irreversible damage to the dentition. Early intervention with release and grafting of the lower and/or upper lips should be carried out as soon as possible. Definitive reconstruction is best carried out at a later period.

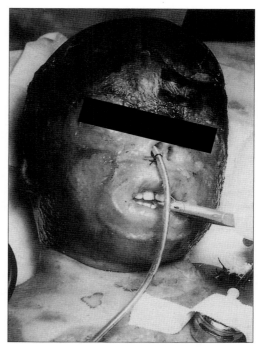

Fig. 54.10 Microstomia during acute phase as a result of circumoral contracture.

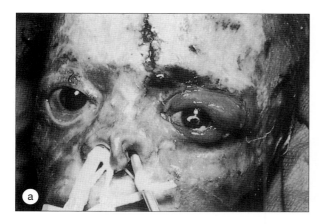

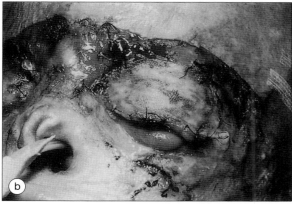

Fig. 54.9 (a) Extreme eyelid ectropion during early acute phase. (b) Successful correction of ectropion with release and graft despite operative wounds.

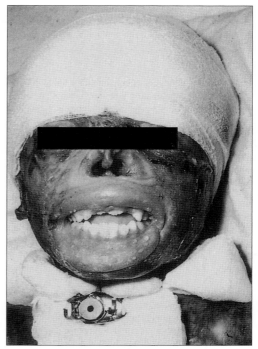

Fig. 54.11 Macrostomia secondary to contracture of open wounds and grafts with lip eversion and loss of oral competence.

Cervical deformities

Anterior neck contractures in the acute period are best prevented by aggressive splinting and incisional releases and grafting when indicated.[21] When severe anterior neck flexion contractures occur, early release and grafting is necessary to allow for adequate airway access and to minimize hypertrophic scarring as a result of excessive and persistent tension (Figure 54.12). Although secondary releases and grafts are often necessary, permanent correction of neck contractures with split-thickness skin grafts is frequently possible when

postoperative management includes proper splinting and pressure[21] (Figure 54.12).

Intermediate-phase reconstruction

The intermediate phase of plastic surgical intervention consists of scar modification designed to favorably influence the healing process in the early months to years following acute wound closure. The treatment options during this period are multifaceted and are continuing to evolve. Significant progress is being made with these types of interventions.

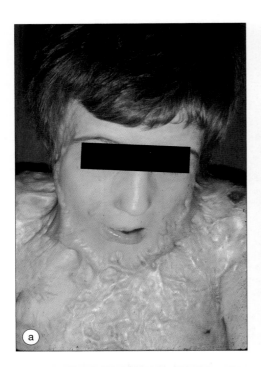
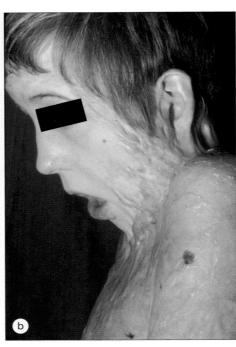
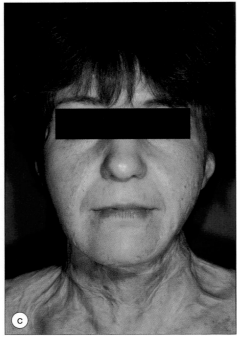
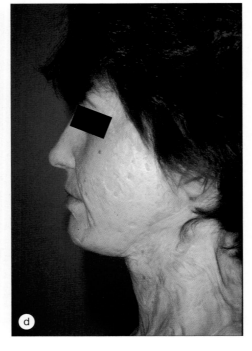

Fig. 54.12 (a, b) Extreme anterior cervical contracture secondary to burns of the entire chest and neck. (c, d) Twenty-three years postburn after release and split-thickness skin grafting. Two additional releases and grafts were required.

It is often recommended that definitive reconstructive surgery be carried out after facial scars and skin grafts are mature, soft, and supple. This process takes at least a year and frequently takes many years to fully occur. The maturation of facial burn scars takes much longer than is generally appreciated by patients and reconstructive surgeons alike. If scars are continuing to improve, it is usually best to allow them to continue to mature. If scars are not maturing favorably, well-timed and well-conceived surgical intervention to favorably influence the scar maturation process can be beneficial. The scar maturation process after facial burns is influenced by multiple factors. The most important factor other than the initial severity of the injury is the amount of tension present in the face and acting on the scars. Surgical procedures to decrease tension and to favorably alter the direction and contour of scars can achieve significant improvement in scar maturation for many years following a burn. Whenever healing burns cross concave surfaces, there is a tendency for hypertrophic scarring to develop. Examples in the face are the glabella, the nasojugal groove, the crus helicis of the ear, and the infracommissural folds. Relieving tension with z-plasties without scar excision is very effective in correcting hypertrophy (Figure 54.13). Steroids, both topically and intralesionally, can be helpful during this period but must be used sparingly

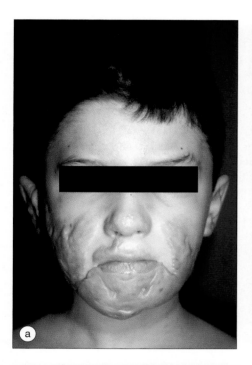
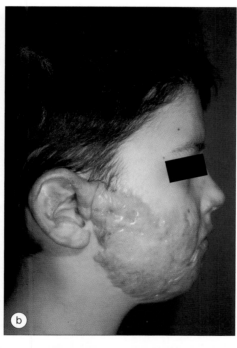
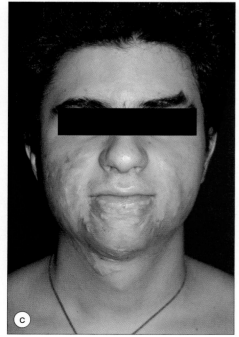
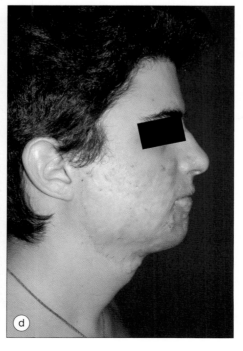

Fig. 54.13 (a, b) Diffuse, hypertrophic scarring of cheeks, chin, and lips 8 months following flame burn injury. (c, d) Twelve years postburn after treatment with pressure therapy, steroid injections, and multiple z-plasties within the scar tissue. No scar tissue was excised.

to avoid atrophy, telangiectasias, and erythema. Tension can also be relieved by judiciously placed releases and skin grafts. The skin grafts can be of either split-thickness or full-thickness variety. Split-thickness skin grafts are best used where the location of the graft will be inconspicuous or where large amounts of skin are required to relieve the contractures. This is frequently indicated when there are associated neck contractures. Tension from the neck must be eliminated as much as possible to allow for favorable maturation of facial burn scars. The use of full-thickness skin grafts during the intermediate phase of reconstruction should be rare and limited to circumstances where definitive repair is being carried out and there is little chance that further skin will be required in that region. The pulsed-dye laser is a promising adjunctive therapy which can decrease erythema and speed the rate of scar maturation (Figure 54.6).

Late-phase reconstruction

Late-phase reconstructive surgery takes place when scars are mature and the patient's deformities are essentially stable. In some patients, scars will be soft and supple, but in others, even long-standing scars may be hypertrophic and hyperemic many years following the burn injury because of persisting tension or unfavorable orientation. Scars can remain indurated and hyperemic for decades following a facial burn. Reorientation in this late phase with z-plasties and treatment with the pulsed-dye laser can result in remarkable improvement (Figure 54.14). Scar excision can often be avoided with its concomitant increase in facial skin tension and distortion of facial features.

Reconstruction of specific areas of the head and neck

Eyebrows

Eyebrow reconstruction following complete loss is an unsolved surgical problem. Composite grafts of hair-bearing scalp from carefully selected sites in the retroauricular area can satisfactorily transfer hair.[22-24] Unfortunately, the hair is scalp hair which grows rapidly and is more projecting than the tangential delicate hair of the normal eyebrow. For complete eyebrow replacement, the technique of composite grafting as described by Brent[22] is most useful. For partial eyebrow loss, micro- and mini-grafting of scalp hair can be efficacious. Occasionally, borrowing composite grafts from a contralateral unburned eyebrow is appropriate. Temporal artery island flaps for eyelid or eyebrow reconstruction have been used for many years.[23,25,26] When used for eyebrow reconstruction, they can be bushy and conspicuous and should be used with caution, particularly when carrying out unilateral eyebrow reconstruction.

Eyelids

Correction of upper and lower eyelid contractures in the late reconstructive period can be a daunting and humbling challenge. The periorbital region is made up of complex three-dimensional anatomy and requires abundant skin to appropriately drape the contours of both the upper and lower eyelids. The slightest amount of excessive tension from either the eyelid skin itself or contractures in adjacent regions such as the forehead or cheek can profoundly and adversely effect

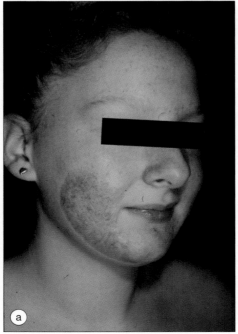
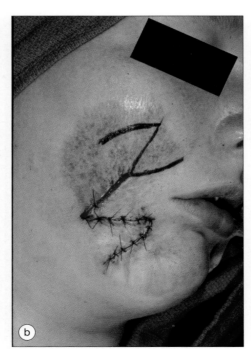
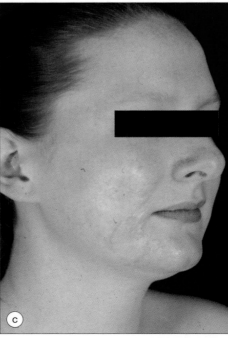

Fig. 54.14 (a) Sixteen-year-old female 11 years following contact burn. Right cheek scar remains erythematous, indurated, and conspicuous. (b) Relaxation and reorientation of scar tissue with z-plasty. (c) Five years later after six treatments with the pulsed-dye laser.

eyelid function and appearance. Reconstructive goals should be restoration of a normally shaped palpebral fissure with appropriate orientation of upper and lower eyelashes at rest and in the open position whenever possible. This often requires extensive releasing incisions extending medial to the medial canthus and lateral to the lateral canthus in order to adequately release all the contracted tissues. When ectropion is the result of a distant contracture, the normal eyelid skin should always be returned to its normal location. Incisions should not be made at the eyelid margin, thereby separating the normal eyelid skin from the ciliary line and replacing it with a graft. When overlying scar is released, care must be taken to prevent injury to the underlying orbicularis oculi muscle. This is often rolled up and contracted and is rarely completely lost. It must be unfolded to its normal flat broad shape and the resulting defect resurfaced with abundant skin graft. Upper eyelid resurfacing is best carried out with split-thickness skin grafts from the best available donor site.[23] Full-thickness skin grafts in the upper eyelid usually transfer a thick dermal component which compromises the delicate contour of the supratarsal fold. Lower eyelid resurfacing may be done with either split-thickness skin grafts or appropriate full-thickness grafts when indicated. For minor contractures of either upper or lower eyelids, the perfect reconstructive material can be obtained from an unburned contralateral upper eyelid. Medial canthal folds are best corrected with z-plasties when there is not a significant tissue deficiency.[27]

Lower lip and chin

Deformities of the lower lip and chin usually occur in combination. Contracting forces result in inferior dislocation and eversion of the lower lip. In addition, there is compression of the soft-tissue contours of the chin prominence. Release should be carried out at the vermillion scar junction and the lower lip carefully unfurled taking care to prevent iatrogenic injury to the underlying orbicularis oris muscle.[12] The resulting defect is then resurfaced with split-thickness skin grafts or full-thickness grafts when indicated. Restoration of chin contour can be improved with chin implants.

Upper lip deformities

The upper lip is usually shortened and retruded by severe facial burn injuries. Releasing and grafting should be carried out, taking care not to overcorrect the deformity and create a long upper lip.[12] Full-thickness grafts from the best available donor sites are usually the best option for resurfacing. Reconstruction of the philtrum when indicated is best performed by the technique of Schmid[28] using a composite graft from the triangular fossa of the ear (see Figures 54.8 and 54.17).

Electrical burns of the oral commissure

Electrical burns of the oral commissure constitute a unique and challenging burn injury to the head and neck. The injury occurs in small children and usually results from placing a live extension cord outlet in the mouth. Most of these injuries are minor and all should be treated conservatively in the acute period. If there has been minimal tissue loss, reconstructive

surgery using local flaps can improve aesthetics.[29–31] When there has been extensive full-thickness loss of skin, vermillion, mucosa, and muscle, as shown in Figure 54.15, reconstruction with a ventral tongue flap can be advantageous.[32] Releasing the contracture associated with the deformity can help restore normal mobility and facial expression (Figure 54.16).

Nasal deformities

Burn injuries to the nose result in a broad range of deformities which can be focal and minor or can result in complete nasal amputation. Minor deformities are best dealt with by local scar revision, particularly with z-plasties to relieve contractures, or releases in combination with full-thickness skin grafting. Shortening of the nose with flaring or partial loss of the alar rims is common in more severe facial burns. Local release of the alar lobules with full-thickness skin grafts is a useful technique for minor to moderate contractures. Complete excision of dorsal scar and graft in an aesthetic unit with a full-thickness skin graft is useful for more severe shortening. When the lower third of the nose has been amputated by the burn injury,

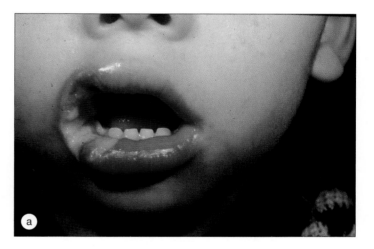

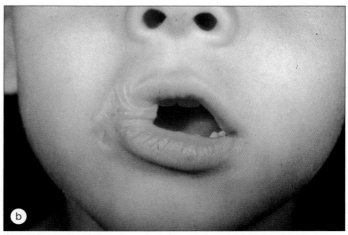

Fig. 54.15 (a) Severe oral commissure burns destroy vermillion, mucosa, muscle, and the skin of the lip and cheek. (b) Extensive contracture results with thickening of the leading edge of the commissure.

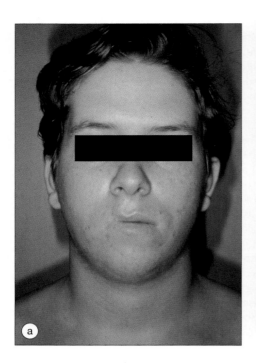

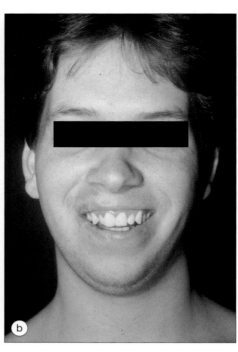

Fig. 54.16 (a) Sixteen years following devastating right oral commissure electrical burn. Forty-percent of lip circumference is lost and the commissure is thick and immobile. (b) Following tongue flap reconstruction, the commissure is thin and mobile and facial expression is restored.

inferiorly-based, turn-down flaps of the dorsal nasal tissues can provide satisfactory lengthening and improved contour to the tip and alar lobules. More severe cases of nasal deformity can be treated by either dorsal turn-down flaps or other forms of total nasal reconstruction. The dorsal turn-down flap usually requires at least two stages but can be effective in even near total nasal amputation (Figure 54.17). Forehead flaps are usually unavailable in patients who have sustained facial burns severe enough to result in total nasal amputation. Distant flaps can be used with either microsurgical transfer using a radial forearm flap or using the frequently unburned skin of the upper inner arm for a Tagliacozzi flap. If the face is otherwise composed of burn scar and graft, these distant flap nasal reconstructions have the disadvantage of appearing to be 'stuck on' and stand out in the midst of the otherwise mosaic appearance of the face. When the face has required resurfacing with flaps, a nasal reconstruction with flap tissue is the best option (Figure 54.18).

Ear deformities

Improved care in the acute phase of burn injury has greatly decreased the incidence of helical chondritis and the resulting associated deformities of crumpled or lost cartilage. Minor ear deformities are often seen in patients with little or no hair loss and can easily be camouflaged. Larger defects can be treated by myriad local reconstructive techniques.[10,33–35] Subtotal ear amputation (Figure 54.19) often lends itself to reconstruction with a conchal transposition flap and skin graft.[36] Complete ear loss can be masked by the use of a prosthesis. Fixation has been improved by the use of osteo-integrated implants but cost and color changes remain problematic. Selected patients can be appropriate candidates for total ear reconstruction using

autologous cartilage and soft-tissue coverage from either temporalis fascia flaps, or expanded local tissue.[37] Alloplastic materials should not be used in the reconstruction of postburn ear deformities due to an acceptably high extrusion rate.[38]

Burn neck contractures

Prevention

Cervical contractures are a major problem in burns involving the chest, neck, and face. The anterior neck skin is thin and the neck is a highly mobile flexion area easily prone to contracture. As noted previously, severe neck flexion neck contractures in the acute phase often require early reconstruction to aid in airway management. Neck contractures should usually be dealt with prior to carrying out facial burn reconstruction as the extrinsic contractile forces from the neck cause facial deformities and can adversely affect the maturation of scars on the face. Preventive methods to minimize cervical contractures during the acute period as burn scars and grafted areas contract include splinting, physical therapy, neck collars, and the use of a three-quarter mattress to encourage neck extension.

Release and grafting

The majority of anterior neck contractures can be satisfactorily treated with release and skin grafting. Extensive contractures usually require split-thickness skin grafting. Focal contractures can be appropriate for full-thickness grafting, which will result in a superior outcome from both a functional and aesthetic standpoint. When neck contractures are exten-

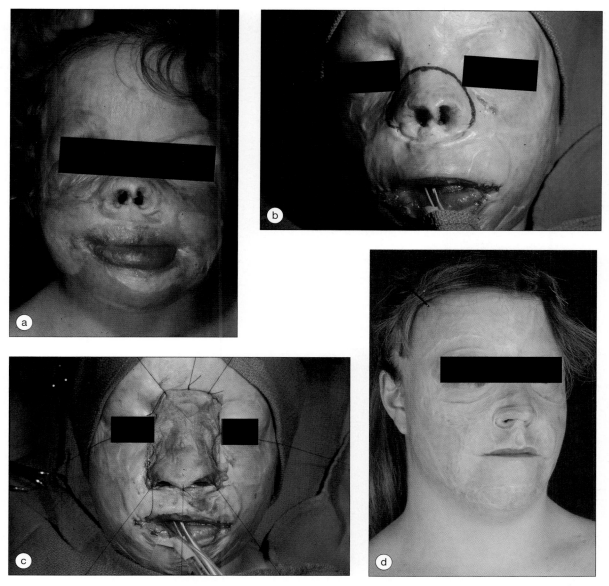

Fig. 54.17 (a) Three-year-old female 10 months following severe facial burn with subtotal nasal amputation. (b) Intraoperative design of a nasal turn-down flap. (c) Split-thickness skin grafting to nasal dorsum following turn-down flap and contracture releases. (d) Fourteen years following turn-down flap after second release and graft.

sive, the lower face and chest are usually a combination of healed skin graft and scar. Split-thickness skin grafts represent 'like tissue' and will blend into the area (Figure 54.12).

Local flap reconstruction

When split-thickness skin grafting is unsuccessful because of recurrent contracture or does not provide a satisfactory aesthetic result, local flap reconstruction of the anterior neck is an excellent technique if there is available tissue. Flaps can either be unilateral or bilateral. When bilateral flaps are available, midline z-plasties secondarily can help to improve neck contour (Figure 54.20). Donor site morbidity is usually minimal

as the upper chest in these patients has frequently been disfigured to some degree by the burn injury.

Distant flap reconstruction

Free flaps have been advocated for the treatment of anterior neck contractures.[39] Excellent outcomes can be obtained but require microsurgical technique and create the possibility of complete flap loss. Another potential negative of free flaps to the anterior neck is that they can be thick and bulky, requiring multiple defattings and secondary revisions. The free flap can also appear to be an island in the midst of a broad area of healed graft and burn scar.

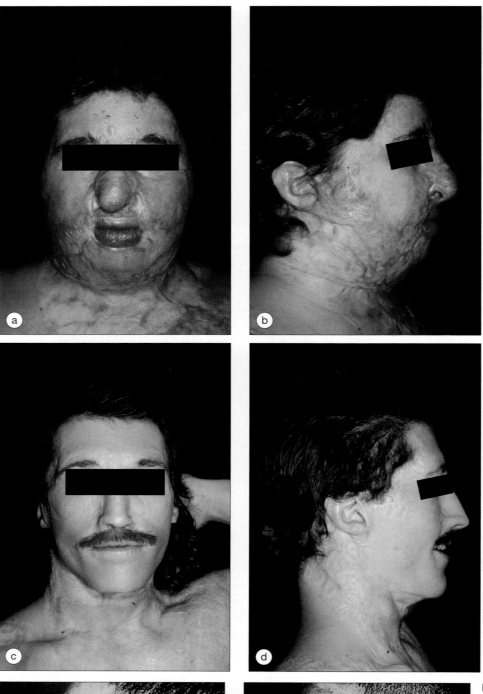

Fig. 54.18 (a, b) Pan-facial burn deformity in a 14-year-old male. Cervicopectoral flap resurfacing was chosen for reconstruction of the cheeks and chin. (c, d) Nasal appearance following reconstruction with a Tagliacozzi flap. A scalp flap was used to reconstruct the upper lip and create a mustache.

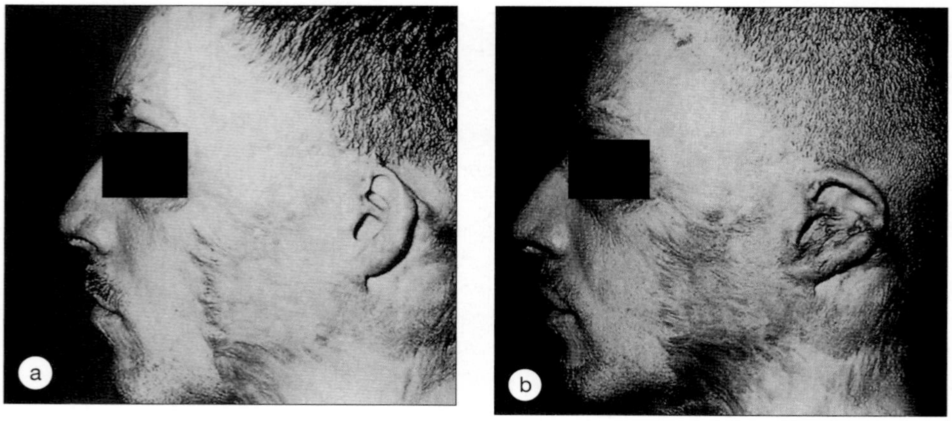

Fig. 54.19 (a) Typical postburn pattern of peripheral helical loss. (b) Reconstructed ear following expansion with conchal transposition flap and skin grafts.

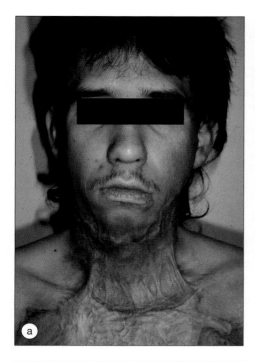

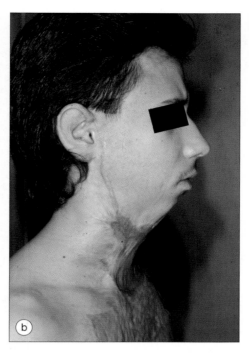

Fig. 54.20 (a, b) Persistent, anterior neck contracture following repeated inadequate split-thickness skin grafting. (c, d) Release and anterior neck resurfacing was carried out with bilateral shoulder flaps. Secondary midline z-plasties improved the vertical release and created an aesthetic neck contour. Chin augmentation improved the patient's profile.

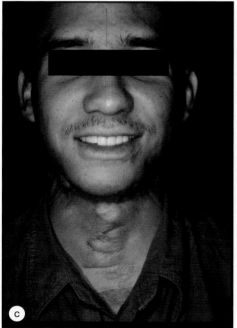

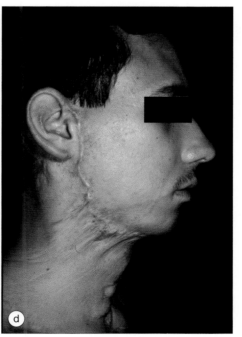

References

1. Donelan MB. Facial burn treatment principles. In: McCarthy JG, Galiano RD, Boutros S, eds. Current therapy in plastic surgery. Philadelphia: Elsevier Science; 2006:184–193.

2. McIndoe A. Total facial reconstruction following burns. Postgrad Med 1949; 6:187.

3. Engrav L, Donelan MB. Face burns: acute care and reconstruction. Oper Tech Plast Reconstr Surg 1997; 4:53–85.

4. Cope O, Langohr JL, Moore FD, et al. Expeditious care of full-thickness burn wounds by surgical excision and grafting. Ann Surg 1947; 125:1–22.

5. Jackson D, Topley E, Cason JS, et al. Primary excision and grafting of large burns. Ann Surg 1960; 152:167–189.

6. Janzekovic A. A new concept in early excision and immediate grafting of burns. J Trauma 1970; 10:1103–1108.

7. Engrav LH, Heimbach DM, Walkishaw MD, et al. Excision of burns of the face. Plast Reconstr Surg 1986; 77:744.
8. Neale HW, Billmire DA, Carey JP. Reconstruction following head and neck burns. Clin Plast Surg 1986; 13:119–136.
9. Cole J, Engrav LH, Heimbach DM, et al. Early excision and grafting of face and neck burns in patients over 20 years. Plast Reconstr Surg 2002; 109:1266–1273.
10. Feldman J. Facial burns. In: McCarthy JG, ed. Plastic surgery. Philadelphia: WB Saunders; 1990:2153–2236.
11. Achauer, B. Reconstructing the burned face. Clin Plast Surg 1992; 19:623–636.
12. Engrav LH, Donelan MB. Acute care and reconstruction of facial burns. In: Mathes SJ, Hentz VR, eds. Plastic surgery. The head and neck. Philadelphia: Saunders Elsevier; 2006:3(2)45–76.
13. Gonzalez-Ulloa M, Castillo A, Stevens E, et al. Preliminary study of the total restoration of the facial skin. Plast Reconstr Surg 1954; 13:151.
14. Ivy RH. Who originated the Z-plasty? Plast Reconstr Surg 1971; 47:67–72.
15. Davis J. The relaxation of scar contractures by means of the z-, or reversed z- type incision: * stressing the use of scar infiltrated tissues. Ann Surg 1931; 94:871–884.
16. Longacre J, Berry HK, Basom CR, et al. The effects of z-plasty on hypertrophic scars. Scand J Plast Reconstr Surg 1976; 10:113–128.
17. Donelan M, Silverman RP. Full-thickness skin grafts for elective facial burn reconstruction; review of 237 consecutive cases. J Burn Care Rehabil 2002; 23(2):S68.
18. Neale H, High RM, Billmore DA, et al. Complications of controlled tissue expansion in the pediatric burn patient. Plast Reconstr Surg 1988; 82(5):840.
19. Pisarski G, Mertens D, Warden GD, et al. Tissue expander complications in the pediatric burn patient. Plast Reconstr Surg 1998; 102:1008.
20. Friedman R, Ingram AE, Rohrich RJ, et al. Risk factors for complications in pediatric tissue expansion. Plast Reconstr Surg 1996; 98:1242.
21. Cronin T. The use of a molded splint to prevent contracture after split-skin grafting on the neck. Plast Reconstr Surg 1961; 27:7.
22. Brent B. Reconstruction of ear, eyebrow and sideburn in the burned patient. Plast Reconstr Surg 1975; 55:312–317.
23. Sloan DF, Huang TT, Larson DL, et al. Reconstruction of the eyelids and eyebrows in burned patients. Plast Reconstr Surg 1976; 58:240–346.
24. Pensler JM, Dillan B, Parry SW. Reconstruction of the eyebrow in the pediatric burned patient. Plast Reconstr Surg 1985; 76:434–439.
25. Monks GH. The restoration of a lower eyelid by a new method. Boston Med Surg J 1898; 139:385–387.
26. Conway H, Stark RB, Kavanaugh JD. Variations of the temporal flap. Plast Reconstr Surg 1952; 9:410–423.
27. Converse JM, McCarthy JG, Dobhovsky M, et al. Facial burns. In: Converse JM, ed. Reconstructive plastic surgery. Philadelphia: WB Saunders; 1977:1628–1631.
28. Schmid E. The use of auricular cartilage and composite grafts in reconstruction of the upper lip, with special reference to reconstruction of the philtrum. In: Broadbent TR, ed. Transactions of the Third International Congress of Plastic Surgery. Amsterdam, The Netherlands: Excerpta Medica; 1964:306.
29. Kazanjian VH, Roopenian A. The treatment of lip deformities resulting from electrical burns of the mouth. Plast Reconstr Surg 1954; 88:884.
30. Gilles H, Millard DR Jr. The principles and art of plastic surgery. Boston: Little, Brown; 1957.
31. Converse JM. Technique of elongation of the oral fissure and restoration of the angle of the mouth. In: Kazanjian JM, Converse JM, eds. The surgical management of facial injuries. Baltimore: Williams and Wilkins; 1959:795.
32. Donelan MB. Reconstruction of electrical burns of the oral commissure with ventral tongue flap. Plast Reconstr Surg 1995; 95:1155–1164.
33. Antia NH, Buch VJ. Chondrocutaneous advancement flap for the marginal defect of the ear. Plast Reconstr Surg 1967; 39:472.
34. Brent B. Reconstruction of the auricle. In: McCarthy JG, ed. Plastic surgery. Philadelphia: WB Saunders; 1990:(3)2094–2152.
35. Davis J. Aesthetic and reconstructive otoplasty. New York: Springer–Verlag; 1987.
36. Donelan MB. Conchal transposition flap for post-burn ear deformities. Plast Reconstr Surg 1989; 83:641–652.
37. Brent B, Byrd HS. Secondary ear reconstruction with cartilage grafts covered by axial, random and free flaps of temporoparietal fascia. Plast Reconstr Surg 1983; 72:141–151.
38. Lynch JB, Pousti A, Doyle J, et al. Our experiences with silastic ear implants. Plast Reconstr Surg 1972; 49:283–285.
39. Angrigiani C. Aesthetic microsurgical reconstruction of anterior neck burn deformities. Plast Reconstr Surg 1994; 93:507.

Reconstruction of the burned scalp using tissue expansion

Robert L. McCauley

Abstract

The involvement of the head and neck can occur in 25–45% of patients with burn injuries. Unfortunately, scalp burns can result in significant burn alopecia. The management of these problems depends on the location and extent of the alopecia. Tissue expansion has become an important part of the armamentarium for correction of this problem with acceptable complication rates. The results of correction of burn alopecia with tissue expansion are an important part of our surgical strategy in the aesthetic reconstruction of cicatricial alopecia.

Introduction

Clinical studies involving soft tissue injuries in patients with large total body surface burns document involvement of the head and neck from 25% to 45%.[1,2] Scarring is the normal end result of any deep traumatic injury to the skin. Burn injury only represents a segment of traumatic injuries in which scarring may become problematic. Scarring can limit function and can be aesthetically unpleasing. The long-term effects of deep burns to the scalp is cicatricial alopecia. The management of this problem depends on these facts:
- the size of the defect,
- its location, and
- the status of the remaining hair-bearing scalp.

The scalp has been a popular donor site for coverage of patients with large total body surface area (TBSA) burns. In 1989, Brou et al. reported a 61% incidence of alopecia in patients with existing scalp burns in which skin grafts were subsequently harvested for wound closure.[3] However, only a 2.2% incidence

of alopecia is noted in patients without burns to the scalp who underwent harvesting of scalp grafts for closure of burn wounds.[4] Yet, regardless of the etiology, burn scar alopecia can pose a significant problem for reconstructive surgeons.

The extensive use of skin grafts, local skin flaps, distant flaps and microvascular free tissue transfer has given plastic surgeons significant tools in the reconstruction of burn patients. However, inherent in each of these techniques are problems with color match and texture. In addition, donor site disfigurement may also play a role. Skin expansion is based on the dynamic nature by which living tissue responds to mechanical stress. Controlled soft tissue expansion offers many advantages over other modalities in the reconstruction of burn patients. The color and texture of expanded skin is a better match to the surrounding tissues than skin grafts or even distant flaps. Donor site morbidity can be minimized. In addition, expanded skin maintains sensibility. Although tissue expansion has numerous advantages, it is not recommended in all situations. Yet, it is such a valuable technique that it has become an integral part of the armamentarium in the reconstruction of burn patients.

Approaches to the correction of burn alopecia

Reconstruction of scalp defects with the use of excision and primary closure has proven to be applicable in regions with small defects.[5,6] Indeed, serial excisions have been reported to be successful in the correction of burn alopecia if less than 15% of the hair-bearing scalp in involved. Huang et al. reported the successful use of primary excision and/or rotation flaps in the correction of defects covering 15% of the hair-bearing scalp.[7] Although, these methods remain useful in the correction of small scalp defects, larger defects often require more involved surgical techniques.

Ortichochea introduced the four-flap technique for reconstruction of scalp defects. This technique was subsequently modified to a three-flap scalp reconstruction in 1971.[8,9] These methods have been quite useful in the correction of moderate-size alopecia defects. The primary disadvantage of these techniques relates to extensive blood loss and the excessive scarring which results from mobilization of multiple scalp flaps. In addition, very large defects may not be closed completely.[10] Subsequently, Juri et al., taking advantage of the profuse blood supply of the scalp, used a variety of monopedicled scalp flaps to cover segmental areas of alopecia, especially in the frontal region.[11–13] The use of this pedicled flap was limited unless the size of the alopecia segment to be corrected was small. However, Feldman showed increased coverage of patients with significant burn alopecia when horizontal scalp reduction was used in combination with the Juri flap.[14] More recently, Barrera has shown that the use of micrografts and minigrafts can be very successful in the correction of large alopecia segments in 32 burn patients.[15] Because of the size of micrografts (1–2 hair follicles) and minigrafts (3–4 hair follicles), the metabolic rate is quite low, thereby allowing them to survive in scar tissue. This technique may be used in combination with tissue expansion. However, the clinical application of tissue expansion to the closure of large scalp defects without excessive scarring has revolutionized our approach to this problem.

Tissue expansion: historical aspects

Skin expansion is based on the dynamic nature in which living tissue responds to a constant mechanical stress load. Our ability to gain or lose massive amounts of weight demonstrates the ability of the skin to develop independently. Tissue expansion represents a medical application of the normal physiological process for the correction of significant traumatic defects using identical tissue.

As part of the exotic aesthetics of various cultures, tissue expansion has achieved significant social implications in a variety of societies throughout the world. The enlarged lips of the Acaridan women were primarily developed to accentuate their own sense of beauty. The elongated necks that were subsequently produced in the Padaung women of Burma also attest to the exotic aesthetics associated with tissue expansion.[16]

However, clinical uses of soft tissue expansion did not gain significance until 1905 when bone lengthening by distraction also resulted in the expansion of soft tissue.[1] These experiments were initially conducted by Codivilla with subsequent follow-up by Putti in 1921.[2] The first reported clinical case of pure soft tissue expansion was reported in 1957 by Neumann for the reconstruction of a traumatic ear defect by expansion of post-auricular skin using a subcutaneous balloon.[17] This expanded flap was then advanced to cover the cartilaginous framework. Yet the concept of soft tissue expansion to correct traumatic defects did not resurface for another 20 years. In 1975, Radavan and Austed, working independently, re-introduced the concept of soft tissue expansion using a silicone implant.[18–20] Although Radavan became the first surgeon to gain extensive experience in the use of silicone expanders, Austed first reported the laboratory and research experience with tissue expanders prior to subsequent clinical use.[18,19]

Biology of tissue expansion

Histological studies of skin

Experimental data on the biology of tissue expanders have resulted from animal experimentation.[20–22] Subsequent human studies were noted to be similar to the animal data.[23] Initial studies by Pasyk et al. showed that the epidermis lost rete and became thicker. These changes persisted 2 years after expansion. Histological examination of the dermis revealed a thinner dermis, with the most significant thinning occurring in the reticular dermis. In addition, it was noted that was an increase in dermal collagen content with disruption of elastic fibers. However, no significant changes in skin appendages were seen. Electron microscopy did not show any significant physiological changes in the skin associated with soft tissue expansion.

Vascular supply of expanded skin

Several investigators have observed a significant increase in vascularity associated with soft tissue expansion both histologically and clinically.[24–26] Several investigators have noted a significant proliferation of blood vessels associated with tissue expansion.[24–26] This vascular proliferation occurs primarily at the junction of the capsule and the host tissues. Within days of expansion, small capillaries become distended and the number of arterioles and venules increase. Cherry et al. showed an increase in the surviving length of expanded skin flaps when compared to delayed skin flaps.[24] Sasaki et al., using labeled microspheres, confirmed these earlier studies while also documenting an increase in blood flow associated with expanded skin flaps.[25] Lantieri et al. believed that vascular endothelial growth factor (VEGF) may play a role in the development of the increased vascularity noted in expanded flaps. This conclusion was based on the fact that the immuno-localization of VEGF only occurred in expanded skin when compared to unexpanded skin.[26] The ability of soft tissues to expand is based on several physiological properties. The skin has a constant ability to adapt, although this depends primarily on the amount and distribution of structural proteins and tissue fluids. Collagen fibers become parallel with the stretching of the tissue. Although elastin fibers are important for recoil after stretching, collagen fibers lengthen permanently.

Molecular basis for tissue expansion

Initial studies by several investigations documented an increased mitotic index in the epidermal layer of the skin with expansion.[20,27] Takei et al. felt that a number of growth factors were involved in this strain-induced cellular activity.[28] The process of expansion not only affects adjacent tissue but also a number of cell types. This group postulated that platelet-derived growth factor (PDGF), as well as other growth factors, could stimulate cutaneous cells. While it is well known that transforming growth factor-beta (TGF-β) can influence extra-cellular matrix production, TGF-β can also enhance fibroblast proliferation. Lastly, membrane-bound molecules may also play a role in the regulation of intercellular signal transduction pathways (Figures 55.1 and 55.2). However, the exact mechanism by which strain influences skin biology is still unclear. Whether we can modulate this response in other ways remains to be seen.

Clinical application of tissue expansion in burn alopecia

The role of tissue expansion in the correction of burn alopecia has slowly become recognized as the gold standard with which other reconstructive methods must be compared. With the increased survival of patients with large total body surface area burns, reconstruction of significant scalp defects has become quite a challenge.

As previously noted, prior to expansion, burn alopecia was managed with serial excision and coverage using local flaps. Huang et al. reported his series of patients with varying degrees of burn alopecia managed with serial incision.[7] This group classified the extent of burn alopecia in children in an attempt to not only guide our surgical interventions but also to give us some expectations as to what to tell our patients. Patients classified as Group A had alopecia that was less than 15% of the hair-bearing scalp; Group B, the alopecia exceeded 15% but was less than 30% of the hair-bearing scalp; Group C, the alopecia exceeded 30% but was less than 50% of the hair-bearing scalp; Group D, the alopecia was more than 50% of the scalp. Using this classification system, scar excision is possible to remove alopecia segments up to 15% of the hair-bearing scalp. Currently, if complete excision of the alopecia segment can be carried out in two or three operations, this approach is preferred by many surgeons. If more operations are deemed necessary, alternative approaches are available.

Manders et al. provided a major thrust in the clinical application of tissue expansion for the correction of burn alopecia. This group demonstrated the efficacy and safety of soft tissue expansion in the correction of scalp defects in pediatric patients.[29] Despite moderately high complication rates, later reports confirmed the feasibility of tissue expansion in the correction of burn alopecia.[29–32] Later, McCauley et al. classified burn alopecia based on not only the pattern of the alopecia but also the extent of the alopecia.[33] This classification was designed as a means by which reconstructive efforts could be designed to correct specific types of burn alopecia (Table 55.1)

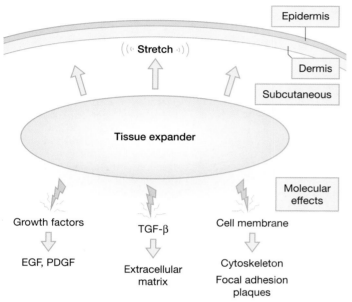

Fig. 55.1 Influence of tissue expansion on the expression of growth factors and the production of extracellular matrix. EGF, epidermal growth factor; TGF-β, transforming growth factor-β; PDGF, platelet-derived growth factor. (Reproduced with permission from: Takei et al. Plast Reconstr Surg 1998; 102:247–258.[28])

TABLE 55.1 CLASSIFICATION OF BURN ALOPECIA	
Type I	Single alopecia segment A Less than 25% of the hair-bearing scalp B 20–50% of the hair-bearing scalp C 50–75% of the hair-bearing scalp D 75% of the hair-bearing scalp
Type II	Multiple alopecia segments amendable to tissue expansion placement
Type III	Patchy burn alopecia not amendable to tissue expansion
Type IV	Total alopecia
(Reproduced with permission from McCauley RL. Correction of burn alopecia. In: Herndon DN, ed. Total burn care, 3rd edn. 2007:690–694. London, Saunders.)	

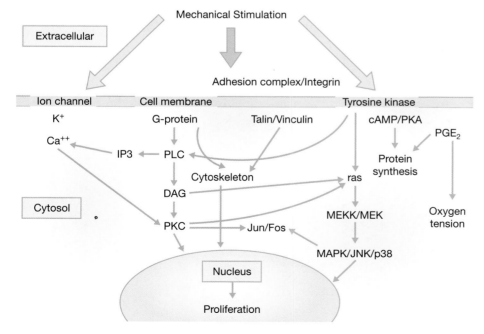

Fig. 55.2 Illustration of possible signal transduction pathways induced by mechanical strain to increase flap length. CTGF, connective tissue growth factor; IGF, insulin-like growth factor; phospholipase C; IP3, inositol phosphate 3; PKC, protein kinase C; DAG, diacyglycerol; MAPK, mitogen-activated kinases; MEKK, MAPK kinase; MEK, MAPK kinase; JNK, c-jun amino terminal kinase. (Reprinted with permission from: McCauley RL. Correction of burn alopecia. In: Herndon DN, ed. Total burn care, 2nd edn. 2001:691. London, WB Saunders.)

In this report, patients with types IA and IB burn alopecia were corrected via a single expansion, although overinflation of the scalp expander may be required (Figure 55.3). Patients with type IC and ID burn alopecia required sequential expansion in order to obtain complete coverage (Figures 55.4 and 55.5). Patients that presented with type II burn alopecia were corrected with a single expanded scalp flap. Lastly, patients with type IIB, C or D required multiple expanders if the adjacent alopecia segment could accommodate an expander. Obviously patients with type III and type IV burn alopecia were not candidates for tissue expansion.

The rate at which expansion occurs postoperatively varies. Expansion has been recommended anywhere from 1 week to 2½ weeks after placement. Injection fractions vary, but 10% of the volume per week is required to complete expansion within a 3-month period. However, individual variations exist, one must be aware of pressure changes which occur with expansion so that flap ischemia and subsequent exposure of the expander does not become a problem. Pietila et al. addressed the issue of accelerated expansion with the 'over filling' technique.[34] This group defined overexpansion as expansion to the point where dermal capillary flow is zero by

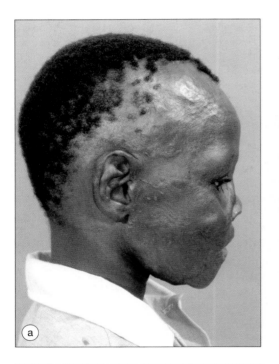

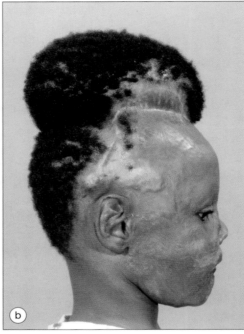

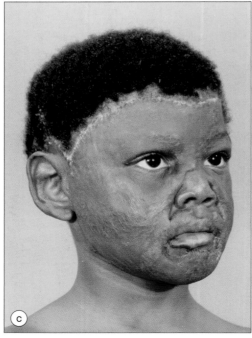

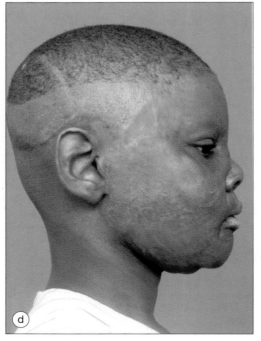

Fig. 55.3 (a) Seven-year-old male with type IB burn alopecia. (b) Complete inflation of a 500 mL tissue expander. (c) One week after correction of alopecia with a single flap advancement. (d) Follow-up 1 year later. (Reprinted with permission from: Garavito E, McCauley RL, Verbitzky J. Reconstruction of the burned scalp. In: McCauley RL, ed. Functional and aesthetic reconstruction of the burn patient. New York: Taylor & Francis; 2005:217–226.)

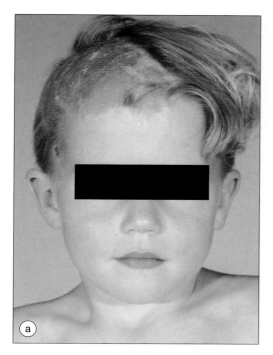

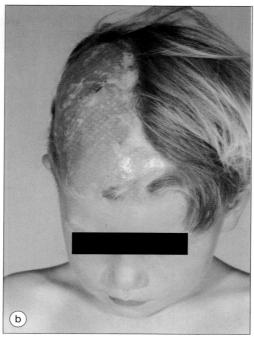

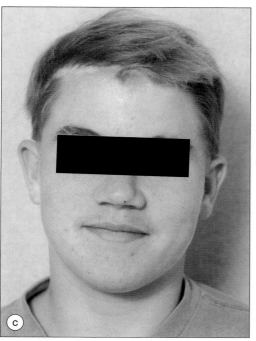

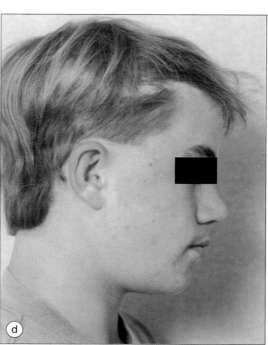

Fig. 55.4 (a, b) Six-year-old white male with type 1B front temporal burn alopecia. (c, d) Same patient at age 14; 7 years after scalp expansion. (Reprinted with permission from: McCauley RL. Tissue expansion reconstruction of the scalp. Semin Plast Surg 2005; 19(2):152.)

laser Doppler flow and patient discomfort is high. Reportedly, fluid was then removed until capillary refill returned and the patient no longer experiences discomfort. They confirmed an average increase of 59% using this technique. However, complications in these patients were not addressed.

Complications of tissue expansion

A number of site-specific studies lends crucial insight into complications associated with expansion of different regions in the body. Scalp expansion for correction of burn alopecia is well documented.[32,33,35] As noted in these reviews, the use of tissue expanders for the correction of burn alopecia has revolutionized our thinking about the correction of this problem.[9,13,36] Of major concern is flap advancement to maintain proper orientation of the hair follicles. Whether or not these wounds are drained does not seem to affect the complication rate of 12–20%.

Complications associated with tissue expanders can be subdivided into those that are major and those that are minor.

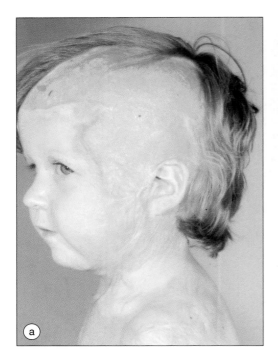

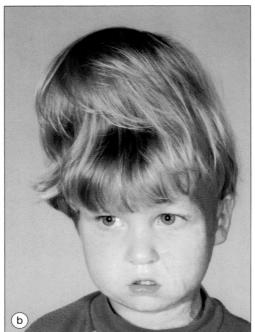

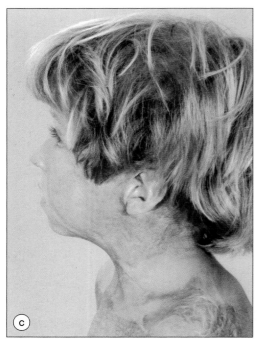

Fig. 55.5 (a) Type IC burn alopecia (b) Complete inflation of an 800 mL tissue expander. (c) Three-year follow-up after correction of alopecia. (Reprinted with permission from: Garavito E, McCauley R L, Verbitzky J. Reconstruction of the burned scalp. In: McCauley RL, ed. Functional and aesthetic reconstruction of the burn patient. New York: Taylor & Francis; 2005:217–226.)

Major complications have been reported to be as low as 3% and as high as 49%.[30–33,37] The major complications are usually defined as those which require removal of the expander (Table 55.2). Such complications may be secondary to infection, exposure of the expander from traumatic extrusion, wound dehiscence, or erosion of the envelope fold or port through the skin.[38] Implant failure, which requires removal of the implant, is also considered a major complication as would be ischemia and flap necrosis. Manders et al. reported a major complication rate of 24%.[10] Other investigators have reported similar complications ranging from 17% to 24%.[31,33] Neale et al.

have shown that with proper protocols and patient selection, the major complication rate (those requiring additional surgery for expander replacement of additional procedures) has decreased from 22% to 12 %.[24] Minor complications have been documented with these patients and have been defined as poor compliance, intolerance of the injection to fill the expanders, and alterations in the early preoperative plans secondary to incomplete coverage following expansion (Table 55.3). Rates of such minor complications have been reported to be between 17% and 40%, with a mean still in the range of 20%.[9,31]

TABLE 55.2 MAJOR COMPLICATIONS OF SOFT TISSUE EXPANSION

Complication	Number of patients
Infection	3
Expander exposure	
Dehiscence of incision	5 (two more
Erosion of envelope fold through skin	incipient exposure)
Erosion of envelope of reservoir	1
through inadequate covering tissue	
Manipulated by psychotic patients	1 (two incipient)
	2
Implant failure	
Remote port connector	1
Physician assembly may be faulty	1
Injection port may lack proper back	1
Envelope may be perforated by needle	1
Induced ischemia	
Flaps may become ischemic when expanded	1 (recognized and
Irradiated tissue may not survive elevation	no problem)
	1

Twenty-four percent of expansions were attended by a major complication. Reproduced with permission from: Manders et al. Plast Reconstr Surg 1984; 74:493–504.[10]

TABLE 55.3 MINOR COMPLICATIONS OF SOFT TISSUE EXPANSION

Complication	Number of patients
Pain on expansion	3
Seroma and drainage after expander inflation	2
Dog-ears after advancement	1
Widening of scar time	1

Seventeen percent of expansions were attended by a minor complication. Reproduced with permission from: Manders et al. Plast Reconstr Surg 1984; 74:493–504. [10]

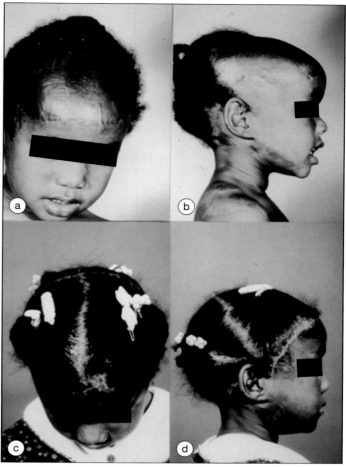

Fig. 55.6 (a, b) Preoperative views of a 6-year-old black female patient with type IC burn alopecia. (c, d) Postoperative views after correction using sequential. (Reprinted with permission from McCauley RL. Correction of burn alopecia. In: Herndon DN, ed. Total burn care, 2nd edn. 2001 Pg 693. London, WB Saunders.)

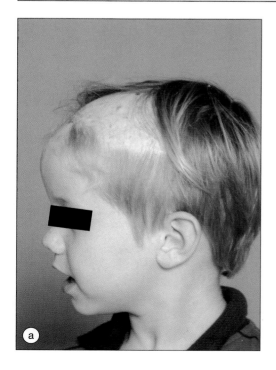

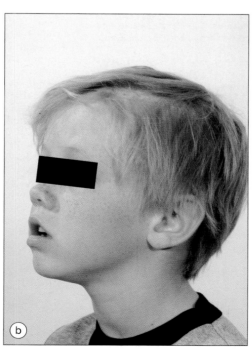

Fig. 55.7 (a) Preoperative view of a 6-year-old white male with type 1A burn alopecia. (b) Postoperative view after correction of alopecia with a single expansion. (Reprinted with permission from: McCauley RL. Correction of burn alopecia. In: Herndon DN, ed. Total burn care, 2nd edn. 2001:692. London, WB Saunders.)

Conclusion

Tissue expanders have a permanent place in the armamentarium of reconstructive surgery for correction of soft tissue defects, especially burn alopecia. It also brings a new perspective for correction of complex problems. The techniques have been refined, and although complication rates have improved, they remain moderately high. Yet, the role of tissue expansion in the correction of burn alopecia has been one with tremendous impact. With so many burn injuries occurring to the head and neck, reconstructive procedures, such as those designed to correct alopecia, are becoming more common. The advantages of tissue expansion are numerous: excellent color and texture match and minimal donor site morbidity (Figures 55.6 and 55.7). The disadvantages are well known and include a protracted time period for completion of the expansion process and a significant complication rate. All patients who are victims of trauma, especially burn injury, want to look and function at their best. Tissue expansion in certain patients offers the chance to replace unstable and unsightly scars with normal adjacent tissue. None of our current reconstructive techniques offer this advantage. As we continue to refine our approach to certain problems using tissue expansion, it is important to communicate to our patients that although the process may be protracted, the end results can be exceptional.

References

1. Codivilla A. On the means of lengthening, in the lower limbs, the muscles and tissues which are shortened through deformity. Am J Orthop Surg 1905; 2:353–369.
2. Putti V. Operative lengthening of the femur. JAMA 1921; 77:937.
3. Brou JA, Vu T, McCauley RL, et al. The scalp as a donor site: revisited. J Trauma 1990; 30(5):579–581.
4. Barret JP, Dziewulski P, Wolf, SE, et al. Outcome of scalp donor sites in 450 consecutive pediatric burn patients. Plast Reconstr Surg 1999; 103(4):1139–1142.
5. Paletta C. Surgical management of the burned scalp. Clin Plast Surg 1982; 9:167.
6. Vallis CP. Surgical management of cicatricial alopecia of the scalp. Clin Plast Surg 1982; 9:179.
7. Huang TT, Larson DL, Lewis SR. Burn alopecia. Plast Reconstr Surg 1977; 60:762.
8. Ortichochea M. Four flap scalp reconstruction technique. Br J Plast Surg 1967; 20:159–171.
9. Ortichochea M. New three flap scalp reconstruction technique. Br J Plast Surg 1971; 24:184–188.
10. Manders EK, Schendon MJ, Fussey JA, et al. Soft tissue expansion: concepts and complications. Plast Reconstr Surg 1984; 74:493–504.
11. Juri J. Use of parieto-occipital flaps in the surgical treatment of baldness. Plast Reconstr Surg 1975; 55:456.
12. Juri J, Juri C, Arufe HN. Use of rotation scalp flaps for the treatment of occipital baldness. Br J Plast Surg 1978; 61:23.
13. Juri J, Juri C. Aesthetic aspects of reconstructive scalp surgery. Clin Plast Surg 1981; 8:243–254.
14. Felman G. Post-thermal burn alopecia and its treatment using extensive horizontal reduction in combination with a Juni flap. Plast Reconstr Surg 1994; 93:1268–1273.
15. Barrera A. The use of micrografts and minigrafts for the treatment of burn alopecia. Plast Reconstr Surg 1999; 103:581–589.
16. Sasaki G. Tissue expansion. In: Jurkiewicz MJ, Krizek TJ, Mathes S, et al., eds. Plastic surgery: principles and practice. St Louis: CV Mosby; 1990:Ch 50, 1608.
17. Neumann CG. The expansion of an area of skin by progressive distention of a subcutaneous balloon. Plast Reconstr Surg 1957; 19:124–130.
18. Austed ED, Thomas SV, Pasyk K. Tissue expansion: dividend or loan? Plast Reconstr Surg 1986; 78:63.
19. Radavan C. Tissue expansion in soft tissue reconstruction. Plast Reconstr Surg 1984; 74:491.
20. Austed ED, Pasyk KA, McClatchey KD, et al. Histomorphometric evaluation of guinea pig skin and soft tissue after controlled tissue expansion. Plast Reconstr Surg 1982; 70:704–710.
21. Pasyk KA, Austed ED, McClatchey KD, et al. Electron microscopic evaluation of guinea pig skin and soft tissues expanded with a self-inflating silicone implant. Plast Reconstr Surg 1982; 70:37.
22. Pasyk KA, Argenta LC, Hasseh C. Quantitative analysis of the thickness of human skin and subcutaneous tissue following controlled expansion with a silicone implant. Plast Reconstr Surg 1988; 81:516.
23. Pasyk KA, Argenta LC, Austed ED. Histopathology of human expanded tissue. Clin Plast Surg 1987; 14:435–445.
24. Cherry GW, Austed GD, Pasyk KA, et al. Increased survival and vascularity of random pattern skin flaps elevated in controlled, expanded skin. Plast Reconstr Surg 1983; 72:680–685.
25. Sasaki GH, Pang CY. Pathophysiology of skin flaps raised on expanded skin. Plast Reconstr Surg 1984; 79:59–65.
26. Lantieri LA, Martin-Garcia N, Wechsler J, et al. Vascular endothelial growth factor expression in expanded tissue: a possible mechanism of angiogenesis in tissue expansion. Plast Reconstr Surg 1998; 101:392–398.
27. Squier CA. The stretching of mouse skin in vivo: effect on epidermal proliferation and thickness. J Invest Dermatol 1980; 74:68–71.
28. Takei T, Mills I, Katsuyuki A, et al. Molecular basis for tissue expansion: clinical implementation for the surgeon. Plast Reconstr Surg 1998; 102:247–258.
29. Manders EK, Graham WP, Schendon MT, et al. Skin expansion to eliminate large scalp defects. Ann Plast Surg 1984; 12:305–312.
30. Ortega MT, McCauley RL, Robson MC. Salvage of an avulsed expanded scalp flap to correct burn alopecia. South Med J 1988; 23:220–223.
31. Neale HW, High RM, Billmon DA, et al. Complications of controlled tissue expansion in the pediatric burn patient. Plast Reconstr Surg 1988; 82:840–845.
32. Buhrer DP, Huang TT, Yee HD. Treatment of burn alopecia with tissue expanding in children. Plast Reconstr Surg 1988; 82:840–845.
33. McCauley RL, Oliphant JR, Robson MC. Tissue expansion in the correction of burn alopecia: classification and methods of correction. Ann Plast Surg 1990; 25:103–115.
34. Pietila JP, Nordstrom RE, Virkkunen PJ, et al. Accelerated tissue expansion with the "overfilling" technique. Plast Reconstr Surg 1988; 81:204–207.
35. Marks M, Argenta LC, Thornton JW. Burn management: the role of tissue expansion. Clin Plast Surg 1987; 14:453–548.
36. Pitanguy I, Gontijo de Amorim NF, Radwanski HN, et al. Repeated expansion in burn sequela. Burns 2002; 28:494–499.
37. Zellweger G, Künzi W. Tissue expanders in reconstruction of burn sequelae. Ann Plast Surg 1991; 26:380–388.
38. Governa M, Bortolani A, Beghini D, et al. Skin expansion in burn sequelae: results and complications. Acta Chir Plast 1996; 38(4):147–153.

Management of contractural deformities involving the axilla (shoulder), elbow, hip, knee, and ankle joints in burn patients

Ted Huang

Chapter contents

Burn injuries, regardless of the etiology, rarely involve a joint. However, the joint function is often impaired because of burns. The joint problems and joint deformities noted in burn patients are mostly due to physical inactivity combined with limitation of joint movement because of scar contracture.

The regimen of burn management, especially during the period immediately following the injury, seldom includes plans to care for the joint; instead, the treatment is focused upon resuscitative efforts to restore fluid balance and to maintain functional integrity of the circulatory and the pulmonary systems. The consequence of joint dysfunction is usually left for later reconstruction.

Contractural deformities of the axilla (shoulder), elbow, wrist, knee, and ankle joints

The factors leading to formation of the contractural deformities

Folding bodily joints in flexion (a so-called posture of 'comfort') is a characteristic body posture seen commonly in a distressed individual. Although the exact reasons are not entirely clear, contraction of muscle fibers at rest and the contractile force difference between the flexor muscle and the extensor muscle may play an important role in the genesis of this body posture. The magnitude of joint flexion, furthermore, increases as an individual loses voluntary control of muscle movement, as frequently occurs in a burn victim (Figure 56.1). Prolonged periods of physical inactivity, associated with burn treatment, and scar tissue contraction around the joint structures as the recovery ensues further impedes the joint mobility.

Incidence of burn contracture involving the axilla (shoulder), elbow, and knee joints

Burn treatment requiring a long period of bed confinement and physical inactivity as well as restriction of joint movement will lead to joint dysfunction. Consequently, every bodily joint (e.g. the vertebral, mandibular, shoulder, elbow, finger, hip, knee and toe) is susceptible to the change. Of various bodily joints involved, the contractural deformities of the axilla (shoulder), elbow, hip, and the knee are relatively common. Factors such as a wide range of joint movement and an asynchronous muscular control are characteristic features of these joints, and, when combined with a high vulnerability to burn injuries, are the probable reasons accounting for the high incidence of deformity encountered. Recent review of the records of 1005 patients treated at the Shriners Burns Hospital in Galveston, Texas over the past 25 years indicated that the elbow was the joint most commonly affected. There were 397 patients with elbow joint deformity, 283 knee contractures, and 248 axillary deformities. The hip joint contracture was the deformity least encountered and was noted in only 77 patients (Table 56.1).

The efficacy of splinting in controlling burn contractures of axilla (shoulder), elbow, and knee joints

Although Cronin in 1955 demonstrated that the neck splint was effective in preventing recurrence of neck contracture following surgical release,[1] the routine use of splinting for burn patients did not become a part of the regimen of burn wound care in Galveston until 1968, when Larson, the former Surgeon-in-Chief, and Willis, the former Chief Occupational Therapist at the Shriners Burns Institute, began to fabricate splints with thermoplastic materials to brace the neck and extremities.[2-5]

For more than three decades, a neck brace, a three-point extension splint, and a molded brace fabricated from thermoplastic materials, the prototypes of devices used to splint the neck, elbow and the knee joints, were used in the management of burn patients at the Shriners Burns Hospital and the University of Texas Medical Branch Hospitals in Galveston, Texas. An 'airplane splint' similarly made of thermoplastic materials was also used to splint the axilla during the period where the use of other splinting and bracing techniques, such as a 'figure-of-eight' bandage, is not feasible.

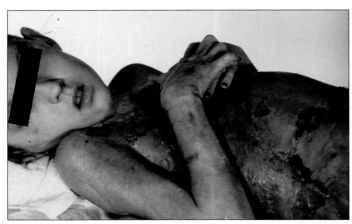

Fig. 56.1 The posture of 'comfort' characterized by flexion of shoulder (axilla) and elbow joints, plus hip and knee joints, is assumed by patients under distress, as in burn patients.

TABLE 56.1 THE DISTRIBUTION OF JOINT DEFORMITIES	
Joint involved	No.
Shoulder (axilla)	248
Elbow	397
Hip	77
Knee	283
Total	**1005**

A study was conducted in 1977 to determine the efficacy of splinting across large joint structures such as the elbow, axilla and knee joints by reviewing the records of 625 patients. There were 961 burns over these joints in this group of patients. Of these, 356 had involved the axillae while 357 and 248, respectively, involved the elbow and the knee joint. The incidence of contractural deformities encountered in these splinted joints was, as expected, low. The incidence of contractures in these joints was 7.3%, provided the patients had worn the splints for 6 months. The effectiveness of splinting was diminished to 55% if splinting was discontinued within 6 months. For comparison, the incidence of contractural deformity ascertained in 219 patients who had never worn the splint was 62% (Table 56.2).

Although splinting and bracing were shown to be effective in minimizing joint contracture, it was not entirely clear if restriction of joint movement would affect the quality of scar tissues formed across the joint surface. The effects were assessed by determining the frequency of secondary surgery performed in this group of patients. Over 90% of 219 individuals who did not use the splint/bracing required reconstructive surgery. In contrast, the need for surgical reconstruction in individuals who wore splints was 25%.[6]

Management of axilla (shoulder), elbow, wrist, knee, and ankle joints

The acute phase of recovery

It is believed that inadequate physical exercise and lack of joint splinting and bracing, while allowing a patient to assume the

TABLE 56.2 THE INCIDENCE OF CONTRACTURES ACROSS THE SHOULDER (AXILLA), ELBOW, AND KNEE JOINTS			
Without splint		With splint	
		<6 months	>6months
Shoulder			
Severe/moderate	137	24	23
Mild/none	37	6	129
Elbow			
Severe/moderate	75	17	10
Mild/none	61	33	161
Knee			
Severe/moderate	26	4	2
Mild/none	45	16	155

posture of 'comfort,' are the main factors responsible for the genesis of contractural deformities seen in burn patients during the acute phase of recovery from burn injuries. The deformities, furthermore, are made worse because of skin involvement and burn scar contracture. In order to minimize this undesirable consequence of burn injury, proper body positioning and splinting of the joint structures must be incorporated into the regimen of burn treatment. The treatment should be implemented as soon as the patient's condition becomes stable.

Bodily positioning and joint splinting

Bodily position: Although a supine position is preferred, the patient may be placed in a lateral decubitus position while confined in bed. The head should be placed in a neutral position with the neck slightly extended. For a patient placed in a supine position, neck extension is achieved by placing a small pad between the scapulae to facilitate the scapular traction. A neck brace may be used if the patient is placed in any other position.

Axillary (shoulder) joint: The axillary (shoulder) joint is kept at 90–120° of abduction and 15–20° of flexion. This generally results in 60–80° of arm elevation. The position is not only useful in protecting the brachial plexus from traction injury but is also effective in maintaining the stability of the glenohumeral joint. The position is best kept with the use of either a foam wedge, trough or airplane splint. A 'figure-of-eight' wrapping over a pad around the axilla, more frequently used for patients during the intermediate phase of recovery from the injury, is effective in maintaining shoulder abduction (it is also useful in preventing excess shoulder flexion).

Elbow joint: Rigid flexion contracture of the elbow is a common sequela in the joint if it is left unattended. In burns of the skin around the olecranon, exposure of the elbow joint is a common sequela if the elbow is allowed to contract freely. Maintaining the elbow in full extension therefore is essential. An extension brace (Figure 56.2), or a three-point extension splint across the elbow joint, is effective for this purpose (Figure 56.3).

Wrist joint: A contractural deformity of the wrist joint is relatively common in individuals with hand burns that were not splinted properly. A cock-up hand splint should be applied to maintain a 30° wrist extension (Figure 56.4).

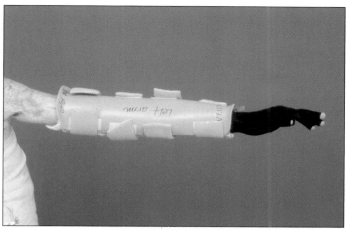

Fig. 56.2 A splint made of thermoplastic material is used to limit joint flexion.

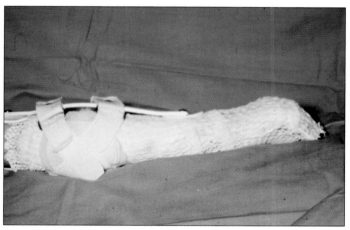

Fig. 56.3 A 'three-point' extension splint manufactured similar to an orthotic device is used either to extend a contracted elbow joint or to immobilize the joint in full extension.

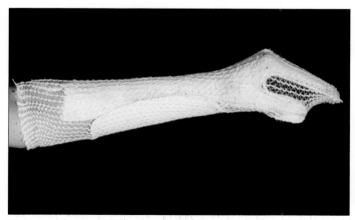

Fig. 56.4 Cock-up hand splint is effective to maintain 30 degree wrist extension.

Knee joint: Flexion of the knee is another posture commonly assumed by a burned victim. Similar to the elbow, uncontrolled flexion of the knee joint will lead to exposure of the joint structure, especially in instances where the injuries involve the patella surface. Maintenance of full extension of

the knee is an essential component of the therapeutic regimen — this is accomplished by means of a knee brace or a three-point extension splint (Figure 56.5).

Ankle joint: In order to minimize a plantar flexion contracture deformity, a common consequence of ankle burns, the joint should be maintained at 90° by applying a posterior splint.

Exercise

Although exercising a burned victim is an integral part of burn therapy, it is seldom implemented until the resuscitative measures are completed and the condition of the patient is considered stable. The primary goal of an exercise routine is the maintenance of the joint's functional integrity and muscle strength. This is attained by, in most instances, manually moving the joint and muscles — passive movement. The frequency and intensity of an exercise regimen, however, may vary depending upon the magnitude of the injury and the extent of joint involvement. The treatment, if possible, should be intensive and is rendered as frequently as possible.

The intermediate phase of recovery

The period from the second month through the fourth month following the injury is considered as *the intermediate phase* of recovery from burn injuries. The burn victims typically have full physiological functions and integumental integrity restored by this time. The cicatricial processes around the injured sites, on the other hand, are still physiologically active — though healing of the burned wound is considered satisfactory. That is, the process is characterized by, in addition to a maximal rate of collagen synthesis, a steady increase in the myofibroblast fraction of the fibroblast population in the wound[7] (the cellular change believed to account for contraction of the scar tissues). Continuous use of splinting and pressure to support the joints and burned sites, in this sense, is essential in order to control changes caused by the scar tissue formation and contraction.

Bodily positioning and joint splinting

Joint splinting and bodily positioning are similar to the regimen used during the acute phase of burn recovery. That is, the shoulder is kept at 15–20° flexion and 80–120° abduction. A 'figure-

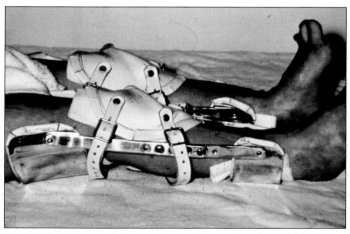

Fig. 56.5 A 'three-point' extension splint can be also used to manage the flexion contractures of a knee joint.

of-eight' wrapping over an axillary pad is used to maintain this shoulder joint position (Figure 56.6). The elbow and knee joints are maintained in full extension by means of a three-point extension splint or brace. A pressure dressing or garment is incorporated into the splint. In instances where the use of a 'figure-of-eight' bandage, pressure dressing and/or garment is not feasible because of recent surgery, devices such as an 'airplane splint' (Figure 56.7), or a three-point extension splint, may be used to splint the axilla, elbow, and the knee joints.

Pressure dressing

A compression dressing, originally incorporated into the treatment of burn wounds of the upper and lower extremities at the Shriners Burns Hospital in 1968 as a means of providing mechanical support to healing wounds, is effective in reducing tissue swelling and in promoting softening of a burn scar. Compression of a burn wound, even though healing is still in progress, is most easily achieved by means of wrapping the extremity in an elasticized bandage. Wrapping of the extremity should begin at the hand or foot. The bandage is moved cephalad in a crisscross fashion. The splint is reapplied over the bandage. It is important to rewrap the extremity three to four times daily. Wrapping an extremity with an elasticized bandage can produce a pressure ingredient of 10–25 mmHg.[5,8] Pressure dressing should be continued for 12–18 months.

Surgical management of established contractural deformities

Patient evaluation

There are numerous factors that will affect joint movements in burn patients. Although hypertrophy and contraction of

scar tissues and/or contracted skin graft around a joint are the most common causes of joint impairment, changes in the ligamentous structures or the joint itself due to burn injuries can also limit joint mobility. Detailed examination that includes radiographic assessment of the joint structures is essential in order to formulate a definitive treatment plan.

Non-operative or minimally invasive approaches to correcting a contracted and/or stiff joint

Restoration of movements in a contracted and/or stiff joint could be attained by minimally invasive or non-surgical means.[2–6] 'Pushing' and 'pulling' of an extremity that, in turn, 'stretches' contracted scars and tissues around an affected joint is the principle behind this modality of managing a contracted and/or stiff joint. The treatment is found to be especially effective in mobilizing a contracted joint caused by a long period of physical inactivity or, in some instances, of scar contracture.

Although the morbidities associated with this modality of treatment are minimal, breakdown of the skin due to pressure and/or friction resulting from 'pushing' and 'pulling' of a limb can occur.

Axillary (shoulder) contracture: Tight scars formed across the shoulder joint, usually in the area along the axillary folds, often limit the joint movement. The joint stiffness caused by scar contracture may be further aggravated by physical inactivity, especially if the patient is allowed to remain in the posture of 'comfort.'

There are two non-surgical methods commonly used to mobilize a contracted axilla (shoulder) joint. One is 'figure of eight' compression dressing technique and the other is an 'airplane' splinting technique:

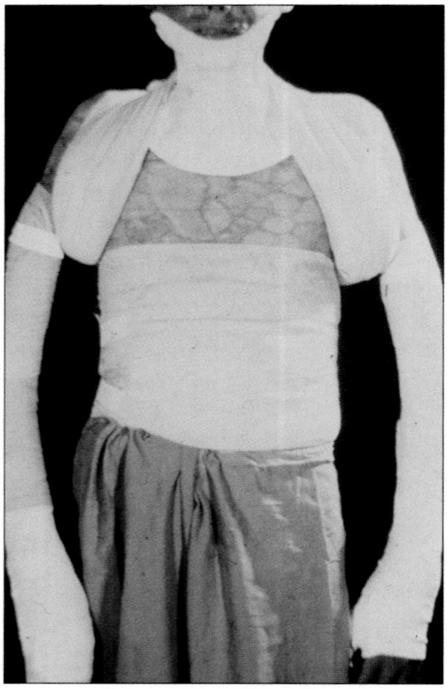

Fig. 56.6 An elasticized bandage is used to wrap around the shoulder (axilla) joints in a 'figure-of-eight' fashion to extend and to abduct the shoulder joints. An axillary pad is included in the wrapping to increase the pressure upon the axillary fold.

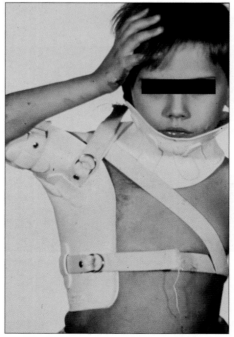

Fig. 56.7 An 'airplane' splint made of thermoplastic materials is used to maintain the shoulder abduction. The angle of separation may be increased, as the joint becomes more mobile.

- A *'figure-of-eight' compression dressing*: An elasticized bandage is used to wrap over a pad placed in the axillary fold around the shoulder joint in a 'figure-of-eight' fashion to extend and abduct the shoulder. Continuous wear of the dressing for a period of 3–6 months is necessary to obtain the release — the dressing is removed only for cleansing. The mobility of the joint increases as the scar tissues across the axilla softens but the extent of relief may be limited if the scar is thick and unyielding to the pressure (Figure 56.8).

- An *airplane splint*: The splint is fabricated with a thermoplastic material. The spreading angle is conformed to the extent of the axilla (shoulder) joint held at maximum abduction plus 10–15° of extension. Abduction and extension of the joint, that is elevation of the arm, will be maintained by 'pushing' the arm away from the upper thorax. Care is needed to protect the skin over the inner aspect of the arm and the side of the chest. The splint is changed regularly as the angle of joint abduction increases. One to 3 months of continu-

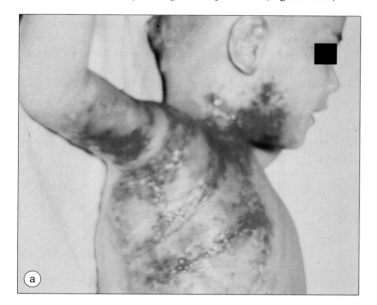

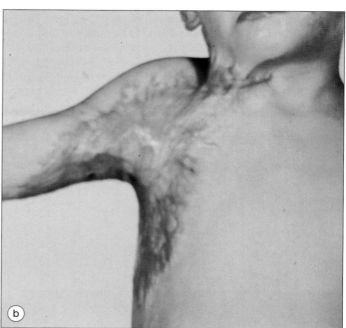

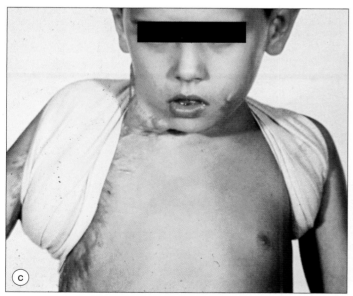

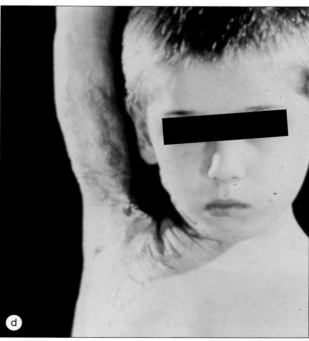

Fig. 56.8 (a) A 6-year-old boy sustained burns of the right side of his body extending from the lower neck to the upper thorax that included the axillary crease. (b) He experienced difficulty in extending both the neck and the right arm because of ensuing contraction of scar tissues around the neck and the axilla. (c) A 'figure-of-eight' dressing was used to maintain the shoulder extension and abduction. The dressing was used for 12 months. (d) He regained the shoulder extension and mobility with the use of pressure dressing.

ous use of this device is usually necessary to achieve the needed release in most instances (Figure 56.7).

Elbow and knee contracture: Flexion contracture is the most common deformity encountered in these two joints. The scar formed across the antecubital and the popliteal fossae frequently aggravates the magnitude of contractural problems in these joints. The following techniques are frequently utilized before surgery to obtain joint movement and joint extension:

- *A three-point extension splint*: The splint is assembled similarly to a prosthetic/orthotic device. Two sidebars hinged at the middle are connected with a bracing trough at the end. A cap pad is attached at the midsection of the sidebar to fit over the elbow or the kneecap. The splint is placed across the antecubital fossa or the popliteal fossa. Fitting of the splint is adjusted using Velcro straps (Figures 56.2 and 56.3).

  Extending the amount of movement of the joint is determined by the extent of the preexisting joint stiffness. The angle of extension is initially determined by the angle of joint contracture. The magnitude of extension is controlled by tightening the olecranon or patella pad. It is increased gradually as the joint gains its mobility. Problems encountered with the use of the 'three-

point extension splint' are uncommon. However, breakdown of the skin can occur. Leverage attainable from three-point pressure application may be limited in a young individual because of the inadequate leverage afforded by the shortness of limb length. The skeletal traction technique, in such instances, may be used.

- *A skeletal traction technique*: Utilizing a skeletal traction technique to restore movements in a contracted joint typically requires percutaneous insertion of a Steinmann pin through the radius for the elbow joint and the tibia for the knee joint. The pin is inserted through both cortices at the junction of the proximal two-thirds and the distal third of the radius or tibia. A contracted joint can be mobilized by the continuous and constant 'pull' on the long bone of a gravitational force generated by a 10–15 pound weight placed on a pulley device.

  For a flexion deformity of the elbow, the patient is placed in a supine position. The pulley traction device will provide a horizontal and then a vertically downward pull (Figure 56.9).

  Instead of utilizing a skeletal traction device to loosen a contracted knee, a weight placed around the ankle,

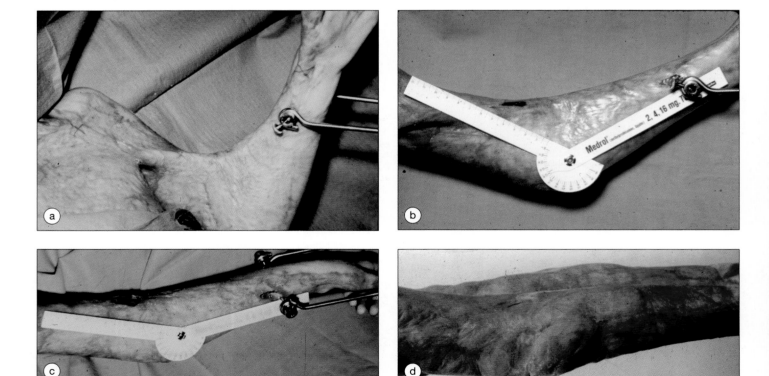

Fig. 56.9 (a) A skeletal traction technique may be used to extend a contracted joint as in this 8-year-old girl. A Steinmann pin was inserted percutaneously through the distal one-third of the radius. The direction of pull was horizontal using 10–15 pound weight. (b) The elbow joint was mobilized in 30–36 hours of constant pull. (c) A near full extension of the elbow joint was achieved in 6 days. (d) This was the appearance of the elbow 2 years after the traction extension treatment for elbow contracture. A minor procedure was, however, needed to release a tight band across the elbow surface.

with the patient in a prone position, may be used to pull on the foreleg. This technique is especially useful in treating individuals with a limited knee flexion contracture. Traction is continued for a period of time and is repeated several times a day (Figure 56.10).

Although morbidities due to infection are uncommon, a continuous and constant force of pull can cause breakdown of the skin located across the joint surface. Any wound thus formed can be temporarily covered with surgical or biological dressings and its closure contemplated once the joint contracture is fully corrected.

Surgical treatment of a contracted joint

Surgical treatment of a contracted joint is contemplated in individuals where the use of non-surgical treatment is ineffective and where functional integrity of a joint is in jeopardy. Surgical intervention, in this regard, is relatively unusual during the acute phase of recovery. Instead, the reconstruction is delayed until the scar tissue becomes fully 'matured,' i.e. flattened and soft.

Pre-surgical evaluation

The patient is seen and the involved joint is examined before surgery. The following features are assessed:

- *The extent of joint contracture* is determined and the passive and active range of joint motion is assessed. Radiographic evaluation may be obtained to delineate the structural integrity of the joint.
- *The magnitude of scarring and scar thickness* is assessed. The scar is usually the thickest across the joint surface.
- *The location and the size of uninjured skin* are delineated. The availability of uninjured skin frequently determines the technique of reconstruction. Skin graft and skin flap donor sites are also ascertained.
- *The point and the axis of joint rotation* are located. The line of incisional release is in alignment with the axis of joint movement.

Reconstruction of contracted joints
Releasing the contracture deformity of the joint

Despite a detailed examination before surgery, the exact cause of joint stiffness can only be delineated with surgery. In practice, contraction of the scar tissues across the joint structure is the most common cause of contractural joint deformities.

- Release of joint contracture by incising the scarred tissue — A contracted joint is freed by making an incision in the scar across the joint surface. The incision is placed in line with the axis of joint rotation and initially confined within the width of the scar. It is lengthened as necessary to achieve the intended release. Prior infiltration of the area with lidocaine containing epinephrine in 1:400 000 concentration is useful in obtaining hemostasis and later pain control. The incision, however, must be made with caution to avoid injuring major vessels and nerves. This is

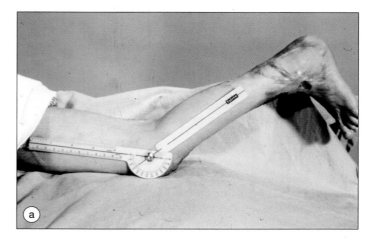

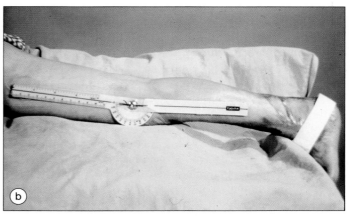

Fig. 56.10 (a) A knee contracture developed in an 8-year-old male youth due to improper positioning and immobilization of the knee joint. There was no direct injuries involving the knee area. With the patient being placed in a prone position, the ankle was strapped with a 10–15 pound weight. (b) The flexion contracture was relieved in 3 days.

achieved by a 'pushing' instead of a 'slicing' motion of the surgical blade to free the scarred tissues. The extent of release is assessed by the improvement of joint motion gained as the scarred tissue is severed. In rare instances, cicatricial changes could involve the joint capsule and reconstruction of the capsular structure prove necessary.

- The use of z-plasty technique[9] — A contracted area can be lengthened by use of the z-plasty technique. The technique utilizes the principle that a contracted wound is lengthened by interposing two triangular skin flaps mobilized from an unburned area immediately adjacent to the area of release. The lengthening of the wound is maximally attained by interposing two triangular flaps of 60° angle. While the z-plasty technique is an excellent means to ameliorate the problem of wound contracture, it is not possible if the amount of uninjured skin adjacent to the wound is limited.
- Wound coverage — there are six basic techniques of wound coverage:
  (1) Primary closure of the wound.
  (2) A full-thickness or partial-thickness skin graft.

(3) An interposition skin flap mobilized from the adjacent area.

(4) Combination of an interposition skin flap and skin grafting.

(5) A muscle or skin-muscle flap mobilized from the adjacent area.

(6) A free skin or skin-muscle flap harvested from a distant site and transferred via a microsurgical technique.

Primary closure of the wound

Wound closure *per primum* following burn scar excision is difficult if not entirely impossible. Inelasticity of the skin surrounding the wound and an inadequate amount of uninjured skin available for mobilization and closure preclude the use of this method. Closure of a resultant wound following release, in practice, would defeat the original objective of the contractural reconstruction.

Skin grafting technique

The use of a piece of skin graft, full or partial thickness, to cover a wound is the most fundamental technique of wound coverage that is technically simple and results in minimal morbidity.

- Operative technique: A partial-thickness skin graft of $^{15}/_{1000}$ to $^{20}/_{1000}$ in thickness is harvested from an unburned area using a dermatome. The scalp, lower abdomen, and the anterior surface of the upper thigh are the common donor sites. A piece of full-thickness skin graft can be harvested from the lower abdomen, above the suprapubic or inguinal area, without leaving unsightly donor site defects. The subdermal fatty tissues are removed but attempts should be made to preserve the subdermal capillary plexus (Figure 56.11). The donor defect is usually closed primarily. The graft is cut to fit the defect and the edges are anchored with 3–0 silk sutures. The ends are left sufficiently long to tie over a bolster to immobilize the graft. Several anchoring 'mattress' stitches using 4–0 or 5–0 chromic catgut sutures may be placed in the center of the graft to immobilize the skin graft against the base. Hemostasis around the recipient site is essential. Hematoma formed underneath the graft will hinder the 'take' of the graft.

- After care: The bolster is usually removed 4–5 days after the procedure. Bodily fluid or blood elements accumulated underneath the graft, i.e. seroma and/or hematoma, are evacuated. This is achieved by making a small 'nick' in the graft with a pair of surgical scissors. The fluid is 'rolled' out with a cotton tip applicator. The joint is immobilized immediately and pressure dressing is used to minimize the consequence of contracture. Physical exercise is resumed 3 weeks after the surgery.

An interposition flap technique: alias ³/₄ z-plasty technique

This technique, known by various names such as 'three-quarter z-plasty' technique, a 'banner' flap interposition technique, etc., is the most useful method of wound coverage following a releasing procedure for a contracted joint. The technique is based on the principle that an open wound consequential to surgical release may be covered with a skin flap mobilized from an adjacent area. While designing of a flap is technically simple, it requires an area of unburned skin adjacent to the released wound.

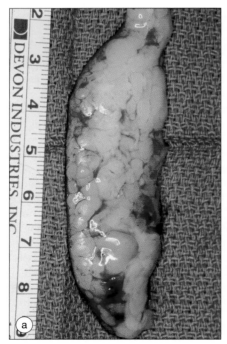
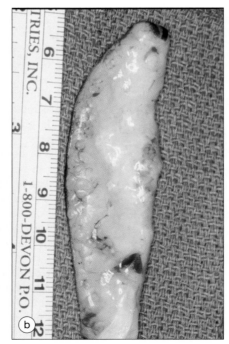
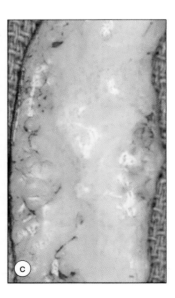

Fig. 56.11 (a) A piece of skin with subcutaneous tissues is removed from the abdomen that will be used as a full-thickness skin graft. (b) The subcutaneous fatty tissues were sharply removed with a pair of fine scissors. The capillaries were left undisturbed. (c) A close-up view to show the capillaries that are left in the graft.

• Operative technique: A triangular skin flap is designed in an unburned area adjacent to the wound following release. A vertical limb of the flap, begun at the end of the released wound edge, is set at a 90° angle to the end of the wound. The limb length is equal to the wound length. A triangular flap is formed by making the width of the flap at the mid-section the same width as the wound. The flap can be based either proximally or distally depending upon the direction of the triangular flap designed (Figure 56.12a). The flap is dissected out and is rotated 90° to cover the defect (Figure 56.12b,c). The flap donor

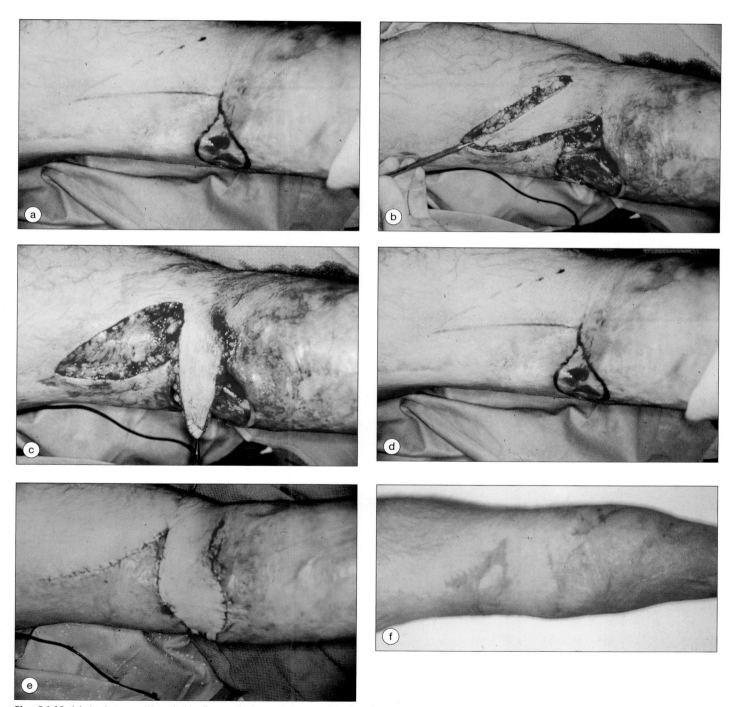

Fig. 56.12 (a) An interpositional skin flap technique, i.e. a modified z-plasty technique, is useful in reconstructing a flexion deformity around the joint, as seen in this 42-year-old individual who had sustained burn injuries around the upper extremity. A triangular flap based distally on the lateral side of the elbow was designed in an uninjured area adjacent to the scarred joint surface. The length of the flap was equal to the length of scar release. (b) The triangular flap was fabricated. (c) The skin flap was rotated 90° to make up the tissue defect. (d) The donor site was closed primarily. (e) The appearance of the wound 1 year following the reconstruction.

defect is closed primarily (Figure 56.12d,e). The width of flap may be narrow in instances where the size of unburned skin is not enough to fabricate a triangular skin flap sufficiently to cover the wound. The flap, in such an instance, is anchored in the middle of the wound. The two sides not covered by the flap are closed with a piece of skin graft (Figure 56.13).

• After care: The wound edges are kept clean with antibiotic ointment. Sutures may be removed at day 10. Splinting of the joint is resumed within 4–5 days and joint exercise in 10–14 days.

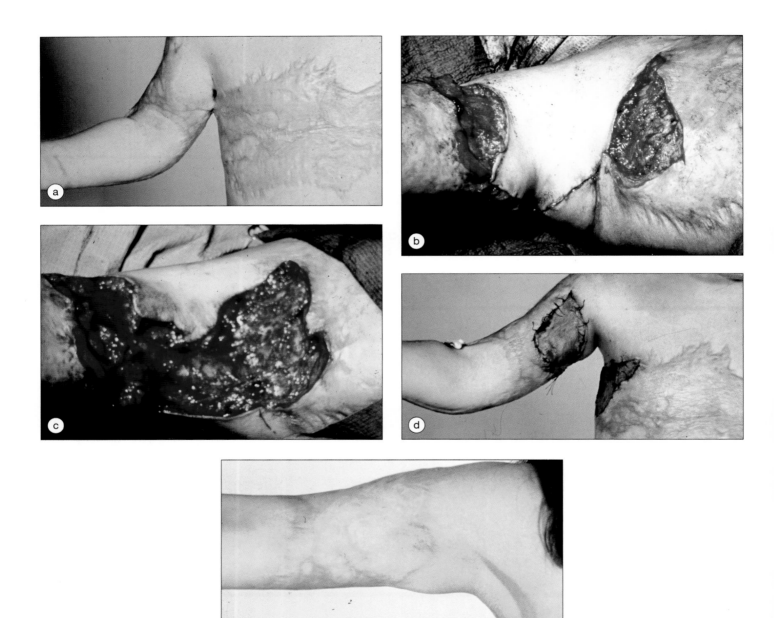

Fig. 56.13 (a) An interpositional skin flap technique of wound closure may be modified as in this 5-year-old girl who had sustained burns around the right axilla that caused contracture of the axillary joint. (b) The skin defect was so extensive that it could not be covered completely with a single flap. (c) The uninjured skin, raised as a flap, was transferred to the middle of the wound, leaving the areas proximal and distal to the flap to be covered with skin grafts. (d) The appearance of the wound 10 days following the surgery. (e) The appearance of the wound 10 years after the surgery. The flap placed in the middle of the wound had increased in size because of body growth and stretching of the scar tissues.

A muscle flap or skin-muscle flap technique

The technique is utilized in instances when the resultant defect following release is so extensive that coverage of the wound with a skin flap or a skin graft is not feasible.

The latissimus dorsi muscle harvested either as a muscle flap or as a musculocutaneous flap may be used to cover the axilla. The soleus muscle flap or the gastrocnemius muscle-skin flap may be used to cover the wound around the knee joint coverage (Figure 56.14).

Muscle or muscle-skin flap, in practice, is seldom used to reconstruct burn deformities unless vital structures such as the brachial or popliteal neurovasculatures become exposed consequential to releasing procedures. Similarly, microsurgical composite tissue transfer technique is limited in burn scar release. Donor site limitation and technical difficulties encountered in pediatric patients probably account for the infrequent use of this method.

The use of a modified fasciocutaneous (FC) z-plasty technique; alias ¾ FC z-plasty technique to reconstruct contracted axilla, elbow, and knee joints

Reconstruction of a contracted joint involving the axilla, elbow, and the knee may be carried out according to the fol-lowing scheme in most instances once the surgical intervention is determined to be the most appropriate approach in providing relief.

- Ascertain that the scar contracture is the primary reason for the joint contraction.
- Determine the axis of joint rotation.
- A line is drawn to connect the axial point of joint rotation and the center point of contracted scar across the joint.
- A second line that is equal and perpendicular to the length of the release line is drawn. This is the cathetus for the first right-angled triangle.
- A second right-angled triangle (sharing the cathetus with the first one), with the hypotenuse drawn to a 30–45° angle, forms a Z pattern of 90° and 30–45° angles (Figure 56.15a).
- The contracted scar is incised to free the joint. An incision is then made along the drawn common cathetus line. Separation of skin and subcutaneous tissues should be sufficiently deep to identify the fascial layer (Figure 56.15b). The fascial layer is sutured to the skin edge to prevent accidental separation of the skin and the fascia. Dissection is continued underneath the fascia but above

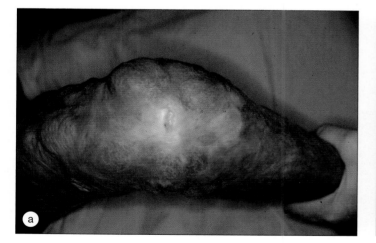
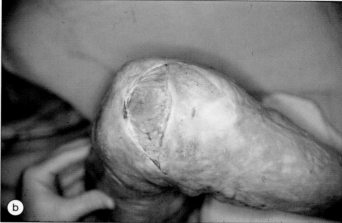
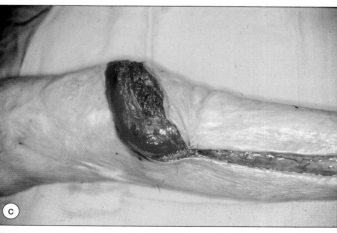
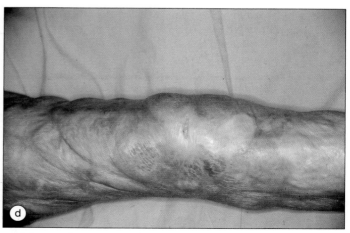

Fig. 56.14 (a) Flexion of the knee was limited because of tight scars around the patella. (b) An incisional release of the tight area across the patella provided the relief of knee contracture. However, it resulted in an open wound of 4–5 cm in size. (c) A medial segment of the soleus muscle was used to cover the defect. (d) The appearance of the knee area 3 months following the procedure.

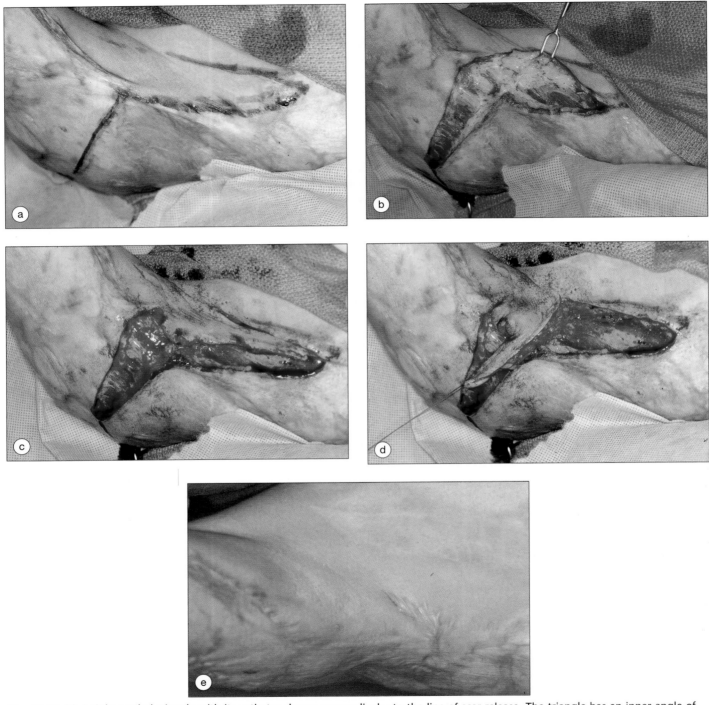

Fig. 56.15 (a) A right-angled triangle with its cathetus drawn perpendicular to the line of scar release. The triangle has an inner angle of 35°. (b) The fascia layer is identified and is separated from the muscle fibers underneath to fabricate a fasciocutaneous (FC) flap. (c) A right-angled triangle FC flap is fabricated. (d) The defect in the right axilla consequential to the releasing procedures is made up with the flap rotated 90°. (e) The appearance of the axilla 2 years following the releasing procedure.

the muscle fibers to fabricate a fasciocutaneous flap triangular in shape. The extent of proximal subfascial dissection is determined by the mobility of the fabricated triangular flap. The proximal tissue dissection ends once the 90° rotation of the flap, without undue tension, is possible (Figure 56.15c).

- The defect resulting from moving a triangular skin-fascia flap is closed in layers as direct closure of the defect is difficult, especially if the flap donor site is scarred or previously grafted. The wound then may be covered with a skin graft (Figure 56.15d,e).

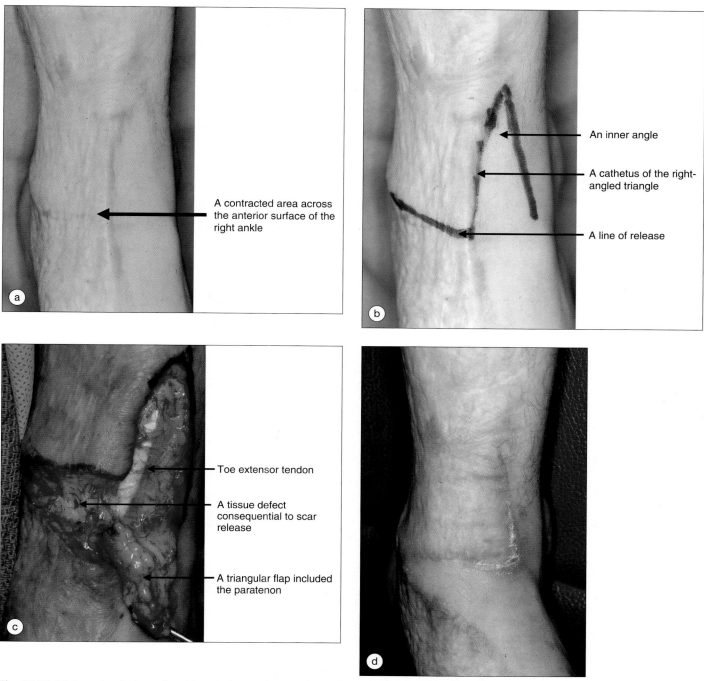

Fig. 56.16 (a) A contracted scar band is noted over the anterior surface of the left ankle. (b) A right-angled triangle is drawn with its cathetus made perpendicular to the contracted area of the ankle. (c) The paratenon is included in the flap fabrication. (d) The ankle surface with the wound healed and the contracture released.

The technique of reconstructing contracted wrist and ankle joints

The indications and the approach in drawing skin lines for z-plasty technique is identical to the maneuver used for other joints. The paratenon instead of the fascia is included in the composite skin flap fabrication (Figure 56.16).

Summary

Contractural deformities of the axilla (shoulder), elbow, wrist, knee, and ankle joints are not uncommon sequelae of burn injuries. Although the injury involving the limbs and the joint structures could account for the deformities encountered, lack of proper positioning and inadequate physical exercise while recovering from the injuries could further contribute to the genesis of the problems.

The use of appropriate brace, splint and/or pressure dressings is important in minimizing such an undesirable consequence of burn injuries. The treatment for an established joint deformity, on the other hand, requires surgical release of the contracted skin and scars. Various methods of reconstruction have been described to manage the problems encountered. Specific approaches to managing contractural deformities involving the axilla (shoulder), elbow, hip, and the knee joints have been outlined.

References

1. Cronin TD. Successful corrections of extensive scar contractures of the neck using split thickness skin grafts. In: Trans First International Congress on Plastic Surgery. Baltimore: Williams & Wilkins; 1957:123.
2. Willis B. The use of orthoplast isoprene in the treatment of the acutely burned child. A follow-up. Am J Occup Ther 1970; 24:187.
3. Larson DL, Evans EB, Abston S, et al. Techniques for decreasing scar formation and scar contractures in the burn patient. J Trauma 1971; 11:807–823.
4. Larson DL, Abston S, Evans EB, et al. Contractures and scar formation in the burn patient. Clin Plast Surg 1974; 1:653–666.
5. Larson D, Huang T, Linaris H, et al. Prevention and treatment of scar contracture. In: Artz CP, Moncrief JA, Pruitt BA, eds. Burns. A team approach. Philadelphia: WB Saunders; 1979:466.
6. Huang TT, Blackwell SJ, Lewis SR. Ten years of experience in managing patients with burn contractures of axilla, elbow, wrist, and knee joints. Plast Reconstr Surg 1978; 61:70–76.
7. Bauer PS, Larson DL, Stacy TR. The observation of myofibroblasts in hypertrophic scar. Surg Gynecol Obstet 1975; 141:22–26.
8. Linaris HA, Larson DL, Willis-Galstaum BA. Historical notes on the use of pressure in the treatment of hypertrophic scars or keloids. Burns 1993; 19:17–21.
9. McCarthy JG. Introduction to plastic surgery. In: McCarthy JG, ed. Plastic surgery. Philadelphia: WB Saunders; 1990:55.

Chapter 57

Reconstruction of the burned breast

Robert L. McCauley

Introduction

Currently, studies have documented that burns of the torso and lower extremities eventually result in a significant number of problems.[1-3] Burvin et al. evaluated 421 female patients admitted to their institution over a 3-year period, focusing on female patients with breast burns. Of the 138 female burn patients identified, only 9% had non-isolated breast burns. Interestingly, 66% of the breast burns were secondary to scald injuries.[1] In 1989, Brou et al. evaluated 25 patients with a mean total body surface area burn of 71%.[2] In this series of patients, 512 reconstructive problems were identified. In the trunk and perineal regions, 70 problems were identified. In 1993, Burns et al. analyzed reconstruction issues associated with 28 patients who survived burns of at least 80% of the total body surface area. In this series, 564 reconstructive problems were noted.[3] In each series, approximately 20 reconstructive problems were identified per patient. In the series by Burns et al., the trunk was the most frequently injured area in the torso/lower extremity section. However, the trunk was only second to the hand as the most frequently injured anatomic section. In addition, the breasts were the most frequently injured region within the truncal/perineal region. McCauley et al. noted that subsequent analysis of the donor sites usually revealed that the tissue available for reconstruction was often less than optimal.[4] Consequently, it became quite clear that a stepwise plan of action for reconstruction could not be followed. Indeed, patient and family desires must be combined with realistic outcomes in order to determine the most judicious and efficacious use of available donor sites. Without question, these issues are of significant concern since it has been recognized that 71% of female patients with burns to the anterior chest wall with involvement of the nipple-areola complex (NAC) will require surgical intervention to assist with breast development.

Historical issues

Evaluation of the management of burns to the truncal region requires longitudinal analysis of parameters of growth and development in order to assess the efficacy of variations in acute burn wound management. Recently, an increase in the survival of burned patients has been associated with better resuscitation, control of the hypermetabolic response, improved antimicrobial therapy and early excision with closure of the burn wound. Such data are well documented in the burn literature and remain the standard of care today.[5-9] Longitudinal assessment of earlier methods of burn care, which included delayed excision and épluchage, exhibited an increase in hospital morbidity and mortality of burned patients. Yet, the conservative management of tissue over the torso proved to be quite beneficial in female patients who survived this type of management. In 1989, McCauley et al. documented that with conservative management of burn tissue over the anterior chest wall, involving the NAC it is possible for normal breast development to occur even with nipple loss[4] (Figure 57.1). This retrospective study, which analyzed burn therapy nearly 20 years earlier, noted that, conservative management of the NAC in these patients was uniformly beneficial. On the other hand, 71% of these patients required incisional releases of the anterior chest wall to assist in breast development. The importance of these studies lies in the observation that, even with loss of the NAC, the breast bud itself is rarely injured.

Several investigations have previously shown that even with the destruction of the NAC, the breast bud may be uninjured.[4,10] In prepubescent females, since the majority of burns to the anterior chest wall are scald injuries, it is believed that the subcutaneous tissue is still quite viable.[13,14] This is significant since the mammary gland in children is believed to be located 4–8 mm in the subcutis. It is believed to be attached to the overlying nipple by the epithelium of the parsinfundibularis of the milk ducts.[11] Although burn management prior to 1970 was quite conservative, the longitudinal effects of blunt eschar separation resulted in maximum tissue preservation, which produced flexible, mature burn scars.

Often it is difficult to evaluate the development of young females who have lost their NAC as they proceed to develop in their adolescent years. Many of these patients require fre-

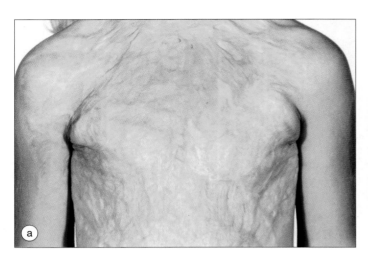

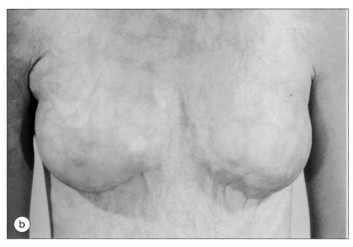

Fig. 57.1 (a) A 5-year-old girl after conservative debridement of burns to the anterior chest wall involving both nipple-areolar complex: subsequent split-thickness skin grafts placed over the chest wall. (b) Breast development noted in teenage years. (Reprinted with permission from: McCauley et al. Functional and Aesthetic Reconstruction of the Burn Patient. New York, Taylor and Francis 2005; 379–392.[22])

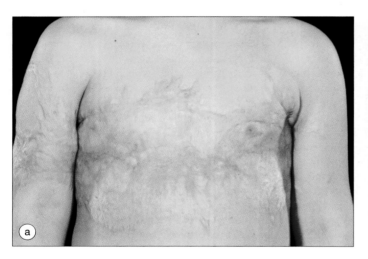

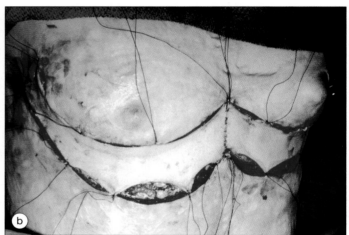

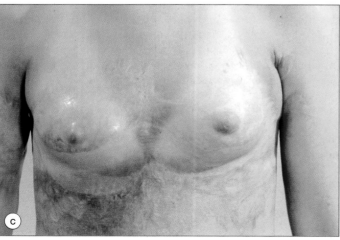

Fig. 57.2 (a) A 6-year-old girl after recovery of anterior chest wall burns treated with conservative debridement and coverage with skin grafts. (b) Six years later with breast development, the patient required bilateral inframammary releases and coverage with skin grafts. (c) Symmetric breast development noted 2 years later. (Reprinted with permission from: McCauley et al. Functional and Aesthetic Reconstruction of the Burn Patient. New York, Taylor and Francis 2005; 379–392.[22])

quent follow-up in order to assess the early stages of breast development and to plan surgical correction should entrapment of the breast in burn scar become a problem. During this period of time, pressure garments are often worn in order to assist the maturity of burn scars over developing breast. Many of these patients may require an incisional release to allow the breasts to develop without distortion (Figure 57.2). Subsequent maturation of skin grafts not only results in blending in with injured tissue but also allows the tissue over the breast to immediately become more relaxed.

Reconstruction of the burned breast

Reconstruction of the burned breast encompasses a variety of techniques.[12-19] Most reconstructive surgeons view this issue in two parts:

* reconstruction of the breast mound, and
* reconstruction of the NAC.

Choosing the best option available is dependent upon the age at which the patient sustained injury, the type of injury, and the extent of surgical management during the acute phase of treatment. Obvious restriction in the breast development as a result of scar contracture has been the standard indication for surgical intervention. However, the timing for such intervention may vary with each patient.

Traditional methods of breast reconstruction after mastectomy for breast cancer may not be an option in these young girls during their developmental years. Areas of significant burn injury and the lack of tissue bulk may prevent the use of the transverse rectus abdominus myocutaneous (TRAM) flap as a method for reconstruction. The need for bilateral breast reconstruction in many of these patients further complicates the issue. The use of the latissimus dorsi myocutaneous flap is an option and has been utilized by a number of plastic surgeons.[15,20,21] Some success has been achieved with the use of tissue expansion and subsequent placement of submuscular breast implants.[22] Because of significant scarring in the inframammary region in many of these patients, the transaxillary approach may be the best operative approach.

The burned male breast represents a challenge due to a decrease in subcutaneous tissue and lack of desirable outcomes for those who undergo reconstruction of the NAC. Most male patients opt not to undergo NAC reconstruction, thus making the opportunity to reconstruct the male breast rare.[23] Literature on the subject of male breast and NAC reconstruction is limited and significant data are not available. The initial surgical reconstruction of the burned male breast centers on scar excision and contracture release by multiple W-plasty and z-plasties.[24] The male NAC can either be reconstructed using a full-thickness graft from non-hair-bearing scrotal skin or from full-thickness skin grafts from the thigh. Tattooing of the areola should be adequate to define the areola.[23] If attempting to raise the nipple, stacked cartilage grafts can be placed beneath the areolar graft.[1] Although many men opt to forego aesthetic treatment for breast and NAC reconstruction, the option should be made available.

In patients who require global fascial excision of the anterior chest wall, breast development will not occur.

Bilateral breast burns: amastia

As previously stated, patients who have sustained injuries to the underlying breast bud may not develop breasts. During the adolescent years, this becomes a significant issue to young girls. The latissimus dorsi myocutaneous flap may be an option with implant placement in breast reconstruction. The author's approach has been to release the scar contractures using thick split-thickness skin grafts with an inverted T incision. Once the new grafts have matured, a transaxillary approach is then used for placement of submuscular tissue expanders. Once expansion is completed, the expanders are removed and breast implants are then inserted using the transaxillary approach.[22]

The use of the transaxillary incision avoids problems which may develop with wound healing if the inframammary approach is undertaken.

The use of tissue expansion and placement of an implant is employed in reconstruction of the burned breast when it is believed that there is adequate skin to result in primary coverage of the prosthesis after placement. Becker introduced the permanent breast expander implant in 1984.[24] Tissue expanders are placed in the subglandular or submuscular plane and are expanded incrementally until the desired growth is obtained.[14] In burned patients, who have undergone fascial excisions, placement in the submuscular plane is the only option. Some authors have recommended that reconstruction be delayed several months to allow for scar softening to take place.[13] Afterwards, the expander can be temporarily deflated to assess tissue laxity.[16,25] At this point, insertion with a subpectoral breast implant proportional in volume to the tissue expander provides a breast mound that is not under tension. Some common complications that are seen with the use of tissue expander and implants include exposure of the injection port, infections, spontaneous deflation, and capsule formation.[25] In such patients, maturity of the tissue over the anterior chest wall is of paramount importance if reconstructive methods are to be successful at a later date. Many of these patients will require tissue expansion and subsequent placement of a muscular prosthesis to give the appearance of developed breasts (Figure 57.3).

The unilateral chest wall burn presents a significant problem. In children, the uninjured side will proceed with uninhibited breast development whereas the burned side may require surgical procedures in order to assist the developing breast.

Mastopexy/reduction mammoplasty

Symmetry of the burned breast is desired and should be the driving force behind breast reconstruction. Correction of asymmetry is complicated and must address skin contractures, nipple dystopia and volume asymmetry.[26] The most difficult technical problem has been that of achieving volumetric and geometric equality.[27] Assessment of proper volume status between the two breasts can be closely approximated perioperatively, but geometric equality will change over time.

In patients with unilateral breast burns, the uninjured breast serves as a guide for shape and symmetry. Unfortunately, in some patients achieving breast symmetry may be challenging. Occasionally, even as breast development proceeds with the injured breast, its subsequent development may still pose a problem with respect to shape and size when compared to the normal breast. The choices of reduction mammoplasty or a mastopexy on the uninjured breast versus augmentation of the injured breast depends on the extent of the asymmetry and patient desires (Figures 57.4 and 57.6). Sometimes different procedures may be required on each breast to achieve symmetry.

Burns to the breast even after extensive releases with skin grafts maintain a very strong outer envelop for breast support. Thai et al. noted that the thick inelasticity of skin grafts creates a sling that does not become ptotic with age.[28] In patients with unilateral breast burns, over time, the contralateral uninjured breast may become ptotic when compared to the reconstructed

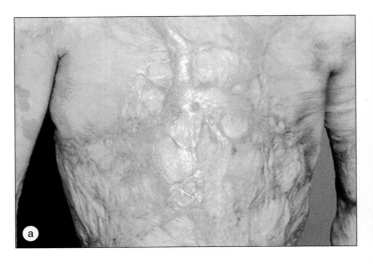

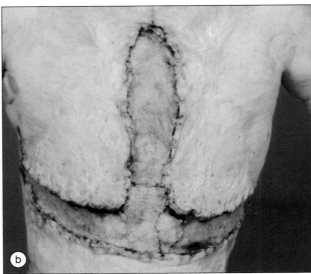

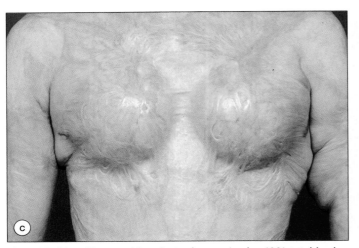

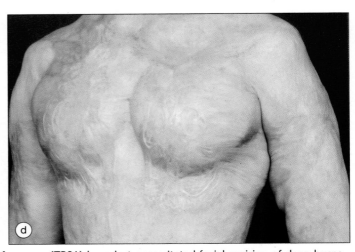

Fig. 57.3 (a) A 15-year-old patient who survived a 60% total body surface area (TBSA) burn but necessitated facial excision of deep burns over anterior chest wall. Note lack of breast development. (b) Inverted T incision performed to release chest contractures. (c) Final appearance after removal of expanders, insertion of saline implants and bilateral revision of lateral redundant tissue over the breasts. (d) Right oblique view. (Reprinted with permission from: McCauley et al. Functional and Aesthetic Reconstruction of the Burn Patient. New York, Taylor and Francis 2005; 379–392.[22])

burned breast (Figures 57.4). In cases where at least a grade II ptosis is present, a mastopexy of the uninjured breast may be necessary. This procedure not only improves breast symmetry but also improves superior pole fullness.

The development of breast asymmetry and contour deformities are quite common. The burned breast tends to be fuller and does not have the natural ptosis associated with a matured female breast. Mastopexy of the uninjured breast may be performed in order to relieve the grade II or greater ptosis, to realign the NAC, and to give the uninjured breast a fuller appearance. Mudge and McCauley documented significant improvement in breast symmetry and aesthetics using this approach.[29]

Multiple operations to release the breast from entrapment of burn scars may result in contour deformities. The lack of fullness and accentuated asymmetry of the infraclavicular may require reconstruction using pedicled fasciocutaneous flaps or a latissimus dorsi musculocutaneous flap. Even if the

level of the NACs is similar, medial or lateral displacement of the nipple may be of significant concern to the patient. If breast contracture is a problem, medial or lateral incisional releases and coverage with skin grafts will allow better nipple positioning. On the other hand, if breast contracture is not a problem, isolated repositioning of NAC is indicated. Clearly in patients with macromastia and breast deformities correction of the breast contracture prior to reduction mammaplasty assures optimal results.[27]

Reconstruction of the nipple-areola complex

Reconstruction of the NAC constitutes the second stage of breast reconstruction. The literature has numerous articles to address this issue.[30–34] The NAC reconstruction is often delayed until the reconstructed breast mound has had time for scars to mature. This may be 9–12 months after breast mound recon-

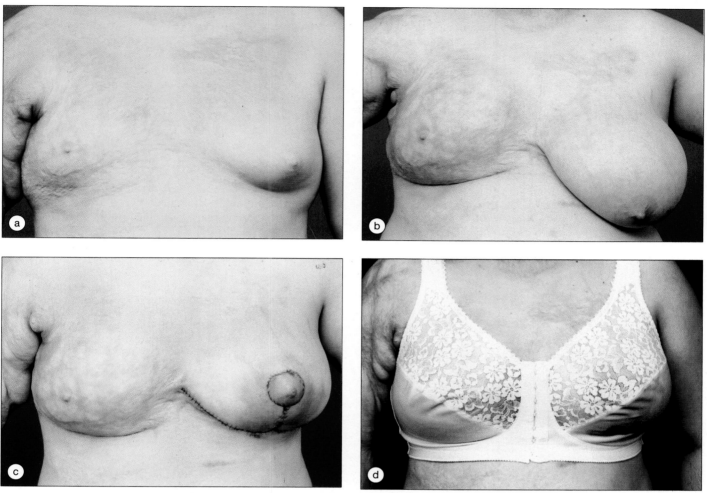

Fig. 57.4 (a) A 10-year-old girl with unilateral right breast burns with preservation of the nipple areolar complex. (b) Same patient at age 17 with unilateral macromastia on the left. Note normal breast shape without ptosis on the right side. (c) Postoperative appearance after left unilateral reduction mammaplasty. (d) Patient is satisfied with results, being able to wear a brassiere for adequate support for both breasts. (Reprinted with permission from: McCauley et al. Functional and Aesthetic Reconstruction of the Burn Patient. New York, Taylor and Francis 2005; 379–392.[22])

struction. As a rule, reconstruction of the NAC is undertaken when the breasts have fully developed. In the reconstructed breast, several problems may exist: malpositioning of the NAC and partial or total absence of the NAC. In cases of malpositioning of the NAC in the burned breast, Mohmand and Nassan suggested the use of two double U-plasty for correction.[30] This technique is quite similar to a z-plasty in which the NAC is transposed inferiorly or superiorly to match the contralateral unburned breast. Of course, the technique can only be performed in patients with no evidence of breast contraction and in patients in which there is minimal displacement of the NAC. Reportedly, there is minimal interference with the sensation of the NAC with this technique.

In situations where the nipple is present but the areola is partially or totally lost, treatment alternatives differ. Partial loss of the areola can be addressed with tattooing of the region to blend in with the color of the remaining areola. In situations where the entire areola is lost, tattooing of the areola or resurfacing with full-thickness skin grafts is useful. The upper inner thigh as a donor site produces excellent contrast with the surrounding tissues in this situation.[35] In unilateral breast burns, the technique utilized may be guided by the color match of the unaffected side. However, in bilateral breast burns with areola loss, either technique provides acceptable results.

Total loss of the NAC presents a difficult problem in the burned patient. Although numerous techniques are available, their role in the reconstruction of the burned breast has yet to be fully evaluated.[30–32] In the absence of the native NAC, a nipple can be reconstructed from numerous composite graft donors, including toe pulp, postauricular cartilage and skin or the opposite nipple.[12] The use of labial skin to reconstruct the NAC has been replaced with more current procedures. Reconstruction of the NAC using auricular skin and cartilage can be used in patients when nipple sharing is not an option. This technique can yield fair to good results.[35] The conchal cartilage is used to simulate Montgomery glands. Free toe pulp grafts as well as composite grafts taken from the second to fourth toe has been utilized in NAC reconstruction. Pensler et al. reviewed different results of various techniques in reconstructing the burned NAC. They recommended the use of full-thickness skin grafts from the superomedial thigh for reconstruction of the areola. This group also recommended the use of the quadrapod flap for nipple reconstruction if there is adequate surrounding dermis.[31] This technique appeared to be superior to the composite grafts and the 'double-bubble' technique over a 1-year period. Several authors have been skeptical with respect to the use of skin flaps in reconstruction of the NAC.[10] Since these flaps require normal dermal elements and subcutaneous tissue to maintain viability to the skin, it was felt that the role of skin flaps in the reconstruction of the NAC in the burned patient was limited.

In 1984, Little described the 'skate' flap for NAC reconstruction[36] (Figure 57.5). Its use in reconstruction of burn patients has received little attention. However, McCauley and Robson reported the successful use of the 'skate' flap in reconstruction of the nipple in the burned breast.[37] This finding clearly demonstrates the re-establishment of an adequate subdermal plexus in burned patients after resurfacing with skin grafts (Figure 57.6). Virtually all techniques that involve the projection of a nipple will succumb to some degree of flattening. Several factors have been cited for this phenomenon, including surface tension of skin, lack of normal infrastructure, and centrifugal forces.[25,38,39]

Summary

Problems associated with reconstruction of burns to the truncal region continue to represent a challenge. Entrapment of breast tissue in burn scars in female patients can be eliminated with

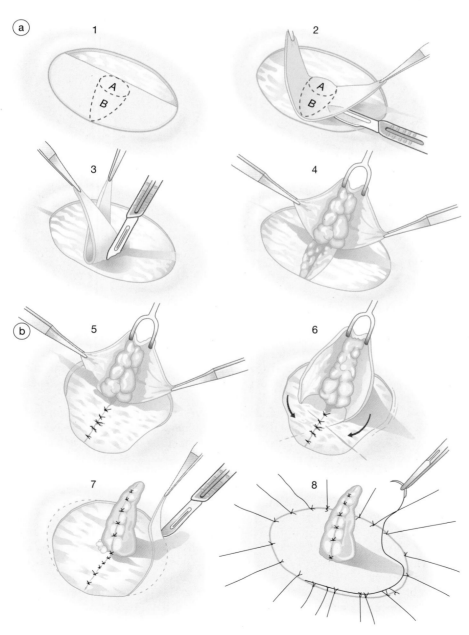

Fig. 57.5 (a) Design of the skate flap as described by Little with elevation of the pedicle. (b) Design of the skate flap as described by Little with reconstruction of the areolar and coverage with a full-thickness skin graft. (Reprinted with permission from: Little[36])

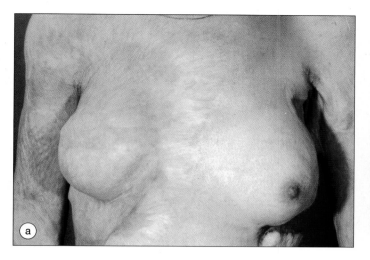

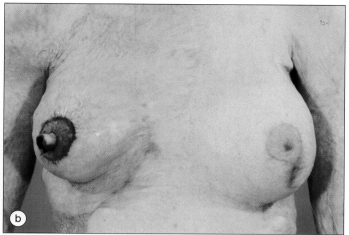

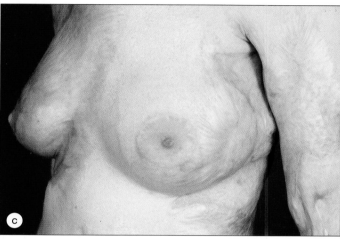

Figures 57.6 (a) A 17-year-old female with right-sided breast burns with a slightly smaller right breast noted. Skin grafts were used in the past to assist right-sided breast development. (b) Left pericresant mastopexy performed to lift the nipple-areolar complex with right-sided augmentation. The right nipple-areolar complex reconstructed with a skate flap and inner thigh full-thickness skin graft. (c) Two-year follow-up. Note projection still of the skate flap. (Reprinted with permission from: McCauley et al. Functional and Aesthetic Reconstruction of the Burn Patient, New York. Taylor and Francis 2005; 379–392.[22])

skin grafts. Contour problems which are associated with developing breasts may be corrected with the use of skin grafts and/or fasciocutaneous flaps. Improved symmetry of the breast is of significant importance for patients who have unilateral burns of the breast. Reconstructive techniques, including mastopexy and reduction mammaplasty, may be required in order to obtain symmetry. In patients requiring fascial excision of full-thickness burns over the anterior chest wall, tissue expansion and subsequent placement of submuscular saline implants have been quite successful for breast reconstruction.

References

1. Burvin R, Robinpour M, Milo Y, et al. Female breast burns: conservative treatment with a reconstructive aim. Isr J Med Sci 1996; 32(12):1297–1301.
1a. Watson EJ, Johnson AM. The emotional significance of acquired physical disfiguration in children. Am J Orthopsychiatry 1958; 28:85–97.
2. Brou JA, Robson MC, McCauley RL, et al. Inventory of potential reconstructive needs in the patient with burns. J Burn Care Rehabil 1989; 10(6):555–560.
3. Burns BF, McCauley RL, Murphy FL, et al. Reconstructive management of patients with greater than 80 per cent TBSA burns. Burns 1993; 19(5):429–433.
4. McCauley RL, Beraja V, Rutan RL, et al. Longitudinal assessment of breast development in adolescent female patients with burns involving the nipple-areolar complex. Plast Reconstr Surg 1989; 83(4):676–680.
5. Burke JF, Bandoc CC, Quinby WC. Primary excision and immediate grafting. A method for shortening illness. J Trauma 1974; 14:389–395.
6. Herndon DN, Parks DH. Comparison of serial debridement and autografting and early massive excision with cadaveric skin overlay in the treatment of large burns in children. J Trauma 1986; 26:149–152.
7. Herndon DN, Gore DC, Cole M, et al. Determinants of mortality in pediatric patients with greater than 70% full thickness total body surface area thermal injury treated by early total excision and grafting. J Trauma 1987; 27:208–212.
8. Herndon DN, Barrow RC, Rutan RL, et al. A comparison of conservative versus early excisional therapies in severely burned patients. Ann Surg 1989; 209:547–553.
9. Desai MH, Herndon DN, Broemeling L, et al. Early burn wound excision significantly reduces blood loss. Ann Surg 1990; 211:753–762.
10. MacLennon SE, Wells MD, Neale HW. Reconstruction of the burned breast. Clin Plast Surg 2000; 27(1):113–119.
11. Kunert P, Schneider W, Flory J. Principles and procedures in female breast reconstruction in the young child's burn injury. Aesth Plast Surg 1988; 12:101–106.

12. Guan W, Jin Y, Cao H. Reconstruction of post-burn female breast deformity. Ann Plast Surg 1988; 21(1):65–69.

13. Pakhomov SM, Dmitriev GI. Scar deformities of the mammary glands – surgical treatment. Acta Chir Plast 1984; 26(3):150–157.

14. Versaci AD, Balkovich ME, Goldstein SA. Breast reconstruction by tissue expansion for congenital and burn deformities. Ann Plast Surg 1986; 16(1):20–30.

15. Kalender V, Aydim H, Karabulut AB, et al. Breast reconstruction with the internal mammary artery pedicle fasciocutaneous island flap: description of a new flap. Plast Reconstr Surg 2000; 106(7):1494–1498.

16. McCauley R. Reconstruction of the trunk and genitalia. In: Herndon DN, ed. Total burn care. Philadelphia: Elsevier; 2001:707–709.

17. Ozgur F, Gokalan I, Mavili E, et al. Reconstruction of post-burn breast deformities. Burns 1992; 18(6):504–509.

18. Psillakis JM, Woisky R. Burned breasts: treatment with a transverse rectus abdominis island musculocutaneous flap. Ann Plast Surg 1985; 14(5):437–442.

19. Slator RC, Phil D, Wilson GR, et al. Post-burn breast reconstruction: tissue expansion prior to contracture release. Plast Reconstr Surg 1992; 90(4):668–674.

20. Bishop JB, Fisher J, Bostwick J, III. The burned female breast. Ann Plast Surg 1980 4(1):25–30.

21. Spence RJ. Bilateral reconstruction of the male nipple. Ann Plast Surg 1992; 28:288–291.

22. McCauley RL, Bowen K, Killyon GW. Reconstruction of the burned breast and nipple-areolar complex. In: McCauley RL, ed. Functional and aesthetic reconstruction of the burn patient. New York: Taylor & Francis; 2005:379–392.

23. Lewis JR. Reconstruction of the breasts. Surg Clin N Am 1971; 51:429–440.

24. Becker H. Breast reconstruction using an inflatable breast implant with detectable reservoir. Plast Reconstr Surg 1984; 73:678–683.

25. Loss M, Infanger M, Kunzi W, Meyer VE. The burned female breast: a report on four cases. Burns 2002; 28:601–605.

26. Payne CE, Malata CM. Correction of post-burn deformity using the Lejour mammoplasty technique. Plast Reconstr Surg 2003; 111:805–809.

27. Corso PF. Plastic surgery for the unilateral hypoplastic breast. Plast Reconstr Surg 1972; 50:134–141.

28. Thai KN, Mertens D, Warden G, Neale HW. Reduction mammaplasty in postburn breasts. Plast Reconstr Surg 1999; 103(7):1882–1886.

29. Mudge B, McCauley RL. Correction of asymmetry in the unilaterally burned breast. Proc Am Burns Assoc. 2000 Vol 21(1 Part 2): S177

30. Mohmand H, Nassan A. Double U-plasty for correction of geometric malposition of the nipple-areola complex. Plast Reconstr Surg 2002; 109(6):2019–2022.

31. Pensler JM, Haab RL, Perry SW. Reconstruction of the burned nipple-areola complex. Plast Reconstr Surg 1986; 78(4):480–485.

32. Adams WM. Labial transplant for correction of loss of the nipple. Plast Reconstr Surg 1979; 4:295–298.

33. Broadbent PR, Wool RH, Metz PS. Restoring the mammary areola by a skin graft from the upper inner thigh. Br J Plast Surg 1977; 30:220–222.

34. Becker H. Nipple-areola tattooing using intradermal tattooing. Plast Reconstr Surg 1988; 81:450.

35. Brent B, Bostwick J. Nipple-areolar reconstruction with auricular tissues. Plast Reconstr Surg 1977; 60:353–361.

36. Little JW. Nipple-areolar reconstruction. Clin Plast Surg 1984; 11:351–364.

37. McCauley RL, Robson MC. Reconstruction of the nipple-areola complex in the burned breast using the 'skate' flap. Proc Am Burn Assoc 1994; 26:14.

38. Kneafsey B, Brawford DS, Jhoo C TK, et al. Correction of developmental breast abnormalities with a permanent expander/implant. Br J Plast Surg 1996; 49:302–306.

39. Becker H. The permanent tissue expander. Clin Plast Surg 1987; 14:519–527.

Chapter 58

Management of burn injuries of the perineum

Ted Huang

Burns of the perineal area are quite uncommon even though the lower trunk and the lower extremities are vulnerable to burn injury. According to Alghanem and Herndon et al., the incidence of perineal burns was about 12 per 1000 admissions.[1] The incidence was reassessed recently by reviewing the records of 5651 patients admitted to the Shriners Burns Hospital between 1976 and 1998. There were only 91 patients identified to have burn injuries of the perineal area. While overall incidence of perineal burns has remained unchanged, boys were found to sustain the injury four times more often than girls in this group of patients. Among 44 boys with genital burns, there were 35 penile burns and 9 with scrotal injuries. In contrast, there were only four patients who had burns of the labial structures. Burns of the vaginal vault were not encountered in this group of patients.

Management of burns of the perineum during acute phase of injury

A conservative approach is used to manage perineal burns:[1,2] i.e. the perineal area is cleansed daily and the wound is covered with antibiotic dressings. The urethral tract is stented with an indwelling Foley catheter which also decompresses the urinary bladder. The perineal area is neither splinted nor braced. The thighs are maintained at 15° of abduction using a wedge splint to minimize contracture of the hip joint. The burn is given time to demarcate and the wound is often left to heal spontaneously. A non-healing wound is managed with the use of a partial-thickness or a full-thickness skin graft. On rare occasions, a skin flap may be mobilized from the area adjacent to reconstruct defects consequential to full-thickness skin loss of the penis and the scrotum.

Other possible problems seen in the acute phase include necrosis of the penile shaft, testicular necrosis, urethral stricture, and rectal prolapse. Although the Shriners Burns Hospital and the University of Texas Medical Branch Hospitals in Galveston, Texas, have adopted a relatively conservative

regimen to the management of perineal burns, wound care approach, in practice, is quite variable and the exact regimen is often modified depending upon the structures involved.

Burns of the penis

Burn injuries limited to the penis, though possible, are quite rare (Figure 58.1). Concomitant involvement of the penis with burn injuries of the lower trunk and the perineal area, on the other hand, is quite common. The initial regimen of patient management, in addition to resuscitative measures, consists of wound care and urethral stenting. An indwelling Foley catheter of appropriate size is inserted into the urinary bladder to stent the urethral tract and at the same time to monitor the urinary output. The catheter is removed once the swelling around the penile shaft subsides and the wound becomes delineated. No attempt is made to debride the wound at this stage. Instead, it is allowed to demarcate and is often allowed to heal spontaneously.

Loss of skin over the penile shaft and the scrotum

Spontaneous healing is expected in most instances with burn injuries of the penis and scrotum since full-thickness injury of the penile and scrotal skin is relatively uncommon. Skin grafting, a partial thickness or a full thickness, could be used to cover the wound if healing is delayed (Figure 58.2).

In rare instances, a skin flap may be needed to reconstruct structures such as the urethral tract and/or scrotal sac because of the loss of skin coverage. An inguinopudendal skin flap mobilized from the inguinal crease area may be used if a skin graft is judged not to be feasible.[3] The use of muscle-skin flaps, such as a gracilis MC flap, is not recommended because such flaps have a high tissue temperature which may interfere with spermatogenesis.

Burn wound of labia majora

Isolated burns of the labial structures are rare. In fact, labial burns are often associated with injuries of the surrounding areas such as the abdomen and inguinal folds. As in the management of male genitalia burns, the injured areas are allowed to heal spontaneously (Figure 58.3). Distortion of the labial structures, mostly due to contraction of the scar tissues in the pubic and inguinal areas, is left for later reconstruction.

Perineal wound coverage

An isolated burn injury of the perineal area is extremely rare. On the other hand, the area will become involved if the lower

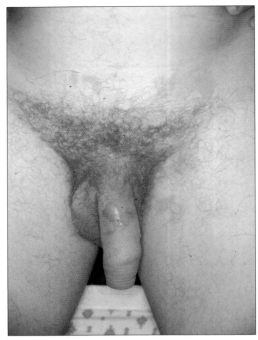

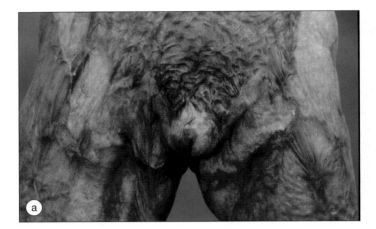

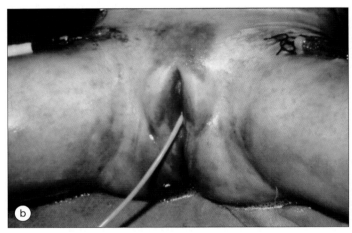

Fig. 58.1 An isolated burn injury of the penis is relatively uncommon. This 27-year-old man sustained scalding burns of the penis from an accidental spillage of hot coffee onto the lap.

Fig. 58.3 (a) Burn injuries involving the lower trunk, thighs, and labia. While the lower abdomen and the thighs required skin grafting, the labial injury was left to heal spontaneously. (b) The appearance of genitalia 5 years after the injury.

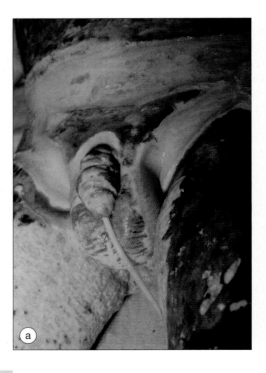

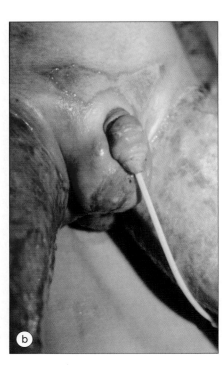

Fig. 58.2 (a) Burns of the penis are more commonly associated with injuries of the lower trunk/lower extremities. (b) Although skin grafting was needed for wound closure around the perineum, the major bulk of the penile wounds healed spontaneously.

trunk/buttock is injured. The extent of scar contracture varies depending upon the depth of burn. While it may heal spontaneously with minimal scarring, contracture of the perineal area is a common sequela, regardless of methods used to care for the wound (Figure 58.4). The natural inclination to keep the thighs together and hips adducted during the recovery phase of acute burn injuries seems to aggravate scar contraction.

Anal burns

Burns of the anus are rare, although the anus could become involved in extensive burns of the perineum. If the skin injury around the anal opening is full thickness, the use of a skin flap may be necessary to minimize the consequential of stricture. A piece of skin flap mobilized from the adjacent area will be necessary in grafting the perianal area. Wound coverage with a skin graft is not only technically difficult but also leads to anal stricture when the graft contracts.

Rectal prolapse

Rectal prolapse occurs occasionally in young children with extensive burn injuries with or without perineal involvement. The exact reasons for rectal prolapse occurring in these burned infants remain unclear. However, rectal prolapse may be due to:

* redundant rectal mucosa,
* the structural relationship of the rectum to other pelvic organs, such as sacrum and coccyx, urinary bladder and uterus,
* the lack of muscular support provided by the pelvic musculatures, and
* the anatomical features uniquely special to infants of 1–3 years of age.

A sudden increase in intra-abdominal pressure and malnutrition due to burn injuries could conceivably aggravate the magnitude of the descent of the rectal mucosa through the anal opening.[4]

Clinically, in addition to eversion of rectal mucosa, edematous swelling around the buttocks and perianal area is quite commonly found, even when these areas are burn free. The onset can be quite sudden without any obvious precipitating event. However, it has been observed that an infant's grunting or performance of the Valsalva maneuver can precipitate an eversion of the rectal canal through the anal opening.

The treatment regimen consists of rectal padding and daily cleansing of the perineal and perianal area. Stool softener is added to the dietary regimen to facilitate bowel movement. Spontaneous regression of the prolapse is likely as nutrition improves and tissue swelling subsides (Figure 58.5). Surgical intervention, though in most instances unnecessary, is indicated if the prolapse is not readily reducible due to anal sphincteric dysfunction and/or intussusception.[4,5]

Reconstruction of established deformities of the perineum and the perineal structures

Cicatricial contracture around the perineum is the most common sequela of perineal burns.[1,6] In our group of 91 patients, over one-half of them suffered contractural deformity in the perineal area. The magnitude of contracture, furthermore, was exaggerated with the contraction of burn scars in the inguinal crease and inferomedial gluteal folds. Other problems, though relatively uncommon, included complete loss of the penis, anal stenosis, and intractable rectal prolapse.

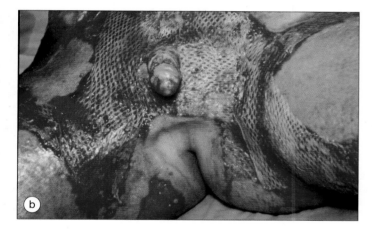
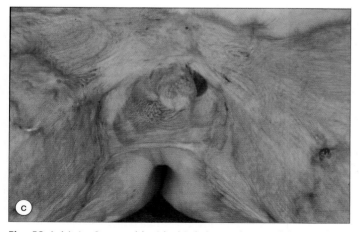

Fig. 58.4 (a) An 8-year-old with third-degree burns of the trunk and the lower extremities, including the penis and the scrotum. (b) The wound, including the scrotum, was debrided and grafted with a meshed partial-thickness skin graft. (c) The ensuing changes in the genitoperineal area were characterized by scar hypertrophy and contracture. Tight scars formed across the perineum and interfered with thigh movement.

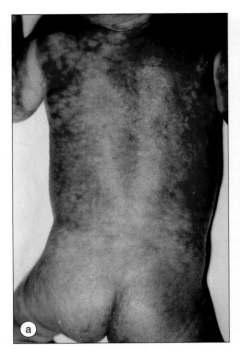

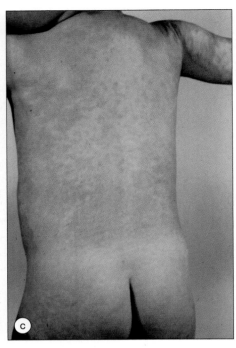

Fig. 58.5 (a) A 2-year-old girl with 65–70% total body surface burns. (b) Prolapse of the rectum appeared 12 days after the accident. The problem was managed non-surgically. (c) The prolapse receded spontaneously 2 months later as she recovered from the burn injury.

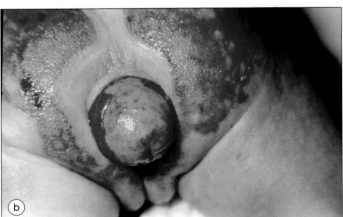

There are numerous methods (z-plasty technique, interpositional skin flap technique, incisional release of scarred tissues closed with local skin flap, skin graft) available to reconstruct the deformities. In practice, the technique used to reconstruct perineal and genital deformities varies depending upon the magnitude of scarring, scarred deformity around the perineum, and the extent of functional impediment encountered.

Reconstruction of penile deformity

The task of assessing the exact extent of penile deformities can be difficult. Distortion of the penile configuration attributable to scar contracture could be due to loss of skin or a combination of skin and Buck's fascia loss. In addition, the scarring in the pubic area and/or the inguinal fold could further exaggerate the extent of penile deformity.

Engorging the penile shaft is necessary to assess precisely the extent of penile deformity, as the gross appearance of a flaccid penis can be misleading. That is, it is necessary to make the penile shaft engorged; i.e. creating an artificial penile erec-

tion, in order to determine the extent and the location of scar involvement. Artificial penile erection is created under anesthesia by placing a tourniquet (a piece of 1/4 inch Penrose drain) at the base of the penile shaft. A sufficient amount of physiological saline solution is injected into the corpus cavernosum to induce congestion. The shaft deformity, attributable to the skin loss and/or fascial loss, is delineated once the corpus becomes engorged.

When Buck's fascia is spared injury, the skin defect, resulting from incisional release of the scar, is covered with a full-thickness skin graft. Rarely, when Buck's fascia is involved, surgical release of the facial deformity is necessary. A dermal graft harvested from the lower abdomen may be used to reconstruct the fascial defect and a skin flap (mobilized from the area along the groin crease, as an island skin pedicle flap) used to cover the skin defect.

A complete loss of the penis, although devastating, is extremely rare (Figure 58.6). Reconstruction of the penis is delayed until puberty. The delay is often necessary due to the

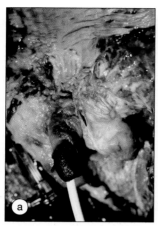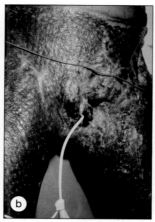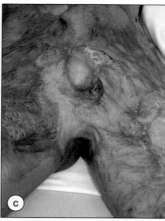

Fig. 58.6 (a) A full-thickness burn of the penis, though uncommon, can occur and the outcome is devastating, as seen in this 10-year-old boy. No attempt was made to remove the penile tissue even though it appeared grossly necrotic. Instead, the wound was allowed to demarcate itself. An indwelling Foley catheter was used to stent the urethra. (b) The patient had lost the phallus entirely. (c) The patient was able to urinate through a short remnant of the penis. Reconstruction of the penile shaft is being planned.

limited amount of soft tissue that can be harvested for genital reconstruction soon after the accident.

There are several methods currently available to reconstruct a neo-phallus. A segment of rectus abdominis MC flap, for instance, may be mobilized from the lower abdomen to form a neo-phallus. In recent years, a forearm osteocutaneous flap transferred to the pubic area via microsurgical technique has been found to be useful in reconstructing a phallus. At the time of phallus reconstruction a urethral tract can be reconstructed either using a piece of full-thickness skin graft or a forearm osteocutaneous flap (utilizing a tube-within-a-tube technique)[7] (Figure 58.7).

Reconstruction of scrotal deformities

Full-thickness burn injuries of the scrotum result in scar encasement of testicular structures. Reconstruction, therefore, requires surgical release of the scarred areas. A thin skin flap, such as the inguinopudendal flap or a flap mobilized from the adjacent area, however, is needed to cover the resultant defect. A musculocutaneous flap, such as a gracilis MC flap, is not suitable for scrotal reconstruction because of the thickness of the flap and the possible impediment of spermatogenesis (due to the high tissue temperature of the flap). Even though contractural deformity is likely to recur, a skin graft may be used to cover the defect.

Reconstruction of labial deformity

An isolated contour deformity of the labia majora is relatively uncommon. On the other hand, scar contracture occurring in the suprapubic and pubic area, as well as the inguinal fold, could distort the normal configuration of the labia. Therefore, surgical release of the contracted scar tissues is essential to determine the extent of labial deformity. Then the method of reconstructing the deformed labia can be chosen.

To restore a contour deformity caused by skin and subcutaneous tissue loss, a skin flap may have to be mobilized from the adjacent area and to reconstruct a contour deformity due to parenchymal tissue loss, injection of free fat cells (lipoinjec-

tion) could be useful. To inject free fat cells to augment the labial contour, the cells are aspirated from the lower abdomen using the inner cannula of #14 Intracath® needle attached to a 3cc syringe. The syringe is moved in a 'back-and-forth' piston-like manner. The fat cells are injected into the labia using the same syringe but connected with a 19 gauge blunt needle.

Reconstruction of band deformity around the perineum

Scarring and scar contracture of the perineum is a common sequela of perineal burns, especially if allowed to heal spontaneously. Although seldom causing difficulty at a young age, the scars around the perineum could eventually interfere with sitting because of tightness or contraction developed around the buttock. In addition, the patient may encounters difficulty with bowel movement because of gluteal contracture and cicatricial changes involving the anal opening.

The deformity in the perineal area usually results from a tight band in the suprapubic area, or between the ischial tuberosities. Inelastic scars cause inadequate spreading of the buttock and are responsible for the discomfort experienced on sitting (Figure 58.8).

Although a contracted perineal band may be incised to gain release, the task of closing the resultant wound with a skin graft can be difficult as recurrence of contracture is a common sequela. Therefore, a multiple z-plasty technique is the preferred method of reconstruction in such cases.

The technique of multiple z-plasty

The patient is placed in the lithotomy position. Tightness and scar band can be delineated with abduction of the hip joint (Figure 58.9a). A line is drawn in the scar band along the horizontal direction of the band. The length of the horizontal line may extend from one side of the scarred area to the other. A triangular flap with its apex at the end of horizontal line is marked. The angle may vary between 30° and 60° depending upon the uninjured tissues available at both ends of the

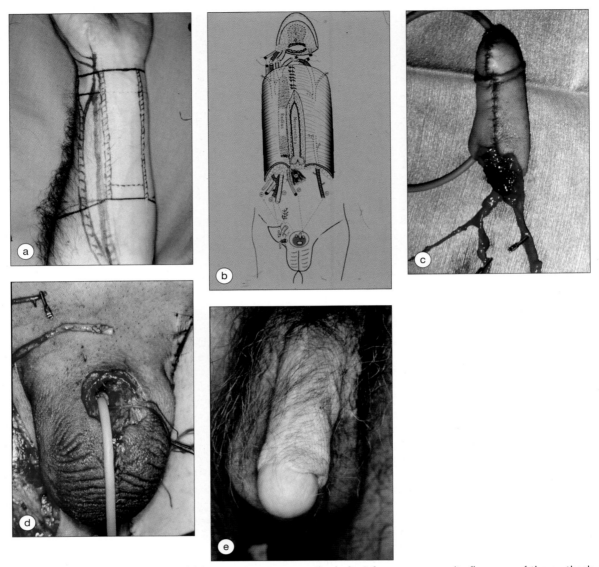

Fig. 58.7 (a) There are various techniques available to reconstruct a penile shaft. A forearm composite flap, one of the methods currently in use, was chosen to reconstruct a phallus structure for a 51-year-old man who had lost his penis because of cancer. (Courtesy of Dr Kenji Sasaki. Reprinted with permission from: Sasaki et al.[7]) (b) As shown in a schematic drawing, a section of the skin with radial artery attached is harvested from the volar surface of the forearm and utilized for penile reconstruction. A tube-inside-the-tube was used to reconstruct the urethral tract. In addition, the pulp from the big toe was used to reconstruct the glans penis. (Courtesy of Dr Kenji Sasaki. Reprinted with permission from Sasaki et al.[7]) (c) The tissues assembled with vessels and nerve structures set for 'hook up.' (d) The appearance of genitalia before reconstruction. (e) A reconstructed penis in a 50-year-old man who had lost the penis because of cancer. (Courtesy of Dr. Kenji Sasaki. Reprinted with permission from: Sasaki et al.[7])

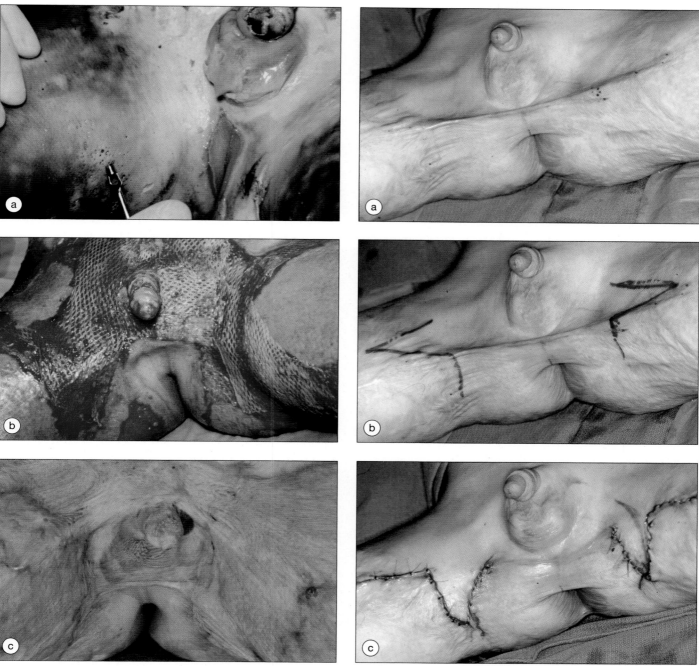

Fig. 58.8 (a) This 11-year-old boy sustained burns in the lower trunk, thigh areas, lateral scrotal skin, and the proximal penile shaft. (b) Debridement and grafting of the burned wound resulted in tight scar bands across the suprapubic and inter-ischial areas. (c) Tight bands developed in the perineal area.

Fig. 58.9 (a) A tight scar band in the perineal area consequential to burn injuries involving the perineum and the lower extremities. (b) Releasing incisions were placed in the areas away from the anal opening to avoid injuring the anal sphincter. A triangular flap was designed in the uninjured area at each end of the scar band. A releasing incision was set perpendicularly to the direction of the scar band. (c) Each triangular flap was rotated 90° to close the open wound resulting from incisional release.

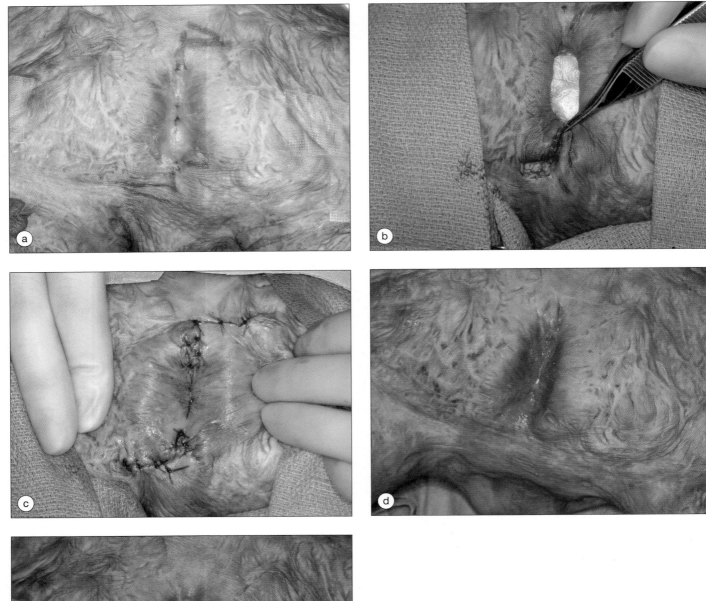

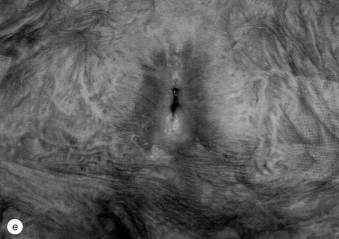

Fig. 58.10 (a) This 4-year-old boy developed, in addition to a tight scar band across the perineum, anal incontinence because of cicatricial changes that involved the entire perineal area. (b) A modified multiple z-plasty technique was utilized to reconstruct the perineal contracture and anal stenosis. (c) Skin flaps were rotated into the areas to reconstruct the deformity following the surgical release. (d) The appearance of the anal area before release. (e) The appearance of the anal area 9 months following release.

horizontal line. The length of the limb of each triangle will be the same as the incision made perpendicular to the horizontal line to release the tight band (Figure 58.9b). Two z-plasties – i.e. two triangular flaps with 30–60° and 90° angles, respectively – are formed as the flaps are raised along the skin markings made. Release of a contracted scar band is achieved by rotating these two flaps at each end (Figure 58.9c).

Although the extent of perineal release may be limited because of scarred tissues surrounding the triangular flaps fashioned, the z-plasty technique is useful in changing the pulling direction of scar tissue, thus diminishing tightness around the perineum.

Reconstruction of anal stricture

While burn injuries rarely involve the entire anorectal canal, it is not unusual that they involve the perianal skin and the external sphincter ani muscle. Stricture of the anal opening due to scar contracture and the cicatricial involvement of the

external sphincter ani muscle are common sequelae. Cicatricial changes around the anal opening can and will interfere with bowel movement.

Treatment requires surgical release of constricted scar bands around the anal opening. An interpositional skin flap fashioned as an island flap, or a modified z-plasty with skin flaps mobilized from the adjacent area, is used to make up the tissue defect (Figure 58.10). The method of using a piece of skin graft to reconstruct the defect is not useful. Application of the graft is difficult and recurrence of stricture is common because of scar contracture.

Reconstruction of rectal prolapse

Although the problem, in most instances, is self-limiting and the prolapse will recede spontaneously as the nutritional status of the patient improves and the burned perineum heals, surgical intervention will be necessary if the rectal prolapse becomes intractable[4,5] (Figure 58.11).

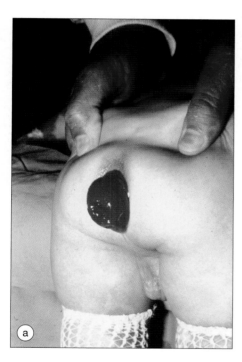
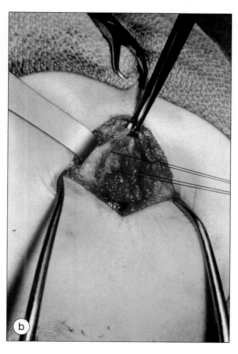
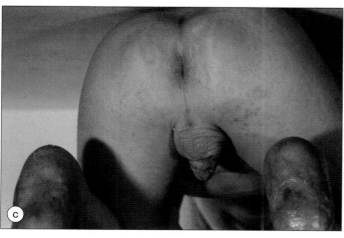

Fig. 58.11 (a) This 2-year-old boy sustained a third-degree scalding burn that mostly involved the lower extremities. He developed rectal prolapse 10 days after the accident. (b) He underwent a rectopexy procedure because of persistent eversion of the rectal mucosa. (c) The patient regained anal continence 6 months after the surgery.

Summary

Burn injury of the perineum is relatively uncommon. The regimen of treatment during the acute phase of recovery is conservative. The urethral tract is stented with an indwelling Foley catheter and the wound is cleaned daily. Neither a splint nor a brace is used to immobilize the perineal area. The wound is usually left to heal spontaneously. With the rare exception when there is total loss of the penis, the resultant deformity is limited. Disfigurement of the scrota/labial contour and/or scar bands around the genitalia is the common complaint presented by such patients.

As they interfere with sitting and/or bowel movement, reconstructing scarred deformities is centered upon the release of tight scar bands around the perineal structures. Incisional release and reconstruction utilizing a z-plasty technique or an interpositional skin flap technique is effective in correcting the deformities.

References

1. Alghanem AA, McCauley RL, Robson RC, et al. Management of pediatric perineal and genital burns: twenty-year review. J Burn Care Rehabil 1990, 11:308–311.
2. Rutan RL. Management of perineal and genital burns. JET Nurs 1993, 20:169–176.
3. Huang T. Twenty years of experience in managing gender dysphoric patients: I. Surgical management of male transsexuals. Plast Reconstr Surg 1995, 96:921–930.
4. Stafford PW. Other disorders of the anus and rectum, anorectal function. In: O'Neill JA, Rowe MI, Grosfield JL, et al., eds. Pediatric surgery, 5th edn. St. Louis: Mosby; 1998:Ch 96,1453.
5. Aschcraft KW, Garred JL, Holder TM, et al. Rectal prolapse: 17-year experience with the posterior repair and suspension. J Pediatr Surg 1990; 25(9):992–995.
6. Pisarski GP, Greenhalgh DG, Warden GD. The management of perineal contractures in children with burns. J Burn Care Rehabil 1994, 15:256–259.
7. Sasaki K, Nozaki M, Morioka K, et al. Penile reconstruction: combined use of an innervated forearm osteocutaneous flap and big toe pulp. Plast Reconstr Surg 1998, 104:1054–1058.

Reconstruction of burn deformities of the foot and ankle

Ted Huang

Although the exact number of incidents is unknown, the lower section of the lower limb, that is foot and ankle, is frequently burned, especially in individuals who suffer extensive burn injuries. The management of foot burns is similar to the regimen used for other bodily sites — the principle of debridement and wound coverage is followed. The technique of tangential excision of the burned wound with skin grafting, though a preferred surgical modality for burn management, may not be effective because of the difference in integumental make-up of the foot and ankle area. The thinness of the skin overlying the dorsum of the foot and ankle area renders the area more vulnerable to injury while full-thickness burns of the sole of the foot are less likely.

Skin grafting is the most common technique used to cover burn wounds. It is also used to release joint contraction. Despite the troublesome consequences of a deformed foot contour and stiffness of the toe and ankle joints affecting the gait cycle and ambulatory movements, the functional disturbance attributable to a burned foot, in practice, is surprisingly limited.

Consequences of foot and ankle burns

Deformities of the foot and ankle depend on the extent of the initial burn: for example, the scarring and contractural deformities of the toes and the ankle joint are minimal if the burn depth is superficial. The contractural problems, more commonly seen in individuals with extensive burns, have been traditionally managed with the skin grafting technique and splinting and physiotherapy are essential components of the therapeutic reconstruction regimen of burn foot deformities.

Reconstruction of the foot and ankle deformities

General principles

Releasing contracted joint structures to restore the usefulness of the foot is the fundamental approach to reconstruction. The resultant tissue defect, consequential to scar release, can be covered with skin grafts and/or skin flaps. A Kirschner wire (0.025–0.035 inch) is usually needed to immobilize the joint structures for alignment. The position of the released joint is maintained for a period of 10–14 days. Then the wires are removed and external appliances or shoes are used to maintain the foot position. The techniques of skin grafting and/or skin flap wound coverage, on the other hand, are not infrequently plagued with problems of graft and flap loss because of tissue congestion and altered vascular supplies to the harvested flap.

Scar deformities involving the dorsum of the foot and the ankle
Hypertrophic scar deformities

Formation of a hypertrophic scar over the dorsal surface of the foot and/or ankle is probably the most common problem encountered with burn injuries that are confined to the dorsum of the foot. Contractural deformities of the foot and/or ankle are uncommon because the intrinsic skeletal rigidity of the tarsal and metatarsal bones oppose the pulling force of the scar. Although total or partial surgical removal of symptomatic and unsightly scars may be considered, a non-surgical regimen that would provide proper joint splinting and scar compression by using a high-top shoe, for example, would probably provide the same, if not a better outcome.

Contractural deformities involving the toes

An extension deformity of the toes at the metatarsophalangeal (MTP) joint level, with or without associated dorsiflexion contracture of the ankle, is common if the burns involve the dorsum of the foot and the ankle. This deformity is largely due to scarring and scar contracture following the destruction of the skin over the dorsum of the foot.

Reconstruction of dorsally contracted toes

The contracted toes are released by incising the scar at the level of the MTP joint and/or proximal interphalangeal (PIP) joint. Releasing the scar tissues at the webspace is delayed to minimize the morbidities associated with delayed wound healing.

In children, and in instances where the onset of toe extension contracture is recent, surgical manipulation of the volar plate of the MTP joint capsule is unnecessary. A Kirschner wire (0.020–0.035 inch) is inserted through the proximal phalanx to keep the digit in full extension while maintaining the MTPJ in 45°–60° plantar flexion. The wires are removed 10–14 days later, once the take of skin graft or flap is established (Figure 59.1).

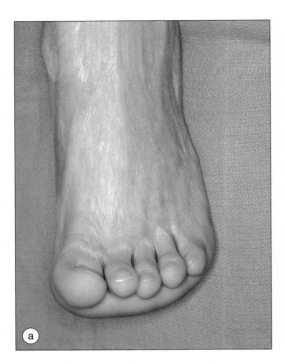

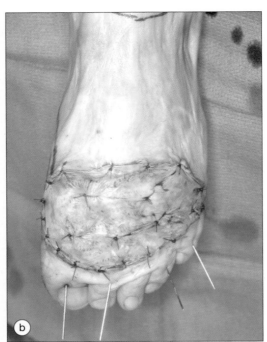

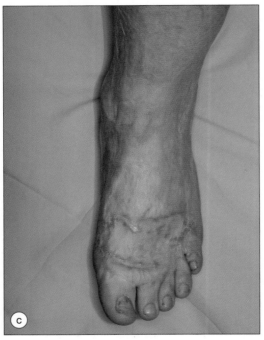

Fig. 59.1 (a) A dorsiflexion deformity of the toes caused by burns involved the dorsum of the left foot. (b) The defect, consequential to a releasing incision made across the level of metatarsophalangeal (MTP) joints, measured 10 cm × 6–7 cm. The MTP joints were flexed and were maintained for 10 days. A piece of split-thickness skin graft of $^{14}/1000$ inch in thickness was used to cover the wound. (c) The appearance of the grafted wound 10 months following the procedure.

While it is seldom indicated in children, volar capsuloplasty, involving the volar plate of the MTP joint, may be necessary in adults or in instances where a joint has been subluxed for a long time. Merely releasing and skin graft/flap covering of the wound over the joint structures may not be enough to restore the joint alignment.

In order to minimize recurrent contracture of the toe joints, commonly associated with the use of skin grafting technique, a skin flap mobilized from the area adjacent may be used, particularly in instances where the joint structure is exposed. A $^3/4$ paratenocutaneous z-plasty technique achieves coverage of both the joint structures and the wound defect (Figure 59.2).

Contractural deformities of the anterior ankle

Tightness of the ankle joint in foot dorsiflexion is the usual deformity encountered in instances where the burn injury is limited to the anterior surface of the ankle. As in other deformities noted, improper splinting of the foot and the ankle joint, plus scar contracture, are the probable culprits. Although the deformity could be amended with proper foot/ankle splinting,

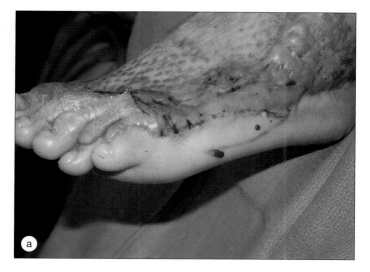

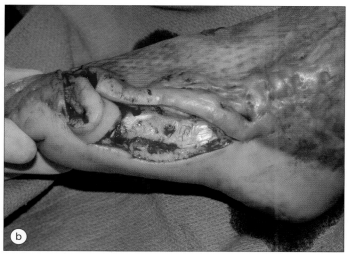

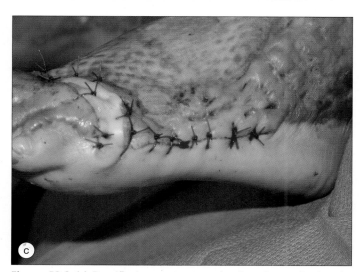

Figure 59.2 (a) Dorsiflexion contracture developed over the fourth and fifth MTP joint level. An incision was made to achieve needed release. (b) A triangular skin flap with an inner angle of 25°–30° was fabricated from the lateral aspect of the foot. (c) The fascial layer of the abductor digiti V was included in the flap formation. The flap was rotated medially and caudally to cover the defect resulting from release.

surgical intervention may be necessary. Of course, correction of an extremely deformed ankle joint may require, in addition to releasing of contracted scar tissues, reconstruction of deformed periarticular structures. Capsuloplasty and re-routing of the tendons around the ankle joint are oftentimes necessary.

Reconstruction of dorsiflexion contracture of the ankle

Although the skin graft is most commonly used to cover wounds around the ankle, the problem of wound contracture is ever present. It is, furthermore, not a useful means of repairing a wound with an exposed joint and tendons, commonly associated with joint realignment procedures requiring elaborate joint structure reconstruction. However, there are two approaches that are useful for scar release and wound coverage:

- A z-plasty technique is used to release a contractile scar across the ankle joint. However, the conventional approach in which triangular skin flaps are elevated tends to cause vascular supply impairment to the flap, thus causing flap necrosis. Instead, the technique of fabricating a composite skin flap, namely a paratenocutaneous flap, may be used to minimize this undesirable consequence (Figure 59.3).
- The technique of 3/4 paratenocutaneous (PC) z-plasty, a variant of the PC z-plasty technique, is useful for instances where scarring is more extensive and uninjured skin available for flap fabrication is scarce. A right-angled triangular skin flap is marked with its cathetus perpendicular to the line of scar release. The paratenon is included in the fabrication of the flap, identical to fabricating a PC flap in a z-plasty technique. The flap is rotated 90° to fill the defect resulting from release (Figure 59.4).

Scar deformities involving the sole of the foot

Deep burns, though uncommon, could involve the plantar surface of the foot and the toes. In such instances, plantar flexion of the toes at all joint levels (claw toe deformities) is the most common problem encountered, especially when burns do not involve the dorsal surface of the toes. Plantar flexion of the toes, compounded by contraction of the scar formed in the area, is the most likely cause of this deformity.

Reconstruction of the plantar flexion deformities of the toe

Surgical release of the contracted scar at the level of maximal contraction is usually unnecessary unless the magnitude of contraction is severe enough to render wearing a shoe difficult and/or ambulation is arduous. (A non-surgical regimen of toe-splinting in these cases is not effective.)

The use of a composite skin flap mobilized from the dorsum of the foot, if it is uninvolved, may be feasible. Skin grafting technique, however, is the best modality for reconstruction. Splinting of the foot and toes immediately following surgery is an essential component of the post-surgical care plan as recurrence of the contracture is very likely without this.

Reconstruction of deformities involving the plantar surface of the foot

The problems are mostly related to the breakdown of the graft caused by pressure and shearing when walking. Although a local composite skin flap, if a flap fabrication is possible, could be used to reconstruct a small defect, breakdown of the skin with ulcer formation is inevitable unless the flap is sensate. Restoration of skin sensation to the pressure points is, in this sense, a prerequisite for successful patient rehabilitation regardless of the techniques used.

Reconstruction of specific ankle deformities

Extensive burns of the foot and ankle area, although partially dependant of the magnitude of the burns and scar contracture, could lead to a talipes-like deformity of the foot (talipes equines, varus and valgus). To restore the joint normality, reconstructive procedures will involve not only the release of the capsular structure around the ankle joint but also the lengthening of the tendon of Achilles (for an equines deformity, for example). In practice, the extent of ankle restoration may be limited because of the difficulty in closing an open wound that has resulted from the release of the soft tissues. Use of a skin flap in conjunction with a skin graft may be considered to cover a wound with exposed tendinous and capsular elements.

Reconstructing a talipes equines-like deformity

Plantar flexion deformity is most commonly caused by an injury involving the heel. While scar contraction could be the main factor responsible for the deformity, tendo-Achilles shortening (an undesirable consequences of inadequate splinting of the ankle) can further aggravate the deformity. Surgical restoration of ankle mobility will require lengthening of the Achilles tendon. Successful closure of the resulting heel wound with exposed tendon structures necessitates measures such as fasciocutaneous (FC) z-plasty or 3/4 FC z-plasty techniques (Figures 59.3 and 59.4).

Reconstructing a talipes vera and valgus-like deformity

Although delineation of the exact extent of tissue destruction and scarring causing the joint deformity may be difficult, by releasing the wound, tendon and joint structures are exposed. Inclusion of a surgical plan for wound coverage, in this sense, is essential to minimize the morbidities. A transpositional FC flap technique, alias 3/4 FC z-plasty, is useful. The technical details of the FC z-plasty and the 3/4 FC z-plasty technique are described as follows:

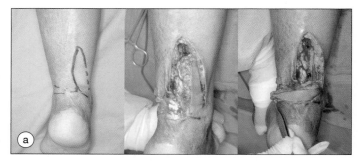

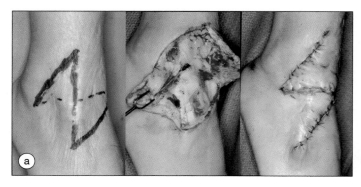

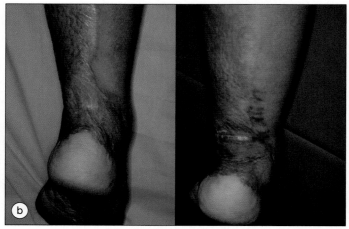

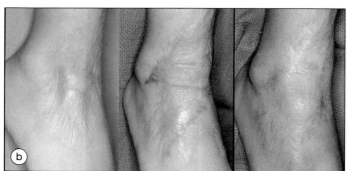

Fig. 59.3 (a) (Left) Two equilateral triangular flaps are marked over the tight anterior surface of the right ankle. (Center) Two flaps that included the paratenon underneath were fabricated. (Right) Two paratenocutaneous (PC) flaps were interposed to achieve the needed release. (b) (Left) The scar located over the anterior surface of the right ankle as noted in (a), indicated joint contracture. (Center) The appearance of right ankle 3 months following the releasing procedure. (Right) The ankle remained free of contraction 2 years after the operation.

Fig. 59.4 (a) (Left) A varus deformity developed in the right ankle due to scar contracture and a tight heel cord. A right-angled triangular skin marking was made in the posterior ankle area in preparation for wound coverage. (Center) A skin flap containing the fascia underneath was fabricated. (Right) The flap was rotated medially to cover a wound resulting from release of the scar and Achilles tendon. (b) (Left) The appearance of the right ankle before release. (Right) The patient is able to maintain the ankle joint properly while walking.

Modified z-plasty technique (includes the paratenon in the flap fabrication): alias ³/₄ paratenocutaneous z-plasty technique

Both techniques are essentially identical to the FC z-plasty and ³/₄ FC z-plasty. They are so termed because the paratenon of the underlying tendon structures is included in the flap fabrication to insure a vascular supply; therefore, in fabricating a flap, the dissection of the tissue must include the paratenon overlying the tendinous structures. A composite triangular skin flap (the skin and the paratenon located underneath) are transposed in a manner identical to other techniques (Figures 59.5 and 59.6).

Comments

The task of managing foot and ankle deformities consequential to burn injuries can be difficult. In recent years there has been a paucity of literature about foot and ankle reconstruction in burn patients. Factors such as patients' lack of desire to undergo reconstruction and/or the advent of physical problems causing a change in treatment priority and the consequential difficulties in patient management may account for the lack of interest shown by physicians in foot and ankle reconstruction in burned patients. The care of these patients, in practice, has been assumed by non-surgical services; a physical therapist is given the task of providing care that will lead

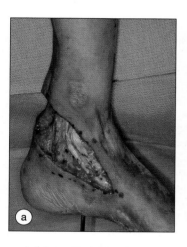
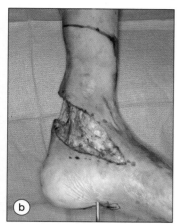
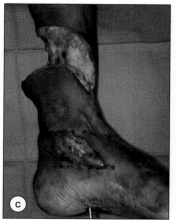
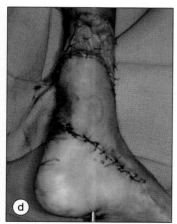
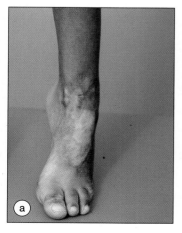
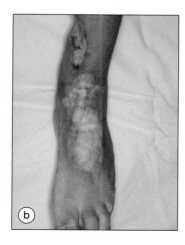

Fig. 59.5 (a) The patient developed a varus deformity of the left ankle. Incisional release of the contracted scar plus tendon transfer was needed to restore the ankle joint alignment. (b) A distally based FC flap was fabricated in the anteromedial aspect of the lower leg and the ankle. (c) The flap was moved caudad to cover the wound where the joint structures and tendons were exposed. (d) The flap donor site defect was covered with a piece of partial-thickness skin graft.

Fig. 59.6 (a) The appearance of left ankle before release. (b) The ankle joint alignment was judged at 9 months after the surgery to be proper.

to the regaining of muscle strength and joint mobility.[1] However, therapeutic goals using physical therapy alone may be unattainable in individuals with permanent structural destruction of the foot and ankle joints — that is, the foot and ankle will remain stiff and walking will be difficult regardless of the intensity and the duration of therapy rendered. It is, therefore, essential that surgeons continue to involve themselves in the care of these patients.

Scar contracture is the most common cause of stiff foot and ankle joints. Surgical release of contracted scar around the joint is, in this sense, the most fundamental and the most common approach used to restore mobility of joints. In practice, maintaining a proper joint alignment is difficult even though the release of scar tissues and surrounding joint structures is complete. This difficulty in restoring joint alignment could be due to structural alteration within the joint capsule caused by the burn injuries and/or protracted abnormal positioning of the joint. Release of ligamentous structures surrounding the joint, however, is seldom needed. Instead, the joint alignment can be maintained easily with the use of Kirschner wires (0.025–0.035 inch) inserted percutaneously, causing 're-shaping' of the altered capsular elements.

Skin grafting is the technique most commonly used to cover an open wound resulting from scar release or joint realignment. However, its usefulness may be compromised if the wound is located in a pressure-bearing area of the foot, e.g. the sole of the foot. Incomplete or inadequate graft sensory re-innervation in a pressure-bearing area, furthermore, will lead to breakdown of the graft. Although various techniques to resurface burned sole have been advocated,[2–4] their usefulness in burn foot reconstruction is limited. Similarly, the skin materials suitable for covering an exposed tendon and joint structure must have the components of subcutaneous fatty tissue. A skin flap, with an assured vascular supply, that can be mobilized from an adjacent area, is ideal material for wound coverage. (Obviously, if the burn has damaged not only the foot but also the adjacent tissues, this negates the possibility of using the tissues from the area as a flap donor site.) A composite tissue transfer via a microsurgical technique for reconstruction, though clinically appealing, may not be feasible because of a lack of suitable donor sites.[5,6] In contrast, a local flap technique – e.g. a rotational flap technique and/or an interpositional flap technique – has a logistic advantage over other techniques. However, a flap fabricated in the leg, especially in the area below the knee, can be plagued with problems of necrosis. Separation of the subcutaneous fatty layer, an essential maneuver in flap fabrication, would inevitably cause disruption of the vascular supplies to the skin. More recently advocated techniques utilizing a musculocutaneous (MC) flap, a perforator flap or reverse flow skin flap,[7–9] appeared to have technical advantages over a random skin flap. The tissue mobilized, however, is, generally speaking, bulky for the wound coverage and excursion of the flap may be limited. A random FC flap and a random PC flap (a composite skin flap that includes the underlying fascia and/or paratenon) appeared to circumvent the anatomical limitation in flap fabrication. Skin located almost anywhere in the foot and in the lower leg could be used for designing a skin flap for wound coverage. (As we have noted, the use of this technique is possible in a scarred area unless the underling fascia and/or paratenon has been destroyed.)

Releasing a contracted scarred area is achieved most efficiently by interposing two equilateral triangular skin flaps sharing a common side, the geometric basis for z-plasty technique. A 3/4 z-plasty technique of tissue release, also known as an interpositional flap technique, a banner flap technique, though it may not be as efficient, is based upon the similar principle that a right-angled triangle is formed with its cathetus made perpendicular to the line of scar release. The internal angle of this triangle may be set at 45° or less. The triangular flap is rotated 90° to make up the tissue defect resulting from releasing of the contracted scar. Although mobilization of the skin flap is simple, surgical dissection of the subcutaneous tissue may compromise the viability of the triangular skin flap. Inclusion of the fascia and/or paratenon in flap design and fabrication, in this sense, assures flap viability and is particularly useful in fabricating a triangular flap with a long cathetus and a narrow internal angle.

Summary

Although the task of reconstructing contractural deformities developed in the foot and ankle is difficult, the basic technique of incisional release with skin graft may be useful. On the other hand, the use of a local rotational skin flap technique, alias 3/4 z-plasty, is preferred, especially in instances where a flap is needed to cover a wound with exposed tendon and joint structure. The viability of a skin flap is enhanced by including the fascia and/or paratenon in flap design.

References

1. Serhgiou MA, Evans EB, Ott S, et al. Comprehensive rehabilitation of the burned patient. In: Herndon D, ed. Total burn care, 2nd edn. Philadelphia: WB Saunders; 2002:Ch 45.
2. Dahl TD, LeMaster JE, Cram AE. Effectiveness of split thickness skin grafts of plantar aspect of the feet. J Burn Care Rehabil 1984; 5:463.
3. Rooks MD. Coverage problems of the feet and ankle. Orth Clin N Am 1989; 20:723.
4. Barclay TL, Sharp DT, Chisholm EM. Cross-leg fasciocutaneous flaps. Plast Reconstr Surg 1983; 72:843.
5. May JW, Gatello GG, Lukash FN. Microvascular transfer of free tissue for closure of burn wounds of the distal lower extremity. N Engl J Med 1982; 306:253.
6. Hallock GG. Simultaneous bilateral foot reconstruction using a single radial forearm flap. Plast Reconstr Surg 1987; 80:836.
7. Reiffel RS, McCarthy JG. Coverage of heel and sole defects: a new subfascial arterialized flap. Plast Reconstr Surg 1981; 66:250.
8. Land A, Soragni O, Monteleone M. The extensor digitorum brevis muscle island flap for soft tissue loss around the ankle. Plast Reconstr Surg 1985; 75:892.
9. Hong G, Steffens K, Wang FB. Reconstruction of the lower leg and foot with the reverse pedicled posterior tibial fasciocutaneous flap. Br J Plast Surg 1989; 42:512.

Chapter 60

The ethical dimension of burn care

Arthur P. Sanford

Chapter contents

Introduction

In seeking optimum health for each patient, 'total burn care' aspires to integrated excellence in multiple dimensions. It is a 'bio-psycho-social-economic-legal-and ethical' enterprise, and the many hyphens indicate that all the dimensions of care are connected. Too often, the bio-psycho-social-etc. dimensions are assumed to be interconnected like railway cars, with the biological dimension in front, and the ethical hooked on only if necessary at the end, like an optional caboose. This is a misleading assumption. In our experience, 'total burn care' is most frequently achieved when it is assumed that *all* the dimensions of burn care are *always* present and in need of regular attention. Moreover, highly integrated, team-oriented, interdisciplinary[1] burn centers practice as if *all* the dimensions of care are *always* interpenetrating, like the length, width, and height of a solid object. In their daily work they assume that no one dimension may be changed without affecting all the others, and they depend on frequent detailed rounds, interdisciplinary staff meetings, and ongoing interviews with patients and families to keep all the dimensions of care ever coordinated and up to date.

In part because the multiple dimensions of burn care are so intimately interrelated, decisions involving the ethical dimension of burn care are extremely common. They are so common, in fact, that care-providers are usually unaware of them. Ethics, after all, is critical thinking about right and wrong, what should or should not be done, etc.[2] The words 'should', 'should not' and so forth indicate that ethical matters are being addressed. For example, whenever we decide which of several therapeutic alternatives *should* be recommended, we are making an ethical decision.[3] Should we spend more time with patient A than with patient B? Should we catch up on our journal reading as opposed to getting more sleep? Should we spend more time with our families and less at work? All are ethical decisions. Ethical decision making is therefore like breathing:[4] ever necessary and ongoing, but regularly automatic unless the problem is serious enough to be singled out for explicit attention.

What is 'an ethical problem?' when is it serious?

Often, significant ethical problems are trivialized by mislabeling them as 'merely problems in communication'.[a] A formal yet practical definition is therefore necessary: an ethical problem is present when it involves a conflict of two or more of the following: rights or rights-claims, obligations, goods and/or values.[b] For example, disputes about writing a 'comfort-measures-only' order for a patient without decision-making capacity and with a very low probability of survival commonly involve a conflict between an obligation and a good: the obligation not to abandon aggressive therapy prematurely, and the good of a maximally pain-free and unprotracted death. In such a case, *the burn team and the patient/surrogate* are ordinarily the major stakeholders and appropriate decision-makers, and we say they are addressing 'a problem in *clinical* ethics'. On the other hand, consider the burn center's or healthcare organization's (HCO's) responsibility to ICU patients when a safe nurse:patient ratio cannot be consistently met despite the burn center's best efforts? If discerning 'what should be done' in such circumstances requires decision-making at the *managerial level* of the burn center or HCO, a 'problem in *organizational ethics*'[5] is the correct term to use.

As indicated, conflicts among rights, obligations etc., are *very* common and vary greatly in difficulty. When should they be taken seriously? An ethical problem is serious when there are stakeholders involved who stand to be affected seriously by the problem or its outcome. Stakeholders working

---

[a] As we shall explain in detail, 'ethical problems' shared by stakeholders are, in fact, optimally resolved by communication . . . but by a very challenging, particular, uncommon, and decidedly untrivial species of communication called ethical dialogue.
[b] Modified slightly from: May WW. Discerning what's right in health care at the clinical level. Lecture at U.S.C. Los Angeles, CA: Keck School of Medicine; May 8, 2000. As used here and elsewhere in this chapter, the term 'values' refers to considerations (e.g. principles, laws, rules, roles, assumptions, preferences, goals, etc.) giving direction and/ or impetus to decision making.

collaboratively without outside help can successfully manage the vast majority of such problems. When are such problems so serious that assistance should be sought from a healthcare ethics committee/consultant (HEC) or its equivalent? There are two answers: the first short and crude, the second longer and more precise. An ethical problem is serious enough to refer to an HEC:

- When you suspect the 'New York Times sniff-test' would be positive,[c] i.e. you think a hypothetical newspaper reporter might be interested in making the problem or its solution public.
- When there is persistent disagreement among the major stakeholders; and codes, rules, laws and more discussions fail to lead to a resolution within generally acceptable ethical boundaries.

How should 'clinical ethics' problems be managed?

In the United States, the 'informed consent process' was developed by the American judiciary to safeguard the legal rights and welfare of all the stakeholders participating in 'bedside' or 'clinical' decision-making. Throughout the USA, this legal process has become the foundation of the healthcare-provider's approach to avoiding and managing serious ethical problems at the bedside. Its application in the burn center was explained and diagrammed in detail in the first edition of this book,[6] and what follows should be considered an update and development of what is stated there.

On the vast majority of occasions, there is little or no difficulty achieving agreement and patient consent about a proposed course of burn management. Occasionally, however, the process of obtaining informed consent leads to problems involving disagreements, anxieties and/or controversies about 'what should be done'. At this point, the participants must give careful attention to the quality of the discussion or 'ethical discourse' being used in attempting to resolve the problem. Ethical discourse is a skill requiring practice, like playing a musical instrument. No one becomes good at playing the violin or participating in ethical discourse simply by reading books about the subject, or by letting a consultant take over when things get difficult. Avoidance of, or reluctance to participate in, discourse with stakeholders about ethical problems is like a violin player who avoids practice, or won't go near the concert hall: both will perform suboptimally when at last forced by circumstances to act.

Contrary to very common practice, ethical discourse at its best is not merely filling your 'opponent's' heads with what you want them to know so they will say what you want hear. Nor is it simply getting your discourse partners to effectively 'get things off their chests' so they will feel better and then say what you want to hear. Least of all is it engaging in verbal warfare in an effort to 'be victorious over your opponents'. At its best, ethical discourse begins by building a 'safe place for ethical dialogue', i.e. establishing an interpersonal 'relation-

ship' made safe for transparent and self-critical honesty by making active listening and openness-to-learning the norm.[7]

The role of the care-provider in ethical dialogue

The care-provider should *develop the trust* necessary to establish the 'safe place for ethical dialogue' described above. To do this, the care-provider should learn the bio-psycho-social-economic- and cultural/religious information required to approach the patient and their family and/or surrogate with empathy for their lives and values. Some religious backgrounds teach us that we have certain limitations to this life and look to the future beyond. Others teach us that within our lives we'll come back and reflect on what our previous lives have been and also place extreme respect on the departed spirit. Finally, there are people who do not have a religious background and live for different goals and different aspirations. All of these must be considered early on when determining what the caregiver's relationship and position will be with the patients and their families. Many patients will decide against extremes of treatment and continuing care with the hope of not burdening their family with large hospital bills. Often these issues must be explored with patients before one can feel comfortable with the decision and its justification.

The care-provider must *discover if the patient has 'decision-making capacity'* sufficient to participate meaningfully in deliberation. To have decision-making capacity, the patient's (or if necessary, the patient's/surrogate's) consent to or refusal of the care-provider's recommendations must be: *informed* (i.e. comprehending and appreciating relevant information); *free* (substantially free of distorting non-rational/emotional influences); *deliberate* (decided after weighing pros versus cons in the light of his or her value system); *voluntary* (reflecting his or her own intentions); and *expressed* (communicated verbally or non-verbally).[8] Decision-making capacity is enhanced by optimizing the patient's physiological stability, consciousness, and pain control as much as possible. It is typically verified by ascertaining orientation, and by asking patients to rephrase the information provided to them in their own words and to say why they have made the decision they have. Determination of decision-making capacity by judicial process (i.e. determination of 'legal competency') is rarely necessary. If despite all efforts, the patient is found to be without decision-making capacity, an appropriate surrogate is commonly available among the patient's family or friends.

The care-provider should *provide appropriate information* about the patient's diagnosis and the therapy proposed, its nature, prognosis, pros and cons, and similar information about plausible alternatives including forgoing the therapy proposed. Prior investigation of the *patient's and/or surrogate's bio-psycho-social-economic-cultural-etc. background* is particularly helpful in the effort to assure clear communication and a common understanding among dialogue partners.

The role of the patient or surrogate

The initial task of the patient is to assimilate the information given by the caregivers. One cannot expect a patient in burn shock to understand or have complete background to understand what medical information is being given to them. There are limitations in their understanding and assimilation of

---

[c]Comment made at the 5th Annual Conference of the Los Angeles County Bioethics Network, Marina del Rey, CA: 18 April, 1998.

information that must be taken into account. Also, the patients have the right within their own value system to make a decision with their own best interest at heart. This includes their aforementioned religious or non-religious background, their family and what the needs and wants of their family are. It becomes an obligation of the patient or their surrogate to become a member of the team responsible for the individual. This obligation includes the necessity to reveal information completely and honestly, to become actively involved in their care, and participate constructively and sincerely in ethical dialogue about the issues at hand.

We must also consider previous life experiences. For example, the patient may have had family members or relatives with severe or terminal illnesses, themselves. Such experiences may influence their decision-making. Religious belief may also be a large factor in people's decisions. A clergyman might be involved at any step of the way to involve the patient's religious resources or spiritual support background in order to try to make the decisions about care and continuing treatments. Finally, there is the perception of what it would be like to survive a significant burn. Many people feel that this is not something that one would wish on anyone, let alone suffer through oneself. Patients may feel that they are not going to be a functional member of society, or that they will lose out on many of the things that they had been previously involved in or hope to achieve. Shriners Burns Hospital-Galveston has performed investigations in this area, looking at children as an example of this outcome; the essence is that children who survive large burn injuries end up at least as well off as their peers.[9] Boys, when they reach maturity, perform better scholastically and have a better self-image than their peers; girls perform at least on an average level with their peers. So, what we are finding is that these people do not become shutins but they do survive and thrive. The philosophy is that if you help the person get through the crisis, their own internal tools dictate whether they are going to fail or succeed. If the patient was going to succeed, they will succeed. If the patient fails, they were going to fail regardless of the burn injury. This can be employed and recognized by these data.

How should persistent ethical conflict be managed?

Even when participants make a sincere effort to establish a 'safe place', 'put relationship before decision-making', and perform their roles well, disagreements about conscientiously held positions occasionally persist. At this point, patience and setting aside adequate time to walk through carefully considered steps in ethical decision-making are necessary, Often, to build up their own skills and enhance chances of success, the patient/surrogate or care-providers will ask an HEC to coach them in pursuing a consensus collaboratively arrived at.

In any serious ethical inquiry, three questions must be answered: What seems to be the problem? What can be done? What should be done?[3] A seven-step decision-making model (illustrated in Table 60.1) has been found helpful in answering these questions.

In arranging a conference designed to achieve a consensus resolving ethical conflict at the clinical level, every effort should be made to have all the major stakeholders present to work collaboratively. To discover their current perceptions and level of understanding, to help equalize power, and to model civil discourse, the patient/surrogate and their significant others are asked to speak first as the care-providers listen carefully and respectfully. As indicated by step 1 (see Table 60.1), patients are asked to introduce themselves, explain the conflict as they see it, and indicate what they hope to achieve by the discussion. Thereafter, the care-providers do the same. This step typically takes the most time, but is the most important of all the seven. It 'lets off steam', makes the patient/surrogate and allies feel 'listened to', and optimally leads them to ask for the corrective and supplementary information they need from the care-providers, which (in step 2) they usually can provide or obtain[d]. If successfully carried out, steps 1 and 2 transform a potential or actual power struggle into a collaborative search for the answers to the next and then the final question listed on Table 60.1.

The conversation of step 3 may address principles (like respect for persons, beneficence, etc.) but more typically cites relevant laws and rules of the community and or institution, and/or other values ('no unnecessary pain', 'what the patient would want if able to speak', etc.). Step 4 is usually best carried out using a blackboard or equivalent to brainstorm and record all the plausible alternative courses of action. In step 5, the group collaboratively may find a principle, rule, value, etc., or some combination thereof so compelling that the proper alternative is clear; e.g. because it is considered unlawful homicide in most locations, large doses of narcotic primarily intended to stop breathing rather than control pain will be found unacceptable. If the decision is still not clear, steps 6 and 7 will usually lead to a mutually acceptable decision within boundaries acceptable institutionally, legally, and ethically.

Rarely, consensus will elude the most sincere adherence to the seven-step process. If 'time to sleep on the problem', further discussion, efforts to transfer care of the patient, etc.,

---

TABLE 60.1 THREE QUESTIONS TO BE ADDRESSED WHEN A CLINICAL ETHICS PROBLEM IS SERIOUS AND PERSISTENT, AND THE STEPS APPROPRIATE FOR ANSWERING EACH QUESTION

Question to be answered	Steps for answering each question
A. What seems to be the problem?	Step 1: Disclose/discover conflicting values of stakeholders Step 2: Disclose/discover the relevant information
B. What should be done?	Step 5: Compare alternatives and values: is decision clear? Step 6: If not, assess consequences Step 7: Make decision, collaboratively if possible

Modified with permission from: May WW. Ethics in the accounting curriculum: cases and readings. Sarasota, FL: American Accounting Association; 1990:1.

---

[d]Note the similarity of these early steps to those of the 'S-P-I-K-E-S' protocol for delivering 'bad news' described by Buckman as quoted by Foley K. A 44-year-old woman with severe pain at end-of-life. JAMA 1999; 281:1937–1945.

fail, appeal to the courts, or (in at least one US state[10]) appeal to relevant legislation for relief from responsibility for care of the patient may be necessary.

The patient without decision-making capacity, surrogate or advance directive

In such cases, care-providers typically have no way of knowing or deducing with confidence what the patient's wishes might be in a given set of circumstances. In general, the decision must seek the 'best interest of the patient', but the process required may vary. In some jurisdictions, consultation with another physician, the healthcare institution's administration, and/or HEC, is mandatory. In others, a court-appointed conservator might be required. In all such cases:

- the search for a surrogate should be diligent;
- all relevant medical information must be obtained and reviewed;
- real or apparent conflicts of interest must be disclosed;
- the opinions of the healthcare team, and of one or more physicians in addition to the responsible attending, should be reviewed;
- burden versus benefit must be weighed from the patient's point of view; and
- steps should be taken to ensure the benefit of continued life to a disabled patient is not devalued or underestimated.[11]

Some institutions also require that consideration of economic impact on healthcare-providers and the healthcare institution be excluded from consideration in such cases. Eventually, a surrogate decision-maker is identified and, hopefully, this is a person who has previously known the patient and their values prior to the accident, who has possibly had discussions about extreme end-of-life issues and can speak on the patient's behalf. The surrogate decision-maker must not make the decision based on what they would want for the patient. However, the surrogate decision-maker must know what that patient would prefer and act as an advocate in this situation since the patient is not able to participate in the decision.

How should 'organizational ethics' problems be managed?

Currently, healthcare decision-making affecting burn care occurs at three levels: in the clinic, in the organization, and in society.[5] The disciplines designed to improve ethical decision-making at the first and last levels are called 'clinical' and 'societal' ethics, respectively. They discern facts and values for guiding *clinical* or *societal* decisions that affect patient care and have received wide attention in both the media and scholarly journals for years. Recently, attention has been called to the need for discernment of facts and values for guiding *managerial* decisions that affect patient care.[5,12] For example, at times problems present as difficulties in clinical decision-making, but have their 'root causes' in areas that require decision-making at the managerial level. With dwindling numbers of nurses entering training, fewer and fewer nurses will be available to provide intensive care, and managerial decisions will be required to produce or recruit more nurses and to judge just when it is no longer safe to admit

new patients to beds without adequate staffing. Perhaps rehabilitation services in a given geographical area have not kept up with the ever increasing numbers of patients with large burns who survive but require more, longer, and more expert rehabilitation. Managerial decisions about the distribution of scarce resources will have to be made if adequate rehabilitation is to be available.

Such decisions are ethical: they involve conflicts of rights, obligations, goods, and/or other values. They tend to be less dramatically immediate and more deferrable, but they usually affect more persons and require more resources and follow-up than clinical ethics decisions.[12] They sometimes appear to be made 'in the front office', apparently without satisfactory input from care-providers, patients or other stakeholders, and without availability of extensive literature or assistance from a committee or consultant skilled in ethical analysis and critique applied at the organizational level.

The development of the discipline of 'organizational ethics' is just beginning, and is overdue in the judgment of JACHO[13] and other authorities.[14] We believe the obligation to be ethical at every level of healthcare decision-making and will become increasingly obvious and pressing with continuing changes in the ways healthcare is delivered. We hope that future editions of this book will report significantly increasing awareness of, and progress in, this level of healthcare ethics. Without such progress, the ability of healthcare ethics to make a difference in practice even at the clinical level will be significantly limited.

Specific problems

Human research

Many of the modern improvements in healthcare, particularly burns, have come through active research protocols. Many advances, including fluid resuscitation, excision and grafting, temperature and nutritional control, and modulation of hypermetabolic response, are based on active research in a clinical setting on human patients. It must be remembered that these are volunteers first and patients must not be coerced into the treatment. Institutions involved in human research must have Institutional Review Boards in place to monitor approved protocols and follow-up on patients and complaints with their research-driven caregivers. Childhood research is an even more scrutinized area because it is the parent, as a surrogate, who is giving consent for the research. It is a difficult area to approach, however, with the thorough monitoring of Institutional Review Boards and the realization children have a great deal to benefit from advances in healthcare. Children should be included in research so that they can get the benefits of progress in medicine and science at the earliest possible opportunity. However, this should not be at the expense of their own rights. Many patients feel that, when asked to participate in research protocols, they have a duty to those who proceeded them and who helped the physicians reach their current level of care. Patients often feel they should try to give something back to the science of medicine. Patients realize that they cannot fully repay their caregivers and may feel they must participate in research in order to help future victims.

Futility

The concept of futility and hopelessness in the care of a patient has changed drastically over the recent past. At one point any burn over a significant size offered no hope for survival.[15] Through efforts in resuscitation, physicians have pushed this survivability to current levels where even in the youngest of age groups extremely large burn victims can function and survive. At the same time, we are finding that there is no simple definition of futility,[16] making simple pronouncements of futility impossible.

Do not resuscitate versus comfort-measures-only versus active withdrawal of treatment

Once the goals of treatment have been agreed upon, decisions about the end-of-life care of an individual patient are to be made. End-of-life care should be a mutual and agreeable choice from the patient with the understanding by the healthcare team that treatment has become inappropriate to the goals agreed upon. Even if these conditions are met, it is important to realize that there is a duty to care for the patient. A do not resuscitate order (DNR) is not equivalent to a do not care (DNC) order.

An allocation of scarce resources

In its simplest terms, this becomes a question of who should survive and what is the price of life in an area where healthcare dollars are less and less available to all people. There is progressive improvement in survival given the concerted efforts of all members of the healthcare team. However, the reality is that society is providing limited funds for the care of burned patients. It becomes a very difficult personal decision of whether the burn unit should focus on saving money and decline treatment of one burn victim to prepare for the next burn or should resources be expended on a patient who perhaps has a poorer possibility of survival. The only problem with holding back on resources is that this next big burn may never come, and one has not provided the full open access of healthcare to the first patient. It can always be said that saving for the future in this situation does not benefit either, and one must advocate the use of the resource; once resources are exhausted, the patient should be redirected. Arguments can be made for both sides; however, if there is no other alterna-tive for the patient, clearly they must be cared for in their current setting.

A final note: 'ethical preposterism[17] in burn care'

As conceived in ancient Athens and during most of its history, Western ethics has been an effort to:

(1) achieve 'the ethical life', i.e. life in all its important dimensions lived at its most flourishing; and
(2) solve any problems about 'what should or should not be done' during that quest.

The sustained pursuit of excellence in 'total burn care' first achieved momentum in the USA in the mid-20th century. It has always drawn its most primal motivation from the fact that burn patients are arguably the most severely injured and utterly vulnerable of human beings, and therefore deserving of the most tender, skillful, and comprehensive care. Commitment to the safety, healing, rehabilitation, and growth of patients during their return to as flourishing a life as possible, has been the spearhead of the quest since its beginning, and both the fire in its belly and the steel in its resolve ever since. Clearly, burn care is an ethical endeavor through and through, not just when and where 'difficult patients' or 'ethical problems' become evident.

In our introduction we observed that the bio-psycho-social-economic-legal-and ethical dimensions of 'total burn care' are often seen as interconnected like railway cars, with 'bio-' (i.e. the biological dimension) in front, and 'ethical' hooked on only if necessary at the end, like an optional caboose. We believe this to be not only misleading but also an example of 'preposterism'.[17] Taken from the Latin *pre-* (before) and *posterus* (following), that is 'preposterous' which puts the first last, and what should follow first.[18] We believe the ethical dimension of burn care should be habitually seen not as a sometimes-tacked-on caboose, but as a leading and driving locomotive which extends its influence back through all dimensions of the enterprise like a steel backbone. Were that image actually lived out as dreamed by the early founders of the effort, the providers and receivers of burn care could confidently expect to experience a continually improving 'ethical climate' and fewer 'ethical problems', no matter where history might take the train.

References

1. Fulginiti VA. The right issue at the right time. In: Holmes DE, Osterweis M, eds. Catalysts in interdisciplinary education. Washington DC: Association of Academic Health Centers; 1999:7–24.
2. Gillon R. Philosophical medical ethics. Chichester: John Wiley; 1985:2.
3. Pellegrino E, Thomasma DC. A philosophical basis of medical practice. New York: Oxford University Press; 1981:119–152.
4. Maguire DC. The moral choice. Garden City, New York: Doubleday; 1978:113.
5. Potter RL. On our way to integrated bioethics: clinical/organizational/communal. J Clin Ethics 1999; 10:171–177.
6. Zawacki BE. Ethically valid decision-making. In: Herndon DN, ed. Total burn care, 1st edn. London: WB Saunders; 1996:575–582.
7. Zawacki BE, Imbus S. Enhancing trust and subjective individual dialogue in the burn center. In: Orlowski JP, ed. Ethics in critical care medicine. Haggerstown MD: University Publishing Group; 1999:489–512.
8. Faden RR, Beauchamp TL. A history and theory of informed consent. New York: Oxford University Press; 1986:235–381.
9. Blakeney P, Herndon D, Desai M, et al. Long-term psychological adjustment following burn injury. J Burn Care Rehabil 1988; 9(6):661–665.
10. Alquist. Health care decisions. (California) Assembly Bill No. 891, Chapter 4, sections 4730–4736; operative July 1, 2000.
11. Ad hoc drafting committee. Guidelines for forgoing life-sustaining treatment for adult patients at the LAC+USC Medical Center. Los Angeles, CA: LAC+USC Medical Center; May 5, 1993.
12. Hirsch NJ. All in the family — siblings but not twins: the relationship of clinical and organizational ethics analysis. J Clin Ethics 1999; 10:210–215.

13. Joint Commission on Accreditation of Healthcare Organizations. Ethical issues and patient rights. Oakbrook Terrace ILL: Joint Commission on Accreditation of Healthcare Organizations; 1998:67–90.

14. Society for Health and Human Values – Society for Bioethics Consultation Task Force on Standards for Bioethics Consultation. Care competencies for health care ethics consultation. Glenview, IL: American Society for Bioethics and Humanities; 1998; 24–26.

15. Herndon D, et al. Teamwork for total burn care: Achievements, directions and hopes. In: Herndon DN, ed. Total burn care, 1st edn. London: WB Saunders; 1996; 1–4.

16. Emmanuel L, et al. Medical futility in end of life care: Report of the council on ethical and judicial affairs. JAMA 1999; 281(10):937–941.

17. Haack S. Manifesto of a passionate moderate. Chicago: University of Chicago Press; 1998:180–208.

18. Modified from: Barzun J. The American University. New York: Harper and Row; 1968:221.

Chapter 61

Maltreatment by burning

Rhonda Robert, Patricia Blakeney, and David N. Herndon

Chapter contents

Introduction

As a subject of scientific investigation, violence, including that occurring within the family, has received much attention from professionals in sociology, mental health, medicine, and law.[1] Yet most health professionals, themselves devoted to healing and comforting others, are reluctant to believe that human beings will cause serious injury to others, especially to those who are significant members of their own family circle and most especially to those who are helpless such as young children or elderly parents. Caregiving professionals value the role of supportive others, and assessing for maltreatment can run counter to career training, values, and interests. The degree of uncertainty in identifying abuse or neglect is uncomfortable, and the family members typically do not validate suspicion. However, the evidence is overwhelming that people do cause injury even to close family members. Sometimes the maltreatment involves burning. Maltreatment to children involving burning has been identified and discussed in the professional literature for many years.[2] Types of maltreatment include neglect, physical abuse, sexual abuse, and emotional abuse. Although any of the forms of maltreatment may be found separately, they often occur in combination. Neglect is the most common form of maltreatment, occurring in 60% of maltreatment cases, followed by physical abuse, which occurs

in 20% of maltreatment cases.[1] More than one-third of child fatalities are attributed to neglect. Burn injury is common to both neglect and physical abuse. The Federal Child Abuse Prevention and Treatment Act (CAPTA) (42 U. S. C. A. 5106 g), as amended by the Keeping Children and Families Safe Act of 2003, defines child abuse and neglect as, at minimum: Any recent act or failure to act, *regardless of intent*, on the part of a parent or caretaker which results in death, serious physical or emotional harm, sexual abuse or exploitation, or an act or failure to act which presents an imminent risk of serious harm.

Maltreatment of adults by burning is a recognized concern, though infrequently documented in empirical studies.[2–7] Burning as a form of violence against adults likely occurs with much greater frequency than reflected in the literature and has often been unrecognized. Unless adult patients are asked about maltreatment, they are unlikely to volunteer the information.[5] As burn care professionals become increasingly sensitive to the problem of maltreatment to adults, the reported incidence will probably increase dramatically, replicating the pattern observed with child maltreatment, i.e. the more we ask, the more we will discover.[7]

The authors share the guilt of failing to be attuned to maltreatment in adults in the same way we are alert to that possibility with children. Therefore, our clinical experience with known adult maltreatment by burning is limited to a few flagrant cases. Our experience with child maltreatment is extensive. Since the literature and our own experience are heavily weighted with information about child maltreatment, this chapter also represents that bias. The reader may, at times, be led to believe that the pediatric population is the only target for maltreatment. That is not an intention but rather a reflection of our current knowledge, and we caution the reader, as we remind ourselves, to avoid that misconception.

In this chapter, we have integrated our experience with available information to identify risk factors in the total population and to suggest therapeutic approaches to treating, in addition to the burn wounds, the complex social, interpersonal, and familial issues that both produce injury and complicate the recovery and rehabilitation of the patient. Because burn care professionals are likely to be the only entrée to help for the victims and the perpetrators and because we know what the 'worst case' outcomes can be, we bear the responsibility of finding ways to prevent further harm while maintaining a trusting relationship with the patient and with the patient's family.

Prevalence of maltreatment

During our pediatric hospital's staff orientation, participants are asked to estimate the percentage of children abused and neglected in the United States annually, as well as to estimate the percentage of children abused and neglected by burning. Well-seasoned healthcare professionals routinely underestimate the prevalence. Approximately one and a half million people in the United States are believed maltreated.[8] Of children in the US suspected to have been abused or neglected, 80% of the injuries involved the skin.[9] Maltreatment is suspected in as many as 30% of admissions to pediatric burn units, and, the majority of the suspected cases are confirmed by investigating officials to have been caused by maltreatment.[8-20] This institution's referral rate to investigating officials is 22%. Adult maltreatment by burning is reported less frequently. In one sample of adult burns, 4% of injuries were attributed to maltreatment.[6]

Without intervention, abuse persists. Hultman et al.[2] found that 36% of the children with suspicious burn injury had been investigated for abuse or neglect prior to the child's burn injury. In addition, 55% of the children with suspicious burn injury had been followed by physicians for significant medical problems: mental retardation, failure to thrive, chronic respiratory infections and otitis media, hypopituitarism, pulmonary stenosis, attention deficit disorder, previous trauma that included skull fractures, and probable Munchausen syndrome by proxy. Given the intense and chronic history reported in Hultman's study, it is hard to hold in mind that the average patient age was 5.[2]

Thirty percent of the children suffering recurrent maltreatment are eventually mortally injured.[13] Thus, many children are injured repeatedly in escalating severity, perhaps over years, until they die from maltreatment. At this institution, 43% of the children who had been referred to investigating officials due to suspicious burn injury had additional unrelated reports for suspected maltreatment. Given that the majority of the population is of pre-school age, the children's futures held many more years of potential vulnerability to victimization.

Dynamics of maltreatment

Maltreatment usually occurs as a multigenerational characteristic that is symptomatic of relationships impoverished of nurturance. Central to understanding maltreatment is to understand that perpetrators typically are individuals who were denied adequate parenting and who experienced severe emotional deprivation. The infantile needs of the perpetrator were unmet; the perpetrator has not learned that it is possible to assert oneself appropriately and to meet one's own needs autonomously. Rather, the perpetrator looks to external sources to meet those needs to be cared for and comforted.

In some situations there are two 'perpetrators': i.e. the actor and the overtly passive observer who does not stop maltreatment. Both persons are elements of a psychosocial system that supports maltreatment, and usually both are from similar backgrounds with similar needs.[21]

Maltreatment grows from a non-thinking, passive life position. Abuse can be thought of as expressions of desperation from immature individuals who feel lost and helpless, incompetent to care for themselves, and who are in a constant quest for some external source of comfort. Their own experiences of parental maltreatment have taught them to mistrust others so that, as adults, they are typically socially isolated. This further decreases opportunities for comfort or for developing self-efficacy. Feeling helpless and inadequate, and predicting rejection in every interpersonal contact, such people also experience more difficulty in seeking and securing employment, thus frequently incurring a further stress of financial instability.

In an environment devoid of emotional support, perpetrators passively wait for comfort from a spouse, a lover, or a child. When those 'others' fail to gratify the perpetrators' needs or when a change in the situation imposes additional stress, these needful persons react in a child-like, non-thinking way to resolve frustration. Acts or failures to act that result in burn injury are often the end results of intense frustration.[22] A child, an elderly person, or a physically dependent adult is commonly an immediate precipitator of stress as well as an easily available target for maltreatment.[3,22,23]

This perceived helplessness and desperate needfulness also explains some of the other behaviors commonly attributed to perpetrators. They often fail to seek appropriate and timely medical treatment for an injured child, not only because they fear punishment but also because of their learned helplessness and passivity. They discount the seriousness of the injury, as well as their ability to take care of the injury. 'I didn't think it was that bad' is an explanation often given for delay in seeking treatment. By diminishing the significance, they relieve themselves of responsibility to act. When the perpetrator does take the child for help, the perpetrator commonly seeks first a relative or neighbor rather than a physician because perpetrators do not believe in their own ability to decide whether to seek medical treatment. Perpetrators are observed to interact inappropriately with their children because they are preoccupied with having their own needs met. A child who is hurt and demanding is unlikely to reward the perpetrator with feelings of comfort that the perpetrator seeks, and so the perpetrator withdraws from the child. If the child is quiet and compliant, the perpetrator may be observed to ignore the child and sit passively, watching television for long periods until some external force acts as a stimulus to motivate the adult into action.

Justice and Justice,[24] in their work with families who mistreat children, identified several erroneous belief systems that are commonly held by perpetrators; these are listed in Box 61.1. Since, as most authorities believe, violence is a multi-generation intra-family pattern, then it is likely that the belief systems attributed to child perpetrators can be extrapolated to perpetrators of adults as well. The issues of dependency, lack of trust, felt inadequacy, frustration, and emotional pain recur in situations describing maltreatment spanning age groups.[3,24,25]

Assessment begins at admission

As with all patients and families, the therapeutic relationship with patients and families in which maltreatment is suspected is initiated at admission and developed through the process of assessment and treatment. Perpetrators are aware that some-

ERRONEOUS BELIEF SYSTEMS COMMONLY CONTRIBUTING TO THE FAMILY SYSTEM IN WHICH ABUSE OCCURS (JUSTICE AND JUSTICE, 1990)[24]

- If my child cries, misbehaves or does not do what I want, he or she does not love me and I am a bad parent
- My child should know what I want and want to do it
- My child should take care of me like I took care of my parents
- My spouse/lover should know what I want and meet all of my needs
- If I have to ask, it does not count
- You cannot trust anyone

TABLE 61.1 EXPOSURE TIME TO RECEIVE A SEVERE BURN IN HOT WATER

Degrees in Celsius	Degrees in Fahrenheit	Time to second-degree burn	Time to third-degree burn
45	113.0	120 minutes	180.0 minutes
47	116.6	20 minutes	45.0 minutes
48	118.4	15 minutes	20.0 minutes
49*	120.0*	8 minutes	10.0 minutes
51	124.0	2 minutes	4.2 minutes
55	131.0	17 seconds	30 seconds
60	140.0	3 seconds	5 seconds

*Voluntary standard published by Consumer Product Safety Commission, American Journal of Public Health, and the plumbing industry. Downward adjustments to time needed for young children.

thing is wrong in their lives, although they may be at an impasse in changing their behavior or limited in degree of personal awareness. The need for medical attention and the visible nature of the burn injury have the potential to heighten the caregiver's sense of vulnerability. This crisis can be utilized to bring positive changes for the family. Risk assessment should be discussed with the family members, including the suspected perpetrator. Once the concerns are presented, the individuals have the opportunity to engage in services from which the family could potentially benefit. The family should be apprised of any report to a protective agency and the events to expect thereafter. Remembering that an important factor in the typical perpetrator's character is reluctance to trust, hospital staff are more effective when truthful and forthcoming. Frequent follow-up sessions with the family throughout the course of hospitalization and outpatient treatment are essential to maximizing family change (Figure 61.1). To facilitate a positive relationship, the helping professional must be sensitive to the fear, pain, and sadness that are often the sources of the perpetrators' maltreatment.[13]

Maltreatment indicators

Most non-accidental burn injuries to children occur to the very young, aged 3 years and under, and are scald (Table 61.1) or contact burns[13–15,17] Maltreated children live in poverty-level households headed by a young, single parent who has two or more children.[13,14,17,26] Maltreated burned children are reported to require longer hospitalization and to have higher rates of morbidity and mortality from their burns than non-maltreated children.[27–29]

Suspicion of maltreatment may be prompted by observations of parental behavior. Parents who are not abusive or neglectful typically report the details of the child's injury spontaneously and express concern about the treatment and prognosis. They exhibit a sense of guilt, ask questions about discharge data and follow-up care, visit the child frequently, and bring gifts. In contrast, perpetrators usually do not volunteer information, but are evasive or contradictory; they seem critical of the child and angry with the patient for being hurt. They do not seem to feel guilty or show remorse. They show no concern about the injury, treatment or prognosis. They seldom visit or play with the child, do not ask about discharge

date or follow-up care, and appear to be preoccupied with themselves and unconcerned about the child.[22]

Prospective studies of abuse do not exist, and the ability to predict future injury is limited. However, factors associated with maltreatment have been reviewed retrospectively in a number of studies.[11,13,15,26,30,31] A comprehensive list of indicators of child maltreatment gleaned from these studies and our own experience is presented in Box 61.2. Utilizing these indicators provides an informed framework from which to begin assessing risk for maltreatment.[32] A semi-structured assessment makes for more thorough interview and documentation at minimum. As the information base is enhanced, risk assessment might eventually assist in accurate identification of maltreatment. Hammond and colleagues[19] forwarded this possibility. They demonstrated that two or more endorsed risk factors of their 13-factor assessment significantly increased the likelihood of abuse.

At this institution, number and type of risk factors have been associated with greater risk for maltreatment. The study design was based on comparison between two groups. One group consisted of children with one report to investigating officials, with that report being the one initiated by the burn center staff regarding the burn injury. The other group consisted of children with additional, unrelated reports to investigating officials. The rationale for groupings was that if different people, in different contexts, across time had concern enough to place a report on the child's behalf, the likelihood of accurate identification and an established pattern of maltreatment was greater for those with more than one report to investigating officials. Thus, the characteristics of children with multiple reports may guide professionals regarding level of concern and type of intervention.

Regarding total numbers of risk factors, children with two or more reports to investigating officials averaged 3 more risk factors than those with one report. Those with two or more reports had an average of 8.4 risk factors and as many as 18.

Attention was drawn to 4 risk factors associated with repeated reports to investigating officials: prior burn injury, blaming the child, lack of external support, and acute family

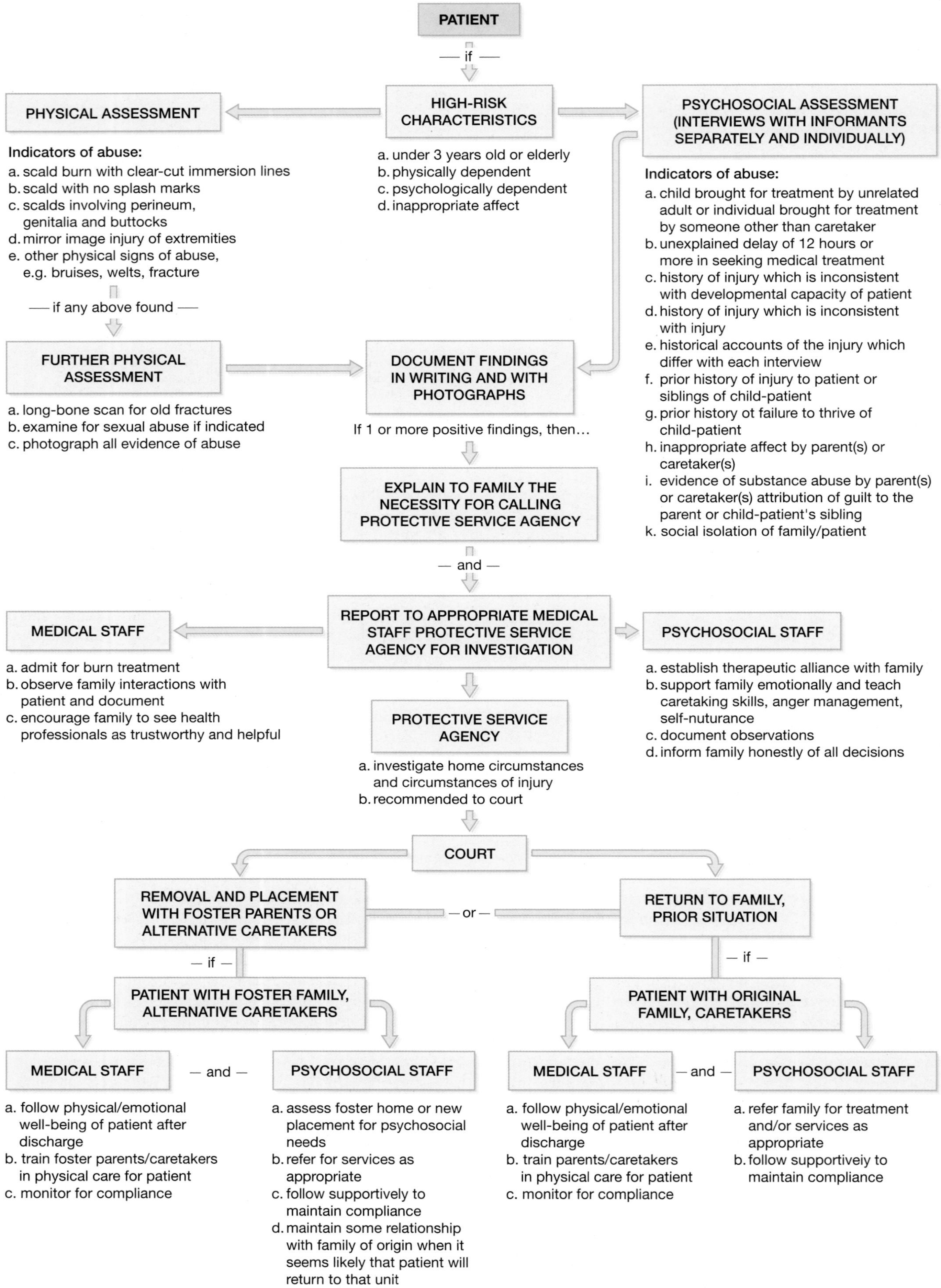

PATIENT

— if —

HIGH-RISK CHARACTERISTICS

a. under 3 years old or elderly
b. physically dependent
c. psychologically dependent
d. inappropriate affect

PHYSICAL ASSESSMENT

Indicators of abuse:

a. scald burn with clear-cut immersion lines
b. scald with no splash marks
c. scalds involving perineum, genitalia and buttocks
d. mirror image injury of extremities
e. other physical signs of abuse, e.g. bruises, welts, fracture

— if any above found —

FURTHER PHYSICAL ASSESSMENT

a. long-bone scan for old fractures
b. examine for sexual abuse if indicated
c. photograph all evidence of abuse

PSYCHOSOCIAL ASSESSMENT (INTERVIEWS WITH INFORMANTS SEPARATELY AND INDIVIDUALLY)

Indicators of abuse:

a. child brought for treatment by unrelated adult or individual brought for treatment by someone other than caretaker
b. unexplained delay of 12 hours or more in seeking medical treatment
c. history of injury which is inconsistent with developmental capacity of patient
d. history of injury which is inconsistent with injury
e. historical accounts of the injury which differ with each interview
f. prior history of injury to patient or siblings of child-patient
g. prior history of failure to thrive of child-patient
h. inappropriate affect by parent(s) or caretaker(s)
i. evidence of substance abuse by parent(s) or caretaker(s) attribution of guilt to the parent or child-patient's sibling
k. social isolation of family/patient

DOCUMENT FINDINGS IN WRITING AND WITH PHOTOGRAPHS

If 1 or more positive findings, then…

EXPLAIN TO FAMILY THE NECESSITY FOR CALLING PROTECTIVE SERVICE AGENCY

— and —

REPORT TO APPROPRIATE MEDICAL STAFF PROTECTIVE SERVICE AGENCY FOR INVESTIGATION

MEDICAL STAFF

a. admit for burn treatment
b. observe family interactions with patient and document
c. encourage family to see health professionals as trustworthy and helpful

PSYCHOSOCIAL STAFF

a. establish therapeutic alliance with family
b. support family emotionally and teach caretaking skills, anger management, self-nuturance
c. document observations
d. inform family honestly of all decisions

PROTECTIVE SERVICE AGENCY

a. investigate home circumstances and circumstances of injury
b. recommended to court

COURT

REMOVAL AND PLACEMENT WITH FOSTER PARENTS OR ALTERNATIVE CARETAKERS

— or —

RETURN TO FAMILY, PRIOR SITUATION

— if —

PATIENT WITH FOSTER FAMILY, ALTERNATIVE CARETAKERS

— if —

PATIENT WITH ORIGINAL FAMILY, CARETAKERS

MEDICAL STAFF — and — **PSYCHOSOCIAL STAFF**

a. follow physical/emotional well-being of patient after discharge
b. train foster parents/caretakers in physical care for patient
c. monitor for compliance

a. assess foster home or new placement for psychosocial needs
b. refer for services as appropriate
c. follow supportively to maintain compliance
d. maintain some relationship with family of origin when it seems likely that patient will return to that unit

MEDICAL STAFF — and — **PSYCHOSOCIAL STAFF**

a. follow physical/emotional well-being of patient after discharge
b. train parents/caretakers in physical care for patient
c. monitor for compliance

a. refer family for treatment and/or services as appropriate
b. follow supportively to maintain compliance

Fig. 61.1 Flow of activities toward treating victims of abuse.

BOX 61.2 Risk factors for abuse/neglect by burning

FORCED — IMMERSION DEMARCATION

- Symmetrical, mirror image burn of extremities
- Glove-like (burned in web spaces)
- Circumferential
- Minimal splash marks
- Uniform depth
- Full-thickness
- Clear line of demarcation, crisp margin
- Doughnut-shaped scars on buttocks/perineum (spared area forcibly compressed against container, decreasing contact with hot liquid, if container is not a heated element)
- Flexion burns, 'zebra' demarcation to popliteal fossa, anterior hip area, or lower abdominal wall
- Injuries of restraint (e.g. bruises mimicking fingers and hands on upper extremities)[16]

INJURY DEMARCATION, OTHER

- In congruent with history of event
- Pattern of household appliance — note whether even pattern versus brushed, imperfect mark
- Scald
- Location of injury: palms, soles, buttocks, perineum, genitalia, posterior upper body
- Cigarette burn, if more than one on normally clothed body parts and if impetigo ruled out

HISTORY OF INJURY

- Evasive, implausible explanation
- Incompatible with child's developmental age
- Changes in story; discovered to be burned — rule out dermatologic epidermolysis bullosa (EB), dermatitis herpetiformis, chemical burn due to analgesic cream, phytophotodermatitis,[17] and birth marks, including Mongolian spots[18]
- Under-supervised — inadequate monitoring, impaired person supervising, inordinately young baby-sitter (<12 years of age)
- Burn is older than history given
- Water outlet temperature greater than 120°F
- Mechanism of burn is incompatible with injury (e.g. exposure time, history of event, and degree burn are inconsistent)
- Patient's per-event behavior displeasing to caregiver (e.g. inconsolable, failed to meet caregiver's expectations)
- Toileting events related to history of injury[19]
- Burn attributed to:
  Child or patient, as per caregiver
  Caregiver who is not present at the healthcare facility
  Caregiver, as per patient
  Delay in seeking medical treatment — note estimated time of delay

DEVELOPMENTAL ASSOCIATIONS

- Pre-verbal, non-verbal person
- Vulnerable person (e.g. special need, failure to thrive, elderly)
- Caregiver expectations are inconsistent with patient's development; caregiver overestimates child's developmental skills and safety knowledge; caregiver unaware of patient's developmental capacity
- Patient has symptoms of mental disorder (e.g. ruminating, aggressive)
- Patient displays disturbing behaviors related to attachment (e.g. excessive crying, clinging, apathy/lethargy, excessively withdrawn, listless, unemotional, submissive, polite, fearful, vacant stare)
- Hyper-sexualized language or behavior, as compared to same age peers

CAREGIVER–PATIENT RELATIONS

- History of interrupted caregiver–child bonding
- Adolescent caregiver(s) (e.g. child–child versus adult–child interactions)
- Strained interactions; inappropriate expectations of the patient by the caregiver
- Role reversal (rely on patient for support)
- Inappropriate or lack of caregiver concern:
  Detached
  Lack of sympathy
  Lack of physical contact (e.g. fails to hold or pick up child)
  Inebriated during visits
  Infrequent visits

OTHER PHYSICAL SIGNS OF ABUSE OF NEGLECT

- Unrelated injuries:
  Fractures, dislocations; rupture to spleen, liver, or pancreas; point tenderness; impaired range of motion or function
  Signs of poisoning
  Ocular insult (edema, scleral hemorrhage, hyphema, bruise, blue sclera)
  Swelling, bogginess, depressions, cephalohematomas palpable on head or increased intracranial pressure at fontanel
  Blood, infection, or foreign body in ear
  Edema, bleeding, septal deviation of nose; foreign bodies in nose; cerebrospinal fluid rhinorrhea from nose
- Unrelated injuries involving the skin: hematomas, soft tissue swelling, lacerations, fingernail markings, scars, bruises (check behind ear), welts, rope burns, strangulation marks, bites, alopecia — note color, size, shape, and location of each (scalp most visible while shampooing)
- Abdominal tenderness, guarding, rebound tenderness, or bruises
- Cardiac instability, tachycardia, murmurs, flow murmurs secondary to anemia, or palpable rib fractures
- Dehydration or malnutrition — note weight, height, and head circumference
- Previous burns
- Unkempt, e.g. severe diaper rash, dirt under nails or in axillae, odoriferous, dirt on plantar surfaces of feet in cold weather
- Inadequate or no immunization record
- Inadequate dental care (e.g. caries); trauma to lips, tongue, gums, frenula, palate, pharynx, or teeth
- Inadequate medical care
- Inappropriate dress
- Assess prior to invasive medical procedures
- Genital, urethral, vaginal, or anal bruising, bleeding
- Swollen, red vulva or perineum
- Foreign body in genital area
- Positive cultures for sexually transmitted diseases — if herpes develops, note whether lesions are on unburned body surface area, on genitals of type II
- Pregnant minor
- Recurrent urinary tract infections, streptococcus pharyngitis, abdominal pain

FAMILY

- Caregiver abused or emotionally deprived during childhood
- Limited disciplinary practices (e.g. only physical punishment)
- Lack of external supports; isolation
- Mental illness; substance abuse; criminal history
- Lack of financial self-sufficiency
- Poor employment history
- Dependent caregiver; unable to cope with daily responsibilities; unorganized
- Violent couples; impulsive; easily frustrated
- Previous Department of Protective and Regulatory Services involvement[20]
- Prior accidents to dependents
- Acute family stressors
- No primary caregiver

stress. In this sample, having had a prior burn injury was associated with greater risk for recurrent reports to investigating officials. Thus, repeated burn injury to a child should increase the clinician's suspicion of abuse.

Blaming the child describes caregiver's reporting style, in which the caregiver addresses the child's role in the history of injury and minimizes the caregiver role in the history of injury. A commonly stated history of injury involves the bathing routine: the caregiver leaves the bathroom to get a towel, hears the child's cries, and returns to the bath. Some caregivers present an explanation for injury and divert to what the child might have done while not being supervised. For example, caregiver behavior may be justified, e.g. 'I needed a towel' and accompanied by a supposition about the child's behavior, e.g. 'He must have turned on the faucet.' This type of history is associated with limited disclosure and guardedness.

In comparison, other caregivers rehearse the situation, consider their decision-making, express feelings of responsibility, speak of the child in terms of being vulnerable, and consider new home safety practices. For the most part, the caregiver is making 'I' statements, e.g. 'I was not watching my baby.' Presentation style is unguarded and the parent is actively planning.

Lack of external support was associated with repeated reports to investigating officials. Fractious relationships, failure to establish alliances, and isolation are typically described. External support is observable to some extent across the period of hospitalization. Given that hospital staff is in the role to assist with accessing resources, caregivers tend to disclose support system information.

Acute family stress was associated with repeated reports to investigating officials. Acute family stress dominates the caregiver's disclosure. The crises described are presently occurring. However, the pattern of being in a crisis is chronic and not acknowledged by the reporter. The family environment is chaotic, and the caregiver is commonly 'putting out a fire.' When evaluating risk factors, consideration should be given to the cultural standards of the family's home community. Folk-healing practices should be queried, as well as use of traditional healers.[11,33] We have seen in the past year two newborns who were burned in hospitals in a country where improperly trained hospital personnel were tending to the infants (Figure 61.2).

Adult maltreatment and indicators

Maltreatment of adults by burning is, as noted earlier, much more rarely reported, probably because the index of suspicion for abuse of an adult is low and therefore injuries are more rarely questioned. Adult victims are also noted to be reluctant

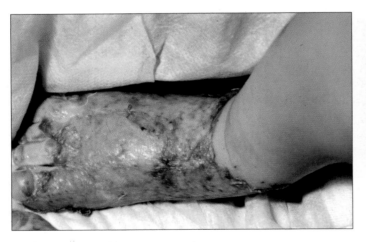
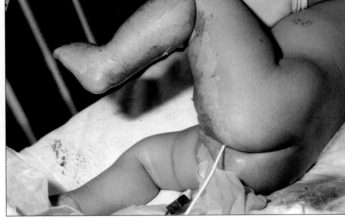
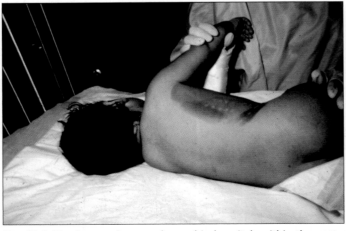
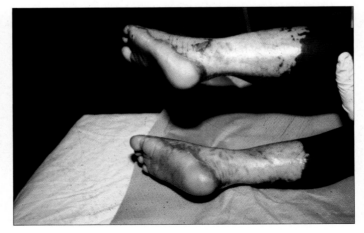

Fig. 61.2 Newborns who were burned in hospitals within the past year.

to report the circumstances of their injuries because of their fear of retaliation or because of shame and embarrassment.[23] Spousal[34] and elder maltreatment[4] are subpopulations within the adult population who are at risk for maltreatment by burning. Two studies describe burn injuries of adults due to violent assault.[5,6] Associated risk factors in these reports were substance abuse and domestic violence. Although Purdue and Hunt[6] report that there was no identifiable burn pattern, Krob et al.[5] described a pattern of scald injury to the anterior trunk and upper extremity. Males and females seem equally at risk for burning by assault.

Bowden et al.[2] describe a population of older adults made vulnerable by physical or mental impairment who were burned from maltreatment. All but three of their 26 subjects were burned while living in healthcare facilities or institutions. Although this single article identifies maltreatment of the elderly by burning as a problem, frequency of maltreatment is likely greater than presently documented, and maltreatment likely occurs within family settings as well as the institutional settings which dominate this Michigan sample.

Elder maltreatment has been identified as a public concern in the United States only in the last 15 years. Relatively little, however, has been written about the subject in spite of the estimated 2.5 million persons who suffer annually.[35] When elder maltreatment does occur within the family, the perpetrator is often an adult child or spouse of the victim. The perpetrators are often intoxicated and were themselves maltreated children.[3] Some perpetrators of elder maltreatment are individuals with no prior history of pathology who have become exhausted by the demands of their lives, e.g. caring for an aged parent as well as a spouse and children of their own.[7,23] Gross neglect is frequently the type of maltreatment sustained by elderly or vulnerable persons, particularly if that person is disoriented or is reluctant to ask for attention and physical care.[35] Risk factors of maltreatment for adults are similar to those for children and are listed in Box 61.3.[2,3,7,23,35]

Reporting and documenting suspected maltreatment

State legislatures in the United States first enacted reporting laws in 1963, and by 1967 every state had laws mandating professionals who work with children to report suspected maltreatment to designated authorities. A federal law, the Child Abuse Prevention and Treatment Act, was passed in 1974. The laws require professionals to report suspected maltreatment of a child when there is evidence that 'would lead a competent professional to believe maltreatment is reasonably likely'.[36] In the case of maltreatment, privileged communication typically only exists for attorney and client. If local laws are not known, staff at the governing protective agency, sourcebooks,[37] or the hospital attorneys will be able to provide necessary legal references.

There are no federal programs to specifically address reporting of suspected abuse in adults. Each state has its own set of definitions, reporting laws, and penalties.[23] Professionals who suspect adult maltreatment should be guided by the same principles as in reporting suspicious injury to a child. When maltreatment is suspected, a report must be made to the proper governing adult protective agency. In the United States, the protective agencies operate under the purview of the State Department of Health and Human Welfare. Most states' referrals are made to a statewide intake office. The numbers are located in all phone books. The National Center on Elder Abuse provides information and assistance on elder abuse, including a listing of state elder abuse hotlines. The website is www.elderabusecenter.org and phone number is (202)-898-2586. Child Help USA is a private charity that established and maintains the National Child Abuse Hotline (800)-4-A-CHILD (800-422-4453) and provides a listing of statewide reporting numbers at their website http://www.childhelpusa.org/report. Telecommunications Device for the Deaf number is (800)-2-A-CHILD. The US Department of Health and Human Services Administration for Children and Families provides a listing of statewide reporting phone numbers at their website http://nccanch.acf.hhs.gov/topics/reporting/report.Cfm. .

Healthcare professionals are often reluctant to report suspicious injuries because they feel as if they are condemning a person with uncertain evidence and because they have been trained to maintain patients' confidentiality. However, the medical professional is the sole point of possible intervention for most victims. The purpose of reporting a suspicious injury is to prevent further harm. Making a report is an official trigger requesting further investigation. The ultimate decision about whether maltreatment has actually occurred is left to the investigating officials; however, the professionals reporting the incident must document the observed data to provide the investigating officials and/or the courts the information necessary to intervene appropriately. Professionals should document, for example, observations that render the caretaker's professed ignorance of the cause of injury questionable or that an explanation of cause is implausible given the nature of the injury. Observations of inappropriate behavior or lack of interest in the child's treatment must be documented. Although any single observation may seem unimportant, the pattern of behaviors described by multiple observations may be very significant in obtaining protection for the victim and help for the perpetrator.[36] In addition to the documentation of first-hand observations, the following tasks should be delegated:

- Examine the patient for other signs of maltreatment, including a skull and long-bone radiological scan.

BOX 61.3 Indicators of abuse/neglect of adults

- Physical dependence
- Psychological dependence
- Accessibility as a target for abuse as in institutional living or living with a 'caretaker'
- Caretaker(s) with a history of substance abuse, and/or other psychopathology
- Social isolation
- An injury that is not consistent with the story described
- Conflicting reports of the injury
- Scalds with clear-cut immersion lines and no splash marks
- Scalds that involve the anterior or posterior half of an extremity and/or the buttocks and genitals, or a flexion pattern
- Other physical signs of abuse/neglect
- History of related incidents

Clearly state that the radiology consultation is for assessment of occult trauma.

- Photograph any possible evidence.
- If the patient has been referred from another hospital, access information from the staff at that hospital to determine whether they identified suspicious aspects of the injury and whether the injury was reported to an investigating agency. If so, ascertain the number assigned to the patient's case by the investigating agency. This number is needed for subsequent calls related to the patient.
- Interview the patient.
- Interview the family members or caretakers individually and together for thorough histories of the event, sensitive to the differences in the story or changes across time.
- Obtain a thorough family history, the patient's medical history and the developmental capacity of the patient.
- Gather other available collateral information, e.g. medical records from other places of treatment.[20]

Understanding that abuse does occur and is an expression of the perpetrators pain and sadness can enable the healthcare professional to begin the process of assessment as a critical observer and empathetic interviewer. The interviewer must not respond personally to off-putting behavior from the informant(s) but recognize the behavior as a form of self-protection. Each informant should be interviewed separately, not only to check for conflicting stories but also because there are likely to be tensions between the informants that inhibit the interviewer's ability to establish a relationship with each individual. The informants should also be interviewed together to provide the opportunity to observe tensions, conflicts, and alliances within the family group.

Interviewing the pediatric patient with suspicious injury

Interviews with the child–patient are especially important in cases of suspicious injury. Even children as young as 29 months often relate information with remarkable accuracy.[38] An interview with the child alone should be conducted by a professional who has established rapport with the child. The professional can first ask the child to recall specific past experiences which are thought to have no relationship to the current suspected abuse, such as a birthday party or Christmas celebration. The descriptions of these events provide some indication of the child's ability to recall and to describe memories either verbally or in drawings. Questions about the specific events leading to injury should initially be very general: e.g. 'how did you get hurt?' and the child should be encouraged to tell the story freely. Specific questions for clarification should be asked only after the child has told the story. If the child seems unwilling to talk about what happened, the interviewer can suggest the child raise a hand or wiggle a finger to signal that they know something but do not yet want to talk about it. Interviews with a young child are best conducted in several short sessions, giving the child an opportunity to feel safe in the hospital and with the interviewer (Figure 61.3).[39]

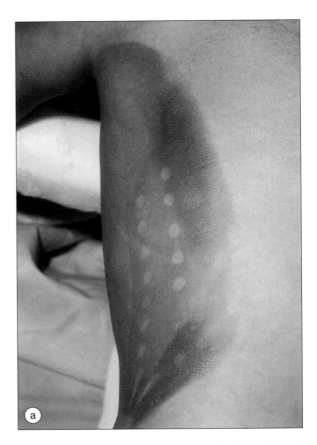

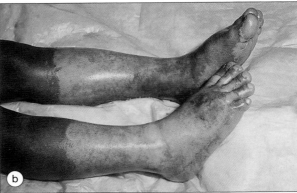

Fig. 61.3 (a) Abuse. Contact burn in which the markings of an iron are clearly visible. (b) Abuse. Classic 'stocking' pattern resulting from feet being immersed in very hot water. The initial history given by the mother of the 21-month-old infant was that an older sibling had turned on the hot water, and the patient herself dipped her feet into the tub.

Interviews with the elderly or handicapped adult patient

When interviewing vulnerable patients, special care must be taken to help them feel safe and comfortable with the interviewer and the hospital setting. The vulnerable adult may be frightened of retribution by the caretaker(s) or afraid of being placed in an institutional setting. The abused adult also may be embarrassed and ashamed of their victimization. If the perpetrator is an adult child, the victim may attempt to protect the perpetrator from detection and punishment. The interviewer must assess the circumstances of the injury and establish a relationship in which the patient can trust the hospital staff to act in the best interest of all concerned, i.e. the patient and the perpetrator(s).

Maintaining professional relationships with patient and family

Working therapeutically with a family suspected of abusing or mistreating the patient requires skill and diplomacy, not only because of a strong tendency on the part of healthcare professionals to align with the victim or be angry with a perpetrator of maltreatment but also because suspected perpetrators often appear off-putting toward the professional staff. Yet, establishing a therapeutic alliance with these families is extremely important, for, no matter how serious the injury, the patient will probably return to that same family, if not at the time of discharge from the hospital, then at a future time.

Therapeutic interventions with perpetrators

Ironically, the professionals of the burn team who identify and report suspected maltreatment also have an exceptional opportunity to intervene in the dynamic process that has led to the maltreatment. During the days or weeks of the patient's hospitalization, the family is placed in a situation of coerced interaction with the burn team. At this time, the family is also in a state of crisis, i.e. their customary defenses have failed to protect them from external scrutiny. In a state of crisis, when their usual belief systems and defensive behaviors are failing, people are more likely to be amenable to new learning and change than during times of equilibrium.[41] Thus, if members of the burn team can interact with the abusive family in ways that invalidate, or at least cast serious doubt upon, the family beliefs, the family system may begin to change. As change is initiated, continued positive support for change can lead to further change.

In order to take advantage of this therapeutic opportunity, the members of the team must relate to perpetrators with honesty and compassion. This does not mean that the team should approve of the behaviors of the perpetrator(s) nor advocate for the perpetrator(s) to be given another opportunity to harm a victim. However, the team members can work with perpetrators in a manner that encourages them to trust professional help. The team members' behavior can demonstrate that relating to others can lead to gratification of their needs for nurturance and comfort. Beneath the hostile suspicious facade of the perpetrator is a frightened and lonely child who feels hopelessly unworthy of kindness. The clinician who is consistently honest, firm, and compassionate can develop a therapeutic alliance with a perpetrator even while explaining that a report is being made to the appropriate agency. The clinician then must assist the family during the process of investigation by honestly informing the family of decisions that are made as a result of the investigation.

Even while explaining that parental rights are terminated or that criminal charges are being filed, a skillful clinician can maintain a therapeutic relationship with the perpetrator(s). By helping the perpetrator(s) perceive the situation, as one in which there is hope and opportunity to receive help, the clinician can continue a therapeutic relationship that greatly enhances the likelihood that the abusive family will accept further assistance to continue the process of change.

The burn team can work with the community agencies to obtain help for abusive families. Many communities have programs that provide foster grandparents or parent aides, i.e. lay therapists who teach parenting skills and nurture the parent(s).[22,24] Local self-help groups or telephone crisis intervention services are commonly available If the burn team has succeeded in developing and maintaining the trust of the abusive family, they are in an advantageous position to encourage families whose prior experiences with social service agencies may have left them suspicious. Even when parental rights are terminated or the patient is removed from the home, the burn team's continued therapeutic support of the perpetrator(s) is advisable since the victim will likely return to that family eventually. In any event, perpetrators of violence against others are a risk to society, and health professionals have an obligation to use their knowledge and skills to diminish that risk.

Future direction for establishing child safety

Accidental attribution for cause of burn injury is easy. Establishing evidence for maltreatment by burning beyond a reasonable doubt is difficult.[3] The more that can be known about maltreatment, the more children will be protected. As burn care professionals increase their expertise in the area of child maltreatment, the more they will be able to assist investigating officials. Historically, physician reporting has had an important impact on determinations made by investigating officials.[4]

A primary step toward increasing the knowledge base of maltreatment by burning is the establishment of a national or international database. When events occur infrequently, large sampling is needed. Some of the most dangerous signs of maltreatment occur infrequently. A national database established under a public safety initiative would allow for larger sampling and greater disclosure of information between agencies. One initial step has been accomplished. As of 1995, the American Burn Association initiated collaboration with the American College of Surgeons and created the TRACS/ABA Burn Registry. Ninety burn centers participate and by 2002, the National Burn Repository (NBR) was well established and generated a report. The NBR collects data on some behavioral parameters of burn injury, including suspected self-inflected injury, child abuse, assault or abuse of adult, and arson. The total of all behavioral parameters monitored through NBR accounts for 4.9% of burn injuries.

Optimally, those participating in a national or international database would develop procedures for consistent assessment and reporting methods. Different forms of maltreatment should be assessed, and at minimum both neglect and physical abuse should be included. Burn centers at which formalized assessment and reporting procedures have been established consistently report high incident rates of suspicious injury. For example, Loyola University Medical Center created thorough procedures for assessment and reporting at 30% of the injuries to the state agency for potential abuse.[5]

Another direction of investigation that may lead to greater expertness would be multidisciplinary studies in which forensic experts, fire dynamics experts, and mechanical engineers work with the experts in burn injury pathophysiology, the burn care professionals.[6]

References

1. Hansen JC, Barnhill LR. Clinical approaches to family violence. Rockville, Maryland: Aspen; 1982:157.
2. Bowden M, Grant S, Vogel B, et al. The elderly, disabled and handicapped adult burned through abuse and neglect. Burns 1988; 14(6):447–450.
3. Rathbone-McCuan E. Elderly victims of family violence and neglect. Social Casework: The J Contemporary Social Work 1980; 296–304.
4. Rathbone-McCuan E, Goodstein R. Elder abuse: clinical considerations. Psychiatric Annals 1985; 15(5):331–339.
5. Krob M, Johnson A, Jordan M. Burned and battered adults. J Burn Care Rehabil 1986; 7(6):529–531.
6. Purdue G, Hunt J. Adult assault as a mechanism of burn injury. Arch Surg 1990; 125:268–269.
7. Pedrick-Cornell C, Gelles RJ. Elder abuse: the status of current knowledge. Family Relations 1982; 31:457–465.
8. Kessler D. Physical, sexual, and emotional abuse of children. Clin Symp 1991; 43(1):1–32.
9. Johnson CF, Showers J. Injury variables in child abuse. Child Abuse Neglect 1985; 9:207–215.
10. Meagher DP. Burns. In: Raffensperger JG, ed. Swenson's pediatric surgery, 5th edn. Norwalk, CT: Appleton & Lange; 1990: 317–337.
11. Giardino A, Christian C, Giardino E. A practical guide to the evaluation of child physical abuse and neglect. Thousand Oaks, CA: Sage; 1997:74–96.
12. Herndon D, Rutan R, Rutan T. Management of the pediatric patient with burns. J Burn Care Rehabil 1993; 14(1):3–8.
13. Weimer C, Goldfarb I, Slater H. Multidisciplinary approach to working with burn victims of child abuse. J Burn Care Rehabil 1988; 9(1):79–82.
14. Showers J, Garrison K. Burn abuse. A four-year study. J Trauma 1988; 28(11):1581–1583.
15. Hight D, Bakalar H, Lloyd J. Inflicted burns in children. Recognition and treatment. JAMA 1979; 242(6):517–520.
16. Hobbs C. When are burns not accidental? Arch Dis Child 1986; 61:357–361.
17. Kumar P. Child abuse by thermal injury – a retrospective survey. Burns 1984; 10:344–348.
18. Rossignal A, Locke J, Burke J. Paediatric burn injuries in New England, USA. Burns 1990; 16(1):41–48.
19. Hammond J, Perez-Stable A, Ward C. Predictive value of historical and physical characteristics for the diagnosis of child abuse. South Med J 1991; 84(2):166–168.
20. Rosenberg N, Marino D. Frequency of suspected abuse/neglect in burn patients. Pediatr Emerg Care 1989; 5(4):219–221.
21. Kempe CH. Paediatric implications of the battered baby syndrome. Arch Dis Child 1971; 46:28–37.
22. Justice B, Justice R. The abusing family. New York: Human Services Press; 1976.
23. Fulmer T. Elder mistreatment: progress in community detection and intervention. Family Community Health 1991; 14(2):26–34.
24. Justice R, Justice B. Crisis intervention with abusing families: short-term cognitive coercive group therapy using goal attainment scaling. In: Roberts AR, ed. Crisis intervention handbook. Belmont, CA: Wadsworth; 1990:153–172.
25. Goldberg H. The dynamics of rage between the sexes in a bonded relationship. In: Hansen JC, Barnhill LR, eds. Clinical approaches to family violence. Rockville, MD: Aspen; 1982:61–67.
26. Bakalar H, Moore J, Hight DW. Psychosocial dynamics of pediatric burn abuse. Health Soc Work 1981; 6(4):27–32.
27. Watkins A, Gagan R, Cupoli J. Child abuse by burning. J Florida Med Assoc 1985; 72(7):497–502.
28. Campbell J, LaClave L. Clinical depression in pediatric burn patients. Burns 1987; 13(3):213–217.
29. Purdue G, Hunt J, Prescott P. Child abuse by burning — an index of suspicion. J Trauma 1988; 28(2):221–224.
30. Rivara F. Developmental and behavioral issues in childhood injury prevention. Dev Behav Pediatr 1995; 16(5):362–370.
31. Ayoub C, Pfeiffer D. Burns as a manifestation of child abuse and neglect. Am J Dis Children 1979; 133:910–914.
32. Doctor M. Abuse through burns. In: Carrougher G, ed. Burn care and therapy. St Louis, MO: Mosby; 1998:359–380.
33. Forjuoh S. Pattern of intentional burns to children in Ghana. Child Abuse Neglect 1995; 19(7):837–841.
34. Hendriks JH, Black D, Kaplan T. When father kills mother: guiding children through trauma and grief. New York: Routledge; 1993.
35. Sukosky DG. Elder abuse: a preliminary profile of abusers and the abused. Family Violence and Sexual Assault Bulletin 1992; 8(4):23–26.
36. Myers JEB. Legal issues in child abuse and neglect. Newbury Park, CA: Sage; 1992:102.
37. Hays JR, Costello R, eds. Texas law and the practice of psychology. Austin, TX: Texas Psychological Association; 1994.
38. Fivush R. Developmental perspectives on autobiographical recall. In: Goodman GS, Bottoms BL, eds. Child victims, child witness: understanding and improving testimony. New York: Guilford; 1993:1–24.
39. Yuille JC, Hunter R, Joffe R, et al. Interviewing children in sexual abuse cases. In: Goodman GS, Bottoms BL, eds. Child victims, child witness: understanding and improving testimony. New York: Guilford; 1993:95–115.
40. Runyan DK. The emotional impact of societal intervention into child abuse. In: Goodman GS, Bottoms BL, eds. Child victims, child witness: understanding and improving testimony. New York: Guilford; 1993:263–277.
41. Roberts AR. An overview of crisis theory and crisis intervention. In: Roberts AR, ed. Crisis intervention handbook. Belmont, CA: Wadsworth; 1990:3–16.
42. Kolko D. Juvenile firesetter intervention clinical training. Pittsburg, PA: University of Pittsburgh School of Medicine, Department of Psychiatry; 2000.
43. Keith-Spiegel P, Koocher G. Ethics in psychology: professional standards and cases. New York: Random House; 1985.

Further reading

Bennett B, Gamelli R. Profile of an abuse burned child. J Burn Care Rehabil 1998; 19(1 Pt 1):88–94.

Dressler D, Hozid J. Thermal injury and child abuse: the medical evidence dilemma. J Burn Care Rehabil 2001; 22(2):180–185.

Hultman CS, Priolo D, Cairns B, et al. Return to jeopardy: the fate of pediatric burn patients who are victims of abuse and neglect. J Burn Care Rehabil 1998; 19(4):367–374.

National Clearinghouse on Child Abuse and Neglect Information (2004). What is child abuse and neglect? US Department of Health and Human Services Administration for Children and Families. Online. Available at: http://nccanch.acf.hhs.gov/pubs/factsheets/ whatiscan.cfm.

Peck M, Priolo-Kapel D. Child abuse by burning: a review of the literature and an algorithm for medical investigations. J Trauma 2002; 53(5):1013–1022.

Ruth G, Smith S, Bronson M, et al. Outcomes related to burn-related child abuse: a case series. J Burn Care Rehabil 2003; 24(5): 318–321.

Chapter 62

Functional sequelae and disability assessment

Glenn D. Warden and Petra M. Warner

Introduction

Advances in acute burn care during the past 25 years, in terms of decreased mortality and decreased length of hospital stay, have been truly outstanding and amazing. In 1971, survival statistics at the Institute of Surgical Research in San Antonio demonstrated an LD_{50} (lethal dose resulting in a 50% survival rate) with approximately 40% TBSA (total body surface area) burn. Thus 50% of the patients with burns of only 40% died. Now, the LD_{50} approaches 80% TBSA, and, if no inhalation injury is involved, patients with burn injuries greater than 80–90% of their TBSA routinely survive. In almost every burn unit in the United States, the length of stay has decreased from nearly 3 days/percent burn to less than 1 day/percent burn. The success can be stated simply: patients with larger, more severe burns are surviving; however, are these patients returning to society to become productive citizens? What is the real outcome of massively burned patients? Do pediatric burned patients become functional adults? How do they function socially later in life? What is the long-term effect on the patient's families and society? Are survival and decreased length of stay really the measure of productivity for our specialty? The real product or measurements of customer service is a patient who can successfully return to society and, even more importantly, be a useful, productive individual who can successfully interact socially within a community. Yes, patients with larger and more severe burns are surviving, but this has created new problems for patients' quality of life. Although the problems are magnified in massively burned patients, they exist even in smaller burns. These problems are best demonstrated in a pediatric burn patient with a 95% TBSA burn (Figure 62.1). Cultured keratinocytes were utilized to achieve wound coverage. The child survived; however, when we examined the patient's current and future reconstructive needs, they totaled 33 potential reconstructive procedures. Thus, the reconstructive problems are monumental in a child with very few donor sites.[1] With regard to survival, the results of this patient are impressive; however, we must ask the question: 'Has the medical expertise in terms of survival progressed past the ability to reconstruct and rehabilitate patients?' Unfortunately, the answer is clearly 'yes'. Are we returning our patients to a society which is not ready financially, psychologically, or socially, to accept them? Again, unfortunately, the answer is clearly 'yes'.

Although the American Burn Association has made rehabilitation a major emphasis, quality work still remains to be done. It is important and imperative that burn centers evaluate the functional outcome of a thermally injured patient. This is important not only for disability assessment but also for evaluation of our medical management. Outcome studies in the 20th century will not only emphasize survival and hospital stay but also patient satisfaction and ability to return to work. The purpose of this chapter is to review the functional sequelae and disability assessment following thermal injury.

Basic considerations — impairment — disability — handicap

The various terms such as 'impairment', 'disability', and 'handicap' appear in laws, regulations, and policies of diverse origin without proper coordination of the ways in which they are used. 'Impairment' refers to an alteration of an individual's physiological, psychological, and anatomical structure or function that interferes with activities of daily living.

'Disability', which is assessed by non-medical means, means an alteration in an individual's capacity to meet personal, social, or occupational demands or to meet statutory or regulatory requirements. Simply stated, impairment is what is wrong with the health of an individual; disability is a gap between what the individual can do and what the individual needs or wants to do. An individual who is impaired is not necessarily disabled. Impairment gives rise to disability only when the medical condition limits the individual's capacity to meet the demands which pertain to non-medical fields and activities. On the other hand, if an individual is able to meet a particular set of demands, the individual is not disabled with respect to those demands, even though a medical evaluation may reveal impairment.

The concept of 'handicap' is independent of both impairment and disability, although it is sometimes used interchangeably with either of those terms. Under the provision of federal laws, an individual who is defined as handicapped has an impairment that substantially limits one or more life activities, including work, has a record of such impairment, or is regarded

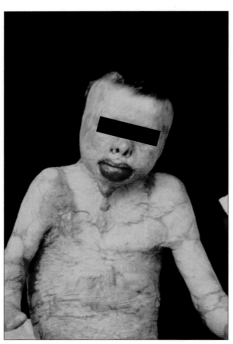

Fig. 62.1 A pediatric burn patient with a 95% TBSA burn.

Impairment assessment

Before discussing the medical aspects of evaluating thermally injured individuals, it must be pointed out that no Social Security and Worker's Compensation disability program medical listing exists for burns. Instead, burns must be evaluated under the appropriate body system. Often, more than one system is involved: in other words, musculoskeletal, respiratory, and skin all must be considered in the final decision. Claims must be aimed primarily at resolving the question of onset, whether the impairment can be expected to last 12 months or end in death. The medical evidence needed to document the existence and severity of a medically determinable impairment due to burns must include a history of the impairment, which describes the origin and course of the condition, dates of confinement, nature of treatment, and the claimant's response; current objective findings such as results of examinations, laboratory tests such as blood pressure, electrocardiogram, x-rays, blood tests, range of motion, medical factual data upon which diagnoses are based; and a description of the objective findings of the claimant's limitations and remaining capacities. In other words, how far can the patient walk, which activities cause breath or chest pain, what extent of motion is there in affected parts of the body. Regional specialized burn centers treat many serious burns annually. These centers are excellent sources of medical evidence as they maintain complete detailed records regarding the nature of an injury, treatment, complications, and prognosis. Advances in burn care have improved the survival rate in major burns. Efforts to rehabilitate these survivors and improve their quality of life represent a significant challenge for those involved in their care. The rehabilitation of these survivors is unique and multifaceted, and rarely limited to one system. Many individuals will experience some type of long-term physical impairment or mental limitation, and the rehabilitation process may take years to complete. It must be emphasized that impairments resulting from a burn are not restricted to the skin. Complications may affect any body system; thus, the examiner who is assessing individuals for disability must be attentive to the systemic sequelae of burn injury. The evaluation of a burn victim has some unique features. The necessity to consider such subjective factors as heat and cold intolerance, sensitivity to sunlight, pain, chemical sensitivity, and changes in sweating pattern, as well as the more objective considerations of decreased coordination, sensation, strength, and contracture, lends itself to a unique evaluation.

Disfigurement from scarring, a frequent sequelae of burns, may not affect performance and thereby, in and of itself, causes no impairment. Scarring represents a special type of disfigurement. Again, no percentage of impairment is assigned for the existence of a scar *per se*; however, scars affect sweat glands, hair growth, and nail growth, and cause pigment changes or contractures and may affect loss of performance and cause impairment. Sensory deficit, pain or discomfort from scars needs to be evaluated, as well as the loss of motion of a scar area. An impairment due to disfigurement from scarring may also create behavioral or psychological impairments which subsequently may be rated. The need for intermittent or continuous treatment of the skin with topical agents and pressure garments can impair a person's function and needs to be considered. There is a surprising lack of published literature

as having such an impairment. As a matter of practicality, however, a handicap may be operationally understood as being manifest in association with a barrier obstacle to functional activity. An individual of limited functional capacity is handicapped if there are barriers to accomplishment of tasks or life activities that can be overcome only by compensating in some ways for the effect of an impairment. If an individual is not able to accomplish a task or activity despite accommodation, or if there is no accommodation that will enable the accomplishment, then in addition to being handicapped, the individual is also disabled. On the other hand, an impaired individual who is able to accomplish a task or activity without accommodation is, with respect to the task or activity, neither handicapped nor disabled. The concept of 'employability' deserves special attention, for, in an occupational setting, if an individual within the boundaries of medical condition has the capacity, with and without accommodation, to meet a job's demands and conditions of employment as designed by the employer, the individual is employable and consequently not disabled. On the other hand, an individual who does not have the capacity or who is unwilling to travel to and from work, to be at work, and to perform assigned tasks and duties, is not employable.

The first critical task in carrying out a medical determination related to employability is to learn about a job, specifically the expectations of the incumbent, with respect to performance, physical activity, reliability, availability, productivity, expected duration of useful service life, and any other criteria associated with qualifications and suitability. Sufficient detailed information from a job analysis will provide a basis upon which a physician determines exactly what kinds of medical information are needed and to what degree of detail to assess an individual's health with respect to demand criteria.

which relates to the impairment evaluation of a burned patient. The following are concepts which must be kept in mind when evaluating a postburn patient for impairment and resulting deformities.

Skin

Scars and cutaneous abnormalities which result from the healing of burned tissue may represent a special type of disfigurement. Scars should be described by giving their dimensions in centimeters, and by describing their shape, color, anatomical location, and evidence of ulceration; their depression or elevation, which relates to whether they are soft and pliable or hard and indurated, thin or thick and smooth or rough; and their attachment, if any, to underlying bone, joints, muscle and other tissues. Good color photography with multiple views of a defect enhances the description of scars.

The tendency of a scar to disfigure should be considered in evaluating whether impairment is permanent or whether the scar can be changed, made less visible, or concealed. Function may be restored without improving appearance and appearance may be improved without altering anatomical or physiological function. If a scar involves loss of sweat gland function, hair growth, nail growth, or pigment formation, the effect of such loss on performance of an activity of daily living should be evaluated. Furthermore, any loss of function due to sensory pain, any sensory defect, pain or discomfort in a scar should be evaluated.

Burn scar contracture is probably the most frequently seen cause of impairment in a postburn individual. Every burn, regardless of the depth of injury, heals with some element of contracture. Contractile forces continue long after a wound is healed and can result in severe skin shortage. Inadequate skin prohibits movement to a joint's normal arc of motion and will influence not only the joint underlying the contracture but also those adjacent to the scar. In the early stages of development, burn scar contractures may often be corrected through the use of splints and pressure garments designed to force developing scar tissue into more normal configurations. In spite of the benefits derived from these modalities, they may also function as a type of impairment, both physically and cosmetically. Understanding the splints which individuals must wear and their limitations are important factors in the assessment of disability. Often, surgical means must be employed in order to restore function. When a surgical release of a contracture is performed, the resultant defect can be of considerable size and will require closure by means of a skin graft or flap of tissue. Burn scar contracture frequently requires a series of staged surgical procedures before optimal function and cosmesis are achieved. Recovery from surgical intervention must be followed by an extensive rehabilitation program. If an individual does not participate in a rehabilitation program, contractures will reoccur.

The definition of functional impairment should not be limited to an individual's ability or inability to perform joint range of motion. An extremity can exhibit full active range of motion and still be considered impaired due to poor skin quality. Although much can be done to restore function, the skin is never restored to normal. Scar tissue is less tolerant of the everyday stress imposed on it than normal skin. Scar epithelium is thin, fragile, and prone to chronic ulceration.

Regardless of the location, these chronic open areas will not heal and eventually require skin grafting. This type of lesion can occur at any time, even years after the initial hospitalization. Skin grafts have the same abnormalities as burn scars in that they all involve contracture formation, have loss of sweat gland function, hair growth, and altered pigment formation. Although frequently cosmetically more acceptable, skin grafts are still not normal skin. Physical limitations such as cold and heat intolerance, difficulty with sun exposure, altered sensation, or painful scars may prohibit individuals from performing their past work or other work.

Musculoskeletal

Functional limitation secondary to burn injury usually results from an anatomical alteration about a major joint. The degree to which the function of a joint is affected is greatly influenced by the amount of soft-tissue loss and the degree of pain associated with movement. Full-thickness burns, those involving all layers of skin, may also result in secondary damage to muscle, bone, tendon, and ligaments. In the acute phase of treatment of such injuries, a joint may be exposed, making it vulnerable, and susceptible to a chronic infection (osteomyelitis), instability, and arthritic changes. Ectopic calcification, the abnormal deposition of calcium around the joints, is usually seen in the elbow, but it can occur in any joint. Symptoms include pain with a significant decrease in motion. These changes in joint structure can be verified by x-ray and will require surgery at a later date for correction. Extensive soft-tissue destruction involving the loss of muscle mass, as seen in electrical injuries, will require numerous staged procedures in order to restore function. An individual may never be restored to full function and may be excluded from performing certain types of work which exist in the national economy.

Restriction of normal movement by contracture is not limited to the extremities. When a scar occurs over the trunk or anterior chest, severe and chronic postural changes can result which may cause secondary spinal deformity or altered respiratory functions. Amputations are another leading contributor to postburn impairment. Unlike amputations which are performed for other medical conditions such as peripheral vascular disease, amputation following an extensive thermal injury will often require several staged surgical procedures in order to produce a stump capable of accommodating a prosthesis. It is also important to realize that amputations are not confined to the extremities alone but may also involve skin appendages such as the ears and nose. Complicated stage procedures using local or distant full-thickness skin or muscle-skin flaps are required in order to restore function and cosmesis in these areas. An understanding of how long it will take for an individual's function to be restored is an important factor in deciding about the issue of disability.

Special senses and speech

Impairment to the senses of hearing or vision can occur as a result of a thermal insult, secondary to life-sustaining treatments or as a complication of a healing burn. The loss of central or peripheral vision may begin at the time of contact with a burning agent and can cause the destruction of the eyelids and damage to the cornea. A series of surgical procedures must be performed in order to create a functional eyelid.

Contracture of the eyelids, more commonly the lower, may develop quickly, resulting in incomplete closure of the eyelid, and potential damage to the cornea can result in conjunctivitis or corneal ulceration. In spite of adequate surgical correction, it is common for such injured individuals to have repetitive episodes of recontracture for up to 2 years post-healing, due to ongoing scar contracture process. Perioral burns that result in lip eversion and microstomia, or contracture of the mouth, may eventually impair mastication and result in drooling as well as inhibiting an individual from producing speech which can be heard or understood. Hearing impairment due to the acute burn is rare, but there may be a loss of the external ear, or deafness secondary to the treatment of life-threatening infections with antibiotics.

Respiratory system

Burns that occur in an enclosed space, such as a building structure, often result in some form of inhalation injury to the respiratory system. Impairment may be limited to a temporary need for ventilatory support or extend to permanent respiratory disease. Chronic and recurrent respiratory infections and pulmonary insufficiency may limit an individual's ability to perform their past work or other work in the national economy, especially when toxic chemicals or dust are present in the workplace. Exposure to irritating gases can also worsen pre-existing asthma or result in irritant-induced asthma. Although this form of reactive airway disease usually resolves with time, some individuals may have persistent respiratory impairment that also may require a change in vocation in order to avoid continued exposure to irritants and exacerbation of symptoms.

Furthermore, patients with severe inhalation injuries may require a tracheostomy long after the burn has healed. Closure of the stoma is often delayed for the purpose of intubation and anesthesia in future reconstructive surgeries. Pulmonary function tests are essential in determining respiratory impairment.

Cardiovascular system

A cardiovascular evaluation should include a good history and electrocardiogram. Patients complaining of chest discomfort thought to be of cardiac origin should have a more extensive work-up. There is some evidence of increased incidence of cardiovascular disease in the long-term follow-up of survivors of large thermal injuries.

Neurological system

Neurological impairment caused by a burn may be obvious at the time of admission to a burn center or become clinically apparent up to 2 years following the injury. Patients who are considered at risk include those who have sustained an electrical injury, are predisposed to stroke, or who exhibit signs of peripheral neuropathies secondary to thermal damage. Such patients should be closely monitored for signs of progressive neurological deficit. Electromyography studies will chart the development of degenerative peripheral nerve or spinal cord dysfunction. Dysfunction may be demonstrated in the form of paresis, paralysis, tremor, involuntary movement, or ataxia. Individuals who have suffered an electrical injury may develop a condition characterized by progressive degeneration of fine and gross motor coordination. Resultant complications can range from inability to perform work-related tasks safely to an inability to perform the routine activities of daily living. It is a disease process which takes place over a significant period of time, and may worsen after an individual has returned to work. In addition to the motor deficits caused by electrical injury, those individuals in whom a current passed above the level of the clavicle have a high incidence of cataract formation with the first 3 years post-injury.

Aside from electrical injury, peripheral nerve injury can also result from deep to full-thickness burns. Symptoms of sensory deficits and pain from nerve injury include anesthesia, dysesthesia, paresthesia, hyperesthesia, cold intolerance, and an intense, burning pain. However, behavioral and psychological issues can make it difficult to assess a patient's true impairment and disability due to peripheral nerve injury. To minimize the subjectiveness of pain-related impairment, only persistent pain that leads to permanent loss of function, in spite of maximum effort toward medical rehabilitation and physiological adjustment, can be classified as permanent impairment.[2]

Heme and lymphatic

Full-thickness or deeper burns, particularly of the lower extremities, will also cause damage to the lymphatic system. Such injured individuals often demonstrate a lack of normal lymphatic drainage, resulting in chronic edema and the development of stasis ulcers. There can be little or no improvement expected post-healing. External support in the form of elastic garments is necessary to help replace the normal activity of the lymphatic system in reabsorption of fluid. These individuals frequently have difficulty in standing for long periods of time or working in a hot and humid environment.

Digestive system

The digestive system is not usually a problem except in those individuals who have had superior mesenteric artery syndrome, cholecystitis, or peptic ulcer disease during the acute admission. The post-discharge clinical course of these individuals is never predictable; if affected individuals become symptomatic, they should be followed up by a specialist.

Genitourinary system

The genitourinary system may be a problem if deep perineal or buttock burns occurred. Aside from the obvious psychological problems, partial loss of the penis or scarring of the external genitalia may result in difficulty voiding. A badly scarred perineum or buttocks may make sitting in one position for prolonged periods painful and difficult.

Psychological

The advances of surgical techniques involving early excision and grafting as well as the increased ability to prevent infection allow many patients who would otherwise perish to face life shattered by psychological problems as a result of disfigurement. The onset of a thermal injury is a sudden and frightening experience not only to a patient but also to his family members. Because of the unexpected nature of onset, all phases of the patient's lifestyle are abruptly changed. Often, the full emotional impact is not felt until the time a patient is discharged from the protected environment of a hospital. At this time, the reality of the emotional, physical, and financial burden of a thermal injury are apparent and must be faced. The extent to which a person can psychologically deal with his injuries varies, as do individual personalities. Each case is unique and must be evaluated as such. Studies on the psychological adjustment of survivors of burns generally reflect a biased adjustment to moderate injuries. Few quantifiable data are available concerning the psychological well-being of long-term survivors of severe injuries. Although most authors conclude that victims of burns make satisfactory adjustments, others report symptoms of the psychopathological sort which contradict this optimism.[3] Public acceptance is an important problem facing a burn patient. Goffman, in 1963, stated that the way that burn disfigured patients have dealt with the world has generally been shown to be affected by society showing negative responses to visible scars. The burn-disfigured person has to contend with their body image as well as the attitudes of the people and the culture around them. TV and radio have altered not only family standards, but standards of self-perception as well. The young and the beautiful are emphasized. Everyone must be a 'ten'. Patients with burns, like paraplegic or quadriplegic persons, have injuries which can be seen and understood by the public; however, there is also marked ambivalence about a patient with burns as emphasized by the movie industry which has frequently characterized the evil person as being deformed. The 'Phantom of the Opera' is a burn victim, while 'A Nightmare on Elm Street' depicts Freddie Krueger as evil, deformed, and scarred. The burned patient must deal not only with his burn injury but also with society's built-in impressions which are fostered early in life through cartoons, advertising, television, and movies. This is especially important in the pediatric burned patient for whom returning to school can be difficult, to say the least. Recent studies from the Shriners Burns Institutes in Boston and Galveston emphasize that, in pediatric patients with large thermal injuries, most children appear to be satisfied with their quality of life.[4–6] This finding was especially true in children with supportive families who had consistent clinical follow-up and early reintegration into society. However, outcome studies on psychosocial impairment are difficult to assess. It is encouraging to see that the Galveston study reported psychosocial adjustment scores within normal limits, with only diminished social competency skills as issues of concerns among their patient group. Unfortunately, in-depth feelings regarding disfigurement and social integration may not surface with the use of present medical evaluation, and further refining and modification, in addition to our current techniques, may be needed to bring out the latent fears and detrimental feelings in these patients.

Impairment evaluation

The physical examination of a burn victim is much the same as the disability evaluation for any patient. With the information gathered from the history and physical examination, and using the tables in the American Medical Association's Guide to the Evaluation of Permanent Impairment,[2] the physician can arrive at an impairment rating. In addition to the usual range of motion form, a questionnaire regarding the special prob-

lems related to burns is useful (Table 62.1). The American Medical Association's Guide to the Evaluation of Permanent Impairment is difficult, complex, and time-consuming. It is helpful to have members of a rehabilitation department, namely physical therapy and/or occupational therapy, be familiar with this evaluation. A combined approach with either an occupational therapist or a physical therapist to evaluate actual objective determination such as range of motion, and a burn surgeon performing the subjective rating for the skin or psychological status, is useful. The objective measurements due to restriction of active motion and amputations are well outlined in the Guide to the Evaluation of Permanent Impairment. The techniques of measurement are simple, practical, and scientifically sound. For the examination of upper and lower extremities, a large and small portable goniometer are used. The upper extremity, lower extremity, the spine, and the pelvis are considered a unit of the whole person; and tables are available in the manual to determine impairment ratings of the whole person. The subjective rating for skin or psychological determination is not precise. The criteria for evaluating permanent impairment of the skin is divided into five classes:

- *Class I impairment of the whole person is 0–9%.* A patient belongs in class I when (a) signs or symptoms of skin disorder are present, and (b) with treatment, there is no limitation or minimal limitation in the performance of the activity of daily living, although exposure to certain physical and chemical agents might increase limitation temporarily.
- *Class II impairment of the whole person is 10–24%.* A patient belongs in class II when (a) signs and symptoms of skin disorder are present, and (b) intermittent skin treatment is required, and (c) there is limitation in the performance of some of the activities of daily living.
- *Class III impairment of the whole person is 25–54%.* A patient belongs in class III when (a) signs and symptoms of skin disorder are present, and (b) continuous treatment is required, and (c) there is limitation in performance of many of the activities of daily living.
- *Class IV impairment of the whole person is 55–84%.* A patient belongs in class IV when (a) signs and symptoms of skin disorder are constantly present, and (b) continuous treatment is required which may include periodic confinement to the home or other domicile, and (c) there is limitation of performance of many of the activities of daily living.
- *Class V impairment of the whole person is 85–95%.* A patient belongs in class V when (a) signs and symptoms of skin disorder are constantly present, and (b) continuous treatment is required which may include constant confinement to the home or other domicile, and (c) there is limitation of performance of most activities of daily living.

The impairment evaluation is somewhat subjective; however, individual patients can be placed into various categories. The final impairment rating is a combination of the actual objective determinations and the subjective rating for skin and psychological impairment.

TABLE 62.1 PATIENT QUESTIONNAIRE RELATED TO BURN SEQUELAE

Decreased sensation	Yes _____	No _____	Areas involved _____	
Heat intolerance	Yes _____	No _____	Areas involved _____	
Cold intolerance	Yes _____	No _____	Areas involved _____	
Sensitivity to sunlight	Yes _____	No _____	Areas involved _____	
Sensitivity to chemicals	Yes _____	No _____	Areas involved _____	
Area of increased perspiration _____				
Area of decreased perspiration _____				
Restricted chest motion	Yes _____	No _____		
Restricted abdominal motion	Yes _____	No _____		
Loss of hair	Yes _____	No _____		
Loss of nails or malformed nails	Yes _____	No _____		
Dysesthesias	Yes _____	No _____	Where _____	
Hypopigmentation	Yes _____	No _____	Where _____	
Hyperpigmentation	Yes _____	No _____	Where _____	
Drug use	Yes _____	No _____		
Increased alcohol use	Yes _____	No _____	Amount _____	
Donor site scarring	None _____	Minor _____	Moderate _____	Severe _____
Approximate body surface area of donor	_____%			
Gastric pain	Yes _____	No _____		
Joint pain	Yes _____	No _____	Where _____	
Tearing, photophobia	Yes _____	No _____		
Decreased vision	Yes _____	No _____		
Shortness of breath	Yes _____	No _____		
Lack of endurance	Yes _____	No _____		
Hoarseness or other vocal cord problem	Yes _____	No _____	Describe _____	

Functional outcome

Outcome from thermal injury depends upon many factors other than severity of illness; this may include social status, family support, and patient motivation. A determination of impairment combined with disability is an excellent modality to determine outcome. Presently, we perform formal impairment ratings only when asked by insurance companies, social security, worker's compensation, or the legal system. With emphasis on continuous quality improvement and insurance companies evaluating care by outcome determinations, it is important for burn surgeons to document their outcome. Impairment ratings are time consuming; however, they are an excellent way to evaluate outcomes of care. A systematic approach to evaluating outcomes in this manner should be initiated.

Summary

Disability determination is a difficult and by no means objective procedure. It is not within the scope of this chapter to present all the possible complications and resulting impairments secondary to burn injury.[5,7,8] There are certain concepts which must be kept in mind when evaluating a postburn patient for impairment and resulting deformity. Most burn injuries which are significant enough to require admission to a specialized burn care facility will likely result in some type of temporary or permanent disability. Concepts unique to burn patients include:
- the most common complications arise from burn scar contracture and cosmetic deformity, and will require staged surgical procedures for correction;
- rehabilitation may take several years to return a patient to an acceptable level of functioning;
- postburn cosmetic deformity needs to be confined to areas which are socially visible;
- resulting disabilities are not proportional to the extent of cutaneous injury; and
- certain complications, such as neurological degeneration, may not arise until a few years following an injury and are fairly unpredictable.

Many burned patients will have limitations which, individually, fall short of the criteria needed for evaluating disability. It is important to evaluate the comprehensive result of all limiting factors in order to accurately assess the level of disability.

References

1. Warden GD. Burn patients: coming of age, the 1993 Presidential Address of the American Burn Association. J Burn Care Rehabil 1993; 14:581–588.
2. Cocchiarella L, Andersson GBJ, eds. Guides to the evaluation of permanent impairment, 5th edn. Chicago, IL: American Medical Association; 2001.
3. Herndon DN, LeMaster J, Beard S, et al. The quality of life after major thermal injury: an analysis of 12 survivors with greater than 80% total body, 70% third degree burns. J Trauma 1986; 26:609–619.
4. Salisbury RE, Carr-Collins J, eds. Disability evaluation of the thermally injured patient. New York: Rehabilitation Committee, American Burn Association; 1988.
5. Abdullah A, Blakeney P, Hunt R, et al. Visible scars and self-esteem in pediatric patients with burns. J Burn Care Rehabil 1993; 15:164–168.
6. Stolov WC, Clower MR. Handbook of severe disability. Washington, DC: Government Printing Office; 1981.
7. Fisher SV. Disability determination. In: Fisher FV, Helm RA, eds. Comprehensive rehabilitation of burns. Baltimore: Williams and Wilkins; 1984:401–411.
8. Salisbury RE. Burn rehabilitation: our unanswered challenge, the 1992 Presidential Address to the American Burn Association. J Burn Care Rehabil 1992; 13:495–505.

Chapter 63

Cost-containment and outcome measures

Juan P. Barret

Chapter contents

Introduction

Several developments in medicine and burn care have occurred during the last six decades. Patient care, clinical observation, and research have produced important advances in the understanding of the pathophysiology of burns and in the treatment of burn injuries and their complications. As described in the first chapter of this book, the nature of burn injury seemed to require the participation of many different specialties, thus leading to the development of 'burn teams' and 'burn centers'. The result of such collegial effort is state-of-the-art burn care that gathers well-trained personnel with ultimate technology. The drawback of such evolution, though, is complex treatment and a climb in hospital costs. The complexity of burn care in the context of the current health economic era has made outcome measurement, quality assurance, and cost-containment in the burn unit extremely important components of burn care. During the last decade, evidence-based medicine has irrupted in the horizon of outcome measurement and cost-containment in an era of financial restraints and in-depth critical evaluation of the provision of health in modern society. The continuous appraisal that this new approach has introduced in current medicine evidences the lack of available data in many, otherwise, widely accepted therapies.

The present chapter gives an insight into the relevance of outcome measurement as an objective reflection of the quality of care that is provided in burn centers. The development of quality assurance programs is necessary to maintain excellent outcomes while improving cost-containment. Evidence-based burn therapy is reviewed, with a focus on available epidemiological data on approved therapies for the burned population. How programs of quality assurance function and how costs are contained with overall improvement of the quality of care are explained below.

Socioeconomic impact of burns

The first step for any system of self-evaluation and control of the quality of care provided is the recognition of the scope of the problem being evaluated. Incidence and prevalence of the disease or condition investigated are necessary to put the health impact in perspective and to determine the background from which all interventions will be instituted and the efficacy of all treatment or interventions developed to improve or treat the condition or conditions. Data acquisition and epidemiological and statistic treatment of such data are necessary although not always available in the burn population.

Burn injuries continue to plague the economic systems of both developed and underdeveloped countries. In developed countries, severe disabilities secondary to burns produce significant financial losses; in the developing world, loss of life from burns is extremely high. In the United States, there are 1.2 million burns each year, resulting in 60 000 hospitalizations and approximately 6000 deaths. The death toll is highest at the extremes of age; young adults more frequently survive with disabilities that truncate their production in society.[1] Minor burns represent economic loss in the form of sick leaves, and their sequelae sometimes interfere with the productivity of the survivor. Survivors of massive burns are more prone to develop long-term sequelae, and consequences to their families and to society can be devastating.[2,3]

The overall incidence of burns in developed countries is still relatively high, while the numbers of persons who die from burns is remarkably low. It is reported that 820 per 100 000 persons/year are burned, with 30 per 100 000 persons/year requiring specialized treatment. Admissions to burn centers account for 6.5 per 100 000 persons/year. The gross burn mortality in developed countries (people who die at the scene of the accident plus people who die in specialized units) is only 0.6 per 100 000 persons/year. LD_{50} (the body surface area burned that kills 50% of people) in the pediatric population[4,5] and in young adults[6] is over 90% total body surface area (TBSA) full-thickness burns, and over 40% TBSA full-thickness burns in the elderly.[6] Burn mortality indices under 4% are common among inpatient populations.

The social cost of minor burns in developed countries is significant. In Western Europe, these costs, including the loss of production at work of the individual, social security cost, and the cost of the entire treatment, are around 7000 euros. For severe burns, social costs are much higher and are to be estimated over 40 000 euros per patient.[8] These are underestimates because the true social costs of long-term disabilities resulting from burn injuries are not yet well determined.

The impact of even the low burn mortality in developed countries is relevant. Beyond the cost of the acute treatment of these severe injuries are the costs of the permanent loss of the individual's productivity at work, social security costs, and insurance costs. When these costs are added, the estimated cost to society upon losing one middle class worker in Western Europe is around 1.1 million euros.[8]

The world view is more dismal. World statistics put burn injuries to the level of a major health problem. Burns described as 'minor' in developed countries produce severe disabilities and even death in developing countries. There are more than 150 000 fire deaths every year in the world, and approximately 30 000 000 people in the world require admission to specialized units. In developing countries, survival of patients with burns over 40% TBSA burned is minimal.[7]

Outcome measures

Outcome measures are the cornerstone of cost-containment and continuous quality improvement in any given health system. They serve to evaluate what works and what does not; they are used for research and for the improvement of clinical practice and to provide higher-quality care in a cost-effective manner.

For a long time, burn mortality has been considered a major outcome measure of the quality of burn care. With the improved survival rates over the last three decades, virtually all pediatric and young adult burn patients should be considered candidates for survival.[5,9] Improvement in burn mortality has produced a change in the expectations of burn care providers. No longer is survival *per se* a sufficient outcome measure (mortality is being questioned as a true outcome measure in current burn practice[10]), but psychosocial adaptation and physical rehabilitation are of prime importance. Rehabilitation, psychology services, and social support departments are now important members of the burn team. Their care, like that of physicians and nurses, begins with the admission of the patient to the burn center and extends for a long period of time after the patient is discharged. The need for some supportive services may extend throughout the patient's lifetime.

Paralleling the development of modern societies, outcome measurements in healthcare systems focus more on rehabilitation and quality of life than on raw incidence, prevalence, and survival rates. When this principle is applied to trauma and burn care systems, there are four main outcome measurements that are to be considered:
1. Burn mortality (raw and relative mortality).
2. Length of stay (LOS).
3. Modulation of the hypermetabolic response.
4. Quality of life.

Burn mortality

As previously mentioned, burn mortality is still one of the major outcome measures in burn centers. It is the most frequently used measure, the data are easily retrieved, and easy to compare among different centers. Although every burn center has its own particular limitations, it is clear that there exists a minimum standard of burn survival (i.e. LD$_{50}$ of

90% TBSA burned in children and young adults) that should be met given the social and economic situations are provided. In order to achieve the minimal standards of care, it is important to analyze the comparability of results of every burn center. Since local geographic and social parameters vary, the generation of models of probability of death or probit analysis[11,12] with statistical logistic regression[13] has proven useful for surveying the outcome of burn victims (Figure 63.1). It has the benefit of comparability,[11] but it presents also the benefit of internal control of the burn center, since the logistic model represents the standard of care for that given center. The probability for survival that the model assigns to patients represents the minimum standard. Patients admitted to the burn center with a determined burn injury are plotted in the graphic of probit analysis, and are assigned a probability of death. Afterwards, the real outcome of the patient is compared to the probability for that outcome, and disparities are analyzed on a case per case basis. Relevant data for every new patient are introduced into the logistic regression model, so the probability of survival for the following patient is more accurate. Ideally, the probability of survival should increase with time, reflecting the continuous improvement of the quality of care. The responsibility of the burn team is to continuously improve those results and generate new revised models of probit analysis. The advantage of this analysis is that it includes all the particular social and economic situations of the local geographic area, and on the other hand it is comparable with the results of other centers. One of the main disadvantages is that the prediction is based only on age and TBSA burned.

Other indices, such as the abbreviated burn severity index (ABSI),[14] include the patient's sex, depth of the injury, and

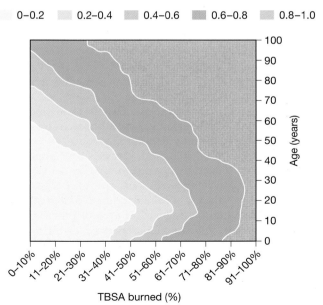

Fig. 63.1 The generation of computer models of death probabilities helps in decision-making and in quality assurance programs. Mortality, though, should not be used alone as an outcome measure, but together with rehabilitation parameters and quality of life.

inhalation injury as risk factors that determine the severity of the burn, achieving a more accurate predictive factor. If additional factors are considered, such as preexisting disease or the abuse of toxic substances, the specificity and sensitivity of the predictors improve.[15] However, even though survival after burn trauma is one of the primary objectives of burn centers, raw mortality and relative mortality (mortality index corrected per age and sex groups in the general population) are no longer the only outcome measures in burn health systems.[10]

Length of stay

Length of stay (number of days admitted to hospital) is a relevant indicator for hospital administrators. It is a direct indicator of cost of treatment and its relevance applies to all patients, regardless of their final outcome. As pointed out by Pereira et al.,[10] data on burn survival have been available for decades, but less information has been published on LOS. Length of stay is an indirect indicator of morbidity (uncomplicated patients should leave hospital sooner than complicated patients), although it must be interpreted with caution. Patients may stay longer for rehabilitation despite being healed completely, or, conversely, patients may be discharged home and readmitted soon after as rehabilitation patients to change insurance coding and reimbursement. The best way to standardize LOS to allow easy access and comparison is to express it as a function of burn size (days/%TBSA). It can then be used as an efficiency of burn care provided, with the ratio below 1 (less than 1 day per 1% burn) as a goal for burn treatment. However, it works very efficiently and as good comparison method for massive burns, but it can produce important bias when considering small burns with specific locations (hands, face, genitalia, feet), depths (deep burns requiring flaps), or age (pediatric or geriatric population). We have to assume that certain populations will stay longer than the 'ideal' ratio and administrators and insurance companies should be aware of that.

Modulation of the hypermetabolic response

Burn patients exhibit a florid inflammatory and hypermetabolic response that is more intense and prolonged than the response of similar critical care and trauma patients. The metabolic rate of a burned person is twice that of an injured one. It causes an hyperdynamic circulatory response with increased body temperature, oxygen and glucose consumption and carbon dioxide production, glycogenolysis, proteolysis, lipolysis and futile substrate cycling. This will lead to wasting of lean body mass, muscle weakness, immunodepression and poor wound healing. It has been an area of intense research in the past decade, and the modulation of this response and the maintenance of lean body mass, a competent immune system, and muscle tone and strength are current outcome measures that can be quantified during hospital course and late in the recovery phase. They are important endpoints that indicate the efficacy of the treatment received and are predictive tools for the assessment of new therapeutic interventions. Furthermore, the modulation of the hypermetabolic response is one of the few areas in burn care with evidenced-based data (see below).

Quality of life measures
Grade of disability

Currently, the grade of disability and the quality of life achieved by burn survivors are also main outcome measures. In modern society, it is not only survival that is important but also the quality of life achieved. Survival at any price may lead to subtotal or total disability, which may be not acceptable for all persons. The latest reports of psychosocial adaptation of patients surviving severe or massive injuries show an optimal response and adaptation in society.[2,3] Moreover, most burn survivors achieve social adjustment that is within normal limits. It is not unusual for people surviving these catastrophic injuries to develop and attain goals such that the resultant quality of life is better than the pre-morbid condition. In other words, some people would never have carried out important and relevant projects in society had the injury not happened. Physical disabilities are certainly common. In particular, patients whose injuries and sequelae are located in important functional areas, such as hands, elbows and feet, present with important restrictions in day-to-day activities. Nevertheless, social adaptation is also good, and some patients develop lives that are very close to 'normal' living. This is particularly true in pediatric patients, whose capacity for adaptation is great. Rehabilitation services, social services, and psychology departments play an important role in the preparation of patients for day-to-day activities and for coping with society in general. These services are involved early on, during the acute phase, and in the overall treatment plan of patients, so that they can help patients through the acute phase and to make a smooth transition to the reintegration into society (Box 63.1). (For more information see 'Organization of Burn Care' In: Barret JP, Herndon DN, eds. A color atlas of burn care. London: WB Saunders; 2001.)

The physical examination of a burn victim is much the same as the disability evaluation for any patient. With history and physical examination, and using the tables of the American Medical Association's Guide to the Evaluation of Permanent Impairment, a rating of impairment can be made.[16] The techniques of measuring, although complex and time-consuming,

---

BOX 63.1 Members of the burn team

- Burn surgeons (plastic surgeons and general surgeons)
- Nurses (ICU, acute and reconstructive wards, scrub nurses, anesthesia nurses)
- Case managers (acute and reconstructive)
- Anesthesiologists (experienced in burn anesthesia)
- Respiratory therapists
- Rehabilitation therapists
- Nutritionists
- Psychosocial experts
- Social workers
- Volunteers
- Microbiologists
- Research nurses
- Support services (secretaries, environmental services, medical records, material management, informatics, technicians, etc.)

Adapted from: Barret JP, Herndon DN, eds. A colour atlas of burn care. London: WB Saunders; 2001.

are practical and scientifically sound. A combined approach, with an occupational or physical therapist who makes the objective determination of physical impairment and a burn surgeon who makes the subjective determinations, is advisable. A systematic approach should be followed, including skin assessment, musculoskeletal system, special senses and speech, respiratory system, cardiovascular system, neurological system, hemic and lymphatic systems, digestive system, genitourinary system, and psychological system. After a thorough assessment has been performed, the patient will be placed in one of the categories for permanent impairment and disability (Box 63.2). This evaluation is very important to determine the outcome of burn patients. Impairment and disability assessments are most relevant for insurance companies, social security, worker's compensation, and the legal system. Since the burn team is not only responsible for the acute care but also for continuous quality improvement and the evaluation of outcome characteristics, disability determination is an integral part of modern burn care. Only with such evaluation can the quality of outcomes be improved.

Quality of life

Although disability and impairment assessment is one of the main outcome measures, it alone does not describe the quality of life that patients achieve after burns are healed and all formal treatment is finished. One of the measures that adapts to healthcare systems is the quality adjusted life years (QALY) introduced by Torrance in 1986.[17] One QALY is a measure of all benefits of health treatment that include increase in life expectancy and enhanced quality of life. The increase in life expectancy is measured in number of years, while quality of life is measured on a scale with a maximum of 1 (perfect health). On this scale, 0 corresponds to death. There are negative numbers, since there are health situations that are considered by patients to be worse than death. The QALY are, therefore, the number of years with perfect health which are also compared to the number of years lived in a specified state of health. For example, if a person lived for 70 years in perfect health and died, they would accomplish 70 QALY. Conversely, if a person lived 45 years in perfect health, and then acquired

chronic renal failure, with a quality of life of 0.4 and died at age 70, they would accomplish 55 QALY [45 QALY + 25(0.4)]. There are two sorts of methods to calculate QALY, the 'standard gamble'[18] and the 'time trade-off'.[19] The second method is the simplest and the most used. Patients are confronted with two situations: the situation of disease and/or sequelae for t years and the situation of perfect health for x years followed by death. The utility of any treatment of a chronic condition is represented by x/t. Life expectancy under a certain chronic condition is compiled from medical literature. This time is converted to QALY under perfect health, and the risks of the medical treatment are then evaluated in terms of the effectiveness in producing QALY.

When QALY are applied to burn patients, it is easy to assume that the treatment of severe injuries, which will result in death without treatment, will produce an important number of QALY. Nevertheless, many burn injuries heal with sequelae, so that the quality of life achieved is not that of perfect health, but sometimes quite less than that. Patients that survive life-threatening injuries acquire a high number of years in terms of life expectancy, whereas the total number of QALY is often less than the optimal number. This is confusing since the overall assessment of quality of life that burn patients express in the long run is usually higher than expected.[2,3] As an example, at the Vall d'Hebron Burn Center in Barcelona, Spain, the overall QALY acquired by all patients (minor and major burns) during 1996, based on an estimation of time trade-off, was 3 QALY per patients.[8] QALY acquired by burn patients were less than expected, especially in severely burned patients. One of the main problems of QALY assessment as a measure of cost-efficacy and cost-utility is that patients tend to make a short-term estimation of life expectancy and quality of life.[20] Burn sequelae are more dramatic in the first months and years after the injury, resulting in a low estimation of QALY.

Other widely used tools are the Short Form 36 (SF-36),[21] that measures global reintegration and socialization and the Vineland Adaptive Behavior Scales – Survey Form,[22] which measures a broad range of functioning in communication, daily living skills, socialization, and motor skills.

Quality assurance

Quality assurance (QA) means a critical appraisal of data collected in the specific system to give assurance to users and to healthcare providers that quality is achieved. Such appraisal should also result in better management, lower complication rates, and better outcomes. The essence of QA is the idea that real quality improvements involve the continuous search for opportunities for all processes to get better.[23] Quality assurance is essential in the modern healthcare system where cost-containment and cost-efficacy are primary endpoints. QA programs provide data to support requests for funding of burn patient care at an appropriate level. They are primordial to suffice the minimal requirements that are to be met by burn centers in order to be endorsed by national societies and state agencies.

The standard QA program is depicted in Figure 63.2 All members of the multidisciplinary burn team (Box 63.1) join together to satisfy common goals and to target all possible

---

BOX 63.2 Categories of burn impairment and disabilities

- Class I: Impairment of 0–10%. No limitation or minimal limitation in the performance of the activity of daily living. Exposure to certain physical and chemical agents might increase limitation temporarily. Skin disorders are present, but no treatment is necessary
- Class II: Impairment of 10–25%. There is limitation in the performance of some of the activities of daily living. Skin disorders are present and intermittent skin treatment is required
- Class III: Impairment of 25–50%. There is limitation in performance of many of the activities of daily living. Skin disorders are present, and continuous treatment is required
- Class IV: Impairment of 55–80%. There is limitation in performance of many of the activities of daily living. Skin disorders are present, and continuous treatment is required, which includes periodic confinement to home or healthcare institution
- Total impairment

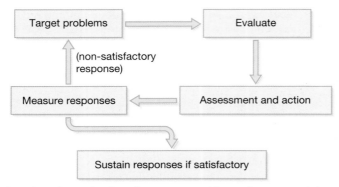

Fig. 63.2 The cycle of quality assurance. The performance of the unit is continuously assessed. When problems are detected, an action is taken after complete evaluation of the situation. The responses and the new performance of the unit are measured again. If the response is deemed adequate, the action is sustained. Should the response not be appropriate, a new cycle begins.

problems encountered in day-to-day work. Should problems arise, an assessment is made; and committees are organized to respond if such a formal response is needed. Actions are carried out in order to solve the problem, and the results of such actions measured. When responses are shown to be effective, the actions and changes in protocols are sustained. Otherwise any new problem that was encountered with the process is targeted for improvement, and actions carried out to address those problems.

Developing a functional QA program requires that the burn team develop clinical protocols and critical care pathways. Although time-consuming at first, this planning saves much time in the long term. Members of the burn team are well acquainted with clinical protocols that begin at the exact time point during patient care. Time points, red flags, and self-stopping parameters are necessary. Protocols are essential for a QA program, since deviations from protocols are easily detected, facilitating evaluation and assessment of the deviations.

Clinical indicators of the overall performance of the unit must be established. It is the responsibility of every member and every department involved in the burn care system to provide the burn team and the QA program with indicators of the well-functioning unit, essentially defining what the unit would be if everything goes very well. Deviation from these performance goals is detected and included in the evaluation system. Outcome measures are the main clinical indicators of the performance of the burn unit as a whole and should be evaluated periodically. Changes in outcomes must be evaluated carefully to detect any malfunction or deviation and develop an appropriate action. Mortality, probit analysis, disability, and quality of life are outcome measures that need to be surveyed constantly. Every specialty involved in burn care must develop their own specific outcome measures that contribute to overall outcome in order to assess, maintain, and constantly improve their contribution to care. Examples of these secondary outcome measures are graft take, pain control, or infection control.

At the Shriners Burns Hospital in Galveston, Texas, QA staff are active and indispensable members of the burn team. Their constant surveillance helps burn patients and burn team

members by assisting to develop protocols and by monitoring achievements according to protocols. They promptly detect deviations so that adequate action can be immediately taken. Their effort assures that no variables will be left to flow without control, so the expected outcome will result. The author finds QA staff to be important back-up aids helping to prevent unwanted surprises.

Finally, QA programs help to maintain cost-efficacy in the burn center. By maintaining outcomes, the investment that society and insurance companies make in the expensive treatment of burn patients is rewarded by provision of state-of-the-art treatment and excellent outcomes. Documentation of such standard of care should result in reimbursement and funding that are maintained if not increased.

Cost-containment in the burn unit

Over the last two decades there has been a continuous change and evolution in health economy. The continuous increase in world population has been joined with an increase in life expectancy, which, along with the decrease in births, has led to an increase in the mean age of population. This is particularly true in developed countries where the population pyramids have reversed their shape. The increasing population of 'elders', along with the economic crisis and the expected increase in costs of healthcare technology and specialists, have provoked an exponential increase in health costs. Economical analysis and cost-containment with an emphasis on cost-efficacy and cost-utility are principal pillars of health economy.

Assessing the maintenance of good outcomes assures that all economic efforts invested in burn centers produce the expected benefits with a positive cost-efficacy effect. Our resources in contemporary society have become limited, so the best outcomes with good cost-efficacy and cost-utility ratios are essential. It is clear that insurance companies and society, in general, seek healthcare systems where less investment still results in the best outcome. It is particularly true in burn centers; reimbursement will peak in centers that provide the best functional outcome in a standard period of time. Contracts flow when good return to productive life is achieved.

Burn treatment presents some particularly relevant differences that make it unique in health economy. In contrast with general costs of tertiary hospital treatments, whose costs peak in human resources, burn treatment costs peak in technology and material costs. These can be as high as 70% of all costs in burn centers, leaving the remaining 30% for wages and salaries of personnel. Materials used in the day-to-day care of burn patients are extremely expensive. However, with cost-containment measures, QA programs, and continuous outcome measures, burn centers can benefit the hospital budget via reimbursement from third-party providers.

In order to maintain a dynamic and viable center, a cost-containment program must be instituted. These programs are defined as all measures directed to produce the best cost-efficacy and -utility ratios; i.e. to maintain costs within expected margins and optimize burn care providing the best outcomes. The main steps of cost-containment programs are:
- data acquisition and outcome measurement;
- treatment protocols; and
- optimization of resources.

Data acquisition and outcome measurement

The first step to control costs in burn centers is the development of a QA program, as previously described, to include data acquisition and outcome measurement. The flow of economic efforts is then bidirectional, from society to patient care and from burn centers to society. All investments made in the burn center are returned to society in the form of excellent outcomes and social reintegration. On the other hand, the knowledge of the most recent outcome figures for the burn unit alert the burn team to know the point of futility of treatment. Expensive efforts to save patients whose burn injuries are fatal increase costs exponentially, decreasing the resources available for other burn patients. It is particularly true in developing countries, where all efforts need to be concentrated only in those patients who will survive.

However, the equal responsibility of the burn team to improve the outcome of burn patients mandates that they push ahead to achieve better survival and better quality of life for their patients. The line that separates futility from constant improvement is vague. The only way to define it and to improve outcomes without increasing futile efforts is with burn research. Experimental and clinical burn research produces new data, which, after critical evaluation of results, will impact and change clinical protocols and pathways.

Evidence-based medicine in burn care

As it has been outlined in previous sections, there has been a burst in wound technology, critical care, and biotechnology during the past two decades. It is not uncommon to be confronted on a daily basis with new technology, pharmaceutical novelties, and expensive new treatments. There has been an exponential improvement in burn care when we compare current survival outcomes with those published 30 years ago. However, paralleling this exponential improvement there is an escalation in treatment expenses, which is not always accompanied by clear data supporting the use of such new technology. In the new era of healthcare, we are confronted with the necessity of providing state-of-the-art burn care while containing burn care expenses. The answer to this ethical and pragmatic dilemma consists of the rationalization of treatment provided supported by clear outcome data. Evidence-based medicine plays a central role in this model of new healthcare, and consists of the provision of treatment based on clear protocols supported by data that warrants cost-efficiency of the therapy used.

Unfortunately, few treatments are evidence-based in burn care, and, most surprisingly, some evidence-based burn care that presents with strong data supporting outcome are not followed by burn practitioners.[24] 'The basis of care should be that simple things should always be performed well.' It is not always so, and even in pre-hospital medicine and accident retrieval we find important differences throughout the world, despite being important outcome data supporting what should be done at the accident scene and transport.[9,25] Another of the few areas where evidence-based burn care has exploded is resuscitation of burn shock. Resuscitation endpoints and monitoring strategies have produced data determining when futility of treatment has been reached, by shifting from fluids and urine output to adequate endpoint monitoring, edema control, adjuvant therapies, and tissue perfusion and oxygenation, supporting the idea that traditional methods of monitoring are not supported by scientific data, and that it should be performed by constant physiological monitoring.[26,27] However, despite emerging data on the necessity of shifting to a more monitor-based resuscitation, most burn centers in the world continue to resuscitate based on tradition and old-based resuscitation formulas. Similar behaviors are encountered in the use of human albumin solutions and hyperbaric oxygen treatment. Strong epidemiological data suggest an increase in mortality with the use of albumin among patients with burns,[28] and the beneficial effect of hyperbaric oxygen in several surgical conditions is an evidence-based therapy.[29] In spite of all this data, albumin is liberally used, and few facilities use hyperbaric oxygen therapy. It seems that tradition and personal belief is stronger that evidence-based therapy in the burn community. A shift in burn treatment towards evidence-based practice is necessary to become cost-effective and provide optimal care.

Treatment protocols and rationalization of pharmaceutical costs

Burn care treatment is expensive. State-of-the-art technology, pharmacological treatments, and skin substitutes are at the top of the price ladder in health treatment. A judicious and clear use of these technologies is clearly indicated for such costs to provide benefit. Clinical protocols and critical care pathways are essential elements to control costs. Protocols and pathways are tools developed after consensus conferences over treatments and diagnostic tests. Experts review the quality and effectiveness of these treatments and techniques, and a consensus is generated about the rationale for the use of old, current, and new technology. Consensus declarations are included in clinical pathways. In this way, well-thoughtout methodology with predicted costs is used to generate outcomes. If no deviations are made and new techniques are not tried without thoughtful consideration, the overall costs of the burn center are contained — provided the annual number of admissions is maintained.

The introduction and testing of new techniques need to be carried out within well-controlled research protocols, and all results need to be critically reviewed. New treatments must be tested versus the standard of care at any given time, and results compared. When better outcomes are achieved with good cost-efficacy results, the new treatment protocol can be general and become standard. As an example, advances that were possible thanks to research supported by the Shriners of North America are prompt eschar excision and immediate wound closure, pressure garments, fluid resuscitation, bacterial translocation control, early enteral nutrition, and improvements in inhalation injury treatment among others. This research was conducted as a comprehensive program of experimental research followed by clinical application in clinical research protocols. Positive results were then applied to routine clinical protocols, improving standard patient care.

Cost-containment, besides QA programs and clinical protocols, is based on rationalization of pharmaceutical costs and optimization of resources. Since more than 60% of all costs in burn centers result from the use of topical and systemic treatments, it is of paramount importance that tight control on the use of such treatments exists. In order to reduce and control costs, it is necessary to use generic drugs in place of trademark (proprietary) drugs when feasible with the same drug activity. The least-expensive trademark should be used when no generic suffices. However, an expensive treatment should be used if such practice reduces the length of hospital stay. For instance, when the treatment of superficial second-degree burns in children is done with Biobrane™, a more expensive treatment alternative than the traditional treatment with 1% silver sulfadiazine, a significant reduction in pain and hospital stay is achieved. Thus, the overall cost of treatment is reduced, and yet there is a significant improvement in outcome.[30] In this situation, the initial treatment with a much more expensive alternative method results in a better outcome, providing a better cost-efficacy ratio.

Optimization of resources

The optimization of resources begins with the organization and calculation of burn unit requirements. In order to calculate the number of personnel required to treat all burns in a determined area, the *method of necessity* is very helpful. To determine the desired number of personnel (RT), one must obtain the catchment population (P), the incidence of burns (I) in persons/year, the number of hours of treatment per day (A), the mean hospital stay in days (L), and the mean number of hours that personnel work in the burn unit (W).[31] The basic formula is as follows:

$$RT = \frac{P \times I \times A \times L}{W}$$

For example, in a geographic area with a population of 5 million people, a raw burn incidence (patients admitted to the burn center) of 6.5 per 100 000 persons/year, and 1 admission per patient per year, a mean hospital stay per patient of 16.5 days with full time (40 hours/week) personnel working a total of 1960 hours per year to provide continuous care of a patient per 24 hours, the total number of personnel required for the complete treatment of burn patients is 65.6, calculated as follows:

$$RT = \frac{\begin{array}{c} 5\,000\,000 \text{ people} \times 6.5/100\,000 \text{ persons}/\text{year} \times \\ 24 \text{ hours} \times 16.5 \text{ days} \end{array}}{1960 \text{ hours}}$$

$$= 65.6$$

The number of beds (NB) dedicated to burn treatment is based on the incidence of burn injuries (I), the mean hospital stay (L), and the ideal index of admissions (IO) estimated as 0.85 (85% of beds used for burn treatment, 15% of beds unoccupied).[32] The formula is as follows:

$$NB = \frac{I \times L}{365 \times IO}$$

When this formula is applied to the same example, the number of beds required are 17.3 beds for a geographic area with 5 000 000 population and a burn incidence (admissions to burn center) of 6.5 per 100 000 persons/year:

$$NB = \frac{5\,000\,000 \text{ people} \times 6.5/100\,000 \text{ persons}/\text{year} \times 16.5 \text{ days}}{365 \times 0.85}$$

$$= 17.3$$

Although all parameters are well known for all countries and the theoretical burn care needs can be calculated with them, it is common knowledge that burn incidence and the index of admissions suffer important oscillations throughout the year. The calculation of an optimal burn center occupation

at 0.85, which is the index for optimal outcome and cost-efficacy, means that the index of admissions may decrease fewer than 40% in certain periods of the year. Even though it does not affect the actual function of the burn center (it does affect if the index is calculated at 1, with periods of bed occupation over 100%), it makes an important impact in cost-containment, since the maintenance of a full functioning burn center with minimal admissions reduces all benefits, and may produce an important financial loss.

In order to optimize the index of occupation of the burn center, and maintain it at 0.85, it is possible to admit patients at the burn center who present with a spectrum of injuries suitable for treatment at the burn center. Given the nature of burn injuries, the burn team is capable of managing patients with a spectrum of trauma and extensive cutaneous or soft-tissue losses. Box 63.3 compiles all patients suitable to be treated at the burn center. Patients that can be successfully treated and benefit from the technology and expertise of the burn team are trauma patients (general multitrauma and neurological trauma, facial trauma), TEN and dermatoses, plastic surgery patients including free flap reconstruction, and chronic wounds. It must be borne in mind, however, that the burn center is a super-specialized unit created for the care of burns, and that, as such, it may be the only facility for such injuries in that particular area. It is imperative to reach a balance between optimal function and cost-containment with optimal treatment of burn injuries. To achieve that, a set of priorities have to be created for admission to the burn center so the treatment of other injuries and patients do not challenge the admission of severe burn injuries. In Box 63.4, all patients suitable for treatment in the burn unit are divided into three types of priorities. Priority 1 patients include all burn patients whose injuries are categorized as major injuries by ABA standards. These patients have priority over all other patients. Patients included in priority 2 are patients who may be treated in other specialized units of the hospital, but also can be treated with the same standard of care in the burn unit and will benefit from care by the burn team. These patients are admitted on a bed availability basis, with the main idea of maintaining an optimal IO. Patients included in priority 3 are patients who do not present with acute injuries but who may

---

BOX 63.3 Patients suitable for treatment in a burn center

- Acute burns
- Rehabilitation and reconstructive burn patients
- Toxic epidermal necrolysis and other life-threatening dermatosis
- Blunt and penetrating trauma patients
- Brain trauma
- Maxillofacial injuries
- Upper and lower limb reconstruction
- Craniofacial surgery
- Free flap reconstruction
- Traumatic soft-tissue avulsions
- Pressure sores
- Chronic wounds
- Diabetic and vascular ulcers

Adapted from: Barret JP, Herndon DN, eds. A colour atlas of burn care. London: WB Saunders; 2001.

BOX 63.4 Priority of admissions to the burn center

PRIORITY 1

1. Severe burns
2. Electrical injuries
3. Burns with inhalation injury
4. Burns in infants
5. Burns in the elderly
6. Burns in patients with chronic or debilitating disease
7. Toxic epidermal necrolysis

PRIORITY 2

1. Multiple blunt or penetrating trauma
2. Brain trauma
3. Maxillofacial injuries
4. Upper and lower limb reconstruction following trauma

PRIORITY 3

1. Free flap surgery
2. Craniofacial surgery
3. Other plastic surgery procedures

Adapted from Barret JP, Herndon DN, eds. A colour atlas of burn care. London: WB Saunders; 2001.

Another important change in modern healthcare is the development of day care programs, i.e. major wound care on an outpatient basis and day surgery. Both types of programs diminish the need of admission to the burn center, thereby decreasing costs and increasing performance. This also allows the treatment of other injuries in the burn center, which increases reimbursement via third-party payers and via the budgets of other departments. Patients who present with burn wounds, even large wounds, that do not need admission for other causes and whose injuries at not at risk of infection at home may be treated as outpatients with daily or periodic dressing changes in the day care unit of the burn center. On the other hand, minor burns, with the advent of new and safer techniques of anesthesia, can be successfully treated surgically in day surgery. These two programs require a strict standardization of protocols so only patients who fit the program are included in the day care unit protocol. Patients must be able to reach the burn center at any time, and all risk factors and warning signs need to be explained verbally and provided in writing to the patient and/or to the person who will take responsibility for the care of the patient. Every effort should be made by the burn team to start a program of day care, since the benefits in patient care, quality of life, and cost-containment are spectacular when the program is fully functioning.

benefit from treatment in the burn center. These patients are admitted as elective cases.

When a conflict arises, i.e. there is a shortage of beds and patients included in priority 1 need to be admitted to the burn center, the priority 1 patients have priority over all other patients. Patients included in priority 3 should be moved to another ward in the hospital, followed by patients included in priority 2 if the need for beds is very acute. (Generally, this occurs in response to a major disaster, and the disaster plan will be activated.) It must be borne in mind that all flow of patients must maintain the required standards of care for all patients. The program of optimization should not be carried out until the required standards of care, as demonstrated via QA programs, can be provided.

Other programs of cost-containment that are very effective in maintaining low costs and improving the quality of care are programs to optimize human resources and programs of day care. Human resources in the burn center can be optimized by planning nurses' shifts. Morning shifts are usually the busiest and 8-hour shifts are the most effective. Therefore, morning shifts can be scheduled with the largest number of nurses, while afternoon and night shifts can be staffed by fewer. On the other hand, nurses' shifts with flow capabilities increase the overall performance of personnel in the burn center. Personnel that can staff the nursing wards, outpatient clinics, and social services provide more freedom in the organization and optimization of resources, diminishing costs in the burn center.

Summary

The relevant socioeconomic impact of burns and the particular characteristics of burn injuries made necessary the development of teams to provide dedicated and specialized treatment of burn injuries. The achievement of total burn care and the current excellent outcomes in burn patients have paralleled a continuous increase in the complexity of treatment of burn victims and concomitant increase in costs of treatment. To contain costs and to prevent decline in standard of treatment, it is necessary to develop clinical protocols providing strict guidelines to healthcare providers. Thus, quality assurance programs are developed. Outcome measurement is also a part of quality improvement, since it is the main indicator of the quality of care that is performed at the burn center. Outcome data are part of the data acquisition of QA programs, and outcomes are also improved by the actions of such programs. The climb in costs must be contained with specific measures following an overall plan and by implementation of evidence-based medicine. QA programs provide the tools to assure that measures to control expenses are applied while maintaining the quality of care so excellent cost-efficacy can be obtained. In the modern era of healthcare management, programs of day care, admission of patients without burn injuries to the center, and optimization of resources (technical and human) are of paramount importance to maintain the gold standard of burn care while containing costs.

References

1. Ramzy PI, Barret JP, Herndon DN. Thermal injury. Crit Care Clin 1999; 15:333–352.
2. Blakeney P, Meyer W III, Robert R, et al. Long-term psychosocial adaptation of children who survive burns involving 80% or greater total body surface area. J Trauma 1998; 44:625–632.
3. Haddadin KJ, Kurdy KA, Haddad AI. Long-term psychological effects of burn unit admission among paediatric patients with minor burns. Ann Burn Fire Dis 1999; 12:168–173.
4. Barret JP, Desai MH, Herndon DN. Survival in paediatric burns involving 100% total body surface area. Ann Burn Fire Dis 1999; 12:139–141.

5. Barret JP, Wolf SE, Desai MH, et al. Cost-efficacy of cultured epidermal autografts in massive pediatric burns. Ann Surg 2000; 231:869–876.

6. Barret JP, Gomez P, Solano I, et al. Epidemiology and mortality of adult burns in Catalonia. Burns 1999; 25:325–330.

7. Munster AM. The 1996 presidential address. Burns of the world. J Burn Care Rehabil 1996; 17:477–484.

8. Barret JP, Solano I. Socio-economic impact of adult burns in Catalonia. Proceedings of the 2nd meeting of the Spanish Burns Association, Barcelona, 1996.

9. Wolf SE, Rose JK, Desai MH, et al. Mortality determinants in massive pediatric burns. Ann Surg 1997; 225:554–559.

10. Pereira C, Murphy K, Herndon D. Outcome measures in burn care. Is mortality dead?. Burns 2004; 30:761–771.

11. Gomez-Cia T, Mallen J, Marquez T, et al. Mortality according to age and burned body surface in the Virgen del Rocio University Hospital. Burns 1999; 25:317–323.

12. Finney DJ. Probit analysis, 3rd edn. Cambridge: Cambridge University Press; 1971.

13. Hosmer DW, Lemeshow S. Applied logistic regression. New York: John Wiley; 1989.

14. Tobiasen J, Hiebert J, Edlich RF. The abbreviated burn severity index. Ann Emerg Med 1982; 11:260–262.

15. Germann G, Barthold U, Lefering R, et al. The impact of risk factors and preexisting conditions on the mortality of burn patients and the precision of predictive admission-scoring systems. Burns 1997; 23:195–203.

16. American Medical Association Committee on Rating of Mental and Physical Impairment. Guide to the evaluation of permanent impairment. Chicago: American Medical Association; 1988.

17. Torrance GW. Measurement of health state utilities for economic appraisal: a review. J Health Econ 1986; 5:1–30.

18. Von Neumann J, Morgenstern D. Theory of games and economic behavior. Princeton: Princeton University Press; 1947.

19. Torrance GW, Thomas WH, Sackett DL. A utility maximation model for evaluation of health care programmes. Health Serv Res 1972; 7:118.

20. Ortun-Rubio V. La economia en sanidad y medicina: instrumentos y limitaciones. Euge, Barcelona; 1991.

21. McHorney CA, Ware JE Jr, Raczek AE. The MOS 36-item short-form health survey (SF-36), II. Med Care 1993; 31:247–263.

22. Sparrow SS, Balla DA, Cicchatti DV. Interview edition survey form manual for the Vineland adaptive behavior scales. Minnesota: American Guidance Service; 1984.

23. Wood FM. Quality assurance in burn patient care: the James Laing Memorial Essay, 1994. Burns 1995; 21:563–568.

24. Childs C. Is there and evidence-based practice for burns?. Burns 1998; 24:29–33.

25. Allison K, Porter K. Consensus on the pre-hospital approach to burns patient management. Injury 2004; 35:734–738.

26. Ahrns KS. Trends in burn resuscitation: shifting the focus from fluids to adequate endpoint monitoring, edema control, and adjuvant therapies. Crit Care Nurs North Am 2004; 16:75–98.

27. Holm C. Resuscitation in shock associated with burns. Tradition or evidence-based medicine? Resuscitation 2000; 44:157–164.

28. Pulimood TB, Park GR. Albumin administration should be avoided in the critically ill. Crit Care 2000; 4:151–155.

29. MacFarlane C, Cronje FS, Benn CA. Hyperbaric oxygen in trauma and surgical emergencies. J R Army Med Corps 2000; 146: 185–190.

30. Barret JP, Dziewulski P, Ramzy PI, et al. Biobrane versus 1% silver sulfadiazine in second degree pediatric burns. Plast Reconstr Surg 2000; 105:62–65.

31. Hornby R, Ray K. Guidelines for health manpower. Geneva: WHO; 1980.

32. Cuervo JL, Varela J, Belenes R. Gestion de Hospitales. Barcelona: Vicens Vives; 1994.

Chapter 64

Management of pain and other discomforts in burned patients

Walter J. Meyer III, David R. Patterson, Mary Jaco, Lee Woodson, and Christopher Thomas

Introduction

The words 'burn injury' trigger, for almost any adult in the world, immediate and vivid images of excruciating pain and suffering. Children are conditioned from early childhood that burn injuries are painful and can cause great harm. Certainly there can be no doubt that complaints of pain are ubiquitous in a burn unit. Burn care professionals should be especially conscious of the management of the pain and suffering endured by their patients. Working to make a patient with burns comfortable is never ending and fraught with frustration. The experience of pain is complex and dependent upon an interaction of dynamic physical and psychological variables. Beecher[1] observed that soldiers burned in battle could perform heroic feats without apparent pain; yet as soon as they were in a safe place their pain was significant. As noted by Choinière the pain expressed by patients with burn injuries varies from day to day and hour to hour (see Figure 64.1).[2] Such fluctuations make it difficult to dose pain medication appropriately so that under- or over-medicating are avoided.

Although pain is not directly observable, it can be inferred from the patient's behavior and physical signs such as blood pressure and pulse of the patient, particularly if that patient is a child. The burn care professional must monitor patient behaviors to determine pain level, be they overt indices such as flinching, crying or screaming, or verbal reports of pain level. More interpretation is required to tease out how much of the discomfort is due to pain and how much is a reflection of fear or anxiety. Adding to this confusion is the fear often

expressed by family members, patients themselves, and even well-trained medical professionals that patients will become addicted to opioid analgesics if they are given 'too much.' Then, just when the professionals seem to have found a good management plan to facilitate comfort for a particular patient, something often changes to upset the balance of factors, and the patient suffers again. Thus, frustrated caregivers understandably might concede defeat to the issue of pain and focus on working to heal the patient with the certain knowledge that, as the patient heals, the pain and other discomforts will also diminish.

Pathology of a burn injury as it relates to pain

All burn injuries are painful. First-degree or very superficial partial-thickness burns may damage only the outer layers of the skin, the epidermis; but they do produce at least mild pain and discomfort, especially when something such as clothing rubs against the burned area. Second-degree or moderate to deep partial-thickness burns result in variable amounts of pain depending on the amount of destruction to the dermis. Superficial dermal burns are the most painful initially. Even the slightest change in air currents moving past the exposed superficial dermis usually causes a patient to experience excruciating pain. Without the protective covering of the epidermis, nerve endings are sensitized and exposed to stimulation. In addition, as the inflammatory response progresses with the increase in swelling and the release of vasoactive substances, pain is increased.[3]

Areas of deeper partial-thickness burns may display a confusing pattern of pain over the first few days. These areas may show little or no response to sharp stimuli such as a pinprick; yet a patient may complain of deep achy pain related to the inflammatory response. These wounds are more similar to full-thickness burns with respect to the pain they cause. In a full-thickness burn, the dermis, with its rich network of nerve endings is completely destroyed. This leads to an initial response of a completely anesthetic wound when a sharp stimulus is present. Yet, patients often complain of a dull or pressure type of pain in these areas. Once the devitalized tissue, i.e. eschar, sloughs and is replaced by granulation tissue, a patient again experiences the sensation of sharp pain to noxious stimuli. It is unclear, but increasingly suspect, that some deep burn injuries carry with them a neuropathic pain component; that is, regenerations of nerves and or nerve damage create a form of pain different from tissue damage

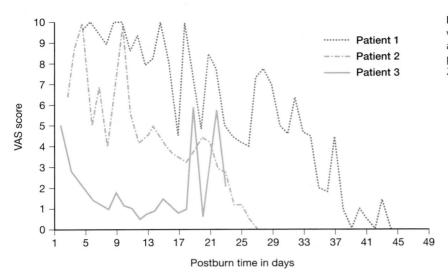

Fig. 64.1 VAS scores for different patients show how variable expressions of pain can be from day to day and from one patient to the next. (Reproduced with permission from: Choinière et al. J Trauma 1989; 29:1531–1539.[2])

known to be a large part of burn injury pain. Two separate patients have described this pain as an insect walking across their skin with spikes on its shoes.

Pain-generating mechanisms during an initial injury

The dearth of information on the mechanisms of pain perception specific to burn injuries leaves many unanswered questions. Some of the best work is that done by Meyer and Campbell[3,4] who attempted to study this in monkeys and humans exposed to a series of thermal stimuli before and after a 53°C 30-second burn to the glabrous skin of the hand. The nociceptors in the skin stimulate both A and C afferents. Both types of fibers are widely distributed in skin and deeper tissues. Their work indicated that the burn injury resulted in increased sensitivity of the A fibers, decreased sensitivity of the C fibers, and increased pain sensitivity (hyperalgesia) in human subjects. This study would suggest that A fibers rather than C fibers are chiefly responsible for the hyperalgesia related to burn injury. Later studies by Coderre and Melzack[5] confirm that burn injuries not only make an injured area and surrounding tissue more painful but also cause hyperalgesia, which is a significant problem for many patients. Sensory nerve damage may also play a role in this difficult-to-treat excessive pain. Burn injury is characterized by release of large amounts of inflamatory factors such as interleukins, which probably add to the perception of pain and the hyperalgesia. The hyperalgesia is further enhanced because the burn wound heals slowly over days or weeks. Some of the various surgical and nonsurgical therapies that are applied to a wound increase pain during the healing phase. Choinière et al.[2] utilized the visual analog scale (VAS) on a daily basis and asked patients to rate their worst pain for each day. Patients' scores varied widely from patient to patient. Even for the same patient, overall pain scores varied widely from day to day, but gradually declined towards the end of hospitalization. In an effort to elucidate the predictor of pain in these patients, Choinière et al. compared pain scores with patient's age, socioeconomic status, and educational level and found no significant correlation. Likewise,

no significant correlation was found between the pain scores and burn size.

When further analysis of the Choinière et al. data included the first-degree areas in total extent of burn and the pain measurements were limited to those obtained during the first week postburn, there was a positive correlation of pain with burn size ($p < 0.02$).[2] In addition they found that pain scores at rest were significantly correlated with extent of first-degree burns ($p < 0.04$) and pain at time of treatments was significantly correlated with extent of second-degree burns ($p < 0.02$). No correlation was found with the extent of third-degree burns. In contrast, Atchison et al.[6] measured pain scores in children and found a significant correlation between pain scores during the procedure and both the extent of total burn injury and the extent of third-degree burn. More recently, Ptacek et al. described the course of pain over 10 days for 47 patients; they found considerable variability over the course of each day.[7] There was a general trend down over days. Psychological factors such as anxiety added greatly to the reporting of pain. Also, persons with large burns showed a higher affective (suffering) component to the pain.

Another source of confusion concerning the amount of pain expressed by burn patients is the role played by psychological problems such as anxiety and depression. Choinière et al.[2] noted that pain at rest was significantly and positively related to levels of anxiety or depression; i.e. with elevated anxiety or depression, pain scores at rest increased. Interestingly, all patients hospitalized more than 3 weeks showed an increase in the depression scores. Although these studies demonstrate the great variability in pain expression in burned patients, they do not identify pain-generating mechanisms, either physiologically or psychologically, in a burn-injured patient. Charlton et al.[8] used the State/Trait Anxiety Inventory to measure anxiety and reported that the study sample of adult burned patients was not particularly anxious. Other studies have suggested that burned patients have increased levels of anxiety, especially related to treatment and outcome, and that these levels may increase over time.[9–11] Anticipation of pain related to treatments that occur at least daily can increase a patient's perception of pain. Anticipatory anxiety related to treatments leads to perception of increased pain, and the increased pain leads to further increases in anxiety. This reaction may explain some findings which suggest that pain increases over time in burned patients.[12–16] Depression also plays a major role in enhancement of pain.[17] Pain leads to depression and depression enhances the perception of pain.[18] In burn care units where very aggressive pain management is practiced, depression is not a major problem.[19] Further work in these areas is needed to better understand the great variability of burn pain.

Pain as a function of the healing process

As a deep dermal or full-thickness burn wound heals, either by primary intention from excision and grafting or by secondary intention through granulation tissue and scar formation, the injured neural tissue is reorganized.[15] Reflex neural function returns to grafted burn skin approximately 5–6 weeks after the burn has been covered by autografted skin.[16] Active vasodilatation, vasoconstriction, and pain sensation all return at this time. These functions also return to the burn wound which heals through scar formation but may take up to 6 months for complete neural reorganization.

Although rare, causalgia, dysesthesia, and phantom pain syndrome can sometimes develop in healing skin. Phantom limb sensation and pain is going to be more common following traumatic amputation, which is usually the case with burn injury. The incidence of these chronic pain syndromes seems to be related to the healing process. Burns that have been excised and grafted on a clean and uniform vascular bed rarely develop one of these chronic pain syndromes. Wounds that heal by granulation and scar formation seem to be more apt to develop a chronic pain problem because of the continued stimulation of nerve fibers in the area with enhancement of the hyperalgesia. Skin biopsies of granulation tissue have clearly shown neuronal tissue entrapment.[16] Pain, in scar tissue, subsides over time as the scar tissue matures.

Types of pain in burned patients during the acute phase of treatment

As already noted, the pain expressed by patients with burn injuries is extremely variable. In many studies, patients have been asked to rate overall pain, pain at rest, overall procedural pain, and worst pain during the procedure. Such perplexing instructions may account for some of the variability in pain reports. For example, if asked to rate one's overall pain for the day, one would expect this rating to include resting pain, pain during normal activity, and pain during painful procedures. A more reasonable approach may be to ask a patient to rate pain as either procedural or non-procedural (background) pain, with each given an operational definition. Procedural pain can be defined as that related to wound care or stretching of the patient's scar tissue, activities that seem to cause the worst pain for burned patients. Background pain is the discomfort experienced at rest or during mild activity. As the therapies for pain management are discussed later in this chapter, the importance of differentiating procedural and background pain will become increasingly clear.

For many years it was thought that infants did not feel pain because of incomplete myelinization of the sensory nerves. Anand and colleagues published data in 1987[20] and 1988[21] to suggest that infants do experience pain as evidenced by a variety of physiological and metabolic responses. Anand and Hickey[22] hypothesize that although A fibers are not completely myelinated and may not be efficient in transmission of pain, unmyelinated C fibers take over the transmission of noxious stimuli. This research has demonstrated the need for pain assessment and management in infants and preverbal children as well as older children.

Measurement of pain in burned patients

Although pain cannot be measured directly, it can be quantified by using one of the standardized tools described below. Using reliable and valid tools allows us to gauge the effectiveness of our treatment for any one patient. Assessing pain on a scheduled basis and using the same tool for each assessment gives us information about how pain is experienced by a single patient throughout the burn treatment; we can note patterns that emerge and schedule medications accordingly. Further, standardized tools allow us to compare pain management of one patient with another as well as one burn unit pain management with that of other burn units in order to determine, for example, the effectiveness of a new protocol for pain management. Another important reason for assessing pain regularly and in a standardized way is that it communicates to the patient that we believe she/he has pain, and we are trying to do something about it. This communication reassures the patient, thereby reducing the likelihood that the patient will escalate pain, anxiety, and other related behaviors.

What is the gold standard for the measurement of pain? Gracely[23] reviewed a number of objective modalities for the measurement of experimental pain. He notes that 'pain arises from and is modulated by, a number of mechanisms. These mechanisms are not static but change over time and involve all levels of the central nervous system. In an attempt to understand these mechanisms, several experimental tools have been employed to further elucidate the exact pathways involved in pain transmission and to better understand the therapies used to relieve pain.'

Some of these tools are: cortical evoked potentials; functional brain imaging (PET or positive emission tomography); functional magnetic resonance imaging (fMRI); source analysis of evoked activity; and electrophysiological recording from the human brain. As noted by Gracely, comparing them with verbal judgments of pain magnitude validates these physiological measures: 'This implicitly elevates subjective judgment to the level of a validation standard.'[23] Clinical measurements of pain must continue to rely on standard subjective measures. A tool to use in the clinical setting must be quick and easy to use and useful for frequently repeated assessments.

A major concern in the clinical setting is the use of a consistent pain measurement tool before and 1–2 hours after the administration of a pain-relieving medication. For procedural pain management, the same tool should be used to measure pain at the beginning of a procedure, during the procedure, and post-procedure in order to measure the effectiveness of the pain management regimen used for procedural pain.

Pain measurement techniques for an adult burned patient

A variety of pain measurement techniques have been used with adult burned patients. The more common measures include adjective scales (Table 64.1), numeric scales (i.e. rating pain on a scale of 0–5, 0–10 or 0–100), and visual analog scales (Figure 64.2). Each of these scales measures the sensory component of a patient's pain. Adjective scales and numeric scales are quick and easy to administer because they do not require a visual representation of the scale. The visual analog scale requires a visual representation of the scale to be presented to a patient. Patients must mark or point to the place on the scale that represents their level of pain. This presents a problem for a burned patient whose hands are burned, so some investigators have used a technique of sliding a line or color strip along the scale with instructions to a patient to direct the movement of the slide, stopping at the point representative of the patient's pain. The visual analog scale has been used in a number of studies with a variety of patient samples and has been shown to be a valid method of measuring the sensory component of a patient's pain. The demonstrated validity of the scale allows for comparisons of visual analog pain assessments between studies with different patient samples.

Motivational-affective and cognitive-evaluative components of pain are most frequently measured using the McGill Pain Questionnaire (MPQ).[24] The MPQ consists of 20 sets of adjectives which describe all three components of pain: sensory, affective, and evaluative. Qualitative profiles and quantitative scores for each dimension as well as a total pain score can be derived from the selected adjectives. The MPQ has been translated into several languages and has been shown to be a reliable and valid measurement tool. Since it takes 10–20 minutes to administer, it may not be as useful for frequent, repeated measurements. Many studies have employed this measurement on a daily basis to measure either overall or resting pain. Gordon et al.,[25] in a prospective multicenter study, asked 40 adult burned patients to rate their pain on 4 scales. These scales were: a visual analog scale, an analog chromatic scale,[26] an adjective scale, and a faces scale.[27] At the end of the study patients were asked to choose their preferred scale. Patients preferred the faces and analog chromatic scales. Although further research is needed to validate these findings, the preference of patients is another variable to be considered.

TABLE 64.1 ADJECTIVE SCALES IN ENGLISH AND SPANISH	
0 No pain	0 Nada de dolor
1 Slight pain	1 Dolor leve (ligero)
2 Moderate pain	2 Dolor moderado
3 Severe pain	3 Dolor severo

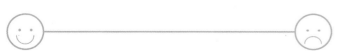

Fig. 64.2 Visual analog scale (VAS) for children to rate their levels of pain. (from the Varni/Thompson Pediatric Pain Questionnaire. with permission from the American Society for Clinical Pharmacology and Therapeutics.[50])

Pain measurement techniques for pediatric burned patients

The measurement of children's pain is much more complex than it is for adults, especially for preverbal children. The American Academy of Pediatrics and the American Pain Society issued a joint statement in 2001 that included the recommendation that in a hospital setting 'ongoing assessment of the presence and severity of pain and the child's response to treatment is essential.'[28] The assessment of pain in children has included physiological measurements, behavioral assessment, and patient reports of pain. The physiological indicators which have been evaluated are heart rate,[29] respiratory rate,[29] blood pressure,[29] endocrine changes,[29,30] and changes in PO_2.[31] None of these shows promise as an indicator for measuring pain in sick children, since all are affected by a variety of stressors, metabolic changes related to a burn, and medications, in addition to pain.

Behavior scales have been devised to measure pain by providing standardized instructions and guidelines for observing behaviors thought to be specific to pain. A number of investigators[32–37] have looked at infants' cries as measurable behaviors that can be observed in order to evaluate pain. Although these studies demonstrate that length of cry, pitch, intensity, and other characteristics of crying may be used to evaluate pain in infants, the analyses of cry are very time consuming and require elaborate audio equipment. Izard et al.,[38] Craig et al.,[39] and Granau and Craig[36] have attempted to code facial expressions as measures of pain in infants. Their system characterizes nine facial actions involved in the expression of pain, but its use requires videotaping and detailed analyses of an infant's facial movements. Although this method offers excellent research applications, it, like the detailed analyses of crying, is too cumbersome and not appropriate for the clinical setting. On the other hand, the studies do provide clinicians with information about various facial actions, as categorized by Granau and Craig, which may be helpful in the clinical identification of pain in infants. Other investigators have devised multidimensional scales that include length of cry, facial expressions, and behavioral states in order to measure pain in infants.[40–42] These scales are easier to use and allow an observer to assess pain as either present or absent without further quantification.

Examples of observational scales which allow for quantification and may be used with toddlers and preverbal children are the CHEOPS (Children's Hospital of Eastern Ontario Pain Scale)[43] and The Observer Scale.[44] The CHEOPS is a scale of six behaviors, each scored on a numeric range; it yields a total numeric score for pain. This scale has been shown to be valid and to have good interrater reliability. The Observer Scale is another standardized instrument that categorizes overall pain or comfort behaviors on a scale of 1–5. The five categories are: laughing, euphoric; happy, contented, playful; calm or asleep; mild-moderate pain — crying, grimacing, restlessness, but can be distracted with toy, food, or parent; and severe pain — crying, screaming, inconsolable.

A burn-specific observational tool was recently developed by Barone et al. at Shriners Hospitals for Children, Cincinnati.[45] The OPAS (Observational Pain Assessment Scale) is useful in children 0–3 years of age. The scale is depicted in Table 64.2.

TABLE 64.2 OBSERVATIONAL PAIN ASSESSMENT SCALE (OPAS)[136]

Observed behavior	0	1	2
Restlessness	Calm, cooperative	Slightly restless, consolable	Very restless agitated, inconsolable
Muscle tension	Relaxed	Slight tenseness	Extreme tenseness
Facial expression	No frowning or grimacing, composed	Slight frowning or grimacing	Constant frowning or grimacing
Vocalization	Normal tone, no sound	Groans, moans, cries out in pain	Cries out, sobs
Wound guarding	No negative response to wound	Reaching/gently touching wound	Grabbing vigorously at wound

Used with permission of authors.
Assess each of the areas identified in the 'observed behavior' column, rating each behavior using 0, 1 or 2 rating. Add the ratings together for each observed behavior. Document your total score.

Research suggests that simple self-report scales can be used with preschool children. Examples of such scales include the Oucher Scale (photographs of children with various facial expressions).[46–48] Drawings of faces[27,49] have also been used with preschool-aged children[50] and school-aged children (8 years).[51] Preschool children have also used the Poker Chip Tool,[52] color scales,[53,54] and a thermometer[54] to report the degree of pain or hurt. These simple tools allow a preschooler to report pain and are easy to use. One caution with the face scales is that a practitioner must help a child differentiate between physical pain and sadness unrelated to pain. Since there is no evidence that any one of these is more valid than another, it is recommended to pick one and use it consistently. When self-report scales are used in conjunction with observational scales, a practitioner gets a better picture of a child's response to pain and pain therapies.

A school-aged child's cognitive development allows more abstract thinking. In addition to the Faces Pain Rating Scales which they enjoy,[55] they can use simple numeric scales, 0–5, in the early school years (ages 7–8)[56] and more complex scales, 0–10 or 0–100, in the later years (age 9–12). Visual analog scales anchored with happy and sad faces[54] and simple adjective scales[54,57] also can be used with this age group. In addition to self-reports of pain, observational scales such as the CHEOPS,[43] or the Procedure Behavior Check List[58] can be used with a school-aged child. Again, the important issue is to use one selected scale consistently since no one has been shown to be more valid than others.

Adolescents can think abstractly and can quantify and qualify phenomena and so can use the same scales as adults. One concern with adolescents is that, when they are ill, they tend to regress and thus may require the use of a simpler scale during such times.[59]

Intubated and sedated children provide more challenges in the assessment of pain. The more disabilities that a child has and the more medications that are being given to the patient creates challenges to the clinician. A 2-year-old child who is blind, with only one extremity that is functioning and on numerous medications, presents a huge assessment challenge to the clinician.

'Pain is what the child says it is' reported McCaffery and Beebe in 1989.[60] What about the case where the nurse documents a lower number than the child says it is because the nurse believes the child is over-rating the score? During a morning assessment while the 10-year-old patient lays in bed,

BOX 64.1 Recommended pain measurement tools for burned patients

INFANTS AND TODDLERS
- OPAS
- CHEOPS[43]
- The Observed Pain Scale

PRESCHOOLER
- Faces Pain Rating Scale[46,47]
- Oucher[41–43]
- Pediatric Pain Questionnaire[50]
- CHEOPS[39]

SCHOOL-AGED CHILD
- Faces Pain Rating Scale[46,47]
- Visual analog
- Numeric scale
- Pediatric Pain Questionnaire[50]
- Procedure Behavior Checklist[54]

ADOLESCENTS AND ADULTS
- Visual analog
- Numeric scales
- Adjective scales
- McGill Questionnare[23]

the nurse asks him to rate his pain on a scale of 1–10 with 10 being the worst possible pain. The child's response is 10. Are we giving the right message if any number other than 10 is documented? Is pain really what the child says it is? In summary, there are many measurement tools for pain assessment across the life span which can be useful to the researcher and the clinician. Box 64.1 presents a list of clinically useful tools according to patient age.

Symptom assessment and management are very important in burn care. The experience of pain may affect the perceptions of other symptoms, including anxiety, fear or itch. Each symptom should be assessed within the context of other symptoms assessments.

Measurement of anxiety

Anxiety is measured in a variety of ways. In 2000, Robert et al. surveyed 64 burn treatment centers to determine how they evaluated and treated anxiety, especially in children.[61] They found that most centers did not use standardized measures of anxiety. Based on that survey and other information, the Shriners Burns Hospital in Galveston has begun using the Fear Thermometer adapted by Silverman and Kurtines[62] from the Walk's Fear Thermometer.[63] That instrument is illustrated in Figure 64.3.

Taal and Faber introduced a tool to measure burn specific pain anxiety (BSPAS).[64] This tool is a 5-item scale used to measure anxiety associated with anticipated procedural pain in adult patients.[65] Initial reliability, validity, and utility studies have been completed.[65,66] A similar tool is needed for children.

Measurement of itching

The severe itching of burn scars and wounds has not been discussed much in the literature, but clinicians can testify that this phenomenon is a very serious problem. Patients who experience such itching often excoriate new grafts or recently healed skin, thus enhancing their susceptibility to infections. When the pruritus is severe, patients can focus on nothing else. Until very recently there have not been any tools for measuring itch. Now, Field et al.[67] reported using a visual analog scale of 1–10 to assess itching. Pat Blakeney and Janet Marvin at the Shriners Burns Hospital in Galveston developed an instrument to measure itch called 'itch man' (Figure 64.4). This instrument was based on a patient's drawing of his experience in the hospital.[68] Children seem to be able to relate to 'itch man,' but validation studies have not been completed. Matheson et al. used a 5-point descriptive itch rating scale in a study comparing effectiveness of shower and bath oil treatments for severe itch.[69] Validation of this tool was not done but it seemed easily understood by the staff and patients. Clearly, validation studies need to be completed on itch measurement scales just as they have been completed on pain and anxiety measurement scales.

Treatment considerations

Once the pain has been assessed and quantified, treatment can be considered. Three modalities of treatment are effective with pain secondary to burn injury: surgical, pharmacological, and behavioral treatment.

Surgical treatment of pain

The pain is predominately related to the open wound. Once the wound is closed, the pain subsides. The use of resection and grafting of open burn wounds significantly reduces the burn pain. Open wounds should be grafted as soon as they are clean enough to do so. Even temporary coverage with cadaver skin or pigskin reduces pain in the area of the burn. In the case of second degree wounds, the use of Biobrane®, OpSite®, Tegaderm® or other wound-covering dressings almost immediately eliminates pain in the burn wound site.[70–73] Duinslaeger et al.[74] compared methods of treatment of open donor sites. Cultured allogeneic keratinocyte sheets accelerated healing and thereby reduced pain and suffering compared to OpSite® treatment. The cultured keratinocyte sheets cut healing time in half. Pain assessment as early as day 3 revealed lower pain scores in those sites treated with keratinocyte sheets.

Pharmacological management of pain

Pharmacological management of burn pain is the mainstay of therapy. General rules are helpful in governing the use of pain medication. The first tenet is that if the patient says he/she is having pain, he/she is suffering. The second tenet is that analgesics are most effective when given on a regular scheduled basis (not 'as needed' or PRN). Thirdly, pain medication should not be given as an intramuscular injection since injections themselves cause pain and anxiety, and almost never present an advantage over other routes of administration. Lastly, dose and type of medication should be reevaluated frequently to make sure pain is continuously controlled and that the patient is experiencing no serious side effects. The dosing of medication should be adjusted for the general clinical condition of the patients, considering factors of nutritional state, shock, sepsis, age extremes, and concurrent illnesses such as hepatitis. Review articles[75–84] during the last 10 years recommend a variety of therapeutic modalities for background and

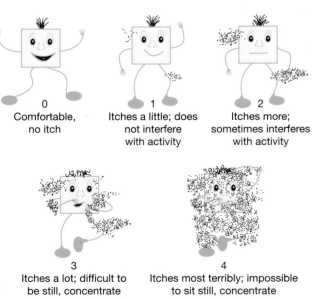

0	1	2
Comfortable, no itch	Itches a little; does not interfere with activity	Itches more; sometimes interferes with activity
3	4	
Itches a lot; difficult to be still, concentrate	Itches most terribly; impossible to sit still, concentrate	

Fig. 64.4 Itch man scale to rate itching intensity in children designed by Blakeney and Marvin.[68] © 2000 Shriners Hospitals for Children. (Reprinted with permission of Shriners Hospitals for Children.)

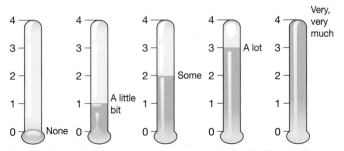

Fig. 64.3 Fear Thermometer to rate anxiety level. (from: Silverman and Kurtines W. Anxiety and phobic disorders: a pragmatic approach. New York: Plenum; 1996 with kind permission of Springer Science and Business Media.[62])

procedural pain during the stages of burn treatment. The three stages are:

- the emergency or resuscitative phase (0–72 hours after injury);
- the acute phase (72 hours to 3 or 5 weeks, until the wounds are closed); and
- the rehabilitative phase (from the time of wound closure to scar maturity), a phase that may last months to years.

Table 64.3 provides a matrix summary of therapies that are recommended for procedural and background pain over the three phases of burn care. A variety of routes or methods of administration are also suggested. The routes or methods recommended include the intravenous bolus (IVB), intravenous continuous infusion (IVCI), patient-controlled analgesia (PCA), and orally administered agents on a time interval rather than pain contingent (non-pain contingent; NPC) basis.

Patterson et al. attempted to examine the question if opioid analgesics PRN (i.e. as needed pain contingent) was better or worse than regularly scheduled opioids for young pediatric patients. The study was inconclusive; he found essentially no difference in pattern of medications administered and pain control.[85] The results were contaminated by a change in practice by the staff when they realized that the scheduled medication could be safely given. This did not require the patient to have pain in order to receive the medication.

Many patients also require anxiolytic medication along with the analgesic medication. Therefore, included in this table are the anxiolytic agents which are suggested for use by several authors.

Emergency phase

For pain management therapy, the emergency or resuscitative phase applies only to patients with burns greater than 10% total body surface area (TBSA). During the emergency phase, the preferred route for most medications is the intravenous route because of potential problems with absorption from the intramuscular site and stomach due to decreased perfusion. Of the agents recommended for the relief of procedural pain, morphine is the most widely used. For procedures, IVB and IVCI are the most common methods of administration used. For extremely painful procedures in both the emergency and acute phase, fentanyl has a major advantage in that it is shorter acting and avoids oversedation following a procedure as might occur with repeated doses of morphine.

In addition to opioid analgesics, anesthetic agents such as ketamine and nitrous oxide may be used for procedural pain. These two agents, along with anxiolytic agents to be used as adjuncts to pain management, will be discussed later in this chapter.

TABLE 64.3 PHARMACOLOGICAL THERAPIES FOR BURN PAIN RELIEF EMERGENT PHASE

EMERGENCY PHASE		
Procedural analgesics	**Background analgesics**	**Anxiolytics**
Morphine (IVB, IVCI)	Morphine (IVCI, PCA)	Diazepam (IV) (Valium)
Meperidine (IVB)	Meperidine (PCA)	Lorazepam (IV) (Ativan)
Fentanyl (IVB, IVCI)	Methadone (PO, NPC)	Midazolam (IV, IVCI) (Versed)
Hydromorphone (IVB, PO) (Dilaudid)		
Nalbuphine (IVB) (Nubain)		
Ketamine (IV) (Ketalar)		
ACUTE PHASE		
Procedural analgesics	**Background analgesics**	**Anxiolytics**
Morphine (IVB, IVCI, PCA)	Morphine (IVCI, PCA)	Diazepam (PO) (Valium)
Roxanol (oral morphine)	Codeine (PO)	
Meperidine (IVB, IM)	Meperidine (IVCI, PCA)	Lorazepam (PO) (Ativan)
Fentanyl (IVB, IM)	Methadone (PO, NPC)	
Hydromorphone (PO) (Dilaudid)	Sustained release morphine (PO, NPC) (MS Contin)	
Nalbuphine (IVB) (Nubain)	Acetaminophen (PO, NPC)	
Ketamine (IV, IM) (Ketalar)	NSAIDs (PO, NPC)	
Oxycodone (PO) (Percocet)	Choline magnesium trisalicylate	
Nitrous oxide (IH)		
REHABILITATIVE PHASE		
For severe pain	**For mild to moderate pain**	**Anxiolytics**
Hydromorphone (PO) (Dilaudid)	Oxycodone (PO) (Percocet)	Diazepam (PO) (Valium)
Fentanyl (transmucosal)	Non-steroidal anti-inflammatory drugs (NSAIDs) with or without narcotics (hydrocone)	Lorazepam (PO) (Ativan)
Morphine (IVB, IVCI, PCA)	Usually not necessary: acetaminophen, NSAIDs	

Acute phase

During the acute phase, the choice of pharmacological agents used to manage procedural pain encompasses a number of orally administered opioid analgesics. To control background pain during the acute phase, the use of PCA of NPC medication regimens are far superior to the PRN method. PRN regimens often result in undermedication by one nurse and overmedication by the next nurse. A patient may become angry and confused about what to expect regarding pain control and may feel realistically helpless in an environment where others decide whether relief is necessary. Allowing a patient to medicate himself as needed usually results in better and smoother pain control as well as better staff and patient relationships. For a burned patient with extensive hand burns, the control cord can be fitted with a padded pedal-type apparatus that can be positioned so that the patient can press it with a foot, elbow, etc. Occasionally, patients will use the highest dose allowed in order to withdraw from the entire treatment setting. If this occurs, confrontation and negotiation are important to get the patient back to the task at hand.

As noted above, we have few studies of the pharmacokinetics of opioids and antianxiety drugs in burned patients. Martyn,[86] in a review of pharmacological studies in burned patients, describes a variety of pathophysiological changes accompanying burn injury which can alter drug deposition. These changes include cardiovascular changes, alteration in renal and hepatic function, and fluctuations in plasma protein concentration, which may render pharmacokinetic studies of non-burned patients not applicable to burned patients. Since it is difficult to predict precisely how drug responses will be altered, it is important to monitor responses on drug levels more closely so that dosage can be titrated to the individual patient's needs.

Ventilator patient

Special consideration should be given to managing the pain of a patient on the respirator. In these patients analgesia must also provide relief from significant discomfort due to the endotracheal tube. If the patient is fighting the respirator and needs to be sedated to provide adequate function of the respirator and prevention of ventilator-induced lung injury,[87] then frequent and high doses of intravenous morphine can be given such as 0.03–0.1 mg/kg every hour or higher in order to ensure pain control with adequate sedation. The use of other forms of sedation without opiates may provide sedation without adequate control of pain. This would lead to being able to assess pain only with blood pressure, pulse rate, and respiratory effort. When muscle relaxants are used to facilitate mechanical ventilation it is necessary to assure that adequate sedation and analgesic medications are continuously administered.

Rehabilitative phase

During the rehabilitative phase, most patients complain more of an aching type of pain, similar to arthritic pain. In this case, mild opioid analgesics, acetaminophen, or non-steroidal anti-inflammatory drugs (NSAIDs) may be used for either procedural (exercise) or background pain. Ibuprofen has been used at 10 mg/kg with some positive effect, but many individuals have gastrointestinal upset with this type of medication. If a procedure will cause severe pain, fentanyl, morphine, hydromorphone, or one of the other oral opiates should be used.

Age of patient and pain management

Since the pharmacological management of burn pain not only spans the phases of burn care but also must be tailored to meet the needs of all age groups, it is important to comment on pain management in both the very young and the elderly. There is a tendency to give less medication to young children because 'they don't complain of pain'. This opinion is supported by the fact that some children become very withdrawn rather than screaming when they are receiving painful stimuli (e.g. abused children). It is unlikely that a burn is any less painful in a 3-month-old infant than in a 30-year-old adult; thus, the same therapeutic modalities adjusted for age and size are appropriate for burned children. A major issue of treating pain in young children is the safety risk of using opiates. One example is a 1998 report of the Seattle group concerning respiratory depression in 3 children treated with standard doses per kilogram of opiates given to other age groups.[88] There has been a similar experience at the Shriners Burns Hospital in Galveston. In all cases the respiratory depression responded well to an opiate antagonist such as naloxone. Young children may have an increased sensitivity to the respiratory depressive effects of opiates.[89]

Many times with children it is very difficult to separate out pain complaints from anxiety, post-traumatic stress or even itching. In this case, the first step is to make sure that the pain medication dose and type is appropriate based on the response of most patients, and that it is actually being administered. After ensuring that the pain medication drug and dosage are adequate, then one can begin to examine carefully for the other associated problems that can mimic pain.

At the other extreme of age is the elderly patient. Again, the tendency is to give less medication, either because these patients do not complain as much or because they are thought to be 'more sensitive' to pain medications. A realistic and important concern with the elderly is oversedation. Studies in non-burned elderly people have shown that, with increased age, the efficiency of the clearance mechanism for certain drugs is decreased, and repeated doses may lead to drug accumulation. This would suggest that, when managing pain in an elderly burned patient, it is not that the dose *per se* should be decreased, but that the interval between dosing should be lengthened so as to prevent accumulation and oversedation.

Neuropathic or phantom pain

Some severely burned patients have partial loss of digits or limbs associated with their burns. This adds a different dimension to the management of their pain since these individuals often have sensations of the existence of these digits or limbs for many years after their loss. This type of pain usually does not respond to traditional pain management with non-steroidal acetaminophen or opioid analgesics. This pain is usually neuropathic in nature, and often does respond to the use of tricyclics or anticonvulsants. Doses of imipramine or amitriptyline of 1 mg/kg body weight often are effective. In a recent study, Thomas et al. reviewed 29 patients who had amputations for either burn or electrical injury.[90] Phantom limb pain was more common in those with electrical injury than following flame injury. Of the 33% who experienced phantom limb pain, all but one patient's pain responded to amitriptyline. If the pain does not respond to this, then carbinazapine might be utilized in doses which are therapeutic for seizures. Recently gabapentin has been used for neuropathic pain with good effect.[91] Over time, this neuropathic pain seems to become more tolerable and slowly dissipates.

Pharmacological agents used in management of pain

The preceding discussion has focused on the reviews and reports of 'how we do it' or the 'bias' of healthcare professionals in treating burn pain. The following focuses on specific pharmacological modalities in burn pain management.

Lidocaine and related agents

Pedersen et al.[92] reported the use of EMLA cream, a prilocaine and lidocaine mixture, to burn wounds in a double-blind randomized manner for 8 hours to reduce pain but it did not reduce late hyperalgesia. Beausang et al. in 1999 recommended adding bupivacaine to the epinephrine solution used in preparing the burn wound eschar site and the grafting site.[93] Their clinical impression was a reduction of pain. In a similar open-label study of 14 teenage patients, a long-acting local anesthetic (bupivacaine up to 1.9 mg/kg) was infiltrated into their donor sites to reduce pain.[94] Bupivacaine plasma levels were monitored and found to peak around 8 hours later and stay in a very safe range. Bussolin et al. used a 0.05–0.1% lidocaine with 1:1 000 000 epinephrine solution as a tumescent local anesthesia up to a maximum dose of lidocaine of 7 mg/kg to infiltrate into the operative area of both the burn excision and the donor sites.[95] The postoperative pain was essentially non-existent when compared to pain in historic controls who required opiates and/or ketamine to control their pain.

Sympathetic nerve blocks with the same medication are effective for blocking thermal pain.[96] Cuignet et al. showed with a double-blind design that facia iliaca compartment block with ropivacaine was very effective in reducing pain at thigh donor sites for burn grafting.[97] Other similar medications such as lidocaine (1 mg/kg) given intravenously has been reported to cause significant relief of pain for up to 3 days.[98] Similiarly, Cassuto and Tarnow used intravenous lidocaine for generalized pain control without oversedation.[99] Seizures have been reported following the use of this class of medication even when given topically.[100]

One additional issue concerning procedures is the amount of pain created from removing a dressing over the burned area. These removals are usually facilitated by soaking the dressings off but the soaks are sometimes painful. Special dressings such as lipidocolloid dressing[101] and moist exposed burn ointment dressing[102] are being developed to reduce that pain.

Opioid analgesics

Of these agents, morphine has continued to be the mainstay for both background and procedural pain management. Long-term use of morphine has several inherent problems. Morphine binds to more than one receptor class. Morphine use is associated with side effects (respiratory depression and constipation) that limit its use. An additional problem is the rapid development of tolerance to morphine and poor pain control that is seen in a small group of burn patients. Tolerance to morphine is associated with activation of central glutamate pathways (NMDA receptors) and hyperalgesia. Changing to other opiates, such as methadone, or other compounds, such as ketamine, which block the NMDA receptor pathways improves the management of pain no longer controlled with morphine.[103,104,179] In fact each opiate binds a slightly different pattern of receptors, and therefore it is often useful to rotate opiates in the long-term patient to keep control over the pain.

Other opiates such as hydromorphone (Dilaudid), levorphanol (Levo-Dromoran), fentanyl, and methadone are all excellent oral agents for the relief of moderate to severe pain when given in equianalgesic doses to morphine. Fentanyl comes in a convenient flavored oralet, especially attractive for use with children. The period of peak hydromorphone effect varies widely from 45 to 90 minutes; the combination of lorazepam given 1 hour alone or with hydromorphone given 45–60 minutes before a procedure results in reasonable pain control for the majority of adult patients. As with other opioid analgesics, tolerance may develop rapidly, so the dose of hydromorphone may need to be adjusted frequently. Methadone has a longer half-life than morphine and therefore can provide coverage for a longer time between doses. Also methadone has been noted to give smoother pain relief for children postoperatively than morphine.[105] Methadone is different from morphine both pharmacokinetically and pharmacodynmically. In addition to opioid receptor interaction, methadone also possesses NMDA receptor antagonism activity as well as amine uptake inhibition (similar to imipramine). Methadone has been reported to be effective in patients tolerant to and poorly controlled by morphine. In addition, methadone is a fraction of the cost of most other opioid analgesics.[106] Perry and Inturrisi[107] reported that the pharmacokinetics of morphine in patients with burn injuries were not significantly altered in comparison to non-burned individuals. They found that the $t_{1/2a}$ (apparent distribution half-life in minutes) was 4.3 ± 3.4 (SD) in burned patients vs. $t_{1/2a}$ 1.7 ± 1.2 in normal subjects and that the $t_{1/2b}$ (apparent elimination half-life in minutes) was 98.8 ± 20.8 (SD) in burned patients vs. 176.8 ± 70.3 in normal subjects. Likewise, the apparent central volume of distribution, clearance, hepatic extraction, and plasma binding were similar for burned patients and normals. Osgood and Syzfelbein[108] described a group of acutely burned children in whom the distribution and elimination half-lifes of morphine were markedly shortened [$t_{1/2a} = 1.2 \pm 0.39$ (SEM) for burned children vs. 2.2 ± 0.49 minutes in normals; $t_{1/2b} = 36.9 \pm 6.40$ for burned children vs. 126 ± 38.18 minutes in normals ($p < 0.05$)].

Bloedow et al.[109] reported on the pharmacokinetics of meperidine in 11 acute patients (1 week post-injury) and in 5 convalescent patients with burn injuries (about 6 weeks postburn). The meperidine steady-state distribution volume (L/kg) during both the acute and convalescent phases was about half the distribution volume reported in the literature for meperidine in healthy subjects. The meperidine clearance in burned patients (acute 420 mL/min and convalescent 600 mL/min) was slower than would be anticipated in the presence of known marked increases in hepatic blood flow in burned patients.

Pain associated with dressing change is very important to manage well. In a randomized double-blind placebo-controlled study of 26 adults, Finn et al. concluded that intranasal fentanyl was as effective and safe as oral morphine.[110] Also Prakash et al. recently reported using PCA with fentanyl as an effective alternative.[111]

From the published literature concerning the use of opioids in patients with burn injury, one would have difficulty making decisions about the best drug, the best dosage range, or the best route or method (i.e. PCA, PRN, or continuous infusion) of administration of these drugs.[107–114] Morphine or other opioid analgesics are considered mainstays of pain relief for burned patients, but many reviewers report less than adequate pain relief for burned patients with the use of such agents. The line between enough opioid analgesics to provide pain relief and too much causing respiratory depression is difficult to find. Also experience of the authors has shown that even a PCA regimen must be individualized and frequently adjusted. Important caveats for the use of PCA should include:

- an initial bolus in adults of 0.1mg/kg of morphine or equivalent dose of other drugs;
- increasing the patient-controlled dose as needed to achieve pain relief (recognizing that tolerance develops at varying rates in individual patients);
- planning for a change in dosing regimens at night to include: (a) giving a bolus dose at bedtime; (b) doubling the patient-controlled dose and lengthening the time interval between doses so that when a patient awakens in pain, he or she does not have to lie awake to push a button several times in order to get adequate medication; and (c) if the increased intermittent dosing is not adequate, being lenient with bolus doses or to start a patient on a continuous morphine drip at night.

The role of synthetic opioid analgesics such as fentanyl deserves special notice. It is becoming more popular since transmucosal fentanyl citrate is now available in a flavored oralet. Fentanyl has desirable pharmacokinetic properties because it acts rapidly, has short duration, and involves no histamine release. It can cause some emesis, however, even with the fentanyl lozenges.[115] In non-burned patients the pharmacokinetic data show great variability, especially with the parent compound fentanyl.[116] Thus, further pharmacokinetic studies, in non-burned as well as burned patients, need to be completed in order to better understand the efficacy and safety of this class of drugs. In 1998, Sharar et al. did a double-blind study comparing their use at a fentanyl dose of 10µg/kg with the more classic oral hydromorphone (60µg/kg).[117] They found in a double-blind crossover design study that the fentanyl oralets provided safe and effective control of pain. In fact, the pain scores were improved before wound care and anxiolysis was improved during wound care; at other times, the two treatments were identical. Robert et al. confirmed these findings with a study of 8 children and similar design.[118] Later, Sharar's group compared oral transmucosal fentanyl citrate with oral oxycodone and again found the oral transmucosal fentanyl superior.[119]

α₂ Adrenergic agonists

Recent years have witnessed a dramatic increase in the use of α_2 adrenergic agonists (clonidine and dexmedetomidine) for their sedative, anxiolytic, analgesic, and sympatholytic properties. Noradrenergic pathways within the locus ceruleus of the brainstem help regulate vigilance, wakefulness, and sleep. The locus ceruleus contains one of the highest densities of α_2 adrenergic receptors in the body. Administration of α_2 adrenergic agonists produces decreased brainstem norepinephrine turnover, resulting in increased activity of inhibitory (GABA) neurons, which mediates the sedative and anxiolytic effect of these drugs.[120,121] α_2 Adrenergic agonists are potent anxiolytics and have been used effectively to treat post-traumatic stress syndrome.[122] Clonidine is also used in controlling attention deficit disorder.[123]

α_2 Adrenergic agonists can produce profound analgesia through central mechanisms.[124] Clonidine and dexmedetomidine have both been found to reduce anesthetic and postoperative analgesic requirements.[120,121] Dexmedetomidine has been found effective as the sole analgesic in ventilated postoperative patients.[125,126] Orally administered dexmedetomidine (2.5µg/kg given 20–30 minutes pre-procedure) produced suitable sedation and allowed placement of peripheral venous catheters in pediatric patients with neurobehavioral problems.[127] Clonidine is useful in pain and anxiety management, either alone or in conjunction with opioids.[128–130] It has the advantage of not causing pruritus or respiratory depression. Much data exist concerning its use in adults and children in the preoperative and postoperative setting.[131–133] Dexmedetomidine has been used to facilitate withdrawal of opioids in critically ill patients.[134] When administered in higher doses, dexmedetomidine has been used by itself as a general anesthetic.[135]

These drugs are distinguished by several unique features. Profound sedation is possible with minimal effects on respiration.[135] Patients sedated with dexmedetomidine can often be aroused. The α_2 adrenergic agonists are not controlled substances and there are no reports of substance abuse with clonidine or dexmedetomidine. Use in the ICU has not been associated with withdrawal symptoms even when dexmedetomidine was infused for up to 168 hours at 0.21–0.49µg/kg/h.

A combination of ketamine and an α_2 adrenergic agonist is particularly effective for procedures. The analgesic effect of ketamine is enhanced by the α_2 adrenergic agonist, allowing lower ketamine doses while at the same time increased heart rate and blood pressure produced by ketamine are moderated.[137] Clonidine has also been found to reduce emergence problems associated with ketamine sedation.[138]

In most burn patients a combination of morphine and a benzodiazepine (e.g. lorazepam) is effective in providing sedation and analgesia in patients with acute burns. Occasionally, burn patients are poorly controlled with morphine despite geometric increases in doses. In these cases rapidly developing tolerance and a hyperalgesic state make pain management difficult. Clonidine or dexmedetomidine have been found effective in such clinical situations and provided suitable sedation and dramatic reductions in morphine dose.[139,140]

In our institution pediatric burn patients poorly controlled with morphine and lorazepam have been found to respond to orally administered (nasogastric tube) clonidine in doses of 2–5 μg/kg (unpublished observations). When more profound sedation of intubated patients is required we have used continuous infusion of dexmedetomidine 0.3–0.7 μg/kg/h after a loading dose of 1 μg/kg intravenously over several minutes.

Non-steroidal anti-inflammatory drugs

Two reports[141,142] were found concerning the use of NSAIDs in burned patients. Neither of these studies reported on the use of NSAIDs for pain management, but one study by Wallace et al.[141] reported a significant reduction in body temperature (0.67°C ($p <0.01$)) and a decrease in metabolic rate (11.4%; $p <0.01$) with the administration of ibuprofen, suggesting that this drug may attenuate the metabolic response to thermal injury by blunting the temperature elevation associated with burn injuries. The second study of the pharmacokinetics of ibuprofen when given enterally to burned patients reports the half-life to vary from 1.4 to 5.1 hours, depending on whether the drug was given by enteral tube with tube feeding ($t_m = 1$ hour) or orally with a regular diet ($t_m = 5.1$ hours).[143] Although ibuprofen was not given for pain control in either study, the results might lead one to ask, concerning the first study, was the decrease in metabolic rate solely related to a decrease in body temperature or was some of the effect a result of better pain control? The second study is important if one is going to use ibuprofen as part of pain management regimen. The results would suggest that different dosing schedules might be necessary if a patient is receiving tube feedings or a regular diet. Non-steroidals, such as ibuprofen, have, in addition to analgesic effects, anti-inflammatory activity, which, in some instances, may be advantageous due to the ability to inhibit prostaglandin biosynthesis. This activity is, however, directly associated with some of the side effects of these drugs which include gastrointestinal bleeding, hypertension, and congestive heart failure. There is disagreement between providers concerning the risk of bleeding from grafts.

Acetam inophen

Because of the significant side-effect profile of non-steroidal and anti-inflammatory drugs such as ibuprofen, acetaminophen has been considered for the management of chronic pain. In 1991, Bradley et al. reported that acetaminophen at a dose of 10–15 mg per kg of body weight given every 4 hours (up to a maximum of 4000 mg/day) was equal in efficacy to ibuprofen at a dose of 10 mg/kg of body weight given every 4 hours (up to a maximum of 2400 mg/day).[143] In addition, acetaminophen is well tolerated and causes almost no side effects, most particularly gastrointestinal side effects as with ibuprofen. There is some concern about long-term liver problems with this medication when used in high doses such that blood levels reach 50 μg/mL.[144]

Meyer at al.,[145] at the Shriners Burns Hospital in Galveston, reported an analysis of 395 consecutive acutely burned pediatric patients who were treated in 1993 and 1994 with a pain management protocol that utilized acetaminophen scheduled at 15 mg/kg every 4 hours as background management with morphine added for breakthrough pain and procedures such as tubbing. The best response was with the younger children

and the smaller burns. Acetaminophen can be easily monitored in the blood, and in the authors' experience, 15 mg/kg every 4 hours did not cause blood levels to exceed 10 μg/mL except in very young children or extremely ill children receiving multiple types of other medications that are metabolized by the liver. One should be aware that, because acetaminophen is packaged in conjunction with hydrocodone in the form of Vicodin® and Loratab®, one should be careful *not* to give acetaminophen in addition to either one of these combination medications.

Medications for anxiety

As mentioned above, anxiety medication should be considered *only* after the patient's pain has been aggressively treated. The medical staff can inappropriately attribute the patient's complaint to anxiety ('just anxious' is a frequently used phrase) when, in fact, the patient is really experiencing pain. The three main antianxiety drugs used in the treatment of burn-related anxiety are lorazepam, diazepam, and midazolam.

Martyn et al.[146] studied the pharmacokinetics of lorazepam in burned patients. After a single dose, there was a rapid decline in concentration due to the high lipid solubility and rapid tissue uptake, leading to a shorter hypnotic effect of the drug. The study compared burned patients to controls matched for age and weight. Interestingly, the elimination half-life was significantly prolonged for burned patients (72 hours vs. 36 hours for control subjects). Therefore, burn patients often need higher than expected doses. Thus, with repeated administration, the tissue could become saturated and then the termination of the effect would depend more on biotransformation by hepatic enzymes. Hepatic enzyme activity has been shown to be quite depressed in patients with burn injuries. Patterson et al.[147] reported that, in a double-blind placebo-controlled study of 79 patients, 1 mg lorazepam did significantly reduce procedural pain ratings in those patients with high baseline pain, but did not reduce baseline trait anxiety.

Based on Martyn's work, we would conclude that lorazepam would be superior to diazepam in treating anxiety in burned patients.[146] Martyn suggests that, in addition to the fact that the clearance of lorazepam is faster than diazepam in burned patients, two other features of lorazepam make it a more acceptable drug for burned patients. First, it is metabolized by conjugation (a cytochrome P450-independent pathway) to a pharmacologically inactive glucuronide metabolite; and, secondly, the unbound volume of distribution is much less than for diazepam that causes clinically effective blood concentrations to persist for many hours, resulting in longer-lasting sedation. Additionally, unlike diazepam, lorazepam is not affected by the concomitant administration of cimetidine. In a recent survey of the use of antianxiety drugs in burned children, 72% received lorazepam at a dose of 0.03–0.05 mg/kg or higher every 4 hours for much of their initial hospitalization.[84] Lorazepam provided aid in anxiety control with essentially no side effects. Fewer than 1% of the children had hallucinations or delirium associated with rapid changes in dose. The occasional child responds with increased agitation or delirium rather than sedation, an occurrence we have also noticed infrequently.[148]

Although the pharmacokinetics of midazolam have not been reported in burned patients, it has characteristics in non-burned patients that would seem to make it an attractive anxiolytic agent for procedures used to clean burn wounds for those with thermal injury. Midazolam has a more rapid onset than either diazepam or lorazepam; thus, it allows for more rapid titration for effect in an individual patient. The elimination half-life of 2.5 hours is considerably shorter than that of lorazepam (13 hours) or diazepam (36 hours) and should result in a shorter recovery time after a procedure.[149] It is better tolerated when given intravenously. The oral dose is very high and expensive. The anesthetic effect of midazolam is greater than diazepam.[150,151] Elderly patients have a more consistent response to a given dose.[152] Of the three benzodiazepines reviewed, either lorazepam or midazolam would seem to be more appropriate than diazepam for repeated use in burn care. However, in our experience, we have found diazepam to be very useful in providing background anxiety control when muscle relaxation is desired (for example, to facilitate rehabilitative exercise) in addition to attenuating anxiety. Because of its long half-life, it is ideal for treating the patient during the rehabilitative period when the healing burn wound is very uncomfortable and seems to inhibit doing any activities, including sleep.

Anesthetic agents used in analgesic doses for procedural pain

Nitrous oxide

Nitrous oxide analgesia is now being used in pediatric surgery as an effective alternative to other forms of sedation.[153] To make it safer, a preset mixture of nitrous oxide and oxygen (Nitonox®) has been developed and shown to be effective in a variety of painful procedures.[154] Filkin et al.[155] reported results from both a retrospective study and a prospective study on the use of 50% nitrous oxide and 50% oxygen for debridement pain. In the retrospective study, the charts of 52 adult male patients, mean TBSA 19% (range 2–85%), were reviewed for the number of treatments, the effectiveness of pain relief, and the frequency of side effects. Only one patient reported no pain relief and requested to discontinue the use of the nitrous oxide. Side effects noted were dizziness, giddiness, increased verbalizations, euphoria, dream-like state, nausea, and non-specific tremors, but they were clinically significant in only two patients. In the prospective double-blind study, all patients were given a standard dose of morphine (0.2 mg/kg) pre-procedure and then randomized to receive either a 50% nitrous oxide–50% oxygen mixture or compressed air for a given study treatment. The study was aborted when 80% of the planned 30 patients requested to withdraw from the study because they did not feel that they were getting consistent pain relief on study days, preferring to use nitrous oxide for all treatments.

A retrospective study by Marvin,[156] in which charts from 130 patients (65 who received nitrous oxide and 65 patients matched for % TBSA burned who did not) were reviewed, found excellent patient acceptance and few side effects. In the study by Marvin, the frequency of specific side effects related to peripheral neuropathy, changes in liver function, and anemia were noted; no patient in either group showed changes in liver function tests while receiving the nitrous oxide mixture. None

of these disorders were similar to the polyneuropathies previously reported in relation to chronic nitrous oxide exposure.[157–160] Hayden et al.[160] reported one case of progressive myeloneuropathy in burns related to the use of nitrous oxide. The PRN use reported for this patient varies from the once- or twice-daily use reported by Basket,[161,162] Filkin,[155] and Marvin.[156] It would seem from the report that the patient consumed vastly larger doses. This may well explain the neurological problems seen in this case, which were similar to those described with chronic abuse of nitrous oxide.[157–160]

The major drawback to the use of nitrous oxide has been its possible toxicity to the staff administering the medication. Adequate gas scavenging equipment should be available to reduce trace gas exposure to caregivers. This is particularly important for pregnant caregivers, since in animals it has been documented to cause spontaneous abortion.[163,164]

Ketamine

Ketamine is used often with children to manage their pain, particularly for protracted wound debridement. Ketamine also blocks the NMDA receptor which mediates the hyperalgesia associated with morphine tolerance. Therefore it is effective in morphine-tolerant patients. The route of administration has been usually oral, IV or IM. In general it is best to avoid IM injections in treating a child since that causes initial pain. Recently Heinrich et al. has suggested rectal administration in conjunction with midazolam.[165] In adults and adolescent males, ketamine causes considerable dysphoria with unpleasant hallucinations and flashbacks even after complete recovery. However, it is very safe because it preserves airway reflexes. In children, these side effects occur much less often. Simultaneous administration of benzodiazpines seems to reduce these side effects.

Slogoff et al.[166] reported their clinical experience with the use of subanesthetic doses of ketamine for 150 debridement and dressing change procedures in 40 burned patients. Fourteen patients had only one exposure and the remainder had 2–13 exposures. The initial dose was 1.6 mg/kg of ketamine given intravenously. The results showed that patients with one or two exposures had coherent conversation or no vocalization 60% of the time; screaming or vocalization unrelated to stimulation occurred 34% of the time; and vocalizations in response to stimulation, 5%. In the group that received two or more exposures, coherent vocalizations dropped to 40%, while screaming or vocalization unrelated to stimulation increased to 49%; and vocalizations related to stimulation increased to 11%. Involuntary movement was rare in either group: 7% in <2 exposures and 8% in >2 exposures. One patient developed upper airway obstruction, which responded to manipulation of the mandible, and one patient experienced unpleasant emergence reactions after each of four procedures but did not refuse further treatment with ketamine. Significant findings in this study were:

- all patients who had more than two procedures required higher doses ($p < 0.001$);
- the duration of analgesia per dose, min/mg/kg, was less with subsequent doses ($p < 0.001$); and
- the time to complete orientation was less with subsequent doses ($p < 0.01$).

With the increase in dosage after the second exposure, the actual time of analgesia remained constant at about 15 minutes. All patients had complete amnesia for all procedures.

Martinez et al.[167] described a dream state of burned patients treated with ketamine for dressing changes. Twelve of 15 subjects stated that they experienced dreams while under the effects of ketamine. Eight of the 12 described their dreams as pleasant. Subjects were also asked to rate their ketamine experience according to a list of descriptions: seven chose 'frightening', eleven chose 'floating', two chose 'beautiful', eight chose 'helpless', two chose 'powerful', and eleven chose 'confusing'.

Several protocols for the use of ketamine in burned patients have been published.[168–170] Some use nurse-administered intramuscular ketamine 2–3 mg/kg body weight for dressing changes under the order and immediate supervision of a physician.[168] Others use ketamine as an anesthetic, not an analgesic agent.[169] The doses used were 1–2 mg/kg body weight, intravenously, or 8–10 mg/kg body weight given intramuscularly. The procedures required administration by an anesthesiologist. Some use low-dose (1–3 mg/kg body weight) of ketamine administered rectally or orally to produce short periods of analgesia (5–30 minutes) for dressing changes. Repeated use may produce tolerance, so increased doses are required over time. The side effects of ketamine include the production of copious upper airway secretions (necessitating the use of drying agents: atropine or glycopyrrolate), hypertension, pulmonary and systemic arterial hypertension, tachycardia, and postoperative emergency reactions. Ketamine is contraindicated for patients with systemic or pulmonary arterial hypertension, myocardial infarction, ventricular failure, history of cerebral injuries, or psychiatric disorders. Ketamine can produce hallucinations post administration, particularly in adolescent boys. Simultaneous administration of benzodiazepines are thought to reduce this side effect.

More recently, Dimick et al.[171] reported on the use of anesthesia-assisted procedures in burned patients. They reported on 109 procedures in 46 patients for staple removal from grafts (34 procedures), massive dressing changes or vigorous debridement (74 procedures), or facial moulage (one procedure). Within 2 hours after the procedure, 72% of patients were able to cooperate fully; and within 4 hours, all were able to cooperate fully. They concluded that anesthesia-assisted procedures in a burn intensive care unit could be performed safely with appropriate professional care and monitoring.

Propofol (Diprivan®)

Propofol is a non-barbiturate hypnotic agent without analgesic activity.[172] It is administered intravenously and is most commonly used as a general anesthesia induction agent. Since it lacks analgesic activity, propofol must be given in doses large enough to cause loss of consciousness to prevent response to painful procedures. It has also been given by continuous infusion in combination with analgesics such as opiates or ketamine. Coimbra et al. reported its use as an adjunct to morphine in a patient-controlled sedation protocol for dressing changes.[173] They used bispectral index monitoring to follow the patients and found it to provide a safe level of sedation/unconsciousness. It is particularly useful for sedation

and pain control during procedures such as line placement or staple removal. Its onset of action is extremely rapid even with a dose as low as 1.5 mg/kg intravenously.[174,175] Having non-anesthesiologists administer propofol is not considered a safe practice in some institutions because if depresses blood pressure, respiratory effort, and decreases airway tone and reflexes. Propofol is considered highly effective for procedural sedation. Its use is still approved in the operating room for anesthesia and it is widely used in the ICU for ordinary procedures when proper precautions for airway management are assured.[176]

Advantages include a rapid onset of action and a rapid emergence with little cumulative effect after prolonged infusion periods.[177,178] In addition, there are no reports of drug dependence associated with propofol and, because its abuse liability is low, propofol is not a controlled substance.

Disadvantages include pain on injection. Along with loss of consciousness, propofol causes loss of pharyngeal motor tone which often causes airway occlusion.[179] Propofol also causes depressed respiratory drive, loss of airway reflexes, and hypotension. These changes increase the risk of respiratory complications. As a result, propofol sedation in non-intubated patients should be used only when practitioners skilled at airway management are available. Due to its low aqueous solubility propofol is formulated in a lipid emulsion. At room temperature this lipid emulsion is an ideal growth medium for bacteria. Endotoxic shock and wound infection have been reported in patients after administration of propofol left at room temperature for prolonged periods of time.[180,181]

Use over 5 days is associated with renal toxicity. This serious complication is referred to as propofol infusion syndrome (including severe metabolic acidosis, rhabdomyolysis, cardiac and renal failure) and has been reported usually after prolonged infusion of high doses in children.[182] There have also been reports of similar problems after shorter periods of infusion and in adults.[183] As a result of these observations, propofol infusion in the ICU is usually limited to shorter periods (24–48 hours) in older patients. In the pediatric ICU environment, infusions of propofol are limited to 6–12 hour periods.[174,176] Propofol infusion has been effective during short periods (overnight) as a bridge during the weaning process from other sedatives needed during mechanical ventilation of pediatric burn patients.[87]

Itch medications

Itch is one of the most common sequelae of burn injury. Field et al. reported that pruritus occurs in 87% of patients who have a burn injury.[184] Although it is thought to be secondary to the injury of the skin, the possibility that morphine is adding to the itch needs to be kept in mind. Itch can definitely influence the quality of life and duration of rehabilitation required. Scratching further injures the skin, leading to graft loss and skin breakdown that sometimes requires further grafting. In addition, it is very common for the patient to have a significant problem exercising or sleeping if the itching is intense. Several classes of medications can be used to treat itch. The approaches to treatment are as varied as the presumed causes of the itching.[185] Pruritus associated with burns is poorly understood, so blocking histamine, kinins, proteases, prostaglandins, substance P and 5-HT release and receptors have all been tried. The first line of defense is a series of moisturizing body shampoos and lotions to alleviate itching due to dry scaly skin. Then, failing that, Preparation H, which contains a caine has been advocated. Topical steroids are not usually used because of the infection risk, until the skin is well healed. They are effective in controlling the itching. Only a small area of skin should be treated with steroids in order to reduce the risk of systemic adrenal suppression. Antihistamine creams such as Benadryl® (diphenylhydramine) cream are available. Other topical medications include colloid and oatmeal baths.[186] Newer topicals are tricyclic antidepressants such as doxipin.[187,188] The major side effect of this preparation is that too much is absorbed, with resultant oversedation. Recently, gabapentin (10–35 mg/kg/day in divided doses) has been found in a pilot study to help with itching produced by burns.[189] Typical individual: dose is 5 mg/kg during the day and 10 mg/kg for bedtime.

Several non-medication approaches have been used. Massage seems to have a very beneficial effect.[184] In addition, Hettrick et al. reported that transcutaneous electrical nerve stimulations (TENS) considerably reduced the perception of itching in 9 adult patients compared to controls.[190] The most recent method involves the use of laser to reduce pruritus in burn scars.[191]

Usually the antihistamines are given orally. Using only one antihistamine results in complete relief for only 10% of the patients.[192] Diphenhydramine PO 1.25 mg/kg q 6h is often the first oral medicine used because of its sedative effect as well as helping control the itch. A few children respond better to loratodine, which is much longer lasting. If itch is not well controlled using only one, then another class of antihistamines can be added such as hydroxyzine PO 0.5/kg q 6h. Lastly, if the itch is still not well controlled, an antiseritonic agent, such as cyproheptadine 0.1 mg/kg q 6h, can be added, scheduled so that one of the medications is given every 2 hours. This is targeted against the 5-HT$_3$ receptors. Care must be made to not use the cyproheptadine with patients who are on serotonergic antidepressants.

Development of protocols for comfort

Interest in pain management of burned patients has been a high priority in the treatment of burns only in the last 10–15 years. Several institutions have developed pain and anxiety management protocols. In 1995, the Journal of Burn Care and Rehabilitation published a special issue devoted to then current practices of systematic treatment of burn pain. In the first edition of this book in 1996, we reported the initial use of a burn pain protocol used at the Shriners Burns Hospital in Galveston.[193] In 1997 the Boston group, headed by Tompkins, published a 3-year history with a similar protocol.[75] They incorporated a distinction in treating ventilated acute patients differently from non-ventilated acute patients. Most recently a national consensus on pain management has been reached. Ulmer[194] brought these to the attention of the burn community in a 1998 article. The protocol currently used in the Shriners Burns Hospital in Galveston is being reviewed and updated every few years.[84] The most recent version is in Box 64.2 and includes management of the most common discomforts of burned patients. It is extremely important to keep trying to improve these protocols as more is learned about the treatment of pain of burn injury.

BOX 64.2 Shriners Burns Hospital (Galveston) comfort protocol for children

BACKGROUND PAIN

Note: Begin bowel prep program simultaneously with beginning opioids

Pre-tub
First choice
PO midazolam 0.3 mg/kg and PO acetaminophen 15 mg/kg
If inadequate,
add PO morphine sulfate solution 0.3–0.6 mg/kg (if >15 kg) or fentanyl lollipop 10 μg/kg
If NPO,
IV midazolam 0.03 mg/kg and IV morphine 0.05–0.1 mg/kg (if >15 kg)

PRE-REHAB THERAPY

On request of therapist,
PO morphine sulfate solution 0.1–0.3 mg/kg or IV morphine 0.02–0.05 mg/kg
If child is very anxious add 0.1 mg/kg diazepam or 0.03–0.05 mg/kg lorazepam

POSTOPERATIVE PAIN

Option A
IV morphine infusion via PCA pump (if >5 years), total dose 10–20 mg/kg/4h

Option B
Attendant-administered bolus, slow IV push morphine 0.03–0.05 mg/dose q 2h (hold if level of responsiveness is decreased)

BACKGROUND PAIN FOR OUTPATIENT

Oral acetaminophen 15 mg/kg q 4h
If inadequate,
add oral morphine solution 0.1–0.3 mg/kg q 4h or MS Contin 0.5 mg/kg PO q 8–12 h

ANXIETY

Lorazepam PO 0.05 mg/kg q 4–6 h
or if muscle relaxation is also desired, diazepam 0.1 mg/kg q 8 hr
Note: taper benzodiazepines slowly by reducing dose by 50% every 2 days

ACUTE STRESS DISORDER OR POST-TRAUMATIC STRESS DISORDER SYMPTOMS[229]

Imipramine 1 mg/kg and increase slowly to 3 mg/kg as needed or fluoxetine 5 mg if under 6 years of age; for older person begin with 5 mg and increase slowly to 20 mg as needed

ITCH

Use skin moistening shampoos and lotions, topical ointments (not hydrocortisone creams)
Begin with diphenhydramine PO 1.25 mg/kg q 6h; if itch not well controlled, add hydroxyzine PO 0.5/kg q 6h; if itch still not well controlled, add cyproheptadine 0.1 mg/kg q 6h so that one of the medications is given every 2 hours

Non-pharmacological therapies in burned patients

As has been discussed, there is a strong interaction between psychological and physiological factors contributing to the pain experience. Anxiety in particular is prevalent among patients with burn injuries and is known to exacerbate acute pain. Non-pharmacological therapies play an important role in addressing the psychological factors that exacerbate pain as well as having a direct impact on the pain itself.[195]

In understanding how non-pharmacological approaches can be used with burn pain, it is important to discuss how behavioral principles contribute to the patient's experience.[196] In terms of classical (stimulus–response) conditioning, patients (particularly children) often will develop a conditioned anxiety response to stimuli associated with painful burn procedures. One study demonstrated that the simple event of a healthcare worker wearing scrubs was enough to elicit a fearful response in burn children.[197] In terms of operant (reinforcement) conditioning, patients can be thought to gain reinforcement by avoiding or escaping painful procedures, perhaps by screaming enough to terminate treatment or to obtain some sort of reinforcement from the staff by showing pain behaviors. Between the stimulus that precedes pain and the pain response that follows, there is the cognitive processing of pain. Such cognitions can be modified as can behavior and influence how much pain a patient experiences. Classical and operant conditioning principles, and modifying internal cognitions, have bearing on how non-pharmacological approaches are applied to burn pain. A series of articles by Thurber and Martin-Herz and colleagues[198,199] provides an extensive discussion of the theory and application of such principles of pain from pediatric wound care.

Classical conditioning

If the stimuli associated with a painful procedure can be conditioned to evoke anxiety or pain, then a logical goal is to reduce the impact that pre-tubbing stimuli have on the fear/pain response. An obvious environmental intervention is to make the wound care procedure setting as minimally threatening as possible. For children this might involve making the hydrotherapy tank a 'bath tub play area' with age-appropriate floating toys, etc. Our understanding is that some clever children's hospital staffs have turned their MRI scan into a 'cave in a jungle'; obviously such a setting will be less threatening to a child than will be the typical location of such radiological procedures. Similar principles can certainly be applied to burn care.[198,199]

There are other implications of classical conditioning. The best way to prevent a conditioned pain response is to optimize pain control in the first place. By aggressively and proactively treating pain, the contributions of conditioned anxiety will be minimized. Conversely, once a patient undergoes a procedure with inadequate analgesia, concomitant anxiety can be extremely difficult to treat.

Psychological preparation plays an important role in minimizing anticipatory anxiety. Patients can be provided with procedural or sensory preparatory information.[200] With procedural-based preparatory information, patients are explained the mechanics of their procedure (e.g. 'we will unwrap your bandages, wash your wounds and debride necrotic skin, apply silver sulfadiazine cream and then rewrap your dressings'). With sensory information, patients are prepared as to what they might feel during a procedure ('You will likely feel a pulling sensation as we remove your dressings and a stinging sensation when we wash your wounds with an antiseptic'). Such information is usually helpful to patients, but we should stress that some patients prefer to have as little information as possible, given their particular coping styles.[196]

Another approach based on classical conditioning is relaxation training. Patients can be taught deep relaxation and imagery prior to undergoing painful procedures. The rationale is to counteract the anxiety stimulated by pre-procedural stimuli with the relaxation response. If anticipatory anxiety is minimized with deep relaxation, the potential for a cyclical interaction between anxiety and acute pain is reduced. A number of studies have applied relaxation training and stress inoculation techniques, as well as some of the behavioral techniques discussed below to reduce burn pain.[201–204]

Operant conditioning

The consequences that patients receive for showing pain can have implications for pain control. Since almost all burn procedures are extremely aversive, it will be the natural tendency of patients, particularly children, to be motivated to escape such events. Staff members who allow patients to terminate procedures might be reinforcing, and potentially exacerbating, such escape behaviors. When left unchecked this process can lead to a distressed patient becoming combative rather than tolerating procedures. While such avoidance behavior should (more importantly) alert the staff that analgesia is inadequate, and the many potential pharmacological protocols discussed above should be invoked, it can also occasionally suggest a need for further limit setting. Rewarding a patient with rest once a stage of wound care is completed rather than based on pain behavior can be a useful means to minimize such escalating behavior. Again, however, the goal of a burn team should be to provide enough preparation and analgesia in a pre-emptive fashion that the need for such escape behaviors do not develop in the first place.

Operant conditioning also has implications for the manner in which patients receive pain medication. When patients are medicated in response to pain behaviors they are potentially receiving social reinforcement in terms of attention from the staff as well as the euphoric effects that the drugs might cause. This is one reason that, as mentioned earlier, it is far preferable that patients are medicated at regular time intervals rather than in response to their pain; the latter encourages them to complain more often in order to get the reward.[205] A similar application of operant principles is particularly important for the patient who excessively complains about pain out of emotional dependency needs, attention seeking, or in seeking euphorigenic properties of the pain medications. In such patients, provided that adequate levels of pharmacological analgesia have indeed been established, it may be important to extinguish pain behavior, ignoring pain behavior, and simultaneously engaging the patient in distraction unrelated to pain. This is a model more consistent with that used for chronic pain, but one that is occasionally useful for patients with burns that seem to overact independent of how aggressive pain is managed.[206]

A final application of operant principles has to do with token economies for children. It can be extremely useful to reward children for successful completion of procedures by using star charts or reinforcement schedules of this nature. Thus, a child, upon completing a procedure, may receive a star in a grid that covers a week of burn care. Older children can use an accumulation of points to purchase a desired reward. It is important that children are rewarded for completing procedures rather than for 'being brave' as the latter can serve as a subtle form of punishment to children; in other words, reinforcement should not be withheld if children act out and have a bad day during wound care, as long as wound care is completed.[198,199]

A particularly useful application of operant principles is to increase therapy activity in patients that are overwhelmed by therapies or appear to have poor motivation. The quota system uses operant principles to reward activity with rest. Patients complete predetermined quotas of activity that are within their capacity, and then are allowed to rest. A baseline determines what is within their capacity. For example, a patient who is trying to walk with burned legs might be instructed to walk until tired for three therapy sessions. The distance walked is recorded for those three sessions, the average is taken, and 80% of that average becomes the starting point. For example, the patient walks 50, 150 and 100 feet during three sessions: 80% of that 100 foot average is 80 feet; 80 feet becomes the starting point. Patients start at 80 feet and increase that amount by 5% (about 5 feet) each session. If they fail to meet a quota, they return to the last successful one. However, they also quit when they reach a program. They do not keep exercising even when they are having a 'good day.' This addresses the problem of pacing and overfatigue. Ehde and Patterson have reported the successful use of the quota with a number of patients with burn injury, both in terms of increasing therapy performance and reducing depression.[207]

Cognitive interventions

How patients think about their pain can be regarded as a behavior that can be modified and, in turn, can influence the degree of suffering they experience. As such, an important non-pharmacological approach is to draw out the thoughts patients have about their pain and teach them to modify accordingly. A particularly salient example is catastrophizing about pain. Catastrophizing thoughts include those such as 'I cannot stand this pain,' 'I will never get better,' or 'The pain means I will die.' Such catastrophizing thoughts have been associated with greater amounts of pain and less-favorable health outcomes in a variety of studies. Patients can be taught to challenge and reinterpret such thoughts. Along the same lines, it can be useful to teach patients to reinterpret the meaning of their pain sensations. For example, the appearance of skin buds and enhanced pain sensation may indicate that a wound is healing and skin grafts may not be necessary.[196]

Under the rubric of cognitive interventions patients may be taught techniques to enhance their ability to cope with pain. Positive self-talk and imagery designed to facilitate coping during periods of pain are examples of this. Thurber and colleagues have described the Two-Process Model of Control as it relates to controlling pediatric burn pain.[199] In terms of primary control, the patient attempts to modify the objective conditions of the painful procedure, such as negotiating how and when a dressing change will take place. In secondary control, the patient makes adjustments so that he or she can better tolerate the difficult procedures (e.g. positive self-talk, catastrophizing). Thurber et al.[199] and Martin-Herz et al.[198] have published a two-part series on a conceptualization of psychological approaches to burn pain, as well as specific examples for treatment.

Another example of enhancing coping is to give the patient more control during painful procedures. Kavanaugh et al. have described how giving children more control during procedures can reduce the effects of learned helplessness and enhance pain tolerance.[208] They reported that children who were provided with the opportunity to participate in and make decisions about their wound care showed lower depression, anxiety, hostility, and stress scores than did controls. Such findings fit well into the paradigm described by Thurber et al.[199]

Distraction is another cognitively based approach to pain control. Processing pain requires a certain amount of conscious attention and distracting such patients' attention can enable patients to tolerate pain better. Movies, music therapy, and games have all been used with some success as distraction techniques for burn pain.[209,210] Music has the additional benefit of inducing a relaxation response. More recently, Hoffman and colleagues have reported on the use of immersive virtual reality (VR) as a powerful analgesic.[210–212] Virtual reality can immerse patients' attention in a computer-generated world, and engage them in interaction with that world. These investigators indicate that VR can significantly reduce pain during wound care and physical therapy,[211,212] even relative to computer game distraction.[213]

Hypnosis

Hypnosis involves a blend of relaxation, imagery, and cognitive-based approach. The technique deserves special attention because there are a number of reports on its use with burn pain and, when it is effective, its impact on burn pain can be quite dramatic. There are over a hundred anecdotal reports in the literature that indicate that hypnosis can dramatically reduce pain and at least a dozen have been done with pain from burn injuries; such studies however lack control groups, standard measures of pain or information about pain medications.[214] More recently, tightly controlled studies with reliable measures of pain have supported hypnosis as an effective non-pharmacological approach to burn pain.[215,216] Patterson and Jensen have reported 12 controlled studies on chronic pain and 17 with acute pain indicating pain reduction; indeed, this modality is becoming far more scientifically acceptable.[217] Patients with burn injuries are ideal candidates for hypnosis for a number of reasons. In a review of such factors, Patterson et al. listed motivation, regression, dissociation, and hypnotizability as factors that promote hypnotic analgesia on the burn unit.[213] Specifically, patients who are faced with the excruciating nature of burn pain are motivated to engage in techniques such as hypnosis. The nature of a burn and its resulting care can cause a patient to become emotionally regressed (i.e. more dependent on the burn staff) and dissociated (i.e. removed from their emotions), and both of these factors seem to be associated with hypnotizability. Such factors likely account for the frequent dramatic effects that are seen with hypnosis and burn care. On the other hand, hypnosis clearly will not benefit some burn patients, and the degree to which patients are inherently hypnotizable (or not hypnotizable) almost certainly has some bearing on this issue.[218]

Ewin[219,220] has strongly argued for providing hypnosis within 2–4 hours after a patient sustains a burn injury. He maintains that this approach can serve to impede the progression of the burn as well as facilitate pain control. Unfortunately it is difficult to have a clinician available during this stage of burn care, and Ewin's findings have yet to be tested in other settings. The protocol used by Patterson and colleagues[216–221] is to provide hypnosis prior to wound care and have nurses provide standard post-hypnotic suggestions during wound care. This approach is efficient for both the hypnotist and the nurses. Patterson et al. have recommended that hypnosis used in this fashion be an adjunct to, rather than replacement for, pain medication.[216] More recently, investigators have combined immersive virtual reality with hypnosis in order to control burn pain. This approach has the advantage of not requiring a trained hypnotist to be present and appears to work as well as 'live hypnosis.'[222,223]

Other approaches

There is some evidence that TENS can be effective with burn pain,[224] but we are aware of only one study of this nature. Massage therapy has been reported to be useful in reducing burn pain.[225] We are unaware of any studies on the efficacy of acupuncture on burn pain, although this modality has been useful with pain from a variety of different etiologies. The acute nature and variable distribution of burn pain, may make acupuncture a challenging modality to apply to this problem.

For patients in the post-hospital, long-term rehabilitation phase, non-pharmacological approaches from physical and occupational therapists become critical. Stretching, strengthening, increasing activity, and hot/cold therapy may all become instrumental in enhancing pain control during the rehabilitative stage.

Summary

The state of the art in burn pain management would seem to be based more on personal bias and tradition than on a systematic, scientific approach. In addition, the number of pharmacokinetic studies of pain-relieving drugs of any kind in young children is virtually nil. Since approximately 35% of all burn injuries occur in children under 16 years, with a great majority of these occurring in children under 2 years, we have almost no information on which to base the use of pain-relieving drugs in burned children. It is no wonder that Perry and Heidrick[226] found great disparity in what burn care staff would order or administer to a young child as compared to an adult with burns of similar size and area of distribution on the body. More pharmacokinetic studies in both adults and children with burn injuries must be initiated.

Similar to the lack of conclusive data about the use of the various opioids or anxiolytic agents, is the scarcity of scientific data to recommend any of the non-pharmacological

techniques. However, significant progress has been made just since the last edition of this book 5 years ago. Most burn centers recognize anxiety as contributing to patient discomfort and are beginning to treat both anxiety and pain. Standardized protocols such as the guidelines (see Box 64.2) for starting doses of medication from the Shriners Burn Hospital in Galveston are being put forth.[84] Non-pharmacological techniques are more frequently included in a center's repertoire of tools for managing anxiety, recognized as a definite adjunct to pharmacotherapy. The major problem currently with these techniques is that they are personnel intensive and therefore are often not offered or reimbursed in the current managed care environment in the USA.

How, then, can we provide the 'best' pain management for a burned patient? Probably the first answer to that question is vigilance in assessment and flexibility in treatment. Patients show great individual variation in their responses to the variety of agents and modalities presented. A successful approach with a burned patient requires that healthcare personnel understand the pain associated with the different depths of wounds, the phase of the healing process, and the components of the pain response. For the burned patient during the initial 3–7 days, the more superficial areas give rise to moderate or severe pain, while the full-thickness areas contribute less to the overall pain response.[2] Although moderate to severe pain is usually related to procedures or physical therapy, background pain (or pain at rest) is usually described as mild, or very mild, but may be exacerbated by emotional concerns and anxiety. By the second week postburn, the moderately deep partial-thickness burn with its multitude of skin buds accounts for the majority of the moderate to severe pain. In many burn centers, deep dermal and full-thickness burns are excised and grafted between the 3rd and 10th days postburn. Although this often eliminates the severe pain associated with wound debridement during the 2nd and 3rd week, donor sites are often as painful as the areas of more superficial burns were initially. Dressing changes 3–5 days post-grafting also may be accompanied by the removal of sutures or staples which is usually described by patients as an excruciatingly painful procedure. By the 3rd or 4th week, if the wounds are not mostly healed, anxiety and depression may cause a patient to perceive increased levels of pain. And, within a single phase of recovery and within a single patient, pain frequency and intensity will vary from day to day. A fixed and inflexible approach to treatment is likely to overmedicate on one day and undermedicate the next.

To avoid over- and undermedication in adults, regimens which allow patients to control their own therapy seem most appropriate. This is very important for adults and teenagers, but children also can benefit from having this control. PCA can be used safely by many children and should not be disregarded as a tool on the basis of age alone. For procedural pain, patient-controlled regimens may include self-administered nitrous oxide, PCA, hypnosis, a variety of behavioral approaches, or a combination of these approaches. For background pain, the best control seems to be the use of slow-release opioids or other pain cocktails given on a non-pain contingent basis (i.e. scheduled every 4–6 hours) with the flexibility to supplement this with PRN or 'as desired' medication. Another approach would be to use PCA with or without a continuous low-dose infusion of narcotics. A variety of non-pharmacological therapies may also help relieve background pain. The most important aspect to remember with all of these regimens, as mentioned before, is flexibility. The other obvious aspect is to remember that a patient is not only the best person to assess his pain but also the best to evaluate the success of the therapies provided.

As challenging as managing comfort is for the healthcare provider, it is equally important to the burned patients. Recent studies suggest both physiological and psychological reasons to successfully manage pain. Kavanagh et al.[228] demonstrated that pain in a burned patient adds significantly to the physiological demands caused by stress. Schreiber and Galai-Gat[229] as well as Ptacek et al.[19] have shown that successful pain management can significantly reduce the occurrence of psychological disorders such as post-traumatic stress syndrome.

Burn care professionals who desire to keep their patients as comfortable as possible can perhaps best prepare themselves by learning to:

- watch and listen to their patients with vigilance;
- use a standardized assessment tool for measuring discomfort on a scheduled basis as well as during moments when the patient is complaining, either verbally or behaviorally, pre- and post-administration of treatment;
- know how discomforts are likely to change as the patient recovers;
- include a variety of pharmacological and non-pharmacological methods for managing discomforts and be prepared to change as the patients' needs change;
- feel comfortable with a process that never ends, but which can bring many moments of relief for the patient and satisfaction for the caregivers.

References

1. Beecher HK. Relationships of significance of wound to pain experience. JAMA 1958; 161:1609–1612.
2. Choinière M, Melzack R, Rondeau J, et al. The pain of burns: characteristics and correlates. J Trauma 1989; 29:1531–1539.
3. Meyer RP, Campbell JN. Myelinated nociceptive afferent account for hyperalgesia that follows a burn to the hand. Science 1981; 213:1527–1529.
4. Campbell JN, Meyer RA, Roya SN. Hyperalgesia: new insights. Pain 1984; Suppl 2:Abst 3.
5. Coderre T, Melzack R. Increase pain sensitivity following heat injury involves a central mechanism. Behav Brain Res 1985; 15:259–262.
6. Atchison NE, Osgood PE, Carr DB, et al. Pain during burn dressing change in children: relationship to burn area, depth and analgesia regimens. Pain 1991; 47:41–45.
7. Ptacek J, Patterson D, Doctor J. Describing and predicting the nature of procedural pain after thermal injuries: implications for research. J Burn Care Rehabil 2000; 21:318–326.
8. Charlton JE, Klein R, Gagliardi G. Factors affecting pain in burned patients: a preliminary report. Postgrad Med 1983; 59:604–607.
9. Andreasen NJC, Noyes R, Hartford CE, et al. Management of the emotional reactions in seriously burned adults. N Engl J Med 1972; 286:65–69.
10. West DA, Schuck JM. Emotional problems of the severely burned patient. Surg Clin North Am 1978; 58:1189–1204.
11. Goodstein RK. Burns: an overview of the clinical consequences afflicting patient, staff and family. Compr Psychiatry 1985; 26:43–57.
12. Savedra M. Coping with pain: strategies of severely burned children. Canadian Nurse 1977; 73:28–29.
13. Beales JG. Factors influencing the expectation of pain among patients in a children's burn unit. Burns 1983; 9:187–192.
14. Mannon JM. Caring for the burned: life and death in a hospital burn center. Springfield, IL: CC Thomas; 1985.
15. Ponten B. Grafted skin: observations on innervation and other qualities. Acta Clin Scand (Suppl) 1960; 257:1–5.
16. Freund PR, Brengelmann GL, Rowell LB, et al. Vasomotor control in healed grafted skin in humans. J Appl Physiol 1981; 51:168–171.
17. Ulmer JF. An exploratory study of pain, coping, and depressed mood following burn injury. J Pain Symptom Manage 1997; 13:148–157.
18. Pruzinsky T, Rice LD, Himel HN, et al. Psychometric assessment of psychologic factors influencing adult burn rehabilitation J Burn Care Rehabil 1992; 13:79–88.
19. Ptacek J, Patterson D, Heimbach D. Inpatient depression in persons with burns. J Burn Care Rehabil 2002; 23:1–9.
20. Anand KJS, Sippel WG, Aynsley-Green A. Randomized trial of fentanyl anesthesia in preterm neonates undergoing surgery: effects on the stress response. Lancet 1987; 1:243–238.
21. Anand KJS, Aynsley-Green A. Does the newborn infant require potent anesthesia during surgery? Answers from a randomized trial of halothane anesthesia. In: Dubner R, Gebhart G, Bond M, eds. Pain research & clinical management. Amsterdam: Elsevier; 1988:vol. 3:329–335.
22. Anand KJS, Hickey PR. Pain and its effects in the human neonate and fetus. N Engl J Med 1987; 317:1321–1329.
23. Gracely RH. Pain measurement. Acta Anaesthesiol Scand 1999; 43:897–908.
24. Melzack R. The McGill pain questionnaire: major properties and scoring methods. Pain 1975; 1:277–299.
25. Gordon M, Greenfield E, Marvin J, et al. Use of pain assessment tools: is there a preference? J Burn Care Rehabil 19:451–454.
26. Grossi E, Broghi C, Cerchiari EL. Analogic Chromatic Continuous Scale (ACCS): a new method for pain assessment. Clin Rheumatol 1983; 1:337–340.
27. Wong D, Baker C. Pain in children: comparison of assessment scales. Pediatr Nurs 1988; 14:9–17.
28. American Academy of Pediatrics and American Pain Society. Joint policy statement on pain in children. Pediatrics 2001; 108:793–797.
29. Attia J, Amiel-Tison C, Mayer N-N, et al. Measurement of postoperative pain and narcotics administration in infants using a new clinical scoring system. Anesthesiology 1987; 67:A532.
30. Szyfelbein SK, Osgood PF, Carr DB. The assessment of pain and plasma β-endorphin immunoactivity in burned children. Pain 1985; 22:173–182.
31. Williamson PS, Williamson ML. Physiologic stress reduction by a local anesthetic during newborn circumcision. Pediatrics 1983; 71:36–40.
32. Fuller B. FM signals in infant vocalizations. Cry 1985; 6:5–10.
33. Fuller B, Horii Y. Differences in fundamental frequency, jitter and shimmer among four types of infant vocalizations. J Commun Dis 1986; 18:111–118.
34. Fuller B, Horii Y. Spectral energy distribution in four types of infant vocalizations. J Commun Dis 1988; 20:111–121.
35. Franck LS. A new method to quantitatively describe pain behavior in infants. Nurse Res 1986; 35:28–31.
36. Granau RVE, Craig KD. Pain expression in neonates: facial action and cry. Pain 1987; 28:395–410.
37. Johnston C, O'Shaughnessy D. Acoustical attributes of infant pain cries: discriminating features. In: Dubner R, Gebhart G, Bond M, eds. Pain research & clinical management. Amsterdam: Elsevier; 1988:vol.3:341–347.

38. Izard CE, Heubner RR, Risser D, et al. The young infant's ability to produce discrete emotional expressions. Dcu Psychol 1980; 19:132–140.

39. Craig KD, McMahon RJ, Morison JD, et al. Developmental changes in infant pain expression during immunization injections. Soc Sci Med 1984; 19:1331–1337.

40. Johnston CC, Strada ME. Acute pain response in infants: a multidimensional description. Pain 1986; 24:373–382.

41. Katz ER, Kellerman J, Siegel SE. Behavioral distress in children with cancer undergoing medical procedures: developmental considerations. J Consult Clin Psychol 1980; 48:356–365.

42. Mills N, Preston A. Acute pain behaviors in infants/toddlers. In: Funk S, Tomquist E, Champagne M, et al., eds. Key aspects of comfort: management of pain, fatigue and nausea. New York: Springer; 1989:52–59.

43. McGrath PJ, Johnson G, Goodman JT, et al. CHEOPS: a behavioral scale for rating postoperative pain in children. In: Fields HL, Dubner R, Cerrera F, eds. Advances in pain research and therapy. New York: Raven; 1985:395–402.

44. Tyler DC, Tu A, Douthit J, et al. Toward validation of pain measurement tools for children: a pilot study. Pain 1993; 52:301–309.

45. Barone M, McCall J, Jenkins M, et al. The development of a observational pain scale (OPAS) for pediatric burns. Abst 230. Presented at the 32nd Annual Meeting of the American Burn Association, Las Vegas, Nevada: March 14–17, 2000.

46. Beyer J, Aradine C. Content validity of an instrument to measure young children's perceptions of the intensity of their pain. Pediatr Nurs 1986; 1:386–395.

47. Beyer J, Aradine C. Patterns of pediatric pain intensity: a methodological investigation of self-report scale. Clin J Pain 1987; 3:130–141.

48. Beyer J, Aradine C. The convergent and discriminant validity of a self report measure of pain intensity for children. Children's Health Care 1981 16:274–282.

49. McGrath PA, de Veber L, Hearn M. Multidimensional pain assessment in children. In: Fields H, Dubner R, Cerrera F, eds. Advances in pain research and therapy. New York: Raven; 1985:387–393.

50. Maunuksela EL, Ollkola KT, Korpela R. Measurement of pain in children with self-reporting and behavioral assessment. Clin Pharmacol Ther 1987; 42:137–141.

51. Bieri D, Reeve RA, Champion GD, et al. The face pain scale for the self-assessment of the severity of pain experienced by children: development, initial validation, and preliminary investigation of ratio scale properties. Pain 1980; 41:139–160.

52. Hester NO. The pre-operational child's reaction to immunization. Nurse Res 1979; 28:250–254.

53. Varni JW, Thompson KL, Hanson V. The Varni/Thompson Pediatric Pain Questionnaire. I. Chronic musculoskeletal pain in juvenile arthritis. Pain 1987; 28:27–38.

54. Eland J. Minimizing pain associated with pre-kindergartner intramuscular injections. Issues Compr Pediatr Nurs 1981; 5:361–372.

55. Wong D, Baker C. Pain in children: comparison of assessment scales Pediatr Nurs 1988; 14:9–17.

56. McGrath PJ, Unruh AM. Pain in children and adolescents. Amsterdam: Elsevier; 1987:351.

57. Sevedra M, Gibbons P, Tesler M, et al. How do children describe pain? A tentative assessment. Pain 1982; 14:95–104.

58. LeBaron S, Zettzer L. Assessment of acute pain and anxiety in children and adolescents by self-report, observer reports, and behavior checklist. J Consult Clin Psychol 1984; 52:729–738.

59. Beyer J, Wells N. The assessment of pain in children. Pediatr Clin North Am 1987; 36:837–854.

60. McCaffery M, Beebe KD. Pain: clinical manual for nursing practice. St. Louis: Mosby; 1989.

61. Robert R, Blakeney P, Villarreal C, et al. Anxiety: current practices in assessment and treatment of anxiety of burn patients. J Burn Care Rehabil 2000; 26:549–552.

62. Siverman W, Kurtines W. Anxiety and phobic disorders: a pragmatic approach. New York: Plenum; 1996.

63. Walk RD. Self-ratings of fear in a fear invoking situation. J Abnorm Social Psychol 1956; 52:171–178.

64. Taal LA, Faber AW. The burn specific pain anxiety scale: introduction of a reliable and valid measure. Burns 1997; 23:147–150.

65. Taal LA, Faber AW, van Loey NEE, et al. The abbreviated burn specific pain anxiety scale: a multicenter study. Burns 1999; 25:493–497.

66. Aaron LA, Patterson DR, Finch CP, et al. The utility of a burn specific measure of pain anxiety to prospectively predict pain and function: a comparative analysis. Burns 2001; 27:329–334.

67. Field T, Peck M, Hernandez-Reif M, et al. Postburn itching, pain, and psychological symptoms are reduced with massage therapy. J Burn Care Rehabil 2000; 21:189–193.

68. Blakeney P, Marvin J. Itch man scale. Copyright, Shriners Hospital for Children.

69. Matheson JD, Clayton J, Muller MJ. Reduction of itch during burn wound healing. J Burn Care Rehabil 2001; 22:76–81.

70. Gerding RL, Imbembo AL, Fratianne RB. Biosynthetic skin substitute vs. 1% silver sulfadiazine for treatment of inpatient partial-thickness thermal burns. J Trauma 1988; 28:1265–1269.

71. Demling RH. Use of Biobrane in management of scalds. J Burn Care Rehabil 1995; 16:329–330.

72. Ou LF, Lee SY, Chen YC, et al. Use of Biobrane in pediatric scald burns – experience in 106 children. Burns 1998; 24:49–53.

73. Barret JP, Dziewulski P, Ramzy PI, et al. Biobrane versus 1% silver sulfadiazine in second-degree pediatric burns. Plast Reconstr Surg 2000; 105:62–65.

74. Duinslaeger LAY, Verbeken G, Vanhalle S, et al. Cultured allogeneic keratinocyte sheets accelerate healing compared to op site treatment of donor sites in burns. J Burn Care Rehabil 1997; 18:545–551.

75. Sheridan R L, Hinson M, Nackel A, et al. Development of a pediatric burn pain and anxiety management program. J Burn Care Rehabil 1997; 18:455–459.

76. Beushausen T, Mucke K. Anesthesia and pain management in pediatric burn patients. Pediatr Surg Int 1997; 12:327–333.

77. MacLennan N, Heimbach DM, Cullen BF. Anesthesia for major thermal injury. Anesthesiology 1998; 89:749–770.

78. Hedderich R, Ness TJ. Analgesia for trauma and burns. Crit Care Clin 1999; 15:167–184.

79. Stoddard FJ, Sheridan RL, Saxe GN, et al. Treatment of pain in acutely burned children J Burn Care Rehabil 2002; 23:135–156.

80. Seidlova D, Zemanova J, Cundrle I, et al. Pain management in children with burn injuries. Acta Chir Plast 2003; 45:81–82.

81. Martin-Herz SP, Patterson DR, Honari S, et al. Pediatric pain control practices of North American burn centers. J Burn Care Rehabil 2003; 24:26–36.

82. Patterson DR, Hoflund H, Espey K, et al. Pain management. Burns 2004; 30:A10–A15.

83. Meyer WJ, Woodson L. Management of burn pain in children. In: Schmidt RE, Willis WD, eds. Encyclopedia of pain. New York: Springer; 2006:in press.

84. Ratcliff SL, Brown A, Rosenberg L, et al. The effectiveness of a pain and anxiety protocol to treat the acute pediatric burn patient. Burns 2006; 32:554–562.

85. Patterson DR, Ptacek JR, Carrougher G, et al. PRN vs regularly scheduled opioid analgesics in pediatric burn patients. J Burn Care Rehabil 2002; 23:424–430.

86. Martyn JAS. Clinical pharmacology and drug therapy in the burn patient. Anesthesiology 1986; 65:67–75.

87. Sheridan RL, Keaney T, Stoddard F, et al. Short-term propofol infusion as an adjunct to extubation in burned children. J Burn Care Rehabil 2003; 24:356–360.

88. Gibbons J, Honari SR, Sharar SR, et al. Opiate-induced respiratory depression in young pediatric burn patients. J Burn Care Rehabil 1998; 19:225–229.

89. Lynn AM, Slattery JT. Morphine pharmacokinetcs in early infancy. Anesthesiology 1987; 66:136–139.

90. Thomas CR, Brazeal BA, Rosenberg L, et al. Phantom limb pain in pediatric burn survivors, Burns 2003; 29:139–142.

91. McGraw T, Stacey BR. Gabapentin for treatment of neuropathic pain in a 12-year-old girl. Clin J Pain 1998; 14:354–356.

92. Pedersen JL, Callesen T, Moiniche S, et al. Analgesic and anti-inflammatory effects of lignocaine-prilocaine (EMLA) cream in human burn injury. Br J Anaesth 1996; 76:806–810.

93. Beausang E, Orr D, Shah M, et al. Subcutaneous adrenaline infiltration in pediatric burn surgery. Br J Plast Surg 1999; 52:480–481.

94. Fischer CG, Lloyd S, Kopcha R, et al. The safety of adding bupivacaine to the subcutaneous infiltration solution used for donor site harvest. J Burn Care Rehabil 2003; 24:361–364.

95. Bussolin L, Busoni P, Giorgi L, et al. Tumescent local anesthesia for the surgical treatment of burns and postburn sequelae in pediatric patients. Anesthesiology 2003; 99:1371–1375.

96. Pedersen JL, Rung GW, Kehlet H. Effect of sympathetic nerve block on acute inflammatory pain and hyperalgesia. Anesthesiology 1997; 86:293–301.

97. Cuignet O, Pirson J, Boughrouph J, et al. The efficacy of continuous fascia iliaca compartment block for pain management in burn patients undergoing skin grafting procedures. Anesth Analg 2004; 98:1077–1081.

98. Jonsson A, Cassuto J, Hanson B. Inhibition of burn pain by intravenous lidocaine infusion. Lancet 1991; 338:151.

99. Cassuto J, Tarnow P. Potent inhibition of burn pain without use of opiates. Burns 2003; 29:163–166.

100. Wehner D, Hamilton GC. Seizures following application of local anesthetics to burn patients. Ann Emerg Med 1984; 13:456–458.

101. Letouze A, Volnchet V, Hoecht B, et al. Using a new lipidocolloid dressing in paediatric wounds: results of French and German clinical studies. J Wound Care 2004; 13:221–225.

102. Ang EST, Lee ST, Gan CS, et al. Pain control in a randomized, controlled, clinical trial comparing moist exposed burn ointment and conventional methods in patients with partial-thickness burns. J Burn Care Rehabil 2003; 24:289–296.

103. Kissin I, Bright CA, Bradley EL. The effect of ketamine on opioid-induced acute tolerance: can it explain reduction of opioid consumption with ketamine-opioid analgesic combinations? Anesth Analg 2000; 91:1483–1488.

104. Callahan RJ, Au JD, Paul M, et al. Functional inhibition by methadone of N-methyl-D-aspartate receptors expressed in Xenopus oocytes: stereospecific and submit effects. Anesth Analg 2004; 98:653–659.

105. Berde CB, Beyer JE, Bournaki MC, et al. Comparison of morphine and methadone for prevention of postoperative pain in 3 to 7 year old children. J Pediatr 1994; 119:136–141.

106. Williams PI, Sarginson RE, Ratcliffe JM. Use of methadone in the morphine-tolerant burned paediatric patient. Br J Anaesth 1998; 80:92–95.

107. Perry SW, Inturrisi LE. Analgesia and morphine deposition in burn patients. J Burn Care Rehabil 1983; 4:276–279.

108. Osgood PF, Syzfelbein SK. Management of burn pain in children. Pediatr Clin North Am 1989; 36:1001–1013.

109. Bloedow DC, Goodfellow LA, Marvin J, et al. Meperidine disposition in burn patients. Res Commun Chem Pathol Pharmacol 1986; 54:87–89.

110. Finn J, Wright J, Fong J, et al. A randomized crossover trial of patient controlled intranasal fentanyl and oral morphine for procedural wound care in adult patients with burns. Burns 2004; 30:262–268.

111. Prakash S, Fatima T, Pawar M. Patient-controlled analgesia with fentanyl for burn dressing changes. Anesth Analg 2004; 99:552–555.

112. Concilus R, Denson DD, Knarr D, et al. Continuous intravenous infusion of methadone for control of burn pain. J Burn Care Rehabil 1989; 10:406–409.

113. Lee JJ, Marvin JA, Heimbach DM. Effectiveness of nalbuphine for relief of burn debridement pain. J Burn Care Rehabil 1989; 10:241–246.

114. Kinsella J, Galvin R, Reid WH. Patient-controlled analgesia for burn patients: a preliminary report. Burns Incl Therm Inj 1988; 14:500–503.

115. Krauss B, Green SM. Sedation and analgesia for procedures in children. N Engl J Med 2000; 13:938–956.

116. Mather LE, Phillips GD. Opioids and adjuvants: principles of use. Clin Crit Care Med 1986; 8:77–103.

117. Sharar SR, Bratton SL, Carrougher GJ, et al. A comparison of oral transmucosal fentanyl citrate and oral hydomorphone for inpatient pediatric burn wound care analgesia. J Burn Care Rehabil 1998; 19:516–521.

118. Robert R, Brack A, Blakeney P, et al. A double-blind study of the analgesic efficacy of oral transmucosal fentanyl citrate and oral morphine in pediatric patients undergoing burn dressing change and tubbing. J Burn Care Rehabil 2003; 24:351–355.

119. Sharar SR, Carrougher GJ, Selzer K, et al. A comparison of oral transmucosal fentanyl citrate and oral oxycodone for pediatric outpatient wound care. J Burn Care Rehabil 2002; 23:27–31.

120. Gertler R, Brown HC, Mitchell DH, et al. Dexmedetomidine: a novel sedative-analgesic agent. BUMC Proc 2001; 14:13–21.

121. Ebert T, Maze M. Dexmedetomidine: another arrow for the clinicians quiver. Anesthesiology 2004; 101:568–570.

122. Lange JT, Lange CL, Cabaltica RB. Primary care treatment of post-traumatic stress disorder. Am Fam Physician 2000; 62:1035–1040.

123. Connor DF, Barkley RA, Davis HT. A pilot study of methylphenidate, clonidine, or the combination in ADHD comorbid with aggressive oppositional defiant or conduct disorder. Clin Pediatr (Phila) 2000; 39:15–25.

124. Jaakola ML, Salonen M, Lehtinen R, et al. The analgesic agent of dexmedetomidine — a novel α_2-adrenoceptor agonist — in health volunteers. Pain 1991; 46:281–285.

125. Tobias JD, Berkenbosch JW. Sedation during mechanical ventilation in infants and children: dexmedetomidine versus midazolam. South Med J 2004; 97:451–455.

126. Venn RM, Karol MD, Grounds RM. Pharmacokinetics of dexmedetomidine infusions for sedation of postoperative patients requiring intensive care. Br J Anaesth 2002; 88:669–675.

127. Zub D, Berkenbosch JW, Tobias JD. Preliminary experience with oral dexmedetomidine for procedural and anesthetic premedication. Pediatr Anesth 2005; 15:932–938.

128. Ramesh VJ, Bhardwah N, Batra YK. Comparative study of oral clonidine and diazepam as premedicants in children. Int J Clin Pharmacol Ther 1997; 35:218–221.

129. Joshi W, Reuben SS, Kilaru PR, et al. Postoperative analgesia for outpatient arthroscopic knee surgery with intraarticular clonidine and/or morphine. Anesth Analg 2000; 90:1102–1106.

130. Quan DB, Wandres DL, Schroeder DJ. Clonidine in pain management. Response: is clonidine effective in the treatment of pain? Ann Pharmacother 1993; 27:313–315.

131. Freeman KO, Connelly NR, Schwartz D, et al. Analgesia for paediatric tonsillectomy and adenoidectomy with intramuscular clonidine. Paediatr Anaesth 2002; 12:617–620.

132. Goyagi T, Tanaka M, Nishikawa T. Oral clonidine premedication enhances postoperative analgesia by epidural morphine. Anesth Analg 1999; 89:1487.

133. Mikawa K, Nishina K, Maekawa N, et al. Oral clonidine premedication reduces postoperative pain in children. Anesth Analg 1996; 82:225–230.

134. Finkel JC, Johnson YJ, Quezado ZM. The use of dexmedetomidine to facilitate acute discontinuation of opioids after cardiac transplantation in children. Crit Care Med 2005; 33:2110–2112.

135. Ramsay MAE, Luterman DL. Dexmedetomidine as a total intravenous anesthetic agent. Anesthesiology 2004; 101:787–790.

136. Riker RR, Ramsay MAE, Prielipp RC, et al. Long-term dexmedetomidine infusions for ICU sedation: a pilot study. Anesthesiology 2001; 95:A383.

137. Handa F, Tanaka M, Nishikawa T, et al. Effects of oral clonidine premedication on side effects of intravenous ketamine anesthesia: a randomized, double-blind, placebo-controlled study. J Clin Anesth 2000; 12:19–24.

138. Levanan J, Makela ML, Scheinin H. Dexmedetomidine premedication attenuates ketamine-induced cardiostimulatory effects and postanesthetic delirium. Anesthesiology 1995; 82:1117–1125.

139. Lyons B, Casey W, Doherty P, et al. Pain relief with low-dose intravenous clonidine in a child with severe burns. Intensive Care Med 1996; 22:249–251.

140. Kariya N, Shindoh M, Nishi S, et al. Oral clonidine for sedation and analgesia in a burn patient. J Clin Anesth 1998; 10:514–517.

141. Wallace BH, Caldwell FT, Cone JB. Ibuprofen lowers body temperature and metabolic rate of humans with burn injury. J Trauma 1992; 32:154–157.

142. Cone JB, Wallace BH, Olsen KM, et al. The pharmacokinetics of ibuprofen after burn injury. J Burn Care Rehabil 1993; 14:666–669.

143. Bradley JA, Brandt KD, Katz BP, et al. Comparison of an antiinflammatory dose of ibuprofen, an analgesic dose of ibuprofen, and acetaminophen in the treatment of patients with osteoarthritis of the knee. N Engl J Med 1991; 325:87–91.

144. Temple AR. Pediatric dosing of acetaminophen. Pediatr Pharmacol (New York) 1983; 3:321–327.

145. Meyer WJ 3rd, Nichols RJ, Cortiella J, et al. Acetaminophen in the management of background pain in children post-burn. J Pain Symptom Manage 1997; 13:50–55.

146. Martyn JA, Greenblatt DS, Quinby WC. Diazepam kinetics following burns. Anesth Analg 1983; 62:293–297.

147. Patterson DR, Ptacek JT, Carrougher GJ, et al. Lorazepam as an adjunct to opioid analgesics in the treatment of burn pain. Pain 1997; 72:367–374.

148. Stanford GK. Postburn delirium associated with use of intravenous lorazepam. J Burn Care Rehabil 1988; 9:160–161.

149. Greenblatt DJ, Locniskar A, Ochs HR, et al. Automated gas chromatography for studies of midazolam pharmacokinetics. Anesthesiology 1981; 55:176–179.

150. McClure JH, Brown DT, Wildsmith JAW. Comparison of the IV administration of midazolam and diazepam as sedation during spinal anaesthesia. Br J Anaesth 1983; 55:1089–1093.

151. Driessen JJ, Booij LH, Vree TB, et al. Midazolam as a sedative on regional anesthesia. Arzneim Forscl V Drug Res 1981; 31:2245–2247.

152. Brophy T, Dundee JW, Heazelwood V, et al. Midazolam, a water-soluble benzodiazepine, for gastroscopy. Anaesth Intensive Care 1982; 10:334–347.

153. Burnweit C, Diana-Zerpa JA, Nahmad MH, et al. Nitrous oxide analgesia for minor pediatric surgical procedures: an effective alternative to conscious sedation? J Pediatr Surg 2004; 39:495–499.

154. Annequin D, Carbajal R, Chauvin P, et al. Fixed 50% nitrous oxide oxygen mixture for painful procedures: a French survey. Pediatrics 2000; 105:1–6.

155. Filkin SA, Cosgrav P, Marvin JA, et al. Self-administered anesthesia: a method of pain control. J Burn Care Rehabil 1981; 2:33–34.

156. Marvin JA, Engrav LH, Heimbach DM. Self-administered nitrous oxide analgesia for debridement: a five year experience. Presented at the 16th Annual Meeting of the American Burn Association, San Francisco, California: April 11–14, 1984.

157. Layzer RH. Myeloneuropathy after prolonged exposure to nitrous oxide. Lancet 1978; 2:1227–1230.

158. Layzer RB, Fishman RA, Schafer JA. Neuropathy following abuse of nitrous oxide. Neurology 1978; 28:504–506.

159. Paulson GW. Recreational misuse of nitrous oxide. J Am Dent Assoc 1979; 98:410–411.

160. Hayden PJ, Hartemink RJ, Nicholson GA. Myeloneuropathy due to nitrous oxide. Burns 1983; 9:267–270.

161. Baskett PJE, Hyland J, Deane M, et al. Analgesia for patient dressing in children. Br J Anaesth 1969; 41:684–688.

162. Baskett PJE. Analgesia for the dressing of burns in children: a method using neuroleptanalgesia and Entonox. Postgrad Med J 1972; 48:138–142.

163. Vieira E, Cleaton-Jones P, Austin JC. Effects of low concentrations of nitrous oxide on rat fetuses. Anesth Analg 1980; 59:175–177.

164. Vieira E. The effect of the chronic administration of nitrous oxide 0.54 to gravid rats. Br J Anaesth 1979; 51:283–287.

165. Heinrich M, Wetzstein V, Muensterer OJ, et al. Conscious sedation: off-label use of rectal s(+)-ketamine and midazolam for wound dressing changes in paediatric heat injuries. Eur J Pediatr Surg 2004; 14:235–239.

166. Slogoff S, Allen GW, Wessels JV, et al. Clinical experience with subanesthetic ketamine. Anesth Analg Curr Res 1974; 53:354–358.

167. Martinez S, Achauer B, Dobkin de Rios M. Ketamine use in a burn center: hallucinogen or debridement facilitator. J Psychoactive Drugs 1985; 17:45–49.

168. Handrop M, Spinella J. Ketamine: featured protocol. J Burn Care Rehabil 1987; 8:148–149.

169. Parker J. Ketamine: review of featured protocol. J Burn Care Rehabil 1987; 8:149.

170. Martyn JAJ. Ketamine pharmacology and therapeutics. J Burn Care Rehabil 1987; 8:146–148.

171. Dimick P, Helvig E, Heimbach D, et al. Anesthesia assisted procedures in a burn intensive care unit procedure room: benefits and complications. J Burn Care Rehabil 1993; 14:446–449.

172. Sebel PS, Lowdon JD. Propofol: a new intravenous anesthetic. Anesthesiology 1989; 71:260–277.

173. Coimbra C, Choinière M, Hemmerling RM. Patient-controlled sedation using propofol for dressing changes in burn patients: a dose-finding study. Anesth Analg 2003; 97:839–842.

174. Cravero JP, Manzi DJ, Rice LJ. The management of procedure-related pain the child. In: Ashburn MA, Rice LJ, eds. The management of pain. New York: Churchill Livingston; 1998.

175. Wolf AR, Potter F. Propofol infusion in children: when does an anesthetic tool become an intensive care liability? Pediatr Anesth 2004; 14:435–438.

176. Tobias JD. Sedation and analgesia in the pediatric intensive care unit. Pediatr Ann 2005; 34:636–645.

177. Ronan KP, Gallagher TJ, George B, et al. Comparison of propofol and midazolam for sedation in intensive care unit patients. Crit Care Med 1995; 23:286–293.

178. Hughes MA, Glass PS, Jacobs JR. Context-sensitive half-time in multicompartment pharmacokinetics models for intravenous anesthetic drugs. Anesthesiology 1992; 76:334–341.

179. Mathru M, Esch O, Lang J, et al. Magnetic resonance imaging of the upper airway. Effect of propofol anesthesia and nasal continuous positive airway pressure in humans. Anesthesiology 1996; 84:253–255.

180. Veber B, Gachot B, Bedos JP, et al. Severe sepsis after intravenous injection of contaminated propofol. Anesthesiology 1994; 80:712–713.

181. Nichols RL, Smith JW. Bacterial contamination of an anesthetic agent. N Engl J Med 1995; 333:184–185.

182. Parke TJ, Stevens JE, Rice AS, et al. Metabolic acidosis and fatal myocardial failure after propofol infusion in children: five case reports. Br Med J 1992; 305:613–616.

183. Burow BK, Johnson ME, Parker DL. Metabolic acidosis associated with propofol in the absence of other causative factors. Anesthesiology 2004; 101:239–243.

184. Field T, Peck M, Hernandez-Reif M, et al. Post-burn itching, pain, and psychological symptoms are reduced with massage therapy. J Burn Care Rehabil 2000; 21:189–193.

185. Odom RB, James WD, Berger TG. Pruritus and neurocutaneous dermatoses. In: Andrews' diseases of the skin. New York: WB Saunders; 2000.

186. Matheson JD, Clayton J, Muller MJ. Reduction of itch during burn wound healing. J Burn Care Rehabil 2001; 22:76–81.

187. Bernstein JE, Whitney DH, Keyoumars S. Inhibition of histamine-induced pruritus by topical tricyclic antidepressants. J Am Acad Dermatol 1981; 5:582–585.

188. Demling R, DeSanti L. Doxepin cream significantly decreases itching and erythema in the healed burn wound compared to oral antihistamines. J Burn Care Rehabil 2002; 23:581.

189. Mendham JE. Gabapentin for the treatment of itching produced by burns and wound healing in children: a pilot study. Burns 2004; 30:851–853.

190. Hettrick H, O'Brien K, Laznick H, et al. Effect of transcutaneous electrical nerve stimulation for the management of burn pruritus: a pilot study. J Burn Care Rehabil 2004; 25:236–240.

191. Allison KP, Kiernan MN, Waters RA, et al. Pulsed dye laser treatment of burn scars. Alleviation or irritation? Burns 2003; 29:207–213.

192. Vitale M, Fields-Blache C, Luterman A. Severe itching in the patient with burns. J Burn Care Rehabil 1991; 12:330–333.

193. Marvin JA, Muller MJ, Blakeney PE, et al. Pain response and pain control. In: Herndon DN, ed. Total burn care. Philadelphia: WB Saunders; 1996.

194. Ulmer JF. Burn pain management: a guideline-based approach. J Burn Care Rehabil 1998:19:151–159.

195. Patterson D, Sharar S. Burn pain. In: Loeser J, ed. Bonica's management of pain, 3rd edn. Baltimore: Lippincott, Williams & Wilkins; 2003:778–787.

196. Patterson DR. Nonopioid based approaches to burn pain. J Burn Care Rehabil 1995; 16:372–376.

197. Meyer D. Children's responses to nursing attire. Pediatr Nurs 1992; 18:157–160.

198. Martin-Herz SP, Thurber CA, Patterson DR. Psychological principles of burn wound pain in children. II: Treatment applications. J Burn Care Rehabil 2000; 21:458–472.

199. Thurber CA, Martin-Herz SP, Patterson DR. Psychological principles of burn wound pain in children. I. Theoretical framework. J Burn Care Rehabil 2000; 21:376–387.

200. Everett JJ, Patterson DR, Chen AC. Cognitive and behavioral treatments for burn pain. The Pain Clin 1990; 3:133–145.

201. Fagerhaugh SY. Pain expression and control on a burn care unit. Nurs Outlook 1974; 22:645–650.

202. Knudson-Cooper MS. Relaxation and biofeedback training in the treatment of severely burned children. J Burn Care Rehabil 1981; 2:102–110.

203. Kueffner M. Passage through hospitalization of severely burned, isolated school-age children. Commun Nurs Res 1976; 7:181–97.

204. Wernick RL, Jaremko ME, Taylor PW. Pain management in severely burned adults: a test of stress inoculation. J Behav Med 1981; 4:103–109.

205. Melzack R. The tragedy of needless pain. Sci Am 1990; 262(2): 27–33.

206. Fordyce WE. Behavioral methods for chronic pain and illness. St. Louis: Mosby Year Book; 1976.

207. Ehde DM, Patterson DR, Fordyce WE. The quota system in burn rehabilitation. J Burn Care Rehabil 1998; 19:436–439.

208. Kavanagh CK, Lasoff E, Eide Y, et al. Learned helplessness and the pediatric burn patient: dressing change behavior and serum cortisol and β-endorphin. Adv Pediatr 1991; 38:335–363.

209. Elliott CH, Olson RA. The management of children's distress in response to painful medical treatment for burn injuries. Behav Res Ther 1983; 21:675–683.

210. Kelley ML, Jarvie GJ, Middlebrook JL, et al. Decreasing burned children's pain behavior: impacting the trauma of hydrotherapy. J Appl Behav Anal 1984; 17:147–158.

211. Hoffman H, Patterson D, Nakamora D, et al. Use of virtual reality for adjunctive treatment of adult burn pain during physical therapy: a case study. Int J Hum Comp Interact.

212. Hoffman HG, Patterson DR, Carrougher GJ. Use of virtual reality for adjunctive treatment of adult burn pain during physical therapy: a controlled study. Clin J Pain 2000; 16: 244–250.

213. Hoffman HG, Doctor JN, Patterson DR, et al. Use of virtual reality as an adjunctive treatment of adolescent burn pain during wound care: a case report. Pain 2000; 85:305–309.

214. Patterson DR, Questad KA, Boltwood MD. Hypnotherapy as a treatment for pain in patients with burns: research and clinical considerations. J Burn Care Rehabil 1987; 8:263–268.

215. Patterson DR, Everett JJ, Burns GL, et al. Hypnosis for the treatment of burn pain. J Consul Clin Psychology 1992; 60:713–717.

216. Patterson DR, Ptacek JT. Baseline pain as a moderator of hypnotic analgesia for burn injury treatment. J Consul Clin Psychology 1997; 65:60–67.

217. Patterson DR, Jensen M. Hypnosis and clinical pain. Psychol Bull 2003; 129:495–521.

218. Patterson DR, Adcock RJ, Bombardier CH. Factors predicting hypnotic analgesia in clinical burn pain. Int J Clin Exp Hypn 1997; 45:377–395.

219. Ewin DM. Emergency room hypnosis for the burned patient. Am J Clin Hypn 1983; 26:5–8.

220. Ewin DM. Hypnosis in surgery and anesthesia. In: Wester WC II, Smith AH Jr, eds. Clinical hypnosis: a multidisciplinary approach. Philadelphia: JB Lippincott; 1984.

221. Patterson DR, Questad KA, DeLateur BJ. Hypnotherapy as an adjunct to narcotic analgesia for the treatment of pain for burn debridement. Am J Clin Hypn 1989; 31:156–163.

222. Patterson DR, Tininenko JR, Schmidt AE, et al. Virtual reality hypnosis: a case report. Int J Clin Exp Hypn 2004; 52: 27–38.

223. Patterson D, Wiechman S, Jensen M, et al. Hypnosis delivered through immersive virtual reality for burn pain. Int J Clin Exp Hypn 2006; in press.

224. Kimball KL, Drews JE, Walker S, et al. Use of TENS for pain reduction in burn patients. J Burn Care Rehabil 1987; 8:28–31.

225. Field T, Peck M, Krugman S, et al. Burn injuries benefit from massage therapy. J Burn Care Rehabil 1998; 19:241–244.

226. Perry S, Heidrick G. Management of pain during debridement: a survey of US burn units. Pain 1982; 13:267–280.

227. Kavanagh CK, Lasoff E, Eide Y, et al. Learned helplessness and the pediatric burn patient: dressing change behavior and serum cortisol and beta-endorphin. Adv Pediatr 1991; 38:335–363.

228. Schreiber S, Galai-Gat T. Uncontrolled pain following physical injury as the core-trauma in post-traumatic stress disorder. Pain 1993; 54:107–110.

229. Tcheung WJ, Robert R, Rosenberg L, et al. Early treatment of acute stress disorder in children with major burn injury. Pediatr Crit Care Med 2005; 6:676–681.

Chapter 65

Psychiatric disorders associated with burn injury

Christopher R. Thomas, Walter J. Meyer III, and Patricia E. Blakeney

Chapter contents

Introduction

The knowledge and skills of a psychiatrist are often needed in the pharmacological management of psychiatric symptoms which commonly occur in conjunction with burn injuries.[1] Psychiatric expertise is also an asset to a burn team in addressing multitudes of psychological issues concomitant to burn injuries. Although a psychiatrist is usually sought as a consultant, a psychiatrist is most helpful to patients and to burn teams as an integrated member of the medical staff.

Preexisting psychiatric disorders and symptoms are relatively common in the histories of burned patients, and frequently appear to have contributed significantly to the etiology of the injury itself.[2–7] Substance abuse,[8] organic brain dysfunction, attention deficit hyperactivity disorder,[9] conduct disorder, and personality disorders have been reported as frequently occurring premorbid conditions. One study found alcohol use disorder in 11% of hospitalized burn patients with almost all of those injuries considered preventable.[10] Patients intoxicated at the time of burn injury also suffer a higher rate of complications in their treatment.[11] Those abusing flammable inhalants are at particular risk for burn injury.[12–14] A small, but important, number of patients are admitted with serious burn injuries resulting from purposeful self-immolation.[15–18] In one study of 67 patients with self-inflicted burns, 75% had a prior psychiatric illness and 20% had a previous suicide attempt.[19] A separate study of 11 patients with self-inflicted burns reported that 10 had a prior psychiatric illness with 2 attempting suicide and 2 motivated by hallucinations.[20] Of patients with self-inflicted burns, those attempting suicide are more likely to have larger burns and longer hospitalizations than those with the intent of self-mutilation.[21] As described by Stoddard and Cahners[17] and by Raskind,[22] burn patients with suicidal intent present emotional, as well as physical, challenges to a treatment team. A suspected suicide attempt will almost invariably elicit requests for psychiatric involvement in management and treatment of a patient. Less dramatic indicators

of premorbid psychiatric disorders are also identifiable early in a patient's admission and signal the need for psychiatric consultation. Burn patients with a history of any premorbid psychiatric disorders are more likely to have preventable injuries,[23] require longer hospitalization,[24,25] and have problems with adjustment early in their recovery.[26,27] The risk of psychiatric complications following burn injury is greater in those patients with a previous history of affective, alcohol or substance use disorders.[28] It is therefore important to screen for any preexisting psychiatric disturbance in burn patients.

In addition to premorbid psychiatric illness, other psychological factors have been found to be associated with an increased risk for psychiatric symptoms following burn injury. Taal and Faber[29] reported that dissociation and anxiety experienced during the burn injury predicted later psychopathology. Tedstone and colleagues[30] found that certain coping styles were predictive of later psychological difficulties. Patients with coping patterns of helplessness, emotion focused, problem focused, focusing on the positive and seeking social support were all at increased risk for subsequent emotional distress. A coping style of acceptance appears to be a protective factor against later anxiety and post-traumatic distress symptoms. In a separate study, avoidant coping or symptoms of anxiety or depression following burn injury were predictive of psychological problems 3 months later, but burn severity was not.[31] While it is understandable to expect patients with major burns to be at risk, even minor burns can result in significant psychological distress and psychiatric symptoms.[32] At the present time, there is no profile that can reliably predict which patients will suffer psychiatric symptoms following burn injury. All patients should be carefully assessed as part of their care.

This chapter will focus on the psychiatric treatment of common mental disturbances that can be expected to occur as part of a symptom complex experienced by any patient who is suffering a serious burn injury. Although preexisting psychopathology alters the expression of a patient's distress and complicates medical management of the patient, the common symptoms described in this chapter are not necessarily indicative of premorbid psychopathology. These symptoms can be very distressing to patient, family, and staff if not well managed by both psychological and pharmacological interventions. The most commonly occurring psychiatric symptoms discussed in this chapter are delirium, organic psychoses, burn encephalopathy, post-traumatic symptoms, sleep disturbances, pain, and depression, which occur during the critical care phase of burn treatment. Psychiatric problems are often noted as part of the long-term process of recovery from burn injury, i.e. phobias and other anxiety disorders, acute stress disorder (ASD), post-traumatic stress disorder (PTSD), major depression, and dysthymia.

Common psychiatric symptoms

Critical care phase
Delirium, organic psychoses, and burn encephalopathy

Organic factors and premorbid conditions contribute to symptoms during the initial part of treatment. Disorientation, confusion, sleep disturbance, transient psychosis, and delirium are commonly observed among adolescent and adult patients.[3,33–36] Causes of these symptoms are usually unclear and multifactorial. Hypertension, hypoglycemia, electrolyte imbalance, sepsis, and/or a variety of organic problems can contribute to delirium. The unusual physical surroundings of an intensive care unit heighten the probability of psychoses. The altered state of consciousness may be transitory, wax and wane over several days, or, with large burns, persist for weeks. The picture may be confused further by a suspected occurrence of anoxia. Delirium has been found to occur more often in males who have a history of substance abuse and with burn injuries over 30% TBSA.[34] A past history of substance abuse is often suspected as contributing to delirium, particularly with adolescent and adult patients. Inhalant abuse or intoxication at the time of a fire are factors to be considered. Another potential cause of disorientation, hallucinations and agitation may be medications used in the treatment of the acute burn patient. Morton and colleagues[37] reported severe psychotic symptoms in a patient following treatment with anabolic steroids. Hallucinations can also be a side effect of anesthesia, especially with ketamine.

In an altered state of consciousness, patients may misinterpret their surroundings, resulting in potentially frightening illusions of reality. Patients may misperceive lines and hoses as snakes. A patient may shout about the fire or the accident, describe symbols of death, monsters, or the devil. A patient may misidentify the people in the room, seeing instead absent friends or dead people, or may identify a treatment team as prison guards. The content of the illusions or hallucinations may be so bizarre and morbid as to suggest a schizophrenia, a brief reactive psychosis, or a psychotic depression (e.g. dead bodies, dead people, or angels). Sometimes patients are so frightened by these visions that they try to escape or become combative. Such psychotic symptoms are understandably frightening to the family of the patient and disconcerting to even experienced staff. Hallucinations are uncommon in children, but when they do occur, the most likely cause is stress, followed by pain and medications.[38] Sepsis and metabolic conditions can also result in hallucinations, and are a more frequent cause of this than psychiatric disorder in young burn patients.

In our experience, symptoms of delirium and transient psychosis occur rarely among children under the age of 10 years;[36] however, burn encephalopathy, as characterized by lethargy, withdrawal, or coma, is a condition observed in children as well as adults.[39,40] EEGs in such cases typically reveal diffuse, non-specific slow waves.[39,41] Causative factors probably are the same as those for delirium.[42] Although Andreasen et al.[43] report long-term neurological impairment following burn delirium in adults, other studies (and our own experience) do not find residual neurological effects following delirium or encephalopathy.[33–36,39,40] These symptoms, though apparently short-lived, are upsetting to a patient's family and treatment team when they do occur. Proper treatment must first address organic causes of delirium and/or encephalopathy. Vital signs must be stabilized and blood chemistries and glucose normalized. Also, oxygenation should be checked and sepsis investigated and treated. Pain must be addressed. Then psychotropic medications may be administered.

The use of antipsychotic phenothiazines in an acute burn unit is a common approach to address delirium and/or combative, uncooperative behavior such as pulling off dressings, attempting to get out of bed, or striking out at caretakers.[44–47] Pharmacological control is preferable to physical restraints, which tend to exacerbate a patient's distress and worsen the symptoms.[1] Haloperidol (Haldol®) is the phenothiazine of choice for adult patients, as it does not have significant cholinergic side effects. The initial dose is 1 or 2 mg of haloperidol, but doses as high as 5 or 10 mg may be administered. Since phenothiazines do not cause respiratory depression, they may be repeated hourly until symptoms begin to come under control. Usually, phenothiazines are administered in two or three doses per day. Pediatric burn patients appear to have a much higher rate of adverse reactions to haloperidol and alternative management of agitation should be considered. In a clinical review of 26 pediatric burn survivors that received haloperidol during acute treatment, 23% had serious side effects.[48]

Chlorpromazine (Thorazine®) and thioridazine (Mellaril®) may be used in place of haloperidol in the dosage range of 25–100 mg per dose. Chlorpromazine and thioridazine have strong sedative effects and interfere with learning, but are less likely than haloperidol to produce associated dystonia, pseudo-parkinsonism, and akathisia. If more than 2 mg of haloperidol per day are used, attention must be given to simultaneous administration of 1 or 2 mg/day of benztropine (Cogentin®) or 2–5 mg/day of trihexyphenidyl (Artane®) in divided doses. Benztropine or trihexyphenidyl are used to avoid dystonia, pseudo-parkinsonism, and akathisia.[45] Occasionally, dystonia takes the form of an oculogyric crisis, which resembles an acute neurological catastrophe[49] and can be a true medical emergency if respiration is impaired. These reactions are usually alleviated by 50 mg IV diphenhydramine (Benadryl®).

There are two severe side effects for which the patient on phenothiazine must be monitored: neuroleptic malignant syndrome[50] and tardive dyskinesia.[45] Neuroleptic malignant syndrome is a potentially life-threatening crisis characterized by fever, muscle rigidity, mental status changes, and autonomic dysfunction. Neuroleptics should be discontinued, and symptoms must be treated aggressively with supportive therapy, as well as benzodiazepines, dantrolene, bromocriptine and anticholinergics. The long-term side effect of greatest concern for patients who receive phenothiazine is tardive dyskinesia. This reaction can be permanent and is characterized by abnormal, involuntary, irregular choreiform and athetoid movements. Usually, a patient is unaware of the writhing and twisting movements that most often involve the tongue, but can also involve the limbs and the trunk as well. The reaction typically occurs only in individuals who have received phenothiazines for extended periods of time, i.e. longer than 6 months. The risk of occurrence is 2–4% per year over the first 7 years in which phenothiazines are taken. Although it is a very unusual complication in individuals who receive phenothiazines for short periods of time, it has been reported.

Due to the problems which have been associated with phenothiazines, benzodiazepines have been used to a greater extent in recent years for the combative, delirious patient.[45,51,52] The two most commonly used benzodiazepines are diazepam (Valium®) and lorazepam (Ativan®). Lorazepam (0.03 mg/kg) orally or intravenously, can usually be given every 4–8 hours; for a very combative patient it can be given hourly. A third benzodiazepine which is frequently used is midazolam (Versed®) at 0.05 mg/kg IV, typically used in conjunction with morphine for procedures such as tubbing and staple removal. Midazolam (Versed) is also used for sedation as a continuous infusion for intubated patients. When using the benzodiazepine class of medications, a clinician must balance the desired effects of relaxation with oversedation. Visual and auditory hallucinations may occur if the dose of benzodiazepine is too high. In those cases, it should be reduced or replaced by another type of medication. In cases of excessive anxiety in the presence of adequate pain control, lorazepam can be added to a patient's treatment. Nighttime doses usually enhance sleep. Diazepam in doses of 2–10 mg per dose, depending on the size of an individual, may be used in place of lorazepam if simultaneous muscle relaxation is desired.[53] Diazepam has an extremely long half-life, 40 hours, and therefore should be used sparingly (see Chapter 54). To avoid excessive sedation by benzodiazepines, a patient should not be awakened for the next dose.

Acute stress and post-traumatic stress disorder symptoms

A significant number of burn survivors will experience post-traumatic stress disorder symptoms, including intrusive memories of the injury, during their acute recovery.[54,55] If anxiety is associated with other symptoms of post-traumatic stress, such as hypervigilance or poor sleep, an antidepressant such as a selective serotonin re-uptake inhibitor (SSRI) like fluoxetine (Prozac®)[56] or a tricyclic antidepressant (TCA) like imipramine (Tofranil®)[36,57] should be considered. The SSRIs have the advantage of being safer drugs for outpatient treatment since an overdose is unlikely to cause significant cardiac problems as have been attributed to the TCAs.[58] The usual starting dose of fluoxetine (Prozac) is 10–20 mg for adults, 5 mg for children <40 kg and 10 mg for children between 40 and 60 kg. Typically, the SSRIs are given in the morning rather than the evening as they may interfere with sleep onset. Side effects of SSRIs include gastrointestinal upset, increased agitation, headaches, and sweating. They have, however, fewer instances of anticholinergic side effects such as constipation. A rare but potentially life-threatening side effect is serotonin syndrome,[59] characterized by at least three of the following symptoms: delirium, agitation, sweating, fever, hyperreflexia, myoclonus, tremor, incoordination, diarrhea and shivering. Severe cases can result in hyperpyrexia, shock or death. The risk of sero-

tonin syndrome increases when patients are on multiple medications that potentiate central nervous system serotonin, such as an SSRI and a monoamine oxidase inhibitor. There is a reported case of serotonin syndrome in a pediatric burn patient who was receiving fluoxetine (Prozac) and linezolid (Zyvox®), a broad-spectrum antibiotic with monoamine oxidase inhibition.[60]

The usual starting dose of imipramine (Tofranil) is 25 mg/day unless the patient weighs less than 25 kg. The beginning dose is 12.5 mg for those under 25 kg. The dose can be increased rapidly over the next few days to a dose of 1 mg/kg. If the symptoms are still uncontrolled, the dose may be increased stepwise to 3 mg/kg, but only with frequent checking of the plasma level and EKG changes with each increment of dose. A steady state is usually not reached until a given dose is maintained for 3–5 days. A dose can be divided and given twice a day, but such division is usually unnecessary. The preferable time of administration is in the evening to aid with sleep. Major side effects of the TCAs are anticholinergic effects (dry mouth and dry nasal passages, constipation, urinary hesitance, and occasional esophageal reflux).[45] Autonomic complications such as orthostatic hypotension, palpitations, and hypertension have been reported in adolescents with this medication.[44] Cardiac arrhythmias, associated with a prolonged PR interval, can be life-threatening.[58,61,62] Sudden death has been reported for teenagers and children receiving desipramine and other TCAs.[63] Amitriptyline or doxepin may be used in place of imipramine. The dosages are similar; however, both these medications may cause more sedation than imipramine.[45]

Following clinical reports of increased suicidal ideation in pediatric patients treated with certain antidepressant medications and a review of clinical trial data, the US Food and Drug Administration instructed all manufacturers to include a 'black box' warning with all antidepressant medications.[64] Pediatric patients and their caretakers must be aware of these risks and clinicians should closely monitor children and adolescents on these medications for possibly increased suicidal ideation and behavior.[65]

Sleep disturbances

Patients with significant sleep problems are common in an acute burn unit.[66–68] When sleep disturbance with nightmares is associated with post-traumatic anxiety, as described above, antidepressant medications are the drugs of choice. Imipramine (Tofranil)[69] and doxepin are both sedating antidepressants that are effective treatments for sleep problems in burn patients. Trazodone and nefazodone are alternative medications for insomnia and do not appear to alter sleep architecture as much as other antidepressants. Mirtazapine (Remeron®) is another antidepressant that has been used for insomnia although little is known about its effects on sleep architecture. Sleep problems may be associated with stimulation from the caretaking staff who awaken a patient while checking vital signs and well-being throughout the night. Sometimes lights and televisions are left on throughout the day and night in a patient's room. These environmental factors can be destructive to a patient's sleep-wake cycle. As soon as physiological conditions allow, a patient should be given as much undisturbed sleep time at night as possible, so as to allow natural sleep cycles to reestablish, and to maintain a normal circadian rhythm. Pain and itch are other problems that can interfere with sleep and should be addressed with appropriate analgesic or antipruritic medications.[70] If a patient continues to have significant sleep problems, sleep can be induced with diphenhydramine. Diphenhydramine doses of 1.5 mg/kg are often used throughout the day for itching and may be used alone for sleep at night or as an adjunct to other sleep medications. Usually, doses of 25 or 50 mg in the evening are adequate.

Often, post-traumatic symptoms other than sleep disturbances are not evident. In such cases, chloral hydrate may also be used in doses of 1.5 mg/kg, up to a maximum of 1 g per single dose.[52] Doses of 250 mg are usually adequate for a child; however, we prefer to use benzodiazepine, imipramine (Tofranil), and/or diphenhydramine for sedation and sleep with pediatric patients because deaths have been reported in children taking chloral hydrate for sedation,[52] Also, in our experience, chloral hydrate does not alleviate nightmares as does imipramine (Tofranil).

Depression

Fluoxetine (Prozac) and the other SSRIs are the first-line medications for treatment of patients with depressive symptoms.[58,62] TCAs should also be considered in the treatment of depression if the patient does not respond or cannot tolerate treatment with an SSRI. They should be used as described above by following symptoms and monitoring blood levels. Patients should be monitored for hypomania or mania induced by antidepressant medications. When this occurs, the antidepressant dose should be lowered and lithium therapy or other mood stabilizer medication, such as valproic acid (Depakote®) or carbamazepine (Tegretol®) should be considered. Lithium is usually not used in patients recovering from burns because of its effect on sodium concentration.

Pain

Symptoms of depression and agitation are often related to excessive pain and subside with adequate pain management (see Chapter 59). A patient's experience of pain is related to the extent and depth of injury and influenced by individual responses to analgesia, pain threshold, emotional state, cognitive functioning, cultural beliefs, interpersonal interactions, and expectations.[42,71–76] The experience of pain has been found to be an important mediating risk factor for PTSD in pediatric burn patients.[77] Chemical analgesics and anesthetics are as important in managing pain with burns as they are with other medical/surgical conditions. Care must be taken to consider the appropriate doses of medication and the most efficacious schedule of administration. Modifications should be continued until good control is achieved.[78,79] Around-the-clock or continuous administration of analgesics achieves better pain control than PRN administration.[80,81] This avoids the period of less than therapeutic levels of the drug with increased discomfort prior to the request for medication and ameliorates a patient's anxiety about whether the medication will be allowed. Postoperatively, patient-controlled analgesia (PCA) pumps are very effective in achieving around-the-clock pain control with minimal undesired side effects for adults and for children.[82,83] The addition of amitriptyline (Elavil®), a TCA, can be effective in controlling neuropathic or phantom limb pain.

In-hospital recuperation

After the initial postburn period, a patient progresses through a series of operative procedures interspersed with days of physical therapy in order to maintain physical activity and range of motion. Immediate operative sites (those grafted and those which donate) are painful. In addition, exercises are painful. A patient's world is one of pain or concern about possible pain in the near future. It must be remembered that many of the treatments and experience of hospitalization may be as traumatic psychologically as the original burn injury, especially for young children.[84] The patient's expectations for treatment are also very important. Those patients who have low expectation for further improvement and attach higher importance to outcome are at greater risk for psychological distress during recovery.[85] The major goal of therapy from the psychiatrist's point of view is to control the pain and maximize a patient's participation in recovery, rehabilitation, and other aspects of care.

In addition to the pharmacological treatment described above, designing a psychological milieu that supports comfort and security is a primary task.[36] A specific daily treatment schedule is crucial to achieving these goals. The schedule provides specific times for pain medication to insure coverage at times of expected pain (e.g. tubbing and physical therapy), but avoids sedation during family, social, and educational activities. Time should be provided in the schedule for fun and diversionary activities. A pediatric patient must have time scheduled for school and play. Patients must be allowed to have expected 'safe' periods without procedures. Whenever possible, the patient, even a young child, should be included in planning the schedule. The schedule should be posted and followed as closely as possible. In order to motivate a patient to participate at a maximum level in rehabilitation, a reward system can be incorporated with rewards consisting of special treats as designated by the patient, such as extra videos or going out of the hospital.

As a latency age child, adolescent, or adult recovers, he/she often wants to talk about the accident. A patient begins a long process of 'understanding' what has happened. Part of this process is learning to look at a 'new' self, literally and metaphorically. As part of the treatment plan, a regularly scheduled meeting with a psychotherapist is established. This special time for 'talking' therapy may vary in content from play therapy with a child or light banter with an adult to serious confrontation with the most difficult emotionally charged issues. The reliability of this safe time in which a patient can complain about everybody and everything, express anger, express fear and sadness, can be very therapeutic. It is important for a patient to have someone other than family who is accepting, safe, and neutral with whom to talk. Communication with the therapist and others may be difficult if the patient is suffering with symptoms of post-traumatic stress disorder or alexithymia, a condition characterized by problems in describing feeling and thoughts.[86,87] It is also important to take into account the cognitive and emotional development of the patient as it determines the level of ability to use reflection and verbalization in processing what has happened. Younger patients may understandably regress in the face of severe trauma and loss.

A patient's experience in adapting to burn injury can be thought of as a grieving process. A patient has experienced a loss of self. Using a familiar paradigm, we can describe a patient as moving through several stages of adjustment to loss: shock, denial, anger, depression, and finally acceptance.[88] This formulation is useful in working with a patient about his/her injury. In our experience, shock and denial predominate during the initial hospitalization; anger and depression often last for years as a patient continues in treatment, faces reconstructive surgeries, and confronts a series of social experiences.

Psychiatric problems beyond acute hospitalization

The novice usually expresses a belief that all burned persons need to see a psychiatrist due to the nature of the injury. A number of approaches have been used to determine the incidence of psychiatric difficulties among survivors of major burns. These studies report with surprising consistency that large numbers of survivors do not suffer long-term major psychiatric disorders or psychosocial impairment.[89,90] Longitudinal studies have found about one-third of burn survivors develop post-traumatic stress disorder within 2 years of their injury.[91,92] It might be expected that the appearance of the burn scar might influence long-term adjustment, and Fukunishi[93] did find cosmetic disfigurement predictive for post-traumatic stress disorder symptoms of avoidance and emotional numbing in women with burn injuries. In contrast, Taal and Farber[94] found that neither the severity nor the visibility of burn scars influence long-term adjustment, but rather social introversion, which predicted the development of pathological shame.

Our own work has focused on children and adolescents who are at least 1 year postburn and are either outpatients or have returned for further reconstructive surgery. One method we have used has been to survey patients with questionnaires pointed at specific psychiatric symptom complexes. For instance, Koon et al.[95] surveyed adolescents with the Piers-Harris Children's Self-concept Scale and found that male pediatric burn survivors had significantly higher scores than the normative population. Females described themselves as less popular, although otherwise equal to the norm. Self-esteem did not appear to be related to other burn-related variables (i.e. age at burn or size of burn). With a similar goal of looking for specific symptoms, we hypothesized significant depression and utilized several standardized instruments, including the Suicide Probability Scale (SPS),[96] to assess depressive symptoms. This study revealed no increase above norm in depression or suicidality, but did reveal significant anger among adolescent burn survivors.

We use a variety of instruments to detect general psychiatric needs among the children that we follow. The Achenbach series of standardized behavioral checklists are useful screening tools.[97–99] They offer validity, reliability, and convenience of administration in a setting such as ours where we must assess many clinical variables in a brief period of time. The Child Behavior Checklist (CBCL)[97] is a 113-item rating of each child's current behavior problems and competencies as perceived by a parent. Complementary to the CBCL are the Teacher Report Form (TRF)[98] and the Youth Self-Report (YSR),[99] which provide assessments of the same behaviors by different observers. Our data from these instruments indicate that about 20–25% of the children and adolescents who survive major thermal injury may develop a variety of significant behavioral problems as indicated, but good adjustment is achieved by the majority of individuals.[100,101] Blakeney et al.[102] and Zeitlin[103] reported similar findings of only modest psychological sequelae to pediatric burns in their long-term follow-up study.

Parents usually report more problems than do the children themselves or the teachers.[100,104] In one study, 60 children with burns (35 boys, 25 girls) were surveyed with the Achenbach instruments at least 1 year after burn injury. The parental perception on the CBCL revealed a statistically significant ($p < 0.05$) increase in problems and decrease in competency for most age groups and both sexes when compared with the normal reference population. In contrast, the TRF and the YSR revealed very few differences from the reference population. Burn size did not account for any of the differences. Item analysis of individual questions revealed excessive endorsement by parents of specific items on all scales compared to their respective reference populations.[105] These results could be explained by increased problems of the children following severe burns that would not be easily observed by persons who do not live with the patient, e.g. nocturnal enuresis or nightmares. Or, perhaps, the parents reporting increased behavioral problems are overly sensitive to any indication of difficulty for their children.

Our investigations have also considered outcomes for the parents of youth burn survivors. The Parental Stress Index (PSI)[106] revealed that parents who reported their children as troubled were themselves more stressed than the normal reference population, not only by their children's behaviors but also in areas unrelated to their children.[107] In addition, on a measure of mood state, the Eight-state Questionnaire (8SQ),[108] mothers who reported troubled children more often felt depressed and guilty than did mothers of well-adjusted children.[107] In a separate study of mothers of children with burns, 52% met criteria for a diagnosis of post-traumatic stress disorder; larger burns were strongly correlated with symptoms in the mother.[109] Fukunishi[110] found higher rates of depressive and post-traumatic stress symptoms in the mothers of children with burns than in their offspring. These studies emphasize the need for psychological attention to parents of burned children, as well as to the children themselves.

Using a standardized psychiatric interview for children, Stoddard et al. reported a very high incidence of psychiatric disorders among 30 pediatric burn survivors.[111,112] In order to make a fair comparison with other populations, these authors compared the burn survivors with a group of survivors of flood trauma and a community sample. Burned children had significantly more phobic disorders, overanxious disorders, enuresis, encopresis, major depression, PTSD, and substance/ethanol abuse than the comparison groups.[112] Sleep disorders and psychotic disorders were also slightly more common among the burned children. Even though most burn survivors eventually make good adjustments, they can be expected, at some time during the adjustment process, to suffer psychiatric sequelae which might be attenuated by psychiatric treatment.

Phobias and other anxiety disorders

Many patients continue beyond acute hospitalization to have periods during which they appear extremely anxious and express fear. These periods often recur in association with return to a hospital for reconstructive surgeries. Some are so anxious that they are constantly soliciting their families or others for comfort. Generalized anxiety disorder or overanxious disorder of childhood is characterized in the Diagnostic and Statistical Manual of Mental Disorders (DSM-IV) by the following criteria:

- excessive worry occurring more days than not for at least 6 months about a number of events;
- difficulty in controlling the anxiety;
- the anxiety causes clinically significant distress or impairment in social, occupation, or other important areas of functioning;
- anxiety and worry associated with three or more (only one for children) of the following symptoms (with some symptoms present for more days than not for the past 6 months): restlessness, feeling on edge, easily fatigued, difficulty concentrating or mind going blank, irritability, muscle tension, sleep disturbances.

In a burned patient, difficulty controlling anxiety which is so distressful that it interferes with important functioning, restlessness, and difficulty in concentrating are diagnostic of anxiety disorders since some other symptoms can be related to burn injuries specifically, e.g. being easily fatigued.

Not infrequently, anxiety spills over to other situations and/or becomes focused on specific objects; thus, phobias develop that are characterized by excessive persistent fear in response to specific stumuli. Although adults may express anxiety through 'panic' symptoms such as sweating, palpitations, trembling, or nausea, children may express anxiety by crying, tantrums, freezing, or clinging. A differential diagnosis of these anxiety disorders distinct from PTSD is difficult and requires a careful interview. Burned patients suffering from post-traumatic stress often see the fire or aspects of their accidents whenever they close their eyes; they dream about their traumas. An overanxious patient is afraid of what might happen; the PTSD patient fears what has happened. Most burn patients, certainly those who qualify for the diagnosis of generalized or overanxious disorder, benefit from lorazepam therapy in addition to supportive psychotherapy.

Acute stress disorder and post-traumatic stress disorder

Acute stress disorder and PTSD are the most common psychiatric disorders seen in survivors of major burns.[113] The two disorders are very similar, differing only in how long the symptoms persist. Acute stress disorder symptoms appear immediately following the trauma, last for at least 2 days and resolve within 4 weeks after the trauma. If symptoms persist or appear more than 4 weeks after the trauma, then the appropriate diagnosis is PTSD. These disorders are characterized in the DSM-IV by the following criteria:

- The person has experienced, witnessed, or was confronted with an event which involved actual or threatened death or serious injury to self or others, and the person's response involved intense fear, helplessness, or horror.
- The traumatic event is persistently re-experienced. Recurrent and intrusive thoughts of the event occur. Burned patients often complain of seeing the fire whenever they close their eyes or when they try to go to sleep. Young children may relive the event over and over again in repetitive play. Nightmares about the event are common; in young children, frightening dreams occur without recognizable content. Feeling as if the event were recurring (e.g. flashback) is reported often. Intense reactivity, psychological and/or physiological, occurs at exposure to internal or external cues that trigger associations with the traumatic incident, e.g. seeing a fire on television.
- There is continued avoidance of stimuli associated with the trauma or numbing of general responsiveness. Persons suffering from PTSD develop flat affect, memory problems, and withdrawal from others. Children's behavior may be regressed; children may lose recently acquired developmental skills such as toilet training or language skills.
- Persistent symptoms of increased arousal, which were not present before the trauma, may develop. These symptoms include sleep disturbance, irritability/anger, difficulty concentrating, hypervigilance, exaggerated startle response, and panic attacks. Patients have periods of feeling afraid and not knowing why.

Nightmares and altered sleep patterns are usually the symptoms first noted. Although one study found no correlation between psychiatric diagnosis emerging during acute hospitalization and later development of post-traumatic disorder,[114] the presence of avoidant post-traumatic disorder symptoms during the acute phase of recovery is reported to predict chronic post-traumatic disorder in burn patients.[91,115–118] In a study of pediatric burn patients, a high resting heart rate, lowered body image, and parental stress symptoms were found to be significant risk factors in development of ASD.[119] Many of the other symptoms are described when a more complete history is taken. Patients should be given ample opportunity to explore their feelings and fears about the traumatic event. This process may persist for months. In addition, medications such as the SSRIs and TCAs are helpful in reducing the nightmares and improving the sleep pattern. A study comparing the treatment of ASD symptoms with either fluoxetine (Prozac) or imipramine (Tofranil) among 128 pediatric burn survivors found them to be equally effective, with about 80% response overall, and that the non-responders to one antidepressant usually responded to the other.[56] Treatment with an SSRI or TCA should be continued for at least 9 months to 1 year following the improvement of symptoms because of the risk of relapse. When medication is discontinued, it should be reduced over time, for suddenly stopping the medicine might cause uncomfortable discontinuation symptoms, although they are not medically threatening. The relatively long half-life of fluoxetine (Prozac) usually protects patients from any discontinuation symptoms, but requires extended vigilance for any drug–drug interactions.

Major depression and dysthymia

Although depression is a reaction most observers would expect of burned patients, it is a rare long-term sequela of burn injury. According to Stoddard,[110] fewer than 50% of the children he surveyed had ever suffered major depression; dysthymia, another depressive disorder, occurred in only 10%. Outcome studies of adult burn survivors show a similar prevalence of major depression.[33,43,120-123]

To diagnose major depression, a patient must have five or more of the following DSM-IV symptoms *for a period of at least 2 weeks, and they must represent a change from previous functioning:*

- depressed mood most of the day (may be an irritable mood in children and adolescents);
- markedly diminished interest or pleasure in most activities;
- significant change in appetite, resulting in either weight loss or gain (for children, failure to make expected weight gains);
- insomnia or hypersomnia;
- feelings of worthlessness or excessive/inappropriate guilt nearly every day;
- fatigue or loss of energy nearly every day;
- diminished concentration or enhanced indecisiveness nearly every day;
- psychomotor agitation or retardation observable by others;
- recurrent thoughts of death, suicidal ideation, suicide attempt or plan.

This is an extremely difficult diagnosis to make during the acute burn period since many of the criteria are linked to physical symptoms. Even beyond the acute phase, the diagnosis is often complicated by grief following the loss of a loved one during a fire, and by sadness at one's altered body. The critical symptoms in a burned patient are depressed mood and anhedonia. Many times a patient's expressed interest in play or plans for the future rule out the diagnosis.

Major depression, with or without grief reaction, should be treated by a team approach. A patient should be involved in scheduled daily activities. Psychotherapy should begin to identify and address appropriate issues. Medication with SSRIs or TCAs, as described for acute and post-traumatic stress, is often helpful. Once the symptoms have responded to medication, treatment should continue for 9 months to 1 year in order to avoid relapse on discontinuation. When discontinuing medication, it should be slowly reduced rather than stopped suddenly so as to prevent discontinuation side effects.

A smaller percentage of burned patients will develop a milder but more protracted type of depression called dysthymia. This condition must be present for *at least 2 years* in *adults,* or 1 year in *children* and *adolescents in order to be diagnosed.* It is characterized by the following:

- depressed or irritable mood,
- appetite changes, sleep difficulties, fatigue, low self-esteem,
- poor concentration or difficulty making decisions,
- feelings of hopelessness.

The same combination of medication and psychotherapy is recommended for dysthymic patients as for major depression.

Summary

Psychiatric symptoms occur commonly as part of the complex systemic response to burn injuries. Psychological and pharmacological treatment are important in the successful recovery of a burned person, and perhaps mitigate against long-term psychiatrical sequelae of post-injury. It is important to note that psychological adaptation is a lengthy process occurring over months or years. During the postburn years, it is imperative that the burn team assess the mental and affective states of patients while assessing their physical recovery. Although most burned patients eventually make satisfactory adjustments, many continue for a long time to struggle with self-image, anger, and sadness. These disturbances often seem to be expressed through symptoms that are not easily observed by other than intimate friends and family of a patient.[124] Sleep disturbance, fear or withdrawal from previous activities are not behavioral disturbances which necessarily insure that a patient will attract psychiatric attention and treatment. They are, however, unhappy responses which can be ameliorated by treatment. It then becomes a responsibility of the expert in burn care and recovery to be aware of frequently occurring disturbed responses, to ask the right questions in order to assess a patient's status, and to assist a patient in receiving psychological and psychiatric assistance.

References

1. Mendelsohn IE. Liaison psychiatry and the burn center. Psychosomatics 1983: 24(3):235–243.
2. Ochitill H. Psychiatric consultation to the burn unit: the psychiatrist's perspective. Psychosomatics 1984; 25(9):689, 697–689, 701.
3. Andreasen NJC, Nayes P, Haraford C. Factors influencing adjustment of burn patients during hospitalization. Psychosom Med 1972; 34(6):517–525.
4. Noyes R, Frye S, Slymen D, et al. Stressful life events and burn injuries. J Trauma 1979; 19(3):141–144.
5. Darko D, Wachtel T, Ward H, et al. Analysis of 585 burn patients hospitalized over a six-year period. Part III: Psychosocial data. Burns 1986; 12:395–401.
6. Vogtsberger K, Taylor E. Psychosocial factors in burn injury. Texas Med 1984; 80:43–46.
7. Patterson DR, Finch CP, Wiechman SA, et al. Premorbid mental health status of adult burn patients: comparison with a normative sample. J Burn Care Rehabil 2003; 24(5):347–350.
8. Barillo DJ, Goode R. Substance abuse in victims of fire. J Burn Care Rehabil 1996; 17:71–76.
9. Thomas CR, Ayoub M, Rosenberg L, et al. Attention deficit hyperactivity disorder and pediatric burn injury: a preliminary retrospective study. Burns 2004; 30(3):221–223.
10. Powers PS, Stevens B, Arias F, et al. Alcohol disorders among patients with burns: crisis and opportunity. J Burn Care Rehabil 1994; 15:386–391.
11. Grobmyer SR, Maniscalco SP, Purdue GF, et al. Alcohol, drug intoxication, or both at the time of burn injury as a predictor of complications and mortality in hospitalized patients with burns. J Burn Care Rehabil 1996; 17:532–539.

12. Ho WS, To EWH, Chan ESY, et al. Burn injuries during paint thinner sniffing. Burns 1998; 24:757–759.

13. Sheridan RL. Burns with inhalation injury and petrol aspiration in adolescents seeking euphoria through hydrocarbon inhalation. Burns 1996; 22(7): 566–567.

14. Oh SJ, Lee SE, Burm JS, et al. Explosive burns during abusive inhalation of butane gas. Burns 1999; 25:341–344.

15. Nielson JA, Kolman PBR, Wachtel TL. Suicide and parasuicide by burning. J Burn Care Rehabil 1984; S(4):335–338.

16. Davidson T, Brown L. Self-inflicted burns: a 5-retrospective study. Burns Incl Therm Inj 1985; 11:157–160.

17. Stoddard FJ, Cahners SS. Suicide attempted by self-immolation during adolescence. II. Psychiatric treatment and outcome. Adolesc Psychiatry 1985; 12:266–280.

18. Krummen DM, James K, Klein RL. Suicide by burning: a retrospective review of the Akron Regional Burn Center. Burns 1998; 24:147–149.

19. Garcia-Sanchez V, Palao R, Legarre F. Self-inflicted burns. Burns 1994; 20(6):537–538.

20. Erzurum VZ, Varcellotti J. Self-inflicted burn injuries. J Burn Care Rehabil 1999; 20:22–24.

21. Tuohig GM, Saffle JR, Sullivan JJ, et al. Self-inflicted patient burns: suicide versus mutilation. J Burn Care Rehabil 1995; 16:429–436.

22. Raskind SM. Suicide by burning: emotional needs of the suicidal adolescent on the burn unit. Issues Compr Pediatr Nurs 1986; 9:369–382.

23. Powers PS, Cruse CW, Boyd F. Psychiatric status, prevention, and outcome in patients with burns: a prospective study. J Burn Care Rehabil 2000; 21:85–88.

24. Van Der Does AJ, Hinderink EM, Vloemans AF, et al. Burn injuries, psychiatric disorders and length of hospitalization. J Psychosom Res 1997; 43(4):431–435.

25. Tarrier N, Gregg L, Edwards J, et al. The influence of preexisting psychiatric illness on recovery in burn injury patients: the impact of psychosis and depression. Burns 2005; 31(1):45–49.

26. Fauerbach JA, Lawrence J, Haythornthwaite J, et al. Preinjury psychiatric illness and postinjury adjustment in adult burn survivors. The Academy of Psychosomatic Medicine 1996; 37(6): November–December.

27. Fauerbach JA, Lawrence J, Stevens S, et al. Work status and attrition from longitudinal studies are influenced by psychiatric disorder. J Burn Care Rehabil 1998; 19:247–252.

28. Fauerbach JA, Lawrence J, Haythornthwaite J, et al. Preburn psychiatric history affects posttrauma morbidity. Psychosomatics 1997; 38:374–385.

29. Taal LA, Faber AW. Dissociation as a predictor of psychopathology following burns injury. Burns 1997; 23(5):400–403.

30. Tedstone JE, Tarrier N, Faragher EB. An investigation of the factors associated with an increased risk of psychological morbidity in burn injured patients. Burns 1998; 24:407–415.

31. Willebrand M, Andersson G, Ekselius L. Prediction of psychological health after an accidental burn. J Trauma 2004; 57(2): 367–374.

32. Tedstone JE, Tarrier N. An investigation of the prevalence of psychological morbidity in burn-injured patients. Burns 1997; 23(7/8):550–554.

33. Steiner H, Clark W. Psychiatric complications of burned adults: a classification. J Trauma 1977; 17:134–143.

34. Perry S, Blank K. Relationships of psychological processes during delirium to outcome. Am J Psychiatry 1984; 141:843–847.

35. Patterson D, Everett J, Bombardier C, et al. Psychological effects of severe burn injuries. Psychol Bull 1993; 113(2):362–378.

36. Blakeney P, Meyer WJ III. Psychological aspects of burn care. Trauma Q 1994; II(2):166–179.

37. Morton R, Gleason O, Yates W. Psychiatric effects of anabolic steroids after burn injuries. Psychosomatics 2000; 41:1 January–February.

38. Thomas AB. A presentation on hallucinations.

39. Haynes B, Bright R. Burn coma: a syndrome associated with severe burn wound infection. J Trauma 1967; 7:46F75.

40. Antoon A, Volpe J, Crawford J. Burn encephalopathy in children. Pediatrics 1972; 50:609–616.

41. Hughes JR, Cayaffa JJ, Boswick JA Jr. Seizures following burns to the skin: III. Electroencephalographic recordings. Dis Nerv Syst 1975; 36:443–447.

42. Stoddard E. Psychiatric management of the burned patient. In: Martyn JAJ, ed. Acute care of the burn patient. Orlando, FL: Grune and Stratton; 1990:256–272.

43. Andreasen NJC, Norris A, Hartford C. Incidence of long-term psychiatric complications in severely burned adults. Ann Surg 1971; 174(5):785–793.

44. Teicher MH, Glod CA. Neuroleptic drags: indications and guidelines for their rational use in children and adolescents. J Child Adolesc Psychopharmacol 1990; 1:33–56.

45. Schatzberg AF, Cole JO. Manual of clinical psychopharmacology, 2nd edn. Washington, DC: American Psychiatric Press; 1991.

46. Kiely WE. Psychiatric syndromes in critically ill patients. JAMA 1976; 23S:2759–2761.

47. Moore DP. Rapid treatment of delirium in critically ill patients. Am J Psychiatry 1977; 134:1431–1432.

48. Ratcliff S, Meyer W, Cuervo L, et al. The use of haloperidol and associated complications in the agitated, acutely ill pediatric burn patient. J Burn Care Rehabil 2004; 25:472–478.

49. Huang V, Figge H, Demling R. Haloperidol in burn patients. J Burn Care Rehabil 1987; 8:269–273.

50. Still J, Friedman B, Law E, et al. Neuroleptic malignant syndrome in a burn patient. Burns 1998; 24:573–575.

51. Coffey BJ. Anxiolytics for children and adolescents. Traditional and new drugs. J Child Adolesc Psychopharmacol 1990; 1:57–83.

52. USP DI Volume I: Drug Information for the health care professional. Rockville, MD: United States Pharmacopeial Convention; 1994.

53. Martyn JAJ, Greenblatt DJ, Quinby WC. Diazepam kinetics in patients with severe burns. Anesth Analg 1983; 62:293–297.

54. Ehde DM, Patterson DR, Wiechman SA, et al. Post-traumatic stress symptoms and distress following acute burn injury. Burns 1999; 25:587–592.

55. Yu BH, Dimsdale JE. Posttraumatic stress disorder in patients with burn injuries. J Burn Care Rehabil 1999; 20:426–433.

56. Tcheung W, Robert R, Rosenberg L, et al. Early treatment of acute stress disorder in children suffering from major burn injury. Pediatr Crit Care Med 2005; 6(6):676–681.

57. Robert R, Blakeney P, Villarreal C, et al. Imipramine treatment in pediatric burn patients with symptoms of acute stress disorder: a pilot study. J Am Acad Child Adolesc Psychiatry 1999; 38(7):873–882.

58. Glassman AH. The newer antidepressant drugs and their cardiovascular effects. Psychopharmacol Bull 1984; 20:272–279.

59. Chiu S, Leonard HI. Antidepressants I: selective serotonin reuptake inhibitors. In: Martin A, Scahill L, Charney DS, et al., eds. Pediatric psychopharmacology: principles and practice. New York: Oxford University; 2003:Ch 22:274.

60. Thomas C, Rosenberg M, Blythe V, et al. Serotonin syndrome with linezolid. J Am Acad Child Adolesc Psychiatry 2004; 43(7): 790.

61. Glassman AH, Bigger JT Jr. Cardiovascular effects of therapeutic doses of tricyclic antidepressants. Arch Gen Psychiatry 1981; 38:815–820.

62. Ryan ND. Heterocyclic antidepressants in children and adolescents. J Child Adolesc Psychopharmacol 1990; 1:21–31.

63. Popper CW, Elliott GR. Sudden death and tricyclic antidepressants: clinical considerations for children. J Child Adolesc Psychopharmacol 1990; 1:125–132.

64. Kondro W. FDA urges 'black box' warning on pediatric antidepressants. CMAJ 2004; 171(8):837–838.

65. Bridge JA, Salary CB, Birmaher B, et al. The risks and benefits of antidepressant treatment for youth depression. Ann Med 2005; 37(6):404–412.

66. Lawrence JW, Fauerbach J, Eudell E, et al. The 1998 Clinical Research Award. Sleep disturbance after burn injury: a frequent yet understudied complication. J Burn Care Rehabil 1998; 19:480–486.

67. Rose M, Sanford A, Thomas C, et al. Factors altering the sleep of burned children. Sleep 2001; 24(1):45–51.

68. Boeve SA, Aaron LA, Martin-Herz SP, et al. Sleep disturbance after burn injury. J Burn Care Rehabil 2002; 23:32–38.

69. Robert R, Meyer WJ III, Villarreal C, et al. An approach to the timely treatment of acute stress disorder. J Burn Care Rehabil 1999; 20:250–258.

70. Raymond I, Ancoli-Israel S, Choiniere M. Sleep disturbances, pain and analgesia in adults hospitalized for burn injuries. Sleep Med 2004; 5:551–559.

71. Szyfelbein S, Osgood P, Catr D. The assessment of pain and plasma B-endorphin immunoactivity in burned children. Pain 1985; 22:173–182.

72. Beales J. Factors influencing the expectation of pain among patients in a children's burns unit. Burns 1983; 9(3):187–192.

73. Charlton J, Gragliardi G, Klein R, et al. Factors affecting pain in burned patients — a preliminary report. Postgrad Med J 1983; 59:604–607.

74. Difede J, Jaffe AB, Musngi G, et al. Determinants of pain expression in hospitalized burn patients. Pain 1997; 72:245–251.

75. Taal LA, Faber AW. Burn injuries, pain and distress: exploring the role of stress symptomatology. Burns 1997; 23(4):288–290.

76. Taal LA, Faber AW. Post-traumatic stress, pain and anxiety in adult burn victims. Burns 1998; 23 (7/8):545–549.

77. Saxe GN, Stoddard F, Hall E, et al. Pathways to PTSD, part I: children with burns. Am J Psychiatry 2005; 162(7):1299–1304.

78. Perq S. Undermedication for pain on a burn unit. Gen Hosp Psychiatry 1984; 6:308–316.

79. Watkins P, Cook E, May R, et al. Psychological stages in adaptation following burn injury: a method for facilitating psychological recovery of burn victims. J Burn Care Rehabil 1988; 9(4):376–384.

80. Yaster M, Deshpande J, Maxwell L. The pharmacologic management of pain in children. Therapy 1989; 15(10):14–26.

81. Colditz R. Management of pain in the newborn infant. J Pediatr Child Health 1991; 27:11–15.

82. Webb C, Stergios D, Rodgers B. Patient-controlled analgesia as postoperative pain treatment for children. J Pediatr Nurs 1989; 4(3):162–171.

83. Gaukroger PB, Chapman MJ, Davey RB. Pain control in pediatric burns – the use of patient-controlled analgesia. Burns 1991; 17(5): 396–399.

84. Wintgens A, Boileau B, Robaey P. Posttraumatic stress symptoms and medical procedures in children. Can J Psychiatry 1997; 42:611–616.

85. Blalock SJ, Bunker BJ, DeVellis RF. Psychological distress among survivors of burn injury: the role of outcome expectations and perceptions of importance. J Burn Care Rehabil 1994; 15: 421–427.

86. Fukunishi I, Yasunori C. Posttraumatic stress disorder and alexithymia in burn patients. Psychol Rep 1994; 75:1371–1376.

87. Fukunishi I, Sasaki K, Chishima Y, et al. Emotional disturbances in trauma patients during the rehabilitation phase. Gen Hosp Psychiatry 1996; 18:121–127.

88. Knudson-Cooper M. Emotional care of the hospitalized burned child. J Burn Care Rehabil 1982; 3:109–116.

89. Shakespeare V. Effect of small burn injury on physical, social and psychological health at 3–4 months after discharge. Burns 1998; 24:739–744.

90. Kimmo T, Jyrki V, Sirpa AS. Health status after recovery from burn injury. Burns 1998; 24:293–298.

91. Bryant RA. Predictors of post-traumatic stress disorder following burns injury. Burns 1996; 22(2):89–92.

92. Taal LA, Faber AW. Posttraumatic stress and maladjustment among adult burn survivors 1–2 years postburn. Burns 1998; 24:285–292.

93. Fukunishi I. Relationship of cosmetic disfigurement to the severity of posttraumatic stress disorder in burn injury or digital amputation. Psychother Psychosom 1999; 68:82–86.

94. Taal L, Faber AW. Posttraumatic stress and maladjustment among adult burn survivors 1 to 2 years postburn. Part II: the interview data. Burns 1998; 24:399–405.

95. Koon K, Blakeney P, Broemeling L, et al. Self-esteem in pediatric burn patients. Proc Am Burn Assoc 1992; 24:112.

96. Cull JG, Gill WS. Suicide probability scale manual. Los Angeles: Western Psychological Services; 1982.

97. Achenbach TM. Manual for child behavior checklist 4/18 and 1991 profile. Burlington, VT: University of Vermont Department of Psychiatry; 1991.

98. Achenbach TM. Manual for the teachers report forms and 1991 profile. Burlington, VT: University of Vermont Department of Psychiatry; 1991.

99. Achenbach TM. Manual for the youth self-report and 1991 profile. Burlington, VT: University of Vermont Department of Psychiatry; 1991.

100. Blakeney P, Meyer W, Moore P, et al. Social competence and behavioral problems of pediatric survivors of burns. J Burn Care Rehabil 1993; 14:65–72.

101. LeDoux J, Blakeney P, Meyer W, et al. Relationships between parental emotional states, family environment and the behavior adjustment of pediatric burn survivors. Proc Am Burn Assoc 1994; 26:134.

102. Blakeney P, Meyer III W, Robert R, et al. Long-term psychosocial adaptation of children who survive burns involving 80% or greater total body surface area. J Trauma 1998; 44(4):625–634.

103. Zeitlin REK. Long-term psychosocial sequelae of paediatric burns. Burns 1997; 23(6):467–472.

104. Blakeney P, Meyer W, Moore P, et al. Psychosocial sequelae of pediatric burns involving 80% or greater total body surface area. J Burn Care Rehabil 1993; 14:684–689.

105. Meyer WJ 3rd, Blakeney PE, Holzer CE, et al. Inconsistencies in psychosocial assessment of children after severe burns. J Burn Car Rehabil 1995: 16(5):559–568.

106. Abidin RR. Parental stress index manual. Charlottesville, VA: Pediatric Pathology Press; 1983.

107. Meyer WJ, Blakeney P, Moore P, et al. Parental well-being and behavioral adjustment of pediatric burn survivors. Burn Care Rehabil 1994; 15:62–68.

108. Curran JP, Cattell RB. Manual for the eight-state questionnaire (85Q). Champaign, IL: Institute for Personality and Ability Testing; 1976.

109. Rizzone LP, Stoddard FJ, Murphy JM, et al. Posttraumatic stress disorder in mothers of children and adolescent with burns. J Burn Care Rehabil 1994; 15:158–163.

110. Fukunishi I. Posttraumatic stress symptoms and depression in mothers of children with severe burn injuries. Psychol Rep 1983; 331–335.

111. Stoddard FJ, Nomzan DK, Murphy M. A diagnosis outcome study of children and adolescents with severe burns. J Trauma 1989; 29:471–477.

112. Stoddard FJ, Nomzan DK, Murphy M, et al. Psychiatric outcome of burned children and adolescents. J Am Acad Child Adolesc Psychiatry 1989; 28:589–595.

113. Baur KM, Hardy PE, Van Dorsten B. Posttraumatic stress disorder in burn populations: a critical review of the literature. J Burn Care Rehabil 1998; 19:230–240.

114. Powers PS, Cruse CW, Daniels S, et al. Posttraumatic stress disorder in patients with burns. J Burn Care Rehabil 1994; 15:147–153.

115. Lawrence JW, Fauerbach J, Munster A. Early avoidance of traumatic stimuli predicts chronicity of intrusive thoughts following burn injury. Behav Res Ther 1996; 34(8):643–646.

116. Difede J, Barocas D. Acute intrusive and avoidant PTSD symptoms as predictors of chronic PTSD following burn injury. J Trauma Stress 1999; 12(2):363–369.

117. Van Loey NE, Maas CJ, Faber AW, et al. Predictors of chronic posttraumatic stress symptoms following burn injury: results of a longitudinal study. J Trauma Stress 2003; 16(4):361–369.

118. Lawrence JW, Fauerbach JA. Personality, coping, chronic stress, social support and PTSD symptoms among adult burn survivors: a path analysis. J Burn Care Rehabil 2003; 24(1):63–72.

119. Saxe G, Stoddard F, Chawla N, et al. Risk factors for acute stress disorder in children with burns. J Trauma Dissociation 2005; 6(2):37–49.

120. Ward H, Moss R, Darko D, et al. Prevalence of post-burn depression following burn injury. J Burn Care Rehabil 1987; 8(4):294–298.

121. Malt U. Long-term psychosocial follow-up studies of burned adults: review of the literature. Burns 1980; 6:190–197.

122. Malt UF, Ugland OM. A long-term psychosocial follow-up study of burned adults. Acta Psychiatr Scand Suppl 1989; 80(355):94–102.

123. Faber A, Klasen H, Sauer E, et al. Psychological and social problems in burn patients after discharge: a follow-up study. Scand J Plast Reconstr Surg 1987; 21(3):307–309.

124. Meyer WJ, LeDoux J, Blakeney P, et al. Diminished adaptive behaviors among pediatric burn survivors. Proc Am Burn Assoc 1994; 26:133.

Chapter 66

Psychosocial recovery and reintegration of patients with burn injuries

Patricia E. Blakeney, Laura Rosenberg, Marta Rosenberg, and James A. Fauerbach

Introduction

Burn treatment extends beyond patient survival to include recovery of optimal function for the whole person. Increased likelihood of physical survival[1] heightens concern for potential psychological morbidity for the burn survivor.[2–8] Even in emergency circumstances, burn care providers enact treatment plans based on an assumption of future life for the patient. Decisions about treatment are influenced by concerns for preserving function, optimizing cosmetic appearance, and restoring psychological well-being. Psychological and social issues are integral parts of burn treatment from the time of injury through recovery and rehabilitation.

Burn survivors experience a series of traumatic assaults to the body and mind and the fabric of their social network which present extraordinary challenges to psychological resilience. Empirical data regarding the long-term sequelae of burn injury indicate that many adult burn survivors do achieve a satisfying quality of life and that most are judged to be well-adjusted individuals.[3,4] Similarly, most pediatric burn survivors, even those with the most extensive and disfiguring injuries, do not exhibit serious behavioral problems.[5–12]

However, 30% of any given sample of adult burn survivors consistently demonstrate moderate to severe psychological and/or social difficulties.[3,4] The incidence of psychopathology among children is approximately the same as that for adults.[5–12] A significant minority of adult burn survivors report a diminished quality of life, including dissatisfaction with appearance and social or occupational difficulties.[13–17] Burn injury often leads to at least temporary reduction in social involvement[16] and vocational activity, with 50–60% of individuals requiring a change in employment status.[14] Decreased sexual satisfaction, particularly for women, may also occur and appears to relate to physical changes and body image more than burn size or location.[15]

Postburn adjustment is affected by quality of adjustment prior to injury, notably preburn psychiatric disorder.[19] It has been demonstrated that even subclinical levels of post-traumatic distress[20] and body image dissatisfaction[21] during the acute hospitalization can independently reduce health-related quality of life for prolonged periods. Importantly, baseline indices of psychosocial strength (absence of preburn psychopathology) and support (marital status and living arrangement) predicts psychological adjustment after a severe burn injury while burn severity (TBSA, burn location, trips to OR) does not.[18,22,23] For children and adolescents, several studies have found that postburn adjustment is determined primarily by the quality of parental and family support. Family cohesion, organization, and emphasis on spiritual/moral concerns have all been found to relate to positive adjustment of pediatric burn survivors.[18,23] For adolescent survivors, families of well-adjusted individuals valued and encouraged autonomy within the context of family cohesion.[18]

Empirical studies, as well as clinical observations and patient self-reports, support the idea that burn care incorporating psychosocial expertise can facilitate positive psychological adaptation to the challenges of traumatic injury, painful treatment, and permanent disfigurement.[10,26] This chapter considers aspects of burn treatment that assist the individual in attaining optimal function psychologically, emotionally, and socially (Figures 66.1 and 66.2).

Psychological treatment concurrent with physical treatment

Burn injury treatment and rehabilitation requires interdisciplinary participation, with a complete spectrum of specialists involved to a greater or lesser extent at each phase of treatment. Specialists focus on specific systems or functional domains of each patient at each stage of treatment but the overall approach of the team is integrated and organized both vertically and horizontally throughout the entire process. The *horizontal organization* flows longitudinally, such that variables assessed in earlier phases impact in measurable ways the variables assessed in later phases. We categorize those factors

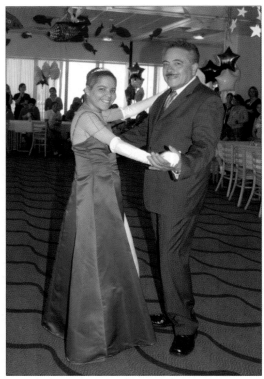

Fig. 66.1 Burn survivor at her Quinceañera shares the traditional first dance with parent.

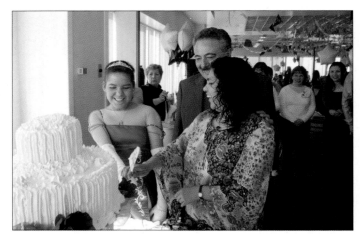

Fig. 66.2 Quinceañera cutting cake with parents.

which influence burn injury and recovery in terms of six horizontal (i.e. longitudinal) time phases (pre-injury, admission, critical care, in-hospital recuperation, reintegration, and rehabilitation). Burn care also has a *vertical organization* in which each phase is further categorized by the domains of function directly related to health-related quality of life (physiological/anatomical, cognitive, psychological, social). The assessment and intervention provided in these domains involve the entire patient from the cellular level upwards in complexity of organization to the organ system level, then to the cognitive and psychological level and finally to the social system level. The individual's functional ability within each domain is bi-directionally related to the other domains. Each specialist interacts with the patient, with significant others in the patient's social system, and with the other members of the burn care and rehabilitation team. The burn care and rehabilitation team comprises a true interdisciplinary system that operates over six time phases (i.e. horizontal organization) and across four functional domains (i.e. vertical organization).

Clinicians with expertise in human behavior should be involved in the treatment program for all burned patients throughout the process.[27–31] In this chapter, these experts are called psychotherapists. Every person, however, who interacts with a patient impacts the psychosocial world of the patient. Any caregiver, including the patient's family, may be the instrument of psychotherapeutic intervention.[26] The role of the psychotherapist is to consult with caregivers about psychological and social issues and to suggest therapeutic interventions that any or all can act upon.[27–32] Furthermore, the psychotherapist on a burn team provides direct treatment to patients as

appropriate to their changing concerns. As the needs of the patient evolve, the intensity of direct psychotherapeutic intervention varies according to those changing needs.

The family of a patient will always greatly influence a patient's recovery and must be considered as part of a patient's treatment plan. For the psychotherapist on the burn team, the family unit is often the 'patient'.[30–33] Each individual within a family, including the burn survivor, is an essential element of this unit which must adapt to change. The psychosocial issues and therapeutic tasks for the patient and family are much the same across the spectrum of ages from young children through the elderly, regardless of size and severity of injury.[26,30,31,34,35]

Assisting with death

Treatment plans and programs must be based on an assumption of life beyond the hospital; however, death also occurs on the burn unit, and psychosocial treatment planning includes plans for assisting patients in living to the cessation of life.[26] As part of such a plan, the patient's family must be aided in preparing for and enduring bereavement.[36] In this event, supporting and enhancing whatever coping strengths the family manifests is the primary task for psychotherapy. Most families initially deny the possibility of death, appearing not to hear an unwanted prognosis. Staff can allow the family to maintain hope while subtly preparing them with honest statements which pose death as an outcome that is possible to accept.[26] Comforting the bereft and helping them to care for themselves, physically and spiritually, are essential elements of a plan that facilitates the family's ability to participate in the process. Keeping the family informed about changes in the patient's condition and actively supporting, sometimes instructing, them in continuing their relationships with the dying patient help the patient and family through this difficult event.

At the time of death, the staff can psychologically support the family by assisting them through the necessary paperwork (e.g. signing consents for release of the body or for autopsy) and in allowing them quiet, private time with the deceased loved one before the body is removed. Bereft family members often want to hold on to something belonging to or representing the deceased. Staff should offer to assist in finding or creating such a tangible object for distraught family members who may not think to make the request. At the Shriners Hospital in Galveston, families typically say they do want a 'memory' item. When no such item is readily available, a hand or foot print on paper or a plaster cast model of the patient's hand or foot seems to bring solace.

Sometimes a patient must be informed about the deaths of others involved in the same situation that brought the patient to the burn unit. Families may be reluctant to tell a loved one such news while they are still in critical condition, but patients need to hear honest answers as soon as they ask questions. It is the role of the psychotherapist to assist family and patient in this difficult situation.[37]

A death occurring in the context of family acceptance is more easily accepted by staff. Nevertheless, deaths, especially of a patient, are always sad and may elicit a wide range of strong emotions among the members of the burn team. Allowing a time for debriefing and validating the feelings of the staff can be extremely helpful in maintaining the morale of the team as a whole.

Cultural sensitivity

Burn patients come from diverse cultures, and burn care teams must be sensitive to how cultural issues can affect patients and families in all the phases of the recovery process. 'Culture' refers to the socially transmitted expectations, beliefs, traditions, and behavioral patterns typical of a given community at a point in time. It is influenced by many factors. Country of origin is influential, but also geographical location within the country, ethnicity, and socioeconomic background are among those factors that together distinguish cultures. Staff must also be aware of their own biases, values, and assumptions that stem from their cultures.[38,39]

Acculturation is the process in which individuals from one culture embrace patterns, customs, beliefs, values, and the language of the dominant culture.[40,41] Patients and their families on first arriving at a burn care facility must rapidly adapt to the culture of the hospital environment. Even if the hospital is within their own community, they experience some level of culture shock and acculturation. This process is even more complicated for those who are transported for care to communities far removed from their homes and perhaps in another country. For many, this traumatic situation is also the first time they have traveled to another country, and the first time they have had to deal with differences in language, currency, living accommodations, and foods. Individuals' concepts of time and space, appropriate hospitality, importance of greetings, how non-verbal gestures are interpreted, and ways of expressing gratitude may differ greatly among cultures. Ideas of what caused the burn injury and what is necessary for healing to occur also are determined by cultural values.[42,43]

Coping with such a multitude of unfamiliar experiences in a situation that is traumatic under the best of circumstances presents extraordinary stress that can inhibit a patient's or family's ability to participate in the recovery process. Such difficulties correctly recognized can be addressed by the burn team so that cultural differences are not impediments to recov-

ery. Cultural traditions can be incorporated into treatment plans to enhance participation toward recovery. It is not necessary for providers to know the beliefs and expectations of every culture, but what is necessary are sensitivity and willingness to learn about cultural differences. Staff can acknowledge their lack of familiarity and pose a question to the patient/family of whether there is anything the team can do to help meet their cultural, spiritual, and religious needs. The question conveys respect for cultural differences and a desire to help through the acculturation process.

Approach to assessment and intervention

Our general approach to assessment and care of burn survivors is described throughout this chapter as we suggest interventions to deal with specific difficulties commonly experienced at each phase of recovery. It is basically a behavioral approach based on learning principles (e.g. operant conditioning, cognitive restructuring, and social learning theories) where maladjusted behavior itself (rather than intrapsychic phenomena, for example) is the target of intervention.[44] Assessment and treatment are integrally related and both occur simultaneously throughout the recovery and rehabilitation process.

The longitudinal pattern of psychological recovery

Psychological healing occurs across time commensurate with physical healing in a pattern which is relatively predictable and consistent.[31,45,46] Awareness of this pattern allows caregivers to anticipate the emergence of psychosocial issues and to prepare a patient for coping with those issues. Predicting problematic issues for patients enables them to view their concerns in a context of normal reactions rather than as symptoms of psychological impairment. For convenience in describing this pattern, we have arbitrarily designated a pre-injury phase and five phases of recovery: admission, critical care, in-hospital recuperation, reintegration, and rehabilitation.

Pre-injury adjustment

Psychosocial assessment is begun as quickly as possible upon admission of the patient. However, preburn physical and psychological health, coping skills, and family/social support are closely related to the behavior, distress, and recovery of a patient[19,47–50] Size or severity of burn, age at injury, and gender of the survivor are important variables in treatment, but have little documented influence on the eventual outcome for a survivor.[4,18,49,50] Prior stressful events and coping strategies, risk factors, as well as psychosocial and economic strengths, are included in a good history of a patient's premorbid lifestyle. A patient's history and position in the family as well as the family's strengths and weaknesses are often helpful pieces of information in guiding plans for treatment.

Because patients will be dependent to some extent on family or other caretakers during recovery, it is essential to identify risk factors in the family system.[26] Historical risk factors which may predispose individuals to burn injury and which portend poor prognoses are physical illness, substance abuse, psychiatric illness, behavioral problems, poverty, inadequate social support, and heightened family disruption.[53–55] These factors are often causally related to the burn injury and to post-injury recovery. For example, a lifetime prevalence of psychiatric disorder is much more common among patients with burn injuries relative to published national data from a representative community sample.[56] This is particularly troublesome in that this history of psychiatric disorder is significantly related to postburn psychiatric complications and to poorer postburn health-related quality of life.[56] In addition to these risk factors, every family has its unique difficulties. The trauma of serious injury exacerbates preexisting problems.

Early identification of psychosocial strengths and vulnerabilities, including those which contributed to the circumstances of the burn injury, allow the team to develop treatment and discharge plans which will optimize the patient's recovery. The importance of assessing the circumstances of injury is emphasized in instances of abuse or malignant neglect. In addition, during early assessment interviews with a family, the staff initiates a therapeutic alliance with those who are most likely to be involved in assisting a patient's recovery.

Admission crisis

At the time of admission, patients with burn injuries universally suffer pain and anxiety. Most are experiencing terror, confusion, and psychological shock. Events causing a serious burn injury are frightening, and patients often believe that death is imminent. The hospital environment can also be confusing and frightening. While the physiological emergency is being treated aggressively, the psychological crisis must also be addressed. On admission, the primary psychological tasks are to establish therapeutic rapport, diminish anxiety, and assess the psychosocial strengths and needs of the patient. The first two tasks are addressed immediately by orienting a patient, by assisting the patient to focus on immediate priorities, and by assuring the patient that the burn team is composed of knowledgeable experts who will provide excellent care. The patient's heightened anxiety can be expected to interfere with their comprehension, so it is usually necessary to repeat statements of reassurance. To prevent a patient from becoming emotionally overwhelmed, it may be necessary to — at least temporarily — not talk about trauma-related content perhaps by asking objective, easily answered questions not directly related to the event or injury (e.g. hometown, favorite sports, etc.).[57]

Psychotherapeutic rapport is developed as a patient associates the voice or touch of a therapist with increased comfort. Techniques of hypnotherapy or relaxation with focused imagery can be very helpful in quickly assisting a patient to feel more comfortable. Patients during this crisis can be expected to be cognitively and emotionally regressed, and it may be important to respond to them at that regressed level. Touching patients in a non-threatening manner and in a soothing rhythm is often the most effective way to maintain a regressed patient's focus and communicate reassurance.

Members of the patient's family are also traumatized and may experience difficulty in eating and sleeping for the first several days. They, too, experience difficulty in concentrating and may require frequent repetition of information. They may feel a loss of control, a generalized sense of incompetence and helplessness in providing comfort for the patient. The psychotherapeutic tasks to be accomplished immediately with a

family are similar to those for a patient (i.e. to establish a therapeutic relationship and to diminish anxiety). Both tasks can often be initiated by assisting them in orienting to the hospital and by providing relevant information about the normal responses to trauma. Explaining, for example, that people in this situation often have difficulty for a few days in eating, sleeping, and concentrating, communicates empathy and validates that their distress is acceptable and temporary. Family members are important components of the therapeutic efforts for the patient, and it is important to say this explicitly. This helps to return to them a sense of purpose and control. Even on the day of admission, the staff begins shaping the family behaviors and support network by outlining some immediate concerns. Learning about the injury and its treatment helps to restore a family's sense of competence and provides opportunities for them to experience the reality of their roles in helping the patient.

The manner in which an individual and family will ultimately adjust to long-term sequelae of a burn injury (e.g. deformity, disfigurement) is often determined in the early stages. It is of utmost importance for the treatment team to demonstrate respect for each individual from their first interactions with patients and families.

Critical care phase

From hospital admission until the majority of open wounds are covered, the emphasis in treatment of a burned patient is necessarily on intensive medical and surgical care to resolve physiological crises. This period is psychologically critical as well. A patient experiences great anxiety during much of this time. Fear of death blends into fear of pain and fear of treatment procedures.[31] A multitude of organic factors stemming from both the injury and its treatment, as well as premorbid conditions, can all contribute to psychological symptoms of disorientation, confusion, sleep disturbance, transient psychosis, and delirium, which are commonly observed among adolescent and adult patients.[31,58] Pharmacological interventions to manage pain and anxiety should be instituted and, along with psychological interventions, can diminish anxiety and confusion. Repeated statements of orientation to time, place, and person are mandatory. Objects that are familiar and comforting can be placed in the patient's view or so that the patient can touch them. The patient's environment should be as soothing as possible. A schedule which approximates a regular wake/sleep cycle helps a patient begin to feel normal. Visits from family and friends can provide familiarity and reassurance to a patient.

Staff interacting with patients during this phase must be willing to listen to patients' anxieties and reassure them that the nightmares and vivid memories are normal aspects of recovery. Staff can help patients focus on the present time in which they are safe in the hospital and are healing. When a patient is withdrawn or in a coma, staff must remember that the patient may be hearing, although not responding, and must take care to talk to the patient. They must also be discreet in what is said within a patient's hearing range. Patients are often listening to determine what will happen to them; and, in their altered mental states, they may attribute unexpected meanings to what they hear. Although the staff should persist in attempting to orient a patient, they should not argue with the patient about what is reality. Arguments with a patient who is having vivid illusions, delusions, or hallucinations are usually counterproductive. Psychological interventions are aimed at diminishing anxiety and increasing comfort rather than correcting a patient's perceptions of reality.[26]

Often, the content of the patient's delirium can be used to facilitate reassurance and relaxation. For example, a man in this phase who believed he was on a boat was combative and remained agitated in spite of psychopharmacological attempts to calm him. The psychologist assisted during procedures by talking to the patient about being on the boat in the same manner used to induce hypnotic trance. As the patient engaged in the description of the boat, the psychologist described calming elements of their imaginary surroundings such as the rhythm of the waves, the cool breeze, the warm sun. For these temporary periods the patient could become calm and could follow the psychologist's instructions to allow procedures. Although the patient was, for several days, disoriented and intermittently agitated, the staff were able to provide the care he needed during this critical phase.

During the critical care phase, family members usually become at ease with the routines of the hospital. They may, however, continue to experience some symptoms of acute traumatic stress, such as intrusive thoughts, difficulties with sleep, or avoidance behaviors.[59] They remain anxious about their relative's condition and eager for information about their patient's present and future status.[59,60] In addition, as they accept what has happened, family members begin to think of other concerns which elicit anxiety. They may find themselves thrust by the burn injury into new roles with new responsibilities. Often, especially if the hospital is at some distance from their home, they are without their customary support systems.

It is helpful to provide families with information about what they may expect to observe with their burned relative in the immediate future and to guide family members as they respond to the patient. Families need instruction about how they can be helpful.[59,60] They may be reluctant to touch the burned person for fear of causing pain and are usually relieved when encouraged to do so. They may feel uncomfortable in talking aloud to a non-responsive patient; the staff can suggest that their voices are extremely important to the patient even though the patient does not respond. The staff must find ways to allow family members to nurture their relative and provide instructions so that the family can begin to become comfortable in caring for the patient's needs. Staff members of critical care units are very busy and may, at moments, want to send the family away so that tasks can be completed more efficiently. However, these first instructions to the family are of critical importance to the future of the patient who needs the expressions of care by loved ones. Taking the time to 'treat' the family is a very important part of treating the patient. In addition, this 'treatment' facilitates the family's resumption of feelings of competence and control, desensitizes them to the sights and odors of the burned person, and encourages the family to join with the burn team in the healing and rehabilitation of the patient.

The burn team must also emotionally support the family's defenses. Often, family members appear to deny or to cling to delusions about the critical nature of the patient's status or the extent of the patient's injuries. It is important to give a family honest information while allowing them to protect themselves from overwhelming despair.[61] A family must find reason to hope, and the staff can assist them by suggesting realistic and optimistic outcomes. For example, we display in our offices many photographs of burn survivors engaged in a variety of activities such as swimming, going to a prom, wedding pictures, pictures of survivors with their children. The snapshots convey a hopeful message even if nothing is said explicitly about them. Family members of acute patients usually can be observed looking at the photos, and at that point it is easy to discuss which of those survivors had injuries comparable to their relative. The message to be conveyed is that there is hope for a good outcome and that successful recovery requires arduous and painful work over a period of time.

Psychotherapeutic work with the family must also identify and plan for management of those family issues which may impede a patient's recovery and rehabilitation. Some of the common issues are financial support, family alliances, historical family events, and beliefs which influence current perceptions and behaviors. Management plans must support, to the extent possible, the physical and emotional well-being of all the members of the family during a period of time in which the burned patient's needs place unusual and urgent demands on the family system.[60–62]

Psychological factors play a significant role in pain and anxiety management. Scheduling of pain and anxiety assessments and the choice of assessment tools used have psychological relevance. Regular, routine assessments of discomfort imply to a patient and a patient's family that the medical staff consider discomfort a valid issue that will be treated. This not only validates a patient's concerns but also sets an expectancy of relief when pain or anxiety is a problem. The use of standardized scales provides the message that to experience a range of pain and comfort responses is normal and allows the patient to participate to some degree in mastering discomfort. When staff assess comfort as routinely as vital signs and indicate that they believe the patients, patients are less likely to feel that they must complain loudly in order to convince the staff that their need for pain relief is legitimate. They also are less likely to feel hopeless and helpless and become depressed.

A supportive milieu that diminishes anxiety also enhances a patient's ability to gain increased comfort with both background and procedural pain. The presence of a supportive person is effective in decreasing pain.[63] Encouraging patient participation in self-care has been demonstrated to be effective in assisting a patient to become more comfortable.[64] In particular, patients who are hypervigilant and reluctant to trust seem to gain mastery over pain when they remove their own dressings or debride their own wounds. Behavioral interventions that enhance a patient's mastery or control, in general, decrease pain and anxiety. For example, adults and children who are developmentally capable of understanding the relationship of treatment to healing better tolerate procedures when told the reason for each procedure.[65] The choice of words used in explanations of procedures can ameliorate anxiety and reduce the expectancy of pain; for example, one can say 'some people feel a poke; others feel a prick or a tingle — you tell me what you feel' rather than saying 'This is going to hurt now.' Touch can be used as a distraction and to induce relaxation; continuous, rhythmic repetitive stroking of a non-injured and non-threatening body part accompanied by comforting sounds assists relaxation of many adults as well as children, including infants.[66] Music therapy can be an excellent adjunct to analgesia. Verbal praise and other tangible reinforcers facilitate learning to cope with painful stimuli by relaxing.[67]

Modeling for and instructing a family in soothing their patient is important. Outside the hospital, family members may know well how to calm their relative, but they may need instruction and/or encouragement from the staff to be comforting within the hospital. Once involved, family members can be valuable assets in providing the 'placebo' that relieves a patient's distress.

Other non-pharmacological interventions also can facilitate comfort. Distraction, deep breathing, progressive relaxation, biofeedback, and virtual reality have all been reported to be effective in decreasing pain and distress associated with burn treatment.[68,69] Hypnosis induces a relaxed and focused state of awareness which can be extremely helpful in facilitating comfort for adults and pediatric patients and may offer other benefits as well, such as: to increase appetite, to decrease regressive behavior, and to enhance a patient's sense of well-being, self-confidence, and body image.[70,71] An inflexible protocol for hypnosis, however, will be no more effective than an inflexible regimen of medications. With each patient, hypnotic inductions and suggestions must be modified to facilitate a patient's use of imagery. Some patients will respond well to suggestions of imagining a 'favorite place'; others can more easily imagine switches to 'turn off' sensation in selected body parts. Children aged 3 and over respond well to storytelling, with suggestions for comfort and mastery interwoven into the story.[72]

Providing good pain control enhances the burn care staff's effectiveness in promoting psychological recovery of a patient by allowing the staff to interact in more pleasant ways with happier patients. Comfortable patients who perceive themselves to have some power are less prone to regressive behavior. They are perceived by staff as more likable which, in turn, reinforces the positive self-regard of the patients.

In-hospital recuperation phase

Paradoxically, as burned patients become physically stronger, open wounds almost healed, and grafting near completion, their continued treatment presents additional and perhaps more difficult challenges to the burn team. Treatment at this stage cannot simply be imposed upon a relatively helpless patient; now the team must succeed in motivating the patient to participate in treatments and to assume responsibility for recovery. The patient who desires optimal recovery must comply with the medical team's orders and instructions, many of which require significant physical discomfort.

In this phase, patients are just beginning to comprehend the extent of their injury and to realize that their body, changed forever, is no longer congruent with their premorbid self-image. Their anxieties now are increasingly about the future and less about the past and present. Pain continues to be a concern; new experiences of pain must be addressed as patients become increasingly active in rehabilitative exercises. Patients are confronted with the new physical limitations imposed by their injuries; they experience their bodies now as incompetent and disfigured. Patients involved in this struggle shift rapidly in affective behaviors reflecting rapid shifts in cognition. Much of the time, patients experience themselves as the 'preburn self' (i.e. the 'real self'). When the body will not move as it did in the past or when the scarred skin is viewed, a patient remembers and grieves. Patients become aware of their changed appearance as they observe the responses of others and note these responses invalidate their former body image. Their concepts about their social roles may no longer fit with society's beliefs. Their premorbid identities no longer exist intact and new identities must incorporate remnants of the old, as well as the changed, physical body, thus further stripping them of their identities. In this confusing state, the patient may be expected to act out anger and fear.

In addition to physical limitations, the role of 'hospital patient' imposes a loss of control and autonomy on the survivor. After a period of realistic dependence on others, a patient may be frightened and ambivalent about resuming self-care.[47] The demanding schedule necessary for treatment during this period heightens a patient's feelings of inadequacy. A patient becomes easily fatigued yet must continue in a schedule of tasks determined primarily by the burn team, thus providing additional evidence of the patient's loss of autonomy and ability.

Emotional lability and cognitive and behavioral regression are typically observed in patients of all ages during this trying time. Perhaps the most difficult behavior for patient, family, and staff is the patient's expression of anger. Patients, of course, have many reasons to be angry, and they need to express that anger in order to define and direct it adaptively; however, there are significant limitations upon the availability of situations in which they can express anger. Patients have almost no privacy, nor can they relieve tension through physical activities such as running. Typically, family members and patient care staff, having devoted much time and energy to the patient, are prone to perceive the patient's angry behavior as a personal and unjust attack by an ungrateful patient. Certainly, the patient will direct rageful temper tantrums toward those who are the safest targets, usually a spouse or parent first and then a nurse or therapist. Angry attacks are best understood as necessary ventilation by the patient rather than sincere evaluations of family or staff.

Expressions of rage are not only upsetting to family and staff; they also frighten patients who themselves perceive this loss of control as evidence of potential destruction of self or others on whom they are dependent. Following an outburst, a patient typically feels guilty and fears withdrawal of love and support by those who were earlier subjugated to the angry behavior. These fears are added to the patient's fears of being rejected because of the changed appearance. Turning anger now toward self, the patient may feel overwhelmed, hopeless, depressed, and even suicidal. If the hospitalization continues over several weeks, patients experience repetitive frustrations, and tend to feel hopeless and depressed more often. Hopelessness is more likely to result when patients feel as if they have no control over aversive events and eventually give up trying to control what happens to them; such hopelessness over time can lead to chronic depression.[73]

Psychotherapeutic work at this phase intensifies and is largely focused on working with the rest of the team to help patients combat feelings of hopelessness and helplessness.

Important toward this end is structuring treatment sessions to promote patients' experience of control, achieving success, and feeling rewarded while progressing through difficult procedures. Positive feelings, generated by achieving the goals one has established, increase one's likelihood of repeating the effort. For example, a rehabilitation exercise session based on a work to quota versus work to tolerance basis establishes clear expectations, rewards adequate performance and consistently builds on prior achievements.[74] Desired behaviors (e.g. pressure garment use, walking on treadmill, reassuring self-statements when looking in a mirror at one's scars) must be reinforced, e.g. by verbal praise or by a time for rest. Since success breeds success it is helpful to begin and end sessions with manageable tasks that generate positive feelings of achievement and mastery. In addition, it can be helpful to 'Always Leave 'em Laughing'. Relaxation, humor, and ending on a good note in general are methods of following the desired response with a rewarding experience.

Much psychotherapeutic work during this phase is accomplished with patient and family together. Families must learn how to assist a patient in adjusting to the new situation, and the family system itself must accommodate to the changed situation. Research has shown the high importance of strengthening the family unit, facilitating family closeness, and supporting their attempts to organize their lives to incorporate the additional duties involved in providing continued care for their patient.[22–24,50] They must plan and implement adjustments in the family and home environment that will be necessary for the continuation of the patient's recovery and rehabilitation after discharge. Maintaining the integrity of the family unit while making needed adjustments is of high priority and is a challenge. Parents of a burned child must learn to advocate for their injured child but to avoid overprotection by themselves or others. They must encourage the child to perform independently to the limits of physical and age-appropriate ability. Parents and spouses even of adult patients often struggle against desires to protect and infantilize their recovering loved one. Staff can model for the family behaviors that demonstrate respect and courtesy for each family member including the patient.

A psychotherapeutic challenge of this phase is to accept and validate the patient's emotional demonstrations as normal behaviors in the recovery process while also setting limits on the ways in which the emotional upheaval will be expressed. Early in this phase, as the patient begins to ask about the future, the psychotherapist can describe the predictable pattern of emotional vicissitudes indicating that, should such occur, they are normal; they can be endured and managed. The staff must demonstrate positive regard and acceptance of the patient while also helping the patient to exercise control over destructive behaviors. At times, they must impose external limits to protect the patient.

Another psychotherapeutic task with both patient and family is to titrate their denial with graded presentations of reality.[47] Staff can anticipate and assist a patient in asking questions about future disfigurement and functional abilities, including sexual activity. Without evading questions, psychotherapists give honest but hopeful appraisals that emphasize ability and minimize deformity and disability. For example, as a patient voices an unrealistic belief that time and/or plastic surgery will return the former appearance, one can state that burned skin will never look like unburned skin and that there will always be some scarring, but that appearance will change with time. Allowing patients to hope, even for unrealistic outcomes, protects them from despair and enables them to continue to believe that there are reasons to endure the pain of rehabilitation.[30,31] Patients and families should be given the information that rehabilitation may require several years to achieve optimal satisfaction, but that the painful efforts usually obtain good results.[26]

The therapeutic message to be delivered is that survivors can find ways of achieving whatever goals they set for themselves; the process is lengthy and difficult, and survivors will often feel overwhelmed and hopeless. Expressing sadness and anger is to be expected and accepted; however, such feelings can never be allowed to stop a patient from participating in the necessary regimen to achieve full recovery. Being burned does not relieve a survivor of the responsibility of competence.

Many survivors have endured the process and discovered that they can enjoy their lives even though their early expectations were not, and could not have been, realized. Introducing such a recovered survivor to the recuperative burned patient can be a very helpful intervention at this point.[31] The more experienced survivor can be heard as a trustworthy authority in a way the unburned professional cannot. Visual images of burn survivors telling their stores and presenting themselves in daily life activities on film or video can aid in accomplishing this purpose.[75] Groups of patients and/or families of burned patients at varying stages of recovery and rehabilitation have been helpful in providing information, emotional validation, and support as well as reinforcing the concept that it is possible to survive burns and live acceptably happy lives.[60]

Reintegration phase

Although plans for a patient's discharge to outpatient status are developed from the time of admission, very specific plans must be made in the final days of hospitalization. A major objective at this time is to facilitate a patient's reentry and reintegration into life at home. Returning home signifies social interactions with the larger community of extended family, friends, and strangers. Patients as well as family must prepare for those encounters. Goodstein[47] appropriately labels this the 'social emergency' phase of treatment.

Families and patients alike are often ambivalent about leaving the safe environment of the hospital. Patients, including very young children, fear social rejection or ridicule because of their changed abilities or appearance.[76,77] Family members will probably feel, and may express, a desire to protect their patient from rejection or ridicule. Family members may also express concerns about their ability to continue the time-consuming physical care of the patient while resuming their usual responsibilities. Patients may doubt their abilities to resume former activities. As discharge approaches, anxieties intensify, and patients can be expected to evidence some regressive behaviors that, in turn, can reinforce the family's doubts.

Psychotherapeutic activities of this phase involve education and preparation of patient and family about the difficulties that can be anticipated at discharge. Patients and families may deny that they will have problems. Rather than accepting their assurance that problems will not arise, the psychotherapist can characterize such events as normal and 'usual', and proceed, without condescending or judging, to offer suggestions for developing a repertoire of alternative behaviors to address those problems 'just in case' they do experience difficulties. Issues such as recurrence of symptoms of post-traumatic stress, sleep disturbance, irritability, or fear of resuming sexual activities should be discussed during the days prior to discharge. This preparatory verbal rehearsal enhances the probability that the patient/family will be less reluctant to ask for help if problems do occur; if problems do not occur, the staff has the opportunity to congratulate the patient/family on their strengths or skills in coping.

Toward the end of inpatient treatment, patients are expected to resume increased autonomy; caretakers are supported in withdrawing assistance to the degree possible. It is helpful at this point to develop with patients/families a daily schedule to guide them in accomplishing necessary tasks. The burn team relinquishes performance of daily care so that the patient/family can assume care to the extent that they will be required to conduct it at home. The patient and family can benefit from the opportunity to rehearse outpatient care while still able to consult with the burn team for direction and support. Rehearsals are opportunities for all involved to experience difficulties in a safe environment and to plan corrective actions.

Important among these rehearsals are those of interpersonal interactions outside the hospital. Burn survivors have reported their most difficult experience at discharge involved observing the reactions of others.[78] Patients benefit from the opportunity to experience such reactions before discharge from the hospital. They may leave the hospital for brief outings and return to the hospital for reassurance, encouragement, and praise.[79] James Partridge of Changing Faces, an organization dedicated to assisting persons with facial disfigurement, recommends a brief social skills training program called '3-2-1-GO!' The program can be provided in the hospital by staff who regularly interact with patients. The patient is asked to plan for uncomfortable social situations by thinking of 3 things to do when someone stares at them, 2 things to say when someone asks them what happened (to cause the scars), and 1 thing to think if someone turns away from them.[80] Patient/family groups can be extremely helpful in the process of anticipating difficulties at discharge and rehearsing solutions while also providing emotional support.

In addition to preparing a patient and family for discharge, the burn team may also prepare the 'community' to which a patient will return. The 'community' may include extended family, neighbors, church groups, social clubs, a patient's workplace or, in the case of a school-age pediatric patient, the school. Instructing those unfamiliar with burns in what to say or do to ease a survivor's reentry may facilitate reintegration.[78,79,81]

A few well-organized reentry programs for pediatric burned patients have been described in the literature.[78,81] Although there is no evidence that adult burn survivors are in less need of assistance with reintegrating into their social worlds, published information about organized reentry programs for adults is scarce.[79,82] Reentry programs for adults and children involve the same fundamental elements and address the same issues. They educate the community in a developmentally sensitive fashion. They address both the intellectual and emotional aspects of burn injury, provide generic information about burn injuries and burn treatment, and emphasize a survivor's abilities as well as clarify the ways in which a survivor may need assistance. Homemade videotapes can be sent to target groups ahead of a patient, thus allowing a community the opportunity to see and hear the burn survivor, to anticipate difficulties, and to plan coping responses. Educational information presented in pamphlets or letters can be directed to those who will play key roles in facilitating a patient's transition from hospital to home community. If possible, one or more members of a burn team may visit the home community and speak to targeted groups, answering questions which people may be reluctant to ask of the patient or family. Although there are no empirical data to demonstrate that reentry programs do, in fact, facilitate reintegration, anecdotal reports and clinical experience suggest that survivors have benefited from such efforts.[83]

Rehabilitation phase, post-discharge

Discharge from acute inpatient treatment does not signify that a patient is well. A burn survivor's wounds are covered with sensitive and fragile skin which is vulnerable to breakdown and requires special care. Dressing changes, exercises, and application of special splints and pressure garments continue. Patients must confront anew their losses and may experience a delayed grief reaction. Upon leaving the protective hospital environment, symptoms of post-traumatic stress that had remitted in the hospital may recur. A survivor must continue the arduous process of tedious, uncomfortable physical treatments while struggling to comprehend and incorporate the multitude of changes into an image of 'self' which the survivor can accept and value.

The process of rehabilitation requires months to years, and patients as well as those around them can become discouraged. It would be extremely valuable to patients leaving the hospital, as well as their social network, employers, and care providers, if there were a set of predictors that could reliably estimate when and to what degree functional improvement could be expected over time. A recent investigation used markers for injury severity (TBSA) and psychological distress (Brief Symptom Inventory's Global Severity Index: GSI) available at discharge to generate benchmarks for postburn impairment.[84] The objectives were to track functional impairment from discharge and across 2 years of follow-up, and, to predict it using only data available at time of discharge. Participants were from a multisite cohort of adult burn survivors with major burns in a prospective study. To set impairment benchmarks, separate logistic regressions related TBSA (TBSA = 30% versus <30%) and GSI (T-score = 63 versus <63) to SF-36 Physical (PCS) and Mental (MCS) Composite Scales. The PCS benchmark (T-score = 37.25) was strongly related to injury group (TBSA), and, interestingly, corresponded to the mean impairment score in a sample with severe lower limb injury. Similarly, the MCS benchmark (= 32.40) was strongly related to distress group (GSI), and, of note, was equivalent to the mean impairment score in a sample with severe major depressive disorder.

At the time of discharge from the acute hospitalization, the prevalence rates of psychological and physical impairment were quite elevated. The data showed that, in general, physical impairment rates remained high among those with larger burns (TBSA = 30%). The rate of impairment for this group was 7%, 85%, 49%, 38%, and 29% at preburn, discharge, and at 6, 12, and 24 months postburn, respectively. The rate of physical impairment among those with smaller burns (TBSA <30%) was 9%, 77%, 21%, 16%, and 16% at preburn, discharge, and at 6, 12, and 24 months postburn, respectively. Physical impairment at all 3 postburn follow-ups was predicted by age, number of operations, and by level of physical health and function both before the burn and at discharge.

The data also revealed that, after an initial increase at 6 months, psychological impairment rates then receded over time. The rate of psychological impairment among those with higher distress at the time of discharge (GSI T-score = 63) was 28%, 50%, 38%, 29%, and 35% at preburn, discharge, and at 6, 12, and 24 months postburn, respectively. The rate of psychological impairment among those with lower distress at discharge (GSI T-score <63) was 3%, 10%, 11%, 9%, and 5% at preburn, discharge, and at 6, 12, and 24 months postburn, respectively. Psychological impairment at all 3 postburn follow-ups was predicted by prior alcohol abuse, in-hospital psychological distress, and by psychological function both before the burn and at discharge. The latter information, available at discharge, may help providers inform patients about modifiable factors effecting functional outcome.[84]

The 'enabling-disabling process' and the paradigm of rehabilitation research

The key terms in rehabilitation science are: injury, impairment, functional limitation, disabling condition, and disability. Uniform definitions of these terms are provided in an Institute of Medicine (IOM) report:[85]

- *Injury* (i.e. pathology) is any interference of normal bodily processes or structures.
- *Impairment* is a loss or abnormality of mental, emotional, physiological, or anatomical structure or function.
- A *functional limitation* is a restriction in the ability to perform an action or activity in the manner or within the range considered 'normal' and which is attributable to impairment.
- *Disability* is a limitation in performing socially defined roles expected of individuals within the social and physical environments.

Impairments and functional limitations represent potentially disabling conditions, while disability itself is a function of the interaction between the person's limits and the environment.[85] The IOM model describes the pathway along which a person with potentially disabling conditions may decline (i.e. experience less access and/or less integration) from injury to impairment, and from impairment to functional limitation. Factors that moderate the relations among these include: biology (e.g. genetic, congenital, pathology), environment (e.g. physical, social, psychological), and lifestyle (e.g. behavior).

- *Enablement* (i.e. the absence of disability) is represented by full social-environmental integration, including access to social opportunities (i.e. roles) and physical space (i.e. absence of physical barriers).

A model for rehabilitation-related research based on the IOM model has been incorporated into the long-range plan of the National Institute on Disability and Rehabilitation Research (NIDRR).[86] NIDRR espouses a paradigm for conceptualizing and conducting rehabilitation research that places environmental factors on an equal footing with person factors. The complex interaction of impairments and functional limitations with environmental structure is understood to determine the degree of disability that results from any given potentially disabling condition. Environmental structure is broadly understood as composed of physical space (e.g. architecture, transportation systems), intrapersonal structure (e.g. personality), interpersonal structure (e.g. social support), and socioeconomic structure (e.g. insurance coverage, work, and training opportunities). It is important to note that one's abilities may interact with aspects of the physical and social environments to enable full function in certain environments or at certain times, but allow for only partial integration into other environments and/or at other times.

The goals of rehabilitation science are to develop basic and applied programs of research that preserve or restore function either directly or via technological accommodation, and to enhance access to the physical and social environment by removing barriers to full integration in the community and the workplace.

Regarding burn injury, there are some data to suggest that the most important long-term (more than 2 years post-injury) disability is at the interface of the burn survivor and social environment. A recent study of young adult survivors of childhood burns (mean time since injury, 14 years) found that, although on standardized behavioral scales the young people were rated by others to be doing well, in individual standardized psychiatric interviews, an unexpected high percentage reported symptoms severe enough to warrant diagnoses, especially of anxieties related to social situations.[87] Similar results were found in a study of adolescents (mean time since injury, 10 years).[88] In both studies, the young people were rated by a physical therapist to have no physical limitations that prevented their abilities to care for themselves and to participate in ordinary activities, but their anxieties were severe enough to limit their achievement to full capacity. Even if most burn survivors eventually function satisfactorily by external criteria, clinically they may be suffering significant *distress* that is not easily observable. A goal of psychosocial care providers in working with survivors is to understand the sources of survivors' distress and to develop interventions that enable survivors to become full participants in society.

Manifestations of psychosocial distress

Among the most common manifestations of psychosocial distress are: sleep disturbance,[89,90] depression,[91] body image dissatisfaction,[21] acute and post-traumatic distress,[90,92] as well as more heterogeneous symptoms.[93] The mean level of psychological distress among those with major burn injuries (37) is reported to be significantly higher than that of a normative sample.[22] Evidence indicates that psychological distress in the hospital can have an enduring impact on health and function.[22,92,94] Psychological distress is closely correlated with poor global quality of life; accounting for substantial variance in concurrently assessed quality of life at 2 (58%), 6 (68%), and 12 (51%) months following a burn injury.[93] Psychological distress while in hospital was found to be associated with significantly greater impairment of physical and psychological function and slower rates of recovery over the course of the first year following a major burn injury even when preburn physical and psychological health and function were statistically controlled.[94]

Acute and post-trauma distress

As described in Chapter 65, acute stress disorder (ASD) and post-traumatic stress disorder (PTSD) following exposure to trauma are common, with a lifetime prevalence in the USA of 7.8%.[95] Severe burn injury is particularly likely to yield PTSD.[56,96] ASD and PTSD are characterized by three symptom clusters:

- re-experiencing trauma — intrusive distressing thoughts of the traumatic event or vivid flashbacks of the event;
- avoidance — suppression of trauma-related stimuli;
- hyperarousal — persistent symptoms such as inability to sleep, chronic anxiety, and irritability.

Between 25 and 38% of burn survivors meet criteria for PTSD in the first postburn year, and almost 50% of survivors meet criteria for at least one of the PTSD symptom clusters.[56,97–99] Post-trauma distress has been found to be associated with greater lengths of acute hospitalization,[56] enhanced sense of distress, and impaired adjustment to injury.[20] It might be assumed that PTSD is related to greater initial injury; however, PTSD among burn survivors has not been found to be related to severity of injury.[100] On the other hand, high levels of acute post-trauma stress symptomatology have been shown to be positively related to perception of more intense pain among hospitalized burn patients.[96,101]

PTSD can impair long-term adjustment following severe burn injury.[19] Certain aspects of pretrauma adjustment (e.g. history of mood disorder) can influence the risk of developing PTSD following trauma exposure.[19,102] Individuals with high levels of trait neuroticism appear to be at greater risk of PTSD symptomatology following burn injury while high levels of extraversion appear protective against PTSD.[97]

Body image dissatisfaction

Scarring, disfigurement, deformity, and loss of function that often result from a severe burn injury are likely to lead to significant perceptual and subjective body image changes.[103] Deformities or disfigurement of the face and other exposed areas may be obvious sources of distress. Disfigurement of areas such as the genitalia may be less apparent, but still highly relevant to body image satisfaction or self-esteem. In any case, changes in appearance or function may result in altered body image perception, a decrease in body image satisfaction, and behavioral avoidance. The association of larger TBSA and facial involvement with body image dissatisfaction of adult survivors may represent the influence of physical injury on psychological disturbance (i.e. physical condition affecting psychological disturbance).[21] Perhaps those individuals who appraise their injuries as worse because of location (i.e. more physically unattractive because of facial burns) or severity (i.e. larger TBSA) are at greater risk of developing body image dissatisfaction. Conversely, it has been suggested that cognitive and affective factors may interact with objective

aspects of the burn to worsen the appraisal of physical impairment and disability following a burn injury (i.e. psychological disturbance affecting physical condition).

Interestingly, three studies of self-regard by adolescent and adult burn survivors indicate that survivors developed positive feelings of global self-worth even while rating themselves low on the characteristic of physical appearance.[104–106] They also ranked physical appearance as a less-important domain in their value structures than job competence, romantic appeal, scholastic competence, and a number of other domains. Apparently, the burn survivors in these studies developed the ability to focus on positive characteristics over which they had some control and deemphasize those factors over which they had little or no control. As one young survivor said when explaining why she wanted no further reconstructive surgeries, 'I'll just have to get by with my *great* personality!'

Stigmatization and social anxiety

Burn survivors often report stigmatizing behaviors on the part of unburned individuals. The behaviors may be obvious such as staring, teasing, or bullying; or they may be subtle such as avoiding eye contact, ignoring, or expressing pity, but all result in the burn survivors feeling discredited and/or demeaned by others because of their scars.[107] Bull and Rumsey hypothesized that experiencing stigmatization has three specific effects on people with appearance distinctions: poor body-esteem, a sense of social isolation, and a violation of privacy effect.[108] The violation of privacy effect refers to the inability of the person to be anonymous, unnoticed, without undue attention. People of non-impaired appearance do not expect to walk down a street receiving intrusive looks or being approached by strangers who attempt to engage them in conversation regarding their traumatic history. Yet, burned individuals can rarely be anonymous; even the act of ignoring is a form of recognition and rejection. Sometimes the extraordinary attention is meant to be positive, but is none-the-less intrusive and dehumanizing.

Unburned children who are rejected (i.e. actively disliked) or neglected (i.e. socially excluded) by their peers report substantially more social anxiety than their accepted classmates[109] and it is likely true that adults who feel rejected experience social anxiety as well. Social anxiety is a promising construct which may serve as a marker for early identification of risk for developing anxiety disorders[110] such as those reported by long-term (more than 2 years post injury) burn survivors in the Meyer et al.[87] and in the Blakeney et al.[88] studies. It seems likely that the gestalt of visible distinction, body image dissatisfaction, stigmatization, and social anxiety are keys to understanding the etiology of burn survivors' distress and to the development of interventions to enable survivors to live with less suffering.

Distress of families of burn survivors

Long-term impact on families of burn survivors has not been well studied, but clinical experience and scanty empirical data indicate the sequelae to be significant. Family members may continue to experience symptoms of post-traumatic stress after a patient has returned home.[59] Parents of survivors of massive injuries appear extraordinarily stressed even several years after their children's recoveries.[6,8] A series of studies at the Shriners Hospital for Children in Galveston found that parents of recovering pediatric burned patients reported significant depressive symptoms at 2 years post-injury, and they attributed their distress to their burned children.[111,112] Although parental distress appears to improve with time for most, parents of the most troubled burned children continued across time to be troubled themselves.[112] Parents also express concern for their unburned children whom some felt had been slighted of attention and time while the burned sibling presented an extensive drain on the family system. Even free medical and surgical care did not eliminate the burden of direct and indirect costs of burn injury, and many families experience financial difficulties attendant to the injury and treatment of their child.[6]

Long-term outcome: quality of life

After survival is assured, quality of life is arguably the most important outcome to individuals who are seriously ill or injured. Health-related quality of life has been defined as a multifactorial construct that involves an individual's degree of satisfaction and level of health and functioning in several core domains, including: physical-behavioral (e.g. ability to perform self-care behaviors) and psychological well-being (i.e. subjective sense of contentment and the absence of emotional distress), social and role functioning (e.g. ability to fulfill family, work, and community responsibilities), and personal perception of health (i.e. satisfaction with one's health status).[113] Although most attempts to assess outcomes following burns have focused on either physical or psychological status, recent research has begun to focus on the overall quality of life.[10,17] As with self-report behavioral scales, most long-term (over 2 years) burn survivors appear to have eventually developed satisfactory adjustment and are within normal range on domain subscales of the SF36, a widely used quality of life assessment tool.[10,113,114] Rosenberg et al.,[17] however, examined the same patients as Baker et al.[114] using the Quality of Life Questionnaire[115] rather than the SF36 and found that on this questionnaire burn survivors rated their quality of life lower than the normal population in most areas, including general well-being, interpersonal relations, occupational activities, leisure activities, and participation in organized outside activities. These differences obviously reflect a difference in the instruments chosen, but generalizability of the results of the latter study is questionable.

Distresses prolong rates of recovery to satisfactory quality of life. Body image dissatisfaction at time of discharge is associated with prolonged periods of poorer mental health-related quality of life among adult patients following disfiguring injuries.[97] The impact of body image dissatisfaction on psychosocial quality of life independent of distress, injury, and pre-injury adjustment variables suggests the importance of early identification of populations at risk and the development of early intervention programs.

Post-trauma distress during the reintegration phase is also related to significant extended problems with adjustment during subsequent phases of recovery.[20,99] These problems are greater for those with post-trauma distress relative both to other burn survivors without significant post-trauma distress and to normative data. Moreover, the effect of post-trauma distress on physical and psychological health-related quality of life is felt even after controlling for pre-injury level of adjustment, baseline state negative affectivity (e.g. depression, body image dissatisfaction), generalized optimistic-pessimistic expectancies, and injury severity (face burn, TBSA full-thickness). On the other hand, the influence of post-trauma distress on physical adjustment appears to be moderated by generalized optimistic-pessimistic expectancies as well as by aspects of the burn injury itself.[99] This is consistent with the literature, indicating that negative affectivity or neuroticism (which covaries with state distress and generalized optimism-pessimism expectancies) may exacerbate symptom reporting and disability in physical illness.[116]

Interventions for burn survivors beyond acute care

Burn survivors and families may need psychotherapeutic attention for months or years as they adapt to new roles. Regular monitoring for psychosocial problems is important, especially for pediatric patients who continue to experience new problems related to burn scars as they mature. Psychotherapists must help patients to define new self-images, incorporating and going beyond body image. In the early months, patients may be encouraged to overcompensate and enjoy the positive identification of 'hero'. Survivors are commended for rehabilitation gains and social accomplishments. Each victory is celebrated. As patients' physical and psychological adaptation stabilizes, psychotherapists must assist patients in resisting the temptation to remain satisfied with the identity of 'heroic survivor'. This role invites survivors to achieve expectations which are unrealistic and to deny unhappiness or anger or pain. The task for psychotherapists is to make explicit the expectation that each burn survivor is a human individual who can be strong and competent, optimistic and autonomous, and also can have moments of sadness, despair, or rage. Guiding patients to accept vulnerabilities and flaws without detracting from the overall positive evaluation of 'self', psychotherapists insist that the person who has been the 'heroic burn survivor' can become a competent, interesting individual who also once survived a serious burn injury.

Most burn survivors who suffer psychological symptoms of distress following discharge from a burn center and who desire treatment must rely on mental health professionals in the community. However, it may be difficult for them to find helpful resources. Of the young adults in the Meyer et al.[87] study, none were receiving professional help for their difficulties. Such treatment is expensive and often not affordable by the individual, at least in the USA, without insurance or other financial assistance. Many burn survivors do not have insurance either because they are classified as 'uninsurable' or because they cannot afford the premiums. Burn survivors do not always qualify for financial assistance because their 'disabilities' are declared insufficient to require such aid. Even when they can afford such treatment, they may be unable to find a mental health professional to work with them. Mental health professionals who are naïve regarding burn survivors' needs sometimes believe that it is inevitable that scarred survivors will feel depressed and/or anxious; thus, they act as if the survivor (and the helper) cannot expect much in the way of improvement.

As the group of mental health professionals with expertise in burns has increased and psychosocial research has become more proficient, specific troubles common to many burn survivors have been identified, as enumerated in this chapter. Equally important has been the finding that survivors of even massive burns can achieve potentially satisfying quality of life. Within recent years psychologically based treatment programs with empirically demonstrated efficacy for burned adults and adolescents have been described to treat PTSD,[117] acute stress disorder,[118] and social skills training for coping with disfigurement.[119,120] In addition, a number of cognitive-behavioral treatments have been developed and demonstrated to be efficacious for treating or preventing body image dissatisfaction in other populations;[121] and two recent volumes contribute to understanding how disfigurement impacts the individual and the group.[103,122]

Support groups for burn survivors and their families are ongoing in many burn centers. Additionally, the Phoenix Society, an organization founded by burn survivors for burn survivors, has established a wide-ranging support network for burn survivors and their significant others. A visit to their website[123] can be inspiring and informative, providing support, guidance, and accurate information.

Summary

Most burn survivors do eventually adapt well and resume lives of productive activity with satisfactory self-esteem and social interactions. Empirical data indicate that the first year or so postburn is fraught with discomfort and distress, but much of the difficulty is transient. The process of psychological adaptation continues for several months or even several years. Symptoms of disturbance that linger among burn survivors are likely to be such that only intimate friends and family members will observe them (e.g. nightmares, flashbacks, body image dissatisfaction, social anxiety), so it is valuable for persons with expertise in burn adaptation to periodically assess survivors (especially pediatric survivors who change constantly) to ask about such common symptoms and to provide an opportunity for intervention.

That most burn survivors do amazingly well should never be interpreted as indicative of ease in adaptation. We would never want to diminish the pain and suffering they endure from physical and psychological wounds. As psychotherapists to a large number of burn survivors, we know very well the struggles of survivors. They have moments of true despair and hopelessness, moments of rage, and moments of joy. Probably at some level, burn survivors always feel some sadness about their scars; eventually they attend to other things most of the time and do not obsess over their scars. Fortunate psychotherapists can know them through all extremes – looking for glimmers of hope, validating anger, celebrating victories, and gaining deep respect for resilience of human beings (Figure 66.3).

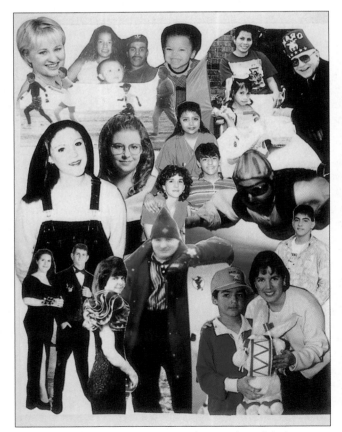
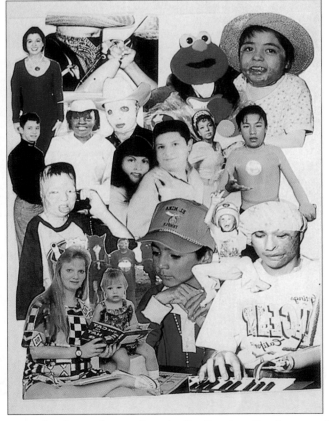

Fig. 66.3 Color collage. Survivors of severe burn injuries can return to active, interesting, and productive lives in spite of scars and amputations. Recovery is a long and difficult process, challenging the physical and psychological resilience of the individual. Burn care professionals must provide guidance and support to survivors and to their families during the years of recovery. (Reprinted from: Herndon DN, ed. Total burn care. London: WB Saunders; 2002.)

References

1. Ryan CM, Schoenfeld DA, Thorpe WP, et al. Objective estimates of the probability of death from burn injuries. N Engl J Med 1998; 338:362–366.

2. Blakeney P, Meyer WJ. Psychological aspects of burn care. Trauma Q 1994; 11(2):166–179.

3. Malt U. A long-term psychosocial follow-up study of burned adults. Acta Psychiatr Scand Suppl 1989; 80(355):94–102.

4. Faber A, Klasen H, Sauer E, et al. Psychological and social problems in burn patients after discharge: a follow-up study. Scand J Plast Reconstr Surg 1987; 21(3):307–309.

5. Tarnowski K, Rasnake L, Linscheid T, et al. Behavioral adjustment of pediatric burn victims. J Pediatr Psychol 1989; 14:607–615.

6. Blakeney P, Meyer W, Moore P, et al. Psychosocial sequelae of pediatric burns involving 80% or greater TBSA. J Burn Care Rehabil 1993; 14:684–689.

7. Moore P, Moore M, Blakeney P, et al. Competence and physical impairment of pediatric survivors of burns of more than 80% total body surface area. J Burn Care Rehabil 1996; 17:547–551.

8. Blakeney P, Meyer W 3rd, Robert R, et al. Long-term psychosocial adaptation of children who survive burns involving 80% or greater total body surface area. J Trauma 1998; 44(4):625–634.

9. Meyers-Paal R, Blakeney P, Murphy L, et al. Physical and psychological rehabilitation outcomes for pediatric patients who suffer >80% total body surface area burn and >70% 3rd degree burns. J Burn Care Rehabil 2000; 21(1, Pt. 1):43–49.

10. Sheridan RL, Hinson MI, Liang MH, et al. Long-term outcome of children surviving massive burns. JAMA 2000; 283(1):69–73.

11. Meyer WJ III, Blakeney P, Russell W, et al. Psychological problems reported by young adults who were burned as children. J Burn Care Rehabil 2004; 25:98–106.

12. Stoddard F, Norman D, Murphy M. A diagnosis outcome study of children and adolescents with severe burns. J Trauma 1989; 29:471–477.

13. Blumenfield M, Reddish P. Identification of psychologic impairment in patients with mild-moderate thermal injury: small burn, big problem. Gen Hosp Psychiatry 1987; 9:142–146.

14. Korloff B. Social and economic consequences of deep burns. In: Wallace AB, Wilkinson AW, eds. Research in burns: transactions of the 2nd International Congress on Research in Burns. Edinburgh, Scotland: Livingstone; 1996.

15. Tudahl LA, Blades BC, Munster AM. Sexual satisfaction in burn patients. J Burn Care Rehabil 1987; 8:292–293.

16. Bernstein NR. Objective bodily damage: disfigurement and dignity. In: Cash TF, Pruzinsky T, eds. Body images; development, deviance, and change. New York: Guilford; 1990.

17. Rosenberg M, Blakeney P, Robert R, et al. Quality of life of young adults who survived pediatric burns. Submitted for publication, 2006.

18. Blakeney P, Herndon D, Desai M, et al. Long-term psychological adjustment following burn injury. J Burn Care Rehabil 1988; 9(6):661–665.

19. Fauerbach JA, Lawrence JW, Haythornthwaite J, et al. Preinjury psychiatric illness and postinjury adjustment in adult burn survivors. Psychosomatics 1996; 37(6):547–555.

20. Fauerbach J, Lawrence J, Munster A, et al. Prolonged adjustment difficulties among those with acute post trauma distress following burn injury. Behav Med 1999; 22:359–378.

21. Fauerbach JA, Heinberg LJ, Lawrence JW, et al. Effect of early body image dissatisfaction on subsequent psychological and physical adjustment after disfiguring injury. Psychosom Med 2000; 62:576–582.

22. Patterson D, Ptacek J, Cromes F, et al. Describing and predicting adjustment in burn survivors. J Burn Care Rehabil 2000; 21(6):490–498.

23. Blakeney P, Portman S, Rutan R. Familial values as factors influencing long-term psychosocial adjustment of children after severe burn injury. J Burn Care Rehabil 1990; 11(6):472–475.

24. LeDoux J, Meyer W, Blakeney P, et al. Relationship between parental emotional states, family environment and the behavioral adjustment of pediatric burn survivors Burns 1998; 24:425–432.

25. Rosenberg L, Blakeney P, Thomas CR, et al. The value of family support for young adults burned during childhood. Submitted for publication, 2006.

26. Blakeney P, Meyer WJ. Psychological aspects of burn care. Trauma Q 1994; 11(2):166–179.

27. Kjaer G. Psychiatric aspects of thermal burns. Northwest Med 1969; 68:537–541.

28. Morris J, McFadd A. The mental health team on a burn unit. A multidisciplinary approach. J Trauma 1978; 18(9):658–663.

29. Ochitill H. Psychiatric consultation to the burn unit: the psychiatrist's perspective. Psychosomatics 1984; 25(9):689, 697–698, 701.

30. Knudson-Cooper M. Emotional care of the hospitalized burned child. J Burn Care Rehabil 1982; 3:109–116.

31. Watkins P, Cook E, Mary R, Ehleben C. Psychological stages in adaptation following burn injury: a method for facilitating psychological recovery of burn victims. J Burn Care Rehabil 1988; 9(4):376–384.

32. Tucker P. Psychosocial problems among adult burn victims. Burns 1987; 13(1):7–14.

33. Shenkman B, Stechmiller J. Patient and family perception of projected functioning after discharge from a burn unit. Heart Lung 1987; 16(5):490–496.

34. Luther S, Price J. Burns and their psychological effects on children. J School Health 1981; 51:419–422.

35. Davidson T, Bowden M, Feller I. Social support and post-burn adjustment. Arch Phys Med Rehabil 1981; 62:274–277.

36. Stoddard F. Psychiatric management of the burned patient. In: Martyn JAJ, ed. Acute care of the burn patient. Orlando, FL: Grune and Stratton; 1990:256–272.

37. Rosenberg L, Robert R, Meyer W, et al. Helping Hispanic families cope with the loss of family members. Proceedings of the American Burn Association 31st Annual Meeting, Vol. 20(1, part 2), Abstract #95. Buena Vista, FL (3/26/99).

38. Sue DW, Bernier JE, Durran A, et al. Position paper: cross-cultural counseling competencies. Counseling Psychologist 1982; 10:45–52.

39. Battaglia B. Meeting the demands of cross cultural counseling. Cross Cultural Connections 2001; 6(4):3.

40. Paniagua FA. Assessing and treating culturally diverse clients, 2nd edn. Thousand Oaks, CA: Sage; 1998:5–19.

41. Cuellar I. Acculturation and mental health: ecological transactional relations of adjustment. In: Cuellar I, Paniagua FA, eds. Handbook of multicultural mental health. New York: Academic Press; 2000:45–62.

42. Angel RJ, Williams R. Cultural models of health and illness. In: Cuellar I, Paniagua FA, eds. Handbook of multicultural mental health. New York: Academic Press; 2000:25–44.

43. Gomez-Beloz A, Chavez N. The botánica as a culturally appropriate health care options for Latinos. J Altern Complement Med 2001; 7(5):537–546.

44. Brockway JA, Fordyce WE. Psychological assessment and management. In: Kottke FJ, Lehmann JF, eds. Krusen's handbook of physical medicine and rehabilitation, 4th edn. Philadelphia: WB Saunders; 1990:153–170.

45. Blakeney P, Moore P, Meyer W, et al. Early identification of long-term problems in the behavioral adjustment of pediatric burn survivors and their parents. Proc Am Burn Assoc, Albuquerque, NM. 1995:vol. 27.

46. Meyer W, Murphy L, Robert R, et al. Changes in adaptive behavior among pediatric burn survivors over time. Proc Am Burn Assoc 1998; 19(1, part 2), Abstract #84.

47. Goodstein R. Burns: an overview of clinical consequences affecting patient, staff, and family. Compr Psychiatry 1985; 26(1):43–57.

48. Roberts J, Browne G, Streiner D, et al. Analyses of coping responses and adjustment: stability of conclusions. Nurs Res 1987; 36(2):94–97.

49. Byrne C, Love B, Browne G, et al. The social competence of children following burn injury: a study of resilience. J Burn Care Rehabil 1986; 7:247–252.

50. Blakeney P, Meyer W, Moore P, et al. Social competence and behavioral problems of pediatric survivors of burns. J Burn Care Rehabil 1993; 14:65–72.

51. Blakeney P, Moore P, Meyer W, et al. Early identification of long-term problems in the behavioral adjustment of pediatric burn survivors and their parents. Proc Am Burn Assoc 27, Albuquerque, NM: 1995.

52. Meyer W, Murphy L, Robert R, et al. Changes in adaptive behavior among pediatric burn survivors over time. Proc Am Burn Assoc 1998; 19(1, part 2), Abstract #84.

53. Darko D, Wachtel T, Ward H, et al. Analysis of 585 burn patients hospitalized over a 6-year period. Part III: psychosocial data. Burns 1986; 12:395–401.

54. Knudson-Cooper M, Leuchtag A. The stress of a family move as a precipitating factor in children's burn accidents. J Hum Stress 1982; June:32–38.

55. Noyes R, Frye S, Slyment D, et al. Stressful life events and burn injuries. J Trauma 1979; 19(3):141–144.

56. Fauerbach JA, Lawrence J, Richter D, et al. Preburn psychiatric history affects posttrauma morbidity. Psychosomatics 1997; 38(4):374–385.

57. Blank K, Perry S. Relationship of psychological process during delirium to outcome. Am J Psychiatry 1984; 141:843–847.

58. Haynes B, Bright R. Burn coma: a syndrome associated with severe burn wound infection. J Trauma 1967; 7:464–475.

59. Cella D, Perry S, Kulchycky S, et al. Stress and coping in relatives of burn patients: a longitudinal study. Hosp Comm Psychiatry 1988; 39(2):159–166.

60. Rivlin E, Forshaw A, Polowyj G, et al. A multidisciplinary group approach to counseling the parents of burned children. Burns 1986; 12(7):479–483.

61. Goodstein R. Burns: an overview of clinical consequences affecting patient, staff, and family. Compr Psychiatry 1985; 26(1):43–57.

62. Terry D. The needs of parents of hospitalized children. Children's Health Care 1987; 16(1):18–20.

63. Kelley M, Jarvie G, Middlebrook J, et al. Decreasing burned children's pain behavior: impacting the trauma of hydrotherapy. J Appl Behav Anal 1984; 17(2):147–158.

64. Kavanagh C. Psychological intervention with the severely burned child: report of an experimental comparison of two approaches and their effects on psychological sequelae. J Am Acad Child Psychiatry 1983; 22(2):145–156.

65. Beales J. Factors influencing the expectation of pain among patients in a children's burns unit. Burns 1983; 9(3):187–192.

66. Baker C, Wong D. Q.U.E.S.T.: a process of pain assessment in children. Orthop Nurs 1987; 6(1):11–21.

67. Elliot C, Olson R. The management of children's distress in response to painful medical treatment for burn injuries. Behav Res Ther 1983; 21(6):675–683.

68. Knudson-Cooper M. Relaxation and biofeedback training in the treatment of severely burned children. J Burn Care Rehabil 1981; 2:103–110.

69. Hoffman HG, Doctor JN, Patterson DR, et al. Virtual reality as an adjunctive pain control during burn wound care in adolescent patients. Pain 2000; 85(1–2):305–309.

70. Wakeman R, Kapan J. An experimental study of hypnosis in painful burns. Am J Clin Hypn 1978; 21(1):3–12.

71. May S, DeClement F. Effects of early hypnosis on the cardiovascular and renal physiology of burn patients. Burns 1983; 9(4):257–266.

72. Kuttner L. Favorite stories: a hypnotic pain-reduction technique for children in acute pain. Am J Clin Hypn 1985; 28:289–295.

73. Abramson LY, Metalsky GI, Alloy LB. Hopelessness depression: a theory-based subtype of depression. Psychol Rev 1989; 96:358–372.

74. Ehde DH, Patterson DR, Fordyce WE. The quota system in burn rehabilitation. J Burn Care Rehabil 1998; 19:436–440.

75. Doctor ME, Burne B, Jarecke D. Through the eyes of a child: burn recovery. Denver, CO: Children's Hospital, videotape, 1993.

76. Langlois JH, Downs AC. Peer relations as a function of physical attractiveness: the eye of the beholder or behavioral reality? Child Dev 1979; 50:409–418.

77. Barden RC. The effects of crania-facial deformity, chronic illness, and physical handicaps on patient and familial adjustment: research and clinical perspectives. In: Lahey BB, Kazdin AE, eds. Advances in clinical child psychology. New York: Plenum; 1990: vol 13:343–375.

78. Blakeney P. School reintegration. In: Tarnowski KJ, ed. Behavioral aspects of pediatric burns. New York: Plenum; 1994:217–241.

79. Dobner D, Mitani M. Community reentry program. J Burn Care Rehabil 1988; 9(4):420–421.

80. James Partridge of Changing Faces. Personal communication, 2005.

81. Doctor ME. Returning to school after a severe burn. In: Boswick JA Jr, ed. The art and science of burn care. Rockville, MD: Aspen; 1987:323–328.

82. Blumenfield M, Schoeps M. Reintegrating the healed burned adult into society: psychological problems and solutions. Clin Plast Surg 1992; 19(3):599–605.

83. Blakeney P, Moore P, Meyer W, et al. Efficacy of school of reentry programs. J Burn Care Rehabil 1995; 16:469–472.

84. Fauerbach JA, Heltshe S, Lezotte DL, et al. Early predictors of long term impairment following burn injury. Proc Am Burn Assoc 2006, U Burn Care Rehabil 2006; 27(2): Abstract 30, S64.

85. Institute of Medicine. Enabling America: assessing the role of rehabilitation science and engineering. Washington, DC: National Academy; 1997.

86. National Institute on Disability and Rehabilitation Research. Long range plan and the new paradigm. Washington DC, Department of Education, USA. 1999.

87. Meyer WJ, Russell W, Blakeney P, et al. Incidence of major psychiatric illness in young adults who were burned as children. 35th Annual Meeting for the American Burn Association, Miami, FL (04/2/2003).

88. Blakeney P, Thomas C, Berniger F, et al. Long term psychiatric disorder in adolescent burn survivors. Proceedings of the ABA 33rd Annual Meeting, Vol. 22, Abstract #99, Boston, 2001.

89. Ehde DM, Patterson DR, Wiechman SA, et al. Post-traumatic stress symptoms and distress following acute burn injury. Burns 1999; 25:587–592.

90. Ehde DM, Patterson DR, Wiechman SA, et al. Post-traumatic stress symptoms and distress 1 year after burn injury. J Burn Care Rehabil 2000; 21:105–111.

91. Wiechman SA, Ptacek JT, Patterson DR, et al. Rates, trends, and severity of depression after burn injuries. J Burn Care Rehabil 2001; 22(6):417–424.

92. Difede J, Ptacek JT, Roberts J, et al. Acute stress disorder after burn injury: a predictor of posttraumatic stress disorder? Psychosom Med 2002; 64(5):826–834.

93. Cromes GF, Holavanahalli R, Kowalske K, et al. Predictors of quality of life as measured by the Burn Specific Health Scale in persons with major burn injury. J Burn Care Rehabil 2002; 23(3):229–234.

94. Fauerbach JA, Lezotte D, Cromes GF, et al. 2004 American Burn Association Clinical Research Award. Burden of burn: a norm-based inquiry into the influence of burn size and distress on recovery of physical and psychosocial function. J Burn Care Rehabil 2005; 26(1):21–32.

95. Kessler RC, Sonnega A, Bromet E, et al. Postraumatic stress disorder in the National Comorbidity Sample. Arch Gen Psychiatry 1995; 52:1048–1060.

96. Taal LA, Faber AW. Post traumatic stress, pain and anxiety in adult burn victims. Burns 1998; 23:545–549.

97. Fauerbach J, Lawrence J, Schmidt C, et al. Personality predictors of injury-related PTSD. J Nerv Ment Dis 2000; 188:510–517.

98. Powers PS, Cruse CW, Daniels S, et al. Posttraumatic stress disorder in patients with burns. J Burn Care Rehabil 1994; 15(2):147–153.

99. Saxe G, Stoddard F, Sheridan R. PTSD in children with burns: a longitudinal study. J Burn Care Rehabil 1998; 19(1, part 2): S206.

100. Bryant RA. Predictors of post-traumatic stress disorder following burn injury. Burns 1996; 22:89–92.

101. Williams D, Kiecolt-Glaser J. Self-blame, compliance and distress among burn patients. J Person Soc Psychol 1987; 53:187–193.

102. Smith EM, North CS, McCool RE, et al. Acute postdisaster psychiatric disorders: identification of persons at risk. Am J Psychiatry 1990; 147(2):202–206.

103. Heinberg LJ. Theories of body image: perceptual, developmental, and sociocultural factors. In: Thompson JK, ed. Body image, eating disorders, and obesity: an integrative guide to assessment and treatment. Washington, DC: American Psychological Association; 1996.

104. LeDoux JM, Meyer W, Blakeney P, et al. Positive self-regard as a coping mechanism for pediatric burn survivors. J Burn Care Rehabil 1996; 17:472–476.

105. Clyne W, Turner S. Perceived changes and adaptations in self-concept following burn injury. Proc Am Burn Assoc Sci Meeting, #23. 1995.

106. Robert R, Bishop S, Murphy L, et al. The evolution of self-perception in children and adolescents post-burn injury. 8th Congress of the European Burns Association, Marathon-Attica, Greece, 1999.

107. Pruzinsky T, Doctor ME. Body images and pediatric burn injury. In: Tarnowski, K, ed. Behavioral aspects of pediatric burns. New York: Plenum; 1994:169–191.

108. Bull RHC, Rumsey N. The social psychology of facial appearance. New York: Springer-Verlag; 1988.

109. La Greca AM, Dandes SK, Wick P, et al. The social anxiety scale for children-revised: factor structure and concurrent validity. J Clin Child Psychol 1993; 22:17–27.

110. Ginsburg GS, La Greca AM, Silverman WK. Social anxiety in children with anxiety disorders: relation with social and emotional functioning. J Abnorm Child Psychol 1998; 26(3):175–185.

111. Blakeney P, Moore P, Broemeling L, et al. Parental stress as a cause and effect of pediatric burn injury. J Burn Care Rehabil 1993; 14(1):73–79.

112. Meyer W, Blakeney P, Moore P, et al. Parental well-being and behavioral adjustment of pediatric burn survivors. J Burn Care Rehabil 1994; 15:62–68.

113. Ware JE, Snow KK, Kosinski M, et al. SF-36 health survey: manual and interpretation guide. Boston, MA: Nimrod; 1993.

114. Baker C, Mossberg K, Meyer W III, et al. Perceived health status of young adults burned as children. Poster presented at 2003 APTA Combined Sections Meeting in Tampa, FL; 2002 TPTA Annual Conference in Austin, TX; 2002 ISBI Conference in Seattle, WA and 2002 ABA Annual Conference in Chicago, IL.

115. Evans DR, Cope WE. Quality of life questionnaire (QLQ). North Tonawanda, NY: Multi-Health Systems; 1989.

116. Watson D, Pennebaker JW. Health complaints, stress and distress: exploring the role of negative affectivity. Psychol Rev 1989; 96:234–254.

117. Foa EB, Keane TM, Friedman MJ. Effective treatments for PTSD. New York: Guilford; 2000.

118. Bryant RA, Harvey AG. Acute stress disorder: a handbook of theory, assessment and treatment. Washington, DC: Proc Am Psychol Assoc; 2000.

119. Robinson E, Rumsey N, Partridge J. An evaluation of the impact of social interaction skills training for facially disfigured people. Br J Plast Surg 1996; 49:281–289.

120. Blakeney P, Thomas C, Holzer C, et al. Efficacy of a short-term social skills training program for burned adolescents. J Burn Care Rehabil 2005; 26(6):546–555.

121. Rohe DE. Psychological aspects of rehabilitation. In: DeLisa JA, Gans BM, eds. Rehabilitation medicine: principles and practice, 3rd edn. Philadelphia: Lipincott-Raven; 1998:189–212.

122. Heatherton TF, Kleck RE, Hebl MR, et al. The social psychology of stigma. New York: Guilford; 2000.

123. The Phoenix Society's. Online. Available at: www.phoenix-society.org

Index

Please note that page references relating to non-textual content such as Figures, Photographs or Tables are in *italic* print, while page numbers relating to main discussion are in **bold**.

AAG (α-acid glycoprotein), 207
AATB (American Association of Tissue Banks), 232, 234, 246
Abbreviated burn severity index (ABSI), 789
Abdomen, electrical injuries, 525–526
Abdominal compartment syndrome (ACS), 101–102, 201, 204, 448
Abdominal infections, 152–153
ABI (ankle-brachial index), 503
ABLS (Advanced Burn Life Support), 50, 52
ABO incompatibility, 221
ABSI (abbreviated burn severity index), 789
AC (alternating current), 90
Acalculous cholecystitis, 438, 505–506
Accidents
    boating, 21
    and disasters, 45
    industrial, 123
    prevention of injuries, 33
    radioactive, 543
    traffic, 21, 123, 502–503
Acculturation, 831
Ace bandage, 76
Acetaminophen, 71, 84, 162, 804, **807**
Acetic acid, 23, 170, 538
Acetylcholine receptors, 208, 209
Acetylcysteine, 7, 266, 284, 299
Aciclovir sodium IV (Zovirax), 169
Acid burns *see* Chemical injuries: acids
Acid labile subunit (ALS), 353
Acid-base abnormalities, blood transfusions, 220–221
α-acid glycoprotein (AAG), 207
Acidosis
    evaluation of wound, 124
    history of treatment, 4
    hypophosphatemia, 392
    metabolic, 102, 113, 220, 250
    wound care, 133
Acinetobacter, 145, 156, 571, 612
ACLS (Advanced Cardiac Life Support), 456
ACS (abdominal compartment syndrome), 101–102, 201, 204, 448
ACSM (American College of Sports Medicine), 642, 647
ACTH (adrenocorticotrophic hormone), 343, 351
Acticoat dressing, 133, 173, 184, 186
α-actin, 584
Activated partial thromboplastin time (APTT), 327
Active-assistive exercises, 639
Activities of daily living (ADL), 620, 645
Acute burns, hemodynamic consequences, 101–102
Acute lung damage (ALD), 327
Acute lung injury (ALI), 468, 469
Acute phase proteins, 158, 327–328
Acute phase response
    growth factors, 369
    hematologic, 336–337
    hepatic, 366–375
    hepatocyte growth factor, 370
    insulin, 371, *373, 374*
    insulin-like growth factor, 370–371
    propranolol, 371–372, *374*
    proteins, 366–367
    recombinant human growth hormone, 369–370
    sepsis, 393
Acute radiation syndrome (ARS), 545

Acute renal failure (ARF), 204–205, 465, 466, 467
Acute renal insufficiency, diagnosis, 449–450
Acute respiratory distress syndrome (ARDS)
    ARDSNet trial, 274, 277, 278
    barotrauma, 273, 274, 276
    fat, 425
    high frequency oscillatory ventilation, 461
    mechanical ventilation, 285
    nursing, 477
    pathophysiology of inhalation injury, 263
    pulmonary system, 469
    radiation injuries, 546
    renal failure, 468, 469
    tidal volumes, 287
    time-cycled pressure control ventilation, 459
Acute Respiratory Distress Syndrome Network, of National Heart, Lung and Blood Institute, 285
Acute stress disorder (ASD), 824, 838
Acute tubular necrosis (ATN), 465
Acyclovir, 146
Adaptic, 71
Adenosine diphosphate (ADP), 439
Adenosine triphosphate (ATP), 98, 108, 379, 393, 439
Adenylyl cyclase, 346
ADH (antidiuretic hormone), 100, 115
ADHR (autosomal dominant hypophosphatemic rickets), 380
ADL (activities of daily living), 620, 645
Adnexal structures, 120
Adolescents
    Coconut Grove Nightclub disaster, 2
    fuels, and flammable liquids, misuse, 20
    mortality rates, 9, 496
    nursing, 482
    pain measurement, 801
    as parents, child abuse by, 23
    work-related burns, 21
    see also Children
ADP (adenosine diphosphate), 439
Adrenal cortical steroids
    bone metabolism, 353
    C₁₉ steroids, release, 351
    glucocorticoids
        and glucose metabolism, 352
        and protein metabolism, 352–353
        release, 350–351
    immune suppression, 353–354
    metabolic pathways, influence on, 351–352
Adrenal medulla, 346
Adrenalectomy, 352
α-2 adrenergic agonists, pain management, 806–807
Adrenergic blockade, 346
Adrenocorticotrophic hormone (ACTH), 343, 351
Advanced Burn Life Support (ABLS), 50, 52
Advanced Cardiac Life Support (ACLS), 456
Advanced Trauma Life Support (ATLS), 502, 510
Aerobic training, 639, 642–643
Aesthetic units, head and neck reconstruction, 705–706
Afterload, cardiovascular system, 471
Age factors
    burn mortality, 27
    chemical injuries, 21
    outcome analysis, 25
    outpatient care, 67
    pain management, 804
    wound healing, 587
    see also Adolescents; Children; Elderly